Dietary Reference Intakes (DRIs): RECOMMENDED DIETARY ALLOWANCES AND ADEQUATE INTAKES, VITAMINS
Food and Nutrition Board, Institute of Medicine, National Academies

Life Stage Group	Vitamin A (μg/d)[a]	Vitamin C (mg/d)	Vitamin D (μg/d)[b,c]	Vitamin E (mg/d)[d]	Vitamin K (μg/d)	Thiamin (mg/d)	Riboflavin (mg/d)	Niacin (mg/d)[e]	Vitamin B_6 (mg/d)	Folate (μg/d)[f]	Vitamin B_{12} (μg/d)	Pantothenic Acid (mg/d)	Biotin (μg/d)	Choline (mg/d)[g]
Infants														
0 to 6 mo	400*	40*	10	4*	2.0*	0.2*	0.3*	2*	0.1*	65*	0.4*	1.7*	5*	125*
6 to 12 mo	500*	50*	10	5*	2.5*	0.3*	0.4*	4*	0.3*	80*	0.5*	1.8*	6*	150*
Children														
1-3 y	**300**	**15**	**15**	**6**	30*	**0.5**	**0.5**	**6**	**0.5**	**150**	**0.9**	2*	8*	200*
4-8 y	**400**	**25**	**15**	**7**	55*	**0.6**	**0.6**	**8**	**0.6**	**200**	**1.2**	3*	12*	250*
Males														
9-13 y	**600**	**45**	**15**	**11**	60*	**0.9**	**0.9**	**12**	**1.0**	**300**	**1.8**	4*	20*	375*
14-18 y	**900**	**75**	**15**	**15**	75*	**1.2**	**1.3**	**16**	**1.3**	**400**	**2.4**	5*	25*	550*
19-30 y	**900**	**90**	**15**	**15**	120*	**1.2**	**1.3**	**16**	**1.3**	**400**	**2.4**	5*	30*	550*
31-SOY	**900**	**90**	**15**	**15**	120*	**1.2**	**1.3**	**16**	**1.3**	**400**	**2.4**	5*	30*	550*
51-70 y	**900**	**90**	**15**	**15**	120*	**1.2**	**1.3**	**16**	**1.7**	**400**	**2.4**[h]	5*	30*	550*
>70 y	**900**	**90**	**20**	**15**	120*	**1.2**	**1.3**	**16**	**1.7**	**400**	**2.4**[h]	5*	30*	550*
Females														
9-13 y	**600**	**45**	**15**	**11**	60*	**0.9**	**0.9**	**12**	**1.0**	**300**	**1.8**	4*	20*	375*
14-18 y	**700**	**65**	**15**	**15**	75*	**1.0**	**1.0**	**14**	**1.2**	**400**[i]	**2.4**	5*	25*	400*
19-30 y	**700**	**75**	**15**	**15**	90*	**1.1**	**1.1**	**14**	**1.3**	**400**[i]	**2.4**	5*	30*	425*
31-50 y	**700**	**75**	**15**	**15**	90*	**1.1**	**1.1**	**14**	**1.3**	**400**[i]	**2.4**	5*	30*	425*
51-70 y	**700**	**75**	**15**	**15**	90*	**1.1**	**1.1**	**14**	**1.5**	**400**	**2.4**[h]	5*	30*	425*
>70 y	**700**	**75**	**20**	**15**	90*	**1.1**	**1.1**	**14**	**1.5**	**400**	**2.4**[h]	5*	30*	425*
Pregnancy														
14-18 y	**750**	**80**	**15**	**15**	75*	**1.4**	**1.4**	**18**	**1.9**	**600**[j]	**2.6**	6*	30*	450*
19-30 y	**770**	**85**	**15**	**15**	90*	**1.4**	**1.4**	**18**	**1.9**	**600**[j]	**2.6**	6*	30*	450*
31-50 y	**770**	**85**	**15**	**15**	90*	**1.4**	**1.4**	**18**	**1.9**	**600**[j]	**2.6**	6*	30*	450*
Lactation														
14-18 y	**1,200**	**115**	**15**	**19**	75*	**1.4**	**1.6**	**17**	**2.0**	**500**	**2.8**	7*	35*	550*
19-30 y	**1,300**	**120**	**15**	**19**	90*	**1.4**	**1.6**	**17**	**2.0**	**500**	**2.8**	7*	35*	550*
31-50 y	**1,300**	**120**	**15**	**19**	90*	**1.4**	**1.6**	**17**	**2.0**	**500**	**2.8**	7*	35*	550*

NOTE: This table (taken from the DRI reports, see www.nap.edu) presents Recommended Dietary Allowances (RDAs) in **bold type** and Adequate Intakes (AIs) in ordinary type followed by an asterisk (*). An RDA is the average daily dietary intake level; sufficient to meet the nutrient requirements of nearly all (97-98 percent) healthy individuals in a group. It is calculated from an Estimated Average Requirement (EAR). If sufficient scientific evidence is not available to establish an EAR, and thus calculate an RDA, an AI is usually developed. For healthy breastfed infants, an AI is the mean intake. The AI for other life stage and gender groups is believed to cover the needs of all healthy individuals in the groups, but lack of data or uncertainty in the data prevent being able to specify with confidence the percentage of individuals covered by this intake.

[a]As retinol activity equivalents (RAEs). 1 RAE = 1 μg retinol, 12 μg β-carotene, 24 μg α-carotene, or 24 μg β-cryptoxanthin. The RAE for dietary provitamin A carotenoids is two-fold greater than retinol equivalents (RE), whereas the RAE for preformed vitamin A is the same as RE.

[b]As cholecalciferol. 1 μg cholecalciferol = 40 IU vitamin D.

[c]Under the assumption of minimal sunlight.

[d]As α-tocopherol. α-Tocopherol includes *RRR*-α-tocopherol, the only form of α-tocopherol that occurs naturally in foods, and the *2R*-stereoisomeric forms of α-tocopherol (*RRR*-, *RSR*-, *RRS*-, and *RSS*-α-tocopherol) that occur in fortified foods and supplements. It does not include the *2S*-stereoisomeric forms of α-tocopherol (*SRR*-, *SSR*-, *SRS*-, and *SSS*-α-tocopherol), also found in fortified foods and supplements.

[e]As niacin equivalents (NE). 1 mg of niacin = 60 mg of tryptophan; 0-6 months = preformed niacin (not NE).

[f]As dietary folate equivalents (DFE). 1 DFE = 1 μg food folate = 0.6 μg of folic acid from fortified food or as a supplement consumed with food = 0.5 μg of a supplement taken on an empty stomach.

[g]Although AIs have been set for choline, there are few data to assess whether a dietary supply of choline is needed at all stages of the life cycle, and it may be that the choline requirement can be met by endogenous synthesis at some of these stages.

[h]Because 10 to 30 percent of older people may malabsorb food-bound B_{12}, it is advisable for those older than 50 years to meet their RDA mainly by consuming foods fortified with B_{12} or a supplement containing B_{12}.

[i]In view of evidence linking folate intake with neural tube defects in the fetus, it is recommended that all women capable of becoming pregnant consume 400 μg from supplements or fortified foods in addition to intake of food folate from a varied diet.

[j]It is assumed that women will continue consuming 400 μg from supplements or fortified food until their pregnancy is confirmed and they enter prenatal care, which ordinarily occurs after the end of the periconceptional period—the critical time for formation of the neural tube.

SOURCES: *Dietary Reference Intakes for Calcium, Phosphorous, Magnesium, Vitamin D, and Fluoride* (1997); *Dietary Reference Intakes for Thiamin, Riboflavin, Niacin, Vitamin B_6, Folate, Vitamin B_{12}, Pantothenic Acid, Biotin, and Choline* (1998); *Dietary Reference Intakes for Vitamin C, Vitamin E, Selenium, and Carotenoids* (2000); *Dietary Reference Intakes for Vitamin A, Vitamin K, Arsenic, Boron, Chromium, Copper, Iodine, Iron, Manganese, Molybdenum, Nickel, Silicon, Vanadium, and Zinc* (2001); *Dietary Reference Intakes for Water, Potassium, Sodium, Chloride, and Sulfate* (2005); and *Dietary Reference Intakes for Calcium and Vitamin D* (2011). These reports may be accessed via www.nap.edu.

Dietary Reference Intakes (DRIs): RECOMMENDED DIETARY ALLOWANCES AND ADEQUATE INTAKES, ELEMENTS
Food and Nutrition Board, Institute of Medicine, National Academies

Life Stage Group	Calcium (mg/d)	Chromium (μg/d)	Copper (μg/d)	Fluoride (mg/d)	Iodine (μg/d)	Iron (mg/d)	Magnesium (mg/d)	Manganese (mg/d)	Molybdenum (μg/d)	Phosphorus (mg/d)	Selenium (μg/d)	Zinc (mg/d)	Potassiunl (g/d)	Sodium (g/d)	Chloride (g/d)
Infants															
0 to 6 mo	200*	0.2*	200*	0.01*	110*	0.27*	30*	0.003*	2*	100*	15*	2*	0.4*	0.12*	0.18*
6 to 12 mo	260*	5.5*	220*	0.5*	130*	11	75*	0.6*	3*	275*	20*	3	0.7*	0.37*	0.57*
Children															
1-3 y	700	11*	340	0.7*	90	7	80	1.2*	17	460	20	3	3.0*	1.0*	1.5*
4-8 y	1,000	15*	440	1*	90	10	130	1.5*	22	500	30	5	3.8*	1.2*	1.9*
Males															
9-13 y	1,300	25*	700	2*	120	8	240	1.9*	34	1,250	40	8	4.5*	1.5*	2.3*
14-18 y	1,300	35*	890	3*	150	11	410	2.2*	43	1,250	55	11	4.7*	1.5*	2.3*
19-30 y	1,000	35*	900	4*	150	8	400	2.3*	45	700	55	11	4.7*	1.5*	2.3*
31-50 y	1,000	35*	900	4*	150	8	420	2.3*	45	700	55	11	4.7*	1.5*	2.3*
51-70 y	1,000	30*	900	4*	150	8	420	2.3*	45	700	55	11	4.7*	1.3*	2.0*
>70 y	1,200	30*	900	4*	150	8	420	2.3*	45	700	55	11	4.7*	1.2*	1.8*
Females															
9-13 y	1,300	21*	700	2*	120	8	240	1.6*	34	1,250	40	8	4.5*	1.5*	2.3*
14-18 y	1,300	24*	890	3*	150	15	360	1.6*	43	1,250	55	9	4.7*	1.5*	2.3*
19-30 y	1,000	25*	900	3*	150	18	310	1.8*	45	700	55	8	4.7*	1.5*	2.3*
31-50 y	1,000	25*	900	3*	150	18	320	1.8*	45	700	55	8	4.7*	1.5*	2.3*
51-70 y	1,200	20*	900	3*	150	8	320	1.8*	45	700	55	8	4.7*	1.3*	2.0*
>70 y	1,200	20*	900	3*	150	8	320	1.8*	45	700	55	8	4.7*	1.2*	1.8*
Pregnancy															
14-18 y	1,300	29*	1,000	3*	220	27	400	2.0*	50	1,250	60	12	4.7*	1.5*	2.3*
19-30 y	1,000	30*	1,000	3*	220	27	350	2.0*	50	700	60	11	4.7*	1.5*	2.3*
31-50 y	1,000	30*	1,000	3*	220	27	360	2.0*	50	700	60	11	4.7*	1.5*	2.3*
Lactation															
14-18 y	1,300	44*	1,300	3*	290	10	360	2.6*	50	1,250	70	13	5.1*	1.5*	2.3*
19-30 y	1,000	45*	1,300	3*	290	9	310	2.6*	50	700	70	12	5.1*	1.5*	2.3*
31-50 y	1,000	45*	1,300	3*	290	9	320	2.6*	50	700	70	12	5.1*	1.5*	2.3*

NOTE: This table (taken from the DRI reports, see www.nap.edu) presents Recommended Dietary Allowances (RDAs) in **bold type** and Adequate Intakes (AIs) in ordinary type followed by an asterisk (*). An RDA is the average daily dietary intake level; sufficient to meet the nutrient requirements of nearly all (97-98 percent) healthy individuals in a group. It is calculated from an Estimated Average Requirement (EAR). If sufficient scientific evidence is not available to establish an EAR, and thus calculate an RDA, an AI is usually developed. For healthy breastfed infants, an AI is the mean intake. The AI for other life stage and gender groups is believed to cover the needs of all healthy individuals in the groups, but lack of data or uncertainty in the data prevent being able to specify with confidence the percentage of individuals covered by this intake.

SOURCES: *Dietary Reference Intakes for Calcium, Phosphorous, Magnesium, Vitamin D, and Fluoride* (1997); *Dietary Reference Intakes for Thiamin, Riboflavin, Niacin, Vitamin B_6, Folate, Vitamin B_{12}, Pantothenic Acid, Biotin, and Choline* (1998); *Dietary Reference Intakes for Vitamin C, Vitamin E, Selenium, and Carotenoids* (2000); and *Dietary Reference Intakes for Vitamin A, Vitamin K, Arsenic, Boron, Chromium, Copper, Iodine, Iron, Manganese, Molybdenum, Nickel, Silicon, Vanadium, and Zinc* (2001); *Dietary Reference Intakes for Water, Potassium, Sodium, Chloride, and Sulfate* (2005); and *Dietary Reference Intakes for Calcium and Vitamin D* (2011). These reports may be accessed via www.nap.edu.

Dietary Reference Intakes (DRIs): RECOMMENDED DIETARY ALLOWANCES AND ADEQUATE INTAKES, TOTAL WATER AND MACRONUTRIENTS
Food and Nutrition Board, Institute of Medicine, National Academies

Life Stage Group	*Total* Water[a] (L/d)	Carbohydrate (g/d)	Total Fiber (g/d)	Fat (g/d)	Linoleic Acid (g/d)	α-Linolenic Acid (g/d)	Protein[b] (g/d)
Infants							
0 to 6 mo	0.7*	60*	ND	31*	4.4*	0.5*	9.1*
6 to 12 mo	0.8*	95*	ND	30*	4.6*	0.5*	11.0
Children							
1-3 y	1.3*	130	19*	ND[c]	7*	0.7*	13
4-8 y	1.7*	130	25*	ND	10*	0.9*	19
Males							
9-13 y	2.4*	130	31*	ND	12*	1.2*	34
14-18 y	3.3*	130	38*	ND	16*	1.6*	52
19-30 y	3.7*	130	38*	ND	17*	1.6*	56
31-50 y	3.7*	130	38*	ND	17*	1.6*	56
51-70 y	3.7*	130	30*	ND	14*	1.6*	56
>70 y	3.7*	130	30*	ND	14*	1.6*	56
Females							
9-13 y	2.1*	130	26*	ND	10*	1.0*	34
14-18 y	2.3*	130	26*	ND	11*	1.1*	46
19-30 y	2.7*	130	25*	ND	12*	1.1*	46
31-50 y	2.7*	130	25*	ND	12*	1.1*	46
51-70 y	2.7*	130	21*	ND	11*	1.1*	46
>70 y	2.7*	130	21*	ND	11*	1.1*	46
Pregnancy							
14-18 y	3.0*	175	28*	ND	13*	1.4*	71
19-30 y	3.0*	175	28*	ND	13*	1.4*	71
31-50 y	3.0*	175	28*	ND	13*	1.4*	71
Lactation							
14-18	3.8*	210	29*	ND	13*	1.3*	71
19-30 y	3.8*	210	29*	ND	13*	1.3*	71
31-50 y	3.8*	210	29*	ND	13*	1.3*	71

NOTE: This table (take from the DRI reports, see www.nap.edu) presents Recommended Dietary Allowances (RDA) in **bold type** and Adequate Intakes (AI) in ordinary type followed by an asterisk (*). An RDA is the average daily dietary intake level; sufficient to meet the nutrient requirements of nearly all (97-98 percent) healthy individuals in a group. It is calculated from an Estimated Average Requirement (EAR). If sufficient scientific evidence is not available to establish an EAR, and thus calculate an RDA, an AI is usually developed. For healthy breastfed infants, an AI is the mean intake. The AI for other life stage and gender groups is believed to cover the needs of all healthy individuals in the groups, but lack of data or uncertainty in the data prevent being able to specify with confidence the percentage of individuals covered by this intake.

[a]*Total* water includes all water contained in food, beverages, and drinking water.

[b]Based on g protein per kg of body weight for the reference body weight, e.g., for adults 0.8 g/kg body weight for the reference body weight.

[c]Not determined.

SOURCE: *Dietary Reference Intakes for Energy, Carbohydrate, Fiber, Fat, Fatty Acids, Cholesterol, Protein, and Amino Acids* (2002/2005) and *Dietary Reference Intakes for Water, Potassium, Sodium, Chloride, and Sulfate* (2005). The report may be accessed via www.nap.edu.

Krause's Food & the Nutrition Care Process

Edition 13

L. Kathleen Mahan, MS, RD, CDE
Nutrition Counselor and Certified Diabetes Educator
Nutrition by Design, Inc.
Seattle, WA;
Affiliate Assistant Professor
Department of Pediatrics
School of Medicine
University of Washington
Seattle, WA

Sylvia Escott-Stump, MA, RD, LDN
Director, Dietetic Internship
Department of Nutrition and Dietetics
East Carolina University
Greenville, NC;
Consulting Nutritionist
Nutritional Balance
Winterville, NC

Janice L. Raymond, MS, RD, CD
Clinical Nutrition Manager, Sodexo
Providence Mount St. Vincent
Seattle, WA;
Adjunct Faculty
Bastyr University
Kenmore, WA

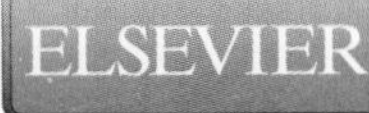

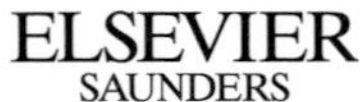

3251 Riverport Lane
St. Louis, Missouri 63043

KRAUSE'S FOOD & THE NUTRITION CARE PROCESS, THIRTEENTH EDITION 978-1-4377-2233-8

Notices

Knowledge and best practice in this field are constantly changing. As new research and experience broaden our understanding, changes in research methods, professional practices, or medical treatment may become necessary.

Practitioners and researchers must always rely on their own experience and knowledge in evaluating and using any information, methods, compounds, or experiments described herein. In using such information or methods they should be mindful of their own safety and the safety of others, including parties for whom they have a professional responsibility.

With respect to any drug or pharmaceutical products identified, readers are advised to check the most current information provided (i) on procedures featured or (ii) by the manufacturer of each product to be administered, to verify the recommended dose or formula, the method and duration of administration, and contraindications. It is the responsibility of practitioners, relying on their own experience and knowledge of their patients, to make diagnoses, to determine dosages and the best treatment for each individual patient, and to take all appropriate safety precautions.

To the fullest extent of the law, neither the Publisher nor the authors, contributors, or editors, assume any liability for any injury and/or damage to persons or property as a matter of products liability, negligence or otherwise, or from any use or operation of any methods, products, instructions, or ideas contained in the material herein.

International Standard Book Number: 978-1-4377-2233-8

Sr. Editor: Yvonne Alexopoulos
Sr. Developmental Editor: Danielle M. Frazier
Publishing Services Manager: Jeff Patterson
Sr. Project Manager: Tracey Schriefer
Design Direction: Maggie Reid
Cover Image: David Scharf/Photo Researchers, Inc.

Vitamin C. Colored Scanning Electron Micrograph (SEM) of the surface of a crystal of ascorbic acid (vitamin C).

Printed in the United States of America

Last digit is the print number: 9 8 7 6 5 4 3 2 1

This 13th edition is dedicated to the students, professors and practitioners who use this text and consider it their "nutrition bible."
We are most grateful to them for their learning, writing, and insights and dedication to the field of nutrition and dietetic practice.

—The Authors, 13th Edition

and

To Robert for his unending love, respect, and loving humor, Carly and Justin for their encouragement, and Ana for whom the "book" is like a sibling and who doesn't know life without it.

—Kathleen

To my husband, children and family for their support and my interns for their insights.

—Sylvia

To my husband, Greg and my sons, Erik and George who are always there for me when I need them. And most of all to Kathy and Sylvia who have allowed me the great honor of working on this book.

—Janice

Contributors

Diane M. Anderson, PhD, RD, CSP, FADA
Associate Professor
Department of Pediatrics
Baylor College of Medicine
Houston, Texas

Cynthia Taft Bayerl, MS, RD, LDN
Nutrition Coordinator
Coordinator Massachusetts Fruit & Vegetable Nutrition Coordinator
Nutrition and Physical Activity Unit
Division of Health Promotion and Disease Prevention
Massachusetts Department of Public Health
Boston, Massachusetts

Peter L. Beyer, MS, RD
Associate Professor
Dietetics & Nutrition
University of Kansas Medical Center
Kansas City, Kansas

Karen Chapman-Novakofski, PhD, RD, LDN
Professor
Department of Food Science & Human Nutrition
University of Illinois
Champaign, Illinois

Pamela Charney, PhD, RD
Lecturer, Nutrition Sciences
Affiliate Associate Professor
Pharmacy, MS Student
Clinical Informatics and Patient Centered Technology
Biobehavioral Nursing
University of Washington
Seattle, Washington

Harriet Cloud, MS, RD, FADA
Nutrition Matters, Owner
Professor Emeritus, Department of Nutrition Sciences
School of Health Related Professions
University of Alabama at Birmingham
Birmingham, Alabama

Sarah C. Couch, PhD, RD, LD
Associate Professor
Department of Nutritional Sciences
University of Cincinnati
Cincinnati, Ohio

Sister Jeanne P. Crowe, PharmD, RPh, RPI
Author/Lecturer/Co-Author 16th Edition Food-Medication Interactions
Former Director of Pharmacy
Camilla Hall Nursing Home
Immaculata, Pennsylvania

Ruth DeBusk, PhD, RD
Geneticist and Clinical Dietician
Private Practice
Tallahassee, Florida

Sheila Dean, DSc, RD, LD, CCN, CDE
Adjunct Faculty, University of Tampa
Dietitians in Integrative & Functional Medicine
Professional Advancement Chair
Tampa, Florida

Nora Decher, MS RD, CNSC
Nutrition Specialist
University of Virginia Health System
Charlottesville, Virginia

Judith L. Dodd, MS, RD, LDN, FADA
Adjunct Assistant Professor
Department of Sports Medicine and Nutrition
School of Health and Rehabilitation Sciences
University of Pittsburgh
Pittsburgh, Pennsylvania

Kimberly R. Dong, MS, RD
Project Manager/Research Dietitian
Department of Public Health & Community Medicine
Nutrition & Infectious Disease Unit
Tufts University School of Medicine
Boston, Massachusetts

Lisa Dorfman, MS, RD, CSSD, LMHC
Director of Sports Nutrition and Performance
Uhealth Department of Sports Medicine
University of Miami
Miami, Florida

Miriam Erick, MS, RD, CDE, LDN
Senior Clinical Dietitian
Department of Nutrition
Brigham and Women's Hospital
Boston, Massachusetts

Sharon A. Feucht, MA, RD, CD
Nutritionist, LEND Program
Center on Human Development and Disability
University of Washington
Seattle, Washington

Marion J. Franz, MS, RD, LD, CDE
Nutrition/Health Consultant
Nutrition Concepts by Franz, Inc.
Minneapolis, Minnesota

Margie Lee Gallagher, PhD, RD
Professor and Senior Scientist
East Carolina University
Greenville, North Carolina

F. Enrique Gómez, PhD
Head, Laboratory of Nutritional Immunology
Department of Nutritional Physiology
Instituto Nacional de Ciencias Médicas y Nutrición Salvador Zubirán (INCMNSZ)
México City, México

Barbara L. Grant, MS, RD, CSO, LD
Oncology Clinical Dietitian
Saint Alphonsus Regional Medical Center
Cancer Care Center
Boise, Idaho

Kathryn K. Hamilton, MA, RD, CSO, CDN
Outpatient Clinical Oncology Dietitian
Carol G Simon Cancer Center
Morristown Memorial Hospital
Morristown, New Jersey

Kathleen A. Hammond, MS, RN, BSN, BSHE, RD, LD
Continuing Education Nurse Planner/Clinical Nutrition Specialist
Corporate Education and Development
Gentiva Health Services, Inc.
Atlanta, Georgia;
Adjunct Assistant Professor
Department of Food and Nutrition
College of Family and Consumer Sciences
Athens, Georgia

Jeanette M. Hasse, PhD, RD, LD, CNSC, FADA
Manager, Transplant Nutrition
Baylor Regional Transplant Institute
Baylor University Medical Center
Dallas, Texas

David H. Holben, PhD, RD, LD
Professor and Director, Didactic Program in Dietetics
College of Health Sciences and Professions
Ohio University
Athens, Ohio

Cindy Mari Imai, MS, RD
Research Coordinator
Tufts University School of Medicine
Department of Public Health and Community Medicine
Nutrition/Infection Unit
Boston, Massachusetts

Carol S. Ireton-Jones, PhD, RD, LD, CNSD, FACN
Nutrition Therapy Specialist/Consultant
Executive Vice President, Professional Nutrition Therapists
Carrollton, Texas

Donna A. Israel, PhD, RD, LD, LPC, FADA
President, Principal, Professional Nutrition Therapists, LLC
Adjunct Professor
Dallas County Community College District
Dallas, Texas

Veena Juneja, MSc, RD
Senior Renal Dietitian
Nutrition Services
St. Joseph's Healthcare
Hamilton, Ontario, Canada

Barbara J. Kamp, MS, RD
Adjunct Professor
Johnson and Wales University
Miami, Florida

Martha Kaufer-Horwitz, DSc, NC
Researcher in Medical Sciences
Obesity and Food Disorders Clinic
Department of Endocrinology and Metabolism
Instituto Nacional de Ciencias Médicas y Nutrición Salvador Zubirán
México City, México

Joseph S. Krenitsky, MS, RD
Nutrition Support Specialist
University of Virginia Health System
Charlottesville, Virginia

Nicole Larson, PhD, MPH, RD
Research Associate
Division of Epidemiology and Community Health
University of Minnesota
Minneapolis, Minnesota

Mary Demarest Litchford, PhD, RD, LDN
President
Case Software & Books
Greensboro, New Carolina

Betty L. Lucas, MPH, RD, CD
Nutritionist
Center on Human Development and Disability
University of Washington
Seattle, Washington

Lucinda K. Lysen, RD, RN, BSN
Medical Editor and Assistant Publisher
Southwest Messenger Press Newspapers
Chicago, Illinois

Ainsley M. Malone, MS, RD, CNSC
Nutrition Support Dietitian
Department of Pharmacy
Mt. Carmel West Hospital
Columbus, Ohio

Laura E. Matarese, PhD, RD, LDN, CNSC, FADA
Director of Nutrition, Assistant Professor of Surgery
Intestinal Rehabilitation and Transplantation Center
Thomas E. Starzl Transplantation Institute
University of Pittsburgh Medical Center
Pittsburgh, Pennsylvania

Kelly N. McKean, MS, RD, CD
Clinical Pediatric Dietitian
Seattle Children's Hospital
Seattle, Washington

Donna H. Mueller, PhD, RD, FADA, LDN
Associate Professor
Department of Biology
Drexel University
Philadelphia, Pennsylvania

Deborah H. Murray, MS, RD, LD
Assistant Professor
Human Consumer Sciences
Athens, Ohio

Diana Noland, MPH, RD, CCN
IFM Nutrition Coordinator
Institute for Functional Medicine
Functional Nutrition Practitioner
Owner, FoodFax
Los Angeles, California

Beth N. Ogata, MS, RD, CD, CSP
Nutritionist, Department of Pediatrics
Center on Human Development and Disability
University of Washington
Seattle, Washington

Zaneta M. Pronsky, MS, RD, LDN, FADA
Author/Speaker/Consultant
Food Medication Interactions
Immaculata, Pennsylvania

Diane Rigassio Radler, PhD, RD
Assistant Professor
Department of Nutritional Sciences
University of Medicine and Dentistry of New Jersey
School of Health Related Professions
Newark, New Jersey

Valentina M. Remig, PhD, RD, LD, FADA
Consultant/Author
Nutrition, Food Safety, & Healthy Aging
Kansas State University
Manhattan, Kansas

Janet E. Schebendach, PhD, RD
Director of Research Nutrition
Eating Disorders Research Unit
New York State Psychiatric Institute
Columbia University Medical Center
New York, New York

Elizabeth Shanaman, RD, BS
Renal Dietitian
Northwest Kidney Centers
Seattle, Washington

Jamie S. Stang, PhD, MPH, RD, LN
Chair, Public Health Nutrition Program
University of Minnesota, School of Public Health
Division of Epidemiology and Community Health
Minneapolis, Minnesota

Tracy Stopler, MS, RD
President, NUTRITION ETC, Inc.
Plainview, New York;
Adjunct Professor
Adelphi University
Garden City, New York

Kathie Madonna Swift, MS, RD, LDN
Owner, SwiftNutrition
Curriculum Designer, Food As Medicine Professional Training Program, Center for Mind Body Medicine
Washington DC;
Faculty, Saybrook University, Graduate College of Mind Body Medicine, California;
Nutritionist, Kripalu Center for Yoga and Health
Stockbridge, Massachusetts;
Nutritionist, UltraWellness Center
Lenox, Massachusetts

Cynthia A. Thomson, PhD, RD
Associate Professor
College of Agriculture & Life Sciences (Department of Nutritional Sciences)
College of Public Health, College of Medicine
University of Arizona
Tucson, Arizona

Cristine M. Trahms, MS, RD, CD, FADA
Cristine M. Trahms Program for Phenylketonuria
PKU/Biochemical Genetics Clinic
Center on Human Development and Disability
University of Washington
Seattle, Washington

Gretchen K. Vannice, MS, RD
Nutrition Research Consultant
Omega-3 RD™ Nutrition Consulting
Portland, Oregon

Allisha Weeden, PhD, RD, LD
Assistant Professor
Idaho State University
Pocatello, Idaho

Susan Weiner, MS, RD, CDE
Registered Dietitian, Masters of Science,
Certified Diabetes Educator, Certified Dietitian Nutritionist
Masters of Science in Applied Physiology and Nutrition
Teachers College, Columbia University New York
New York, New York

Nancy S. Wellman, PhD, RD, FADA
Former Director, National Resource Center on Nutrition
Physical Activity and Aging
Florida International University
Miami, Florida

Katy G. Wilkens, MS, RD
Manager
Nutrition & Fitness Services
Northwest Kidney Centers
Seattle, Washington

Marion F. Winkler, PhD, RD, LDN, CNSC
Surgical Nutrition Specialist
Rhode Island Hospital
Nutritional Support Service
Senior Clinical Teaching Associate of Surgery
Alpert Medical School of Brown University
Providence, Rhode Island

Reviewers

Peter L. Beyer, MS, RD
Associate Professor
Dietetics & Nutrition
University of Kansas Medical Center
Kansas City, Kansas

Rachel K. Johnson, PhD, MPH, RD
Professor of Nutrition
Associate Provost
University of Vermont
Burlington, Vermont

Diana Noland, MPH, RD, CCN
IFM Nutrition Coordinator
Institute for Functional Medicine
Functional Nutrition Practitioner
Owner, FoodFax
Los Angeles, California

Foreword

For more than 80 years the Krause nutrition textbook has been used in colleges to teach nutrition and diet therapy. The first edition was published in 1952! The title has changed during the past 60 years, as have the editors and authors, but the 13th edition of *Krause's Food and the Nutrition Care Process* remains the comprehensive textbook for the beginner as well as a treasured resource for the competent dietetic practitioner. Kathleen Mahan remains the key editor, along with Sylvia Escott-Stump, 2011-2012 President of the American Dietetic Association, and this edition adds a new editor, Janice Raymond.

Historically, one or two or three authors could together write a fundamental book on nutrition, metabolism, nutrients needs and sources, lifespan issues, medical nutrition therapy, and the steps of the nutrition care process. Today, however, the depth and breadth of knowledge of the field requires experts writing the chapters to pass on their knowledge to the novices and beginners and to mentor the next generation. Although the students may not recognize the strengths of the chapter authors (I can remember being a new student!), I look at these authors and see a "Who's Who" of nutrition research and practice. All are prominent specialists or experts in their content area. I am fortunate to personally know approximately two thirds of them, and many could have written or in fact have written texts in their specialties. To distill this knowledge into a chapter for the emerging professional is a labor of love, and makes this a great book for students of all ages. I will add it to my own bookshelf and use it to improve my competence in those areas in which I have limited knowledge. I will use it with confidence, knowing that these authors have summarized the key points using the most up-to-date scientific evidence.

The content of the book combines the nutrition care process and its terminology in a useable way. It is essential for the standardized method of documenting what we do in nutritional care and for developing methodologies to describe the care we give individuals. It also allows multisite evaluation groups to demonstrate or improve our effectiveness in caring for clients and the public. The keys of assessment, diagnosis, and intervention are incorporated into the first 15 chapters. The book covers the fundamentals of nutrition: digestion, absorption, metabolism, the role of genomics, nutrient metabolism, inflammation, and integrated care. This is followed by six chapters on life span issues and five chapters on nutrition for optimal health and performance.

Finally, the book is best known for its complete discussion of medical nutrition therapy (MNT). The book covers MNT for the key chronic diseases plus emerging areas such as rheumatic, thyroid, neurologic, and psychiatric disorders; pediatric needs for neonates; metabolic disorders; and developmental disorders.

This new edition includes more on inflammation; a chapter on thyroid and related disorders; and an emphasis on assessment, including laboratory analysis and physical assessment. The book is as current as a new book can be, even covering the new U.S. Department of Agriculture MyPlate system and new World Health Organization growth charts.

I congratulate the publishers and editors for including experts who can share their knowledge with dietetic students and practitioners. I thank the authors for being mentoring resources to the practitioner of the future—our entry-level dietetics students—and for providing a quick reference for areas that are not key focus areas for many of us. I encourage other allied health and nursing professionals, especially those in advanced practice programs, to use the book to help them understand what registered dietitians do as part of the team and to ground them in the science and practice of nutrition care.

Congratulations on the longevity of the book and on the new 13th edition!

Julie O'Sullivan Maillet, PhD, RD, FADA
Professor, Department of Nutritional Sciences
Interim Dean
University of Medicine and Dentistry of New Jersey,
School of Health Related Professions
American Dietetic Association President 2002-2003

Preface

The 13th edition of this classic text supports the Nutrition Care Process as the standard for dietetics. Students and practitioners will embrace the standardized language for their own settings, whether for individuals, families, groups, or communities, and all readers are encouraged to use the most recent edition of the International Nutrition and Diagnostic Terminology in their practice.

AUDIENCE

Scientific knowledge and clinical information is presented in a form that is useful to students in dietetics, nursing, and other allied health professions in an interdisciplinary setting. It is valuable as a reference for other disciplines such as medicine, dentistry, child development, health education, and lifestyle counseling. Nutrient and assessment appendixes, tables, illustrations, and clinical insight boxes provide practical hands-on procedures and clinical tools for students and practitioners alike.

This textbook accompanies the graduating student into clinical practice as a treasured shelf reference. The popular features remain: having basic information on nutrients all the way through to protocols for clinical nutrition practice in one place, clinical management algorithms, focus boxes that give "nice to know" detailed insight, sample nutrition diagnoses for clinical scenarios, useful websites, and extensive appendices for patient education. All material reflects current evidence-based practice as contributed by authors, experts in their fields. This text is the first choice in the field of dietetics for students, educators, and clinicians.

ORGANIZATION

This edition follows the Conceptual Framework for Steps of the Nutrition Care Process (see inside of back cover). All nutritional care process components are addressed to enhance or improve the nutritional well-being of individuals, their families, or populations. New to this edition is a flow of chapters according to the steps of assessment, nutrition diagnosis, intervention, monitoring, and evaluation. Also new is the separation of the pediatric medical nutrition therapy (MNT) chapters into their own section to assist with that specialty practice.

Part 1, Nutrition Assessment, organizes content for an effective assessment. Chapters here provide an overview of the digestive system as well as calculation of energy requirements and expenditure, macronutrient and micronutrient needs, nutritional genomics, and food intake. A thorough review of biochemical tests, acid-base balance issues, and medications promote the necessary insight for provision of excellent care. A new approach for this edition is a chapter titled "Clinical: Inflammation, Physical, and Functional Assessments," which addresses the latest knowledge about inflammation as a cause of chronic disease and the necessity of assessing for it. The final chapter in this section addresses the behavioral aspects of an individual's food choices within the community, a safe food supply, and available resources for sufficiency in food accessibility.

Part 2, Nutrition Diagnosis and Intervention, describes the critical thinking process from assessment to selection of relevant, timely, and measurable nutrition diagnoses. These nutrition diagnoses can be resolved by the registered dietitian or trained health professional. The process is generally used for individuals, but can be applied when helping families, teaching groups, or when evaluating the nutritional needs of a community or a population. A nutrition diagnosis requires an intervention and interventions relate to food and nutrient delivery (including nutrition support), use of bioactive substances and integrative medical nutrition, education, counseling, and referral when needed.

Part 3, Nutrition in the Life Cycle, presents in-depth information on the nutrition for life stages from nutrition in the womb and pregnancy and through lactation and infancy. There is a chapter on nutrition in adolescence and another that deals with the nutrition issues and chronic disease that usually start appearing in adulthood. Finally, nutrition and the aging adult is discussed in detail because much of the employment of nutrition professionals in the future is going to be in providing nutrition services to this growing population.

Part 4, Nutrition for Health and Fitness, provides nutrition concepts for the achievement and maintenance of health and fitness, as well as the prevention of many disease states. Weight management, problems with eating disorders, dental health, bone health, and sports nutrition focus on the role of nutrition in promoting long-term health.

Part 5, Medical Nutrition Therapy, reflects evidence-based knowledge and current trends in nutrition therapies. All of the chapters are written and reviewed by specialists in their fields who present nutritional aspects of conditions such as cardiovascular disorders; diabetes; liver disease; renal disease; pulmonary disease; infectious disease; endocrine disorders, especially thyroid disease; and rheumatologic, neurologic, and psychiatric disorders.

Part 6, Pediatric Specialties, describes the role of nutrition therapies in childhood. Chapters provide details for low-birthweight, neonatal intensive care conditions, genetic metabolic disorders, and developmental disabilities.

NEW TO THIS EDITION

- **New Title:** The new title reflects the profession's move to the "nutrition care process" while providing current, cutting-edge information upon which instructors and students alike have come to rely.
- **Newest Recommendations:** The dietary reference intakes are provided, with the new recommended dietary allowances for calcium and vitamin D that were published in 2010. The new MyPlate from the USDA in 2011, is also included.
- **Nutrition Care Process Tools:** The chapters are organized by the steps in the nutrition care process. In streamlined appendixes, the reader will find the essential clinical references and tools.
- **Medical Nutrition Therapy:** A new chapter is added to the Medical Nutrition Therapy section: "Medical Nutrition Therapy for Thyroid and Related Disorders." In addition, the three cardiovascular chapters on hypertension, atherosclerosis and congestive heart failure from past editions have been merged into one chapter for easier care understanding of the chronic disease and MNT planning.

PEDAGOGY

- **UNIQUE Pathophysiology and Care Management Algorithms:** Pathophysiology related to nutrition care continues to be a basic highlight of the text. Newly edited algorithms illustrate pathophysiology and relevant medical and nutritional management. These algorithms equip the reader with an understanding of the illness as background for providing optimal nutritional care.
- **Focus On Boxes:** Focus On boxes provide thought-provoking information on key concepts for well-rounded study and to promote further discussion within the classroom.
- **New Directions Boxes:** New Directions boxes suggest areas for further research by spotlighting emerging areas of interest within the field.
- **Clinical Insight Boxes:** Clinical Insight boxes present information for better understanding that enriches the student's interaction with the patient around his or her nutritional care.
- **Key Terms:** Terms are bolded and defined within the text.
- **Useful Websites:** A list of websites in each chapter direct the reader to online resources that relate to the chapter topics.
- **Chapter References:** References are current and extensive, with the purpose of giving the student and instructor lots of opportunity for further reading and understanding.

ANCILLARIES

Accompanying this edition is the Evolve website which includes updated and invaluable resources for instructors and students. These materials can be accessed by going to http://evolve.elsevier.com/Mahan/nutrition/.

INSTRUCTOR RESOURCES

- **Power Point presentations:** More than 900 slides to help guide classroom lectures.
- **Image Collection:** Approximately 200 images from the text are included in the PowerPoint presentations, as well as more illustrations that can be downloaded and used to develop other teaching resources.
- **Audience Response System Questions (for use with iClicker and other systems):** Three to five questions per chapter help aid incorporation of this new technology into the classroom.
- **Testbank:** Each chapter includes NCLEX-formatted questions with page references specific to that chapter's content to bring you more than 900 multiple-choice questions.
- **Animations:** Approximately 50 animations have been developed to visually complement the text and the processes described.
- **Nutrition Care Process Tools:** Consisting of assessment and monitoring tools and intervention tools, this information can be used by the new student and practitioner in teaching and guiding the client in his or her specific nutritional care.

STUDENT RESOURCES

Study Exercises with Answers: With more than 20 questions per chapter, these exercises give instant feedback on questions related to the chapter's content.

We hope that instructors and students find this text as intriguing to study from as we find it in updating and keeping it current and relevant.

L. Kathleen Mahan, MS, RD, CDE
Sylvia Escott-Stump, MA, RD, LDN
Janice L. Raymond, MS, RD, CD

Acknowledgments

We sincerely thank the contributors of this edition who have devoted hours and hours of time and commitment to researching the book's content for accuracy, reliability and practicality. We are greatly in debt to them and realize that we could not continue to produce this book without them. Thank you!

The contributors would like to thank Diana Noland, MPH, RD, CCN who reviewed Chapter 6 on Inflammation, Physical and Functional Assessments; Jillian Pollock, Simmons College Dietetic Intern, who assisted with updating the Nutrition in Adulthood chapter; Jean Cox, MS, RD who reviewed Chapter 16 on Pregnancy and Lactation; Russell Jaffe, MD, PhD, CCN, and Jean E. Lloyd, National Nutritionist, US Administration on Aging, for their review of the Nutrition in Aging chapter; Emily Mohar for research assistance in writing and Janice V. Joneja, PhD, CDR for review of Chapter 27 on Adverse Reactions to Foods; Carol Parrish, MS, RD, for her review of the MNT in Gastrointestinal Disorders chapters; Kwai Y. Lam, RD, and Erica Kasuli, RD for help and the deceased Victor Herbert, MD, JD, for inspiration in the writing of the MNT in Anemia chapter; Kathie Swift, MS, RD and Jeff Bland, PhD for their review of the MNT in Thyroid and Related Disorders chapter; Debra Clancy, RD with her expertise on transplantation, Ann Lipkin, MS, RD, expert in continuous renal replacement therapy (CRRT) and Peggy Solan, RD with her expertise in renal pediatric for help in the preparation of the MNT in Renal Disease chapter; Marta Mazzanti, MS, RD, CD, for her assistance in writing the chapter on MNT in Neurological Disease; Scot G Hamilton for his review of the MNT in Cancer Prevention, Treatment and Recovery chapter; and Michael Hahn for his review and editing of many chapters.

We also wish to acknowledge the hard work of Yvonne Alexopoulos, Senior Editor, who keeps the vision; Danielle Frazier, Senior Developmental Editor, who along with Editorial Assistant, Kit Blanke, can get the "hot off the press" items we'd like included; and most of all Tracey Schriefer, Senior Project Manager, who accommodated our deadline misses, endless editing requests, and made this edition and us, all look good. Thank you!

Contents

PART 4
Nutrition for Health and Fitness

PART 5
Medical Nutrition Therapy

PART 6
Pediatric Specialties

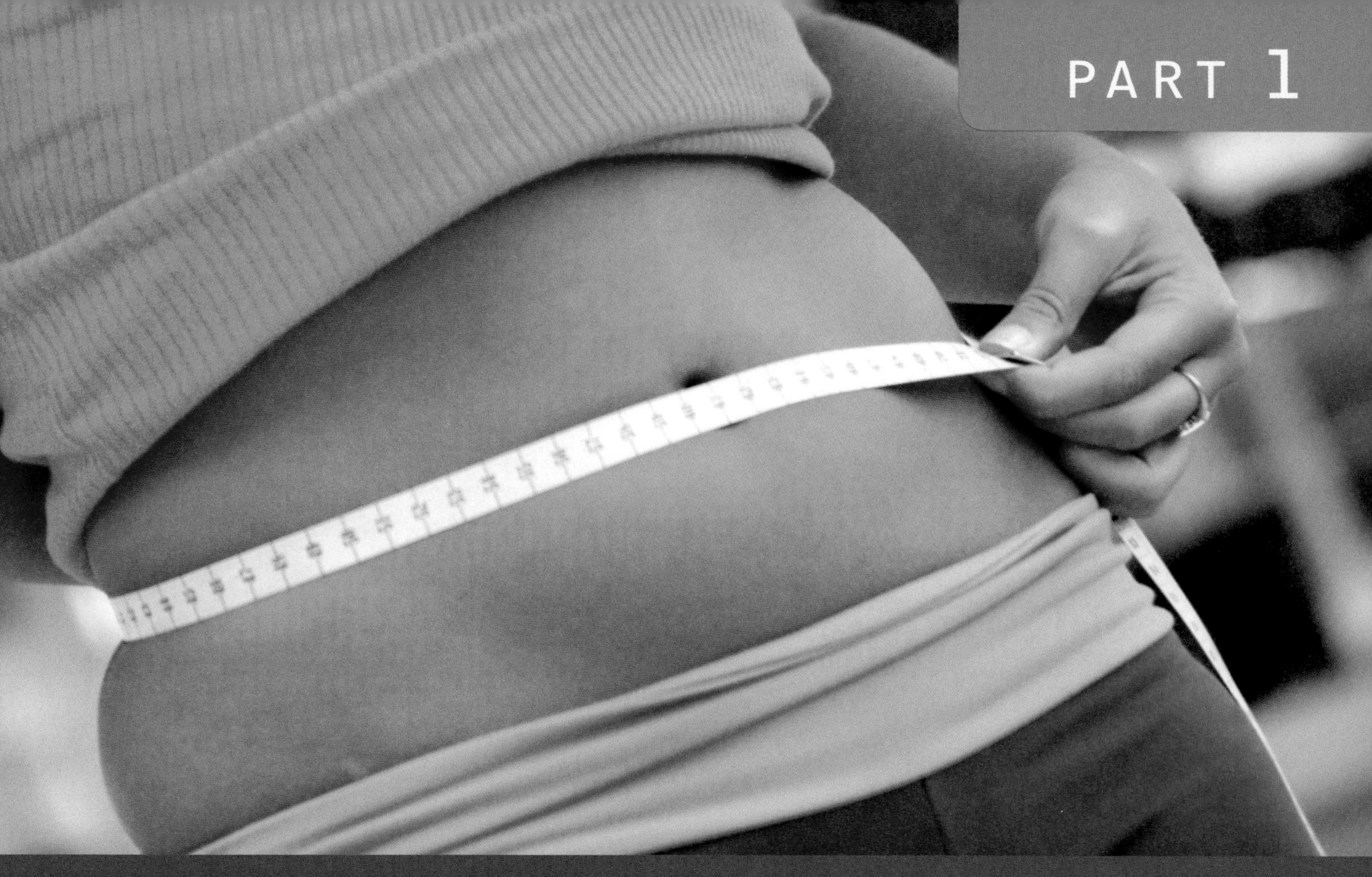

PART 1

Nutrition Assessment

Food provides energy and building materials for countless substances that are essential for the growth and survival of every human being. This section opens with a brief overview of the digestion, absorption, transportation, and excretion of nutrients. These remarkable processes convert myriads of complex foodstuffs into individual nutrients ready to be used in metabolism. Macronutrients (proteins, fats, and carbohydrates) each contribute to the total energy pool, but ultimately the energy they yield is available for the work of the muscles and organs of the body. Release of energy for synthesis, movement, and other functions requires the micronutrients (vitamins and minerals), which function as coenzymes, co-catalysts, and buffers in the miraculous, watery arena of metabolism. The way nutrients become integral parts of the body and contribute to proper functioning depends heavily on the physiologic and biochemical processes that govern their actions.

For the health provider, nutrition assessment is the first step in the nutrition care process. To implement a successful nutrition plan, the assessment must include key elements of the patient's clinical or medical history, current complaint, anthropometric measurements, biochemical and laboratory values, information on medication and herbal supplement use for potential food-drug interactions, plus a thorough food and nutrition intake and history. Thus, the chapters in Part 1 provide an organized way to develop the skills needed to fulfill the remainder of the nutrition care process.

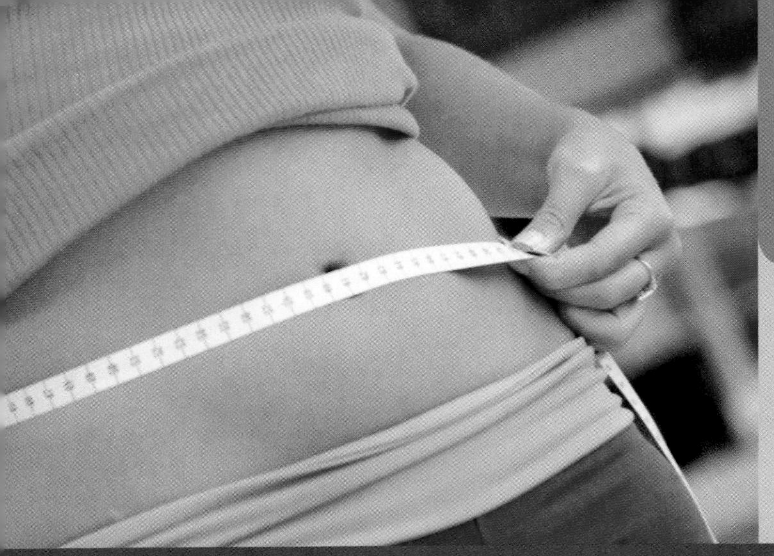

CHAPTER 1

Peter L. Beyer, MS, RD

Intake: Digestion, Absorption, Transport, and Excretion of Nutrients

KEY TERMS

active transport
amylase
brush border
chelation
cholecystokinin (CCK)
chyme
colonic salvage
enterohepatic circulation
facilitated diffusion
gastrin
lactase
maltase
micelle
microvilli
motilin
pancreatic lipase
parietal cells
passive diffusion
pepsin
peristalsis
prebiotic
probiotic
proteolytic enzymes
secretin
somatostatin
sucrase
synbiotic
villi

THE GASTROINTESTINAL TRACT

One of the primary considerations for a complete nutrition assessment is to consider the three-step model of "ingestion, digestion, and utilization." In this model, consideration is given to each step to identify all areas of inadequacy or excess. If there is any reason why a step is altered from physical, biochemical, or behavioral-environmental causes, the astute nutrition provider must select an appropriate nutrition diagnosis for which intervention is required. Intake and assimilation of nutrients should lead to a desirable level of nutritional health.

The gastrointestinal tract (GIT) is designed to (1) digest protein, carbohydrates, and lipids from ingested foods and beverages; (2) absorb fluids, micronutrients, and trace elements; and (3) provide a physical and immunologic barrier to microorganisms, foreign material, and potential antigens consumed with food or formed during the passage of food through the GIT. In addition, the GIT participates in many other regulatory, metabolic, and immunologic functions that affect the entire body.

The human GIT is well suited for digesting and absorbing nutrients from a tremendous variety of foods, including meats, dairy products, fruits, vegetables, grains, complex starches, sugars, fats, and oils. Depending on the nature of the diet consumed, 90% to 97% of food is digested and absorbed; most of the unabsorbed material is of plant origin. Compared with ruminants and animals with a very large cecum, humans are considerably less efficient at extracting energy from grasses, stems, seeds, and other coarse fibrous materials. Humans lack the enzymes to hydrolyze the chemical bonds that link the molecules of sugars that make up plant fibers. Fibrous foods and any undigested carbohydrates are fermented to varying degrees by bacteria in the human colon, but only 5% to 10% of the energy needed by humans can be derived from this process (Engylst and Englyst, 2005).

The GIT extends from the mouth to the anus and includes the oropharyngeal structures, esophagus, stomach, liver and gallbladder, pancreas, and small and large intestine. It is one of the largest organs in the body, has the greatest surface area, has the largest number of immune cells, and is one of the most metabolically active tissues in the body (Figure 1-1). The human intestine is about 7 m long and configured in a pattern of folds, pits, and fingerlike projections called **villi**. The villi are lined with epithelial cells and even smaller, cylindrical extensions called **microvilli**. The result is a tremendous increase in surface area compared with that expected from a smooth, hollow cylinder (Figure 1-2). The cells lining the intestinal tract have a life span of approximately 3 to 5 days, and then they are sloughed into the lumen and "recycled," adding to the pool of available nutrients. The cells are fully functional only for the last 2 to 3 days as they migrate from the crypts to the distal third of the villi.

The health of the body depends on a healthy, functional GIT. Because of the unusually high metabolic activity and requirements of the GIT, the cells lining it are more susceptible than most tissues to micronutrient deficiencies; protein-energy malnutrition; and damage resulting from toxins, drugs, irradiation, or interruption of its blood supply. Approximately 45% of the energy requirement of the small intestine and 70% of the energy requirement of cells lining the colon are supplied by nutrients passing through its lumen. After only a few days of starvation, the GIT atrophies (i.e., the surface area decreases and secretions, synthetic functions, blood flow, and absorptive capacity are all reduced). Resumption of food intake, even with less than adequate calories, results in cellular proliferation and return of normal GI function after only a few days. Optimum function of the human GIT seems to depend on a constant supply of foods rather than on consumption of large amounts of foods interrupted by prolonged fasts.

BRIEF OVERVIEW OF DIGESTIVE AND ABSORPTIVE PROCESSES

The sight, smell, taste, and even thought of food start the secretions and movements of the GIT. In the mouth, chewing reduces the size of food particles, which are mixed with salivary secretions that prepare them for swallowing. A small amount of starch is degraded by salivary amylase, but this overall carbohydrate digestion is minimal. The esophagus transports food and liquid from the oral cavity and pharynx to the stomach. In the stomach, food is mixed with acidic fluid and proteolytic and lipolytic enzymes. Small amounts of lipid digestion take place, and some proteins

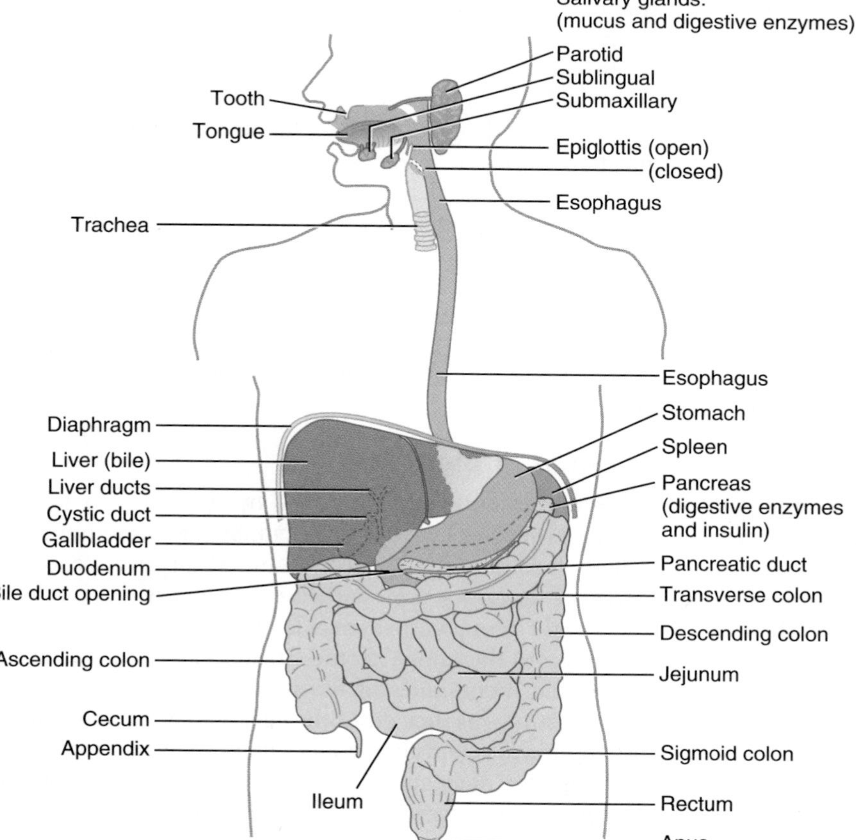

FIGURE 1-1 The digestive system.

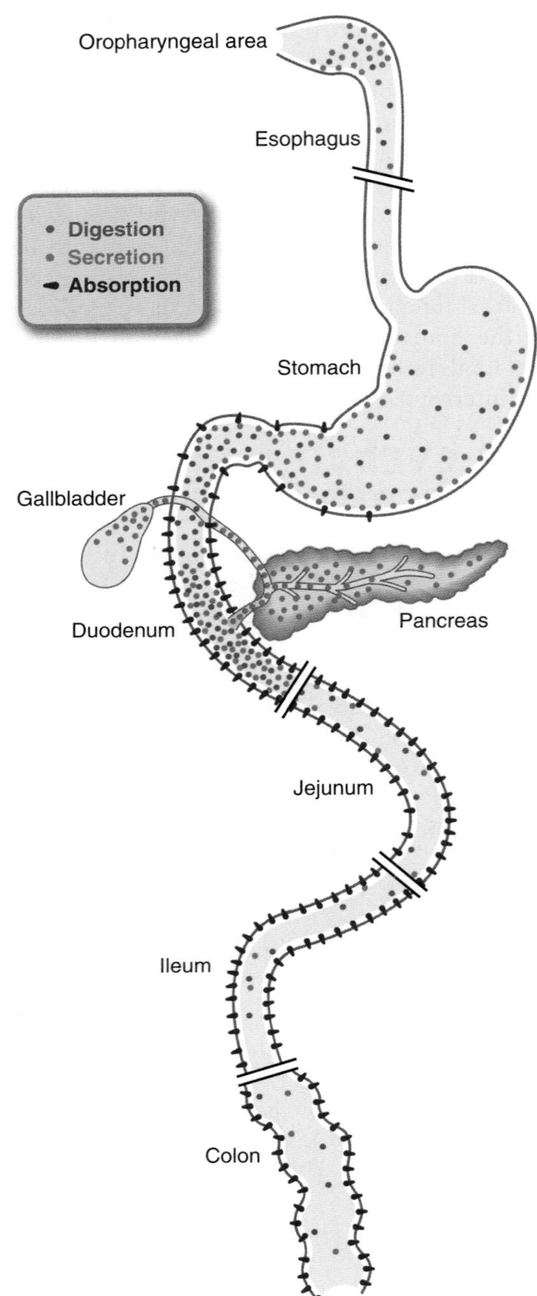

FIGURE 1-2 Sites of secretion, digestion, and absorption.

are changed in structure or partially digested to large peptides (Soybel, 2005). When food reaches the appropriate consistency and concentration, the stomach allows its contents to pass into the small intestine, where most digestion takes place. Alcohol, the exception, is absorbed through the stomach.

In the first 100 cm of small intestine, a flurry of activity occurs, resulting in the digestion and absorption of most ingested food. Here the presence of food stimulates the release of hormones that stimulate the production and release of powerful enzymes from the pancreas and small intestine and bile from the liver and gallbladder. Starches and proteins are reduced to smaller-molecular-weight carbohydrates and small to medium-size peptides. Dietary fats are reduced from visible globules of fat to microscopic droplets of triglycerides, then to free fatty acids and monoglycerides. Enzymes from the brush border of the small intestine further reduce the remaining carbohydrates to monosaccharides and peptides to single amino acids, dipeptides, and tripeptides (Keller and Layer, 2005). Together with salivary and gastric secretions, secretions from the pancreas, small intestine, and gallbladder contribute 7 to 9 L of fluid in a day, approximately three to four times more fluid than is normally consumed orally. All but 100 to 150 mL of the total fluid entering the lumen is reabsorbed.

The movement of ingested and secreted material in the GIT is regulated primarily by peptide hormones, nerves, and enteric muscles. Along the remaining length of the small intestine, almost all the macronutrients, minerals, vitamins, trace elements, and fluid are absorbed before reaching the colon. The colon and rectum absorb most of the remaining fluid delivered from the small intestine. The colon absorbs electrolytes and only a small amount of remaining nutrients.

Most nutrients absorbed from the GIT enter the portal vein for transport to the liver, where they may be stored, transformed into other substances, or released into circulation. End products of most dietary fats are transported into the bloodstream via the lymphatic circulation.

Remaining fiber, resistant starch, sugar, and amino acids are fermented in the brush border of the colon. Fermentation of the remaining carbohydrates results in the production of short-chain fatty acids (SCFAs) and gas. SCFAs help maintain normal mucosal function, salvage a small amount of energy from some of the residual carbohydrates and amino acids, and facilitate the absorption of salt and water (Englyst and Englyst, 2005). Some of the carbohydrate and fiber resistant to digestion in the upper GIT serve as "prebiotic" material by producing SCFAs, decreasing the colonic pH, and increasing the mass of "helpful" bacteria (Macfarlane et al., 2008). Prebiotic substances support the symbiotic relationship between the GIT and its microbiological environment.

The large intestine provides temporary storage for waste products. The distal colon, rectum, and anus control defecation.

Enzymes in Digestion

Digestion of food is accomplished by enzymatic hydrolysis. Cofactors such as hydrochloric acid, bile, and sodium bicarbonate facilitate the digestive and absorptive processes. Digestive enzymes are synthesized in specialized cells in the mouth, stomach, pancreas, and small intestine and are released into the lumen. Some enzymes are localized in the lipoprotein membranes of the mucosal cells and attach to their substrates as they enter the cell. Table 1-1 summarizes the GI enzymes and their functions in the small intestine.

Except for fiber and some carbohydrates, digestion and absorption are essentially completed in the small intestine. No digestive enzymes are secreted from the large intestine.

TABLE 1-1

Summary of Enzymatic Digestion and Absorption

Secretion and Source	Enzymes	Substrate	Action and Resulting Products	Final Products Absorbed
Saliva from salivary glands in mouth	Ptyalin (salivary amylase)	Starch	Hydrolysis to form dextrins and branched oligosaccharides	—
Gastric juice from gastric glands in stomach mucosa	Pepsin	Protein (in the presence of hydrochloric acid)	Hydrolysis of peptide bonds to form polypeptides and amino acids	—
	Gastric lipase	Fat, especially shorter chain	Hydrolysis to form free fatty acids	—
Exocrine secretions from pancreas	Lipase	Fat (in the presence of bile salts)	Hydrolysis to form monoglycerides and fatty acids; incorporated into micelles	Fatty acids into mucosal cells; reesterified as triglycerides
	Cholesterol esterase	Cholesterol	Hydrolysis to form esters of cholesterol and fatty acids; incorporated into micelles	Cholesterol into mucosal cells; transferred to chylomicrons
	α-Amylase	Starch and dextrins	Hydrolysis to form dextrins and maltose	—
	Trypsin (activated trypsinogen)	Proteins and polypeptides	Hydrolysis of interior peptide bonds to form polypeptides	—
	Chymotrypsin (activated chymotrypsinogen)	Proteins and peptides	Hydrolysis of interior peptide bonds to form polypeptides	—
	Carboxypeptidase	Polypeptides	Hydrolysis of terminal peptide bonds (carboxyl end) to form amino acids	Amino acids
	Ribonuclease and deoxyribonuclease	Ribonucleic acids and (RNA) deoxyribonucleic acids (DNA)	Hydrolysis to form mononucleotides	Mononucleotides
	Elastase	Fibrous protein	Hydrolysis to form peptides and amino acids	—
Small intestine enzymes (primarily in brush border)	Carboxypeptidase, aminopeptidase, and dipeptidase	Polypeptides	Hydrolysis of carboxyl terminus, amino terminus, or internal peptide bonds	Amino acids
	Enterokinase	Trypsinogen	Activates trypsin	Dipeptides and tripeptides
	Sucrase	Sucrose	Hydrolysis to form glucose and fructose	Glucose and fructose
	α-Dextrinase (isomaltase)	Dextrin (isomaltose)	Hydrolysis to form glucose	Glucose
	Maltase	Maltose	Hydrolysis to form glucose	Glucose
	Lactase	Lactose	Hydrolysis to from glucose and galactose	Glucose and galactose
	Nucleotidases	Nucleic acids	Hydrolysis to form nucleotides and phosphates	Nucleotides
	Nucleosidase and phosphorylase	Nucleosides	Hydrolysis to form purines, pyrimidines, and pentose phosphate	Purine and pyrimidine bases

Although water, monosaccharides, vitamins, minerals, and alcohol are usually absorbed in their basic form, often they must be unbound from other molecules or attached to carriers before absorption. Generally, the carbohydrates, lipids, and proteins must be converted to their simple constituents by digestive enzymes before they are absorbed (see Chapter 3).

Regulators of Gastrointestinal Activity: Nerves, Neurotransmitters, and Neuropeptide Hormones

Neural Mechanisms

GI movement, including contraction, mixing, and propulsion of luminal contents, is the result of the coordinated activity of enteric nerves, extrinsic nerves, endocrine cells, and smooth muscle. The neural mechanisms include (1) an intrinsic system consisting of two layers of nerves embedded in the gut wall and (2) an external system of nerve fibers running to and from the central and autonomic nervous systems. Mucosal receptors in the gut wall are appropriately sensitive to the composition of the **chyme** (a semiliquid substance of acid, fatty acids, and amino acids) and lumen distention (i.e., fullness) and send impulses through submucosal and mesenteric nerves.

Neurotransmitters and neuropeptides with small molecular weights signal nerves to contract or relax muscles, increase or decrease fluid secretions, or change blood flow. The GIT then largely regulates its own motility and secretory activity. However, signals from the central nervous system can override the enteric system and affect GI function. Hormones, neuropeptides, and neurotransmitters in the GIT not only affect GI function but also have an effect on other nerves and tissues in many parts of the body. Some examples of neurotransmitters released from enteric nerve endings are listed in Table 1-2. In people with GI disease (e.g., infections, inflammatory bowel disease, irritable bowel syndrome), the enteric nervous system may be overstimulated, resulting in abnormal secretion, altered blood flow, increased permeability, and altered immune function.

Autonomic innervation is supplied by the sympathetic fibers that run along blood vessels and by the parasympathetic fibers in the vagal and pelvic nerves. In general, sympathetic neurons, which are activated by fear, anger, and stress, tend to slow transit of GI contents by inhibiting neurons affecting muscle contraction and inhibiting secretions. The parasympathetic nerves innervate specific areas of the alimentary tract. For example, the sight or smell of food stimulates vagal activity and subsequent secretion of acid from **parietal cells** scattered along the walls of the stomach. The GIT also sends signals that are perceived as colicky pain, sharp pain, nausea, urgency or gastric fullness, or gastric emptiness by way of the vagal and spinal nerves. Inflammation, dysmotility, and various types of intestinal damage may intensify these perceptions.

Primary Neuropeptide Hormones

Regulation of the GIT involves numerous peptide hormones that can act locally or distally. These regulators can act locally in an autocrine, paracrine, or endocrine role by traveling through the blood to their target organs. More than 100 peptide hormones and hormone-like growth factors have been identified. Their actions are often complex and extend well beyond the GIT. Some of the hormones (e.g., of the cholecystokinin [CCK] and somatostatin family) also serve as neurotransmitters between neurons.

The GIT secretes more than 30 families of neuropeptide hormones and is the largest endocrine organ in the body (Rehfeld, 2004). GI hormones are involved in initiating and terminating feeding, bringing on sensations of hunger and satiety, increasing or decreasing movements of the GIT, enhancing or retarding esophageal and gastric emptying, regulating blood flow and permeability, regulating immune functions, and stimulating the growth of cells (within and beyond the GIT). Ghrelin, a neuropeptide secreted from the stomach, and motilin, a related hormone secreted from the duodenum, send a "hungry" message to the

TABLE 1-2

Examples of Neurotransmitters and Their Actions

Neurotransmitter	Site of Release	Primary Action
GABA	Central nervous system	Relaxes lower esophageal sphincter.
Norepinephrine	Central nervous system, spinal cord, sympathetic nerves	Decreases motility, increases contraction of sphincters, inhibits secretions.
Acetylcholine	Central nervous system, autonomic system, other tissues	Increases motility, relaxes sphincters, stimulates secretion.
Neurotensin	GI tract, central nervous system	Inhibits release of gastric emptying and acid secretion.
Serotonin (5-HT)	GI tract, spinal cord	Facilitates secretion and peristalsis.
Nitric oxide	Central nervous system, GI tract	Regulates blood flow, maintains muscle tone, maintains gastric motor activity.
Substance P	Gut, central nervous system, skin	Increases sensory awareness (mainly pain), and peristalsis.

5-HT, 5-hydroxytryptamine; *GABA*, α-aminobutyric acid; *GI*, gastrointestinal.

brain. Once food has been ingested, hormones *PYY 3-36*, CCK, glucagon-like polypeptide-1 (GLP-1), oxyntomodulin, pancreatic polypeptide, and gastrin-releasing polypeptide (bombesin) send signals to decrease hunger and increase satiety (Stanley et al., 2005). Some of the GI hormones, including some of those that affect satiety, also tend to slow gastric emptying and decrease secretions (e.g., somatostatin). Other GI hormones (e.g., motilin) increase motility.

The signaling agents of the GIT are also involved in several metabolic functions. The neuropeptides glucose-dependent insulinotropic polypeptide (GIP) and GLP-1 are called *incretin hormones* because they help lower blood sugar by facilitating insulin secretion, decreasing gastric emptying, and increasing satiety. Several of these neuropeptide hormones and analogs are used in management of obesity, inflammatory bowel disease, diarrhea, diabetes, GI malignancies, and other conditions. This area of research is critically important.

Some functions of the hormones that affect GI cell growth, deoxyribonucleic acid (DNA) synthesis, inflammation, proliferation, secretion, movement, or metabolism have not been fully identified (Kahn and Ghia, 2010). Knowledge of major hormone functions becomes especially important when the sites of their secretion or action are diseased or removed in surgical procedures or when hormones and their analogs are used to suppress or enhance some aspect of GI function. The key GIT hormones are summarized in Table 1-3.

Gastrin, a hormone that stimulates gastric secretions and motility, is secreted primarily from endocrine "G" cells in the antral mucosa of the stomach. Secretion is initiated by (1) distention of the antrum after a meal; (2) impulses from the vagus nerve such as those triggered by the smell or sight of food; and (3) the presence in the antrum of secretagogues such as partially digested proteins, fermented alcoholic beverages, caffeine, or food extracts (e.g., bouillon). When the lumen gets more acidic, feedback involving other hormones inhibits gastrin release (Schubert, 2009). Gastrin binds to receptors on parietal cells and histamine-releasing cells to stimulate gastric acid, to receptors on chief cells to release pepsinogen, and to receptors on smooth muscle to increase gastric motility.

Secretin, the first hormone to be named, is released from "S" cells in the wall of the proximal small intestine into the

TABLE 1-3

Functions of Major Gastrointestinal Hormones

Hormone	Site of Release	Stimulants for Release	Organ Affected	Effect on Organ
Gastrin	Gastric mucosa, duodenum	Peptides, amino acids, caffeine Distention of the antrum Some alcoholic beverages, vagus nerve	Stomach, esophagus, GIT in general	Stimulates secretion of HCl and pepsinogen. Increases gastric antral motility. Increases lower esophageal sphincter tone.
			Gallbladder	Weakly stimulates contraction of gallbladder.
			Pancreas	Weakly stimulates pancreatic secretion of bicarbonate.
Secretin	Duodenal mucosa	Acid in small intestine	Pancreas	Increases output of H_2O and bicarbonate; increases some enzyme secretion from the pancreas and insulin release.
			Duodenum	Decreases motility. Increases mucus output.
CCK	Proximal small bowel	Peptides, amino acids, fats, HCl	Pancreas	Stimulates secretion of pancreatic enzymes.
			Gallbladder	Causes contraction of gallbladder.
			Stomach	Slows gastric emptying.
			Colon	Increases motility. May mediate feeding behavior.
GIP	Small intestine	Glucose, fat	Stomach, pancreas	Stimulates insulin release.
GLP-1	Small intestine	Glucose, fat	Stomach, pancreas	Prolongs gastric emptying Inhibits glucagon release. Stimulates insulin release.
Motilin	Stomach, small and large bowel	Biliary and pancreatic secretions	Stomach, small bowel, colon	Promotes gastric emptying and GI motility.

CCK, Cholecystokinin; *GI*, gastrointestinal; *GIP*, glucose-dependent insulinotropic polypeptide; *GIT*, gastrointestinal tract; *GLP-1*, glucagon-like polypeptide; *H_2O*, water; *HCl*, hydrochloric acid.

bloodstream. It is secreted in response to gastric acid and digestive end products in the duodenum, stimulates the pancreas to secrete water and bicarbonate into the duodenum, and inhibits gastric acid secretion and emptying (the opposite of gastrin). Neutralized acidity protects the duodenal mucosa from prolonged exposure to acid and provides the appropriate environment for intestinal and pancreatic enzyme activity. The human receptor is found in the stomach and ductal and acinar cells of the pancreas. In different species, other organs may express secretin, including the liver, colon, heart, kidney, and brain (Chey and Chang, 2003).

Small bowel mucosal "I" cells secrete **cholecystokinin (CCK)**, an important multifunctional hormone released in response to the presence of protein and fat. Receptors for CCK are in pancreatic acinar cells, pancreatic islet cells, gastric somatostatin-releasing D cells, smooth muscle cells of the GIT, and the central nervous system. Major functions of CCK are to (1) stimulate the pancreas to secrete enzymes, some bicarbonate, and water; (2) stimulate gallbladder contraction; (3) increase colonic and rectal motility; (4) slow gastric emptying; and (5) increase satiety (Keller and Layer, 2005). CCK is also widely distributed in the brain and plays a role in neuronal functioning (Deng et al, 2010).

GLP-1 and GIP, released from the intestinal mucosa in the presence of meals rich in glucose and fat, stimulate insulin synthesis and release. GLP-1 also decreases glucagon secretion, delays gastric emptying, and may help promote satiety. GLP-1 and GIP are examples of incretin hormones, which help keep blood glucose from rising excessively after a meal (Nauck, 2009). This may explain why a glucose load received enterally results in less of an increase in blood glucose than when an equal amount of glucose is received intravenously.

Motilin is released by endocrine cells in the duodenal mucosa during fasting to stimulate gastric emptying and intestinal motility. Erythromycin, an antibiotic, has been shown to bind to motilin receptors; thus analogs of erythromycin and motilin have been used as therapeutic agents to treat delayed gastric emptying (De Smet et al., 2009).

Somatostatin, released by D cells in the antrum and pylorus, is a hormone with far-reaching actions. Its primary roles are inhibitory and antisecretory. It decreases motility of the stomach and intestine and inhibits or regulates the release of several GI hormones. Somatostatin and its analog, octreotide, are being used to treat certain malignant diseases (Van Op Den Bosch et al., 2009) as well as numerous GI disorders such as diarrhea, short bowel syndrome, pancreatitis, dumping syndrome, and gastric hypersecretion.

Digestion in the Mouth

In the mouth, the teeth grind and crush food into small particles. The food mass is simultaneously moistened and lubricated by saliva. Three pairs of salivary glands—the parotid, submaxillary, and sublingual glands—produce approximately 1.5 L of saliva daily. A serous secretion containing **amylase** (ptyalin) begins the digestion of starch. This digestion is minimal, and the amylase becomes inactive when it reaches the acidic contents of the stomach. Another type of saliva contains mucus, a protein that causes particles of food to stick together and lubricates the mass for swallowing. The oropharyngeal secretions also contain a lipase that is capable of digesting a minimal amount of fat.

The masticated food mass, or bolus, is passed back to the pharynx under voluntary control, but throughout the esophagus the process of swallowing (deglutition) is involuntary. **Peristalsis** then moves the food rapidly into the stomach (see Chapter 41 for detailed discussion on swallowing).

Digestion in the Stomach

Food particles are propelled forward and mixed with gastric secretions by wavelike contractions that progress forward from the upper portion of the stomach (fundus), to the midportion (corpus), and then to the antrum and pylorus. In the stomach gastric secretions are mixed with food and beverages. An average of 2000 to 2500 mL of gastric juice is secreted daily. The gastric secretions contain hydrochloric acid (secreted by the parietal cells in the walls of the fundus and corpus), a protease, gastric lipase, mucus, intrinsic factor (a glycoprotein that facilitates vitamin B_{12} absorption in the ileum), and the GI hormone gastrin. The protease is **pepsin**, which is also secreted from glands in the fundus and corpus. It is secreted in an inactive form, pepsinogen, which is converted by hydrochloric acid to its active form. Pepsin is active only in the acid environment of the stomach and serves primarily to change the shape and size of some of the proteins in a normal meal.

An acid-stable lipase is secreted into the stomach by chief cells. Although this lipase is considerably less active than pancreatic lipase, it contributes to the overall processing of dietary triglycerides. Gastric lipase is more specific for triglycerides composed of medium- and SCFAs, but the normal diet contains few of these fats. Lipases secreted in the upper portions of the GIT may have a relatively important role in the liquid diet of infants; but, when pancreatic insufficiency occurs, it becomes apparent that lingual and gastric lipases are not sufficient to prevent lipid malabsorption (Keller and Layer, 2005). In the process of gastric digestion, most of the food becomes semiliquid chyme, which is 50% water. Gastric secretions are also important in increasing the availability and downstream absorption of vitamin B_{12}, calcium, iron, and zinc (Soybel, 2005).

When food is consumed, significant numbers of microorganisms are also consumed. The stomach pH is quite low, ranging from about 1 to 4. The combined actions of hydrochloric acid and proteolytic enzymes result in a significant reduction in the concentration of microorganisms ingested. Some microbes may escape and enter the intestine if consumed in sufficient concentrations or if achlorhydria, gastrectomy, GI dysfunction or disease, poor nutrition, or drugs that suppress acid secretions are present. This may increase the risk of bacterial overgrowth in the intestine.

The stomach continuously mixes and churns food and normally releases the mixture in small quantities into the small intestine. The amount emptied with each contraction of the antrum and pylorus varies with the volume and type of food consumed, but only a few milliliters are released at a time. The presence of food in the intestine and regulatory hormones provide feedback to slow gastric emptying.

Most of a liquid meal empties within 1 to 2 hours, and most of a solid meal empties within 2 to 3 hours. When eaten alone, carbohydrates leave the stomach the most rapidly, followed by protein, fat, and fibrous food. In a meal with mixed types of foods, emptying of the stomach depends on the overall volume and characteristics of the foods. Liquids empty more rapidly than solids, large particles empty more slowly than small particles, and concentrated food tends to empty more slowly than low-calorie meals. These factors are important considerations for practitioners who counsel patients with nausea, vomiting, diabetic gastroparesis, or partial obstruction or for practitioners monitoring patients after GI surgery or malnourished patients.

The lower esophageal sphincter (LES) above the entrance to the stomach prevents reflux of gastric contents into the esophagus. The pyloric sphincter in the distal portion of the stomach helps regulate the exit of gastric contents, preventing backflow of chyme from the duodenum into the stomach. Emotional changes, food, GI regulators, and irritation from nearby ulcers may alter the performance of strictures. Certain foods and beverages may alter LES pressure, permitting reflux of stomach contents back into the esophagus (see Chapter 28).

Digestion in the Small Intestine

The small intestine is the primary site for digestion of foods and nutrients. The small intestine is divided into the duodenum, the jejunum, and the ileum (Figure 1-2). The duodenum is approximately 0.5 m long, the jejunum is 2 to 3 m, and the ileum is 3 to 4 m. Most of the digestive process is completed in the duodenum and upper jejunum, and the absorption of most nutrients is largely complete by the time the material reaches the middle of the jejunum. The acidic chyme from the stomach enters the duodenum, where it is mixed with duodenal juices and the secretions from the pancreas and biliary tract. As a result of the secretion of bicarbonate-containing fluid from the pancreas and dilution from other secretions, acid chyme is neutralized. Enzymes of the small intestine and pancreas operate more effectively in a more neutral pH.

The entry of partially digested foods, primarily fats and protein, stimulates the release of several hormones that in turn stimulate the secretion of enzymes and fluids and affect GI motility and satiety. Bile, which is predominantly a mixture of water, bile salts, and small amounts of pigments and cholesterol, is secreted from the liver and gallbladder. Through their surfactant properties, the bile salts facilitate the digestion and absorption of lipids, cholesterol, and fat-soluble vitamins. Bile acids are also regulatory molecules; they activate the vitamin D receptor and cell-signaling pathways in the liver and GIT that alter gene expression of enzymes involved in the regulation of energy metabolism (Hylemon et al., 2009). It is now known that bile acids play an important role in hunger and satiety.

The pancreas secretes potent enzymes capable of digesting all of the major nutrients, and enzymes from the small intestine help complete the process. The primary lipid-digesting enzymes secreted by the pancreas are **pancreatic lipase** and colipase. **Proteolytic enzymes** include trypsin and chymotrypsin, carboxypeptidase, aminopeptidase, ribonuclease, and deoxyribonuclease. Trypsin and chymotrypsin are secreted in their inactive forms and are activated by enterokinase (also known as *enteropeptidase*), which is secreted when chyme contacts the intestinal mucosa. Pancreatic amylase serves to hydrolyze large starch molecules eventually into units of approximately two to six sugars. Enzymes lining the brush border of the villi further break down the carbohydrate molecules into monosaccharides before absorption. Varying amounts of resistant starches and most ingested dietary fiber escape digestion in the small intestine and may add to fibrous material available for fermentation by colonic microbes (Englyst and Englyst, 2005).

Intestinal contents move along the small intestine at a rate of 1 cm per minute, taking from 3 to 8 hours to travel through the entire intestine to the ileocecal valve; along the way, remaining substrates continue to be digested and absorbed. The ileocecal valve, like the pyloric valve, serves to limit the amount of intestinal material passed back and forth from the small intestine to the colon. A damaged or nonfunctional ileocecal valve results in the entry of significant amounts of fluid and substrate into the colon and increased chance for microbial overgrowth in the small intestine (see Chapter 28).

THE SMALL INTESTINE: PRIMARY SITE OF NUTRIENT ABSORPTION

Structure and Function

The primary organ of nutrient and water absorption is the small intestine, which has an expansive absorptive area. The surface area is attributable to its extensive length, as well as to the organization of the mucosal lining. The small intestine has characteristic folds in its surface called *valvulae conniventes.* These convolutions are covered with fingerlike projections called *villi* (Figure 1-3), which in turn are covered by microvilli, or the **brush border**. The combination of folds, villous projections, and microvillous border creates an enormous absorptive surface of approximately 200 to 300 m^2. The villi rest on a supporting structure called the *lamina propria.* Within the lamina propria, which is composed of connective tissue, the blood and lymph vessels receive the products of digestion.

Each day, on average, the small intestine absorbs 150 to 300 g of monosaccharides, 60 to 100 g of fatty acids, 60 to 120 g of amino acids and peptides, and 50 to 100 g of ions. The capacity for absorption in the healthy individual far exceeds the normal macronutrient and caloric requirements. In the small intestine, all but 1 to 1.5 L of the 7 or 8 L of fluid secreted from the upper portions of the GIT, in addition to 1.5 to 3 L of dietary fluids, is absorbed by the time the contents reach the end of the small intestine.

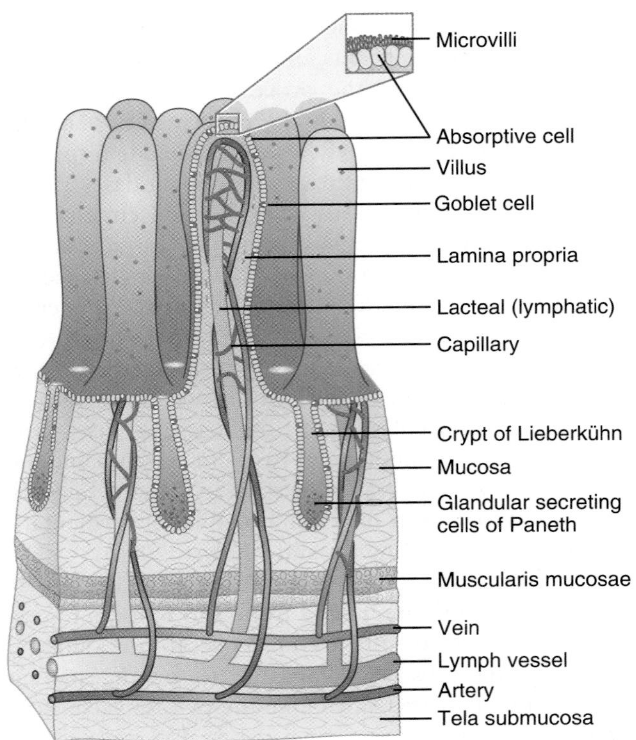

FIGURE 1-3 Structure of the villi of the human intestine showing blood and lymph vessels.

Approximately 95% of the bile salts secreted from the liver and gallbladder are reabsorbed as bile acids in the distal ileum. Without recycling bile acids from the GIT (enterohepatic circulation), synthesis of new bile acids in the liver would not keep pace with needs for adequate digestion. Bile salt insufficiency becomes clinically important in patients who have resections of the distal small bowel and diseases affecting the small intestine, such as Crohn disease, radiation enteritis, and cystic fibrosis. The distal ileum is also the site for vitamin B_{12} (with intrinsic factor) absorption.

Emulsification of fats in the small intestine is followed by their digestion, primarily by pancreatic lipase, into free fatty acids and monoglycerides. Pancreatic lipase typically cleaves the first and third fatty acid, leaving one attached to the middle glycerol carbon. When the concentration of bile salts reaches a certain level, they form **micelles** (small aggregates of fatty acids, monoglycerides, cholesterol, bile salts, and other lipids), which are organized with the polar ends of the molecules oriented toward the watery lumen of the intestine. The products of lipid digestion are rapidly solubilized in the central portion of the micelles and carried to the intestinal brush border (Figure 1-4).

At the surface of the unstirred water layer (UWL), the slightly acidic and watery plate that forms a boundary between the intestinal lumen and the brush border membranes, the lipids detach from the micelles. Remnants of the micelles return to the lumen for further transport. The monoglycerides and fatty acids are thus left to make their way across the lipophobic UWL to the more lipid-friendly membrane cells of the brush border. Lipids are taken up and transported through the endoplasmic reticulum and Golgi apparatus where fatty acids are re-esterified to triglyceride. Triglycerides are packaged, along with other lipids, into chylomicrons, which are released into the lymphatic circulation. Cholesterol absorption is facilitated by a protein transport system specific to cholesterol and not to other sterols (Hui et al., 2008; Lammert and Wang, 2005).

Absorptive and Transport Mechanisms

Absorption is complex, combining the intricate process of active transport with the simple process of passive diffusion. In absorption, nutrients pass through the intestinal mucosal cells (enterocytes or colonocytes) and make their way into the venous system to the liver or into the lymphatic circulation. Diffusion involves random movement through openings in or between the membranes of the mucosal cell walls using channel proteins (**passive diffusion**) or carrier/transport proteins in **facilitated diffusion** (Figure 1-5).

Active transport involves the input of energy to move ions or other substances, in combination with a transport protein, across a membrane against an energy gradient. Some nutrients may share the same carrier and thus compete for absorption. Transport or carrier systems can also become saturated, slowing the absorption of the nutrient. A notable example of such a carrier is intrinsic factor, which is responsible for the absorption of vitamin B_{12} (see Chapters 3 and 33).

Some molecules are moved from the intestinal lumen into mucosal cells by means of pumps, which require a carrier and energy from adenosine triphosphate. The absorption of glucose, sodium, galactose, potassium, magnesium, phosphate, iodide, calcium, iron, and amino acids occurs in this manner.

Pinocytosis has been described as the "drinking in," or engulfing, by the epithelial cell membrane of a small drop of intestinal contents. Pinocytosis allows large particles such as whole proteins to be absorbed in small quantities. The movement of foreign proteins across the GIT into the bloodstream, where they cause allergic reactions, may be the result of pinocytosis. The immunoglobulins from breast milk are probably absorbed through pinocytosis.

THE LARGE INTESTINE

The large intestine is approximately 1.5 m long and consists of the cecum, colon, and rectum. Mucus secreted by the mucosa of the large intestine protects the intestinal wall from excoriation and bacterial activity and provides the medium for binding the feces together. Bicarbonate ions secreted in exchange for absorbed chloride ions help to neutralize the acidic end products produced from bacterial action. Approximately 2 L of fluids are taken in food and beverages during the day, and 7 to 9 L of fluid is secreted along the GIT. Under normal circumstances, most of that fluid is absorbed in the small intestine and approximately 1 to 1.5 L of fluid enters the large intestine. Only approximately 100 mL remain to be excreted in the feces.

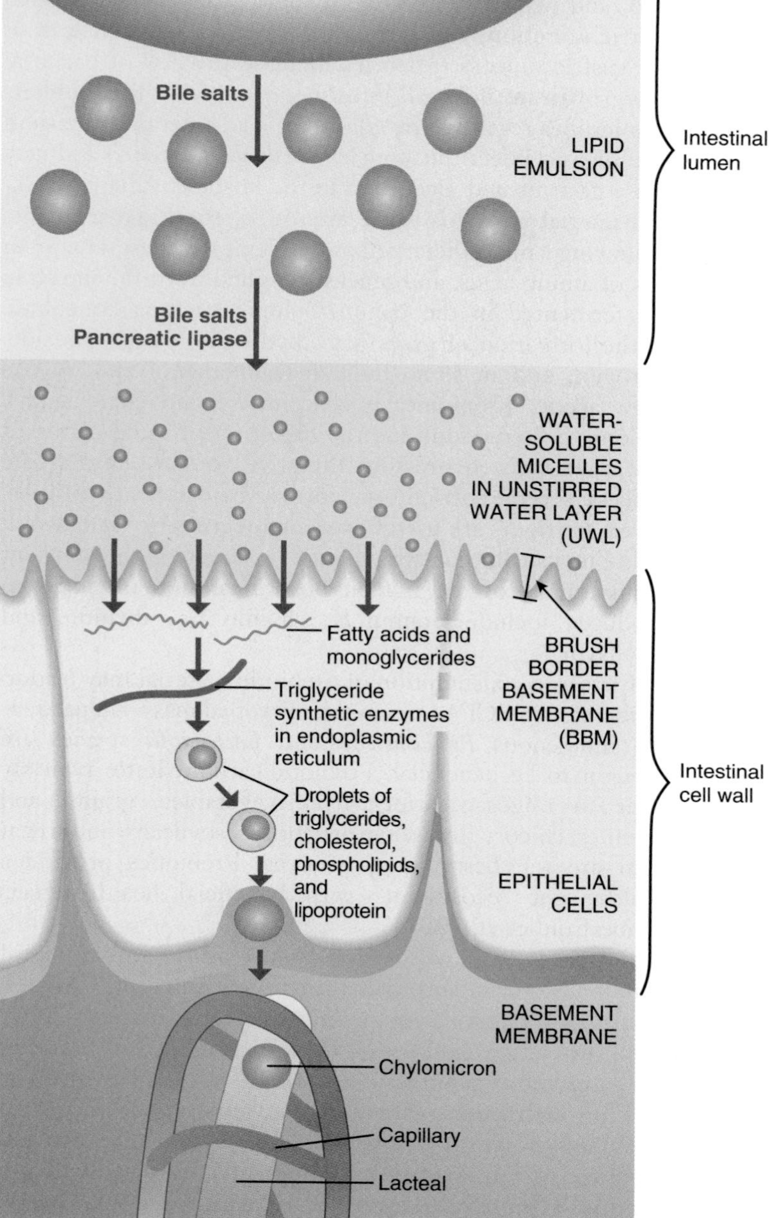

FIGURE 1-4 Summary of fat absorption.

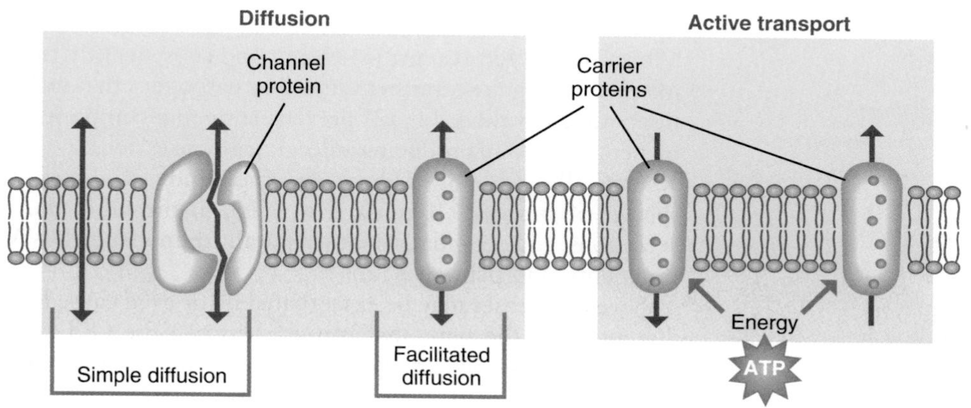

FIGURE 1-5 Transport pathways through the cell membrane, as well as basic transport mechanisms. *ATP*, Adenosine triphosphate.

The large intestine is also the site of bacterial fermentation of remaining carbohydrates and amino acids, synthesis of a small amount of vitamins, storage, and excretion of fecal residues. Colonic contents move forward slowly at a rate of 5 cm/h, and some remaining nutrients may be absorbed.

Defecation, or expulsion of feces through the rectum and anus, occurs with varying frequency, ranging from three times daily to once every 3 or more days. Average stool weight is in the range of 100 to 200 g, and mouth-to-anus transit time may vary from 18 to 72 hours. The feces generally consist of 75% water and 25% solids, but the proportions vary greatly. Approximately two thirds of the contents of the wet weight of the stool is bacteria, with the remainder coming from GI secretions, mucus, sloughed cells, and undigested foods. A diet that includes abundant fruits, vegetables, legumes, and whole grains typically results in a shorter overall GI transit time, more frequent defecation, and larger and softer stools.

Bacterial Action

The gut microflora make up a complex community that is estimated to involve thousands of species of microorganisms (Frank and Pace, 2008). At birth the GIT is essentially sterile, but accumulation of various microorganisms soon takes place. *Lactobacillus* organisms are the chief component of the GIT flora until an infant begins to eat solid foods. *Escherichia coli* then become predominant in the distal ileum, and the primary colonic flora are anaerobic, with species of the genus *Bacteroides* occurring most frequently. Lactobacilli are also present in the stools of most people who consume an ordinary mixed diet; but differences in the host's genome, dietary intake, hygiene, and medical and surgical history affect the kind of flora in the GIT (Table 1-4).

TABLE 1-4

Most Common Microbes Colonizing the Gastrointestinal Tract

Bacteria	Lactobacilli	Fungi
Acinetobacter	*Peptostreptococcus*	*Candida*
Bacteroides	*Porphyromonas*	
Bifidobacterium	*Prevotella*	*Parasites*
Clostridium	*Propionibacterium*	*Blastocystis*
Corynebacterium	*Pseudomonas*	*Endolimax*
Eubacterium	*Staphylococcus*	*Entamoeba coli*
Enterobacteriaceae	*Streptococcus* A, B, C, F, G	*E. hartmanni*
Enterococcus	*Streptococcus bovis*	*E. polecki*
Fusobacterium	*Streptococcus*	*Iodamoeba*
Helicobacter	*Veillonella*	*Trichomonas hominis*

Modified from Walter J. Ecological role of Lactobacilli in the gastrointestinal tract: implications for fundamental and biomedical research, Appl Environ Microbiol 74:4985, 2008.

Normally relatively few bacteria remain in the stomach or small intestine after meals because bile, hydrochloric acid, and pepsin work as germicides. However, decreased gastric secretions can increase the risk of inflammation of the gastric mucosa (*gastritis*), increase the risk of bacterial overgrowth in the small intestine, or increase the numbers of microbes reaching the colon. An acid-tolerant bacterium is known to infect the stomach (*Helicobacter pylori*) and may cause gastritis and ulceration in the host (see Chapter 28).

Bacterial action is most intense in the large intestine. Following a meal, dietary fiber, resistant starches, remaining bits of amino acids, and mucus sloughed from the intestine are fermented in the colon. Colonic bacteria contribute to the formation of gases (e.g., hydrogen, carbon dioxide, nitrogen, and in some individuals methane) and SCFAs (e.g., acetic, propionic, butyric, and some lactic acids). Colonic bacteria continue the digestion of some materials that have resisted previous digestive activity. During the process, several nutrients are formed by bacterial synthesis. These nutrients are used to varying degrees by GI mucosal cells but usually contribute little to meeting the nutrient requirements of the human host. Examples of nutrients produced include vitamin K, vitamin B_{12}, thiamin, and riboflavin.

Increased consumption of prebiotic material may lead to an increase in SCFAs and in the microbial mass—in particular, indigenous *Bifidobacteria* and *Lactobacilli* species are thought to be beneficial. Prebiotic carbohydrates typically refer to oligosaccharides from vegetables, grains, and legumes; chicory, Jerusalem artichokes, soybeans, and wheat bran are the best dietary sources. Prebiotics provide a healthy gut "ecosystem" with beneficial health effects (Roberfroid et al, 2010.)

Bacterial action also may result in the formation of potentially toxic substances such as ammonia, indoles, amines, and phenolic compounds such as indolacetate, tyramine, histamine, and cresol (MacFarlane, 2008). Some of the gases and organic acids contribute to the odor of feces.

The interactions between the innate and acquired immune systems evolve based on one's genetic heritage and exposure to a myriad of environmental substances over a lifetime. Malnutrition, exposure to toxic agents, and disease may affect the relationships among the physical and immunologic components of the GIT and the tremendous number of substances that reside or pass through its lumen (Quigley, 2010). Each individual's GI immune system, therefore, has a formidable task. It must (1) mount and subsequently turn off an attack against transient invading pathogens that make their way into the GIT; (2) prevent antigenic components of peptides from producing allergic responses locally and systemically; and (3) tolerate the thousands of different species of "normal" bacteria that reside in the GIT, their secretions, and degradation into cell wall components, DNA fragments, and peptides.

Several diseases may be exacerbated by or even caused by disruption of the tenuous harmony between the GIT and the contents of its lumen. Interactions among the host immune system, host genome, diet, and GI microflora may be linked with several infectious and inflammatory bowel diseases, allergies, immune disorders, metabolic disorders, and neoplasms (O'Keefe, 2008; Tappenden and Deutsch, 2007). In addition to the therapeutic use of antibiotics and antiinflammatory or immunosuppressive agents, attention is being given to the therapeutic potential of probiotic, prebiotic, and synbiotic products.

Probiotics are foods or concentrates of live organisms that contribute to a healthy microbial environment and suppress potential harmful microbes. Knowledge of their role in preventing and treating a host of GI and systemic disorders has expanded tremendously (Snelling, 2005).

Prebiotics are oligosaccharide components of the diet (e.g., fructo-oligosaccharides, inulin) that are the preferred energy substrates of "friendly" microbes in the GIT. When prebiotics, other sources of soluble dietary fiber, and other carbohydrates resistant to digestion are fermented by bacteria in the distal ileum and colon, they produce SCFAs that serve as fuel for the cells lining the GIT. SCFAs also serve as regulatory agents for several GI and host functions (Roberfroid et al, 2010.)

Synbiotics are a combination of probiotics and prebiotics. Synbiotics are long-chain, inulin-type fructans as compared with short-chain derivatives. These fructans, extracted from chicory roots, are prebiotic food ingredients that are fermented to lactic acid and SCFAs in the gut lumen. Synbiotics may be useful for early prevention or treatment of allergic disease (van de Pol et al, 2011.)

Colonic Salvage of Malabsorbed Energy Sources and Short-Chain Fatty Acids

Normally, varying amounts of some small-molecular-weight carbohydrates and amino acids remain in the chyme after leaving the small intestine. Accumulation of these small molecules could become osmotically important were it not for the action of bacteria in the colon. The disposal of residual substrates through production of SCFAs is called **colonic salvage** (Figure 1-6). SCFAs produced in fermentation are rapidly absorbed and take water with them. They also serve as fuel for the colonocytes and gut microbes, stimulate colonocyte proliferation and differentiation, enhance the absorption of electrolytes and water, and reduce the osmotic load of malabsorbed sugars. SCFAs may also help slow the movement of GI contents and participate in several other regulatory functions.

The ability to salvage carbohydrates is limited in humans. Colonic fermentation normally disposes of 20 to 25 g of carbohydrate over 24 hours. Excess amounts of carbohydrate and fermentable fiber in the colon can cause increased gas production, abdominal distention, bloating, pain, increased flatulence, decreased colonic pH, or even diarrhea. Over time, adaptation seems to occur in individuals consuming diets high in fiber that are resistant to human digestive enzymes. Current recommendations are for the consumption of approximately 24 to 38 g of dietary fiber per day from fruits, vegetables, legumes, seeds, and whole grains for (1) maintaining the health of the cells lining the colon, (2) preventing excessive intracolonic pressure, (3) preventing constipation, and (4) maintaining a stable and healthful microbial population.

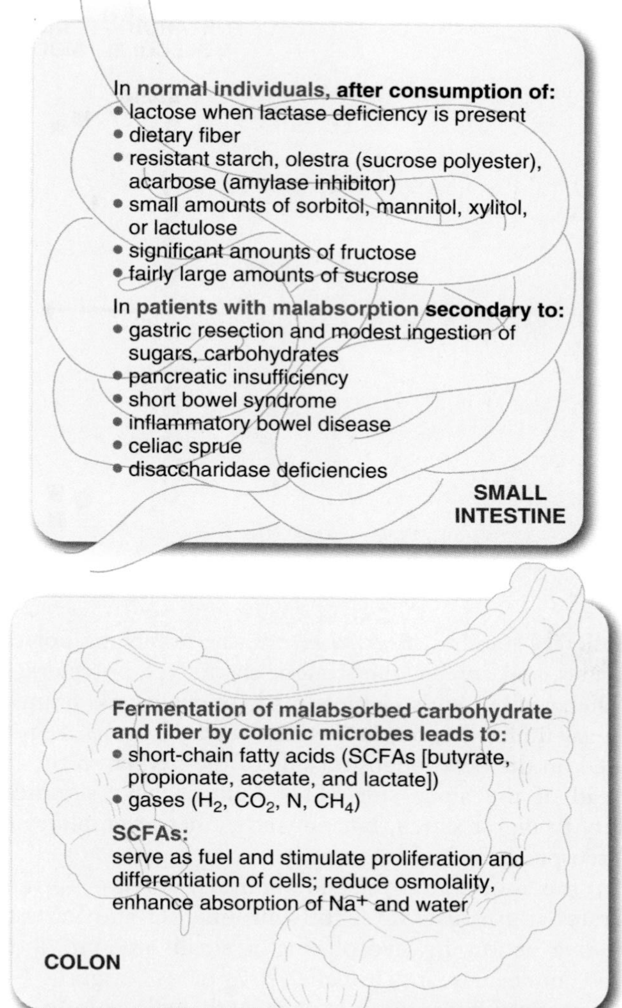

FIGURE 1-6 Colonic fermentation of malabsorbed carbohydrates and fiber.

Digestion and Absorption of Specific Types of Nutrients

Carbohydrates and Fiber

Most dietary carbohydrates are consumed in the form of starches, disaccharides, and monosaccharides. Starches, or polysaccharides, usually make up the greatest proportion of carbohydrates. Starches are large molecules composed of straight or branched chains of sugar molecules that are joined together, primarily in 1-4 or 1-6 linkages. Most of

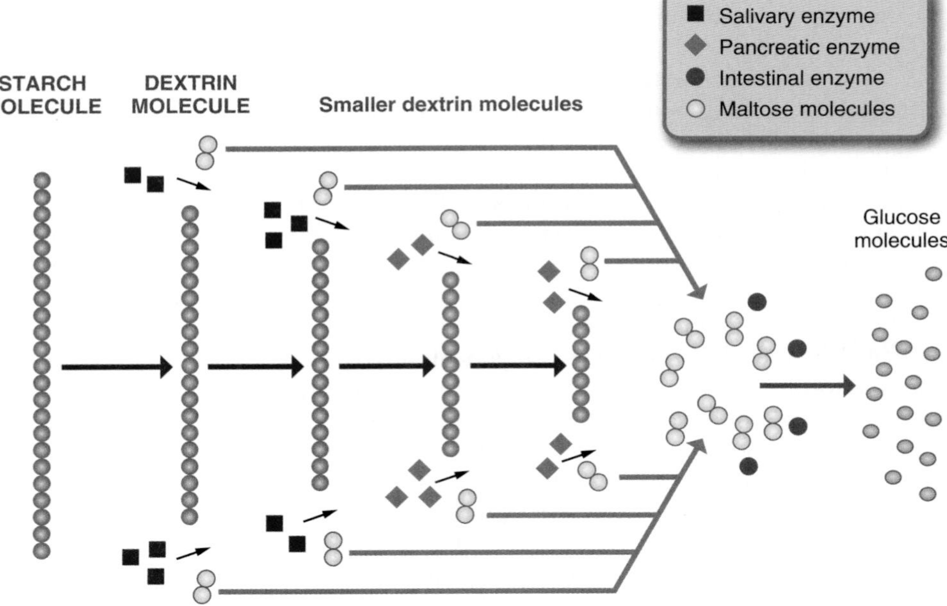

FIGURE 1-7 The gradual breakdown of large starch molecules into glucose by digestion enzymes.

the dietary starches are *amylopectins*, the branching polysaccharides, and *amylose*, the straight chain–type polymers.

Dietary fiber is also largely made of chains and branches of sugar molecules, but in this case the hydrogens are positioned on the beta (opposite) side of the oxygen in the link instead of the alpha side. That humans have significant ability to digest starch, but not most fiber, exemplifies the "stereospecificity" of enzymes.

In the mouth, the enzyme salivary amylase (ptyalin) operates at a neutral or slightly alkaline pH and starts the digestive action by hydrolyzing a small amount of the starch molecules into smaller fragments (Figure 1-7). Amylase deactivates after contact with hydrochloric acid. If digestible carbohydrates remained in the stomach long enough, acid hydrolysis could eventually reduce most of them into monosaccharides. However, the stomach usually empties before significant digestion can take place. By far, most carbohydrate digestion occurs in the proximal small intestine.

Pancreatic amylase breaks the large starch molecules at 1-4 linkages to create maltose, maltotriose, and "alpha-limit" dextrins remaining from the amylopectin branches. Enzymes from the brush border of the enterocytes further break the disaccharides and oligosaccharides into monosaccharides. For example, **maltase** from the mucosal cells breaks down the disaccharide maltose into two molecules of glucose. These outer-cell membranes also contain the enzymes **sucrase**, **lactase**, and isomaltase (or a-dextrinase), which act on sucrose, lactose, and isomaltose, respectively (Figure 1-8).

The resultant monosaccharides (i.e., glucose, galactose, and fructose) pass through the mucosal cells and into the bloodstream via the capillaries of the villi, where they are carried by the portal vein to the liver. At low concentrations, glucose and galactose are absorbed by active transport, primarily by a sodium-dependent transporter called the glucose (galactose) cotransporter. At higher luminal concentrations of glucose, glucose transporter (GLUT) 2 becomes a primary facilitative transporter into the intestinal cell. Fructose is more slowly absorbed and uses GLUT5 and the facilitative transporter from the lumen. GLUT2 is used to transport both glucose and fructose across the intestinal cell membranes into the blood (Kellett and Brot-Laroche, 2005).

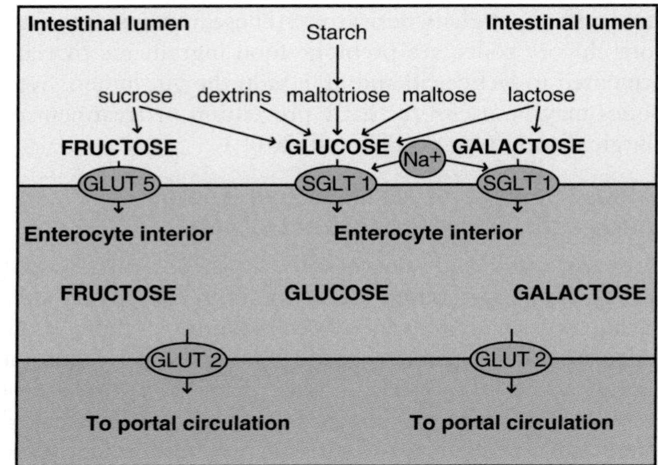

FIGURE 1-8 Starch, sucrose, maltotriose, and galactose are digested to their constituent sugars. Glucose and galactose are transported through the apical brush border membrane of the enterocyte by a sodium-dependent transporter, glucose (galactose) cotransporter; and fructose is transported by glucose transporter (GLUT) 5. Glucose, fructose, and galactose are transported across the serosal membrane by the sodium-independent transporter, GLUT2.

The sodium-dependent transport of monosaccharides is the reason why sodium-glucose drinks are used to rehydrate infants with diarrhea or athletes who have lost too much fluid. Glucose is transported from the liver to the tissues, although some glucose is stored in the liver and muscles as glycogen. Most of the fructose, as in the case of galactose, is transported to the liver, where it is converted to glucose. Consumption of large amounts of lactose (especially in individuals with a lactase deficiency), fructose, stachyose, raffinose, or alcohol sugars (e.g., sorbitol, mannitol, or xylitol) can result in considerable amounts of these sugars passing unabsorbed into the colon (Beyer et al., 2005) and may cause increased gas and loose stools. Fructose is found naturally in many fruits (e.g., in sucrose and high-fructose corn syrup) but is likely to produce symptoms only if consumed as the single monosaccharide or if the food has an abundance of fructose compared with glucose (as in the case of apple juice).

Some forms of carbohydrates (i.e., cellulose, hemicellulose, pectin, gum, and other forms of fiber) cannot be digested by humans because neither their salivary nor pancreatic amylase has the ability to split the linkages connecting the constituent sugars. These carbohydrates pass relatively unchanged into the colon, where they are partially fermented by bacteria in the colon. However, unlike humans, cows and other ruminants can subsist on high-fiber food because of the bacterial digestion of these carbohydrates that takes place in the rumen. Other resistant starches and sugars are also less well digested or absorbed by humans; thus their consumption may result in significant amounts of starch and sugar in the colon. The resistant starches and some types of dietary fiber are fermented into SCFAs and gases. Starches resistant to digestion tend to include plant foods with a high protein and fiber content such as those from legumes and whole grains. One form of dietary fiber, lignin, is made of cyclopentane units and is neither readily soluble nor fermentable.

Proteins

Protein intake in the Western world ranges from approximately 50 to 100 g daily, and a good deal of the protein consumed is from animal sources. Additional protein is added all along the GIT from GI secretions and cells sloughed from GI tissues. The GIT is one of the most active synthetic tissues in the body, and the life span of enterocytes migrating from the crypts of the villi until they are shed is only 3 to 4 days. The number of cells shed daily is in the range of 10 to 20 billion cells. The latter accounts for an additional 50 to 60 g of protein that is digested and "recycled" and contributes to the daily supply. In general, animal proteins are more efficiently digested than plant proteins, but human GI physiology allows for very effective digestion and absorption of large amounts of ingested protein sources.

Protein digestion begins in the stomach, where some of the proteins are split into proteoses, peptones, and large polypeptides. Inactive pepsinogen is converted into the enzyme pepsin when it contacts hydrochloric acid and other pepsin molecules. Unlike any of the other proteolytic enzymes, pepsin digests collagen, the major protein of connective tissue. Most protein digestion takes place in the upper portion of the small intestine, but it continues throughout the GIT (Soybel, 2005). Any residual protein fractions are fermented by colonic microbes.

Contact between chyme and the intestinal mucosa stimulates release of enterokinase, an enzyme that transforms inactive pancreatic trypsinogen into active trypsin, the major pancreatic protein-digesting enzyme. Trypsin in turn activates the other pancreatic proteolytic enzymes. Pancreatic trypsin, chymotrypsin, and carboxypeptidase break down intact protein and continue the breakdown started in the stomach until small polypeptides and amino acids are formed.

Proteolytic peptidases located on the brush border also act on polypeptides, breaking them down into amino acids, dipeptides, and tripeptides. The final phase of protein digestion takes place in the brush border, where some of the dipeptides and tripeptides are hydrolyzed into their constituent amino acids by peptide hydrolases.

End products of protein digestion are absorbed as both amino acids and small peptides. Several transport molecules are required for the different amino acids, probably because of the wide differences in the size, polarity, and configuration of the different amino acids. Some of the transporters are sodium- or chloride-dependent, and some are not. Considerable amounts of dipeptides and tripeptides are also absorbed into intestinal cells using a peptide transporter, a form of active transport (Daniel, 2004). Absorbed peptides and amino acids are transported to the liver via the portal vein for metabolism by the liver and are released into the general circulation.

The presence of antibodies to many food proteins in the circulation of healthy individuals indicates that immunologically significant amounts of large intact peptides escape hydrolysis and can enter the portal circulation. The exact mechanisms that cause a food to become an allergen are not entirely clear, but these foods tend to be high in protein, to be relatively resistant to complete digestion, and to produce an immunoglobulin response (see Chapter 27). With new technology, it is possible to map and characterize allergenic peptides; this will eventually lead to safe immunotherapy treatments (Lin et al., 2009).

Almost all protein is absorbed by the time it reaches the end of the jejunum, and only 1% of ingested protein is found in the feces. Small amounts of amino acids may remain in the epithelial cells and are used for synthesis of new proteins, including intestinal enzymes and new cells.

Lipids

Approximately 97% of dietary lipids are in the form of triglycerides, and the rest are in the form of phospholipids and cholesterol. Only small amounts of fat are digested in the mouth with lingual lipase and in the stomach from the action of gastric lipase (tributyrinase). Gastric lipase hydrolyzes some triglycerides, especially short-chain triglycerides (such as those found in butter), into fatty acids and glycerol. However, most fat digestion takes place in the small intestine as a result of the emulsifying action of bile salts and hydrolysis by pancreatic lipase. As in the case of carbohydrates and protein, the capacity for digestion and absorption of dietary fat is in excess of ordinary needs.

Entrance of fat and protein into the small intestine stimulates the release of CCK and enterogastrone, which inhibit gastric secretions and motility, thus slowing the delivery of lipids. As a result, a portion of a large, fatty meal may remain in the stomach for 4 hours or longer. In addition to its many other functions, CCK stimulates biliary and pancreatic secretions. The combination of the peristaltic action of the small intestine and the surfactant and emulsification action of bile reduces the fat globules into tiny droplets, thus making them more accessible to digestion by the most potent lipid-digesting enzyme, pancreatic lipase (Keller and Layer, 2005).

Bile is a liver secretion composed of bile acids (primarily conjugates of cholic and chenodeoxycholic acids with glycine or taurine), bile pigments (which color the feces), inorganic salts, some protein, cholesterol, lecithin, and many compounds such as detoxified drugs that are metabolized and secreted by the liver. From its storage organ, the gallbladder, approximately 1 L of bile is secreted daily in response to the stimulus of food in the duodenum and stomach.

The free fatty acids and monoglycerides produced by digestion form complexes with bile salts called *micelles*. The micelles facilitate passage of the lipids through the watery environment of the intestinal lumen to the brush border (see Figure 1-4). The micelles release the lipid components and are returned to the gut lumen. Most of the bile salts are actively reabsorbed in the terminal ileum and returned to the liver to reenter the gut in bile secretions. This efficient recycling process is known as the **enterohepatic circulation**. The pool of bile acids may circulate from 3 to 15 times per day, depending on the amount of food ingested.

In the mucosal cells the fatty acids and monoglycerides are reassembled into new triglycerides. A few are further digested into free fatty acids and glycerol and then reassembled to form triglycerides. These triglycerides, along with cholesterol, fat-soluble vitamins, and phospholipids, are surrounded by a lipoprotein coat, forming chylomicrons (see Figure 1-4). The lipoprotein globules pass into the lymphatic system instead of entering portal blood and are transported to the thoracic duct and emptied into the systemic circulation at the junction of the left internal jugular and left subclavian veins. The chylomicrons are then carried through the bloodstream to several tissues, including liver, adipose tissue, and muscle. In the liver, triglycerides from the chylomicrons are repackaged into very low-density lipoproteins and transported primarily to the adipose tissue for metabolism and storage.

The fat-soluble vitamins A, D, E, and K are also absorbed in a micellar fashion, although water-soluble forms of vitamins A, E, and K supplements and carotene can be absorbed in the absence of bile acids.

Under normal conditions approximately 95% to 97% of ingested fat is absorbed into lymph vessels. Because of their shorter length and thus increased solubility, fatty acids of 8 to 12 carbons (i.e., medium-chain fatty acids) can be absorbed directly into colonic mucosal cells without the presence of bile and micelle formation. After entering mucosal cells, they are able to go directly without esterification into the portal vein, which carries them to the liver.

Increased motility, intestinal mucosal changes, pancreatic insufficiency, or the absence of bile can decrease absorption of fat. When undigested fat appears in the feces, the condition is known as *steatorrhea* (see Chapter 29. Medium-chain triglycerides (MCTs) have fatty acids 8 to 12 carbons long; MCTs are clinically valuable for individuals who lack necessary bile salts for long-chain fatty acid metabolism and transport. Supplements for clinical use are normally provided in the form of oil or a dietary beverage with other macronutrients and micronutrients.

For the nutrition care process, several nutrition diagnoses can be identified. The following list provides examples:

Common or Possible Nutrition Diagnoses Related to Digestion or Metabolism

Altered GI function
Imbalance of nutrients
Altered nutrient utilization
Altered nutritional laboratory results
Inadequate or excessive fluid intake
Food-drug interaction

Vitamins and Minerals

Vitamins and minerals from foods are made available as macronutrients and are digested and absorbed across the mucosal layer, primarily in the small intestine (Figure 1-9). Besides adequate passive and transporter mechanisms, various factors affect the bioavailability of vitamins and minerals, including the presence or absence of other specific nutrients, acid or alkali, phytates, and oxalates. Each day approximately 8 to 9 L of fluid is secreted from the GIT and serves as a solvent, a vehicle for chemical reactions, and a medium for transfer of several nutrients.

At least some vitamins and water pass unchanged from the small intestine into the blood by passive diffusion, but several different mechanisms might be used to transport individual vitamins across the GI mucosa. Drugs are absorbed by a number of mechanisms, but often by passive diffusion. Thus drugs may share or compete with mechanisms for the absorption nutrients into intestinal cells (see Chapter 9).

Mineral absorption is more complex, especially the absorption of the cation minerals. These cations, such as selenium, are made available for absorption by the process of **chelation**, in which a mineral is bound to a ligand—usually an acid, an organic acid, or an amino acid, so that it is in a form absorbable by intestinal cells.

Iron and zinc absorption share several characteristics in that the efficiency of absorption partly depends on the needs of the host. They also use at least one transport protein, and each has mechanisms to increase absorption when stores are inadequate. Because phytates and oxalates from plants

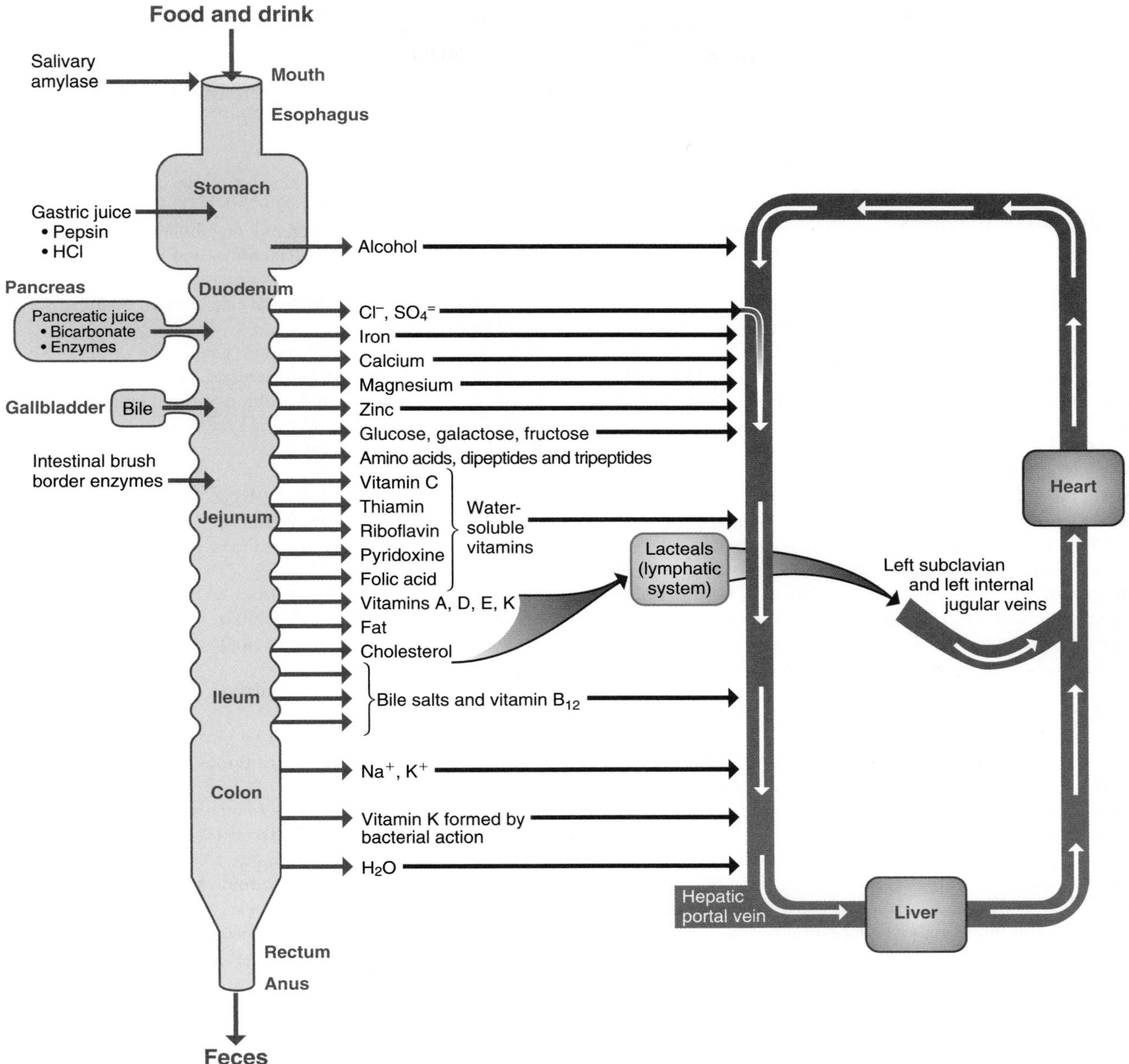

FIGURE 1-9 Sites of secretion and absorption in the gastrointestinal tract.

impair the absorption of both iron and zinc, absorption is better when animal sources are consumed. The absorption of zinc is impaired with disproportionately increased amounts of magnesium, calcium, and iron. Calcium absorption into the enterocyte occurs through channels in the brush border membrane, where it is bound to a specific protein carrier for transportation across the basolateral membrane. The process is regulated by the presence of vitamin D. Phosphorus is absorbed by a sodium phosphorus cotransporter, which is also regulated by vitamin D or low phosphate intake.

The GIT is the site of important interactions among minerals. Supplementation with large amounts of iron or zinc may decrease the absorption of copper. In turn, the presence of copper may lower iron and molybdenum absorption. Cobalt absorption is increased in patients with iron deficiency, but cobalt and iron compete and inhibit one another's absorption. These interactions are probably the result of an overlap of mineral absorption mechanisms.

Minerals are transported in blood bound to protein carriers. The protein binding is either specific (e.g., transferrin, which binds with iron, or ceruloplasmin which binds with copper) or general (e.g., albumin, which binds with a variety of minerals). A fraction of each mineral is also carried in the serum as amino acid or peptide complexes. Specific protein carriers are usually not completely saturated; the reserve capacity may serve as a buffer against excessive exposure.

Toxicity from minerals usually results only after this buffering capacity is exceeded.

USEFUL WEBSITES

American Gastroenterological Association
http://www.gastro.org/
NIH Digestive Diseases
http://digestive.niddk.nih.gov/

REFERENCES

Beyer P, et al: Fructose intake at current level in the United States may cause gastrointestinal distress in normal adults, *J Am Diet Assoc* 105:1559, 2005.

Chey WY, Chang TM: Secretin, 100 years later, *J Gastroenterol* 38:1025, 2003.

Daniel H: Molecular and integrative physiology of intestinal peptide transport, *Ann Rev Physiol* 66:361, 2004.

Deng PY, et al: Cholecystokinin facilitates glutamate release by increasing the number of readily releasable vesicles and releasing probability, *J Neurosci* 30:5136, 2010.

De Smet B, Mitselos A, Depoortere I: Motilin and ghrelin as prokinetic drug targets, *Pharmacol Ther* 123:207, 2009.

Englyst KN, Englyst HN: Carbohydrate bioavailability, *Br J Nutr* 94:1, 2005.

Frank DN, Pace NR: Gastrointestinal microbiology enters the metagenomics era, *Curr Opin Gastroenterol* 1:4, 2008.

Hui DY, et al: Development and physiological regulation of intestinal lipid absorption. III. Intestinal transporters and cholesterol absorption, *Am J Physiol Gastrointest Liver Physiol* 294:G839, 2008.

Hylemon PB, et al: Bile acids as regulatory molecules, *J Lipid Res* 50:1509, 2009.

Kahn WI, Ghia JE: Gut hormones: emerging role in immune activation and inflammation, *Clin Exp Immunol* 161:19, 2010.

Keller J, Layer P: Human pancreatic endocrine response to nutrients in health and disease, *Gut* 54:1, 2005.

Kellett G, Brot-Laroche E: Apical GLUT 2: a major pathway of intestinal sugar absorption, *Diabetes* 54:3056, 2005.

Lammert F, Wang DO: New insights into the genetic regulation of intestinal cholesterol absorption, *Gastroenterology* 128:718, 2005.

Lin J, et al: Microarrayed allergen molecules for diagnostics of allergy, *Methods Mol Biol* 524:259, 2009.

Macfarlane GT, et al: Bacterial metabolism and health-related effects of galacto-oligosaccharides and other prebiotics, *Ann Microbiol* 104:305, 2008.

Nauck MA: Unraveling the science of incretin biology, *Am J Med* 122S:S3, 2009.

O'Keefe SJ: Nutrition and colonic health: the critical role of the microbiota, *Curr Opin Gastroenterol* 24:51, 2008.

Quigley EM: Prebiotics and probiotics: modifying and mining the microbiota, *Pharmacol Res* 61:213, 2010.

Rehfeld JF: A centenary of gastrointestinal endocrinology, *Horm Metab Res* 36:735, 2004.

Roberfroid M, et al: Prebiotic effects: metabolic and health benefits, *Brit J Nutr* 104:1S, 2010.

Schubert ML: Hormonal regulation of gastric acid secretion, *Curr Gastroenterol Rep* 10:523, 2009.

Snelling AM: Effects of probiotics on the gastrointestinal tract, *Curr Opin Infect Dis* 18:420, 2005.

Soybel DI: Anatomy and physiology of the stomach, *Surg Clin North Am* 85:875, 2005.

Stanley S, et al: Hormonal regulation of food intake, *Physiol Rev* 85:1131, 2005.

Tappenden KA, Deutsch AS: The physiological relevance of the intestinal microbiota—contributions to human health, *J Am Coll Nutr* 26:679S, 2007.

van de Pol MA, et al: Synbiotics reduce allergen-induced T-helper 2 response and improve peak expiratory flow in allergic asthmatics, *Allergy* 66:39, 2011.

Van Op Den Bosch J, et al: The role of somatostatin, structurally related peptides and somatostatin receptors in the gastrointestinal tract, *Regul Pept* 156:1, 2009.

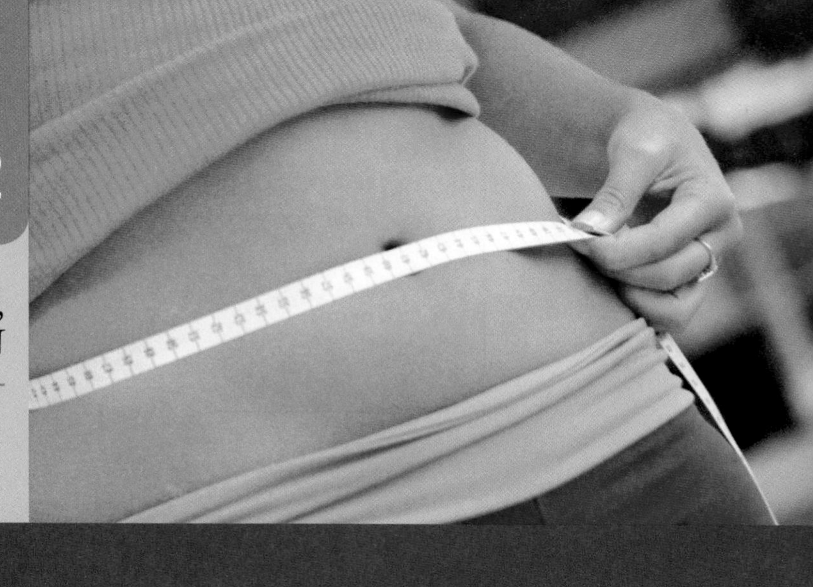

CHAPTER 2

Carol S. Ireton-Jones, PhD, RD, LD, CNSD, FACN

Intake: Energy

KEY TERMS

activity thermogenesis (AT)
basal energy expenditure (BEE)
basal metabolic rate (BMR)
direct calorimetry
energy expenditure
estimated energy requirement (EER)
excess postexercise oxygen consumption (EPOC)
facultative thermogenesis
fat-free mass (FFM)
high-metabolic-rate organ (HMRO)
indirect calorimetry (IC)
kilocalorie (kcal)
metabolic equivalents (METs)
nonexercise activity thermogenesis (NEAT)
obligatory thermogenesis
physical activity level (PAL)
resting energy expenditure (REE)
resting metabolic rate (RMR)
respiratory quotient (RQ)
thermic effect of food (TEF)
total energy expenditure (TEE)

Energy may be defined as "the capacity to do work." The ultimate source of all energy in living organisms is the sun. Through the process of photosynthesis, green plants intercept a portion of the sunlight reaching their leaves and capture it within the chemical bonds of glucose. Proteins, fats, and other carbohydrates are synthesized from this basic carbohydrate to meet the needs of the plant. Animals and humans obtain these nutrients and the energy they contain by consuming plants and the flesh of other animals.

The body makes use of the energy from dietary carbohydrates, proteins, fats, and alcohol; this energy is locked in chemical bonds within food and is released through metabolism. Energy must be supplied regularly to meet needs for the body's survival. Although all energy eventually takes the form of heat, which dissipates into the atmosphere, unique cellular processes first make possible its use for all of the tasks required for life. These processes involve chemical reactions that maintain body tissues, electrical conduction of the nerves, mechanical work of the muscles, and heat production to maintain body temperature.

Sections of this chapter were written by Rachel Johnson, PhD, RD and Carol D. Frary, MS, RD for the previous edition of this text.

ENERGY REQUIREMENTS

Energy requirements are defined as the dietary energy intake that is required for growth or maintenance in a person of a defined age, gender, weight, height, and level of physical activity. In children and pregnant or lactating women, energy requirements include the needs associated with the deposition of tissues or the secretion of milk at rates consistent with good health (Institute of Medicine, 2002, 2005). In ill or injured people, the stressors have an effect by increasing or decreasing **energy expenditure** (Joffe, 2009).

Body weight is one indicator of energy adequacy or inadequacy. The body has the unique ability to shift the fuel mixture of carbohydrates, proteins, and fats to accommodate energy needs. However, consuming too much or too

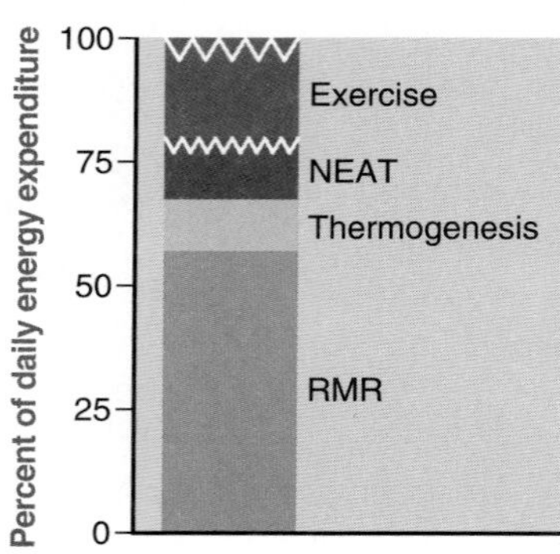

FIGURE 2-1 The components of total energy expenditure: activity, diet-induced thermogenesis, and basal or resting metabolic rate.

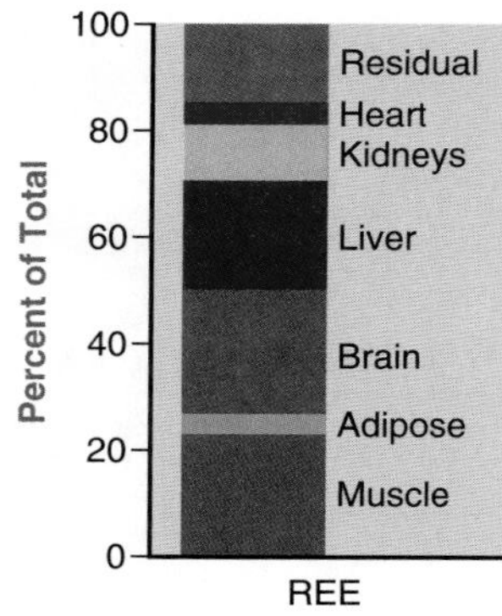

FIGURE 2-2 Proportional contribution of organs and tissues to calculated resting energy expenditure. *(Modified and used with permission from Gallagher D et al: Organ-tissue mass measurement allows modeling of REE and metabolically active tissue mass, Am J Physiol Endocrinol Metab 275:E249, 1998. Copyright American Physiological Society.)*

little energy over time results in body weight changes. Thus body weight reflects adequacy of energy intake, but it is not a reliable indicator of macronutrient or micronutrient adequacy. Additionally, because body weight is affected by body composition, a person with a higher lean mass to body fat mass or body fat mass to lean mass may require differing energy intakes compared with the norm or "average" person.

COMPONENTS OF ENERGY EXPENDITURE

Energy is expended by the human body in the form of **basal energy expenditure (BEE)**, thermic effect of food (TEF), and activity thermogenesis (AT). These three components make up a person's daily **total energy expenditure (TEE)** (Figure 2-1).

Basal and Resting Energy Expenditure

BEE, or **basal metabolic rate (BMR)**, is the minimum amount of energy expended that is compatible with life. An individual's BEE reflects the amount of energy used during 24 hours while physically and mentally at rest in a thermoneutral environment that prevents the activation of heat-generating processes, such as shivering. Measurements of BEE should be done before an individual has engaged in any physical activity (preferably on awakening from sleep) and 10 to 12 hours after the ingestion of any food, drink, or nicotine. The BEE remains remarkably constant on a daily basis, typically representing 60% to 70% of TEE (see Figure 2-1).

Resting energy expenditure (REE), or **resting metabolic rate (RMR)**, is the energy expended in the activities necessary to sustain normal body functions and homeostasis. These activities include respiration and circulation, the synthesis of organic compounds, and the pumping of ions across membranes. It includes the energy required by the central nervous system and for the maintenance of body temperature. For practical reasons the BEE is now rarely measured. REE measurements are used in its place, which in most cases are higher than the BEE by 10% to 20% (Institute of Medicine, 2002, 2005). The terms *REE* and *RMR* and *BEE* and *BMR* can be used interchangeably, but *REE* and *BEE* are used in this chapter.

Factors Affecting Resting Energy Expenditure

Numerous factors cause the REE to vary among individuals, but body size and composition have the greatest effect. See Chapter 4 for discussion of methods used to determine body composition.

Age. Because REE is highly affected by the proportion of lean body mass (LBM), it is highest during periods of rapid growth, especially the first and second years of life (Butte et al., 2000). The additional energy required for synthesizing and depositing body tissue is approximately 5 kcal/g of tissue gained (Roberts and Young, 1988). Growing infants may store as much as 12% to 15% of the energy value of their food in the form of new tissue. As a child becomes older, the energy requirement for growth is reduced to approximately 1% of TEE. After early adulthood there is a decline in REE of 1% to 2% per kilogram of fat-free mass (FFM) per decade (Keys et al., 1973; Van Pelt, 2001). Fortunately, exercise can help maintain a higher LBM and a higher REE. Decreases in REE with increasing age may be partly related to age-associated changes in the relative size of LBM components (Gallagher et al., 2006).

Body Composition. **Fat-free mass (FFM)**, or LBM, comprises the majority of metabolically active tissue in the body and is the primary predictor of REE. FFM contributes to approximately 80% of the variations in REE (Bosy-Westphal et al., 2004). Because of their greater FFM, athletes with greater muscular development have approximately a 5% higher resting metabolism than nonathletic individuals. Organs in the body contribute to heat production (Figure 2-2). Approximately 60% of REE can be accounted for by the heat produced by **high-metabolic-rate organs (HMROs)**, that is, the liver, brain, heart, spleen, and kidneys (Gallagher et al., 1998). Indeed, differences in FFM between ethnic groups may be related to the total mass of these HRMOs (Gallagher et al, 2006). Relatively small individual variation in HMRO mass significantly affects REE (Javed et al., 2010).

Body Size. Larger people generally have higher metabolic rates than smaller people, but tall, thin people have higher metabolic rates than short, wide people. For example, if two people weigh the same but one person is taller, the taller person has a larger body surface area and a higher metabolic rate (Cereda, 2009). The amount of LBM is highly correlated with total body size. For example, obese children have higher REEs than nonobese children, but, when REE is adjusted for body composition, FFM, and fat mass, no REE differences are found (Byrne, 2003).

Climate. The REE is affected by extremes in environmental temperature. People living in tropical climates usually have REEs that are 5% to 20% higher than those living in temperate areas. Exercise in temperatures greater than 86° F imposes a small additional metabolic load of approximately 5% from increased sweat gland activity. The extent to which energy metabolism increases in extremely cold environments depends on the insulation available from body fat and protective clothing (Dobratz et al., 2007).

Gender. Gender differences in metabolic rates are attributable primarily to differences in body size and composition. Women, who generally have more fat in proportion to muscle than men, have metabolic rates that are approximately 5% to 10% lower than men of the same weight and height. However, with aging, this difference becomes less pronounced (Poehlman, 1993).

Hormonal Status. Hormones affect metabolic rate. Endocrine disorders, such as hyperthyroidism and hypothyroidism, increase or decrease energy expenditure, respectively. Stimulation of the sympathetic nervous system during periods of emotional excitement or stress causes the release of epinephrine, which promotes glycogenolysis and increased cellular activity. Ghrelin and peptide YY are gut hormones involved in appetite regulation and energy homeostasis (Larson-Meyer et al., 2010). The metabolic rate of women fluctuates with the menstrual cycle. During the luteal phase (i.e., the time between ovulation and the onset of menstruation), metabolic rate increases slightly (Ferraro, 1992). During pregnancy, growth in uterine, placental, and fetal tissues, along with the mother's increased cardiac workload, contributes to gradual increases in BEE (Butte et al., 2004).

Temperature. Fevers increase REE by approximately 7% for each degree of increase in body temperature more than 98.6° F or 13% for each degree more than 37° C as noted by classic studies (Hardy and DuBois, 1937). Studies in hospitalized patients have demonstrated increases in energy expenditure during fever as well as during cooling, varying according to the patient's condition (Bruder et al., 1998).

Other Factors. Caffeine, nicotine, and alcohol use stimulate metabolic rate. Caffeine intakes of 200 to 350 mg in men or 240 mg in women may increase mean REE by 7% to 11% and 8% to 15%, respectively (Compher et al., 2006). Nicotine use increases REE by approximately 3% to 4% in men and by 6% in women; alcohol consumption increases REE in women by 9% (Compher et al., 2006). Under conditions of stress and disease, energy expenditure may increase or decrease, based on the clinical situation. Energy expenditure may be higher in people who are obese (Dobratz et al., 2007), but depressed during starvation or chronic dieting and in people with anorexia nervosa (Sedlet and Ireton-Jones, 1989).

Thermic Effect of Food

The **thermic effect of food (TEF)** is the increase in energy expenditure associated with the consumption, digestion, and absorption of food. The TEF accounts for approximately 10% of TEE (Institute of Medicine, 2002). The TEF may also be called *diet-induced thermogenesis, specific dynamic action*, or the *specific effect of food*. TEF can be separated into obligatory and facultative (or adaptive) subcomponents. **Obligatory thermogenesis** is the energy required to digest, absorb, and metabolize nutrients, including the synthesis and storage of protein, fat, and carbohydrates. Adaptive or **facultative thermogenesis** is the "excess" energy expended in addition to the obligatory thermogenesis and is thought to be attributable to the metabolic inefficiency of the system stimulated by sympathetic nervous activity.

The TEF varies with the composition of the diet, with energy expenditure increasing directly after food intake, particularly after consumption of a meal higher in protein compared with a meal higher in fat (Tentolouris et al., 2008). Fat is metabolized efficiently, with only 4% wastage, compared with 25% wastage when carbohydrate is converted to fat for storage. These factors are thought to contribute to the obesity-promoting characteristics of fat (Prentice, 1995). Although the extent of TEF depends on the size and macronutrient content of the meal, TEF decreases after ingestion over 30 to 90 minutes. Furthermore, the macronutrient oxidation rate is not different in lean and obese individuals (Tentolouris et al., 2008).

Spicy foods enhance and prolong the effect of the TEF. Meals with chili and mustard may increase the metabolic rate as much as 33% over that after an unspiced meal, and this effect may last for more than 3 hours (McCrory et al., 1994). Caffeine, capsaicin, and different teas such as green, white, and oolong tea may also increase energy expenditure and fat oxidation (Hursel and Westerterp-Plantenga, 2010). The role of TEF in weight management is discussed in Chapter 22.

Actual measurement of the TEF is appropriate only for research purposes. Thus to measure the TEF, it would be necessary to determine BEE and the energy expended in excess of BEE every 30 minutes for at least 5 hours after a meal. For practical purposes, it is calculated as no more than an additional 10% of the REE added to the sum of the REE and the activity thermogenesis.

Activity Thermogenesis

Beyond REE and TEF, energy is expended in activity, either exercise related or part of daily work and movement.

Although it can be broken down into two categories, for most individuals, additional kilocalorieskcals are allocated for the more general term *"activity,"* which includes **activity thermogenesis (AT)** and **nonexercise activity thermogenesis (NEAT)**. *AT* is the energy expended during sports or fitness exercise; the energy expended during activities of daily living is referred to as *NEAT* (Levine and Kotz, 2005). The contribution of physical activity is the most variable component of TEE, which may be as low as 100 kilocalories (kcal)/day in sedentary people or as high as 3000 kcal/day in athletes. NEAT represents the energy expended during the work day and during leisure-type activities (e.g., shopping, fidgeting, even gum chewing), which may account for vast differences in energy costs among people (Levine and Kotz, 2005); see Appendix 28.

Individual AT varies considerably, depending on body size and the efficiency of individual habits of motion. The level of fitness also affects the energy expenditure of voluntary activity because of variations in muscle mass. AT tends to decrease with age, a trend that is associated with a decline in FFM and an increase in fat mass (Roubenoff et al., 2000). In general, men have a greater skeletal muscle than women, which may account for their higher AT (Janssen et al., 2000).

Excess postexercise oxygen consumption (EPOC) affects energy expenditure. The duration and magnitude of physical activity increase EPOC, resulting in an elevated metabolic rate even after exercise has ceased (Bahr et al., 1992). Habitual exercise does not cause a significantly prolonged increase in metabolic rate per unit of active tissue, but it has been shown to cause an 8% to 14% higher metabolic rate in men who are moderately and highly active, respectively, because of their increased FFM (Horton and Geissler, 1994). These differences seem to be related to the person, not to the activity.

Measurement of Energy Expenditure

The standard unit for measuring energy is the *calorie*, which is the amount of heat energy required to raise the temperature of 1 ml of water at 15° C by 1° C. Because the amount of energy involved in the metabolism of food is fairly large, the **kilocalorie (kcal)**, 1000 calories, is used to measure it. A popular convention is to designate kilocalorie by *Calorie* (with a capital *C*). In this text, however, *kilocalorie* is abbreviated *kcal*. The *joule* (J) measures energy in terms of mechanical work and is the amount of energy required to accelerate with a force of 1 Newton (N) for a distance of 1 m; this measurement is widely used in countries other than the United States. One kcal is equivalent to 4.184 kilojoules (kJ).

Because various methods are available to measure human energy expenditure, it is important to gain an understanding of the differences in these methods and how they can be applied in practical and research settings.

Direct Calorimetry

Direct calorimetry is possible only with very specialized and expensive equipment. An individual is monitored in a room-type structure (a whole-room calorimeter) that permits a moderate amount of activity. It includes equipment that monitors the amount of heat produced by the individual inside. Direct calorimetry provides a measure of energy expended in the form of heat but provides no information on the kind of fuel being oxidized. The method is also limited by the confined nature of the testing conditions. Hence the measurement of TEE using this method is not representative of a free-living (i.e., engaged in normal daily activities) individual in a normal environment because physical activity within the chamber is limited. High cost, complex engineering, and scarcity of appropriate facilities around the world also limit the use of this method.

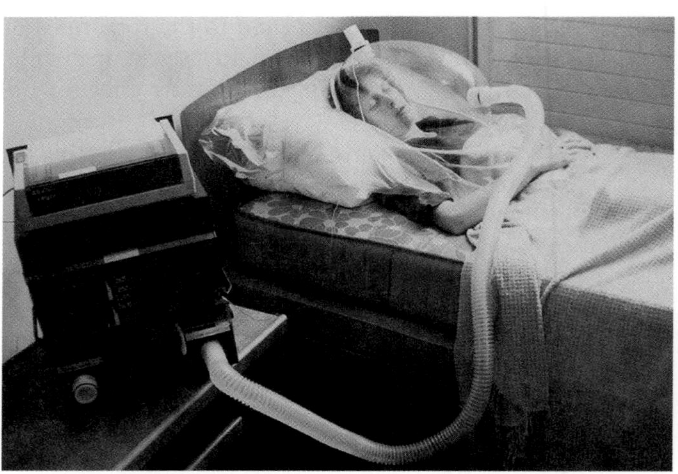

FIGURE 2-3 Measuring resting metabolic rate using a ventilated hood system. *(Courtesy of MRC Mitochondrial Biology Unit, Cambridge, England.)*

Indirect Calorimetry

Indirect calorimetry (IC) is a more commonly used method for measuring energy expenditure. An individual's oxygen consumption and carbon dioxide production are quantified over a given period. The Weir equation (1949) and a constant respiratory quotient value of 0.85 are used to convert oxygen consumption to REE. The equipment varies but usually involves an individual breathing into a mouthpiece (with nose clips), a mask that covers the nose and mouth, or a ventilated hood that captures all expired carbon dioxide (Figure 2-3). Ventilated hoods are useful for short- and long-term measurements.

IC measurements are achieved through the use of equipment called a *metabolic measurement cart* or *monitor*. There are various types of metabolic measurement carts, varying from larger equipment that measures oxygen consumption and carbon dioxide production only to equipment that also has the capability of providing pulmonary function and exercise testing parameters. These larger carts are more expensive because of the expanded capabilities, including measurement interface for IC measurements of hospitalized patients who are ventilator dependent. Metabolic carts are often used at hospitals to assess energy requirements and are most typically found in the intensive care unit (Ireton-Jones, 2010). Individuals and patients who are spontaneously breathing may have their energy expenditure measured with smaller "handheld" indirect calorimeters designed specifically for measuring oxygen consumption while using a static value for carbon dioxide production (St-Onge, 2004). These have easy mobility and relatively low equipment cost.

A strict protocol should be followed before performing IC measurement. For "normal" healthy people, a minimum of a 5-hour fast after meals and snacks is recommended. Caffeine should be avoided for at least 4 hours and alcohol and smoking for at least 2 hours. Testing should occur no sooner than 2 hours after moderate exercise; following vigorous resistance exercise, a 14-hour period is advised (Compher et al., 2006). To achieve a steady-state measurement, there should be a rest period of 10 to 20 minutes before the measurement is taken. An IC measurement duration of 10 minutes with the first 5 minutes deleted and the remaining 5 minutes having a coefficient of variation less than 10% indicates a steady-state measurement (Compher et al., 2006). When the measurement conditions listed here are met and a steady state is achieved, energy expenditure can be measured at any time during the day.

Energy expenditure can be measured for ill or injured individuals as well. Equipment used for the patient who is ventilator dependent may be different from that used for the ambulatory individual; however, a protocol specifying the conditions of measurement should be used for these patients as well (Ireton-Jones, 2010). When these conditions are met, IC can be applied for measuring the energy expenditure of acute or critically ill inpatients, outpatients, or healthy individuals.

Respiratory Quotient

When oxygen consumption and carbon dioxide production are measured, **respiratory quotient (RQ)** may be calculated as noted in the following equation. The RQ indicates the fuel mixture being metabolized. The RQ for carbohydrate is 1 because the number of carbon dioxide molecules produced is equal to the number of oxygen molecules consumed.

$$\text{RQ} = \text{volume of } CO_2 \text{ expired/volume of } O_2 \text{ consumed } (VO_2/VCO_2)$$

RQ values:
1 = carbohydrate
0.85 = mixed diet
0.82 = protein
0.7 = fat
≤0.65 = ketone production

RQs greater than 1 are associated with net fat synthesis; carbohydrate (glucose) intake or total caloric intake that is excessive, whereas a very low RQ may be seen under conditions of inadequate nutrient intake (Elia and Livesey, 1988; Ireton-Jones and Turner, 1987; McClave et al., 2003). Although RQ has been used to determine the efficacy of nutrition support regimens for hospitalized patients, McClave found that changes in RQ failed to correlate to percent calories provided or required, indicating low sensitivity and specificity that limits the efficacy of RQ as an indicator of overfeeding or underfeeding. It is appropriate to use RQ as a marker of test validity (to confirm measured RQ values are in physiologic range) and a marker for respiratory tolerance of the nutrition support regimen.

Other Methods of Measuring Energy Expenditure

Doubly Labeled Water. The doubly labeled water (DLW) technique for measuring TEE is considered the gold standard for determining energy requirements and energy balance in humans. The method was first applied to humans in 1982, and since that time scientists have developed a database that is used to develop recommendations for energy intake (Institute of Medicine, 2002; 2005). The DLW method is based on the principle that carbon dioxide production can be estimated from the difference in the elimination rates of body hydrogen and oxygen. After administering an oral loading dose of water labeled with deuterium oxide (^2H_2O) and oxygen-18 ($H_2{}^{18}O$)—hence the term *doubly labeled water*—the ^2H_2O is eliminated from the body as water, and the $H_2{}^{18}O$ is eliminated as water and carbon dioxide. The elimination rates of the two isotopes are measured for 10 to 14 days by periodic sampling of body water from urine, saliva, or plasma. The difference between the two elimination rates is a measure of carbon dioxide production. Carbon dioxide production can then be equated to TEE using standard IC techniques for the calculation of energy expenditure.

The DLW technique has numerous characteristics that make it a useful method for measuring TEE in various populations (Friedman and Johnson, 2002). First, it provides a measure of energy expenditure that incorporates all the components of TEE, REE, TEF, and AT. The administration is easy, and the person is able to engage in typical activities of daily living throughout the measurement period. Therefore the technique provides a measure of the person's usual daily TEE, which is beneficial for those such as infants, young children, older adults, and disabled individuals who cannot easily withstand the rigorous testing involved in the measurement of oxygen consumption during various activities. DLW also provides a method by which more subjective estimates of energy intakes (e.g., diet recalls, records) and energy expenditure (e.g., physical activity logs) can be validated (Schoeller, 1990). Most important, the method is accurate and has a precision of 2% to 8% (Plasqui and Westerterp, 2007).

The DLW technique is clearly most applicable as a research tool; the stable isotopes are expensive, and expertise is required to operate the highly sophisticated and costly mass spectrometer for the analysis of the isotope enrichments. These disadvantages make the DLW technique impractical for daily use by clinicians. However, DLW research studies have provided the data used to develop some prediction equations to estimate total energy requirements (Institute of Medicine, 2002; 2005). These equations should be used only as a guide or starting point, after which the person must be monitored closely and interventions developed to promote optimal nutrition status. As with most equations, these apply to healthy individuals, not to those who are ill, injured, or requiring intensive nutrition support (Wells et al., 2002).

Measuring Activity-Related Energy Expenditure

Doubly Labeled Water. The caloric value of AT can be estimated by using the DLW method in conjunction with IC. After the postprandial REE (which includes a measure of the TEF) has been measured using IC, an estimated AT can be determined by subtracting the postprandial REE from the TEE that was measured using DLW (Goran et al., 1995). This method is generally used only in research settings but can be used to validate other, more practical and easily administered methods of measuring physical activity.

Uniaxial Monitors. Uniaxial monitors measure the degree and intensity of movement in a vertical plane. Resembling a pager worn on the hip, the uniaxial monitor is a portable device designed for children and adults to estimate activity-related energy expenditure. Among adults, the uniaxial monitor was found to be an effective tool for measuring energy expenditure when compared with the DLW technique (Gretebeck et al., 1991; 1992). It may be acceptable for estimates of activity-related energy expenditure in groups of people, but it has limited use with individuals.

A triaxial monitor has also been used to measure energy related to activity (Philips Research, Eindhoven, The Netherlands). It more efficiently measures multidirectional movement by employing three uniaxial monitors. In a review of numerous articles, Plasqui and Westerterp (2007) found that a triaxial monitor correlated with energy expenditure measured using DLW technique. Application of an easily accessible and useable monitor allows determination of real activity levels, thereby reducing errors related to overreporting or underreporting of actual energy expenditure for weight management.

Physical Activity Questionnaire

Physical activity questionnaires (PAQs) are the simplest and least expensive tools for gaining information about an individual's activity level (Winters-Hart et al., 2004.) DLW allows researchers to determine the validity of these questionnaires. The Seven-Day Recall and the Yale Physical Activity Survey are two questionnaires that are validated (Bonnefoy et al., 2001). The Baecke questionnaire and an adapted version of the Tecumseh Community Health Study questionnaire are useful for determining whether a group or an individual is active or inactive (Philippaerts et al., 1999). Reporting errors are common among PAQs, which can lead to discrepancies between calculated energy expenditure and that determined by DLW (Neilson et al., 2008). For normal individuals, this may account for slowed weight loss or gain and, as such, a need to modify caloric intake.

ESTIMATING ENERGY REQUIREMENTS

Equations for Estimating Resting Energy Expenditure

Over the years several equations have been developed to estimate the REE. Equations are available that allow the estimation of REE as derived from measurement using IC in adults. Until recently, the Harris-Benedict equations were some of the most widely used equations to estimate REE in normal and ill or injured individuals (Harris and Benedict, 1919). The Harris-Benedict formulas have been found to overestimate REE in normal weight and obese individuals by 7% to 27% (Frankenfield, 2003). A study comparing measured REE with estimated REE using the Mifflin-St. Jeor equations, Owen equations, and Harris-Benedict equations for both males and females found that the Mifflin-St. Jeor equations were most accurate in estimating REE in both normal weight and obese people (Frankenfield et al., 2003; Owen et al., 1986; Owen et al., 1987). The Mifflin-St Jeor equations were developed from measured REE using IC in 251 males and 247 females; 47% of these individuals had a body mass index (BMI) between 30 and 42 kg/m^2 (Mifflin et al., 1990). These equations are as follows:

Mifflin-St. Jeor Equations

Males: kcal/day = 10 (wt) + 6.25 (ht) − 5 (age) + 5

Females: kcal/day = 10 (wt) + 6.25 (ht) − 5 (age) −161

Weight = actual body weight in kilograms;
Height = centimeters; Age = years

Although the Harris-Benedict equations have been applied to ill and injured people, these equations, as well as those of Mifflin, were developed for use in "normal" healthy individuals, and their application to any other population is questionable. For energy requirements for critically ill patients, see Chapter 39.

Estimating Energy Requirements from Energy Intake

Traditionally, recommendations for energy requirements were based on self-recorded estimates (e.g., diet records) or self-reported estimates (e.g., 24-hour recalls) of food intake. However, it is now well accepted that these methods do not provide accurate or unbiased estimates of an individual's energy intake. The percentage of people who underestimate or underreport their food intake ranges from 10% to 45%, depending on the person's age, gender, and body composition. Underestimating tends to increase as children age, is worse among women than men, and is more prevalent and severe among obese people (Johnson, 2000).

Multiple online programs are available whereby an individual can enter the food and quantity consumed into a program that will estimate the macronutrient and micronutrient content. These programs allow users to enter data and receive a summary report, often with a detailed report provided to the health professional as well. Widely available programs include Food Prodigy and the MyPlate Tracker from the United States Department of Agriculture.

Energy Requirements Prediction Equations

The National Academy of Sciences, Institute of Medicine, and Food and Nutrition Board, in partnership with Health Canada, developed the estimated energy requirements for men, women, children, and infants and for pregnant and lactating women (Institute of Medicine, 2002; 2005). The **estimated energy requirement (EER)** is the average dietary energy intake that is predicted to maintain energy balance in a healthy adult of a defined age, gender, weight, height, and level of physical activity consistent with good health. In children and pregnant and lactating women, the EER is taken to include the energy needs associated with the deposition of tissues or the secretion of milk at rates consistent with good health. Table 2-1 lists average dietary reference intake (DRI) values for energy in healthy, active people of reference height, weight, and age for each life-stage group (Institute of Medicine, 2002; 2005).

TABLE 2-1

Intensity and Effect of Various Activities on Physical Activity Level in Adults*

Physical Activity	METs†	Δ PAL/10 min‡	Δ PAL/hr‡
Daily Activities			
Lying quietly	1	0	0
Riding in a car	1	0	0
Light activity while sitting	1.5	0.005	0.03
Watering plants	2.5	0.014	0.09
Walking the dog	3	0.019	0.11
Vacuuming	3.5	0.024	0.14
Doing household tasks (moderate effort)	3.5	0.024	0.14
Gardening (no lifting)	4.4	0.032	0.19
Mowing lawn (power mower)	4.5	0.033	0.20
Leisure Activities: Mild			
Walking (2 mph)	2.5	0.014	0.09
Canoeing (leisurely)	2.5	0.014	0.09
Golfing (with cart)	2.5	0.014	0.09
Dancing (ballroom)	2.9	0.018	0.11
Leisure Activities: Moderate			
Walking (3 mph)	3.3	0.022	0.13
Cycling (leisurely)	3.5	0.024	0.14
Performing calisthenics (no weight)	4	0.029	0.17
Walking (4 mph)	4.5	0.033	0.20
Leisure Activities: Vigorous			
Chopping wood	4.9	0.037	0.22
Playing tennis (doubles)	5	0.038	0.23
Ice skating	5.5	0.043	0.26
Cycling (moderate)	5.7	0.045	0.27
Skiing (downhill or water)	6.8	0.055	0.33
Swimming	7	0.057	0.34
Climbing hills (5-kg load)	7.4	0.061	0.37
Walking (5 mph)	8	0.067	0.40
Jogging (10-min mile)	10.2	0.088	0.53
Skipping rope	12	0.105	0.63

Modified from Institute of Medicine of The National Academies: Dietary reference intakes for energy, carbohydrate, fiber, fat, fatty acids, protein, and amino acids, Washington, DC, 2002, The National Academies Press.

MET, Metabolic equivalent; *PAL*, physical activity level.

*PAL is the physical activity level that is the ratio of the total energy expenditure to the basal energy expenditure.

†METs are multiples of an individual's resting oxygen uptakes, defined as the rate of oxygen (O_2) consumption of 3.5 ml of O_2/min/kg body weight in adults.

‡The Δ PAL is the allowance made to include the delayed effect of physical activity in causing excess postexercise oxygen consumption and the dissipation of some of the food energy consumed through the thermic effect of food.

Supported by DLW studies, prediction equations have been developed to estimate energy requirements for people according to their life-stage group. Box 2-1 lists the EER prediction equations for people of normal weight. TEE prediction equations are also listed for various overweight and obese groups, as well as for weight maintenance in obese girls and boys. All equations have been developed to maintain current body weight (and promote growth when appropriate) and current levels of physical activity for all subsets of the population; they are not intended to promote weight loss (Institute of Medicine, 2002; 2005).

The EER incorporates age, weight, height, gender, and level of physical activity for people ages 3 years and older. Although variables such as age, gender, and feeding type (i.e., breast milk, formula) can affect TEE among infants and young children, weight has been determined as the sole predictor of TEE needs (Institute of Medicine, 2002; 2005). Beyond TEE requirements, additional calories are required for infants and young children and children ages 3 through 18 to support the deposition of tissues needed for growth, and for pregnant and lactating women; thus the EER among these subsets of the population is the sum of TEE plus the caloric requirements for energy deposition.

The prediction equations include a physical activity (PA) coefficient for all groups except infants and young children (see Box 2-1). PA coefficients correspond to four **physical activity level (PAL)** lifestyle categories: sedentary, low active, active, and very active. Because PAL is the ratio of TEE to BEE, the energy spent during activities of daily living, the sedentary lifestyle category has a PAL range of 1 to 1.39. PAL categories beyond sedentary are determined according to the energy spent by an adult walking at a set pace (Table 2-2). The walking equivalents that correspond to each PAL category for an average-weight adult walking at 3 to 4 mph are 2, 7, and 17 miles per day, respectively (Institute of Medicine, 2002; 2005).

TABLE 2-2

Physical Activity Level Categories and Walking Equivalence*

PAL Category	PAL Values	Walking Equivalence (miles/day at 3-4 mph)
Sedentary	1-1.39	
Low active	1.4-1.59	1.5, 2.2, 2.9 for PAL = 1.5
Active	1.6-1.89	3, 4.4, 5.8 for PAL = 1.6
		5.3, 7.3, 9.9 for PAL = 1.75
Very active	1.9-2.5	7.5, 10.3, 14 for PAL = 1.9
		12.3, 16.7, 22.5 for PAL = 2.2
		17, 23, 31 for PAL = 2.5

From Institute of Medicine, The National Academies: Dietary reference intakes for energy, carbohydrate, fiber, fat, fatty acids, cholesterol, protein, and amino acids, Washington, DC, 2002/2005, The National Academies Press.

PAL, Physical activity level.

*In addition to energy spent for the generally unscheduled activities that are part of a normal daily life. The low, middle, and high miles/day values apply to relatively heavyweight (120-kg), midweight (70-kg), and lightweight (44-kg) individuals, respectively.

Estimated Energy Expended in Physical Activity

Energy expenditure in physical activity can be estimated using either the method shown in Appendix 28, which represents energy spent during common activities and incorporates body weight and the duration of time for each activity as variables, or using information in the DRI tables (see tables on inside front cover), which represents energy spent by adults during various intensities of physical activity—energy that is expressed as metabolic equivalents (METs) (Institute of Medicine, 2002; 2005).

Estimating Energy Expenditure of Selected Activities Using Metabolic Equivalents

Metabolic equivalents (METs) are units of measure that correspond with a person's metabolic rate during selected physical activities of varying intensities and are expressed as multiples of REE (Institute of Medicine, 2002; 2005). An MET value of 1 is the oxygen metabolized at rest (3.5 mL of oxygen per kilogram of body weight per minute in adults) and can be expressed as 1 kcal/kg of body weight per hour (Ainsworth et al., 1993). Thus the energy expenditure of adults can be estimated using MET values (1 MET = 1 kcal/kg/hour). For example, an adult who weighs 65 kg and is walking moderately at a pace of 4 mph (which is a MET value of 4.5) would expend 293 calories in one hour (4.5 kcal × 65 kg × 1 = 293).

To estimate a person's energy requirements using the Institute of Medicine EER equations, it is necessary to identify a PAL value for that person. A person's PAL value can be affected by various activities performed throughout the day and is referred to as the *change in physical activity level* (Δ PAL). To determine Δ PAL, take the sum of the Δ PALs for each activity performed for 1 day from the DRI tables (Institute of Medicine, 2002; 2005). To calculate the PAL value for 1 day, take the sum of activities and add the BEE (1) plus 10% to account for the TEF (1 + 0.1 = 1.1). For example, to calculate an adult woman's PAL value, take the sum of the Δ PAL values for activities of daily living, such as walking the dog (0.11) and vacuuming (0.14) for 1 hour each, sitting for 4 hours doing light activity (0.12), and then performing moderate to vigorous activities such as walking for 1 hour at 4 mph (0.20) and ice skating for 30 minutes (0.13) for a total of (0.7). To that value include the BEE adjusted for the 10% TEF (1.1) for the final calculation (0.7 + 1.1 = 1.8). For this woman the PAL value (1.8) falls within an active range. The PA coefficient that correlates with an active lifestyle for this woman is 1.27.

To calculate the EER for an adult woman, use the EER equation for women 19 years and older (BMI 18.5-25 kg/m^2); see Box 2-1 (Institute of Medicine, 2002; 2005). The following calculation estimates the EER for a 30-year-old

BOX 2-1

Estimated Energy Expenditure* Prediction Equations at Four Physical Activity Levels†

EER for Infants and Young Children 0-2 Years (Within the 3rd-97th Percentile for Weight-for-Height)

EER = TEE‡ Energy deposition

0-3 months (89 × Weight of infant [kg] − 100) + 175 (kcal for energy deposition)

4-6 months (89 × Weight of infant [kg] − 100) + 56 (kcal for energy deposition)

7-12 months (89 × Weight of infant [kg] −100) + 22 (kcal for energy deposition)

13-35 months (89 × Weight of child [kg] − 100) + 20 (kcal for energy deposition)

EER for Boys 3-8 Years (Within the 5th-85th Percentile for BMI§)

EER = TEE‡ Energy deposition

EER = 88.5 − 61.9 × Age (yr) + PA × (26.7 × Weight [kg] + 903 × Height [m]) + 20 (kcal for energy deposition)

EER for Boys 9-18 Years (Within the 5th-85th Percentile for BMI)

EER = TEE Energy deposition

EER = 88.5 − 61.9 × Age (yr) + PA × (26.7 × Weight [kg] + 903 × Height [m]) + 25 (kcal for energy deposition)

in which

PA = Physical activity coefficient for boys 3-18 years:
PA = 1 if PAL is estimated to be ≥ 1 < 1.4 (Sedentary)
PA = 1.13 if PAL is estimated to be ≥ 1.4 < 1.6 (Low active)
PA = 1.26 if PAL is estimated to be ≥ 1.6 < 1.9 (Active)
PA = 1.42 if PAL is estimated to be ≥ 1.9 < 2.5 (Very active)

EER for Girls 3-8 Years (Within the 5th-85th Percentile for BMI)

EER = TEE Energy deposition

EER = 135.3 − 30.8 × Age (yr) + PA × (10 × Weight [kg] + 934 × Height [m]) + 20 (kcal for energy deposition)

EER for Girls 9-18 Yr (Within the 5th-85th Percentile for BMI)

EER = TEE + Energy deposition

EER = 135.3 − 30.8 × Age (yr) + PA × (10 × Weight [kg] + 934 × Height [m]) + 25 (kcal for energy deposition)

in which

PA = Physical activity coefficient for girls 3-18 years:
PA = 1 (Sedentary)
PA = 1.16 (Low active)
PA = 1.31 (Active)
PA = 1.56 (Very active)

EER for Men 19 Years and Older (BMI 18.5-25 kg/m²)

EER = TEE

EER = 662 − 9.53 × Age (yr) + PA × (15.91 × Weight [kg] + 539.6 × Height [m])

in which

PA = Physical activity coefficient:
PA = 1 (Sedentary)
PA = 1.11 (Low active)
PA = 1.25 (Active)
PA = 1.48 (Very active)

EER for Women 19 Years and Older (BMI 18.5-25 kg/m²)

EER = TEE

EER = 354 − 6.91 × Age (yr) + PA × (9.36 × Weight [kg] + 726 × Height [m])

in which

PA = Physical activity coefficient:
PA = 1 (Sedentary)
PA = 1.12 (Low active)
PA = 1.27 (Active)
PA = 1.45 (Very active)

EER for Pregnant Women

14-18 years: EER = Adolescent EER + Pregnancy energy deposition

First trimester = Adolescent EER + 0 (Pregnancy energy deposition)
Second trimester = Adolescent EER + 160 kcal (8 kcal/wk 1 × 20 wk) + 180 kcal
Third trimester = Adolescent EER + 272 kcal (8 kcal/wk × 34 wk) + 180 kcal

19-50 years: = Adult EER + Pregnancy energy deposition

First trimester = Adult EER + 0 (Pregnancy energy deposition)
Second trimester = Adult EER + 160 kcal (8 kcal/wk × 20 wk) + 180 kcal
Third trimester = Adult EER + 272 kcal (8 kcal/wk × 34 wk) + 180 kcal

EER for Lactating Women

14-18 years: EER = Adolescent EER + Milk energy output − Weight loss

First 6 months = Adolescent EER + 500 − 170 (Milk energy output − Weight loss)
Second 6 months = Adolescent EER + 400 − 0 (Milk energy output − Weight loss)

19-50 years: EAR = Adult EER + Milk energy output − Weight loss

First 6 months = Adult EER + 500 − 70 (Milk energy output − Weight loss)
Second 6 months = Adult EER + 400 − 0 (Milk energy output − Weight loss)

Continued

BOX 2-1

Estimated Energy Expenditure Prediction Equations at Four Physical Activity Levels—cont'd

Weight Maintenance TEE for Overweight and At-Risk for Overweight Boys 3-18 Years (BMI >85th Percentile for Overweight)

TEE = 114 − 50.9 × Age (yr) + PA × (19.5 × Weight [kg] + 1161.4 × Height [m])

in which

PA = Physical activity coefficient:
PA = 1 if PAL is estimated to be ≥ 1.0 < 1.4 (Sedentary)
PA = 1.12 if PAL is estimated to be ≥ 1.4 < 1.6 (Low active)
PA = 1.24 if PAL is estimated to be ≥ 1.6 < 1.9 (Active)
PA = 1.45 if PAL is estimated to be ≥ 1.9 < 2.5 (Very active)

Weight Maintenance TEE for Overweight and At-Risk for Overweight Girls 3-18 Years (BMI >85th Percentile for Overweight)

TEE = 389 − 41.2 × Age (yr) + PA × (15 × Weight [kg] + 701.6 × Height [m])

in which

PA = Physical activity coefficient:
PA = 1 if PAL is estimated to be ≥ 1 < 1.4 (Sedentary)
PA = 1.18 if PAL is estimated to be ≥ 1.4 < 1.6 (Low active)
PA = 1.35 if PAL is estimated to be ≥ 1.6 < 1.9 (Active)
PA = 1.60 if PAL is estimated to be ≥ 1.9 < 2.5 (Very active)

Overweight and Obese Men 19 Years and Older (BMI ≥25 kg/m²)

TEE = 1086 − 10.1 × Age (yr) + PA × (13.7 × Weight [kg] + 416 × Height [m])

in which

PA = Physical activity coefficient:
PA = 1 if PAL is estimated to be ≥ 1 < 1.4 (Sedentary)
PA = 1.12 if PAL is estimated to be ≥ 1.4 < 1.6 (Low active)
PA = 1.29 if PAL is estimated to be ≥ 1.6 < 1.9 (Active)
PA = 1.59 if PAL is estimated to be ≥ 1.9 < 2.5 (Very active)

Overweight and Obese Women 19 Years and Older (BMI ≥25 kg/m²)

TEE = 448 − 7.95 × Age (yr) + PA × (11.4 × Weight [kg] + 619 × Height [m])

where

PA = Physical activity coefficient:
PA = 1 if PAL is estimated to be ≥ 1 < 1.4 (Sedentary)
PA = 1.16 if PAL is estimated to be ≥ 1.4 < 1.6 (Low active)
PA = 1.27 if PAL is estimated to be ≥ 1.6 < 1.9 (Active)
PA = 1.44 if PAL is estimated to be ≥ 1.9 < 2.5 (Very active)

Normal and Overweight or Obese Men 19 Years and Older (BMI ≥18.5 kg/m²)

TEE = 864 − 9.72 × Age (yr) + PA × (14.2 × Weight [kg] + 503 × Height [m])

in which

PA = Physical activity coefficient:
PA = 1 if PAL is estimated to be ≥ 1 < 1.4 (Sedentary)
PA = 1.12 if PAL is estimated to be ≥ 1.4 < 1.6 (Low active)
PA = 1.27 if PAL is estimated to be ≥ 1.6 < 1.9 (Active)
PA = 1.54 if PAL is estimated to be ≥ 1.9 < 2.5 (Very active)

Normal and Overweight or Obese Women 19 Years and Older (BMI ≥18.5 kg/m²)

TEE = 387 − 7.31 × Age (yr) + PA × (10.9 × Weight [kg] + 660.7 × Height [m])

in which

PA = Physical activity coefficient:
PA = 1 if PAL is estimated to be ≥ 1 < 1.4 (Sedentary)
PA = 1.14 if PAL is estimated to be ≥ 1.4 < 1.6 (Low active)
PA = 1.27 if PAL is estimated to be ≥ 1.6 < 1.9 (Active)
PA = 1.45 if PAL is estimated to be ≥ 1.9 < 2.5 (Very active)

From Institute of Medicine, Food and Nutrition Board: Dietary reference intakes for energy, carbohydrate, fiber, fat, fatty acids, cholesterol, protein, and amino acids, Washington, DC, 2002, The National Academies Press, www.nap.edu.

BMI, Body mass index; *EER*, estimated energy requirement; *PA*, physical activity; *PAL*, physical activity level; *TEE*, total energy expenditure.

*EER is the average dietary energy intake that is predicted to maintain energy balance in a healthy adult of a defined age, gender, weight, height, and level of physical activity consistent with good health. In children and pregnant and lactating women, the EER includes the needs associated with the deposition of tissues or the secretion of milk at rates consistent with good health.

†PAL is the physical activity level that is the ratio of the total energy expenditure to the basal energy expenditure.

‡TEE is the sum of the resting energy expenditure, energy expended in physical activity, and the thermic effect of food.

§BMI is determined by dividing the weight (in kilograms) by the square of the height (in meters).

active woman who weighs 65 kg, is 1.77 m tall, with a PA coefficient (1.27):

$$\text{EER} = 354 - 6.91 \times \text{Age (yr)} + \text{PA} \times (9.36 \times \text{Weight [kg]} + 726 \times \text{Height [m]})$$

$$\text{EER} = 354 - (6.91 \times 30) + 1.27 \times ([9.36 \times 65] + [726 \times 1.77])$$

$$\text{EER} = 2551 \text{ kcal}$$

A simplified way of predicting physical activity additions to REE is through the use of estimates of the level of physical activity, which are then multiplied by the measured or predicted REE. To estimate TEE for minimal activity, increase REE by 10% to 20%; for moderate activity, increase REE by 25% to 40%; for strenuous activity, increase REE by 45% to 60%. These levels are ranges used in practice and can be considered "expert opinion" rather than evidence-based at this time.

Physical Activity in Children

Energy spent during various activities and the intensity and impact of selected activities can also be determined for children and teens (see Box 2-1) (Institute of Medicine, 2002; 2005).

CALCULATING FOOD ENERGY

The total energy available from a food is measured with a bomb calorimeter. This device consists of a closed container in which a weighed food sample, ignited with an electric spark, is burned in an oxygenated atmosphere. The container is immersed in a known volume of water, and the rise in the temperature of the water after igniting the food is used to calculate the heat energy generated.

Not all of the energy in foods and alcohol is available to the body's cells because the processes of digestion and absorption are not completely efficient. In addition, the nitrogenous portion of amino acids is not oxidized but is excreted in the form of urea. Therefore the biologically available energy from foods and alcohol is expressed in values rounded off slightly below those obtained using the calorimeter. These values for protein, fat, carbohydrate, and alcohol (Figure 2-4) are 4, 9, 4, and 7 kcal/g, respectively. Fiber is "unavailable carbohydrate" that resists digestion and absorption; its energy intake is minimal.

Although the energy value of each nutrient is known precisely, only a few foods, such as oils and sugars, are made up of a single nutrient. More commonly, foods contain a

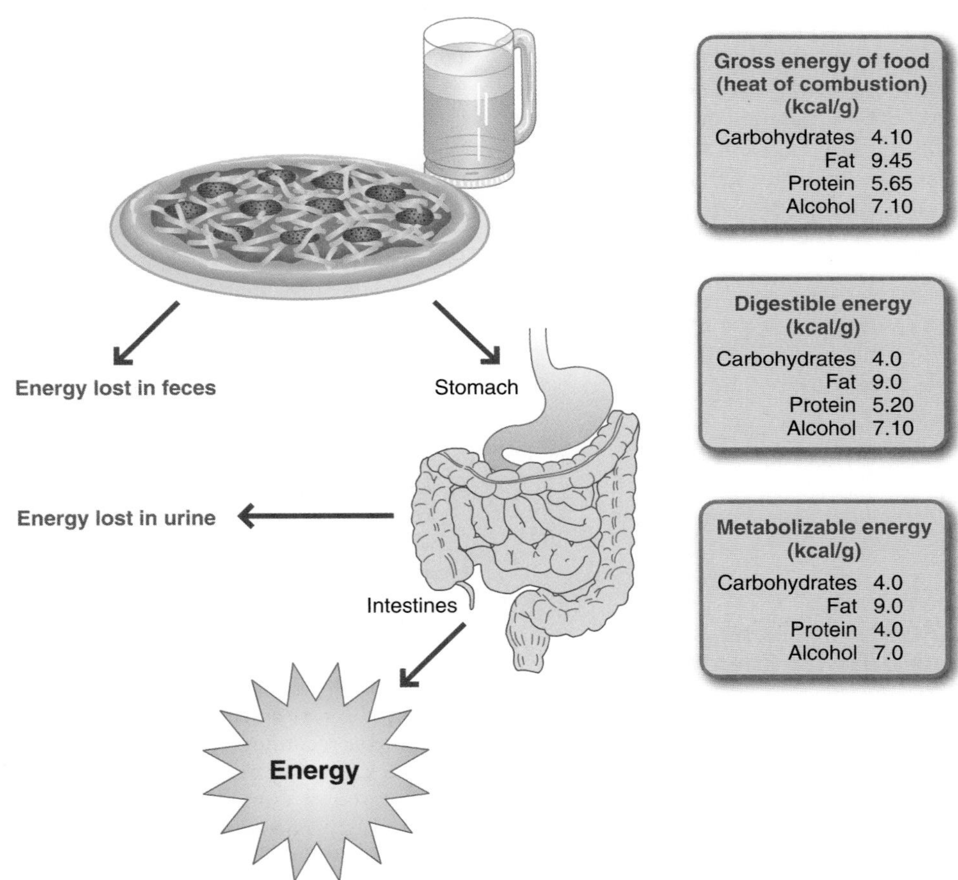

FIGURE 2-4 Energy value of food.

mixture of protein, fat, and carbohydrate. For example, the energy value of one medium (50-g) egg calculated in terms of weight is derived from protein (13%), fat (12%), and carbohydrate (1%) as follows:

$$\textit{Protein}: 13\% \times 50\ \text{g} = 6.5\ \text{g} \times 4\ \text{kcal/g} = 26\ \text{kcal}$$

$$\textit{Fat}: 12\% \times 50\ \text{g} = 6\ \text{g} \times 9\ \text{kcal/g} = 54\ \text{kcal}$$

$$\textit{Carbohydrate}: 1\% \times 50\ \text{g} = 0.05\text{g} \times 4\ \text{kcal/g} = 2\ \text{kcal}$$

$$\textit{Total} = 82\ \text{kcal}$$

The energy value of alcoholic beverages can be determined using the following equation (Gastineau, 1976): Alcohol kcal = Amount of beverage (oz) × Proof × 0.8 kcal/proof/1 oz. *Proof* is the proportion of alcohol to water or other liquids in an alcoholic beverage. The standard in the United States defines 100-proof as equal to 50% of ethyl alcohol by volume. To determine the percentage of ethyl alcohol in a beverage, divide the proof value by 2. For example, 86-proof whiskey contains 43% ethyl alcohol. The latter part of the equation—0.8 kcal/proof/1 oz—is the factor that accounts for the caloric density of alcohol (7 kcal/g) and the fact that not all of the alcohol in liquor is available for energy. For example, the number of kilocalories in 1 1/2 oz of 86-proof whiskey would be determined as follows:

1 1/2 oz × 86% proof × 0.8 kcal/proof/1 oz = 103 kcal. Energy values of foods based on chemical analyses may be obtained from the U.S. Department of Agriculture (USDA) Nutrient Data Laboratory website or from *Bowes and Church's Food Values of Portions Commonly Used* (Pennington and Douglass, 2009). Many computer software programs that use the USDA nutrient database as the standard reference are also available and there are many online websites that can be used. See Appendixes 38 and 44.

USEFUL WEBSITES

American Dietetic Association—Evidence Analysis Library
www.adaevidencelibrary.com

American Society for Parenteral and Enteral Nutrition
www.nutritioncare.org/

Food Prodigy
www.esha.com/foodprodigy

National Academy Press—Publisher of Institute of Medicine DRIs for Energy
www.nal.usda.gov/fnic/foodcomp/

MyPlate Tracker
www.chooseMyPlate.gov/tracker

U.S. Department of Agriculture Food Composition Tables
www.ars.usda.gov/main/site_main.htm?modecode=12-35-45-00

REFERENCES

Ainsworth BE, et al: Compendium of physical activities: classification of energy costs of human physical activities, *Med Sci Sports Exerc* 25:71, 1993.

Bahr R, et al: Effect of supramaximal exercise on excess postexercise O_2 consumption, *Med Sci Sports Exerc* 24:66, 1992.

Bonnefoy M, et al: Simultaneous validation of ten physical activity questionnaires in older men: a doubly labeled water study, *J Am Gerontological Society* 49:28, 2001.

Bosy-Westphal A, et al: Effect of organ and tissue masses on resting energy expenditure in underweight, normal weight and obese adults, *Int J Obes Related Metabol Disord* 28:72, 2004.

Bruder N, et al: Influence of body temperature, with or without sedation, on energy expenditure in severe head-injured patients, *Crit Care Med* 26:568, 1998.

Butte NF, et al: Energy requirements derived from total energy expenditure and energy deposition during the first 2 years of life, *Am J Clin Nutr* 72:1558, 2000.

Butte NF, et al: Energy requirements during pregnancy based on total energy expenditure and energy deposition, *Am J Clin Nutr* 79:1078, 2004.

Byrne NM, et al: Influence of distribution of lean body mass on resting metabolic rate after weight loss and weight regain: comparison of responses in white and black women, *Am J Clin Nutr* 77:1368, 2003.

Cereda E, et al: Height prediction formula for middle-aged (30-55 y) Caucasians, *Nutrition* 26:1075, 2010. [Epub ahead of print 2009.]

Compher C, et al: Best practice methods to apply to measurement of resting metabolic rate in adults: a systematic review, *J Am Diet Assoc* 106:881, 2006.

Dobratz JR, Sibley SD, Beckman TR, et al: Prediction of energy expenditure in extremely obese women, *J Parenter Enteral Nutr* 31:217, 2007.

Elia M, Livesey G: Theory and validity of indirect calorimetry during net lipid synthesis, *Am J Clin Nutr* 47:591, 1988.

Ferraro R, et al: Lower sedentary metabolic rate in women compared with men, *J Clin Invest* 90:780, 1992.

Frankenfield DC, et al: Validation of several established equations for resting metabolic rate in obese and nonobese people, *J Am Diet Assoc* 103:1152, 2003.

Friedman A, Johnson RK: Doubly labeled water: new advances and applications for the practitioner, *Nutr Today* 27:243, 2002.

Gallagher D, et al: Organ-tissue mass measurement allows modeling of REE and metabolically active tissue mass, *Am J Physiol Endocrinol Metab* 275:E249, 1998.

Gallagher D, et al: Small organs with a high metabolic rate explain lower resting energy expenditure in African American than in white adults, *Am J Clin Nutr* 83:1062, 2006.

Gastineau CF: Alcohol and calories, *Mayo Clin Proc* 51:88, 1976.

Goran MI, et al: Energy requirements across the life span: new findings based on measurement of total energy expenditure with doubly labeled water, *Nutr Res* 15:115, 1995.

Gretebeck R, et al: Comparison of the doubly labeled water method for measuring energy expenditure with Caltrac accelerometer recordings, *Med Sci Sports Exerc* 23:60S, 1991.

Gretebeck R, et al: Assessment of energy expenditure in active older women using doubly labeled water and Caltrac recordings, *Med Sci Sports Exerc* 23:68S, 1992.

Hardy JD, DuBois EF: Regulation of heat loss from the human body, *Proc Natl Acad Sci U S A* 23:624, 1937.

Harris JA, Benedict FG: *A biometric study of basal metabolism in man*, Pub no. 279, Washington, DC, 1919, Carnegie Institute of Washington.

Horton T, Geissler C: Effect of habitual exercise on daily energy expenditure and metabolic rate during standardized activity, *Am J Clin Nutr* 59:13, 1994.

Hursel R, Westerterp-Plantenga MS: Thermogenic ingredients and body weight regulation, *Int J Obes (Lond)* 34:659, 2010. [Epub ahead of print 2010.]

Institute of Medicine of the National Academies, Food and Nutrition Board: *Dietary reference intakes: for energy, carbohydrate, fiber, fat, fatty acids, cholesterol, protein, and amino acids*, Washington, DC, 2002, The National Academies Press.

Institute of Medicine of the National Academies, Food and Nutrition Board: *Dietary reference intakes for energy, carbohydrate, fiber, fat, fatty acids, cholesterol, protein, and amino acids*, Washington DC, 2005, The National Academies Press, pp. 107-264.

Ireton-Jones C: Indirect calorimetry. In Skipper A, editor: *The dietitian's handbook of enteral and parenteral nutrition*, ed 3, Sudbury, Mass, 2010, Jones and Bartlett (in press).

Ireton-Jones CS, Turner WW: The use of respiratory quotient to determine the efficacy of nutritional support regimens, *J Am Diet Assoc* 87:180, 1987.

Janssen I, et al: Skeletal muscle mass and distribution in 468 men and women aged 18-88 yr, *J Appl Physiol* 89:81, 2000.

Javed F, et al: Brain and high metabolic rate organ mass: contributions to resting energy expenditure beyond fat-free mass, *Am J Clin Nutr* 91:907, 2010. [Epub ahead of print 2010.].

Joffe A, et al: Nutritional support for critically ill children, *Cochrane Database Syst Rev* 2:CD005144, 2009 Apr 15.

Johnson RK: What are people really eating, and why does it matter? *Nutr Today* 35:40, 2000.

Keys A, et al: Basal metabolism and age of adult man, *Metabolism* 22:579, 1973.

Larson-Meyer DE, et al: Ghrelin and peptide YY in postpartum lactating and nonlactating women, *Am J Clin Nutr* 91:366, 2010.

Levine JA, Kotz CM: NEAT—non-exercise activity thermogenesis —egocentric & geocentric environmental factors vs. biological regulation, *Acta Physiol Scand* 184:309, 2005.

McClave SA, et al: Clinical use of the respiratory quotient obtained from indirect calorimetry, *J Parenter Enteral Nutr* 27:21, 2003.

McCrory P, et al: Energy balance, food intake and obesity. In Hills AP, Wahlqvist ML, editors: *Exercise and obesity*, London, 1994, Smith-Gordon.

Mifflin MD, St. Jeor ST, et al: A new predictive equation for resting energy expenditure in healthy individuals, *Am J Clin Nutr* 51:241,1990.

Neilson HK, et al: Estimating activity energy expenditure: how valid are physical activity questionnaires? *Am J Clin Nutr* 87:279, 2008

Owen OE, et al: A reappraisal of caloric requirements in healthy women, *Am J Clin Nutr* 44:1, 1986.

Owen OE, et al: A reappraisal of the caloric requirements of men, *Am J Clin Nutr* 46:875, 1987.

Pennington JA, Douglass JS: *Bowes and Church's food values of portions commonly used*, ed 19, Philadelphia, 2009, Lippincott Williams & Wilkins.

Philippaerts RM, et al: Doubly labeled water validation of three physical activity questionnaires, *Int J Sports Med* 20:284, 1999.

Plasqui G, Westerterp KR: Physical activity assessment with accelerometers: an evaluation against doubly labeled water, *Obesity* 15:2371, 2007.

Poehlman ET: Regulation of energy expenditure in aging humans, *J Am Geriatr Soc* 41:552, 1993.

Prentice AM: All calories are not equal, *International dialogue on carbohydrates* 5:1, 1995.

Roberts SB, Young VR: Energy costs of fat and protein deposition in the human infant, *Am J Clin Nutr* 48:951, 1988.

Roubenoff R, et al: The effect of gender and body composition method on the apparent decline in lean mass–adjusted resting metabolic rate with age, *J Gerontol Series A: Biol Sci Med Sci* 55:M757, 2000.

St-Onge MP, et al: A new hand-held indirect calorimeter to measure postprandial energy expenditure, *Obes Res* 12:704, 2004.

Schoeller DA: How accurate is self-reported dietary energy intake? *Nutr Rev* 48:373, 1990.

Sedlet KL, Ireton-Jones CS: Energy expenditure and the abnormal eating pattern of a bulimic: a case study, *J Am Diet Assoc* 89:74, 1989.

Tentolouris N, et al: Diet induced thermogenesis and substrate oxidation are not different between lean and obese women after two different isocaloric meals, one rich in protein and one rich in fat, *Metabolism* 57:313, 2008.

Van Pelt RE, et al: Age-related decline in RMR in physically active men: relation to exercise volume and energy intake, *Am J Physiol Endocrinol Metab* 281:E633, 2001.

Weir JB: New methods of calculating metabolic rate with special reference to protein metabolism, *J Physiol* 109:1, 1949.

Wells JC, et al: Energy requirements and body composition in stable pediatric intensive care patients receiving ventilatory support, *Food Nutr Bull* 23:95S, 2002.

Winters-Hart CS, et al: Validity of a questionnaire to assess historical physical activity in older women, *Med Sci Sports Exerc* 36:2082, 2004.

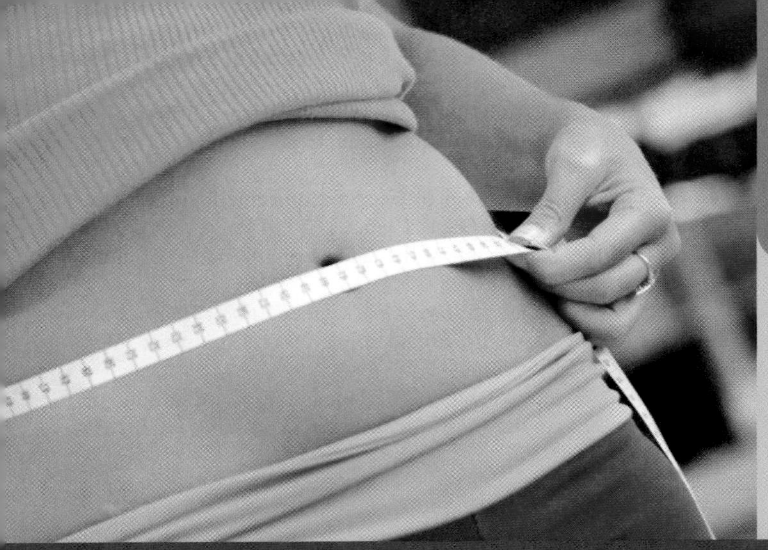

CHAPTER 3

Margie Lee Gallagher, PhD, RD

Intake: The Nutrients and Their Metabolism

KEY TERMS

acetyl coenzyme A (acetyl CoA)
amino acid
amino acid score
amylopectin
amylose
antioxidant
ascorbic acid
beta-glucans (glucopyranose)
beriberi
bioavailability
bioflavonoids
biotin
calbindins
calcitriol
carnitine
carotenoids
ceruloplasmin
cellulose
chiral carbon
cholecalciferol
cholesterol
chylomicrons
cobalamin
coenzyme Q_{10} (CoQ_{10})
conjugated linoleic acid (CLA)
cretinism
deamination
denaturation
dextrins
diacylglycerols (diglycerides)
dietary fiber
disaccharides
essential amino acids
ferritin
folate
free radicals
fructans
fructose
functional fiber
galactose
glucose tolerance factor (GTF)
glutathione peroxidase (GSH-Px)
glycemic index
glycemic load
glycogen
glycolipids
goiter
goitrogens
heme iron
hemoglobin
hemosiderin
hepcidin
hydrogenation
hydroxyapatite
hypercarotenodermia
isoprenoid
ketone
lactose
lecithin (phosphatidylcholine)
lignin
limiting amino acid
macrominerals
maltose
meat-fish-poultry (MFP) factor
medium-chain triglycerides (MCTs)
menadione
menaquinones
metallothionein
microminerals

monoacylglycerols (monoglycerides)
monosaccharides
monounsaturated fatty acids (MFAs)
myoglobin
myo-inositol
niacin
night blindness
nonessential amino acids
nonheme iron
oligosaccharides
omega-3 (ω-3) fatty acid
omega-6 (ω-6) fatty acid
pantothenic acid
pellagra
peptide bond
phospholipid
phytic acid (phytate)
polysaccharides
polyunsaturated fatty acids (PUFAs)
proteins
protein digestibility corrected amino acid score (PDCAAS)
pyridoxine (PN)
resistant starch
retinol
retinol activity equivalents (RAEs)
riboflavin
rickets
saturated fatty acid (SFA)
short-chain fatty acids (SCFAs)
scurvy
structured lipids
sucrose
tetany
thiamin
thyroxine (T_4)
tocopherol
total iron-binding capacity (TIBC)
trace elements
transamination
***trans*-fatty acids**
triglycerides (triacylglycerols TAG)
triiodothyronine (T_3)
ubiquinones
ultratrace elements
ultratrace minerals
urea
vitamer
vitamin
vitamin K
xerophthalmia

MACRONUTRIENTS

CARBOHYDRATES

Carbohydrates are manufactured by plants and are a major source of energy, composing approximately half the total calories in the diet. Carbohydrates are composed of carbon, hydrogen, and oxygen in a ratio of $C:O:H_2$. Important dietary carbohydrates can be categorized as (1) monosaccharides, (2) disaccharides and oligosaccharides, and (3) polysaccharides.

Monosaccharides

Monosaccharides do not normally occur as free molecules in nature but as basic components of disaccharides and polysaccharides. Only a small number of the many monosaccharides found in nature can be absorbed and used by humans. Monosaccharides can have three to seven carbons, but the most important are the six-carbon hexoses: glucose, galactose, and fructose. These hexoses all have the same chemical formula but differ importantly from one another. These differences result from small but significant differences in their chemical structure, some resulting from the presence of **chiral carbons** with four different atoms or groups attached. These groups can occur in different positions (isomers): glucose and galactose (Figure 3-1). The most important monosaccharide is α-D-glucose. *Blood sugar* refers to glucose. Because the brain depends on a regular, predictable supply, the body has highly adapted physiologic mechanisms to maintain adequate blood glucose levels.

Fructose is the sweetest of all monosaccharides (Table 3-1). *High-fructose corn syrup* is intensely sweet, inexpensive, and manufactured enzymatically by changing the glucose in cornstarch to fructose. Epidemiologic evidence suggests that high-fructose diets (including intake from sweetened beverages) may contribute to obesity and other health conditions, such as the metabolic syndrome. Both galactose and fructose are metabolized in the liver by incorporation into metabolic pathways for glucose, but fructose bypasses a major control enzyme in the glycolytic pathway (Figure 3-2). **Galactose** is produced from lactose by hydrolysis during the digestive process. Infants born with an inability to metabolize galactose have galactosemia (see Chapter 44).

Disaccharides and Oligosaccharides

Although a wide variety of disaccharides exist in nature, the three most important **disaccharides** in human nutrition are sucrose, lactose, and maltose. These sugars are formed from monosaccharides joined by a glycosidic linkage between the active aldehyde or **ketone** carbon and a specific hydroxyl on another sugar (Figure 3-3). **Sucrose** occurs naturally in many foods and is also an additive in commercially processed items; it is consumed in large amounts by most Americans. *Invert sugar* is also a natural form of sugar (unlinked glucose and fructose in a 1 : 1 ratio) that is used commercially because it is sweeter than equal concentrations of sucrose. Invert sugar forms smaller crystals than sucrose and is

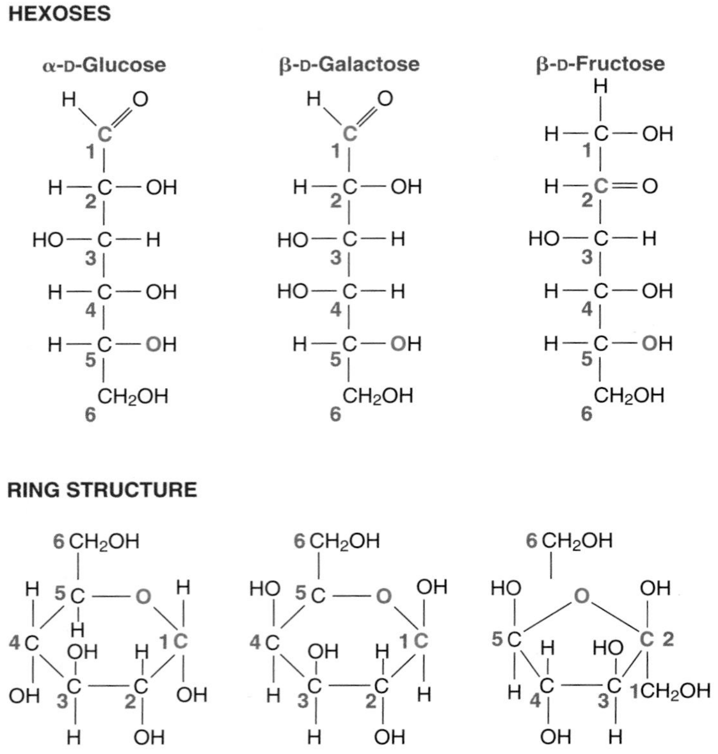

HEXOSES

α-D-Glucose β-D-Galactose β-D-Fructose

RING STRUCTURE

FIGURE 3-1 The three monosaccharides of importance in humans differ from each other in how they are handled metabolically even though they have very similar structures. They are isomers of one another.

TABLE 3-1

Sweetness of Sugars and Sugar Substitutes

Substance	Sweetness Value (% equivalent to sucrose)
Natural Sugar or Sugar Product	
Levulose, fructose	173
Invert sugar	130
Sucrose	100
Xylitol	100
Glucose	74
Sorbitol	60
Mannitol	50
Galactose	32
Maltose	32
Lactose	16
Sugar Substitutes	
Cyclamate—banned in United States	30
Aspartame (Equal)*—FDA approved	180
Acesulfame-K (Sunette)—FDA approved	200
Stevia (Rebiana, Truvia, Purvia—FDA approved	300
Saccharin (Sweet 'n Low)—FDA approved	300
Sucralose (Splenda)—FDA approved	600
Neotame (NutraSweet)*– FDA approved	8000

*Nutritive (has calories).

Note: In the United States, six sugar substitutes have been approved for use; stevia, aspartame, sucralose, neotame, acesulfame potassium, and saccharin. Hundreds of new sweeteners are evaluated each year. New sweeteners on the market, such as Swerve and Just Like Sugar, are considered equal in sweetness to sugar.

For more information, see FDA website at: http://www.fda.gov/Food/FoodIngredientsPackaging/ucm094211.htm#qanatural, accessed 1-14-11.

preferred in the preparation of candies and icings. *Honey* is an invert sugar. **Lactose** is made almost exclusively in the mammary glands of lactating animals. **Maltose** is seldom found naturally in the food supply but is formed by hydrolysis of starch polymers during digestion and is also consumed as an additive in numerous food products. **Oligosaccharides** are small (3-10 monosaccharide units), readily water soluble, and often sweet (Roberfroid, 2005). Enzymes found in the brush border of the intestine (see Chapter 1) break bonds between molecules in disaccharides and are specific to the particular bond. Larger molecules with linkages that are different are not digestible and are classified as **dietary fiber** (American Dietetic Association, 2008).

FIGURE 3-2 Overview of macronutrient metabolism. *1,* Hexokinase/glucokinase (liver) reaction: uses adenosine triphosphate (ATP), is reversed by glucose 6-phosphotase in gluconeogenesis. *2,* Phosphofructokinase reaction: modulated by ATP, positively modified by adenosine monophosphate and adenosine diphosphate (ADP), uses ATP, and is reversed by specific phosphatase in gluconeogenesis. *3,* Pyruvate kinase reaction: second example of substrate level phosphorylation of ADP → ATP is not reversible and must be bypassed for gluconeogenesis. *4,* Pyruvate dehydrogenase enzyme complex reaction: unidirectional and cannot be reversed. *5,* Dehydrogenase reaction: similar to pyruvate dehydrogenase, characterizes the removal of hydrogens in the Krebs cycle. *6,* Glycogenesis uses a glycogenic primer reaction and then glycogen synthetase and branching enzymes to synthesize glycogen. The reactions are not reversible. Glycogen is catabolized by a highly controlled phosphorylase. *ADP,* Adenosine diphosphate; *ATP,* adenosine triphosphate; *cAMP,* cyclic adenosine monophosphate. *(Courtesy Margie Gallagher, PhD, RD, East Carolina University.)*

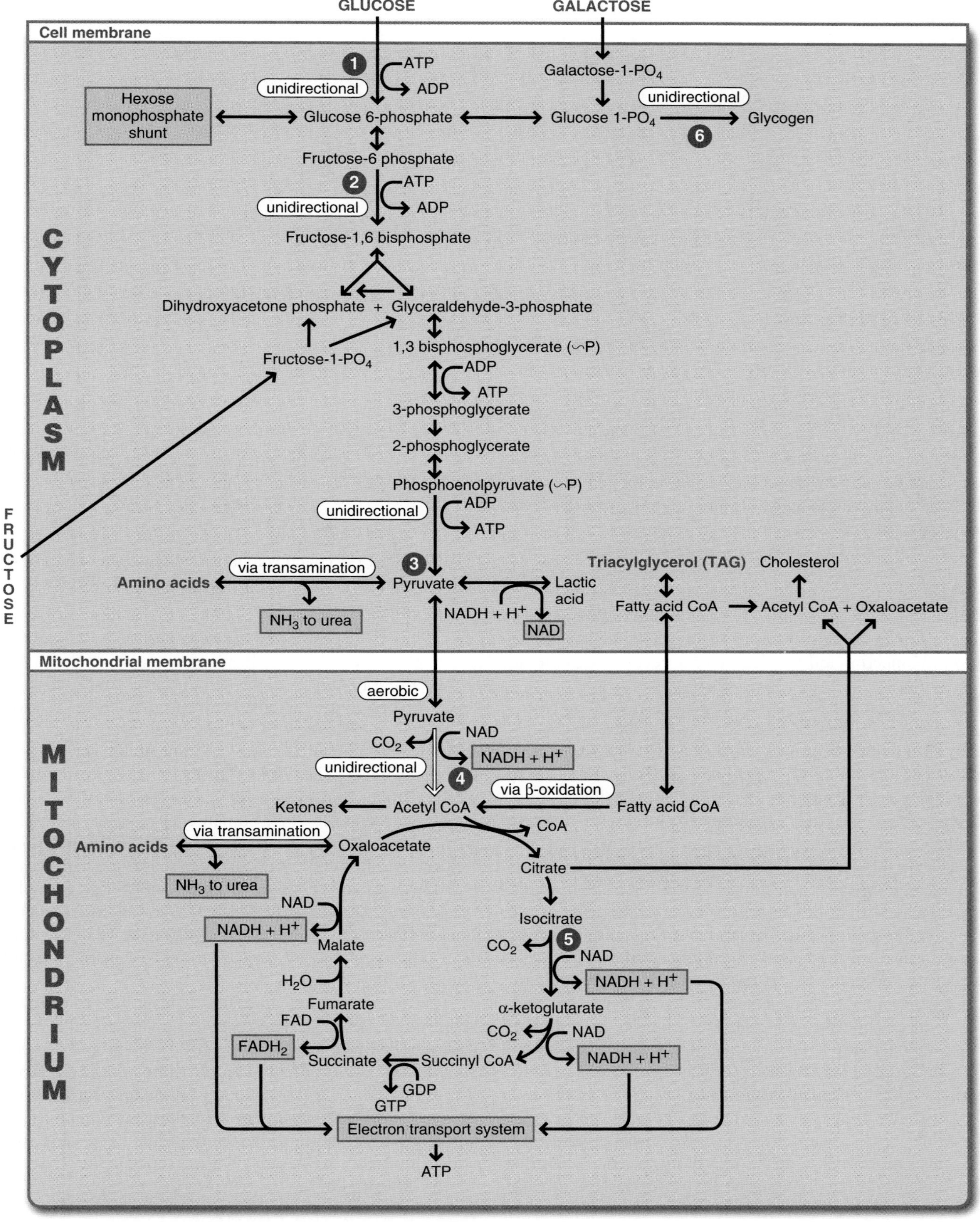
GLUCOSE
GALACTOSE
Cell membrane
1
ATP
ADP
unidirectional
Galactose-1-PO_4
Hexose monophosphate shunt
Glucose 6-phosphate
Glucose 1-PO_4
unidirectional
Glycogen
6
Fructose-6 phosphate
2
ATP
ADP
unidirectional
Fructose-1,6 bisphosphate
CYTOPLASM
Dihydroxyacetone phosphate + Glyceraldehyde-3-phosphate
Fructose-1-PO_4
1,3 bisphosphoglycerate (~P)
ADP
ATP
3-phosphoglycerate
2-phosphoglycerate
Phosphoenolpyruvate (~P)
unidirectional
ADP
ATP
FRUCTOSE
via transamination
3
Amino acids
Pyruvate
Lactic acid
NADH + H^+
NAD
NH_3 to urea
Triacylglycerol (TAG)
Cholesterol
Fatty acid CoA
Acetyl CoA + Oxaloacetate
Mitochondrial membrane
aerobic
Pyruvate
CO_2
NAD
NADH + H^+
unidirectional
4
via β-oxidation
Ketones
Acetyl CoA
Fatty acid CoA
CoA
MITOCHONDRIUM
via transamination
Amino acids
Oxaloacetate
Citrate
NH_3 to urea
NAD
NADH + H^+
Malate
Isocitrate
CO_2
5
NAD
NADH + H^+
H_2O
Fumarate
α-ketoglutarate
FAD
$FADH_2$
CO_2
NAD
NADH + H^+
Succinate
Succinyl CoA
GDP
GTP
Electron transport system
ATP

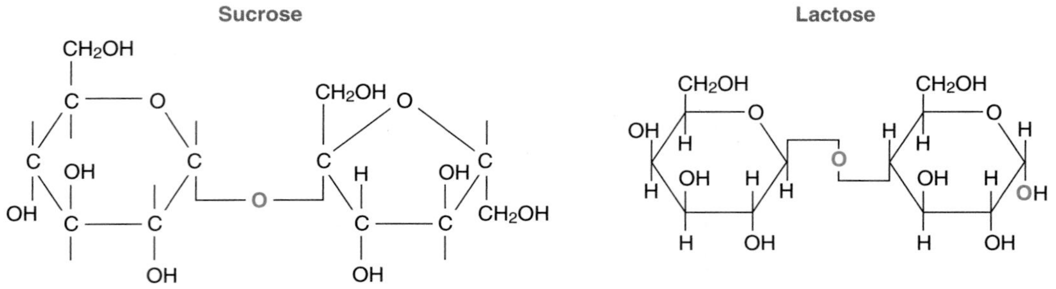

FIGURE 3-3 Disaccharides of importance in humans: sucrose (glucose and fructose) and lactose (glucose and galactose).

Polysaccharides

Polysaccharides are carbohydrates with more than 10 monosaccharide units. Plants store these carbohydrates as *starch* granules formed by linking glucose in straight chains and branching into a complex granular structure. Plants make two types of starch, amylose and amylopectin. **Amylose** is a smaller, linear molecule that is less than 1% branched whereas **amylopectin** is highly branched. Because of its larger size, amylopectin is more abundant in the food supply, especially in grains and starchy tubers.

Starches from corn, arrowroot, rice, potato, tapioca, and other plants are glucose polymers with the same chemical composition. Their unique character, taste, texture, and absorbability are determined by the relative numbers of glucose units in straight (amylase) and branched configurations (amylopectin) and the degree of accessibility to digestive enzymes.

Raw starch from raw potato or grains is poorly digested. Moist cooking causes the granules to swell, gelatinizes the starch, softens and ruptures the cell wall, and makes the starch more digestible by pancreatic amylase. Starch that remains intact throughout cooking, recrystallizes after cooling, resists enzyme breakdown, and yields limited amounts of glucose for absorption is known as **resistant starch**. *Waxy starch*, from corn and rice strains bred for more branched amylopectin chains, forms a smooth paste in water that gels only with a high concentration. Once a gel forms, the product remains thick during freezing and thawing, making it an ideal thickener for commercially frozen fruit pies, sauces, and gravies. *Modified food starch* is chemically or physically modified to change its viscosity, ability to gel, and other texture properties. Pregelatinized starch, dried on hot drums and made into a porous powder, is rapidly rehydrated with cold liquid. This starch rapidly thickens and is used in instant puddings, salad dressings, pie fillings, gravies, and baby food.

Dextrins result from the digestive process and are large, linear glucose polysaccharides of intermediate lengths cleaved from high amylose starch by α-amylase. *Limit dextrins* are cleaved from amylopectin containing branch points and are subsequently digested into glucose by the mucosal enzyme isomaltase.

In contrast to plants, animals use carbohydrates primarily to maintain blood glucose concentrations between feedings.

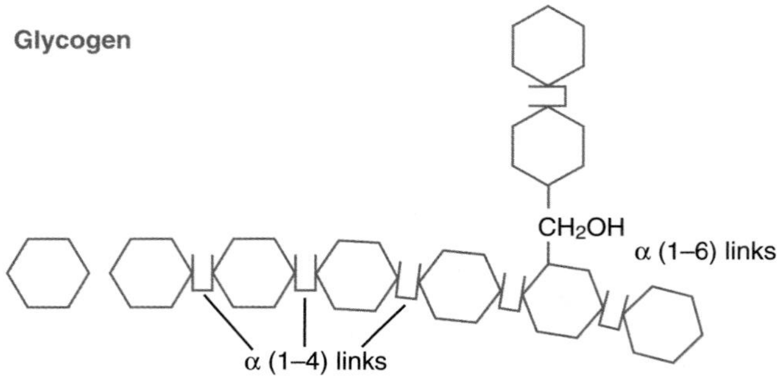

FIGURE 3-4 Glycogen is a branched glucose polymer similar to amylopectin, but the branches in glycogen are shorter and more numerous.

To ensure a readily available supply, liver and muscle cells store carbohydrate as **glycogen** (Figure 3-4). Glycogen is stored hydrated with water; thus the water makes glycogen large, cumbersome, and unsuitable for long-term energy storage. The 70-kg "average" man stores only an 18-hour fuel supply as glycogen, compared with a 2-month supply stored as fat. If all human energy stores were glycogen, humans would need to weigh 60 additional pounds (Alberts et al., 2002). Approximately 150 g of glycogen is stored in muscle, which can be increased fivefold with physical training (see Chapter 24) but is not available to maintain blood glucose directly. It is the glycogen store in the human liver (approximately 90 g) that is involved in the hormonal control of blood sugar.

The recommended amount of digestible carbohydrate required in the diet ranges between 45% and 65% of total calories (Institute of Medicine [IOM], Food and Nutrition Board, 2002). The percent carbohydrate of selected foods is given in Table 3-2. The Dietary Guidelines for Americans recommend that consumers select fruits, vegetables, and whole grains for higher fiber intake while decreasing sugar-added food choices (United States Department of Agriculture [USDA], 2005).

Dietary Fiber and Functional Fiber

Dietary fiber refers to intact plant components that are not digestible by gastrointestinal (GI) enzymes, whereas **functional fiber** refers to nondigestible carbohydrates that

TABLE 3-2

Carbohydrate Content of Foods

Food	Carbohydrate (g/100 g)
Sugar	
Concentrated Sweets	
Sugar: Cane, beet, powdered,	99.5
brown, maple	90-96
Candies	70-95
Honey (extracted)	82
Syrup: Table blends, molasses	55-75
Jams, jellies, marmalades	70
Carbonated, sweetened beverages	10-12
Fruits	
Prunes, apricots, figs (cooked, unsweetened)	12-31
Bananas, grapes, cherries, apples, pears	15-23
Fresh: Pineapples, grapefruits, oranges, apricots, strawberries	8-14
Milk	
Skim	6
Whole	5
Starch	
Grain products	
Starches: Corn, tapioca, arrowroot	86-88
Cereals (dry): Corn, wheat, oat, bran	68-85
Flour: Corn, wheat (sifted)	70-80
Popcorn (popped)	77
Cookies: Plain, assorted	71
Crackers, saltines	72
Cakes: Plain, without icing	56
Bread: White, rye, whole wheat	48-52
Macaroni, spaghetti, noodles, rice (cooked)	23-30
Cereals (cooked): Oat, wheat, grits	10-16
Vegetables	
Boiled: Corn, white and sweet potatoes, lima and dried beans, peas	15-26
Beets, carrots, onions, tomatoes	5-7
Leafy: Lettuce, asparagus, cabbage, greens, spinach	3-4

have been extracted or manufactured from plants. Both of these types of fiber have been shown to have beneficial physiologic functions in the GI tract and in reducing risk of certain disease states. These fibers and their functions are summarized in Table 3-3.

Homopolysaccharides contain repeating units of the same molecule. An example is **cellulose**, which cannot be hydrolyzed by amylase enzymes. Cellulose is the most abundant organic compound in the world, constituting 50% or more of all the carbon in vegetation. The long cellulose molecule folds back on itself and is held in place by hydrogen bonding, thus giving cellulose fibrils great mechanical strength but limited flexibility. Cellulose is found in carrots and other vegetables. Other homopolymers called **beta-glucans (glucopyranose)** occur with branching, which makes them more soluble; examples include oats and barley.

Heteropolysaccharides are made by modifying the basic cellulose structure to form compounds with different water solubilities. *Hemicellulose* is a glucose polymer substituted with different sugar molecules that have different water solubilities. The predominant sugar is used to name the hemicellulose (e.g., xylan, galactan, mannan, arabinose, galactose). *Pectins* and *gums* contain sugars and sugar alcohols that make these molecules more water soluble. The galacturonic acid structure of pectin absorbs water and forms a gel that it is widely used for making jams and jellies. The galacturonic acid backbone has rhamnose units inserted at intervals and side chains of arabinose and galactose. Pectin is found in apples, citrus fruit, strawberries, and other fruits. *Gums and mucilages* (e.g., guar gum) are similar to pectin, except their galactose units are combined with other sugars (e.g., glucose) and polysaccharides. Gums are found in plant secretions and seeds. The specific textural qualities of gums and mucilages are commercially useful when added to processed foods such as ice cream.

Fructans include *fructooligosaccharides (FOSs)*, *inulin*, *inulin-type fructans*, and *oligofructose* and are composed of fructose polymers, often linked with an initial glucose. Inulin is a diverse group of fructose polymers widely distributed in plants as a storage carbohydrate. Oligofructose is a subgroup of inulin with fewer than 10 fructose units. All are poorly digested in the upper GI tract and thus supply only approximately 1 kcal/g (Roberfroid, 2005). Fructans contain fructose; have a sweet, clean flavor; and are half as sweet as sucrose. Major sources of fructans include wheat, onions, garlic, bananas, and chicory; other sources include tomatoes, barley, rye, asparagus, and Jerusalem artichokes. Inulin compounds are widely used to improve the flavor and sweetness of low-calorie foods and to improve the stability and acceptability of fat-reduced foods. Because they are not absorbed in the proximal intestine, fructans have been used as a sugar replacement for diabetic patients.

Prebiotics are nondigestible food substances that selectively stimulate the growth or activity of beneficial bacterial species already resident in the colon (*probiotics*) and are beneficial to the host. Various prebiotics, including inulin, inulin-type fructans, and FOSs, stimulate the growth of intestinal bacteria, principally *bifidobacteria*. Fructans (synthesized or extracted) have prebiotic properties and are considered to be functional fiber (Roberfroid, 2007). Functional fiber is commonly added to liquid nutrition supplements and tube feeding formulas.

Algal polysaccharides (e.g., carrageenan) are extracted from seaweed and algae and are used as thickening and stabilizing agents in infant formulas, ice cream, milk pudding, and sour cream products. Algal polysaccharides are used commercially because they form weak gels with proteins and

TABLE 3-3

Types, Composition, Sources, and Functions of Fibers

Type of Fiber	Major Chemical Components	Sources	Major Functions
Less Soluble Fiber			
Cellulose	Glucose (β-1-4 linkages)	Whole wheat, bran, vegetables	Increase water-holding capacity, thus increasing fecal volume and decreasing gut transit time
Hemicellulose	Xylose, mannose, galactose	Bran, whole grains	
Lignin	Phenols	Fruits and edible seeds, mature vegetables	Fermentation produces short-chain fatty acids associated with decreased risk of tumor formation
More Soluble Fibers			
Gums	Galactose and glucuronic acid	Oats, legumes, guar, barley	Cause gel formation, thus decrease gastric emptying, slow digestion, gut transit time, and glucose absorption
Pectins	Polygalacturonic acid	Apples, strawberries, carrots, citrus	Also binds minerals, lipids, and bile acids increasing excretion of each, thus decreasing serum cholesterol
Functional Fibers*			
Chitin	Glucopyranose	Supplement from crab or lobster shells	Reduces serum cholesterol
Fructans (including inulin)	Fructose polymers	Extracted from natural sources: chicory, onions, etc.	Prebiotic that stimulates growth of beneficial bacteria in gut, used as fat replacer
β-glucans	Glucopyranose	Oat and barley bran	Reduces serum cholesterol
Algal polysaccharides (carrageenan)		Isolated from algae and seaweed	Gel forming—used as thickeners, stabilizers (can be toxic)
Polydextrose, polyols	Glucose and sorbitol, etc.	Synthesized	Used as a bulking agent or sugar substitute
Psyllium		Extracted from psyllium seeds	Has a high water-binding capacity (choking hazard)

*Isolated or extracted.

stabilize food mixtures, preventing suspended ingredients from settling. Tobacman (2001) demonstrated that carrageenan damages human cells in culture and destroys human mammary myoepithelial cells at concentrations as low as 0.00014%. With its wide use in commercial foods and uncertainty about the extent of human sensitivity, further investigation of carrageenan is needed.

Polydextrose and other polyols are synthetic polymers of *sugar alcohols* that are used as sugar substitutes in foods. They are not digestible, contribute to increased fecal bulk, and may be fermented in the small intestine. They are not yet classified as functional fibers (IOM, Food and Nutrition Board, 2002).

Lignin is a woody fiber found in the stems and seeds of fruits and vegetables and the bran layer of cereals. It is not a carbohydrate but is a polymer composed of phenylpropyl alcohols and acids. The phenyl groups contain conjugated double bonds, which make them excellent antioxidants. Flaxseed lignin also has phytoestrogen activity and can mimic estrogen at its receptors on reproductive organs and bone.

Role of Fiber in Digestion and Absorption

The role of fiber in the GI tract varies based on its solubility. Nonabsorbable oligosaccharides and fibers have a significant effect on human physiology. Insoluble fibers such as cellulose increase the water-holding capacity of undigested material, increase fecal volume, increase numbers of stools per day, and decrease GI transit time. On the other hand, soluble fibers form gels, slow GI transit time, bind other nutrients such as cholesterol and minerals, and decrease their absorption. Certain nondigestible oligosaccharides (NDOs), which are fermented by intestinal bacteria, stimulate the intestinal absorption and retention of minerals such as calcium, magnesium, zinc, and iron (Scholz-Ahrens et al., 2001).

Serum lipid concentrations can be modified by both insoluble cellulose and lignin or by soluble pectin and psyllium. They bind fecal bile acids and increase excretion of bile acid–derived cholesterol, thereby reducing lipid absorption. Fermentable oligosaccharides and dietary fiber are converted by intestinal bacteria to **short-chain fatty acids (SCFAs)**, which lower blood lipids. Evidence for the hypocholesterolemic effect of soluble fibers—including FOSs, synthetic polydextrose and polyols, viscous pectin, guar gum, oat bran, psyllium husk, beans, legumes, and fruits and vegetables—is conflicting. Effects vary with the type and amount of fiber (American Dietetic Association, 2008.) Prebiotic modulation by fiber is by fermentation into the SCFAs, acetate, butyrate, and propionate. SCFAs are readily absorbed by the intestinal and colonic mucosa. They enhance sodium and water absorption, colonic blood flow, colonocyte proliferation, GI hormone production, metabolic energy production, and they stimulate the autonomic nervous system via specific receptors in the colon (Tazoe et al., 2008). More than 70% of the fuel for colonocytes is the SCFA butyrate (4C), derived primarily from starch. Propionate (3C) is absorbed and cleared by the liver for hepatic lipid or glucose metabolism. Acetate (2C), produced from undigested carbohydrate, is rapidly metabolized into carbon dioxide by peripheral tissues as a substrate for lipid and cholesterol synthesis (Cummings et al., 2001).

The roles of fiber in the physiology of the GI tract are complex. The adequate intake (AI) of total fiber is set at 38 g/day for men and 25 g/day for women (IOM, Food and Nutrition Board, 2002). Americans' mean intake of fiber is currently less than half this. In addition to fiber, other nonnutrient components of plants, including tannins, saponins, lectins, and phytates, interact with nutrients, and may reduce their absorption. **Phytic acid** or **phytate**, a six-carbon ring with phosphate bound to each carbon, is found in the seed coat of grains and legumes and can bind metal ions, especially calcium, copper, iron, and zinc. Excess phytate can reduce starch hydrolysis if it binds with calcium, which catalyzes the action of amylase.

Glucose Absorption and the Glycemic Index

Dietary carbohydrates are digested into glucose, fructose, and galactose through the actions of α-amylase and brush-border digestive enzymes in the upper GI tract. The ability to digest carbohydrates is modified by the relative availability of the starch to enzyme action, the activity of digestive enzymes at the mucosal brush border, and the presence of other dietary factors (such as fat) that slow stomach emptying. Nonabsorbable oligosaccharides and viscous dietary fibers, such as pectins, β-glucans, and gums dilute enzyme concentration. Thus a diet rich in whole foods, such as fruits, vegetables, legumes, nuts, and minimally processed grains, slows the pace of glucose absorption.

Once digested, glucose is actively absorbed across the intestinal cell and transferred to the portal blood for transport to the liver (see Chapter 1). The liver removes approximately 50% of absorbed glucose for oxidation and storage as glycogen. Galactose (absorbed actively) and fructose (absorbed by facilitated diffusion) are also taken up by the liver and incorporated into glucose metabolic pathways. Glucose exits the liver, enters the systemic circulation, and is available for insulin-dependent uptake by peripheral tissues. Major regulators of blood glucose concentration after a meal are the amount and digestibility of ingested carbohydrate, absorption and degree of liver uptake, insulin secretion, and sensitivity of peripheral tissues to insulin action.

The **glycemic index** is used to rank carbohydrates by their ability to raise blood glucose levels as compared with a reference food. Riccardi et al. (2008) concluded that foods with a low glycemic index have consistently shown beneficial effects on blood glucose control in both the short and long term in diabetic patients. The glycemic index of a diet has a predictable effect on blood glucose levels. However, the Institute of Medicine (IOM) declined to set an upper limit for the glycemic index in the 2002 recommendations because it is difficult to separate the other factors that contribute to blood glucose levels. A metaanalysis by Livesey et al. (2008) concluded that although consumption of diets with reduced glycemic index were followed by positive health markers, fiber (unavailable carbohydrate) was equally important. The **glycemic load** of a food is the glycemic index of the carbohydrate divided by 100 and multiplied by its amount of available carbohydrate content (i.e. carbohydrates minus fiber) in grams. The glycemic load and dietary fiber also have important implications for individuals manifesting the metabolic syndrome. Published data on the glycemic index of individual foods, using white bread and glucose as reference foods, have been consolidated for the convenience of users. Use of the glycemic index to modify diets and prevent and control chronic disease is still under investigation.

Carbohydrate Regulation of Blood Lipids

Carbohydrate-induced hypertriglyceridemia can result from consuming a high-carbohydrate diet. The body regulates macronutrient levels to provide adequate fuel for body tissues. The brain uses the most of the approximately 200 g of glucose required per day. When blood glucose level falls to less than 40 mg/dL, counterregulatory hormones release macronutrients from stores. When blood glucose level rises to more than 180 mg/dL, glucose is spilled into the urine. High intakes of carbohydrate trigger large releases of insulin for compensatory responses, including insulin-dependent glucose uptake by muscle or fat and active synthesis of glycogen and fat. Blood glucose then drops to a normal range. Approximately 2 hours after a meal, intestinal absorption is complete, but insulin effects persist and blood glucose falls. The body interprets this hypoglycemic state as starvation and secretes counterregulatory hormones to release free fatty acids from fat cells (Ludwig, 2002). Fatty acids are packed into transport lipoproteins (very-low-density lipoproteins [VLDLs]) in the liver, thereby elevating serum triglycerides.

FATS AND LIPIDS

Lipid Structures and Functions

Fats and lipids constitute approximately 34% of the energy in the human diet. Because fat is energy rich and provides 9 kcal/g of energy, humans are able to obtain adequate energy with a reasonable daily consumption of fat-containing foods. Dietary fat is stored in *adipose* cells. The ability to store and use large amounts of fat enables humans to survive without food for weeks and sometimes months. Some fat deposits are not used effectively during a fast; they are classified as *structural fat.* Structural fat pads hold the body organs and nerves in position, protecting them against traumatic injury and shock. Fat pads on the palms and buttocks protect the bones from mechanical pressure. A subcutaneous layer of fat insulates the body, preserving body heat and maintaining body temperature.

Dietary fat is essential for the digestion, absorption, and transport of the fat-soluble vitamins and phytochemicals such as carotenoids and lycopenes. Dietary fat depresses gastric secretions, slows gastric emptying, and stimulates biliary and pancreatic flow, thereby facilitating digestion. Fat also conveys important textural properties to foods such as ice creams (smoothness) and baked goods (tenderness—caused by "shortening" strands of gluten). Box 3-1 lists the fat content of some common foods.

Unlike carbohydrates, lipids are not polymers; they are small molecules extracted from animal and plant tissues.

BOX 3-1

Fat Content of Some Common Foods

0 g

Most fruits and vegetables
Nonfat milk
Nonfat yogurt
Plain pasta and rice
Angel food cake
Popcorn, air popped, unbuttered
Soft drinks
Jam or jelly

1 to 3 g

Popcorn, oil popped, unbuttered, 1 cup
Low-calorie salad dressing, 1 tbsp
Baked beans, ½ cup
Soup, chicken noodle, canned, 1 cup
Whole-wheat bread, 1 slice
Dinner roll, 1
Waffle, frozen, 4 inch, 1
Coleslaw, ½ cup
Flounder or sole, baked, 3 oz
Chicken, without skin, baked or roasted, 3 oz
Tuna, canned in water, 3 oz
Cheese, cottage, 2% fat, ½ cup
Ice milk, soft serve, ½ cup

4 to 6 g

Low-fat yogurt, 1 cup
Cheese, mozzarella, part skim, 1 oz
Chicken, baked or roasted with skin, 3 oz
Egg, scrambled, 1
Turkey, roasted, 3 oz
Granola, 1 oz
Muffin, bran, 1 small
Pizza, cheese, ¼ of 12 inch
Burrito, bean, 1
Brownie, with nuts, 1 small
Margarine or butter, 1 tsp
Popcorn, oil popped, buttered, 1 cup
French dressing, regular, 1 tbsp

7 to 10 g

Cheese, cheddar, 1 oz
Milk, whole, 1 cup
Bologna, beef, 1 slice
Sausage, 1 patty
Steak, sirloin, broiled, 3 oz
Potatoes, French fried, 10
Chow mein, chicken, 1 cup
Chocolate candy bar, 1 oz
Corn chips, 1 oz
Doughnut, cake type, plain, 1
Mayonnaise, 1 tbsp

15 g

Hot dog, beef, 2 oz
McDonald's Chicken McNuggets, 6 pieces
Peanut butter, 2 tbsp
Pork chop, broiled, 3 oz
Sunflower seeds, dry roasted, ¼ cup
Avocado, ½ medium
Chop suey, beef and pork, 1 cup
Cinnamon roll, 1

20 g

Lasagna with meat, 1 medium piece
Macaroni and cheese, homemade, 1 cup
Peanuts, dry roasted, ¼ cup
Ground beef, broiled, 3 oz

25 g

Polish sausage, 3 oz
Cheeseburger, large
Pie, pecan, ⅛ of 9 inch
Chicken pot pie, frozen, baked, 1 pie
Quiche, bacon, ⅛ pie

Lipids are composed of a heterogeneous group of compounds characterized by their insolubility in water; they are classified into three major groups (Box 3-2). Figure 3-5 shows some important lipid structures.

Fatty Acids

Fatty acids are rarely free in nature and almost always are linked to other molecules by their *hydrophilic* carboxylic acid head group. Fatty acids occur primarily as unbranched hydrocarbon chains with an even number of carbons and are classified according to the number of carbons, the number of double bonds, and the position of the double bonds in the chain. Chain length and extent of saturation contribute to the melting temperature of a fat. In general, fats with shorter fatty acid chains or more double bonds are liquid at room temperature. Saturated fats, especially those with long chains, are solid at room temperature. A fat such as coconut oil, which is also highly saturated, is semiliquid at room temperature because the predominant fatty acids are short (8 to 14 carbons). Some manufacturers cool oil and filter out solidified lipid particles before sale; the resulting "winterized" oil remains clear when refrigerated. In general, SCFAs are considered to have 4 to 6 carbons, medium-chain fatty acids to have 8 to14, and long-chain fatty acids (LCFAs), to have 16 to 20 or more.

BOX 3-2
Classification of Lipids

Simple Lipids

Fatty Acids

Neutral fats: Esters of fatty acids with glycerol

Monoglycerides, diglycerides, triglycerides

Waxes: Esters of fatty acids with high-molecular-weight alcohols

Sterol esters (e.g., cholesterol ester)

Nonsterol esters (e.g., retinyl palmitate [vitamin A esters])

Compound Lipids

Phospholipids: Compounds of phosphoric acid, fatty acids, and a nitrogenous base

Glycerophospholipids (e.g., lecithins, cephalins, plasmalogens)

Glycosphingolipids (e.g., sphingomyelins, ceramide)

Glycolipids: Compounds of fatty acids, monosaccharides, and a nitrogenous base (e.g., cerebrosides, gangliosides)

Lipoproteins: Particles of lipid and protein

Miscellaneous Lipids

Sterols (e.g., cholesterol, vitamin D, bile salts)

Vitamins A, E, K

From Examples of current and proposed ingredients for fats. J Am Diet Assoc 92:472, 1992.

In a **saturated fatty acid (SFA)**, all carbon binding sites not linked to another carbon are linked to hydrogen and are therefore saturated. There are no double bonds between carbons. **Monounsaturated fatty acids (MFAs)** contain only one double bond, and **polyunsaturated fatty acids (PUFAs)** contain two or more double bonds. In MFAs and PUFAs one or more pairs of hydrogen have been removed, and double bonds form between adjacent carbons. Because fatty acids with double bonds are vulnerable to oxidative damage, humans and other warm-blooded organisms store fat predominantly as saturated palmitic fatty acid (C16:0) and stearic fatty acid (C18:0). Cell membranes must be stable and flexible. To achieve this requirement, membrane phospholipids contain one SFA and one highly PUFA, the most abundant of which is arachidonic acid (C20:4). Commonly occurring fatty acids and a typical food source are listed in Table 3-4.

Fatty acids are also characterized by the location of their double bonds. Two notation conventions are used to describe the location of the double bonds (Table 3-5). Omega notation is used in this chapter. In omega notation, a lowercase omega (ω) or *n* is used to refer to the placement of the first double bond counting from the methyl end (the fatty acid's omega number). Thus arachidonic acid (20:4 ω-6 or 20:4 *n*-6), the major highly polyunsaturated fat in membranes of land animals, is an **omega-6 (ω-6) fatty acid**. It has 20 carbons and four double bonds, the first of which is six carbons from the terminal methyl group. Eicosapentaenoic acid (EPA) (20:5 ω-3 or 20:5 *n*-3) is found in marine organisms and is an **omega-3 (ω-3) fatty acid**. It has five double bonds, the first of which is three carbons from the terminal methyl group. Sources of the longer EPA and docosahexaenoic acid (DHA) ω-3 fatty acids are primarily marine, such as cod liver oil, mackerel, salmon, and sardines (Table 3-6).

Essential Fatty Acids and the Omega-6/Omega-3 Ratio

Only plants (including marine phytoplankton) can synthesize ω-6 and ω-3 fatty acids. Humans and other animals can only place double bonds as low as the ω-9 carbon and cannot produce their own ω-6 and ω-3 fatty acids. But humans can desaturate and elongate linoleic acid (18:2 *n*-6) to arachidonic acid (20:4 *n*-6) and alpha-linoleic acid (ALA) (C18:3 ω-3) to EPA (C20:5 ω-3) and DHA (C22:6 ω-3). Therefore both linoleic (18:2 *n*-6) and ALA (C18:3 ω-3) acids are essential in the diet (IOM, Food and Nutrition Board, 2002).

An *essential fatty acid* refers to the families of ω-6 and ω-3 fatty acids. Yet it is the longer-chain fatty acids made from them that are components of cell membranes and are precursors of eicosanoids such as prostaglandins, thromboxanes, and leukotrienes. *Eicosanoids* act as localized (paracrine) hormones and have multiple local functions. They can alter the size and permeability of the blood vessels, alter the activity of platelets and contribute to blood clotting, and modify the processes of inflammation

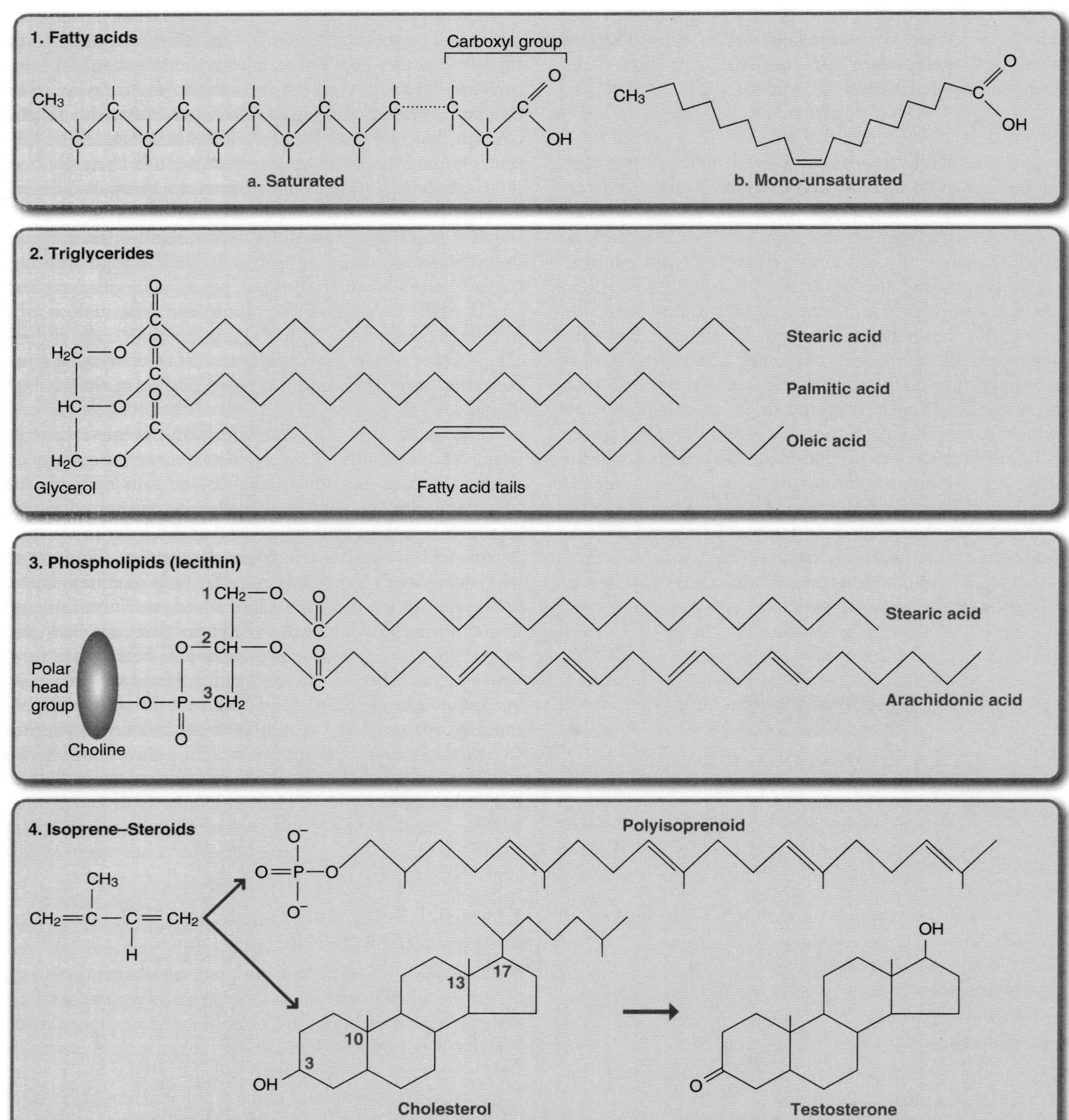

FIGURE 3-5 Structures of physiologically important fats and lipids.

(Figure 3-6). Derivatives of *n*-3 fatty acids from dietary sources or fish oil can have beneficial effects in a number of disease states (Freemantle et al., 2006; McCowen and Bistrian, 2005), including improved brain function during aging. Roles for ω-3 fatty acids are discussed in chapters related to cardiovascular disease, arthritis and inflammatory conditions, and neurologic disorders.

An imbalance between dietary ω-3 and ω-6 fatty acids contributes to a wide range of disease states (Wertz, 2009). Excess amounts of ω-6 fatty acids in the diet saturate the enzymes that desaturate and elongate both ω-3 and ω-6 fatty acids; this prevents conversion of ALA into EPA and DHA (Kris-Etherton, 2000). The optimal ω-6/ω-3 ratio has been estimated to be 2:1 to 3:1, four times lower than

TABLE 3-4

Common Fatty Acids

Common Name	Systematic Name	Number of Carbon Atoms*	Number of Double Bonds	Typical Fat Source
Saturated Fatty Acids				
Butyric	Butanoic	4	0	Butterfat
Caproic	Hexanoic	6	0	Butterfat
Caprylic	Octanolic	8	0	Coconut oil
Capric	Decanoic	10	0	Coconut oil
Lauric	Dodecanoic	12	0	Coconut oil, palm kernel oil
Myristic	Tetradecanoic	14	0	Butterfat, coconut oil
Palmitic	Hexadecanoic	16	0	Palm oil, animal fat
Stearic	Octadecanoic	18	0	Cocoa butter, animal fat
Arachidic	Elcosanoic	20	0	Peanut oil
Behenic	Docosanoic	22	0	Peanut oil
Unsaturated Fatty Acids				
Caproleic	9-Decenoic	10	1	Butterfat
Lauroleic	9-Dodecenoic	12	1	Butterfat
Myristoleic	9-Tetradecenoic	14	1	Butterfat
Palmitoleic	9-Hexadecenoic	16	1	Some fish oils, beef fat
Oleic	9-Octadecenoic	18	1	Olive oil, canola oil
Elaidic	9-Octadecenoic	18	1	Butterfat
Vaccenic	11-Octadecenoic	18	1	Butterfat
Linoleic	9, 12-Octadecadienoic	18	2	Most vegetable oils, especially safflower, corn, soybean, cottonseed
Linolenic	9, 12, 15-Octadecatrienoic	18	3	Soybean oil, canola oil, walnuts, wheat germ oil, flaxseed oil
Gadoleic	11-Eicosaenoic	20	1	Some fish oils
Arachidonic	5, 8, 11, 14-Eicosatetraenoic	20	4	Lard, meats
—	5, 8, 11, 14, 17- EPA	20	5	Some fish oils, shellfish
Erucic	13-Docosenoic	22	1	Canola oil
—	4, 7, 10, 13, 16, 19- DHA	22	6	Some fish oils, shellfish

Modified from Institute of Shortening and Edible Oils: Food fats and oils, ed 6. Washington, DC, 1988, The Institute.

DHA, Docosahexaenoic acid; *EPA*, eicosapentaenoic acid.

*All double bonds are in the cis configuration except for elaidic acid and vaccenic acid, which are trans.

TABLE 3-5

Fatty Acid Families

α-Linolenic Family (Omega-3)	Linoleic Family (Omega-6)	Oleic Family (Omega-9)
18:3 ω-3 → 18:4 ω-3	18:2 ω-6 → 18:3 ω-6	18:1 ω-9 → 18:2 ω-9
linolenic	Linoleic	Oleic
↓	↓	↓
20:4 ω-3 → 20:5 ω-3	20:3 ω-6 → 20:4 ω-6	20:2 ω-9 → 20:3 ω-9
Eicosapentaenoic	Arachidonic	Eicosatrienoic*
↓	↓	
22:5 ω-3 → 22:6 ω-3	22:4 ω-6 → 22:5 ω-6	
Docosahexanoic	Docosapentaenoic	

Elongation, ↓ desaturation, →

*Increases in essential fatty acid deficiency.

TABLE 3-6

Sources of Omega-3 Fatty Acids

Food Source (100 g Edible Portion, Raw)	Total Fat (g)	Omega-3 Fat DHA (22:6 ω-3) EPA (20:5 ω-3)
Sardines, in sardine oil	15.5	3.3
Mackerel, Atlantic	13.9	2.5
Herring, Atlantic	9	1.6
Salmon, Chinook	10.4	1.4
Anchovy	4.8	1.4
Salmon, Atlantic	5.4	1.2
Bluefish	6.5	1.2
Salmon, pink	3.4	1
Pompano, Florida	9.5	0.6
Tuna	2.5	0.5
Trout, brook	2.7	0.4
Shrimp	1.1	0.3
Catfish, channel	4.3	0.3
Lobster, northern	0.9	0.2
Haddock	0.7	0.2
Flounder	1	0.2

Modified from Conner SL, Conner WE: Are fish oils beneficial in the prevention and treatment of coronary artery disease? Am J Clin Nutr (Suppl 4):1020, 1997.

DHA, Docosahexaenoic acid; *EPA*, eicosapentaenoic acid.

the current intake; therefore it is recommended that humans consume more ω-3 fatty acids from vegetable and marine sources. ALA is found in flaxseed (57%), canola oil (8%), soybean oil (7%), and green leaves in a few plants such as purslane.

Trans-Fatty Acids

In natural unsaturated fatty acids, the two carbons participating in a double bond each bind a hydrogen on the *same* side of the bond (the *cis*-isomer form), causing the fatty acid to bend (see Figure 3-5). The more double bonds per fatty acid, the more bends in the molecule. **Hydrogenation** of unsaturated fatty acids is a chemical process that adds hydrogen to oils to form a stable, solid fat such as margarine. Hydrogen can be added both in the natural *cis* position (with two hydrogens on the same side of the double bond) and in the *trans* position (with one hydrogen on opposite sides of the double bond). Membrane function depends on the three-dimensional configuration of membrane fatty acids found in phospholipids. The *cis* double bonds in the membrane bend, allowing the fatty acids to pack loosely, thus making the membrane fluid. Because proteins embedded in a membrane float or sink, depending on the membrane's fluidity, membrane viscosity is important for membrane protein function.

***Trans*-fatty acids** do not bend; they pack into the membrane as tightly as if they were fully saturated. *Trans*-fatty

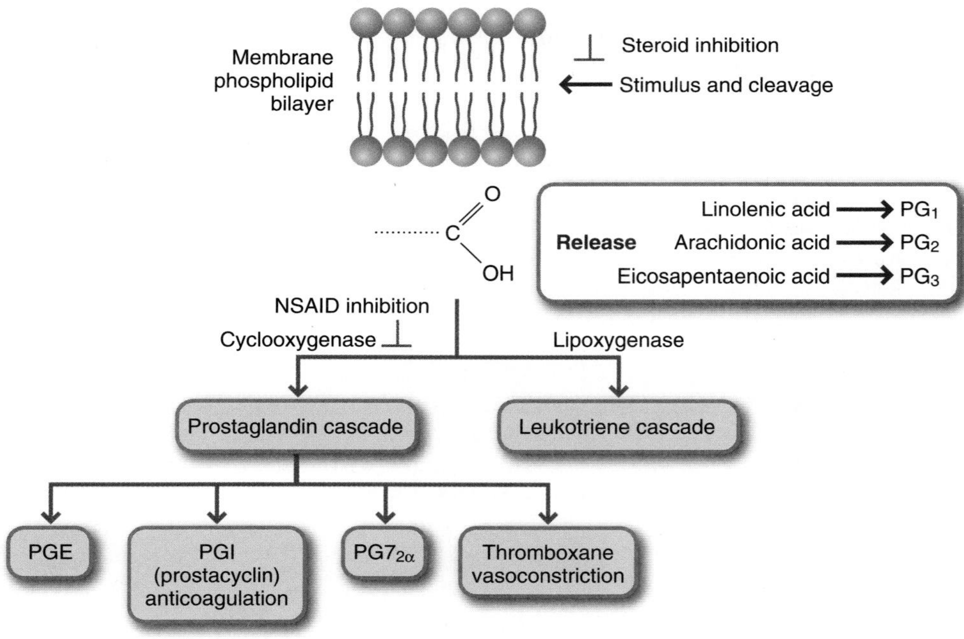

FIGURE 3-6 Eicosanoid synthesis after phospholipid cleavage in the biomembrane. Injury, inflammation, and other stimuli cleave the highly unsaturated fatty acid at the C-2 position of the membrane phospholipid. Arachidonic acid or eicosapentaenoic acid is the major fatty acid released; the pathway entered depends on the degree to which the target tissue expresses the enzyme. The cyclooxygenase pathway leads to prostaglandin, thromboxane, and prostacyclin synthesis. The lipoxygenase pathway, which is common in the lungs and bronchi, leads to leukotriene synthesis and subsequent bronchoconstriction. Note the point at which steroidal and nonsteroidal antiinflammatory drugs act.

acids inhibit the desaturation and elongation of linoleic and ALA, which are critical for fetal brain and organ development. Major sources of *trans*-fatty acids in the American diet are chemically hydrogenated margarine, shortening, commercial frying fats, high-fat baked goods, and salty snacks containing these fats. Butter and animal fat can also contain *trans*-fatty acids from bacterial fermentation in the rumen of cows and sheep.

Higher intakes of *trans*-fatty acids are associated with increased risk for coronary heart disease, cancer, type 2 diabetes, and allergies, possibly because of their potential to influence membrane fluidity (Micha and Mozaffarin, 2009). The U.S. Department of Agriculture Dietary Guidelines for Americans (2005) recommends limiting intake of *trans*-fatty acids and SFAs to as little as possible.

Conjugated Linoleic Acid

Conjugated linoleic acids (CLAs) are positional and geometric isomers of linoleic acid, not separated by a methylene group as occurs in linoleic acid. These isomers are minor components of the lipids from meat and dairy products. CLA isomers are metabolized in the body through different metabolic pathways with different physiologic outcomes. Eighty percent of CLA is the *cis*-9, *trans*-11 isomer. Another notable isomer is *trans*-10, *cis*-12, which is more efficiently oxidized and has different biological outcomes. The *cis*-9, *trans*-11 isomer appears to be responsible for the anticarcinogenic effect of CLAs; the *trans*-10, *cis*-12 isomer reduces body fat and alters blood lipids. Both isomers seem to be responsible for insulin resistance in humans. CLAs are of interest because of these anticarcinogenic, antidiabetogenic, and antiatherogenesis effects. Studies on CLA supplementation demonstrate reduction in body fat percentage and body mass (Baddini et al., 2009; Churrucal et al., 2009).

Triglycerides

The body forms **triglycerides (triacylglycerols TAG)** by joining three fatty acids to a glycerol side chain (see Figure 3-5, *2*), thereby neutralizing reactive fatty acids and making triglycerides water insoluble (hydrophobic). The hydroxyl group on each fatty acid is bound to a hydroxyl group on glycerol, releasing water and forming an ester linkage. Neutral fats can be safely transported in the blood and stored in fat cells (adipocytes) as an energy reserve. Different fatty acids can make up a single triglyceride and depend on the dietary fatty acids and the amount of synthesis taking place. Storage triglycerides from land animals are predominately saturated because SFAs are relatively inert and not susceptible to oxidative damage during storage. Cold-water creatures must maintain their fatty acids in liquid form even at low temperatures; therefore triglycerides in fish oils and marine-derived fats contain longer (C20 and C22), highly unsaturated fatty acids.

Phospholipids

Phospholipids are derivatives of phosphatidic acid, a triglyceride modified to contain a phosphate group at the third position (see Figure 3-5, *3*). Phosphatidic acid is esterified into a nitrogen-containing molecule, usually choline, serine, inositol, or ethanolamine, and named for its nitrogenous base (e.g., phosphatidylcholine, phosphatidylserine). Membrane phospholipids usually contain one SFA (C16 to C18) at C-1 and a highly PUFA (C16 to C20) at C-2, usually one of the essential fatty acids. ALA (C18:3 ω-3), arachidonic acid (C20:4 ω-6), and ω-3 substitutes can be cleaved from the lipid bilayer to provide substrate for synthesis of prostaglandins and other mediators of cell activity.

Because it is polar at physiologic pH, the phosphate-containing portion of the molecule forms hydrogen bonds with water, whereas the two fatty acids have hydrophobic interactions with other fatty acids (Figure 3-6). The polar head groups face outward into the aqueous external and cytoplasmic fluids, whereas the centrally placed fatty acid tails participate in hydrophobic interactions at the membrane center. The barrier formed by this lipid bilayer can be crossed only by very small lipid soluble molecules (e.g., oxygen, carbon dioxide, and nitrogen) and to a limited extent by small, uncharged polar molecules such as water and urea.

Lecithin (phosphatidylcholine) is a major phospholipid, and it is the primary component of lipid in the membrane lipid bilayer. Lecithin is also a major component of lipoproteins (i.e., VLDLs, low-density lipoproteins [LDLs], and high-density lipoproteins [HDLs]) used to transport fats and cholesterol. Lecithin is made by the body with arachidonic acid. Because all cells contain lecithin as a lipid bilayer component, animal products, especially liver and egg yolks, are rich sources of lecithin. Plant products such as soybeans, peanuts, legumes, spinach, and wheat germ are also rich sources. Lecithin is widely distributed in the food supply and is added to food products such as margarine, ice cream, snack crackers, and confections as a stabilizer.

Sphingolipids, Alcohols, Waxes, Isoprenoids, and Steroids

All organisms produce small amounts of complex lipids with specialized, critical functions. Many of these lipids do not contain glycerol and are built from two-carbon **acetyl coenzyme A (acetyl CoA)** units. *Sphingolipids* are lipid esters attached to a sphingosine base rather than a glycerol. They are widely distributed in the nervous systems of animals and the membranes of plants and lower eukaryotes such as yeast. Sphingomyelin includes the nitrogenous base choline and makes up more than 25% of the myelin sheath, the lipid-rich structure that protects and insulates cells of the central nervous system. In addition to phosphatidylcholine, sphingomyelin is found in all membranes. Sphingolipidoses comprise a group of genetic lipid-storage diseases in which normal sphingolipid degradation is blocked. Tay-Sachs disease is an example of such a lipid-storage disease.

Long-chain alcohols are metabolic by-products of lipids. The feces contain cetyl alcohol, a by-product of palmitic acid. Beeswax is rich in the alcohol myricyl palmitate. Waxes consist of LCFAs bound to long-chain alcohols. These molecules are almost completely water insoluble and are often used as water repellants, as they are in the feathers of birds and on the leaves of plants.

Isoprenoids, activated derivatives of isoprene, are an extraordinarily large and diverse group of lipids built from one or more five-carbon units. Isoprene contains alternating single and double (conjugated) bonds, an arrangement that can quench free radicals by accepting or donating electrons. *Terpene* is a generic term for all compounds synthesized from isoprene precursors and includes essential oils of plants (e.g., turpentine from trees and limonene from lemons). Plant pigments that transfer electrons in photosynthesis are also isoprenoids and include lycopene (the red pigment in tomatoes), carotenoids (the yellow and orange pigments in squash and carrots), and the yellow and green chlorophyll group. Fat-soluble vitamins A, D, E, and K and the electron transducer coenzyme Q have isoprenoid structures. Vitamin E, lycopene, and β-carotene are effective antioxidants; nonnutritive phytochemicals with antioxidant function also have an isoprenoid structure.

Steroids constitute a class of lipids derived from a four-membered saturated ring (see Figure 3-5, *4*). **Cholesterol** is the basis for all steroid derivatives made in the body, including glucocorticoids (cortisone) and mineralocorticoids (aldosterone), which are made in the adrenal gland; androgens (testosterone) and estrogens (estradiol), which are made in the testes and ovaries, respectively; and bile acids, which are made in the liver. Vitamin D hormone is made when ultraviolet rays from the sun cleave cholesterol in subcutaneous fat to form cholecalciferol (D_3). Synthetic vitamin D is made by irradiating the plant steroid ergosterol to form ergocalciferol (D_2).

Cholesterol also plays an important role in membrane function. The rigid, four-ringed cholesterol molecule is bound into the hydrophobic membrane by its hydroxyl group. The stiff, planar rings spread apart and partially immobilize the fatty acid chains near the polar region. At the same time, the nonpolar hydrocarbon tail contributes to greater fluidity in the interior of the membrane. Plasma membranes contain large amounts of cholesterol—up to one molecule for every phospholipid molecule.

Glycolipids include the cerebrosides and gangliosides, which are composed of a sphingosine base and very long-chain (22C) fatty acids. Cerebrosides contain galactose; gangliosides also contain glucose and a complex compound containing an amino sugar. Structurally both compounds are components of nerve tissue and cell membranes, where they play a role in lipid transport.

Synthetic Lipids

Medium-chain triglycerides (MCTs) are SFAs with a chain length of between 6 and 12 carbons. Although MCTs occur naturally in milk fat, coconut oil, and palm kernel oil, they are also produced commercially (MCT oil) as a by-product of margarine production. MCT oils provide 8.25 kcal/g and are of value in a number of clinical situations because they are short enough to be water soluble, require less bile salt for solubilization, are not reesterified in the enterocyte, and are transported as free fatty acids, bound to albumin, through the portal system. Because the portal blood flow rate is approximately 250 times faster than the lymph flow, MCTs are digested quickly and not likely to be affected by intestinal factors that inhibit fat absorption. They are not stored in adipose tissue but are oxidized to acetic acid.

Structured lipids include MCT oil esterified with a desired fatty acid such as linoleic acid or an ω-3 lipid. The combined product is absorbed faster than the long-chain triglyceride alone. Clinically, structured lipids have a role in parenteral and enteral formulas, such as to enhance immune function or athletic performance.

Fat replacers (Table 3-7) are structurally different from fats and do not provide readily absorbable nutrients. Their commercial importance is that they imitate the texture and other sensations of fat, especially in the mouth. Fat replacers differ in their macronutrient base and the extent to which they mimic the characteristics of fat. The caloric value of these substitutes varies between 5 kcal/g (e.g., caprenin) and 0 kcal/g (e.g., olestra, carrageenan). Most fat replacers are derived from plant polysaccharides such as gums, cellulose, dextrins, fiber, maltodextrins, starches, and polydextrose. Olestra is a sucrose polyester in which sucrose is esterified with six to eight fatty acids to form esters. The fatty acid chains range in length from 12 to 24 carbons and are derived from edible oils such as soybean, cottonseed, and corn oils. The product has the physical properties of natural dietary fats. Because they are nonabsorbable, sucrose polyesters do not contribute calories to the diet.

Protein-based fat replacers alter the texture of a product in various ways. Microparticulated proteins can act like small ball bearings, providing a fatlike feeling in the mouth. These replacers contribute between 1.3 and 4 kcal/g and augment the protein content of the food. Note that some of these proteins can stimulate an allergic or antigenic response in susceptible individuals (see Chapter 27).

Fat sources can be modified to reduce GI absorption and caloric availability. **Monoacylglycerols (monoglycerides)** and **diacylglycerols (diglycerides)** are used as emulsifiers and contribute to the sensory properties of fat but have fewer calories (approximately 5 kcal/g). Salatrim has SFA and LCFA triglyceride molecules and contains 5 kcal/g because of reduced absorbability. Concerns about the long-term effects of fat substitutes are that they may bind essential fatty acids and fat-soluble vitamins and contribute to their malabsorption or have negative effects on fundamental energy intake regulatory mechanisms (McKiernan et al., 2008). However, under most circumstances they appear to be safe, effective, and feasible alternatives for controlling fat and energy in diets (American Dietetic Association, 2005).

TABLE 3-7

Examples of Fat Replacers and Their Functions and Properties

Class of Fat Replacers	Trade Names	Applications	Functional Properties
Carbohydrate Based			
Polydextrose	Litesse,[a] Sta-Lite[b]	Dairy products, sauces, frozen desserts, salad dressings, baked goods, confections, gelatins, puddings, meat products, chewing gum, dry cake and cookie mixes, frostings and icings	Moisture retention, bulking agent, texturizer
Starch (modified food starch)	Amalean I & II,[c] N-Lite,[d] Instant Stellar,[e] Sta-Slim,[b] OptaGrade,[e] Pure-gel[f]	Processed meats, salad dressings, baked goods, fillings and frostings, condiments, frozen desserts, dairy products	Gelling, thickening, stabilizing, texturizer
Maltodextrins	CrystaLean,[e] Maltrin,[f] Lycadex,[g] Star-Dri,[b] Paselli Excell,[h] Rice-Trim[i]	Baked goods, dairy products, salad dressings, spreads, sauces, fillings and frostings, processed meat, frozen desserts, extruded products	Gelling, thickening, stabilizing, texturizer
Grain based (fiber)	Betatrim,[j] Opta[e] Oat Fibere,[k] Snowite[k] TrimChoice,[b] Fibrim[l]	Baked goods, meats, extruded products, spreads	Gelling, thickening, stabilizing, texturizer
Dextrins	N-Oil,[d] Stadex[b]	Salad dressings, puddings, spreads, dairy products, frozen desserts, chips, baked goods, meat products, frostings, soups	Gelling, thickening, stabilizing, texturizer
Gums (xanthan, guar, locust bean carrageenan, alginates)	Kelcogel,[m] Keltrol,[n] Viscarin,[o] Gel-carin,[o] Fibrex,[p] Novagel,[q] Rohodi-gel,[j] Jaguar[r]	Salad dressings, processed meats, formulated foods (e.g., desserts, processed meats)	Water retention, texturizer, thickener, mouth texture, stabilizer
Pectin	Grindsted,[s] Slendid,[t] Splendid[t]	Baked goods, soups, sauces, dressings	Gelling, thickening, mouth texture
Cellulose (carboxymethyl cellulose, microcrystalline cellulose)	Avicel,[q] cellulose gel, Methocel,[u] Solka-Floc,[v] Just Fiber[w]	Dairy products, sauces, frozen desserts, salad dressings	Water retention, texturizer, stabilizer, mouth texture
Fruit Based (fiber)	Prune paste, dried plum paste, Lighter Bake,[x] WonderSlim[y] fruit powder	Baked goods, candy, dairy products	Moisturizer, mouth texture
Protein Based	Simplesse,[z] K-Blazer[aa] Dairy-lo,[bb] Veri-lo,[bb] Ultra-Bake,[b] Powerpro,[cc] Proplus,[dd] Supro[dd]	Cheese, mayonnaise, butter, salad dressing, sour cream, spreads, bakery products	Mouth texture
Fat Based	Caprenin,[ee] Olean,[ee] Benefat,[bb] Dur-Em[w] Dur-Lo[w]	Chocolate, confections, bakery products, savory snacks	Mouth texture
Combinations	Prolestra,[ff] Nutrifat,[ff] Finesse[ff]	Ice cream, salad oils, mayonnaise, spreads, sauces, bakery products	Mouth texture

From American Dietetic Association: Position of the American Dietetic Association: fat replacers, J Am Diet Assoc 105:266, 2005.

[a]Cultor Food Science, Inc, Ardsley, N.Y.

[b]AE Staley manufacturing Co, Decatur, Ill.

[c]Cerestar USA, Inc, Hammond, Ind.

[d]National Starch and Chemical Co. Bridgewater, N.J.

[e]Opta Food Ingredients, Bedford, Mass.

[f]Grain Processing Corp, Muscatine, Iowa.

[g]Roquette America, Inc, Keokuk, Iowa.

[h]AVEBE America Inc, Princeton, N.J.

[i]Zumbro, Inc, Hayfield, Minn.

[j]Rhone-Poulenc, Inc, Cranbury, N.J.

[k]Canadian Harvest USA, Cambridge, Minn.

[l]Protein Technologies International, Pryor, Okla.

Continued

TABLE 3-7

Examples of Fat Replacers and Their Functions and Properties—cont'd

[m]Monsanto, Chicago, Ill.
[n]Kelco, Division of Merck, Clark, N.J.
[o]FMC Corp, Rockland, Me.
[p]Purity Foods, Okemos, Mich.
[q]FMC Corp, Philadelphia, Pa.
[r]Aston Chemicals, Aylesbury, Buckinghamshire, England.
[s]Danisco, New Century, Ky.
[t]Hercules Inc, Wilmington, Del.
[u]Dow Chemical, Midland, Mich.
[v]Fiber Sales and Development Corp, Green Brook, N.J.
[w]Loders Croklaan, Glen Ellyn, Ill.
[x]Sunsweet Growers, Yuba City, Calif.
[y]The Heart Garden Corporation, Los Angeles, Calif.
[z]Nutrasweet, San Diego, Calif.
[aa]Kraft Food Ingredients, Memphis, Ind.
[bb]Cultor Food Science, Ardsley, N.Y.
[cc]Land O'Lakes Food Division, Arden Hill, Minn.
[dd]Protein Technologies International, St Louis, Mo.
[ee]Procter and Gamble, Cincinnati, Ohio.
[ff]Reach Associates, South Orange, N.J.

Recommendations for Lipid Intake

Recommendations for lipid intake must take into account the documented physiologic and health effects of various lipid components, as well as the worldwide obesity epidemic. For example, SFAs are known to increase LDLs and HDLs, whereas PUFAs decrease the "bad" and "good" lipoproteins. The 2005 Dietary Guidelines for Americans (USDA) recommended the consumption of less than 10% of calories as SFA. SFAs and MFAs, especially those in olive oil, that are similarly thermally stressed do not produce these toxic products. Saturated fat and partially hydrogenated oils have fewer oxygen-binding sites and thereby have increased stability and a longer shelf life; however, their intake is associated with greater risk of cardiovascular disease. On the other hand, too much PUFA can also be dangerous. Double bonds are highly reactive and bind oxygen to form peroxides when exposed to air or heat. When subjected to routine frying or cooking, PUFAs can generate high levels of toxic aldehyde products that promote cardiovascular disease and cancer.

Alcohol (Ethyl Alcohol)

Alcohol has 7 kcal/g and no nutrient value. It is able to permeate all membranes and is absorbed quickly and easily. It is metabolized primarily by the liver enzyme alcohol dehydrogenase (ADH) to acetaldehyde and then to acetyl-CoA, where it can be used to synthesize fat or enter the tricarboxylic acid (TCA) cycle. ADH requires both thiamin and niacin to function. When the amount of alcohol in the cell exceeds the capacity of ADH to metabolize it or when niacin (as NAD^+) is depleted, the microsomal ethanol oxidizing system (MEOS) will also metabolize alcohol to acetaldehyde. Chronic alcohol consumption induces both ADH and certain enzymes in the MEOS system. Because the MEOS system is also responsible for the metabolism of many drugs, chronic ingestion of large amounts of alcohol can alter drug responses in unpredictable ways. For example, overall alcoholism leading to induction of the MEOS causes a person to be tolerant not only of alcohol but other drugs as well. But if at any given time the MEOS is saturated with alcohol, drugs are not metabolized at the expected rate and a drug overdose can occur. In addition the production of acetaldehyde in these pathways may be toxic in itself, leading to cirrhosis of the liver.

AMINO ACIDS AND PROTEIN

Whereas plant structures are composed primarily of carbohydrates, the body structure of humans and animals is built on protein. **Proteins** differ molecularly from carbohydrates and lipids in that they contain nitrogen. Primary roles for proteins in the body include structural protein, enzymes, hormones, transport, and immunoproteins. Proteins are composed of amino acids (Figure 3-7) linked by **peptide bonds** (Figure 3-8).

The sequence of the amino acids determines the ultimate structure and function of the protein and is determined by the genetic code stored in the cell nucleus as deoxyribonucleic acid (DNA). As illustrated in Figure 3-9 and in Chapter 5, protein synthesis is a complex process through which the protein pattern is copied from DNA to ribonucleic acid (RNA). The pattern for protein synthesis is carried to the rough endoplasmic reticulum via messenger RNA (mRNA). New proteins are built by attaching amino acids as dictated by the mRNA in a precise linear sequence. When the protein has been built, it detaches from the message and is ready to be used or further processed for use (see Chapter 5).

Proper folding of the completed linear amino acid chain is essential for a protein to perform its unique functions. The linear sequence of individual amino acids dictates the configuration of the mature protein. R groups protrude from the newly synthesized peptide chain and are in position to react with each other. Folding is accomplished through hydrogen bonding, ionic bonding, and hydrophobic and other interactions between individual R groups on each amino acid. For example, a negative charge on one amino acid R group forms an attraction with a positive charge on another, forming a precise, three-dimensional structure. Proteins have the following four levels of structure:

All amino acids have the same general structure $HOOC{-}C^{\alpha}H(NH_2){-}R$ in which R is different for each.

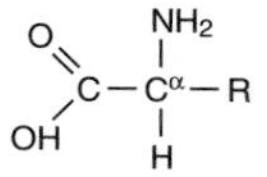

FUNCTIONAL TYPE	AMINO ACID (abbr.)	R GROUP	CHARACTERISTICS OF THE AMINO ACID
Aliphatic	Glycine (Gly) G	H	Tiny R group (H), which allows hairpin bends in the peptide chains
	Alanine (Ala) A	CH_3	Can be deaminated to pyruvate and used for glucose synthesis
	Valine (Val) V*	$-CH(CH_3)_2$	Branched-chain amino acids; metabolized in muscle
	Leucine (Leu) L*	$-CH_2-CH(CH_3)_2$	Branched-chain amino acids more hydophobic; muscle metabolism
	Isoleucine (Ile) I*	$-CH(CH_3)-CH_2-CH_3$	Branched-chain amino acids most hydophobic; muscle metabolism
Sulfur	Cysteine (Cys) C**	$-CH_2-SH$	Essential for glutatione synthesis; synthesis limited in chronic diseases
	Methionine (Met) M*	$-CH_2-CH_2-S-CH_2$	Converted to S-adenosylmethionine (SAM), the universal methyl donor, and cysteine
Hydroxyl	Serine (Ser) S	$-CH_2-OH$	Hydroxyl group phosphorylated to activate and inactivate protein
	Threonine (Thr) T*	$-CH_2-OH-CH_3$	Also site for regulatory phosphorylation
Aromatic	Phenylalanine (Phe) F*	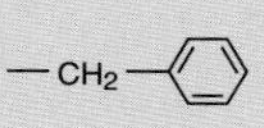 $-CH_2-$(phenyl ring)	Converted to tyrosine for synthesis of norepinephrine, epinephrine, and dopamine
	Tyrosine (Tyr) Y	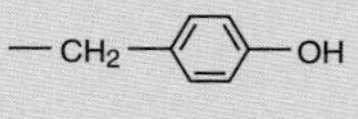 $-CH_2-$(phenyl ring)$-OH$	Converted to neurotransmitters norepinephrine, epinephrine, and dopamine
	Tryptophan (Trp) W*	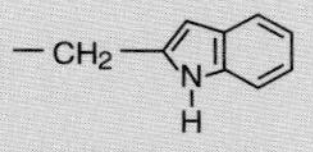 $-CH_2-$(indole ring, N–H)	Converted to neurotransmitter serotonin and to niacin
Cyclic	Proline (Pro) P	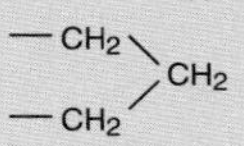 $-CH_2-CH_2-CH_2-$ (ring)	Allows triple helix; proline in collagen to be hydroxylated for cross-linkage
Basic	Lysine (Lys) K*	$-CH_2-CH_2-CH_2-CH_2-\overset{+}{N}H_3$	Site for hydroxylation in proteins; hydrophylic; used in signaling
	Histidine (His) H**	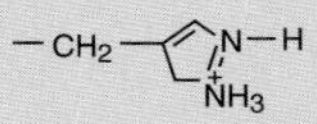 $-CH_2-$(imidazole ring, N–H, $\overset{+}{N}H_3$)	Hydrophilic, binds zinc in signaling proteins
	Arginine (Arg) R	$-CH_2-CH_2-CH_2-NH-C(=\overset{+}{N}H_2)-NH_2$	Formed in the urea cycle; essential for synthesis of nitric oxide signaling pathway
Acidic	Aspartic acid (Asp) D	$-CH_2-C(=O)O^-$	Takes a second nitrogen to form asparagine (Asn) N $-CH_2-C(=O)NH_2$
	Glutamic acid (Glu) E	$-CH_2-CH_2-C(=O)O^-$	Takes a second nitrogen to form glutamine (Gln) Q $-CH_2-CH_2-C(=O)NH_2$

FIGURE 3-7 Structures and functions of the 20 amino acids required by humans. All amino acids have the same general structure, but the R group is different for each. Amino acids are abbreviated using a three-letter and single-letter code. Amino acids marked with an asterisk (*) are essential; those marked with double asterisks (**) are essential for infants and those with certain chronic diseases.

1. *Primary structure:* Peptide bonds are formed between sequential amino acids according to directions on mRNA. The completed protein is a linear chain of amino acids.
2. *Secondary structure:* Attractions between R groups of amino acids create helices and pleated sheet structures.
3. *Tertiary structure:* Helices and pleated sheets are folded into compact domains. Small proteins have one domain, and large proteins have multiple domains.
4. *Quaternary structure:* Individual polypeptides can serve as subunits in the formation of larger

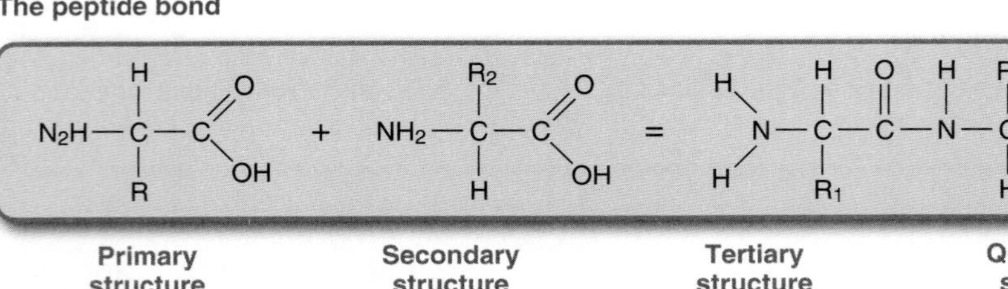

FIGURE 3-8 The peptide bond and protein folding.

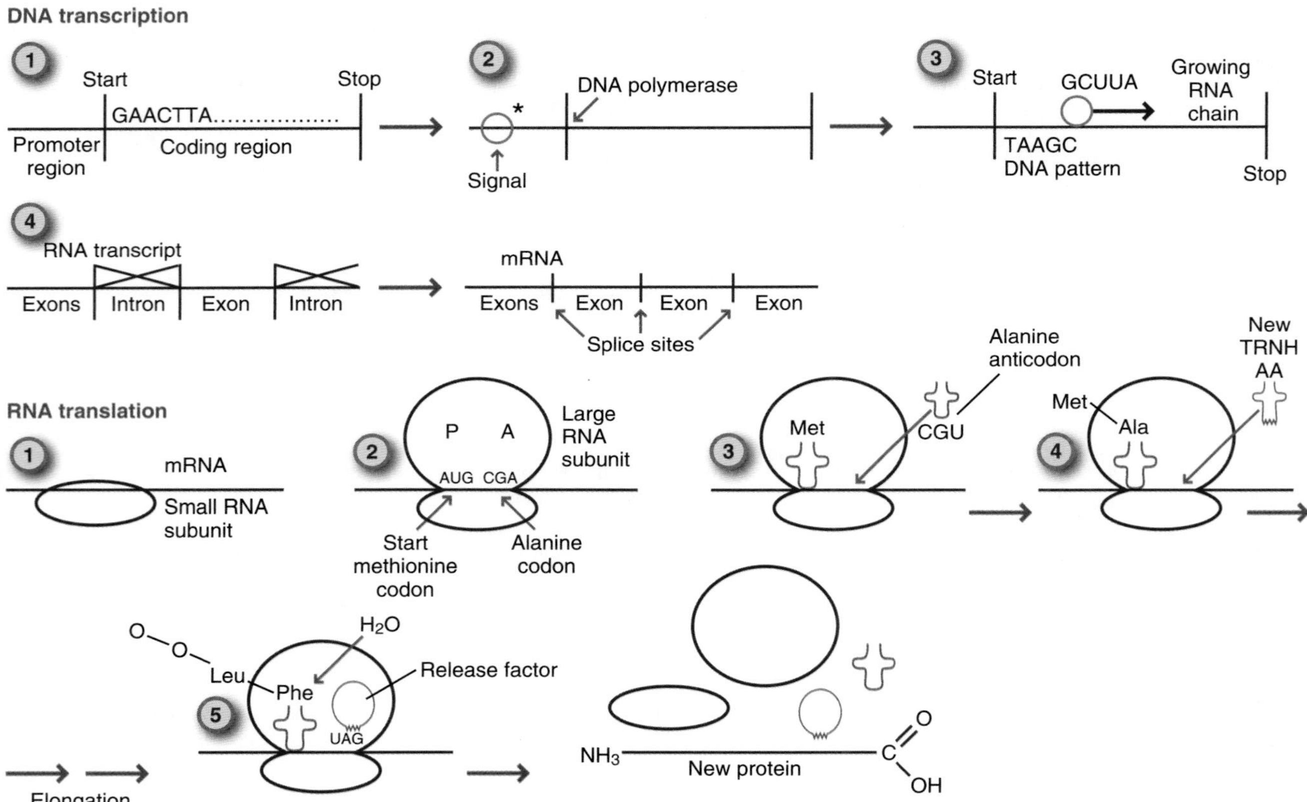

FIGURE 3-9 Summary of deoxyribonucleic acid transcription and ribonucleic acid translation in the eukaryotic cell.

assemblies, or complexes. Subunits are bound together by numerous weak, noncovalent interactions; sometimes they are stabilized by disulfide bonds. For example, four hemoglobin monomers are joined to form the tetramer hemoglobin molecule.

Protein structure is a critical component of protein function. The active and catalytic sites at which protein action occurs are formed by juxtaposing functional groups from nearby but occasionally distant R groups. If the linear protein sequence is altered, as in genetic diseases, the protein is unable to form active sites, and its activity may be reduced or eliminated entirely.

Essential Amino Acids

Synthesis of proteins requires the presence of all necessary amino acids during the process. Chemically, **amino acids** are carboxylic acids with an amino group attached to the α-carbon. All amino acids have this same general structure; the side chain is also attached to the α-carbon (the R group), which dictates the identity and function of each amino acid. Note that the α-carbon is a chiral carbon, and isomers can be formed. The L-isomer is functional in the human body. Many amino acids can be synthesized from carbon skeletons produced as intermediates in the major metabolic pathways by a process called **transamination**, which adds an amino group from another amino acid without actually producing a free amino group. Transamination is an important process because it allows for the production of **nonessential amino acids** from metabolic intermediates while using free amino groups, so that they are not left to produce toxic ammonia. For example, pyruvate formed during glycolysis is easily converted to the amino acid alanine by adding an amino group via the enzyme alanine aminotransaminase. On the other hand, **essential amino acids** have carbon skeletons that humans cannot synthesize in adequate amounts and therefore must obtain from the diet (Table 3-8). Protein can also be an energy source. Proteins contain 5 kcal/g; removal of the amino group and the formation and excretion of urea (**deamination**) has a metabolic cost of 1 kcal/g. Therefore the resulting carbon skeleton product can be used for energy at the rate of 4 kcal/g. These carbon skeletons can also be used to produce glucose. When the diet is low in carbohydrate or an individual is starving, protein is the only good source of de novo synthesis of glucose available; this process is called *gluconeogenesis.* Oxaloacetate is moved out of the mitochondria and converted to phosphoenolpyruvate (PEP) (see Figure 3-2). From PEP, the glycolytic pathway can be reversed because all the enzymes with the exception of phosphofructokinase and glucokinase are reversible. Both of these enzymes can be reversed by specific phosphatase enzyme when there is a need for blood glucose. Because glucokinase is found primarily in the liver, it is only reversed there, making the liver the primary site for gluconeogenesis. Amino acids that produce carbon skeletons that can be converted to glucose are called *glucogenic amino acids.* Only two of the 20 amino acids cannot be used to produce at least some glucose. These amino acids are lysine and threonine. They produce products that are converted to ketones and used for energy; thus they are known as *ketogenic amino acids.*

TABLE 3-8

Estimates of Amino Acid Requirements

Amino Acid	Requirements (mg/kg/day) by Age-Group: Infants, Age 3-4 mo*	Children, Age ~2 yr†	Children, Age 10-12 yr‡	Adults§
Histidine	28	Not determined	Not determined	8-12
Isoleucine	70	31	28	10
Leucine	161	73	44	14
Lysine	103	64	44	12
Methionine plus cystine	58	27	22	13
Phenylalanine plus tyrosine	125	69	22	14
Threonine	87	37	28	7
Tryptophan	17	12.5	3.3	3.5
Valine	93	38	25	10
Total without histidine	714	352	216	84

Modified from World Health Organization: Energy and protein requirements report of a joint FAO/WHO/UNU expert consultation, Technical Report Series 724, p 65, Geneva, 1985, WHO.

*Based on amounts of amino acids in human milk or cow's milk formulas fed at levels that supported good growth.

†Based on achievement of nitrogen balance sufficient to support adequate lean tissue gain (16 mg nitrogen/kg/day).

‡Based on upper range of requirement for positive nitrogen balance.

§Based on highest estimate of requirement to achieve nitrogen balance.

According to current recommendations, a healthy adult human requires 0.8 g of protein per kilogram of healthy body weight (IOM, Food and Nutrition Board, 2002). To obtain this quantity of protein, humans benefit when dietary protein makes up approximately 10% to 15% of total energy intake. Protein requirements increase during times of stress and disease. Protein-rich foods are obtained primarily from animal flesh or animal products such as eggs and milk. Most plant foods are relatively poor sources of protein, with the exception of legumes and beans.

Dietary Protein Quality

Because the synthesis of proteins for the body depends on the availability of all necessary amino acids, the quality of a dietary protein depends on its amino acid makeup and their bioavailability. A number of methods have been used to measure the quality of proteins based on these properties. More than 50 years ago, Block and Mitchel (1946) determined that a protein's biologic value could be determined by the essential amino acid profile compared with human requirements. The essential amino acid that occurred in the least concentration compared with human requirement was the **limiting amino acid**, from which a "chemical score" of protein quality could be calculated.

Protein quality is also determined by measuring the amount of protein actually used by an organism; *net protein utilization (NPU)* is the one method of doing so. Dietary protein is equated with its metabolic products by measuring nitrogen in the diet and biologic samples and converting it to the amount of protein on the basis of the formula (nitrogen [grams] × 6.25 = protein [grams]). The gain in nitrogen is compared with the nitrogen intake, and the proportion of nitrogen retained in the body is computed to obtain the NPU. The NPU ranges from approximately 40 to 94, with protein from animal products scoring higher and protein from vegetables scoring lower. However, care must be taken when using animals in trials for determining the quality of a protein for humans.

The World Health Organization (WHO) and the U.S. Food and Drug Administration (FDA) have adopted a **protein digestibility corrected amino acid score (PDCAAS)** as the official assay for evaluating protein quality in humans. The PDCAAS is based on amino acid requirements of children ages 2 to 5 years and represents the **amino acid score** after correcting for digestibility. After being corrected for digestibility, proteins that provide amino acids equal to or in excess of requirements receive a PDCAAS of 1. Gilani et al. (2008) have identified the need for more accurate, standardized methods that include bioactive peptides.

Digestibility is a major factor affecting protein quality and is affected by multiple factors. Meat preparation procedures often involve wine or vinegar marinades and moist heat to tenderize tough cuts of meat through **denaturation**. Proteins are kept in their functional three-dimensional structure by hydrogen and ionic interactions; these bonds loosen in the presence of acid, salt, and heat. Because they denature proteins, these methods also soften gristle, or connective tissue proteins, and release muscle proteins from their attachments, thereby making all proteins more available to digestive enzymes.

Vegetable protein is less efficient than animal protein; it is encased in carbohydrate and is less available to digestive enzymes. Some plants contain enzymes that interfere with protein digestion and require heat inactivation before consumption. For example, soybeans contain a trypsinase that inactivates trypsin, the major protein-digesting enzyme in the intestine. Although research suggests that plant protein may benefit blood pressure control, little has been published regarding protein sources in diets of U.S. adults and factors influencing these choices (Lin et al., 2010). Protein source frequencies in the lifestyle-changing PREMIER trial were poultry, dairy, refined grains and beef; animal protein was two thirds of intake, and one third was from plant protein, varying by sex, race, age, and body weight status (Lin et al., 2010).

Food processing can damage amino acids and reduce their digestive availability in several ways. Mild heat treatment in the presence of reducing milk sugars (glucose and galactose) during processing causes a loss of available lysine. Lactose reacts with lysine side chains and renders them unavailable. This *browning* (the *Maillard reaction)* causes significant lysine loss at high temperatures. Under severe heating conditions in the presence (or even absence) of sugars or oxidized lipids, all amino acids in food proteins become resistant to digestion. When protein is exposed to severe treatment with alkali, the amino acids lysine and cysteine can react together and form a potentially toxic lysinoalanine. Exposure to sulfur dioxide and other oxidative conditions can result in loss of methionine. Thermal processing and low-moisture storage of proteins can also result in reductive binding of vitamin B_6 to lysine residues, thereby inactivating the vitamin. Therefore proper handling of protein foods is necessary to maintain their integrity and usefulness.

As noted, if the amino acid profile of a food does not match human needs, those in short supply are "limiting." The quality of dietary protein can be improved by combining protein sources with different limiting amino acids. Diets based on a single plant food staple do not foster optimal growth because the diet does not have enough of the limiting amino acid to provide substrates for protein synthesis. If another plant protein that contains an excess of the limiting amino acid is added to the diet, the protein combination is *complemented;* essential amino acids are adequate to support human protein synthesis. The concept of complementary proteins is important for populations without animal protein intake or at risk from insufficiently diverse foods. Complementary foods that, when eaten together, provide all of the essential amino acids are shown in Table 3-9. It is not necessary to eat complementary amino acids during a single meal, but they should be eaten within the same day (American Dietetic Association, 2009). Children, pregnant women, and nursing mothers who have vegan diets need to plan their diets carefully to include a mixture of amino acid–containing foods.

Nitrogen Balance

Homeostatic regulations control the concentrations of specific amino acids in the amino acid pool and the rate at which muscle and plasma proteins are synthesized and broken down. Body protein synthesis and turnover are regulated. In healthy individuals the amount of protein taken in is balanced by protein used for body maintenance and excreted in feces, in urine, and from skin, resulting in a zero protein balance (Figure 3-10). This balance reflects homeostatic regulations within tissues.

TABLE 3-9

Food Combinations Providing All Essential Amino Acids

Excellent Combinations*	Examples
Grains and legumes	Rice and beans, pea soup and toast, lentil curry and rice
Grains and dairy	Pasta and cheese, rice pudding, cheese sandwich
Legumes and seeds	Garbanzo beans and sesame seeds; hummus as dip, falafel, or soup

*Other combinations, such as dairy and seeds, dairy and legumes, grains and seeds, are less effective because the chemical scores are similar and not effectively complementary.

For food lists containing high protein, see http://www.nal.usda.gov/fnic/foodcomp/Data/SR18/nutrlist/sr18w203.pdf

Muscle mass (*somatic protein*) is maintained with the circulating amino acid pool such that similar quantities of muscle protein are destroyed and rebuilt daily. Muscle mass can be estimated using the creatinine/height index and the midarm muscle circumference. Amino acids are also required for synthesis of *visceral proteins* by the liver and other tissues. A person with an infection or a traumatic injury excretes more nitrogen than is ingested; inflammatory cytokines cause nitrogen loss and negative nitrogen balance under these conditions. The pregnant woman and her growing child use ingested protein for growth and to retain more protein than is lost daily (positive nitrogen balance).

Nitrogen in the form of ammonia (NH_3) is highly toxic, easily crosses membranes, and cannot be allowed to travel unbound throughout the body. In the fed state, pyruvate and other carbon skeletons take up nitrogen (via transamination) and transport it to the liver as nonessential amino acids, usually alanine and glutamic acid (from α-ketoglutarate). When these amino acids reach the liver, they are deaminated or transaminated back into the carbon skeleton. A deaminated ammonia ion is combined with carbon dioxide in the presence of high-energy phosphate and magnesium by the enzyme *carbamoyl phosphate synthase* to form carbamoyl phosphate, the first intermediate of the urea cycle. A second amino group enters the urea cycle via aspartic acid. Thus with each urea molecule formed, two excess amino groups can be excreted. **Urea** makes up 90% of urinary nitrogen in the fed state. Arginine, one of the basic amino acids is also a product of the urea cycle. Arginine is required for formation of nitric oxide and other mediators of the inflammatory response (Gropper et al., 2005). Although classified as a *nonessential amino acid*, arginine may be essential for critically ill individuals.

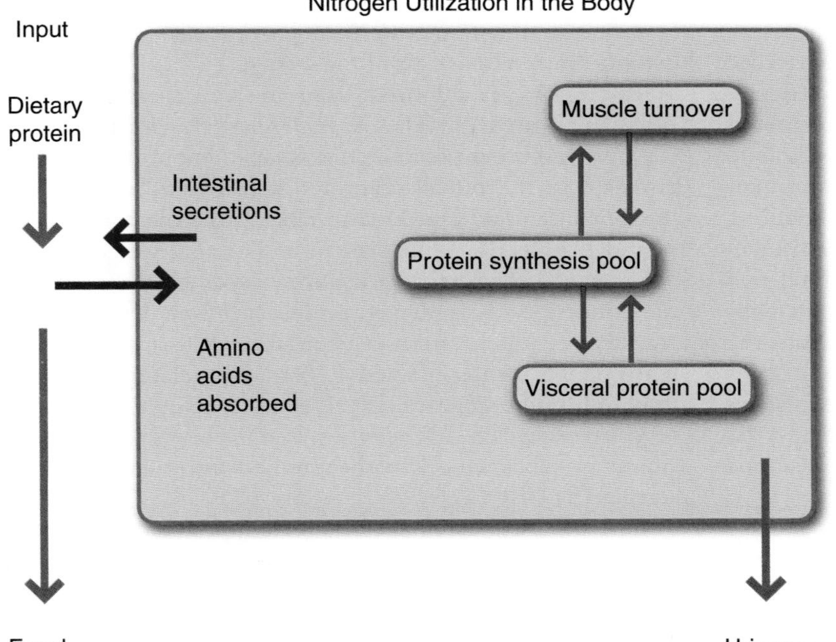

FIGURE 3-10 Nitrogen use in the body. Protein supplies nitrogen in the form of amino acids, according to the formula (nitrogen [grams] = protein [grams] ÷ 6.25). Dietary protein and protein from endogenous secretions are available for absorption across the gastrointestinal tract. More than 95% of protein is normally absorbed and enters the synthetic pool. Muscle proteins and visceral (i.e., plasma) proteins are broken down and built up daily. Nitrogen is converted to urea and excreted in the urine. Minor amounts of nitrogen are lost in the menstrual flow and the normal secretions and turnover of skin and its appendages. In a healthy individual, nitrogen intake equals nitrogen losses; the person is in zero protein balance. *(Modified from Crim MC, Munro HN: Proteins and amino acids. In Shils ME et al., editors: Modern nutrition in health and disease, Philadelphia, 1994, Lea & Febiger.)*

MACRONUTRIENT USE AND STORAGE IN THE FED STATE

Absorbed carbohydrates are transported as plasma glucose in the portal vein. An increase in the glucose level in the portal vein stimulates pre-formed insulin secretion from the pancreas. One of the most dramatic effects of insulin is its effects on the glucose transporters (GLUT 4) in insulin-dependent adipose and muscle. However, the liver is the first organ to receive portal blood glucose. The liver takes up approximately 50% of absorbed glucose via noninsulin-dependent transporters (GLUT 2) and immediately phosphorylates glucose into glucose-6-phosphate using the high-capacity enzyme glucokinase, thereby retaining glucose in the liver cells (see Figure 3-2).

Insulin enhances the oxidation of glucose in the glycolytic pathway by increasing the activity of glucokinase. *Pyruvate dehydrogenase* is also stimulated, increasing glycolysis and acetyl CoA production in both the liver and the muscle to generate adenosine triphosphate (ATP). In addition, insulin increases glycogen synthase activity in the liver and muscle, maximizing glucose storage as glycogen storage under fed conditions. Muscle glycogen is used within the muscle cell to provide ATP for muscle contraction. Its concentration in the muscle depends on the physical activity of the individual and can be greatly increased by physical training.

Liver glycogen serves as a reservoir, providing a readily available supply of glucose to maintain blood glucose levels during the fasting state. If carbohydrate intake exceeds the body's oxidative and storage capacities, the cells convert carbohydrate into fat. Elevated insulin levels increase the activity of fatty acid and triglyceride synthesis enzymes such as acetyl CoA carboxylase in the liver, lipoprotein lipase (LPL) in the adipose tissue, and fatty acid synthetase.

Because they are fat soluble, lipids cannot be transported unbound through the aqueous media of the body. Absorbed fatty acids and monoglycerides are reesterified into triglycerides within mucosal cells, and the fat-soluble center is surrounded with a thin layer of protein and phospholipid for transport. The protein component includes apoproteins (Apo) B, A, C, and E with specific functions. The resulting **chylomicrons** contain only 2% protein; the rest are triglycerides (84%), cholesterol, and phospholipids. The lipid-rich particles leave the mucosal cells and travel through lymphatic channels to the thoracic duct that empties into the right side of the heart. Rapid blood flow in the heart prevents the large, lipid-rich chylomicrons from forming clumps and fat emboli. Chylomicrons transport dietary fat and are found in blood only after meals, making the plasma appear milky after a high-fat meal.

Chylomicrons leave the heart through the aorta and are dispersed into the general circulation and transported to the adipocytes. The enzyme LPL is expressed on the membrane of endothelial cells lining capillaries in the region of the adipocytes. LPL is activated by lipoprotein-bound Apo C to bind chylomicrons and cleave triglycerides, releasing fatty acids and monoglycerides that cross the fatty lipid membrane, enter the adipocytes, and become reesterified into triglyceride for safe and hydrophobic storage. Note that insulin, the predominant hormone in the fed state, activates LPL and facilitates fat storage. The chylomicron remnant, relieved of some of its triglyceride content, is bound to liver receptors and recycled.

The liver receives fat from numerous sources: chylomicron remnants, circulating fatty acids, uptake of intermediate lipoproteins and other lipoproteins, and endogenous synthesis. The liver reesterifies fat from all sources and forms VLDLs, which are richer in cholesterol compared with chylomicrons but still contain a large proportion of triglycerides. VLDLs also contain Apos B, E, and C and adsorb Apo A as they circulate. In the fed state numerous VLDLs are formed and transported to the adipocytes, where triglycerides are again hydrolyzed, reesterified, and stored. Even in fasting, VLDLs are formed to carry endogenous lipids.

Dietary cholesterol is transported via chylomicrons and VLDLs but is not removed by LPL. After LPL has cleaved the maximum triglyceride from VLDLs, the remnant remaining is called an *intermediate-density lipoprotein.* Once the maximum triglyceride is removed, the lipoprotein is known as an *LDL* and primarily carries cholesterol. Although LDLs can be taken up by the liver on receptors for Apo B and Apo E, they are first taken up by specific LDL receptors that bind these cholesterol-rich particles. After uptake, endocytic vesicles containing LDL fuse with a lysosome. The digestive enzymes in the lysosome break down the protein and phospholipids, leaving free cholesterol. Free cholesterol regulates cholesterol synthesis and LDL uptake within the cell by inhibiting 3-hydroxy-3-methylglutaryl (HMG) CoA reductase, the rate-limiting enzyme for cholesterol synthesis from acetyl CoA. It downregulates cellular synthesis of the LDL receptor and reduces receptor expression on the membrane. Free cholesterol also increases the esterification of cholesterol for storage.

Cholesterol is removed from the cell membrane and other lipoproteins by HDLs. HDL particles are formed in the liver and other tissues as disk-shaped lipoproteins. They circulate in the bloodstream and accumulate free cholesterol, which they esterify with fatty acid from their phosphatidylcholine (lecithin) structure. The ability of HDLs to function as a cholesterol transporter depends on the activity of their copper-dependent enzyme lecithin-cholesterol acyltransferase, which esterifies cholesterol and stores it in its hydrophobic center. When it has accumulated sufficient lipid to become spherical, HDL is taken up by the liver and recycled. Recycled cholesterol is used for bile acid synthesis, stored in subcutaneous tissue, formed into vitamin D, or secreted as VLDL.

The LDLs that remain in circulation too long are susceptible to oxidative damage and macrophage scavenging. Macrophages are large cells that engulf other particles. They are distributed throughout the body, play a major role in immune defense, and inhabit the arteries, where they serve as a surveillance mechanism against foreign and microbial agents in the blood. Although macrophages do not recognize and ingest normal lipoproteins, they do recognize as foreign those lipoproteins that have undergone oxidation. Macrophages ingest oxidized LDLs and accumulate ingested fat within their cytoplasm, giving them a foamy appearance (thus the name *foam cells*). LDL ingestion activates macrophages and stimulates them to secrete mediators that trigger multiple inflammatory and proliferative cascades, some of which lead to atherosclerosis.

MACRONUTRIENT CATABOLISM IN THE FASTED STATE

The body has a remarkable ability to withstand food deprivation, allowing humans to survive cycles of feast and famine. Adaptive changes allow the body to access stored macronutrients to provide for routine activities.

Individuals with protein-energy malnutrition (PEM) or protein-calorie malnutrition (PCM) can have varying symptoms, determined by the cause of the malnutrition. Starvation of both protein and calories leads to *marasmus* at one end of the PEM continuum. At the opposite end is protein deprivation that occurs in individuals who are consuming carbohydrates almost entirely. *Kwashiorkor* is the Ghanaian word for the disease that develops when a mother's first child is weaned from protein-rich breast milk to a protein-poor carbohydrate food source. The condition is caused by severe protein deficiency and hypoalbuminemia. In adults, the correct term is *protein-energy malnutrition*, not the pediatric term, *kwashiorkor*. The starving adult has simply "malnutrition" described more fully in Chapter 14.

Glucose is an obligate nutrient for the brain and nervous system, red and white blood cells, and other glucose-requiring tissues. To maintain function, the blood glucose level must be maintained within a normal range at all times. During early fasting, glucose is obtained from glycogen by the action of the hormones glucagon and epinephrine; these stores are depleted in 18 to 24 hours. At this point, new glucose must be synthesized using protein as a substrate. The catabolic hormones epinephrine, thyroxine, and glucagon stimulate the release of muscle protein and other available substrates for gluconeogenesis. The most common amino acid substrate for gluconeogenesis is alanine; when its nitrogen is removed, alanine becomes pyruvate. Note that glycogen is never totally depleted, even during long-term starvation. A small amount of preformed glycogen is carefully guarded as a primer for glycogen resynthesis.

As fasting is prolonged and the body adapts to starvation conditions, liver gluconeogenesis decreases from producing 90% of the glucose to less than 50%, with the remainder being supplied by the kidney. Although the muscle and brain are unable to release free glucose, the muscle can release pyruvate and lactate for gluconeogenesis in the *Cori cycle*. Muscles also release glutamine and alanine. These amino acids can be deaminated or transaminated into α-ketoglutarate or pyruvate, respectively, and converted into oxaloacetate, then to glucose. During prolonged fasting the kidney requires ammonia to excrete acidic metabolic products. Muscle-derived glutamine is used for this purpose; deaminated glutamine (α-ketoglutarate) can then be used to produce glucose. Thus, during starvation, glucose production by the kidney increases while production by the liver decreases.

In addition to glucose, a reliable energy source is required during fasting. The best source is fat that is stored in adipocytes and used primarily by muscles, including the heart muscle, to make ATP. Fatty acid release and use require low insulin levels and an increase of the antiinsulin hormones glucagon, cortisone, epinephrine, and growth hormone. Antiinsulin hormones activate the hormone-sensitive lipase enzyme on the adipocyte membrane. This enzyme cleaves stored triglycerides, releasing fatty acids and glycerol from fat cells. Fatty acids travel to the liver bound to serum albumin and easily enter the liver cells. Once inside the cell, fatty acids enter the liver mitochondria via the carnitine acyltransferase transport system, which carries fatty acid **carnitine** esters across the mitochondrial membrane. Once inside the mitochondria, acetyl CoA is formed from fatty acid CoA via the process of β-oxidation. During starvation, excess acetyl CoA molecules accumulate in the liver because the liver is able to obtain all necessary energy from the process of β-oxidation and form ketones, which then enter the bloodstream and act as a source of energy for the muscles, thus sparing protein.

Adaptation to starvation depends on ketone production. As the blood ketone level rises during fasting, the brain and nervous system, although obligate glucose consumers, begin to use ketones as an energy source. Because the brain is using a fuel other than glucose, the demand on muscle protein for gluconeogenesis declines, thereby reducing the rate of muscle catabolism. Reduced muscle catabolism reduces the amount of ammonia received by the liver. Liver synthesis of urea decreases precipitously, reflecting the slower rate of muscle protein deamination. If the fast extends for weeks, the rate of urea synthesis and excretion is minimized. In an individual who has adapted to starvation, urea is excreted from the kidney at approximately the same rate as uric acid.

Thus, in an individual who is adapting to starvation, protein losses are minimized and lean body mass spared. Although fat cannot be converted into glucose, it does provide fuel for the muscle and brain as ketones. As long as water is available, a normal-weight individual can fast for a month. Relatively normal nutritional indices, immune function, and other system function are maintained. However, when fat stores are exhausted, protein is used, and death is the ultimate consequence.

In certain cases of trauma and sepsis, the individual is not able to adapt to fasting or starvation. If an individual who is fasting develops an infection, inflammatory mediators such as interleukin-1 and tumor necrosis factor stimulate insulin secretion and prevent the development of mild ketosis. Without ketones the brain and other tissues continue to depend on glucose, thereby limiting the person's ability to adapt to starvation. Muscle mass erodes to provide glucose substrates. A fasting person with an infection rapidly develops a negative nitrogen balance. When 50% of the protein stores is exhausted, recovery from infection is poor.

Adaptation to starvation is also not possible for those with protein malnutrition because the carbohydrate intake stimulates insulin production. Insulin is a storage hormone that prevents fat stores from being accessed for fuel. It also inhibits fat from being formed into ketones, thereby limiting adaptation to starvation. Insulin secretion inhibits muscle breakdown. Protein cannot be used to make albumin and other visceral proteins. Edema results because albumin exerts osmotic pressure in the vessels. If the albumin concentration is low, fluid remains in the extracellular spaces and causes edema. Compromised neural function or GI absorption, decreased cardiac output, immune function, fatigue, and other symptoms of malnutrition result from inadequate protein synthesis, inadequate ATP production, and fluid accumulation in the tissues.

Nonadapted malnutrition is dangerous. Not only can unremitting protein loss become life threatening by compromising the muscles of the heart and respiratory system, but it also compromises the immune system. The individual becomes susceptible to a vicious cycle of infections, diarrhea, additional nutrient loss, an even weaker immune system, and finally opportunistic infections and death. Iatrogenic, or "physician-induced," malnutrition was recognized long ago as a danger for hospitalized patients and remains so to this day (Kruizenga et al., 2005). Often lung failure occurs from weakened respiratory muscles. Pneumonia yields the mortal blow, yet malnutrition is the actual underlying cause.

MICRONUTRIENTS: VITAMINS

The discovery of vitamins gave birth to the field of nutrition. The term **vitamin** came to describe a group of essential micronutrients that generally satisfy the following criteria: (1) organic compounds (or class of compounds) distinct from fats, carbohydrates, and proteins; (2) natural components of foods, usually present in minute amounts; (3) not synthesized by the body in amounts adequate to meet normal physiologic needs; (4) essential in minute amounts for normal physiologic function (i.e., maintenance, growth, development, and reproduction); and (5) cause a specific deficiency syndrome by their absence or insufficiency.

The elucidation of these compounds was an exciting and convoluted story (see *Focus On:* Pellagra, Politics, and the Poor).

Vitamers are the multiple forms (all isomers and active analogs) of vitamins. Although the vitamins have few close chemical similarities, their metabolic functions have classically been described in one of four general categories: membrane stabilizers, hydrogen (H^+) and electron donors and

FOCUS ON

Pellagra, Politics, and the Poor

The history of niacin and pellagra is an example of the complicated search for the vitamins. Even though oranges and lemons were used as early as 1601 on the ships of the East India Company to prevent scurvy, the idea that a chemical in the diet could prevent certain diseases eluded the scientific and medical communities for hundreds of years. Pellagra was among these diseases. In 1915, 11,000 deaths from pellagra were reported in the southern United States. By 1917, more than 170,000 cases developed in the South. The situation was so grave that the Public Health Service sent Joseph Goldberger to investigate the deaths. He determined that a nutrient deficiency was the cause of the disease and that it could be cured by a diet containing high-quality protein. In fact, he showed that he could eliminate the disease simply by improving the diet. In 1918, Goldberger published these findings. Considering these facts, why in 1927 were 120,000 cases reported in the South? Between 1927 and 1930 27,103 deaths were recorded.

Why were there so many deaths from a disease that was entirely preventable? Several factors contributed to the situation. First, Pasteur's germ theory of disease was sweeping the scientific community. It was thought that scurvy, beriberi, and rickets were each caused by a microbe rather than by the lack of a nutrient. The antiberiberi actions of whole-grain rice were thought to be caused by a pharmacologic substance that acted against an unknown bacterium rather than a substance that served as a nutrient (thiamin). Even after Goldberger showed that pellagra was not contagious, doubts persisted. The problem was further complicated because (1) high-quality protein does not contain niacin—it contains the **tryptophan** precursor; and (2) the isolation of individual vitamins from the B-complex isolate took many years of painstaking laboratory research. Many more years passed before tryptophan was recognized as an important precursor of niacin.

More significant factors contributed to the numerous deaths from pellagra. The southern United States in the 1940s (with more than 2000 deaths per year) and early 1950s (with more than 500 deaths per year) were afflicted by economic and social factors. All who died from pellagra were poor and got poorer in the Great Depression of the late 1920s and 1930s. Pellagra primarily affected black Americans. In the South, people died from a lack of food, whereas in other parts of the country, farmers burned or threw away food because they could not sell the excess.

acceptors, hormones, and coenzymes. Their functions in human health are much broader and often include roles in gene expression. Subclinical or even less than optimum levels of some vitamins can contribute to disease states that are not normally associated with vitamin status. A number of vitamins and minerals have roles in prevention of the symptoms of deficiency diseases.

Subclinical deficiencies may have important effects on development of chronic disease. For example, folate and B_{12} are critical for both DNA synthesis and repair; low intake levels are common in the general population and in the elderly. Folate also has a role in maintaining the stability of DNA. Individuals who are homozygous for the gene that controls key folate-metabolizing enzymes have decreased risk of colorectal cancer. Similarly, riboflavin and niacin status affect cancer risk by playing an important role in response to DNA damage and genomic stability (Kirkland, 2003). More substantial evidence supports riboflavin's role in iron metabolism

Vitamin D is essential for healthy bones and is protective against bone diseases. Vitamin D also protects against certain types of cancers, multiple sclerosis, and type 1 diabetes (Grant and Holick, 2005). Vitamins A and D and calcium deficits predispose individuals to certain types of cancers, chronic inflammatory and autoimmune diseases, metabolic syndrome, and hypertension (Peterlik and Cross, 2005). Multiple nutrients have also been implicated in the development of osteoporosis (Nieves, 2005) and lung disease (Romieu, 2005). The widespread deficit of these nutrients in the American population is a major challenge for preventive medicine. As the roles of vitamins and minerals in preventing secondary disease become clear, recommended daily intakes may need to be revised for some populations. Currently, data cannot support the benefits of vitamin or mineral supplements to prevent cancer or chronic disease (Lin et al, 2009). An adequate dietary intake is essential, in conjunction with a variety of macronutrients and phytochemicals.

THE FAT-SOLUBLE VITAMINS

The fat-soluble vitamins are absorbed passively and must be transported with dietary lipid. They tend to be found in the lipid portions of the cell such as membranes and lipid droplets. Fat-soluble vitamins need fat for proper absorption and are generally excreted with the feces via enterohepatic circulation.

Vitamin A

Vitamin A (retinoids) refers to three pre-formed compounds that exhibit metabolic activity: the alcohol (retinol), the aldehyde (retinal or retinaldehyde), and the acid (retinoic acid) (Table 3-10). Stored retinol is often esterified to a fatty acid, usually retinyl-palmitate, which is usually found complexed with food proteins. The active forms of vitamin A exist only in animal products.

In addition to pre-formed vitamin A found in animal products, plants contain a group of compounds known as **carotenoids**, which can yield retinoids when metabolized in the body. Although several hundred carotenoids exist in foods naturally as antioxidants, only a few have significant vitamin A activity. The most important of these is β-carotene. The amount of vitamin A available from dietary carotenoids depends on how well they are absorbed and how efficiently they are converted to retinol. Absorption varies greatly (from 5% to 50%) and is affected by other dietary factors such as the digestibility of the proteins complexed with the carotenoids and the level and type of fat in the diet.

Absorption, Transport, and Storage

Before either vitamin A or its carotenoid provitamins can be absorbed, proteases in the stomach and small intestine must hydrolyze proteins that are usually complexed with these compounds. In addition, retinyl esters must be hydrolyzed in the small intestine by lipases to retinol and free fatty acids (Figure 3-11, *A*). Retinoids and carotenoids are incorporated into micelles along with other lipids for passive absorption into the mucosal cells of the small intestine. Once in the intestinal mucosal cells, retinol is bound to a cellular retinol-binding protein (CRBP) and reesterified, primarily by lecithin retinol acyl transferase into retinyl esters. Carotenoids and retinyl esters are then incorporated into chylomicrons for transport into the lymph and eventually the bloodstream. They may also be cleaved into retinal, which is then reduced to retinol and reesterified into retinyl esters to be incorporated into chylomicrons (Figure 3-11, *B*).

The liver plays an important role in vitamin A transport and storage (Figure 3-11, *C*). Chylomicron remnants deliver retinyl esters to the liver. These esters are immediately hydrolyzed into retinol and free fatty acids. **Retinol** in the liver has three major metabolic fates. First, retinol may be bound to CRBP, which controls free retinol concentrations that can be toxic in the cell. Second, retinol may be reesterfied to form retinyl palmitate for storage. Approximately 50% to 80% of the vitamin A in the body is stored in the liver. Adipose tissue, lungs, and kidneys also store retinyl esters in specialized cells called *stellate cells*. This storage capacity buffers the effects of highly variable patterns of vitamin A intake and is particularly important during periods of low intake when a person is at risk for developing a deficiency.

Finally, retinol may be bound to *retinol-binding protein (RBP)*. Retinol bound to RBP leaves the liver and enters the blood, where the *transthyretin (TTR)* protein attaches and forms a complex to transport retinol in the blood to the peripheral tissues. Because hepatic RBP synthesis depends on adequate protein, protein deficiency affects retinol levels along with vitamin A deficiency. Thus individuals with PCM typically have low circulating retinol levels that may not respond to vitamin A supplementation until protein deficiency is also corrected.

The retinol-RBP-TTR complex delivers retinol to other tissues via cell surface receptors. Retinol is transferred from RBP to CRBP with the subsequent release of Apo RBP into binding protein and TTR to the blood. Apo RBP is

TABLE 3-10

Vitamins, Vitamers, and Their Functions

Group	Vitamers	Provitamins	Physiologic Functions
Vitamin A	Retinol Retinal Retinoic acid	β-carotene Cryptoxanthin	Visual pigments; cell differentiation; gene regulation
Vitamin D	Cholecalciferol (D_3) Ergocalciferol (D_2)		Ca homeostasis; bone metabolism
Vitamin E	α-tocopherol γ-tocopherol Tocotrienols		Membrane antioxidant
Vitamin K	Phylloquinones (K_1) Menaquinones (K_2) Menadione (K_3)		Blood clotting; Ca metabolism
Vitamin C	Ascorbic acid Dehydroascorbic acid		Reductant in hydroxylations in biosynthesis of collagen and carnitine and in the metabolism of drugs and steroids
Vitamin B_1	Thiamin		Coenzyme for decarboxylations of 2-keto acids and transketolations
Vitamin B_2	Riboflavin		Coenzyme in redox reactions of fatty acids and the TCA cycle
Niacin	Nicotinic acid Nicotinamide		Coenzymes for several dehydrogenases
Vitamin B_6	Pyridoxol Pyridoxal Pyridoxamine		Coenzymes in amino acid metabolism
Folate	Folic acid Pteroylmonoglutamate Polyglutamyl folacins		Coenzymes in single-carbon metabolism
Biotin	Biotin		Coenzyme for carboxylations
Pantothenic acid	Pantothenic acid		Coenzyme in fatty acid metabolism
Vitamin B_{12}	Cobalamin		Coenzyme in metabolism of propionate, amino acids, and single carbon fragments

TCA, Tricarboxylic acid.

eventually metabolized and excreted by the kidney. In addition to CRBP, cellular retinoic acid–binding proteins (CRABPs) bind retinoic acid in the cell and serve to control retinoic acid concentrations similar to the way CRBP controls retinol concentrations.

Metabolism

In addition to being esterified for storage, the transport form of retinol can also be oxidized into retinal and then into retinoic acid or conjugated into retinyl glucuronide or phosphate. After retinoic acid is formed, it is converted to forms that are readily excreted. Chain-shortened and oxidized forms of vitamin A are excreted in the urine; intact forms are excreted in the bile and feces.

Functions

Vitamin A has essential but separate roles in vision and various systemic functions, including normal cell differentiation and cell surface function (e.g., cell recognition), growth and development, immune functions, and reproduction.

Retinal is a structural component of the visual pigments of the rod and cone cells of the retina and is essential to photoreception. The 11-*cis* isomer, 11-*cis*-retinal, constitutes the photosensitive group of various visual pigment proteins (i.e., the opsins—rhodopsin in the rods and iodopsin in the cones). Photoreception results from light-induced isomerization of 11-*cis*-retinal to the completely all-*trans* form. For example, in the rod, rhodopsin progresses through a series of reactions leading to the dissociation of "bleached" rhodopsin into all-*trans*-retinal and opsin, a reaction that is coupled to nervous stimulation of the visual centers of the brain. All-*trans*-retinal can then be converted back enzymatically to 11-*cis*-retinal for subsequent binding to opsin (Figure 3-12). The movement of retinal into designated sites in the retina is controlled by the proteins and interphotoreceptor retinal-binding protein, which serves a similar function.

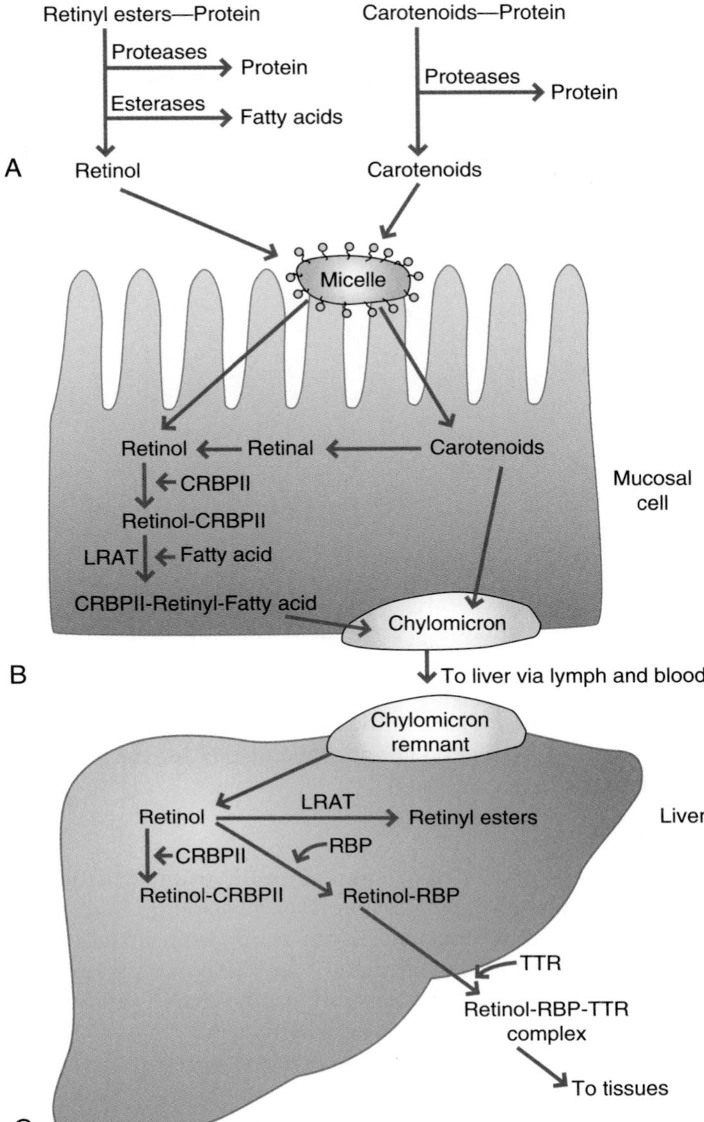

FIGURE 3-11 Retinol and carotenoids. **A,** Digestion. **B,** Absorption. **C,** Transport. *CRBPII,* Cellular retinol-binding protein II; *RBP,* retinol-binding protein; *TRR,* transthyretin.

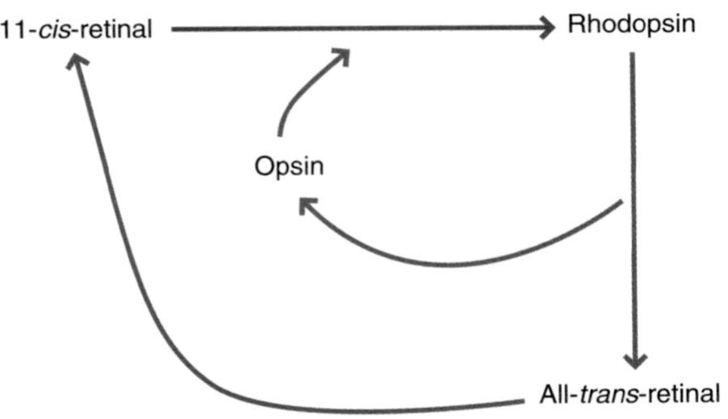

FIGURE 3-12 The visual cycle.

Although the systemic functions of vitamin A are not completely understood, they can be separated into two major categories. First, retinoic acid acts as a hormone to affect gene expression (see Chapter 5). Within the cell, CRABP transports retinoic acid to the nucleus. In the nucleus, retinoic acid and 9-*cis*-retinoic acid bind to retinoic acid receptors or retinoid receptors on the gene (Figure 3-13). Subsequent interactions allow stimulation or inhibition of transcription of specific genes, thus affecting protein synthesis and many body processes. Only a few of these processes are known, and they include morphogenesis in embryonic development and epithelial cell function (including differentiation and production of keratin proteins). The second major role of vitamin A in systemic functions involves glycoprotein synthesis. In a series of reactions, retinol forms retinyl-phosphomannose and then transfers the mannose to the glycoprotein. Glycoproteins are important for normal cell surface functions such as cell aggregation and cell recognition. This role in glycoprotein synthesis may also account for the importance of vitamin A in cell growth because it may increase glycoprotein synthesis for cell receptors that respond to growth factors. Vitamin A (retinol) is also essential for normal reproduction, bone development and function, and immune system function, although its actions in these roles are currently unclear.

Although a consistent body of epidemiologic evidence indicates that higher blood levels of carotenoids reduce the risk of several chronic diseases, the only clear function of the carotenoids is as provitamin A (IOM, Food and Nutrition Board, 2001). β-Carotene can act as an antioxidant. Its other properties include retinoid-dependent signaling, gap junction communications, regulation of cell growth, and induction of enzymes (Stahl et al., 2002).

Dietary Reference Intakes Measurement

The vitamin A content of foods is measured as **retinol activity equivalents (RAEs).** One RAE equals the activity of 1 mcg of retinol (1 mcg of retinol is equal to 3.33 International Units) (Box 3-3). The efficiency of β-carotene absorption is lower (14%) than previously believed (33%). In developed countries, 12 mcg of β-carotene is equal to 1 RAE, and 24 mcg of other carotenoids equal 1 RAE. The rate in developing countries is less efficient, requiring at least 21 molecules of β-carotene to get 1 molecule of vitamin A (Sommer, 2008).

Dietary reference intakes (DRIs) have been determined for vitamin A and are expressed in micrograms per day (mcg/day). The AI for infants is based on the amount of retinol in human milk. The DRIs for adults are based on levels that provide adequate blood levels and liver stores and are adjusted for differences in average body size. Increased amounts of the vitamin during pregnancy and lactation allow for fetal storage and the vitamin A in breast milk.

No DRIs have been established for the carotenoids. Indeed, while supplementation may be harmful, increased

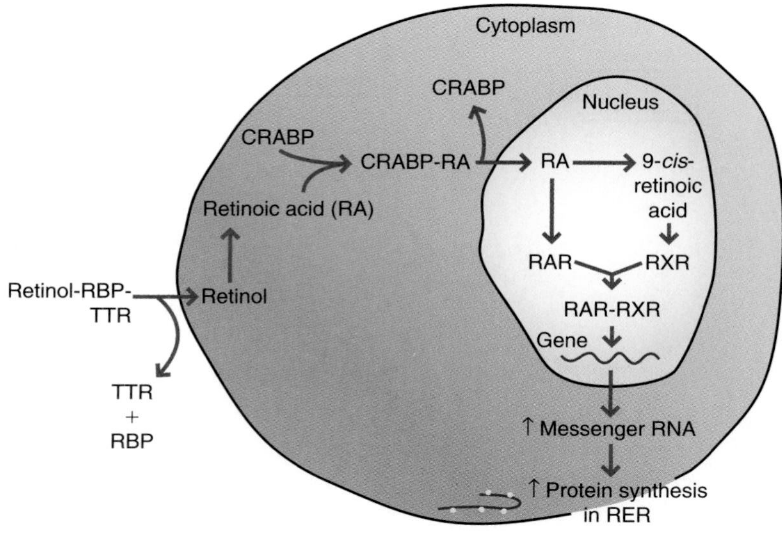

FIGURE 3-13 Role of vitamin A in gene expression. *CRABP*, Cellular retinoic acid-binding protein; *RAR*, retinoic acid receptor; *RBP*, retinol-binding protein; *RXR*, retinoid X receptor; *TTR*, transthyretin.

BOX 3-3

Vitamin A Activity

1 RAE =
  1 mcg of retinol
  12 mcg of β-carotene (from food)
  3.33 IU of vitamin A activity (on a label)*
For example: 5000 IU vitamin A (supplement or food label) =
  1500 RAE = 1500 mcg of retinol

Data from Institute of Medicine, Food and Nutrition Board: Dietary reference intakes for vitamin A, vitamin K, arsenic, boron, chromium, copper, iodine, iron, manganese, molybdenum, nickel, silicon, vanadium, and zinc, Washington, DC, 2001, National Academies Press.

RAE, Retinol activity equivalent.

*The vitamin A activity on a food or supplement label is stated in international units (IU), a term outdated scientifically but still required legally on labels.

consumption of fruits and vegetables containing carotenoids is clearly beneficial (IOM, Food and Nutrition Board, 2001).

Sources

Pre-formed vitamin A exists only in foods of animal origin, either in storage areas such as the liver or in the fat of milk and eggs. Very high concentrations of vitamin A are found in cod and halibut liver oils. Nonfat milk in the United States, which by U.S. law can contain 0.1% fat, is routinely fortified with retinol. Provitamin A carotenoids are found in dark green, leafy and yellow-orange vegetables and fruit; deeper colors are associated with higher carotenoid levels. In much of the world, carotenoids supply most of the dietary vitamin A. The American food supply provides roughly equal amounts of pre-formed vitamin A and provitamin A carotenoids. Carrots, greens, spinach, orange juice, sweet potatoes, and cantaloupe are rich sources of provitamin A. In many of these foods, vitamin A bioavailability is limited by binding of carotenoids to proteins; this can be overcome by cooking, which disrupts the protein association and frees the carotenoid. Table 3-11 and Appendix 47 list the vitamin A content of selected foods.

Deficiency

Primary deficiencies of vitamin A result from inadequate intakes of pre-formed vitamin A or provitamin A carotenoids. Secondary deficiencies can result from malabsorption caused by insufficient dietary fat, biliary or pancreatic insufficiency, impaired transport from abetalipoproteinemia, liver disease, PEM, or zinc deficiency.

An early sign of vitamin A deficiency is impaired vision from the loss of visual pigments. This manifests clinically as **night blindness**, or nyctalopia. This impairment of dark adaptation (the ability to adapt from being in a bright light or glare to being in darkness [e.g., while driving at night or moving from a brightly lighted to a dark room]), results from the failure of the retina to regenerate rhodopsin. Individuals with night blindness have poor visual discriminatory abilities and may not be able to see in dim light or at twilight. In addition to measuring plasma retinol levels, dark adaptation testing is one of the recommended methods for testing for vitamin A adequacy (IOM, Food and Nutrition Board, 2001).

Subsequent vitamin A deficiency leads to impaired embryonic development or spermatogenesis, spontaneous abortion, anemia, impaired immunocompetence (reduced numbers and mitogenic responsiveness of T lymphocytes), and fewer osteoclasts in bone. Vitamin A deficiency also leads to the keratinization of the mucous membranes that line the respiratory tract, alimentary canal, urinary tract, skin, and epithelium of the eye. Clinically these conditions manifest as poor growth, blindness caused by xerophthalmia, corneal ulceration, or occlusion of the optic foramina from periosteal overgrowth of the cranium. **Xerophthalmia**

TABLE 3-11

Vitamin A Content of Selected Foods

Food	RAE*
Turkey, 1 cup	15,534
Sweet potato, baked, 1 small	7,374
Carrots, raw, 1 cup	5,553
Spinach, cooked, 1 cup	6,882
Squash, butternut, 1 cup	2,406
Mixed vegetables, frozen, 1 cup	2,337
Apricots, canned, 1 cup	1,329
Cantaloupe, 1 cup	1,625
Broccoli, cooked, 1 cup	725
Brussel sprouts, 1 cup	430
Tomatoes, 1 cup	450
Peaches, canned, 1 cup	283

DRIs

Infants and young children, AI = 400-500 RAE/day, depending on age
Older children and adolescents, RDA = 600-900 RAE/day, depending on age
Adults, RDA = 700-900 RAE/day, depending on gender
Pregnant, RDA = 750-770 RAE/day, depending on age
Lactating, RDA = 1200-1300 RAE/day, depending on age

From U.S. Department of Agriculture, Agricultural Research Service: Nutrient Database for Standard Reference, Release 18, retrieved 2005, Data Laboratory home page, http://www.nal.usda.gov/fnic/foodcomp/Data/SR18/nutrlist/sr18w318.pdf

DRI, Dietary reference intake; *RAE,* retinol activity equivalents; *RDA,* recommended dietary allowance.

*1 RAE = 1 mcg of retinol; RAE from plant sources calculated based on 12 mcg β-carotene = 1 RAE.

involves atrophy of the periocular glands, hyperkeratosis of the conjunctiva, softening of the cornea (keratomalacia), and blindness. The condition is now rare in the United States (usually associated with malabsorption), but it is more common in developing countries. In fact, vitamin A deficiency is the most significant cause of blindness in the developing world, and an estimated 250 million children are at risk. Between 250,000 and 500,000 cases of blindness from vitamin A deficiency occur annually. Millions of preschool children have xerophthalmia, and two thirds of those newly diagnosed die within months of going blind because of enhanced susceptibility to infections.

Vitamin A deficiency produces characteristic changes in skin texture involving follicular hyperkeratosis (phrynoderma). Blockage of the hair follicles with plugs of keratin causes the distinctive "goose flesh" or "toad skin"; and the skin becomes dry, scaly, and rough. At first the forearms and thighs are affected, but in advanced stages the whole body is affected (Figure 3-14). Loss of mucous membrane integrity increases susceptibility to bacterial, viral, or parasitic infections. The deficiency also leads to impairments in cell-mediated immunity, ultimately increasing the risk for infection, particularly respiratory infections.

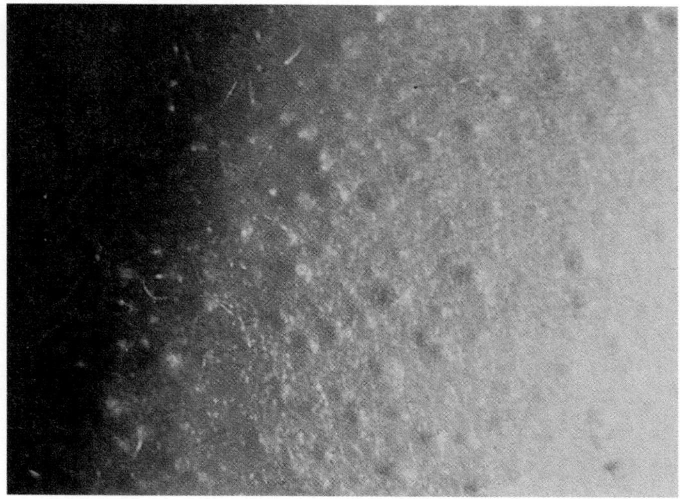

FIGURE 3-14 Follicular hyperkeratosis. Dry, bumpy skin associated with vitamin A or linoleic acid (essential fatty acid) deficiency. Linoleic acid deficiency may also result in eczematous skin, especially in infants. *(From Taylor KB, Anthony LE: Clinical nutrition, New York, 1983, McGraw-Hill.)*

Acute vitamin A deficiency is treated with large oral doses of vitamin A. When the deficiency is part of concomitant PEM, the malnutrition must be treated for the patient to benefit from vitamin A treatment. The signs and symptoms of deficiency respond to vitamin A supplementation in approximately the same order as they appear; night blindness responds very quickly, whereas the skin abnormalities may take several weeks to resolve. Massive, intermittent dosing with large doses of vitamin A has been used in developing countries. Treatments with single doses of 60,000 RAE of vitamin A have reduced child mortality by 35% to 70% (IOM, Food and Nutrition Board, 2001). However, Gogia and Sachdev (2009) recently concluded that that there is no reduction in risk of infant mortality associated with neonatal vitamin A supplementation.

Toxicity

Persistent large doses of vitamin A (>100 times the required amount) overcome the capacity of the liver to store the vitamin, produce intoxication, and eventually lead to liver disease. This intoxication is marked by high plasma levels of retinyl esters associated with lipoproteins. Hypervitaminosis A in humans is characterized by changes in the skin and mucous membranes (Box 3-4). Dry lips (cheilitis) are a common initial sign, followed by dryness of the nasal mucosa and eyes. More advanced signs include dryness, erythema, scaling and peeling of the skin, hair loss, and nail fragility. Headache, nausea, and vomiting have also been reported. Animals with hypervitaminosis A frequently have bone abnormalities involving overgrowth of periosteal bone. An increased incidence of hip fractures was found in women with high vitamin A intakes (Feskanich et al., 2002).

Acute hypervitaminosis A can be induced by single doses of retinol greater than 200 mg (200,000 RAEs) in adults or

BOX 3-4

Signs of Vitamin A Toxicity

Serum vitamin A of 75-2000 RAE/100 mL
Bone pain and fragility
Hydrocephalus and vomiting (infants and children)
Dry, fissured skin
Brittle nails
Hair loss (alopecia)
Gingivitis
Cheilosis
Anorexia
Irritability
Fatigue
Hepatomegaly and abnormal liver function
Ascites and portal hypertension

RAE, Retinol activity equivalent.

greater than 100 mg (100,000 RAEs) in children. Chronic hypervitaminosis A can result from chronic intakes (usually from misuse of supplements) greater than at least 10 times the AI (i.e., 4000 RAEs/day for an infant or 7000 RAEs/day for an adult). Dramatic stories in the literature describe reddening and exfoliation of the skin of Arctic explorers and fishermen who feasted on polar bear or halibut liver, both extremely high in vitamin A.

Retinoids can be toxic to embryos exposed in the womb. This is particularly true for 13-*cis*-retinoic acid (Accutane), a form very effective in treating severe cystic acne but that can cause craniofacial, central nervous system, cardiovascular, and thymic malformations in the fetus. Fetal malformations have also been linked to daily exposures of 6000 to 7500 RAEs of vitamin A from supplements, and pregnant women are advised against exceeding 3000 RAEs/day of vitamin A.

The toxicities of carotenoids are low, and daily intakes of as much as 30 mg of β-carotene have no side effects other than the accumulation of the carotenoid in the skin and consequent yellowing. However, high doses of β-carotene have been implicated as playing a role in some types of lung cancer, especially in smokers. **Hypercarotenodermia** differs from jaundice in that the former affects only the skin, leaving the sclera (white) of the eye clear. Hypercarotenodermia is reversible if excessive carotene intake is decreased.

Vitamin D (Calciferol)

Vitamin D is known as the "sunshine vitamin" because modest exposure to sunlight should be sufficient for most people to produce their own vitamin D using ultraviolet light and cholesterol in the skin. Because the vitamin can be produced in the body, has specific target tissues, and does not have to be supplied in the diet, it performs as a steroid hormone.

Brief and casual exposure of the face, arms, and hands to sunlight should be promoted. Ultraviolet light penetration depends on the amount of melanin in the skin, clothing type, blockage of effective rays by window glass, and use of sunscreens. Holick (2004) described sensible sun exposure as 5 to 10 minutes of exposure of the arms and legs or the hands, arms, and face, two or three times per week. This type of casual exposure seems to provide sufficient vitamin D to last through the winter months except in those unable or unwilling to go outside. For these individuals who get sun exposure in the summer and who live in the United States, the present level of fortification of foods with vitamin D has been thought to be adequate. However, 40% of all Americans may be vitamin-D deficient (Pietras et al., 2009).

Two sterols—one in the lipids of animals (7-dehydrocholesterol) and one in plants (ergosterol)—can serve as precursors of vitamin D. Each of these can undergo photolytic ring opening when exposed to ultraviolet irradiation. Ring opening of 7-dehydrocholesterol yields a provitamin form of 7-dehydrocholesterol, which yields **cholecalciferol**, or vitamin D_3 (Table 3-12). Ergosterol ring opening yields ergocalciferol, or vitamin D_2. Vitamin D_2 requires further metabolism to yield the metabolically active form of 1,25-dihydroxyvitamin D (1,25[OH]$_2$D$_3$; **calcitriol**), vitamin D_3 (Figure 3-15). In this form, vitamin D_3 plays an important role in the maintenance of calcium homeostasis and healthy bones and teeth, as well as influencing hundreds of genes.

Absorption, Transport, and Storage

Dietary vitamin D is incorporated with other lipids into micelles and absorbed with lipids into the intestine by passive diffusion. Inside the absorptive cells, the vitamin is incorporated into chylomicrons, and enters the lymphatic system and finally the plasma, where it is delivered to the liver by chylomicron remnants or to the specific carrier vitamin D–binding protein (DBP), or transcalciferin. The efficiency of this absorption process is approximately 50%. Vitamin D synthesized in the skin from cholesterol enters the capillary system and is transported by DBP and delivered to the peripheral tissues. Little vitamin D is stored in the liver.

Metabolism

Vitamin D must be activated by two sequential hydroxylations. The first occurs in the liver and yields 25-hydroxyvitamin D_3 (25-hydroxycholecalciferol), the predominant circulating form. The second hydroxylation is carried out by the enzyme α-1-hydroxylase in the kidney and yields 1,25(OH)$_2$D$_3$, the most active form. The activity of α-1-hydroxylase is increased by parathyroid hormone (PTH) in the presence of low plasma concentrations of calcium, yielding increased production of 1,25(OH)$_2$D$_3$ (calcitriol). The enzyme decreases when calcitriol levels increase (see Figure 3-15). In supplements and fortified foods, vitamin D is available as D-2 (ergocalciferol) and D-3 (cholecalciferol), yet controversy persists as to the overall effectiveness of D-2 supplementation and whether it can influence the serum level of D-3 (Stiff, 2009).

TABLE 3-12

Summary of Vitamins

	RDA for Adults	Sources	Stability	Comments
Fat-Soluble Vitamins				
Vitamin A (retinol; α-, β-, γ-carotene) 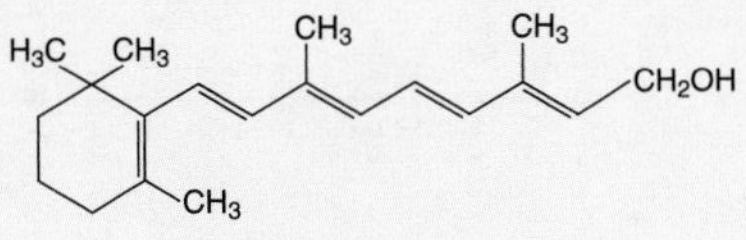 All-*trans*-retinal 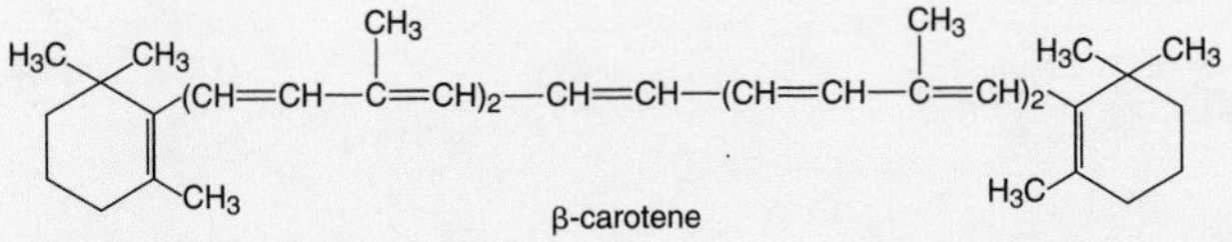 β-carotene	M: 900 RAE F: 700 RAE	Liver, kidney, milk fat, fortified margarine, egg yolk, yellow and dark-green leafy vegetables, apricots, cantaloupe, peaches	Stable in presence of light, heat, and usual cooking methods. Destroyed by oxidation, drying, very high temperature, ultraviolet light.	Essential for normal growth, development, and maintenance of epithelial tissue. Essential for the integrity of night vision. Helps promote normal bone development and influences normal tooth formation. Functions as antioxidant. Toxic in large quantities.
Vitamin D (calciferol) 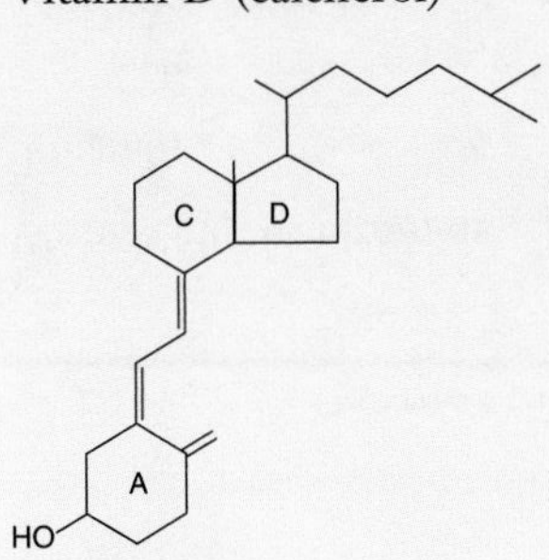 Vitamin D (cholecalciferol)	M & F 600 IU/day. Over age 70, 800 IU/day.	Vitamin D–fortified mild, irradiated foods, some in milk fat, liver, egg yolk, salmon, tuna fish, sardines Sunlight converts 7-dehydrocholesterol to cholecalciferol.	Stable in presence of heat and oxidation.	Is a prohormone. Essential for normal growth and development; important for formation and maintenance of normal bones and teeth. Influences absorption and metabolism of phosphorus and calcium. Toxic in large quantities.
Vitamin E (tocopherols and tocotrienols) 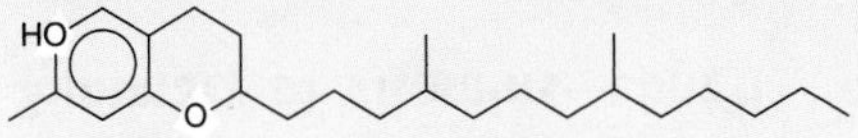 α-tocopheral	M: 15 α-TE F: 15 α-TE	Wheat germ, vegetable oils, green leafy vegetables, milk fat, egg yolk, nuts	Stable in presence of heat and acids. Destroyed by rancid fats, alkali, oxygen, lead, iron salts, and ultraviolet irradiation.	Is a strong antioxidant. May help prevent oxidation of unsaturated fatty acids and vitamin A in intestinal tract and body tissues. Protects red blood cells from hemolysis. Role in reproduction (in animals). Role in epithelial tissue maintenance and prostaglandin synthesis.

Continued

TABLE 3-12

Summary of Vitamins—cont'd

	RDA for Adults	Sources	Stability	Comments
Vitamin K (phylloquinone and menaquinone) 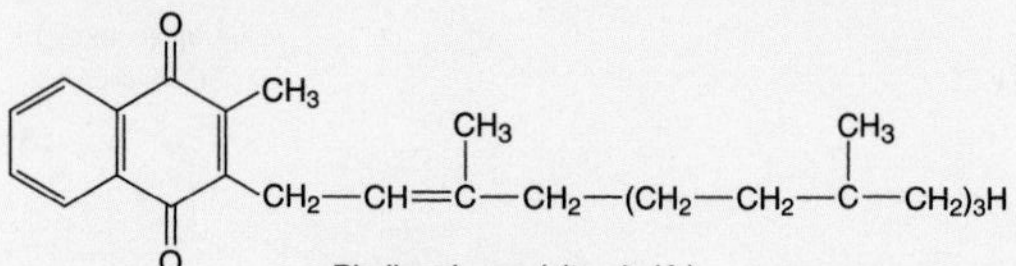 Phylloquinone (vitamin K_1)	M: 120 mcg F: 90 mcg AI	Liver, soybean oil, other vegetable oils, green leafy vegetables, wheat bran Synthesized by intestinal tract bacteria.	Resistant to heat, oxygen, and moisture. Destroyed by alkali and ultraviolet light.	Aids in production of prothrombin, a compound required for normal clotting of blood. Involved in bone metabolism. Toxic in large amounts.
Water-Soluble Vitamins				
Thiamin 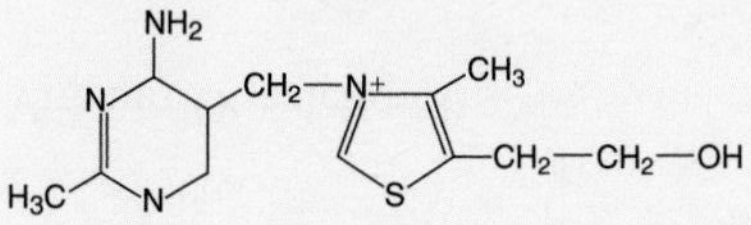 Thiamin	M: 1.2 mg F: 1.1 mg	Pork liver, organ meats, legumes, whole-grain and enriched cereals and breads, wheat germ, potatoes	Unstable in presence of heat, alkali, or oxygen. Heat stable in acid solution.	As part of cocarboxylase, aids in removal of CO_2 from α-keto acids during oxidation of carbohydrates. Essential for growth, normal appetite, digestion, and healthy nerves.
Riboflavin 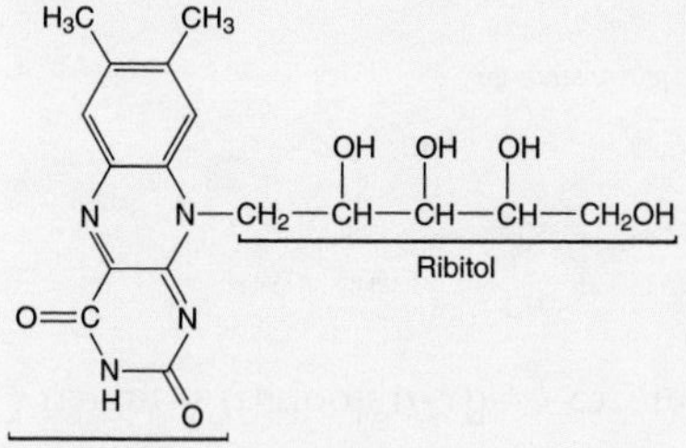 Ribitol Flavin	M: 1.3 mg F: 1.1 mg	Milk and dairy foods, organ meats, green leafy vegetables, enriched cereals and breads, eggs	Stable in presence of heat, oxygen, and acid. Unstable in presence of light (especially ultraviolet) or alkali.	Essential for growth. Plays enzymatic role in tissue respiration and acts as a transporter of hydrogen ions. Coenzyme forms FMN and FAD.
Niacin (nicotinic acid and nicotinamide) 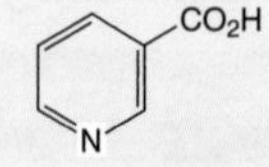 Nicotinic acid (niacin)	M: 16 mg NE F: 14 mg NE	Fish, liver, meat, poultry, many grains, eggs, peanuts, milk, legumes, enriched grains	Stable in presence of heat, light, oxidation, acid, and alkali.	As part of enzyme system, aids in transfer of hydrogen and acts in metabolism of carbohydrates and amino acids. Involved in glycolysis, fat synthesis, and tissue respiration.

Pantothenic acid 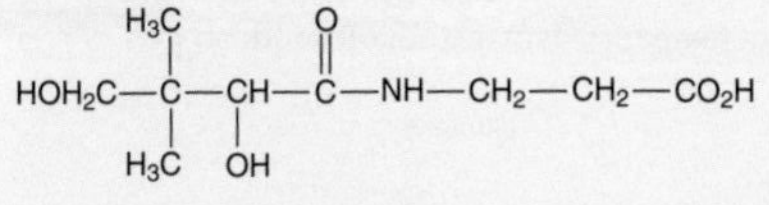 Pantothenic acid	5 mg AI	All plant and animal foods Eggs, kidney, liver, salmon, and yeast are best sources. Possibly synthesized by intestinal bacteria.	Unstable in presence of acid, alkali, heat, and certain salts.	As part of coenzyme A, functions in the synthesis and breakdown of many vital body compounds. Essential in the intermediary metabolism of carbohydrate, fat, and protein.
Vitamin B_6 (pyridoxine, pyridoxal, and pyridoxamine) 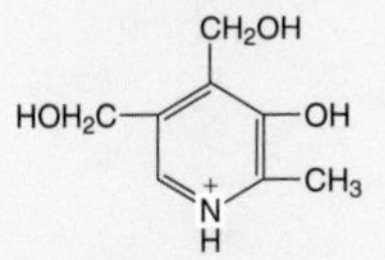 Pyridoxine (PN)	M: 1.3-1.7 mg F: 1.3-1.5 mg	Pork, glandular meats, cereal bran and germ, milk, egg yolk, oatmeal, legumes	Stable in presence of heat, light, and oxidation.	As a coenzyme, aids in the synthesis and breakdown of amino acids and of unsaturated fatty acids from essential fatty acids. Essential for conversion of tryptophan to niacin. Essential for normal growth.
Folate (folic acid, folacins) 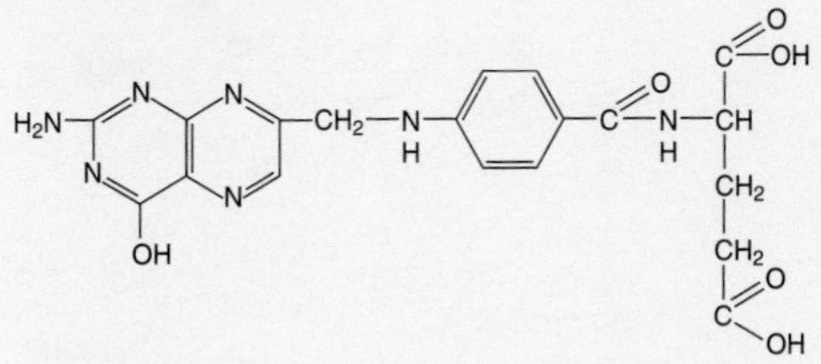 Folate	400 mcg	Green leafy vegetables, organ meats (liver), lean beef, wheat, eggs, fish, dry beans, lentils, cowpeas, asparagus, broccoli, collards, yeast	Stable in presence of sunlight when in solution. Unstable in presence of heat in acid media.	Essential for biosynthesis of nucleic acids—especially important in early fetal development. Essential for normal maturation of red blood cells. Functions as a coenzyme—tetrahydrofolic acid.
Biotin 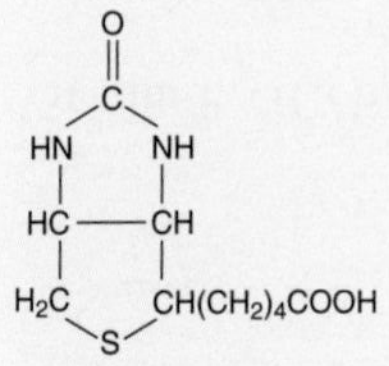 Biotin	30 mcg AI	Liver, mushrooms, peanuts, yeast, milk, meat, egg yolk, most vegetables, banana, grapefruit, tomato, watermelon, strawberries Synthesized by intestinal bacteria.	Stable under most conditions.	Essential component of enzymes. Involved in synthesis and breakdown of fatty acids and amino acids through aiding the addition and removal of CO_2 to or from active compounds and the removal of NH_2 from amino acids.

Continued

TABLE 3-12

Summary of Vitamins—cont'd

	RDA for Adults	Sources	Stability	Comments
Vitamin C (ascorbic acid) 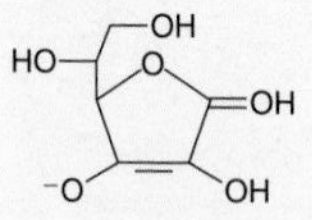 Ascorbate	M: 90 mg F: 75 mg	Acerola (West Indian cherry-like fruit), citrus fruit, tomato, melon, peppers, greens, raw cabbage, guava, strawberries, pineapple, potato, kiwi	Unstable in presence of heat, alkali, and oxidation, except in acids. Destroyed by storage.	Maintains intracellular cement substance with preservation of capillary integrity. Cosubstrate in hydroxylations requiring molecular oxygen. Important in immune responses, wound healing, and allergic reactions. Increases absorption of nonheme iron.
Vitamin B_{12} (Cobalamin) 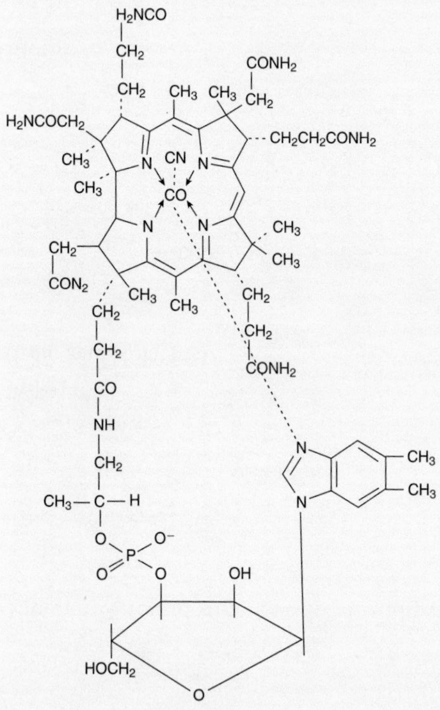 Cobalamin	2.4 mcg	Liver, kidney, milk and dairy foods, meat, eggs Vegans require supplement.	Slowly destroyed by acid, alkali, light, and oxidation.	Involved in the metabolism of single-carbon fragments. Essential for biosynthesis of nucleic acids and nucleoproteins. Role in metabolism of nervous tissue. Involved with folate metabolism. Related to growth.

α-TE, α-Tocopherol equivalents; *AI*, adequate intake; *F*, female; *FAD*, flavin adenine dinucleotide; *FMN*, flavin adenine mononucleotide; *M*, male; *NE*, niacin equivalents; *RAE*, retinol activity equivalents; *RDA*, recommended dietary allowance.

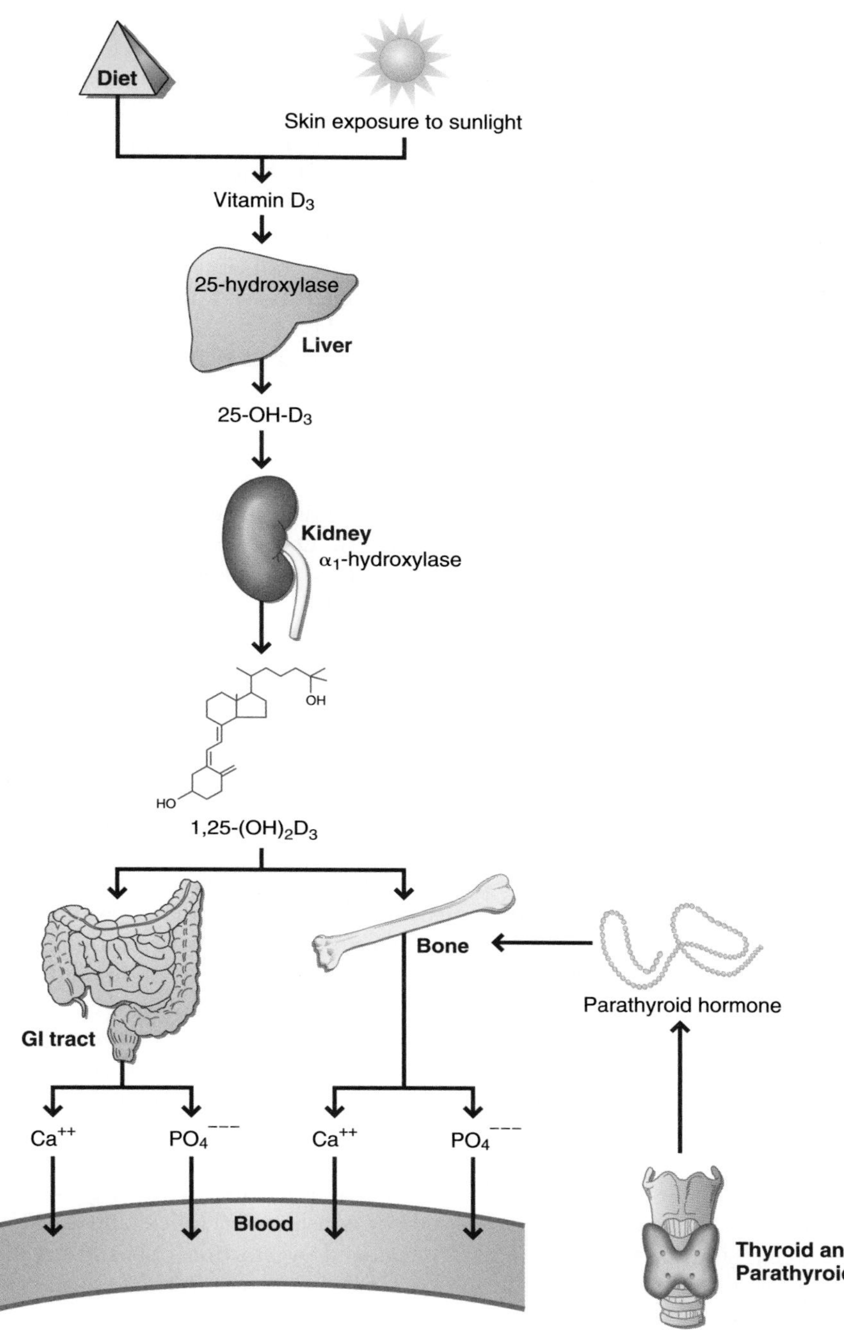

FIGURE 3-15 Metabolism and function of vitamin D. Vitamin D_3 (cholecalciferol) changes into its biologically active forms: 25-(OH)D_3 and 1,25-(OH)2 D_3(calcitriol). Calcitriol increases calcium and phosphate absorption in the intestine, increases calcium and phosphate resorption in bone, and acts on the kidney to decrease calcium loss in urine.

Functions

Calcitriol (1,25[OH]$_2$D$_3$) functions primarily like a steroid hormone. Its major actions involve interaction with cell membrane receptors and nuclear vitamin D receptor (VDR) proteins to affect gene transcription in a wide variety of tissues. When calcitriol binds to VDR proteins in the nucleus, the affinity of the VDR proteins for specific promoter regions of the genes—vitamin D response elements (VDRE)—increases, allowing the VDR-calcitriol complex to bind to the VDRE. Once the VDR-calcitriol complex is attached to the VDRE region, transcription for specific mRNAs for specific proteins is either promoted or inhibited (Figure 3-16).

More than 50 genes are known to be regulated by vitamin D (Omdahl et al., 2002). Although most of the genes regulated by vitamin D are unrelated to mineral metabolism, this is its most widely recognized function. Vitamin D maintains calcium and phosphorus homeostasis in three major ways. First, through gene expression, calcitriol in the small intestine enhances the active transport of calcium across the gut, which stimulates synthesis of calcium-binding proteins (including calbindin) in the mucosal brush border. These

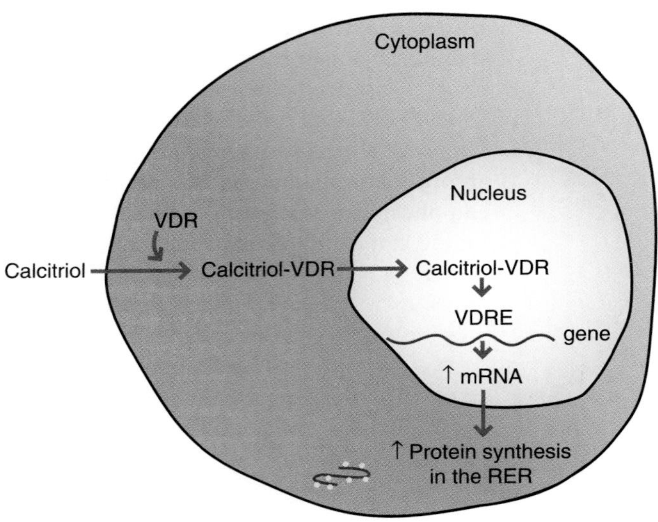

FIGURE 3-16 Role of vitamin D in gene expression. *RER*, Rough endoplasmic reticulum; *VDR*, vitamin D receptor protein; *VDRE*, vitamin D response elements.

proteins then increase calcium absorption. Phosphate absorption is also increased by enhancing acid phosphatase activity, which cleaves phosphate esters and allows increased phosphorus absorption. Second, PTH, along with calcitriol or estrogen, moves calcium and phosphorus from the bone to maintain normal blood levels. The process most probably involves increased osteoclast activity, increased numbers of new osteoclasts through cell differentiation, or both. Third, in the kidney, calcitriol increases renal tubular reabsorption of calcium and phosphate. These activities are coordinated to maintain plasma calcium concentrations within a narrow range. Calcitonin is secreted by the thyroid to counter the activity of calcitriol and PTH; it suppresses bone mobilization and increases the renal excretion of calcium and phosphate.

Calcitriol plays important roles in cell differentiation, proliferation, and growth in the skin, muscles, pancreas, nerves, parathyroid gland, and immune system. It influences the onset of conditions as diverse as multiple sclerosis (Simon et al., 2010), cardiovascular disease (Artaza et al., 2009), proteinuria, and diabetic nephropathy (Agarwal, 2009). Vitamin D has paracrine functions through local activation by 1-alpha-hydroxylase and thus maintains immunity, vascular function, and cardiomyocyte health; it reduces inflammation and insulin resistance (Agarwal, 2009). Randomized, controlled trials are needed to determine whether vitamin D supplements during pregnancy and early in life might protect against these disorders.

Dietary Reference Intakes

The preferred units for quantification of vitamin D are micrograms (mcg) of vitamin D_3. Both vitamins D_2 and D_3 are used to quantify total vitamin D. International Units (IU) are still used on some labels. Vitamin D_3 in 1 IU equals 0.025 mcg of vitamin D_3, and 1 mcg of vitamin D_3 equals 40 IU of vitamin D_3.

The DRIs for vitamin D are a mix of RDA and AIs, set to meet the body's needs when a person has inadequate exposure to sunlight. The tolerable upper intake levels (ULs) are set at those considered to pose no risk of adverse effects. Although 2.5 mcg (100 IU) of vitamin D daily is sufficient to prevent vitamin D–deficiency rickets, higher levels are recommended (AI = 400 IU/day for infants; RDA = 600 IU/day for children) during skeletal development. Adults require continual bone remodeling and adequate calcium and phosphorus homeostasis. The RDA for adults 71 years and older is 800 IU/day.

The UL for vitamin D for infants is 1000-1500 IU/day, 2500-3000 IU/day for children, and 2000-2500 IU/day for adults.

The normal adult is presumed to obtain sufficient vitamin D from exposure to sunlight and incidental ingestion through small amounts in foods. However, increasing evidence suggests that vitamin D status is low (Parks and Johnson, 2005; Pettifor, 2005) and increasing vitamin D intake has been recommended. However, recently the IOM, Food and Nutrition Board (2010) reported that vitamin D deficiencies were likely overestimated and set the RDA for normal individuals at 600 IU.

Pietras et al. (2009) and Holick and Chen (2008) have recommended that the AI for vitamin D be increased (800-1000 IU) in normal individuals and much higher for treatment of individuals with bone disease and a vitamin D deficiency. Supplemental vitamin D is especially appropriate for individuals consistently shielded from sunlight, such as those who are housebound, live in northern latitudes or areas with high atmospheric pollution, wear clothing that completely covers the body, or work at night and stay indoors during the day.

Milk continues to be a food of choice for vitamin D fortification because of its calcium content. Soy milks and other nondairy milks are now often fortified with the same amount of vitamin D and calcium found in cow's milk. However, milk and infant formulas may not always contain the amount stated on the label; fortification of other foods such as pasta and orange juice should be considered (Holick, 2006; 2007). Caution is necessary to avoid overfortification and underfortification; a unified fortification monitoring program is needed (Calvo et al., 2004).

Sources

Vitamin D_3 exists naturally in animal products, and the richest sources are fish liver oils. It is found in only small and highly variable amounts in butter, cream, egg yolk, and liver. Human milk and unfortified cow's milk tend to be poor sources of vitamin D_3, providing only 0.4 to 1 mcg/L. However, approximately 98% of all fluid milk sold in the United States is fortified with vitamin D_2 (usually 10 mcg [400 IU]/qt), as is most dried whole milk, evaporated milk, some margarines, butters, soy milks, certain cereals, and all infant formula products. Vitamin D is very stable and does not deteriorate when foods are heated or stored for long periods (Table 3-13; see also Appendix 51).

TABLE 3-13

Vitamin D Content of Selected Foods

Food	IUs per serving IUs = International Units
Cod liver oil, 1 tablespoon	1360
Salmon (sockeye), cooked, 3 ounces	794
Mackerel, cooked, 3 ounces	388
Tuna fish, canned in water, drained, 3 ounces	154
Milk, nonfat, reduced fat, and whole, vitamin D-fortified, 1 cup	115-124
Orange juice fortified with vitamin D, 1 cup (check product labels, as amount of added vitamin D varies)	100
Yogurt, fortified with 20% of the DV for vitamin D, 6 ounces (more heavily fortified yogurts provide more of the DV)	80
Margarine, fortified, 1 tablespoon	60
Sardines, canned in oil, drained, 2 sardines	46
Liver, beef, cooked, 3.5 ounces	46
Ready-to-eat cereal, fortified with 10% of the DV for vitamin D, 0.75-1 cup (more heavily fortified cereals might provide more of the DV)	40
Egg, 1 whole (vitamin D is found in yolk)	25
Cheese, Swiss, 1 ounce	6
DRIs*	
Infants	10 mcg (400 IU)
Children and adolescents	15 mcg (600 IU)
Adults	15 mcg (600 IU)
Adults > age 70	20 mcg (800 IU)
Pregnant	15 mcg (600 IU)
Lactating	15 mcg (600 IU)

From

(1) Institute of Medicine, Food and Nutrition Board. Dietary Reference Intakes for Calcium and Vitamin D. Washington, DC: National Academy Press, 2010. Accessed 1-14-11.

(2) USDA. http://www.ars.usda.gov/SP2UserFiles/Place/12354500/Data/SR22/nutrlist/sr22w324.pdf; Accessed 1-14-11.

DRI, Dietary reference intake.

*Recalculated in micrograms of D_3: IU = 0.025 mcg; 1mcg = 40 IU.

Deficiency

Vitamin D deficiency manifests as rickets in children and as osteomalacia in adults. Vitamin D deficiency can also precipitate and exacerbate osteoporosis and fractures in adults and is associated with increased risk of common cancers, autoimmune diseases, hypertension, and infectious diseases (Holick and Chen, 2008). Inadequate vitamin D intake is prevalent around the world, regardless of age or health status (Pietras et al., 2009). A level of 30 ng/mL is considered the minimum level for sufficient serum 25-hydroxy vitamin D (Holick, 2007).

Rickets. **Rickets** is a disease involving impaired mineralization of growing bones. It is the result not only of deprivation of vitamin D, but of deficiencies of calcium and phosphorus. Rickets is characterized by structural abnormalities of the weight-bearing bones (e.g., tibia, ribs, humerus, radius, ulna) as in Figure 3-17. Bone pain, muscular tenderness, hypocalcemic tetany, and soft, pliable, rachitic bones occur. This results in bowed legs, "knock knees," beaded ribs (the rachitic rosary), pigeon breast, and frontal bossing of the skull. Radiography reveals enlarged epiphyseal growth plates manifested as enlarged wrists and ankles resulting from their failure to mineralize and continue growth. Increased plasma and serum levels of alkaline phosphatase occur when released by the affected osteoblasts.

Historically, rickets has afflicted poor children in industrialized cities where exposure to sunlight is limited. In North America the vitamin D supplementation of foods virtually eliminated the disease. However, the incidence of vitamin D–dependent rickets is increasing again. The children most at risk have dark skin and are breastfed for long periods without exposure to sunlight or vitamin D supplements (Holick, 2006). Rickets can also develop in children with chronic problems of lipid malabsorption and in those undergoing long-term anticonvulsant therapy (which reduces the circulating levels of $1,25[OH]_2D_3$).

Rickets caused strictly by vitamin D deprivation can be treated effectively with oral preparations of the vitamin or natural sources rich in the vitamin. Vitamin D concentrates of fish-liver oil may be prescribed; 1 teaspoon (4 mL) of cod-liver oil contains 9 mcg (360 IU) of vitamin D. For those with calcium deficiency–related or hypophosphatemic vitamin D–refractory rickets, vitamin D treatment alone may not be effective, and active vitamin D metabolites such as $25\text{-}(OH)D_3$ or $1,25(OH)2D_3$, or a synthetic analog become necessary.

Osteomalacia. Osteomalacia develops in adults whose epiphyseal closures make that portion of the bone resistant to vitamin D deficiency. Therefore the disease involves generalized reductions in bone density and the presence of pseudofractures, especially of the spine, femur, and humerus. Patients experience muscular weakness with associated increase in fall risk as well as bone pain and have a greater risk of fractures, particularly of the wrist and pelvis. These nonspecific symptoms can lead to misdiagnosis of osteomalacia as fibromyalgia, chronic fatigue syndrome, or depression (Holick, 2007).

Prevention of osteomalacia is usually possible with an adequate consumption of vitamin D, calcium, and phosphorus in the diet. It has been estimated that as little as 10 to 15 minutes of sun exposure on a clear summer day two or three times a week is sufficient to prevent osteomalacia among most older adults. Osteomalacia can be treated effectively with vitamin D_3 in doses of 25 to 125 mcg (1000 to

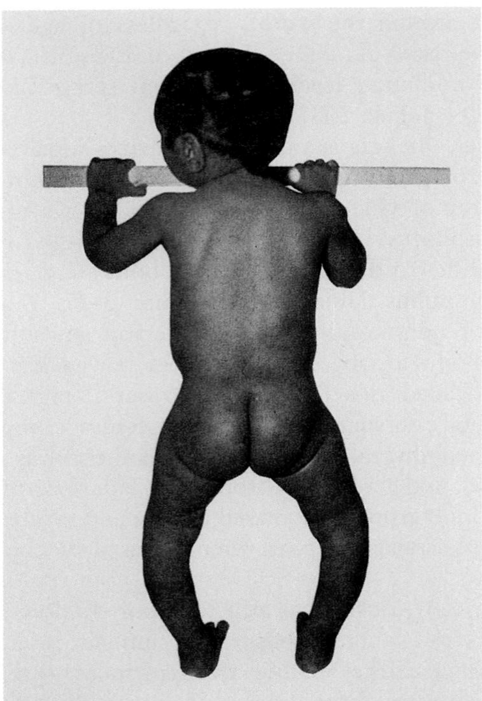

FIGURE 3-17 Severely bowed legs caused by rickets, an indication of vitamin D and calcium deficiencies in children. Rickets is a disorder of cartilage cell growth and enlargement of epiphyseal growth plates. *(From Latham MC et al: Scope manual on nutrition, Kalamazoo, Mich., 1980, The Upjohn Company.)*

1250 IU/day); in those whose conditions are complicated by lipid malabsorption, daily doses as large as 1250 mcg (12,500 IU) have been used.

Osteoporosis. Osteoporosis differs from osteomalacia; it involves diminished bone mass but with retention of a normal histologic appearance. Osteoporosis is a multifactorial disease involving impaired vitamin D metabolism and function, often associated with low or decreasing estrogen levels. It is the most common bone disease of postmenopausal women, but it also develops in older men. Chronic use of the active form $1,25(OH)_2D_3$ by women can delay of the onset and show some reversal of the signs and symptoms of osteoporosis.

Toxicity

Excessive intake of vitamin D can produce intoxication characterized by elevated serum calcium (hypercalcemia) and phosphorus (hyperphosphatemia) levels and ultimately the calcification of soft tissues (calcinosis), including the kidney, lungs, heart, and even the tympanic membrane of the ear, which can result in deafness. Patients often complain of headache and nausea (Box 3-5). Infants given excessive amounts of vitamin D may have GI upset, bone fragility, and retarded growth.

Hypervitaminosis D is progressive; individuals seem to vary in their susceptibility to the condition. The UL for vitamin D is 1000 IU)/day for infants up to age 6 months; 1500 IU/day for infants 6 to 12 months; 2500 IU/day for ages 1-3 years; 3000 IU/day for children aged 4-8 years. Infants and small children are most susceptible to hypervitaminosis D. In children aged 9 through all older age groups, the IU is 4000 IU/day.

BOX 3-5

Signs of Vitamin D Toxicity

- Excessive calcification of bone
- Kidney stones
- Metastatic calcification of soft tissues (kidney, heart, lung, and tympanic membrane)
- Hypercalcemia
- Headache
- Weakness
- Nausea and vomiting
- Constipation
- Polyuria
- Polydipsia

Vitamin E

Vitamin E has a fundamental role in protecting the body against the damaging effects of reactive oxygen species that are formed metabolically or encountered in the environment. Vitamin E includes two classes of biologically active substances: (1) the **tocopherols** and (2) the related but less biologically active compounds, the tocotrienols. The vitamers are named according to the position and number of methyl groups on their ring systems. The most important of these is α-tocopherol (see Table 3-12) in the natural D-isomer form.

Absorption, Transport, and Storage

Vitamin E is absorbed in the upper small intestine by micelle-dependent diffusion; its use depends on the presence of dietary fat and adequate biliary and pancreatic function. The esterified forms of vitamin E found in supplements are more stable and can be absorbed only after hydrolysis by esterases at the duodenal mucosa. However, esters of natural and synthetic α-tocopherol are digested equally well (IOM, Food and Nutrition Board, 2000a). The absorption of vitamin E is highly variable, and efficiencies range from 20% to 70%. Absorbed vitamin E is incorporated into chylomicrons and transported into the general circulation via lymph. Vitamin E delivered to the liver is incorporated into VLDLs using a transport protein specific for vitamin E. In the plasma, tocopherol is also partitioned into LDLs and HDLs, where it may protect the lipoproteins from oxidation.

The cellular uptake of vitamin E can occur either as a receptor-mediated process (in which LDLs deliver the vitamin into the cell) or as a process mediated by lipoprotein lipase (LPL) as vitamin E is released from chylomicrons and

VLDLs by the action of LPL. Within the cell, intracellular transport of the tocopherol requires an intracellular tocopherol-binding protein. In most nonadipose cells, vitamin E is located almost exclusively in membranes. In adipose tissues it is not readily mobilized.

Metabolism

The metabolism of vitamin E is limited. It is primarily oxidized into the biologically inactive tocopheryl quinone, which can be reduced to tocopheryl hydroquinone. Glucuronic acid conjugates of the hydroquinone are secreted in the bile, making excretion in the feces the major route of elimination of the vitamin. With usual intakes of vitamin E, a very small portion is excreted in the urine as water-soluble, side-chain metabolites (tocopheronic acid and tocopheronolactone).

Functions

Vitamin E is the most important lipid-soluble **antioxidant** in the cell. Located in the lipid portion of cell membranes, it protects unsaturated phospholipids of the membrane from oxidative degradation from highly reactive oxygen species and other **free radicals**. Vitamin E performs this function through its ability to reduce such radicals into harmless metabolites by donating a hydrogen to them (Figure 3-18), which is called free *radical scavenging*.

As a membrane free radical scavenger, vitamin E is an important component of the cellular antioxidant defense system, which involves other enzymes (e.g., superoxide dismutases [SODs], glutathione peroxidases [GSH-Pxs], glutathione reductase [GR], catalase, thioredoxin reductase [TR]), and nonenzymatic factors (e.g., glutathione, uric acid), many of which depend on other essential nutrients. For example, GSH-Px and TR depend on adequate selenium status; SODs depend on adequate copper, zinc, and manganese statuses; and the activity of GR depends on adequate riboflavin status. Therefore the antioxidant function of vitamin E can be affected by the levels of many other nutrients.

This antioxidant function suggests that vitamin E and related nutrients may collectively be important in protecting the body against and treating conditions related to oxidative stress. However, care must be taken in making broad statements regarding these antioxidant effects. Although vitamin E is known to inhibit processes related to the development of atherosclerosis, clinical trials using supplements have given variable results, mostly negative (Weinberg, 2005). Recent evidence has indicated that vitamin E also functions in regulation of cell signaling processes and gene expression, particularly of drug metabolizing enzymes (Brigelius-Flohe, 2005).

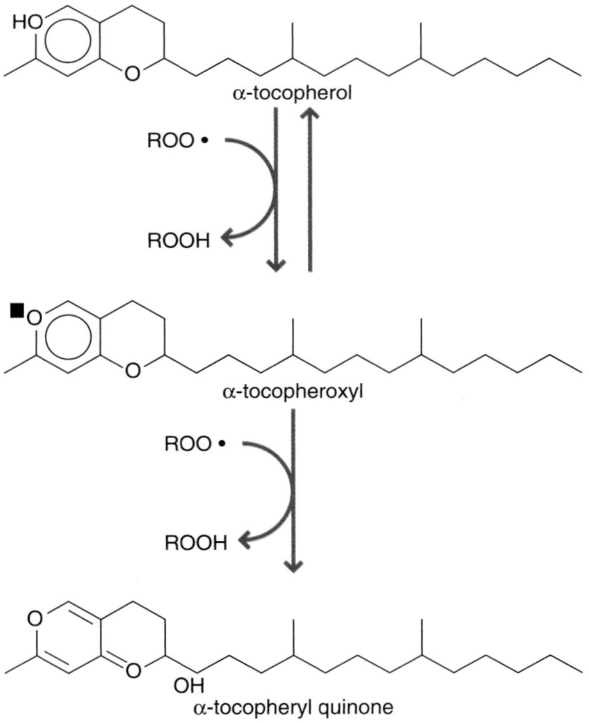

HO
α-tocopherol
ROO •
ROOH
O
α-tocopheroxyl
ROO •
ROOH
O
OH
α-tocopheryl quinone

FIGURE 3-18 Mechanism of vitamin E scavenging oxygen-centered free radicals. *(From Combs GF: The vitamins: fundamental aspects in nutrition and health, ed 2, Orlando, 1998, Academic Press.)*

Dietary Reference Intakes

Vitamin E is quantified in terms of α-tocopherol equivalents (α-TEs); 1 mg of R,R,R-α-tocopherol is defined as 1 α-TE, and 1 mg of the synthetic all-rac-α-tocopherol is defined as 0.5 α-TE. Although outdated, International Units of vitamin E are still found on food labels. An International Unit of vitamin E is equal to 0.67 mg of RRR-α-tocopherol and 1 mg of all-rac-α-tocopherol (IOM, Food and Nutrition Board, 2000a). The DRIs for vitamin E have been established (IOM, Food and Nutrition Board 2000a) with AIs for infants and recommended dietary allowances (RDAs) for children and adults based solely on the α-tocopherol form of the vitamin because other forms are not converted to α-tocopherol in humans. The need for vitamin E depends in part on the amount of PUFAs consumed. For Americans, typical intakes are approximately 0.4 mg α-TE/mg of PUFAs; because the United States does not have significant vitamin E deficiency problems, this ratio is thought to be adequate.

Sources

Tocopherols and tocotrienols are synthesized only by plants; plant oils are the best sources of them, with α- and γ-tocopherols being the forms in most common foods. Nearly two thirds of the vitamin E in the typical American diet is supplied by salad oils, margarines, and shortenings, approximately 11% by fruits and vegetables, and approximately 7% by grains and grain products. Table 3-14 and Appendix 49 list the vitamin E content of selected foods (IOM, Food and Nutrition Board, 2000a).

The free alcohol forms of vitamin E (e.g., tocopherols) are fairly stable but can be destroyed by oxidation. Vitamin E esters (e.g., tocopheryl acetate) are very stable, even in oxidizing conditions. Because the vitamers E are insoluble

TABLE 3-14

Vitamin E Content of Selected Foods

Food	α-TE (mg)
Raisin bran, 1 cup	13.50
Almonds, 1 oz	7.33
Sunflower oil, 1 tbsp	5.59
Mixed nuts 1 oz	3.10
Canola oil, 1 tbsp	2.39
Asparagus, 1 cup	2.16
Peanut oil, 1 tbsp	2.12
Corn oil, 1 tbsp	1.94
Olive oil, 1 tbsp	1.94
Apricots, canned, sweetened, ½ cup	1.55
Margarine, 1 tbsp	1.27
Flounder, 3 oz	0.56
Cashews, 1 oz	0.26
Baked beans, canned with pork, 1 cup	0.25
DRIs	
Infants	4-5 α-TE (mg)/day, depending on age
Young children	6-7 α-TE (mg)/day, depending on age
Older children and adolescents	11-15 α-TE (mg)/day, depending on age
Adults	15 α-TE (mg)/day
Pregnant	15 α-TE (mg)/day
Lactating	19 α-TE (mg)/day

From U.S. Department of Agriculture, Agricultural Research Service: Nutrient Database for Standard Reference, Release 18, Data Laboratory home page: http://www.nal.usda.gov/fnic/foodcomp/Data/SR18/nutrlist/sr18w323.pdf; accessed 2011.

α-TE, α-Tocopherol equivalents; *DRI,* dietary reference intake.

in water, they are not lost by cooking in water but can be destroyed by deep-fat frying.

Deficiency

The clinical manifestations of vitamin E deficiency vary considerably. In general, the targets of deficiency are the neuromuscular, vascular, and reproductive systems. Vitamin E deficiency, which may take 5 to 10 years to develop, manifests with loss of deep tendon reflexes, impaired vibratory and position sensation, changes in balance and coordination, muscle weakness, and visual disturbances (Sokol, 2001). Symptoms in humans have occurred only in those with lipid malabsorption attributable to diseases such as biliary atresia or exocrine pancreatic insufficiency or with lipid transport abnormalities like abetalipoproteinemia.

At the cellular level, a deficiency of vitamin E is accompanied by an increase in lipid peroxidation of the cell membrane. Because of this, vitamin E–deficient cells exposed to an oxidant stress experience more rapid injury and necrosis.

Because there is limited transplacental movement of vitamin E, newborn infants have low tissue concentrations of vitamin E and premature infants may be at risk for vitamin E deficiency (see Chapter 43).

Toxicity

Vitamin E is one of the least toxic of the vitamins. Humans and animals seem to be able to tolerate relatively high intakes—at least 100 times the nutritional requirement. The UL for vitamin E in adults is 1000 mg/day. However, in very high doses, vitamin E can decrease the body's ability to use other fat-soluble vitamins. Animals fed excessive amounts of vitamin E have impaired bone mineralization, hepatic vitamin A storage, and blood coagulation (Traber, 2008). In the last few years, conflicting data regarding high-dose supplementation of vitamin E and increased mortality of patients with cardiovascular disease, inflammatory joint diseases, and cancer have been noted. A causal relationship of vitamin E supplementation and increased mortality is questionable and should have further study (Gerss and Kopcke, 2009).

Vitamin K

Scientists now know that **vitamin K** plays a role in blood clotting, bone formation, and regulation of multiple enzyme systems (Denisova and Booth, 2005). Naturally occurring forms of vitamin K are the phylloquinones (the vitamin K_1 series), which are synthesized by green plants, and the **menaquinones** (the vitamin K2 series), which are synthesized by bacteria. Both of these natural forms have a 2-methyl-1,4-napthoquinone ring and alkylated side chains (see Table 3-12). The synthetic compound **menadione** (vitamin K3) has no side chain but can be alkylated in the liver to produce menaquinones. Menadione is twice as potent biologically as the naturally occurring forms vitamins K_1 and K_2.

Absorption, Transport, and Storage

The phylloquinones (K_1) are absorbed by an energy-dependent process in the small intestine. However, the menaquinones (K_2) and menadione (K_3) are absorbed in the small intestine and colon by passive diffusion. Like the other fat-soluble vitamins, absorption depends on a minimum amount of dietary fat and on bile salts and pancreatic juices. The absorbed vitamers K are incorporated into chylomicrons in the lymph and taken to the liver, where they are incorporated into VLDLs and subsequently delivered to the peripheral tissues by LDLs.

Vitamin K is found in low concentrations in many tissues, where it is localized in cellular membranes. Because of the metabolism of the vitamin, tissues show mixtures of vitamers K even when a single form is consumed. Most tissues contain phylloquinones and menaquinones.

Metabolism

Phylloquinones can be converted to menaquinones by successive bacterial dealkylation and realkylation before absorption. Side-chain shortening and oxidation produce metabolites that are excreted in the feces via the bile, frequently as glucuronic acid conjugates, and catabolize phylloquinones and menaquinones. Menadione is metabolized more rapidly; it is excreted primarily in the urine as a phosphate, sulfate, or glucuronide derivative.

Functions

Vitamin K is essential for the posttranslational carboxylation of glutamic acid residues in proteins to form carboxyglutamate ([GLA] residues); the residues bind calcium. In the process of generating residues, vitamin K is oxidized to an epoxide. It is restored to its hydroquinone form by the enzyme epoxide reductase (Figure 3-19). This process is known as the *vitamin K cycle*. The vitamin K cycle can be disrupted by coumarin-type drugs such as warfarin and dicumarol, which is the basis for their anticoagulant activities. Patients taking these anticoagulant drugs do not need to eliminate vitamin K from their diets but should maintain a consistent level of vitamin K intake.

Four plasma-clotting GLA proteins have been identified, including thrombin, which is necessary for the conversion of fibrinogen to fibrin in blood clotting. In addition, at least three proteins are found in calcified tissues (osteocalcin being one) and at least one protein is found in calcified atherosclerotic tissue (atherocalcin).

Vitamin K regulates enzymes involved in sphingolipid metabolism in the brain, as well as other enzyme systems (Denisova and Booth, 2005). Vitamin K may also play roles in age-related bone loss, cardiovascular disease, and regulation of inflammation (Booth, 2009).

Dietary Reference Intakes

Although the various vitamers K vary widely in their biopotencies, no standardization of means exists for accommodating these differences when quantifying the amounts of the vitamin K in foods or diets. Each vitamer is expressed in terms of its mass in micrograms of vitamin K. The DRIs for vitamin K are given as AIs, and no UL has been determined. However, it should not be assumed that high vitamin K consumption has adverse effects because data on such effects are very limited.

Sources

Vitamin K is found in large amounts in green leafy vegetables, usually at levels greater than 100 mcg/100 g (Table 3-15; see also Appendix 50). The amounts of the vitamin in dairy products, meats, and eggs tend to vary, ranging from 0 to 50 mcg/g, and fruits and cereals usually contain approximately 15 mcg/g. Breast milk tends to be low in vitamin K and does not provide enough of the vitamin for infants younger than 6 months of age. Products that contain plant oils can be a good source of phylloquinone.

TABLE 3-15

Vitamin K Content of Selected Foods

Food	Content (mcg)
Spinach, frozen, cooked, 1 cup	1027
Broccoli, cooked, 1 cup	220
Asparagus, cooked, 1 cup	144
Cabbage, cooked, 1 cup	73
Green beans, raw, 1 cup	47
Carrot, raw, 1 cup	14
Lettuce, iceberg, 1 cup	13
Avocado, raw, 1 oz	6
Turkey, cooked, 3 oz	0.03
Potato, baked, 1 medium	0.5
Ground beef, cooked, 3 oz	1.0
Orange, raw, 1 medium	0
DRIs	
Infants	2.0-2.5 mcg/day, depending on age
Young children	30-55 mcg/day, depending on age
Older children and adolescents	60-75 mcg/day, depending on age
Adults	90-120 mcg/day, depending on gender
Pregnant	75-90 mcg/day, depending on age
Lactating	75-90 mcg/day, depending on age

From U.S. Department of Agriculture, Agricultural Research Service: Nutrient Database for Standard Reference, Release 18, Data Laboratory home page: http://www.nal.usda.gov/fnic/foodcomp/Data/SR18/nutrlist/sr18w430.pdf; accessed 1-14-11.

DRI, Dietary reference intake.

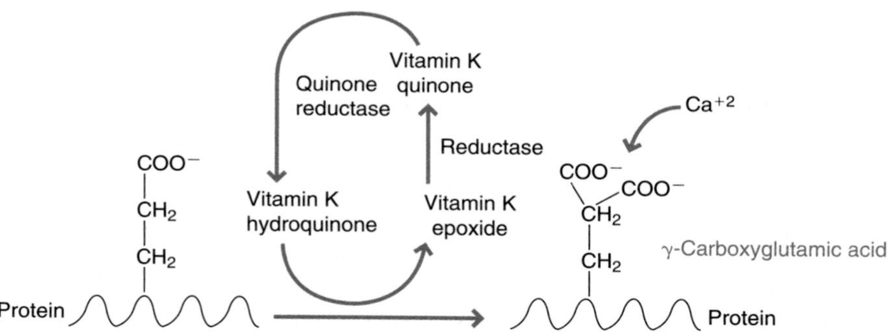

FIGURE 3-19 Function and regeneration of vitamin K in the production of γ-carboxyglutamic acid.

Meat, dairy, and fast foods do contain small amounts of menaquinone, which could be physiologically significant (Elder et al., 2006).

The analytic task of determining the vitamers K in foods is formidable; tabulated vitamin K values for food are often inaccurate. Nevertheless, the absence of evidence of a significant vitamin K deficiency in the general population indicates that adequate amounts of the vitamin can normally be obtained by foods or produced by enteric microflora. Vitamin K is not destroyed by ordinary cooking methods, nor is it lost in cooking water, but it is sensitive to light and alkalis.

Deficiency

The predominant sign of vitamin K deficiency is hemorrhage, which in severe cases can cause fatal anemia. The underlying condition is hypoprothrombinemia, characterized by prolonged clotting time. Vitamin K deficiencies are rare among humans but have been associated with lipid malabsorption, destruction of intestinal flora in those receiving chronic antibiotic therapy, and liver disease. Newborn infants, particularly those who are premature or exclusively breastfed, are susceptible to hypoprothrombinemia during the first few days of life. Poor placental transfer of vitamin K and failure to establish a vitamin K–producing intestinal microflora are problematic. Hemorrhagic disease in the newborn is treated prophylactically by administering menadione intramuscularly at birth.

In older adults, low intakes of vitamin K have been associated with increased incidence of hip fractures. Vitamin K_1 and alendronate are more cost-effective than either risedronate or strontium ranelate; but further research is required because it is unlikely that the present prescribing policy (i.e., alendronate as first-line treatment) will be altered (Stevenson et al., 2009).

Toxicity

Neither the phylloquinones nor the menaquinones have shown any adverse effects by any route of administration. However, menadione can be toxic; excessive doses have produced hemolytic anemia in rats and severe jaundice in infants.

THE WATER-SOLUBLE VITAMINS

Thiamin, riboflavin, niacin, vitamin B_6, pantothenic acid, biotin, folic acid, vitamin B_{12}, and vitamin C are referred to as the *water-soluble vitamins.* Solubility in water is one of the only characteristics that they share. Because they are water soluble, these vitamins tend to be absorbed by simple diffusion when ingested in large amounts and by carrier-mediated processes when ingested in smaller amounts. They are distributed in the aqueous phases of the cell (i.e., the cytoplasm and mitochondrial matrix space) and are essential cofactors or cosubstrates of enzymes involved in various aspects of metabolism. Most are not stored in appreciable amounts, making regular consumption a necessity. The water-soluble vitamins are transported by carriers and are excreted in the urine.

Thiamin

Thiamin (see Table 3-12) plays essential roles in carbohydrate metabolism and neural function. The vitamin must be activated by phosphorylation into thiamin triphosphate, or cocarboxylase, which serves as a coenzyme in energy metabolism and the synthesis of pentoses. Thiamin's role in neural function is unclear, but it probably does not act as a coenzyme (Gropper et al., 2005).

Absorption, Transport, and Storage

Thiamin is absorbed from the proximal small intestine by active transport in low doses and passive diffusion in high doses (>5 mg/day). Active transport is inhibited by alcohol consumption, which interferes with transport of the vitamin, and by folate deficiency, which interferes with the replication of enterocytes. The mucosal uptake of thiamin is coupled to its phosphorylation into thiamin diphosphate (ThDP); activated ThDP is carried to the liver by the portal circulation.

Approximately 90% of circulating thiamin is carried as ThDP by erythrocytes, although small amounts exist primarily as free thiamin and thiamin monophosphate (ThMP) bound chiefly to albumin. Uptake by cells of peripheral tissues occurs by passive diffusion and active transport. Tissues retain thiamin as phosphate esters, mostly bound to proteins. Tissue levels of thiamin vary, with no appreciable storage of the vitamin.

Metabolism

Thiamin is phosphorylated in many tissues by specific kinases into the diphosphate and triphosphate esters. Each of these esters can be catabolized by a phosphorylase to yield ThMP. Small amounts of some 20 other excretory metabolites are also produced and excreted in the urine.

Functions

The major functional form of thiamin is ThDP, which is a coenzyme for several dehydrogenase enzyme complexes essential in the metabolism of pyruvate and other α-keto acids. Thiamin is essential for the oxidative decarboxylation of α-keto acids, including the oxidative conversion of pyruvate to acetyl CoA, which enters the TCA, or Krebs, cycle to generate energy. It is also required for the conversion of α-ketoglutarate and the 2-ketocarboxylates derived from the amino acids methionine, threonine, leucine, isoleucine, and valine. ThDP also serves as the coenzyme for transketolase, which catalyzes 2-carbon fragment exchange reactions in the oxidation of glucose by the hexose monophosphate shunt.

Dietary Reference Intakes

Thiamin is expressed quantitatively in terms of its mass, usually in milligrams. The DRIs for thiamin include AIs for infants and the newly defined RDAs. In general, the RDAs are based on levels of energy intake because of the direct role of thiamin in energy metabolism, whereas the AIs for infants are based on the thiamin levels typically found in human milk.

Sources

Thiamin is widely distributed in many foods, but in low concentrations. The richest sources are yeasts and liver; however, cereal grains are the most important source of the vitamin (Table 3-16). Although whole grains are typically rich in thiamin, most of it is removed during milling and refining. In the United States most refined grain products are supplemented with thiamin and other B vitamins. Plant foods contain thiamin predominantly in the free form, whereas almost all of the thiamin in animal products exists as the more efficient ThDP.

Thiamin can be destroyed by heat, oxidation, and ionizing radiation, but it is stable when frozen. Cooking losses of the vitamin tend to vary widely, depending on cooking time, pH, temperature, quantity of water used and discarded, and whether the water is chlorinated. Thiamin can be destroyed by sulfites added in processing; by thiamin-degrading enzymes (thiaminases) in raw fish, shellfish, and some bacteria; and by certain heat-stable factors in plants such as ferns, tea, and betel nuts.

Deficiency

Thiamin deficiency is characterized by anorexia and weight loss, as well as cardiac and neurologic signs (Table 3-17). In humans thiamin deficiency eventually results in **beriberi**, with mental confusion, muscular wasting, edema (wet beriberi), peripheral neuropathy, tachycardia, and cardiomegaly. The nonedematous (dry beriberi) disease is usually associated with energy deprivation and inactivity, whereas the wet form is usually associated with a high carbohydrate intake along with strenuous physical exertion. The latter is characterized by edema caused by biventricular heart failure with pulmonary congestion. Without ThDP, pyruvate cannot be converted to acetyl CoA and enter the TCA cycle, and energy deprivation of the heart muscle results in heart failure.

Historically, beriberi has been endemic among the poor in areas of the world where polished white rice is the major

TABLE 3-16

Thiamin Content of Selected Foods

Food	Content (mg)
Fortified ready to eat cereal, 1 cup	Up to 9.90
Pork chop, lean, 3 oz	1.06
Ham, lean, 3 oz	0.82
Sunflower seeds, shelled, 1 oz	0.59
Bagel, plain, 4 inch	0.53
Tuna sushi, 6-inch roll	0.46
Green peas, 1 cup	0.45
Beans, baked, 1 cup	0.13
Pasta, spaghetti, cooked, 1 cup	0.29
Rice, white, enriched, cooked, 1 cup	0.26
Potato, mashed, 1 cup	0.23
Doughnut, yeast, 1	0.22
Orange juice, from frozen concentrate, 6 fl oz	0.2

DRI Range

0.2-1.4 mg/day, depending on age and gender

From U.S. Department of Agriculture, Agricultural Research Service: Nutrient Database for Standard Reference, Release 18, Data Laboratory home page: http://www.nal.usda.gov/fnic/foodcomp/Data/SR18/nutrlist/sr18w404.pdf; accessed 2011.

DRI, Dietary reference intake.

TABLE 3-17

Clinical Features of Thiamin Deficiency

Deficiency Type	Features
Early stage of deficiency	Anorexia Indigestion Constipation Malaise Heaviness and weakness of legs Tender calf muscles "Pins and needles" and numbness in legs Anesthesia of skin, particularly at the tibia Increased pulse rate and palpitations
Wet beriberi	Edema of legs, face, trunk, and serous cavities Tense calf muscles Fast pulse Distended neck veins High blood pressure Decreased urine volume
Dry beriberi	Worsening of early-stage polyneuritis Difficulty walking Wernicke-Korsakoff syndrome: possible Encephalopathy • Loss of immediate memory • Disorientation • Nystagmus (jerky movements of eyes) • Ataxia (staggering gait)
Infantile beriberi (2-5 mo of age)	Acute • Decreased urine output • Excessive crying; thin and plaintive whining • Cardiac failure Chronic • Constipation and vomiting • Fretfulness • Soft, toneless muscles • Pallor of skin with cyanosis

staple food and where people also consume raw fish and other sources of thiaminase. Such conditions usually produce not only beriberi but also multiple nutritional deficiencies. Beriberi has also been reported in infants (infantile beriberi) who were fed formulas that were not supplemented with thiamin; deterioration is sudden and characterized by cardiac failure and cyanosis. Beriberi responds to thiamin treatment, particularly if neural damage and cardiac involvement are not great.

Frank thiamin deficiency is not common in the United States because of the thiamin supplementation of rice and other refined cereal products. Subclinical thiamin deficiency develops in those with alcoholism who tend to have inadequate thiamin intake and impaired absorption of the vitamin. In addition, thiamin is required for the metabolism and detoxification of alcohol, so those with alcoholism need more. Some older Americans are at risk for thiamin deficiency because of their poor diets and long-term use of diuretics for high blood pressure or heart failure. In addition, patients who have had gastric bypass may be at risk for deficiency and should be monitored carefully (Welch et al., 2010).

Deficient individuals may have Wernicke-Korsakoff syndrome, the signs of which range from mild confusion to coma. Beginning around 1900, investigators began to recognize a relationship between Korsakoff's psychosis, delirium tremens, peripheral polyneuropathy, and Wernicke encephalopathy (Lanska, 2009).

Others who are deficient in thiamin have an inherited abnormal transketolase incapable of normal ThDP binding. Biochemical changes that reflect thiamin status occur well before the appearance of overt symptoms. Thus thiamin status can be assessed by determining erythrocyte transketolase activity, measuring blood or serum levels of thiamin or measuring urinary thiamin excretion levels (see Appendix 30).

Toxicity

Little information exists about the toxic potential of thiamin, although massive doses (1000 times greater than nutritional needs) of commercial thiamin hydrochloride suppress the respiratory center and cause death (IOM, Food and Nutrition Board, 2000b). Parenteral doses of thiamin at 100 times the recommended levels have produced headache, convulsions, muscular weakness, cardiac arrhythmia, and allergic reactions.

Riboflavin

Riboflavin is essential for the metabolism of carbohydrates, amino acids, and lipids and supports antioxidant protection. It carries out these functions as the coenzymes flavin adenine dinucleotide (FAD) and flavin adenine mononucleotide (FMN). Because of its fundamental roles in metabolism, riboflavin deficiencies are first evident in tissues that have rapid cellular turnover such as the skin and epithelia.

Absorption, Transport, and Storage

Riboflavin is absorbed in the free form by a carrier-mediated process in the proximal small intestine. Because most foods contain the vitamin in its coenzyme forms, FMN and FAD, absorption occurs only after the hydrolytic cleavage of free riboflavin from its various flavoprotein complexes by various phosphatases. Riboflavin absorption is a carrier-mediated process that requires ATP. The mucosal uptake of free riboflavin depends on its phosphorylation into FMN.

Riboflavin is transported in the plasma as free riboflavin and FMN, both of which are mainly bound to plasma albumin. A specific riboflavin-binding protein has also been identified and is thought to function in the transplacental movement of the vitamin. Riboflavin is transported in its free form into cells by a carrier-mediated process, and then it is converted to FMN or FAD. Their protein binding prevents diffusion out of the cell and makes them resistant to catabolism. Although small amounts of the vitamin are found in the liver and kidney, it is not stored in any useful amount and therefore must be supplied in the diet regularly.

Metabolism

Riboflavin is converted to its coenzyme forms by ATP-dependent phosphorylation to yield riboflavin-5'-phosphate, or FMN, by the enzyme flavokinase. Most FMN is then converted to FAD by FAD-pyrophosphorylase. Both steps are regulated by the thyroid hormones adrenocorticotropic hormone and aldosterone.

Most excess riboflavin is excreted as such in the urine. However, free riboflavin can be glycosylated in the liver, and the glycosylated metabolite is excreted. Riboflavin may also have a direct metabolic function. It can also be catabolized by oxidation, demethylation, and hydroxylation of its ring system to yield products that are excreted in the urine with free riboflavin.

Functions

The flavin coenzymes FMN and FAD accept pairs of hydrogen atoms forming $FMNH_2$ or $FADH_2$. As such they can participate in either one- or two-electron redox reactions. FMN and FAD serve as prosthetic groups of several flavoprotein enzymes that catalyze oxidation-reduction reactions in the cells and function as hydrogen carriers in the mitochondrial electron transport system. FMN and FAD are also coenzymes of dehydrogenases (such as in the TCA cycle) that catalyze initial fatty acid oxidation and several steps in glucose metabolism.

FMN is required for the conversion of pyridoxine (PN; vitamin B_6) to its functional form, pyridoxal phosphate (PLP). FAD is required for the biosynthesis of the vitamin niacin from the amino acid tryptophan. In other cellular roles, mechanisms dependent on riboflavin and nicotinamide adenine dinucleotide phosphate (NADPH) seem to combat oxidative damage to the cell. Nutritional supplements that include riboflavin may protect against cataracts (Jacques et al., 2005).

Dietary Reference Intakes

The DRIs for riboflavin include AIs for infants and newly defined RDAs. In general, the RDAs are based on the amount required to maintain normal tissue reserves based on urinary excretion, red blood cell riboflavin contents, and erythrocyte GR activity. Riboflavin requirements are higher during pregnancy and lactation so that they can meet the needs of increased tissue synthesis and the losses of riboflavin secreted in breast milk.

Sources

Riboflavin, measured in milligrams in foods, is widely distributed in foods in a form bound to proteins as FMN and FAD. Rapidly growing, green leafy vegetables are rich in the vitamin; however, meats and dairy products are the most important contributors to the American diet (Table 3-18). More than half of the vitamin is lost when flour is milled; however, most breads and cereals are enriched with riboflavin and contribute appreciably to the total daily intake.

Riboflavin is stable when heated but can be readily destroyed by alkali and exposure to ultraviolet irradiation. Very little of the vitamin is destroyed during the cooking and processing of foods; however, because of its sensitivity to alkali, the practice of adding baking soda to soften dried peas or beans destroys much of their riboflavin content.

TABLE 3-18

Riboflavin Content of Selected Foods

Food	Content (mg)
Liver, beef, 3 oz	2.91
Fortified ready to eat cereal, 1 cup	Up to 1.70
Milk, 2% fat, 1 cup	0.45
Yogurt, fruit flavored, low fat, 1 cup	0.40
Clams, canned, 3 oz	0.36
Cheese, cottage, 1 cup	0.37
Egg, 1	0.25
Custard, baked, ½ cup	0.25
Pork, roast loin, 3 oz	0.27
Bagel, plain, 1	0.22
Hamburger, lean, broiled medium, 3.5 oz	0.21
Spinach, fresh, cooked, ½ cup	0.21
Chicken, dark meat, 3 oz	0.21
Broccoli, 1 cup	0.19
Cheese, American, 1 oz	0.10
Banana, 1	0.09
DRI Range	
0.3-1.6 mg/day, depending on age and gender	

From U.S. Department of Agriculture, Agricultural Research Service: Nutrient Database for Standard Reference, Release 18, Data Laboratory home page: http://www.nal.usda.gov/fnic/foodcomp/Data/SR18/nutrlist/sr18w405.pdf; accessed 2011.

DRI, Dietary reference intake.

Wax-lined paper containers protect milk against riboflavin loss from exposure to sunlight.

Deficiency

Riboflavin deficiency becomes manifest after several months of deprivation of the vitamin. The initial symptoms include photophobia; tearing; burning and itching of the eyes; loss of visual acuity; and soreness and burning of lips, mouth, and tongue. More advanced symptoms include fissuring of the lips (*cheilosis*) and cracks in the skin at the corners of the mouth (*angular stomatitis*). It may manifest as a greasy eruption of the skin in the nasolabial folds, scrotum, or vulva; a purple, swollen tongue (Figure 3-20); capillary overgrowth around the cornea of the eye; and peripheral neuropathy (Box 3-6).

Riboflavin has been implicated in cataract formation when multiple vitamin deficiencies are present (Jacques et al., 2005). Phototherapy for infants with hyperbilirubinemia often leads to riboflavin deficiency (by photodestruction of the vitamin) if the therapy does not also include riboflavin supplementation. Otherwise riboflavin deficiencies usually occur in combination with deficiencies of other water-soluble vitamins such as thiamin and niacin, especially in those who are malnourished. The B vitamins and several gene polymorphisms that affect DNA synthesis and methylation have shown a small, inverse association between riboflavin and gastric cancer risk (Eussen et al., 2010). Riboflavin status is measured by assessment of the activity of erythrocyte GR. This enzyme requires FAD and converts oxidized glutathione to reduced glutathione.

Toxicity

Riboflavin is not known to be toxic; high oral doses are considered essentially nontoxic. However, high doses are not beneficial.

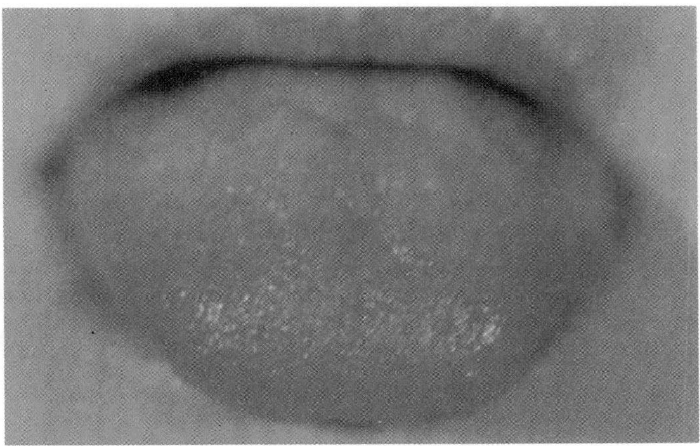

FIGURE 3-20 Magenta tongue, a sign of riboflavin deficiency. In contrast, a person with an iron deficiency often has a pale tongue; and vitamin B–complex deficiency results in a beefy, red-colored tongue. *(From McLaren DS: Colour atlas of nutritional diseases, England, 1981, Yearbook Medical Publishers.)*

BOX 3-6

Signs of Possible Riboflavin Deficiency

Soreness and burning of lips, mouth, and tongue*
Cheilosis*
Angular stomatitis*
Glossitis*
Purplish or magenta tongue*
Hypertrophy or atrophy of tongue papillae*
Seborrheic dermatitis of nasolabial folds, vestibule of nose, and sometimes the ears and eyelids, scrotum, and vulva
Ocular pathologic conditions (sometimes)
- Inflammation of conjunctiva
- Superficial vascularization of cornea
- Ulcerations of cornea
- Photophobia

Anemia—normocytic and normochromic
Neuropathy

Modified from Goldsmith GA: Riboflavin deficiency. In Rivlin RS, editor: Riboflavin, New York, 1975, Plenum Press.

*Tongue and mouth changes are difficult to differentiate from those caused by niacin, folic acid, thiamin, vitamin B_6, or vitamin B_{12} deficiency.

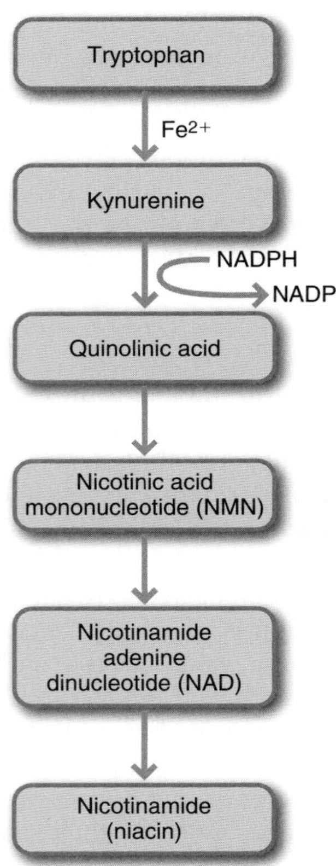

FIGURE 3-21 Synthesis of niacin from tryptophan. *NADPH,* Nicotinamide adenine dinucleotide phosphate in the reduced form.

Niacin

Niacin is the generic term for nicotinamide (Nam) and nicotinic acid (NA). It functions as a component of pyridine nucleotide coenzymes nicotinamide adenine dinucleotide (NAD) and NADPH, which are essential in all cells for energy production and metabolism. NAD and NADPH are the reduced forms of NAD and NADP; they carry a hydrogen ion. Niacin was first identified as a result of the search for the cause and cure of pellagra, a disease common in Spain and Italy in the eighteenth century and that devastated the southern United States in the early twentieth century.

Biosynthesis, Absorption, Transport, and Storage

Niacin can be synthesized from the essential amino acid tryptophan. Even though this process is not efficient, dietary tryptophan intake is important to the overall niacin status of the body (Figure 3-21).

Niacin in many foods, particularly those from animal sources, consists mostly of the coenzyme forms NAD and NADPH, each of which must be digested to release the absorbed forms, Nam and NA. Many foods derived from plants, particularly grains, contain niacin in covalently bound complexes with small peptides and carbohydrates that are not released during digestion. These forms (niacytin) are not biologically available but can become bioavailable through alkaline hydrolysis. Thus the Central American tradition of soaking maize in lime water before preparing tortillas effectively increases the bioavailability of niacin in what otherwise would be considered a low-niacin food.

Ultimately Nam and NA are absorbed in the stomach and small intestine by carrier-mediated facilitated diffusion. Both are transported in the plasma in free solution, and each is taken up by most tissues through passive diffusion. Some tissues like erythrocytes, kidney, and brain require a transport system for NA. Niacin is retained in tissues as NAD but may also be converted to NADPH.

Metabolism

The de novo synthesis of NAD and NADPH occurs from quinolinic acid, a metabolite of the essential amino acid tryptophan. The conversion of tryptophan to niacin depends on such factors as the amount of tryptophan and niacin ingested and PN status (B_6); therefore the body must have adequate levels of riboflavin and, to a lesser extent, vitamin B_6. Humans are moderately efficient at this conversion, and 60 mg of tryptophan is considered equal to 1 mg of niacin.

NAD and NADPH can be produced from NA and Nam obtained from the diet. Nam is deaminated to yield NA. Then two ribose phosphates are attached to the nitrogen in the pyridine ring. Next, adenosine is attached to the ribose. Finally, an amino group is added to the acid group, forming an amide and yielding NAD. NAD can be phosphorylated in the hexose monophosphate shunt to yield NADPH.

NAD and NADPH are catabolized by hydrolysis to yield Nam, which can be deaminated into NA or methylated to yield 1-methylnicotinamide. Dietary protein deficiency changes the profile of urinary metabolites, presumably because of changes in the amount of tryptophan converted to niacin.

Functions

The coenzymes NAD and NADPH are the most central electron carriers of cells, playing essential roles as cosubstrates of more than 200 enzymes for the metabolism of carbohydrates, fatty acids, and amino acids. In general, NAD and NADPH facilitate hydrogen transport by two-electron transfers, which use the hydride ion (H^+) as the carrier but play very different roles in metabolism. The NAD-dependent reactions are involved in intracellular respiration (e.g., beta-oxidation, TCA cycle function [see Figure 3-2], and the electron transport system). NADPH, on the other hand, is important for biosynthetic (e.g., fatty acid, sterol) pathways.

Because of its fundamental role in metabolism, niacin may play an important role in mechanisms for DNA repair and gene stability (Kirkland, 2003). Nam, the amide form, participates in the cellular energy metabolism that directly affects normal physiology, influences oxidative stress, and modulates multiple pathways tied to both cellular survival and death; it is a robust cytoprotectant that holds great potential for multiple disease entities (Maiese et al., 2009). It may have roles in Alzheimer disease, Parkinson disease, aging, diabetes, cancer, and cerebral ischemia (Li et al., 2006).

TABLE 3-19

Pre-formed Niacin Content of Selected Foods*

Food	Content (mg)
Ready-to-eat cereals	Up to 26.43
Chicken, ½ breast	14.73
Tuna, canned in water, 3 oz	11.29
Rice, white, 1 cup	7.75
Mushrooms, cooked, 1 cup	6.96
Beef, ground regular, cooked	4.55
Ham, canned, 3 oz	4.28
Peanuts, dry roasted, 1 oz	3.83
Coffee, 2 fl oz	3.12
Egg bagel, 4 inch	3.06
Pizza with pepperoni	3.05
Noodles, 1 cup	2.68

DRI Range

2-18 mg/day, depending on age and gender

From U.S. Department of Agriculture, Agricultural Research Service: Nutrient Database for Standard Reference, Release 18, Data Laboratory home page: http://www.nal.usda.gov/fnic/foodcomp/Data/SR18/nutrlist/sr18w406.pdf; accessed 2011.

DRI, Dietary reference intake.

*These data do not take into account niacin available from food via synthesis from tryptophan.

Dietary Reference Intakes

Niacin is expressed in total milligrams of niacin or niacin equivalents (NEs), which are calculated from the pre-formed niacin content plus 1/60 of the tryptophan content. The DRIs established for niacin include AIs for infants, RDAs, and the tolerable UL. Requirements are directly related to energy intake because of niacin's role in energy-producing reactions in metabolism; they are expressed as NEs from pre-formed niacin and tryptophan.

Sources

Significant amounts of niacin are found in many foods; lean meats, poultry, fish, peanuts, and yeasts are particularly rich sources. Niacin exists predominantly as protein-bound NA in plant tissues and as Nam, NAD, and NADPH in animal tissues. Milk and eggs contain small amounts of niacin, but they are excellent sources of tryptophan, giving them significant NE contents. The amount of niacin in foods depends on the total milligrams of niacin (NA and Nam) plus 1/60 of the tryptophan content. Table 3-19 lists the pre-formed niacin content of various foods. Many tables of food nutrient composition list only pre-formed niacin and underestimate the total niacin equivalencies of other foods.

Deficiency

Niacin deficiency begins with muscular weakness, anorexia, indigestion, and skin eruptions. Severe deficiency of niacin leads to **pellagra**, which is characterized by dermatitis, dementia, and diarrhea ("the three Ds"); tremors; and a beefy red, sore tongue. The dermatologic changes are usually the most prominent. Skin that has been exposed to the sun develops cracked, pigmented, scaly dermatitis (Figure 3-22). Central nervous system involvement symptoms include confusion, disorientation, and neuritis. Digestive abnormalities cause irritation and inflammation of the mucous membranes of the mouth and the GI tract. Untreated pellagra can cause death, which is often referred to as "the fourth D."

Patients with pellagra may also show clinical signs of riboflavin deficiency, highlighting the metabolic interrelationships of these vitamins. Patients with pellagra are likely to have very poor diets that not only provide little niacin but also lack protein and other nutrients. The most reliable method for assessing niacin status is the measurement of the urinary excretion of the methylated metabolites methylnicotinomide and methylpyridone carboxamide.

Toxicity

In general, niacin toxicity is low. However, high doses of 1 to 2 g of NA three times per day—dosages that have been used in attempts to lower blood cholesterol concentrations (Malik and Kashyap, 2003)—can have untoward side effects. The main side effect is a histamine release that causes flushing and may be harmful to those with asthma or peptic ulcer disease. Nam does not have this effect. High doses of niacin can also be toxic to the liver; risks are greater with

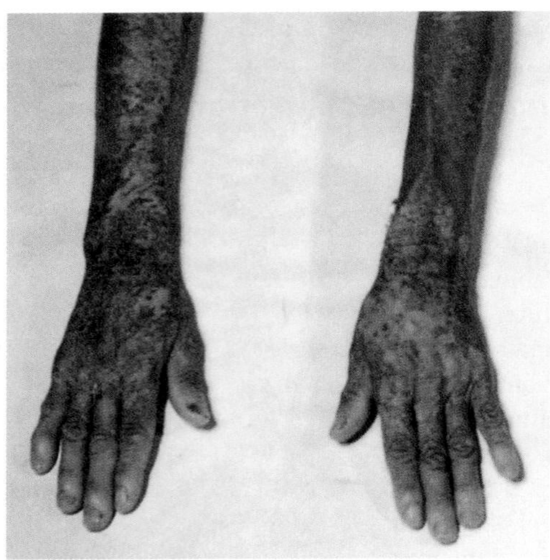

FIGURE 3-22 Pellagra. Pigmented keratotic scaling lesions caused by niacin deficiency. The lesions are especially prominent in areas exposed to the sun, such as the hands, forearms, neck, and legs. *(From Latham MC et al: Scope manual on nutrition, Kalamazoo, Mich., 1980, The Upjohn Company.)*

time-released forms of the vitamin. Megavitamin use should be monitored carefully because high doses act as drugs and not nutritional supplements (Kamanna, 2009; Kamanna and Kashyap, 2008).

Pantothenic Acid

Pantothenic acid is widely distributed in foods; clinical deficiency is rare. The vitamin has critical roles in metabolism. It is an integral part of CoA, which is essential in energy production from the macronutrients, and acyl-carrier protein (ACP), which is used in synthesis reactions.

Absorption, Transport, and Storage

Pantothenic acid exists in foods mostly as CoA and ACP. Therefore absorption requires hydrolysis to phosphopantetheine and then conversion to pantothenic acid. Pantothenic acid is absorbed by both passive diffusion and active transport in the jejunum. It is transported in the free acid form in solution in the plasma and taken up by diffusion into erythrocytes, which carry most of the vitamin in the blood. Pantothenic acid is taken up by cells of peripheral tissues by a sodium-dependent active transport process in some tissues and by facilitated diffusion in others. Within the cell, the vitamin is converted to CoA, which is its predominant form in most tissues, particularly the liver, adrenals, kidney, brain, heart, and testes.

Metabolism

All tissues are capable of synthesizing CoA from pantothenic acid. This multienzyme process takes place in four steps. First pantothenic acid is phosphorylated to yield 4′-phosphopantothenic acid. Then it is condensed with cysteine to yield 4′-phosphopantothenoylcysteine. Next phosphopantothenoylcysteine is decarboxylated to yield 4′-phosphopantetheine, which is finally converted to CoA. ACP contains 4′-phosphopantetheine that is transferred from CoA to bind to the Apo acetyl carrier protein, forming ACP.

CoA and ACP are degraded to yield free pantothenic acid and other metabolites. The vitamin is excreted mainly in the urine as free pantothenic acid but also as 4′-phosphopantothenate. An appreciable amount (some 15% of the daily intake) is oxidized completely and excreted through the lungs as carbon dioxide.

Functions

CoA and ACP function metabolically as carriers of acyl groups. CoA is critical in the formation of acetyl CoA, which condenses with oxaloacetate and enters the TCA cycle to release energy. It is also the compound in the first steps of the synthesis of fatty acids or cholesterol or in the acetylation of alcohols, amines, and amino acids. It also activates fatty acids before their incorporation into triglycerides and acts as an acyl donor for proteins. ACP is a component of the multienzyme complex fatty acid synthase, which is necessary for fatty acid synthesis.

Dietary Reference Intakes

Pantothenic acid is measured in milligrams. DRIs are expressed as AIs. No estimated average requirements (EARs) or RDAs have been established.

Sources

Pantothenic acid is present in all plant and animal tissues. The most important sources in mixed diets are meats (particularly liver and heart). Mushrooms, avocados, broccoli, egg yolks, yeast, skim milk, and sweet potatoes are also good sources of the vitamin (Table 3-20). Pantothenic acid is fairly stable during ordinary cooking and storage, although the vitamin can be lost in frozen meats during thawing. Because it is localized in the outer layers of grains, approximately half of the vitamin is lost in the milling of flour.

Deficiency

Pantothenic acid deficiency results in impairments in lipid synthesis and energy production. Because the vitamin is so widely distributed in foods, deficiencies are rare. However, pantothenic acid deficiency has been observed among severely malnourished humans. Symptoms include paresthesia in the toes and soles of the feet, burning sensations in the feet, depression, fatigue, insomnia, and weakness (IOM, Food and Nutrition Board, 2000b).

Toxicity

The toxicity of pantothenic acid is negligible; no adverse effects after ingestion of large doses of the vitamin have been reported in any species. Massive doses (e.g., 10 g/day)

TABLE 3-20

Pantothenic Acid Content of Selected Foods

Food	Content (mg)
Fortified dry cereal, 1 cup	Up to 10.65
Mushrooms, cooked, 1 cup	3.37
Rice, white, 1 cup	2.10
Tropical trail mix, 1 cup	1.70
Corn, sweet, canned, 1 cup	1.45
Yogurt, plain, 8 oz	1.45
Vanilla shake, 16 fl oz	1.39
Potatoes, mashed, 1 cup	1.20
Chicken breast, 1/2 breast	1.15
Milk, 2% fat, 1 cup	0.78
Salmon, pink, canned, 3 oz	0.47
Banana, 1	0.39
DRI Range	
1.7-7 mg/day, depending on age and gender	

From U.S. Department of Agriculture, Agricultural Research Service: Nutrient Database for Standard Reference, Release 18, Data Laboratory home page: http://www.nal.usda.gov/fnic/foodcomp/Data/SR18/nutrlist/sr18w410.pdf; accessed 2011.

DRI, Dietary reference intake.

administered to humans have produced only mild intestinal distress and diarrhea.

Vitamin B_6 (Pyridoxine)

Vitamin B_6 is the general term for numerous 2-methyl-3, 5-dihydroxymethylpyridine derivatives exhibiting the biologic activity of **pyridoxine (PN)**, the alcohol derivative. The biologically active analogs are the aldehyde pyridoxal (PL) and the amine pyridoxamine (PM). All three compounds are converted to the metabolically active coenzyme form PLP, which is primarily involved in the metabolism of amino acids.

Absorption, Transport, and Storage

Vitamin B_6 is absorbed by passive diffusion of the dephosphorylated forms PN, PL, or PM—primarily in the jejunum and ileum. Absorption is driven by phosphorylation to form PLP and pyridoxamine phosphate (PMP) and then by protein binding of each of these metabolites in the intestinal mucosa and blood.

The predominant form of the vitamin in the blood is PLP, most of which is derived from the liver after metabolism by hepatic flavoenzymes. Small amounts of free PN are also found in the circulation, but most is PLP bound to albumin. However, PLP must be dephosphorylated to PL to be taken up by the cells. On uptake, PL is again phosphorylated to PLP and PMP, with the greatest levels being found in liver, brain, kidney, spleen, and muscle, where they are bound to proteins. Muscle is the largest depot, containing 80% to 90% of the total body vitamin stores in the form of PLP bound to glycogen phosphorylase.

Metabolism

The vitamers of B_6 are readily metabolically interconverted by phosphorylation-dephosphorylation, oxidation-reduction, and amination-deamination reactions. The limiting step during this metabolism is catalyzed by the FMN enzyme PLP oxidase. Thus riboflavin deficiency can reduce the conversions of PN and PM to the active coenzyme PLP. In the liver PLP is dephosphorylated and oxidized by FAD- and NAD-dependent enzymes to yield 4-pyridoxic acid and other inactive metabolites that are excreted in the urine.

Functions

The metabolically active form (PLP) is a coenzyme for numerous enzymes in the metabolism of amino acids. PLP is the cofactor for more than 100 enzyme-catalyzed reactions in the body, including many involved in the synthesis or catabolism of neurotransmitters (Clayton, 2006). It also has roles in the metabolism of glycogen, sphingolipids, heme, and steroids. These roles relate to the ability of the PLP aldehyde group to react with α-amino groups of the amino acid and thus to stabilize the other bonds on the bound carbon. Thus vitamin B_6 is essential for various amino acid transaminases, decarboxylases, racemases, and isomerases.

Vitamin B_6 is needed for the biosynthesis of the neurotransmitters serotonin, epinephrine, norepinephrine, and γ-aminobutyric acid; the vasodilator and gastric secretagogue histamine; and the porphyrin precursors of heme. The vitamin is also required for the metabolic conversion of tryptophan to niacin, the release of glucose from glycogen, the biosynthesis of sphingolipids in the myelin sheaths of nerve cells, and the modulation of steroid hormone receptors.

Dietary Reference Intakes

The DRIs for vitamin B_6 include AIs for infants, the redefined RDAs, and the UL for children and adults. In general, needs for vitamin B_6 increase with increasing intake of protein.

Sources

The vitamin is obtained from two exogenous sources: a dietary source absorbed in the small intestine and a bacterial source synthesized in significant quantities by the normal microflora of the large intestine; the carrier-mediated process for PN uptake by mammalian colonocytes is under study (Said et al., 2008).

Vitamin B_6 is widely distributed in foods, occurring in greatest concentrations in meats, whole-grain products (especially wheat), vegetables, and nuts (Table 3-21). Vitamin B_6 derived from animal sources tends to have superior bioavailability. Much of the vitamin B_6 in foods is bound

TABLE 3-21

Pyridoxine Content of Selected Foods

Food	Content (mg)
Ready-to-eat cereals	Up to 3.6
Potato, baked, 1	0.63
Banana, 1	0.43
Rice, white, cooked, 1 cup	0.30
Chicken, light meat, fried, 3 oz	0.53
Pork chop, baked, 3 oz	0.44
Baked beans, vegetarian, 1 cup	0.34
Beef, hamburger, broiled, 3 oz	0.32
Chicken, dark meat, fried, 3 oz	0.31
Tuna, canned, 3 oz	0.30
Sunflower seeds, kernels, ¼ cup	0.26
Avocado, California, 1 oz	0.08
Whole-wheat bread, 1 slice	0.05
DRI Range	
0.1-2.0 mg/day, depending on age and gender	

From U.S. Department of Agriculture, Agricultural Research Service: Nutrient Database for Standard Reference, Release 18, Data Laboratory home page: http://www.nal.usda.gov/fnic/foodcomp/Data/SR18/nutrlist/sr18w415.pdf; accessed 1-14-11.

DRI, Dietary reference intake.

covalently to proteins or glycosylated. PN in some plants (e.g., potatoes, spinach, beans, and other legumes) is often glycosylated and has a low bioavailability.

Deficiency

Deprivation of vitamin B_6 leads to metabolic abnormalities resulting from insufficient production of PLP. These manifest clinically as dermatologic and neurologic changes such as weakness, sleeplessness, peripheral neuropathies, cheilosis, glossitis, stomatitis, and impaired cell-mediated immunity. Inadequate levels of PLP in the brain cause neurologic dysfunction, particularly epilepsy; treatment with PN or PLP can be lifesaving (Clayton, 2006).

Because of the widespread distribution of the vitamin in foods, cases of vitamin B_6 deficiency are relatively rare. However, deficiency may be precipitated by medications like the antitubercular drug isoniazid that interfere with vitamin B_6 metabolism. An increased requirement for PN or PLP is also found with inborn errors affecting the B_6 pathways, celiac disease with malabsorption, and renal dialysis with increased losses of B_6 vitamers (Clayton, 2006).

Toxicity

Many of the signs of vitamin B_6 toxicity resemble those of deficiency. Toxicity from diet is relatively low. High-dose PN or PLP may have deleterious side effects, particularly peripheral neuropathy (Clayton, 2006). Indeed, a man using 9.6 g/day developed severe sensorimotor neuropathy (Gdynia et al., 2008). With over-the-counter use of B_6 for everything from carpal tunnel to premenstrual syndrome, health providers must ask about the frequency of use and the quantity of vitamins consumed, including those considered to be nontoxic because of water solubility.

Folate

Folate refers generally to pteroylmonoglutamic acid and its derived compounds. The reduced compound, tetrahydrofolic acid (FH_4), functions metabolically as a carrier for single-carbon moieties. Each carrier form is named according to the moiety it carries and each can be used in single-carbon synthesis reactions.

Absorption, Transport, and Storage

Dietary folates are absorbed only as the monoglutamate forms of 5-methyltetrahydrofolic acid and 5-formyltetrahydrofolic acid. Absorption occurs by active transport mainly in the jejunum, but the vitamin can also be absorbed by passive diffusion when ingested in large amounts. Because most folate in foods is present in polyglutamate forms (more than one glutamate residue attached), absorption requires hydrolysis to the monoglutamate form in the brush border and intracellular mucosa.

The bioavailability of folates from fruit, vegetables, and liver is approximately 80% that of folic acid; therefore consumption of a diet rich in food folate can improve the folate status of a population more efficiently than was previously thought (Winkels et al., 2007). Although folic acid has historically been used as the reference folate in human intervention studies, using the reference of 5-methyltetrahydrofolic acid is more desirable and realistic (Wright et al., 2009).

Folate taken up by the intestinal mucosal cell is reduced to FH_4, which can either be transferred to the portal circulation or converted to 5-methyl-FH_4 before entering the circulation. Only monoglutamate derivatives found in plasma are taken up by the cells using an energy-dependent process with a specific folate-binding protein or a carrier-mediated process. Within cells, FH_4 is methylated to 5-methyl-FH_4, which is retained intracellularly by binding to intracellular macromolecules. There is additional conversion to folyl polyglutamates. The liver is the most important depot for folate, containing approximately half of the total body store as polyglutamates of 5-methyl-FH_4 and 10-formyl-FH_4. Tissues with high rates of cell division like the intestinal mucosa tend to have low concentrations of 5-methyl-FH_4 and high concentrations of 10-formyl-FH_4, whereas 5-methyl-FH_4 predominates in tissues with low rates of cell division.

Metabolism

Folates are metabolized in three ways: reduction of the pterin ring by the enzyme reductase in the kidney and liver; reactions of the polyglutamyl side chain by the enzyme polyglutamate synthetase, which add the amino acid glutamate; and acquisition of single-carbon moieties at certain positions on the pterin ring.

Folate is metabolically activated by conversion to one of several derivatives with single-carbon units substituted at the N-5 or N-10 (or both) positions of the pterin ring. The main source of the single-carbon fragments is via serine hydroxymethyltransferase, which uses the dispensable amino acid serine and the single-carbon donor to produce 5,10-methylene-FH_4. Other enzymes also yield other single-carbon metabolites: 5-methyl-FH_4, 5, 10-methenyl-FH_4, 5-formimino-FH_4, 5-formyl-FH_4, and 10-formyl-FH_4.

Tissue folates turn over by cleavage of their pteridine and paraaminobenzoyl polyglutamate moieties. The latter are further degraded to a variety of water-soluble side-chain metabolites that are excreted in the urine and bile (Figure 3-23).

Functions

FH_4, with its moieties attached, functions as an enzyme cosubstrate in many synthesis reactions in the metabolism of amino acids and nucleotides by donating or accepting single carbon units. For example, it functions in new synthesis and repair of DNA by transferring formate (as 5,10-methenyl-FH_4) for purine synthesis and formaldehyde (as 5,10-methylene-FH_4) for thymidylate synthesis. It is required for the conversion of histidine to glutamic acid, impairments of which result in accumulation of the intermediary product, formiminoglutamic acid, which must be excreted in the urine.

FH_4 provides labile methyl groups (as 5-methyl-FH_4) for the synthesis of methionine from homocysteine. This conversion also requires vitamin B_{12}, which passes the methyl group from 5-methyl-FH_4 to homocysteine; therefore deficiencies of either folate or vitamin B_{12} can lead to elevated serum homocysteine levels (homocystinemia). Folate deficiency was initially recognized clinically as a macrocytic anemia in the 1920s, and only clearly separated from pernicious anemia by the mid-twentieth century (Lanska, 2009). Because of this interrelationship, deprivation of vitamin B_{12} alone can produce a functional secondary folate deficiency by interrupting the regeneration of FH_4, effectively trapping the vitamin as 5-methyl-FH_4—a process called the *methyl-folate trap*. For synthesis and repair of DNA, both folate and B_{12} have pivotal roles in maintaining gene stability.

Finally, folate is essential for the formation of red and white blood cells in the bone marrow and for their maturation and is a single-carbon carrier in the formation of heme. The role of folate in normal cell division makes it particularly important in embryogenesis. Periconceptual folate supplementation can reduce the risk of serious birth defects, including cleft palate and neural tube defects.

Dietary Reference Intakes

The DRIs for folate are expressed as dietary folate equivalents (DFEs), which is an attempt to account for known differences in the bioavailability of folates noted previously.

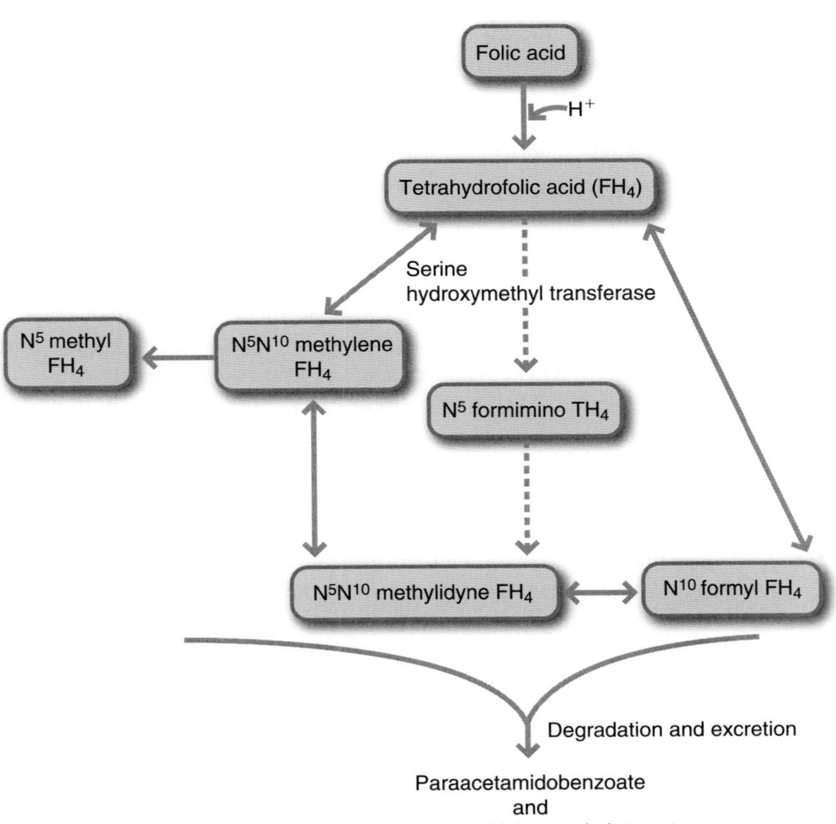

FIGURE 3-23 Metabolism of folates.

One DFE equals 1 mcg of food folate, which is equal to 0.6 mcg of folic acid consumed with food or 0.5 mcg of synthetic folic acid taken as a supplement on an empty stomach. The DRIs for folate include AIs for infants and RDAs for children and adults. The DRIs for women include increased amounts for women who could become pregnant. Although low folate stores are found in approximately 10% of the population, they are not accompanied by overt signs of deficiency.

Sources

Folates exist as reduced folyl polyglutamates (of mostly 5-methyl-FH_4 and 10-formyl-FH_4) in various foods of plant and animal origin. Rich sources include liver, mushrooms, green leafy vegetables ("foliage" such as spinach, asparagus, and broccoli). Lean beef, potatoes, whole-wheat bread, orange juice, and dried beans are good sources (Table 3-22). Although controversial because folic acid can mask a B_{12} deficiency (Osterhues et al., 2009), the United States began fortification of wheat products in 1998. These products are now major sources of folate.

Folate exists in 150 different forms, and their bioavailability varies widely. The reduced forms in foods are easily oxidized. Losses of 50% to 90% typically occur during storage, cooking, or processing at high temperatures. The bioavailability in foods varies considerably because of inherent differences among its forms, the presence or absence of conjugase inhibitors and folate binders, and the nutritional status of the host. Deficiencies of iron and vitamin C can also impair folate use. Analysis of foods for their folate content is complex and difficult, and values in tables of food composition are often too low.

TABLE 3-22

Dietary Folate Equivalents (DFE) of Selected Foods

Food	Content (mcg)
Fortified dry cereal, 1 cup	100-672
Black-eyed peas, boiled, 1 cup	358
Lentils, boiled, 1 cup	358
Beans, white, boiled, 1 cup	263
Spinach, cooked, ½ cup	131
Asparagus, cooked, 1 cup	243
Broccoli, cooked, 1 cup	168
Spaghetti, cooked, enriched, 1 cup	167
Cabbage, Chinese, 1 cup	70
Fresh orange juice, 1 cup	75
Cabbage, raw, 1 cup	30
Egg yolk, 1	27
Banana, 1	24
DRI Range	
65-600 mcg, depending on age and gender	

From U.S. Department of Agriculture, Agricultural Research Service: Nutrient Database for Standard Reference, Release 18, Data Laboratory home page: http://www.nal.usda.gov/fnic/foodcomp/Data/SR18/nutrlist/sr18w435.pdf; accessed 2011.

DRI, Dietary reference intake.

Deficiency

Deficiencies of folate result in impaired biosynthesis of DNA and RNA, thus reducing cell division. This is most apparent in rapidly multiplying cells such as red blood cells, leukocytes, epithelial cells of the stomach, intestine, vagina, and uterine cervix. In blood this is characterized by megaloblastic, macrocytic anemia with large, immature erythrocytes that have excessive amounts of hemoglobin. Initial signs of deficiency in humans include nuclear hypersegmentation of circulating polymorphonuclear leukocytes followed by megaloblastic anemia and then general weakness, depression, and polyneuropathy. Dermatologic lesions and poor growth are also symptoms.

Folate-responsive homocystinemia is related to the role of folate in regeneration of methionine from homocysteine, is a condition associated with elevated risk for occlusive vascular disease, and is prevalent among apparently healthy Americans. Other studies suggest a role for lowering homocysteine in Alzheimer disease, Parkinson disease, amyotrophic lateral sclerosis (ALS), and other neuropsychiatric disorders. This suggests that subclinical folate deficiencies may be more common than previously thought.

There are genetic predispositions for neural tube defects, including both infant and maternal gene polymorphisms for enzymes involved in folate-dependent homocysteine metabolism; the genotype of the mother, the genotype of the unborn child, and environmental factors (e.g., folate intake) can all affect the risk for neural tube defects (Lanska, 2009). Well-designed randomized trials established that folate supplementation prevents more than 70% of neural tube defects (Lanska, 2009). Results from these trials convinced the American government to establish fortification mandates by adding folate to wheat flour.

Where there are genetic polymorphisms in the folate pathway, the bioavailable form (L-methylfolate) can be obtained by prescription for use in pregnancy, cancer prevention, and many neuropsychiatric disorders. Nearly one third of gene-variant cancer associations are statistically significant for variants in genes that encode for metabolizing enzymes; the *MTHFR* gene allele for the C>T phenotype is linked with gastric cancer, for example (Dong et al., 2008). Folate status is assessed by measuring the erythrocyte folate concentration, sometimes in conjunction with plasma homocysteine concentrations and testing for genetic alleles. The interrelationships of B_{12}, folate, and homocysteine continue to intrigue researchers (Varela-Moreiras et al., 2009). Elevated homocysteine levels and low serum folate may play a role in several conditions, including cognitive changes in aging.

High doses of folate may have a positive benefit by reducing arsenic toxicity in genetically susceptible persons. Arsenic-contaminated groundwater is a global environmental health concern known to promote skin and bladder cancers. Arsenic metabolism involves methylation by a folate-dependent process, so folate supplementation may be helpful in excreting more arsenic (Kile and Ronnenberg, 2008).

Toxicity

No adverse effects of high oral doses of folate have been reported in animals, although parenteral administration of amounts some 1000 times the dietary requirement produce epileptiform seizures in the rat. It has been suggested that high levels of folate may render zinc unavailable through the formation of nonabsorbable complexes in the gut, and studies have shown that folate treatment can exacerbate the teratogenic effects of nutritional zinc deficiency in animals. As noted previously, high supplemental doses of folate can mask a B_{12} deficiency if dietary B_{12} is insufficient.

Vitamin B_{12} (Cobalamin)

The term *vitamin B_{12}* (Table 3-23) refers to the family of **cobalamin** compounds containing the porphyrin-like, cobalt-centered corrin nucleus. This family includes analogs containing cobalt-bound methyl groups (methylcobalamin), 5′-deoxyadenosyl groups (adenosylcobalamin), hydroxl (OH^-) groups (hydroxocobalamin), nitrito groups (nitritocobalamin), or water (aquacobalamin). Of the several cobalamin compounds that exhibit vitamin B_{12} activity, cyanocobalamin and hydroxycobalamin are the most active.

TABLE 3-23

Vitamin B12 Content of Selected Foods

Food	Content (mcg)
Liver, beef, 3.5 oz	70.66
Clams, canned, 3 oz	84.06
Oysters, raw, eastern, 6 medium	16.35
Crab, Alaskan king, raw, 3 oz	9.78
Tuna, light, canned, in water, 3 oz	2.54
Beef, hamburger, lean, broiled, 3 oz	2.39
Halibut, baked, ½ filet	2.18
Cottage cheese, 1 cup	1.60
Yogurt with fruit, 8 oz	1.07
Pork chop, boiled, 3.5 oz	0.93
Skim milk, 1 cup	1.30
Bologna, beef and pork, 2 slices	1.03
Ready to eat cereals	0.5-6.00
DRI Range	
0.4-2.8 mcg/day, depending on age and gender	

From U.S. Department of Agriculture, Agricultural Research Service: Nutrient Database for Standard Reference, Release 18, Data Laboratory home page: http://www.nal.usda.gov/fnic/foodcomp/Data/SR18/nutrlist/sr18w418.pdf; accessed 2011.

DRI, Dietary reference intake.

Absorption, Transport, and Storage

Vitamin B_{12} is bound to protein in food and must be released from it by pepsin digestion in the stomach. The vitamin then combines with R proteins (cobalophilins) in the stomach and moves into the small intestine, where the R proteins are hydrolyzed and intrinsic factor (IF), a specific binding protein for B_{12} produced in the stomach, binds the cobalamin. Most vitamin B_{12} is absorbed by this active transport, and IF is essential to the process. Only approximately 1% can be absorbed by simple diffusion even in high amounts. IF can bind any of the four cobalamins in an IF–vitamin B_{12} complex by which the vitamin is taken into the enterocyte by a process involving binding to a specific membrane receptor on the ileal brush border (Figure 3-24). After absorption, cobalamin binds to the plasma R proteins known as transcobalamins (TCs): TCI, TCII, and TCIII. TCII is the main transporter protein for newly absorbed cobalamins as they circulate to peripheral tissues (Gropper et al., 2005). Cellular uptake of vitamin B_{12} seems to be mediated by a specific TC receptor that internalizes the TC-vitamin complex. After lysosomal degradation of TC, the free vitamin is released for binding to vitamin B_{12}–dependent enzymes.

In adequately nourished individuals, vitamin B_{12} is stored in appreciable amounts (≈2000 mcg) mainly in the liver, which typically accumulates a substantial store—some 5 to 7 years' worth—mostly in the form of adenosylcobalamin. Enterohepatic circulation of the vitamin also contributes to these stores.

Metabolism

Vitamin B_{12} is metabolically active only as derivatives that have either a 5″-deoxyadenosine or a methyl group attached covalently to the corrin ring cobalt atom. These conversions are accomplished by vitamin B_{12} coenzyme synthetase and 5-methyl-FH_4:homocysteine methyltransferase, respectively. Little or no metabolism of the corrinoid ring system occurs, and the vitamin is excreted intact by renal and biliary routes. Only the free plasma cobalamins, not the adenosylated or methylated forms, are available for excretion.

Functions

Vitamin B_{12} functions in two coenzyme forms: adenosylcobalamin (with methylmalonyl-CoA mutase and leucine mutase) and methylcobalamin (with methionine synthetase). These forms of the vitamin play important roles in the metabolism of propionate, amino acids, and single carbons, respectively. Because these steps are essential for normal metabolism of cells in the GI tract, bone marrow, and nervous tissue, a deficiency of the vitamin is marked by increases in plasma and urinary levels of methylmalonic acid, aminoisocaproate, homocysteine and losses of FH_4 (via the methyl folate trap).

Dietary Reference Intakes

Vitamin B_{12} is expressed in micrograms. The DRIs for vitamin B_{12} include AIs for infants and defined RDAs. The

FIGURE 3-24 Digestion and absorption of vitamin B_{12}. $B1_2$-R: B_{12}, R Protein complex; B_{12}-IF: B_{12}, intrinsic factor complex; B_{12}-TCII: B_{12}, transcobalamin II complex.

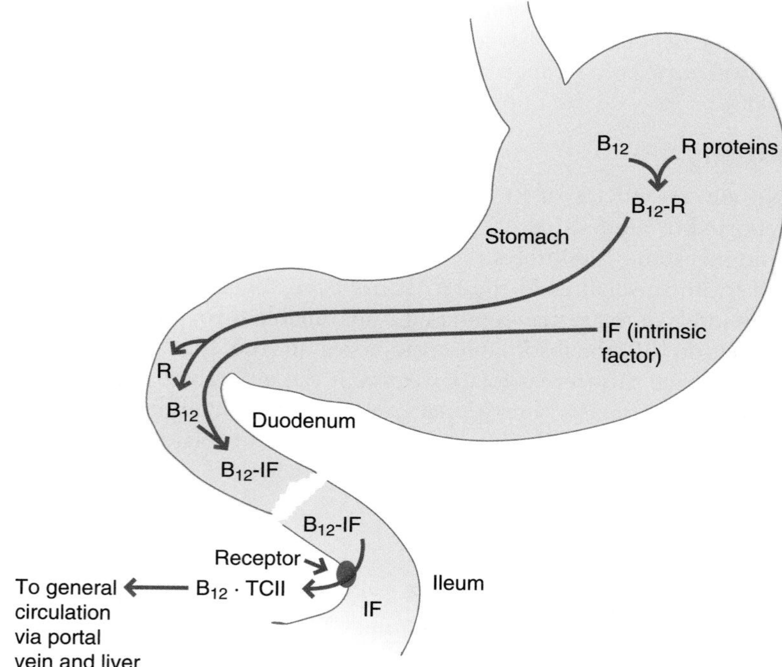

adult RDA provides for substantial body stores because of the prevalences of achlorhydria and atrophic gastritis associated with losses of IF production and of pernicious anemia in those older than 60 years of age.

Sources

Vitamin B_{12} is synthesized by bacteria, but the vitamin produced from the microflora in the colon is not absorbed. The richest sources of the vitamin are liver and kidney, milk, eggs, fish, cheese, and muscle meats (see Table 3-23). Foods of plant origin contain the vitamin only through contamination or bacterial synthesis.

Many people believe that fermented foods contain sufficient vitamin B_{12} to meet their needs; however, this theory is not supported by analysis. Individuals consuming strictly vegetarian (vegan) diets, particularly after 5 to 6 years, typically have lower circulating levels of vitamin B_{12} unless they use supplemental forms. This is not true for ovolactovegetarians whose diets include food sources of vitamin B_{12}.

Because the vitamin is found in food bound to protein, approximately 70% of its activity is retained during the cooking of most foods. However, appreciable amounts of the vitamin can be lost when milk is pasteurized or evaporated.

Deficiency

Vitamin B_{12} deficiency causes impaired cell division, particularly in the rapidly dividing cells of the bone marrow and intestinal mucosa, through arrested synthesis of DNA. The ensuing reduction in mitotic rate results in abnormally large cells and a characteristic megaloblastic anemia. The anemia of B_{12} deficiency relates to a secondary folate deficiency because of the methyl folate trap (see "Folate" earlier in this chapter). Folate supplementation alleviates the anemia caused by B_{12} deficiency; however, other symptoms progress unless B_{12} is provided. Cobalamin deficiency also produces neurologic abnormalities that develop much later than the anemia, with nerve demyelination commencing peripherally and proceeding centrally. Symptoms include numbness, tingling and burning of the feet, stiffness and generalized weakness of the legs, neurologic disorders including impaired mentation, and depression. If prolonged, deficiency causes permanent nerve damage. Finally, B_{12} deficiency symptoms may include a waxy, lemon-yellow tint to the skin and eyes; and a smooth, beefy, red tongue.

Poor vitamin B_{12} status occurs from a low dietary intake of the vitamin from animal-source foods and from malabsorption. Deficiency occurs in 15% of seniors older than age 65 (Andrés et al., 2007). Food-bound cobalamin malabsorption is due to gastric atrophy in the older adults, probably as a result of *Helicobacter pylori* infection (Allen, 2008).

A more common cause of vitamin B_{12} deficiency is malabsorption because of inadequate production and secretion of IF. Clinically a form of pernicious anemia, it may result from atrophy of gastric parietal cells or autoimmune incapacitation of IF. Gene polymorphisms in TCs affect plasma vitamin B_{12} concentrations (Allen, 2008). Although cobalamin injections are commonly prescribed, oral cobalamin therapy is especially useful for food-cobalamin malabsorption (Andrés et al., 2007).

The long-term consumption of strict vegan diets without supplemental vitamin B_{12} leads to very low circulating levels. Vitamin B_{12} deficiency and bone fractures are common in vegetarians and so must be managed carefully (Hermann et al., 2009). In addition, bariatric surgeries may aggravate preexisting B_{12} deficiency or cause one. The Roux-en-Y procedure is more problematic than laparoscopic sleeve gastrectomy (Gehrer et al., 2010).

Serum B_{12} level is not a good indicator of status. Although the methods are expensive, vitamin B_{12} is best assessed by measuring blood levels of the metabolites methylmalonic acid and homocysteine, which are B_{12} dependent.

Toxicity

Vitamin B_{12} has no appreciable toxicity.

Biotin

Biotin (see Table 3-12) consists of a ureido ring joined to a thiophene ring with a valeric acid side chain and is necessary for critical carboxylations in metabolism.

Absorption, Transport, and Storage

Biotin in foods is largely protein bound. It is released by proteolytic digestion to yield free biotin, biocytin, or biotin-peptide. Biotinidase of pancreatic or intestinal origin releases free biotin from the latter two compounds. Free biotin is absorbed in the proximal small intestine by carrier-mediated diffusion or specific transporters (Zempleni, 2009 2008). Smaller amounts of biotin can also be absorbed from the colon, which facilitates the use of the vitamin produced by hindgut microflora. Biotin is transported in the plasma primarily as free biotin, but approximately 12% is also bound to protein and biotinidase. Biotin is taken into cells by a specific carrier-mediated process. Appreciable amounts of the vitamin are stored in the liver; however, these stores do not seem to be mobilized well when the body is deprived of the vitamin.

Metabolism

Little catabolism of biotin occurs, but some of the vitamin is oxidized to biotin sulfoxides. The vitamin is rapidly excreted in the urine (95% of an oral dose is excreted within 24 hours)—half as free biotin and the balance as bisnorbiotin, biotin sulfoxides, and various side-chain metabolites.

Functions

Biotin is a carboxyl carrier covalently bound to the carboxylase enzymes pyruvate carboxylase (which converts pyruvate to oxaloacetate in gluconeogenesis), acetyl CoA carboxylase (which synthesizes malonyl CoA for fatty acid formation), propionyl CoA carboxylase (which allows the use of odd-chain fatty acids by converting propionate to succinate), and 3-methylcrotonyl-CoA carboxylase (which catabolizes leucine). These roles of biotin link it to the metabolic roles of folic acid, pantothenic acid, and vitamin B_{12}. In recent years noncarboxylase roles for biotin have been elucidated, including a direct effect of biotin at the transcription level on glucokinase and phosphoenol pyruvate carboxykinase, as well as other enzymes (Dakshinamurti, 2005; Zempleni et al., 2009).

Dietary Reference Intake

The AIs for biotin have been established. However, because of uncertainty about the amount of biotin provided by intestinal flora and differences in bioavailability of biotin from foods, the establishment of EARs and RDAs is problematic.

Sources

Biotin is widely distributed in foods, but its content varies significantly, it has been determined for relatively few foods, and it may not be very accurate. Peanuts, almonds, soy protein, eggs, yogurt, nonfat milk, and sweet potatoes are sources. Biotin content is not usually reported in food composition tables (IOM, Food and Nutrition Board, 2000b). The bioavailability of biotin varies considerably among different foods because of differences in the digestibility of various biotin-protein complexes. Biotin is unstable in oxidizing conditions and is destroyed by heat, especially in the presence of lipid peroxidation.

In addition to foods, intestinal bacteria can also contribute appreciable amounts of biotin. Fecal and urinary excretions are considerably higher than dietary intake, reflecting the magnitude of the microfloral synthesis of biotin.

Deficiency

Because biotin can be obtained from many foods and gut microbial metabolism, simple biotin deficiency in animals is rare. Biotin deficiency has been induced by feeding raw egg white or its active component—the heat-labile, biotin-binding protein avidin. Avidin impairs biotin absorption, causing such symptoms as seborrheic dermatitis, alopecia, and paralysis. Impaired biotin absorption can also occur in such GI tract disorders as inflammatory bowel diseases or achlorhydria. Zempleni et al., (2009) noted that decreases in the activities of biotinidase and other proteins associated with digestion, absorption, and transport of biotin can cause a deficiency.

The few cases of biotin deficiency that have been described in humans have involved patients receiving incomplete parenteral nutrition and nursing infants whose mothers' milk contained very low amounts of the vitamin. In each case the signs included dermatitis, glossitis, anorexia, nausea, depression, hepatic steatosis, and hypercholesterolemia. Inherited defects in all of the known biotin enzymes have been identified in humans, but they are rare and usually have serious neurologic consequences. Blood levels of biotin are most often used to assess biotin status.

Toxicity

Biotin has no known toxic effects, even in very large doses.

Ascorbic Acid

Vitamin C, or **ascorbic acid** (see Table 3-12), is synthesized from glucose and galactose by plants and most animals. However, humans, other primates, guinea pigs, some bats, and a few species of birds, lack the enzyme l-gulonolactone oxidase and thus cannot biosynthesize the factor; for them, it is a vitamin.

Absorption, Transport, and Storage

Species that cannot biosynthesize ascorbic acid absorb it from the diet by active transport and passive diffusion. The oxidized form of the vitamin, dehydroascorbic acid, is better absorbed than the reduced form, ascorbate, or ascorbic acid. The efficiency of enteric absorption of the vitamin is 80% to 90% at low intakes, but declines markedly at intakes greater than 1 g/day.

Vitamin C is transported in the plasma in the reduced form in free solution. It is taken up by cells via GLUT 1, GLUT 2, and GLUT 3, as well as sodium-coupled transporters (sodium-dependent vitamin C transporter 1 and 2) (Rivas et al., 2008). Each system moves dehydroascorbic acid into cells, where it is readily reduced to ascorbate. The GLUT-based system of uptake is not as fast as the specific system, but it is stimulated by insulin and inhibited by glucose. Thus diabetic patients with high glucose levels typically have high plasma levels and low cellular levels of dehydroascorbic acid. The vitamin is concentrated primarily as dehydroascorbic acid in many vital organs, particularly the adrenals, brain, and eye.

Metabolism

Ascorbic acid is oxidized in vivo by two successive losses of single electrons forming the free radical (monodehydroascorbic acid). This intermediate can be further oxidized to dehydroascorbic acid (Figure 3-25). Subsequently the oxidized product undergoes irreversible hydrolysis to yield 2,3-diketo-l-gulonic acid, which can be decarboxylated to yield carbon dioxide and several five-carbon fragments (e.g., xylose, xylonic acid) or oxidized to yield oxalic acid and several four-carbon fragments (e.g., threonic acid). In addition, the vitamin can be converted to ascorbic acid 2-sulfate.

Functions

Because ascorbic acid easily loses electrons and is reversibly converted to dehydroascorbic acid, it serves as a biochemical redox system involved in many electron transport reactions, including those involved in the synthesis of collagen and carnitine and other metabolic reactions. During collagen and carnitine synthesis, vitamin C acts as a reducing agent to keep iron in its ferrous state, thus enabling hydroxylation enzymes to function. For example, collagen, the major protein in fibrous tissues such as connective tissue, cartilage, bone matrix, and tendons, depends on the posttranslational hydroxylation of proline residues in procollagen to form hydroxyproline.

Cellular vitamin C deficiency may lead to oxidative stress in cells, contributing to an increased risk of ischemic heart disease (McNulty et al., 2007). An important role for vitamin C in atherogenesis is as a vasodilator because of its redox properties (Frikke-Schmidt and Lykkesfeldt, 2009). Vitamin C concentration decreases in periods of stress when adrenal cortical hormone activity is high. During periods of emotional, psychological, or physiologic stress, the urinary excretion of ascorbic acid increases.

Ascorbic acid also acts as an antioxidant as it undergoes single-electron oxidation to the ascorbyl radical and dehydroascorbate. By reacting with potentially toxic reactive oxygen species such as the superoxide or hydroxyl radical, the vitamin can prevent oxidative damage. Vitamin C is essential for the oxidation of phenylalanine and tyrosine, the conversion of folate to FH_4, the conversion of tryptophan to 5-hydroxytryptophan and the neurotransmitter serotonin, and the formation of norepinephrine from dopamine. It also reduces ferric to ferrous iron in the intestinal tract to facilitate iron absorption and is involved in the transfer of iron from plasma transferrin to liver ferritin.

Vitamin C promotes resistance to infection through its involvement with the immunologic activity of leukocytes, the production of interferon, the process of inflammatory reaction, and the integrity of the mucous membranes. The value of large amounts of ascorbic acid to prevent and cure the common cold has been reported, but conclusions from these studies remain controversial (Heimen et al., 2009). It is generally accepted that taking high doses of vitamin C for colds reduces the severity of the symptoms, but it does not prevent them. Vitamin C maintains proper lung function, especially in asthma (Kaur et al., 2009).

Dietary Reference Intakes

The DRIs for vitamin C are expressed quantitatively in milligrams. Although as little as 10 mg of vitamin C can prevent scurvy, this level does not provide acceptable reserves of the vitamin. Because of the lower concentrations of ascorbic acid in the serum of cigarette smokers, it has been recommended that smokers increase their intake. Whereas the average body pool of vitamin C is 1.5 g, of which 40 to

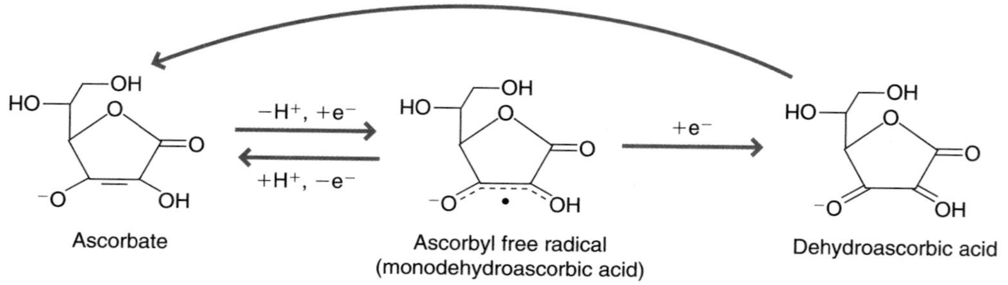

FIGURE 3-25 Oxidation-reduction reaction of vitamin C. *(From Combs GF: The vitamins: fundamental aspects in nutrition and health, ed. 2, Orlando, 1998, Academic Press.)*

TABLE 3-24

Vitamin C Content of Selected Foods

Food	Amount	Content (mg)
Pepper, sweet, yellow	1 cup	283
Orange juice		
Fresh	1 cup	124
Frozen, diluted, canned	1 cup	97
Canned	1 cup	86
Broccoli		
Fresh, boiled	1 cup	116
Frozen, chopped, boiled	1 cup	74
Brussels sprouts, cooked	1 cup	97
Strawberries	1 cup	106
Grapefruit juice, from frozen concentrate, unsweetened	1 cup	83
Cantaloupe	1 cup	68
Mango	1	57
Kale, from raw, cooked	1 cup	53
Tomato juice	1 cup	45
DRI Range		
15-120 mg/day, depending on age and gender		

From U.S. Department of Agriculture, Agricultural Research Service: Nutrient Database for Standard Reference, Release 18, Data Laboratory home page: http://www.nal.usda.gov/fnic/foodcomp/Data/SR18/nutrlist/sr18w401.pdf; accessed 2011.

DRI, Dietary reference intake.

60 mg is used daily, smokers may need as much as 140 mg/day (Berger, 2009).

Sources

Vitamin C is found in plants and animal tissues as ascorbic acid and dehydroascorbic acid. The best sources are fruits, vegetables, and organ meats, but the actual ascorbic acid contents of foods can vary with the conditions of growth and degree of ripeness when harvested. Refrigeration and quick freezing help retain the vitamin. Most commercially frozen foods are processed so close to the source of supply that their ascorbic acid content is often higher than that of fresh foods that have been shipped across the country and spent time in storage and on supermarket shelves. Table 3-24 lists the vitamin C content of selected fruits and vegetables. Citrus fruits and juices are very important sources of the vitamin for many Americans, who tend not to eat many servings of other fruits and vegetables.

Ascorbic acid is easily destroyed by oxidation, and, because it is soluble in water, it is often extracted and discarded in cooking water. Sodium bicarbonate, added to preserve and improve the color of cooked vegetables, destroys vitamin C. The cumulative losses of the vitamin from prepared vegetables refrigerated for 24 hours can be as high as 45% in fresh products and 52% in frozen products. Because consumers are eating out more frequently and more foods are being supplied to restaurants or institutions partially prepared (e.g., shredded lettuce, peeled and diced vegetables) or served from open salad bars, this vitamin loss must be considered when evaluating dietary intake.

Deficiency

Acute vitamin C deficiency results in **scurvy** in individuals unable to synthesize the vitamin. In human adults signs are manifest after 45 to 80 days of vitamin C deprivation. In children the syndrome is called *Moeller-Barlow disease;* it can also develop in infants fed formulas not enriched with vitamin C. In both cases lesions occur in mesenchymal tissues and result in impaired wound healing; edema; hemorrhages; and weakness in bone, cartilage, teeth, and connective tissues. Adults with scurvy may have swollen, bleeding gums with eventual tooth loss, lethargy, fatigue, rheumatic pains in the legs, muscular atrophy, skin lesions, and a variety of psychological changes.

Toxicity

Vitamin C is one of the most commonly used supplements in the United States. The adverse effects of high doses of vitamin C in humans include GI disturbances and diarrhea. Because the catabolism of vitamin C yields oxalate (among other metabolites), it is also reasonable to be concerned about the possibility of high doses of the vitamin increasing the risk of forming renal oxalate stones (see Chapter 36). Individuals with histories of forming renal stones should avoid consuming too much vitamin C. Excess ascorbic acid excreted in the urine can also give a false-positive urinary glucose test. The relationship of vitamin C to cancer is discussed later in the text. Table 3-12 summarizes the information on the known vitamins.

OTHER VITAMIN-LIKE FACTORS

Other food factors have vitamin characteristics but do not meet the criteria of vitamin status. These quasivitamins include those that can be biosynthesized but may be beneficial supplements in certain life stages or medical conditions (e.g., choline and betaine, carnitine) and those yet to be proven to be essential in the diet (e.g., myo-inositol, the ubiquinones, the bioflavonoids).

Choline and Betaine

Choline (2-hydroxy-*N,N,N*-trimethylenthanolamine) is a methyl-rich essential component of animal tissues, where it is a structural component of lecithin (phosphatidylcholine) in membrane phospholipids and the neurotransmitter acetylcholine. Choline is released by the hydrolysis of lecithin by pancreatic and intestinal lipases and is absorbed by a carrier-mediated process and passive diffusion. Absorbed choline is transported via chylomicrons in the lymphatic circulation primarily in the form of lecithin; it is transferred to lipoproteins in this form for distribution to peripheral tissues. Choline can be biosynthesized from ethanolamine by sequential methylations using *S*-adenosylmethionine, but most humans obtain it from dietary phosphatides.

Betaine (*N,N,N*-trimethylglycine) was named for its source, sugar beets.

Functions

Choline and betaine are important components of the one-carbon metabolism cycle, linked with the amino acid homocysteine and lipid metabolism (Bruce et al., 2010). Choline has several other functions as a methyl donor. As phosphatidylcholine it is a structural element of membranes, a precursor to the sphingolipids, and a promoter of lipid transport. As acetylcholine, it is a neurotransmitter and a component of platelet-activating factor. It functions as an emulsifier in bile, thus helping with the absorption of fat, and is also a component of pulmonary surfactant.

Betaine (Cystadane) may be prescribed to treat homocystinuria or homocystinemia; it is a "nutrient" within the drug classification system. Betaine may also be used to protect against ethanol damage in the brain and the liver. Betaine homocysteine methyltransferase catalyzes a methionine pathway. When ethanol intake is prolonged, this enzyme remethylates homocysteine and supports desirable levels of *S*-adenosylmethionine, which is the key methylating agent (Kharbanda, 2009).

Dietary Reference Intakes

The AIs were established for choline as part of the 1998 DRIs. The UL has been set at 3.5 g/day. Mean choline intakes for older children, men, women, and pregnant women are far below the AI level established by the IOM (Zeisel and da Costa, 2009). There are no DRIs or AIs established for betaine.

Sources

Choline is widely distributed in fat as lecithin (eggs, liver, soybeans, beef, milk, and peanuts). Eggs and meats are the richest sources of choline in the North American diet, providing up to 430 mg/100 g (Zeisel and da Costa, 2009). Whole-grain cereal products and products containing cereal bran are excellent dietary sources of free choline and betaine (Bruce et al., 2010). Free choline is also present in liver, oatmeal, soybeans, iceberg lettuce, cauliflower, kale, and cabbage.

Deficiency

Choline deficiency is thought to have an effect on diseases such as liver disease, atherosclerosis, and neurologic disorders (Zeisel and da Costa, 2009). Deficiency during the perinatal period results in "metabolic imprinting," a permanent alteration in the cholinergic organization of the brain (Meck and Williams, 2003). Elevated neural tube defects are associated with lower levels of total choline, despite grain fortification with folic acid in the United States (Shaw et al., 2009).

Metabonomics may become a diagnostic tool in conditions such as ulcerative colitis (UC). In active and quiescent UC, biopsies show lower levels of lipid, glycerophosphocholine, myo-inositol, and betaine (Bjerrum et al., 2010). Oral supplements of choline may increase endurance in athletes, but only if blood choline levels are low (Penry and Manore, 2008). Finally, no correlation has been found from low intakes of choline or betaine with cancers at this time.

Carnitine

Carnitine (β-hydroxy-γ-*N*-trimethylaminobutyrate) helps transport LCFAs into the mitochondria for oxidation as sources of energy in the carnitine palmitoyltransferase system (Rufer et al., 2009). Mammals and birds can synthesize carnitine from the amino acid lysine using a process that requires vitamin C. In some instances carnitine may be a conditionally essential nutrient. Carnitine is efficiently absorbed across the gut by active transport and simple diffusion. Approximately half of carnitine is acetylated during absorption; free and acetylated forms are found in circulation in plasma and erythrocytes. Carnitine is taken up primarily by skeletal peripheral tissues, which contain approximately 90% of the body stores. Foods of plant origin are generally low in carnitine, whereas meats and dairy products are good sources.

Tissue depletion of carnitine has been reported in adults undergoing hemodialysis, adults with liver disease, and preterm infants. Carnitine supplementation improves fatty acid oxidation, which is important in cardiovascular disease and in type 2 diabetes (Mingrone, 2004). Deficiency may also be apparent in some genetic metabolic disorders (see Chapter 44).

Myo-inositol

Myo-inositol (*cis*-1,2,3,5-*trans*-4,6-cyclohexanehexol) functions in metabolism as *phosphatidylinositol* (PI). This provides structural support in membranes and serves as an anchor for membrane proteins through covalent bonding. PI is a source of arachidonic acid for the biosynthesis of eicosanoids. In addition, PI is the source of important intracellular signals and secondary cell messengers in response to hormonal stimuli. For example, hormone-sensitive phospholipase C can act on phosphorylated PI, producing free inositol triphosphate (IP3) and a diacylglycerol (DAG). IP3 activates the release of calcium ions, which in turn stimulate calcium-dependent enzymes. DAG initiates a process that results in the alteration of some cellular enzyme activities

(Gropper et al., 2005). IP is concentrated in the brain and cerebrospinal fluid but also exists in other tissues. Myo-inositol may be useful in the treatment of bipolar disorder caused by abnormalities in the role of PI as a cell messenger, but has not yet been found relevant to other psychiatric disorders (Kim, 2005).

Myo-inositol is efficiently absorbed in its free form by an active transport process. It is transported in the blood primarily in its free form, with some as PI associated with lipoproteins. Free myo-inositol is converted in the tissue to PI, which is metabolized by sequential phosphorylations to the monophosphate and diphosphate forms.

Mammals synthesize myo-inositol from glucose; but it is also obtained from fruits, grains, vegetables, nuts, legumes, and organ meats such as liver and heart. Dietary sources include various inositol phospholipids in animal products and phytic acid (inositol hexaphosphate) in plant materials. Because humans and most other mammals lack an intestinal phytase, phytic acid is not a useful source of myo-inositol. Phytates are not listed in food composition tables, but they may actually have some benefits for lowering blood glucose and lipids (Schlemmer et al., 2009).

Only female gerbils and certain fish have been shown to have a clear dietary need for pre-formed myo-inositol. In these animals deprivation of the factor produced anorexia, dermatologic lesions, and intestinal lipodystrophy. Experimental pharmaceutical treatment alternatives for treatment-resistant depression are being explored; they include inositol along with ω-3 fatty acids, *S*-adenosyl-*L*-methionine, and folic acid (Shelton et al., 2010). In addition, inositol has been studied for its role in sleep management, bipolar disorder, and other neurologic disorders. To date, a daily requirement for inositol has yet to be defined.

Ubiquinones

The **ubiquinones** are a group of substituted 1,4-benzoquinone derivatives with varying lengths of isopentyl side chains. The principal species has 10 such side-chain units and is referred to as **coenzyme Q_{10} (CoQ_{10})**, first isolated in 1957. The ubiquinones are essential components of the mitochondrial electron transport chain, in which they undergo reversible reduction-oxidation reactions to pass electrons from flavoproteins (NAD or succinic dehydrogenases) to the cytochromes via cytochrome b5. In addition, the redox properties of CoQ_{10} enable it to function as a fat-soluble antioxidant, much like α-tocopherol. Relatively high concentrations of the ubiquinones are maintained in tissues, apparently by biosynthesis from endogenous precursors.

The use of CoQ_{10} in clinical situations has been extensively reviewed. Low ubiquinone synthesis may play a role in the causal factors of heart disease; supplemental CoQ_{10} may be useful in treating cardiomyopathy and congestive heart failure. CoQ_{10} and its analogue, idebenone, have also been widely used in the treatment of Parkinson disease, Huntington disease, ALS, Friedreich ataxia, and other mitochondrial disorders (Mancuso et al., 2010). Mitochondrial dysfunction leads to oxidative stress, deletions or damage to mitochondrial DNA, altered morphology, and ultimately neuronal demise (Beal, 2009). Loss of CoQ_{10} after HMG-CoA reductase inhibitor (statin) treatment has been implicated in the associated myotoxicity (Mancuso et al., 2010). CoQ_{10} is found in various foods, most notably fish oils, nuts, fish, and meats.

Bioflavonoids

The **bioflavonoids** (phenolic derivatives of 2-phenyl-1, 4-benzopyrone) have no known immediate metabolic function. They have been shown to reduce capillary fragility and potentiate the antiscorbutic activity of ascorbic acid, both of which may involve their chelation of divalent metal ions (Cu^{++}, Fe^{++}) and their intrinsic antioxidant properties. Epidemiologic studies have shown an association between diets high in bioflavonoids and reduced risks for cardiovascular disease and several cancers. The bioflavonoids are ubiquitous in foods of plant origin; more than 800 different bioflavonoids, such as quercetin, rutin, and hesperidin, have been isolated from plants in which they are the major sources of noncarotenoid red, blue, and yellow pigments.

MICRONUTRIENTS: MINERALS

The mineral nutrients most are traditionally divided into **macrominerals** (≥100 mg/day required) and **microminerals** or trace elements (<15 mg/day required). Studies of patients receiving long-term total parenteral nutrition (TPN) have helped to determine the essentiality of **ultratrace elements** that are necessary in microgram quantities each day. Mineral nutrients are recognized as essential for human function, even though specific requirements have not been established for a few of them.

MINERAL COMPOSITION OF THE BODY

Minerals represent approximately 4% to 5% of body weight, or 2.8 to 3.5 kg in adult women and men, respectively. Approximately 50% of this weight is calcium, and another 25% is phosphorus, existing as phosphates. Almost 99% of the calcium and 70% of the phosphates are found in bones and teeth. The five other essential macrominerals (magnesium, sodium, potassium, chloride, and sulfur) and the 11 established microminerals (iron, zinc, iodide, selenium, manganese, fluoride, molybdenum, copper, chromium, cobalt, and boron) constitute the remaining 25%. The ultratrace elements such as arsenic, aluminum, tin, nickel, vanadium, and silicon, provide a negligible amount of weight.

Macrominerals exist in the body and food chiefly in the ionic state. Sodium, potassium, and calcium form positive ions (cations), whereas other minerals exist as negative ions (anions). The latter include chlorine as chloride, sulfur as sulfate, and phosphorus as phosphates. Minerals also exist as components of organic compounds such as phosphoproteins, phospholipids, metalloenzymes, and other metalloproteins such as hemoglobin.

With the exception of heme iron, minerals are usually absorbed in the ionic state. Therefore minerals that remain bound to organic molecules (chelated) or remain as inorganic complexes after the digestion usually cannot be absorbed and are not bioavailable. However, a few minerals may be absorbed better in a chelated form when they are properly bound to an amino acid in a covalent bond (e.g., selenomethionine). Unabsorbed minerals are excreted in the feces. Once a mineral is absorbed at the brush border of the intestinal epithelial cells, each must transfer through the cytosol and be transported across the basolateral membrane into the blood, usually by an active transport mechanism. If the mineral is not transported across the basolateral membrane, it remains in the intestinal cell bound to proteins. For example, calcium ions bind to calbindins, iron to intestinal ferritin, and zinc to metallothionein; if not transported into the blood, they are excreted when the intestinal cells die and slough off into the intestinal lumen. Such mechanisms may have evolved to protect the body against the potential toxicity of excessive absorption.

Bioavailability also is equated with absorption of a mineral element after its digestion from food and before its use in tissue and cells. Several factors can affect bioavailability of ingested minerals. Low bioavailability may also result from the formation of soaps, from calcium and magnesium binding to free fatty acids in the lumen in fat malabsorption, or from precipitation when one of a pair of ions (e.g., calcium, which combines with phosphates) is present in the lumen in a very high concentration. Mineral-mineral interactions also can result in depressed absorption of elements or reduced bioavailability. For example, the absorption of zinc is typically reduced by nonheme iron supplementation; excessive intake of zinc reduces the absorption of copper; and excessive intake of calcium may reduce the absorption of manganese, zinc, and iron.

Many organic molecules in foods influence bioavailability, either by enhancing absorption or inhibiting absorption. Examples of inhibitors include the binding by phytates and oxalates of calcium and other divalent cations. Enhancers include ascorbate for nonheme iron or the hemoglobin protein for iron. Vegetarians tend to consume foods with higher quantities of many of the inhibiting factors, but they typically also ingest more ascorbic acid, an enhancer. In addition, the bioavailability of elements may be influenced by many physiologic factors such as gastric acidity, homeostatic adaptations, and stress. NDOs fermented by intestinal bacteria stimulate the intestinal absorption and retention of calcium, magnesium, zinc, and iron.

Certain minerals generally have a low bioavailability from foods (e.g., iron, chromium, manganese), whereas others have a high bioavailability (e.g., sodium, potassium, chloride, iodide, fluoride). Calcium and magnesium have a medium bioavailability.

Problem Minerals in the U.S. Diet

A few minerals, such as calcium and iron, continue to be consumed in less than optimal amounts by a large percentage of people in the United States. The intakes of magnesium, zinc, and possibly a couple of other trace minerals are also generally insufficient in the population. In the last decade fortification of foods, especially of ready-to-eat cereals, have improved intakes of iron and zinc but not calcium (Heaney and Rafferty, 2009); the mean intakes still do not meet DRI levels.

Calcium

Calcium, the most abundant mineral in the body, makes up approximately 1.5% to 2% of the body weight and 39% of total body minerals. Approximately 99% of the calcium exists in the bones and teeth. The calcium in teeth, unlike bone, cannot be mobilized back to the blood; the minerals of erupted teeth are fixed. The remaining 1% of calcium is in the blood and extracellular fluids and within the cells of all tissues, where it regulates many important metabolic functions. Figure 3-26 illustrates the pathways of calcium metabolism. Bone is a dynamic tissue that returns calcium and other minerals to the extracellular fluids and blood on demand. Bone also takes up calcium and other minerals from the blood when they are consumed.

Absorption, Transport, Storage, and Excretion

Calcium is absorbed by all parts of the small intestine, but the most rapid absorption after a meal occurs in the more acidic (pH <7) duodenum. Absorption is slower in the remainder of the small bowel because of the alkaline pH, but the amount of calcium absorbed is actually greater in the lower segments of the small intestine, including the ileum. Small amounts of calcium can also be absorbed in the colon. Only approximately 30% of ingested calcium is absorbed by adults, but a few individuals may absorb as little as 10% and some (rarely) as much as 60% of ingested calcium. Late in life, bone retention of calcium from food and supplements is limited unless sufficient vitamin D or a bone-conserving drug is available.

Calcium is absorbed by two mechanisms: active transport, which operates predominantly at low luminal concentrations of calcium ions, and passive transport or paracellular transfer, which operates at high luminal concentrations of calcium ions. The active transport mechanism, mainly in the duodenum and proximal jejunum, has limited capacity. It is controlled through the action of $1,25(OH)_2D_3$. This vitamin-hormone increases calcium uptake at the brush border of the intestinal mucosal cell by also stimulating the production of calcium-binding proteins (**calbindins**) and other mechanisms. The role of calbindins in the intestinal absorbing cells is to store calcium ions temporarily after a meal and ferry them to the basolateral membrane for the final step of absorption. The

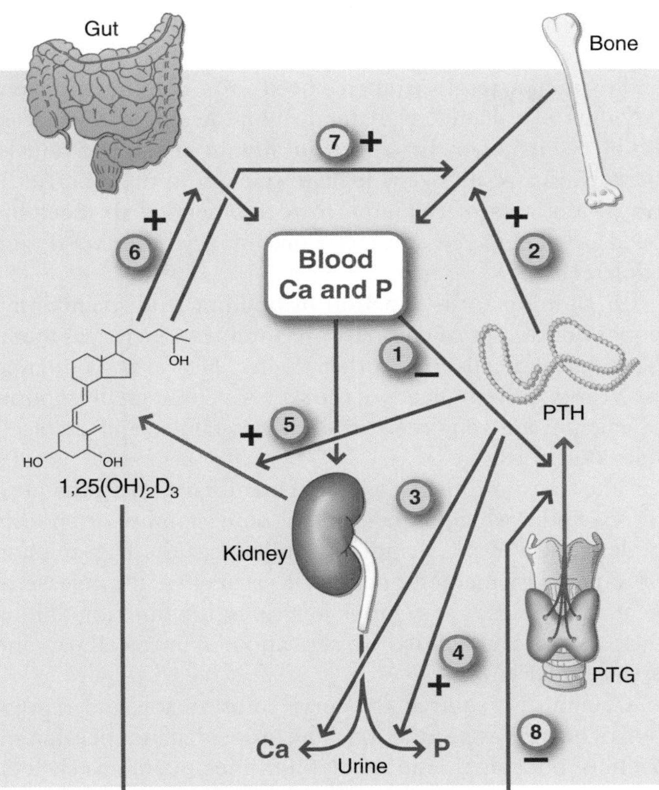

FIGURE 3-26 Pathways of calcium metabolism. The regulation of calcium metabolism involves intestinal absorption (gut), blood calcium, and phosphate concentrations, bone, the kidneys—which produce the hormonal form of vitamin D (1,25[OH]2 D3)—and the parathyroid glands, which secrete parathyroid hormone (PTH). Steps 1 through 8 are specific regulation points. A low serum calcium or high serum phosphate level stimulates PTH secretion (step 1) through negative feedback.

calcium-binding proteins bind two or more calcium ions per protein molecule.

The second absorption mechanism, which is passive, nonsaturable (with no limit), and independent of vitamin D, occurs along the entire length of the small intestine. When large amounts of calcium are consumed in a single meal (e.g., from a dairy food or a supplement), much of the calcium is absorbed by this passive route. The active transport mechanism is more important when calcium intakes are well below recommended intakes and body requirements are not being met.

Numerous factors influence the bioavailability and absorption of calcium within the gut lumen. The greater the need and the smaller the dietary supply, the more efficient is absorption. Increased needs during growth, pregnancy, lactation, calcium-deficient states, or exercise resulting in high bone density enhance calcium absorption. Low vitamin D intake or inadequate exposure to sunlight reduces calcium absorption, especially among older adults. In addition, the efficiency of skin production of vitamin D by older adults is lower than that of younger people. Aging is also characterized by achlorhydria, which results in less gastric acidity and reduced calcium absorption.

Calcium is absorbed only if it is present in an ionic form. Thus calcium is best absorbed in an acidic medium; the hydrochloric acid secreted in the stomach, such as that secreted during a meal, increases calcium absorption by lowering the pH in the proximal duodenum. This also applies to calcium supplements; therefore taking a calcium supplement with a meal improves absorption, especially in older adults. Lactose enhances calcium absorption. Even in adults with lactose intolerance, lactose probably improves calcium absorption.

Calcium is not absorbed if it is precipitated by another dietary constituent such as oxalate or if it forms soaps with free fatty acids. Oxalic acid (oxalate) in rhubarb, spinach, chard, and beet greens forms insoluble calcium oxalate in the digestive tract (see Chapter 36). For example, only 5% of the calcium in spinach is absorbed. Phytic acid (phytate) combines with calcium to form calcium phytate, which is insoluble and cannot be absorbed. These unabsorbed forms of calcium are excreted in the feces as calcium oxalates and calcium soaps.

Dietary fiber may decrease calcium absorption, but this may only be a problem for those who consume more than 30 g/day. Lower intakes of fiber have little effect on calcium availability. Medications can affect bioavailability or increase calcium excretion, both of which may contribute to bone loss. With fat malabsorption, calcium absorption is decreased because of the formation of calcium–fatty acid soaps. Calcium absorption does not seem to be affected by the amount of phosphate in the diet unless the intake of phosphate is excessively high or by the calcium/phosphorus ratio.

Renal Excretion. Approximately 50% of the ingested calcium is excreted in the urine each day, but an almost equivalent amount is also secreted into the intestine and joins unabsorbed calcium in the feces. Calcium resorption from the renal tubules occurs by transport mechanisms similar to those in the small intestine. Urinary calcium excretion varies throughout the life cycle, but it is typically low during periods of rapid skeletal growth. At menopause calcium excretion increases greatly, but in postmenopausal women treated with estrogen, less calcium is excreted. After approximately 65 years of age, calcium excretion decreases, most likely because of decreased intestinal absorption of calcium. In general, urinary calcium levels correlate well with calcium intake. A high sodium intake contributes to lower renal resorption of calcium and higher urinary calcium losses.

Skin Losses. Dermal losses of calcium occur in the form of skin exfoliation and sweat. The amount of calcium lost in sweat is approximately 15 mg/day. Strenuous physical activity with sweating increases the loss, even in persons with a low calcium intake.

Serum Calcium. Total serum calcium consists of three distinct fractions: free, or ionized, calcium; complexes between calcium and anions such as phosphate and citrate;

and calcium that is protein bound with albumin. Serum albumin binds between 70% and 90% of the calcium that is protein bound. Ionized calcium (Ca^{2+}) is regulated and equilibrates rapidly with protein-bound calcium in blood. The serum ionized calcium concentration is controlled primarily by PTH, although other hormones have minor roles in its regulation. These other hormones include calcitonin, vitamin D, estrogens, and others.

Total serum calcium level is maintained within a narrow range of 8.8 to 10.8 mg/dL, of which the ionized calcium concentrations range from 4.4 to 5.2 mg/dL because hypocalcemia and hypercalcemia have significant physiologic effects. Serum levels of calcium are highest early in life, gradually decrease throughout life, and reach the lowest levels during the older years. Several factors affect the relative distribution of calcium in blood serum or plasma. One of these is pH; the ionized calcium fraction is higher in acidosis and lower in alkalosis. Total calcium changes concurrently with changes in plasma protein levels; however, the ionized fraction usually remains within normal limits. The strict regulation of ionized calcium makes it a useful diagnostic tool in assessing parathyroid gland function, monitoring kidney disease, and monitoring sick neonates for whom hypocalcemia could be life threatening.

Regulation of Serum Calcium. Calcium in bones is in equilibrium with calcium in the blood. PTH plays the major role in maintaining serum calcium, as noted previously. When the blood calcium concentration falls below this level, PTH stimulates the transfer of exchangeable calcium from the bone into the blood. At the same time, PTH promotes renal tubular resorption of calcium, and it indirectly stimulates increased intestinal absorption of calcium by increasing kidney production of vitamin D ($1,25[OH]_2D_3$) (see Figure 3-26).

Other hormones—such as glucocorticoids, thyroid hormones, and sex hormones—also have important roles in calcium homeostasis. Glucocorticoid excess leads to bone loss, particularly of trabecular bone, as a result of impaired calcium absorption through both active and passive mechanisms. Thyroid hormones (T_4 and T_3) may stimulate bone resorption; chronic hyperthyroid conditions result in loss of compact and trabecular bone. In women normal bone balance requires serum estrogen concentrations to be within normal limits. The rapid decrease of the serum estrogen concentration during menopause is a major factor contributing to bone resorption. Treating postmenopausal women with estrogen slows the rate of bone resorption; bone reabsorption is also inhibited by testosterone.

Functions

Adequate dietary calcium is needed to permit optimal gains in bone mass and density in the prepubertal and adolescent years. These gains are especially critical for girls because the accumulated bone may provide additional protection against osteoporosis in the years after menopause. Peak calcium retention by girls has been shown to occur in the prepubertal and early pubertal periods and is influenced by race, with black girls having significantly higher retention rates (Wigertz et al., 2005).

Postmenopausal women need to obtain sufficient amounts of calcium to maintain bone health and suppress PTH, which increases later in life in most individuals, perhaps as a result of inadequate calcium in the diet. Additional amounts of calcium are recommended to meet the needs of pregnancy and lactation, infancy, childhood, and adolescence.

In addition to its function in building and maintaining bones and teeth, calcium also has numerous critical metabolic roles in cells in all other tissues. However, compared with the significant needs of the skeleton, only small amounts of calcium are required for all other cellular and extracellular functions.

The transport functions of cell membranes are influenced by calcium, which affects membrane stability in poorly understood ways. Calcium also influences the transmission of ions across membranes of cell organelles, the release of neurotransmitters at synaptic junctions, the function of hormones, and the release or activation of intracellular and extracellular enzymes.

Calcium is required for nerve transmission and regulation of heart muscle function. The proper balance of calcium, sodium, potassium, and magnesium ions maintains skeletal muscle tone and controls nerve irritability. A significant increase in the serum calcium level can cause cardiac or respiratory failure, whereas a decrease results in **tetany** of skeletal muscles. In addition, calcium ions play a critical role in smooth muscle contractility.

Ionized calcium initiates the formation of a blood clot by stimulating the release of thromboplastin from blood platelets. Calcium ions also serve as required cofactors for several enzymatic reactions, including the conversion of prothrombin to thrombin, which aids in the polymerization of fibrinogen to fibrin and the final step in blood clot formation.

High dietary calcium intakes are associated with decreased prevalence of overweight and obesity. The mechanism for this affect appears to be related to (1) depression of the PTH and 1,25 hydroxy vitamin D, which leads to inhibition of lipogenesis and increased lipolysis; and (2) increased excretion of fecal fat caused by soaps formation (Heaney and Rafferty, 2009) (Table 3-25).

Dietary Reference Intakes

The IOM, Food and Nutrition Board (2010) has recently set the RDA for calcium, based on estimates of requirements of both genders throughout the life cycle. The tolerable UL has also been established for this nutrient. During several periods of the female life cycle, calcium intake is critical: prepuberty and adolescence, postmenopause, and during pregnancy and lactation (Kovacs, 2005). In a study of adolescent girls, calcium intakes of 1300 mg or more each day were necessary for maximum calcium retention by the body's skeleton. Abrams (2005) noted that calcium supplementation was helpful to children and adolescents and that catch-up mineralization was possible later in puberty if intakes were adequate.

TABLE 3-25

Minerals in Human Nutrition

	Body Location and Selected Biologic Functions	DRIs	Food Sources	Likelihood of Deficiency
Macronutrients Essential at Daily Levels of 100 mg or More				
Calcium	99% is found in bones and teeth. Ionic calcium in body fluids is essential for ion transport across cell membranes. Calcium may also be bound to protein, citrate, or inorganic acids.	1300 mg ages 9 through 18. 1000 mg for adults 19-50 yr. 1200 mg for females 51+ yr and all adults over age 70.	Milk and milk products, sardines, clams, oysters, kale, turnip greens, mustard greens, tofu	Dietary surveys indicate that many people do not meet AIs for calcium. Because bone serves as a homeostatic mechanism to maintain calcium levels in the blood, many essential functions are maintained, regardless of dietary intake. Long-term dietary deficiency is probably one of the factors responsible for development of osteoporosis later in life.
Phosphorus	Approximately 80% is found in inorganic portion of bones and teeth. Phosphorus is a component of every cell, as well as of important metabolites, including DNA, RNA, ATP, and phospholipids. Phosphorus is also important for pH regulation.	700 mg for adults (RDA)	Cheese, egg yolk, milk, meat, fish, poultry, whole-grain cereals, and almost all other foods	Dietary inadequacy is not likely if protein and calcium intake are adequate.
Micronutrients Essential at Daily Levels of a Few Milligrams or Less				
Magnesium	Approximately 50% is in bone; the remaining 50% is almost entirely inside body cells, with only about 1% located in extracellular fluid.	400-420 mg for men, 310-320 mg for women 14-70+ yr (RDA)	Whole-grain cereals, tofu nuts, meat, milk, green vegetables, legumes, chocolate	Dietary inadequacy is considered unlikely, but conditioned deficiency often develops and is usually associated with surgery, alcoholism, malabsorption, loss of body fluids, and certain hormonal and renal diseases.
Sulfur	Bulk of dietary sulfur is present in sulfur-containing amino acids needed for synthesis of essential metabolites. Sulfur functions in oxidation-reduction reactions, as part of thiamin and biotin.	No DRI; the need for sulfur is satisfied by essential sulfur-containing amino acids.	Protein foods such as meat, fish, poultry, eggs, milk, cheese, legumes, nuts	Dietary intake is chiefly from sulfur-containing amino acids, and adequacy is related to protein intake.
Iron	Approximately 70% is found in hemoglobin; approximately 25% is stored in liver, spleen, and bone. Iron is a component of hemoglobin and myoglobin and is important in oxygen transfer. It is also present in serum transferring and certain enzymes. Almost none exists in ionic form.	8 mg for men, 18 mg for women (after menopause, 8 mg) (RDA)	Liver, meat, egg yolk, legumes, whole or enriched grains, dark green vegetables, dark molasses, shrimp, oysters	Iron deficiency anemia occurs in women of reproductive age and infants and preschool children. Deficiency may be associated with unusual blood loss, parasites, or malabsorption. Anemia is the last state of deficiency.

Continued

TABLE 3-25

Minerals in Human Nutrition—cont'd

	Body Location and Selected Biologic Functions	DRIs	Food Sources	Likelihood of Deficiency
Zinc	Zinc is present in most tissues, with greatest amounts in the liver, voluntary muscle, and bone. A constituent of many enzymes and of insulin, zinc is important for nucleic acid metabolism.	11 mg for men, 8 mg for women (RDA)	Oysters, shellfish, herring, liver, legumes, milk, wheat bran	The extent of dietary zinc inadequacy in the United States is not known. Conditioned deficiency may develop with systemic childhood illnesses and in patients who are nutritionally depleted or have been subjected to severe stress such as surgery.
Copper	Copper is found in all body tissues, with the bulk in the liver, brain, heart, and kidney. Copper is a constituent of enzymes and ceruloplasmin and erythrocuprein in blood. It may be an integral part of DNA or RNA.	900 mcg for men and women (RDA)	Liver, shellfish, whole grains, cherries, legumes, kidney, poultry, oysters, chocolate, nuts	No evidence shows that specific deficiencies of copper occur in humans. Menkes disease is a genetic disorder resulting in copper deficiency.
Iodine	Iodine is a constituent of T_4 and related compounds synthesized by the thyroid gland. T_4 functions in the control of reactions involving cellular energy.	150 mcg for men and women (RDA)	Iodized table salt, seafood, water and vegetables in regions without goiter	Iodization of table salt is recommended, especially in areas where food is low in iodine.
Manganese	The highest concentration of manganese is in bone; relatively high concentrations also exist in pituitary, liver, pancreas, and gastrointestinal tissue. Manganese is a constituent of essential enzyme systems and is rich in mitochondria of liver cells.	2.3 mg for men, 1.8 mg for women (AI)	Beet greens, blueberries, whole grains, nuts, legumes frit, tea	Deficiency is unlikely to occur in humans.
Fluoride	Fluoride exists in bones and teeth. In optimal amounts from water and diet, fluoride reduces dental caries and may minimize bone loss.	4 mg for men, 3 mg for women (AI)	Drinking water (1 ppm), tea, coffee, rice, soybeans, spinach, gelatin, onions, lettuce	In areas where the fluoride content of water is low, fluoridation of water (at 1 ppm) has reduced the incidence of dental caries.
Molybdenum	Molybdenum is a constituent of an essential enzyme (xanthine oxidase) and flavoproteins.	45 mcg for men and women (RDA)	Legumes, cereal, grains, dark green leafy vegetables, organ meats	No available information.

Cobalt	Cobalt is a constituent of cyanocobalamin (vitamin B_{12}), existing bound to protein in foods of animal origin. Cobalt is essential for the normal function of all cells, particularly cells of bone marrow and nervous and gastrointestinal systems.	2.4 mcg vitamin B_{12}	Liver, kidney, oysters clams, poultry, milk	Primary dietary inadequacy is rare except in those who consume no animal products. Deficiency may be associated with lack of gastric intrinsic factor, gastrectomy, or malabsorption syndromes.
Selenium	Selenium is involved in fat metabolism, cooperates with vitamin E, and acts as an antioxidant.	55 mcg for men and women (RDA)	Grains, onions, meats, milk; varied amounts in vegetables depending on selenium content of soil	Keshan disease is a selenium-deficient state. Deficiency has occurred in patients receiving long-term TPN without selenium supplementation.
Chromium	Chromium is associated with glucose metabolism.	35 mcg for men, 25 mcg for women (AI)	Corn oil, clams, whole-grain cereals, brewer's yeast, meats, drinking water (amount varies)	Deficiency is found in those with severe malnutrition and may be a factor in diabetes in older adults and cardiovascular disease.

From Institute of Medicine, The Food and Nutrition Board: Dietary reference intakes for vitamin A, vitamin K, arsenic, boron, chromium, copper, iodine, iron, manganese, molybdenum, nickel, silicon, vanadium, and zinc, Washington, DC, 2001, National Academies Press; Institute of Medicine, Food and Nutrition Board: Dietary reference intakes for vitamin C, vitamin E, selenium, and carotenoids, Washington, DC, 2000b, National Academy Press; and Institute of Medicine, Food and Nutrition Board: Dietary reference intakes for calcium and vitamin D, Washington, DC, 2011, National Academy Press.

AI, Adequate intake; *DRI*, dietary reference intake; *RDA*, recommended dietary allowance; *TPN*, total parenteral nutrition.

Food Sources and Intakes

Cow's milk and dairy products are the most concentrated sources of calcium. Dark green leafy vegetables such as kale, collards, turnip greens, mustard greens, and broccoli; almonds; blackstrap molasses; the small bones of sardines and canned salmon; and clams and oysters are good sources of calcium. Soybeans also contain ample amounts. Oxalic acid limits the availability of calcium in rhubarb, spinach, chard, and beet greens. Fortified foods (orange juice, soy, nut, grain or rice milks) contain as much calcium as cow's milk. Many bottled waters and energy bars have calcium and sometimes vitamin D added. Tofu prepared by calcium precipitation is also a source of calcium. Table 3-26 shows the calcium content of selected foods.

Calcium supplements are now commonly used to increase intake. The most common form is calcium carbonate, which is relatively insoluble, particularly at a neutral pH. Although it has less calcium than calcium carbonate by weight, calcium citrate is much more soluble and would be suitable for patients with a lack of hydrochloric acid in the stomach (achlorhydria). In patients with achlorhydria, the efficiency of calcium absorption is greatly decreased because of the higher pH of the stomach contents; however, calcium absorption is increased by the consumption of a meal, which improves the solubility of calcium ions because of the increased gastric acidity. The selection of the most appropriate calcium supplement depends on several factors, including physical and chemical properties, interactions with other medications being taken concurrently, current medical conditions, and age. Beginning at the age of 11 years, median dietary calcium intakes in the United States are considerably less than the AIs (Figure 3-27). Therefore calcium intakes of Americans are insufficient for the critical ages of bone deposition in both genders, as well as being inadequate at other critical stages.

Deficiency

The development of peak bone mass requires adequate amounts of calcium and phosphorus, vitamin D, and other

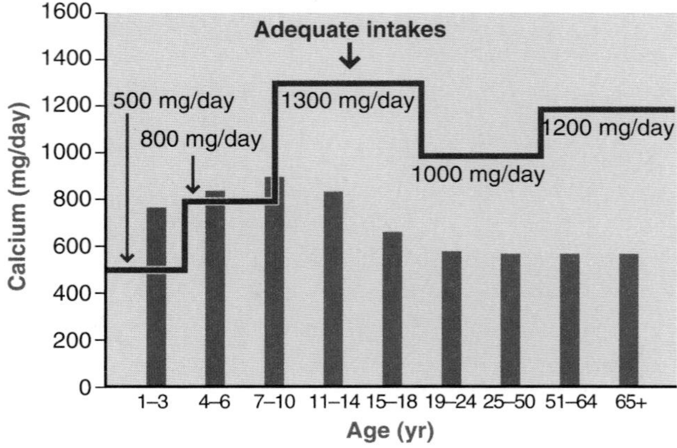

FIGURE 3-27 Comparison of the median daily calcium intake for females in the United States and the adequate intakes established in 1998.

TABLE 3-26

Calcium Content of Selected Foods

Food	Content (mg)
Milkshake, vanilla, 11 oz	457
Yogurt, low fat, with fruit, 1 cup	345
Fast-food enchilada, 1	324
Rhubarb, cooked, ½ cup	318
Spinach, frozen, cooked, 1 cup	291
Milk, 2% milkfat, 1 cup	285
Cheese, cheddar, 1 oz	204
Waffle, frozen, 4-inch diameter, 1	191
Salmon, canned, with bones, 3½ oz	181
Tofu, regular, ¼ block	163
Cheese, cottage, 2% fat, 1 cup	155
Ice cream, vanilla, softserve, ½ cup	113
Almonds, 1oz	70
Baked beans, white, ½ cup	64
Broccoli, cooked from fresh, 1 cup	62
Frankfurter, turkey, 1	58
Orange, 1 medium	52
Halibut, baked, 3 oz	51
Kale, fresh, cooked, ½ cup	47
Bread, whole wheat, 1 slice	20
Banana, 1 medium	7
Ground beef, lean, 3 oz	4
DRIs	
Infants	200-260 mg/day, depending on age
Children aged 1-8 years	700-1000 mg/day, depending on age
Children over age 9 and adolescents	1300 mg/day
Adults (ages 19-50)	1000 mg/day
Adults 51 to 70	1000 mg/day males; 1200 mg/day females
Adults over age 70	1200 mg/day
Pregnant	1000 mg/day; 1300 mg/day aged 14-18 years
Lactating	Same as for pregnancy

From U.S. Department of Agriculture, Agricultural Research Service: Nutrient Database for Standard Reference, Release 18. Data Laboratory home page: http://www.nal.usda.gov/fnic/foodcomp/Data/SR18/nutrlist/sr18w301.pdf; accessed 2011.

AI, Adequate intake; *DRI*, dietary reference intake.

nutrients. Compared with adulthood, greater amounts of calcium and phosphate are required for skeletal development; therefore AIs of these minerals and others have a significant effect on peak bone mass development until the time of puberty and throughout adolescence. After adolescence, bone gains may still occur, but the amounts of calcium required decrease. Vitamin D status may or may not be a problem, depending on the intakes of calcium and phosphorus. When calcium intake is well below the recommended amount, PTH is released; a persistent elevation may contribute to low bone mass. Calcium and vitamin D intakes of many older women are inadequate.

Hogan (2005) suggested that epidemic obesity and subsequent dieting may have a detrimental effect on bone status, leading to osteoporosis. An inadequate intake of calcium, in addition to an inadequate intake of vitamin D, may contribute to osteomalacia, colon cancer, and hypertension. Dietary Approaches to Stop Hypertension studies show that adequate dietary intakes of calcium, magnesium, potassium, and other micronutrients from low-fat dairy foods, fruits, and vegetables can substantially reduce blood pressure in those with hypertension or prevent its development.

Toxicity

A very high intake of calcium (>2000 mg/day) may lead to hypercalcemia. This can be exacerbated by high intakes of vitamin D. Such toxicity may lead to excessive calcification in soft tissues, especially the kidneys, and may be life-threatening. In addition, long-term high intakes of calcium may lead to increased bone fractures in older adults, perhaps because of high bone remodeling rates that lead to exhaustion of osteoblast (Klompmaker, 2005).

High intakes of calcium may also interfere with the absorption of other divalent cations such as iron, zinc, and manganese. Therefore supplements of certain minerals should be taken at different times. Another effect of excessive calcium intake is constipation, common among older women who take calcium supplements.

Physical Immobility

Prolonged bed rest or periods of weightlessness during space travel promote significant calcium losses in response to a lack of tension or gravity on the bones. Older individuals who require a prolonged recovery with limited activity, such as those with hip fractures or other illnesses, also have increased calcium losses. Physical activity, especially weight-bearing exercise, promotes bone health.

Phosphorus

Phosphorus ranks second to calcium in abundance in human tissues. Approximately 700 g of phosphorus exists in adult tissues, and approximately 85% is present in the skeleton and teeth as calcium phosphate crystals. The remaining 15% exists in the metabolically active pool in every cell in the body and in the extracellular fluid compartment. Almost 50% of the inorganic phosphate is present in serum as free ions (i.e., $H_2PO_4^-$ and $H_2PO_4^{2-}$). Smaller percentages are bound to protein (≈10%) or complexed (≈40%).

The serum inorganic phosphorus level is closely maintained by PTH at 3 to 4 mg/100 mL in adults, but it is not as closely regulated as the serum calcium level. Normal blood concentrations in infants are higher. In older adults serum phosphate concentrations are typically lower; hypophosphatemia (<2.5 mg/dL) may be common among older adults. Phosphorus balance is illustrated in Figure 3-28.

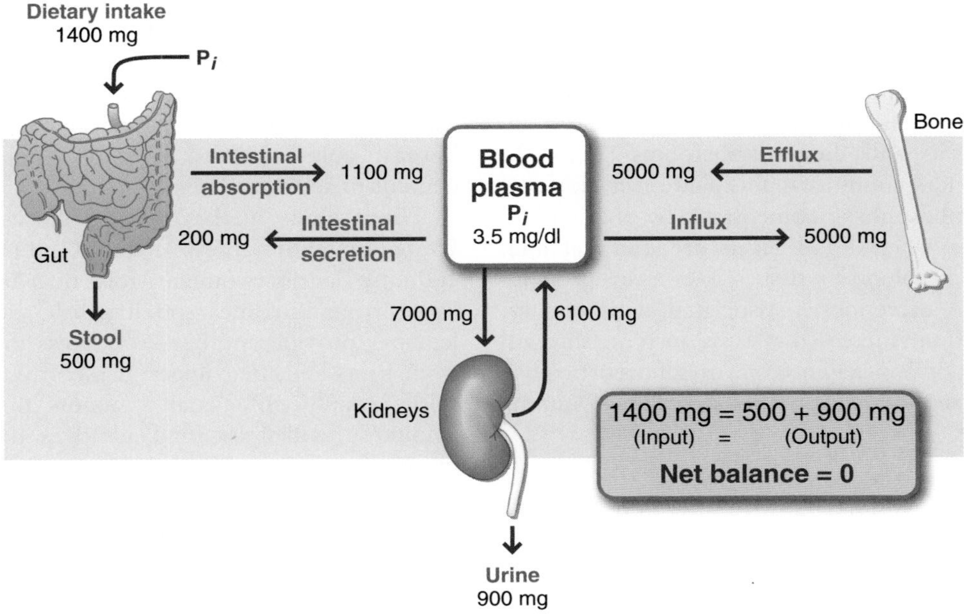

FIGURE 3-28 Phosphorus balance is maintained primarily by the amount of phosphate absorbed versus the amount excreted by the kidneys and intestine. Bone is the major storage site for phosphate, as it is for calcium. The metabolic pathways share many similarities with the calcium pathways.

Absorption, Transport, Storage, and Excretion

The relative amounts of inorganic and organic phosphates in the diet vary with the food or supplement consumed. Regardless of the form, most phosphates are absorbed in the inorganic state. Organically bound phosphate is hydrolyzed in the lumen of the intestine and released as inorganic phosphate, primarily through the action of pancreatic or intestinal phosphatases. Bioavailability depends on the form of the phosphate and the pH. The acidic milieu of the most proximal portion of the duodenum is important in maintaining phosphorus solubility and therefore bioavailability. In vegetarian diets the major portion of the phosphorus exists as phytate, which is poorly digested. Humans do not have the phytase enzyme; however, intestinal bacteria have the enzyme needed to hydrolyze phosphates. The yeast used in making bread contains a phytase, which releases phosphate.

In general, the efficiency of phosphate absorption is 60% to 70% in adults, twice as high as that of calcium. Phosphate absorption is also much more rapid than that of calcium. Peak absorption of phosphates occurs approximately 1 hour after ingestion of a meal; calcium enters the blood 3 to 4 hours after a meal.

The primary route of phosphorus excretion is renal, which also is the primary site of phosphate regulation. Major determinants of urinary phosphorus loss are an increased intake of phosphate, an increase in phosphate absorption, and the plasma phosphorus concentration. Other factors contributing to increased urinary phosphate loss are hyperparathyroidism, acute respiratory or metabolic acidosis, diuretic use, and the expansion of extracellular volume. If PTH levels are high, the urinary route excretes additional phosphate. Starvation or chronic undernutrition typically contributes to most of the alterations in metabolism that result in hypophosphatemia and renal losses of phosphate. According to Berndt and Kumar (2009), long-term regulation of phosphorus homeostasis may be controlled by hormones such as the vitamin D endocrine system and PTH as well as and the phosphatonins (FGF-23, sFRP-4, MEPE). Endogenous fecal phosphate excretion can also contribute to phosphorus homeostasis by eliminating excessive phosphate when PTH levels are elevated and phosphate load in the blood or tissues is excessively high. Reduced phosphate excretion is associated with dietary phosphorus restriction; increased plasma insulin, thyroid hormone, growth hormone, glucagon, or glucocorticoids; metabolic or respiratory alkalosis; and extracellular volume contraction.

Functions

As phosphates, phosphorus participates in numerous essential functions of the body. DNA and RNA are based on phosphate. The major cellular form of energy, ATP, contains high-energy phosphate bonds, as do creatinine phosphate and PEP. Cyclic adenosine monophosphate (cAMP) acts as a secondary signal within cells following peptide hormone activation of many membrane receptors. As part of phospholipids, phosphorus is present in every cell membrane in the body. Numerous phospholipid molecules also act as secondary messengers within the cytosol. Phosphorylation-dephosphorylation reactions control various steps in the activation or deactivation of cytosolic enzymes by kinases or phosphatases. Total intracellular concentrations of phosphate (but not ionic concentrations) are much higher than extracellular concentrations because phosphorylated compounds do not cross cell membranes easily and are trapped within the cell.

The phosphate buffer system is important in intracellular fluid and the kidney tubules, where phosphate functions in the excretion of hydrogen ion. Filtered phosphate reacts with secreted hydrogen ions, releasing sodium in the process. In turn, the sodium can be resorbed under the influence of aldosterone. Finally, phosphate ions combine with calcium ions to form **hydroxyapatite**, the major inorganic molecule in teeth and bones. Bone mineral, but not tooth mineral, provides phosphate ions via homeostatic regulation of serum calcium by PTH.

Dietary Reference Intakes

DRIs for phosphorus are somewhat lower than those for calcium for all age groups. Tolerable ULs are also established.

Food Sources and Intakes

In general, good sources of protein are also good sources of phosphorus. Meat, poultry, fish, and eggs are excellent sources. Milk and milk products are good sources, as are nuts and legumes, cereals, and grains. Phosphorus is bound to serine, threonine, and tyrosine in proteins. In the outer coating of cereal grains, particularly wheat, phosphorus exists in the form of phytic acid, which can form a complex with some minerals to create insoluble compounds. In conventional breads phytic acid is converted to the soluble form of orthophosphate during the leavening process. However, in the unleavened breads commonly eaten in the Middle East, the availability of practically all minerals is much lower. Table 3-27 and Appendix 36 list the phosphorus content of selected foods.

The average intakes of phosphorus by adults in the United States are approximately 1300 mg/day for men and 1000 mg/day for women. More than 60% of phosphorus comes from milk, meat, poultry, fish, and eggs. Cereals and legumes provide another 20%. Less than 10% is derived from fruits and their juices; tea, coffee, vegetable oils, and spices supply only small amounts of phosphorus. The amount provided by food additives to such products as meats, cheeses, dressings, beverages, and bakery products can be significant.

Deficiency

Phosphate deficiency is rare. It could develop in individuals who are taking phosphate binders for renal disease or in older adults because of poor intake in general. The widespread, ultimately fatal consequences of severe phosphorus depletion reflect its ubiquitous roles in body functions.

TABLE 3-27

Phosphorus Content of Selected Foods

Food	Content (mg)
Fast food pancakes, 2	476
Sole (fillet)	246
Fast food hamburger (1)	284
Macaroni and cheese, 1 cup	322
Milk, 2% fat, 1 cup	232
Cheddar cheese, 1oz	146
Ham, 3 oz	210
Ice milk, soft serve, 1 cup	202
Mixed nuts, 1 oz	123
Cheese, cottage, 2% fat, 1 cup	341
Cheese, cheddar, 1 oz	146
Shrimp, boiled, 2 large	137
Baked beans, 1 cup	293
Ground beef, cooked, 3 oz	165
Tofu, regular, ½ cup	120
Potato, baked, with skin, 1	115
Egg, 1	96
Bread, whole wheat, 1 slice	65
Cola beverage, 1 can, 12 oz	46
Potato chips, 14	43
Bread, white, 1 slice	23
Cauliflower, fresh, ½ cup	23
Orange, 1	18
DRIs	
Infants and young children	100-500 mg/day, depending on age
Older children and adolescents	1250 mg/day
Adults	700 mg/day
Pregnant	700-1250 mg/day, depending on age
Lactating	700-1250 mg/day, depending on age

From U.S. Department of Agriculture, Agricultural Research Service: Nutrient Database for Standard Reference, Release 18, retrieved 2005, Data Laboratory home page: http://www.nal.usda.gov/fnic/foodcomp/Data/SR18/nutrlist/sr18w305.pdf; accessed 1-14-11.

DRI, Dietary reference intake.

Symptoms result from decreased synthesis of ATP and other organic phosphate molecules. Neural, muscular, skeletal, hematologic, renal, and other abnormalities occur.

Because phosphorus is so widely available from foods, including processed foods and soda types of soft drinks, a dietary inadequacy is unlikely. Clinical phosphate depletion and hypophosphatemia can result from long-term administration of glucose or TPN without sufficient phosphate, excessive use of phosphate-binding antacids, hyperparathyroidism, or treatment of diabetic acidosis. It may develop in those who have alcoholism, with or without decompensated liver disease. Premature infants who are fed unfortified human milk may also develop hypophosphatemia.

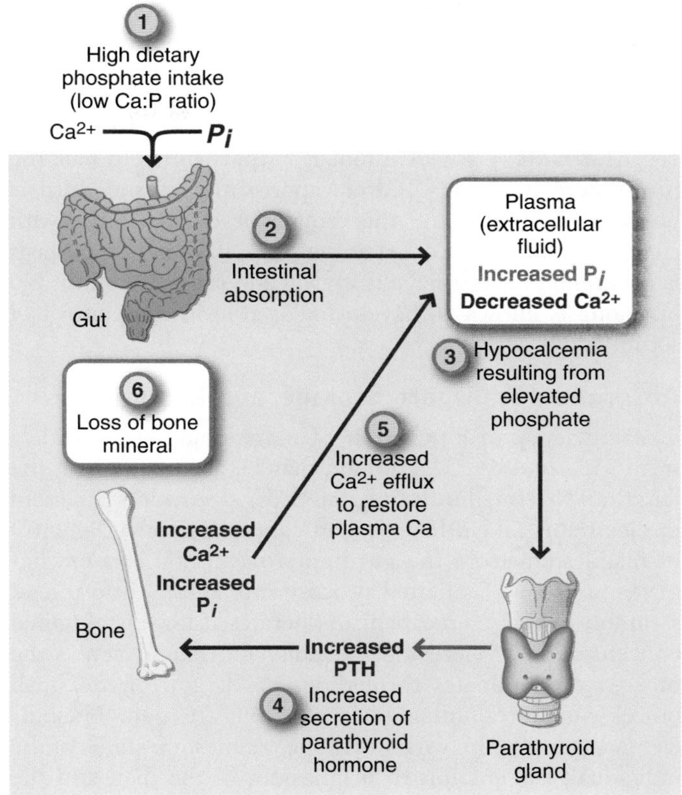

FIGURE 3-29 Mechanism through which a low dietary calcium/phosphorus ratio contributes to the development of a persistently high parathyroid hormone concentration.

Toxicity

A persistently high concentration of PTH may result after chronic consumption of a low-calcium, high-phosphorus diet, called *nutritional secondary hyperparathyroidism.* PTH levels in blood that result from this diet typically remain within a high normal range (Figure 3-29). This persistently high PTH contributes to increased bone turnover, reduction of bone mass and density, and even fragility fractures because of excessive resorption and thinning of trabecular plates at bone sites throughout the skeleton. Individuals with a low calcium/phosphorous ratio benefit from increasing calcium intake from foods or supplements. Adequate calcium intake reduces the serum PTH concentration and may inhibit bone loss. The persistently high PTH level contributes to the limited bone mineralization during growth; this yields inadequate peak bone mass accumulation and the loss of bone mass.

Magnesium

After potassium, magnesium is the second-most abundant intracellular cation in the body. The adult human body contains approximately 20 to 28 g of magnesium, of which approximately 60% is found in bone, 26% in muscle, and the remainder in soft tissues and body fluids. Gender differences in the body content of magnesium begin before puberty. Magnesium in bone is present in exchangeable and nonexchangeable pools. Magnesium ions in the bone fluid compartment are much more exchangeable than magnesium ions that have become part of the crystal lattice. Normal serum levels are usually in the range of 1.5 to 2.1 mEq/L (0.75 to 1.1 mmol/L). Approximately half the magnesium in plasma is free; approximately one third is bound to albumin; and the remainder is complexed with citrate, phosphate, or other anions. Magnesium homeostasis is governed by intestinal absorption and renal excretion. No hormone is known to have a major role in the control of serum magnesium.

Absorption, Transport, Storage, and Excretion

The efficiency of absorption of magnesium varies widely from 35% to 45%. Magnesium may be absorbed along the length of the small intestine, but most absorption occurs in the jejunum. Like other divalent cation minerals, the entry of magnesium from the gut lumen occurs by two mechanisms: a carrier-facilitated process and simple diffusion. A saturable facilitated mechanism operates at low intraluminal concentrations, whereas paracellular movement across the mucosa predominates throughout the length of the small bowel when intraluminal concentrations are high. The efficiency of absorption varies with the magnesium status of the individual, the amount of magnesium in the diet, and the composition of the diet as a whole. Vitamin D has little or no effect on magnesium absorption.

Serum magnesium concentration is remarkably constant. Maintenance of these constant values depends on absorption, excretion, and transmembranous cation flux rather than on hormonal regulation. Once in the cells, magnesium is bound mainly to protein and energy-rich phosphates. The magnesium balance is illustrated in Figure 3-30.

The kidneys control magnesium balance by conserving magnesium efficiently, particularly when intake is low. Supplementing a normal intake increases urinary excretion while serum levels remains stable. Low dietary intake of magnesium results in reduced urinary excretion of magnesium. To allow nursing mothers to meet the increased needs for magnesium, urinary excretion of the mineral tends to decrease during lactation. Renal resorption varies inversely with that of calcium.

Functions

The major function of magnesium is to stabilize the structure of ATP in ATP-dependent enzyme reactions. Magnesium is a cofactor for more than 300 enzymes involved in the metabolism of food, synthesis of fatty acids and proteins, phosphorylation of glucose in the glycolytic pathway, and promoting transketolase reactions. Magnesium is important in the formation of cAMP, the first cytosolic messenger to be identified as a mechanism for transmitting messages from outside the cells in response to hormones, local hormonelike factors, or other molecules.

Magnesium plays a role in neuromuscular transmission and activity, working in concert with and against the effects of calcium, depending on the system involved. In a normal muscle contraction, calcium is a stimulator, and magnesium is a relaxant. Magnesium acts as a physiologic calcium-channel blocker. High magnesium intakes are associated with greater bone density. The reactivity of vascular and other smooth muscle cells depends on the ratio of calcium to magnesium in the blood.

Magnesium also plays a role in learning and memory. A new product, magnesium-L-threonate, leads to the enhancement of learning, working memory, and short and long-term memory in all ages of rats (Slatsky et al., 2010).

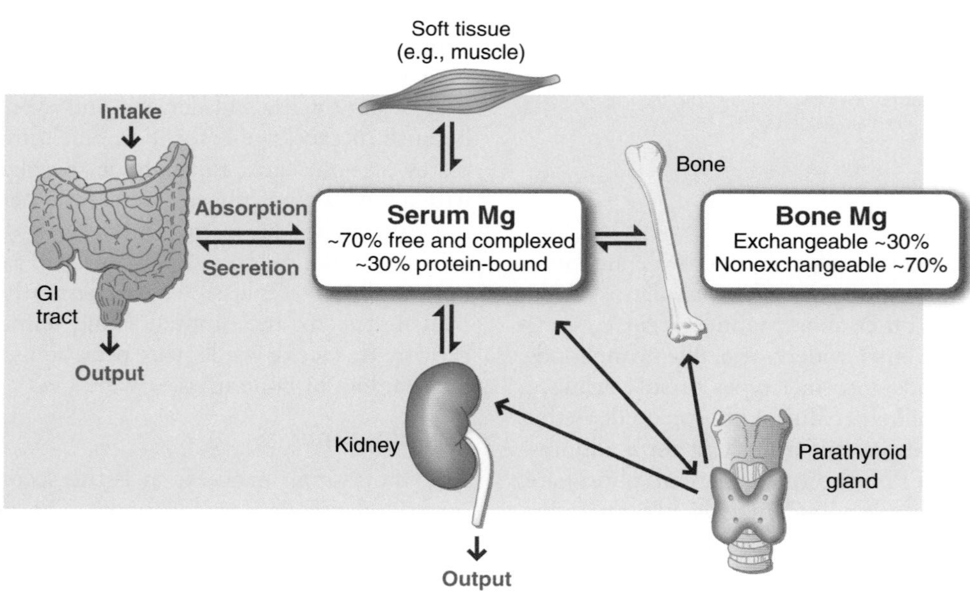

FIGURE 3-30 Magnesium balance is maintained largely by gastrointestinal absorption and renal excretion.

Although it is too early to extrapolate to humans, this is an exciting area of research. Magnesium depletion has been detected in persons with migraine headaches, severe asthma, dysmenorrhea, leg cramps, diabetes mellitus, chronic renal failure, nephrolithiasis, osteoporosis, aplastic osteopathy, and heart and vascular disease (Guerrera et al., 2009; Musso, 2009).

Large doses of magnesium can result in central nervous system depression, anesthesia, or even paralysis, especially in patients with renal insufficiency. Thus patients with renal problems should not be given magnesium supplements.

Dietary Reference Intakes

The RDA for magnesium was increased in 1997; different recommendations were made for boys and girls beginning at puberty. ULs were also established, as were AIs for infants.

Food Sources and Intakes

Magnesium is abundant in many foods. Good sources are seeds, nuts, legumes, and milled cereal grains, as well as dark green vegetables, because magnesium is an essential constituent of chlorophyll. Milk is a moderately good source of magnesium, especially because milk and other dairy products are so widely consumed. Tofu prepared by magnesium precipitation (check the label) is a good source.

Fish, meat, oranges, apples, and bananas, are poor sources of magnesium. Diets high in refined foods, meat, and dairy products are usually lower in magnesium than diets rich in vegetables and unrefined grains (Table 3-28). Magnesium is lost during the processing of foods such as sugar; after refining wheat cereals, it is not generally replaced as enrichment.

The most commonly consumed food sources include milk, bread, coffee, ready-to-eat cereals, beef, potatoes, and dried beans and lentils. Americans have had median intakes of magnesium well below the RDAs, with older adults having the lowest intakes (Figure 3-31). This trend is implicated in development of diseases such as osteoporosis and diabetes (He et al., 2006). High intakes of calcium, protein, vitamin D, and alcohol all increase the requirements for magnesium; physical or psychologic stress may also increase magnesium needs.

TABLE 3-28

Magnesium Content of Selected Foods

Food	Content (mg)
Halibut, baked, ½ fillet	170
Spinach, canned, 1 cup	163
Cow peas, cooked, 1cup	91
Muffin, oat bran 1	89
Rice, brown, cooked, 1 cup	84
Refried beans, 1 cup	83
Cashews, roasted, 1 oz	77
Orange juice, 6 oz	72
Mixed nuts, roasted, 1 oz	67
Baked potato with skin, 1	57
Raisins, 1 cup	46
Tofu, firm, ¼ block	30
Bread, whole wheat, 1 slice	29
Milk, 2% fat, 1 cup	27
Spinach, fresh, 1 cup	24
Ground beef, lean, cooked, 3 oz	18
Fruits	10-25
DRIs	
Infants, AIs	30-75 mg/day, depending on age
Young children, RDAs	80-130 mg/day, depending on age
Older children and adolescents, RDAs	240-410 mg/day, depending on age and gender
Adults	310-400 mg/day, depending on age and gender
Pregnant	350-400 mg/day, depending on age
Lactating	310-360 mg/day, depending on age

From U.S. Department of Agriculture, Agricultural Research Service: Nutrient Database for Standard Reference, Release 18, Data Laboratory home page: http://www.nal.usda.gov/fnic/foodcomp/Data/SR18/nutrlist/sr18w304.pdf; accessed 1-14/11.

AI, Adequate intake; *DRI*, dietary reference intake; *RDA*, recommended dietary allowance.

Deficiency

Although rare, severe magnesium deficiency symptoms include tremors, muscle spasms, personality changes, anorexia, nausea, and vomiting. Tetany, myoclonic jerks, athetoid movements, convulsions, and coma have also been reported. Hypocalcemia and hypokalemia typically occur first, combined with impairment of the individual's responsiveness to PTH and sodium retention.

The effects of severe magnesium depletion on bone metabolism include decreased PTH secretion by the parathyroid glands, very low serum PTH, impaired responsiveness of bone and kidneys to PTH, decreased serum $1,25(OH)_2D_3$, vitamin D resistance, altered hydroxyapatite crystal formation, impaired bone growth in young patients, or the development of osteoporosis in seniors. With continued depletion of magnesium, PTH concentrations drop even further. Intravenous administration of magnesium reverses the clinical signs and symptoms within a short time.

Moderate depletion of magnesium apparently is prevalent in older populations in Western nations (Leenhardt et al., 2005). Such deficiencies are typically precipitated by low dietary intakes, especially in individuals who avoid consuming dark green leafy vegetables, milk, and other good sources of magnesium. An increased loss of electrolytes, especially potassium, or a shift in electrolyte balance also triggers a moderate magnesium deficiency. Conditions and situations that may cause acute deficiencies

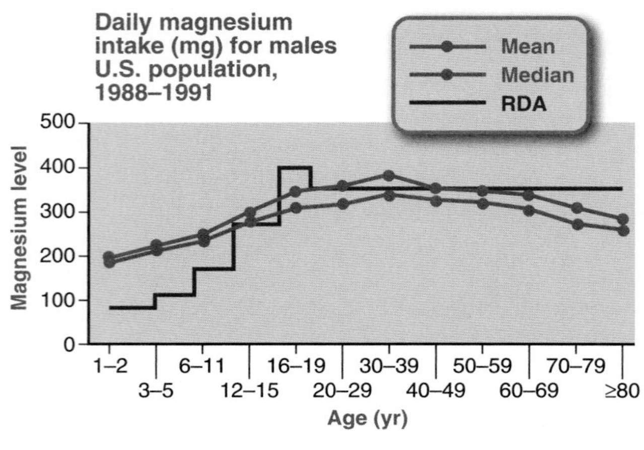

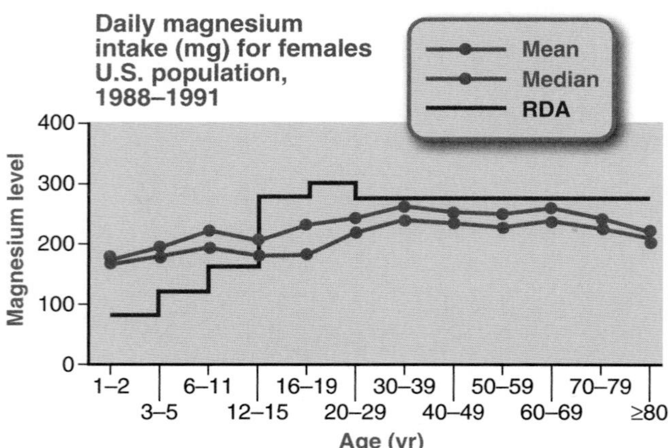

FIGURE 3-31 Comparison of the median daily magnesium intake for Americans and the dietary reference intakes.

include renal disease, diuretic therapy, malabsorption, hyperthyroidism, pancreatitis, protein insufficiency, diabetes, parathyroid gland disorders, postsurgical stress, and vitamin D–resistant rickets. Magnesium deficiency has also been linked to insulin resistance and metabolic syndrome because magnesium is required for carbohydrate metabolism (He et al., 2006).

Magnesium status is difficult to determine from serum measurements of magnesium because the total serum magnesium level remains constant within a wide range of intake levels. Leukocyte magnesium contents are much more sensitive to nutritional status, which makes them a superior marker. Urinary excretion of magnesium (and often of potassium) is less in those with a magnesium deficiency than in those with sufficient magnesium, suggesting that those with magnesium deficiencies have greater retention of magnesium and improved tissue magnesium status throughout the body.

Attention has focused on the interrelationships of magnesium and other electrolytes, particularly potassium, and related effects. For example, a low magnesium intake contributes to hypertension along with inadequate intakes of potassium and calcium. Oral magnesium supplementation may lower systolic and diastolic blood pressure significantly. Low magnesium intakes have also been associated with coronary heart disease, myocardial infarction, and osteoporosis.

Toxicity

Although excess magnesium can inhibit bone calcification, excesses from dietary sources and supplements are unlikely to result in toxicity. However, the ULs for magnesium from supplements or pharmacologic agents were established in 1998. The only cases of toxicity that have been reported involve smelter workers who inhale or otherwise ingest toxic levels of magnesium dust.

Sulfur

Although sulfur has long been studied as a mineral, it functions almost entirely as a component of organic molecules. Sulfur exists in the body as a constituent of three amino acids—cystine, cysteine, and methionine—and as part of organic molecules in all cells and extracellular compartments, such as connective tissue. The tertiary structure of proteins is attributable in part to covalent bonding between cysteine residues in which the SH groups are oxidized to form disulfide bridges. These bridges also provide the three-dimensional structural modifications necessary for the activity of some enzymes, insulin, and other proteins. Sulfhydryl groups of proteins also participate in diverse cellular reactions. For example, the poisonous effects of arsenic are caused by its ability to bind sulfhydryl groups of enzymes. The sulfur of cysteine binds to iron-sulfur clusters in electron transfer proteins involved in basic, life-sustaining processes, such as photosynthesis, nitrogen fixation, and oxidative phosphorylation.

Glutathione, a tripeptide-containing cysteine, acts as a donor of reducing equivalents for the reduction of hydrogen peroxide and organic peroxides by GSH-Px. In the broadest sense, sulfur can be considered an antioxidant. Sulfur is as a component of heparin, an anticoagulant found in liver and tissues, and as chondroitin sulfate in bone and cartilage. Sulfur is also an essential component of three vitamins—thiamin, biotin, and pantothenic acid (Brosnan and Brosnan, 2009).

Sulfur is also part of the molecule, *S*-adenosylmethionine. The transmethylation pathway within cells, especially in the liver, converts methionine to homocysteine while transferring the methyl group to other molecules. This pathway is linked to the metabolism of other important molecules such as cysteine, adenine (a nucleoside), and polyamines.

Sulfur-containing amino acids regulate lipid metabolism (Oda, 2006). Taurine, a sulfur-containing amino acid made by liver cells, is used to conjugate bile acids before secretion. Nonhepatic cells use sulfate bound to an organic donor for the synthesis of iron-sulfur proteins. In addition, structural molecules within cells like proteoglycans contain sulfated monosaccharide (glucose and galactose) residues.

The metabolism of sulfur-containing amino acids generates inorganic acids, especially sulfate anions, in substantial amounts. These sulfates are thought to combine with calcium ions in the glomerular ultrafiltrate, thereby reducing the renal tubular resorption of calcium. This mechanism may explain as much as 50% of the calcium loss associated with protein-induced hypercalciuria, which develops after consumption of meals rich in animal proteins—proteins that are rich in sulfur.

Methionine and cysteine provide almost 100% of the sulfur in the human diet. Food sources of sulfur include meat, poultry, fish, eggs, dried beans, broccoli, and cauliflower. Sulfur deficiency or toxicity is highly unlikely. Excess inorganic sulfur generated as a result of hepatic or renal metabolism is excreted in the urine as sulfates. There are no DRIs for sulfur.

MICROMINERALS/TRACE ELEMENTS

Numerous microminerals or **trace elements** are present in minute amounts in body tissues and are essential for optimum human growth, health, and development. The functions of and deficiency symptoms produced by trace elements are subtle and difficult to identify, partly because many of these effects occur at the cellular or subcellular level. For example, iron deficiency eventually results in a type of anemia that is easy to identify. The cellular effects cannot be identified as easily but may actually be more harmful to the individual.

The knowledge of the various functions of trace and ultratrace minerals continues to grow. DRIs and ULs have been established for nine essential trace elements: chromium, copper, iodine, iron, manganese, molybdenum, selenium, zinc, and fluoride. DRIs for five potentially essential trace elements—arsenic, boron, nickel, silicon, and vanadium—have not yet been published. No DRI exists for cobalt, just for cobalt-containing vitamin B_{12} (cobalamin).

General Characteristics

Trace elements exist in two forms: as charged ions or bound to proteins. Each element has different chemical properties that become critical in its functional role in cells or extracellular compartments. In blood and other tissue and cellular fluids, the trace elements do not exist in the free ionic state; they are typically bound to transporting or holding proteins. Fluoride ions become bound in the hydroxyapatite crystals of bones and teeth.

Functions

Many enzymes require small amounts of one or more trace metals for full activity. Metals function in enzyme systems by participating directly in the catalyzed reaction, by combining with substrates to form complexes on which enzymes act, by forming metalloenzymes that bind substrates, by combining with reaction end products, or by maintaining quaternary structures. Minute concentrations of trace minerals affect the whole body through interactions with the enzymes or hormones that regulate masses of substrate. This ability is amplified if, in turn, the substrate has some regulatory function. Trace minerals may also interact with DNA to control the transcription of proteins important for the metabolism of that particular trace mineral.

Food Sources

Compared with other sources, foods of animal origin are generally superior sources of trace elements because concentrations of the elements tend to be higher and the metals more available for absorption. Seafood in particular is usually rich in nearly all micronutrients except manganese, which is more readily available from plant sources. The trace element content of many plants depend on the minerals content of the soil; in addition, trace elements are not distributed evenly in wheat grains, and the germ and outer layers that contain major amounts of most minerals are removed to a large extent by the milling process. However, the small quantities of minerals that remain in white flour are more biologically available than those in whole-wheat flour, which are in complexes with or bound by molecules in the inner layer such as phytate and fiber. Unless the pH is lowered during product production, these minerals remain unavailable.

Iron

Iron has been recognized as an essential nutrient for more than a century. Nutritional iron deficiency and iron deficiency anemia remain far too common in the twenty-first century given the wide availability of iron-rich foods (see Chapter 33). Indeed, iron-deficiency anemia is the world's most common nutritional deficiency disease. Many advances have been made in the study of iron metabolism and iron deficiency, but questions persist about mechanisms regulating absorption and iron balance. The adult human body contains iron in two major pools: (1) functional iron in hemoglobin, myoglobin, and enzymes; and (2) storage iron in ferritin, hemosiderin, and transferrin. Healthy adult men have approximately 3.6 g of total body iron, whereas women have approximately 2.4 g (Table 3-29). Adult women

TABLE 3-29

Relative Proportions of Iron in Young, Healthy Adults

	Men: Iron Content		Women: Iron Content	
Iron Type	**(mg)**	**(%)**	**(mg)**	**(%)**
Functional				
Hemoglobin	2300	64	1700	73
Myoglobin	320	9	180	8
Heme enzymes	80	2	60	3
Nonheme enzymes	100	3	80	3+
Storage				
Ferritin	540	15	200	9
Hemosiderin	230	6	100	4
Transferrin	5	<1	4	<1
Total	3575	100	2314	100

store much lower amounts of iron than do men. Iron is highly conserved; approximately 90% is recovered and reused every day and the rest is excreted, primarily in bile. If dietary iron is not available to meet this 10% gap, iron deficiency results.

Two concerns about iron nutritional status predominate: the incidence of iron-deficiency anemia and the role of excessive iron intake in coronary heart disease and cancer. Because of food fortification and the use of iron supplements by so many individuals, high iron intakes by men and postmenopausal women may be contributing to the risk of these chronic diseases. In fact, a study of older adults replete with iron in the Framingham Heart Study cohort concluded that increased iron stores are a liability (Fleming et al., 2001).

Absorption, Transport, Storage, and Excretion

Dietary iron exists as **heme iron**, found in hemoglobin, myoglobin, and some enzymes; and as **nonheme iron**, found predominantly in plant foods, but also in some animal foods as nonheme enzymes and ferritin. Heme iron is absorbed across the brush border of intestinal absorbing cells after it is digested from animal sources. After heme enters the cytosol, the ferrous iron is enzymatically removed from the ferroporphyrin complex. The free iron ions combine immediately with apoferritin to form ferritin in the same way that free nonheme iron combines with apoferritin.

Ferritin is an intracellular store, a "ferry" that carries bound iron from the brush border to the basolateral membrane of the absorbing cell. The final step of absorption by which iron ions are moved into the blood involves an active transport mechanism. At this point, it is the same for heme and nonheme iron (Figure 3-32). The absorption of heme iron is affected only minimally by the composition of meals and GI secretions. Heme iron represents only 5% to 10% of the dietary iron in a mixed diet, but absorption may be as high as 25%, compared with only 5% for nonheme iron. Because vegans consume only plant foods, sufficient amounts of nonheme iron must be ingested and absorbed to meet body requirements or supplements would be needed.

Three steps of absorption also precede the entry of nonheme iron into the circulation. Nonheme iron must be digested from plant sources and enter the duodenum and upper jejunum in a soluble, ionized form if it is to be transferred across the brush border. The acid of gastric secretions enhances the solubility and changes iron to the ionic state—either as ferric (+3 oxidation state) or ferrous (+2 oxidation state) iron—within the gut luminal contents. Iron in the reduced, ferrous state is preferred for the entry step of absorption. The brush border iron transporter, divalent metal transporter 1 (DMT1), transports ferrous iron. Ferric iron may be reduced by a brush border enzyme, ferric reductase, for absorption. As chyme moves down the duodenum, pancreatic and duodenal secretions increase the pH of the contents to 7, at which point most ferric iron is precipitated unless it has been chelated. However, ferrous iron is significantly more soluble at a pH of 7, so these ions remain available for absorption in the remainder of the small intestine.

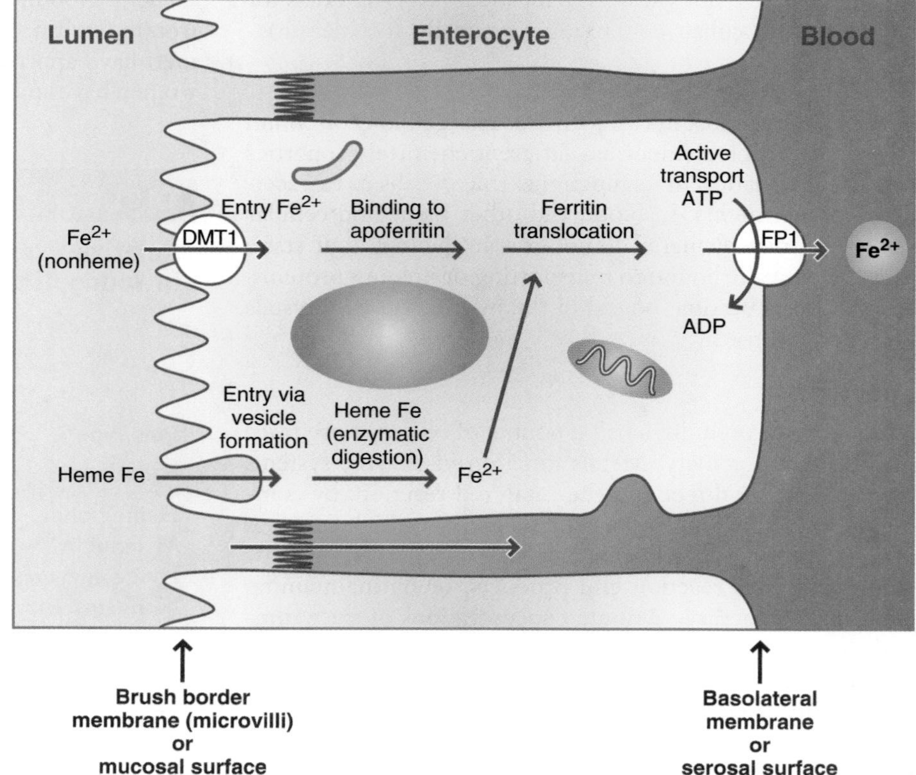

FIGURE 3-32 Intestinal absorption of iron from heme and nonheme sources by an intestinal absorbing cell, or enterocyte. Enterocytes contain two membranes: the brush border membrane and the basolateral membrane. The entry step of nonheme iron at the brush border membrane is different from that of heme iron. Heme iron enters by vesicle formation around the heme, whereas nonheme iron (ionic iron) enters by facilitated diffusion down a concentration gradient. Absorbed ions combine with apoferritin to form ferritin complexes that move across the cell by diffusion to the basolateral membrane for the exit step of absorption by active transport. The iron of heme iron is enzymatically removed, and these ions exit at the basolateral membrane by an unknown mechanism. *ADP*, Adenosine diphosphate; *ATP*, adenosine triphosphate.

The efficiency of nonheme iron absorption seems to be controlled by the intestinal mucosa, which allows certain amounts of iron to enter the blood from the cytosolic ferritin pool according to the body's needs. A small peptide hormone known as **hepcidin** is the main iron regulatory hormone. Production in the liver is responsive to liver iron levels, inflammation, hypoxia, and anemia. Its major action is to act on the mucosa cell and inhibit iron absorption. Therefore chronic inflammation can lead to decreased iron absorption from production of hepcidin (Muñoz et al., 2009).

Other signals from the body to the absorbing cells may be transferrin saturation, or the percentage of iron bound to transferrin (Figure 3-33). Normally transferrin saturation is 30% to 35% in healthy, iron-consuming individuals. The percentage can vary greatly, depending on iron intake and bioavailability. A low percentage (e.g., 15%) of the **total iron-binding capacity (TIBC)** of transferrin would stimulate the absorbing cells to transport iron by the exit step at the basolateral membrane to the blood. Conversely, if the iron concentration in the body is excessive, absorbing cells would be downregulated, and less iron would be absorbed. The latter situation occurs during iron overloads to protect the body against toxicity.

The life span of an intestinal absorbing cell is approximately 3 to 6 days. During this time the cell emerges from the crypt after cell division, passes up the villus to the tip, and eventually sloughs off as a dead cell. During the early life of the individual cell, signals resulting from the saturation percentage of circulating transferrin are sent to the young cells to adjust their number of receptors for transferrin (e.g., to increase iron absorption in a state of iron deficiency). Other cells formed before or after may have different numbers of receptors, depending on the nutritional supply of iron.

In individuals who persistently consume inadequate levels of iron, especially women in their childbearing years, the number of receptors may consistently be upregulated to maximize iron absorption. The efficiency of iron absorption by adults with normal hemoglobin values averages 5% to 15% of the iron, heme and nonheme, from food and supplements. Although absorption may be as high as 50% in those with iron deficiency anemia, this level is not common. Most women with an iron deficiency, but not anemia, probably

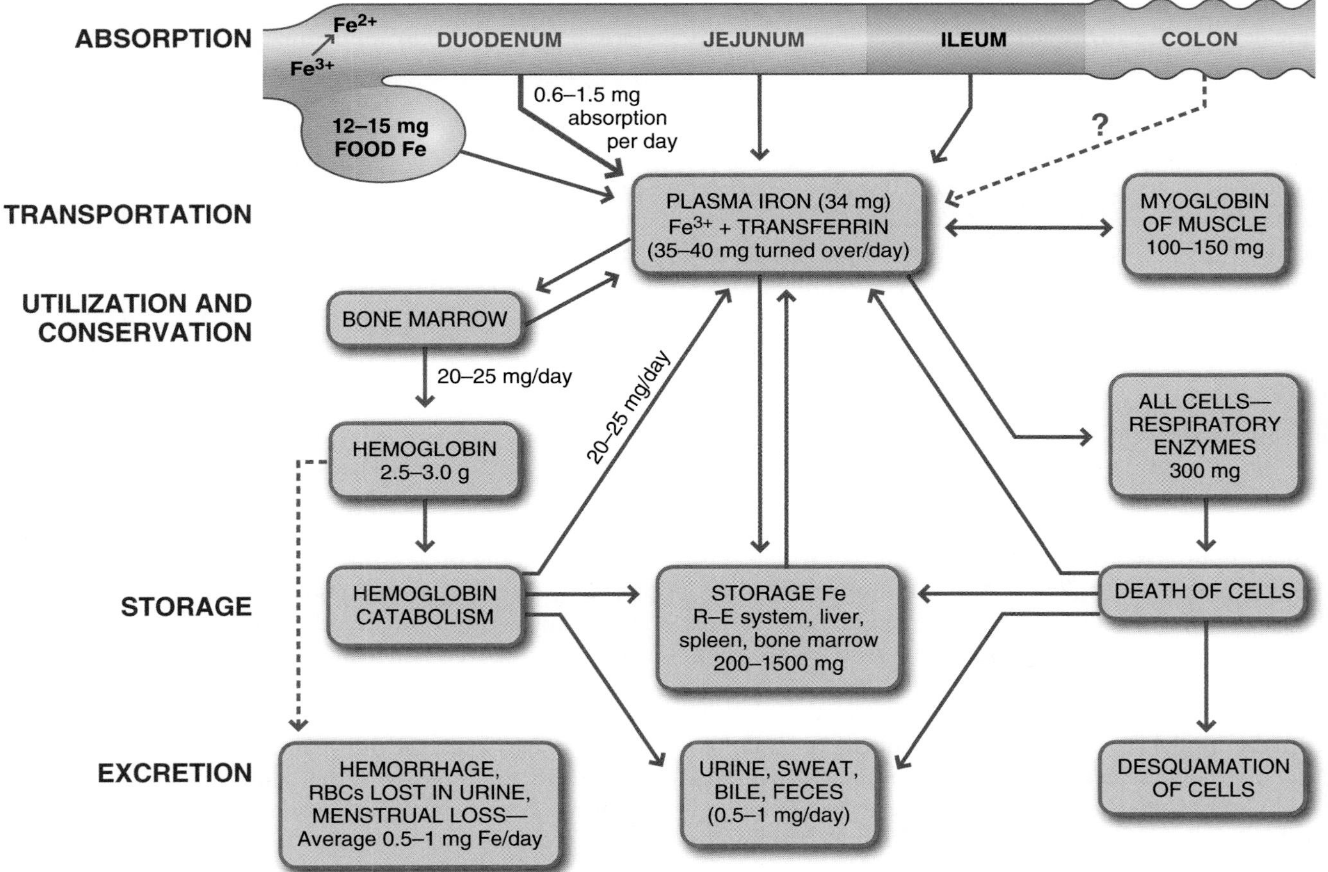

FIGURE 3-33 Iron metabolism in adults. Most iron is absorbed from the duodenum and jejunum, after which it is transported as plasma iron or bound to transferrin. *RBCs*, Red blood cells; *R-E system*, reticuloendothelial system.

have absorption efficiencies of 20% to 30%. From 2% to 10% of nonheme iron in vegetables is absorbed, and from 10% to 30% of iron heme and nonheme from animal sources is typically absorbed.

Several factors affect the intestinal absorption of iron. The efficiency of iron absorption is determined to some extent by the foods from which it is derived or with which it is consumed. Ascorbic acid, the most potent enhancer of iron absorption, reduces ferric to ferrous iron and forms a chelate with iron that remains soluble at the alkaline pH of the lower small intestine. Other food molecules, such as sugars and sulfur-containing amino acids, may also enhance iron entry by forming chelates with ionic iron. In addition, animal proteins from beef, pork, veal, lamb, liver, fish, and chicken enhance absorption. The substance responsible for this improved absorption—the **meat-fish-poultry (MFP) factor**—remains unknown, but specific amino acids or dipeptide digestion products may enhance iron absorption.

Although the iron content of human milk is very low, it is highly bioavailable because of the presence of milk lactoferrin, which enhances iron absorption. Infants retain more iron from human milk than from cow's milk or infant formulas because of the presence of lactoferrin in breast milk. Whey protein (lactalbumin), which constitutes a greater percentage of the total protein in human milk than in cow's milk, may also improve iron absorption.

The degree of gastric acidity enhances solubility and therefore bioavailability of iron derived from foods. Therefore achlorhydria, hypochlorhydria, or administration of alkaline substances such as antacids can interfere with nonheme iron absorption by not permitting the solubilization of iron in gastric and duodenal fluids. Gastric secretions also seem to increase the absorption of heme iron.

Certain physiologic states such as pregnancy and growth that involve increased blood formation stimulate iron absorption. In addition, more iron is absorbed during iron deficiency states because of adaptive mechanisms that enhance nonheme iron absorption.

Foods with high phytate content have low iron bioavailability, but whether phytate is the cause is not clear. Oxalates can inhibit absorption. Tannins, which are polyphenols, in tea also reduce nonheme iron absorption. On the other hand, the presence of an adequate amount of calcium helps to remove phosphate, oxalate, and phytate that would otherwise combine with iron and inhibit its absorption.

The availability of iron from various compounds used for food enrichment or as supplements varies widely according to their chemical composition. Although iron in the ferrous form is most readily absorbed, not all ferrous compounds are equally available. Ferrous pyrophosphate is used frequently in products such as breakfast cereals because it does not add a gray color to the food; however, this compound and others such as ferrous citrate and ferrous tartrate are poorly absorbed. Iron is usually added to baby foods in an elemental form, the absorbability of which depends on the iron particle size. Increased intestinal motility decreases iron absorption by decreasing contact time and rapidly removing the chyme from the area of highest intestinal acidity. Poor fat digestion leading to steatorrhea also decreases iron absorption and the absorption of other cations.

Transport. Iron (nonheme) is transported, bound to transferrin (see Figure 3-33), from the intestinal absorbing cells to various tissues to meet their needs. It rarely exists in the free ionic state in serum.

Storage. Between 200 and 1500 mg of iron is stored in the body as ferritin and hemosiderin; 30% is in the liver, 30% is in the bone marrow, and the rest is in the spleen and muscles. Up to 50 mg/day can be mobilized from storage iron, 20 mg of which is used in hemoglobin synthesis; see estimates in Table 3-29. The amounts of circulating ferritin in blood correlate closely with total body iron stores, which makes this measurement valuable for evaluation of iron status.

Intestinal Excretion. Iron is lost from the body only through bleeding and in very small amounts through defecation, sweat, and the normal exfoliation of hair and skin. Most of the iron lost in the feces could not be absorbed from food. The remainder comes from bile and the cells exfoliated from the GI epithelium. Almost no iron is excreted in the urine. Daily iron loss is approximately 1 mg for men and slightly less for nonmenstruating women. The loss of iron accompanying menstruation averages approximately 0.5 mg/day. However, wide variations exist among individuals, and menstrual losses of more than 1.4 mg of iron daily have been reported in approximately 5% of normal women.

Functions

The functions of iron relate to its ability to participate in oxidation and reduction reactions. Chemically, iron is a highly reactive element that can interact with oxygen to form intermediates with the potential of damaging cell membranes or degrading DNA. Iron must be tightly bound to proteins to prevent these potentially destructive oxidative effects.

Iron metabolism is complex because this element is involved in so many aspects of life, including red blood cell function, myoglobin activity, and the roles of numerous heme and nonheme enzymes. Because of its oxidation-reduction (redox) properties, iron has a role in the blood and respiratory transport of oxygen and carbon dioxide, and it is an active component of the cytochromes (enzymes) involved in the processes of cellular respiration and energy (ATP) generation. Iron is also involved in immune function and cognitive performance; this underscores the importance of preventing iron deficiency anemia throughout the world.

Hemoglobin, which is present in red blood cells, is synthesized in immature cells in bone marrow. Hemoglobin works in two ways: the iron-containing heme combines with oxygen in the lungs; and the heme releases the oxygen in tissues, where it picks up carbon dioxide and then releases it in the lungs after its return from the tissues. **Myoglobin**, also a heme-containing protein, serves as an oxygen reservoir within muscle. Table 3-30 lists the major iron molecules in the body and their functions.

Oxidative production of ATP within the mitochondria involves many heme and nonheme iron-containing enzymes.

TABLE 3-30

Iron Molecules in the Body

Molecule	Function
Metabolic Proteins	
Heme proteins	
Hemoglobin	Oxygen transport from lungs to tissues
Myoglobin	Transport and storage of oxygen in muscle
Enzymes: Heme	
Cytochromes	Electron transport
Cytochrome P-450	Oxidative degradation of drugs
Catalase	Conversion of hydrogen peroxide to oxygen and water
Enzymes: Nonheme	
Iron-sulfur and metalloproteins	Oxidative metabolism
Enzymes: Iron dependent	
Tryptophan pyrolase	Oxidation of tryptophan
Transport and Storage Proteins	
Transferrin	Transport of iron and other minerals
Ferritin	Storage
Hemosiderin	Storage

The cytochromes, present in nearly all cells, function in the mitochondrial respiratory chain in the transfer of electrons and the storage of energy through the alternate oxidation and reduction (redox) of iron (Fe^{2+} to and from Fe^{3+}). Numerous water-insoluble drugs and endogenous organic molecules are transformed by the iron-containing cytochrome P-450 system in the liver into more water-soluble molecules that can be secreted in the bile and eliminated. Ribonucleotide reductase, the rate-limiting enzyme involved in DNA synthesis, is also an iron enzyme. Although these vital enzymes represent only a small portion of the total iron in the body, a severe decrease in their concentrations can have long-term consequences. Other enzymes, including several in the brain, also require iron.

An adequate iron intake is essential for the normal function of the immune system. Iron overloads and deficiencies result in changes in the immune response. Iron is required by bacteria; therefore an iron overload (especially intravenously) may result in an increased risk of infection. Iron deficiency affects humoral and cellular immunity. Concentrations of circulating T-lymphocytes decrease in individuals with an iron deficiency, and the mitogenic response is typically impaired. Natural killer (NK) cell activity also decreases. Production of interleukin-1 is reduced in iron-deficient animals, and depressed interleukin-2 production has been reported.

Two iron-binding proteins—transferrin (in blood) and lactoferrin (in breast milk)—seem to protect the body against infection by withholding iron from microorganisms that need it for proliferation. Iron is used by brain cells for normal function in people of all ages. Iron is involved in the function and synthesis of neurotransmitters and possibly myelin. The detrimental effects of early iron deficiency anemia in children can persist for many years. For example, declines have been found between the scholastic performance, sensorimotor competence, attention, learning, and memory of children with anemia. Iron supplementation in children with iron deficiency anemia has been found to improve learning, as indicated by achievement test scores (Beard, 2001). Changes in iron metabolism occur in Alzheimer disease and other disorders.

Dietary Reference Intakes

DRIs have been established for iron. The RDA for men and postmenopausal women is 8 mg/day. The RDA for women of childbearing age (to replace iron loss from menstruation and provide for iron stores sufficient to support a pregnancy) is 18 mg/day. For teenage boys (ages 14 to 18) the iron RDA is 11 mg/day. Full-term infants are born with a reserve supply of iron from placental transfer during gestation, but normal-term infants still require adequate iron from food sources and fortified milk products during the first year of life. Premature infants have limited iron stores because they lack most of the iron and other trace minerals that are normally transferred during the last trimester of pregnancy. The need for iron to support rapid growth in premature infants becomes apparent at approximately 2 to 3 months of age. The RDAs for ages 1 year and older are (variably) 7, 8, or 10 mg/day until adolescence begins at age 14. Figure 3-34 shows the physiologic requirements for iron in relation to age. Requirements are highest during infancy and adolescence. Iron needs among males decrease after the adolescent growth spurt, whereas the iron needs of their female counterparts continue to be high until the menopause. Iron allowances increase during pregnancy from 15 to 27 mg/day, but not during lactation, although many lactating women are told to continue taking their iron supplements.

Food Sources and Intakes

By far the best source of dietary iron is liver, followed by seafood, kidney, heart, lean meat, and poultry. Dried beans and vegetables are the best plant sources. Some other foods that provide iron are egg yolks, dried fruits, dark molasses, whole-grain and enriched breads, wine, and cereal. Old-fashioned iron skillets used for cooking add to the total iron intake. Table 3-31 presents the iron content of selected foods.

The availability of iron derived from food is important in the consideration of dietary sources. For example, only 50% or less of the iron in whole-grain cereals and in some green vegetables is available in a usable form. Corn is a notoriously poor source of iron; milk and milk products are practically devoid of iron. When dietary intake focuses

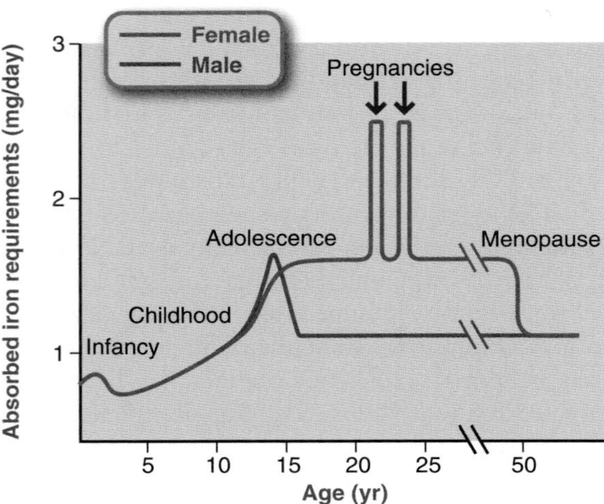

FIGURE 3-34 The absorbed iron requirement for various ages. The greatest requirements for iron occur during infancy. During childhood, requirements are the same for boys and girls. During the adolescent growth spurt, iron needs increase and are greater for boys than girls. However, because of menstruation, the requirements after adolescence remain high for females but decrease for males.

primarily on these foods, anemia levels can be high. Vegetarian or vegan women can obtain enough iron from their plant-based diet, but they must consume sufficient amounts of moderately iron-rich foods, such as legumes and dried fruits. Soy products are typically good sources of both iron and zinc.

Iron fortification of cereals, flours, and bread has added significantly to the total iron intake of the U.S. population. Fortified cereals are a substantial source of iron for infants and children, as well as for adolescents and adults. Concern about potential iron overloading from fortified breakfast foods has been raised because analyzed values of iron content may be considerably greater than labeled values. The foods that supply the greatest amount of iron in the U.S. diet include ready-to-eat cereals fortified with iron; bread, cakes, cookies, doughnuts, and pasta (all fortified with iron); beef; dried beans and lentils; and poultry.

Whereas the median iron intakes of most women are lower than the RDA, the median intakes of men generally exceed the RDA. An adequate diet containing meats and other animal sources typically has high iron content, containing approximately 6 mg of iron per 1000 kcal. Therefore the average omnivorous woman of childbearing age consuming 2000 kcal takes in only 12 mg of iron, or approximately 67% of the RDA of 18 mg/day. This intake level meets the needs of almost no menstruating woman. However, iron intakes totaling much less than 12 mg/day place women at more serious risk for developing deficiency anemia. Women with high daily iron losses compensate with an increased rate of absorption. Even with this adaptation, insufficient stores of iron typically exist and the risk of anemia remains high.

TABLE 3-31

Iron Content of Selected Foods

Food	Content (mg)
Cereal, ready-to-eat, fortified, 1 cup	1-22
Clams, canned, 3 oz	23.7
Rice, white, enriched, 1 cup	9.73
Baked beans, 1 cup	8.2
Braunschweiger, 2 slices	6.35
Oysters, cooked, 3 oz	5.9
Bagel, enriched, 1, 4-inch	5.38
Beef liver, fried, 3 oz	5.24
Fast food roast beef sandwich, 1	4.23
Refried beans, 1 cup	4.18
Potato skin, 1	4.08
Burrito, bean, 1	1.13
Ground beef, lean, 3 oz	1.8
Oatmeal, unfortified, 1 cup	1.6
Spinach, cooked, 1 cup	6.43
Corn dog, 1	6.18
Macaroni and cheese, 1 cup	1.86
Egg, 1	0.92
Peanuts, dry roasted, 3 oz	0.8
Blueberries, frozen, ½ cup	4.5
Chicken, breast, roasted, ½	0.64
Broccoli, fresh, cooked, ½ cup	0.64
Wine, red, ½ cup	0.5
Cheese, cheddar, 1 oz	0.2
Milk, 2% fat, 1 cup	0.07
RDA	
Infants and young children	7-11 mg/day, depending on age
Older children and adolescents	8-15 mg/day, depending on age
Adults	8-18 mg/day, depending on age and gender
Pregnant	27 mg/day
Lactating	9-10 mg/day, depending on age

From U.S. Department of Agriculture, Agricultural Research Service: Nutrient Database for Standard Reference, Release 18, Data Laboratory home page: http://www.nal.usda.gov/fnic/foodcomp/Data/SR18/nutrlist/sr18w303.pdf; accessed 2011.

RDA, Recommended dietary allowance.

Deficiency

Iron deficiency, the precursor of iron deficiency anemia, is the most common of all nutritional deficiency diseases. In the United States and worldwide, iron deficiency anemia is prevalent among children and women of childbearing age. The groups considered to be at greatest risk for iron deficiency anemia are infants younger than 2 years of age, adolescent girls, pregnant women, and older adults. Pregnant teenagers are frequently at high risk because of poor eating habits and continuing growth. Women in their childbearing years who are iron deficient benefit from either a diet rich in iron-containing foods or supplements.

The final stages of iron deficiency include hypochromic, microcytic anemia. Anemia may be corrected by providing high-dose supplements in the form of ferrous sulfate or ferrous gluconate until blood parameters return to normal. To prevent worsening of the iron deficiency, individuals should be counseled regarding a diet that is appropriately rich in iron.

Iron deficiency can be caused by injury, hemorrhage, or illness (e.g., blood loss from hookworms, GI diseases that interfere with iron absorption). Iron deficiency may also be aggravated by an unbalanced diet containing insufficient iron, protein, folate, and vitamin C. Anemia typically develops because of an inadequate amount of dietary iron or faulty iron absorption.

Female athletes, especially cross-country runners and others involved in endurance sports, often have an iron deficiency at some point in their training if they are not taking iron supplements or do not have diets high in iron. The source of the additional iron losses in those with athletic amenorrhea may be through the gut; losses may increase during the stressful conditions of training. It seems that without supplementation, the greater the intensity of training, the lower the iron levels become in women.

Toxicity

The major cause of iron overload is hereditary hemochromatosis, whereas transfusion iron overload is rare. The latter may be seen in individuals with sickle cell disease or thalassemia major who require transfusions for their anemia. Iron overload is linked to a distinct gene that favors excessive iron absorption if the iron is available in the diet. Both are linked to decreased hepcidin levels (Nemeth and Ganz, 2009). The characteristic chemical parameters of iron overload are listed in Box 3-7.

Frequent blood transfusions or long-term ingestion of large amounts of iron can lead to abnormal accumulation of iron in the liver. Saturation of tissue apoferritin with iron is followed by the appearance of **hemosiderin**, which is similar to ferritin but contains more iron and is very insoluble. Hemosiderosis is an iron storage condition that develops in individuals who consume abnormally large amounts of iron or in those with a genetic defect resulting in excessive iron absorption. If the hemosiderosis is associated with tissue damage, it is called *hemochromatosis*. See Chapter 33.

Iron supplements may not be beneficial for postmenopausal women and older men because of increased risks for heart disease and cancer; iron contributes to an environment that favors oxidation of LDL cholesterol, arterial vessel damage, and other adverse effects. In addition, excessive iron may help generate free radicals that attack cellular molecules, thereby increasing the number of potentially carcinogenic molecules within cells. These potential adverse iron-disease linkages need to be confirmed.

BOX 3-7

Iron Overload Symptoms (Hemochromatosis)

Abnormal accumulation of iron in the liver
Excessive tissue ferritin levels
Elevated serum transferrin levels
Oxidation of LDL cholesterol
Cardiovascular complications

LDL, Low-density lipoprotein.

Zinc

Zinc is abundantly distributed throughout the human body, second only to iron among trace elements. The human body has approximately 2 to 3 g of zinc, with the highest concentrations in the liver, pancreas, kidney, bone, and muscles. Other tissues with high concentrations include parts of the eye, prostate gland, spermatozoa, skin, hair, fingernails, and toenails. Zinc is primarily an intracellular ion, functioning in association with more than 300 different enzymes of various classes. Even though zinc is abundant in the cytosol, virtually all of it is bound to proteins, but it is in equilibrium with a small ionic fraction.

The most readily available form of zinc occurs in animal flesh, particularly red meats and poultry. Meat intake is frequently low among preschoolers, usually displaced by cereal foods, milk, and milk products that children tend to prefer. This observation led to the fortification of infant and children's foods, especially cereals, with zinc. Milk is a good source of zinc, but high intakes of calcium from milk may interfere with the absorption of iron and zinc (see the bioavailability discussion. The phytates from whole grains in unleavened breads may limit zinc absorption in some populations. According to the WHO, zinc deficiency is one of the 10 major factors contributing to disease in developing countries (Shrimpton et al., 2005). Deficiencies are less likely to be a problem in Western nations, where breads, breakfast foods, and other cereal-based foods are made primarily from refined grains and are typically fortified.

Absorption, Transport, Storage, and Excretion

Zinc absorption and excretion are controlled by poorly understood homeostatic mechanisms. The mechanism of absorption involves two pathways. A saturable carrier mechanism operates most efficiently at low zinc intakes when luminal zinc concentrations are low; a passive mechanism works when zinc intakes and luminal concentrations are high. Solubility of zinc in the gut lumen is critical. Zinc ions are generally bound to amino acids or short peptides in the lumen, released at the brush border for absorption via the carrier mechanism (hZIPI family). The entry step of absorption across the brush border is followed by the binding of zinc ions to metallothionein and other proteins within the cytosol of the absorbing cell. Metallothionein carries the zinc (via transcellular movement) to the basolateral border for the exit step from the absorbing cell to the blood. The exit step occurs by active transport because the blood concentration of zinc is significantly greater than the cytosolic ion concentration. The process of zinc absorption is illustrated in Figure 3-35.

Zinc absorption is affected not only by the level of zinc in the diet but also by the presence of interfering substances, especially phytates. After the consumption of zinc in a meal, the serum zinc level rises and then decreases in a dose-response pattern. A protein-rich diet promotes zinc absorption by forming zinc–amino acid chelates that present zinc in a more absorbable form. Zinc absorption is slightly higher during pregnancy and lactation. Absorbed zinc is taken up from the portal circulation initially by the liver, but most of the zinc is subsequently redistributed to other tissues. Impaired absorption is associated with a variety of intestinal diseases such as Crohn disease or pancreatic insufficiency.

Several dietary factors affect zinc absorption. Phytate decreases zinc absorption, but other complexing agents (e.g., tannins) do not. Copper and cadmium compete for the same carrier protein; thus they reduce zinc absorption. High calcium or iron intakes reduce zinc absorption and balance. Folic acid may also reduce zinc absorption when zinc intake is low. On the other hand, high doses of zinc can impair absorption of iron from ferrous sulfate, the form in vitamin and mineral supplements. Dietary fiber may also interfere with zinc absorption, but the significance is unclear. Zinc absorption may be enhanced by glucose or lactose and by soy protein consumed alone or mixed with beef. Red table wine also increases zinc absorption, probably because of its congeners. Like iron, zinc is better absorbed from human milk than from cow's milk.

Transport in Blood. Albumin is the major plasma carrier of zinc. The amount of zinc transported in the blood depends not on zinc but also on the availability of albumin. Some zinc is transported by transferrin and by α_2-macroglobulin. Most zinc in the blood is localized in erythrocytes and leukocytes. Plasma zinc is metabolically active and fluctuates in response to dietary intake and physiologic factors such as injury or inflammation. Levels drop by 50% in the acute phase of a response to an injury, probably because of the sequestering of zinc by the liver.

Intestinal Excretion. Excretion of zinc in normal individuals is via the feces. When zinc is administered intravenously, approximately 10% of the dose appears in the intestine within 30 minutes. However, increased urinary excretion has been reported in starvation, nephrosis, diabetes, alcoholism, hepatic cirrhosis, and porphyria. Plasma and urine concentrations of zinc-binding cysteine and histidine, and other urinary metabolites, may have a role in increasing zinc losses in these patients.

Functions

Zinc has structural, catalytic, and regulatory functions in the cell, primarily as an intracellular ion (Tuerk and Fazel, 2009). Zinc plays important structural roles as components of several proteins. It also functions in association with more than 300 different enzymes, in reactions involving either synthesis or degradation of carbohydrates, lipids, proteins, and nucleic acids. It also functions as an intracellular signal in brain cells where it is stored in specific synaptic vesicles and is fundamental to normal central nervous system function (Bitanihirwe and Cunningham, 2009). In addition, zinc is involved in the stabilization of protein and nucleic acid structure and the integrity of subcellular organelles, as well as in transport processes, immune function, and expression of genetic information.

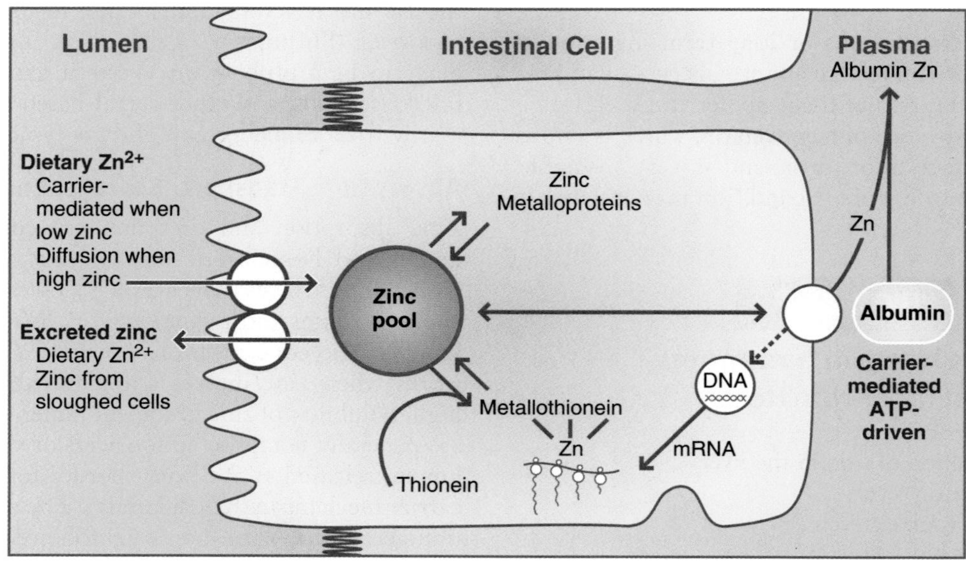

FIGURE 3-35 Model for zinc absorption showing the relationship between metallothionein and cysteine-rich intestinal protein. *ATP*, Adenosine triphosphate; *DNA*, deoxyribonucleic acid; *mRNA*, messenger ribonucleic acid.

Metallothionein is the most abundant, nonenzymatic zinc-containing protein. This low-molecular-weight protein is rich in cysteine and exceptionally high in metals, among which are zinc and lesser amounts of copper, iron, cadmium, and mercury. The biologic role of metallothionein is not clear, but it does have a function in zinc absorption. Metallothionein may function as an intracellular reservoir that can donate zinc ions to other proteins, or it may have a redox role that reduces oxidative stress, especially in cells with high stress. Thus metallothionein may have a role in the detoxification of metals as well as in their absorption.

Zinc is abundant in the nucleus, where it stabilizes RNA and DNA structure, and is required for the activity of RNA polymerases important in cell division. Zinc also functions in chromatin proteins involved in transcription and replication, and it protects against age-related macular degenerative disease. Although widely touted to cure or prevent common colds, zinc gluconate lozenges or nasal sprays are not very effective.

Dietary zinc causes an increase in bone mass. Zinc appears in the crystalline structure of bone, in bone enzymes, and at the zone of demarcation. It is needed for adequate osteoblastic activity, formation of bone enzymes such as alkaline phosphatase, and calcification (see Table 3-25). Beta-alanyl-histidine (carnosine) is a zinc compound that stimulates bone formation intensively and restores bone loss from aging, skeletal unloading, aluminum bone toxicity, calcium and vitamin D deficiency, adjuvant arthritis, estrogen deficiency, diabetes, and fracture healing (Yamaguchi, 2010). Such new zinc compounds may become adjuvant therapy for osteoporosis and other disorders.

Dietary Reference Intakes

The zinc DRI for adolescent and adult males is 11 mg/day. Because of the lower body weight of adolescent and adult women, their DRI is 8 to 9 mg/day. The DRI for preadolescents is estimated to be 8 mg/day. The DRIs for infants are 2 mg/day for the first 6 months and 3 mg/day for the second 6 months of life.

Food Sources and Intakes

For most Americans, most daily intake of zinc is provided by meat, fish, poultry, ready-to-eat breakfast cereals fortified with zinc, and milk and milk products. Oysters are especially high in zinc, and other shellfish, liver, whole-grain cereals, dry beans, and nuts are all good sources (Table 3-32). Soy products may also be fairly good sources of zinc. In general, zinc intake correlates well with protein intake.

The zinc content of typical diets of adults in Western countries ranges between 10 and 15 mg/day; women consume less than men because of lower energy intakes. The zinc density of the American adult's diet is approximately 5.6 mg/1000 kcal.

TABLE 3-32

Zinc Content of Selected Foods

Food	Content (mg)
Oysters, 6 medium	76.7
Beef shanks, cooked, 3 ounces	8.9
Crab, Alaska king, cooked, 3 ounces	6.5
Pork shoulder, cooked, 3 ounces	4.2
Breakfast cereal fortified with 25% of the DV for zinc, ¾ cup serving	3.8
Chicken leg, roasted, 1 leg	2.7
Pork tenderloin, cooked, 3 ounces	2.5
Lobster, cooked, 3 ounces	2.5
Baked beans, canned, ½ cup	1.7
Cashews, dry roasted, 1 ounce	1.6
Yogurt, fruit, low fat, 1 cup	1.6
Raisin bran, ¾ cup	1.3
Chickpeas, ½ cup	1.3
Cheese, Swiss, 1 ounce	1.1
Almonds, dry roasted, 1 ounce	1.0
Milk, 1 cup	0.9
Chicken breast, roasted, ½ breast with skin removed	0.9
Cheese, cheddar or mozzarella, 1 ounce	0.9
Kidney beans, cooked, ½ cup	0.8
Peas, boiled, ½ cup	0.8
Oatmeal, instant, 1 packet	0.8
Flounder or sole, cooked, 3 ounces	0.5
DRIs	
Infants and young children	2-5 mg/day, depending on age
Older children and adolescents	8-11 mg/day, depending on age and gender
Adults	8-11 mg/day, depending on gender
Pregnant	11-13 mg/day, depending on age
Lactating	12-14 mg/day, depending on age

From U.S. Department of Agriculture, Agricultural Research Service: Nutrient Database for Standard Reference, Release 18, Data Laboratory home page: http://www.nal.usda.gov/fnic/foodcomp/Data/SR18/nutrlist/sr18w309.pdf; accessed 1-14-11.

DRI, Dietary reference intake.

Deficiency

The clinical signs of zinc deficiency were first described as short stature, hypogonadism, mild anemia, and low plasma zinc level. This deficiency was caused by a diet high in unrefined cereals and unleavened breads, which contain high levels of fiber and phytate, which chelate with zinc in the intestine and prevent absorption. Additional symptoms of zinc deficiency include hypogeusia (decreased taste acuity), delayed wound healing, alopecia, and diverse forms of skin lesions. Acquired zinc deficiency may occur as the

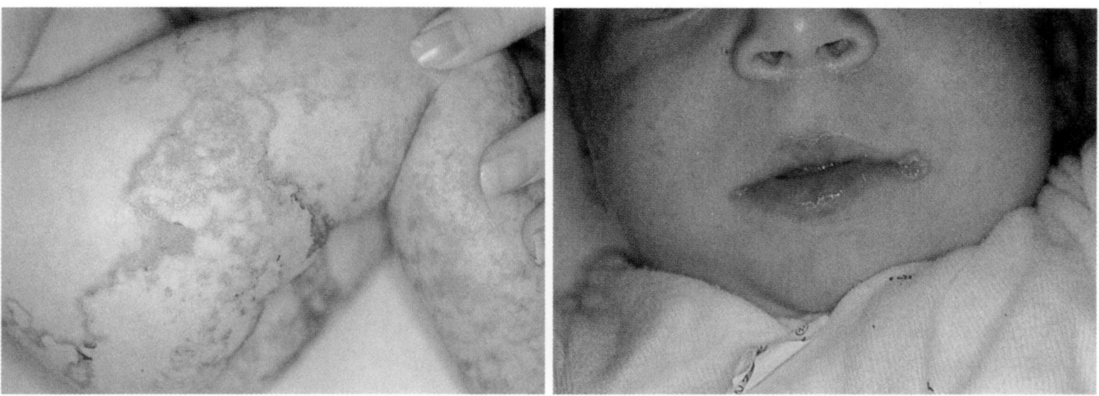

FIGURE 3-36 Cutaneous manifestations of zinc deficiency. *(From Callen WBS et al: Color atlas of dermatology, Philadelphia, 1993, Saunders.)*

result of malabsorption, starvation, or increased losses via urinary, pancreatic, or other exocrine secretions. Patients with alcoholism may have altered zinc metabolism. Pregnant women and older adults are also at increased risk for deficiency. Low-dose zinc supplementation may improve measures of poor zinc status.

Acrodermatitis enteropathica, an autosomal-recessive disease characterized by zinc malabsorption, results in eczematoid skin lesions (Figure 3-36), alopecia, diarrhea, bacterial and yeast infections, and even death if left untreated. Symptoms generally first develop during weaning from human milk to cow's milk. Researchers are working to identify the genetic basis of inherited nutritional deficiencies such as acrodermatitis enteropathica; the hZIP4 gene is involved. Zinc, biotin, protein, or essential fatty acid deficiency should be considered when there are systemic signs of failure to thrive (Gehrig and Dinulos, 2010).

Zinc deficiency results in various immunologic defects. Severe deficiency is accompanied by thymic atrophy, lymphopenia, reduced lymphocyte proliferative response to mitogens, a selective decrease in T-helper cells, decreased NK cell activity, anergy, and deficient thymic hormone activity. Even mild zinc deficiency can reduce immune function, such as impaired interleukin-2 production. Supplementation with zinc may improve immune status, but more studies are needed. Moderate zinc deficiency is associated with anergy and diminished NK cell activity but not with thymic atrophy or lymphopenia. Box 3-8 summarizes the clinical manifestations of human zinc deficiency. Similarities between patients with sickle cell anemia and zinc deficiency suggest the possibility of a secondary zinc deficiency in those with the anemia.

Problems caused by low zinc intakes seem to be increasing, partly because of the low bioavailability of zinc. Athletes may also have an increased risk for developing zinc deficiency. Physical activity may increase mobilization of zinc from bone stores for cellular needs (e.g., for the synthesis of zinc-metalloenzymes). Finally, patients on long-term parenteral nutrition who do not receive zinc will show signs of deficiency; requirements have been estimated to be 3 mg/day in patients without GI losses and a mean of 12 mg/day in patients with diarrhea and fistula losses (Jeejeebhoy, 2009).

BOX 3-8

Zinc Deficiency Symptoms

Growth retardation
Delayed sexual maturation
Hypogonadism and hypospermia
Alopecia
Delayed wound healing
Skin lesions
Impaired appetite
Immune deficiencies
Behavioral disturbances
Eye lesions, including photophobia and night blindness
Impaired taste (hypogeusia)

Toxicity

Oral ingestion of toxic amounts of zinc (100 to 300 mg/day) is rare, but the UL for zinc in adults is 40 mg/day. Excessive zinc supplementation has long been known to interfere with copper absorption. A major form of zinc toxicity develops in patients receiving hemodialysis for renal failure, with contamination of dialysis fluids from the adhesive plastic used on the dialysis coils or from galvanized pipes. The toxic syndrome in these patients is characterized by anemia, fever, and central nervous system disturbances. Zinc sulfate in amounts of 2 g/day or more may cause GI irritation and vomiting. Inhalation of zinc fumes during welding may be toxic, but exposure to fumes can be prevented with proper precautions.

Fluoride

Fluoride is a natural element found in nearly all drinking water and soil, although the fluoride content varies greatly throughout the world. For example, some well water has much more fluoride than other water, so families who use well water need to monitor fluoride levels periodically to make sure that levels are not in the toxic range. Although fluoride is not considered an essential element, this anion is known to be important for the health of bones and teeth. The average skeleton contains 2.5 mg of fluoride.

Functions

Fluoride is considered important, if not essential, because of its benefits for tooth enamel. Its incorporation into enamel produces more stable apatite crystals (Robinson et al., 2004). Fluoride also acts as an antibacterial agent in the oral cavity, serving as an enzyme inhibitor. Fluoride has no known requirement in human metabolic pathways.

The prevalence of dental caries has decreased by 50% in recent decades because of fluoridation of drinking water and the use of topical fluorides. The prevalence of dental caries has also decreased in communities without fluoridated water. This decrease probably results from the use of fluoridated toothpaste, topical fluoride applications, and use of fluoridated water used in food processing, all of which provide fluoride for incorporation into teeth. Soft drinks typically are prepared with fluoridated waters at bottling plants in urban areas.

Fluoride substitutes for the hydroxyl group on the lattice structure of calcium phosphate salts (i.e., hydroxyapatites) of the bones and teeth to form fluoroapatite, which is harder and less readily resorbed than hydroxyapatite (Chachra et al., 2008). After fluoridation, bone tissue formed at high fluoride blood levels is not healthy; it is subject to fractures from too tight binding of the fluoroapatite crystals compared with the hydroxyapatite in unfluoridated bone.

Dietary Reference Intakes

The AIs for fluoride were established for the first time in 1997. AIs for adult men and women are 4 and 3 mg/day, respectively. Depending on age, the AIs range from 2 to 3 mg/day for children and adolescents and from 0.7 to 1 mg/day for young children between the ages of 1 and 8 years. For comparison, an 8-oz glass of fluoridated water (1 ppm or 1 mg/L) provides approximately 0.2 mg of fluoride. ULs have also been established for fluoride.

Food Sources and Intakes

The major dietary sources of fluoride are drinking water and processed foods that have been prepared or reconstituted with fluoridated water. Seafood also is high in fluoride, but the content in freshwater fish is lower than that of saltwater fish. Soups and stews made with fish and meat bones also provide substantial fluoride, as do beef liver and mechanically deboned meat and fowl. Although fluorides exist in fruits and vegetables, the amounts in most foods are not significant.

The amount in tea leaves can be substantial, depending on the brewing strength. One cup of tea may contain as much as 1 mg of fluoride. Fluoridated toothpastes are also a source of fluoride; calcium carbonate–based fluoride toothpastes are effective in reducing caries and provide oral calcium as well (Lynch and Cate, 2005). The standard recommendation is 1 ppm for fluoridated community water supplies. Children who drink fluoridated water typically consume more total fluoride than those who do not. Intakes higher than 2 mg raise concerns about mild fluorosis, which has been reported in a few U.S. communities.

Deficiency

Because no known metabolic function exists for fluoride, fluoride cannot have a true deficiency that results in disease. Fortuitous binding in hydroxyapatite crystals, especially from fluoridated water supplies, reduces dental caries, but it does not seem to have any effect on reducing osteoporotic fractures.

Toxicity

A mild fluorosis can develop from daily doses of 0.1 mg/kg (i.e., greater than approximately 2 to 3 ppm of fluoride in the drinking water). The resulting discoloration of the teeth, or mottling, has no adverse effect except cosmetically. However, higher intakes lead to tooth flaking and more serious dental effects. Some evidence suggests that fluoride intakes are increasing among toddlers and young children because of the proliferating sources of fluoride. When drinking water contained less fluoride, the average intake was lower. Even the highest values did not exceed the recommendation of 0.08 mg/kg daily. Intakes of fluoride by young children may vary greatly from the use of dentifrices, fluoridated water, bottled drinks, and other sources. Some children may ingest total amounts of fluoride that exceed the optimum intake level (0.05 to 0.07 mg/kg daily), possibly causing dental fluorosis.

Copper

Copper, a normal constituent of blood, is another established essential micronutrient. Recent interest in copper has increased because of the many tissue-related functions. Concentrations of copper are highest in the liver, brain, heart, and kidney. Muscle contains a low level of copper, but, because of its large mass, skeletal muscle contains almost 40% of all the copper in the body. Recent investigations have increased the understanding of the physiologic roles of copper, copper homeostasis, and copper needs throughout the life cycle.

Absorption, Transport, Storage, and Excretion

Copper absorption, transport, storage and excretion are highly controlled (Kaplan and Lutsenko, 2009; Lalioti et al., 2009). Copper absorption occurs in the small intestine. Entry at the mucosal surface is by facilitated diffusion, and exit across the basolateral membrane is primarily by active transport; facilitated transfer may also occur. Competition between copper ions and other divalent cations exists at each step. Within the intestinal absorbing cells, copper ions are bound to metallothionein with greater affinity than zinc or other ions; the amount of copper absorbed may be regulated by the amount of metallothionein in the mucosal cells. Net absorption of copper varies from 25% to 60%. Low absorption efficiencies help to regulate the retention of copper in the body; therefore the percentage of absorption decreases with increased intake. Fiber and phytate intakes may slightly inhibit copper absorption.

Copper does not exist as a free ion in the body. Approximately 90% of the copper in serum is incorporated into **ceruloplasmin**, a functional enzyme at the erythrocyte-forming cells of the bone marrow. The remaining 10% is bound loosely to albumin, transcuprein, and other proteins; free amino acids; and possibly histidine. Serum copper and immunoreactive ceruloplasmin levels tend to be higher in women than in men. Serum copper concentration is greatest in the neonate, decreasing gradually during the first year of life.

Copper is transported bound to albumin, which serves as a temporary storage site for copper. In the liver copper binds to metallothionein. It serves as a storage form of copper and is incorporated into ceruloplasmin and secreted into the plasma for the transport of copper to cells. Copper is also secreted from the liver as a component of bile, its major route of excretion. Once in the GI tract, copper becomes part of the pool that may be resorbed or excreted, depending on bodily needs. Biliary excretion increases in response to excessive intakes of copper but may not be able to keep up with intake, sometimes allowing it to reach toxic levels.

Small amounts of copper are found in urine, sweat, and menstrual blood. Copper can be conserved by the kidney if necessary when substantial amounts are filtered through the glomeruli and resorbed in the tubules.

The interaction of copper with other nutrients negates the fallacy that taking vitamin and mineral supplements in amounts in excess of the recommended levels of consumption is good. In amounts of 150 mg/day, zinc induces copper deficiency by overwhelming the capacity of metallothionein in intestinal absorbing cells. High ascorbic acid intake (1500 mg/day) also reduces blood concentrations of copper, which may decrease the role of ceruloplasmin in red cell formation.

Functions

Copper is a component of many enzymes, and symptoms of copper deficiency are attributable to enzyme failures. Copper in ceruloplasmin has a well-documented role in oxidizing iron before it is transported in the plasma. Lysyl oxidase, a copper-containing enzyme, is essential in the lysine-derived cross-linking of collagen and elastin, connective tissue proteins with great tensile strength. Through the involvement of copper-containing electron transport proteins, copper also has roles in mitochondrial energy production. As part of copper-containing enzymes such as SOD, copper protects against oxidants and free radicals and promotes the synthesis of melanin and catecholamines. Other functions of copper-containing enzymes have not yet been completely defined.

Dietary Reference Intakes

An RDA of 900 mcg/day (0.9 mg/day) for adults of both genders has been established for copper (IOM, Food and Nutrition Board, 2001). Adolescents need 890 mcg. Copper intakes should range between 200 and 220 mcg/day for infants and between 340 and 440 mcg for young children. Premature infants are born with low copper reserves and may require additional dietary copper during their first few months of life.

Food Sources and Intakes

Copper is distributed widely in foods, including animal products (except for milk), and most diets provide between 0.6 and 2 mg/day. Foods high in copper are shellfish (oysters), organ meats (liver, kidney), muscle meats, chocolate, nuts, cereal grains, dried legumes, and dried fruits (Table 3-33).

In general, fruits and vegetables contain little copper. Cow's milk, a poor source of copper, contains 0.015 to 0.18 mg/L, whereas the copper in human milk is well absorbed and ranges from 0.15 to 1.05 mg/L. Infants fed cow's milk may be at risk for copper deficiency because of its low copper content.

Copper intakes of individuals in several age categories in the United States have been consistently below recommended amounts, with adolescent girls consuming only approximately 50% of the recommended intakes. Typically

TABLE 3-33

Copper Content of Selected Foods

Food	Content (mg)
Beef liver, fried, 3 oz	12.4
Oysters, 3 oz	3.63
Orange juice, 1 cup	0.11
Cashews, dry roasted, ¼ cup	0.61
Sunflower seeds, ¼ cup	0.59
Baking chocolate, 1 square	0.92
Mushrooms, cooked, 1 cup	0.79
Tropical trail mix, 1 cup	0.74
Beans, white, canned, 1 cup	0.61
Yogurt, 8 oz	0.03
Broccoli, raw, 1 cup	0.04
Peaches, canned, 1 cup	0.05
Milk chocolate, 1 oz	0.16
Milk, 2% fat, 1 cup	0.03
DRI Range	
0.2-1.3 mg/day, depending on age and gender	

From U.S. Department of Agriculture, Agricultural Research Service: Nutrient Database for Standard Reference, Release 18, Data Laboratory home page: http://www.nal.usda.gov/fnic/foodcomp/Data/SR18/nutrlist/sr18w312.pdf; accessed 1-14-11.

DRI, Dietary reference intake.

the copper content of drinking water is not considered in diet surveys. The amount of copper in water from copper pipes is considered insignificant. Copper intakes may be low in U.S. diets because until recently, ready-to-eat cereals typically were not fortified with copper as they were for iron and zinc. Another reason for the potential existence of low copper intakes is the inaccuracy associated with short-term assessments of dietary copper.

Deficiency

Serum copper and ceruloplasmin levels are useful biomarkers to assess copper status in populations. More sensitive indicators of copper status such as copper-containing enzymes in blood cells are needed (Harvey et al., 2009). Copper deficiency is characterized by anemia, neutropenia, and skeletal abnormalities, especially demineralization. Other changes may also develop, including subperiosteal hemorrhages, hair and skin depigmentation, and defective elastin formation. The failure of erythropoiesis, as well as cerebral and cerebellar degeneration, may lead to death. Neutropenia and leukopenia are the best early indications of copper deficiency in children.

Classic cases of copper deficiency were reported among infants who were poorly nourished, had diarrhea, and were fed diluted cow's milk. Other cases of deficiency have been reported. Premature infants are likely to have copper deficiency unless given a supplement because most of the copper is normally transferred across the placenta during the last few months of a full-term pregnancy. Because diets in developing countries continue to be low in copper, pregnancy outcomes need to be monitored (Pathak and Kapil, 2004).

Copper is stored in the liver; deficiency develops slowly as stores become depleted. Deficiencies have not been reported in otherwise healthy humans consuming a varied diet. Low serum copper, ceruloplasmin, and SOD levels provide supportive evidence of copper deficiency, but these markers are not sensitive to marginal copper status. Bone changes, osteoporosis, metaphyseal spur formation, and soft tissue calcification in infants receiving prolonged TPN may resolve with copper supplementation. The only signs of copper deficiency found in adults are neutropenia and microcytic anemia; deficiency is very rare because copper accumulates in the liver throughout life in most individuals.

Wilson disease is an autosomal-recessive disorder of copper metabolism and liver dysfunction (Schilsky, 2009). Menkes syndrome, also known as *kinky-hair syndrome*, is a sex-linked recessive defect caused by at least 160 identified gene mutations (Møller et al., 2009). The syndrome results in copper malabsorption, increased urinary copper loss, and abnormal intracellular copper transport, all of which cause an abnormal distribution of copper among organs and within cells. Affected infants have retarded growth, defective keratinization and pigmentation of the hair, hypothermia, degenerative changes in aortic elastin, abnormalities of the metaphyses of long bones, and progressive mental deterioration. These infants typically do not survive the first few months of life. Many of the features of this disorder result from interference with the cross-linking of collagen and elastin, steps that require one or more copper enzymes. Brain tissue is practically devoid of cytochrome C oxidase, and a marked accumulation of copper occurs in the intestinal mucosa, although serum copper and ceruloplasmin levels remain very low. Many connective tissue defects occur in patients with Menkes syndrome.

Decreased plasma copper levels develop in patients with malabsorption diseases such as celiac disease, tropical sprue, protein-losing enteropathies, and nephrotic syndrome. Like zinc, low copper intakes may also contribute to reduced immune responses in otherwise healthy individuals.

Toxicity

Copper toxicity from food consumption is considered impossible. Excessive supplementation or copper salts used in agriculture may lead to liver cirrhosis and abnormalities in red blood cell formation.

Ceruloplasmin concentrations increase during pregnancy and with the use of oral contraceptives. Serum copper concentrations in pregnant women are approximately twice those in women who are not pregnant. Serum and biliary copper concentrations can be elevated in acute or chronic infections, liver disease, and pellagra. The physiologic significance of these elevations is not known.

Any chronic liver disease that interferes with the excretion of bile may contribute to the retention of copper. Primary biliary cirrhosis, as well as mechanical obstruction of the bile ducts, contributes to a progressive rise in liver copper content.

ULTRATRACE MINERALS

Ultratrace minerals such as iodine, selenium, manganese, molybdenum, chromium, and a few other nonessential minerals are found in the body in small quantities; their amounts are typically measured in micrograms. Each of these elements has one or more essential roles. Because of their small quantities in human tissues, special analytic instrumentation and ultraclean laboratories are necessary for the routine analysis or experimental work relating to the ultratrace minerals.

Iodine

Iodine deficiency in the United States and many Western nations has practically been eliminated with the iodinization of salt. However, people living in many mountainous areas of the world and a few low-lying delta regions still have low iodine intakes because of the low content in soil used for cultivating crops. Others living in lowlands may have high goitrogen consumption that reduces iodine use by the thyroid gland. The body normally contains 20 to 30 mg of iodine, with more than 75% in the thyroid gland and the rest distributed throughout the body, particularly in the lactating mammary gland, gastric mucosa, and blood.

Absorption, Transport, Storage, and Excretion

Iodine is absorbed easily as iodide. In the circulation iodine exists freely and protein bound, but the bound iodide predominates. Excretion is primarily via urine, but small amounts are found in the feces as a result of biliary secretion.

Functions

Dietary iodine is needed for the synthesis of thyroid hormones. Iodine is stored in the thyroid gland, where it is used in the synthesis of **triiodothyronine (T_3)** and **thyroxine (T_4)**. Uptake of iodide ions by the thyroid cells may be inhibited by goitrogens (substances that exist naturally in foods). Thyroid hormone is degraded in target cells and the liver, and the iodine is highly conserved under normal conditions. Selenium is important in iodine metabolism because of its presence in one enzyme responsible for forming active T_3 from thyroglobulin stored in the thyroid gland.

Dietary Reference Intakes

An iodine intake of 150 mcg/day has been suggested as sufficient for all adults and adolescents. The RDA for pregnant and lactating women increases to 220 mcg and 290 mcg, respectively. The AI is 110 mcg for infants up to 6 months of age and 130 mcg for older infants. The RDA for children is between 90 and 120 mcg and increases with age or body size. Urinary iodine, serum thyroxine, or thyroid-stimulating hormone levels are useful biomarkers of iodine status (Ristic-Medic et al., 2009). See Chapter 32.

Food Sources and Intakes

Iodine exists in variable amounts in food and drinking water. Seafood, such as clams, lobsters, oysters, sardines, and other saltwater fish, is the richest source. Saltwater fish contain 300 to 3000 mcg/kg of flesh; freshwater fish contain 20 to 40 mcg/kg, but they are still good sources. The iodine content of cow's milk and eggs is determined by the iodides available in the diet of the animal; the iodide content of vegetables varies according to the iodine content of the soil in which they grow. Iodine also enters the food chain through iodophors, which are used as disinfectants in dairy processing, coloring agents, and dough conditioners. These sources add significant amounts of iodine to the food supply. Table 3-34 lists the iodine content of various foods.

The best way to obtain an AI of iodine is to use iodized salt (approximately 60 mcg of iodine per gram of salt) in food preparation. Sea salt naturally contains variable amounts of iodine and only approximately one-tenth the level of iodized salt. More than 50% of the table salt sold in the United States is iodized; however, iodized salt is not used in processed foods. Mandatory iodinization has been adopted by many nations, including Canada, but is not legally required in the United States, where iodine deficiency is now very rare. The use of iodized salt should still be advocated in certain areas to prevent goiter.

TABLE 3-34

Iodine Content of Selected Foods

Food	Content (mcg)
Ocean fish, 6 oz	650
Salt, iodized, ¼ teaspoon	95
Bread, made with iodate dough conditioner and continuous mix process, 1 slice	142
Yogurt, low fat, 8 oz	87
Bread, made with regular process, 1 slice	35
Cheese, cottage, 2% fat, 4 oz	26-71
Shrimp, 3 oz	21-37
Egg, 1	24
Cheese, cheddar, 1 oz	5-23
Ground beef, 3 oz	8
DRIs	
Infants	110-130 mcg/day, depending on age
Children ages 1-8 years	90 mcg/day
Children 9-13 years	120 mcg/day
Adolescents and Adults	150 mcg/day
Pregnant	220 mcg/day
Lactating	290 mcg/day

From:

(1) U.S. Department of Agriculture: Composition of foods, USDA Handbook No. 8 Series, Washington, DC, 1976-1986, Agricultural Research Service, The Department.

(2) Medline Plus. Website http://www.nlm.nih.gov/medlineplus/ency/article/002421.htm, accessed 1-14-11.

DRI, Dietary reference intake.

The Total Diet Study of the FDA showed that median adult iodine intakes from 1982 to 1991 ranged from 130 to 140 mcg/day for women and 182 to 204 mcg/day for men. The median iodine intake for male and female teenagers was even higher. Intakes of iodine in the United States seem adequate for most people because of iodinization of salt and the use of iodofors. Vegans consume iodine in seaweed or kelp tablets; some individuals may have excessive iodine intakes.

Deficiency

An estimated two billion people worldwide remain at risk for iodine deficiency. Most are in developing countries, especially those who do not have seafood as part of their diets. These individuals may have a moderate iodine deficiency, even when obvious goiter, a severe condition, is not evident. In children, iodine deficiency is associated with poor cognition. Use of iodized salt or the oral administration of a single dose of iodized oil and weekly iodine supplements are effective. Use of iodized salt should be encouraged during pregnancy, especially through the end of the second trimester.

Very low iodine intakes are associated with the development of endemic or simple **goiter**, which is an enlargement of the thyroid gland (Figure 3-37). Deficiency may be nearly total, especially in mountainous areas and regions of high goitrogen intakes, or relative, subsequent to an increased need for thyroid hormones (e.g., by females during adolescence, pregnancy, and lactation).

Although many countries have worked to eliminate iodine deficiency, goiter may affect as many as 200 to 300 million people worldwide (Kusic and Jukic, 2005). In some countries goiter is so common that it is regarded as a normal physical feature. In the United States the prevalence rate of goiter for all ages is 1.9/1000 persons. The rate is higher in women than in men and in older individuals than in younger ones.

Goitrogens, which exist naturally in foods, can also cause goiter by blocking uptake of iodine from the blood by thyroid cells. Foods containing goitrogens include cabbage, turnips, rapeseeds (from rape plants), peanuts, cassava, sweet potatoes, kelp, and soybeans. Goitrogens are inactivated by heating or cooking.

Severe iodine deficiency during gestation and early postnatal growth results in **cretinism** in infants, characterized by mental deficiency, spastic diplegia or quadriplegia, deaf mutism, dysarthria, a characteristic shuffling gait, shortened stature, and hypothyroidism. Less severe variations of this syndrome also exist, manifesting as moderate retardation in intellectual or neuromotor maturation. In some areas, use of iodine supplementation has been found to improve cognitive function in school-aged children who are mildly deficient (Gordon et al., 2009). The WHO has increased the recommended iodine intake during pregnancy from 200 to 250 mcg/day; in regions where less than 90% of households are using iodized salt, iodine supplementation should be used in pregnancy and infancy (Zimmerman, 2009).

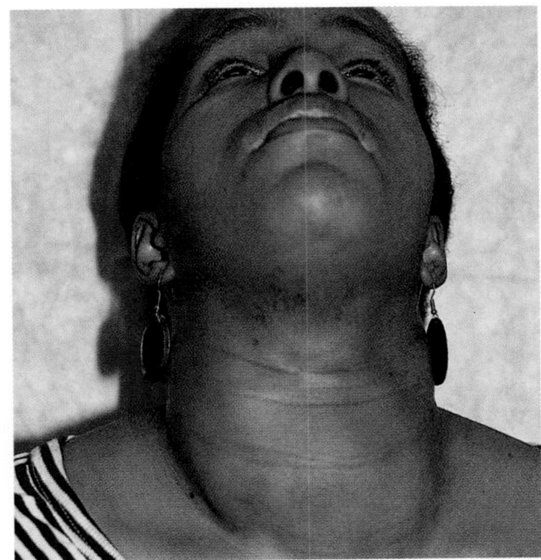

FIGURE 3-37 Goiter caused by iodine deficiency. *(From Swartz MH: Textbook of physical diagnosis history and examination, ed 3, Philadelphia, 1998, Saunders.)*

Toxicity

Even though iodine intakes have a wide margin of safety, tolerable ULs have been established (IOM, Food and Nutrition Board, 2001). Adults have a UL of 1100 mcg/day, and young children have a UL of 200 to 300 mcg/day. In some cases goiter develops slowly as a consequence of long-term iodine intakes that are much higher than physiologic requirements. The role of excessive iodine in thyroid disease or disorder is not clear. Today the level of iodine in foods is not considered a significant public health problem in the United States or Canada. The level of iodine in most American diets is appropriate for good health. For small groups of people with underlying thyroid pathologic conditions, excessive iodine in the diet may result in hypothyroidism, goiter formation, or hyperthyroidism (Mussig et al., 2006).

Selenium

A narrow dietary intake range exists for selenium, below which deficiency occurs and above which toxicity develops. Only in China have these extremes been shown to relate to the selenium content of the soil. A dietary intake of approximately 40 mcg of selenium per day seems to be necessary to maintain **glutathione peroxidase (GSH-Px)**, an enzyme containing selenium (Schrauzer and Surai, 2009). GSH-Px, discovered to be a selenoenzyme in the early 1970s, is considered the major active form of selenium in tissues, although other selenium proteins have since been discovered. Tissue levels are influenced by dietary intake and reflect the geochemical environment. Regions of North America identified as low in selenium content are the Northeast, Pacific, Southwest, and coastal plains of the southeastern region of the United States, as well as north central and eastern Canada. The lowest selenium content of soil exists in a few regions of China, especially Keshan, where severe selenium deficiency was first reported in a human population in 1979. Other areas with low selenium content include parts of Finland and New Zealand.

Absorption, Transport, Storage, and Excretion

Absorption of selenium, which occurs in the upper segment of the small intestine, is more efficient under conditions of deficiency. Increased intake frequently results in increased excretion of selenium in the urine. Selenium status is assessed by measuring selenium or GSH-Px in serum, platelets, and erythrocytes or in whole blood. Erythrocyte selenium measurement is an indicator of long-term intake. Selenium is transported bound to albumin initially and subsequently to α_2-globulin.

Functions

Selenium, as selenomethionine or selenocysteine, exists in several proteins that are widely distributed in the body. Cellular GSH-Px has been found in almost all cells and extracellularly in serum and milk. GSH-Px acts with other antioxidants to reduce cellular peroxides and free radicals in general into water and other harmless molecules. This family of enzymes may help provide a reserve of selenium in proteins that can be drawn on when needed. Many but not all of the pathologic changes caused by selenium deficiency reflect inadequate levels of GSH-Px enzymes.

Phospholipid hydroperoxide GSH-Px is found in lipid-soluble fractions of the cell and has roles in lipid and eicosanoid metabolism. Type 1 iodothyronine 5′-deiodinase, an enzyme capable of converting T_4 to T_3, is a selenoprotein. Moderate selenium intakes (40 mcg/day) seem adequate to maintain activities of these deiodinases. However, high intakes (350 mcg/day) are associated with depressed T_3 levels. GSH-Px enzymes have also been shown to be critical in several endocrine systems (Beckett and Arthur, 2005).

Selenoprotein P may act as a free radical scavenger or a transporter of selenium. Selenium is used in the synthesis of these molecules in the anionic form. In the molecules, selenium is covalently bound, as is sulfur, which it typically replaces in some of these molecules. The antioxidant effects of selenium and vitamin E may reinforce each other by the overlap of their protective actions against oxidative damage. These two antioxidant nutrients may participate in other cooperative activities that help maintain healthy cells. GSH-Px acts in the cytosol and the mitochondrial matrix, whereas vitamin E exerts its antioxidative actions within cell membranes.

The GSH-Px reaction step is illustrated in Figure 3-38. Other selenium-dependent enzymes exist in mammalian systems, but less is known about their requirements for selenium. The selenium-containing enzymes may have an antioxidative role in preventing cancer. Many other selenoproteins have been identified, but their functions have not yet been elucidated.

Dietary Reference Intakes

The RDAs for selenium are 55 mcg/day for women, men, and adolescents (ages 14 to 18), whereas the RDAs for children range from 20 to 30 mcg/day. The AIs for infants is 15 to 20 mcg/day. The RDA during pregnancy is 60 mcg, and the RDA during lactation is 70 mcg/day. Requirements for selenium may increase with a high consumption of unsaturated fatty acids because of the need for higher antioxidant activity. However, low-dose chronic exposure to selenium may be widespread in some populations; the upper safe limit may actually be set too high (Vinceti et al., 2009).

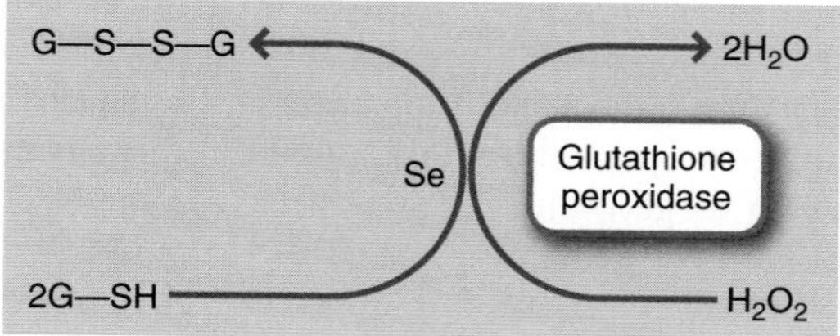

FIGURE 3-38 Enzymatic reaction catalyzed by the selenium-containing enzyme, glutathione peroxidase. Selenium is a prosthetic form of the enzyme that removes highly reactive hydrogen peroxide from within cells by converting it to water while simultaneously converting two molecules of reduced glutathione to oxidized glutathione.

Food Sources and Intakes

No comprehensive table of the selenium content of foods has been published. The selenium concentration in foods depends on the selenium content of the soil and water where the food was grown. Improvements in analytic techniques have resulted in changes being made to many previously published data of the selenium content of foods during the last few decades (Table 3-35).

Major food sources of selenium are Brazil nuts, seafood, kidney, liver, meat, and poultry. Highest intake in the United States is from animal flesh foods. Grains vary in selenium content, depending on where they are grown. Fruits and vegetables are low in selenium content.

Selenium content and GSH-Px activity in human breast milk are influenced directly by maternal intake and by the

TABLE 3-35

Selenium Content of Selected Foods

Food	Content (mcg)
Brazil nuts, 1 oz	543
Fast food fish sandwich, 1	89
Halibut, baked, ½ fillet	74
Tuna , canned, 3oz	68
Oysters, raw, 3 oz	56
Rice, white, long grain, 1 cup	44
Chicken, breast, baked, 3 oz	39
Pie crust, 1	38
Egg noodles, cooked, 1 cup	38
Lobster, 3 oz	36
Wheat germ, toasted, ¼ cup	28
Bagel, 1, 4-inch	27
Sunflower seeds, ¼ cup	25
Egg, 1	16
Bread, whole wheat, 1 slice	10
Asparagus, cooked, 1 cup	7
Milk, 2% fat, 1 cup	6
DRIs	
Infants	15-20 mcg/day, depending on age
Young children	20-30 mcg/day, depending on age
Older children and adolescents	40-55 mcg/day, depending on age
Adults	55 mcg/day
Pregnant	60 mcg/day
Lactating	70 mcg/day

From U.S. Department of Agriculture, Agricultural Research Service: Nutrient Database for Standard Reference, Release 18, Data Laboratory home page: http://www.nal.usda.gov/fnic/foodcomp/Data/SR18/nutrlist/sr18w317.pdf; accessed 2011.

DRI, Dietary reference intake.

form of selenium consumed. Plasma selenium concentrations of infants fed unsupplemented formula are lower than those of infants fed supplemented formula or human milk. Selenium fortification of infant formulas has been shown to improve the status of infants.

Deficiency

Despite a wide range of selenium intakes from food, selenium deficiency is rare in populations throughout the world. Selenium deficiency takes years to develop when food intake is adequate. Severe selenium deficiency in a population has only been reported in China. Keshan disease, a cardiomyopathy that mainly affects children and women, was first observed in the Keshan province of China. Since its discovery, supplementation programs in Keshan have totally eradicated the disease. However, in individuals with established disease, the response to supplementation is poor, probably because of other factors contributing to myopathy; a viral infection combined with selenium deficiency has been suggested (Beck et al., 1995).

The second selenium deficiency disease, discovered in Mongolia, is known as *Kashan-Beck disease* and is common in preadolescent and adolescent children. These two diseases occur in areas where the soil content of selenium is very low. This disease may also have a viral component combined with the selenium deficiency. Illness initially involves symmetric stiffness, swelling, and often pain in the interphalangeal joints of the fingers, followed by generalized osteoarthritis. Here iodine deficiency may be another risk factor.

Patients with some cancers have been shown to have low serum selenium levels, although the underlying mechanisms for this correlation have not been established. One possible explanation lies in the possible failure of GSH-Px to scavenge free radicals efficiently in dividing cells. In addition, patients with cirrhosis have low plasma selenium concentrations, which may predispose them to cancer (Latavayova et al., 2006).

Selenium deficiency has been reported in malnourished patients receiving long-term TPN. Supplementation results in improved serum selenium levels, platelet GSH-Px activity, and reduced clinical symptoms. Selenium deficiency should no longer be a problem in patients receiving long-term TPN or enteral nutrition because these solutions now include a trace element supplement.

Toxicity

Indicators of selenium toxicity have been reported in China and Australia. Signs of toxicity (*selenosis*) include skin and nail changes, tooth decay, and nonspecific GI and neurologic abnormalities. Research also suggests that excessive intakes may be mutagenic or genotoxic, a point that is important to note for pregnant women. In addition, the long-term effects of selenium supplementation on the thyroid hormones have not been clearly identified (Combs et al., 2009). In countries such as New Zealand, where both selenium and iodine levels tend to be low, supplementation with selenium alone will not improve thyroid function; iodine is also required (Thomson et al., 2009).

Manganese

Manganese deficiency in humans was first reported in 1972, and its essentiality in humans is well established. Chronic exposure to excessive manganese levels can result in psychiatric and motor disturbances, referred to as *manganism* (Yin et al., 2010). A healthy balance is required.

Absorption, Transport, Storage, and Excretion

Manganese is absorbed throughout the small intestine. Iron and cobalt compete for common binding sites for absorption. Men absorb less manganese than women, a difference noted by iron status and plasma ferritin levels. Heme iron has no influence on manganese status, but diets high in nonheme iron can be associated with lower serum manganese values, higher urinary manganese losses, and lower activity of manganese-containing enzymes.

Manganese is transported bound to a macroglobin, transferrin, and transmanganin. Excretion occurs mainly in the feces after secretion into the intestine via the bile. The cytoplasmic iron exporter ferroportin (Fpn) functions as a manganese exporter; manganese exposure promotes Fpn protein expression, which reduces manganese accumulation and its related cytotoxicity (Yin et al., 2010). Antioxidants may also play a role in the excretion of toxic levels of manganese.

Functions

Manganese is associated with the formation of connective and skeletal tissues, growth, and reproduction. The 10 to 20 mg of manganese contained in the adult human body tends to be concentrated predominantly in mitochondria. Manganese activates many enzymes, especially in conjunction with magnesium. Manganese is essential for proper metabolism of amino acids, proteins and lipids.

Manganese is a component of many enzymes, including glutamine synthetase, pyruvate carboxylase, and mitochondrial SOD (MnSOD). It catalyzes detoxification of free radicals and may protect against some types of cancer. MnSOD converts superoxide anion into hydrogen peroxide but this must be detoxified by GSH-Px. If that does not occur, hydrogen peroxide forms a hydroxyl radical with iron, which is detrimental for patients with cirrhosis who have an altered SOD gene (Nahon et al., 2009).

Dietary Reference Intakes

The AIs for manganese are 2.3 mg/day for men and 1.8 mg/day for women. For children 9 years of age and older the AIs are 1.9 to 2.2 mg/day for boys and 1.6 mg/day for girls. For children younger than 9 the AIs are 1.2 to 1.5 mg/day, depending on their age.

Food Sources and Intakes

The manganese content of foods varies greatly. The richest sources are whole grains, legumes, nuts, and tea. Fruits and vegetables are moderately good sources. Relatively high amounts exist in instant coffee and tea.

Animal tissues, seafood, and dairy products are poor sources. Human milk is relatively low in manganese. Intakes are often low for adolescent girls.

Deficiency

Manganese deficiency, although rare, affects reproductive capacity, pancreatic function, and aspects of carbohydrate metabolism. Symptoms of deficiency are weight loss, transient dermatitis, occasionally nausea and vomiting, a change in hair color, and slow hair growth. In addition, there is a correlation between low blood manganese and convulsions (Gonzalez-Reyes et al., 2007).

Animal studies have established that manganese is necessary for reproduction. Sterility develops in both sexes; striking skeletal abnormalities and ataxia characterize the offspring of mothers who are manganese deficient. Lower blood manganese levels may be associated with fetal intrauterine growth retardation and lower birth weight in humans (Wood, 2009).

Toxicity

Manganese toxicity has developed in miners as a result of absorption of manganese through the respiratory tract. The excess, which accumulates in the liver and central nervous system, produces Parkinson-like symptoms. Manganese intake in excess leads to neurotoxicity, impairing energy metabolism and causing cell death (Puli et al., 2006). This is especially true for dopaminergic neurons.

Toxicity has also been reported in patients receiving TPN with added manganese. Symptoms include headaches, dizziness, and abnormal magnetic resonance imaging results and hepatic dysfunction (Masumoto et al., 2001).

The ULs of manganese from diet have been difficult to establish. Red wine may be a source of relatively high levels of metal ions, leading to a very high target hazard quotient for those individuals consuming at least 250 mL per day for many years (Hague et al., 2008). The implications for manganese require further study.

Chromium

A biologic role for chromium was proposed in 1954 but not accepted until 1977. Patients receiving parenteral nutrition exhibited abnormalities of glucose metabolism that were reversed with chromium supplementation. The low concentrations of chromium in food, body tissues, and body fluids require careful, appropriate analytic techniques, and new standard reference materials for accurate measurements.

Absorption, Transport, Storage, and Excretion

As with other minerals, organic and inorganic forms of chromium are absorbed differently. Organic chromium is readily absorbed but quickly passes out of the body. Less than 2% of the trivalent chromium consumed is absorbed. Chromium absorption is increased by oxalate and is higher in iron-deficient animals than in animals with adequate iron, suggesting that it shares some similarities with the iron absorption pathway. With dietary intakes of 40 mcg or more per day, chromium absorption reaches and remains at a plateau; at such high intakes, urinary excretion increases to maintain balance.

The type of dietary carbohydrate consumed modifies absorption from chromium chloride. Starch rather than sugar increases absorption. Absorption is also greater from chromium picolinate than from chromium chloride, where absorption is 2% or less.

Chromium and iron are carried by transferrin; however, albumin is also capable of assuming this role if iron transferrin saturation is high. In addition, α- and β-globulins and lipoproteins can also bind chromium.

Primarily the kidney excretes inorganic chromium, with small amounts being excreted through hair, sweat, and bile. Organic chromium is excreted through bile. Strenuous exercise, physical trauma, or an increased intake of simple sugar results in increased chromium excretion.

Functions

Chromium potentiates insulin action and influences carbohydrate, lipid, and protein metabolism. It may have a beneficial effect on serum triglyceride levels. Although the chemical nature of the relationship between chromium and insulin activity has not been clearly identified, a possible chromium-NA (chromium polynicotinate) complex has been identified. Chromium may regulate the synthesis of a molecule that potentiates insulin action; this **glucose tolerance factor (GTF)** is controversial. However, chromium supplementation alone or combined with vitamins C and E minimizes oxidative stress; it also improves glucose metabolism in type 2 diabetes mellitus patients (Lai, 2008). Another possible role for chromium, similar to that of zinc, is in the regulation of gene expression.

Dietary Reference Intakes

The AIs recommended for chromium range from 25 to 35 mcg/day for males 9 years of age and older and 21 to 25 mcg/day for females of the same age. Depending on the age of the child, 11 to 15 mcg/day has been established for children 1 to 8 years of age.

Food Sources and Intakes

Precise assessment of chromium in foods is difficult; biologically available chromium and inorganic chromium cannot be distinguished from each other. Analyses done before 1980 must be considered with caution because determinations were flawed by contamination and analytic problems.

Brewer's yeast, oysters, liver, and potatoes have high chromium concentrations; seafood, whole grains, cheeses, chicken, meats, and bran have medium chromium concentrations. The refining of wheat removes chromium with the wheat germ and the bran; refining sugar fractionates the chromium into the molasses portion. Dairy products, fruits, and vegetables are low in chromium. Table 3-36 and Appendix 52 present the chromium content of selected foods.

TABLE 3-36

Chromium Content of Selected Foods

Food	Content (mcg)
Broccoli, 1/2 cup	11
Grape juice, 1 cup	8
English muffin, whole wheat, 1	4
Potatoes, mashed, 1 cup	3
Garlic, dried, 1 teaspoon	3
Basil, dried, 1 tablespoon	2
Beef cubes, 3 ounces	2
Orange juice, 1 cup	2
Turkey breast, 3 ounces	2
Whole wheat bread, 2 slices	2
Red wine, 5 ounces	1-13
Apple, unpeeled, 1 medium	1
Banana, 1 medium	1
Green beans, ½ cup	1
DRIs = AIs	
Infants	0.2-5.5 mcg/day, depending on age
Young children	11-15 mcg/day, depending on age
Older children and adolescents	21-35 mcg/day, depending on age and gender
Adults	20-35 mcg/day, depending on age and gender
Pregnant	29-30 mcg/day, depending on age
Lactating	44-45 mg/day, depending on age

From:

(1) Anderson RA, Bryden NA, Polansky MM: Dietary chromium intake, Biol Trace Elem Res 32:117, 1992.

(2) Chromium Fact Sheet. http://ods.od.nih.gov/factsheets/chromium/; accessed 1-14-11.

AI, Adequate intake; *DRI*, dietary reference intake.

Usual chromium intakes range between 25 and 35 mcg/day for women and men, respectively. Chromium intakes are not assessed in the USDA, National Health and Nutrition Examination Survey, or Total Diet Study surveys because of inadequate methodology. Human breast milk contains 3 to 8 nmol/L of chromium, which is lower than the recommended intake for infants.

Deficiency

Chromium deficiency results in insulin resistance and a few lipid abnormalities, which can be ameliorated by chromium supplementation. Insufficient chromium may be consumed by some Americans; true deficiency is more likely to occur in populations with very low intakes. Some epidemiologic studies suggest low tissue levels of chromium in patients with diabetes. However, they recommend long-term clinical trials to assess safety of chronic chromium supplementation before it is used in these patients. Claims that the ingestion of high doses of chromium consumed as chromium picolinate improves strength, body composition, endurance, or other characteristics of physical fitness are controversial, with some studies supporting these claims and others not.

Toxicity

Chromium toxicity from food has not been reported. Chromium picolinate taken as a supplement in high doses by athletes and power lifters has resulted in some adverse effects, primarily skin lesions. An increase risk of cancer has been identified in China in a population that was exposed to high chromium levels in drinking water (Smith and Steinmaus, 2009).

Molybdenum

Molybdenum has been established as an essential micronutrient, particularly because of its requirement in the enzyme xanthine oxidase (see Table 3-25). Interrelationships among molybdenum, copper, and sulfate absorption in livestock and between molybdenum intake and copper excretion in humans and animals have been demonstrated. Individuals receiving long-term TPN have displayed symptoms of molybdenum deficiency, including mental changes and abnormalities of sulfur and purine metabolism.

Absorption, Transport, Storage, and Excretion

Molybdenum, which is found in minute amounts in the body, is readily absorbed from the stomach and small intestine, with the rate of absorption being higher in the proximal small intestine than in the distal small intestine. As with other minerals, molybdenum is absorbed by two mechanisms: carrier-mediated and passive diffusion. Molybdenum is excreted primarily in the urine. Excretion rather than absorption is the homeostatic mechanism. Some molybdenum is also excreted in the bile.

Functions

Xanthine oxidase, aldehyde oxidase, and sulfite oxidase, all enzymes that catalyze oxidation-reduction reactions, require a prosthetic group containing molybdenum (Schwarz et al., 2009). Sulfite oxidase is important to the degradation of cysteine and methionine and catalyzes the formation of sulfate from sulfite. Whether molybdenum is involved in the response of some asthmatics to sulfites is not known. Genetic sulfite oxidase deficiency is a fatal disorder of cysteine metabolism. Clinical symptoms include severe brain damage with mental retardation, dislocation of the lens, and increased urinary output of sulfate.

Dietary Reference Intakes

The RDAs for molybdenum throughout the life cycle range from 43 to 45 mcg/day for adolescents and adults. Depending on the child's age, RDAs range from 17 to 34 mcg/day for children.

Food Sources and Intakes

Molybdenum is distributed widely in commonly consumed foods such as legumes, whole-grain cereals, milk and milk products, and dark green leafy vegetables. Estimated intakes, as determined by the Total Diet Study of the FDA, ranged from 50 mcg/day in infants to 80 and 126 mcg/day for 14- to 16-year-old girls and boys, respectively. These intakes were found to decrease slowly over the lifetime.

Deficiency

Molybdenum deficiency has not been established in humans other than patients treated with TPN. Symptoms of molybdenum deficiency include mental changes and abnormalities of sulfur and purine metabolism.

Toxicity

An excessive molybdenum intake of 10 to 15 mg/day is associated with a goutlike syndrome (Nielsen, 2009). However, no good biomarkers are available to assess the presence of molybdenum excess accurately. Nonetheless, plasma molybdenum does seem to reflect molybdenum intake.

Boron

The essentiality of boron for humans has not yet been established, but its essentiality for plants and animals is widely accepted. Boron, an ultratrace element, is obtained from foods such as sodium borate, and it is rapidly and almost completely (90%) absorbed. The highest concentrations of boron are found in bone, spleen, and thyroid, although it is present in all other tissues of the body.

Functions

Boron is associated with cell membranes and in plants is involved with the functional efficiency of cell membranes. Response to boron deprivation is enhanced when other nutrients that alter membrane functions are also deficient. Boron apparently binds to the active site of some enzymes, reducing their ability to function. Boron is also thought to compete with some enzymes for the coenzyme NAD.

Boron influences the activity of many metabolic enzymes and the metabolism of such nutrients as calcium, magnesium, and vitamin D (Devirian and Volpe, 2003). Evidence from animal studies shows that boron deprivation affects two major organs: the brain and bone. Boron deficiency alters brain composition and function and reduces bone composition, structure, and strength. Because of the role of boron in bone, studies in humans have focused on its potential role in the development of osteoporosis. Boron may have actions similar to estrogens on bone (Nielsen, 2009). Boron is also required for normal reproduction and healthy immune response. Other roles of boron in humans have not been well studied.

Dietary Reference Intakes

No DRIs have been established for boron.

Food Sources and Intakes

Foods that are good sources of boron include plant foods, especially noncitrus fruits, vegetables, nuts, and legumes. Wine, cider, and beer are other good sources of boron.

Deficiency and Toxicity

Symptoms of severe boron deficiency have not been established (Nielsen, 2009). No toxicity level has been identified.

Cobalt

Most of the cobalt in the body exists with vitamin B_{12} stores in the liver. Only one enzyme has an established specific requirement for cobalt. Blood plasma contains approximately 1 mcg of cobalt per 100 mL.

Absorption, Transport, Storage, and Excretion

Cobalt may share part of the same intestinal transport mechanism as iron. Absorption is higher in patients with deficient iron intake, portal cirrhosis with iron overload, and idiopathic hemochromatosis. The major route of cobalt excretion is the urine; small amounts are excreted via feces, sweat, and hair.

Functions

The well-known essential role of cobalt is as a component of vitamin B_{12} (cobalamin). This vitamin is essential for the maturation of red blood cells and the normal function of all cells. Methionine aminopeptidase, an enzyme involved in the regulation of translation (i.e., of DNA to RNA), is the only enzyme in humans known to have an established requirement of this trace element.

Dietary Reference Intakes

The dietary requirement for cobalt is expressed in terms of vitamin B_{12}. Approximately 2 to 3 mcg of vitamin B_{12} is needed daily.

Food Sources and Intakes

Cobalt exists in foods; however, only microorganisms are able to synthesize vitamin B_{12}. Ruminant animals obtain cobalamin as the result of a symbiotic relationship with the microorganisms of their GI tract. The microorganisms of monogastric species such as humans have an extremely limited capacity for synthesis; therefore humans must obtain vitamin B_{12}—and thus cobalt—from animal foods such as organ and muscle meats. In some circumstances ordinary bacterial contamination of foods of vegetable origin may supply the minute required amounts of this vitamin. Strict vegetarians who avoid all animal products may develop vitamin B_{12} deficiency, either after 3 to 6 years or not at all.

Deficiency

A cobalt deficiency develops only in relation to a vitamin B_{12} deficiency. Insufficient vitamin B_{12} causes a macrocytic anemia. A genetic defect limiting vitamin B_{12} absorption results in pernicious anemia, which is treated appropriately with massive doses of the vitamin.

Toxicity

A high intake of inorganic cobalt (existing freely from cobalamin) in animal diets produces polycythemia (an overproduction of red blood cells), hyperplasia of bone marrow, reticulocytosis, and increased blood volume.

The information on the microminerals known to be required by humans is summarized in Table 3-36.

OTHER TRACE ELEMENTS

Several other trace elements of uncertain essentiality exist, including aluminum, lithium, nickel, silicon, tin, and vanadium. A few other ultratrace elements, including arsenic, may be added to this list in the future. They are classified as ultratrace elements because of their very low quantities in human tissues. Requirements remain undefined for all of these elements because of their uncertain essentiality. The ultratrace elements continue to be enigmas because of their uncertain roles in human function. It has long been established that these elements exist in human tissues, especially in the skeleton, because of their abundance on the earth's surface, but the essentiality of any of these in humans remains questionable (Nielsen, 2009).

USEFUL WEBSITES

American Society for Bone and Mineral Research
www.asbmr.org
Dietary Guidelines for Americans
http://www.cnpp.usda.gov/dietaryguidelines.htm
Dietary Reference Intakes
http://fnic.nal.usda.gov/nal_display/index.php?info_center=4&tax_level=3&tax_subject=256&topic_id=1342&level3_id=5140
Food and Drug Administration
http://www.fda.gov/Food/default.htm
National Dairy Council
www.nationaldairycouncil.org/
National Institute of Medicine
http://www.iom.edu
USDA Nutrient Database Laboratory (Food Composition Tables)
http://www.ars.usda.gov/Services/docs.htm?docid=8964

REFERENCES

Abrams SA: Calcium supplementation during childhood: long-term effects on bone mineralization, *Nutr Rev* 63:251, 2005.

Agarwal R: Vitamin D, proteinuria, diabetic nephropathy, and progression of CKD, *Clin J Am Soc Nephrol* 4:1523, 2009.

Alberts B, et al: Cell chemistry and biosynthesis, membrane structure, energy conversion, mitochondria and chloroplasts. In *Molecular Biology of the Cell*, ed 4, New York, 2002, Garland Science.

Allen LH: Causes of vitamin B12 and folate deficiency, *Food Nutr Bull* 29:20S, 2008.

American Dietetic Association: Position of the American Dietetic Association: vegetarian diets, *J Am Diet Assoc* 109:1266, 2009.

American Dietetic Association: Position of the American Dietetic Association: fat replacers, *J Am Diet Assoc* 105:266, 2005.

American Dietetic Association: Position of the American Dietetic Association: health implications of dietary fiber, *J Am Diet Assoc* 108:1716, 2008.

Andrés E, et al: Clinical aspects of cobalamin deficiency in elderly patients: epidemiology, causes, clinical manifestations, and treatment with special focus on oral cobalamin therapy, *Eur J Intern Med* 18:456, 2007.

Artaza JN, et al: Vitamin D and the cardiovascular system, *Clin J Am Soc Nephrol* 4:1515, 2009.

Baddini F, et al: Conjugated linoleic acid (CLA): effect modulation of body composition and lipid profile, *Nutr Hosp* 24:422, 2009.

Beal MF: Therapeutic approaches to mitochondrial dysfunction in Parkinson's disease, *Parkinsonism Relat Disord* 15:189S, 2009.

Beard JL: Iron biology in immune function, muscle metabolism, and neuronal functioning, *J Nutr* 131:568, 2001.

Beck M, et al: Rapid genomic evolution of a non-virulent coxsackievirus B_3—in selenium-deficient mice results in selection of identical virulent isolates, *Nat Med* 1:433, 1995.

Beckett GJ, Arthur JR: Selenium and endocrine systems, *J Endocrinol* 184:455, 2005.

Berger MM: Vitamin C requirements in parenteral nutrition, *Gastroenterology* 137:70S, 2009.

Berndt T, Kumar R: Novel mechanisms in the regulation of phosphorus homeostasis, *Physiology (Bethesda)* 24:17, 2009.

Bitanihirwe BK, Cunningham MG: Zinc: the brain's dark horse, *Synapse* 63:1029, 2009.

Bjerrum JT et al. Metabonomics in ulcerative colitis: diagnostics, biomarker identification, and insight into the pathophysiology, *J Proteome Res* 9:954, 2010.

Block RJ, Mitchel HH: The correlation of the amino acid composition of proteins with their nutritive value, *Nutr Abstr Rev* 16:249, 1946.

Booth SL: Roles for vitamin K beyond coagulation, *Annu Rev Nutr* 29:89, 2009.

Brigelius-Flohe R: Induction of drug metabolizing enzymes by vitamin E, *J Plant Physiol* 162:797, 2005.

Brosnan JT, Brosnan ME: The sulfur-containing amino acids: an overview, *J Nutr* 136:1636S, 2009.

Bruce SJ, et al: Quantitative measurement of betaine and free choline in plasma, cereals and cereal products by isotope dilution LC-MS/MS, *J Agric Food Chem* 58:2055, 2010.

Calvo MS, et al: Vitamin D fortification in the United States and Canada: current stats and data needs, *Am J Clin Nutr* 80(6 Suppl):1710S, 2004.

Chachra D, et al: Fluoride and mineralized tissues, *Crit Rev Biomed Eng* 36:183, 2008.

Churrucal I, et al: Conjugated linoleic acid isomers: differences in metabolism and biological effects, *Biofactors* 35:105, 2009.

Clayton PT: B6-responsive disorders: a model of vitamin dependency, *J Inherit Metab Dis* 29:317, 2006.

Combs GF, et al: Effects of selenomethionine supplementation on selenium status and thyroid hormone concentrations in healthy adults, *Am J Clin Nutr* 89:1808, 2009.

Cummings JH, et al: Prebiotic digestion and fermentation, *Am J Clin Nutr* 73:415S, 2001.

Dakshinamurti K: Biotin–a regulator of gene expression, *J Nutr Biochem* 16:419, 2005.

Denisova NA, Booth SL: Vitamin K and sphingolipid metabolism: evidence to date, *Nutr Rev* 63:111, 2005.

Devirian TA, Volpe SL: The physiological effects of dietary boron, *Crit Rev Food Sci Nutr* 43:219, 2003.

Dong LM, et al: Genetic susceptibility to cancer: the role of polymorphisms in candidate genes, *JAMA* 299:2423, 2008.

Elder SJ, et al: Vitamin K contents of meat, dairy, and fast foods in the U.S. diet, *J Agric Food Chem* 54:463, 2006.

Eussen SJ, et al: Vitamins B2 and B6 and genetic polymorphisms related to one-carbon metabolism as risk factors for gastric adenocarcinoma in the European prospective investigation into cancer and nutrition, *Cancer Epidemiol Biomarkers Prev* 19:28, 2010.

Feskanich D, et al: Vitamin A intake and hip fracture among postmenopausal women, *JAMA* 287:47, 2002.

Fleming DJ, et al: Iron status of the free-living, elderly Framingham Heart Study cohort: an iron-replete population with a high prevalence of elevated iron stores, *Am J Clin Nutr* 73:638, 2001.

Freemantle E, et al: Omega-3 fatty acids, energy substrates, and brain function during aging, *Prostaglandins Leukot Essent Fatty Acids* 75:213, 2006.

Frikke-Schmidt H, Lykkesfeldt J: Role of marginal vitamin C deficiency in atherogenesis: in vivo models and clinical studies, *Basic Clin Pharmacol Toxicol* 104:419, 2009.

Gdynia HJ, et al: Severe sensorimotor neuropathy after intake of highest dosages of vitamin B6, *Neuromuscul Disord* 18:156, 2008.

Gehrer S, et al: Fewer nutrient deficiencies after laparoscopic sleeve gastrectomy (LSG) than after laparoscopic Roux-Y-gastric bypass (LRYGB)—a prospective study, *Obes Surg* 20:447, 2010.

Gehrig KA, Dinulos JG: Acrodermatitis due to nutritional deficiency, *Curr Opin Pediatr* 22:107, 2010.

Gerss J, Kopcke W: The questionable association of vitamin E supplementation and mortality—inconsistent results of different meta-analytic approaches, *Cell Mol Biol* 55:1111S, 2009.

Gilani GS, et al: Need for accurate and standardized determination of amino acids and bioactive peptides for evaluating protein quality and potential health effects of foods and dietary supplements, *JAOAC Int* 91:894, 2008.

Gogia S, Sachdev HS: Neonatal vitamin A supplementation for prevention of mortality and morbidity in infancy: systematic review of randomized controlled trials, *BMJ* 338:919, 2009.

Goldberger J, et al: A study of the diet of nonpellagrous and pellagrous households, *JAMA* 71:944, 1918.

Gonzalez-Reyes RE, et al: Manganese and epilepsy: a systematic review of the literature, *Brain Res Rev* 53:332, 2007.

Gordon RC, et al: Iodine supplementation improves cognition in mildly iodine-deficient children, *Am J Clin Nutr* 90:1264, 2009.

Grant WB, Holick MF: Benefits and requirement of vitamin D for optimal health: a review, *Altern Med Rev* 10:94, 2005.

Gropper SS, et al: *Advanced Nutrition and Human Metabolism*. ed 4, Stamford, Conn., 2005, Wadsworth, p 584.

Guerrera MP, et al: Therapeutic uses of magnesium, *Am Fam Physcian* 80:157, 2009.

Hague T, et al: Determination of metal ion content of beverages and estimation of target hazard quotients: a comparative study, *Chm Cent J* 2:13, 2008.

Harvey LJ, et al: Methods of assessment of copper status in humans: a systematic review, *Am J Clin Nutr* 89:2009S, 2009.

He K, et al: Magnesium intake and incidence of metabolic syndrome among young adults, *Circulation* 113:1675, 2006.

Heaney RP, Rafferty K: Preponderance of the evidence: an example from the issue of calcium intake and body composition, *Nutr Rev* 67:32, 2009.

Heimen KA, et al: Examining the evidence for the use of vitamin C in the prophylaxis and treatment of the common cold, *J Am Acad Nurse Pract* 21:295, 2009.

Hermann W, et al: Enhanced bone metabolism in vegetarians—the role of vitamin B12 deficiency, *Clin Chem Lab Med* 47:1381, 2009.

Hogan SL: The effects of weight loss on calcium and bone, *Crit Care Nurs Q* 28:269, 2005.

Holick MF, Chen TC: Vitamin D deficiency: a worldwide problem with health consequences, *Am J Clin Nutr* 87:1080S, 2008.

Holick MF: Vitamin D deficiency, *Med Prog* 357:266, 2007.

Holick MF: Resurrection of vitamin D deficiency and rickets, *J Clin Invest* 116:2062, 2006.

Holick MF: Sunlight and vitamin D for bone health and prevention of autoimmune diseases, cancers and cardiovascular disease, *Am J Clin Nutr* 80:1678S, 2004.

Institute of Medicine, Food and Nutrition Board: *Dietary reference intakes for thiamin, riboflavin, niacin, vitamin B_6, folate, vitamin B_{12}, pantothenic acid, biotin, and choline*, Washington, DC, 2000a, National Academies Press.

Institute of Medicine, Food and Nutrition Board: *Dietary reference intakes for vitamin C, vitamin E, selenium, and carotenoids*, Washington, DC, 2000b, National Academies Press.

Institute of Medicine, Food and Nutrition Board: *Dietary reference intakes for vitamin A, vitamin K, arsenic, boron, chromium, copper, iodine, iron, manganese, molybdenum, nickel, silicon, vanadium, and zinc*, Washington, DC, 2001, National Academies Press.

Institute of Medicine, Food and Nutrition Board: *Dietary reference intakes for energy, carbohydrates, fiber, fat, protein and amino acids (macronutrients)*, Washington, DC, 2002, National Academies Press.

Institute of Medicine, Food and Nutrition Board: *Dietary reference intakes for calcium and vitamin D*, Washington, DC, 2010, National Academies Press.

Jacques PF, et al: Long-term nutrient intake and 5-year change in nuclear lens opacities, *Arch Opthalmol* 123:517, 2005.

Jeejeebhoy K: Zinc: an essential trace element for parenteral nutrition, *Gastroenterology* 137:7S, 2009.

Kamanna VS, et al: Niacin: an old drug rejuvenated, *Curr Atheroscler Rep* 11:45, 2009.

Kamanna VS, Kashyap ML: Mechanism of action of niacin, *Am J Cardiol* 101:20B, 2008.

Kaplan JH, Lutsenko S: Copper transport in mammalian cells: special care for a metal with special needs, *J Biol Chem* 284:25461, 2009.

Kaur B, et al: Vitamin C supplementation for asthma. *Cochrane Databse Syst Rev* 2009 Jan 21;(1):CD000993.

Kharbanda KK: Alcoholic liver disease and methionine metabolism, *Semin Liver Dis* 29:155, 2009.

Kile ML, Ronnenberg AG: Can folate intake reduce arsenic toxicity? *Nutr Rev* 66:349, 2008.

Kim H: A review of the possible relevance of inositol and the phosphatidylinositol second messenger system (PI-cycle) to psychiatric disorder—focus on magnetic resonance spectroscopy (MRS) studies, *Hum Psychopharmacol* 20:309, 2005.

Kirkland JB: Niacin and carcinogenesis, *Nutr Cancer* 46:110, 2003.

Klompmaker TR: Lifetime high calcium intake increases osteoporotic fracture risk in old age, *Med Hypotheses* 65:552, 2005.

Kovacs CS: Calcium and bone metabolism during pregnancy and lactation, *J Mammary Gland Biol Neoplasia* 10:105, 2005.

Kris-Etherton PM, et al: Polyunsaturated fatty acids in the food chain in the United States, *Am J Clin Nutr* 71:179, 2000.

Kruizenga HM, et al: Effectiveness and cost-effectiveness of early screening and treatment of malnourished patients, *Am J Clin Nutr* 82:1082, 2005.

Kusic Z, Jukic T: History of endemic goiter in Croatia: from severe iodine deficiency to iodine sufficiency, *Coll Antropol* 29:9, 2005.

Lai MH: Antioxidant effects and insulin resistance improvement of chromium combined with vitamin C and e supplementation for type 2 diabetes mellitus, *J Clin Biochem Nutr* 43:191, 2008.

Lalioti V, et al: Molecular mechanisms of copper homeostasis, *Front Biosci* 4:4878, 2009.

Lanska DJ: Historical aspects of the major neurological vitamin deficiency disorders: the water-soluble B vitamins, *Handbook Clin Neurol* 95:445, 2009.

Latavayova L, et al: Selenium: from cancer prevention to DNA damage, *Toxicology* 227:1, 2006.

Leenhardt F, et al: Moderate decrease of pH by sourdough fermentation is sufficient to reduce phytate content of whole wheat flour through endogenous phytase activity, *J Agric Food Chem* 53:98, 2005.

Li F, et al: Cell Life versus cell longevity: the mysteries surrounding the NAD+ precursor nicotinamide, *Curr Med Chem* 13:883, 2006.

Lin PH, et al: Factors influencing dietary protein sources in the PREMIER trial population, *J Am Diet Assoc* 110:291, 2010.

Livesey G, et al: Glycemic response and health—a systematic review and meta-analysis: relations between dietary glycemic properties and health outcomes, *Am J Clin Nutr* 87:258S, 2008.

Ludwig DS: The glycemic index: physiological mechanisms relating to obesity, diabetes and cardiovascular disease, *JAMA* 287:2414, 2002.

Lynch RJ, Cate JM: The anti-caries efficacy of calcium carbonate-based fluoride toothpastes, *Int Dent J* 55:175, 2005.

Maiese K, et al: The vitamin nicotinamide: translating nutrition into clinical care, *Molecules* 14:3446, 2009.

Malik S, Kashyap ML: Niacin, lipids, and heart disease, *Curr Cardiol Rep* 5:470, 2003.

Mancuso M et al. Coenzyme Q10 in neuromuscular and neurodegenerative disorders, *Curr Drug Targets* 11:111, 2010.

Masumoto K, et al: Manganese intoxication during intermittent parenteral nutrition: report of two cases, *J Parenter Enter Nutr* 25:95, 2001.

McCowen KC, Bistrian BR: Essential fatty acids and their derivatives, *Curr Opin Gastroenterol* 21:207, 2005.

McKiernan F, et al: Relationships between human thirst, hunger, drinking, and feeding, *Physiol Behav* 94:700, 2008.

McNulty PH, et al: Effect of hyperoxia and vitamin C on coronary blood flow in patients with ischemic heart disease, *J Appl Physiol* 102:2040, 2007.

Meck WH, Williams CL: Metabolic imprinting of choline by its availability during gestation: implications for memory and attentional processing across the lifespan, *Neurosci Biobehav Rev* 27:385, 2003.

Micha R, Mozaffarin D: Trans fatty acids: effects on metabolic syndrome, heart disease and diabetes, *Nat Rev Endocrinol* 5:335, 2009.

Mingrone G: Carnitine in type 2 diabetes, *Ann NY Acad Sci* 1033:99, 2004.

Muñoz M, et al: An update on iron physiology, *World J Gastroenterol* 15:4617, 2009.

Musso CG: Magnesium metabolism in health and disease, *Int Urol Nephrol* 41:357, 2009.

Møller LB, et al: Molecular diagnosis of Menkes disease: genotype-phenotype correlation, *Biochimie* 91:1273, 2009.

Mussig K, et al: Iodine-induced thyrotoxicosis after ingestion of kelp-containing tea, *J Gen Intern Med* 21:666, 2006.

Nahon P, et al: Myeloperoxidase and superoxide dismutase 2 polymorphisms comodulate the risk of hepatocellular carcinoma and death in alcoholic cirrhosis, *Hepatology* 50:1484, 2009.

Nemeth E, Ganz T: The role of hepcidin in iron metabolism, *Acta Haematol* 122:78, 2009.

Nielsen FH: Is boron nutritionally relevant? *Nutr Rev* 66:183, 2009.

Nieves JW: Osteoporosis: the role of micronutrients, *Am J Clin Nutr* 81:1232S, 2005.

Oda H: Functions of sulfur-containing amino acids in lipid metabolism, *J Nutr* 136:1666S, 2006.

Omdahl JL, et al: Hydroxylase enzymes of the vitamin D pathway: expression, function, and regulation, *Annu Rev Nutr* 22:139, 2002.

Osterhues A, et al: Shall we put the world on folate? *Lancet* 374:959, 2009.

Parks S, Johnson MA: Living in low-latitude regions in the United States does not prevent poor vitamin D status, *Nutr Rev* 63:203, 2005.

Pathak P, Kapil U: Role of trace elements zinc, copper and magnesium during pregnancy and it outcome, *Indian J Pediatr* 71:1003, 2004.

Penry JT, Manore MM: Choline: an important micronutrient for maximal endurance-exercise performance? *Int J Sport Nutr Exerc Metab* 18:191-203, 2008.

Peterlik, M Cross HS: Vitamin D and calcium deficits predispose for multiple chronic diseases, *Eur J Clin Invest* 35:290, 2005.

Pettifor JM: Rickets and vitamin D deficiency in children and adolescents, *Endocrinol Metab Clin North Am* 34:537, 2005.

Pietras SM, et al: Vitamin D2 treatment for vitamin D deficiency and insufficiency for up to 6 years, *Arch Intern Med* 169:1806, 2009.

Puli S, et al: Signaling pathways mediating manganese-induced toxicity in human glioblastoma cells (u87), *Neurochem Res* 31:1211, 2006.

Riccardi G, et al: Role of glycemic index and glycemic load in the healthy state, in prediabetes, and in diabetes, *Am J Clin Nutr* 87:269S, 2008.

Ristic-Medic D, et al: Methods of assessment of iodine status in humans: a systematic review, *Am J Clin Nutr* 89:2052S-2069S, 2009.

Rivas CI, et al: Vitamin C transporters, *J Physiol Biochem* 64:357, 2008.

Roberfroid MB: Introducing inulin-type fructans, *Br J Nutr* 93(Suppl 1):S13, 2005.

Roberfroid MB: Inulin-type fructans: functional food ingredients, *J Nutr* 137:2493S, 2007.

Robinson C, et al: The effect of fluoride on the developing tooth, *Caries Res* 38:268, 2004.

Romieu I: Nutrition and lung health, *Int J Tuberc Lung Dis* 9:362, 2005.

Rufer AC et al. Structural insight into function and regulation of carnitine palmitoyltransferase, *Cell Mol Life Sci* 66:2489, 2009.

Said ZM, et al: Pyridoxine uptake by colonocytes: a specific and regulated carrier-mediated process, *Am J Physiol Cell Physiol* 294:1192, 2008.

Schlemmer U, et al: Phytate in foods and significance for humans: food sources, intake, processing, bioavailability, protective role and analysis, *Mol Nutr Food Res* 53:330S, 2009.

Schilsky ML: Wilson disease: Current status and the future, *Biochimie* 91:1278, 2009.

Scholz-Ahrens KE, et al: Effects of prebiotics on mineral metabolism, *Am J Clin Nutr* 73:459S, 2001.

Schrauzer GN, Surai PF: Selenium in human and animal nutrition: resolved and unresolved issues, *Crit Rev Biotechnol* 29:2, 2009.

Schwarz G, et al: Molybdenum cofactors, enzymes and pathways, *Nature* 460:839, 2009.

Shaw GM, et al: Choline and risk of neural tube defects in a folate-fortified population, *Epidemiology* 20:714, 2009.

Shelton RC, et al: Therapeutic options for treatment-resistant depression, *CNS Drugs* 24:131, 2010.

Shrimpton R, et al: Zinc deficiency: what are the most appropriate interventions? *BMJ* 330:347, 2005.

Simon KC, et al: Polymorphisms in vitamin D metabolism related genes and risk of multiple sclerosis, *Mult Scler* 16:133, 2010.

Slatsky I, et al: Enhancement of learning and memory by elevating brain magnesium, *Neuron* 65:165, 2010.

Smith AH, Steinmaus CM: Health effects of arsenic and chromium in drinking water: recent human findings, *Ann Rev Public Health* 30:107, 2009.

Sokol RJ: Antioxidant defenses in metal-induced liver damage, *Semin Liver Dis* 16:39, 2001.

Sommer A: Vitamin A deficiency and clinical disease: an historical overview, *Nutrition* 138:1835, 2008.

Stahl W, et al: Non-antioxidant properties of carotenoids, *Biol Chem* 383:553, 2002.

Stevenson M, et al: Vitamin K to prevent fractures in older women: systematic review and economic evaluation, *Health Technol Assess* 13:iii, 2009.

Stiff L: How should the effectiveness of a nutrition intervention addressing suboptimal intake of vitamin D be evaluated? *J Am Diet Assoc* 109:2120, 2009.

Tazoe H, et al: Roles of short-chain fatty acids receptors, GPR41 and GPR43 on colonic functions, *J Physiol Pharmacol* 59:251S, 2008.

Thomson CD, et al: Selenium and iodine supplementation: effect on thyroid function of older New Zealanders, *Am J Clin Nutr* 90:1038, 2009.

Tobacman JK: Review of harmful gastrointestinal effects of carrageenan in animal experiments, *Environ Health Perspect* 109:983, 2001.

Traber MG: Vitamin E and K interactions—a 50-year-old problem, *Nutr Rev* 66:624, 2008.

Tuerk MJ, Fazel N: Zn deficiency, *Curr Opin Gastroenterol* 25:136, 2009.

United States Department of Agriculture: Dietary guidelines for Americans 2005: http://www.health.gov/dietaryguidelines/dga2005/document/.

Varela-Moreiras G, et al: Cobalamin, folic acid, and homocysteine, *Nutr Rev* 67:S69, 2009.

Vinceti M, et al: Risk of chronic low-dose selenium overexposure in humans: insights from epidemiology and biochemistry, *Rev Environ Health* 24:231, 2009.

Weinberg PD: Analysis of the variable effect of dietary vitamin E supplements on experimental atherosclerosis, *Plant Physiol* 162:823, 2005.

Welch G, et al: Evaluation of clinical outcomes for gastric bypass surgery: results from a comprehensive follow-up study, *Obes Surg* 21:18-28, 2011.

Wertz PW: Essential fatty acids and dietary stress, *Toxicol Ind Health* 25:279, 2009.

Wigertz K, et al: Racial differences in calcium retention in response to dietary salt in adolescent girls, *Am J Clin Nutr* 81:895, 2005.

Winkels RM, et al: Bioavailability of food folates is 80% of that of folic acid, *Am J Clin Nutr* 85:465, 2007.

Wood RJ: Manganese and birth outcome, *Nutr Rev* 67:416, 2009.

Wright AJ, et al: Comparison of (6 S)-5-methyltetrahydrofolic acid v. folic acid as the reference folate in longer-term human dietary intervention studies assessing the relative bioavailability of natural food folates: comparative changes in folate status following a 16-week placebo-controlled study in healthy adults, *Br J Nutr* 26:1, 2009.

Yamaguchi M. Role of nutritional zinc in the prevention of osteoporosis, *Mol Cell Biochem* 338:241, 2010.

Yin Z, et al: Ferroportin is a manganese-responsive protein that decreases manganese cytotoxicity and accumulation, *J Neurochem* 112:1190, 2010.

Zeisel S, da Costa KA: Choline: an essential nutrient for public health, *Nutr Rev* 67:615, 2009.

Zempleni J, et al: Biotin, *Biofactors* 35:36, 2009.

Zimmerman MB: Iodine deficiency in pregnancy and the effects of maternal iodine supplementation on the offspring: a review, *Am J Clin Nutr* 89:668S, 2009.

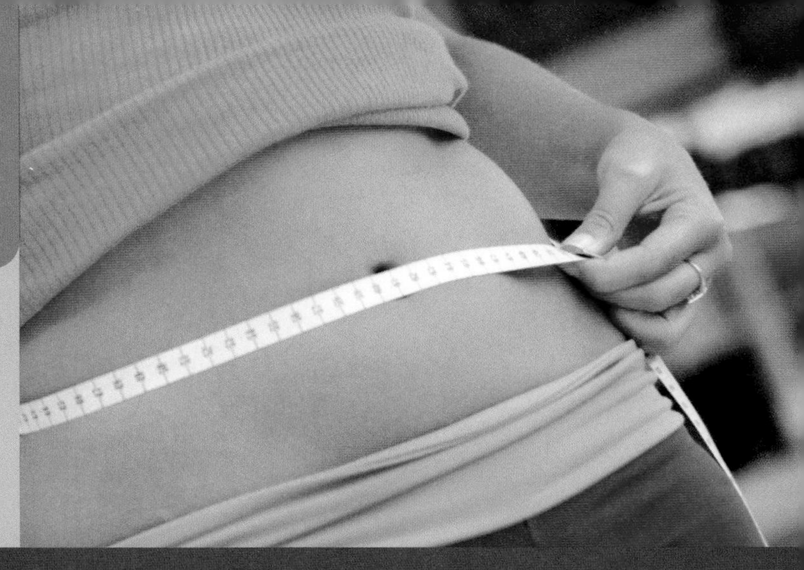

CHAPTER 4

Kathleen A. Hammond, MS, RN, BSN, BSHE, RD, LD

Intake: Analysis of the Diet

KEY TERMS

24-hour recall
ageusia
anosmia
diet history
dietary intake data
dysgeusia
food diary
food frequency questionnaire
Geriatric Nutritional Risk Index (GNRI)
Mini Nutritional Assessment (MNA)
Malnutrition Universal Screening Tool (MUST)
nutrient intake analysis (NIA)
nutrition assessment
nutrition status
overnutrition
Subjective Global Assessment (SGA)
undernutrition

Nutrition status mirrors the degree to which physiologic nutrient needs are met for an individual. The balance between nutrient intake and nutrient requirements equals that nutrition status. When adequate nutrients are consumed to support the body's daily needs, including any increased metabolic demands, the person moves into optimal nutrition status (Figure 4-1). Adequate intake promotes growth and development, maintains general health, supports activities of daily living, and helps protect the body from disease and illness.

Accurate assessment of dietary intake is essential for researchers and public health practitioners to make advancements in public health, especially for population groups that display high disease prevalence rates (Fialkowski et al., 2010). Appropriate assessment techniques can detect a nutritional deficiency in the early stages of development, allowing dietary intake to be improved through nutrition support and counseling before a more severe condition develops. Personal intake is influenced by factors such as economic situation, eating behavior, emotional climate, cultural influences, effects of disease states on appetite, and the ability to acquire and absorb nutrients. Nutrient requirements are influenced by genetics, physiologic stressors such as infection, acute or chronic disease processes, fever, trauma; anabolic states such as pregnancy, childhood, or rehabilitation; overall body maintenance; and psychological stress.

Although a nutrition assessment can be performed routinely for any individual, ideal tools will differ for healthy versus critically ill individuals. Persons at nutritional risk can be identified on the basis of screening information that is routinely obtained at the time of admission to a hospital or nursing home, in a clinic setting, or after returning to home-based care. This information is then used to design an individualized nutrition care plan. A thorough assessment increases the likelihood that effective interventions will be applied to resolve the identified nutritional diagnoses.

NUTRITION IMBALANCE

Nutrition is an important factor in the cause and management of several major causes of death and disability in contemporary society (Table 4-1) (Centers for Disease Control and Prevention [CDC], 2009b; Xu et al., 2009).

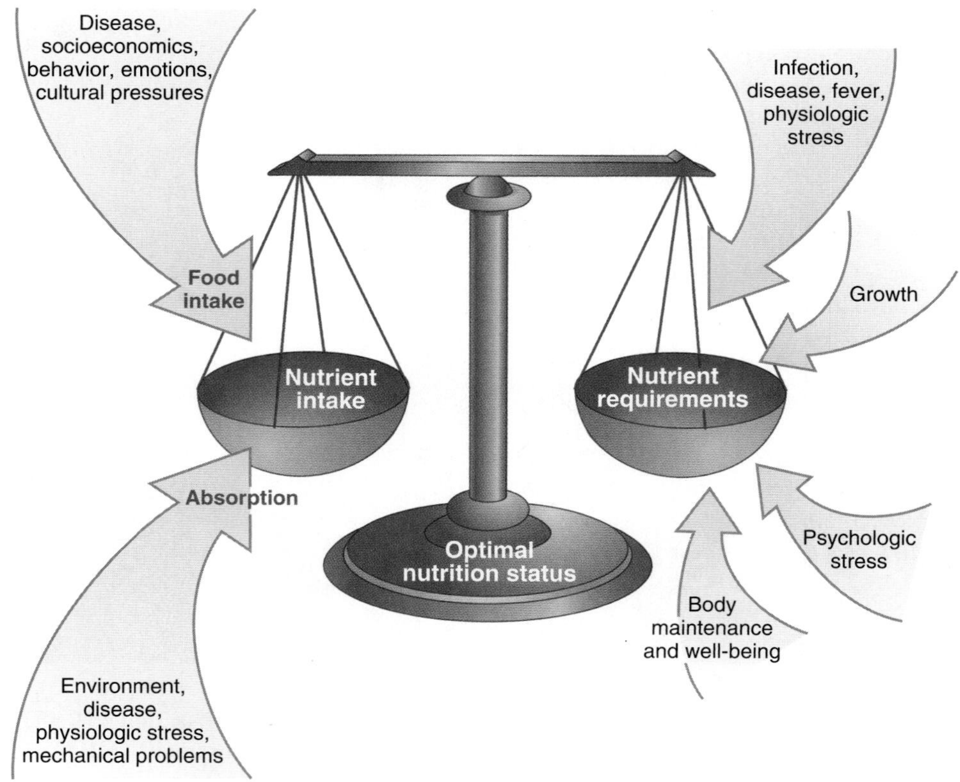

FIGURE 4-1 Optimal nutrition status: a balance between nutrient intake and nutrient requirements.

TABLE 4-1

Ranking of the Leading Causes of Death in the United States, 2005

All Causes	Rank for All Races, Both Sexes, All Ages	Rank for White Race, Both Sexes, All Ages	Rank for Hispanic, Both Sexes, All Ages	Rank for Black, Both Sexes, All Ages	Rank for Native American, Both Sexes, All Ages
Heart diseases	1	1	1	1	1
Malignant neoplasms	2	2	2	2	2
Cerebrovascular diseases	3	3	4	3	5
Chronic lower respiratory	4	4	8	7	7
Accidents, unintentional injuries	5	5	3	4	3
Diabetes mellitus	6	7	5	5	4
Alzheimer disease	7	6	—	—	—
Influenza and pneumonia	8	8	9	—	9
Nephritis, nephritic syndrome, nephrosis	9	9	—	8	10
Septicemia	10	—	—	10	—
Suicide	—	10	—	—	8
Chronic liver disease or cirrhosis	—	—	6	—	6
Assault or homicide	—	—	7	6	—
Conditions originating in prenatal period	—	—	10	—	—
AIDS or HIV infection	—	—	—	9	—

From Heron M, Tejada-Vera B: Deaths: leading causes for 2005: national vital statistics reports, vol 58, no. 8, Hyattsville, Md, 2009, National Center for Health Statistics.

—, a ranking was not in the top 10 causes for the category; *AIDS*, Acquired immunodeficiency syndrome; *HIV*, human immunodeficiency virus.

Heart disease, strokes, diabetes, and most cancers are influenced by the type and amount of food consumed. Nutrition is also significant in major diseases such as obesity, anemia, and osteoporosis. In addition, cirrhosis of the liver and some accidents may be associated with excessive alcohol intake. Modifications in diet can assist in the prevention of disease, particularly for overweight and obese individuals. In addition, nutrition intake affects gene expression and vice versa, with implications for many disorders.

States of nutritional deficiency or excess occur when nutrient intake does not match an individual's requirements for optimal health. Within the safe range of intake, homeostatic mechanisms allow the body to use nutrients equally effectively, with no detectable advantage gained by a specific intake. As deficiencies or excesses develop, adaptations are made to achieve a new steady state without any significant loss in physiologic function. As the intake departs further from the desirable range, the organism accommodates to the changing supply of nutrients by reducing the function, size, or status of the affected body compartments. The nutrition status of an individual is identified by the success or failure of these adaptations. For example, before iron deficiency anemia is diagnosed from measures of hematocrit, hemoglobin, and clinical signs, a gradual diminution in iron stores can be diagnosed on the basis of increased iron absorption, decreased serum ferritin levels, or bone marrow evaluation.

When nutritional reserves are depleted or intake is inadequate to meet daily metabolic needs, a state of **undernutrition** develops. Undernutrition may stem from inadequate ingestion, impaired digestion or absorption, dysfunctional metabolic processing, or increased excretion of essential nutrients. Infants, children, pregnant women, individuals with low incomes, hospitalized persons, and older adults are at the greatest risk for becoming undernourished. Impaired growth and development, lowered resistance to infection, delayed wound healing, poor clinical outcome from disease or trauma, development of chronic disease and increased morbidity and mortality may result.

Critically ill patients who have severe injury and stress can rapidly break down their body protein and energy stores; in such cases, malnutrition and protein wasting can negatively affect patient outcome (Btaiche et al., 2010). Hospital malnutrition was identified more than 30 years ago in a landmark article by Butterworth (1974), yet the problem continues today (DeLegge and Drake, 2007). It is estimated that in academic hospitals in the United States, 25% to 50% of patients show some type of malnutrition, generalized wasting, or protein depletion; this is most detrimental in a lengthy hospital stay.

Overnutrition also presents problems manifesting as obesity, diabetes, atherosclerotic heart disease, hypertension, and the metabolic syndrome. These conditions may also result in poor clinical outcomes. Obesity is associated with low-grade inflammation, high levels of inflammatory markers such as C-reactive protein, and proinflammatory cytokines. Obesity has reached epidemic proportions in the United States and in other parts of the world. One third of all adults are classified as obese and 300,000 deaths per year in the US are related to obesity (CDC, 2009a; USDHHS, 2007; 2009). Assessing the obese injured patient presents an even greater challenge. Screening tools that identify one to be at risk only when undernourished may label the injured obese patient as low risk and less likely to be identified as having the potential for increased morbidity. More appropriate tools are needed to accurately assess this population.

Nutritional well-being and the continuum of nutritional health are essential concepts to understand. Indeed, the best nutrition-based strategy for promoting optimal health and reducing the risk of chronic disease is to choose a wide variety of nutrient-rich foods and to use supplements when necessary (American Dietetic Association [ADA], 2009). Figure 4-2 illustrates the general sequence of steps leading to nutritional decline and the development of a nutritional deficiency, as well as areas in which an assessment can identify problems.

Many factors help measure whether a person is at nutritional risk. Factors to consider include food and nutrient intake patterns, psychosocial factors, medical and health histories, physical conditions associated with particular disease states and disorders, body weight and fatness, physical examination, biochemical abnormalities, medication regimens and use of herbs or botanical products (Table 4-2).

Screening and assessment are integral parts of nutrition care. The accepted nutrition care process (NCP) has four steps: (1) assessment of nutrition status; (2) identification of nutritional diagnoses; (3) interventions such as goal setting, food and nutrient delivery, education, counseling, coordination of care; and (4) monitoring and evaluation of the effectiveness of the interventions (ADA, 2010).

NUTRITION SCREENING

Ideally everyone should undergo periodic nutrition screening throughout life. Just as a medical provider conducts an annual health examination, a trained nutrition provider conducts regular nutritional evaluations. To provide cost-effective nutrition services in today's health care environment, it is important first to screen patients to find those who are at nutritional risk. Screening precedes the NCP provided by a registered dietitian (RD). The purpose of a nutrition screen is to quickly identify individuals who are malnourished or at nutritional risk and determine whether a more detailed assessment is warranted (ASPEN, 2009; Charney, 2005). In most settings the nutrition screen is completed by a dietetic technician, nurse, physician, or other qualified health care professional. Once completed, patients who are at nutritional risk are referred to an RD to perform a more in-depth assessment. Evaluation of intake is truly the specialized role of the dietetics profession, as it requires depth and skills related to nutrition and food sciences, social and behavioral sciences, physiology, and biochemistry.

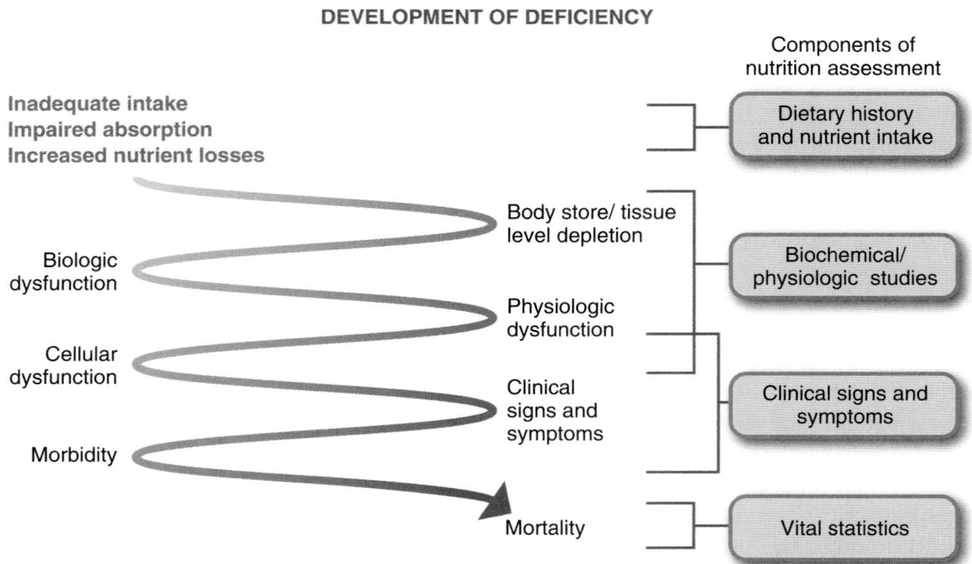

FIGURE 4-2 Development of clinical nutritional deficiency with corresponding dietary, biochemical, and clinical evaluations.

Although the components of nutrition screening may vary slightly from one setting to another, the tool should be simple and easy to complete, inclusive of readily available data, cost-effective, and effective in identifying nutrition problems. The tools must be both *reliable* (consistent between measures of the same factor, such as weight) and *valid* to measure what it is supposed to measure. In a survey of clinical nutrition managers, most common screenings include history of weight loss, current need for nutrition support, skin breakdown, poor intake, and chronic use of modified diets (Chima, 2006). Further information collected during a nutrition screen depends on (1) the setting in which the information is obtained (e.g., home, clinic, hospital), (2) the life stage or disease type, (3) available data, (4) a definition of risk priorities, and (5) the goal for the screening process. Regardless of the information gathered, the goal of screening is to identify individuals who are at nutritional risk, those likely to become at nutritional risk, and those who need further assessment. For example, being 85 years or older, having low nutrient intake, losing the ability to eat independently, having swallowing and chewing difficulties, becoming bedridden, having pressure ulcers or a hip fracture or dementia, and suffering from two or more chronic illnesses are factors of concern in a nutritional screen (Salva et al., 2009).

One useful screening tool is the **Malnutrition Universal Screening Tool (MUST)** developed by Stratton and colleagues (2004) to assess malnutrition rapidly, easily, accurately, and completely (Figure 4-3). MUST is designed to be used by multiple disciplines of professionals. Three independent criteria are used: current weight and height with determination of body mass index (BMI), unintentional weight loss using specific cutoff points, and acute disease effect on nutrition intake for greater than 5 days. These three components work better together to predict outcome rather than the individual components. Once the scores are added, the overall risk of malnutrition can be determined using three categories: 0 = low risk, 1= medium risk, and 2 and above = high risk. Management guidelines can then be followed (Stratton et al., 2004). The MUST tool is more effective than some other available tools (Henderson et al., 2008).

The **Mini Nutritional Assessment (MNA)** is a rapid and reliable method for evaluating nutritional status in older patients (i.e., 65 years and older). This tool includes both a screening section and assessment section. The screening portion contains questions related to food intake, weight loss, mobility, stress, neuropsychological condition, and BMI. Recently, a shorter version was validated using 6 versus 18 questions; this version can be completed in 15 minutes (Kaiser et al., 2009) (Figure 4-4).

Another tool is the **Geriatric Nutritional Risk Index (GNRI)**, which relies on serum albumin and differences between current and previous body weights. With the GNRI, ideal body weight (calculated using the Lorentz formula) is used in place of usual weight because usual or normal weight is often difficult to assess in the older population (Box 4-1). The GNRI can be used to predict the risk of malnutrition from weight loss and low BMI associated with illness and functional decline (Bouillanne et al., 2005).

Regardless of the tool used, the management of undernutrition requires a multidisciplinary approach. Dietary and environmental improvements, managing multiple comorbidities, avoiding polypharmacy, and the need for supplementation or tube feeding should be considered.

NUTRITION ASSESSMENT

Nutrition assessment is a comprehensive evaluation carried out by an RD using medical, and health, social, nutritional, and medication histories; physical examination; anthropometric measurements; and laboratory data. Nutrition

TABLE 4-2

Nutritional Risk Factors

Category	Factors
Food and nutrient intake patterns	• Calorie and protein intake greater or less than that required for age and activity level • Vitamin and mineral intake greater or less than that required for age • Swallowing difficulties • Gastrointestinal disturbances • Unusual food habits (e.g., pica) • Impaired cognitive function or depression • Nothing by mouth for more than 3 days • Inability or unwillingness to consume food • Increase or decrease in activities of daily living • Misuse of supplements • Inadequate transitional feeding, tube feeding or parenteral nutrition, or both • Bowel irregularity (e.g., constipation, diarrhea) • Restricted diet • Feeding limitations
Psychological and social factors	• Low literacy • Language barriers • Cultural or religious factors • Emotional disturbances associated with feeding difficulties (e.g., depression) • Limited resources for food preparation or obtaining food and supplies • Alcohol or drug addiction • Limited or low income • Lack of or inability to communicate needs • Limited use or understanding of community resources
Physical conditions	• Extreme age: adults older than 80 years, premature infants, very young children • Pregnancy: adolescent, closely spaced, or three or more pregnancies • Alterations in anthropometric measurements: marked overweight or underweight for height, age, or both; head circumference less than normal; depressed somatic fat and muscle stores; amputation • Fat or muscle wasting • Obesity or overweight • Chronic renal or cardiac disease and related complications • Diabetes and related complications • Pressure ulcers or altered skin integrity • Cancer and related treatments • Acquired immune deficiency syndrome • Gastrointestinal complications (e.g., malabsorption, diarrhea, digestive or bowel changes) • Catabolic or hypermetabolic stress (e.g., trauma, sepsis, burns, stress) • Immobility • Osteoporosis, osteomalacia • Neurologic impairments, including impairment in sensory function • Visual impairments
Abnormal laboratory values	• Visceral proteins (e.g., albumin, transferrin, prealbumin) • Lipid profile (cholesterol, high-density lipoproteins, low-density lipoproteins, triglycerides) • Hemoglobin, hematocrit, and other hematologic tests • Blood urea nitrogen, creatinine, and electrolyte levels • Fasting serum blood glucose level • Other laboratory indexes as indicated
Medications	• Chronic use • Multiple and concurrent administration (polypharmacy) • Drug-nutrient interactions and side effects

Adapted from the Council on Practice, Quality Management Committee: ADA's definitions for nutrition screening and nutrition assessment, J Am Diet Assoc 94:838, 1994.

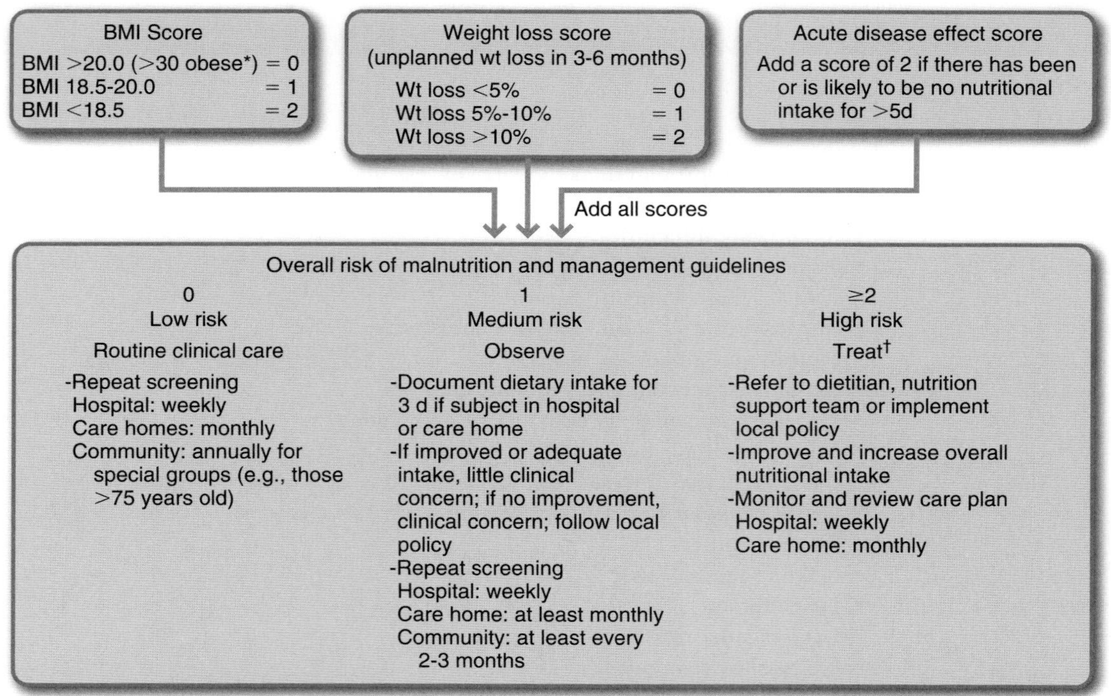

FIGURE 4-3 The Malnutrition Universal Screening Tool ("MUST") for adults. Record malnutrition risk category, presence of obesity and/or need for special diets and follow local policy for those identified at risk.

If unable to obtain height and weight, alternative measurements and subjective criteria are provided (Elia, 2003).

*In the obese, underlying acute conditions are generally controlled before treatment of obesity.

†Unless detrimental or no benefit is expected from nutritional support (e.g., imminent death).

(Courtesy Professor Marinos Elia, Editor; BAPEN, 2003 ISBN 1 899467 70X. Copies of the full report are available from the BAPEN Office, Secure Hold Business Centre, Studley Road, Redditch, Worcs BN98 7LG Tel: 01527 457850.)

BOX 4-1

Geriatric Nutritional Risk Index

GNRI = [1.489 × albumin (g/L) + [41.7 × (weight/WLo*)]

Interpretation: Four grades of nutrition-related risk

Major: (GNRI: <82)

Moderate: (GNRI: 82 to <92)

Low: (GNRI: 92 to ≤98)

None: (GNRI: >98)

*The Lorentz formula to calculate IBW is based on gender and height (Tarnus and Bourdon: Anthropometric evaluations of body composition of undergraduate students at the University of La Reunion, Adv Physiol Educ 30:248, 2006):

Female: IBW (kg) = height (cm) − 100 − {[height (cm) − 150]/2}

Male: IBW (kg) = height (cm) − 100 − {[height (cm) − 150]/4}

Derived from Bouillanne O et al: Geriatric nutrition risk index: a new index for evaluating at-risk elderly medical patients, Am J Clin Nutr 82:777, 2005.

GNRI, Geriatric Nutritional Risk Index; *IBW,* ideal body weight.

assessment interprets data from the nutrition screen and incorporates additional information. The purpose of assessment is to gather adequate information in which to make a professional judgment about nutrition status (ASPEN, 2009). Assessment is the first step in the nutrition care process Table 4-3.

The information gathered depends on the particular setting, the present health status of the individual or group, how data are related to particular outcomes, whether it is an initial or follow-up assessment, and recommended practices (ADA, 2009). Once the nutrition assessment process is complete and a nutrition diagnosis made, the plan of care can be developed. Once interventions are chosen, they can be tailored for the appropriate setting (hospital, clinic, long-term care facility, rehabilitation center, or home). In an intensive care unit, assessment is best administered within 24 hours of admission to the unit. Malnourished patients experience increased morbidity and mortality and prolonged hospital stays; nutrition support measures should begin early (Agency for Healthcare Research and Quality, 2010).

The goals of nutrition assessment are to (1) identify individuals who require aggressive nutrition support, (2) restore or maintain an individual's nutrition wellness, and (3) identify appropriate medical nutrition therapy (MNT). Patients with acute or chronic illnesses who have the potential for malnutrition should be evaluated further. Malnutrition is common in those who are obese, cachexic, or older; who have undergone trauma; and in whom nutritional intervention is neglected. Furthermore, the nutrition status of patients who are hospitalized for longer than 2 weeks deteriorates. With only minimum training in nutrition in many

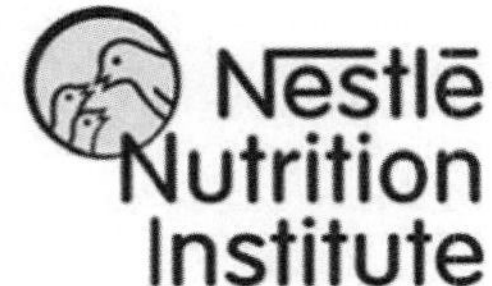

Mini Nutritional Assessment MNA®

Last name: First name:

Sex: Age: Weight, kg: Height, cm: Date:

Complete the screen by filling in the boxes with the appropriate numbers. Total the numbers for the final screening score.

Screening

A Has food intake declined over the past 3 months due to loss of appetite, digestive problems, chewing or swallowing difficulties?
0 = severe decrease in food intake
1 = moderate decrease in food intake
2 = no decrease in food intake ☐

B Weight loss during the last 3 months
0 = weight loss greater than 3 kg (6.6 lbs)
1 = does not know
2 = weight loss between 1 and 3 kg (2.2 and 6.6 lbs)
3 = no weight loss ☐

C Mobility
0 = bed or chair bound
1 = able to get out of bed / chair but does not go out
2 = goes out ☐

D Has suffered psychological stress or acute disease in the past 3 months?
0 = yes 2 = no ☐

E Neuropsychological problems
0 = severe dementia or depression
1 = mild dementia
2 = no psychological problems ☐

F1 Body Mass Index (BMI) (weight in kg) / (height in m^2)
0 = BMI less than 19
1 = BMI 19 to less than 21
2 = BMI 21 to less than 23
3 = BMI 23 or greater ☐

IF BMI IS NOT AVAILABLE, REPLACE QUESTION F1 WITH QUESTION F2.
DO NOT ANSWER QUESTION F2 IF QUESTION F1 IS ALREADY COMPLETED.

F2 Calf circumference (CC) in cm
0 = CC less than 31
3 = CC 31 or greater ☐

Screening score
(max. 14 points) ☐☐

12-14 points: Normal nutritional status
8-11 points: At risk of malnutrition
0-7 points: Malnourished

For a more in-depth assessment, complete the full MNA® which is available at **www.mna-elderly.com**

Ref. Vellas B, Villars H, Abellan G, et al. *Overview of the MNA® - Its History and Challenges.* J Nutr Health Aging 2006;10:456-465.
Rubenstein LZ, Harker JO, Salva A, Guigoz Y, Vellas B. *Screening for Undernutrition in Geriatric Practice: Developing the Short-Form Mini Nutritional Assessment (MNA-SF).* J. Geront 2001;56A: M366-377.
Guigoz Y. *The Mini-Nutritional Assessment (MNA®) Review of the Literature - What does it tell us?* J Nutr Health Aging 2006; 10:466-487.
® Société des Produits Nestlé, S.A., Vevey, Switzerland, Trademark Owners
© Nestlé, 1994, Revision 2009. N67200 12/99 10M
For more information: www.mna-elderly.com

FIGURE 4-4 Mini Nutritional Assessment—Short form. *(Permission by Nestlé Healthcare Nutrition.)*

TABLE 4-3

Nutrition Care Process: Step 1: Nutrition Assessment

Basic definition and purpose	First step of the nutrition care process. Its purpose is to obtain adequate information to identify nutrition-related problems. It is initiated by referral or screening of individuals or groups for nutritional risk factors. Nutrition assessment is a systematic process of verifying and interpreting data to make decisions about the nature and cause of nutrition-related problems. The specific types of data gathered in the assessment vary, depending on (1) practice settings, (2) individual's or group's present health status, (3) how data are related to outcomes to be measured, (4) recommended practices such as the American Dietetic Association's Evidenced-Based Guides for Practice, and (5) whether it is an initial assessment or a reassessment. Requires making comparisons between the information obtained and reliable standards (ideal goals). An ongoing, dynamic process that involves not only initial data collection but also continual reassessment and analysis of patient, client, or group needs. Provides the foundation for the nutrition diagnosis at the next step of the nutrition care process.
Data sources/tools for assessment	Referral information and interdisciplinary records Patient or client interview (across the life span) Community-based surveys and focus groups Statistical reports; administrative data Epidemiologic studies
Types of data collected	Nutritional adequacy (dietary history; detailed nutrient intake) Health status (anthropometric and biochemical measurements, physical and clinical conditions, physiologic and disease status) Functional and behavioral status (social and cognitive function, psychological and emotional factors, quality-of-life measures, change readiness)
Nutrition assessment components	Review dietary intake for factors that affect health conditions and nutrition risk. Evaluate health and disease condition for nutrition-related consequences. Evaluate psychological, functional, and behavioral factors related to food access, selection, preparation, physical activity, and understanding of health condition. Evaluate patient's, client's, or group's knowledge, readiness to learn, and potential for changing behaviors. Identify standards by which data will be compared. Identify possible problem areas for making nutrition diagnoses.
Critical thinking	The following types of critical thinking skills are especially needed in the assessment steps: Observing for nonverbal and verbal cues that can guide and prompt effective interviewing methods. Determining appropriate data to collect. Selecting assessment tools and procedures (matching the assessment methods to the situation). Applying assessment tools in valid and reliable ways. Distinguishing relevant from irrelevant data. Distinguishing important from unimportant data. Validating the data. Organizing and categorizing the data in a meaningful framework that relates to nutrition problems. Determining when a problem requires consultation with or referral to another provider.
Documentation of assessment	Documentation is an ongoing process that supports all of the steps in the nutrition care process. Quality documentation of the assessment step should be relevant, accurate, and timely; inclusion of the following information would further describe quality assessment documentation: Date and time of assessment Pertinent data collected and comparison with standards Patient's/client's/group's perceptions, values, and motivation related to presenting problems Changes in patient's/client's/group's level of understanding, food-related behaviors, and other clinical outcomes for appropriate follow-up Reason for discharge/discontinuation if appropriate
Determination for continuation of care	If on completion of an initial or reassessment it is determined that the problem cannot be modified by further nutrition care, discharge or discontinuation from this episode of nutrition care may be appropriate.

Adapted from Lacey K, Pritchett E: Nutrition care process and model: ADA adopts road map to quality care and outcomes management, J Am Diet Assoc 103(8):1064, 2003.

medical schools physicians often graduate with little practical knowledge about nutrition and the features of malnutrition. To maintain a high level of awareness, physician education programs in nutritional topics should be conducted regularly.

Tools for Assessment of Nutritional Status

Several tools are available for the assessment of nutritional status. The **Subjective Global Assessment (SGA)** is a nutritional assessment tool that has been validated and correlates well with nutrition risk indices and other assessment data in hospitalized patients (DeLegge and Drake, 2007; Kyle et al., 2006) (see Table 6-5). The MNA tool mentioned earlier evaluates independence, medication therapy, pressure sores, number of full meals consumed per day, protein intake, consumption of fruits and vegetables, fluid intake, mode of feeding, self-view of nutritional status, comparison with peers, and mid-arm and calf circumferences (Figure 4-5) (Bauer et al., 2008; Guigoz, 2006).

Histories

The information collected about individuals or populations is used as part of the nutrition status assessment. Frequently the information is in the form of histories—health and medical, social, medication, and dietary.

Medical or Health History

The medical or health history usually includes the following information: chief complaint, present and past illness, current health, allergies, past or recent surgeries, family history of disease, psychosocial data, and a review of problems—by body system—from the patient's perspective (Hammond, 2006). These histories usually provide much insight into nutrition-related problems. Alcohol and drug use, increased metabolic needs, increased nutritional losses, chronic disease, recent major surgery or illness, disease or surgery of the gastrointestinal tract, and recent significant weight loss all may contribute to malnutrition. In older patients, additional review is recommended to detect mental deterioration, constipation or incontinence, poor eyesight or hearing, slowed reactions, major organ diseases, effects of prescription and over-the-counter drugs, and physical disabilities.

Medication History

Food and drugs interact in many ways that affect nutrition status and drug therapy effectiveness; thus a medication history is an important part of any nutrition assessment. Those who are older, are chronically ill, have a history of marginal or inadequate nutritional intake, or are receiving multiple drugs for a long time are susceptible to drug-induced nutritional deficiencies. The effects of drug therapy can be altered by specific foods, the timing of food and meal consumption, and use of herbal products; see Chapter 9.

Social History

Social aspects of the medical or health history may also affect nutrition intake. Socioeconomic status, the ability to purchase food independently, whether the person is living alone, physical or mental handicaps, smoking, drug or alcohol addiction, confusion caused by environmental changes, unsuitable housing conditions, lack of socialization at meals, psychological problems, or poverty may add to the risks for inadequate nutrition intake. Knowledge of various cultures is also important to meet the needs of diverse groups of clients. Factors that affect a person's cultural values include religious beliefs; rituals; symbols; language; dietary practices; education; communication style; views on health, wellness, and illness; and racial identity. Establishing a bond with clients of different cultures is important for positive outcomes (Stein, 2010). See Chapter 12 for more guidance on nutrition and cultural competency.

Nutrition or Diet History

Inadequate nutrient intake and nutritional inadequacy can result from anorexia, **ageusia** (loss of the sense of taste), **dysgeusia** (diminished or distorted taste), **anosmia** (loss of smell), excessive alcohol intake, poor-fitting dentures, fad dieting, chewing or swallowing problems, frequent meals away from home, adverse food and drug interactions, cultural or religious restrictions of diet, an inability to eat for more than 7 to 10 days, intravenous fluid therapy for more than 5 days, or feeding dependence. For many older adults, denture problems, changes in taste and smell, long-established poor food habits, food fads, and inadequate knowledge of nutrition are problems. Alternative nutrition therapies, including use of megadoses of vitamins and minerals, various herbs, macrobiotic diets, probiotics, and amino acid supplements, must be addressed because they have an effect on the person's nutritional and overall health care.

A **diet history** is perhaps the best means of obtaining dietary intake information and refers to a review of an individual's usual patterns of food intake and the food selection variables that dictate the food intake. See Box 4-2 for the kind of information collected from a dietary history. **Dietary intake data** may be assessed either by collecting retrospective intake data as with a 24-hour recall or food frequency questionnaire or summarizing prospective intake data, as with a food record kept for a number of days by an individual or the caretaker. Each method has specific purposes, strengths, and weaknesses. Any self-reported method of obtaining data can be challenging because it is difficult for people to remember what they ate, the content, or even an accurate statement of portion size (Thompson et al., 2010). The choice of data collection depends on the purpose and setting in which the assessment is completed. The goal is to determine the nutrient content of the food and the appropriateness of the intake for a particular individual. The prospective method involves recording data at the time the food is consumed or shortly thereafter.

A daily food record, or **food diary**, involves documenting dietary intake as it occurs and is often used in outpatient clinic settings. The food diary is usually completed by the individual client (Figure 4-6). A food diary or record is usually most accurate if the food and amounts eaten are

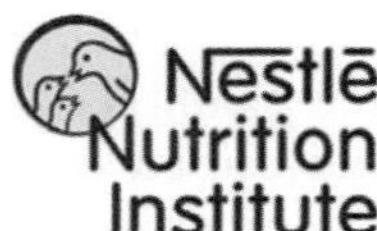

Mini Nutritional Assessment MNA®

Last name: First name:

Sex: Age: Weight, kg: Height, cm: Date:

Complete the screen by filling in the boxes with the appropriate numbers. Add the numbers for the screen. If score is 11 or less, continue with the assessment to gain a Malnutrition Indicator Score.

Screening

A Has food intake declined over the past 3 months due to loss of appetite, digestive problems, chewing or swallowing difficulties?
0 = severe decrease in food intake
1 = moderate decrease in food intake
2 = no decrease in food intake ☐

B Weight loss during the last 3 months
0 = weight loss greater than 3kg (6.6lbs)
1 = does not know
2 = weight loss between 1 and 3kg (2.2 and 6.6 lbs)
3 = no weight loss ☐

C Mobility
0 = bed or chair bound
1 = able to get out of bed / chair but does not go out
2 = goes out ☐

D Has suffered psychological stress or acute disease in the past 3 months?
0 = yes 2 = no ☐

E Neuropsychological problems
0 = severe dementia or depression
1 = mild dementia
2 = no psychological problems ☐

F Body Mass Index (BMI) (weight in kg) / (height in m²)
0 = BMI less than 19
1 = BMI 19 to less than 21
2 = BMI 21 to less than 23
3 = BMI 23 or greater ☐

Screening score ☐☐
(subtotal max. 14 points)

12-14 points:	Normal nutritional status
8-11 points:	At risk of malnutrition
0-7 points:	Malnourished

For a more in-depth assessment, continue with questions G-R

Assessment

G Lives independently (not in nursing home or hospital)
1 = yes 0 = no ☐

H Takes more than 3 prescription drugs per day
0 = yes 1 = no ☐

I Pressure sores or skin ulcers
0 = yes 1 = no ☐

J How many full meals does the patient eat daily?
0 = 1 meal
1 = 2 meals
2 = 3 meals ☐

K Selected consumption markers for protein intake
- At least one serving of dairy products (milk, cheese, yoghurt) per day yes ☐ no ☐
- Two or more servings of legumes or eggs per week yes ☐ no ☐
- Meat, fish or poultry every day yes ☐ no ☐

0.0 = if 0 or 1 yes
0.5 = if 2 yes
1.0 = if 3 yes ☐.☐

L Consumes two or more servings of fruit or vegetables per day?
0 = no 1 = yes ☐

M How much fluid (water, juice, coffee, tea, milk...) is consumed per day?
0.0 = less than 3 cups
0.5 = 3 to 5 cups
1.0 = more than 5 cups ☐.☐

N Mode of feeding
0 = unable to eat without assistance
1 = self-fed with some difficulty
2 = self-fed without any problem ☐

O Self view of nutritional status
0 = views self as being malnourished
1 = is uncertain of nutritional state
2 = views self as having no nutritional problem ☐

P In comparison with other people of the same age, how does the patient consider his / her health status?
0.0 = not as good
0.5 = does not know
1.0 = as good
2.0 = better ☐.☐

Q Mid-arm circumference (MAC) in cm
0.0 = MAC less than 21
0.5 = MAC 21 to 22
1.0 = MAC 22 or greater ☐.☐

R Calf circumference (CC) in cm
0 = CC less than 31
1 = CC 31 or greater ☐

Assessment (max. 16 points) ☐☐.☐

Screening score ☐☐.☐

Total Assessment (max. 30 points) ☐☐.☐

Malnutrition Indicator Score

24 to 30 points	☐	normal nutritional status
17 to 23.5 points	☐	at risk of malnutrition
Less than 17 points	☐	malnourished

Ref. Vellas B, Villars H, Abellan G, et al. *Overview of MNA® - Its History and Challenges.* J Nut Health Aging 2006; 10: 456-465.
Rubenstein LZ, Harker JO, Salva A, Guigoz Y, Vellas B. Screening for Undernutrition in Geriatric Practice: *Developing the Short-Form Mini Nutritional Assessment (MNA-SF).* J. Geront 2001; 56A: M366-377.
Guigoz Y. The Mini-Nutritional Assessment (MNA®) *Review of the Literature – What does it tell us?* J Nutr Health Aging 2006; 10: 466-487.

For more information: www.mna-elderly.com

FIGURE 4-5 Mini Nutritional Assessment—Long form. *(Permission by Nestlé Healthcare Nutrition.)*

recorded at the time of consumption, minimizing error from incomplete memory or attention (Thompson et al., 2010). The individual's nutrient intake is then calculated and averaged at the end of the desired period, usually 3 to 7 days, and compared with dietary reference intakes or guidelines in the MyPlate guide.

The **food frequency questionnaire** is a retrospective review of intake frequency (i.e., food consumed per day, per week, or per month). For ease of evaluation, the food frequency chart organizes foods into groups that have common nutrients. Because the focus of the food frequency questionnaire is the frequency of consumption of food groups rather

BOX 4-2

Diet History Information

Category	
Allergies, Intolerances, or Food Avoidances	Foods avoided and reason for avoidance Length of avoidance Description of problems caused by foods
Appetite	Good, poor, any changes Factors that affect appetite Changes in taste or smell perception
Attitude Toward Food and Eating	Disinterest in food Irrational ideas about food, eating, or body weight Parental interest in child's eating
Chronic Disease	Treatment Length of treatment time Dietary modification: self-imposed or physician prescribed, date of modification Past nutrition and diet education, compliance with diet
Culture and Background	Influence of culture on eating habits Religious practices, holiday rituals Educational background Health beliefs
Dental and Oral Health	Problems with chewing Foods that cannot be eaten Problems with swallowing, salivation, choking, food sticking
Economics	Income: frequency and steadiness of employment Amount of money for food each week or month Individual's perception of financial adequacy for meeting food needs Eligibility for food stamps and cost of stamps Public aid assistance status
Gastrointestinal Factors	Problems with heartburn, bloating, gas Problems with diarrhea, vomiting, constipation, distention Frequency of problems Home remedies Antacid, laxative, or other drug use
Home Life and Meal Patterns	Number in household (eat together?) Person who does shopping Person who does cooking Food storage and cooking facilities (e.g., stove, refrigerator) Type of housing (e.g., home, apartment, room) Ability to shop and prepare foods, disabilities
Medications, Supplements, Herbal Remedies	Vitamin and mineral supplements: frequency of administration, type, amount Medications: type, amount, frequency of administration, length of time on medication Herbal remedies: type, amount, purpose
Nutritional Problems	Concerns as perceived by patient and family Referrals from physician, nurse, other therapist, agency
Physical Activity	Occupation: type, hours/week, shift, energy expenditure Exercise: type, amount, frequency (seasonal?) Sleep: hours/day (uninterrupted?) Handicaps
Weight Pattern and History	Loss or gain: how many pounds and over what length of time? Intentional or nonvolitional % Usual weight; healthy weight; desirable weight

FIGURE 4-6 Food diary format.

Food Diary: DAY ___________

MEAL Foods (list)	AMOUNT EATEN	HOW PREPARED	WHERE EATEN (home, work, etc.)
Breakfast:			
Snack:			
Lunch:			
Dinner:			
Snack:			

Food Supplements Cans/Day: ___________ Name: ___________
Vitamins/Mineral Supplement: ___________

than of specific nutrients, the information obtained is general, not specific, for certain nutrients. During illness, food consumption patterns can change, depending on the stage of illness. Therefore it is helpful to complete food frequency questionnaires for the period immediately before hospitalization and before illness to obtain a complete and accurate history. Box 4-3 shows a food frequency questionnaire. Another more specific, quantified questionnaire is online at http://www.fhcrc.org/science/shared_resources/nutrition/ffq/gsel.pdf.

The **24-hour recall** method of data collection requires individuals to remember the specific foods and amounts of foods they consumed in the past 24 hours. The information is then analyzed by the person or professional gathering the information. Problems commonly associated with this method of data collection include (1) an inability to recall accurately the kinds and amounts of food eaten, (2) difficulty in determining whether the day being recalled represents an individual's typical intake, and (3) the tendency for persons to exaggerate low intakes and underreport high intakes of foods. Concurrent use of food frequency and 24-hour recall questionnaires (i.e., doing a cross-check) improves the accuracy of intake estimates.

Reliability and validity of dietary recall methods are important issues. When attention is directed toward the diet, people may consciously or unconsciously alter their intake either to simplify recording or impress the interviewer, thus decreasing the information's validity. The validity of dietary recall information from obese individuals is often questionable because they tend to underreport their intakes. The same can be true for children, patients with eating disorders, those who are critically ill, those who abuse drugs or alcohol, individuals who are confused, and those whose intake is unpredictable. Table 4-4 describes the advantages and disadvantages of the various methods used to obtain accurate dietary intake data.

Technology is currently being adapted and incorporated into dietary assessment through a variety of means that are found to be very helpful and reduce associated cost. Electronic diaries can be more accurate and useful compared with handwritten entries. There are also recording electronic devices that can link a kitchen scale directly to a computer, and other devices use a bar code reader to transmit data by telephone (Thompson et al., 2010). Sun and associates (2010) describe an electronic system for dietary reporting by a person wearing a device to record food intake. The device contains a camera, a microphone, and other sensors that can be worn around the neck and can collect pictures of the actual meal to identify food items.

Nutrient Intake Analysis

A **nutrient intake analysis (NIA)** may also be referred to as a *nutrient intake record* or *calorie count*, depending on the information collected and the analysis done. The NIA is a tool used in various inpatient settings to identify nutritional inadequacies by monitoring intakes before deficiencies develop. Information about actual intake is collected through direct observation or an inventory of foods eaten based on observation of what remains on the individual's tray or plate after a meal. Intake from tube feeding and intravenous products (enteral and parenteral nutrition) is also recorded.

An NIA should be recorded for at least 72 hours to reflect variations in intake that may occur from day to day. Complete records for this period usually accurately reflect an average intake for most individuals. If the record is incomplete, it may be necessary to extend the duration of the

BOX 4-3

General Food Frequency*

1. Do you drink milk? If so, how much? What kind? Whole Skim Low-fat
2. Do you use fat? If so, what kind? How much?
3. How often do you eat meat? Eggs? Cheese? Beans?
4. Do you eat snack foods? If so, which ones? How often? How much?
5. Which vegetables (in each group) do you eat? How often?
   a. Broccoli Green peppers Cooked greens Carrots Sweet potatoes
   b. Tomatoes Raw cabbage
   c. Asparagus Beets Cauliflower Corn Cooked cabbage Celery Peas Lettuce
6. Which fruits do you eat? How often?
   a. Apples or applesauce Apricots Bananas Berries Cherries Grapes or grape juice Peaches Pears Pineapple Plums Prunes Raisins
   b. Oranges, orange juice Grapefruit Grapefruit juice
7. Bread and cereal products
   a. How much bread do you usually eat with each meal? How much between meals?
   b. Do you eat cereal? (daily? weekly?) What type? Cooked Dry
   c. How often do you eat foods such as macaroni, spaghetti, and noodles?
   d. Do you eat whole-grain breads and cereals? How often?
8. Do you use salt? Do you salt your food before tasting it? Do you cook with salt? Do you crave salt or salty foods?
9. How many teaspoons of sugar do you use daily? Include sugar on cereal, fruit, toast, and in beverages such as coffee and tea.
10. Do you eat desserts? How often?
11. Do you drink sugar-containing beverages such as soda pop or sweetened juice drinks? How often? How much?
12. How often do you eat candy or cookies?
13. Do you drink water? How often during the day? How much each time? How much water do you drink each day?
14. Do you use sugar substitutes in packet form or in drinks? What type do you use? How often?
15. Do you drink alcohol? Which type: beer, wine, liquor? How often? How much?
16. Do you drink caffeinated beverages? How often? How much per day?

*To determine the frequency of food consumption, the following pattern of questions may be useful. However, questions may need to be modified based on information from the 24-hour recall. For instance, if a woman states that she drank a glass of milk the day before, do not ask, "Do you drink milk?" Rather, ask, "How much milk do you drink?" Record answers with the appropriate time frame designated (e.g., 1/day, 1/wk, 3/mo) or as accurately as possible. The frequency may need to be recorded as "occasionally" or "rarely" if the patient cannot be more specific.

TABLE 4-4

Methods of Obtaining Dietary Intake Data

Method	Advantages	Disadvantages
Nutrient intake analysis	Allows actual observation of food in clinical setting	Does not account for possible variation in portion size. Does not reflect intake of free-living individual
Daily food record or diary	Provides daily record of food consumption. Can provide information on quantity of food, how food is prepared, and timing of meals and snacks.	Depends on variable literacy skills of participants. Requires ability to measure or judge portion size. Actual food intake possibly influenced by the recording process. Reliability of records is questionable.
Food frequency	Easily standardized. Can be beneficial when considered in combination with usual intake. Provides overall picture of intake.	Requires literacy skills. Does not provide meal pattern data. Requires knowledge of portion sizes.
24-h recall	Is quick and easy.	Relies on memory. Requires knowledge of portion sizes. May not represent usual intake. Requires interviewing skills.

Data from Diet manual and nutrition practice guidelines: a manual of the Georgia Dietetic Association, Section 5.5-5.3, 2004.

intake until a full 72-hour record can be completed. It should be kept in mind that eating habits or meals consumed during the weekend and during the week may differ.

The record of total intake can then be analyzed for its nutrient content, using one of several available computerized methods. The diet can be analyzed for macronutrient and micronutrient intake. Macronutrients are analyzed to assess total calorie intake along with the carbohydrate, fiber, fat, and protein content of the diet. Micronutrients, vitamins and minerals, can also be analyzed to assess intake to ensure proper body functioning. In addition, it may be advantageous to assess the phytonutrient and prebiotic content of the diet. Determining the oxygen radical absorbance capacity (ORAC) of certain types of fruits, nuts, and vegetables in the diet gives a measure of the anti-inflammatory effect of the diet because inflammation and its downstream effect of oxidative stress is linked to many chronic and degenerative diseases, including cancer, heart disease, Alzheimer disease, Parkinson disease, and also the aging process. A diet rich in fruit, nuts, and vegetables with high ORAC scores is considered to contain good sources of antioxidants. It is possible to search selected foods to obtain the ORAC value of each (U.S. Department of Agriculture, 2007).

Technological advances have been made for processing dietary intake data. Computerized processing of dietary intake data is a common practice in most settings. Several database choices are available for estimation of intake and can vary by the nutrient composition database used to process the data (Thompson et al., 2010).

CLINICAL SCENARIO

Laverne, a 66-year-old black woman, has contacted you to set up an outpatient nutrition screening appointment. She has a 20-year history of diabetes mellitus, a 10-year history of colon cancer, and hypertension. She is 5 ft, 8 in tall and weighs 203 lb. Her current medications are glyburide and a diuretic. (She does not know its name.) She tells you that she eats throughout the day and sometimes at night after going to bed.

Nutrition Diagnostic Statement

Overweight/obesity related to poor food choices as evidenced by a BMI of 31.

Nutrition Care Questions

1. What would you include in a nutrition screening for Laverne?
2. What would you include in a nutrition assessment for Laverne?
3. How could you identify her medications?
4. What additional information is needed for assessment of her dietary and nutrient intake?
5. If you need more details, what questions would you ask her physician?

BMI, Body mass index.

USEFUL WEBSITES

Centers for Disease Control and Prevention—Growth Charts
http://www.cdc.gov/growthcharts/

International Food Information Council
http://www.foodinsight.org/

Malnutrition Universal Screening Tool
http://www.bapen.org.uk/must_tool.html

National Cancer Institute (NCI) Diet History
http://riskfactor.cancer.gov/DHQ/

Automated Self-administered 24-hour Dietary Recall
http://riskfactor.cancer.gov/tools/instruments/asa24/

National Heart, Lung, and Blood Institute
http://www.nhlbi.nih.gov/index.htm

National Health and Nutrition Examination Survey Food Frequency Questionnaire
http://riskfactor.cancer.gov/diet/usualintakes/ffq.html

Nutrition Analysis Tool
http://nat.illinois.edu/

U.S. Department of Agriculture
http://www.nal.usda.gov/fnic/etext/000108.html

U.S. Department of Agriculture Healthy Eating Index
http://www.cnpp.usda.gov/HealthyEatingIndex.htm

U.S. Department of Agriculture Nutrient Content of the Food Supply
http://www.cnpp.usda.gov/USFoodSupply.htm

REFERENCES

Agency for Healthcare Research and Quality (AHRQ): National Quality Measures Clearinghouse. Assessment of risk and prevention of malnutrition: percentage of intensive care unit (ICU) patients who are assessed for risk of malnutrition within 24 hours after admission. Accessed February 1, 2010 at http://www.qualitymeasures.ahrq.gov/content.aspx?id=14394.

American Dietetic Association (ADA): Nutrition assessment. In *ADA Nutrition Care Manual On-line*, Chicago, 2010, American Dietetic Association.

American Dietetic Association (ADA): Position of the American Dietetic Association: nutrient supplementation, *J Am Diet Assoc* 109:2073, 2009.

ASPEN Board of Directors: Guidelines for the use of parenteral and enteral nutrition in adults and pediatric patients, *JPEN J Parenter Enteral Nutr* 33:255, 2009.

Bauer JM, et al: The Mini Nutritional Assessment—its history, today's practice, and future perspectives, *Nutr Clin Pract* 23: 388, 2008.

Bouillanne O, et al: Geriatric nutritional risk index: a new index for evaluating at-risk elderly medical patients, *Am J Clin Nutr* 82:777, 2005.

Btaiche IF, et al: Critical illness, gastrointestinal complications, and medication therapy during enteral feeding in critically ill adult patients, *Nutr Clin Pract* 25:32, 2010.

Butterworth CE: The skeleton in the hospital closet, *Nutr Today* March/April:4, 1974.

Centers for Disease Control and Prevention (CDC): Overweight and obesity, 2009a. Accessed 10 February 2010 at http://www.cdc.gov/obesity/.

Centers for Disease Control and Prevention (CDC): Quickstats: Age-adjusted death rates for the 10 leading causes of death—National Vital Statistics System, United States, 2006 and 2007, *MMWR* 58(46), 2009b. Accessed 10 February 2010 at http://www.cdc.gov/mmwr/preview/mmwrhtml.

Charney P: Nutrition screening and assessment in older adults, *Today's Dietitian* 7:10, 2005.

Chima C: *Nutrition screening practices in health care organizations: a pilot survey, Clinical Nutrition Management*, Chicago, 2006, American Dietetic Association. Accessed 14 February 2010 from http://www.cnmdpg.org/index_875.cfm.

DeLegge M, Drake L: Nutritional assessment, *Gastroenterol Clin North Am* 36:1, 2007.

Elia M: *Screening for malnutrition: a multidisciplinary responsibility: development and use of the "malnutrition universal screening tool" ("MUST") for adults*, Worcester, England, 2003, Redditch.

Fialkowski MK, et al. Evaluation of dietary assessment tools used to assess the diet of adults participating in the Communities Advancing the Studies of Tribal Nations Across the Lifespan Cohort, *J Am Diet Assoc* 109:65, 2010.

Guigoz Y: The Mini nutrition assessment (MNA®) review of the literature—what does it tell us? *JNHA J Nutr Health Aging* 10:6, 2006.

Hammond KA: Physical assessment. In Lysen LK, editor: *Quick reference to Clinical Dietetics*, ed 2, Boston, 2006, Jones and Bartlett.

Henderson S, et al. Do the malnutrition universal screening tool (MUST) and Birmingham nutrition risk (BNR) score predict mortality in older hospitalised patients? *BMC Geriatr* 8:26, 2008.

Heron M, Tejada-Vera B: Deaths: leading causes for 2005. *National Vital Statistics Reports*, vol 58, no. 8, Hyattsville, Md, 2009, National Center for Health Statistics.

Kaiser MJ, et al. The short-form Mini Nutritional Assessment® (MNA-SF): Can it be improved to facilitate clinical use? *J Nutr Health Aging* 13(Suppl 2):S16, 2009.

Kyle UG, et al: Comparison of tools for nutritional assessment and screening at hospital admission: a population study, *Clin Nutr* 25:409, 2006.

Salva A, et al: Nutritional assessment of residents in long-term care facilities (LTCFs): recommendations of the task force on nutrition and ageing of the IAGG European region and the IANA, *J Nutr Health Aging* 13:475, 2009.

Stein K: Moving cultural competency from abstract to act, *JADA* 110(2):180, 2010.

Stratton RJ, et al: Malnutrition in hospital outpatients and inpatients: prevalence, concurrent validity and ease of use of the "malnutrition universal screening tool" ("MUST") for adults, *Br J Nutr* 92(5):799, 2004.

Sun M, et al: A wearable electronic system for objective dietary assessment, *J Am Diet Assoc* 110:45, 2010.

Tarnus E, Bourdon E: Anthropometric evaluations of body composition of undergraduate students at the University of La Reunion, *Adv Physiol Educ* 30:248, 2006.

Thompson F, et al: Need for technological innovation in dietary assessment, *J Am Diet Assoc* 110:48, 2010.

U.S. Department of Agriculture (USDA): *Oxygen radical absorbance capacity (ORAC) of Selected Foods, 2007*, Beltsville, Md, 2007, USDA.

U.S. Department of Health and Human Services (USDHHS): *Healthy people 2020*, Washington, DC, 2009, USDHHS.

U.S. Department of Health and Human Services (USDHHS): *The Surgeon General's call to action to prevent and decrease overweight and obesity*, Rockville, Md, 2007, Office of the Surgeon General.

Xu J, et al: Deaths: preliminary data for 2007. *National Vital Statistics Reports* 58(1):19, August 2009, U.S. Dept. of Health and Human Services, 2009.

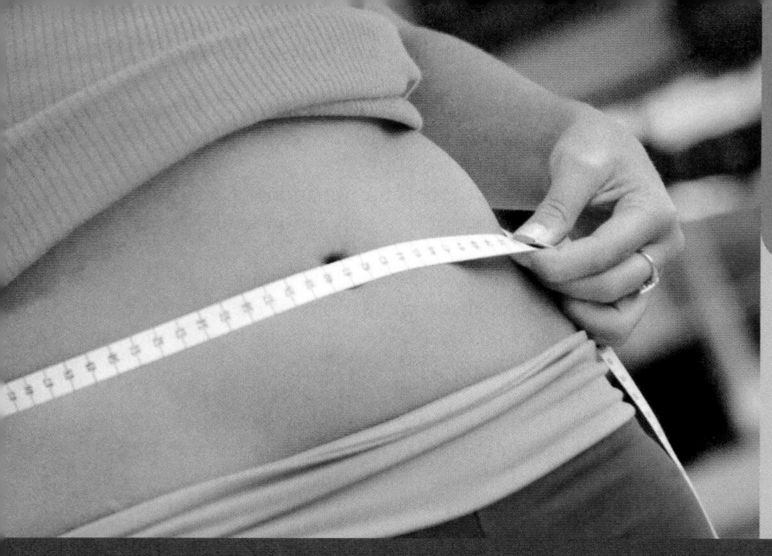

CHAPTER 5

Ruth DeBusk, PhD, RD

Clinical: Nutritional Genomics

KEY TERMS

allele
autosomal dominant
autosomal recessive
autosome
bioactive food components
bioinformatics
coding region
codon
CpG island
deletion
deoxyribonucleic acid (DNA)
DNA methylation
dominant
epigenetics and epigenomics
exon
gene x environment (GxE)
genetic code
genetic engineering
Genetic Information Nondiscrimination Act (GINA)
genetic variation
genome
genomic imprinting
genomics
genotype
heterozygous
histone
homozygous
inborn errors of metabolism (IEM)
intervening sequences
intron
karyotype
ligand
meiosis
Mendelian inheritance
messenger RNA (mRNA)
metabolomics
microarray technology (DNA "chips")
mitochondrial (maternal) inheritance
mitosis
model system
mutation
nucleosome
nucleotide
nutrigenetics
nutrigenomics
nutritional genomics
pedigree
penetrance
peroxisome proliferator-activated receptor (PPAR)
pharmacogenomics
phenotype
polymerase chain reaction (PCR)
polymorphism
posttranscriptional processing
posttranslational processing
promoter region
proteomics
recessive
recombinant DNA
regulatory region
response element
restriction endonuclease (restriction enzyme)
RNA interference (RNAi)
sex chromosome
sex-linked
signal transduction
silent mutation
single nucleotide polymorphism (SNP)
transcription

transcription factor
translation
whole exome capture
xenobiotics
X-linked dominant
X-linked recessive
Y-linked inheritance

Nutrition professionals have long been intrigued and puzzled by the fact that one person can be lean, yet that person's identical twin can be overweight; that the Pima Indians living in northern Mexico are lean, but their genetic counterparts in the American southwest struggle with a high prevalence of obesity and type 2 diabetes mellitus (T2DM); and that a low-fat diet can improve blood lipid levels in many people, but not in everyone. Although our genetic makeup sets the stage, environmental factors such as nutrition and other lifestyle choices determine who among the susceptible actually develops a disease. The interactions among genes, diet, lifestyle factors, and their influence on health and disease are the focus of **nutritional genomics**.

Genetic research is rapidly clarifying how variations are correlated with dysfunction and disease. This appreciation for the central role of genes is having a significant effect on the way health is viewed. As the details of the connections among genes, their protein products, and disease unfold, the focus of the health care system is shifting. During the past 50 years the focus has been on treating overt disease, and physicians have had increasingly sophisticated drugs and technologies available to meet this challenge. However, with the understanding that disease is genetically based but environmentally influenced, the focus is now on targeted intervention and prevention. Although the first applications of this changed focus in health care involved the medical and pharmaceutical aspects of acute care, nutrition therapy is expected to figure prominently as a cornerstone of preventive care and in the management of the chronic, diet- and lifestyle-related diseases.

Genetic research is helping to clarify the pathogenesis of disease with the influence of bioactive components in food. From these advances will come diagnostic tests and assessments of disease susceptibility that, coupled with genetic testing and family history analysis, will allow health care professionals to predict those at risk for particular disorders. Nutrition can mitigate the harmful effects of many genetic changes that predispose to disease, from supplying missing metabolites to altering gene expression.

Nutritional genomics can also offer effective approaches for preventing disease. By analyzing individual genotypes prenatally or at birth, disease susceptibilities will be known from an early age and can be factored into the nutrition and lifestyle choices made throughout life. Armed with extensive knowledge of one's genetic makeup (**genotype**) and how to make lifestyle choices that support that genotype, humans will have the option to live to their full genetic potential throughout a healthy, active life.

The nutrition profession is pivotal in this new era of health promotion and disease prevention. The role includes assessing disease susceptibilities, then recommending preventive therapy and lifestyle approaches. Increasingly, genotyping must be incorporated into the nutrition assessment and recommendations customized to the genetic uniqueness of individuals.

THE HUMAN GENOME PROJECT

The Human Genome Project has been the impetus for this fundamental shift to integrating genetic principles into health care. This project, completed in 2003, was a multinational effort to identify each of the nucleotides in the deoxyribonucleic acid (DNA) that makes up the genetic material (genome) of human beings. Currently the focus is on (1) cataloging the number of genes present in human DNA; (2) identifying the protein encoded within each gene and understanding its function (**proteomics**); (3) associating variations in genes with specific diseases; (4) understanding the way genes, proteins, and environmental factors interact to cause the functional changes that result in disease; (5) identifying metabolites that are useful in monitoring health status (**metabolomics**); and (6) understanding **epigenetics** (changes in single genes caused by environmental factors in utero, from chemicals or diet or aging) and **epigenomics** (population-specific gene changes) and their implications for human development and health. These efforts will lead to an understanding of effective approaches for restoring health and preventing disease.

Additional goals include sequencing the genomes of other organisms that are used as **model systems** in the laboratory to explore the molecular basis of disease, addressing the ethical, legal, and social implications of genetic research, developing genetic technologies useful for clinical applications, educating genetic scientists and clinicians, and integrating the results of genetic research into clinical practice. Sophisticated computer technology that can handle the vast amount of data is the backbone of the field of **bioinformatics**.

Clinical Applications

Much of the knowledge and many of the technologic advances gained from the Human Genome Project have clinical applications. Knowing the gene associated with a particular disease and the gene's DNA sequence, its protein product, and the function of the protein in promoting health or illness provides the basis for diagnostic assays and effective interventions. For example, tumors that appear identical physically can be distinguished by their genetic profiles. This distinction is important for effective therapy because different types of tumors respond to different therapeutic approaches. Not only can such assays be used to definitively reach a diagnosis, they also can be used to detect dysfunction in those without symptoms, which allows interventions to be initiated before the symptoms of a disease become apparent.

Similarly, the information gained has been pivotal in developing diagnostic assays to determine **genetic variations** in drug-metabolizing enzymes (**pharmacogenomics**). Each human being has the same basic set of drug-metabolizing enzymes, but the genes and the resulting enzyme functions can vary. One drug may have the intended effects on one person, be ineffective for another, and actually be harmful to a third. The ability to assess an individual's major drug-metabolizing gene variants helps the physician select the right drug and dosage. Like drugs, food requires enzymatic processes to be digested, absorbed, and used by the body's cells. The ability to tailor food to the genetic makeup of individuals—the science of nutritional genomics—is expected to be an important application of genetic research, similar in concept to pharmacogenomics.

GENOTYPE AND NUTRITION ASSESSMENT

The application expected to have the most dramatic effect on clinical nutrition professionals is the ability to associate a unique genotype with that person's susceptibility to particular diseases. This advance is an important enhancement in the nutrition assessment, diagnosis, and intervention phases of the nutrition care process. As understanding of how genotype influences the ability to function within a particular environment and how environmental factors influence gene expression, nutrition protocols will be developed. Specific counseling and nutrient recommendations will be guided by the client's genetic profile.

Nutrition professionals must be able to translate client genotypes to develop appropriate interventions. If nutrition professionals are going to be prepared for the era of genomic-directed health care, they must build a foundation in genetics, biochemistry, molecular biology, metabolism, and other foundational sciences of 21st century nutrition (Milner, 2008; Panagiotou and Nielsen, 2009; Stover and Caudill, 2008).

GENETIC FUNDAMENTALS

The reader must have a basic understanding of DNA as the genetic material for chromosomal and molecular genetics. Among the key concepts at the chromosomal level are the packaging of DNA into chromosomes within the nucleus, the processes of meiosis and mitosis, autosomal and **sex-linked** inheritance, linkage and the mapping of genes, and chromosomal mutation and its consequences. At the molecular level, key concepts include (1) information stored within DNA must be decoded and converted into proteins through the processes of transcription, posttranscriptional processing, translation, and **posttranslational processing**; (2) genes have a regulatory region with response elements, transcription factors, promoters, and a coding region with exons and introns; and (3) genetic variations within the human genome affect an individual's phenotype, including disease susceptibility.

In addition to the information contained in the nucleotide sequence of DNA (the "DNA code"), there are two other sources of information: the epigenetic code and the environmental factors to which cells are exposed. Epigenetics is nature's "pen-and-pencil set" (Gosden and Feinberg, 2007). Acetyl or methyl groups covalently attached to histone proteins associated with DNA or to the DNA itself, respectively, affect whether DNA is accessible for decoding. These groups can be added and removed as needed, and are influenced by diet. Nutrition counselors will have a great opportunity to affect this. (Kauwell, 2008.)

Molecules in the environment such as traditional nutrients, phytochemicals, toxins, hormones, and drugs communicate information as to the state of the environment and ultimately influence when and whether particular genes are expressed. The science of nutritional genomics encompasses all of these types of interactions between diet and lifestyle factors and DNA and their influence on health outcomes. Figures 5-1 through 5-5 review these fundamental genetic principles.

Genetics and Genomics: Nutritional Genomics, Nutrigenetics, and Nutrigenomics

Genetics is the science of inheritance. Historically genetics focused on identifying the mechanisms by which traits were passed from parent to child, such as eye or hair color, and certain rare diseases that were inherited from generation to generation. Originally, genetic diseases were in a separate category of disease. Today scientists realize that, directly or indirectly, all disease is connected to the information in the genes.

The science of genetics has significantly expanded in scope and includes the whole set of genetic information in

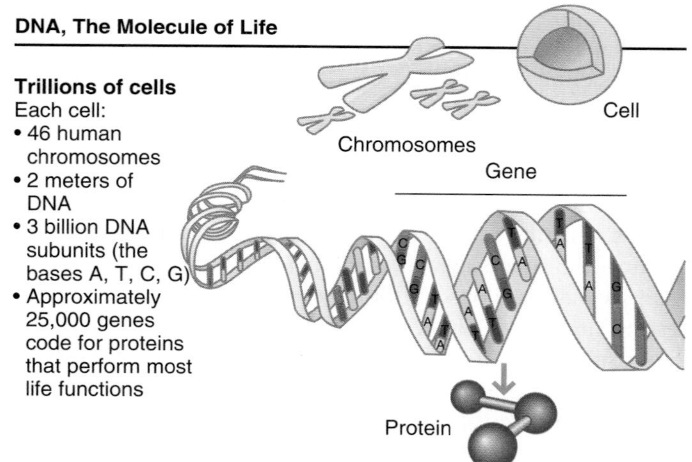

FIGURE 5-1 Cells are the fundamental working units of every living system. All the instructions needed to direct their activities are contained within the chemical deoxyribonucleic acid. *(From U.S. Department of Energy, Human Genome Program: www.ornl.gov/hgmis.)*

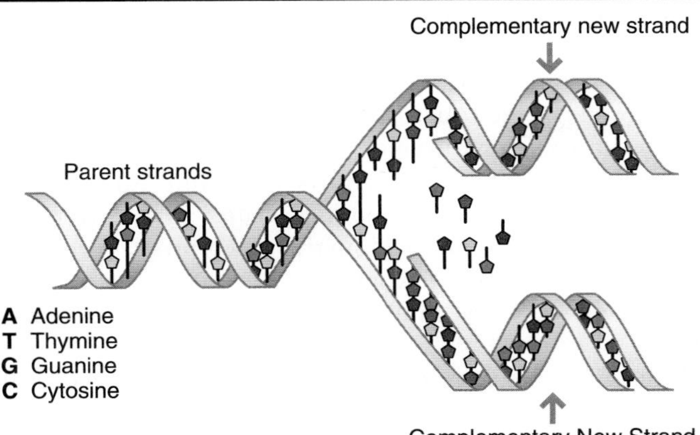

FIGURE 5-2 Each time a cell divides into two daughter cells, its full genome is duplicated; for humans and other complex organisms, this duplication occurs in the nucleus. During cell division the deoxyribonucleic acid (DNA) molecule unwinds, and the weak bonds between the base pairs break, allowing the strands to separate. Each strand directs the synthesis of a complementary new strand, with free nucleotides matching up with their complementary bases on each of the separated strands. Strict base-pairing rules are adhered to (i.e., adenine pairs only with thymine [an A-T pair] and cytosine with guanine [a C-G pair]). Each daughter cell receives one old and one new DNA strand. The cells' adherence to these base-pairing rules ensures that the new strand is an exact copy of the old one. This minimizes the incidence of errors (mutations) that may greatly affect the resulting organism or its offspring. *(From U.S. Department of Energy, Human Genome Program: www.ornl.gov/hgmis.)*

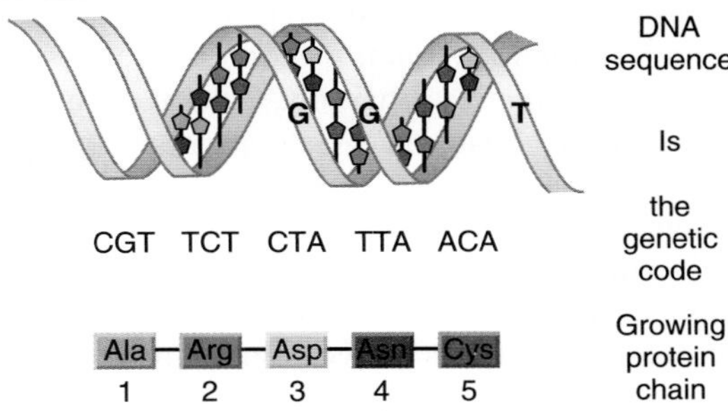

FIGURE 5-3 All living organisms are composed largely of proteins. Proteins are large, complex molecules made up of long chains of subunits called *amino acids.* Twenty different kinds of amino acids are usually found in proteins. Within the gene, each specific sequence of three deoxyribonucleic acid bases (codons) directs the cells protein-synthesizing machinery to add specific amino acids. For example, the base sequence ATG codes for the amino acid methionine. Because three bases code for one amino acid, the protein coded by an average-sized gene (3000 bp) will contain 1000 amino acids. The genetic code is thus a series of codons that specify which amino acids are required to make up specific proteins. *A,* Adenine; *bp,* base pairs; *G,* guanine; *T,* thymine. *(From U.S. Department of Energy, Human Genome Program: www.ornl.gov/hgmis.)*

DNA Sequence Variation in a Gene Can Change the Protein Produced by the Genetic Code

						Protein products
Gene A from person 1	CGT	TCT	CTA	TTA	ACA	
	Ala	Arg	Asp	Asn	Cys	
	1	2	3	4	5	
Gene A from person 2 (Codon made no difference in amino acid sequence)	CGC	TCT	GAT	TTA	ACA	
	Ala	Arg	Asp	Asn	Cys	
	1	2	3	4	5	
Gene A from person 3 (Codon resulted in a different amino acid at position 2)	CGT	TTT	GAT	TTA	ACA	Or
	Ala	Lys	Asp	Asn	Cys	
	1	2	3	4	5	

FIGURE 5-4 Some variations in a person's genetic code will have no effect on the protein that is produced; others can lead to disease or an increased susceptibility to a disease. *(From U.S. Department of Energy, Human Genome Program: www.ornl.gov/hgmis.)*

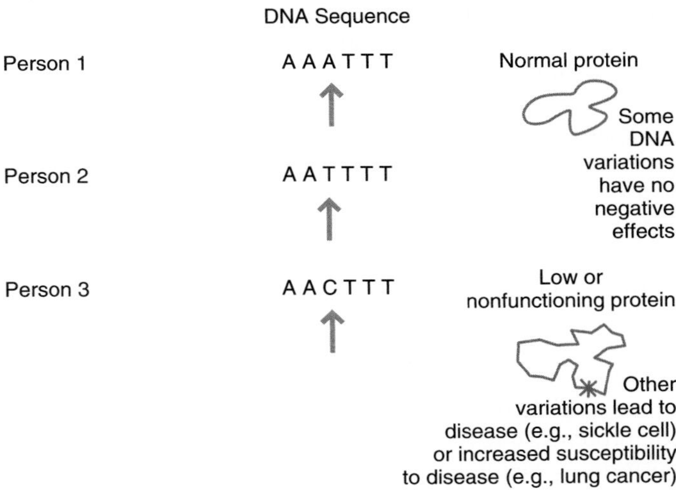

FIGURE 5-5 It is estimated that human beings differ from each other in only 0.1% of the total sequence of nucleotides that compose deoxyribonucleic acid. These variations in genetic information are thought to be the basis for the physical and functional differences between individuals. *(From U.S. Department of Energy, Human Genome Program: www.ornl.gov/hgmis.)*

an organism—its **genome**—and the interactions of the various genes and their protein products with each other and the environment. **Genomics** more accurately describes this complex, interactive situation. Whereas genetics was initially concerned with diseases that arose from a change in a single gene, genomics is more concerned with today's chronic diseases that result from the interaction between gene variants and factors in the environment. Nutritional genomics focuses on diet- and lifestyle-related disorders that result from these interactions. Nutritional genomics is the field itself, and includes *nutrigenetics*, *nutrigenomics*, and *epigenetics* or *epigenomics*.

Nutrigenetics concerns how an individual's particular genetic variations affect function. For example, an individual with a particular variant in the 5,10-methylenetetrahydrofolate reductase (*MTHFR*) gene is likely to require a more bioavailable form of folate for optimal health. **Nutrigenomics** is the study of the influence of specific environmental factors on changes in the expression of particular genes. Epigenetics and epigenomics provide another influence on outcomes by controlling whether genes can be expressed, which in turn determines whether nutrigenetic or nutrigenomic influences can occur. Diet and other lifestyle choices should be geared toward the particular variants of each individual.

Genetic Basics

Deoxyribonucleic acid (DNA) is the genetic material of all living organisms. The molecule is a double helix consisting of two strands of **nucleotide** subunits held together by hydrogen bonds. Each subunit contains the sugar deoxyribose, the mineral phosphorus, and one of four nitrogenous bases: adenine (A), thymine (T), guanine (G), or cytosine (C). The nucleotides are arranged side by side, and it is this linear arrangement that determines the particular information encoded in a stretch of DNA.

Approximately 3 billion nucleotides make up the human genome, which is housed in the nucleus of cells. A gene is a sequence of nucleotides that encodes the information for synthesizing a protein. The human genome contains approximately 20,000 to 25,000 genes, which is only 2% of the total genome (Human Genome Project, 2010). Long stretches of nucleotides are often found between one gene and the next along the chromosome. Such sequences are called **intervening sequences** and compose the majority of the DNA in humans. These sequences do not code for proteins, but they are not "junk DNA." Instead, they perform structural and regulatory functions, such as controlling when, where, and how much of a protein is produced.

To be useful to the cells, information in the DNA must first be decoded and translated into proteins, which perform the work of the organism at the cellular level. Information decoding occurs in two steps: (1) the process of **transcription**, during which the enzyme ribonucleic acid polymerase (RNA polymerase) converts DNA into an intermediate molecule (**messenger RNA [mRNA]**) and (2) a subsequent **translation** step in which the information encoded within the mRNA directs the assembly of amino acids into the protein molecule according to a universal **genetic code**. Genes have a common structure, with a **promoter region** where the binding of the RNA polymerase is controlled, which in turn controls transcription; and a **coding** (informational) **region** where the RNA polymerase transcribes the DNA into mRNA. Within the coding region are sequences of nucleotides (**exons**) that correspond to the order of the amino acids in the gene's protein product. The coding region also contains **introns** (sequences that are interspersed between exons and do not code for amino acids).

Following transcription, the mRNA must be processed (**posttranscriptional processing**) so that the introns are removed before the protein is synthesized. At this point, each set of three nucleotides in the transcribed and processed exon makes up a **codon**, which in turn specifies a particular amino acid and its position within the protein. Some proteins need further posttranslational processing before they are active, such as occurs with glycoproteins, proenzymes, and prohormones that must be cleaved or enzymatically processed before becoming active.

Prior to ("upstream from") the promoter region is the **regulatory region**, where control of transcription takes place. Within this region are **response elements**, DNA sequences that serve as binding sites for regulatory proteins such as **transcription factors** and their bound **ligands**. The binding of transcription factors triggers the recruitment of additional proteins to form a protein complex that in turn changes the expression of that gene by changing the conformation of the promoter region, increasing or decreasing the ability of RNA polymerase to attach and transcribe (express) the gene. The array of response elements within the promoter region can be quite complex, allowing for the binding of multiple transcription factors that in turn fine-tune the control of gene expression. It is through the binding of transcription factors to response elements that environmental factors such as the bioactive components in food essentially "talk" to a gene, conveying information that more or less of its protein product is needed.

The proteins coded for by the genes provide the metabolic machinery for the cells, such as enzymes, receptors, transporters, antibodies, hormones, and communicators. Changes within a gene can alter the amino acid sequence of the DNA protein. Such changes are called **mutations**, which historically have been associated with the concept of severely impairing the function of that protein and creating dysfunction within the cells and, ultimately, the organism. A single nucleotide change may be all that is needed to cause a debilitating disease. For example, in those with sickle cell disease a single nucleotide change causes a single amino acid change in the hemoglobin molecule, resulting in severe anemia (see Chapter 33).

Changes in the DNA are the basis for evolution; thus clearly not all mutations are harmful. Some changes actually improve function, and many **silent mutations** have no effect. The effect of the mutation on the functioning of the encoded protein is what determines the outcome, from debilitating disease to no effect at all. All changes to the DNA are technically mutations. However, at this point in the development of genomics, the term mutation tends to be applied to those changes that sufficiently influence function such that a measurable outcome results. In contrast, the term *genetic variation* (or *gene variant*) is reserved for those mutations with an effect on function that is not strong enough to lead to a disease or other measurable outcome by itself. Nutritional genomics is primarily concerned with those variations that interact with environmental factors.

Thus a gene can exist in slightly different forms as a result of a seemingly minor change, such as a substitution of a single nucleotide with another (e.g., guanine can replace cytosine). The term for the different forms of a gene is an **allele** or **polymorphism**. As a result, genes have protein products with differing amino acid sequences (isoforms) and often different functions. Polymorphism (allelism) is an important concept because it explains why human beings, although 99.9% alike genetically, are distinctively different. The 0.1% difference is sufficient to explain the obvious physical variations among humans. It is also the basis for more subtle differences that may not be readily observable, such as in the functional ability of a key metabolic enzyme to catalyze its characteristic reaction. Such variations are thought to underlie many of the inconsistencies that are observed in therapeutic outcomes and in nutritional intervention research.

The **single nucleotide polymorphism (SNP)** is the structural variant best studied to date. However, ongoing analysis of the human genome suggests that other structural variations may also play an important role in the genotypic and phenotypic variation among humans (Feuk et al., 2006). Loss or gain of nucleotides, duplication of nucleotide sequences, and copy number variants also have important consequences.

Understanding the prevalence and significance of genetic variation is a primary focus of 21st-century nutrition, which represents a major departure from nutrition research and therapy to date. Each person is susceptible to a different set of diseases, handles environmental toxins differently, metabolizes molecules somewhat differently, and has slightly unique nutritional requirements. These exciting discoveries are revolutionizing the way people think about the clinical aspects of medicine, pharmacology, and nutrition. Personalized therapy using individualized dietary requirements will be the practice of future dietitians.

Modes of Inheritance

Traits are transmitted from one generation to the next in three ways: Mendelian inheritance, mitochondrial inheritance, and epigenetic inheritance.

Mendelian Inheritance

Each cell's nucleus contains a complete set of genetic material (genome), divided among 22 pairs of chromosomes (called **autosomes**) and 2 **sex chromosomes** for a total of 46 chromosomes. During cell division (**mitosis**) all 46 chromosomes are duplicated and distributed to each new cell. During **meiosis**, one member of each of the autosome and sex chromosome pairs is distributed to each egg or sperm; the full set of 46 chromosomes is then restored upon fertilization.

Because genes are carried on chromosomes, the rules governing the distribution of chromosomes during mitosis and meiosis govern the distribution of genes and any changes (mutations, variations) they contain. These rules describe the **Mendelian inheritance** of a gene, named after Gregor Mendel, who first deduced that the inheritance of traits was governed by a predictable set of rules. It is possible to track a mutation through multiple generations by knowing these rules of inheritance. This transmission is typically depicted as a **pedigree** and can be used to predict the probability of a genetic change being inherited by a particular family member. When the change causes a disease, a pedigree can be helpful in predicting the probability that another family member will inherit the disease. The Family History Initiative, implemented by the U.S. Surgeon General, helps people construct their family pedigree.

Mendelian transmission can be autosomal or sex-linked, dominant or recessive. There are five classic modes of Mendelian inheritance: autosomal dominant, autosomal recessive, X-linked dominant, X-linked recessive, and Y-linked. An individual's genotype obeys the laws of inheritance, but the **phenotype** (the measurable expression of the genotype) may not. Each gene in an individual is present in two copies (alleles), one on each chromosome. When the alleles are the same (either both are the common or usual version or both are the mutant or variant form), the individual is said to be **homozygous**. If the alleles are different, the individual is **heterozygous** (also called a *carrier*).

Dominance and *recessiveness* refer to whether a trait is expressed in a heterozygous individual that has one common allele and one variant allele. If a trait is expressed when only a single copy of a variant allele is present, the allele is said to be **dominant** (i.e., the phenotype of the variant allele is the predominant one). Alleles that do not dominate the genotype when only a single copy is present are called **recessive**. The variant allele is present in the genome but the trait is not expressed unless two copies of the variant allele are present.

Further confounding the nomenclature is the concept of **penetrance**. Even when a pedigree suggests that a gene is present that should lead to the individual displaying a certain phenotype, the disease may not be evident. Such a gene is said to have *reduced penetrance*, meaning that not everyone who has the gene expresses it in a measurable form. An interesting side note is that "measurable form" very much depends on what is able to be measured. Many alleles that were thought to be recessive 50 years ago can be detected today as the result of new and more sensitive technologies. Penetrance is of interest to nutrition professionals because it reflects the inability of a genetic variation to impair function and cause disease unless the individual is exposed to specific environmental triggers, such as diet and lifestyle factors. Modifying these factors can potentially improve outcomes for those with such variants. Terminology may change as understanding advances in the field.

Mitochondrial Inheritance

In addition to genetic material in the nucleus, the mitochondria in each cell also contain DNA that codes for a limited number of proteins. The majority of these genes are involved in maintenance of the mitochondrion and its energy-producing activities. As with nuclear DNA, changes in mitochondrial DNA (mtDNA) can lead to disease. Traits resulting from mitochondrial genes have a characteristic inheritance pattern; they are non-Mendelian because mitochondria and their genetic material typically pass from mother to child, called **mitochondrial** or **maternal inheritance**. This biologic principle has become the basis for anthropologic studies that trace lineage and population migration patterns through the centuries. It also has provided a way to trace familial diseases caused by changes in mtDNA. However, as with other biologic processes, occasional mistakes occur; reports exist of some mtDNA being passed from father to child.

Epigenetic Inheritance, Genomic Imprinting

Epigenetic inheritance illustrates another mechanism by which genetic information is passed between generations. Epigenetics provides an additional set of instructions beyond that contained in the DNA nucleotide sequence. It affects gene expression but does not change the nucleotide sequence itself (van der Maarel, 2008; Villagra et al., 2010). At least three mechanisms are involved: histone modification, DNA modification, and RNA interference (RNAi).

Histones are proteins associated with DNA. Units of histones form a scaffolding around which DNA is wrapped to create the **nucleosome**, similar to thread wrapped around a spool. Similar in concept to condensing data on a hard drive, this mechanism helps to fit the large amount of DNA into the small space of the nucleus. When DNA is condensed, it is not available for transcribing into mRNA. The attachment and removal of acetyl groups is an important mechanism for controlling whether DNA is relaxed and available for transcription to proceed or condensed and closed to transcription, respectively.

Similarly, DNA itself can be modified by the covalent attachment and removal of functional groups, such as methyl groups. Methylation takes place at cytosine residues that occur within CpG islands found near a gene's promoter region. **CpG islands** (the *p* refers to the phosphodiester bond between (C) cytosine and (G) guanine nucleotides) are DNA sequences enriched in cytosine and guanine that, when methylated, interfere with transcription and therefore gene expression. In general, methylation silences gene expression and demethylation promotes gene expression.

DNA methylation and histone modification can contribute to genomic imprinting and affect gene expression. **Genomic imprinting** is an unusual phenomenon in which only one of the two alleles of a gene is expressed, either the allele contributed by the mother or by the father. If each allele contains a different mutation that leads to a measurable phenotype, the individual's phenotype will differ depending on whether the mother's or the father's allele is the one expressed. Prader-Willi syndrome and Angelman syndrome provide examples of genomic imprinting; they involve DNA on chromosome 15. When the father's allele is expressed, the child develops Prader-Willi syndrome. When the mother's allele is expressed, the child develops Angelman syndrome. Both syndromes are characterized by intellectual disabilities, but Prader-Willi individuals also experience a lack of perception of satiety, which leads to overeating and morbid obesity. The suspected underlying basis for the phenotypic differences is the different pattern of epigenetic markings (either histone acetylation or **DNA methylation**) between the two parents rather than differences in the DNA sequence itself. Genomic imprinting has important clinical implications (Butler, 2009; Das et al., 2009).

The third mechanism, **RNA interference (RNAi)**, is a posttranscriptional mechanism whereby short pieces of single-stranded RNA (21-23 nucleotides) attach to DNA or mRNA. Attaching to mRNA interferes with gene expression by preventing translation of the gene into its encoded protein. Attaching to DNA leads to silencing of whole regions of chromosomes, a phenomenon called *epigenetic gene silencing*, which is the basis for X-inactivation in mammalian females in which one of the two X-chromosomes is silenced. In this way the amount of information contributed by the X-chromosome is equalized between females and males, the latter having only a single X-chromosome (Kloc and Martienssen, 2008; Suzuki and Kelleher, 2009).

Epigenetics is of interest to nutrition professionals because diet has been found to influence at least one epigenetic mechanism, DNA methylation, and the effects can be inherited. The mouse has been used as a mammalian model system for dissecting this complex process. In a landmark study by Waterland and Jirtle (2003), a strain of mice with a mutation in the *agouti* gene was used. The wild-type (normal) *agouti* allele causes the mouse's coat color to be brown. The Avy mutation (*agouti viable yellow* allele) causes the coat color to be yellow and, because this allele is dominant, all mice with at least one copy of Avy have the potential to develop the yellow coat color. The researchers bred genetically identical female mice with brown coats (two copies of the normal *agouti* allele) with genetically identical males that had two copies of the Avy mutation and had yellow coats. On a standard mouse chow diet, the coat color of the mothers would be brown, that of the fathers would be yellow, and the coat color of the offspring, who have one *agouti* allele and one Avy allele, would be yellow because the Avy allele is dominant. In this study, half of the females were fed the usual diet and half were fed a methyl-rich diet in which methyl donors such as folate, vitamin B_{12}, choline, and betaine were added to the diet. Most of the unsupplemented mothers had offspring with yellow coats. Most of the offspring from the mothers on the methyl-rich diet, however, had a mottled coat with a mix of brown and yellow (called *pseudo-agouti*). Clearly, the mother's diet affected the coat color of the offspring and this effect persisted into adulthood. There was a correlation between mottled coat and degree of methylation of the *agouti* gene, suggesting that the methyl-rich diet led to epigenetic silencing of the Avy allele.

Furthermore, this effect of diet could be inherited. Cropley and associates (2006) found that feeding the females of the "grandmother" generation a methyl-rich diet but not enriching the daughter offspring's diet with methyl donors still produced a number of offspring with mottled brown coats, suggesting that the effect the diet had on coat color could be transmitted between generations. Diet and possibly other environmental factors may have a transgenerational effect through their influence on epigenetic "markings" that affect gene expression without altering the DNA sequence. This type of gene-diet epigenetic mechanism could explain why identical twins, although having the exact same genotype, typically do not have identical phenotypes.

Inheritance and Disease

Changes to the genetic material, whether to the chromosomal DNA, mtDNA, or even a single nucleotide, have the potential to alter one or more proteins that may be critical to the operation of the cells, tissues, and organs of the body. There are important consequences from changes to the genetic material at each of these levels.

Disease at the Chromosomal Level

Change in the number of chromosomes, or the arrangement of the DNA within a chromosome, is almost always detrimental or fatal to the individual. Chromosomal disorders are detected by means of a **karyotype**, a visualization of all the chromosomes in picture form. An example of a nonfatal chromosomal abnormality is trisomy 21 (Down syndrome), which results from an addition to chromosome 21.

Some syndromes are caused by the loss of a portion of a chromosome (a partial **deletion**). In Beckwith-Wiedemann syndrome (a chromosome 11 deletion), changes are characterized by organ overgrowth, including an oversized tongue, which leads to feeding difficulties and hypoglycemia. Nutrition professionals play an important role in the therapy of those with chromosomal disorders because these individuals often have oral-motor problems that affect their nutritional status and cause growth problems in early life. Later in development, obesity may become an issue, and nutrition therapy is helpful in controlling weight, diabetes, and cardiovascular complications. In people with such abnormalities, varying degrees of mental retardation often complicate therapy. A knowledgeable nutrition professional can mitigate the detrimental effects of these disorders on nutritional status (see Chapter 45).

Disease at the Mitochondrial Level

Mitochondria are subcellular organelles that are thought to have originated from bacterium; they function primarily to produce adenosine triphosphate. Human mtDNA codes for 13 proteins, 2 ribosomal RNAs, and 22 transfer RNAs to synthesize these proteins; the remainder of the proteins are coded for by nuclear DNA. In contrast to nuclear DNA, mtDNA is small (16,569 base pairs), circular, and exists in hundreds to thousands of copies in each mitochondrion. As noted earlier, mtDNA is passed from the mother to her offspring.

Not surprisingly, alterations in mtDNA are typically degenerative and primarily affect tissues with a high demand for oxidative phosphorylation. They also have varied clinical manifestations because of the multiple copies of mtDNA, not all of which may contain the genetic change. Mutations in mtDNA can manifest at any age and include neurologic diseases, cardiomyopathies, and skeletal myopathies (MITOMAP, 2009). For example, Wolfram syndrome, a form of diabetes with associated deafness, was one of the earliest disorders to be traced to mtDNA. More than 60 diseases that result from changes in mtDNA have been identified thus far (Tuppen et al., 2009.)

Disease at the Molecular Level

The majority of disease conditions associated with nutritional genomics involve changes at the molecular level. Changes to the DNA typically involve a single nucleotide change or several nucleotides within a single gene through substitutions, additions or deletions. In addition, larger-scale changes involving the deletion or addition of multiple nucleotides can also occur in the regulatory or protein coding regions of a gene. Alterations in the regulatory region may increase or decrease the quantity of protein produced or alter the ability of the gene to respond to environmental signals. Alterations in the coding region may affect the amino acid sequence of the protein, which in turn can affect the conformation and function of the protein and thereby the functioning of the organism. Because the vast majority of human genes reside on nuclear chromosomes, gene variations are transmitted according to Mendelian inheritance and are subject to modification from epigenetic markings.

Autosomal dominant single-gene disorders that have nutritional implications include several that may result in oral-motor problems, growth problems, susceptibility to weight gain, and difficulties with constipation. Examples include Albright hereditary osteodystrophy, which commonly results in dental problems, obesity, hypocalcemia, and hyperphosphatemia; chondrodysplasias, which often result in oral-motor problems and obesity; and Marfan syndrome, which promotes cardiac disease, excessive growth, and increased nutritional needs. Familial hypercholesterolemia results in a defective low-density lipoprotein (LDL) receptor, elevated levels of cholesterol, and susceptibility to atherosclerosis.

Autosomal recessive disorders are much more common and include metabolic disorders of amino acid, carbohydrate, and lipid metabolism. Traditionally these disorders were detected because the mutation had a detrimental effect on the newborn infant that led to serious developmental consequences or death. These disorders were heritable, ultimately associated with a particular mutation, and designated **inborn errors of metabolism (IEM)**.

IEM disorders are the earliest known examples of nutritional genomics, and dietary modification is the primary treatment modality (see Chapter 44). A brief overview of IEM from a genetic perspective is included here to emphasize the important role of the nutrition professional in restoring health to these individuals and to contrast the IEM with chronic disorders that result from the same type of genetic change but that affect function less severely.

A classic example of an IEM of amino acid metabolism is phenylketonuria (PKU). PKU results from a mutation in the gene coding for the enzyme phenylalanine hydroxylase, leading to an inability to convert phenylalanine to tyrosine. Lifelong dietary restriction of phenylalanine enables individuals with PKU to live into adulthood and enjoy a quality life. In maple syrup urine disease, the metabolic defect is branched-chain alpha-keto acid decarboxylase, an enzyme complex encoded by six genes. A mutation in any one of these genes can result in accumulation of alpha-keto acids in the urine, which produces an odor similar to maple syrup. Failure to limit branched-chain amino acid intake can lead to mental retardation, seizures, and death.

Hereditary fructose intolerance is an example of an autosomal recessive IEM of carbohydrate metabolism. A mutation in the gene encoding aldolase B (fructose-1, 6-biphosphate aldolase) impairs the catalytic activity of the enzyme and prevents fructose from being converted to glucose. Breast-fed infants are typically asymptomatic until fruit is added to the diet. Nutrition therapy involves the elimination of fructose and the fructose-containing disaccharide sucrose.

Autosomal recessive disorders of lipid metabolism include the deficiency of medium-chain acyl-coenzyme A (acyl-CoA) dehydrogenase, which prevents medium-chain fatty acids from being oxidized to provide energy during periods of fasting. Nutrition therapy focuses on preventing the accumulation of toxic fatty acid intermediates that, when not controlled, can lead to death (Isaacs and Zand, 2007). Recent guidelines for expanded newborn screening for IEM in the United States use tandem mass spectrometry and provide information on approximately 40 diseases (Dietzen et al, 2009).

The **X-linked dominant** fragile X syndrome also affects nutritional status. Fragile X syndrome is characterized by developmental delays, mental impairment, and behavioral problems. The lesion occurs within the *FMR1* gene on the X chromosome in which a CGG segment is repeated more times than normal. The multiple repeats of this trinucleotide make the X chromosome susceptible to breakage.

X-linked recessive conditions include nephrogenic diabetes insipidus, adrenoleukodystrophy, and Duchenne muscular dystrophy (DMD) disorders. Individuals with X-linked recessive nephrogenic diabetes insipidus are unable to concentrate urine and exhibit polyuria and polydipsia. This disorder is usually detected in infancy and can manifest as dehydration, poor feeding, vomiting, and failure to thrive. X-linked recessive adrenoleukodystrophy results from a defect in the enzyme that degrades long-chain fatty acids. These fats accumulate and lead to brain and adrenal dysfunction and ultimately motor dysfunction. X-linked recessive DMD is characterized by fatty infiltration of muscles and extreme muscle wasting. Children are typically confined to a wheelchair by the time they reach their teens and need assistance with feeding.

Y-linked inheritance disorders involve male sex determination and physiologic "housekeeping functions." To date no nutrition-related disorders have been conclusively assigned to the Y chromosome.

In summary, any gene can potentially undergo mutation, which can affect the function of its protein and the health of the individual. Its location within the nuclear or mtDNA determines the mode of inheritance.

Genetic Technologies

Progressing beyond knowing the chromosomal location of a disease trait to associating the disease with a particular mutation and understanding its functional consequences has required the development of sophisticated molecular genetic technologies. One of the most critical technologic advances occurred in the early 1970s with the introduction of **recombinant DNA** technology, which allowed major progress in terms of studying genes, their functions, and the regulation of their expression. Using bacteria-derived **restriction endonucleases (restriction enzymes)**, researchers could cut the DNA in precise, reproducible locations along the nucleotide chain, isolate the fragments and, using **polymerase chain reaction (PCR)** technology, make unlimited copies of the DNA for various applications. This basic approach has been the cornerstone of many routine techniques, such as **genetic engineering** and the production of therapeutic proteins such as insulin and growth hormone as well as new genetic strains of crops and food for animals.

Recombinant DNA technology paved the way for DNA sequencing, which is used to identify the sequence of nucleotides within a gene, pinpoint the exact location of any change, and identify each of the nucleotides in an individual's genome. A recent improvement to DNA sequencing, **whole exome capture**, promises to be an efficient way to identify the DNA sequences that constitute genes (Choi et al., 2009). Recombinant DNA is also the basis for detecting variations in DNA sequences that can be used to identify individuals for forensic and paternity purposes and to predict disease susceptibilities. Another important application is gene therapy, by which a corrected gene sequence can be introduced into the cells of an individual with a disease-causing mutation.

One of the outgrowths of these earlier technologies is **microarray technology.** Microarrays, also called **DNA "chips,"** are used to determine which genes are expressed at a particular time under particular conditions, such as during the different developmental stages. They can also be used to determine which genes are turned on (or off) in response to environmental factors, such as nutrients. A useful clinical application is the comparison of gene expression between normal and diseased cells, with important implications in cancer.

Another type of genetic technology involves interfering with a gene's expression to determine the function of that gene and its encoded protein. The concept was originally exploited in model systems involving transgenic animals, particularly the laboratory mouse ("knockout mouse"). Because the mouse and human share many of the same genes, the ability to manipulate the genetic material of the mouse and examine the effect on metabolism and physiologic function has been valuable for understanding humans.

In the knockout mouse, a gene is altered ("knocked out") so that the normal protein is no longer made. Alternatively, a gene can be altered so that it expresses too much or too little of its product. Regulatory sequences can be altered so that a gene no longer responds appropriately to environmental signals. In these ways the normal function of a gene can be determined, the effects of over-expressing or under-expressing a gene can be studied, and details of the communication process between signals outside the organism and the genetic material inside the organism can be determined. Transgenic mice are particularly valuable for studying gene-diet interactions. A recent application of this concept involves RNAi. Short sequences of RNA bind to mRNA and interfere with translation of the mRNA into protein ("knock down"). By measuring the outcome of a decrease in a particular protein, researchers can gain insight into the role of the protein and its contribution to the organism's function.

GENETICS AND NUTRITION THERAPY

Chromosomal or single-gene mutations alter nutrition status and illustrate the importance of nutrition therapy. The rapid development of molecular nutrition and nutritional genomics expands the role of the nutrition professional beyond rare disorders and into more prevalent chronic diseases such as cardiovascular disease (CVD), cancer, diabetes, inflammatory disorders, osteoporosis, and even obesity.

Progress in identifying gene variants associated with particular chronic disorders and understanding the interaction of **bioactive food components** with these variants requires that nutrition professionals be able to interpret genetic screening information and integrate the findings into their services. Nutrition professionals will be needed at an advanced practice level to assist individuals in making gene-directed diet and lifestyle choices (DeBusk, 2009; DeBusk and Joffe, 2006; Jones et al., 2010).

Nutritional genomics is unique in its focus on how the interactions between genetic variations and environmental factors influence the genetic potential of individuals and populations, the "**gene x environment**" **(GxE)** premise (Ordovas and Tai, 2008). Here, *environment* broadly encompasses the typical toxins to which humans are exposed, as well as diet and lifestyle choices that also influence genetic potential. Nutrigenetics is concerned with how an individual's unique set of genetic variations affects the ability to function optimally in a particular environment. Nutrigenomics identifies how the environment affects gene expression.

Nutrigenetic Influences on Health and Disease

The interplay between nutrition and genetics varies from being straightforward to being highly complex. The most straightforward is the direct correlation between a faulty gene, a defective protein, a deficient level of a metabolite, and a resultant disease state that is passed on through Mendelian inheritance and is responsive to nutrition therapy. The IEM are good examples of such interactions and have been referred to as *genetic diseases*. As our understanding of disease at the molecular level has become more sophisticated, this terminology is no longer appropriate. The IEM are characterized as rare mutations that result in protein dysfunction that leads to metabolic disorders. The distinguishing characteristic is the rare occurrence of these particular mutations.

All humans have mutations that result in protein dysfunction that leads to metabolic disease. The human species requires certain amino acids, fatty acids, vitamins, and mineral, and there are mutations that limit the ability to synthesize these important nutrients. The diet must supply them to prevent dysfunction and disease. For example, humans lack the gene for the enzyme gulonolactone oxidase and cannot synthesize vitamin C. If dietary vitamin C intake is below needed levels, individuals are at risk for developing scurvy, which can be fatal.

New is the understanding of the genetic basis for nutrient requirements, the realization that nutrition therapy can circumvent genetic limitations by supplying the missing nutrients, and that each individual may require a different level of nutrient because of his or her particular set of genetic variations. More than 50 metabolic reactions that involve enzymes with decreased affinities for their cofactors and that require high levels of a nutrient to restore function have been identified. Many of the supplementation levels are well in excess of the usual recommended nutrient levels, which highlights the importance of remembering that each individual is genetically unique and has distinct metabolic needs.

Although generalized guidelines for recommended nutrient levels are helpful, individuals may have genetic variations that require them to consume significantly more or less of certain nutrients than the general recommendation. Nutritional genomics has changed the thinking about global dietary recommended intakes, from an age- and sex-related orientation to incorporating nutrigenetic makeup and its influence on protein function (Stover, 2006). Nutrition therapy, then, is a critical tool for compensating for changes in the DNA that can lead to increased risk of disease.

The inborn error of amino acid metabolism, classic homocystinuria, is of interest because it led to the realization that an elevated blood level of homocysteine is an independent risk factor for CVD. A defect in the vitamin B_6–requiring enzyme cystathionine beta-synthase prevents the conversion of homocysteine to cystathionine. Homocysteine accumulates, promotes atherosclerosis, and forms the dipeptide homocystine, which leads to abnormal collagen crosslinking and osteoporosis. Nutrition therapy is multipronged, depending on the specific genetic defect. Some individuals have an enzyme defect that requires a high concentration of the vitamin B_6 cofactor for activity. Others are not responsive to B_6 and need a combination of folate, vitamin B_{12}, choline, and betaine to convert homocysteine to methionine. Others must limit their methionine intake. At least three forms of homocystinuria exist, each requiring a different nutritional approach. The ability to use genetic analysis to distinguish these similar disorders has been a useful technologic advance (see Chapters 6 and 33).

Genetic variation in the *MTHFR* gene provides an excellent example of nutrigenetics as well as how genetic variation can influence nutrient requirements. This gene codes for the enzyme 5,10-methyltetrahydrofolate reductase that produces the biologically active form of folate (5-methyltetrahydrofolate). Folate is essential for the conversion of homocysteine to *S*-adenosylmethionine, a critical methyl donor to numerous metabolic reactions, including those involved in synthesizing nucleic acids (see Chapter 33). A common variation in the *MTHFR* gene is the 677C>T gene variant, which involves substitution of thymine (T) for cytosine (C) at nucleotide position 677 within the coding region of the *MTHFR* gene. The resultant enzyme has reduced activity, which leads to decreased production of active folate and accumulation of homocysteine. In addition to the increased risk of CVD, elevated serum homocysteine increases the risk of neural tube defects in developing fetuses. As a result of these risks, in the United States cereal grains are now fortified with folic acid to ensure adequate levels in women of childbearing age (see Chapter 16).

Studies indicate that homocysteine levels can be lowered through supplementation with one or more of the B vitamins folate, B_2, B_6, and B_{12} (Albert et al., 2008; Ebbing et al., 2008; Shidfar et al., 2009; Varela-Moreiras et al., 2009). The genotype of the individual is an important factor in this response, supporting the need for tailoring nutrient recommendations accordingly.

Disease-causing changes can also occur in genes coding for other types of proteins such as transport proteins, structural proteins, membrane receptors, hormones, and transcription factors. Mutations that increase the transport of iron (hereditary hemochromatosis) or copper (Wilson disease) to higher-than-normal levels have nutritional implications (see Chapter 30). Mutations in vitamin D receptors are not only associated with deleterious effects on bone health, but throughout the body because vitamin D is a hormone involved in hundreds of metabolic and regulatory processes. Changes in the gene coding for insulin can result in structural changes in the insulin hormone and lead to dysglycemia, as can mutations in the insulin receptor. Many proteins such as kinases, cytokines, and transcription factors that are involved in critical signaling cascades are subject to mutational changes, altered activities, and health consequences.

Nutrigenomic Influences on Health and Disease

In addition to compensating for metabolic limitations, nutrients and other bioactive components in food can influence gene expression. This ability has long been known from studies with lower organisms, such as is seen with the *lac* and *trp* operons of bacteria. In these situations the organism "senses" the presence of a nutrient in its external environment and alters its gene expression accordingly. In the case of lactose, the proteins required to use lactose as an energy source are induced by transcriptional regulation of the genes that code for the lactose transport system and for the enzyme that initially metabolizes lactose. The opposite occurs when tryptophan is present in the environment: the organism inhibits the endogenous biosynthesis of tryptophan by inhibiting transcription of the genes that encode tryptophan biosynthetic proteins. GxE interactions, such as monitoring and responding to environmental signals by changing gene expression, are fundamental processes of living systems, allowing them to use resources efficiently.

Higher organisms such as humans have similar mechanisms by which they monitor the environment that bathes their cells and alter cellular or molecular activities as needed. An example is the response of cells to the presence of glucose. Insulin is secreted and binds to its receptor on the surface of skeletal muscle cells and initiates a stepwise biochemical signaling cascade (**signal transduction**). Signaling results in the translocation of glucose transporter type 4 (GLUT4), a receptor involved in glucose entry into cells, from the interior of the cell to the cell surface. Exercise also promotes the translocation of GLUT4, which is helpful in controlling blood sugar levels. A drop in blood sugar levels triggers the release of epinephrine and glucagon that, in turn, bind to cell surface receptors in the liver and skeletal muscle and, through signal transduction, stimulate glycogen breakdown to glucose to restore blood sugar levels.

Nutrients and other bioactive food components can also serve as ligands, molecules that bind to specific nucleotide sequences (response elements) within a gene's regulatory region. Binding results in a change in gene expression through the regulation of transcription. Examples of such food components are the polyunsaturated ω-3 fatty acids. These fats decrease inflammation. They serve as precursors for the synthesis of antiinflammatory eicosanoids and decrease the expression of genes that lead to the production of inflammatory cytokines, such as tumor necrosis factor–alpha and the interleukin-1 genes (Calder, 2009).

The ω-3 and ω-6 fatty acids have also been found to serve as ligands for the **peroxisome proliferator-activated receptor (PPAR)** family of transcription factors. The PPARs function as lipid sensors and regulate lipid and lipoprotein metabolism, glucose homeostasis, adipocyte proliferation and differentiation, and the formation of foam cells from monocytes during atherogenic plaque formation. They are important components in the sequence of events by which a high-fat diet promotes insulin resistance and obesity (Christodoulides and Vidal-Puig, 2009).

To influence the expression of the genes under its control, a PPAR transcription factor must complex with a second transcription factor, the retinoic X receptor (RXR). Each has its ligand attached—polyunsaturated fatty acid and retinoic acid (vitamin A derivative), respectively. The PPAR-RXR complex can then bind to the appropriate response element within the regulatory region of a gene under its control. Binding results in a conformational change in the structure of the DNA molecule that allows RNA polymerase to bind and transcribe the PPAR-regulated genes, leading to a host of lipogenic and proinflammatory activities. A large number of transcription factors have been identified and the mechanisms of action are under investigation.

The bioactive components that serve as ligands for these transcription factors are either provided by the diet or made endogenously, such as ω-3 and ω-6 fatty acids, cholesterol, steroid hormones, bile acids, **xenobiotics** (foreign chemicals, or "new-to-nature" molecules), the active form of vitamin D, and numerous phytonutrients, to name just a few (Wise, 2008). In all cases these bioactives must communicate their presence to the DNA sequestered within the nucleus. Depending on their size and lipid solubility, some bioactives can penetrate the various membrane barriers and interact directly with the DNA, as in the fatty acid example discussed previously. Others, including phytochemicals found in the cruciferous vegetables, may not be able to cross the cell membrane and will instead interact with a receptor on the cell surface and set into motion the cascade of signal transduction events that results in a transcription factor being translocated to the nucleus. See *Focus On:* Phytochemical and Bioactive Food Components.

Identification of the genetic and biochemical mechanisms underlying health and disease provides the basis for developing individualized intervention and prevention strategies. In the case of the ω-3 fatty acids, researchers are actively seeking conditions under which dietary ω-3s can be used to decrease inflammation and increase insulin sensitivity. An understanding of the mechanisms by which gene expression is controlled is also helpful in developing drugs that can target various aspects, including gene expression. For example, the thiazolidinedione class of antidiabetic drugs targets the PPAR mechanism described previously to improve insulin sensitivity.

Identifying bioactive components in fruits, vegetables, and whole grains that are responsible for positive health effects and the mechanisms by which they influence gene expression is of considerable interest. Small-molecular-weight lipophilic molecules can penetrate the cellular and nuclear membranes and serve as ligands for transcription factors that control gene expression. Depending on the gene and the particular bioactive, expression may be turned on or off or increased or decreased in magnitude in keeping with the information received. Examples include resveratrol from purple grape skins; along with a large number of flavonoids such as the catechins found in tea, dark chocolate, and onions and the isoflavones genistein and daidzein from soy.

For bioactive phytochemicals that are too large or too hydrophilic to penetrate the cell's membrane barriers, communication occurs by means of signal transduction. The bioactive interacts with a receptor protein at the cell surface and initiates a cascade of biochemical reactions that ultimately results in one or more transcription factors interacting with DNA and modulating gene expression. Examples of this type of indirect communication are seen with the organosulfur compounds such as sulforaphane and other glucosinolates from the cabbage family vegetables. As a result of the signaling pathway, transcription factors (e.g., *nrf*) are activated and increase transcription of the

FOCUS ON

Phytochemical and Bioactive Food Components

Bioactive food components are molecules in food that influence biological responses in living tissues, including gene expression. Bioactives may be an integral part of a food or they may be contaminants that have entered the food supply. They serve as molecular sensors, communicating valuable information to cells about the surrounding environment and influencing health outcomes.

Phytochemicals are a major source of bioactives that occur naturally in plants; many have been found to positively affect health. They may be traditional nutrients such as vitamins that have been documented to be essential for health or they may be more recently discovered compounds with health effects under investigation, such as resveratrol in red wine for its heart and longevity benefits and lutein in spinach for protection against macular degeneration in the eye. Although numerous studies have positively associated various phytochemicals with health, how they work remains to be defined. Various roles that are emerging include protection against oxidative stress (antioxidant properties,) promotion of cancer cell death (apoptosis), alteration of hormone metabolism, enhancement of the immune response or cell-cell communication, protection against the effects of environmental toxins, and promotion of a healthy mix of microorganisms in the digestive tract.

Phytochemicals are classified by their chemical structure into alkaloids (e.g., caffeine), carotenoids (alpha- or beta-carotene, lutein, zeaxanthin, and lycopene), nitrogen-containing compounds (some alkaloids and organosulfur compounds), organosulfur compounds (e.g., glucosinolates), and phenolics. Phenolics include numerous flavonoids and stilbenes and are abundant in plant foods, especially fruits and vegetables and are of particular interest for their possible protection against heart disease and cancer.

glutathione-S-transferases needed for phase II detoxification, which helps to protect against cancer. Flavonoids such as naringenin found in citrus fruits and quercetin from onions and apples activate signaling pathways, leading to increased apoptosis of cancer cells.

It can be challenging to communicate the specifics of phytochemicals to consumers because they do not think about the bioactive substances in the food they eat. Attempts have been made to simplify the message, such as focusing on thinking of food in terms of its dominant color and understanding that each color contributes different valuable phytochemicals. For example, eating one to two servings from a wide variety of fruits, vegetables, legumes, grains, nuts, and seeds within the red, orange, green, purple, and white color categories daily will supply a variety of healthy phytochemicals. Individuals with particular disease susceptibilities or environmental challenges should increase the number of servings within a particular category to meet their specific health needs. Practitioners can provide a valuable service by translating these research findings into practical food solutions for consumers (Keijr et al., 2010; Kim et al., 2009).

Epigenetic Influences on Health and Disease

Epigenetics, including gene silencing and genomic imprinting, is under active investigation presently (Butler, 2009; Mathers, 2008; Waterland, 2009). Inappropriate gene expression can have serious consequences. During development, for example, specific genes are turned on or off with precise timing. Alterations in that timing can impair fetal development and may cause death. Cancer is another example. Certain genes (oncogenes) promote uncontrolled cell growth; others (tumor suppressor genes) help to put the brakes on such growth. Inappropriate methylation of these genes can result in oncogenes being expressed when they should be silent and tumor suppressor genes being silenced when they would normally be expressed. Either situation can promote uncontrolled cell growth and the development of cancer.

As the significance of epigenetics and the critical nature of epigenetic reprogramming during germ cell development and early embryogenesis is increasingly appreciated, researchers have begun to ask how reproductive technologies such as in vitro fertilization might affect fetal development (Dupont et al., 2009; Grace et al., 2009; Swanson et al., 2009).

Nutritional Genomics and Chronic Disease

Chronic disorders (e.g., CVD, cancer, diabetes, osteoporosis, inflammatory disorders) are typically more complex than single-gene disorders in which the change in the DNA is known, the abnormal protein can be identified and analyzed, and the resulting phenotype is clearly defined. Multiple genes, each with multiple variations, contribute in small ways to the overall chronic condition rather than a single variant having a dramatic effect. The genes involved with chronic disease are influenced by environmental factors in addition to the genetic variation. An individual might have gene variants that predispose to a particular chronic disorder, but the disorder may or may not develop.

Genetic Variability

Given the genetic variability among individuals in a population, the high degree of variability in client response to nutrition therapy should not be surprising. Although a change in a gene—including diet- and lifestyle-related genes—can affect function severely enough to cause disease outright, the majority of these genes appear to affect the magnitude of response and do not pose a life-threatening situation. They confer an increased susceptibility. Many of these variants are responsive to diet and other lifestyle parameters, providing the opportunity to minimize their effect through informed lifestyle choices.

The major focus of nutritional genomics research is on identifying (1) gene-disease associations, (2) the dietary components that influence these associations, (3) the mechanisms by which dietary components exert their effects, and (4) the genotypes that benefit most from particular diet and lifestyle choices. The practical applications of this research include a new set of tools that nutrition professionals can use. The growing body of knowledge will support strategies for disease prevention and intervention that are specifically targeted to the underlying mechanisms.

The following section takes a brief look at some of the key diet-related genes, their known variants, and how these variants affect a person's response to diet. Chronic disease involves complex interactions among genes and bioactive food components, and unraveling the details will require population and intervention studies large enough to have the statistical power needed to draw meaningful conclusions.

Cardiovascular Disease

CVD remains the number one disease plaguing developed countries. Not surprisingly, a major focus of nutritional genomics has been to identify gene-diet associations for CVD and to study the influence of diet and exercise parameters in managing and preventing this chronic disease. Nutrition professionals who work with clients with dyslipidemia know firsthand the high degree of individual variability of responses to standard dietary interventions. These therapies are used primarily to lower elevated blood levels of LDL cholesterol (LDL-C), raise high-density lipoprotein cholesterol (HDL-C), and lower triglycerides (TGs). The standard approach is a diet low in saturated fat, with increased content of polyunsaturated fats (PUFAs). Response across a population varies, ranging from reduced LDL-C levels and TGs in some to decreased HDL-C levels or elevated TGs in others. Furthermore, some have had their LDL-C levels respond dramatically to dietary oat bran and other soluble fibers, whereas others have had more modest responses. In some a low-fat diet has caused a shift to a lipid pattern that is more atherogenic than the original. Genotype is an important factor; dietary interventions must be matched to genotypes to accomplish the intended lipid-lowering response.

A number of contributing genes have already been identified and include those involved with postprandial lipoprotein and TG response, homocysteine metabolism, hypertension, blood-clotting, and inflammation (Lovegrove and Gitau, 2008; Minihane, 2009). Gene-diet interactions are noted for those that code for apolipoprotein E (*APOE*), apolipoprotein A-1 (*APOA1*), cholesterol esteryl transport protein (*CETP*), hepatic lipase (*LIPC*), lipoxygenase-5 (*ALOX5*), *MTHFR*, angiotensinogen (*AGT*), angiotensin-converting enzyme (*ACE*), the interleukin-1 family (*IL1*), interleukin-6 (*IL6*), and tumor necrosis factor-alpha (*TNF*). Five new SNPs that appear to be common among multiple populations have been identified from the Atherosclerosis Risk in Communities Study by using the genome-wide association study technique (Bressler et al., 2010).

Data from the Framingham Study provided an early example of how knowing the client's genetic variants could be helpful in developing effective nutritional interventions. The *APOA1* gene codes for apolipoprotein A-1, the primary protein in HDL (see Chapters 15 and 34). One variant that is diet-related is –75G>A, in which guanine has been replaced with an adenine at position 75 within the regulatory region of the *APOA1* gene (the "–" sign indicates the site for the variation comes prior to the first nucleotide—position "0"—of the gene's coding region). In women with two copies of the more common G allele, increasing dietary PUFA was accompanied by declining HDL levels. However, in women with at least one copy of the A allele, increasing PUFA concentrations increased HDL levels. Manipulating PUFA levels will have different effects on HDL levels, depending on which variant an individual has and how many copies.

A sampling of other diet- and lifestyle-responsive gene variants that have implications for nutrition therapy related to preventing and treating CVD include *APOE* gene variants and the responses to dietary fat, soluble fiber, and alcohol (Corella and Ordovas, 2005); *CETP* variants and effects on HDL levels, lipid-modifying response to statin drugs, and response of lipid parameters to physical activity (Ayyobi et al., 2005); *APOE*, *CETP*, and *APOA-IV* gene variants and low HDL levels (Miltiadous et al., 2005); effect of *LIPC* gene variants on HDL levels and modification by saturated fat (Zhang et al., 2005); *APOA2*, dietary fat, and body mass index (Corella et al., 2009); and *APOA5* and TGs (Lai et al., 2006; Tai and Ordovas, 2008). The possibilities for nutritional intervention are endless (Afman and Müller, 2006).

CVD is also an inflammatory disorder (Rocha and Libby, 2009), and variants of *TNF*, *IL1*, and *IL6* are being investigated for their effect on CVD susceptibility. Knowing the genotype of clients provides additional important information as to how they are likely to respond to particular dietary interventions (Ordovas, 2007).

Inflammatory Disorders

Inflammation is now recognized as an underlying factor in chronic disorders, from heart disease to cancer to diabetes to obesity to more traditional inflammatory disorders such as arthritis and the inflammatory bowel disorders. Inflammation is a normal and desirable response to insult by the body. Typically, inflammation is an acute phase response; once the threat has passed, inflammation subsides and healing ensues. Certain genetic variations predispose individuals to be proinflammatory, making them more reactive to inflammatory triggers and extending the inflammation phase so that inflammation becomes a chronic state. The regular assault of proinflammatory mediators such as the cytokines and eicosanoids on tissues leads to oxidative stress and cellular degeneration rather than the healing that is characteristic of the acute phase.

Among the genes known to be of particular importance to the inflammatory response are *IL1*, which encodes the interleukin-1β cytokine (also known as IL-1F2), *IL6* (encoding the interleukin-6 cytokine), and *TNF*. Variants in each of these genes have been discovered that increase the susceptibility of humans to be in a proinflammatory state, which in turn increases the risk of developing one or more chronic disorders. Certain diet and lifestyle approaches can minimize susceptibility and dampen existing inflammation (Massaro et al., 2008). Examples include the inclusion of fish and foods that contain ω-3 fatty acids and plant foods rich in various polyphenols.

Immune Health and Cancer

The relationship of gene variants and gene-diet interactions to immune health and cancer is of considerable interest to researchers around the world (Milner, 2008; Trottier et al., 2010; Villagra et al., 2010). One of the key mechanisms by which the body protects against cancer is detoxification, the process of neutralizing potentially harmful molecules. Among the better-characterized genes involved in various aspects of detoxification are the cytochrome P450 isozymes (*CYPs*), glutathione *S*-transferases (*GSTs*), and superoxide dismutases (*SOD1*, *SOD2*, *SOD3*). The *CYP* and *GST* genes are part of the phase I and phase II detoxification system, respectively, found in the liver and the gut. The *SOD* genes code for proteins that dismantle the reactive oxygen species superoxide. Each of these genes has nutritional implications, and variants have been identified that result in decreased detoxification. Nutritional genomics provides the basis for directing nutrition therapy to protect against cancer by augmenting endogenous detoxification activity.

Epidemiologic studies have suggested that consuming plant foods is cancer-protective. Numerous dietary factors play a role in protecting against cancer. Examples include curcumin from the spice turmeric (Aggarwal and Shishodia, 2006; Surh and Chun, 2007; Trottier et al., 2009), resveratrol from purple grape skins (Athar et al., 2009; Udenigwe et al., 2008), glucosinolates in cruciferous vegetables (Ambrosone and Tang, 2009), epigallocatechin gallate catechins from green tea (Na and Surh, 2008), isoflavones from soybeans (Steiner et al., 2008), folic acid (Ebbing et al., 2009; Fife et al., 2009; Oaks et al., 2009), and vitamin D (van der Rhee et al., 2009). Numerous labs are investigating the underlying mechanisms by which these phytochemicals exert their protective effects (Surh et al., 2008; Tan and Spivack, 2009).

Blood Sugar Regulation

Glucose is the preferred source of energy for the body's cells. Accordingly, blood glucose levels are carefully controlled through an intricate system of checks and balances. When glucose levels are higher than normal (hyperglycemia), the hormone insulin is secreted from the beta-cells of the pancreas, glucose is taken up by the cells, and a normal blood sugar level (euglycemia) is restored. When blood glucose levels fall (hypoglycemia), the hormone glucagon is secreted by the liver, glycogen is hydrolyzed to glucose, and euglycemia is again restored. When this process goes awry, the stage is set for the chronic conditions of insulin resistance, metabolic syndrome, and, ultimately, T2DM.

Identification of gene variants that lead to T2DM would allow individuals with this susceptibility to be identified early in the lifespan so that intervention could be initiated. A few rare mutations have been associated with the development of T2DM, but they do not explain the high prevalence of the disease. It is likely that multiple gene variants contribute to the development of this condition. One promising variant is the transcription factor 7-like 2 (*TCF7L2*) identified by Grant and colleagues (2006). The variant occurs frequently within multiple populations. Evidence suggests the gene is involved in insulin secretion from pancreatic beta-cells (Villareal et al, 2010).

Bone Mineralization and Maintenance

Healthy bone tissue depends on a balance between the action of the osteoblasts that synthesize new bone tissue and resorption by osteoclasts. Important components in this dynamic balance are vitamin D, calcium, other nutrients, and hormones such as parathyroid hormone and estrogen. When resorption predominates, bones become fragile, are subject to fracture, and osteoporosis results. Osteoporosis can occur in men and women as they age; it is prevalent among older postmenopausal women.

Numerous genes and their protein products are involved in the overall process. Variants are being investigated, including the *VDR* gene, which codes for the vitamin D receptor present on the surface of many cell types. Vitamin D has multiple roles in metabolism, but its control of the absorption of dietary calcium from the digestive tract truly affects bone health. Four *VDR* variants have been studied over several years (ApaI, BsmI, FokI, and TaqI), but no clear association has emerged (Gennari et al., 2009). Two of the more promising variants at this time are *COL1A1*, which encodes the major protein in bone (α1 peptide of Type 1 collagen) and *LRP5*, which encodes a protein that forms a cell surface receptor and activates the signaling pathway. Further research is imperative.

Weight Management

The ability to maintain a healthy weight is another challenge of modern society. As with the other chronic disorders, the regulation of body weight is a complex process and offers multiple points at which a gene variant can give rise to an impaired protein that, when combined with the appropriate environmental trigger, promotes body fat storage. Similar to T2DM, variations in single genes have been associated with excess weight, but these genetic changes are not likely the basis for the rapid rise in prevalence of excess body weight during the past several generations (Hetherington and Cecil, 2010).

A variant in the *FTO* gene has been identified and found to occur frequently among multiple populations (Chu et al, 2008; Dina et al., 2007). An SNP in the *FTO* gene is associated with increased risk of obesity, and the effect was directly correlated with the number of copies of the SNP. That is, those with one copy of the risk allele weighed more than those with no copies, and those with two copies weighed the most of the three groups (Frayling et al., 2007). In 2009, two large genome-wide association studies found the *FTO* variant to be associated with BMI (Thorleifsson et al., 2009; Willer et al., 2009). The mechanism of action of the *FTO* gene is not yet known. A number of other gene variants have been implicated in weight management, including *ADRB3*, *FABP2*, *POMC*, and *PPARG*, but none so dramatically as *FTO*. The *FTO* variant may also increase risk for T2DM and CVD through its effect on susceptibility to increased body fat.

Adipose tissue is dynamic tissue that is highly vascularized and produces hormones, inflammatory peptides (cytokines), and new adipocytes in addition to storing excess calories as TGs and hydrolyzing them as energy is needed. The multistep process of transporting free fatty acids into the adipocyte, esterifying them into TGs, and mobilizing the TGs potentially provides many proteins that could be affected by genetic variation such that fat is stored more readily or mobilized more slowly than normal. Adipocytes have cell surface receptors that respond to various environmental factors, such as catecholamines produced during exercise, to mobilize stored fat. An example is the receptor encoded by the *ADRB2* gene, which has a greater propensity to store dietary fat as body fat. Individuals with either of these variants will find it more challenging to maintain a healthy weight and may need to restrict their dietary fat intake or engage in regular, vigorous exercise to achieve and maintain a healthy weight.

Other Chronic Diseases

Candidate genes, gene variants, and diet-gene interactions are being investigated for many chronic disorders. Populations differ in the types and frequencies of the gene variants; dietary approaches that are most appropriate will vary accordingly. As gene variants and their health implications are identified, attention is also being paid to examining the frequency of particular variants among populations.

ETHICAL, LEGAL, AND SOCIAL IMPLICATIONS

If nutritional genomics is to realize its potential as a valuable tool, genetic testing is an essential component of identifying the variations in each individual. Such testing is not, however, without controversy. Consumers worry that genetic testing for any purpose could be used against them, primarily to deny insurance coverage or employment; they are particularly uncomfortable with insurers and employers having access to their personal genetic information (Genetics & Public Policy Center, 2010.)

Although theoretically possible, according to existing case law such discrimination has rarely occurred. Furthermore, identifying gene variants that increase susceptibility to diet- and lifestyle-related diseases that can be addressed through readily available diet and lifestyle measures may also lead to legal debate. Many legislators and legal experts believe the Americans with Disabilities Act sufficiently protects against discrimination, but, as an added measure of protection, the **Genetic Information Nondiscrimination Act (GINA)** was passed by Congress and went into effect on November 21, 2009. GINA defines genetic testing and genetic information, bans discrimination based on genetic information, and penalizes those who violate the provisions of this law. Consumers and health care professionals can feel comfortable in adopting this new service.

Consumers and health care professionals should ask critical questions prior to consent for genetic testing. The laboratory itself should have the appropriate credentials and state licensing, if required (at a minimum, Clinical Laboratory Improvement Amendment (CLIA) certification according to the CLIA of 1988) and should have an appropriately credentialed health professional available for assistance in interpreting the test results. The laboratory should have written, readily available policies concerning how it will protect the privacy of the individual being tested and whether the DNA sample will be retained by the lab or destroyed following testing. Transparency in each of these areas will increase consumer comfort.

A second concern on the part of consumers and health care professionals is that nutritional genomics is elitist by nature, in that only the wealthy will be able to benefit. At this early stage in its development, the cost of nutritional genomics testing precludes its use as a public health measure and effectively restricts access to those with sufficient disposable income. However, like any other new technology, as the sales volume increases, the cost will decrease.

Numerous additional issues need to be thoroughly discussed in the course of integrating genetic technologies into health care. Box 5-1 lists key questions to be answered in the development of nutritional genomics practices. These and other ethical, legal, and social issues relating to nutritional genomics in particular have been explored. Authors address ethical treatment of research participants (Bergman et al., 2008), consumer versus health care professional testing (Foster and Sharp, 2008; Royal et al, 2010); the capacity gap in terms of health care professionals trained in nutritional genomics (Farrell, 2009); and various other aspects of the ethical, legal, and social implications of nutritional genomics (Reilly and DeBusk, 2008; Ries and Castle, 2008).

CLINICAL SCENARIO

Jared and Matthew are identical twins who grew up together but have lived apart since college. Jared lives in New York City and is a certified public accountant in a high-profile accounting firm, working long hours in a stressful environment. Matthew attended college in California, where he studied nutrition and exercise physiology and now manages the wellness program at a large fitness center. At age 30 the two brothers are noticeably different in weight and body shape. Jared has a body mass index of 29 compared with Matthew's 23. Jared has developed central obesity, hypertension, and problems with blood sugar regulation, all signs of a tendency toward developing type 2 diabetes. In contrast, Matthew is lean and has normal blood pressure and normal blood sugar levels.

Nutrition Diagnostic Statement

Overweight related to possible genetic susceptibility, limited physical activity, overeating with snacks and consumption of large meals as evidenced by diet history, central obesity, and body mass index

Nutrition Care Questions

1. Because they are identical twins, would you have expected the two brothers to have similar health profiles?
2. How would you expect their diets to be different?
3. What is going on? Does Matthew not have the same genetic susceptibilities that Jared has? If not, why not? If so, why doesn't Matthew exhibit the same phenotype as Jared? This question is complex: think about the twins' deoxyribonucleic acid, but also their environmental influences and their epigenetic markings.
4. How could you confirm your suspicion that Jared is genetically predisposed to type 2 diabetes?
5. What would you advise Jared to do to decrease his genetic susceptibility to diabetes?
6. As part of the nutrition assessment, Jared is found to be homozygous for IL1 -511C>T and heterozygous for IL6 -174G>C. These genes code for the proinflammatory cytokines interleukin-1 and interleukin-6 and these particular single nucleotide polymorphisms have been strongly associated with chronic inflammation. What would you discuss with Jared about the implications of these genotype findings and his susceptibility to chronic disease?

BOX 5-1

Important and Ethical Questions Related to Genetics Testing

Which laboratory will analyze the deoxyribonucleic acid?
What measures are in place in that laboratory to protect privacy?
What is the total cost of the test?
Which gene variants are tested?
Is there is a lifestyle action that can be taken for each variant?
Has the test has been scientifically validated for accuracy and reliability?
When will the test results be received?
How and to whom will the test results be presented?
Who should be tested?
Should individuals be tested for a disease for which there is no cure?
Do parents have the right to have their minor children tested for a genetic susceptibility?
Do parents have the right to withhold the results from the children?
Should gene therapy be allowed on reproductive cells so that any corrected genes can be inherited by subsequent generations?
Should human cloning be allowed?
What is the best way to educate those who are already in practice as health care professionals?
What changes are needed so that future health care practitioners can be properly educated?

USEFUL WEBSITES

CDC Genomics
www.cdc.gov/genomics
Center for Nutritional Genomics
www.nutrigenomics.nl
Ethical, Legal, and Social Issues
http://www.ornl.gov/sci/techresources/Human_Genome/elsi/elsi.shtml
Family History Initiative
http://www.hhs.gov/familyhistory
Genetics and Genomics
http://www.genome.gov/Education/
Genetics Core Competencies
http://www.nchpeg.org/core/Core_Comps_English_2007.pdf
Genetic Information Nondiscrimination Act (GINA)
www.gpo.gov/fdsys/pkg/PLAW-110publ233/pdf/PLAW-110publ233.pdf
Genetics Glossary
www.ornl.gov/TechResources/Human_Genome/glossary
Human Genome Project
www.ornl.gov/hgmis/project/info.html
NUGO for Dietitians
http://www.nugo.org/everyone/28182
Nutrigenomics—New Zealand
www.nutrigenomics.org.nz
Nutrigenomics—University of California–Davis
http://nutrigenomics.ucdavis.edu

REFERENCES

Afman L, Müller M: Nutrigenomics: from molecular nutrition to the prevention of disease, *J Am Diet Assoc* 106:569, 2006.

Aggarwal BB, Shishodia S: Molecular targets of dietary agents for prevention and therapy of cancer, *Biochem Pharmacol* 71:1397, 2006.

Albert CM, et al: Effect of folic acid and B vitamins on risk of cardiovascular events and total mortality among women at high risk for cardiovascular disease: a randomized trial, *JAMA* 299:2027, 2008.

Ambrosone CB, Tang L: Cruciferous vegetable intake and cancer prevention: role of nutrigenetics, *Cancer Prev Res (Phila Pa)* 2:298, 2009.

Athar M, et al: Multiple molecular targets of resveratrol: anti-carcinogenic mechanisms, *Arch Biochem Biophys* 486:95, 2009.

Ayyobi AF, et al: Cholesterol ester transfer protein (CETP) Taq1B polymorphism influences the effect of a standardized cardiac rehabilitation program on lipid risk markers, *Atherosclerosis* 181:363, 2005.

Bergman MM, et al: Bioethical considerations for human nutrigenomics, *Annu Rev Nutr* 28:447, 2008.

Bressler J, et al: Genetic variants identified in a European genome-wide association study that were found to predict incident coronary heart disease in the atherosclerosis risk in communities study, *Am J Epidemiol* 171:14, 2010.

Butler MG: Genomic imprinting disorders in humans: a mini-review, *J Assist Reprod Genet* Oct 21, 2009. [Epub ahead of print.]

Calder PC: The 2008 ESPEN Sir David Cuthbertson lecture: fatty acids and inflammation—From the membrane to the nucleus and from the laboratory bench to the clinic, *Clin Nutr* 2009. [Epub ahead of print.]

Choi M, et al: Genetic diagnosis by whole exome capture and massively parallel DNA sequencing, *Proc Natl Acad Sci U S A* 106:19096, 2009.

Christodoulides C, Vidal-Puig A: PPARS and adipocyte function, *Mol Cell Endocrinol* 318:61, 2010.

Chu X, et al: Association of morbid obesity with FTO and INSIG2 allelic variants, *Arch Surg* 143:235, 2008.

Cropley JE, et al: Germ-line epigenetic modification of the murine Avy allele by nutritional supplementation, *Proc Natl Acad Sci USA* 103:17308, 2006.

Corella D, et al: APOA2, dietary fat, and body mass index: replication of a gene-diet interaction in 3 independent populations, *Arch Intern Med* 169(20):1897, 2009.

Corella D, Ordovas JM: Single nucleotide polymorphisms that influence lipid metabolism: interaction with dietary factors, *Annu Rev Nutr* 25:341, 2005.

Das R, et al: Imprinting evolution and human health, *Mamm Genome* 20:563, 2009.

DeBusk R: Diet-related disease, nutritional genomics, and food and nutrition professionals, *J Am Diet Assoc* 109:410, 2009.

DeBusk R, Joffe Y: *It's not just your genes!*, San Diego, 2006, BKDR.

Dietzen DJ, et al: National academy of clinical biochemistry laboratory medicine practice guidelines: follow-up testing for metabolic disease identified by expanded newborn screening using tandem mass spectrometry: executive summary, *Clin Chem* 55:1615, 2009.

Dina C, et al: Variation in FTO contributes to childhood obesity and severe adult obesity, *Nat Genet* 39:724, 2007.

Dupont C, et al: Epigenetics: definition, mechanisms and clinical perspective, *Semin Reprod Med* 27:351, 2009.

Ebbing M, et al: Cancer incidence and mortality after treatment with folic acid and vitamin B12, *JAMA* 302:2119, 2009.

Ebbing M, et al: Mortality and cardiovascular events in patients treated with homocysteine-lowering B vitamins after coronary angiography: a randomized controlled trial, *JAMA* 300:795, 2008.

Farrell J: Health care provider capacity in nutrition and genetics—a Canadian case study. In Castle D, Ries N, editors: *Nutrition and genomics: issues of ethics, law, regulation and communication*, Toronto, 2009, Elsevier.

Feuk L, et al: Structural variation in the human genome, *Nat Rev Genet* 7:85, 2006.

Fife J, et al: folic acid supplementation and colorectal cancer risk: a meta-analysis, *Colorectal Dis* Oct 27, 2009. [Epub ahead of print.]

Foster MW, Sharp RR: Out of sequence: how consumer genomics could displace clinical genetics, *Nat Rev Genet* 9:419, 2008.

Frayling TM, et al: A common variant in the FTO gene is associated with body mass index and predisposes to childhood and adult obesity, *Science* 316:889, 2007.

Gennari L, et al: Update on the pharmacogenetics of the vitamin D receptor and osteoporosis, *Pharmacogenomics* 10:417, 2009.

Genetics & Public Policy Center, Johns Hopkins University: http://www.dnapolicy.org/images/reportpdfs/GINAPublic_Opinion_Genetic_Information_Discrimination.pdf. Accessed Jan 22, 2010.

Gosden RG, Feinberg AP: Genetics and epigenetics—nature's pen-and-pencil set, *N Engl J Med* 356:731, 2007.

Grace KS, Sinclair KD: Assisted reproductive technology, epigenetics, and long-term health: a developmental time bomb still ticking, *Semin Reprod Med* 27:409, 2009.

Grant SF, et al: Variant of transcription factor 7-like 2 (*TCF7L2*) gene confers risk of type 2 diabetes, *Nat Genet* 38:320, 2006.

Hetherington MM, Cecil JE: Gene-environment interactions in obesity, *Forum Nutr* 63:195, 2010.

Human Genome Project: www.ornl.gov/hgmis/project/info.html. Accessed Jan 22, 2010.

Isaacs JS, Zand DJ: Single-gene autosomal recessive disorders and Prader-Willi syndrome: an update for food and nutrition professionals, *J Am Diet Assoc* 107:466, 2007.

Jones DS, et al: *21st century medicine: a new model for medical education and practice:* http://www.functionalmedicine.org. Accessed Jan 2, 2010.

Kauwell GP: Epigenetics: what it is and how it can affect dietetics practice, *J Am Diet Assoc* 108:1056, 2008.

Keijr J, et al: Bioactive food components, cancer cell growth limitation and reversal of glycolytic metabolism, *Biochim Biophys Acta* 1807:697, 2011.

Kim YS, et al: Bioactive food components, inflammatory targets, and cancer prevention, *Cancer Prev Res (Phila Pa)* 2:200, 2009.

Kloc A, Martienssen R: RNAi, heterochromatin and the cell cycle, *Trends Genet* 24:51, 2008

Lai CQ, et al: Dietary intake of ω-6 fatty acids modulates effect of apolipoprotein A5 gene on plasma fasting triglycerides, remnant lipoprotein concentrations, and lipoprotein particle size: the Framingham Heart Study, *Circulation* 113:2062, 2006.

Lovegrove JA, Gitau R: Personalized nutrition for the prevention of cardiovascular disease: a future perspective, *J Hum Nutr Diet* 21:306, 2008.

Massaro M, et al: ω-3 fatty acids, inflammation and angiogenesis: nutrigenomics effects as an explanation for anti-atherogenic and anti-inflammatory effects of fish and fish oils, *J Nutrigenet Nutrigenomics* 1:4, 2008.

Mathers JC: Session 2: Personalised nutrition. Epigenomics: a basis for understanding individual differences? *Proc Nutr Soc* 67:390, 2008.

Milner JA: Nutrition and cancer: essential elements for a roadmap, *Cancer Lett* 269;189, 2008.

Miltiadous G, et al: Gene polymorphisms affecting HDL-cholesterol levels in the normolipidemic population, *Nutr Metab Cardiovas Dis* 15:219, 2005.

Minihane AM: Nutrient gene interactions in lipid metabolism, *Curr Opin Clin Nutr Metab Care* 12:357, 2009.

MITOMAP: map of the mitochondrial genome: http://www.mitomap.org/. Accessed 2009.

Na HK, Surh YJ: Modulation of Nrf2-mediated antioxidant and detoxifying enzyme induction by the green tea polyphenols EGCG, *Food Chem Toxicol* 46:1271, 2008.

Oaks BM, et al: Folate intake, post-folic acid grain fortification, and pancreatic cancer risk in the Prostate, Lung, Colorectal, and Ovarian Cancer Screening Trial, *Am J Clin Nutr* December 2009. [Epub ahead of print.]

Ordovas J: Diet/genetic interactions and their effects on inflammatory markers, *Nutr Rev* 65(12 Pt 2):S203, 2007.

Ordovas JM, Tai ES: Why study gene-environment interactions? *Curr Opin Lipidol* 19:158, 2008.

Panagiotou G, Nielsen J: Nutritional systems biology: definitions and approaches, *Annu Rev Nutr* 29:329, 2009.

Reilly PR, DeBusk RM: Ethical and legal issues in nutritional genomics, *J Am Diet Assoc* 108:36, 2008.

Ries NM, Castle D: Nutrigenomics and ethics interface: direct-to-consumer services and commercial aspects, *OMICS* 12:245, 2008.

Rocha VZ, Libby P: Obesity, inflammation and atherosclerosis, *Nat Rev Cardiol* 6:399, 2009.

Royal CD, et al: Inferring genetic ancestry: opportunities, challenges, and implications. *Am J Hum Genet* 86:661, 2010.

Shidfar F, et al: Effect of folate supplementation on serum homocysteine and plasma total antioxidant capacity in hypercholesterolemic adults under lovastatin treatment: a double-blind randomized controlled clinical trial, *Arch Med Res* 40:380, 2009.

Steiner C, et al: Isoflavones and the prevention of breast and prostate cancer: new perspectives opened by nutrigenomics, *Br J Nutr* 99:ES78, 2008.

Stover PJ: Influence of human genetic variation on nutritional requirements, *Am J Clin Nutr* 83:436S, 2006.

Stover PJ, Caudill MA: Genetic and epigenetic contributions to human nutrition and health: managing genome-diet interactions, *J Am Diet Assoc* 108:1480, 2008.

Surh YJ, Chun KS: Cancer chemopreventive effects of curcumin, *Adv Exp Med Biol* 595:149, 2007.

Surh YJ, et al: Nrf2 as a master redox switch in turning on the cellular signaling involved in the induction of cytoprotective genes by some chemopreventive phytochemicals, *Planta Med* 74:1526, 2008.

Suzuki K, Kelleher AD. Transcriptional regulation by promoter targeted RNAs, *Curr Top Med Chem* 9:1079, 2009.

Swanson JM, et al: Developmental origins of health and disease: environmental exposures, *Semin Reprod Med* 27:391, 2009.

Tai ES, Ordovas JM: Clinical significance of apolipoprotein A5. *Curr Opin Lipidol* 19:349, 2008.

Tan XL, Spivack SD: Dietary chemoprevention strategies for induction of phase II xenobiotic-metabolizing enzymes in lung carcinogenesis: a review, *Lung Cancer* 65:129, 2009.

Thorleifsson G, et al: Genome-wide association yields new sequence variants at seven loci that associate with measures of obesity, *Nat Genet* 41:18, 2009.

Trottier G, et al: Nutraceuticals and prostate cancer prevention: a current review, *Nat Rev Urol* Dec 8, 2009. [Epub ahead of print.]

Tuppen HA, et al: Mitochondrial DNA mutations and human disease, *Biochim Biophys Acta* 2009. [Epub ahead of print.]

Udenigwe CC, et al: Potential of resveratrol in anticancer and anti-inflammatory therapy, *Nutr Rev* 66:445, 2008.

Van der Maarel SM: Epigenetic mechanisms in health and disease, *Ann Rheum Dis* 67(Suppl 3):iii97, 2008.

Van der Rhee H, et al: Sunlight, vitamin D and the prevention of cancer: a systematic review of epidemiological studies, *Eur J Cancer Prev* 18:458, 2009.

Varela-Moreiras G, et al: Cobalamin, folic acid, and homocysteine, *Nutr Rev* 67(Suppl 1):S69, 2009.

Villagra A, et al: Histone deacetylases and the immunological network: implications in cancer and Inflammation, *Oncogene* 29:157, 2010.

Villareal DT, et al: TCF7L2 variant rs7903146 affects the risk of type 2 diabetes by modulating incretin action, *Diabetes* 59:479, 2010.

Waterland RA: Is epigenetics an important link between early life events and adult disease? *Horm Res* 71:13S, 2009.

Waterland RA, Jirtle RL: Transposable elements: targets for early nutritional effects on epigenetic gene regulation, *Mol Cell Biol* 23:5293, 2003.

Willer CJ, et al: Six new loci associated with body mass index highlight a neuronal influence on body weight regulation, *Nat Genet* 41:24, 2009.

Wise A: Transcriptional switches in the control of macronutrient metabolism, *Nutr Rev* 66:321, 2008.

Zhang C, et al: Interactions between the −514C>T polymorphism of the hepatic lipase gene and lifestyle factors in relation to HDL concentrations among U.S. diabetic men, *Am J Clin Nutr* 81:1429, 2005.

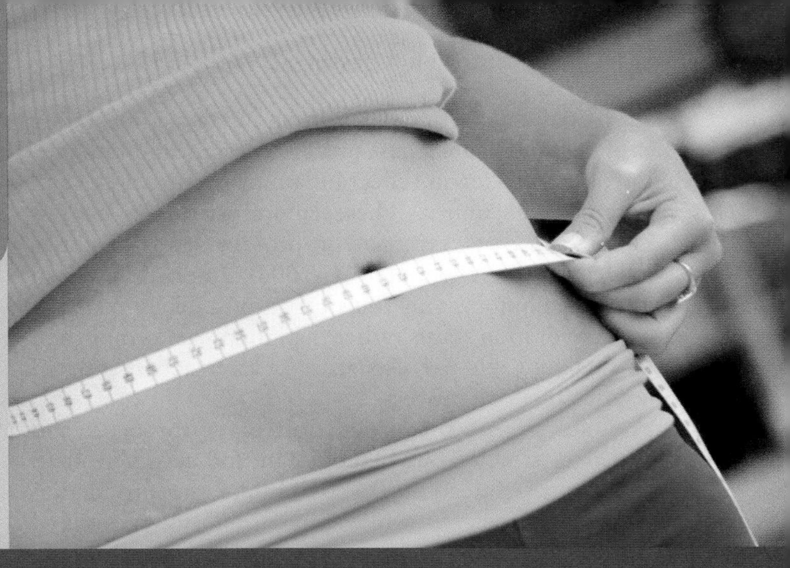

CHAPTER 6

Kathleen A. Hammond, MS, RN, BSN, BSHE, RD, LD
Mary Demarest Litchford, PhD, RD, LDN

Clinical: Inflammation, Physical, and Functional Assessments

KEY TERMS

air displacement plethysmogram (ADP)
anthropometry
bioelectrical impedance analysis (BIA)
body composition
body mass index (BMI)
functional laboratory testing
functional medicine
Functional Nutrition Assessment (FNA)
head circumference
height-for-age curve
length-for-age curve
ideal body weight
inflammation
malabsorption
midarm circumference (MAC)
statiometer
Subjective Global Assessment (SGA)
usual body weight (UBW)
waist circumference
waist-to-hip circumference ratio (WHR)
weight-for-age curve
weight-for-length curve

NUTRITION AND INFLAMMATION

Nutrition assessment would be incomplete if the effects of inflammation on health status were not noted. **Inflammation** is a protective response by the immune system to infection, acute illness, trauma, toxins, many chronic diseases, and physical stress. Acute inflammation reactions are short term because of the involvement of negative feedback mechanisms (Calder et al., 2009). These acute inflammatory mediators have short half-lives and are quickly degraded.

Chronic inflammation begins as a short-term process, but is not extinguished. The body continues to synthesize inflammatory mediators, which alter normal physiological processes and affect innate immunity (Germolec, 2010). Loss of barrier function, responsiveness to a normally benign stimulus, infiltration of large numbers of inflammatory cells, overproduction of oxidants, cytokines, chemokines, eicosanoids, and matrix metalloproteinases all contribute to disease onset and progression (Calder et al., 2009). For example, insulin resistance in the setting of obesity results from a combination of altered functions of insulin target cells and the accumulation of macrophages that secrete proinflammatory mediators, which can promote the metabolic syndrome (Olefsky and Glass, 2010). The chronic inflammatory process also contributes to allergy, asthma, cancer, diabetes, autoimmune disease and some neurodegenerative disorders and infectious diseases.

Inflammatory conditions trigger the immune response to release eicosanoids and cytokines, which mobilize nutrients required to synthesize positive acute-phase proteins and white blood cells. Cytokines (interleukin 1β [IL-1β], tumor necrosis factor alpha [TFN-α], interleukin-6 [IL-6]) and eicosanoids (prostaglandin E2 [PGE2]) influence whole-body metabolism, body composition, and nutritional status. Cytokines reorient hepatic synthesis of plasma proteins and increase the breakdown of muscle protein to meet the demand for protein and energy during the inflammatory response. Moreover, there is a redistribution of albumin to the interstitial compartment, resulting in edema. Declining values of negative acute-phase proteins, serum albumin, prealbumin, and transferrin reflect inflammatory processes and severity of tissue injury. These laboratory values do not reflect current dietary intake or protein status (Dennis, 2008; Devakonda, 2008; Ramel, 2008). Improvements in albumin, prealbumin, and transferrin most likely reflect a change in hydration status rather than increased protein and energy intake. Table 6-1 lists acute phase reactants related to the inflammatory process.

Cytokines impair the production of erythrocytes and reorient iron stores from hemoglobin and serum iron to ferritin. During infection IL-1β inhibits the production and release of transferrin while stimulating the synthesis of ferritin. Therefore laboratory test results used to predict the risk of nutritional anemias are not useful in assessing the patient with an inflammatory response. The effects of cytokines on organ systems are noted in Table 6-2.

TABLE 6-1

Acute Phase Reactants

Positive Acute-Phase Reactants	Negative Acute-Phase Proteins
C-reactive protein	Albumin
a-1 antichymotrypsin	Transferrin
a_1-antitrypsin	Prealbumin (transthyretin)
Haptoglobins	Retinol-binding protein
Ceruloplasmin	
Serum amyloid A	
Fibrinogen	
Ferritin	
Complement and components C3 and C4	
Orosomucoid	

As the body responds to acute inflammation, TFN-α, IL-1β, IL-6, and PGE2 increase to a set threshold, then IL-6 and PGE2 inhibit TFN-α synthesis and IL-1β secretion, creating a negative feedback cycle. Hepatic synthesis of positive acute-phase proteins diminishes and synthesis of negative acute-phase proteins increases. Albumin shifts from interstitial compartment to the extravascular space. Iron stores shift from ferritin to transferrin and hemoglobin (Northrop-Clewes, 2008).

Inappropriate synthesis of inflammatory mediators can be triggered by an injury, reactive oxygen species, or abnormal levels of a body component such as glucose or visceral adipose tissue. Treatment with ω-3 fatty acids is associated with reductions in TNF-α and IL-1β in healthy subjects and reduction in TNF-α in subjects with diabetes (Riediger et al., 2009). Yet overall reduction in inflammatory biomarkers through increased consumption of fruits, vegetables, or nutrient supplements has generated mixed results (Bazzano et al., 2006; Ridker, 2008). More research is needed to identify how various dietary components modulate the predisposition to chronic inflammatory conditions (Calder et al., 2009).

Chronic inflammation is present in Crohn disease, rheumatoid arthritis, cardiovascular disease, diabetes, and obesity (Hye, 2005). Factors that have an important role in disease management decrease inflammatory mediator production through effects on cell signaling and gene expression (ω-3 fatty acids, vitamin E, plant flavonoids), reduce the production of damaging oxidants (vitamin E and other antioxidants), and promote gut barrier function and anti-inflammatory responses (prebiotics and probiotics) (Calder et al., 2009).

Inflammation and Immune Regulation

B cells help to regulate cellular immune responses and inflammation. There are phenotypically diverse B-cell subsets with regulatory functions related to inflammation and autoimmunity (Dililo et al., 2010). Total lymphocyte count (TLC) is an indicator of immune function reflective

TABLE 6-2

Cytokine Actions and Nutritional Consequences

Organ System	Cytokine-Modulated Behavior	Nutritional Consequences
Brain	Sickness syndrome, including fatigue, apathy, cognitive dysfunction, anorexia, sleepiness	↓ food intake weight loss
Endocrine	Euthyroid sick syndrome, anorexia, ↑ in metabolic rate	↓ food intake muscle wasting
Liver	↑ synthesis of positive acute phase proteins, ↓ synthesis of negative acute phase proteins, ↑ fatty acid synthesis, ↑ lipolysis, ↓ LPL	↑ edema hypertriglyceridemia
Muscles	↑ insulin resistance	Hyperglycemia
Blood	↓ product RBC, redistribution of albumin, prealbumin, and iron	anemia ↑ edema
GI Tract	↓ gastric secretion, ↓ GI motility, ↓emptying time, ↑ protein degradation	↓ food intake weight loss ↓ protein reserves

GI, Gastrointestinal; *LPL*, lipoprotein lipase, *RBC*, red blood cell.

Litchford MD: Inflammatory biomarkers and metabolic meltdown, Greensboro, NC, 2009, Case Software and Books.

of B and T cells (see Chapter 27). Skin testing, or delayed cutaneous hypersensitivity (DH) reactivity, measures cell-mediated immunity. DH and TLC are affected by inflammatory metabolism, chemotherapy, and steroids, and thus are most useful in cases of uncomplicated nutrition depletion.

DH involves the intradermal injection of small amounts of antigen (tuberculin, *Candida* organisms, mumps, or trichophytin) just under the skin to determine the person's reaction. A healthy person reacts with induration, indicating that exposure has probably taken place and that immunocompetence is intact. Because electrolyte imbalance, infection, cancer and its treatments, liver disease, renal failure, trauma, and immunosuppression can alter results, DH is not always used for the nutrition assessment of hospitalized patients (Russell and Mueller, 2007). Therapeutic approaches that alter the innate immune system response to inflammatory and microbial insults are exciting areas of study in both nutrition science and medical practice. See Chapter 8 for more details on biochemical assessment.

PHYSICAL AND FUNCTIONAL ASSESSMENTS

Anthropometry

Anthropometry involves obtaining physical measurements of an individual, then relating them to standards that reflect the growth and development of that individual. These physical measurements are another component of the nutrition assessment that are useful for evaluating overnutrition or undernutrition. They can also be used to monitor the effects of nutrition interventions. Individuals conducting these measurements should be trained in the proper technique; if more than one professional is conducting these measurements, measures of accuracy between them should be established. Measurements of accuracy can be established by several clinicians taking the same measurement and comparing results. Anthropometric data are most valuable when they reflect accurate measurements recorded over time. Valuable measurements are height, weight, skinfold thicknesses, and girth measurements. Head circumference and length are used in pediatric populations. Birth weight and ethnic, familial, and environmental factors affect these parameters and should be considered when anthropometric measures are evaluated.

Interpretation of Height and Weight

Currently, reference standards are based on a statistical sample of the U.S. population. Therefore an individual measurement shows how a person's measurement compares with that of the total population. Height and weight measurements of children are evaluated against various norms. They are recorded as percentiles, which reflect the percentage of the total population of children of the same sex who are at or below the same height or weight at a certain age. Children's growth at every age can be monitored by mapping data on growth curves, known as **height-for-age**, **length-for-age**, **weight-for-age**, and **weight-for-length curves**. Appendixes 9 through 16 provide pediatric growth charts and percentile interpretations. Height and weight are also useful for evaluating nutrition status in adults. Both should be measured because the tendency is to overestimate height and underestimate weight, resulting in an underestimation of the relative weight or body mass index (BMI). In addition, many adults are shrinking as a result of osteoporosis, joint deterioration, and poor posture, and this should be noted (Box 6-1).

Length and Height

Height measurements are valuable when used in conjunction with other assessment measurements. Various methods may be used to measure length and height. Measurements of height can be obtained using a direct or an indirect approach. The direct method involves a measuring rod, or **statiometer**, and the person must be able to stand or recline flat. Indirect methods, including knee-height measurements, arm span, or recumbent length using a tape measure, may be options for those who cannot stand or stand straight such as individuals with scoliosis, kyphosis (curvature of the spine), cerebral palsy, muscular dystrophy, contractures, paralysis, or who are bedridden (see Appendix 20). Recumbent height measurements made with a tape measure while the person is in bed may be appropriate for individuals in institutions who are comatose, critically ill, or unable to be moved. However, this method can only be used with patients who do not have musculoskeletal deformities or contractures.

Sitting heights are used for children who cannot stand (see Chapter 45). Recumbent length measurements are used for infants and children younger than 2 or 3 years of age. Ideally these young children should be measured using a length board as shown in Figure 6-1. Recumbent lengths in children ages 2 and younger should be recorded on the birth to 24-month growth grids, whereas standing heights of children ages 2 to 3 years should be recorded on the 2- to 20-year growth grids, as in Appendixes 9 through 16. Recording on the proper growth grids provides a record of a child's gain in height over time and compares the child's height with that of other children of the same age. The rate of length or height gain reflects long-term nutritional adequacy.

BOX 6-1

Using Height and Weight to Assess a Hospitalized Patient's Nutritional Status

- Measure. Do not just ask a person's height.
- Measure weight (at admission, current, and usual).
- Determine percentage of weight change over time (weight pattern).
- Determine percentage above or below usual or ideal body weight.

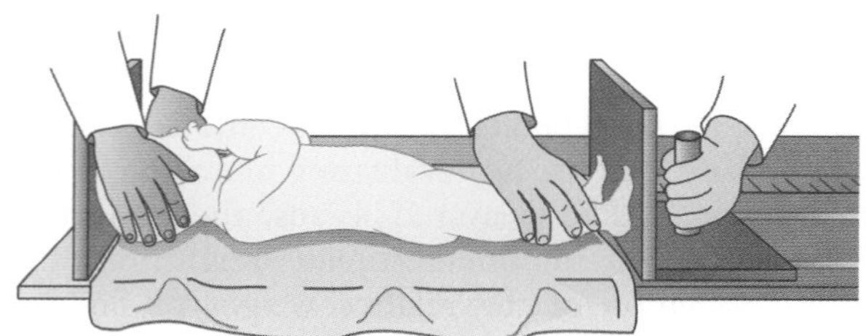

FIGURE 6-1 Measurement of the length of an infant. Crown-to-heel length of children 3 years and younger should be measured as follows: (1) Lay the child on a ruled board that has an attached piece of wood at one end and a movable piece at the other. (2) Stretch the child out on the board for the most accurate measurement. (3) Place the movable end flat against the bottom of the child's foot and read the length from the side of the board.

Weight

Weight is another measure that is important to obtain. In children it is a more sensitive measure of nutritional adequacy than height because it reflects recent nutritional intake. Weight also provides a rough estimate of overall fat and muscle stores. For those who are obese or have edema, weight alone makes it difficult to assess overall nutritional status. Body weight is obtained and interpreted using various methods, including BMI, usual weight, and actual weight. Ideal weight for height reference standards such as the Metropolitan Life Insurance Tables from 1959 and 1983 or the National Health and Nutrition Examination Survey percentiles are no longer used. A commonly used method of determining ideal body weight is the Hamwi Equation (Hamwi, 1964). It does not adjust for age, race, or frame size and its validity is questionable. Nonetheless, it is in widespread use by clinicians as a quick method of estimation:

Men: 106 lbs for first 5 feet of height and 6 lbs per inch over 5 feet; or 6 lbs subtracted for each inch under 5 feet.

Women: 100 lbs for first 5 feet of height and 6 lbs per inch over 5 feet; or 5 lbs subtracted for each inch under 5 feet.

Actual body weight is the weight measurement obtained at the time of examination. This measurement may be influenced by changes in the individual's fluid status. Weight loss can reflect dehydration but can also reflect an immediate inability to meet nutrition requirements; this may indicate nutritional risk. The percentage of weight loss is highly indicative of the extent and severity of an individual's illness. The Blackburn formula (1977) is useful for determining the percentage of recent weight loss:

Significant weight loss: 5% loss in 1 month, 7.5% loss in 3 months, 10% loss in 6 months

Severe weight loss: >5% weight loss in 1 month, >7.5% weight loss in 3 months, >10% weight loss in 6 months

Another method for evaluating the percentage of weight loss is to calculate an individual's current weight as a percentage of usual weight. **Usual body weight (UBW)** is a more useful parameter than **ideal body weight** for those who are ill. Comparing present weight to the UBW allows weight changes to be assessed. However, one problem with using UBW is that it may depend on the patient's memory.

Body Mass Index

Another method to determine whether an adult's weight is appropriate for height is the Quetelet index (W/H^2) or the **body mass index (BMI)** (Lee and Nieman, 2003). The BMI calculation requires weight and height measurements and can indicate overnutrition or undernutrition. BMI accounts for differences in body composition by defining the level of adiposity and relating it to height, thus eliminating dependence on frame size (Stensland and Margolis, 1990). The BMI has the least correlation with body height and the highest correlation with independent measures of body fat for adults. The BMI does not measure body fat directly, but correlates with the direct body fat measures such as underwater weighing and dual x-ray absorptiometry (Keys et al., 1972; Mei et al., 2002). BMI is calculated as follows:

$$\text{Metric: BMI} = \text{Weight (kg)} \div \text{Height (m)}^2$$

$$\text{English: BMI} = \text{Weight (lb)} \div \text{Height [in]}^2 \times 703$$

Nomograms are also available to calculate BMI, as are various charts (see Appendix 23). *Clinical Insight:* Calculating BMI and Determining Appropriate Body Weight gives an example of the BMI calculation for a woman.

Standards classify a BMI for an adult at less than 18.5 as underweight, a BMI between 25 and 29 as overweight, and a BMI greater than 30 as obese. A healthy BMI for adults is considered between 18.5 and 24.9 (CDC, 2009). Although a strong correlation exists between total body fat and BMI, individual variations need to be recognized before making conclusions (Russell and Mueller, 2007).

Differences in race, sex, and age must be considered when evaluating the BMI (Yajnik and Yudkin, 2004). BMI values tend to increase with age (Vaccarino and Krumholz, 2001). Although studies report an association between really high and low BMIs and mortality, the data suggest that a higher BMI range is protective in older adults (see Chapter 21). The standards for ideal weight (BMI of 18.5 to 25) may be too restrictive in the elderly. Therefore careful interpretation of risk factors must be part of the total assessment.

The method of calculation of BMI in children and teens is the same as that for adults, but the interpretation is different. Appendixes 11 and 15 allow for the plotting of the BMI on a growth grid used with children ages 2 to 20 years. Appendixes 12 and 16 provide sample grids for recording BMI measurements and changes for children and

CLINICAL INSIGHT

Calculating BMI and Determining Appropriate Body Weight

Example: Woman who is 5′8″ (68 in) tall and weighs 185 pounds (lb)

Step 1: Calculate current BMI:

Formula: (Metric)	Weight (kg) 84 kg ÷ Height (m^2) (1.72 m) × (1.72 m) = 84 ÷ 2.96 m^2 = BMI = 28.4 = overweight

Step 2: Appropriate weight range to have a BMI that falls between 18.5 and 24.9

18.5	(18.5) × (2.96) = 54.8 kg = 121 pounds
24.9	(24.9) × (2.96) = 73.8 kg = 162 pounds

Appropriate weight range = 121 – 162 lb or 54.8 – 73.8 kg

Formula (English) Weight (lb) ÷ (Height [in] × Height [in]) × 703 = BMI

BMI, Body mass index.

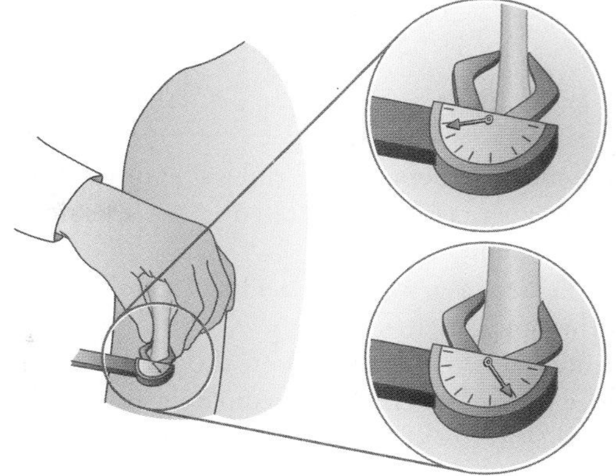

FIGURE 6-2 Skinfold calipers measuring the thickness of subcutaneous fat (in millimeters), giving a rough measurement of adiposity. Measurements are read counterclockwise. *(Courtesy Dorice Czajka-Narins, PhD.)*

adolescents over time. For example, a BMI of only 17 is very appropriate for a 10-year-old girl (see Appendix 19), but would be a concern in an older adult.

Body Composition

Body composition is used along with other assessment factors to provide an accurate description of one's overall health. Differences in skeletal size and the proportion of lean body mass can contribute to body weight variations among individuals of similar height. For example, muscular athletes may be classified as overweight because their excess muscle mass, not their adipose mass, increases their weight. Older adults tend to have lower bone density and reduced lean body mass and therefore may weigh less than younger adults of the same height. Variation in body composition exists among different population groups as well as within the same group (Deurenberg and Deurenberg-Yap, 2003). The majority of body composition studies that were performed on whites may not be valid for other ethnic groups. There are differences and similarities between blacks and whites relative to fat-free body mass, fat patterning, and body dimensions and proportions; blacks have greater bone mineral density and body protein as compared with whites (Wagner and Heyward, 2000). In addition, BMIs for Asian populations need to be in the lower ranges for optimal health to reflect their higher cardiovascular risks (Zheng et al., 2009). These factors must be considered to avoid inaccurate estimation of body fat and interpretation of risk.

Indirect methods for measuring body composition include triceps skin fold, midarm muscle circumference, and midarm circumference (MAC) (Russell and Mueller, 2007). The health professional must realize that these measures are useful in the assessment of individuals over time but not in critical- and acute-care settings; changes in body fluid and composition may skew the results. When conducting body composition measurements, strict adherence to established protocols must be followed to yield accurate results. For example, most North American investigators use the right side of the body to take skinfold measurements, and the standards are based on this. The methods used to gather meaningful data should be considered carefully.

Subcutaneous Fat in Skinfold Thickness

The fat-fold or skinfold thickness measurement is a means of assessing the amount of body fat in an individual. It is practical in clinical settings, although its validity depends on the accuracy of the measuring technique (see Box 6-2) and repetition of measurements over time. If changes are going to occur, they take 3 to 4 weeks to develop. Skinfold measurement assumes that 50% of body fat is subcutaneous (Figure 6-2).

Accuracy decreases with increasing obesity. The skinfold sites identified as most reflective of body fatness are over the triceps and the biceps, below the scapula, above the iliac crest (suprailiac), and on the upper thigh. The triceps skinfold (TSF) and subscapular measurements are the most useful because the most complete standards and methods of evaluation are available for these sites (Figures 6-3 and 6-4; see Appendixes 24-26). Figure 6-5 shows the measurement of the suprailiac crest skinfold.

Circumference Measurements

If more complete information on actual body composition is needed, additional measurements can be obtained. For

BOX 6-2

Skinfold Measurement Techniques

1. Take measurement on the right side of the body.
2. Mark the site to be measured and use a flexible, nonstretchable tape.
3. The tape measure can be used to locate the midpoints on the body.
4. Firmly grasp the skinfold with the thumb and index finger of the left hand approximately 1 cm or ½ inch proximal to the skinfold site, pulling it away from the body.
5. Hold the caliper in the right hand, perpendicular to the long axis of the skin fold and with the caliper's dial face up. Place the caliper tip on the site and approximately 1 cm or ½ inch distal to the fingers holding the skinfold. (Pressure from the fingers does not affect the measurement.)
6. Do not place the caliper too deeply into the skinfold or too close to the tip of the skinfold.
7. Read the caliper approximately 4 seconds after pressure from the measurer's hand has been released from the lever. Exerting force longer than 4 seconds results in smaller readings because fluids are forced from the compressed tissue. Measurements should be recorded to the nearest 1 mm.
8. Take a minimum of two measurements at each site to verify results. Wait 15 seconds between measurements to allow the skinfold site to return to normal. Maintain pressure with thumb and index finger during measurements.
9. Do not take measurements immediately after the person has exercised or if the person is overheated because the shift in body fluid makes the result larger.
10. When measuring obese clients, it may be necessary to use both hands to pull the skin away while a second person makes the measurement. If the calipers do not fit, another technique may be required.

Data from Lee RD, Nieman DC: Nutritional assessment, ed 3, New York, 2003, McGraw-Hill.

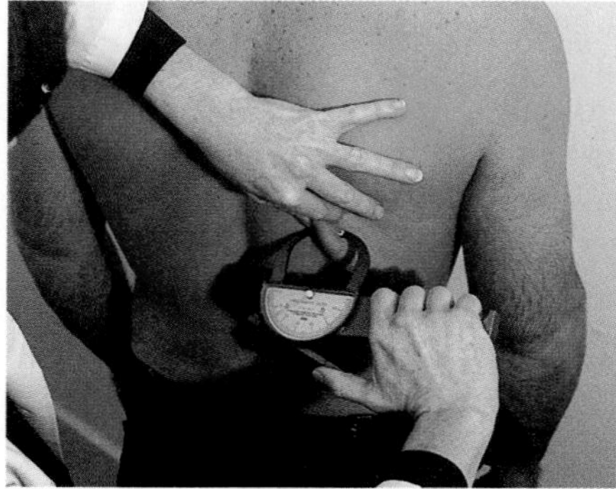

FIGURE 6-3 Measurement of the subscapular skinfold thickness.

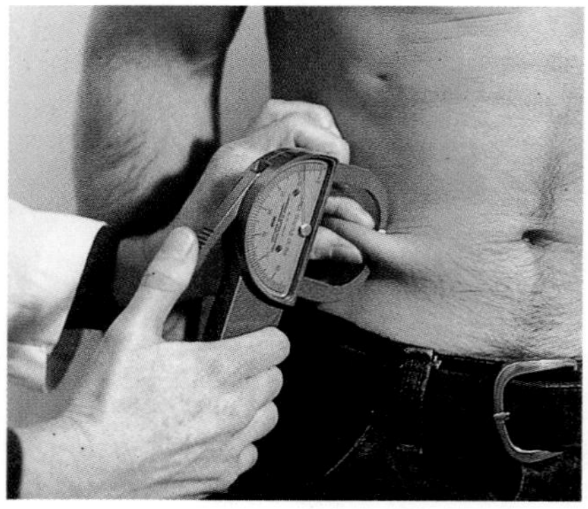

FIGURE 6-5 Measurement of the suprailiac crest skinfold (in mm) above the bony prominence of the iliac crest and across from the navel.

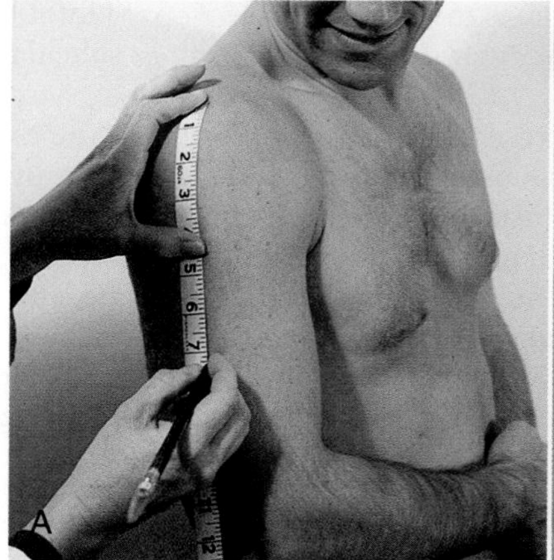

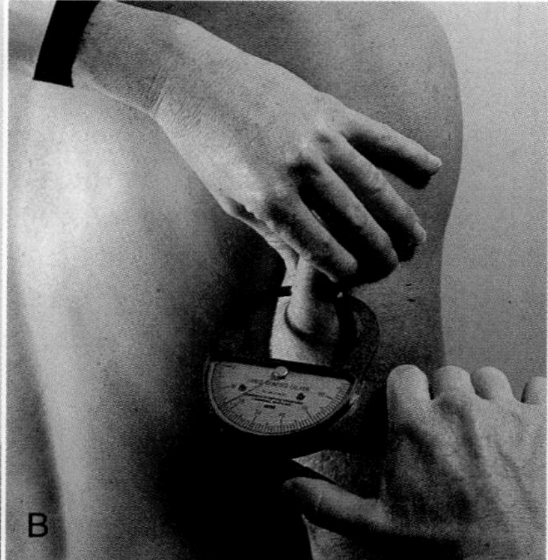

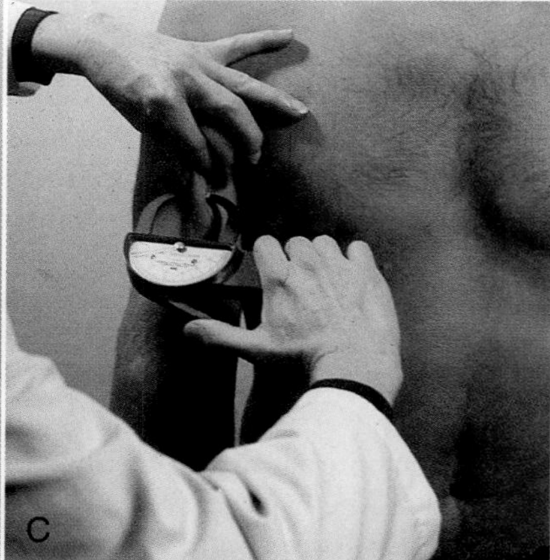

FIGURE 6-4 A, Measurement and marking of the midpoint between the acromion process at the shoulder and the olecranon process at the elbow. **B,** Measurement of the triceps skinfold (in mm) at the marked midpoint, and **C,** measurement of the biceps skinfold (in mm) at the marked midpoint.

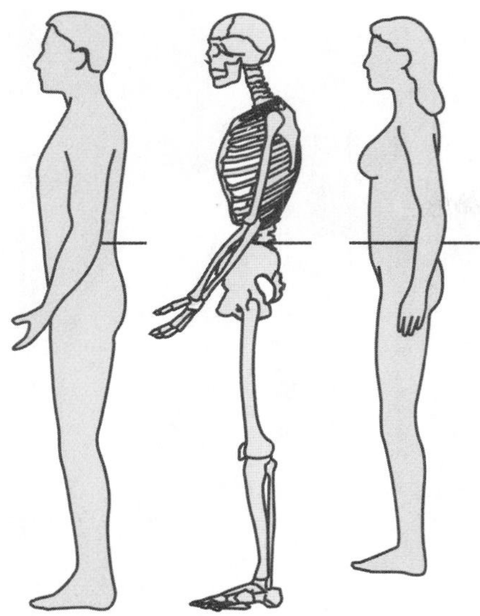

FIGURE 6-6 Measuring tape position for waist (abdominal) circumference measurement. *(From www.nhlbi.nih.gov/guidelines/obesity/e_txtbk/txgd/4142.htm.)*

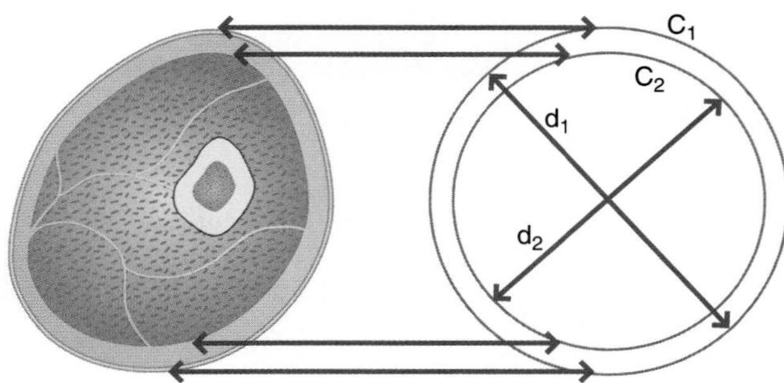

$$AA\ (mm^2) = \pi/4 \times d_1^2 \text{ where } d_1 = C_1/\pi$$
$$AMA\ (mm^2) = (C_1 - \pi T)^2/4\pi = (C_1 = \pi T)^2/12.56$$
$$AFA\ (mm^2) = AA - AMA$$
Bone-free AMA = AMA − 10 for males
Bone-free AMA = AMA − 6.5 for females

FIGURE 6-7 Upper arm area (AA), upper arm muscle area (AMA), and upper arm fat area (AFA) are derived from measurements of upper arm circumference in centimeters (C1) and triceps skinfold (T) in millimeters.

example, in the acute-care setting where the patient experiences more acute pathophysiologic changes such as daily fluid shifts, measures of arm circumference and TSF measurements are not usually performed. But in the long-term care setting, sports clinic, or home environment, these measurements can be tracked over time (e.g., monthly or quarterly) to provide valuable information on overall nutrition status.

Because fat distribution is an indicator of risk, circumferential or girth measurements may be used. The presence of excess body fat around the abdomen out of proportion to total body fat is a risk factor for chronic diseases associated with obesity and the metabolic syndrome. **Waist-to-hip circumference ratio (WHR)** is used to detect possible signs of excess fat deposition (lipodystrophy) in those infected with HIV. It also detects cardiovascular risk somewhat better than BMI (Elsayed et al., 2008). A ratio of 0.8 or above indicates risk in a woman, and 1 or more indicates risk in a man.

Waist circumference is obtained by measuring the distance around the smallest area below the rib cage and above the umbilicus with the use of a nonstretchable tape measure. A measurement of greater than 40 inches (102 cm) for men and greater than 35 inches (88 cm) for women is an independent risk factor for disease (CDC, 2009). These measurements may not be as useful for those less than 60 inches tall or with a BMI of 35 or above (CDC, 2009). Figure 6-6 shows the proper location to measure waist (abdominal) circumference.

Midarm circumference (MAC) is measured in centimeters halfway between the acromion process of the scapula and the olecranon process at the tip of the elbow (see Figure 6-4, *A*). Combining MAC with TSF measurements allows indirect determination of the arm muscle area (AMA) and arm fat area (see Appendixes 25 and 26). Bone-free AMA is calculated by using the formula shown in Figure 6-7. For men, a factor of 10 is subtracted from the AMA, whereas for women a factor of 6.5 is subtracted (Frisancho, 1984). The bone-free muscle area (AMA) is a good indication of lean body mass and skeletal protein reserves. The AMA is important in growing children and in evaluating possible protein-energy malnutrition as a result of chronic illness, stress, eating disorders, multiple surgeries, or an inadequate diet.

Head circumference measurements are useful in children younger than 3 years of age, primarily as an indicator of nonnutritional abnormalities. Undernutrition must be very severe to affect head circumference; see Box 6-3, Measuring Head Circumference.

Other Methods of Measuring Body Composition

Air Displacement Plethysmogram. **Air displacement plethysmogram (ADP)** relies on measurements of body density to estimate body fat and fat-free masses. Performing an ADP with the BOD-POD device is a densitometry technique found to be an accurate method to measure body composition. ADP appears to be a reliable instrument in body composition assessment; it is of particular interest in the pediatric and obese individual. ADP does not rely on body water content to determine body density and body composition, which makes it potentially useful in those adults with end-stage renal disease (Flakoll et al., 2004). However, further research is needed in understanding possible sources of measurement error (Fields et al., 2005). The use of a BOD-POD is usually based on budget, the patient population, and the experience of the clinician (Figure 6-8).

Bioelectrical Impedance Analysis. **Bioelectrical impedance analysis (BIA)** is a body composition analysis technique based on the principle that, relative to water, lean

BOX 6-3

Measuring Head Circumference

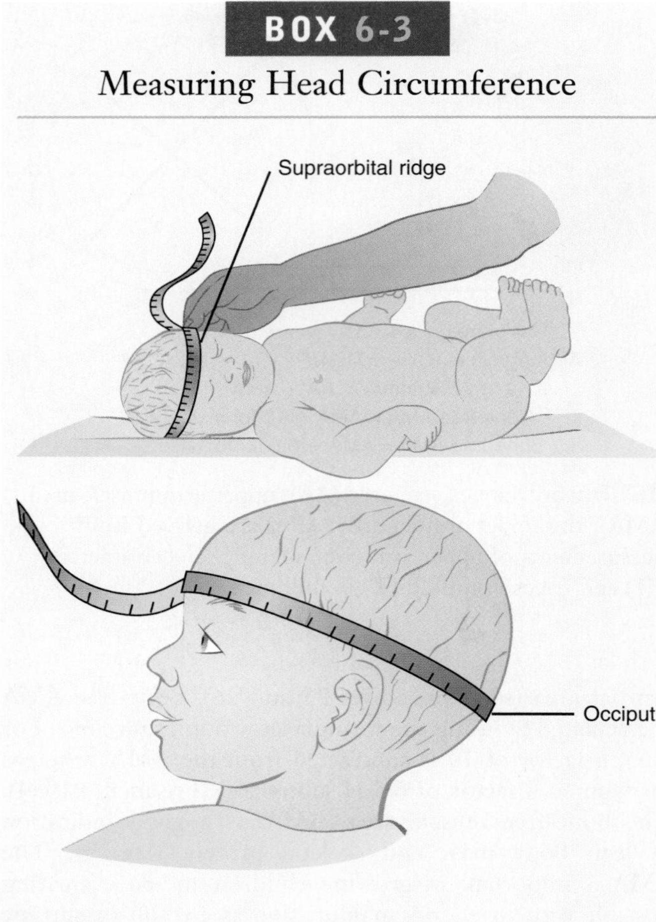

Indications

Head circumference is a standard measurement for serial assessment of growth in children from birth to 36 months and in any child whose head size is in question.

Equipment

Paper or metal tape measure (cloth can stretch) marked in tenths of a centimeter because growth charts are listed in 0.5-cm increments

Technique

1. The head is measured at its greatest circumference.
2. The greatest circumference is usually above the eyebrows and pinna of the ears and around the occipital prominence at the back of the skull.
3. More than one measurement may be necessary because the shape of the head can affect the location of the maximum circumference.
4. Compare the measurement with the National Center for Health Statistics standard curves for head circumference (see Appendixes 10 and 14).

Data from Hockenberry MJ, Wilson D: Wong's nursing care of infants and children, ed 8, St Louis, 2007, Mosby.

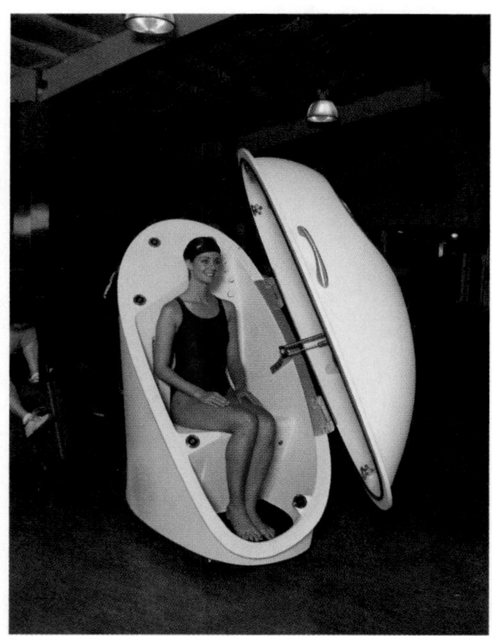

FIGURE 6-8 The BOD-POD measures body fat and fat-free mass. *(Courtesy COSMED USA, Inc., Concord, CA.)*

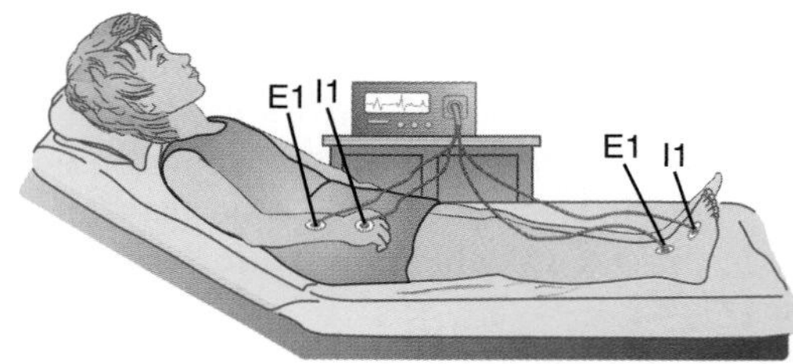

FIGURE 6-9 Bioelectrical impedance analysis.

tissue has a higher electrical conductivity and lower impedance than fatty tissue because of its electrolyte content. BIA has been found to be a reliable measurement of body composition (fat-free mass and fat mass) when compared with BMI or skinfold measurements or even height and weight measurements. BIA involves attaching electrodes to the right hand, wrist, ankle, and foot of a patient and passing a small electrical current through the body (Figure 6-9). The BIA method is popular because it is safe, noninvasive, portable, and rapid. For accurate results the patient should be well hydrated; have not exercised in the previous 4 to 6 hours; and have not consumed alcohol, caffeine, or diuretics in the previous 24 hours. If the person is dehydrated, a higher percentage of body fat than really exists is measured. Fever, electrolyte imbalance, and extreme obesity may also affect the reliability of measurements.

Dual-Energy X-Ray Absorptiometry. Dual-energy x-ray absorptiometry (DEXA) assesses bone mineral density and can be used for measuring fat and boneless lean tissue. The energy source in DEXA is an x-ray tube that contains an energy beam. The amount of energy loss depends on

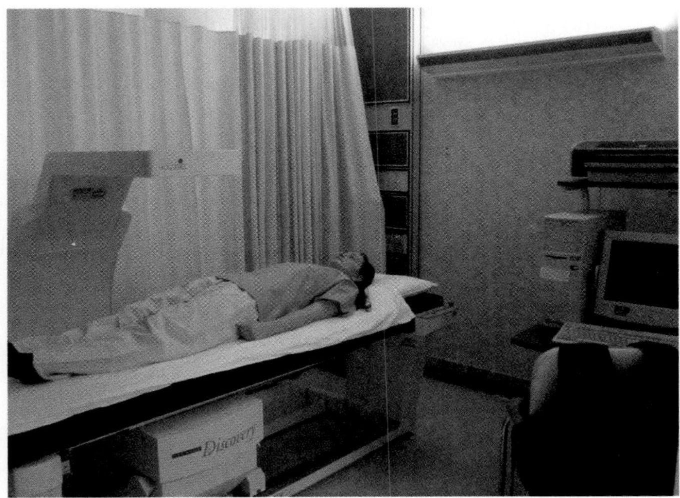

FIGURE 6-10 A patient undergoing a dual-energy x-ray absorptiometry scan. *(Courtesy of the Division of Nutrition, University of Utah.)*

the type of tissue through which the beam passes; the result can be used to measure mineral, fat, and lean tissue compartments (Russell and Mueller, 2007). DEXA is easy to use, emits low levels of radiation, and is relatively available in the hospital setting, making it a useful tool. However, the patient must remain still for more than a few minutes, which may be difficult for older adults and those in chronic pain. Differences in hydration status and the presence of bone or calcified soft tissue can result in inaccurate measurements (Lee and Nieman, 2003). Figure 6-10 illustrates a DEXA scan.

Neutron Activation Analysis. Neutron activation analysis allows measurement of lean body mass. This analysis also distinguishes between intracellular and extracellular components of the body by creating unstable isotopes of calcium, nitrogen, and sodium, and then measuring gamma radiation from the same isotopes (Russell and Mueller, 2007). This type of measurement is expensive and impractical in a daily clinical setting.

Total Body Potassium. Total body potassium can be used to study body composition because more than 90% of the body's potassium is found in fat-free tissues. Measurements are made with a special counter that is fitted with multiple gamma-ray detectors interfaced with a computer that is expensive and not always readily available. Not all researchers agree on the exact concentration of potassium in fat-free tissue and the differences between sexes, during the aging process, and in obese individuals.

Underwater Weighing. Underwater weighing is a direct measure of determining whole-body density. Densitometry includes underwater (hydrostatic) weighing based on Archimedes' principle: the volume of an object submerged in water equals the volume of water the object displaces. Once the volume and mass are known, the density can be calculated. Although this method is considered the gold standard it is not always practical, involves significant training to perform, and requires considerable cooperation on the part of those being measured. Subjects must be submerged under water and remain motionless long enough for the measurements to be made (Lee and Nieman, 2003).

Ultrasound and Magnetic Resonance Imaging. Magnetic resonance imaging (MRI) can be used to measure the size of visceral organs, the size of the skeleton, and the amount and distribution of intraabdominal fat. MRI has several advantages, two of which are that it is noninvasive and involves no ionizing radiation, which makes it safe for children, females of childbearing age, and multiple studies on the same individual. The disadvantages of MRI include expense and limited availability (Russell and Mueller, 2007).

THE NUTRITION-FOCUSED PHYSICAL EXAMINATION

The nutrition-focused physical examination is an important component of overall assessment because some nutritional deficiencies may not be identified by other approaches. Some signs of nutritional deficiency are not specific and must be distinguished from those with nonnutritional causal factors.

Approach

A systems approach is used when performing the examination, which should be conducted in an organized, logical way that progresses from head to toe to ensure efficiency and thoroughness. The examination moves from a global to a more defined or focused examination based on the results of the medical and nutrition histories. The nutrition-focused physical examination is tailored for each patient. In short, every body system may not have to be assessed; clinical judgment guides this decision according to the problems, history, and current complaints of the individual (Hammond, 2006).

Equipment

The extent of the nutrition-focused physical examination dictates the necessary equipment. Any or all of the following may be used: a stethoscope, a penlight or flashlight, a tongue depressor, scales, a reflex hammer, calipers, a tape measure, a blood pressure cuff, and an ophthalmoscope.

Examination Techniques and Findings

Four basic physical examination techniques are used during the nutrition-focused physical examination. These techniques include inspection, palpation, percussion, and auscultation (Table 6-3). Appendix 29 discusses the nutrition-focused physical examination in more detail.

Some nutritional findings from the physical examination that should alert the clinician to the need for further assessment and intervention include temporal wasting, proximal muscle weakness, depleted muscle bulk, dehydration, overhydration, poor wound healing, and chewing or swallowing difficulties. The appearance of the skin should be evaluated for any pallor, scaly dermatitis, wounds, quality of wound healing, bruising, and hydration status.

Membranes such as in the conjunctiva or pharynx should be examined for integrity, hydration, pallor, and bleeding. Special attention should be given to the areas where signs of nutritional deficiencies appear most often, such as the skin, hair, teeth, gums, lips, tongue, and eyes. The hair, skin, and mouth are susceptible because of the rapid cell turnover of epithelial tissue. Symptoms of nutrient deficiencies may or may not be apparent during the physical examination, or may result from a lack of several nutrients or from nonnutritional causes.

TABLE 6-3

Physical Examination Techniques

Technique	Description
Inspection	General observation that progresses to a more focused observation using the senses of sight, smell, and hearing; most frequently used technique
Palpation	Tactile examination to feel pulsations and vibrations; assessment of body structures, including texture, size, temperature, tenderness, and mobility
Percussion	Assessment of sounds to determine body organ borders, shape, and position; not always used in a nutrition-focused physical examination
Auscultation	Use of the naked ear or a stethoscope to listen to body sounds (e.g., heart and lung sounds, bowel sounds, blood vessels)

From Hammond K: Nutrition focused physical assessment, Support Line 18(4):4, 1996.

Other Assessment Measures and Tools

Biochemical Analysis

Biochemical tests are the most objective and sensitive measures of nutrition status. Not all of them are purely related to nutrition. Caution must be used when interpreting results because they can be affected by disease state and therapies; see Chapter 8.

FUNCTIONAL NUTRITION ASSESSMENT

Functional medicine is an evolving, evidence-based discipline that treats the body with its mutually interactive systems as a whole, rather than as a set of isolated signs and symptoms. The Institute of Functional Medicine (IFM) promotes an evaluation process that recognizes the biochemical, genetic, and environmental individuality of each person. The focus is patient-centered, not just disease-centered. Lifestyle and health-promoting factors include nutrition, exercise, adequate sleep, healthy relationships, and a positive mind-body-belief system. Assessment in the functional medicine mode identifies the following factors: pattern recognition, under- and overnutrition, reduction of toxin exposures, and antecedents or events in a person's history that may act as triggers for a response beginning a disease process. IFM has established an interdisciplinary Functional Medicine Matrix Model to guide this holistic assessment process (Figure 6-11).

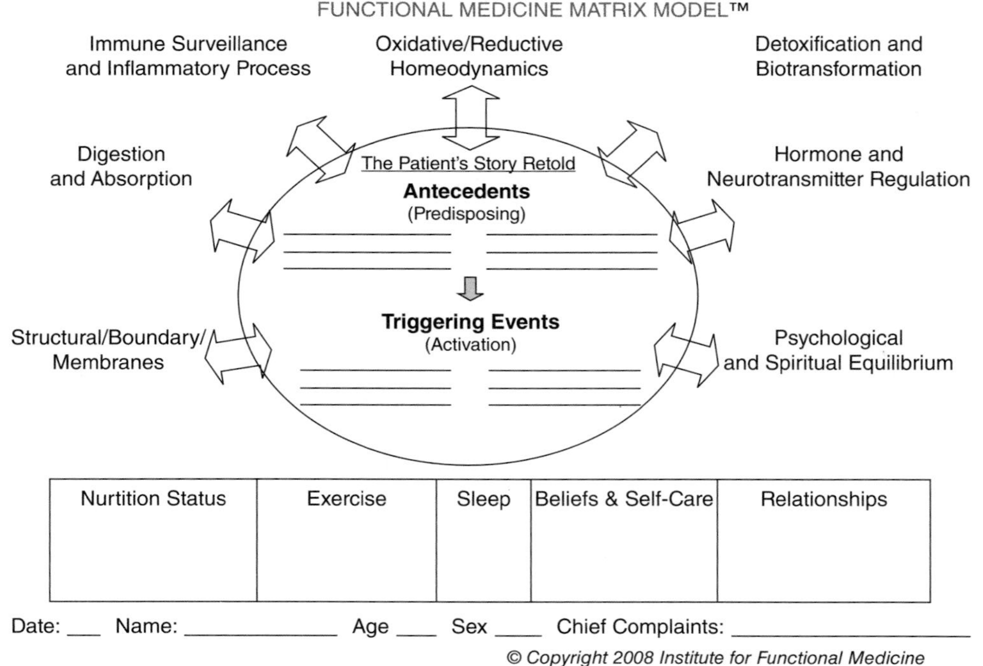

FIGURE 6-11 The Functional Medicine Matrix for assessment. *(Courtesy Institute of Functional Medicine, 2010.)*

For dietitians, the **Functional Nutrition Assessment (FNA)** expands traditional assessment by adding cellular, molecular, and genomic data to the process. This expanded determination of nutrition status quantifies the tissue nutrient reserves, cellular function, and genetic potential influenced by the interaction of diet, environment and lifestyle. See *New Directions:* Functional Nutrition Assessment.

Gastrointestinal Function

Assessment of the capacity for digestion, absorption, and transport as well as the hormonal status provides critical background information as to why a patient may be malnourished. **Malabsorption** syndrome, in which several nutrients are abnormally absorbed, is the most dramatic. Constipation, diarrhea, excessive vomiting, or flatulence also warrant further analysis. Mucosal changes in the gastrointestinal (GI) tract are indicated by problems such as diarrhea and anorexia. Tests may be done on a stool sample and can reveal excessive amounts of fat, an indication of malabsorption, the status of the GI flora and the amounts and types of bacteria present in the gut. The acidity of the stomach, important for maintaining an optimal milieu for digestion and absorption, can be assessed using manual intragastric titration, which gives an indication of gastric hydrochloric acid secretion.

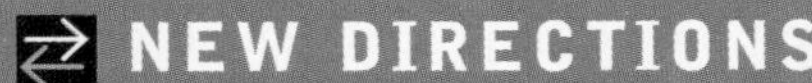

Functional Nutrition Assessment

by Diana M. Noland, MPH, RD, CCN

The expense of dealing with the global epidemic of chronic disease is forcing national health care systems to refocus on early diagnosis and treatment of these conditions. It is becoming critical for practitioners to understand the prominent role played by diet and lifestyle factors, as well as the interaction between genes and environmental factors. Following the recent recognition of the role of long-latency nutritional insufficiencies, there is also a growing appreciation for the understanding of the molecular mechanisms that underlie chronic disease. These considerations are an important part of the Functional Nutrition Assessment (FNA) approach.

This assessment technique is uniquely suited to the identification of the root causes of chronic disease by integrating traditional dietetic practice with nutritional genomics, the restoration of gastrointestinal function, the quelling of chronic inflammation, and the interpretation of nutritional biomarkers of cellular and molecular dysfunction. The Functional Nutrition Practitioner organizes the data collected from ingestion, digestion and utilization (IDU) factors, leading to identification of the root causes for each individual. Some factors related to chronic disease risk that are examined in the FNA include:

Ingestion

Food, fiber, water, supplements, medication
Intake patterns affected by emotional or disordered eating
Toxins entering the body via food, skin, inhalants, water, environment (including pesticides and chemicals)

Digestion

Adequate microflora
Allergies
Genetic enzyme deficits
Hydration
Infection
Lifestyle—sleep, exercise, stressors

Utilization—Cellular and Molecular Functional Relationships

Antioxidants—water-soluble vitamin C, phytonutrients
Methylation and acetylation—dependence on adequate B complex and minerals
Oils and fatty acids—prostaglandin balance, cell membrane function, vitamin E function
Protein metabolism—connective tissue, enzymes, immune function, etc.
Vitamin D—in concert with functional metabolic partner nutrients vitamins A and K

The ability to assess a person's nutrition status has benefited from recent, rapid advances in the science of nutrition, genomics and measurement technologies. A more thorough evaluation of cellular function is possible today. The identification of the human genome and the understanding of epigenetic effects of environment on gene expression have been especially informative. Nutrition assessment has been facilitated by additions to the nutritionist's tool kit, including bioelectric impedance analysis, **functional laboratory testing**, and a more comprehensive health history with triggering events and genetic predisposition.

Thus the FNA method is rapidly gaining acceptance for guidance in the relief of many chronic diseases and conditions with nutritional implications (Jones et al., 2009). By using an IDU approach, dietitians can develop more personalized intervention plans, support the body's natural mechanisms, and restore balance and health (Noland, 2010). In the future, the clinical encounter will require a collaborative, healing partnership. Phytonutrients, personalized dietary advice, exercise and energy requirements, meditation, and yoga may all one day be part of that therapeutic dialogue.

Handgrip Dynamometry

Handgrip dynamometry can provide a baseline nutritional assessment of muscle function by measuring grip strength and endurance, and is useful in serial measurements. Measurements of handgrip dynamometry are expressed as a percentage of a standard. The assumption is that strong hands reflect strength elsewhere. Decreased grip strength is an important sign of frailty, especially in older adults. The Groningen Fitness Test for the Elderly was developed by Koen and colleagues (2001) for a longitudinal study in the Netherlands of age-related fitness and it continues to be useful. Low grip strength is consistently associated with a greater likelihood of premature mortality, the development of disability, and an increased risk of complications or prolonged length of stay after hospitalization or surgery in middle-aged and older adults (Bohannon, 2008).

Hydration

It is important to recognize the fluid volume status of an individual during the nutrition-focused physical examination. Fluid disturbances can be associated with other imbalances such as electrolyte imbalance.

Dehydration

Note excessive loss of water and electrolytes from vomiting, diarrhea, excessive laxative abuse, fistulas, GI suction, polyuria, fever, excessive sweating, edema (third-space fluid shifts), or decreased intake caused by anorexia, nausea, depression, or inadequate access to fluids. Characteristics include weight loss that occurs over a short period, decreased skin and tongue turgor, dry mucous membranes, postural hypotension, a weak and rapid pulse, slow-filling peripheral veins, a decrease in body temperature (95°-98° F), decreased urine output, elevated hematocrit , cold extremities, disorientation, or a blood urea nitrogen (BUN) level elevated out of proportion to serum creatinine.

Overhydration

Note any history of renal failure, congestive heart failure, cirrhosis of the liver, or Cushing syndrome, excess use of sodium-containing intravenous fluids, and excessive intake of sodium-containing food or medication products. Characteristics of fluid volume excess include weight gain that occurs over a short period, peripheral edema, distended neck veins, slow emptying of peripheral veins, rales in the lungs, polyuria, ascites, pleural effusion, a bounding and full pulse, decreased BUN, and low hematocrit. Pulmonary edema may occur in severe cases.

Physical Activity Assessment

Because diet and physical activity are lifestyle and behavioral factors that play a role in the cause and prevention of chronic diseases, inclusion of a physical activity assessment is part of a full nutrition assessment. Many instruments used to measure activity are difficult to use, and are prone to reporting errors. However, dietetic professionals can ask a few questions to gain insight into the activity levels of their clients. Box 6-4 provides a series of questions that can be

BOX 6-4

Physical Activity Assessment Questionnaire

To be considered physically active, **you must get at least:**

- ☐ 30 minutes of moderate physical activity on 5 or more days a week, **OR**
- ☐ 20 minutes of vigorous physical activity on 3 or more days a week

How physically active do you plan to be over the next 6 months? *(Choose the best answer.)*

- ____ I am not currently active and do not plan to become physically active in the next 6 months.
- ____ I am thinking about becoming more physically active.
- ____ I intend to become more physically active in the next 6 months.
- ____ I have been trying to get more physical activity.
- ____ I am currently physically active and have been for the last 1-5 months.
- ____ I have been regularly physically active for the past 6 months or more.

Compared to how physically active you have been over the last 3 months, how would you describe the last 7 days: *(Check one)*

______ More active ______ Less active ______ About the same

Recall your participation in activities or in sedentary behaviors, over the past 24 hours:

- Reading, watching TV, or computer time _____ minutes/day
- Fast walking ____ minutes/day
- Physical activity (swimming, tennis, racquetball, similar) ______ minutes/day
- Other physical activity (describe _________________) _______ minutes/day

BOX 6-4

Physical Activity Assessment Questionnaire—cont'd

What are the 3 most important reasons why you would consider increasing your physical activity?
- ☐ Improve my health ☐ Control my weight ☐ Lower my stress
- ☐ Look better ☐ Improve my fitness ☐ Feel better
- ☐ Lower my risk of disease ☐ Other: __________

How confident are you that you could increase your physical activity if you decided to do so? *(Check one)*
- ☐ Very confident ☐ Fairly confident
- ☐ Somewhat confident ☐ Not at all confident

Would you consider using a pedometer to count your steps per day? Yes ____ No ____

Record all of your activity—what you did and amount of time spent, for the next two days and review with counselor.

asked to identify the current levels and interest in future activity levels for ambulatory patients and clients.

Subjective Global Assessment

The **Subjective Global Assessment (SGA)** is a tool based on history, dietary data, GI symptoms, functional capacity, effects of disease on nutritional requirements, and physical appearance. This tool has been validated and more recently has been shown to correlate well with the nutrition risk index and other assessment data in hospitalized patients (DeLegge and Drake, 2007). Documentation of assessment data using the SGA allows other providers to identify the same factors as problematic, and provides a baseline for comparison in that individual over time (Box 6-5).

Once the nutrition assessment process is complete, the extent of nutritional adequacy, deficiency, or excess should be apparent. Severity of malnutrition can then be classified based on body weight, body fat, somatic and visceral protein stores, and laboratory values. When nutrition problems are noted, the appropriate nutrition diagnoses can be selected and the other steps in the nutrition care process may be implemented accordingly (see Chapter 11). Refer to the most current *International Dietetics and Nutrition Terminology Reference Manual* for updates and guidelines (American Dietetic Association, 2009).

CLINICAL SCENARIO

Carl is a 32-year-old man who is 5 ft, 9 in tall. He was diagnosed as having acquired immune deficiency syndrome 1 year ago. In the past year his weight has gradually decreased from a usual weight of 175 lb to the current low of 130 lb. His visceral proteins are depleted, and a triceps skinfold measurement reveals a body fat value that is 55% of standard. Carl's oral intake ability has gradually decreased; he can only take sips of an enteral supplement and occasional bites of food.

Nutrition Diagnostic Statement

Inadequate oral food/beverage intake related to poor appetite and inability to eat as evidenced by loss of 45 lb in 12 months and intake much less than requirements.

Nutrition Care Questions

1. Is Carl exhibiting a degree of undernutrition? If so, how severe is his malnutrition?
2. Carl's current weight is what percentage of his usual body weight?
3. What is Carl's body mass index?
4. Develop a nutrition assessment questionnaire for Carl.

BOX 6-5

The Subjective Global Assessment

Directions: Select appropriate category with a checkmark, or enter numerical values where indicated by #.

A. History

1. Weight change:
   Overall loss in past 6 months: amount = # ________ kg, %loss = #________
   Change in past 2 weeks: ________ increase, ________ no change, ________ decrease.
2. Dietary intake change (relative to normal)
   _____ No change
   _____ Change Duration = # __________ weeks.
   Type: _______ suboptimal solid diet ______ full liquid diet _____ hypocaloric liquids ________ starvation.
3. Gastrointestinal symptoms (that persisted for >2 weeks)
   ________ none, ________ nausea, ________ vomiting, _______ diarrhea, _______ anorexia

Continued

BOX 6-5

The Subjective Global Assessment—cont'd

4. Functional capacity
_________ No dysfunction (e.g., full capacity),
_________ Dysfunction __________ duration = # _________ weeks __________
type: _________ working suboptimally, _________ ambulatory, _________ bedridden.
5. Disease and its relation to nutritional requirements
Primary diagnosis (specify) ____________________
____
Metabolic demand (stress): ______ no stress, ______ low stress, ______ moderate stress, ______ high stress.

B. Physical (for each trait specify: 0 = normal, 1+ = mild, 2+ = moderate, 3+ = severe)

#______________ loss of subcutaneous fat (triceps, chest)
#______________ muscle wasting (quadriceps, deltoids)
#______________ ankle edema
#______________ sacral edema
#______________ ascites
SGA rating (select one): ________ A = Well nourished
______ B = Moderately for suspected of being malnourished
______ C = Severely malnourished

With permission. Detsky AS et al: What is subjective global assessment of nutritional status? JPEN J Parentral Enteral Nutrition 11:55, 1987.

SGA, Subjective Global Assessment.

USEFUL WEBSITES

American Dietetic Association, Evidence Analysis Library
http://www.adaevidencelibrary.com/topic.cfm?cat=1225

Assessment Tools for Weight-Related Health Risks
http://www.columbia.edu/itc/hs/medical/nutrition/dat/dat.html

Body Mass Index Assessment Tool
http://www.nhlbisupport.com/bmi/

Centers for Disease Control and Prevention—Growth Charts
www.cdc.gov/ growthcharts/

Centers for Disease Control and Prevention—Weight Assessment
http://www.cdc.gov/healthyweight/assessing/index.html

Institute of Functional Medicine
http://www.functionalmedicine.org/

REFERENCES

American Dietetic Association: *International dietetics and nutrition terminology reference manual*, Chicago, 2009, American Dietetic Association.

Bazzano LA, et al: Effect of folic acid supplementation on risk of cardiovascular diseases: a meta-analysis of randomized controlled trials, *JAMA* 296:2720, 2006.

Blackburn GL: Nutritional and metabolic assessment of the hospitalized patient, *JPEN J Parenter Enteral Nutr* 1:11, 1977.

Bohannon R: Hand-grip dynamometry predicts future outcomes in aging adults, *J Geriatr Phys Ther* 31:3, 2008.

Buchman AL: *Handbook of nutritional support*, Baltimore, 1997, Williams & Wilkins.

Calder PC, et al: Inflammatory disease processes and interactions with nutrition, *Br J Nutr* 101:S1, 2009.

Centers for Disease Control (CDC) and Prevention: Overweight and obesity, 2009, http://www.cdc.gov/obesity/.

DeLegge M, Drake L: Nutritional assessment, *Gastroenterol Clin North Am* 36:1, 2007.

Dennis RA, et al: Changes in prealbumin, nutrient intake, and systemic inflammation in elderly recuperative care patients, *J Am Geriatric Soc* 56:1270, 2008.

Devakonda A, et al: Transthyretin as a marker to predict outcome in critically ill patients, *Clin Biochem* 41:1126, 2008.

Deurenberg P, Deurenberg-Yap M: Validity of body composition methods across ethnic population groups, *Acta Diabetol* 40:246S, 2003.

Dililo DJ, et al: B10 cells and regulatory B cells balance immune responses during inflammation, autoimmunity, and cancer, *Ann N Y Acad Sci* 1183:38, 2010.

Elsayed EF, et al: Waist-to-hip ratio and body mass index as risk factors for cardiovascular events in CKD, *Am J Kidney Dis* 52:49, 2008.

Fields DA, et al: Air-displacement plethysmography: here to stay, *Curr Opin Clin Nutr Metabol Care* 8:624, 2005.

Flakoll PJ, et al: Bioelectrical impedance vs air displacement plethysmography and dual-energy X-ray absorptiometry to determine body composition in patients with end-stage renal disease, *JPEN J Parenter Enteral Nutr* 28:13, 2004.

Frisancho AR: New standards of weight and body composition by frame size and height for assessment of nutritional status of adults and the elderly, *Am J Clin Nutr* 40:808, 1984.

Germolec DR, et al: Markers of inflammation, *Methods Mol Biol* 598:53, 2010.

Hammond, KA: Physical assessment. In Lysen LK, editor: *Quick reference to clinical dietetics*, ed 2, Boston, 2006, Jones and Bartlett.

Hamwi GJ: *Diabetes mellitus, diagnosis and treatment*, New York, 1964, American Diabetes Association.

Hye SP, et al: Relationship of obesity and visceral adiposity with serum concentrations of CRP, TNF-a and IL-6, *Diabetes Res Clin Pract* 69:29, 2005.

Jones D, et al: *21st century medicine: a new model for medical education and practice*, Gig Harbor, WA, 2009, Institute for Functional Medicine.

Keys A, et al: Indices of relative weight and obesity, *J Chronic Dis* 25:329, 1972.

Koen A, et al: Reliability of the Groningen Fitness Test for the elderly, *J Aging Phys Act* 9:194, 2001.

Lee RD, Nieman DC: *Nutritional assessment*, ed 3, New York, 2003, McGraw-Hill.

Litchford MD: *Inflammatory biomarkers and metabolic meltdown*, Greensboro, NC, 2009, Case Software and Books.

Mei Z, et al: Validity of body mass index compared with other body-composition screening indexes for the assessment of body fatness in children and adolescents, *Am J Clin Nutr* 75:978, 2002.

Noland D: *Functional nutrition therapy: principles of assessment*, Gig Harbor, WA, 2010, Institute for Functional Medicine.

Northrop-Clewes C: Interpreting indicators of iron status during an acute phase response—lessons from malaria and human immunodeficiency virus, *Ann Clin Biochem* 45:18, 2008.

Olefsky JM, Glass CK: Macrophages, inflammation, and insulin resistance, *Annu Rev Physiol* 72:219, 2010.

Ramel A, et al: Anemia, nutritional status and inflammation in hospitalized elderly, *Nutrition* 24:1116, 2008.

Ridker PM, et al. for the JUPITER Study Group: Rosuvastatin to prevent vascular events in men and women with elevated C-reactive protein, *N Engl J Med* 359:2195, 2008.

Riediger N, et al: A systemic review of the roles of ω-3 fatty acids in health and disease, *J Am Diet Assoc* 109:668, 2009.

Russell M, Mueller C: Nutrition screening and assessment. In Gottschlich M, et al., editors: *The science and practice of nutrition support: American Society for Parenteral and Enteral Nutrition*, Dubuque, IA, 2007, Kendall/Hunt.

Stensland SH, Margolis S: Simplifying the calculation of body mass index for quick reference, *J Am Diet Assoc* 90:856, 1990.

Vaccarino HA, Krumholz HM: An evidence-based assessment of federal guidelines for overweight and obesity as they apply to elderly persons, *Arch Intern Med* 161:1194, 2001.

Wagner D, Heyward V. Measures of body composition in blacks and whites: a comparative review, *Am J Clin Nutr* 71:1392, 2000.

Yajnik CS, Yudkin JS: Appropriate body mass index for Asian populations and its implications for policy and intervention strategies, *Lancet* 363:157, 2004.

Zheng Y, et al: Evolving cardiovascular disease prevalence, mortality, risk factors, and the metabolic syndrome in China, *Clin Cardiol* 32:491, 2009.

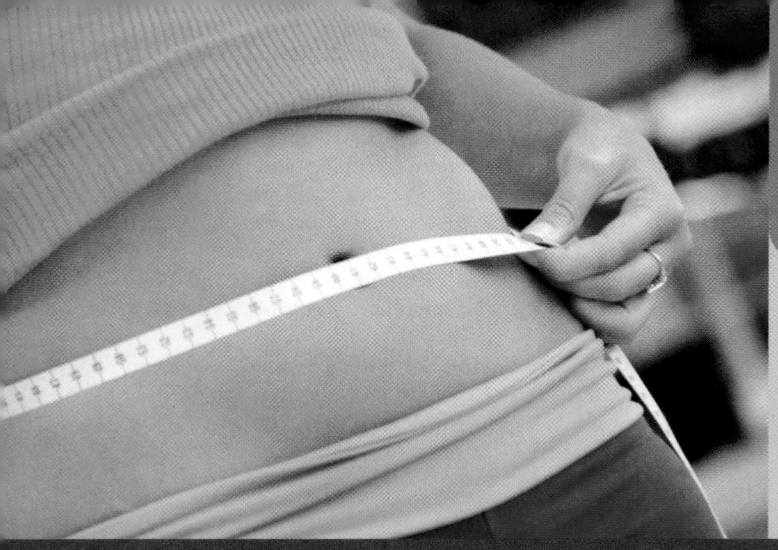

CHAPTER 7

Pamela Charney, PhD, RD

Clinical: Water, Electrolytes, and Acid-Base Balance

KEY TERMS

acid-base balance
acidemia
alkalemia
anion gap
buffer
colloidal osmotic pressure
compensation
contraction alkalosis
corrected calcium
dehydration
edema
electrolytes
extracellular fluid
extracellular water
insensible water loss
interstitial fluid
intracellular fluid
intracellular water (ICW)
metabolic acidosis
metabolic alkalosis
metabolic water
oncotic pressure
osmolality
osmolarity
osmotic pressure
renin-angiotensin system
respiratory acidosis
respiratory alkalosis
sensible water loss
sodium-potassium adenosine triphosphatase (Na/K ATPase) pump
syndrome of inappropriate antidiuretic hormone secretion (SIADH)
"third space" fluid
vasopressin
water intoxication

The volume, composition, and distribution of body fluids have profound effects on cell function. A stable internal environment is maintained through a sophisticated network of homeostatic mechanisms that are focused on ensuring that water intake and water loss are balanced. Protein-energy malnutrition, disease, trauma, and surgery can disrupt fluid, electrolyte, and acid-base balance and alter the composition, distribution, or amount of body fluids. Even small changes in pH, electrolyte concentrations, and fluid status can adversely affect cell function. If these derangements are not corrected, severe consequences or death can ensue (Bartelmo and Terry, 2008.)

BODY WATER

Water is the largest single component of the body. At birth, water accounts for approximately 75% to 85% of total body weight; this proportion decreases with age and adiposity. Water accounts for 60% to 70% of total body weight in the lean adult but only 45% to 55% in the obese adult.

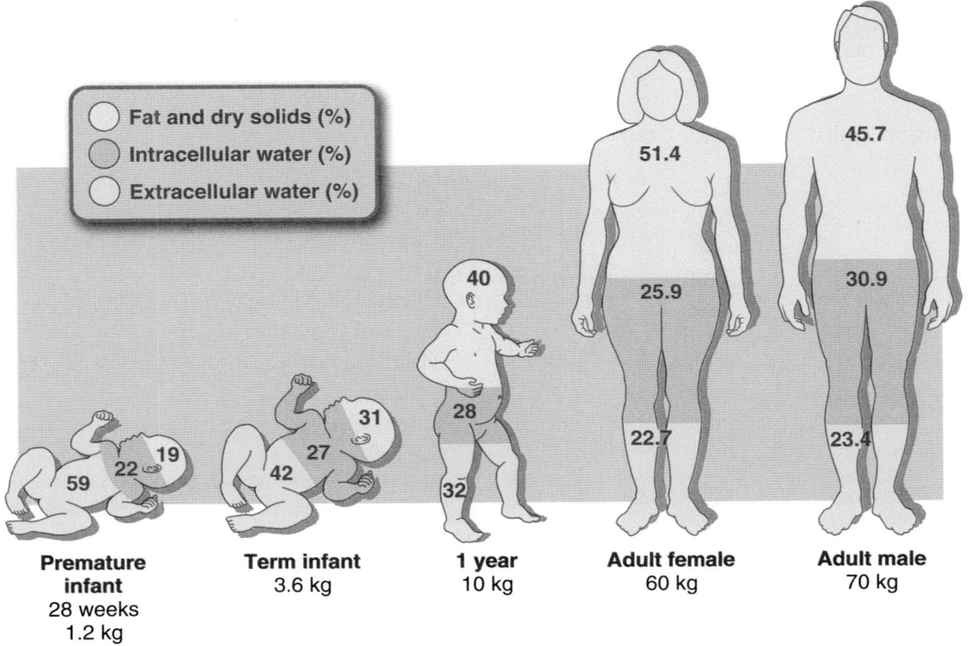

FIGURE 7-1 Distribution of body water as a percentage of body weight.

Metabolically active cells of the muscle and viscera have the highest concentration of water; calcified tissue cells have the lowest. Total body water is higher in athletes than in non-athletes and decreases with age and diminished muscle mass (Figure 7-1). Although the proportion of body weight accounted for by water varies with age and body fat, there is little day-to-day variation in the percentage of body water in the individual.

Functions

Water makes solutes available for cellular reactions. It is a substrate in metabolic reactions and a structural component, providing form to cells. Water is essential for the processes of digestion, absorption, and excretion. It also plays a key role in the structure and function of the circulatory system and acts as a transport medium for nutrients and all body substances.

Water maintains the physical and chemical constancy of intracellular and extracellular fluids and has a direct role in maintaining body temperature. Evaporation of perspiration cools the body during warm weather, preventing or delaying hyperthermia. Loss of 20% of body water (**dehydration**) may cause death; loss of only 10% may lead to damage to essential body systems (Figure 7-2). Healthy adults can live up to 10 days without water, and children can live up to 5 days, whereas one can survive for several weeks without food.

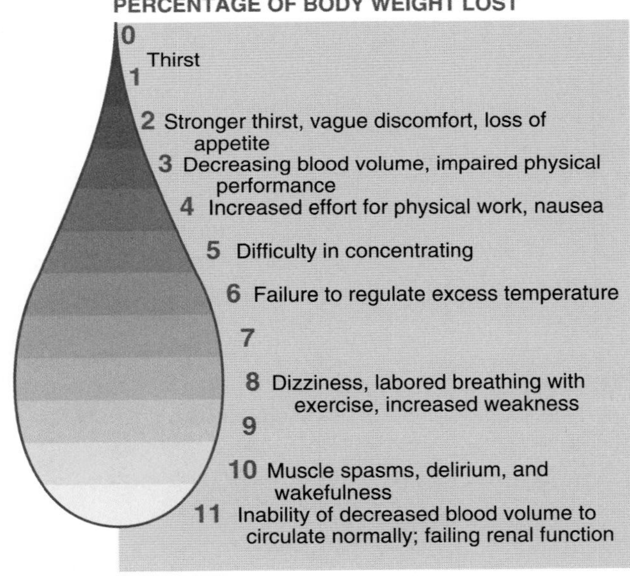

FIGURE 7-2 Adverse effects of dehydration.

Distribution

Intracellular water (ICW) is contained within cells and accounts for two thirds of total body water. **Extracellular water** in plasma, lymph, secretions, and spinal fluid equals one third of total body water or 20% of body weight. **Extracellular fluid** is the water and dissolved substances in the plasma, lymph, spinal fluid, and secretions; this includes the **interstitial fluid**, which is the fluid between and around the cells in tissues. While the distribution of body water varies under different circumstances, the total amount in the body remains relatively constant. Water consumed during the day through intake of foods and beverages is balanced by water lost through urination, perspiration, feces, and respiration. **Edema** is the abnormal accumulation of fluid in the intercellular tissue spaces or body cavities.

TABLE 7-1

Water Balance

Water Intake and Output (mL)*	Water Source
Water Intake	
1400	Fluids
700	Food
200	Cellular oxidation of food
2300	TOTAL
Water Output	
Normal Temperature	
1400	Urine
100	Feces
100	Skin (perspiration)
	Insensible loss
350	Skin
350	Respiratory tract
2300	TOTAL
Hot Weather	
1200	Urine
100	Feces
1400	Skin (perspiration)
	Insensible loss
350	Skin
250	Respiratory tract
3300	TOTAL
Prolonged Exercise	
500	Urine
100	Feces
5000	Skin (perspiration)
	Insensible loss
350	Skin
650	Respiratory tract
6600	TOTAL

Modified from Guyton AC: Textbook of medical physiology, ed 9, Philadelphia, 1996, Saunders.

*Average values.

TABLE 7-2

Percentage of Water in Common Foods

Food	Percentage
Lettuce, iceberg	96
Celery	95
Cucumbers	95
Cabbage, raw	92
Watermelon	92
Broccoli, boiled	91
Milk, nonfat	91
Spinach	91
Green beans, boiled	89
Carrots, raw	88
Oranges	87
Cereals, cooked	85
Apples, raw, without skin	84
Grapes	81
Potatoes, boiled	77
Eggs	75
Bananas	74
Fish, haddock, baked	74
Chicken, roasted, white meat	70
Corn, boiled	65
Beef, sirloin	59
Cheese, Swiss	38
Bread, white	37
Cake, angel food	34
Butter	16
Almonds, blanched	5
Saltines	3
Sugar, white	1
Oils	0

From U.S. Department of Agriculture, Agricultural Research Service: Nutrient database for standard reference, Release 16. Accessed April 18, 2010 from http://www.nal.usda.gov/fnic/foodcomp/Data/SR18/sr18.html.

Water Balance

Shifts in water balance can have adverse consequences. Therefore homeostatic regulation by the gastrointestinal (GI) tract, kidneys, and brain keeps body water content fairly constant. The amount of water taken in daily is approximately equivalent to the amount lost (Table 7-1).

Hormonal Regulation

Changes in cellular water content are sensed by baroreceptors in the central nervous system that provide feedback to the hypothalamus, close to the centers that regulate the antidiuretic hormone, **vasopressin**. Increased serum osmolality or decreased blood volume lead to its release, signaling the kidneys to conserve water. When vascular baroreceptors are stimulated by decreased extracellular fluid volume, the kidneys release renin to produce angiotensin II (the **renin-angiotensin system**). Angiotensin II has several functions, including stimulation of vasoconstriction and the thirst centers.

Water Intake

The sensation of thirst is a powerful signal to consume fluids. In fact, it controls water intake in healthy individuals. Both cellular dehydration and decreased extracellular fluid volume play a role in stimulating thirst. Sensitivity to thirst is decreased in older individuals, leading to higher risk for water deficits and ensuing dehydration.

Water is ingested as fluid and as part of food (Table 7-2). The oxidation of foods in the body also produces **metabolic water** as an end product. The oxidation of 100 g of fat, carbohydrate, or protein yields 107, 55, or 41 g of water, respectively, for a total of approximately 200 to 300 mL/day from consumption of the usual diet. When water cannot be ingested via the GI system it must be administered intravenously in the form of salt (saline) solutions, which closely resemble the electrolyte content of body fluids; dextrose solutions; parenteral nutrition; or in blood or plasma as transfusions. Water is absorbed rapidly because it moves freely through membranes by diffusion. This movement is controlled mainly by osmotic forces generated by inorganic ions in solution in the body (see *Clinical Insight:* Osmotic Forces).

Water Intoxication

Water intoxication occurs as a result of water intake in excess of the body's ability to excrete water. The increased **intracellular fluid** volume is accompanied by osmolar dilution. The increased volume of intracellular fluid causes the cells, particularly the brain cells, to swell, leading to headache, nausea, vomiting, muscle twitching, blindness, and convulsions with impending stupor. If left untreated, water intoxication can be fatal. Water intoxication is not commonly seen in normal, healthy individuals. It may be seen in endurance athletes who consume large amounts of electrolyte-free beverages during events, individuals with psychiatric illness, or as a result of water drinking contests (Goldman, 2009; Rogers and Hew-Butler, 2009).

Water Elimination

Water loss normally occurs through the kidneys as urine and through the GI tract in the feces (measurable, **sensible water loss**), as well as through air expired from the lungs and water vapor lost through the skin (nonmeasurable, **insensible water loss**) (see Table 7-1). The kidney is the primary regulator of sensible water loss. Under normal conditions the kidneys have the ability to adjust to changes in body water composition by either decreasing or increasing water loss in the urine. Natural diuretics are substances in the diet that increase urinary excretion, such as alcohol, caffeine and some herbs.

Insensible water loss is continuous and usually unconscious. High altitude, low humidity, and high temperatures can increase insensible fluid loss through the lungs and

CLINICAL INSIGHT

Osmotic Forces

Osmotic pressure is directly proportional to the number of particles in solution and usually refers to the pressure at the cell membrane. It is convenient (although not entirely accurate) to consider the osmotic pressure of intracellular fluid as a function of its potassium content because potassium is the predominant cation there. In contrast, the osmotic pressure of extracellular fluid may be considered relative to its sodium content because sodium is the major cation present in extracellular fluid. Although variations in the distribution of sodium and potassium ions are the principal causes of water shifts between the various fluid compartments, chloride and phosphate also influence water balance. Proteins cannot diffuse because of their size and thus also play a key role in maintaining osmotic equilibrium.

Oncotic pressure, or **colloidal osmotic pressure**, is the pressure at the capillary membrane. It is maintained by dissolved proteins in the plasma and interstitial fluids. Oncotic pressure helps to retain water within blood vessels, preventing its leakage from plasma into the interstitial spaces. In patients with an exceptionally low plasma protein content, such as those who are under physiologic stress or have certain diseases, water leaks into the interstitial spaces, causing edema or third spacing; and the fluid is called **"third space" fluid**.

Osmoles and Milliosmoles

Concentrations of individual ionic constituents of extracellular or intracellular fluids are expressed in terms of milliosmoles per liter (mOsm/L). One mole equals the gram molecular weight of a substance; when dissolved in 1 L of water, it becomes 1 osmole (osm). One milliosmole (mOsm) equals 1/1000th of an osmole. The number of milliosmoles per liter equals the number of millimoles per liter multiplied by the number of particles into which the dissolved substance dissociates. Thus 1 mmol of a nonelectrolyte (e.g., glucose) equals 1 mOsm; similarly, 1 mmol of an electrolyte containing only monovalent ions (e.g., sodium chloride) equals 2 mOsm. One mOsm dissolved in 1 L of water has an osmotic pressure of 17 mm Hg.

Osmolality is a measure of the osmotically active particles per kilogram of the solvent in which the particles are dispersed. It is expressed as milliosmoles of solute per kilogram of solvent (mOsm/kg). **Osmolarity** is the term formerly used to describe concentration—milliosmoles per liter of the entire solution; but osmolality is now the measurement for most clinical work. However, in reference to certain conditions such as hyperlipidemia, it makes a difference whether osmolality is stated as milliosmoles per kilogram of solvent or per liter of solution.

The average sum of the concentration of all the cations in serum is approximately 150 mEq/L. The cation concentration is balanced by 150 mEq/L of anions, yielding a total serum osmolality of approximately 300 mOsm/L. An osmolar imbalance is caused by a gain or loss of water relative to a solute. A key point is that an osmolality of less than 285 mOsm/L generally indicates a water excess; an osmolality of greater than 300 mOsm/L indicates a water deficit.

through sweat. Athletes can lose 3 to 4 lb from fluid loss when exercising in a temperature of 80° F and low humidity or even more at higher temperatures.

The GI tract can be a major source of water loss. Under normal conditions the water contained in the 7 to 9 L of digestive juices and other extracellular fluids secreted daily into the GI tract is almost entirely reabsorbed in the ileum and colon, except for approximately 100 mL that is excreted in the feces. Because this volume of reabsorbed fluid is approximately twice that of the blood plasma, excessive GI fluid losses through diarrhea may have serious consequences, particularly for very young and very old individuals.

Fluid loss through diarrhea is responsible for thousands of children's deaths in developing countries. Oral rehydration therapy with a simple mixture of water, sugar, and salt is highly effective in reducing the number of deaths if instituted early. Other abnormal fluid losses may occur as a result of emesis, hemorrhage, fistula drainage, burn and wound exudates, gastric and surgical tube drainage, and the use of diuretics.

When water intake is insufficient or water loss is excessive, healthy kidneys compensate by conserving water and excreting more concentrated urine. The renal tubules increase water reabsorption in response to the hormonal action of vasopressin. However, the concentration of the urine made by the kidneys has a limit: approximately 1400 mOsm/L. Once this limit has been reached, the body loses its ability to excrete solutes. The ability of the kidneys to concentrate urine may be compromised in older individuals or in young infants, resulting in increased risk of developing dehydration or hypernatremia, especially during illness.

Signs of dehydration include headache, fatigue, decreased appetite, light-headedness, poor skin turgor (although this may be present in well-hydrated older persons), skin tenting on the forehead, concentrated urine, decreased urine output, sunken eyes, dry mucous membranes of the mouth and nose, orthostatic blood pressure changes, and tachycardia (Armstrong, 2005). In a dehydrated person the specific gravity, a measure of the dissolved solutes in urine, increases above the normal levels of 1.010 where the urine becomes remarkably darker (Cheuvront et al, 2010.) High ambient temperature and dehydration adversely affect exercise performance; changes may be mediated by serotonergic and dopaminergic alterations in the central nervous system (Maughan et al., 2007). Fluids of appropriate composition in appropriate amounts are essential. See *Clinical Insight:* Water Requirements—When Eight Cups Is Not Enough.

ELECTROLYTES

Electrolytes are substances that dissociate into positively and negatively charged ions (cations and anions) when dissolved in water. Electrolytes can be simple inorganic salts of sodium, potassium, or magnesium or complex organic molecules; they play a key role in a host of normal metabolic functions (Table 7-3). One milliequivalent (mEq) of any substance has the capacity to combine chemically with 1 mEq of a substance with an opposite charge. For univalent ions (e.g., Na^+) 1 millimole (mmol) equals 1 mEq; for divalent ions (e.g., Ca^{++}) 1 mmol equals 2 mEq (see Appendix 3 for conversion guidelines).

The major extracellular electrolytes are sodium, calcium, chloride, and bicarbonate (HCO_3^-). Potassium, magnesium,

CLINICAL INSIGHT

Water Requirements—When Eight Cups Is Not Enough

The body has no provision for water storage; therefore the amount of water lost every 24 hours must be replaced to maintain health and equilibrium. Under ordinary circumstances, a reasonable allowance based on recommended caloric intake is 1 ml/kcal for adults and 1.5 ml/kcal for infants. This translates into approximately 35 ml/kg of usual body weight in adults, 50 to 60 ml/kg in children, and 150 ml/kg in infants.

In most cases a suitable daily allowance for water from all sources, including foods, is approximately 3.7 L (15.5 cups) for men and 2.7 L (11+ cups) for women, depending on body size (Institute of Medicine, 2004). Because solid food provides 19% of total daily fluid intake, this equals 750 ml of water or approximately 3 cups daily. When this is added to the 200-300 mL (approximately 1 cup) of water contributed by oxidative metabolism, men should consume approximately 11.5 cups of fluid daily and women need 7 cups of fluids daily. Total fluid intake comes from drinking water, other liquids, and food; the AI values for water are for total daily water intake and include all dietary water sources.

Infants need more water because of the limited capacity of their kidneys to handle a large renal solute load, their higher percentage of body water, and their large surface area per unit of body weight. A lactating woman's need for water also increases to approximately 600-700 mL (2.5-3 cups) per day for milk production.

Thirst is a less effective signal to consume water in infants, heavily exercising athletes, sick individuals, and older adults who may have a diminished thirst sensation. Anyone sick enough to be hospitalized, regardless of the diagnosis, is at risk for water and electrolyte imbalance. Older adults are particularly susceptible because of factors such as impaired renal concentrating ability, fever, diarrhea, vomiting, and a decreased ability to care for themselves. In situations involving extreme heat or excessive sweating, thirst may not keep pace with the actual water requirements of the body.

TABLE 7-3

Normal Electrolyte Concentration of Serum

Electrolyte	Normal Range
Cations	
Sodium	136-145 mEq/L
Potassium	3.5-5 mEq/L
Calcium	4.5-5.5 mEq/L (9-11 mg/dL)
Magnesium	1.5-2.5 mEq/L (1.8-3 mg/dL)
Anions	
Chloride	96-106 mEq/L
CO_2 (content)	24-28.8 mEq/L
Phosphorus (inorganic)	3-4.5 mg/dL (1.9-2.85 mEq/L as HPO_4^{2-})
Sulfate (as S)	0.8-1.2 mg/dl (0.5-0.75 mEq/L as SO_2^{2-})
Lactate	1.8 mEq/L (6-16 mg/dL)
Protein	6 g/dl (14-18 mEq/L); depends on albumin level

CO_2, Carbon dioxide; *HPO_4^2*, monohydrogen phosphate; *SO_2^2*, sulfate.

and phosphate are the major intracellular electrolytes. These elements, which exist as ions in body fluids, are distributed throughout all body fluids. They maintain physiologic body functions, including osmotic equilibrium, acid-base balance, and intracellular and extracellular concentration differentials. Changes in either intracellular or extracellular electrolyte concentrations can have a major effect on bodily functions. The **sodium-potassium adenosine triphosphatase (Na/K ATPase) pump** closely regulates cellular electrolyte contents by actively pumping sodium out of cells in exchange for potassium. Other electrolytes follow ion gradients.

Calcium

Although approximately 99% of the body's calcium (Ca^{++}) is stored in the bone, the remaining 1% has important physiologic functions. Ionized calcium within the vascular compartment is a cation with a positive charge. Approximately half of the calcium found in the intravascular compartment is bound to the serum protein albumin. Thus when serum albumin levels are low, total calcium levels decrease because of hypoalbuminemia. The **corrected calcium** formula, often used in renal disease is

$$\text{serum calcium} + 0.8\,(4 - \text{serum albumin}).$$

The binding ability of calcium and its ionized content in blood have implications for normal homeostatic mechanisms. Blood tests for calcium levels often measure both total and ionized calcium levels. This is because ionized (or free, unbound) calcium is the active form of calcium and is not affected by hypoalbuminemia. In healthy adults, normal levels for serum total calcium are approximately 8.5 to 10.5 mg/dL, whereas normal levels for ionized calcium are 4.5 to 5.5 mEq/L.

Ionized calcium levels are inversely altered by changes in acid-base balance; as serum pH rises, calcium binds with protein, leading to decreased ionized calcium levels. As pH is lowered, the opposite occurs. Because calcium has an important role in cardiac, nervous system, and skeletal muscle function, both hypocalcemia and hypercalcemia can become life-threatening.

Functions

Calcium is found in bones as part of the compound hydroxyapatite. Outside of the bone, calcium is a second messenger in responding to changes in intracellular calcium content following binding of hormones or proteins to the cell surface (the first messenger). Calcium is also an important factor in regulating cell electroconductivity and in blood clotting.

Calcium content is carefully regulated by the actions of parathyroid hormone (PTH), calcitonin, vitamin D, and phosphorus. When serum calcium levels are low, PTH causes release of calcium from the bones and stimulates increased absorption from the GI tract. Calcitonin works in the opposite direction, shutting off bone calcium release and decreasing GI absorption. Vitamin D stimulates while phosphorus inhibits calcium absorption in the GI tract.

Absorption and Excretion

Approximately 20% to 60% of dietary calcium is absorbed and is tightly regulated because of the need to maintain steady serum calcium levels in the face of fluctuating intake. The ileum is the most important site of calcium absorption. Calcium is absorbed via passive transport and through a vitamin D–regulated transport system. See Chapter 3.

The kidney is the main site of calcium excretion. The majority of serum calcium is bound to proteins and not filtered by the kidneys; only approximately 100 to 200 mg is excreted in the urine in normal adults.

Sources

Dairy products are the main source of calcium in the American diet, with some green vegetables, nuts, canned fish including bones, and calcium-extracted tofu having moderate amounts of calcium. Food manufacturers fortify many foods with additional calcium.

Recommended Intakes

Recommended intakes of calcium range from 1000 to 1300 mg/day, depending on age and gender. An upper limit for daily calcium intake has been estimated to be approximately 2500 mg (see inside cover).

Sodium

Sodium (Na^+) is the major cation of extracellular fluid. Normal serum concentration is 136 to 145 mEq/L. Secretions such as bile and pancreatic juice contain substantial amounts of sodium. Approximately 35% to 40% of the total body sodium is in the skeleton; however, most of it is only slowly exchangeable with that in body fluids. Contrary to common belief, sweat is hypotonic and contains a relatively small amount of sodium.

TABLE 7-4

Dietary Reference Intakes for Sodium, Potassium, and Chloride Daily Intake

Age	Sodium	Potassium	chloride	Salt (sodium Chloride)
Adult 19-49	1.5 g (65 mmol)	4.7 g (120 mmol)	2.3 g (65 mmol)	3.8 g (65 mmol)
Adult 50-70	1.3 g (55 mmol)	4.7 g (120 mmol	2.0 g (55 mmol)	3.2 g (55 mmol)
Adult 71	1.2 g (50 mmol)	4.7 g (120 mmol)	1.8 g (50 mmol)	2.9 g (50 mmol)
UL	2.3 g (100 mmol)			

Institute of Medicine, Food and Nutrition Board: Dietary reference intakes for water, potassium, sodium, chloride, and sulfate, Washington, DC, 2004, National Academies Press.

UL, Tolerable upper intake level.

Functions

As the predominant ion of the extracellular fluid, sodium thus regulates both extracellular and plasma volume. Sodium is also important in neuromuscular function and maintenance of acid-base balance. Maintenance of serum sodium levels is vital, because severe hyponatremia can lead to seizures, coma and death.

Extracellular sodium concentrations are much higher than intracellular levels (normal serum sodium is approximately 135 mEq/L whereas intracellular levels are approximately 10 mEq/L). The Na/K ATPase pump is an active transport system that works to keep sodium outside the cell through exchange with potassium. The Na/K ATPase pump requires carriers for both sodium and potassium along with energy for proper function. Exportation of sodium from the cell is the driving force for facilitated transporters that import glucose, amino acids, and other nutrients into the cells.

Absorption and Excretion

Sodium is readily absorbed from the intestine and carried to the kidneys, where it is filtered and returned to the blood to maintain appropriate levels. The amount absorbed is proportional to the intake in healthy adults.

Approximately 90% to 95% of normal body sodium loss is through the urine; the rest is lost in feces and sweat. Normally the quantity of sodium excreted daily is equal to the amount ingested. Sodium excretion is maintained by a mechanism involving the glomerular filtration rate, the cells of the juxtaglomerular apparatus of the kidneys, the renin-angiotensin-aldosterone system, the sympathetic nervous system, circulating catecholamines, and blood pressure.

Sodium balance is regulated in part by aldosterone, a mineralocorticoid secreted by the adrenal cortex. When blood sodium levels rise, the thirst receptors in the hypothalamus stimulate the thirst sensation. Ingestion of fluids returns sodium levels to normal. Under certain circumstances, sodium and fluid regulation can be disrupted, resulting in abnormal blood sodium levels. The **syndrome of inappropriate antidiuretic hormone secretion (SIADH)** is characterized by concentrated, low-volume urine and dilutional hyponatremia as water is retained. SIADH can result from central nervous system disorders, pulmonary disorders, tumors, and certain medications. See Chapter 36.

Estrogen, which is slightly similar to aldosterone, also causes sodium and water retention. Changes in water and sodium balance during the menstrual cycle, during pregnancy, and while taking oral contraceptives are partially attributable to changes in progesterone and estrogen levels.

Dietary Reference Intakes

Actual minimum requirements for sodium are not known but have been estimated to be as low as 200 mg/day. Estimated adequate intakes (AIs) for sodium were published in the 2004 Dietary Reference Intakes (Institute of Medicine, 2004). The mean daily salt intake in Western societies is approximately 10 to 12 g (4 to 5 g of sodium) per capita, far in excess of the estimated minimum requirements and even in excess of the AIs for sodium of 1.2 to 1.5 g per day, depending on age, with lower amounts recommended for the elderly (Table 7-4).

Approximately 3 g of the daily salt intake exists naturally in foods, 3 g is added during processing, and 4 g is added by the individual. Increased reliance on restaurants, fast food, and commercially prepared convenience foods has contributed to this high per capita salt and thus sodium intake.

Healthy kidneys are usually able to excrete excess sodium intake; however, there is concern about persistent excessive sodium intake, which has been implicated in development of hypertension. See Chapter 34. In addition to its role in hypertension, excessive salt intake has been associated with increased urinary calcium excretion (Teucher and Fairweather-Tait, 2003) (see Chapter 36) and some cases of osteoporosis (He and MacGregor, 2010). The dietary reference intakes (DRI) give an upper limit of 2.3 g of sodium per day (or 5.8 g sodium chloride per day), given the potential role of sodium in hypertension (Joint National Committee, 2003).

Sources

The major source of sodium is sodium chloride, or common table salt, of which sodium constitutes 40% by weight. Protein foods generally contain more naturally existing sodium than do vegetables and grains, whereas fruits contain little or none. The addition of table salt, flavored salts, flavor enhancers, and preservatives during food processing accounts for the high sodium content of most convenience and fast-food products. For instance, ½ cup of frozen vegetables prepared without salt contains 10 mg of sodium, whereas ½ cup of canned vegetables contains approximately 260 mg of sodium. Similarly, 1 ounce of plain meat contains 30 mg of sodium, whereas 1 ounce of luncheon meat contains approximately 400 mg of sodium. The larger-portion sizes that are being offered by dining establishments to consumers are increasing the sodium intake even more.

Magnesium

The adult human body contains approximately 24 g of magnesium, which is the second most prevalent intracellular cation. Approximately half of the body's magnesium is located in bone, whereas another 45% resides in soft tissue; only 1% of the body's magnesium content is in the extracellular fluids (Rude, 2000). Normal serum magnesium levels are approximately 1.7 to 2.5 mEq/L; however, approximately 70% of serum magnesium is free or ionized. The remainder is bound to proteins and is not active.

Function

Magnesium (Mg^{++}) is an important cofactor in many enzymatic reactions in the body and is also important in bone metabolism as well as central nervous system and cardiovascular function. Many of the enzyme systems regulated by magnesium are involved in nutrient metabolism and nucleic acid synthesis, leading to the body's need to carefully regulate magnesium status. As with calcium, severe hypomagnesemia or hypermagnesemia can have life-threatening sequelae.

Intakes of Mg^{++}, potassium, fruits, and vegetables have been associated with higher alkaline status and a subsequent beneficial effect on bone health; enhanced mineral-water consumption may be an easy, inexpensive way to reduce the onset of osteoporosis (Wynn et al., 2010). See *Clinical Insight:* Urinary pH—How Does Diet Affect It? in Chapter 36.

Absorption and Excretion

Approximately one third of ingested magnesium is absorbed. Although magnesium absorption occurs throughout the GI tract, absorption is optimized in the ileum and distal jejunum through both passive and active mechanisms. Magnesium absorption is regulated to maintain serum levels; if levels drop, more is absorbed and if levels increase, less is absorbed. The kidney is the major regulator of magnesium excretion.

Sources

Magnesium is found in a wide variety of foods, making an isolated magnesium deficiency unlikely in otherwise healthy individuals. Highly processed foods tend to have lower magnesium content, whereas green leafy vegetables, legumes, and whole grains are good sources. The high magnesium content of vegetables helps to alleviate some concerns about the potential for phytate binding.

Dietary Reference Intakes

The recommended intake of magnesium ranges from 310 to 420 mg/day, depending on age and gender (see tables on inside front cover).

Phosphorus

Phosphorus is an important constituent of the intracellular fluid and in its role in ATP is vital in energy metabolism. In addition, phosphorus is important in bone metabolism. Approximately 80% of the body's phosphorus is found in bones. Phosphorus is found in the body as phosphate—the terms are often used interchangeably. Normal levels for serum phosphorus are between 2.4 and 4.6 mg/dL.

Functions

Large amounts of free energy are released when the phosphate bonds in ATP are split. In addition to this role, phosphorus is vital for cellular function in phosphorylation and dephosphorylation reactions, as a buffer in acid-base balance, and in cellular structure as part of the phospholipids membrane. Because of the vital role that phosphorus plays in energy production, severe hypophosphatemia can be a life-threatening event.

Absorption and Excretion

Phosphorus absorption is fairly efficient and is related to intake at most intake levels. The kidney is the major site of phosphorus excretion.

Sources

Phosphorus is mainly found in animal products, including meats and milk; some dried beans are also good sources.

Dietary Reference Intakes

The recommended intake of phosphorus is approximately 700 mg/day, depending on age and gender, with an upper limit of 3500 to 4000 mg. See tables on inside front cover.

Potassium

Potassium (K^+), the major cation of intracellular fluid, is present in small amounts in extracellular fluid. The normal serum potassium concentration is 3.5 to 5 mEq/L.

Functions

With sodium, potassium is involved in maintaining a normal water balance, osmotic equilibrium, and acid-base balance. In addition to calcium, it is important in the regulation of neuromuscular activity. Concentrations of sodium and potassium determine membrane potentials in nerves and muscle. Potassium also promotes cellular growth. The potassium content of muscle is related to muscle mass and glycogen storage; therefore, if muscle is being formed, an adequate supply of potassium is essential. Potassium has an integral role in the Na/K ATPase pump. Both hypokalemia and hyperkalemia can have devastating cardiac implications.

Absorption and Excretion

Potassium is readily absorbed from the small intestine. Approximately 80% to 90% of ingested potassium is excreted in the urine; the remainder is lost in the feces. The kidneys maintain normal serum levels through their ability to filter, resorb, and excrete potassium under the influence of aldosterone. Ionized potassium is excreted in place of ionized sodium through the renal tubule exchange mechanism.

Sources

As a rule, fruits, vegetables, fresh meat, and dairy products are good sources of potassium. Box 7-1 categorizes select foods according to their potassium content.

Dietary Reference Intakes

The AI level for potassium for adults is 4700 mg/day. No upper limit has been set. Potassium intake is inadequate in a as many as 50% of adult Americans. The reason for the poor potassium intakes is simply inadequate consumption of fruits and vegetables. Insufficient potassium intakes have been linked to hypertension and cardiac arrhythmia.

ACID-BASE BALANCE

An acid is any substance that tends to release hydrogen ions in solution, whereas a base is any substance that tends to accept hydrogen ions in solution. The hydrogen ion concentration $[H^+]$ determines acidity. Because the magnitude of hydrogen ion concentration is small compared with that of other serum electrolytes, acidity is more readily expressed in terms of pH units. A low blood pH indicates a higher hydrogen ion concentration and greater acidity, whereas a high pH value indicates a lower hydrogen ion concentration and greater alkalinity.

Acid-base balance is the dynamic equilibrium state of hydrogen ion concentration. Maintaining the arterial blood pH level within the normal range of 7.35 to 7.45 is crucial for many physiologic functions and biochemical reactions. Regulatory mechanisms of the kidneys, lungs, and buffering systems enable the body to maintain the blood pH level despite the enormous acid load from food consumption and tissue metabolism. A disruption of the acid-base balance occurs when acid or base losses or gains exceed the body's regulatory capabilities, or when normal regulatory mechanisms become ineffective. These regulatory disturbances may develop in association with certain diseases, toxin ingestion, shifts in fluid status, and certain medical and surgical treatments (Table 7-5). If a disrupted acid-base balance is left untreated, multiple detrimental effects ranging from electrolyte abnormalities to death can ensue.

Acid Generation

Acids are introduced exogenously through the ingestion of food, acid precursors, and toxins. They are also generated endogenously through normal tissue metabolism. Fixed acids such as phosphoric and sulfuric acids are produced from the metabolism of phosphate-containing substrates and sulfur-containing amino acids, respectively. Organic acids such as lactic and keto acids typically accumulate only during exercise, acute illness, or fasting. Carbon dioxide (CO_2), a volatile acid, is generated from the oxidation of carbohydrates, amino acids, and fat. Under normal conditions, the body is able to maintain normal acid-base status through a wide range of acid intake from foods. See *Clinical Insight:* Urinary pH—How Does Diet Affect It? in Chapter 36 for the acid and alkaline effects of foods.

Regulation

Various regulatory mechanisms maintain the pH level within very narrow physiologic limits. At the cellular level, **buffer** systems composed of weak acids or bases and their corresponding salts minimize the effect on pH of the addition of a strong acid or base. The buffering effect involves formation of a weaker acid or base in an amount equivalent to the strong acid or base that has been added to the system (Figure 7-3).

Proteins and phosphates are the primary intracellular buffers, whereas the HCO_3^- and carbonic acid (H_2CO_3) system is the primary extracellular buffer. The acid-base balance is also maintained by the kidneys and lungs. The kidneys regulate hydrogen ion (H^+) secretion and HCO_3^- resorption. The lungs control alveolar ventilation by altering either the depth or rate of breathing. In turn, changes in breathing alter the amount of carbon dioxide expired.

ACID-BASE DISORDERS

Acid-base disorders can be differentiated based on whether they have metabolic or respiratory causes. The evaluation of acid-base status requires analysis of serum electrolytes and arterial blood gas (ABG) values (Table 7-6). Metabolic acid-base imbalances result in changes in HCO_3^- (i.e., base) levels, which are reflected in the total carbon dioxide (TCO_2) portion of the electrolyte profile. TCO_2 includes HCO_3^-, H_2CO_3, and dissolved carbon dioxide; however, all but 1 to 3 mEq/L is in the form of HCO_3^-. Thus, for ease of interpretation, TCO_2 should be equated with HCO_3^-. Respiratory acid-base imbalances result in changes in the partial pressure of dissolved carbon dioxide (Pco_2). This is reported in the ABG values in addition to the pH, which reflects the overall acid-base status.

Metabolic Acidosis

Metabolic acidosis results from increased generation or accumulation of acids or loss of base (i.e., HCO_3^-) in the extracellular fluids. Simple, acute metabolic acidosis results in a low blood pH, or **acidemia**. Examples of metabolic acidosis include diabetic ketoacidosis, lactic acidosis, toxin ingestion, uremia, and excessive HCO_3^- loss via the kidneys or intestinal tract. Multiple deaths have previously been attributed to lactic acidosis caused by administration of parenteral nutrition devoid of thiamin. In patients with metabolic acidosis, the anion gap is calculated to help determine cause and appropriate treatment. The **anion gap** is a measurement of the interval between the sum of "routinely measured" cations minus the sum of the "routinely measured" anions in the blood.

BOX 7-1

Classification of Select Foods by Potassium Content

Low (0-100 mg/serving)*	Medium (100-200 mg/serving)*	High (200-300 mg/serving)*	Very High (>300 mg/serving)*
Fruits	**Fruits**	**Fruits**	**Fruits**
Applesauce	Apple, 1 small	Apricots, canned	Avocados, ¼ small
Blueberries	Apple juice	Grapefruit juice	Banana, 1 small
Cranberries	Apricot nectar	Kiwi, ½ medium	Cantaloupe, ¼ small
Lemon, ½ medium	Blackberries	Nectarine, 1 small	Dried fruit, ¼ cup
Lime, ½ medium	Cherries, 12 small	Orange, 1 small	Honeydew melon, ⅛ small
Pears, canned	Fruit cocktail	Orange juice	Mango, 1 medium
Pear nectar	Grape juice	Peach, fresh, 1 medium	Papaya, ½ medium
Peach nectar	Grapefruit, ½ small	Pear, fresh, 1 medium	Prune juice
	Grapes, 12 small		
	Mandarin oranges		
	Peaches, canned		
	Pineapple, canned		
	Plum, 1 small		
	Raspberries		
	Rhubarb		
	Strawberries		
	Tangerine, 1 small		
	Watermelon, 1 cup		
Vegetables	**Vegetables**	**Vegetables**	**Vegetables**
Cabbage, raw	Asparagus, frozen	Asparagus, fresh, cooked, 4 spears	Artichoke, 1 medium
Cucumber slices	Beets, canned	Beets, fresh, cooked	Bamboo shoots, fresh
Green beans, frozen	Broccoli, frozen	Brussels sprouts	Beet greens, ¼ cup
Leeks	Cabbage, cooked	Kohlrabi	Corn on the cob, 1 ear
Lettuce, iceberg, 1 cup	Carrots	Mushrooms, cooked	Chinese cabbage, cooked
Water chestnuts, canned	Cauliflower, frozen	Okra	Dried beans
Bamboo shoots canned	Celery, 1 stalk	Parsnips	Potatoes, baked, ½ medium
	Corn, frozen	Potatoes, boiled or mashed	Potatoes, French fries, 1 oz
	Eggplant	Pumpkin	Spinach
	Green beans, fresh raw	Rutabagas	Sweet potatoes, yams
	Mushrooms, fresh raw		Swiss chard, ¼ cup
	Onions		Tomato, fresh, sauce, or juice; tomato paste, 2 tbsp
	Peas		Winter squash
	Radishes		
	Turnips		
	Zucchini, summer squash		
		Miscellaneous	**Miscellaneous**
		Granola	Bouillon, low sodium, 1 cup
		Nuts and seeds, 1 oz	Cappuccino, 1 cup
		Peanut butter, 2 tbsp	Chili, 4 oz
		Chocolate, 1½-oz bar	Coconut, 1 cup
			Lasagna, 8 oz
			Milk, chocolate milk, 1 cup
			Milkshakes, 1 cup
			Molasses, 1 tbsp
			Pizza, 2 slices
			Salt substitutes, ¼ tsp
			Soy milk, 1 cup
			Spaghetti, 1 cup
			Yogurt, 6 oz

*One serving equals ½ cup unless otherwise specified.

TABLE 7-5

Four Major Acid-Base Imbalances

Acid-base Imbalance	Plasma pH	Primary Disturbance	Compensation	Possible Causes
Respiratory				
Respiratory acidosis	Low	Increased Pco_2	Increased renal net acid excretion with resulting increase in serum bicarbonate	Emphysema, COPD, neuromuscular disease in which respiratory function is impaired, excessive retention of CO_2
Respiratory alkalosis	High	Decreased Pco_2	Decreased renal net acid excretion with resulting decrease in serum bicarbonate	Aftermath of intense exercise, anxiety, early sepsis, excessive expiration of CO_2 and H_2O
Metabolic				
Metabolic acidosis	Low	Decreased HCO_3^-	Hyperventilation with resulting low Pco_2	Diarrhea; uremia; ketoacidosis from uncontrolled diabetes mellitus; starvation; high-fat, low-carbohydrate diet; drugs
Metabolic alkalosis	High	Increased HCO_3^-	Hypoventilation with resulting increase in Pco_2	Diuretics use, increased ingestion of alkali, loss of chloride, vomiting

CO_2, Carbon dioxide; *COPD*, chronic obstructive pulmonary disease; *H_2O*, water; *HCO_3^-*, bicarbonate; *Pco_2*, carbon dioxide pressure.

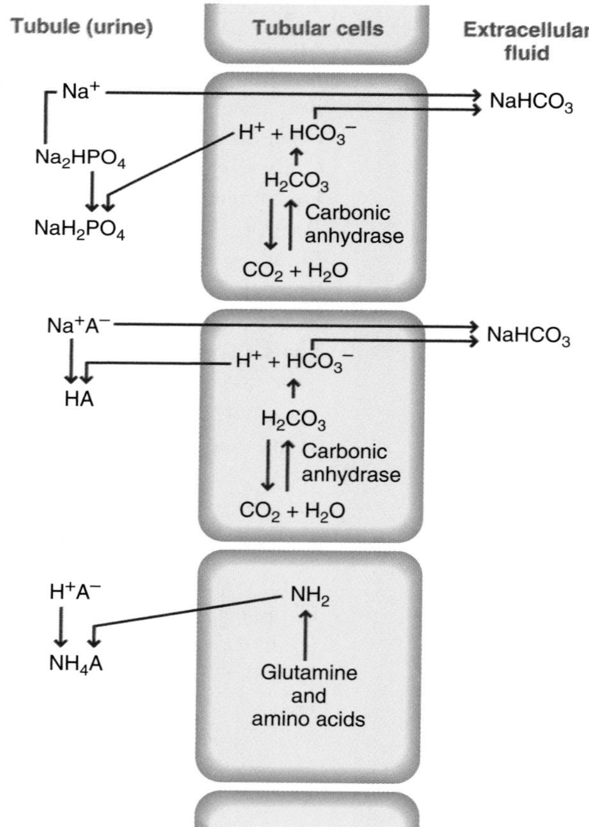

FIGURE 7-3 Generation of sodium bicarbonate and clearance of hydrogen ion concentration by the three buffer systems that function in the kidney. *HA*, Any acid in the body.

TABLE 7-6

Normal Arterial Blood Gas Values

Clinical Test	ABG Value
pH	7.35-7.45
Pco_2	35-45 mm Hg
Po_2	80-100 mm Hg
HCO_3^-	22-26 mEq/L
O_2 saturation	>95%

ABG, Arterial blood gas; *HCO_3^-*, bicarbonate; *O_2*, oxygen; *Pco_2*, carbon dioxide pressure; *Po_2*, oxygen pressure.

$$\text{Anion gap} = (Na^+ + K^+) - (Cl^- + HCO_3^-)$$

in which Na^- is sodium, K^+ is potassium, Cl^- is chloride, and HCO_3^- is bicarbonate. Normal is 12 to 14 mEq/L.

Anion gap metabolic acidosis occurs when a decrease in HCO_3^- concentration is balanced by increased acid anions other than chloride. This causes the calculated anion gap to exceed the normal range of 12 to 14 mEq/L. This normochloremic metabolic acidosis may develop in association with the following conditions, represented by the acronym MUD PILES (Wilson, 2003):

- *M*ethanol ingestion
- *U*remia
- *D*iabetic ketoacidosis
- *P*araldehyde ingestion
- *I*atrogenic
- *L*actic acidosis
- *E*thylene glycol or ethanol ingestion
- *S*alicylate intoxication

Nongap metabolic acidosis occurs when a decrease in HCO_3^- concentration is balanced by an increase in chloride concentration, resulting in a normal anion gap. This hyperchloremic metabolic acidosis, may develop in association with the following, represented by the acronym USED CARP) (Wilson, 2003):

*U*reterosigmoidostomy
*S*mall bowel fistula
*E*xtra chloride ingestion
*D*iarrhea
*C*arbonic anhydrase inhibitor
*A*drenal insufficiency
*R*enal tubular acidosis
*P*ancreatic fistula

Metabolic Alkalosis

Metabolic alkalosis results from the administration or accumulation of HCO_3^- (i.e., base) or its precursors, excessive loss of acid (e.g., during gastric suctioning), or loss of extracellular fluid containing more chloride than HCO_3^- (e.g., from villous adenoma or diuretic use). Simple, acute metabolic alkalosis results in a high blood pH, or **alkalemia**. Metabolic alkalosis may also result from volume depletion; decreased blood flow to the kidneys stimulates reabsorption of sodium and water, increasing HCO_3^- reabsorption. This condition is known as **contraction alkalosis**. Alkalosis can also result from severe hypokalemia (serum potassium concentration <2 mEq/L). As potassium moves from the intracellular to the extracellular fluid, hydrogen ions move from the extracellular to the intracellular fluid to maintain electroneutrality. This process produces intracellular acidosis, which increases hydrogen ion excretion and HCO_3^- reabsorption by the kidneys.

Respiratory Acidosis

Respiratory acidosis is caused by decreased ventilation and consequent carbon dioxide retention. Simple, acute respiratory acidosis results in a low pH, or acidemia. Acute respiratory acidosis can occur as a result of sleep apnea; asthma; aspiration of a foreign object; or acute respiratory distress syndrome, also known as *adult respiratory distress syndrome*. Chronic respiratory acidosis is associated with obesity hypoventilation syndrome, chronic obstructive pulmonary disease or emphysema, certain neuromuscular diseases, and starvation cachexia.

Respiratory Alkalosis

Respiratory alkalosis results from increased ventilation and elimination of carbon dioxide. The condition may be mediated centrally (e.g., from head injury, pain, anxiety, cerebrovascular accident, or tumors) or by peripheral stimulation (e.g., from pneumonia, hypoxemia, high altitudes, pulmonary embolism, congestive heart failure, or interstitial lung disease). Simple, acute respiratory alkalosis results in a high pH, or alkalemia.

Compensation

When an acid-base imbalance occurs, the body attempts to restore the normal pH by developing an opposite acid-base imbalance to offset the effects of the primary disorder, a response known as **compensation**. For example, the kidneys of a patient with a primary respiratory acidosis (decreased pH) compensate by increasing HCO_3^- reabsorption, thereby creating a metabolic alkalosis. This response helps to increase the pH. Similarly, in response to a primary metabolic acidosis (decreased pH), the lungs compensate by increasing ventilation and carbon dioxide elimination, thereby creating a respiratory alkalosis. This compensatory respiratory alkalosis helps to increase pH.

Respiratory compensation for metabolic acid-base disturbances occurs quickly—within minutes. In contrast, renal compensation for respiratory acid-base imbalances may take 3 to 5 days to be maximally effective. Compensation does not always occur; and when it does, it is not completely successful (i.e., does not result in a pH of 7.4). The pH level still reflects the underlying primary disorder. It is imperative to distinguish between primary disturbances and compensatory responses because treatment is always directed toward the primary acid-base disturbance and its underlying cause. As the primary disturbance is treated, the compensatory response corrects itself. Predictive values for compensatory responses are available to differentiate between primary acid-base imbalances and compensatory responses (Whitmire, 2002). Clinicians may also use tools such as clinical algorithms.

CLINICAL SCENARIO

Mary has been admitted to your hospital through the Emergency Room. She was running in the local marathon and collapsed. Her labs are, as follows: plasma sodium 120 mEq/L, other electrolytes are normal. Mary states that she drank a liter of water during her run. The doctor indicates that Mary is suffering from exercise-induced hyponatremia.

Nutrition Diagnostic Statement

Altered nutritional labs related to excessive fluid intake as evidenced by low plasma sodium (120 mEq/L) and collapse during a marathon.

Nutrition Care Questions

1. Would you offer Mary a sports drink? Why or why not?
2. What happens to the body when the kidneys cannot excrete excess fluid?
3. What tips would you suggest to Mary for her next marathon?

USEFUL WEBSITES

Acid-Base Tutorial
http://www.acid-base.com/

The Beverage Institute Hydration Calculator
http://www.weather.com/outlook/health/fitness/tools/hydration

The Merck Manual of Diagnosis and Therapy
http://www.merckmanuals.com/professional/index.html
The Weather Channel—Hydration Calculator
http://www.weather.com/outlook/health/fitness/tools/hydration

REFERENCES

Armstrong LE: Hydration assessment techniques, *Nutr Rev* 63:S40, 2005.

Bartelmo J, Terry DP: *Fluids and Electrolytes Made Incredibly Easy*, ed 4, Philadelphia, 2008, Wolters Kluwer/Lippincott Williams & Wilkins.

Cheuvront SN, et al. Biological variation and diagnostic accuracy of dehydration assessment markers, *Am J Clin Nutr* 92:565, 2010.

Goldman MB: The mechanism of life-threatening water imbalance in schizophrenia and its relationship to the underlying psychiatric illness, *Brain Res Rev* 61:210, 2009.

He FJ, MacGregor GA: Reducing population salt intake worldwide: from evidence to implementation, *Prog Cardiovasc Dis* 52:363, 2010.

Institute of Medicine, Food and Nutrition Board: *Dietary reference intakes for water, potassium, sodium, chloride, and sulfate*, Washington, DC, 2004, National Academies Press.

Joint National Committee (JNC): *The Seventh Report of the Joint National Committee on Prevention, Detection, Evaluation, and Treatment of High Blood Pressure*, NIH Pub No 03-5233, 2003.

Maughan RJ, et al: Exercise, heat, hydration and the brain, *J Am Coll Nutr* 26:604S, 2007.

Rogers IR, Hew-Butler T: Exercise-associated hyponatremia: overzealous fluid consumption, *Wilderness Environ Med* 20:139, 2009.

Rude RK: Magnesium. In Stipanuk MH, editor: *Biochemical and physiological aspects of human nutrition*, Philadelphia, 2000, Saunders.

Teucher B, Fairweather-Tait S: Dietary sodium as a risk factor for osteoporosis: where is the evidence? *Proc Nutr Soc* 62:859, 2003.

Whitmire SJ: Fluids, electrolytes, and acid-base balance. In Matarese LE, Gottschlich MM, editors: *Contemporary nutrition support practice: a clinical guide*, ed 2, Philadelphia, 2002, Saunders.

Wilson RF: Acid-base problems. In Tintinalli JE, Krome RL, Ruiz E, editors: *Emergency medicine: a comprehensive study guide*, ed 6, New York, 2003, McGraw-Hill.

Wynn E, et al: Postgraduate symposium: positive influence of nutritional alkalinity on bone health, *Proc Nutr Soc* 69:166, 2010.

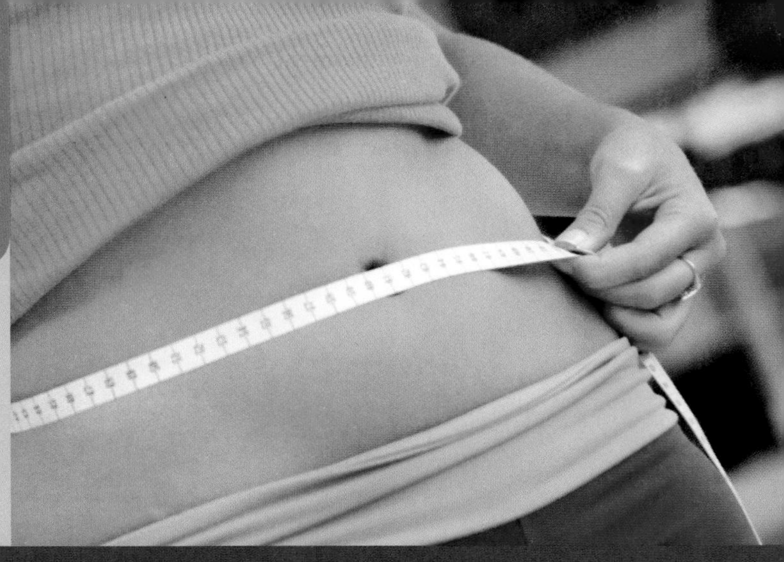

CHAPTER 8

Mary Demarest Litchford, PhD, RD, LDN

Clinical: Biochemical Assessment

KEY TERMS

25-hydroxy vitamin D (25-[OH]D_3)
albumin
analyte
anemia of chronic and inflammatory diseases (ACD)
apolipoprotein E (apoE) phenotype
basic metabolic panel (BMP)
complete blood count (CBC)
comprehensive metabolic panel (CMP)
C-reactive protein (CRP)
creatinine
differential count
ferritin
functional assay
hematocrit (Hct)
hemoglobin (Hgb)
hemoglobin A1C (Hgb A1C)
high-sensitivity CRP (hs-CRP)
homocysteine
macrocytic anemia
microcytic anemia
negative acute-phase proteins
nutrition-specific laboratory data
osteocalcin
oxidative stress
positive acute-phase proteins
prealbumin (PAB)
reactive oxygen species (ROS)
retinol
retinol-binding protein (RBP)
static assay
total iron-binding capacity (TIBC)
transferrin
transthyretin (TTHY)
urinalysis

Laboratory tests are ordered to diagnose diseases, support nutrition diagnoses, monitor medication effectiveness, and evaluate nutrition care process (NCP) interventions. Acute illness or injury can trigger dramatic changes in laboratory test results, including rapidly deteriorating nutrition status. However, chronic diseases that develop slowly over time also influence these results, making them useful in preventive care. Laboratory test results provide objective data to use in the NCP. Furthermore, because numeric values do not themselves connote personal judgment, this data can often be shared with a patient without implicit or perceived blame.

DEFINITIONS AND USEFULNESS OF NUTRITION LABORATORY DATA

Laboratory assessment is a stringently controlled process. It involves comparing control samples with predetermined substance or chemical constituent (**analyte**) concentrations with every patient specimen. The results obtained must compare favorably with predetermined acceptable values before the patient data can be considered valid. Laboratory data are the only objective data used in nutritional assessment that are "controlled"—that is, the validity of the

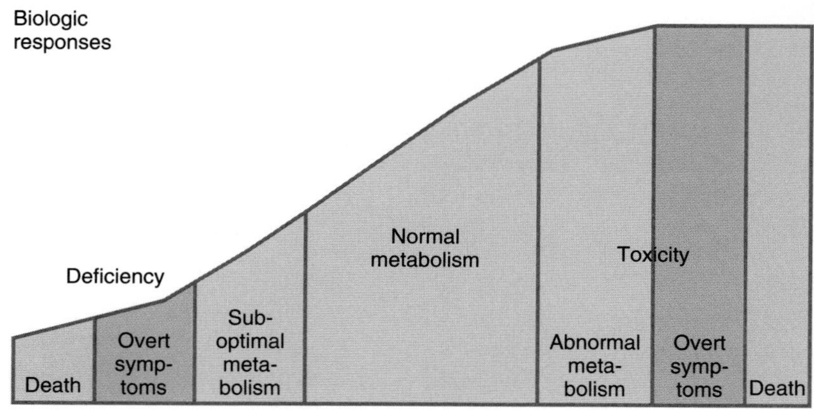

FIGURE 8-1 The size of a nutrient pool can vary continuously from frankly deficient, to adequate, to toxic.

method of its measurement is checked each time a specimen is assayed by also assaying a sample with a known value.

Laboratory-based nutritional testing, used to estimate nutrient availability in biologic fluids and tissues, is critical for assessment of both clinical and subclinical nutrient deficiencies. As shown in Figure 8-1, the size of a nutrient pool can vary continuously from frankly deficient to adequate to toxic. Most of these states can be assessed in the laboratory so that nutritional intervention can occur before a clinical or anthropometric change or a frank deficiency occurs (Litchford, 2009). Single test results must be evaluated in light of the patient's current medical condition, medications, lifestyle choices, age, hydration status, fasting status at the time of specimen collection, and reference standards used by the clinical laboratory. Single test results are useful for screening or to confirm an assessment based on changing clinical, anthropometric, and dietary status. Comparison of current test results to historic baseline test results from the same laboratory is desirable, when available. Changes in laboratory test results that occur over time are often an objective measure of nutrition or pharmacologic interventions.

Specimen Types

Ideally the specimen to be tested reflects the total body content of the nutrient to be assessed. However, the best specimen may not be readily available. The most common specimens for analysis for nutrients and nutrient-related substances include:

- Whole blood: Collected with an anticoagulant if entire content of the blood is to be evaluated; none of the elements are removed; contains red blood cells (RBCs), white blood cells(WBCs), and platelets suspended in plasma
- Serum: The fluid obtained from blood after the blood has been clotted and then centrifuged to remove the clot and blood cells
- Plasma: The transparent (slightly straw-colored) liquid component of blood, composed of water, blood proteins, inorganic electrolytes, and clotting factors
- Blood cells: Separated from anticoagulated whole blood for measurement of cellular analyte content
- Erythrocytes: RBCs
- Leukocytes: WBCs and leukocyte fractions
- Blood spots: Dried whole blood from finger or heel prick that is placed on paper and can be used for selected hormone tests and other tests such as infant phenylketonuria screening
- Other tissues: Obtained from scrapings or biopsy samples
- Urine (from random samples or timed collections): Contains a concentrate of excreted metabolites
- Feces (from random samples or timed collections): Important in nutritional analyses when nutrients are not absorbed and therefore are present in fecal material or to determine composition of gut flora

Less commonly used specimens include the following:

- Breath tests: Noninvasive tool to evaluate nutrient metabolism, use, and malabsorption, particularly of sugars
- Hair and nails: Easy-to-collect tissue for determining exposure to toxic metals; poor indicator of actual body levels of nutrients
- Saliva: Noninvasive medium with a fast turnover; currently is used to evaluate functional adrenal stress and hormone levels
- Sweat: Electrolyte test used to detect sweat chloride levels to determine presence of cystic fibrosis

The hair and nails specimens have significant drawbacks, including potential environmental contamination. Lack of standardized procedures exist for processing, assay, and quality control. Nutrient levels or indices may be less than the amounts that can be measured accurately. However, because these specimens can be collected at the point of care, considerable research is being done to improve their usefulness.

Hair analysis is not particularly useful for assessing levels of minerals such as sodium, magnesium, phosphorus, potassium, calcium, iron, and iodine and good tests already exist for evaluating body functions related to these minerals. However, hair analysis may be helpful in assessing levels of trace elements such as zinc, copper, chromium, and manganese—for which measurements of functional status are not well developed—and levels of mercury, cadmium, and lead, which have negative biologic effects. Hair can be used for deoxyribonucleic acid (DNA) testing and may be useful in the future as a noninvasive methodology to predict genetic predisposition to disease and effectiveness of medical nutrition therapy (see Chapter 5 for more information).

Assay Types

The two fundamental types of laboratory assays are static assays and functional assays. **Static assays** measure the actual level of nutrient in the specimen. Examples of this kind of assay include serum iron and white blood cell ascorbic acid. Although this kind of assay is absolutely specific for the nutrient of interest, specimen nutrient concentrations do not reflect the amount of that substance stored in body pools that are not sampled. Another major limitation of static assays is that recent dietary intake influences the amount of a nutrient found in serum, plasma, or any other fluid or tissue. This problem can be overcome, at least partially, by collecting the specimen following an overnight (8-12 hour) fast.

Functional assays quantitatively measure a biochemical or physiologic activity that depends on the nutrient of interest. This type of assay can be very sensitive for a nutrient at its functional site. A good example of a functional assay is serum ferritin. The concentration of ferritin released into the blood is a function of the iron present in the cellular storage pool. Unfortunately functional assays are not always specific for the nutrient of interest because many physiologic and biochemical functions depend on various biologic factors in addition to the specific nutrient.

NUTRITION INTERPRETATION OF ROUTINE MEDICAL LABORATORY TESTS

Clinical Chemistry Panels

Laboratory tests are ordered as panels or groupings of tests or as individual tests. The most commonly ordered groups of tests are the **basic metabolic panel (BMP)** and the **comprehensive metabolic panel (CMP)** that include groups of laboratory tests defined by the Centers for Medicare and Medicaid Services for reimbursement purposes. The BMP includes eight tests used for screening, and the CMP includes all the tests in the BMP and six additional tests (Box 8-1). Table 8-1 briefly explains these tests, but the information is not exhaustive and reference norms may vary; see Appendix 30 to obtain more detailed information. Clinical chemistry panels provide **nutrition-specific laboratory data** that are used in conjunction with health history, physical examination findings, anthropometric data, nutrition-focused physical assessment and dietary intake data to identify nutrition diagnoses. Follow-up data are used to monitor and evaluate outcomes of various NCP interventions.

BOX 8-1

Two Common Groups of Laboratory Tests

BMP Includes

Glucose
Calcium
Sodium
Potassium
CO_2 (carbon dioxide, bicarbonate)
Chloride
BUN
Creatinine

CMP Includes

Glucose
Calcium
Sodium
Potassium
CO_2 (carbon dioxide, bicarbonate)
Chloride
BUN
Creatinine
Albumin
Total protein
ALP
ALT
AST
Bilirubin

ALP, Alkaline phosphate; *ALT*, alanine aminotransferase; *AST*, aspartate aminotransferase; *BMP*, basic metabolic panel; *BUN*, blood urea nitrogen; *CMP*, comprehensive metabolic panel.

Complete Blood Count

The **complete blood count (CBC)** provides a count of the cells in the blood and description of the RBCs. A hemogram is a CBC with a white blood cell **differential count** (often called a *differential* or *diff*). Table 8-2 provides a list of the basic elements of the CBC and differential, with reference ranges and explanatory comments.

Stool Testing

Fecal samples may be tested for the presence of blood, pathogens, and gut flora. The fecal occult blood test is routinely ordered for adults older than age 50 and younger adults with unexplained anemia. Stool culture testing may be ordered in patients with prolonged diarrhea, especially if food-borne illness is suspected. If pathogenic bacteria are isolated in stool culture, appropriate pharmacologic interventions are initiated. Patients with chronic gastrointestinal (GI) symptoms such as maldigestion or unexplained weight loss or gain may benefit from gut flora testing to identify

TABLE 8-1

Constituents of the Common Serum Chemistry Panels

Analytes	Reference Range*	Significance
Serum Electrolytes		
Na^+	135-145 mEq/L†	Of general interest in monitoring various patients, such as those receiving total parenteral nutrition or who have renal conditions, chronic obstructive pulmonary disease, uncontrolled DM, various endocrine disorders, ascitic and edematous symptoms, or acidotic or alkalotic conditions; decreased K^+ associated with diarrhea, vomiting, or nasogastric aspiration, some drugs, licorice ingestion, and diuretics; increased K^+ associated with renal diseases, crush injuries, infection, and hemolyzed blood specimens
K^+	3.6-5 mEq/L†	
Cl^-	101-111 mEq/L†	
HCO_3^- (or total CO_2)	21-31 mEq/L†	
Glucose	70-99 mg/dL ; 3.9-5.5 mmol/L(fasting)	Fasting glucose >125 mg/dL indicates DM (oral glucose tolerance tests are not needed for diagnosis); fasting glucose >100 mg/dL is indicator of insulin resistance Monitor levels along with triglycerides in those receiving total parenteral nutrition for glucose intolerance
Creatinine	0.6-1.2 mg/dL; 53-106 μmol/L (males) 0.5-1.1 mg/dL; 44-97 μmol/L (females)	Increased in those with renal disease and decreased in those with PEM (i.e., BUN/creatinine ratio >15 : 1)
BUN or urea	5-20 mg urea nitrogen/dL 1.8-7 mmol/L	Increased in those with renal disease and excessive protein catabolism; decreased in those with liver failure and negative nitrogen balance and in females who are pregnant
Albumin	3.5-5 mg/dL; 30-50 g/L	Decreased in those with liver disease or acute inflammatory disease
Serum Enzymes		
ALT	4-36 units/L at 37° C; 4-36 units/L	Increased in those with any of a variety of malignant, muscle, bone, intestinal, and liver diseases or injuries
γ-glutamyltransferase	4-27 units (females) 8-38 units (males)	AST and ALT useful in monitoring liver function in those receiving total parenteral nutrition
ALP	30-120 units/L; 0.5-2 μKat/L	
AST	10-35 IU/L; 0-0.58 μKat/L	
Bilirubin	Total bilirubin 0.3-1 mg/dL; 5.1-17 μmol/L Indirect bilirubin 0.2-0.8 mg/dL; 3.4-12 μmol/L Direct bilirubin 0.1-0.3 mg/dL; 1.7-5.1 μmol/L	Increased in association with drugs, gallstones, and other biliary duct diseases; intravascular hemolysis and hepatic immaturity; decreased with some anemias
Total calcium	8.5-10.5 mg/dL; 2.15-2.57 mmol/L Normal dependent on albumin level	Hypercalcemia associated with endocrine disorders, malignancy, and hypervitaminosis D Hypocalcemia associated with vitamin D deficiency and inadequate hepatic or renal activation of vitamin D, hypoparathyroidism, magnesium deficiency, renal failure, and nephrotic syndrome
Phosphorous (phosphate)	3-4.5 mg/dL; 0.75-1.35 mmol/L	Hyperphosphatemia associated with hypoparathyroidism and decreased intake; hypophosphatemia associated with hyperparathyroidism, chronic antacid ingestion, and renal failure
Total cholesterol	<200 mg/dL; 5.15 mmol/L	Decreased in those with protein-calorie malnutrition, liver diseases, and hyperthyroidism
Triglycerides	<100 mg/dL; <1.13 mmol/L (age and gender dependent)	Increased in those with glucose intolerance (e.g., in those receiving total parenteral nutrition who have combined hyperlipidemia) or in those who are not fasting

*Reference ranges may vary slightly among laboratories.

†mEq/L = 1 mmol/L.

ALP, Alkaline phosphate; *ALT*, alanine aminotransferase; *AST*, aspartate aminotransferase; *BUN*, blood urea nitrogen; *Cl^-*, chlorine; *CO_2*, carbon dioxide; *DM*, diabetes mellitus; *HCO_3^-*, bicarbonate; *K^+*, potassium; *Na^+*, sodium; *PEM*, protein-energy malnutrition.

TABLE 8-2

Constituents of the Hemogram: Complete Blood Count and Differential

Analytes	Reference Range*	Significance
Red blood cells	4.7-6.1 × 10^6/μL (males); 4.7-6.1 10^{12}/L 4.2-5.4 × 10^6/μL (females); 4.2-5.4 10^{12}/L	In addition to nutritional deficits, may be decreased in those with hemorrhage, hemolysis, genetic aberrations, marrow failure, or renal disease or who are taking certain drugs; not sensitive for iron, vitamin B_{12}, or folate deficiencies
Hemoglobin concentration	14-18 g/dL; 8.7-11.2 mmol/L (males) 12-16 g/dL; 7.4-9.9 mmol/L (females) >11 g/dL; >6.8 mmol/L (pregnant females) 14-24 g/dL; 8.7-14.9 mmol/L (newborns)	In addition to nutritional deficits, may be decreased in those with hemorrhage, hemolysis, genetic aberrations, marrow failure, or renal disease or who are taking certain drugs; not sensitive for iron, vitamin B_{12}, or folate deficiencies
Hematocrit	42%-52% (males) 35%-47% (females) 33% (pregnant females) 44%-64% (newborns)	In addition to nutritional deficits, may be decreased in those with hemorrhage, hemolysis, genetic aberrations, marrow failure, or renal disease or who are taking certain drugs; not sensitive for iron, vitamin B_{12}, or folate deficiencies
MCV	80-99 fl 96-108 fl (newborns)	Decreased (microcytic) in presence of iron deficiency, thalassemia trait and chronic renal failure, anemia of chronic disease; increased (macrocytic) in presence of vitamin B_{12} or folate deficiency and genetic defects in DNA synthesis; neither microcytosis nor macrocytosis sensitive to marginal nutrient deficiencies
MCH	27-31 pg/cell 23-34 pg (newborns)	Causes of abnormal values similar to those for MCV
MCHC	32-36 g/dL; 32-36% 32-33 g/dL; 32-33% (newborns)	Decreased in those with iron deficiency and thalassemia trait; not sensitive to marginal nutrient deficiencies
WBC	5-10 × 10^9/L; 5,000-10,000/mm^3 (2 yr-adult) 6-17 × 10^9/L; 6,000-17,000/mm^3 (<2 yr) 9-30 × 10^9; 9,000-30,000/mm^3 (newborns)	Increased (leukocytosis) in those with infection, neoplasia, and stress decreased (leucopenia) in those with PEM, autoimmune diseases, or overwhelming infections or who are receiving chemotherapy or radiation therapy
Differential	55%-70% neutrophils 20-40% lymphocytes 2-8% monocytes 1%-4% eosinophils 0.5%-1% basophils	*Neutrophilia:* Ketoacidosis, trauma, stress, pus-forming infections, leukemia *Neutropenia:* PEM, aplastic anemia, chemotherapy, overwhelming infection *Lymphocytosis:* Infection, leukemia, myeloma, mononucleosis *Lymphocytopenia:* Leukemia, chemotherapy, sepsis, AIDS *Eosinophilia:* Parasitic infestation, allergy, eczema, leukemia, autoimmune disease *Eosinopenia:* Increased steroid production *Basophilia:* Leukemia *Basopenia:* Allergy

*Reference ranges may vary slightly among laboratories.

AIDS, Acquired immune deficiency syndrome; *DNA*, deoxyribonucleic acid; *MCH*, mean corpuscular hemoglobin; *MCHC*, mean corpuscular hemoglobin concentration; *MCV*, mean corpuscular volume; *PEM*, protein-energy malnutrition.

pathologic flora or an imbalance of physiologic flora. In addition, stool tests may be helpful to evaluate the effectiveness of probiotic, prebiotic, and synbiotic use.

Urinalysis

The **urinalysis** test is used as a screening or diagnostic tool to detect substances or cellular material in the urine associated with different metabolic and kidney disorders. Some urinalysis data have broader medical and nutritional significance e.g., glycosuria suggests abnormal carbohydrate use and possibly diabetes. The full urinalysis includes a record of (1) the appearance of the urine, (2) the results of basic tests done with chemically impregnated reagent strips (often called dipsticks) that can be read visually or by an

TABLE 8-3

Chemical Tests in a Urinalysis

Analyte	Expected Value	Significance
Specific gravity	1.010-1.025	Can be used to test and monitor the concentrating and diluting abilities of the kidney and hydration status; low in those with diabetes insipidus, glomerulonephritis, or pyelonephritis; high in those with vomiting, diarrhea, sweating, fever, adrenal insufficiency, hepatic diseases, or heart failure
pH	4.6-8 (normal diet)	Acidic in those with a high-protein diet or acidosis (e.g., uncontrolled DM or starvation), during administration of some drugs, and in association with uric acid, cystine, and calcium oxalate kidney stones; alkaline in individuals consuming diets rich in vegetables or dairy products and in those with a urinary tract infection, immediately after meals, with some drugs, and in those with phosphate and calcium carbonate kidney stones
Protein	2-8 mg/dL	Marked proteinuria in those with nephrotic syndrome, severe glomerulonephritis, or congestive heart failure; moderate in those with most renal diseases, preeclampsia, or urinary tract inflammation; minimal in those with certain renal diseases or lower urinary tract disorders
Glucose	Not detected (2-10 g/dL in DM)	Positive in those with DM; rarely in benign conditions
Ketones	Negative	Positive in those with uncontrolled DM (usually type 1); also positive in those with a fever, anorexia, certain GI disturbances, persistent vomiting, or cachexia or who are fasting or starving
Blood	Negative	Indicates urinary tract infection, neoplasm, or trauma; also positive in those with traumatic muscle injuries or hemolytic anemia
Bilirubin	Not detected	Index of unconjugated bilirubin; increase in those with certain liver diseases (e.g., gallstones)
Urobilinogen	0.1-1 units/dL	Index of conjugated bilirubin; increased in those with hemolytic conditions; used to distinguish among hepatic diseases
Nitrite	Negative	Index of bacteriuria
Leukocyte esterase	Negative	Indirect test of bacteriuria; detects leukocytes

DM, Diabetes mellitus; *GI*, gastrointestinal.

automated reader, and (3) the microscopic examination of urine sediment. Table 8-3 provides a list of the chemical tests performed in a urinalysis and their significance.

ASSESSMENT OF HYDRATION STATUS

Disorders of fluid balance include dehydration and overhydration. Dehydration is a state of negative fluid balance caused by decreased intake, increased losses, and fluid shifts. Overhydration, or edema, occurs when there is an increase in the extracellular fluid volume. The fluid shifts from the extracellular compartment to the interstitial fluid compartment. Overhydration is caused by an increase in capillary hydrostatic pressure or capillary permeability, a decrease in colloid osmotic pressure, or physical inactivity. Laboratory measures of hydration status include serum sodium, blood urea nitrogen, serum osmolality, and urine specific gravity. Although the laboratory tests are important, decisions regarding hydration should only be made in conjunction with other information from physical examination, nutrition-focused physical assessment, and the clinical condition of the patient (see the discussion of acid-base balance in Chapter 7).

Bioelectrical Impedance Analysis

Bioelectrical impedance analysis (BIA) estimates body composition based on the difference in electrical conductive properties of various body tissues. BIA instruments automatically calculate total body water, fat-free mass, and percent body fat. Normal hydration is critical for results to be valid. Individuals who are overhydrated have a lower percent of body fat and a dehydrated individual has an elevated reading for percent body fat.

ASSESSMENT OF STRESS-RELATED PROTEIN-ENERGY MALNUTRITION

Acute illness or trauma causes inflammatory stress. Hormones and cell-mediated responses trigger the breakdown of lean body mass to synthesize cytokines, **positive**

acute-phase proteins, lactic acid, and white blood cells (see Chapter 39). Evaluation of nutrition status of acutely ill patients exhibiting inflammatory stress is difficult because none of the standard laboratory test results consistently reflect changes in protein status at either the onset of illness or with refeeding. It is clear that the acutely ill patient loses protein rapidly because of the inflammatory process. However, increasing exogenous protein intake alone does not attenuate the loss of endogenous protein. Nutrition therapy must be combined with physical therapy to reduce loss of muscle mass (Campbell, 2007; Hays et al., 2009). The following measures should be interpreted cautiously as components of nutritional status because stress changes parameters and values may not reflect nutritional intake of protein accurately.

C-Reactive Protein

Use of inflammatory biomarkers such as **C-reactive protein (CRP)** helps to identify when the acute hypermetabolic period of the inflammatory response wanes. **High-sensitivity CRP (hs-CRP)** is a sensitive measure of chronic inflammation seen in patients with atherosclerosis and other chronic diseases (Bajpai et al., 2010). Both CRP and hs-CRP are nonspecific markers and reflect any type of inflammation. Although the exact function of CRP is unclear, it increases in the initial stages of acute stress—usually within 4 to 6 hours of surgery or other trauma. Furthermore, its level can increase as much as 1000-fold, depending on the intensity of the stress response. When the CRP level begins to decrease, the patient has entered the anabolic period of the inflammatory response when more intensive nutrition therapy may be beneficial. Ongoing assessment and follow-up is required to address changes in nutrition status.

Creatinine

Creatinine is formed from creatine, found almost exclusively in muscle tissue. Serum creatinine is used along with BUN to assess kidney function. Urinary creatinine has been used to assess somatic (muscle) protein status. Creatine is synthesized from the amino acids glycine and arginine with addition of a methyl group from the folate- and cobalamin-dependent methionine–S-adenosylmethionine (SAM)–**homocysteine** cycle. Creatine phosphate is a high-energy phosphate buffer that provides a constant supply of adenosine triphosphate (ATP) for muscle contraction. When creatine is dephosphorylated, some of it is spontaneously converted to creatinine by an irreversible, nonenzymatic reaction. Creatinine has no specific biologic function; it is continuously released from the muscle cells and excreted by the kidneys with little reabsorption.

The use of urinary creatinine to assess somatic protein status is confounded by omnivorous diets. Because creatine is stored in muscle, muscle meats are rich sources. The creatinine formed from dietary creatine cannot be distinguished from endogenously produced creatinine. When a patient follows a meat-restricted diet, the size of the somatic (muscle) protein pool is directly proportional to the amount of creatinine excreted. Therefore men generally have higher serum levels and excrete larger amounts of creatinine than women, and individuals with greater muscular development have higher serum levels and excrete larger amounts than those who are less muscular. Total body weight is not proportional to creatinine excretion, but muscle mass is.

Daily creatinine excretion varies significantly within individuals, probably because of losses in sweat. In addition, the test is based on 24-hour urine collections, which are difficult to obtain. Because of these limitations, urinary creatinine concentration as a marker of muscle mass has limited use in health care settings and is typically used only for doing research. Creatinine excretion rate is related to muscle mass, and is expressed as a percentage of a standard value as shown by the following equation for creatinine-height index (CHI):

$$\text{CHI} = (24 \text{ hr urine creatinine (mg)} \times 100) \div \text{expected 24 hr urine creatinine/cm height}$$

Calculated CHI >80% normal, 60-80% suggests mild skeletal muscle depletion, 40-60% suggests moderate depletion and <40% suggests severe depletion. See Table 8-4. (Blackburn, 1977)

Another predictive equation used to estimate skeletal muscle that does not account for height or gender was proposed by Wang (1996),

$$\text{Skeletal muscle mass (kg)} = 4.1 + 18.9 \times \text{24-hr creatinine excretion (g/day)}$$

Although this equation works well for some individuals, it is not used for sick or injured patients, older adults or for body builders.

TABLE 8-4

Expected Urinary Creatinine Excretions for Adults Based on Height

Adult Males*		Adult Females**	
Height (cm)	Creatinine (mg)	Height (cm)	Creatinine (mg)
157.5	1288	147.3	830
160.0	1325	149.9	851
162.6	1359	152.9	875
165.1	1386	154.9	900
167.6	1426	157.5	925
170.2	1467	160.0	949
172.7	1513	162.6	977
175.3	1555	165.1	1006
177.8	1596	167.6	1044
180.3	1642	170.2	1076
182.9	1691	172.7	1109
185.4	1739	175.3	1141
188.0	1785	177.8	1174
190.5	1831	180.3	1206
193.0	1891	182.9	1240

*Creatinine coefficient males 23 mg/kg "ideal" body weight.

**Creatinine coefficient females 18 mg/kg "ideal" body weight.

Immunocompetence

Protein-energy malnutrition (PEM) is associated with impaired immunocompetence, including depressed cell-mediated immunity, phagocyte dysfunction, decreased levels of complement components, reduced mucosal secretory antibody responses, and lower antibody affinity. Assessing immunocompetence in critically ill patients may be useful in determining the extent of the inadequate nutrition and disease. Assessing immunocompetence is also useful in the patient who is being treated for allergies.

There is no single marker for immunocompetence except for the clinical outcome of infection or allergic response. Laboratory markers with a high degree of sensitivity include vaccine-specific serum antibody production, delayed-type hypersensitivity response, vaccine-specific or total secretory immunoglobulin A in saliva, and the response to attenuated pathogens. Less sensitive markers include natural killer cell cytotoxicity, oxidative burst of phagocytes, lymphocyte proliferation, and the cytokine pattern produced by activated immune cells. Using a combination of markers is currently the best approach to measure immunocompetence (Albers et al., 2005).

Nitrogen Balance

Nitrogen balance studies are used primarily in research studies to estimate the balance between exogenous nitrogen intake (orally, enterally, or parenterally) and renal removal of nitrogen-containing compounds (urinary, fecal, wound), and other nitrogen sources. These studies are not a measure of protein anabolism and catabolism because true protein turnover studies require consumption of labeled (stable isotope) protein to track protein use. Even if useful, nitrogen balance studies are difficult because valid 24-hour urine collections are tedious unless the patient has a catheter. In addition, changes in renal function are common in patients with inflammatory metabolism, making standard nitrogen balance calculations inaccurate without calculation of nitrogen retention (Gottschlich et al., 2001). Clinicians using nitrogen balance to estimate protein flux in critically ill patients must remember the limitations of these studies and that positive nitrogen balance may not mean that protein catabolism has decreased, particularly in inflammatory (disease and trauma) conditions. Adequate nutrition cannot circumvent the inflammatory metabolism.

Hepatic Transport Proteins

Unlike nitrogen balance measurements that assess only short-term changes in whole-body protein status, plasma protein levels integrate protein synthesis and degradation over longer periods. Albumin, prealbumin (PAB); transthyretin [TTHY]), retinol-binding protein, transferrin, and other transport proteins are synthesized in the liver and represent approximately 3% of total body protein. Serum levels of albumin and PAB have traditionally been used as part of nutrition assessment; however, levels may not reflect the patient's protein status. Albumin, PAB, retinol binding protein, and transferrin are **negative acute-phase proteins**; they plummet during inflammatory stress, injury, and illness. Serum levels reflect the severity of illness, but may not reflect current protein status or the effects of nutrient-dense supplemental nutrition. Levels of both albumin and PAB remain nearly normal during uncomplicated starvation as redistribution from the interstitium to the plasma occurs. For these reasons, a well-nourished but stressed patient may have low levels of the hepatic transport proteins, whereas a patient who has had significant weight loss and undernutrition may have normal or close to normal levels.

Albumin

Albumin accounts for approximately 60% of total serum proteins. Albumin transports major blood constituents, hormones, enzymes, medications, minerals, ions, fatty acids, amino acids, and metabolites. However, its major purpose is to maintain colloidal osmotic pressure; providing approximately 80% of colloidal osmotic pressure of the plasma. When serum albumin levels decrease, the water in the plasma moves to the interstitial compartment and promotes edema. The loss of plasma fluid results in hypovolemia; this triggers renal retention of water and sodium. Albumin has a half-life of 18-21 days, and thus does not reflect current protein intake.

Prealbumin (Transthyretin)

Prealbumin (PAB), officially **transthyretin (TTHY)**, is a hepatic protein transported in the serum as a complex of retinol-binding protein and vitamin A. It transports the thyroid hormones triiodothyronine and thyroxine (T_4), along with T_4-binding globulin. Because PAB has a short half-life ($t_{1/2}$ = 2 days), it has been used as an indicator of protein status. Levels of PAB fall precipitously in inflammatory stress and often do not improve with aggressive nutrition support. Serum levels decrease with inflammation, malignancy, and protein-wasting diseases of the intestines or kidneys. Serum levels also decrease in the presence of a zinc deficiency because zinc is required for hepatic synthesis and secretion of PAB. Consider zinc status from dietary intake and medical history, in addition to inflammation, when interpreting low plasma PAB levels.

PAB levels are often maintained in "uncomplicated" malnutrition and decreased in well-nourished individuals who have undergone recent stress or trauma. During pregnancy, the changed estrogen levels stimulate PAB synthesis and serum levels may increase. In nephrotic syndrome, PAB levels may also be increased. Proteinuria and hypoproteinemia are common in nephrotic syndrome; because PAB is rapidly synthesized, a disproportionate percentage of PAB can exist in the blood, whereas other proteins take longer to produce (Litchford, 2010).

Retinol-Binding Protein

The hepatic protein with the shortest half-life ($t_{1/2}$ = 12 hr) is **retinol-binding protein (RBP)**, a small plasma protein that does not pass through the renal glomerulus because it circulates in a complex with PAB. As implied by its name, RBP binds retinol, and transport of this vitamin A metabolite seems to be its exclusive function. RBP is synthesized in the liver and released with retinol. After RBP releases retinol in peripheral tissue, its affinity for PAB decreases, leading to dissociation of the PAB-RBP complex and filtration of apoprotein (apo)-RBP by the glomerulus. The protein is then catabolized in the renal tubule.

The plasma RBP concentration has been shown to decrease in uncomplicated protein calorie malnutrition. However, as a negative acute-phase protein, RBP levels fall in the presence of inflammatory stress and may not improve with refeeding. RBP may not reflect protein status in acutely stressed patients; however, it is not as affected by inflammatory stress as albumin, transferrin, or PAB. Simultaneous secretion of RBP and retinol from the liver means that retinol status also complicates the interpretation of reduced RBP values. RBP cannot reliably be used to assess protein status when the vitamin A status is compromised.

The use of RBP in assessing PEM is complicated by the normal catabolism of apo-RBP by the kidney. Patients with renal failure are likely to have elevated RBP levels, regardless of their protein-energy status, because the RBP is not being catabolized by the renal tubule.

RBP4 is an adipocyte-derived peptide of RBP that influences glucose homeostasis and may play a role in lipoprotein metabolism. Human clinical trials have demonstrated increased RBP4 levels in obesity, insulin resistance, gestational diabetes, proliferative diabetic retinopathy, and nondiabetic stage 5 chronic kidney disease, suggesting a possible relationship between these conditions. Larger clinical trials are needed (Axelsson, 2009; Choi, 2008; Klein, 2010; Li, 2010).

Transferrin

Transferrin is a globulin protein that transports iron to the bone marrow for production of hemoglobin (Hgb). The plasma transferrin level is controlled by the size of the iron storage pool. When iron stores are depleted, transferrin synthesis increases. It has a shorter half-life ($t_{1/2}$ = 8 days) than albumin. Levels diminish with acute inflammatory reactions, malignancies, collagen vascular diseases, and liver diseases. Although the half-life of transferrin is shorter than that of albumin, it still does not respond rapidly enough to changes in nutrient intake to be useful as a measure of protein status in acute-care settings.

LABORATORY DATA TO ASSESS FOR NUTRITIONAL ANEMIAS

Anemia is a condition characterized by a reduction in the number of erythrocytes per unit of blood volume or a decrease in the Hgb of the blood to below the level of usual physiologic need. By convention, anemia is defined as a Hgb concentration below the 95th percentile for healthy reference populations of men, women, or age-grouped children. Anemia is not a disease but a symptom of various conditions, including extensive blood loss, excessive blood cell destruction, or decreased blood cell formation. It is observed in many hospitalized patients and is often a symptom of a disease process; its cause should be investigated. Clinical nutritionists must distinguish between anemia caused by nutritional inadequacies and that caused by other factors. See Chapter 33 for discussion of the management of anemias. For example, hydration problems can mask nutritional anemias or may result in falsely low blood values.

Classification of Anemia

Nutritional deficits are a major cause of decreased Hgb and erythrocyte production. The initial descriptive classification of anemia is derived from the hematocrit (Hct) value or CBC as explained in Table 8-2. Anemias associated with a mean RBC volume of less than 80 fl (femtoliters) are microcytic; those with values of 80 to 99 fl are normocytic; those associated with values of 100 fl or more are macrocytic. (See Chapter 33 on Anemias.) Data from the CBC are helpful in differentiating any nutritional causes of anemia. **Microcytic anemia** is most often associated with iron deficiency, whereas **macrocytic anemia** is generally caused by either folate- or vitamin B_{12}–deficient erythropoiesis. However, because of the low specificity of these indexes, additional data are needed to distinguish between the various nutritional causes and nonnutritional causes, such as thalassemia trait and chronic renal insufficiency. Normocytic anemia is associated with the **anemia of chronic and inflammatory diseases (ACD)**. This type of anemia is associated with rheumatic diseases, chronic heart failure, chronic infection, cancer, severe tissue injury, multiple fractures, and Hodgkin disease. ACD does not respond to iron supplementation.

Other information from the CBC that helps to differentiate the nonnutritional causes of anemia includes leukocyte, reticulocyte, and platelet counts. When these levels are low, marrow failure is indicated; high counts are associated with anemia caused by leukemia or infection. Erythrocyte sedimentation rate testing is ordered when symptoms are nonspecific and if inflammatory autoimmune diseases are suspected. Reticulocytes are large, nucleated, immature RBCs that are released in small numbers with mature cells. When RBC production rates increase, reticulocyte counts also increase. Any time anemia is accompanied by a high reticulocyte count, elevated erythropoietic activity in response to bleeding should be considered. In such cases, stool specimens can be tested for occult blood to rule out chronic GI blood loss. Other causes of a high reticulocyte count include intravascular hemolysis syndromes and an erythropoietic response to therapy for iron, vitamin B_{12}, or folic acid deficiencies.

Normocytic or microcytic anemia may be caused by chronic or acute blood loss, such as from recent surgery, injury, or positive occult stool tests. Note that in those with hemolytic anemias and early iron deficiency anemia, the RBC size may still be normal. Macrocytic anemias include megaloblastic anemia or folate deficiency and pernicious anemia or vitamin B_{12} deficiency. The presence of macrocytic RBCs requires evaluation of both folate and vitamin B_{12} status. Both nutrients arrest DNA synthesis resulting in impaired RBC synthesis and maturation of RBCs. These changes cause large, nucleated cells to be released into the circulation. Although pernicious anemia is categorized as a macrocytic normochromic anemia, approximately 40% of the cases are normocytic.

Tests for Iron Deficiency Anemias

Hematocrit or Packed Cell Volume and Hemoglobin

Hematocrit (Hct) and **hemoglobin (Hgb)** are part of a routine CBC and are used together to evaluate iron status. Hct is the measure of the percentage of RBCs in total blood volume. Usually the Hct percentage is three times the Hgb concentration in grams per deciliter. The Hct value is affected by an extremely high WBC count and hydration status. Individuals living in high altitudes often have increased values. It is common for individuals older than age 50 to have slightly lower levels than younger adults.

The Hgb concentration is a measure of the total amount of Hgb in the peripheral blood. It is a more direct measure of iron deficiency than Hct because it quantifies total Hgb in RBCs rather than a percentage of total blood volume. Hgb and Hct are below normal in the four types of nutritional anemias and should always be evaluated in light of other laboratory values and recent medical history.

Serum Ferritin

Ferritin is the storage protein that sequesters the iron normally gathered in the liver (reticuloendothelial system), spleen, and marrow. As the iron supply increases, the intracellular level of ferritin increases to accommodate iron storage. A small amount of this ferritin leaks into the circulation. This ferritin can be measured by assays that are available in most clinical laboratories. In individuals with normal iron storage, 1 ng/mL of serum ferritin equals approximately 8 mg of stored iron. In healthy adults, the measurement of ferritin that has leaked into the serum is an excellent indicator of the size of the body's iron storage pool.

Ferritin is a positive acute-phase protein, meaning that synthesis of ferritin increases in the presence of inflammation. Ferritin is not a reliable indicator of iron stores in patients with acute inflammation, uremia, metastatic cancer or alcoholic-related liver diseases. Cytokines and other inflammatory mediators can increase ferritin synthesis, ferritin leakage from cells, or both. Elevations in ferritin occur 1 to 2 days after the onset of the acute illness and peak at 3 to 5 days. If iron deficiency also exists, it may not be diagnosed because the level of ferritin would be falsely elevated.

ACD is the primary condition in which ferritin fails to correlate with iron stores. ACD, a common form of anemia in hospitalized patients, occurs in those with cancer or inflammatory or infectious disorders (Thomas and Thomas, 2005). It occurs during inflammation because red cell production decreases as the result of inadequate mobilization of iron from its storage sites. This is caused by the release of cytokines such as interleukin-1 and tumor necrosis factor (TNF), which also inhibit division of erythroid progenitors and may inhibit erythropoietin production. In those with arthritis, depletion of stored iron develops partly because of reduced absorption of iron from the gut. Also the regular use of nonsteroidal antiinflammatory drugs can cause occult GI blood loss. This form of anemia is usually mild and normocytic.

In 30% to 50% of patients, hypochromic (i.e., having inadequate amounts of Hgb), microcytic red cells are made, serum iron levels and total iron-binding capacity (TIBC) are low, and iron stores are normal or elevated. Because iron stores do not decrease, normal amounts of ferritin should be present in the plasma. Although iron stores may be depleted, inflammatory mediators may cause ferritin levels to remain normal. Patients with chronic inflammatory diseases such as rheumatoid arthritis may have reduced or deficient stores. ACD has many forms and must be distinguished from iron deficiency anemia so that inappropriate iron supplementation is not initiated.

Serum Iron

Serum iron measures the amount of circulating iron that is bound to transferrin. However, it is a relatively poor index of iron status because of large day-to-day changes, even in healthy individuals. Diurnal variations also occur, with the highest concentrations occurring midmorning (from 6 AM to 10 AM), and a nadir, averaging 30% less than the morning level, occurring midafternoon. Serum iron should be evaluated in light of other laboratory values and recent medical history to assess iron status.

Total Iron-Binding Capacity and Transferrin Saturation

Total iron-binding capacity (TIBC) is a direct measure of all proteins available to bind mobile iron and depends on the number of free binding sites on the plasma iron-transport protein transferrin. Each transferrin molecule binds ferric ions at each of two binding sites and two bicarbonate ions at separate sites. Intracellular iron availability regulates the synthesis and secretion of transferrin. Therefore the plasma transferrin concentration increases in those with iron deficiency. In addition, when the amount of stored iron available for release to transferrin decreases and dietary iron intake is low, saturation of transferrin decreases.

There are exceptions to the general rule that transferrin saturation decreases and TIBC increases in patients with iron deficiency. For example, TIBC increases in those with hepatitis. It also increases in people with hypoxia, women who are pregnant, or those taking oral contraceptives or receiving estrogen replacement therapy. On the other hand, TIBC decreases in those with malignant disease, nephritis, and hemolytic anemias. Furthermore, the plasma level of transferrin may be decreased in those with PEM, fluid overload, and liver disease. Thus, although TIBC and transferrin saturation are more specific than Hct or Hgb values, they are not perfect indicators of iron status.

An additional concern about the use of serum iron, TIBC, and transferrin saturation values is that normal values persist until frank deficiency actually develops. Thus these tests cannot detect decreasing iron stores and preanemic iron deficiencies.

Tests for Macrocytic Anemias from B Vitamin Deficiencies

Macrocytic anemias include megaloblastic anemia from folate deficiency and pernicious anemia with vitamin B_{12} deficiency. The nutritional causes of macrocytic anemia are related to the availability of folate and vitamin B_{12} (cobalamin) in the bone marrow and require evaluation of both nutrient levels. Both nutrients arrest DNA synthesis by preventing the formation of thymidine monophosphate. Folate and vitamin B_{12} are used at different steps of the synthetic pathway. Impaired RBC synthesis occurs and large, nucleated RBCs are then released into the circulation.

Assessing Folate and Vitamin B_{12} Status

Evaluation for macrocytic anemia includes static measurement of folate and vitamin B_{12} deficiency in blood. They can be assayed using tests of the ability of the patient's blood specimen to support the growth of microbes that require either folate or vitamin B_{12}, radiobinding assays, or immunoassays.

Serum Homocysteine. Folate and vitamin B_{12} are required for the synthesis of SAM, the biochemical precursor involved in the transfer of one-carbon (methyl) groups during many biochemical syntheses. SAM is synthesized from the amino acid methionine by a reaction that includes the addition of a methyl group and the purine base adenine (from ATP). For example, when SAM donates a methyl group for the synthesis of thymine, choline, creatine, epinephrine, and protein and DNA methylation, it is converted to S-adenosylhomocysteine. After losing the adenosyl group, the remaining homocysteine can either be converted to cysteine by the vitamin B_6–dependent transsulfuration pathway or converted back to methionine in a reaction that depends on adequate folate and vitamin B_{12}.

When either folate or vitamin B_{12} is lacking, the homocysteine-to-methionine reaction is virtually blocked, causing homocysteine to build up in the affected tissue and spill into the circulation. The vitamin B_6–dependent transsulfuration pathway can metabolize excess homocysteine. Homocysteine has been shown to be very sensitive to folate and vitamin B_{12} deficiency.

Therefore an elevated homocysteine level indicates either genetic defects involved in the enzymes that catalyze these reactions or a deficiency in folate, vitamin B_{12}, or vitamin B_6. Research indicates that several folate gene polymorphisms contribute risk for several chronic cardiovascular and neurologic disorders (Albert et al., 2009; Fan et al., 2010).

Folate Assessment. Folate is most often simultaneously measured in whole blood with its combined plasma and blood cells, and in the serum alone. The difference between whole-blood folate and serum folate levels is then used to calculate total RBC folate concentration. RBC folate concentration is a better indicator of folate status than serum folate, because folate is much more concentrated in RBCs than in the serum. RBC folate measurement more closely reflects tissue stores and is considered the most reliable indicator of folate status. Folate is absorbed in the jejunum, and its malabsorption has several causes, but a specific test for folate absorption is not available. The presence and extent of deficiency should be assessed in patients with celiac disease, those who have had bariatric surgery, those with a history of long-term use of medications such as anticonvulsants and sulfasalazine, and chronic alcohol consumption. Chapter 5 discusses genetic markers affecting folate absorption and metabolism.

Vitamin B_{12} Assessment. Vitamin B_{12} is measured in the serum, and all indications are that the serum level gives as much information about vitamin B_{12} status as does the RBC level. If vitamin B_{12} status is compromised, intrinsic factor antibodies and parietal cell antibodies are measured; the presence of antibodies suggests the main cause of pernicious anemia. Historically the Schilling test was used to detect defects in vitamin B_{12} absorption; it is rarely used today because the test requires that the patient be given radioactive vitamin B_{12}. Methylmalonic acid (MMA) levels in serum or urine are also useful to assess B_{12} status.

Vitamin B_{12} and Methylmalonic Acid. Once a genetic cause is ruled out, the most straightforward biochemical method for differentiating between folate and vitamin B_{12} deficiencies is to monitor the hyperhomocysteinemia by measuring the serum or urinary MMA level. MMA is formed during the degradation of the amino acid valine and odd-chain fatty acids. MMA is the side product in this metabolic pathway that increases when the conversion of methylmalonic coenzyme A (CoA) to succinyl CoA is blocked by lack of vitamin B_{12}, a coenzyme for this reaction. Therefore deficiency leads to an increase in the MMA pool, which is reflected by the serum or urinary MMA level. The urinary MMA test is more sensitive than the serum B_{12} test because it indicates true tissue B_{12} deficiency. The serum MMA test may give falsely high values in renal insufficiency and intravascular volume depletion. The urinary MMA test is the only B_{12} deficiency assay that has been validated as a screening tool (Morris et al., 2005). Homocysteine and MMA tend to detect impending vitamin deficiencies better than the static assays. This is especially important when assessing the status of certain patients such as vegans or older adults, who could have vitamin B_{12} deficiency associated with central nervous system impairment.

FAT-SOLUBLE VITAMINS

Fat malabsorption often results in impaired absorption of vitamins A, E, D, and K. Factors including low luminal pH, bile salts below the critical micellar concentration, and inadequate triglyceride hydrolysis can interfere with normal bile salt micelle formation, causing impaired absorption of fat-soluble vitamins. Individuals with fat malabsorptive disorders, including those who have had bariatric surgery, are at greatest risk of deficiencies of fat-soluble vitamins. See Appendix 30 for further discussion of tests for assessing specific vitamin adequacy.

Vitamin A

Vitamin A status can be estimated using serum **retinol** and the normal level in adults is 30-80 mcg/dL. A primary deficiency of vitamin A can result from inadequate intake, fat malabsorption, or liver disorders. A secondary deficiency of vitamin A may be due to decreased bioavailability of provitamin A carotenoids or interference with vitamin A absorption, storage, or transport (e.g., celiac disease, cystic fibrosis, pancreatic insufficiency, malabsorptive weight loss surgery, or bile duct obstruction). Vitamin A deficiency is common in prolonged PEM. Because of shared absorptive mechanisms with vitamin D, serum retinol should always be assessed in the presence of vitamin D supplementation (see Chapter 3). Acute or chronic vitamin A toxicity is defined as retinol levels greater than 100 mcg/dL. Chronic vitamin A toxicities are associated with loss of hair; dry mucous membranes; dry, rough skin; and even cortical bone loss and fractures.

Vitamin D

Individual vitamin D status can be estimated by measuring plasma **25-hydroxy vitamin D (25-[OH]D_3)** levels. Current clinical practice reference ranges have been updated by the 2011 IOM (IOM, 2011). Traditional levels defining vitamin D sufficiency have been based on the lowest threshold value for plasma 25-(OH)D_3 (approximately 80 nmol/L or 32 ng/mL) that prevents secondary hyperparathyroidism, increased bone turnover, bone mineral loss, or seasonal variations in plasma parathyroid hormone. The IOM review concluded that individuals are at risk of deficiency at serum 25(OH)D_3 levels below 30 nmol or 12 ng/mL and that practically all persons have sufficient serum levels at 50 nmol or 20 ng/mL. Current clinical practice reference ranges define insufficiency as 50-80 nmol/L or 20-31 ng/mL, and deficiency is defined as less than 50 nmol/L or 20 ng/mL. Serum levels even higher at 90-100 nmol/L (36-40 ng/mL) are recommended by some (Bischoff-Ferrari et al., 2006). Optimal levels of 25(OH)D_3 have not been defined and the measurement of serum levels lacks standardization and calibration.

A deficiency may be caused by inadequate dietary intake, inadequate exposure to sunlight, or malabsorption. Deficiency of vitamin D can also lead to secondary malabsorption of calcium. Calcium malabsorption occurs in chronic renal failure because renal hydroxylation is required to activate vitamin D, which promotes synthesis of a calcium-binding protein in intestinal absorptive cells (Mosekilde, 2005). See Chapter 36.

Vitamin K

Vitamin K status can be estimated using prothrombin time (PT). PT is used to evaluate the common pathway of blood clotting. The synthesis of clotting factors II, VII, IX, and X are vitamin K–dependent. **Osteocalcin** or bone G1a protein (BGP), a bone turnover marker, may also be used to assess vitamin K status. BGP is a vitamin K–dependent protein that is increased with bone formation and depressed with increased bone loss. A reduced vitamin K status is associated with reduced BGP or serum osteocalcin levels. The relationship may explain the pathophysiologic findings of vitamin K–deficiency osteoporosis.

WATER-SOLUBLE VITAMINS AND TRACE MINERALS

Vitamin B_{12} and folate are the most common water-soluble vitamin deficiencies reported in adults. Frank deficiencies of other water-soluble vitamins and trace minerals are uncommon in populations that consume a variety of whole foods and fortified foods. Thiamin deficiency has been reported in individuals who chronically consume high levels of alcohol with inadequate thiamin intake, in those with persistent vomiting, and in those with impaired absorption because of disease or surgery. To assess thiamin status, thiamin diphosphate in whole blood is measured because plasma and serum levels reflect recent dietary changes and may be misleading. Subclinical deficiencies of water-soluble vitamins and other trace minerals may be present in some individuals. However the current methodologies for evaluating nutritional status of these components are both expensive and controversial. See Appendix 30 for further discussion of tests for assessing specific vitamin and trace mineral adequacy.

CHRONIC DISEASE RISK ASSESSMENT

Lipid Indices of Cardiovascular Risk

Serum lipoprotein and cholesterol levels are directly implicated in the development of atherosclerosis and are affected by modifiable factors, including diet. Patients undergoing lipid assessments should be fasting for 12 hours at the time of blood sampling. Fasting is necessary primarily because triglyceride levels rise and fall dramatically in the postprandial state, and low-density lipoprotein (LDL) cholesterol values are calculated from measured total serum cholesterol and high-density lipoprotein cholesterol concentrations. This calculation, based on the Friedewald equation, is most accurate when triglyceride concentrations are less than 400 mg/dL. The Friedewald equation gives an estimate of fasting LDL cholesterol levels that is generally within 4 mg/dL of the true value when triglyceride concentrations are less than 400 mg/dL.

Risk for cardiovascular disease (CVD) appears to be more related to the number of atherogenic lipoprotein particles in the serum than it is to the total volume of cholesterol. Differentiating subparticles of LDL by size and grouping by pattern has been used; however, the subparticle testing is costly and findings do not serve as independent markers for risk (Box 8-2). In patients with metabolic syndrome, lowering LDL does not reflect similar reductions in LDL particle levels (Rosenson, 2008). LDL contains the atherogenic apolipoprotein B (apoB). Some researchers propose that

BOX 8-2

Lipid and Lipoprotein Cardiovascular Disease Risk Factors

LDL: Elevated levels are atherogenic
VLDL density: Remnants are atherogenic
Triglyceride concentrations: Elevated levels are atherogenic
Lp(a): Elevated levels are atherogenic
apoprotein B: Increased concentration is atherogenic
apoprotein A-I: Decreased concentration is atherogenic
hs-CRP: Elevated levels, without acute or chronic inflammatory condition, are atherogenic
Serum homocysteine: Increased; greater risk
RBP4: Elevated levels may identify early insulin resistance and associated cardiovascular risk factors

HDL, High-density lipoprotein; *hs-CRP*, high-sensitivity C-reactive protein; *IDL*, intermediate-density lipoprotein; *LDL*, low-density lipoprotein; *Lp(a)*, lipoprotein little a; *RBP4*, retinol-binding protein 4; *VLDL*, very low–density lipoprotein.

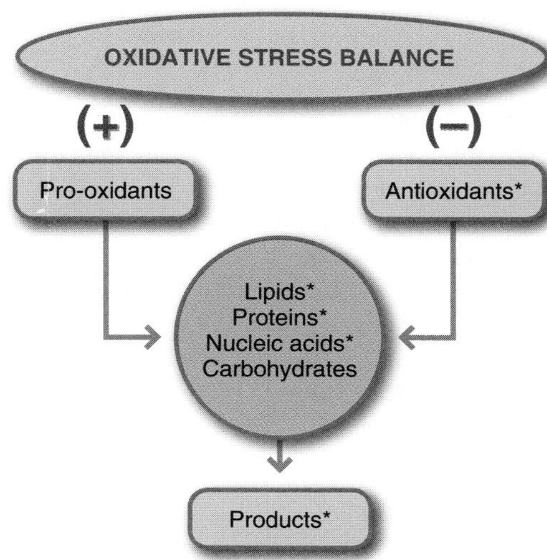

FIGURE 8-2 Steps in maintaining the balance between prooxidants (reactive oxygen species) and antioxidants. The compounds marked with an asterisk (*) have been used as markers of oxidative stress balance.

measuring the concentration of apoB provides a direct measure of the number of circulating atherogenic lipoprotein particles and is superior to LDL for predicting probability of CVD (Barter, 2006; Brunzell, 2008). Clinicians may suggest testing the genetic profile for the **apolipoprotein E (apoE) phenotype**, which precedes CVDs in some populations (Chasman et al., 2009). Other inflammatory genes are under study. See Chapter 34 for further discussion of the lipid profile and cardiovascular risk.

Hemoglobin A1C and Diabetes

In adults with normal glucose control, approximately 4% to 6% of the total Hgb is glycosylated. The percent of glycohemoglobin in the blood is directly related to the average blood glucose levels for the preceding 2-3 months. **Hemoglobin A1C (Hgb A1C)** does not reflect more recent changes in glucose levels. It is useful in differentiating between short-term hyperglycemia in individuals under stress or who have had an acute myocardial infarction and diabetes. It has been added as a diagnostic criteria for diagnosis of diabetes mellitus once the initial value is confirmed by a repeat Hgb A1C >6.5% or plasma glucose >200 mg/dL (11 mmol/L). Hgb A1C is not used as a diagnostic criterion for gestational diabetes because of changes in red cell turnover (American Diabetes Association [ADA], 2011).

Hgb A1C can be correlated with daily mean plasma glucose. Each 1% change in Hgb A1C represents approximately 35 mg/dL change in mean plasma glucose. Test results are useful to provide feedback to patients about changes they have made in their nutritional intakes (ADA, 2011). See Chapter 31 for further discussion of Hgb A1C and diabetes management.

Oxidative Stress

Aging and many diseases, including CVD, Alzheimer disease, Parkinson disease, inflammatory bowel disease, and cancer, are initiated in part by **oxidative stress** as evidenced by free radical oxidation of lipids, nucleic acids, or proteins (Figure 8-2). Oxidative stress is imposed on cells as a result of three factors: (1) an increase in oxidant generation, (2) a decrease in antioxidant protection, or (3) a failure to repair oxidative damage. Cell damage is caused by **reactive oxygen species (ROS)**. ROS are either free radicals, reactive anions containing oxygen atoms, or molecules containing oxygen atoms that can either produce free radicals or are chemically activated by them (Blanck et al., 2003). These products include the superoxide radical (O_2^-) hydroxyl radical (OH), and hydrogen peroxide. The formation of ROS is sometimes, but not always, mediated by certain essential trace elements (e.g., iron, copper, chromium, and nickel).

In the case of CVD, the ROS react with unsaturated fatty acids in LDL, creating lipid peroxides, another free radical species. Like all free radicals, lipid peroxides initiate the oxidation of other compounds, including apolipoprotein, the protein present in lipoproteins. This oxidation leads to the formation of free radical products throughout the large, heterogeneous lipoprotein particle. Cells associated with the arterial wall ingest the resulting oxidized lipoproteins. Once present in these cells, additional metabolism of this modified complex does not seem to occur. Over time, other pathophysiologic responses stabilize the deposited oxidized lipoprotein as atherosclerotic plaque.

Antioxidant Status

An indirect way of assessing the level of oxidative stress is to measure the levels of antioxidant compounds present in body fluids. Oxidative stress is related to levels of the following:

- Antioxidant vitamins (tocopherols and ascorbic acid)
- Dietary phytochemicals with antioxidant properties (e.g., carotenoids)
- Minerals with antioxidant roles (e.g., selenium)
- Endogenous antioxidant compounds and enzymes (e.g., superoxide dismutase, glutathione)

More precisely, the concentration of these compounds correlates with the balance between their intake and production and their use during the inhibition of free radical compounds.

Markers of Oxidative Stress

Biomarkers of oxidative stress status and inflammation have been associated with many chronic conditions and risk factors. Measurement of intracellular antioxidant thiols such as glutathione can be estimated using the free oxygen radical test via spectrophotometric techniques on specimens obtained from finger sticks. However, further standardization of protocols for assays and methods of combining and integrating multiple panels of biomarkers of oxidative stress and inflammation are needed to facilitate evaluation of biomarkers for risk factor prediction. Although some intervention studies examining the effects of dietary supplements, diet, and exercise on biomarkers of oxidative stress and inflammation have been done, the data have been inconclusive, and more studies are needed to understand the underlying mechanisms.

The most commonly used chemical markers of oxidative stress are presented in Table 8-5. Some tests measure the presence of one class of free radical products, and others measure the global antioxidant capacity of plasma or a plasma fraction. These tests have been promoted on the assumption that knowledge of the total antioxidant capacity of the plasma or plasma fraction might be more useful than knowledge of the individual concentrations of free radical markers or antioxidants. This total antioxidant activity is determined by a test that assesses the combined antioxidant capacities of the constituents. Unfortunately, the results of these tests include the antioxidant capacities of compounds such as uric acid and albumin, which are not compounds of interest. In other words, no one type of assay is likely to provide a global picture of the oxidative stress to which an individual is exposed. A new noninvasive method that may become useful in the future is a method that uses Raman spectroscopy in the biophotonic antioxidant laser scanner (see *New Directions:* Raman Spectroscopy Used to Measure Antioxidant Capacity).

Despite this lack of correlation or specificity of assays of oxidative stress, two assays seem promising. One is the immunoassay myeloperoxidase used in conjunction with CRP to predict CVD mortality risk (Heslop, 2010). The second assay is the measurement of the compounds F_2

NEW DIRECTIONS

Raman Spectroscopy Used to Measure Antioxidant Capacity

Noninvasive measurements of clinical parameters are always preferable to those requiring blood, urine, or tissue. Raman spectroscopy is just such a measurement technique and may become widely used in the future. A laser light is pointed toward the fat pad of the palm. As the laser light penetrates the skin, the amount of carotenoids (all-trans-beta-carotene, lycopene, alpha-carotene, gamma-carotene, phytoene, phytofluene, sepapreno-betacarotene, dihydro-beta-carotene, astaxanthin, canthaxanthin, zeaxanthin, lutein, beta-apo-8′ carotenal, violaxanthins, and rhodoxanthin) is measured at the cellular level. Because all carotenoids have a carbon backbone with alternating carbon double and single bonds, the vibration of these bonds can be detected with Raman spectroscopy. Raman spectroscopy has been used to assess carotenoids in precancerous skin lesions as well as in the retina to assess early stages of macular degeneration (Ermakov et al., 2005).

Carotenoids are powerful antioxidants, and because they are part of the "antioxidant network," a measure of their presence can give a good assessment of the antioxidant capacity of the cell. The Raman spectroscopy score also correlates inversely with urinary isoprostanes, a measure of oxidative stress (Carlson et al., 2006).

Serum carotenoids significantly correlate with skin carotenoids, as measured using Raman spectroscopy and the biophotonic laser scanner (Smidt et al., 2004; Zidichouski et al., 2004). Serum carotenoids are a good measure of the absorptive capacity of the individual (see Chapters 1 and 3). Thus an individual with a diet high in fruits and vegetables, and therefore large amounts of dietary carotenoids, usually has a high carotenoids antioxidant score. The antioxidant score, or the numeric result from this scan, can be used to determine how well a person is processing carotenoid antioxidants and whether the antioxidants are reaching the cell where they exert their protective functions. The number, which seems to be in the range of 40,000 and higher in those with optimal health, increases with greater consumption of carotenoid-containing fruits and vegetables, consumption of carotenoid-containing nutritional supplements, smoking cessation, and loss of excess body fat (Carlson et al., 2006). The measurement is quick, easy, and inexpensive, making it a possible assessment tool for nutrition professionals in the future.

TABLE 8-5

Markers of Oxidative Stress

Class	Functions	Comment
Class I: Antioxidant Markers		
Vitamin C (plasma or leukocyte)	Specific inhibitor of water-soluble radicals	Measured by chromatography, capillary electrophoresis, or an automated enzymatic assay
α-Tocopherol	Inhibitor of lipid peroxidation	Measured by chromatography or capillary electrophoresis
γ-Tocopherol	An inhibitor of the nitrous oxide radical	Measured by chromatography or capillary electrophoresis
Carotenoids	Primarily inhibitors of lipid peroxidation	Measured by chromatography and spectroscopy; includes α- and β-carotenes, lycopene, cryptoxanthin, zeaxanthin, and lutein
Class II: Endogenous Systems		
Glutathione assay	Detoxifies the ROS H_2O_2	Measured by plasma or erythrocyte glutathione or ratio of reduced to oxidized glutathione
Class III: Global Tests of Antioxidant Capacity		
LDL oxidative susceptibility	Reflects the concentration of antioxidants in LDLs	In vitro determination of the rate of formation of LDL oxidation products called *conjugated dienes*
ORAC	NA	Measures decrease in fluorescence over time; reflects the total antioxidant capacity of the specimen
TRAP	NA	Measures total antioxidant capacity; reflects the levels of uric acid and albumin
ABTS	NA	ABTS assay in commercial by available kit; also called *total antioxidant status*
8-OH-d-G	Reflects ongoing oxidative stress in body	Emerging biomarker; elevated levels associated with inadequate intake of carotenoids, antioxidant rich foods and supplemental antioxidants
Class IV: Products of Free Radical Reactions		
Myeloperoxidase	NA	Used in conjunction with hs-CRP to predict CVD risk
Isoprostane	No known function	Primary form, isoprostane $F_{2\alpha}$, measured by chromatography or an immunoassay that is available commercially and can be rapidly performed
TBARS	NA	A colorimetric assay that is easy to perform but not specific for oxidation products; measures products of lipid peroxidation called *aldehydes* (e.g., malondialdehyde)

ABTS, 2,2′-Azino-bis (3-ethyl benzytiazoline-sulfonic acid); *CVD*, cardiovascular disease; H_2O_2, hydrogen peroxide; *hs-CRP*, high-sensitivity C-reactive protein; *LDL*, low-density lipoprotein; *ORAC*, oxygen radical absorbance capacity; *NA*, not applicable; *ROS*, reactive oxygen species; *TBARS*, thiobarbituric acid reactive substances; *TRAP*, total peroxyl radical trapping parameter; *8-OH-d-G*, urinary 8-hydroxy-2′deoxyguanosine.

isoprostanes either in plasma or urine (Harrison and Nieto, 2004). This test measures the presence of a continuously formed free radical compound that is produced by free radical oxidation of specific polyunsaturated fatty acids. Isoprostanes are prostaglandin-like compounds that are produced by free radical mediated peroxidation of lipoproteins. Elevated isoprostane levels are associated with oxidative stress, and clinical situations of oxidative stress such as hepatorenal syndrome, rheumatoid arthritis, atherosclerosis, and carcinogenesis (Roberts and Fessel, 2004).

CLINICAL SCENARIO 1

Clara is seen at County Hospital emergency room. She has a long history of yo-yo dieting and alcohol abuse. In the last 6 months she has had the stomach flu that lasted 4 days, seasonal flu, and colitis. She works at a retirement community as a kitchen assistant. One of the benefits of her job is one free meal the days she works. Clara keeps snack foods, beer, and soft drinks in her apartment and eats most meals at fast-food restaurants when she is not at work. Clara has called in sick to work for the past 3 days. She has a poor work history, and her employer questions her motives for missing work.

Continued

CLINICAL SCENARIO 1—cont'd

Her employer told her if she is really too sick to come to work, she must see her doctor for a medical release to return to work. The emergency department doctor orders laboratory tests and Clara is admitted to the hospital. She tells the doctor that she cannot remember what has happened in the last few days. Her medical profile today is:

Age	32 years old
Height	5′9″
Weight	285 lb
Frame	Large
Glucose	142 mg/dL; 7.8 mmol/L
Calcium	9.1 mg/dL; 2.27 mmol/L
Sodium	149 mEq/L; 149 mmol/L
Potassium	3.8 mEq/L; 3.8 mmol/L
CO_2	25 mEq/L/ 25 mmol/L
Chloride	106 mEq/L; 106 mmol/L
BUN	30 mg/dL; 10.7 mmol/L
Creatinine	0.9 mg/dL; 79.6 μmol/L
Albumin	4.8 g/dL; 48 g/L
Total protein	8.5 g/dL; 85 g/L
ALP	35 U/L; 0.5 μkat/L
ALT	28 units/L; 28 units/L
AST	23 units/L; 0.38 μkat/L
Bilirubin, total	1.5 mg/dL; 25.65 μmol/L
RBC	5.1×10^6 mL; 5.1×10^{12} L
Hgb	11.5 g/dL; 7.1 mmol/L
Hct	28%; 0.28
MCV	102 mm^3; 102 fL
MCH	33 pg
MCHC	26 g/dL; 26%
WBC	12×10^9

Clara is referred for medical nutrition therapy. Assess her nutrition status using the data provided. Note that Clara is scheduled for a series of tests. She is given intravenous fluids, a blood transfusion and is made NPO which means no food or fluid by mouth. The preliminary findings indicate several tumors obstructing the gall bladder. Exploratory surgery is scheduled tomorrow.

Nutrition Diagnostic Statement

Altered laboratory values related to disordered eating pattern as evidenced by signs of nutritional anemia and dehydration.

Nutrition Care Questions

1. Estimate Clara's energy and protein needs based on her anthropometric data.
2. Considering Clara's medical history, what does her laboratory report for hemoglobin, hematocrit, mean corpuscular volume, mean corpuscular hemoglobin, and mean corpuscular hemoglobin concentration suggest?
3. What does her laboratory report for ALP, AST, and ALT values suggest?
4. What does her laboratory report for sodium, blood urea nitrogen, and creatinine suggest about her hydration status?
5. What does her laboratory report for blood urea nitrogen and creatinine suggest about her renal status?
6. How would you expect Clara's laboratory tests to change 24 hours after major surgery?
7. What additional laboratory tests would be helpful for a comprehensive nutrition assessment?

ALP, Alkaline phosphate; *ALT*, alanine aminotransferase; *AST*, aspartate aminotransferase; *BUN*, blood urea nitrogen; CO_2, carbon dioxide; *Hct*, hematocrit; *Hgb*, hemoglobin; *MCH*, mean corpuscular hemoglobin; *MCHC*, mean corpuscular hemoglobin concentration; *MCV*, mean corpuscular volume; *RBC*, red blood cell; *WBC*, white blood cell.

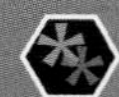

CLINICAL SCENARIO 2

Omar is seen at the Western Medical Clinic today complaining of fatigue, fluttery heart beat, and tightness in his chest after he walks up two flights of steps. He works in a high-stress job as a computer software engineer. Omar has a history of high blood pressure and takes medication daily. He is concerned about his risk for heart disease. He has gained 18 pounds after quitting smoking and getting married a year ago. Omar eats breakfast and lunch at fast-food restaurants. His favorite foods are sweet rolls and fast foods. His wife prepares the evening meal. Omar reports drinking three to five beers nightly while watching television. He does not get any regular exercise except walking up two flights of steps at his office building. His medical profile is a follows: 39-year-old male; height: 5′10″; weight: 225 lb, large frame.

Laboratory Report

Glucose	155 mg/dL; 8.6 mmol/L
Calcium	10.1 mg/dL; 2.52 mmol/L
Sodium	142 mEq/L; 142 mmol/L
Potassium	3.2 mEq/L; 3.2 mmol/L
CO_2	22 mEq/L; 22 mmol/L
Chloride	103 mEq/L; 103 mmol/L
BUN	46 mg/dL; 16.4 mmol/L
Creatinine	0.6 mg/dL; 53 μmol/L
Albumin	2.8 g/dL; 28 g/L
Total protein	6.0 g/dL; 60 g/L
ALP	30 U/L; 0.5 μkat/L
ALT	48 units/L; 48 units/L
AST	40 units/L; 0.67 μkat/L

CLINICAL SCENARIO 2—cont'd

Bilirubin, total	1.0 mg/dL; 17.1 µmol/L
RBC	5.5 × 10^6 mL; 5.5 × 10^{12} L
Hgb	15.5 g/dL; 9.6 mmol/L
Hct	45%; 0.45
MCV	92 mm^3; 92 fl
MCH	30 pg
MCHC	31 g/dL; 31%
WBC	7 × 10^9

Other Labs

Total serum cholesterol	250 mg/dL; 6.5 mmol/?
HDL cholesterol	40 mg/dL; 1.03 mmol/L
LDL cholesterol	140 mg/dL; 3.6 mmol/L
Triglycerides	350 mg/dL; 3.95 mmol/L
Homocysteine	18 mmol/L
Blood pressure	186/99 mm Hg

Nutrition Diagnostic Statement

Altered laboratory values related to recent weight gain and smoking cessation as evidenced by elevated blood pressure, symptoms of metabolic syndrome, and dietary history.

Nutrition Care Questions

1. Based on the health history, social history, fasting laboratory report, and medical profile, what risk factors does Omar have for chronic diseases?
2. Considering Omar's medical profile, what does his laboratory report for glucose, blood urea nitrogen, sodium, potassium, and creatinine suggest?
3. What does his laboratory report for alkaline phosphate, aspartate aminotransferase, and alanine aminotransferase suggest?
4. What does his lipid profile and homocysteine suggest?
5. Omar is referred for medical nutrition therapy. Assess his nutrition status based on the data provided.

ALP, Alkaline phosphate; *ALT*, alanine aminotransferase; *AST*, aspartate aminotransferase; *BUN*, blood urea nitrogen; CO_2, carbon dioxide; *Hct*, hematocrit; *HDL*, high-density lipoprotein; *Hgb*, hemoglobin; *LDL*, low-density lipoprotein; *MCH*, mean corpuscular hemoglobin; *MCHC*, mean corpuscular hemoglobin concentration; *MCV*, mean corpuscular volume; *RBC*, red blood cell; *WBC*, white blood cell.

USEFUL WEBSITES

National Center for Health Statistics, National Health and Nutrition Examination Survey
http://www.cdc.gov/nchs/nhanes.htm

National Cholesterol Education Program—ATPIII Guidelines
http://www.nhlbi.nih.gov/guidelines/cholesterol/index.htm

The Merck Manual of Diagnosis and Therapy Section I—Nutritional Disorders
www.merck.com/pubs/mmanual/section1/sec1.htm

REFERENCES

Albers R, et al: Markers to measure immunomodulation in human nutrition intervention studies, *Br J Nutr* 94:452, 2005.

Albert MA, et al: Candidate genetic variants in the fibrinogen, methylenetetrahydrofolate reductase, and intercellular adhesion molecule-1 genes and plasma levels of fibrinogen, homocysteine, and intercellular adhesion molecule-1 among various race/ethnic groups: data from the Women's Genome Health Study, *Am Heart J* 157:777, 2009.

American Diabetes Association (ADA): Diagnosis and classification of diabetes mellitus, *Diabetes Care* 34(3):62, 2011.

Axelsson J, et al: Serum retinol-binding protein concentration and its association with components of the uremic metabolic syndrome in nondiabetic patients with chronic kidney disease stage 5, *Am J Nephrol* 29:447, 2009.

Bajpai A, et al: Should we measure C-reactive protein on earth or just on JUPITER? *Clin Cardiol* 33:190, 2010.

Barter PJ, et al: Apo B versus cholesterol in estimating cardiovascular risk and in guiding therapy: report of the thirty person/ten-country panel, *J Intern Med* 259:247, 2006.

Bischoff-Ferrari HA, et al: Estimation of optimal serum concentrations of 25-hydroxyvitamin D for multiple health outcomes, *Am J Clin Nutr* 84:18, 2006.

Blackburn G, et al: Nutritional and metabolic assessment of the hospitalized patient, *JPEN* 1:11-21, 1977.

Blanck HM, et al: Laboratory issues: use of nutritional biomarkers, *J Nutr* 133:888S, 2003.

Brunzell JD, et al: Lipoprotein management in patients with cardiometabolic risk: consensus conference report from the American Diabetes Association and the American College of Cardiology Foundation, *J Am Coll Cardiol* 51:1512, 2008.

Campbell WW: Synergistic use of higher-protein diets or nutritional supplements with resistance training to counter sarcopenia, *Nutr Rev* 65:416, 2007.

Carlson JJ, et al: Associations of antioxidant status, oxidative stress with skin carotenoids assessed by Raman spectroscopy (RS), *FASEB J* 20:1318, 2006.

Chasman DI, et al: Forty-three loci associated with plasma lipoprotein size, concentration, and cholesterol content in genome-wide analysis, *PLoS Genet* 5:e1000730, 2009.

Choi S, et al: High plasma retinol binding protein-4 and low plasma adiponectin concentrations are associated with severity of glucose intolerance in women with previous gestational diabetes mellitus, *J Clin Endocrinol Metab* 93:3142, 2008.

Ermakov IV, et al: Resonance Raman detection of carotenoids antioxidants in living human tissue, *J Biom Opt* 10:064028, 2005.

Fan AZ, et al: Gene polymorphisms in association with emerging cardiovascular risk markers in adult women, *BMC Med Genet* 11:6, 2010.

Gottschlich MM, et al, editors: *The science and practice of nutrition support: a case-based core curriculum*, Dubuque, Ia, 2001, Kendall/Hunt Publishing.

Harrison DG, Nieto FJ: *NHLBI Workshop on Oxidative Stress/Inflammation meeting proceedings*, Bethesda, Md, 29 November 2004. Accessed 18 April 2010 from http://www.nhlbi.nih.gov/meetings/workshops/oxidative-stress.htm.

Hays NP, et al: Effects of whey and fortified collagen hydrolysate protein supplements on nitrogen balance and body composition in older women, *J Am Diet Assoc* 109:1082, 2009.

Heslop C, et al: Myeloperoxidase and C-reactive protein have combined utility for long-term prediction of cardiovascular mortality after coronary angiography, *J Am Coll Cardiol* 55:1102, 2010.

IOM (Institute of Medicine): *Dietary Reference Intakes for Calcium and Vitamin D*, Washington, DC, 2011, The National Academies Press.

Klein K, et al: Retinol-binding protein 4 in patients with gestational diabetes mellitus, *J Women's Health* Feb 2010. (E-pub ahead of print.)

Li Z, et al: Serum retinol-binding protein 4 levels in patients with diabetic retinopathy, *J Int Med Res* 38:95, 2010.

Litchford, MD: *Common denominators of declining nutritional status*, Greensboro, N.C., 2009, CASE Software & Books.

Litchford MD: *Laboratory assessment of nutritional status: bridging theory and practice*, Greensboro, N.C., 2010, CASE Software & Books.

Morris MC, et al: Dietary folate and B_{12} intake and cognitive decline among community-dwelling older persons, *Arch Neurol* 62:641, 2005.

Mosekilde L: Vitamin D and the elderly, *Clin Endocrinol* 62:265, 2005.

Roberts LJ, Fessel JP: The biochemistry of the isoprostane, neuroprostane, and isofuran pathways of lipid peroxidation, *Chem Phys Lipids* 128:173, 2004.

Rosenson R, et al: Lipoprotein particles identify residual risk after lipid goal achievement in patients with the metabolic syndrome, *Circulation* 118:S1151, 2008.

Smidt CR, et al: Non-invasive Raman spectroscopy measurement of human carotenoid status, *FASEB J* 18:A480 (Abstract), 2004.

Thomas C, Thomas L: Anemia of chronic disease: pathophysiology and laboratory diagnosis, *Lab Hematol* 11:14, 2005.

Wang, ZM, Gallagher, D, Nelson, M Total-body skeletal muscle mass: evaluation of 24-h urinary creatinine excretion by computerized axial tomography. *AJCN* 1996, 63(6); 863-869.

Zidichouski, et al: Clinical validation of a novel Raman spectroscopic technology to non-invasively assess carotenoid status in humans, *Am Coll Nutr* 23:468, 2004.

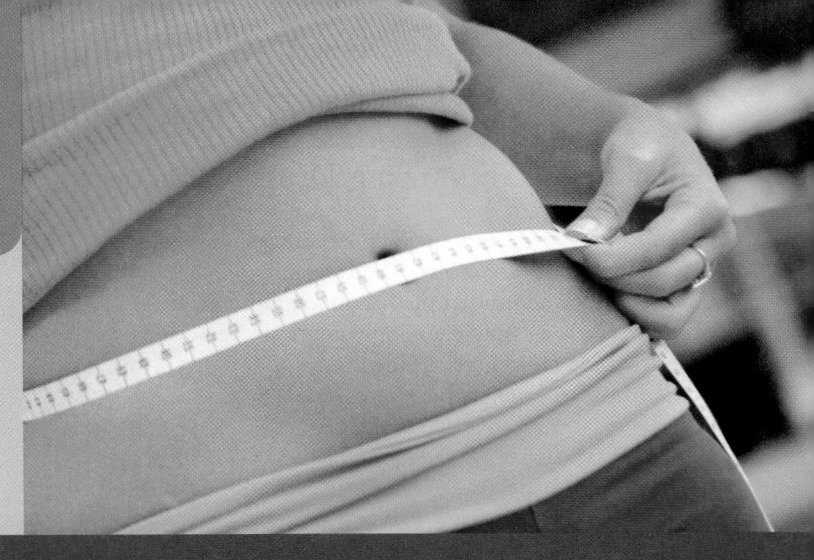

CHAPTER 9

Zaneta M. Pronsky, MS, RD, LDN, FADA
Sr. Jeanne P. Crowe, PharmD, RPh, RPI

Clinical: Food-Drug Interactions

KEY TERMS

absorption
acetylation
adsorption
bioavailability
biotransformation
black box warning
cytochrome P-450 enzyme system
distribution
drug-nutrient interaction
excipient
excretion
food-drug interaction
gastrointestinal pH
half-life
metabolism
pharmacodynamics
pharmacogenomics
pharmacokinetics
physical incompatibility
polypharmacy
pressor agents
side effect
therapeutically important
unbound fraction

The management of many diseases requires drug therapy, frequently involving the use of multiple drugs. Food-drug interactions can change the effects of drugs, and the therapeutic effects or side effects of medications can affect the nutrition status of an individual. Alternatively, the diet and use of supplements, genetic makeup, or the nutritional status of the patient can decrease the efficacy of a drug or increase its toxicity.

The terms *drug-nutrient interaction* and *food-drug interaction* are often used interchangeably. In actuality, drug-nutrient interactions are some of the many possible food-drug interactions. **Drug-nutrient interactions** include specific changes to the pharmacokinetics of a drug caused by a nutrient or nutrients or changes to the kinetics of a nutrient caused by a drug. **Food-drug interaction** is a broader term that also includes the effects of a medication on nutritional status. Nutritional status may be affected by the side effects of a medication, which could include an effect on appetite or the ability to eat.

For clinical, economic, and legal reasons, it is important to recognize food-drug interactions. Food-drug interactions that reduce the efficacy of a drug can result in longer or repeated stays in health care facilities, the use of multiple drugs, and deterioration of the patient because of the effects of the disease. Additional health problems can occur because of long-term drug-nutrient interactions. An example of this type of interaction is the long-term effects of corticosteroids on calcium metabolism and the resulting osteoporosis. Medical team members should be aware that **therapeutically important** food-drug interactions can do the following:

- Alter the intended response to the medication
- Cause drug toxicity
- Alter normal nutritional status

BOX 9-1

Benefits of Minimizing Drug Interactions

Medications achieve their intended effects.
Patients do not discontinue their drug.
The need for additional medication is minimized.
Fewer caloric or nutrient supplements are required.
Adverse side effects are avoided.
Optimal nutritional status is preserved.
Accidents and injuries are avoided.
Disease complications are minimized.
The cost of health care services is reduced.
There is less professional liability.
Licensing agency requirements are met.

From Pronsky ZM, Crowe JP: Food-medication interactions, ed 16, Birchrunville, Pa, 2010, Food-Medication Interactions.

Awareness of these interactions enables the health care professional and patient to work together to avoid or minimize problems (Box 9-1).

PHARMACOLOGIC ASPECTS OF FOOD-DRUG INTERACTIONS

Medication is administered to produce a pharmacologic effect in the body or, more specifically, in a target organ or tissue. To achieve this goal, the drug must move from the site of administration into the bloodstream and eventually to the site of drug action. In due course the drug may be changed to active or inactive metabolites and is ultimately eliminated from the body. An interaction between the drug and food, a food component, or a nutrient can alter this process at any point. Food-drug interactions may be divided into two broad types: (1) pharmacodynamic interactions, which affect the pharmacologic action of the drug; and (2) pharmacokinetic interactions, which affect the movement of the drug into, around, or out of the body.

Pharmacodynamics

Pharmacodynamics is the study of the biochemical and physiologic effects of a drug. The mechanism of action of a drug might include the binding of the drug molecule to a receptor, enzyme, or ion channel, resulting in the observable physiologic response. Ultimately this response may be enhanced or attenuated by the addition of other substances with similar or opposing actions. **Pharmacokinetics** is the study of the time course of a drug in the body involving the absorption, distribution, metabolism (biotransformation), and excretion of the drug. **Absorption** is the process of the movement of the drug from the site of administration to the bloodstream. This process depends on (1) the route of administration, (2) the chemistry of the drug and its ability to cross biologic membranes, (3) the rate of gastric emptying (for orally administered drugs) and gastrointestinal (GI) movement, and (4) the quality of the product formulation. Food, food components, and nutrition supplements can interfere with the absorption process, especially when the drug is administered orally.

Distribution occurs when the drug leaves the systemic circulation and travels to various regions of the body. Body areas of distribution vary with different drugs, depending on the drug's chemistry and ability to cross biologic membranes. The rate and extent of blood flow to an organ or tissue strongly affect the amount of drug that reaches the area. Many drugs are highly bound to plasma proteins such as albumin. The bound fraction of drug does not leave the vasculature and therefore does not produce a pharmacologic effect. Only the **unbound fraction** is able to produce an effect at a target organ.

A drug is eliminated from the body as either an unchanged drug or a metabolite of the original compound. The major organ of **metabolism**, or **biotransformation**, in the body is the liver, although other sites, such as the intestinal membrane, contribute to variable degrees. One of the more important enzyme systems that facilitate drug metabolism is the **cytochrome P-450 enzyme system**. This is a multienzyme system in the smooth endoplasmic reticulum of numerous tissues that is involved in phase I of liver detoxification (see Chapter 20). Food or dietary supplements may either increase or inhibit the activity of this enzyme system, which can significantly change the rate or extent of drug metabolism. The general tendency of the process of metabolism is to transform a drug from a lipid-soluble to a more water-soluble compound that can be handled more easily by the kidneys and excreted in the urine.

Renal **excretion** is the major route of elimination for drugs and drug metabolites either by glomerular filtration or tubular secretion. To a lesser extent drugs may be eliminated in feces, bile, and other body fluids. Under certain circumstances, such as a change in urinary pH, drugs that have reached the renal tubule may pass back into the bloodstream. This process is known as *tubular resorption.* The recommended dose of a drug generally assumes normal liver and kidney function. The dose and dosing interval of an excreted drug or active metabolite must be adjusted to meet the degree of renal dysfunction in patients with kidney disease (see Chapter 36).

RISK FACTORS FOR FOOD-DRUG INTERACTIONS

Patients must be assessed individually for the effect of food on drug action and the effect of drugs on nutrition status. Interactions can be caused or complicated by **polypharmacy**, nutrition status, genetics, underlying illness, special diets, nutrition supplements, tube feeding, herbal or phytonutrient products, alcohol intake, drugs of abuse, nonnutrients in food, excipients in drugs or food, allergies, or intolerances. Poor patient compliance and physicians' prescribing patterns further complicate the risk. Drug-induced malnutrition occurs most commonly during long-term treatment for chronic disease, and older patients are at a particularly high risk for many reasons (see *Focus On:* Polypharmacy in Older Adults).

◎ FOCUS ON

Polypharmacy in Older Adults

Older patients are more likely to take multiple drugs, both prescription and over-the-counter, than are younger patients. They have a higher risk of food-drug interactions because of physical changes related to aging, such as the increase in the ratio of fat tissue to lean body mass, a decrease in liver mass and blood flow, and impairment of kidney function. Illness, cognitive or endocrine dysfunction, and ingestion of restricted diets also increase this risk. Malnutrition and dehydration affect drug kinetics. The use of herbal or phytonutrient products has increased significantly in all developed countries, including use by older adults. Drugs of abuse or excessive alcohol intake are often missed in the older patient.

Central nervous system side effects of drugs can interfere with the ability or desire to eat. Drugs that cause drowsiness, dizziness, ataxia, confusion, headache, weakness, tremor, or peripheral neuropathy can lead to nutritional compromise, particularly in older patients. Recognition of these problems as a drug side effect rather than a consequence of disease or aging can be overlooked. An old list known as the Beers criteria lists some medications that can cause cardiac, gastrointestinal or urinary effects, although the usefulness of the Beers criteria is now controversial (Steinman et al., 2009).

Care must be taken to evaluate intake of interacting nutrients (in the oral diet, supplements, or tube feedings) when specific drugs are used. Examples are vitamin K with warfarin (Coumadin); calcium and vitamin D with tetracycline; and potassium, sodium, and magnesium with loop diuretics such as furosemide (Lasix). Patients with Parkinson disease may be concerned with the amount and timing of protein intake because of interaction with levodopa (Sinemet, Dopar). The interdisciplinary team, which includes the physician, pharmacist, nurse, and dietitian, must work together to plan and coordinate the medication regimen and diet and nutritional supplements to preserve optimal nutrition status and minimize food-drug interactions (Figure 9-1).

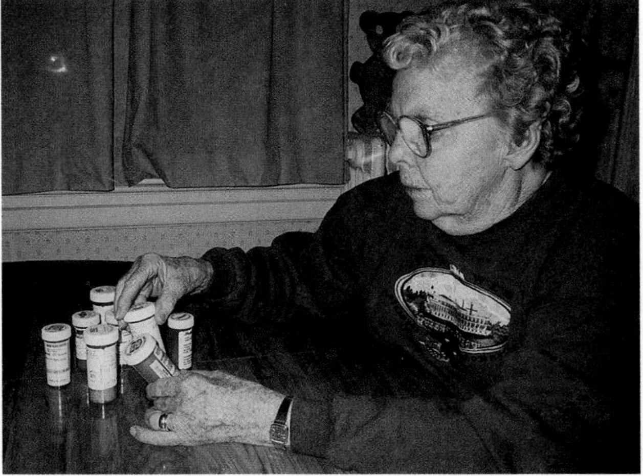

FIGURE 9-1 As a result of the increased potential for illness with aging, older adults often take multiple drugs, both prescription and over-the-counter preparations. This places them at increased risk for drug-drug and food-drug interactions.

Existing malnutrition places patients at greater risk for drug-nutrient interactions. Protein alterations—specifically low albumin levels—and changes in body composition secondary to malnutrition can affect drug disposition by altering protein binding and drug distribution. Patients with active cancer or human immunodeficiency virus (HIV) infection who have significant anorexia and wasting are at special risk because of the high prevalence of malnutrition and reduced intakes. Treatment modalities such as chemotherapy and radiation may also exacerbate nutritional disturbances. For example, cisplatin (Platinol-AQ) and other cytotoxic agents commonly cause mouth sores, nausea, vomiting, diarrhea, anorexia, and reduced food intake.

Drug disposition can be affected by alterations in the GI tract, such as vomiting, diarrhea, hypochlorhydria, mucosal atrophy, and motility changes. Malabsorption caused by intestinal damage from disease such as cancer, celiac disease, or inflammatory bowel disease creates greater potential for food-drug interactions. Body composition is another important consideration in determining drug response. In obese or older patients, the proportion of adipose tissue to lean body mass is increased. In theory, accumulation of fat-soluble drugs such as the long-acting benzodiazepines (e.g., diazepam [Valium]) is more likely to occur. Accumulation of a drug and its metabolites in adipose tissue may result in prolonged clearance and increased toxicity (Spriet et al., 2009). In older patients this interaction may be complicated by decreased hepatic clearance of the drug.

The developing fetus, infant, and pregnant woman are also at high risk for drug-nutrient interactions. Many drugs have not been tested on these populations, making it difficult to assess the risks of negative drug effects, including food-drug interactions.

Pharmacogenomics

Gene-nutrient interactions reflect the genetic heterogeneity among humans, environmental factors and dietary chemicals, and diverse physiologies (Wise and Kaput, 2009). Because the efficacy and safety disparity of drugs varies according to race and genetic variants, pharmacogenetic knowledge is important for the interpretation and prediction of drug interaction-induced adverse events (Bai, 2010). **Pharmacogenomics** involves genetically determined variations that are revealed solely by the effects of drugs and can be a driver for nutrigenomics, as discussed in Chapter 5

(Ghosh et al., 2007). Food-drug interaction ramifications are seen in glucose-6-phosphate dehydrogenase (G6PD) enzyme deficiency, slow inactivation of isoniazid (INH) or phenelzine (Nardil), and warfarin (Coumadin) resistance. Warfarin resistance affects individual requirements for and response to warfarin.

Slow inactivation of INH used in tuberculosis (TB) represents the effect of slow **acetylation**, a conjugation reaction that metabolizes and inactivates amines, hydrazines, and sulfonamides. "Slow acetylators" are persons who metabolize these drugs more slowly than average because of inherited lower levels of the hepatic enzyme acetyl transferase. Therefore unacetylated drug levels remain higher for longer periods in these persons than in those who are "rapid acetylators." For example, the **half-life** of INH for fast acetylators is approximately 70 minutes, whereas the half-life is more than 3 hours for slow acetylators. A dose of drug prescribed normally for fast acetylators can be toxic for slow acetylators. Elevated blood levels of affected drugs in slow acetylators increase the potential for food-drug interactions. Slow inactivation of INH increases the risk of pyridoxine deficiency and peripheral neuropathy. Slow inactivation of phenelzine, a monoamine oxidase (MAO) inhibitor, increases the risk for hypertensive crisis if foods high in tyramine are consumed. Dapsone (DDS) and hydralazine (Apresoline) are also metabolized by acetylation and are affected by inherited differences in acetylase enzymes.

Deficiency of G6PD is an X-chromosome–linked deficiency of G6PD enzyme in red blood cells that can lead to neonatal jaundice, hemolytic anemia, or acute hemolysis. Most common in African, Middle Eastern, and Southeast Asian populations, it is also called *favism*. Intake of fava beans, aspirin, sulfonamides, and antimalarial drugs can cause hemolysis and acute anemia in G6PD-deficient persons. The potential exists for food-drug interactions in G6PD deficiency resulting from the ingestion of fava beans (broad beans), as well as vitamin C or vitamin K.

Another factor that affects drug metabolism is genetically different activity of cytochrome P450 (CYP) enzymes. Therapeutic proteins affect the disposition of drugs that are metabolized by these enzymes (Lee et al., 2010). "Slow metabolizers" may have less of a specific enzyme or their enzymes may be less active. Such individuals have a higher risk of adverse drug effects. Slow CYP2D6 metabolizers make up approximately 5% to 10% of whites, whereas approximately 20% of Asians are CYP2C19 poor metabolizers. Tests are now available to analyze deoxyribonucleic acid (DNA) to determine variations in the activity of these two enzymes. CYP2D6 and CYP2C19 metabolize approximately 25% of all drugs, including many antipsychotics, antidepressants, and narcotics. Slow metabolizers achieve a higher blood level with usual doses of such drugs, whereas fast metabolizers may have an unpredictable response as a result of rapid metabolism of the drug (*Medical Letter*, 2005).

Drug response genotyping helps to determine which drugs will be effective, depending on an individual's genetic makeup (see Chapter 5). The ability to predict response to specific drugs determines more effective treatments for cancer, mental illness, and even pain management. Genotyping will help reduce adverse drug reactions, including food-medication interactions.

EFFECTS OF FOOD ON DRUG THERAPY

Drug Absorption

The presence of food and nutrients in the stomach or intestinal lumen may reduce the absorption of a drug. **Bioavailability** describes the fraction of an administered drug that reaches the systemic circulation. If a medication is administered intravenously, its bioavailability is 100%, but bioavailability decreases because absorption and metabolism are incomplete when taken orally. Examples of a critically significant reduction in drug absorption are the antiosteoporosis drugs alendronate (Fosamax), risedronate (Actonel), or ibandronate (Boniva). Absorption is negligible if these drugs are given with food and reduced by 60% if taken with coffee or orange juice. The manufacturer's instructions for alendronate or risedronate are to take the drug on an empty stomach with plain water at least 30 minutes before any other food, drink, or medication. Ibandronate must be taken at least 60 minutes before any other food, drink, or medication. The absorption of the iron from supplements can be decreased by 50% if taken with food. Iron is best absorbed when taken with 8 oz of water on an empty stomach. If iron must be taken with food to avoid GI distress, it should not be taken with bran, eggs, high-phytate foods, fiber supplements, tea, coffee, dairy products, or calcium supplements, because each of these can decrease iron absorption (see Chapter 3).

Various mechanisms may contribute to the reduction in the rate or extent of drug absorption in the presence of food or nutrients. The presence and type of meal or food ingested influence the rate of gastric emptying. Gastric emptying may be delayed by the consumption of high-fiber meals and meals with high fat content. In general, a delay in drug absorption is not clinically significant as long as the extent of absorption is not affected. However, delayed absorption of antibiotics or analgesics may be clinically significant. Chelation reactions occur between certain medications and divalent or trivalent cations, such as iron, calcium, magnesium, zinc, or aluminum, and the absorption of drugs may be reduced by chelation with one of these metal ions.

The Parkinson disease drug entacapone (Comtan) chelates with iron; therefore the iron must be taken 1 hour before or 2 hours after taking the drug. The antibiotics ciprofloxacin (Cipro) and tetracycline (Achromycin-V or Sumycin) form insoluble complexes with calcium in dairy products or calcium-fortified foods and beverages; calcium, magnesium, zinc, or iron supplements; or aluminum in antacids, thus preventing or reducing the absorption of both drug and nutrient (Neuhofel et al., 2002). The optimal approach to avoid this interaction is to stop noncritical supplements for the duration of the antibiotic prescription. If this is not possible, particularly with magnesium or with long-term antibiotic use, it is advisable to give the drug at least 2 hours before or 6 hours after the mineral.

Adsorption, or the adhesion to food or a food component, is another mechanism by which drug absorption is slowed or reduced. A high-fiber diet may decrease the absorption of tricyclic antidepressants such as amitriptyline (Elavil), leading to loss of therapeutic effect of the antidepressant because of the adsorption of the drug to the fiber. Likewise, the cardiovascular drug digoxin (Lanoxin) should not be taken with high-phytate foods such as wheat bran or oatmeal.

Gastrointestinal pH is another important factor in the absorption of drugs. Any situations resulting in changes in gastric acid pH, such as achlorhydria or hypochlorhydria, may reduce drug absorption. An example of such an interaction is the failure of ketoconazole (Nizoral) to clear a *Candida* infection in patients with HIV infection or in persons taking potent acid-reducing agents for gastroesophageal reflux disease (GERD). Ketoconazole achieves optimal absorption in an acid medium. Because of the high prevalence of achlorhydria in HIV infected patients, dissolution of ketoconazole tablets in the stomach is reduced, leading to impaired drug absorption. This is also a concern with hypochlorhydria in persons receiving chronic acid suppression therapy, such as antacids, histamine 2 (H_2) receptor antagonists (e.g., famotidine [Pepcid]), or proton-pump inhibitors (e.g., omeprazole [Prilosec]). Ingestion of ketoconazole with an acidic liquid such as cola or a dilute hydrochloric acid (HCl) solution may improve bioavailability in these patients.

The presence of food in the stomach enhances the absorption of some medications, such as the antibiotic cefuroxime axetil (Ceftin) or the antiretroviral drug saquinavir (Invirase). These drugs are prescribed to be taken after a meal to reduce the dose that must be taken to reach an effective level. The bioavailability of cefuroxime axetil is substantially greater when taken with food, compared with taking it in the fasting state.

Medication and Enteral Nutrition Interactions

Continuous enteral feeding is an effective method of providing nutrients to patients who are unable to swallow or eat adequately. However, use of the feeding tube to administer medication can be a problem. When liquid medications are mixed with enteral formulas, incompatibilities may occur. Types of **physical incompatibility** include granulation, gel formation, and separation of the enteral product; these frequently clog feeding tubes and interrupt delivery of nutrition to the patient. Examples of drugs that can cause granulation and gel formation are ciprofloxacin suspension (Cipro), chlorpromazine (Thorazine) concentrate, ferrous sulfate elixir, guaifenesin (Robitussin expectorant), and metoclopramide (Reglan) syrup (Wohlt et al., 2009). Emulsion breakage occurs when acidic pharmaceutical syrups are added to enteral formulas, more commonly in enteral formulas with intact protein and less so with hydrolyzed protein or free amino acids.

Most compatibility studies of medication and enteral products have focused on the effect of the drug on the integrity of the enteral product. More important is the effect of the enteral product on the bioavailability of the drug. This area requires much more research as feeding tube placement becomes a more common practice. Bioavailability problems are common with phenytoin (Dilantin) suspension and tube feeding. Because blood levels of phenytoin are routinely performed to monitor the drug, much information exists about the reduction of phenytoin bioavailability when given with enteral feedings. Stopping the tube feeding before and after the phenytoin dose is generally suggested; a 2-hour feeding-free interval before and after the dose of phenytoin is administered can safely be recommended.

Information may not be readily available concerning a drug and enteral product interactions even though the manufacturer may have unpublished information about their drug's interaction with enteral products. Checking with the manufacturer's medical information department may yield more information for the clinician.

Drug Distribution

Albumin is the most important drug-binding protein in the blood. Low serum albumin levels, often the result of inadequate protein intake and poor nutrition, provide fewer binding sites for highly protein-bound drugs. Fewer binding sites mean that a larger free fraction of drug will be present in the serum. Only the free fraction (unbound fraction) of a drug is able to leave the vasculature and exert a pharmacologic effect at the target organ. Patients with albumin levels below 3 g/dL are at increased risk for adverse effects from highly protein-bound drugs. Usual adult doses of highly protein-bound drugs in such persons may produce more pronounced pharmacologic effects than the same dose in persons with normal serum albumin levels. A lower dose of such drugs is often recommended for patients with low albumin levels. In addition, the risk for displacement of one drug from albumin-binding sites by another drug is greater when albumin levels are less than 3 g/dL.

The anticoagulant warfarin, which is 99.9% serum protein–bound, and the anticonvulsant phenytoin, which is greater than 90% protein-bound, are common drugs used in older patients. Low albumin levels tend to be more common in older patients and in critically ill patients. In the case of warfarin, higher levels of free drug lead to risk of excessive anticoagulation and bleeding. Phenytoin toxicity can result from higher serum levels of free phenytoin.

Drug Metabolism

Enzyme systems in the intestinal tract and the liver, although not the only sites of drug metabolism, account for a large portion of the drug metabolizing activity in the body. Food can both inhibit and enhance the metabolism of medication by altering the activity of these enzyme systems. A diet high in protein and low in carbohydrates can increase the hepatic metabolism of the antiasthma drug theophylline (Theo-Dur).

Conversely, a substance found in grapefruit and grapefruit juice can inhibit the intestinal metabolism of drugs such as calcium channel blockers that are dihydropyridine derivatives (felodipine [Plendil]) (Sica, 2006) and some 3-hydroxy-3-methylglutaryl (HMG)–coenzyme A (CoA) reductase inhibitors such as simvastatin (Zocor). Grapefruit inhibits the cytochrome P-450 3A4 enzyme system responsible for the oxidative metabolism of many orally administered drugs. This interaction appears to be clinically significant for drugs with low oral bioavailability, which are substantially metabolized and inactivated in the intestinal tract by the cytochrome P-450 3A4 enzyme in the intestinal wall. When grapefruit or grapefruit juice is ingested, the metabolizing enzyme is irreversibly inhibited, which reduces the normal metabolism of the drug. This reduction in metabolism allows more of the drug to reach the systemic circulation; the increase in blood levels of unmetabolized drug results in a greater pharmacologic effect and possible toxicity. Unfortunately, the effects of grapefruit on intestinal cytochrome P-4503A4 last up to 72 hours, until the body can reproduce the enzyme. Therefore separating the ingestion of the grapefruit and the drug does not appear to alleviate this interaction.

Seville oranges (used in some marmalades but not in commercial orange juice), pomelos, and tangelos may also cause similar reactions (Egashira et al., 2003). Even a small amount of these foods may be dangerous and should be totally avoided with some drugs such as the immunosuppressant tacrolimus (Prograf) or simvastatin (Zocor). These foods may be taken in small amounts with other drugs such as fluvoxamine (Luvox). The interaction is not significant in drugs that are not metabolized by cytochrome P-450 3A4 in the intestinal wall, such as the HMG-CoA reductase inhibitors pravastatin (Pravachol) or fluvastatin (Lescol).

Competition between food and drugs such as propranolol (Inderal) and metoprolol (Lopressor) for metabolizing enzymes in the liver may alter the first-pass metabolism of these medications. Drugs absorbed from the intestinal tract by the portal circulation are first transported to the liver before they reach the systemic circulation. Because many drugs are highly metabolized during this first pass through the liver, only a small percentage of the original dose is actually available to the systemic circulation and the target organ. In some cases, however, this percentage can be increased by concurrent ingestion of food with the drug. When food and drug compete for the same metabolizing enzymes in the liver, more of the drug is likely to reach the systemic circulation, which can lead to a toxic effect if the dose of the drug is titrated to an optimal level in the fasting state.

Drug Excretion

Food and nutrients can alter the resorption of drugs from the renal tubule. Resorption of the antimanic agent lithium (Lithobid or Eskalith) is closely associated with the resorption of sodium. When sodium intake is low or when a patient is dehydrated, the kidneys resorb more sodium. In the person treated with lithium, the kidney resorbs lithium as well as sodium under these conditions. Higher lithium levels and possible toxicity result. When excess sodium is ingested, the kidneys eliminate more sodium in the urine and likewise more lithium. This produces lower lithium levels and possible therapeutic failure.

Drugs that are weak acids or bases are resorbed from the renal tubule into the systemic circulation only in the nonionic state. An acidic drug is largely in the nonionic state in urine with an acidic pH, whereas a basic drug is largely in a nonionic state in urine with an alkaline pH. A change in urinary pH by food may change the amount of drug existing in the nonionic state, thus increasing or decreasing the amount of drug available for tubular resorption. Foods such as milk, most fruits (including citrus fruits), and most vegetables are urinary alkalinizers (see *Clinical Insight*: Urinary pH—How Does Diet Affect It? in Chapter 36). This change can affect the ionic state of a basic drug such as the antiarrhythmic agent quinidine gluconate (Quinaglute Dura-Tabs). In alkaline urine the drug will be predominately in the nonionic state and available for resorption from the urine into the systemic circulation, which may lead to higher blood quinidine levels. The excretion of memantine (Namenda), a drug used to treat Alzheimer dementia, is also decreased by alkaline pH, thus raising the drug blood levels. Higher drug levels increase the risk of toxicity. This interaction is most likely to be clinically significant when the diet is composed exclusively of a single food or food group. Patients should be cautioned against initiating major diet changes without consulting their physician or dietitian.

Licorice, or glycyrrhizic acid, is an extract of glycyrrhiza root used in "natural" licorice candy. Approximately 100 g of licorice (the amount in two or more twists of natural licorice) can increase cortisol concentration, resulting in pseudohyperaldosteronism with increased sodium resorption, water retention, increased blood pressure, and greater excretion of potassium. The action of diuretics and antihypertensive drugs may be antagonized. The resultant hypokalemia may alter the action of some drugs (Pronsky and Crowe, 2010).

EFFECTS OF DRUGS ON FOOD AND NUTRITION

Many of the interactions discussed in this section are the opposite of those discussed previously under the Effects of Food on Drug Therapy. For instance, the chelation of a mineral with a medication not only decreases the absorption and therefore the action of the drug, but also decreases the absorption and availability of the nutrient.

Nutrient Absorption

Medication can decrease or prevent nutrient absorption. Chelation reactions between medications and minerals (metal ions) reduce the amount of mineral available for absorption. An example is tetracycline (Achromycin-V or Sumycin) and ciprofloxacin, which chelates calcium found in supplements or in dairy products such as milk or yogurt. This is also true for other divalent or trivalent cations such as iron, magnesium, and zinc found in individual mineral supplements or multivitamin-mineral supplements.

Standard advice is to take the minerals at least 2 to 6 hours apart from the drug.

Adsorption also can decrease nutrient absorption. Antihyperlipidemic, bile acid sequestrant cholestyramine (Questran) is also used to treat diarrhea. It adsorbs fat-soluble vitamins A, D, E, and K. Vitamin supplementation is recommended with long-term use of this drug, especially when it is taken more than once a day. More than 2 tbsp (30 ml) of mineral oil per day decreases absorption of fat-soluble vitamins A, D, E, and K. It is advised to take the mineral oil in the morning and the vitamins at least 2 hours later, primarily with chronic mineral oil use.

Drugs can reduce nutrient absorption by influencing the transit time of food and nutrients in the gut. Cathartic agents and laxatives reduce transit time and may cause diarrhea, leading to losses of calcium and potassium. Diarrhea may be induced by drugs containing sorbitol, such as syrup or solution forms of furosemide (Lasix), valproic acid (Depakene), carbamazepine (Tegretol), trimethoprim/sulfamethoxazole (Septra), or by drugs that increase peristalsis such as the gastric mucosa protectant misoprostol (Cytotec).

A drug also can prevent nutrient absorption by changing the GI environment. H_2-receptor antagonists, such as famotidine (Pepcid) or ranitidine (Zantac), and proton-pump inhibitors, such as omeprazole (Prilosec) or esomeprazole (Nexium), are antisecretory drugs used to treat ulcer disease and GERD. They inhibit gastric acid secretion and raise gastric pH. These effects may impair absorption of vitamin B_{12} by reducing cleavage from its dietary sources. Cimetidine (Tagamet) is an antagonist that also reduces intrinsic factor secretion; this can be a problem for vitamin B_{12} absorption and can result in vitamin B_{12} deficiency with long-term use. Because of the hypothesized effect on calcium absorption, protein pump inhibitors were thought to raise the risk of osteoporosis (Fourniet et al., 2009) but recent information refutes this hypothesis (Targownik et al., 2010).

Drugs with the greatest effect on nutrient absorption are those that damage the intestinal mucosa. Damage to the structure of the villi and microvilli inhibits the brush-border enzymes and intestinal transport systems involved in nutrient absorption. The result is general or varying degrees of specific malabsorption, which can alter the ability of the GI tract to absorb minerals, especially iron and calcium. Damage to the gut mucosa commonly results from chemotherapeutic agents, nonsteroidal antiinflammatory drugs (NSAIDs), and long-term antibiotic therapy. NSAIDs may adversely affect the colon by causing a nonspecific colitis or by exacerbating a preexisting colonic disease (Valley et al., 2006). Patients with NSAID-induced colitis present with bloody diarrhea, weight loss, and iron deficiency anemia; the pathogenesis of this colitis is still controversial.

Drugs that affect intestinal transport mechanisms include (1) colchicine, an antiinflammatory agent used to treat gout; (2) paraaminosalicylic acid, an anti-TB drug; (3) sulfasalazine (Azulfidine), used to treat ulcerative colitis; and (4) trimethoprim (antibiotic in sulfamethoxazole-trimethoprim [Bactrim]) and antiprotozoal agent pyrimethamine (Daraprim). The first two agents impair absorption of vitamin B_{12}; the others are competitive inhibitors of folate transport mechanisms.

Nutrient Metabolism

A drug may increase the metabolism of a nutrient, causing it to pass through the body faster, resulting in higher requirements; or a drug may cause vitamin antagonism by blocking conversion of a vitamin to the active form. Anticonvulsants phenobarbital and phenytoin induce hepatic enzymes and increase the metabolism of vitamins D and K, and folic acid (Crawford, 2005; Nicolaidou et al., 2006). Supplements of these vitamins are often prescribed with these drugs. Carbamazepine (Tegretol) has been reported to affect the metabolism of biotin, vitamin D, and folic acid, leading to possible depletion. Measurement of vitamin D levels and supplementation if indicated are recommended with these anticonvulsants (Holick, 2007).

The anti-TB drug INH blocks the conversion of pyridoxine (vitamin B_6) to its active form, pyridoxal 5-phosphate. Particularly in patients with low pyridoxine intake, this interaction may cause pyridoxine deficiency and peripheral neuropathy. Pyridoxine supplementation (25 to 50 mg/day) is generally recommended with the prescription of INH because it is prescribed for at least 6 months at a time. Some other drugs that function as pyridoxine antagonists are hydralazine (Apresoline), penicillamine, levodopa (Dopar), and cycloserine (Seromycin).

Methotrexate (MTX; Rheumatrex) is a folic acid antagonist used to treat cancer and rheumatoid arthritis. Without folic acid, DNA synthesis is inhibited, cell replication stops, and the cell dies. Pyrimethamine (Daraprim), used to treat malaria and ocular toxoplasmosis, is also a folic acid antagonist. These drugs bind to and inhibit the enzyme dihydrofolate reductase, preventing conversion of folate to its active form (see Chapter 3), which could lead to megaloblastic anemia from folate deficiency (see Chapter 33). Leucovorin (folinic acid, the reduced form of folic acid) is used with folic acid antagonists to prevent anemia and GI damage, especially with chemotherapy such as high-dose MTX. Leucovorin does not require reduction by dihydrofolate reductase; thus, unlike folic acid, it is not affected by folic acid antagonists. Therefore leucovorin may "rescue" normal cells from MTX damage by competing for the same transport mechanisms into the cells. Administration of daily folic acid supplements or folinic acid can lower toxicity without affecting efficacy of the drug. See also Chapter 8, "Clinical: Biochemical Assessment," for more information on the assessment for folic acid.

Statin drugs (HMG-CoA reductase inhibitors) such as atorvastatin (Lipitor) affect the formation of coenzyme Q_{10} (CoQ_{10}; ubiquinone) See Box 9-2 on the mechanism of this effect. When HMG-CoA reductase is inhibited by statins, the production of cholesterol is significantly decreased. It is reasonable to conclude that the production of CoQ_{10} is also decreased (Ghirlanda, 1993). Studies have shown that circulatory, platelet, and lymphocyte levels of CoQ_{10} are also diminished. Although reports and small studies suggest that

BOX 9-2

Steps in the Hepatic Production of Cholesterol

Acetyl CoA

↓ + *HMG-CoA synthase*

HMG-CoA

↓ + *HMG-CoA reductase* (site of statin action)

Production of cholesterol interrupted at this point in the presence of a statin drug

Mevalonate

↓

Isopenterylpyrophosate

↓

Geranylpyrophosate

↓

Dolichol ← Farnesylpyrophosate → CoQ_{10} (ubiquinone)

↓

Squalene

↓

Cholesterol

CoA, Coenzyme A; *CoQ_{10}*, coenzyme Q_{10}; *HMG*, 3-hydroxy-3-methylglutaryl.

muscle pain and weakness can be relieved by CoQ_{10} supplementation (Littarru 2007), further large-scale studies are still needed. It may be worthwhile to supplement patients taking HMG-CoA reductase inhibitors with at least 100 mg CoQ_{10} daily for the preventive effect.

Nutrient Excretion

Some drugs can either increase or decrease the urinary excretion of nutrients. Drugs can increase the excretion of a nutrient by interfering with nutrient resorption by the kidneys. For instance, most clinicians know that loop diuretics such as furosemide (Lasix) or bumetanide (Bumex) increase the excretion of potassium; but these diuretics also increase the excretion of magnesium, sodium, chloride, and calcium. Potassium supplements are routinely prescribed with loop diuretics. In addition, clinicians need to consider supplements of magnesium and calcium, especially with long-term drug use, high doses of the diuretics, or poor dietary intake. Electrolyte and magnesium blood levels should be monitored. Prolonged use of high-dose diuretics, particularly by older patients on low-sodium diets, can cause sodium depletion. Hyponatremia may be overlooked in older patients because the mental confusion that is symptomatic of sodium depletion may be misdiagnosed as organic brain syndrome or dementia. Thiazide diuretics such as hydrochlorothiazide (HCTZ) increase the excretion of potassium and magnesium but reduce the excretion of calcium by enhancing renal resorption of calcium. High-dose HCTZ plus calcium supplementation may result in hypercalcemia.

Potassium-sparing diuretics such as spironolactone (Aldactone) or triamterene (Dyrenium) increase excretion of sodium, chloride, and calcium. Blood levels of potassium can rise to dangerous levels if patients also take potassium supplements or suffer from renal insufficiency. Antihypertensive angiotensin-converting enzyme (ACE) inhibitors such as enalapril (Vasotec) or fosinopril (Monopril) decrease potassium excretion, leading to increased serum potassium levels. *The combination of a potassium-sparing diuretic and an ACE inhibitor increases the danger of hyperkalemia.*

Corticosteroids such as prednisone decrease sodium excretion, resulting in sodium and water retention. Conversely, enhanced excretion of potassium and calcium is caused by these drugs; so a low-sodium, high-potassium diet is recommended. Calcium and vitamin D supplements are generally recommended with long-term corticosteroid use to prevent osteoporosis, such as might be the case for a person with asthma, lupus, or rheumatoid arthritis. With corticosteroid use this risk is important because it appears that not only is calcium lost in the urine, but corticosteroids may impair intestinal calcium absorption.

Phenothiazine-class antipsychotic drugs such as chlorpromazine (Thorazine) increase excretion of riboflavin and can lead to riboflavin deficiency in those with poor dietary intake. A complication associated with the use of another drug, cisplatin, is the development of acute hypomagnesemia resulting from nephrotoxicity; hypocalcemia, hypokalemia, and hypophosphatemia are also common. Both intravenous magnesium supplementation via rectal treatment or post-treatment hydration and oral magnesium supplements taken between chemotherapeutic courses have been used to prevent magnesium depletion. Hypomagnesemia can result from cisplatin use even with high-dose magnesium replacement therapy. Hypomagnesemia can persist for months or even years after the final course. When any drugs known to cause hypomagnesemia are administered, preventive treatment is warranted (Atsmon and Dolev, 2005).

MODIFICATION OF DRUG ACTION BY FOOD AND NUTRIENTS

Food or nutrients can alter the intended pharmacologic action of a medication by enhancing the medication effects or by opposing it. The classic example of an enhanced drug effect is the interaction between monoamine oxidase inhibitors (MAOIs) such as phenelzine sulfate (Nardil) or tranylcypromine (Parnate) and **pressor agents** such as dopamine, histamine, and especially tyramine. These biologically active amines are normally present in many foods (Box 9-3), but they rarely constitute a hazard because they are deaminated rapidly by MAO and diamine oxidases. Inhibition of MAO by medication prevents the breakdown of tyramine and other pressor agents. Tyramine is a vasoconstrictor that raises blood pressure. Significant ingestion of high-tyramine foods such as aged cheeses and cured meats while being

BOX 9-3

Pressor Agents in Foods and Beverages (Tyramine, Dopamine, Histamine, Phenylethylamine)

Avoid with MAOI medications: phenelzine (Nardil), tranylcypromine (Parnate), isocarboxazid (Marplan), selegiline (Eldepryl) in doses >10 mg/day, and the antibiotic linezolid (Zyvox).

Foods That Must Be Avoided

- Aged cheeses (e.g., cheddar, blue, Gorgonzola, Stilton)
- Aged meats (e.g., dry sausage such as salami, mortadella, Chinese dried duck)
- Soy sauce
- Fermented soya beans, soya bean paste, teriyaki sauce
- Tofu/fermented bean curd, tempeh
- Miso
- Fava (broad) beans or pods, snow pea pods (contain dopamine)
- Sauerkraut, kim chee
- Tap beer, Korean beer
- Concentrated yeast extracts (Marmite)
- Banana peel
- All casseroles made with aged cheese
- Meats, fish or poultry stored longer than 3-4 days in the refrigerator

Foods That May Be Used with Caution

- Red or white wine 2-4 oz per day
- Coffee, cola*
- Pizza (homemade or gourmet pizzas may have higher content)
- Bottled beer, two 12-oz bottles, maximum
- Alcohol-free beer, two 12-oz bottles, maximum
- Liquers or distilled spirits (two 1½-oz servings per day)

Foods Not Limited (based on current analyses)

- Unfermented cheeses (cream, cottage, ricotta, mozzarella, processed American if refrigerated less than 2-3 weeks)
- Smoked white fish, salmon, carp, or anchovies
- Pickled herring
- Fresh meat poultry or fish
- Canned figs, raisins
- Fresh pineapple
- Beetroot, cucumber
- Sweet corn, mushrooms
- Salad dressings, tomato sauce
- Worcestershire sauce
- Baked raised products, English cookies
- Boiled egg, yogurt, junket, ice cream
- Avocado, figs, banana, raspberries
- Brewer's yeast (vitamin supplements)
- Curry powder
- Peanuts, chocolate
- Packaged or processed meats (e.g., hot dogs, bologna, liverwurst), although they should be stored in refrigerator immediately and eaten as soon as possible; histamine content is highest in improperly stored or spoiled fish, tuna

From Pronsky ZM & Crowe JP: Food medication-interactions, ed 16, Birchrunville, Pa, 2010, Food-Medication Interactions.

MAOI, Monoamine oxidase inhibitor.

*Contains caffeine, a weak pressor agent; in quantities >500 mg/day may exacerbate reactions.

treated with an MAOI antidepressant can cause a hypertensive crisis with increased heart rate, flushing, headache, stroke, and even death. This reaction may be avoided with use of a transdermal administration method that bypasses the GI tract and omits contact with the indicated foods (Blob et al., 2007).

Caffeine in foods or beverages (see Appendix 39) increases the adverse effects of stimulant drugs such as amphetamines, methylphenidate (Ritalin, Concerta), or theophylline, causing nervousness, tremor, and insomnia. Conversely, the central nervous system (CNS) stimulatory properties of caffeine can oppose or counteract the antianxiety effect of tranquilizers such as lorazepam (Ativan).

Warfarin (Coumadin) is an oral anticoagulant that reduces the hepatic production of four vitamin K–dependent clotting factors by inhibiting the conversion of vitamin K to a usable form. Because this is a competitive interaction, the ingestion of vitamin K in the usable form will oppose the action of warfarin and allow the production of more clotting factors. To achieve an optimal level of anticoagulation, a balance must be maintained between the dose of the drug and the ingestion of vitamin K. Counseling of a person taking oral anticoagulation therapy should include nutrition therapy to maintain a consistent dietary vitamin K intake rather than prohibiting all high–vitamin K foods, such as dark green leafy vegetables (Johnson, 2005). CoQ_{10}, St. John's wort, or avocado may also counteract the effect of warfarin.

Ingestion of other substances may enhance the anticoagulant effect of warfarin. These substances include onions, garlic, quinine, papaya, mango, or vitamin E supplements in doses greater than 400 IU. Certain herbal products such as dong quai, which contain coumarin-like substances, or ginseng, which is a platelet inhibitor, also enhance the effect of the warfarin. Enhancement of the anticoagulation effects of warfarin may lead to serious bleeding events (Greenblatt and von Moltke, 2005). Recently there has been concern about an interaction with cranberry and warfarin (Coumadin) and the Food and Drug Administration (FDA) required a label warning change because of anecdotal reports.

However, several studies found no evidence-based information to support this warning (Ansell, 2009).

Alcohol

Ethanol combined with certain medications produces additive toxicity, affecting various body organs and systems. Ethanol combined with CNS-depressant medications such as a benzodiazepine (e.g., diazepam [Valium]) or a barbiturate (e.g., phenobarbital) may produce excessive drowsiness, incoordination, and other signs of CNS depression.

In the GI tract ethanol acts as a stomach mucosal irritant. Combining ethanol with drugs that cause the same effect such as aspirin or other NSAIDs (ibuprofen [Advil or Motrin]) may increase the risk of GI ulceration and bleeding. Because of the hepatotoxic potential of ethanol, it should not be combined with medications that also exhibit a risk of hepatotoxicity such as acetaminophen (Tylenol), amiodarone (Cordarone), or methotrexate (Rheumatrex).

Ethanol can inhibit gluconeogenesis, particularly when consumed in a fasting state. Inhibition of gluconeogenesis will prolong a hypoglycemic episode caused by insulin or an oral hypoglycemic agent such as glyburide (Diabeta, Micronase).

The combination of disulfiram (Antabuse) and ethanol produces a potentially life-threatening reaction characterized by flushing, rapid heartbeat, palpitations, and elevation of blood pressure. Disulfiram inhibits aldehyde dehydrogenase, an enzyme necessary for the normal catabolism of ethanol by the liver. As a result of this enzyme inhibition, high levels of acetaldehyde accumulate in the blood. Symptoms such as flushing, headache, and nausea appear within 15 minutes of alcohol ingestion. Because these symptoms are unpleasant, the drug is sometimes used as an aid to prevent alcoholics from returning to drinking. However, because these symptoms may also be life threatening, candidates for this drug must be chosen carefully. Other medications, when ingested concurrently with ethanol, may produce disulfiram-like reactions. Some of these medications are the antibiotics metronidazole (Flagyl) and cefoperazone (Cefobid), the oral hypoglycemic agent chlorpropamide (Diabinese), and the antineoplastic agent procarbazine (Matulane).

Ethanol can also affect the physical characteristics of a medication. The FDA recently required a change in the labeling of the extended-release capsules of morphine sulfate (Avinza, Kadian). The label now includes a **black box warning** that patients must not consume alcoholic beverages or take morphine sulfate with medications containing alcohol. If taken with alcohol, the extended-release beads of morphine can dissolve rapidly, delivering a potentially fatal dose of morphine.

EFFECTS OF DRUGS ON NUTRITION STATUS

The desired effects of medications often are accompanied by effects that are considered undesirable, or **side effects**. Side effects are often an extension of the desired effects, such as bacterial overgrowth as a result of use of an antibiotic. Overgrowth of *Clostridium difficile* causes pseudomembranous colitis. Suppression of natural oral bacteria may lead to oral yeast overgrowth, or candidiasis (see Chapter 26).

Oral, Taste, and Smell

Many drugs affect the ability to taste or smell foods (Box 9-4). Drugs can cause an alteration in taste sensation (dysgeusia), reduced acuity of taste sensation (hypogeusia), or an unpleasant aftertaste, any of which may affect food intake. The mechanisms by which drugs alter the chemical senses are not well understood. They may alter the turnover of taste cells or interfere with transduction mechanisms inside taste cells; or they may alter neurotransmitters that process chemosensory information. Common drugs that cause dysgeusia include the antihypertensive drug captopril (Capoten), the antineoplastic cisplatin (Platinol-AQ), and the anticonvulsant phenytoin. When exploring taste changes related to medication use it is always important to consider changes in zinc absorption related to the medication. An underlying zinc deficiency may affect the sense of taste (Heckmann and Lang, 2006).

Captopril (Capoten) may cause a metallic or salty taste and the loss of taste perception. The antibiotic clarithromycin (Biaxin) enters the saliva. The drug itself has a bitter taste that stays in the mouth as long as the drug is present in the body. An unpleasant or metallic taste has been reported by up to 34% of patients taking the sleep aid eszopiclone (Lunesta).

Antineoplastic drugs, used in chemotherapy for cancer, affect cells that reproduce rapidly, including the mucous membranes. Inflammation of the mucous membranes, or mucositis, occurs and is manifest as stomatitis (mouth inflammation), glossitis (tongue inflammation), or cheilitis (lip inflammation and cracking). Mucositis can be extremely painful to the point that patients are not able to eat or even drink (see Chapter 38.) Aldesleukin, also called interleukin-2 (Proleukin), paclitaxel (Taxol), and carboplatin (Paraplatin), are examples of antineoplastic agents that commonly cause severe mucositis.

Anticholinergic drugs (Box 9-5) compete with the neurotransmitter acetylcholine for its receptor sites, thereby inhibiting transmission of parasympathetic nerve impulses. This results in decreased secretions, including salivary secretions, causing dry mouth (xerostomia). Tricyclic antidepressants such as amitriptyline (Elavil), antihistamines such as diphenhydramine (Benadryl), and antispasmodic bladder control agents such as oxybutynin (Ditropan) are particularly problematic. Dry mouth immediately causes loss of taste sensation. Long-term dry mouth can cause dental caries and loss of teeth, gum disease, stomatitis, and glossitis, as well as nutritional imbalance and undesired weight loss (Friedlander et al., 2003) (see Chapter 26).

Gastrointestinal Effects

GI irritation and ulceration are serious problems with many drugs. The antiosteoporosis drug alendronate is contraindicated in patients who are unable to sit upright for at

BOX 9-4

Examples of Drugs That Cause Altered Taste, or Dysgeusia

Antiasthmatics

Beclomethasone (Beconase, Vancenase)
Terbutaline (Brethine, Bricanyl)

Antineoplastics

Carboplatin (Paraplatin)
Cisplatin (Platinol-AQ)
Dactinomycin (Actinomycin-D)
Fluorouracil (5-FU) (Adrucil)
Interferon α-2a (Roferon-A)
Methotrexate (Methotrexate, Rheumatrex)
Oxaliplatin (Eloxatin)

Antiinfectives

Cefuroxime (Ceftin, Zinacef)
Clarithromycin (Biaxin)
Clotrimazole (Mycelex)
Didanosine (Videx)
Ethionamide (Trecator-SC)
Metronidazole (Flagyl)
Pyrimethamine (Daraprim)
Pentamidine isethionate (NebuPent, Pentam 300)
Rifabutin (Mycobutin)

Cardiac Drugs

Acetazolamide (Diamox)
Captopril (Capoten)
Gemfibrozil (Lopid)
Quinidine (Quinaglute Dura, Quinidex Extentabs, Quinora)

Central Nervous System Drugs

Clomipramine (Anafranil)
Eszopiclone (Lunesta)
Levodopa (Dopar, Larodopa)
Phenytoin (Dilantin)
Phentermine (Adipex-P, Fastin, Ionamin)
Sumatriptan succinate (Imitrex)

Miscellaneous

Disulfiram (Antabuse)
Docusate sodium (Colace)
Etidronate disodium (Didronel)
Selenium (Se)

From Pronsky ZM & Crowe JP: Food-medication interactions, ed 16, Birchrunville, Pa, 2010, Food-Medication Interactions.

BOX 9-5

Examples of Drugs with Anticholinergic Effects

Antiemetics, Antivertigo Agents

Dimenhydrinate (Dramamine)
Meclizine (Bonine, Antivert)
Scopolamine (Transderm Scop)

Antihistamines

Clemastine (Tavist)
Cyproheptadine (Periactin)
Diphenhydramine (Benadryl)
Hydroxyzine HCl (Atarax)
Hydroxyzine pamoate (Vistaril)
Promethazine (Phenergan)

Antiparkinson Agents

Benztropine (Cogentin)
Trihexyphenidyl (Artane)

Bladder Anticholinergics

Flavoxate (Urispas)
Oxybutynin (Ditropan)
Tolterodine (Detrol)
Trospium (Sanctura)

Gastrointestinal Antispasmodics

Atropine
Dicyclomine (Bentyl)
Glycopyrrolate (Robinul)
L-Hyoscyamine (Levsin)
Propantheline (Pro-Banthine)

Inhalation Solution

Ipratropium (Atrovent)

Psychotropics

Antipsychotics, Phenothiazines
Chlorpromazine (Thorazine)
Mesoridazine (Serentil)
Thioridazine HCl (Mellaril)

Antipsychotics, Atypical

Clozapine (Clozaril)
Olanzapine (Zyprexa)

Antipsychotics, Typical

Haloperidol (Haldol)
Perphenazine (Trilafon)
Thiothixene (Navane)

Antidepressants, Tricyclic

Amitriptyline (Elavil)
Clomipramine (Anafranil)
Doxepin (Sinequan)
Imipramine (Tofranil)

Antidepressants, Monoamine Oxidase Inhibitors

Isocarboxazide (Marplan)
Phenelzine (Nardil)
Tranylcypromine (Parnate)

From Pronsky ZM & Crowe JP: Food medication interactions, ed 16, Birchrunville, Pa, 2010, Food Medication Interactions.

BOX 9-6

Examples of Drugs That Cause Gastrointestinal Bleeding and Ulceration

Antiinfectives

Amphotericin B (Abelcet, AmBisome, Amphotec, Fungizone)
Ganciclovir sodium (Cytovene)

Antineoplastics

Aldesleukin interleukin-2 (Proleukin)
Erlotinib (Tarceva)
Fluorouracil (5-FU) (Adrucil)
Leuprolide acetate (Lupron)
Imatinib mesylate (Gleevec)
Leuprolide (Lupron)
Mitoxantrone (Novantrone)
Methotrexate (Methotrexate, Rheumatrex)
Vinblastine sulfate (Velban)

Bisphosphonates

Alendronate (Fosamax)
Ibandronate (Boniva)
Pamidronate (Aredia)
Risedronate (Actonel)

Immunosuppressants

Corticosteroids (Prednisone)
Myophenolate mofetil (CellCept)

Miscellaneous

Bromocriptine (Parlodel)
Donepezil (Aricept)
Fluoxetine (Prozac)
Fluvoxamine (Luvox)
Levodopa (Dopar)
Paroxetine (Paxil)
Sertraline (Zoloft)
Trazodone HCl (Desyrel)

NSAIDs, Analgesics, Antiarthritics

Aspirin/acetylsalicylic acid (Bufferin, Ecotrin)
Celecoxib (Celebrex)
Diclofenac sodium (Cataflam, Voltaren)
Etodolac (Lodine)
Ibuprofen (Advil, Motrin)
Indomethacin (Indocin)
Ketoprofen (Orudis)
Meloxicam (Mobic)
Nabumetone (Relafen)
Naproxen (Naprosyn, Anaprox, Aleve)
Sulindac (Clinoril)

From Pronsky ZM & Crowe JP: Food-medication interactions, ed 16, Birchrunville, Pa, 2010, Food-Medication Interactions.

NSAID, Nonsteroidal antiinflammatory drug.

least 30 minutes after taking it because of the danger of esophagitis. NSAIDs such as ibuprofen or aspirin can cause stomach irritation, dyspepsia, gastritis, ulceration, and sudden serious gastric bleeding, sometimes leading to fatalities. Fluoxetine (Prozac) and other selective serotonin reuptake inhibitors can also cause serious gastric irritation, leading to hemorrhage, especially when aspirin or NSAIDs are also used (Yuan et al., 2006) (Box 9-6).

Antineoplastic drugs, used to treat cancer, often cause severe nausea and vomiting. Severe, prolonged nausea and vomiting, lasting as long as a week, have been reported with cisplatin (Platinol-AQ). Dehydration and electrolyte imbalances are of immediate concern. Weight loss and malnutrition are common long-term effects of these drugs, although it is often difficult to distinguish these effects from the complications of the disease itself (see Chapter 37). Serotonin antagonists such as ondansetron (Zofran) help to reduce these GI side effects.

Drugs can cause changes in bowel function that can lead to constipation or diarrhea. Narcotic agents such as codeine and morphine (MS Contin, MSIR, Avinza) cause a nonproductive increase in smooth muscle tone of the intestinal muscle wall, thereby decreasing peristalsis and causing constipation. A new parenteral drug methylnaltrexone (Relistor) is a laxative, administered subcutaneously, specifically indicated for severe opioid-induced constipation.

Drugs with anticholinergic effects decrease intestinal secretions, slow peristalsis, and cause constipation. The atypical antipsychotic clozapine (Clozaril), tricyclic antidepressant amitriptyline (Elavil), and antihistamine diphenhydramine (Benadryl) cause constipation and possibly impaction. Patients should be closely monitored and kept adequately hydrated.

Some drugs are used to inhibit intestinal enzymes, such as the diabetic drugs acarbose (Precose) and miglitol (Glyset), which are α-glucosidase inhibitors. Such action leads to a delayed and reduced rise in postprandial blood glucose levels and plasma insulin responses. The major adverse effect is GI intolerance, specifically diarrhea, flatulence, and cramping secondary to both the osmotic effect and bacterial fermentation of undigested carbohydrates in the distal bowel.

Prescription orlistat (Xenical, or over-the-counter [OTC] Alli), is a lipase inhibitor for weight loss that reduces the absorption of fat by binding to lipase in the intestine, thereby inhibiting its action. Consequently, fecal fat excretion is increased, a factor that contributes to the GI complaints associated with the drug, specifically oily spotting, increased fecal urgency, and possible fecal incontinence. A low-fat diet of no more than 30% of calories from fat is essential. Fat intake should be distributed among all three meals. Orlistat is not an appetite suppressant, and some persons may find it difficult to maintain a low-fat diet. Sufficient counseling and support is needed for success with this medication. Attention should also be given to potential malabsorption of fat soluble vitamins A, D, E, and K and carotenoids

BOX 9-7

Examples of Drugs That Cause Diarrhea

Antibiotics

Amoxicillin (Amoxil)
Amphotericin B (Abelcet, AmBisome, Amphotec, Fungizone)
Ampicillin
Atovaquone (Mepron)
Azithromycin (Zithromax)
Cefdinir (Omnicef)
Cefixime (Suprax)
Cefuroxime (Ceftin Zinacef)
Cephalexin (Keflex)
Clofazimine (Lamprene)
Clindamycin (Cleocin)
Levofloxacin (Levaquin)
Linezolid (Zyvox)
Meropenem (Merrem IV)
Metronidazole (Flagyl)
Quinine sulfate (Quinine)
Rifampin (Rifadin)
Penicillin
Pyrimethamine (Daraprim)
Tetracycline HCl (Achromycin-V, Sumycin)

Antigout Agents

Colchicine (Colchicine)

Antineoplastics

Aldesleukin/interleukin-2 (Proleukin)
Capecitabine (Xeloda)
Carboplatin (Paraplatin)
Fluorouracil (5-FU) (Adrucil)
Imatinib mesylate (Gleevec)
Irinotecan (Camptosar)
Methotrexate (Methotrexate, Rheumatrex)
Mitoxantrone (Novantrone)
Paclitaxel (Taxol)

Antiviral Agents

Didanosine (Videx)
Lopinavir (Kaletra)
Nelfinavir (Viracept)
Ritonavir (Norvir)
Stavudine (Zerit)
Foscarnet (Foscavir)

Gastrointestinal Agents

Lactulose (Chronulac)
Magnesium magonate (Milk of Magnesia)
Metoclopramide HCl (Reglan)
Misoprostol (Cytotec)
Casanthranol and docusate sodium (Peri-Colace)
Sorbitol
Orlitstat (Xenical, Alli)

Oral Hypoglycemic Agents

Acarbose (Precose)
Metformin (Glucophage)
Miglitol (Glyset)

From Pronsky ZM & Crowe JP: Food-medication interactions, ed 16, Birchrunville, Pa, 2010, Food-Medication Interactions.

requiring the presence of fat for optimal absorption. Obviously any of these problems, from dry mouth, to GI irritation, to constipation or diarrhea, can negatively affect food intake and nutrient absorption and nutrition status (see Chapter 22).

The use of antibiotics, particularly broad-spectrum antibiotics (Box 9-7) for long periods, destroy all sensitive bacteria of the gut flora. Intestinal flora that are not sensitive to the antibiotic will continue to grow because they are no longer inhibited by the bacteria that have been destroyed. An example of this situation is the overgrowth of *C. difficile*, causing pseudomembranous colitis with very strong-smelling yellow diarrhea (see also Chapter 29).

Appetite Changes

Drugs can suppress appetite (Box 9-8), leading to undesired weight changes, nutritional imbalance, and growth retardation in children. In the past the stimulant drug dextroamphetamine (Dexedrine) was used as an appetite suppressant. Because of the potential for abuse, the use of amphetamines for appetite suppression is no longer legal. Dextroamphetamine (part of Adderall) is now only indicated for treatment of attention-deficit hyperactivity disorder (ADHD) or narcolepsy.

In general, most CNS stimulants, including the amphetamine mixture (Adderall) and methylphenidate (Ritalin, Concerta, Metadate, Daytrana), suppress appetite or cause frank anorexia. These drugs are used extensively to treat ADHD in children and may cause weight loss and inhibit growth (see Chapter 18).

Sibutramine (Meridia) and phentermine (Adipex-P, Ionamin), structurally related to amphetamines, are used as appetite suppressants. These drugs are indicated for short-term use, along with a reduced-calorie diet and exercise, in obese patients (i.e., patients with a body mass index [BMI] greater than 30) or in overweight patients (BMI greater than 27) with additional risk factors such as hypertension, diabetes, or hyperlipidemia.

A major side effect of stimulant drugs is hypertension. Thus they are often contraindicated for hypertensive patients or those who have seizures or cardiac disease. Because hypertension is common among obese persons, these contraindications may limit the use of stimulants in obese or overweight hypertensive patients.

BOX 9-8
Examples of Drugs That Cause Anorexia

Antiinfectives

Amphotericin B (Abelcet, AmBisome, Amphotec, Fungizone)
Atovaquone (Mepron)
Cidofovir (Vistide)
Didanosine (ddI) (Videx)
Ethionamide (Trecator-SC)
Fomivirsen (Vitravene)
Foscarnet sodium (Foscavir)
Hydroxychloroquine sulfate (Plaquenil)
Metronidazole (Flagyl)
Pentamidine isethionate (NebuPent, Pentam 300)
Pyrimethamine (Daraprim)
Sulfadiazine
Zalcitabine (HIVID)

Antineoplastics

Aldesleukin/interleukin-2 (Proleukin)
Bleomycin sulfate (Blenoxane)
Capecitabine (Xeloda)
Carboplatin (Paraplatin)
Cytarabine (ara-C) (Cytosar-U)
Dacarbazine (DTIC-Dome)
Fluorouracil (Adrucil) (5-FU)
Hydroxyurea (Hydrea)
Imatinib mesylate (Gleevec)
Irinotecan HCl (Camptosar)
Methotrexate (MTX)
Vinblastine sulfate (Velban)
Vinorelbine tartrate (Navelbine)

Bronchodilators

Albuterol sulfate (Proventil, Ventolin)
Theophylline (Elixophyllin, Slo-Phyllin, Theo-24, Theobid, Theolair, Uniphyl)

Cardiovascular Drugs

Amiodarone HCl (Cordarone)
Acetazolamide (Diamox)
Hydralazine HCl (Apresoline)
Quinidine (Quinaglute Dura, Quinidex Extentabs, Quinora)

Stimulants

Amphetamines (Adderall, Dexedrine)
Methylphenidate HCl (Ritalin, Concerta, Metadate, Daytrana)
Phentermine (Adipex-P)

Miscellaneous

Fluoxetine (Prozac, Sarafem)
Galantamine (Reminyl)
Naltrexone HCl (ReVia)
Oxycodone (OxyContin)
Rivastigmine (Exelon)
Sibutramine HCl (Meridia)
Sulfasalazine (Azulfidine)
Topiramate (Topamax)

From Pronsky ZM & Crowe JP: Food-medication interactions, ed 16, Birchrunville, Pa, 2010, Food-Medication Interactions.

CNS side effects can interfere with the ability or desire to eat. Drugs that cause drowsiness, dizziness, ataxia, confusion, headache, weakness, tremor, or peripheral neuropathy can lead to nutritional compromise, particularly in older or chronically ill patients. Recognition of these problems as a drug side effect rather than a consequence of disease or aging is often overlooked.

Many medications stimulate appetite and lead to weight gain (Box 9-9). Antipsychotic drugs such as clozapine (Clozaril), olanzapine (Zyprexa), tricyclic antidepressant drugs such as amitriptyline (Elavil), and the anticonvulsant divalproex (Depakote) often lead to weight gain. Patients complain of a ravenous appetite and the inability to "feel full." Weight gains of 40 to 60 lb in a few months are not uncommon. Corticosteroid use is associated with dose-dependent weight gain in many patients. Sodium and water retention, as well as appetite stimulation, causes weight increases with corticosteroids. Medical nutrition therapy (MNT) is essential, as is routine exercise.

Appetite stimulation is desirable for patients suffering from wasting (cachexia) resulting from disease states such as cancer or HIV or the acquired immunodeficiency (AIDS) virus (Tisdale, 2006). Drugs indicated as appetite stimulants or antiwasting agents are the hormone megestrol acetate (Megace, Megace ES), human growth hormone somatropin (Serostim), the anabolic steroid oxandrolone (Oxandrin), and the marijuana derivative dronabinol (Marinol). Drugs also used as appetite stimulants, although not FDA-indicated as such, are the anabolic steroids oxymetholone (Anadrol-50) and nandrolone (Deca-Durabolin), the antihistamine cyproheptadine (Periactin), and the hormone testosterone (Androderm, Virilon). The ω-3 fatty acid, eicosapentaenoic acid has been suggested as an appetite stimulant. Although some studies have not shown improvement in appetite or weight gain (Fearon et al., 2006), one has shown improvement in cachexia (Stehr and Heller, 2006). Obviously this is an area of further study. With the successful advent of highly active antiretroviral therapy (HAART), lipodystrophy is often a problem for patients with HIV/AIDS. Debate about an accurate definition of lipodystrophy is ongoing. Redistribution of body fat, fat wasting, glucose intolerance, hypertension, and hyperlipidemia are common aspects of this syndrome. Antidiabetic drugs such as metformin (Glucophage) and rosiglitazone (Avandia) are used to

BOX 9-9

Examples of Drugs That Increase Appetite

Psychotropics

Alprazolam (Xanax)
Benzodiazepine antianxiety agents
Chlordiazepoxide (Librium)

Antipsychotics, Typical

Haloperidol (Haldol)
Perphenazine (Trilafon)
Thiothixene (Navane)
Thioridazine HCl (Mellaril)

Antipsychotics, Atypical

Clozapine (Clozaril)
Olanzapine (Zyprexa)
Quetiapine Fumarate (Seroquel)
Risperidone (Risperdal)

Antidepressants, Tricyclic

Amitriptyline HCl (Elavil)
Clomipramine HCl (Anafranil)
Doxepin HCl (Sinequan)
Imipramine HCl (Tofranil)
Selegiline (Eldepryl) only in doses >10 mg/day

Antidepressants, MAOI

Isocarboxazide (Marplan)
Phenelzine sulfate (Nardil)
Tranylcypromine sulfate (Parnate)

Antidepressants, Other

Mirtazapine (Remeron)
Paroxetine (Paxil)

Anticonvulsants

Divalproex/valproic acid (Depakote/Depakene)
Gabapentin (Neurontin)

Hormones

Corticosteroids (cortisone, methylprednisolone, prednisone)
Human growth hormone/somatropin (Serostim)
Medroxyprogesterone acetate (Provera, Depo-Provera)
Megestrol acetate (Megace)
Oxandrolone (Oxandrin)
Oxymetholone (Anadrol-50)
Testosterone (Androderm, Testoderm)

Miscellaneous

Cyproheptadine (Periactin)
Dronabinol (Marinol)

From Pronsky ZM & Crowe JP: Food-medication interactions, ed 16, Birchrunville, Pa, 2010, Food-Medication Interactions.

normalize glucose and insulin levels. Antihyperlipidemic drugs such as atorvastatin (Lipitor), pravastatin (Pravachol), or fenofibrate (Tricor) are used to control elevated triglycerides and cholesterol.

Organ System Toxicity

Drugs can cause specific organ system toxicity such as hepatotoxicity, nephrotoxicity, pulmonary toxicity, neurotoxicity, ototoxicity, ocular toxicity, pancreatitis, or cardiotoxicity. MNT may be indicated as part of the treatment of these toxicities. Although all toxicities are of concern, hepatotoxicity and nephrotoxicity are addressed here because drugs are eliminated from the body predominately through the liver and kidney.

Examples of drugs that cause hepatotoxicity (liver damage) leading to hepatitis, jaundice, hepatomegaly, or even liver failure are amiodarone (Cordarone), amitriptyline (Elavil), lovastatin (Mevacor) and other "statin" antihyperlipidemic drugs, divalproex (Depakote), carbamazepine (Tegretol), methotrexate, kava, niacin, and sulfasalazine (Azulfidine). Monitoring of hepatic function through routine blood work for liver enzyme levels is generally prescribed with use of these drugs (see Table 8-1).

Nephrotoxicity (kidney damage) may change the excretion of specific nutrients or cause acute or chronic renal insufficiency, which may not resolve with cessation of drug use. Examples of drugs that often cause nephrotoxicity are antiinfectives amphotericin B (especially with intravenous desoxycholate form [Fungizone]) and cidofovir (Vistide), as well as antineoplastics cisplatin (Plaquenil-AQ), gentamicin (Garamycin), ifosfamide (Ifex), methotrexate, and pentamidine (Pentam 300). Adequate or extra prehydration, often administered intravenously, is prescribed to reduce renal toxicity. For example, with cidofovir, 1 L of intravenous normal saline (0.9% sodium chloride [NaCl]) is infused 1 to 2 hours before infusion of the drug. If tolerated, up to an additional liter may be infused after the drug infusion. Oral probenecid (Benemid) is also prescribed with cidofovir to reduce nephrotoxicity.

Glucose Levels

Many drugs affect glucose metabolism, causing hypoglycemia or hyperglycemia and in some cases frank diabetes (Box 9-10). The mechanisms of these effects vary from drug to drug and from individual to individual. Drugs may stimulate glucose production or impair glucose uptake. They may inhibit insulin secretion, decrease insulin sensitivity, or increase insulin clearance.

Glucose levels may be affected by changes in parameters, such as hypokalemia induced by thiazide diuretics or weight

BOX 9-10

Examples of Drugs That Affect Glucose Levels

Antidiabetes (Lower or Normalize Glucose Levels)

Acarbose (Precose)
Exenatide (Byetta)
Glimepiride (Amaryl)
Glipizide (Glucotrol)
Glyburide (DiaBeta)
Insulin (Humulin)
Metformin (Glucophage)
Miglitol (Glyset)
Nateglinide (Starlix)
Pioglitazone HCl (Actos)
Pramlintide (Symlin)
Repaglinide (Prandin)
Rosiglitazone maleate (Avandia)

Drugs That Can Cause Hypoglycemia

Disopyramide (Norpace) antiarrhythmic
Pentamidine isethionate (Pentam 300) antiprotozoal
Quinine antimalarial
Ethanol

Drugs That Can Increase Glucose Levels

Antiretroviral agents, protease inhibitors
Nelfinavir mesylate (Viracept)
Ritonavir (Norvir)
Saquinavir (Invirase, Fortovase)

Diuretics, Antihypertensives

Furosemide (Lasix)
Hydrochlorothiazide (HCTZ, HydroDIURIL, Microzide)
Indapamide (Lozol)

Hormones

Corticosteroid (cortisone, prednisone)
Danazol (Danocrine)

Estrogen or Estrogen/Progesterone (Hormone Replacement Therapy)

Medroxyprogesterone (Cycrin, Provera, Depo-Provera)
Megestrol acetate (Megace)
Nandrolone decanoate (Deca-Durabolin)
Octreotide acetate (Sandostatin)

Oral Contraceptives

Oxandrolone (Oxandrin)
Oxymetholone (Anadrol-50)

Miscellaneous

Niacin (nicotinic acid) antihyperlipidemic
Baclofen (Lioresal) skeletal muscle relaxant
Caffeine (No-Doz) stimulant
Clofazimine (Lamprene) antibiotic
Clozapine (Clozaril) antipsychotic
Olanzapine (Zyprexa) antipsychotic
Cyclosporine (Neoral, Sandimmune) immunosuppressant
Interferon alfa-2a (Roferon-A) antineoplastic

From Pronsky ZM & Crowe JP: Food-medication interactions, ed 16, Birchrunville, Pa, 2010, Food-Medication Interactions.

gain induced by antipsychotic medications (Izzedine et al., 2005). Corticosteroids, particularly prednisone, prednisolone, and hydrocortisone, are diabetogenic because of increased gluconeogenesis, but they also cause insulin resistance and therefore inhibit glucose uptake. Second-generation antipsychotics, particularly clozapine (Clozaril) or olanzapine (Zyprexa), have been reported to cause treatment-emergent hyperglycemia. Recently the FDA added a labeling requirement on all second-generation antipsychotics to warn of the possibility of developing hyperglycemia and diabetes.

EXCIPIENTS AND FOOD-DRUG INTERACTIONS

An **excipient** is added to drug formulations for its action as a buffer, binder, filler, diluent, disintegrant, glidant, flavoring, dye, preservative, suspending agent, or coating. Excipients are also called inactive ingredients (Box 9-11). Hundreds of excipients are approved by the FDA for use in pharmaceuticals. Several common excipients have potential for interactions in persons with an allergy or enzyme deficiency. Often just one brand of a drug or one formulation or strength of a particular brand may contain the excipient of concern. For example, tartrazine, listed as yellow dye No. 5, is used in a brand of clindamycin (Cleocin) capsules in the 75- and 150-mg strengths but not in the 300-mg strength. A brand of metoclopramide (Reglan) 5-mg tablets contain lactose, but the 10-mg tablets do not. Micronized progesterone (Prometrium) capsules contain peanut oil and lecithin, whereas other progesterone forms do not. Micronized progesterone labeling includes a warning that anyone allergic to peanuts should not use the drug (see Chapter 27).

Lactose is commonly used as a filler in many pills and capsules. The amount of lactose may be significant enough to cause GI problems for lactase-deficient patients, particularly those on multiple drugs throughout the day (see Chapter 29). Product information on prescription drugs and labeling on OTC drugs contain information on excipients, usually called “inactive ingredients,” including lactose.

BOX 9-11

Examples of Potential Interactive Drug Excipients

Albumin (egg or human): May cause allergic reaction. Human albumin is a blood product.

Alcohol (ethanol): CNS depressant used as a solvent. All alcohol and alcohol-containing products and drugs must be avoided with medications such as disulfiram (Antabuse) or limited with other drugs to prevent additive CNS or hepatic toxicity. Most elixirs contain 4% to 20% alcohol. Some solution, syrup, liquid, or parenteral forms contain alcohol.

Aspartame: A nonnutritive sweetener composed of the amino acids aspartic acid and phenylalanine. Patients with PKU lack the enzyme phenylalanine hydroxylase. If patients with PKU ingest aspartame in significant quantities, accumulation of phenylalanine causes toxicity to brain tissue.

Lactose: Lactose is used as a filler. The natural sweetener in milk, lactose is hydrolyzed in the small intestine by the enzyme lactase to glucose and galactose. Lactose intolerance (caused by lactase deficiency) results in gastrointestinal distress when lactose is ingested. Lactose in medications may cause this reaction.

Mannitol: The alcohol form of the sugar mannose, used as a filler. Mannitol is absorbed more slowly, yielding half as many calories per gram as glucose. Because of slow absorption, mannitol can cause soft stools and diarrhea.

Saccharin: Nonnutritive sweetener. Extensive human research has found no evidence of carcinogenicity.

Sorbitol: The alcohol form of sucrose. Absorbed more slowly than sucrose, sorbitol inhibits the rise in blood glucose. Because of slow absorption, sorbitol can cause soft stools or diarrhea.

Starch: Starch from wheat, corn, or potato is added to medication as a filler, binder, or diluent. Celiac disease patients have a permanent intolerance to gluten, a protein in wheat, barley, rye, and a contaminant of oat. In celiac disease, gluten causes damage to the lining of the small intestine.

Sucrose: Sweetener. Significant source of simple carbohydrate and calories.

Sulfites: Sulfiting agents are used as antioxidants. Sulfites may cause severe hypersensitivity reactions in some people, particularly asthmatics. They include sulfur dioxide, sodium sulfite, and sodium and potassium metabisulfite. The FDA requires the listing of sulfites when present in foods or drugs.

Tartrazine: Tartrazine is a yellow dye No. 5 color additive, which causes severe allergic reactions in some people (1 in 10,000). The FDA requires the listing of tartrazine when it is present in foods or drugs.

Vegetable oil: Soy, sesame, cottonseed, corn, or peanut oil is used in some parenteral drugs as a nonaqueous vehicle. Hydrogenated vegetable oil is a tablet or capsule lubricant. May cause allergic reactions in sensitive people.

Modified from Pronsky ZM & Crowe JP: Potential interactive ingredients. In Pronsky ZM: Food-medication interactions, ed 16, Birchrunville, Pa, 2010, Food-Medication Interactions.

CNS, Central nervous system; *FDA*, Food and Drug Administration; *PKU*, phenylketonuria.

Patients with celiac disease have gluten sensitivity and must practice lifelong abstinence from wheat, barley, rye, and oats (which may be contaminated with gluten; see Chapter 29). They are particularly concerned with the composition and source of excipients such as wheat starch or flour, which might contain gluten. Only a few pharmaceutical companies guarantee their products to be gluten-free. Excipients such as dextrin and sodium starch glycolate are usually made from corn and potato, respectively, but can be made from wheat or barley. For example, the excipient dextrimaltose, a mixture of maltose and dextrin, is produced by the enzymatic action of barley malt on corn flour (Crowe and Falini, 2001; Kibbe, 2000). The source of each drug ingredient, if not specified, should be checked with the manufacturer.

Finally, some drug brands may contain enough excipient to be nutritionally significant (see Table 9-1), magnesium in quinapril (Accupril), calcium in calcium polycarbophil (Fibercon, Fiber-Lax), and soybean oil lipid emulsion in propofol (Diprivan). Propofol is commonly used in the long term for sedation of patients in the intensive care unit. Its formulation includes 10% emulsion, which contributes 1.1 kcal/mL. When infused at doses up to 9 mg/kg/hr in a patient weighing 70 kg, for instance, it may contribute an additional 1663 kcal/day from the emulsion. For a patient receiving total parenteral nutrition, limiting the use of long-chain fatty acids and using medium-chain triglyceride (MCT) oil may be recommended while he or she is taking propofol (Dubey and Kumar, 2005). Specific brands or formulations of a specific brand provide significant amounts of sodium and therefore may be contraindicated for patients who need to limit sodium.

MEDICAL NUTRITION THERAPY

MNT can be divided into prospective and retrospective care. Prospective MNT occurs when the patient first starts a drug. A diet history must be obtained, including information about the use of OTC (nonprescription) drugs, alcohol, vitamin and mineral supplements, and herbal or

TABLE 9-1

Examples of Drugs That Contain Nutritionally Significant Ingredients

Trade Name	Generic Name	Ingredient	Nutritional Significance
Accupril	Quinapril	Magnesium carbonate Magnesium stearate	Provides 50-200 mg magnesium daily
Accutane	Isotretinoin	Drug is related to vitamin A; contains soybean oil	Avoid vitamin A or β-carotene May cause allergic reaction
Atrovent (inhaler)	Ipratropium Bromide	Soya lecithin	May cause allergic reaction
Fibercon/ Fiber-Lax	Calcium polycarbophil	Calcium polycarbophil	100 mg Ca/tablet; up to 6 tablets/day = 600 mg calcium total
Marinol	Dronabinol	Sesame oil	May cause allergic reaction
Phazyme	Simethicone	Soybean oil in capsule	May cause allergic reaction
Prometrium	Micronized progesterone	Peanut oil	May cause allergic reaction
Diprivan	Propofol	10% soybean oil emulsion Egg yolk phospholipids	Oil is significant caloric source May cause allergic reaction
Videx	Didanosine	Sodium buffer in powder	≥2760 mg Na/adult daily dose
Zantac	Ranitidine	Sodium in *prescription* granules and tablets; Zantac 75 (nonprescription) is sodium free	350-730 mg Na/adult daily dose

Data from Pronsky ZM & Crowe JP: Food-medication interactions, ed 16, Birchrunville, Pa, 2010, Food-Medication Interactions.

phytonutrient supplements. The patient should be evaluated for genetic characteristics, weight and appetite changes, altered taste, and GI problems (see Chapter 6).

Prospective drug MNT provides basic information about the drug: the name, purpose, and duration of prescription of the drug plus when and how to take the drug. This information includes whether to take the drug with or without food. Specific foods and beverages to avoid while taking the drug and potential interactions between drug and vitamin or mineral supplements need to be emphasized. For instance, the patient taking tetracycline (Achromycin-V or Sumycin) or ciprofloxacin (Cipro) should be warned not to combine the drug with milk, yogurt, or supplements containing divalent cations, calcium, iron, magnesium, zinc, or vitamin-minerals containing any of these cations.

Potential significant side effects must be delineated, and possible dietary suggestions to relieve the side effects should be described. For instance, information about a high-fiber diet with adequate fluids should be part of MNT about an anticholinergic drug such as oxybutynin (Ditropan), which often causes constipation. Conversely, diarrhea can be controlled by the use of psyllium (Metamucil) or probiotics, such as *Lactobacillus acid-ophilus* (Lactinex), particularly for antibiotic-associated diarrhea even in children (Szajewska et al., 2006). Probiotics may be contraindicated for some individuals and should be prescribed and monitored by the physician.

Patients should be warned about potential nutritional problems, particularly when dietary intake is inadequate, such as hypokalemia with a potassium-depleting diuretic. Dietary changes that may alter drug action should be included, such as the effect of an increase in foods high in vitamin K on warfarin action. Special diet information, such as a low-cholesterol, low-fat, limited-sugar diet with atorvastatin (Lipitor) or other antihyperlipidemic drugs, is essential information. Written information should list medication ingredients such as nonnutrient excipients in the medication. Examples include lactose, starch, tartrazine, aspartame, and alcohol. Patients with lactose intolerance, celiac disease, allergies, phenylketonuria, or alcoholism need to avoid or limit one or more of these ingredients.

Prospective MNT should also cover potential concerns with OTC drugs and herbal and natural products (Herr, 2005). It is important to emphasize that the pharmacokinetic and pharmacodynamic interactions explained in this chapter occur with all medications, whether obtained by prescription, OTC, or as natural or herbal products.

Retrospective MNT evaluates symptoms to determine if medical problems might be the result of food-drug interactions. To determine whether a patient's symptoms are the result of a food-drug interaction, a complete medical and nutrition history is essential, including prescription and nonprescription drugs, vitamin-mineral supplements, and herbal or phytonutrient products. The date of beginning to take the drugs versus the date of symptom onset is significant information. It is important to identify the use of nutrition supplements such as enteral products or significant dietary changes such as fad diets during the course of drug prescription. Finally it is important to investigate the reported incidence of side effects (by percentage as compared with a placebo). For example, vomiting occurs in 1.5% of those taking omeprazole (Prilosec) compared with

4.7% of those taking a placebo. Therefore in a patient treated with omeprazole, it would be appropriate to consider other causes for vomiting. A rare drug effect is less likely to be the reason for a negative symptom than an effect that is common.

In summary, although food provides energy for sustenance and physiological benefits for good health, and drugs prevent or treat many diseases, together the synergistic effects can be very positive (MacDonald et al., 2009). The nutrition therapist must assess, intervene, and evaluate the mixtures with care.

CLINICAL SCENARIO

Henry is a 31-year-old man who began to suffer seizures after a head trauma injury from a motorcycle accident at the age of 18. For the first 2 years after the accident, he was prescribed various anticonvulsant regimens. The combination of phenytoin (Dilantin), 300 mg daily, and phenobarbital, 120 mg daily, has proven to be the most effective therapy to control his seizures. Henry has been stabilized on this regimen for the last 11 years.

Henry is a senior computer programmer for a large corporation. He is 6 feet 2 inches tall and weighs 182 lb. Henry admits to having an aversion for exercise and athletics. In his free time, he enjoys reading, playing computer games, and watching television. During the past year, Henry has broken his left femur and tibia on two separate occasions. He broke his femur when he missed the bottom step on the stairway in his office building. Several months later he broke his tibia when he tripped over a broken branch in his yard. Henry recently complained to his orthopedic surgeon about hip and pelvic pain of several weeks' duration. An orthopedic examination with x-ray examination, bone scan, and Dexa scan revealed that Henry is suffering from osteomalacia. A review of Henry's typical diet reveals a nutritionally marginal diet that commonly includes fast foods and frozen dinners. His diet is generally deficient in fresh fruits, vegetables, and dairy products.

Nutrition Diagnostic Statement

Food-medication interaction related to inadequate calcium and vitamin D intake while taking anticonvulsant medications as evidenced by osteomalacia.

Nutrition Care Questions

1. Is osteomalacia common in young men?
2. How does Henry's lifestyle contribute to the development of osteomalacia?
3. What vitamin or mineral deficiency may have contributed to the current state of Henry's bones?
4. Describe the food-drug interaction that has contributed to Henry's osteomalacia.
5. What medical nutritional therapy would you recommend for Henry?

USEFUL WEBSITES

Access to MedLine
www.pubmed.com

Food and Drug Administration Center for Drug Evaluation and Research
www.fda.gov/cder/

Food and Nutrition Information Center
www.nal.usda.gov/fnic/

Food Medication Interactions
www.foodmedinteractions.com

Grapefruit-Drug Interactions
www.powernetdesign.com/grapefruit

National Institutes of Health Patient Handouts
www.cc.nih.gov/ccc/patient_education/

Project Inform's Drug Interactions (HIV/AIDS)
www.projinf.org/fs/drugin.html

REFERENCES

Ansell J, et al: The absence of an interaction between warfarin and cranberry juice: a randomized, double-blind trial, *J Clin Pharmacol* 49:824, 2009.

Atsmon J, Dolev E: Drug-induced hypomagnesemia: Scope and management, *Drug Saf* 28:763, 2005.

Bai JP: Ongoing challenges in drug interaction safety: from exposure to pharmacogenomics, *Drug Metab Pharmacokinet* 25:62, 2010.

Blob LF, et al: Effects of a tyramine-enriched meal on blood pressure response in healthy male volunteers treated with selegiline transdermal system 6 mg/24 hr, *CNS Spectr* 12:25, 2007.

Crawford P: Best practice guidelines for the management of women with epilepsy, *Epilepsia* 46:117, 2005.

Crowe JP, Falini NP: Gluten in pharmaceutical products, *Am J Health Syst Pharmacol* 58:396, 2001.

Dubey PK, Kumar A: Pain on injection of lipid-free propofol and propofol emulsion containing medium-chain triglyceride: a comparative study, *Anesth Analg* 101:1060, 2005.

Egashira K, et al: Pomelo-induced increase in the blood level of tacrolimus in a renal transplant patient, *Transplantation* 75:1057, 2003.

Fearon KC, et al: Double-blind, placebo-controlled, randomized study of eicosapentaenoic acid diester in patients with cancer cachexia, *J Clin Oncol* 24:3401, 2006.

Fourniet MR, et al: Proton pump inhibitors, osteoporosis, and osteoporosis-related fractures, *Maturitas* 64:9, 2009.

Friedlander AH, et al: Late-life depression: its oral health significance, *Int Dent J* 53:41, 2003.

Ghosh D, et al: Pharmacogenomics and nutrigenomics: synergies and differences, *Eur J Clin Nutr* 61:567, 2007.

Ghirlanda G, et al: Evidence of plasma CoQ10-lowering effect by HMG-CoA reductase inhibitors: a double blind, placebo-controlled study, *J Clin Pharmacol* 33:226, 1993.

Greenblatt DJ, Von Moltke LL: Interaction of warfarin with drugs, natural substances and foods, *J Clin Pharmacol* 45:127, 2005.

Heckmann JG, Lang CJ: Neurological causes of taste disorders, *Adv Otorhinolaryngol* 63:255, 2006.

Herr SM: *Herb-drug interaction handbook*, ed 3, Nassau, NY, 2005, Church Street Books.

Holick MF: Vitamin D deficiency, *N Engl J Med* 357:266, 2007.

Izzedine H, et al: Drug-induced diabetes mellitus, *Expert Opin Surg Saf* 4:1097, 2005.

Johnson MA: Influence of vitamin K on anticoagulant therapy depends on vitamin K status and the source and forms of vitamin K, *Nutr Rev* 63:91, 2005.

Kibbe AH, editor: *Handbook of pharmaceutical excipients*, ed 3, Washington, DC, 2000, American Pharmaceutical Association.

Lee JI, et al: CYP-mediated therapeutic protein-drug interactions: clinical findings, proposed mechanisms and regulatory implications, *Clin Pharmacokinet* 49:295, 2010.

Littarru GP, Langsjoen P: Coenzyme Q10 and statins: biochemical and clinical implications, *Mitochondrion* 7:S168, 2007.

MacDonald L, et al: Food and therapeutic product interactions—a therapeutic perspective, *J Pharm Pharm Sci* 12:367, 2009.

Medical Letter: AmpliChip CYP450 tes, *Med Lett Drugs Ther* 47:71, 2005.

Neuhofel AL, et al. Lack of bioequivalence of ciprofloxacin when administered with calcium-fortified orange juice: a new twist on an old interaction, *J Clin Pharmacol* 42:461, 2002.

Nicolaidou P, et al: Effects of anticonvulsant therapy on vitamin D status in children: prospective monitoring study, *J Child Neurol* 21:2005, 2006.

Pronsky ZM, Crowe JP: *Food medication interactions*, ed 16, Birchrunville, Pa, 2010, Food Medication Interactions.

Sica DA: Interaction of grapefruit juice and calcium channel blockers, *Am J Hyperts* 19:768, 2006.

Spriet I, et al: Mini-series: II. Clinical aspects. Clinically relevant CYP450-mediated drug interactions in the ICU, *Intensive Care Med* 35:603, 2009.

Stehr SN, Heller AR: ω-3 fatty acid effects on biochemical indices following cancer surgery, *Clin Chim Acta* 373:1, 2006.

Steinman MA, et al: Agreement between drugs-to-avoid criteria and expert assessments of problematic prescribing, *Arch Int Med* 169:1326, 2009

Szajewska H, et al: Probiotics in the prevention of antibiotic associated diarrhea in children: a meta-analysis of randomized controlled trials, *J Pediatr* 149:367, 2006.

Targownik LE, et al: Proton-Pump inhibitor use is not associated with osteoporosis of accelerated bone miner density loss, *Gastroenterology* 138:896, 2010.

Tisdale MJ: Clinical anticachexia treatments, *Nutr Clin Pract* 21:168, 2006.

Valley M, et al: Emerging peptide therapeutics for inflammatory diseases, *Curr Pharm Biotechnol* 7:241, 2006.

Wise C, Kaput J: A strategy for analyzing gene-nutrient interactions in type 2 diabetes, *J Diabetes Sci Technol* 3:710, 2009.

Wohlt PD, et al: Recommendations for use of medications with continuous enteral nutrition, *Am J Health-Syst Pharm* 66:1458, 2009.

Yuan Y, et al: Selective serotonin reuptake inhibitors and risk of upper GI bleeding: confusion or confounding? *Am J Med* 119:719, 2006.

CHAPTER 10

Judith L. Dodd, MS, RD, LDN, FADA
Cynthia Taft Bayerl, MS, RD, LDN

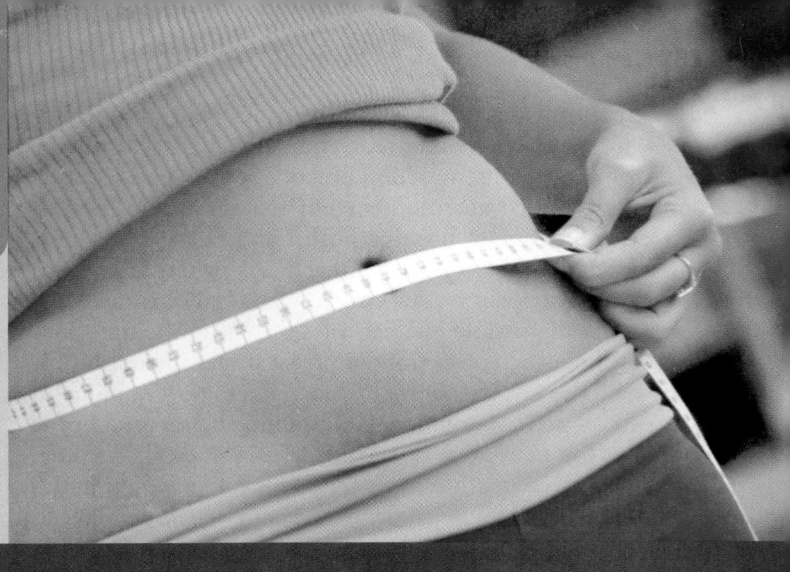

Behavioral-Environmental: The Individual in the Community

KEY TERMS

- biosecurity
- bioterrorism
- community needs assessment
- Department of Homeland Security (DHS)
- Federal Emergency Management Agency (FEMA)
- foodborne illness
- food security
- Hazard Analysis Critical Control Points (HACCP)
- National Food and Nutrition Survey (NFNS)
- National Health and Nutrition Examination Survey (NHANES)
- National Nutrient Databank
- National Nutrition Monitoring and Related Research (NNMRR) Act
- organic foods
- pandemic
- primary prevention
- public health assurance
- risk assessment
- risk management
- secondary prevention
- Special Supplemental Nutrition Program for Women Infants and Children (WIC)
- Supplemental Nutrition Assistance Program (SNAP; formerly the food stamp program)
- tertiary prevention
- U.S. Department of Health and Human Services (USDHHS)

Community nutrition is an evolving area of practice with the broad focus of serving the population at large. Although this practice area encompasses the goals of public health, in the United States the current model has been shaped and expanded by prevention and wellness initiatives that evolved in the 1960s. Because the thrust of community nutrition is to be both proactive and responsive to the needs of the community, current emphasis areas include disaster and **pandemic** control, food and water safety, and controlling environmental risk factors related to obesity.

Historically *public health* was defined as "the science and art of preventing disease, prolonging life, and promoting health and efficiency through organized community effort" (Winslow, 1920). The public health approach, also known as a *population-based* or *epidemiologic* approach, differs from the clinical or patient care model generally seen in hospitals and other clinical settings. In the public health model the client is the community, a geopolitical entity. The focus of the traditional public health approach is **primary prevention** with health promotion, as opposed to **secondary prevention** with the goal of risk reduction, or **tertiary prevention** with rehabilitation efforts. Changes in the health care system, technology, and attitudes of the nutrition consumer have influenced the expanding responsibilities of community nutrition providers.

In 1988, the Institute of Medicine published a landmark report that promoted the concept that the scope of community nutrition is a work in progress. This report defined a mission and delineated roles and responsibilities for practicing community nutrition that are still the basis for community nutrition practice today. The scope of community-based nutrition encompasses efforts to prevent disease and promote positive health and nutritional status for individuals and groups in settings where they live and work. The focus is on well-being and building potential for the best possible quality of life. "Well-being" goes beyond the usual constraints of physical and mental health and includes other factors that affect the quality of life within the community. Community members need a safe environment and adequate housing, food, income, employment, and education. The mission of community nutrition is to promote the conditions in which people can be healthy.

Programming and services can be for any segment of the population. The program or service should reflect the diversity of the designated community, such as politics, geography, culture, ethnicity, ages, genders, socioeconomic issues, and overall health status. Along with primary prevention, community nutrition provides links to programs and services with goals of disease risk reduction and rehabilitation.

In the traditional model, funding sources for public health efforts were monies allocated from official sources (government) at the local, state, or federal level. Currently nutrition programs and services are funded alone or in partnership with a broad range of sources, including public (government), private, and voluntary health sectors. As public source funding has declined, the need for private funding has become more crucial. The potential size and diversity of a designated "community" makes collaboration critical. A single agency may be unable to fund or deliver the full range of services. In addition, it is likely that the funding will be services or product (in-kind) rather than cash. Creative funding and management skills are crucial for a community practitioner.

NUTRITION PRACTICE IN THE COMMUNITY

Nutrition professionals recognize that successful delivery of food and nutrition services involves actively engaging people in their own community. The pool of nutrition professionals delivering medical nutrition therapy (MNT) and nutrition education in community-based or public health facilities continues to expand. In addition, the objectives of *Healthy People 2020* offer a common framework of measurable public health outcomes that can be used to assess the overall health of a community. Although the settings may vary, there are three core functions in community nutrition practice.

The three "core" functions of public health are community assessment, policy development, and public health assurance. These areas are also the components of community nutrition practice, especially community needs assessment as it relates to nutrition. The findings of these needs assessments shape policy development and protect the nutritional health of the public.

Although there is shared responsibility for completion of the core functions of public health, official state health agencies have primary responsibility for this task. Under this model, state public health agencies, community organizations, and leaders have responsibility for assessing the capacity of their state to perform the essential functions and to attain or monitor the goals and objectives of *Healthy People 2020*. Local health agencies are charged with protecting the health of their population groups by ensuring that effective service delivery systems are in place. The federal government can support the development and dissemination of public health knowledge and provide funding. See Box 10-1 for a list of various government agencies.

Typical settings for community nutrition include public health agencies (state and local) and the **Special Supplemental Nutrition Program for Women Infants and Children (WIC)**, a federal program that allocates funds to states for specific foods, health care referrals, and nutrition education for low-income, nutritionally at-risk pregnant, breastfeeding, and non-breastfeeding postpartum women, infants and children up to age five. The expansion of community-based practice beyond the scope of traditional public health has opened new employment opportunities for nutrition professionals.

Nutrition professionals often serve as consultants or may establish community-based private practices. Nutrition services also occur in programs for senior adults, community health centers, early intervention programs, Head Start (a federal program for low-income preschool children and their families), health maintenance organizations, food pantries and shelters, physicians' offices, and schools. Effective practice in the community requires a nutrition professional who understands the effect of economic, social, and political issues on health. Because many community-based efforts are funded or guided by legislation and the resulting regulations and policies, community practice requires an understanding of the legislative process and an ability to translate policies into action. In addition, community practice requires a working knowledge of funding sources and resources at the federal, state, regional, and local level.

NEEDS ASSESSMENT FOR COMMUNITY-BASED NUTRITION SERVICES

Nutrition services should be organized to meet the needs of a "community." Once that community has been defined, a **community needs assessment** is developed to shape the planning, implementation, and evaluation of nutrition services. An assessment is a current snapshot of the community and is used to identify the health risks or areas of greatest

BOX 10-1

Government Agencies Related to Food and Nutrition

Centers for Disease Control and Prevention (Department of Health and Human Services)	http://www.cdc.gov/
Central website for Access to All U.S. Government Information on Nutrition	http://www.nutrition.gov
Environmental Protection Agency	http://www.epa.gov/
Federal Trade Commission	http://www.ftc.gov
Food and Agriculture Organization of the United Nations	http://www.fao.org
Food and Drug Administration	http://www.fda.gov
Food and Drug Administration Advisory Committees	http://www.fda.gov/nctr/
Food and Drug Administration Center for Food Safety and Applied Nutrition	http://www.vm.cfsan.fda.gov
Food and Nutrition Service—Assistance Programs	http://www.fns.usda.gov/fns/Default.htm
Indian Health Service—Medical and Nutrition	http://www.his.gov/MedicalPrograms/Nutrition/
National Cancer Institute (Department of Health and Human Services)	http://www.nci.nih.gov
National Health Information Center	http://www.health.gov/nhic
National Institutes of Health (Department of Health and Human Services)	http://www.nih.gov
National Institutes of Health- Office of Dietary Supplements	http://ods.od.nih.gov
National Marine Fisheries Service	http://www.nmfs.noaa.gov/
USDA Center for Nutrition Policy and Promotion	http://www.usda.gov/cnpp
USDA Food and Nutrition Service	http://www.fns.usda.gov/fns
USDA Food Safety and Inspection Service	http://www.fsis.usda.gov
USDA National Agriculture Library	http://www.nal.usda.gov/fnic

concern to community well-being. To be effective, the needs assessment must be a dynamic document that is responsive to changes in the community. A plan is only as good as the research used to shape the decisions, so a mechanism for ongoing review and revision should be built into the planning.

A needs assessment is based on objective data, including demographic information and health statistics. Information should represent the community's diversity and be segmented by such factors as age, gender, socioeconomic status, disability, and ethnicity. Examples of information to be gathered include current morbidity and mortality statistics, number of low-birth-weight infants, deaths attributed to chronic diseases with a link to nutrition, and health-risk indicators such as incidence of smoking or obesity. *Healthy People 2020* outlines the leading health indicators that can be used to create target objectives. Subjective information such as input from community members and leaders and health and nutrition professionals can be useful in supporting the objective data or in emphasizing questions or concerns. The process mirrors what the business world knows as *market research.*

Accessible community resources and services should also be catalogued. Environmental, policy, and societal changes have contributed to the rapid rise in obesity over the past few decades; walkable neighborhoods, good access to recreation facilities, and ready access to healthy foods are important measures to assess (Sallis and Glanz, 2009). In nutrition planning the goal is to determine who and what resources are available to community members when they need food- or nutrition-related products or services. For example, what services are available for nutrition therapy, nutrition and food education, and child care or homemaker skills training? Are there safe areas for exercise or recreation? Is there access to transportation? Is there compliance with disability legislation? Are mechanisms in place for emergencies that might affect access to adequate and safe food and water?

At first glance some of the data gathered in this process may not appear to relate directly to nutrition, but an experienced community nutritionist or a community-based advisory group with public health professionals can help connect this information to nutrition- and diet-related issues. Often the nutritional problems identified in a review of nutrition indicators are associated with dietary inadequacies, excesses, or imbalances that can be triggers for disease risk. Examples of trigger areas are presence of risk factors for cardiovascular disease; diabetes and stroke, including elevated blood cholesterol and lipids, inactivity, smoking, elevated blood glucose, high body mass index (BMI), and elevated blood pressure; risk factors for osteoporosis; evidence of eating disorders; high levels of teenage pregnancy; and evidence of hunger and food insecurity. Careful attention should be paid to the special needs of adults and children with disabilities or other lifestyle-limiting conditions. Access to safe and adequate amounts of food and water can be interrupted by something as simple as a power outage or as complex as a disaster. Once evaluated, the information is used to propose needed services, including MNT as discussed in other chapters, as part of the strategy for improving the overall health of the community.

Sources for Assessment Information

It is critical that community practitioners know how to locate relevant resources and evaluate the information for validity and reliability. Knowing the background and intent of any data source and identifying the limitations and the dates when the information was collected are critical points to consider when selecting and using such sources. Census information is a starting point for beginning a needs assessment. Morbidity and mortality and other health data collected by state and local public health agencies, the Centers for Disease Control and Prevention (CDC), and the National Center for Health Statistics (NCHS) are useful. Federal agencies and their state program administration counterparts are data sources; these agencies include the **U.S. Department of Health and Human Services (USDHHS)**, U.S. Department of Agriculture (USDA), and the Administration on Aging. Local providers such as community hospitals, WIC and child care agencies, health centers, and universities with a public health or nutrition department are additional sources of information. Volunteer organizations such as the March of Dimes, the American Heart Association (AHA), the American Diabetes Association, and the American Cancer Society (ACS) maintain population statistics. Health insurers are a source for current information related to health care consumers and geographic area.

NATIONAL NUTRITION SURVEYS

Nutrition and health surveys at the federal and state level provide information on the dietary status of a population, the nutritional adequacy of the food supply, the economics of food consumption, and the effects of food assistance and regulatory programs. Public guidelines for food selection are usually based on survey data. The data are also used in policy setting; program development; and funding at the national, state, and local levels. Until the late 1960s, the USDA was the primary source of food and nutrient consumption data. Although much of the data collection is still at the federal level, other agencies and states are now generating information that provides comprehensive information on the health and nutrition of the public.

National Health and Nutrition Examination Survey

The **National Health and Nutrition Examination Survey (NHANES)** provides a framework for describing the health status of the nation. Sampling the noninstitutionalized population, the initial study began in the early 1960s, with subsequent studies on a periodic basis from 1971 to 1994. NHANES has been collected on a continuous basis since 1999. The process includes interviewing approximately 6000 individuals each year in their homes and following up with approximately 5000 individuals with a complete health examination. Since its inception, each successive NHANES has included changes or additions that make the survey more responsive as a measurement of the health status of the population. NHANES I to III included medical history, physical measurements, biochemical evaluation, physical signs and symptoms, and diet information using food frequency questionnaires and a 24-hour recall. Design changes added special population studies to increase information on under-represented groups. NHANES III (1988-1994) included a large proportion of persons age 65 years and older. This information enhanced understanding of the growing and changing population of senior adults. Currently, reports are released in 2-year cycles. Sampling methodology is planned to over-sample high-risk groups not previously covered adequately (low income, those older than the age of 60, blacks, and Hispanic Americans).

Continuing Survey of Food Intake of Individuals: Diet and Health Knowledge Survey

The Continuing Survey of Food Intake of Individuals (CSFII) was a nationwide dietary survey instituted in 1985 by the USDA. In 1990 CSFII became part of the USDA National Nutrition Monitoring System. Information from previous surveys is available from the 1980s and 1990s. The Diet and Health Knowledge Survey (DHKS), a telephone follow-up to CFSII, began in 1989. The DHKS was designed as a personal interview questionnaire that allowed individual attitudes and knowledge about healthy eating to be linked with reported food choices and nutrient intakes. Early studies focused on dietary history and a 24-hour recall of adult men and women ages 19 to 50. The 1989 and 1994 surveys questioned men, women, and children of all ages and included a 24-hour recall (personal interview) and a 2-day food diary. Household data for these studies were determined by calculating the nutrient content of foods reported to be used in the home during the survey. These results were compared with nutrition recommendations for persons matching in age and gender. The information derived from the CSFII and DHKS is still useful for decision makers and researchers in monitoring the nutritional adequacy of American diets, measuring the effect of food fortification on nutrient intakes, tracking trends, and developing dietary guidance and related programs. In 2002, both surveys merged with NHANES to become the **National Food and Nutrition Survey (NFNS)** or What We Eat in America.

National Food and Nutrition Survey: What We Eat in America

The integrated survey, What We Eat in America, is collected as part of NHANES. Food-intake data are linked to health status from other NHANES components, allowing for exploration of relationships between dietary indicators and health status. The USDHHS is responsible for sample design and data, whereas the USDA is responsible for the survey's collection and maintenance of the dietary data. Data are released at 2-year intervals and are accessible from the NHANES website (U.S. Department of Agriculture [USDA] and Agricultural Research Service, 2009).

National Nutrition Monitoring and Related Research Act

In 1990 Congress passed Public Law 101-445, the **National Nutrition Monitoring and Related Research (NNMRR) Act**. The purpose of this law is to provide organization, consistency, and unification to the survey methods that monitor the food habits and nutrition of the U.S. population, and to coordinate the efforts of the 22 federal agencies that implement or review nutrition services or surveys. Data obtained through NNMRR are used to direct research activities, develop programs and services, and make policy decisions regarding nutrition programs such as food labeling, food and nutrition assistance, food safety, and nutrition education. Reports of the various activities are issued approximately every 5 years and provide information on trends, knowledge, attitudes and behavior, food composition, and food supply determinants. They are available from the National Agricultural Library database.

National Nutrient Databank

The **National Nutrient Databank**, maintained by the USDA, is the United States' primary resource of information from private industry, academic institutions, and government laboratories on the nutrient content of foods. Historically the information was published as the series *Agriculture Handbook 8*. Currently, the databases are available to the public on tapes and on the Internet. The bank is updated frequently and includes supplemental sources, international databases, and links to other sites. This databank is a standard and updated source of nutrient information for commercial references and data systems. When using sources other than the USDA site, it is important to check the sources and the dates of the updates for evidence that these sources are reliable and current.

The Centers for Disease Control and Prevention

The CDC is a component of the USDHHS. It monitors the nation's health, detects and investigates health problems, and conducts research to enhance prevention. The CDC is also a source of information on health for international travel. Housed at CDC is the NCHS, the lead agency for NHANES, morbidity and mortality, BMI, and other health-related measures. Public health threats, such as the H1N1 virus, are also monitored by CDC.

NATIONAL NUTRITION GUIDELINES AND GOALS

Policy development describes the process by which society makes decisions about problems, chooses goals, and prepares the means to reach them. Such policies may include health priorities and dietary guidance.

Early dietary guidance had a specific disease approach. The 1982 National Cancer Institute (NCI) landmark report, *Diet, Nutrition and Cancer*, evolved into *Dietary Guidelines for Cancer Prevention.* These were updated and broadened, combining recommendations on energy balance, nutrition, and physical activity in 2004. The ACS and the American Institute for Cancer Research (AICR) are excellent resources along with materials from the NCI. Another federal agency, the National Heart, Lung, and Blood Institute provided three sets of landmark guidelines for identifying and treating lipid disorders between 1987 and 2010.

The AHA guidelines focused on persons at risk for hypertension and coronary artery disease; they were written in 2000 and revised in 2006 to include environmental influences on food choices. Another consumer-friendly, single health guideline was released in 1991 as a part of the "5-A-Day for Better Health" program sponsored by the NCI, the National Institutes of Health, and the Produce for Better Health Foundation. This guidance was built around fruits and vegetables being naturally low in fat and good sources of fiber, several vitamins and minerals, and phytonutrients. In keeping with evidence-based messages, the quantity was expanded to five to nine servings of fruits and vegetables a day to promote good health under the name of "Fruits and Veggies: More Matters" (U.S. Department of Health and Human Services [USDHHS], 2009).

Dietary Guidelines for Americans

Senator George McGovern and the Senate Select Committee on Nutrition and Human Needs presented the first

Dietary Goals for the United States in 1977. In 1980 the goals were modified and issued jointly by the USDHHS and the USDA as the *Dietary Guidelines for Americans (DGA).* The original guidelines were a response to an increasing national concern for the rise in overweight, obesity, and chronic diseases such as diabetes, coronary artery disease, hypertension, and certain cancers. The approach continues to be one of health promotion and disease prevention, with special attention paid to specific population groups.

The release of the DGA led the way for a synchronized message to the community. The common theme has been a focus on a diet lower in sodium and saturated fat, with emphasis on foods that are sources of fiber, complex carbohydrates, and lean or plant-based proteins. The message is based on food choices for optimal health using appropriate portion sizes and calorie choices related to a person's physiologic needs. Exercise, activity, and food safety guidance are standard parts of this dietary guidance. Fortunately, the current DGA are evidence-based rather than just "good advice." The expert committee report provides scientific documentation that is widely used in health practice. The DGA have become a central theme in community nutrition assessment, program planning, and evaluation; they are incorporated into programs such as *School Lunch and Congregate Meals.* Updated every 5 years, the DGA have recently undergone revision in 2010.

Food Guides

In 1916 the USDA initiated the idea of food grouping in the pamphlet, *Food for Young Children.* Food grouping systems have changed in shape (wheels, boxes, and pyramids) and numbers of groupings (four, five, and seven groups), but the intent remains consistent: to present an easy guide for healthful eating. In 2005, an Internet-based tool called *MyPyramid.gov: Steps to a Healthier You* was released. In 2011, MyPyramid.gov was replaced with chooseMyPlate.gov along with a version for children called chooseMyPlate.gov/kids. These food guidance systems focus on health promotion and disease prevention, and are updated whenever DGA guidance changes.

Healthy People and the Surgeon General's Report on Nutrition and Health

The 1979 report of the Surgeon General, *Promoting Health/Preventing Disease: Objectives for the Nation,* outlined the prevention agenda for the nation with a series of health objectives to be accomplished by 1990. In 1988, *The Surgeon General's Report on Nutrition and Health* further stimulated health promotion and disease prevention by highlighting information on dietary practices and health status. Along with specific health recommendations, documentation of the scientific basis was provided. Because the focus included implications for the individual as well as for future public health policy decisions, this report remains a useful reference and tool. *Healthy People 2000: National Health Promotion and Disease Prevention Objectives* and *Healthy People 2010* were the next generations of these landmark public health efforts. Both reports outlined the progress made on previous objectives and set new objectives for the next decade.

During the evaluation phase for setting the 2010 objectives, it was determined that the United States made progress in reducing the number of deaths from cardiovascular disease, stroke, and certain cancers. Dietary evaluation indicated a slight decrease in total dietary fat intake. However, during the previous decade there has been an increase in the number of persons who are overweight or obese, a risk factor for cardiovascular disease, stroke, and other leading chronic diseases and causes of death.

Objectives for *Healthy People 2020* have specific goals that address nutrition and weight, heart disease and stroke, diabetes, oral health, cancer, and health for seniors. These goals are important for consumers and health care providers alike. The website for *Healthy People 2020* offers an opportunity to monitor the progress on past objectives as well as on the shaping of future health initiatives.

National School Lunch Program

The National School Lunch Program (NSLP) is a federal assistance program that provides free or reduced-cost meals for low-income students in public, nonprofit private and residential institutions. It is administered at a state level through the education agencies that generally employ dietitians. In 1998 the program was expanded to include after-school snacks in schools with after-hours care. Currently the guidelines for calories, percent of calories from fat, percent of saturated fat, and the amount of protein and key vitamins and minerals must meet the DGA.

A requirement for wellness policies in schools that participate in the NSLP is in place (Edelstein et al., 2010). However, the School Nutrition Dietary Assessment Study, a nationally representative study fielded during school year 2004-2005 to evaluate nutritional quality of children's diets, identified that 80% of children had excessive intakes of saturated fat and 92% had excessive intakes of sodium (Clark and Fox, 2009). An increase in whole grains, fresh fruits, and a greater variety of vegetables is needed (Condon et al., 2009). The state of Texas made changes to their school lunches by restricting portion sizes of high-fat and high-sugar snacks and sweetened beverages, fat content of foods, and high-fat vegetables like french fries; this led to a desired reduction in energy density (Mendoza et al., 2010). For current information and updates to these programs, check the USDA website.

The Recommended Dietary Allowances and Dietary Reference Intakes

The recommended dietary allowances (RDAs) were developed in 1943 by the Food and Nutrition Board of the National Research Council of the National Academy of Sciences. The first tables were developed at a time when the U.S. population was recovering from a major economic depression and World War II; nutrient deficiencies were a concern. The intent was to develop intake guidelines that would promote optimal health and lower the risk of nutrient deficiencies. As the food supply and the nutrition needs of the population changed, the intent of the RDAs was adapted to prevention of nutrition-related disease. Until 1989 the RDAs were revised approximately every 10 years.

The RDAs have always reflected gender, age, and life-phase differences. There have been additions of nutrients and revisions of the age-groups. However, recent revisions are a major departure from the single list some professionals still view as the RDAs. Beginning in 1998 an umbrella of nutrient guidelines known as the dietary reference intakes (DRIs) was introduced. Included in the DRIs are RDAs, as well as new designations, including guidance on safe upper limits of certain nutrients. As a group the DRIs are evaluated and revised at intervals, making these tools reflective of current research and population base needs (see Chapter 12).

FOOD ASSISTANCE AND NUTRITION PROGRAMS

Public health assurance addresses the implementation of legislative mandates, maintenance of statutory responsibilities, support of crucial services, regulation of services and products provided in both the public and private sector, and maintenance of accountability. This includes providing for food security, which translates into having access to an adequate amount of healthful and safe foods.

In the area of **food security**, or access by individuals to a readily available supply of nutritionally adequate and safe foods, programs such as the **Supplemental Nutrition Assistance Program (SNAP)** for food stamps, food pantries, and home-delivered meals, child nutrition programs, supermarkets, and other food sources should be available and used. For example, research on neighborhood food access indicates that low availability of healthy food in area stores is associated with low-quality diets of area residents (Rose et al., 2010). See Table 10-1 for a list of food and nutrition assistance programs.

FOODBORNE ILLNESS

Each year there are an estimated 76 million cases of foodborne illness in the United States. The majority of foodborne illness outbreaks reported to the CDC result from bacteria, followed by viral outbreaks, chemical causes, and parasitic causes. Segments of the population are particularly susceptible to foodborne illnesses; vulnerable individuals are more likely to become ill and experience complications. Some of the nutritional complications associated with foodborne illness include reduced appetite and reduced nutrient absorption from the gut.

The 2000 edition of the DGA was the first to include food safety, important for linking the safety of the food and water supply with health promotion and disease prevention. This acknowledges the potential for **foodborne illness** to cause both acute illness and long-term chronic complications. Since 2000 all revisions of the DGA have made food safety a priority. Persons at increased risk for foodborne illnesses include young children; pregnant women; older adults; persons who are immunocompromised because of human immunodeficiency virus or acquired immunodeficiency syndrome, steroid use, chemotherapy, diabetes mellitus, or cancer; alcoholics; persons with liver disease, decreased stomach acidity, autoimmune disorders, or malnutrition; persons who take antibiotics; and persons living in institutionalized settings. Costs associated with foodborne illness include those related to investigation of foodborne outbreaks and treatment of victims, employer costs related to lost productivity, and food industry losses related to lower sales and lower stock prices (American Dietetic Association, 2009). Table 10-2 describes common foodborne illnesses and their signs and symptoms, timing of onset, duration, causes, and prevention.

All food groups have ingredients associated with food safety concerns. There are concerns about microbial contamination of fruits and vegetables especially those imported from other countries. An increased incidence of foodborne illness occurs with new methods of food production or distribution, and with increased reliance on commercial food sources (ADA, 2009). Improperly cooked meats can harbor organisms that trigger a foodborne illness. Even properly cooked meats have the potential to cause foodborne illness if the food handler allows raw meat juices to contaminate other foods during preparation. Sources of a foodborne illness outbreak vary, depending on such factors as the type of organism involved, the point of contamination and the duration and temperature of food during holding.

Targeted food safety public education campaigns are important. However, the model for food safety has expanded beyond the individual consumer and now includes government, the food industry, and the general public. Several government agencies provide information through websites with links to the CDC, the USDA Food Safety and Inspection Service (FSIS), the Environmental Protection Agency (EPA), the National Institute of Allergy and Infectious Diseases, and the Food and Drug Administration (FDA). A leading industry program, ServSafe®, provides food safety and training certification and was developed and administered by the National Restaurant Association. Because our food supply comes from a global market, food safety concerns are worldwide. The 2009 Country of Origin Labeling (COOL) legislation requires that retailers provide customers with the source of foods such as meats, fish, shellfish, fresh and frozen fruits and vegetables, and certain nuts and herbs. The USDA Agricultural Marketing Service has responsibility for COOL implementation. Future practice must include awareness

Text continued on p. 244

TABLE 10-1

U.S. Food Assistance and Nutrition Programs

Program Name	Goal/Purpose	Services Provided	Target Audience	Eligibility	Funding	Level of Prevention*
After-School Snack Program	Provides reimbursement for snacks served to students after school.	Provides cash reimbursement to schools for snacks served to students after the school day. Snacks must contain two of four components: fluid milk, meat/meat alternate, vegetable or fruit or full-strength juice, whole-grain or enriched bread.	Children younger than 18 whose school sponsors a structured, supervised after-school enrichment program and provides lunch through the NSLP.	School programs located within the boundaries of eligible low-income areas may be reimbursed for snacks served at no charge to students.	USDA	Primary, secondary
Child and Adult Care Food Program	Provides nutritious meals and snacks to infants, young children, and adults receiving day care services, as well as infants and children living in emergency shelters.	Provides commodities or cash to help centers serve nutritious meals that meet federal guidelines.	Infants, children, and adults receiving day care at childcare centers, family day care homes, and homeless shelters		USDA FNS	Primary, secondary
Commodity Supplemental Food Program	Provides no-cost monthly supplemental food packages composed of commodity foods to populations perceived to be at nutritional risk.	Provides food packages; nutrition education services are available often through Extension Service Programs; program referrals provided.	Generally children ages 5-6, postpartum nonbreastfeeding mothers from 6-12 months' postpartum, seniors	Between 130% and 185% of the poverty guideline	USDA FNS	Primary, secondary
Disaster Feeding Program	Makes commodities available for distribution to disaster relief agencies.	Commodities are provided to disaster victims through congregate dining settings and direct distribution to households.	Those experiencing a natural disaster	Those experiencing a natural disaster	USDA FNS	Primary
TEFAP	Commodities are made available to local emergency food providers for preparing meals for the needy or for distribution of food packages.	Surplus commodity foods are provided for distribution.	Low-income households	Low-income households at 150% of the federal poverty income guideline	USDA FNS	Primary

EFSP	Funds are used to purchase food and shelter to supplement and extend local services.	EFSP provides funding for the purchase of food products, operation costs associated with mass feeding and shelter, limited rent or mortgage assistance, providing assistance for first month's rent, limited off-site emergency lodging, and limited utility assistance.	Those in need of emergency services	Primary	FEMA	Primary
Head Start	Provides agencies and schools with support and guidance for half- and full-day child development programs for low-income children.	Programs receive reimbursement for nutritious meals and snacks and USDA-donated commodities, support for curriculum, social services, and health screenings.	Low-income children ages 3-5; parents are encouraged to volunteer and be involved	Same as NSLP	USDA (food) USDHHS (health)	Primary Secondary
National School Breakfast Program	Provides nutritionally balanced, low-cost or free breakfasts to children enrolled in participating schools.	Participating schools receiving cash subsidies and USDA-donated commodities in return for offering breakfasts that meet same criteria as school lunch and offering free and reduced-price meals to eligible children.	Children preschool age through grade 12 in schools; children and teens 20 years of age in residential childcare and juvenile correctional institutions	Same as NSLP	USDA FNS	Primary, secondary
NSLP	Provides nutritionally balanced, low-cost or free lunches to children enrolled in participating schools.	Participating schools receive cash subsidies and USDA-donated commodities in return for offering lunches that meet dietary guidelines and ⅓ of RDA for protein, iron, calcium, vitamins A and C, and calories and for offering free and reduced-price meals to eligible children.	Children preschool age through grade 12 in schools; children and teenagers 20 years of age and younger in residential childcare and juvenile correctional institutions	185% of federal poverty income guideline for reduced-price lunches; 130% for free lunches	USDA FNS	Primary, secondary

Continued

TABLE 10-1

U.S. Food Assistance and Nutrition Programs—cont'd

Program Name	Goal/Purpose	Services Provided	Target Audience	Eligibility	Funding	Level of Prevention*
Nutrition Program for the Elderly/ Area Agencies on Aging	Provides commodity and cash assistance to programs providing meal services to older adults.	Provides nutritious meals for older adults through congregate dining or home-delivered meals.	Older adults	No income standard applied	USDHHS administers through state and local agencies; USDA cash and commodity assistance	Primary
Seniors' Farmers Market Nutrition Program	Provides fresh, nutritious, unprepared, locally grown fruits, vegetables, and herbs from farmers' markets, roadside stands, and community-supported agriculture programs to low-income seniors.	Coupons for use at authorized farmers' markets, roadside stands, and community-supported agriculture programs (Foods that are not eligible for purchase with coupons by seniors are dried fruits or vegetables, potted plants and herbs, wild rice, nuts, honey, maple syrup, cider and molasses.)	Low-income adults older than age 60	Low-income seniors with household incomes not exceeding 195% of the federal poverty income guideline	USDA FNS	Primary
SNAP	Provides benefits to low-income people that they can use to buy food to improve their diets.	Provides assistance such as food stamps.	Any age	For households in the 48 contiguous states and the District of Columbia. To get SNAP benefits, households must meet certain tests, including resource and income tests.	USDA FNS	Primary Secondary
Special Milk Program	Provides milk to children in participating schools who do not have access to other meal programs.	Provides cash reimbursement for milk with vitamins A and D at RDA levels served at low or no cost to children; milk programs must be run on nonprofit basis.	Same target audience as school lunch and school breakfast programs	Eligible children do *not* have access to other supplemental foods programs.	USDA FNS	Primary, secondary

Summer Food Service Program	Provides healthy meals (per federal guidelines) and snacks to eligible children when school is out, using agriculture commodity foods.	Reimburses for up to two or three meals and snacks served daily free to eligible children when school is not in session; cash based on income level of local geographic area or of enrolled children.	Infants and children 18 years of age and younger served at variety of feeding sites		USDA FNS	Primary, secondary
WIC	Provides supplemental foods to improve health status of participants.	Nutrition education, free nutritious foods (protein, iron, calcium, vitamins A and C), referrals, breastfeeding promotion.	Pregnant, breastfeeding and postpartum women up to 1 year Infants, children up to 5 yrs	185% of federal poverty income guideline nutritional risk	UDSA FNS, home state support	Primary, secondary, tertiary
WIC FMNP	Provides fresh, unprepared, locally grown fruits and vegetables to WIC recipients, and to expand the awareness, use of and sales at farmers' markets.	FMNP food coupons for use at participating farmers' markets stands; nutrition education through arrangements with state agency.	Same as WIC recipients	Same as WIC recipients	USDA FNS	Primary

EFSP, Emergency Food and Shelter Program; *FEMA*, Federal Emergency Management Agency; *FMNP*, Farmers Market Nutrition Program; *FNS*, Food and Nutrition Service; *NSLP*, National School Lunch Program; *RDA*, recommended daily allowance; *SNAP*, Special Nutrition Assistance Program; *USDA*, U.S. Department of Agriculture; *USDHHS*, U.S. Department of Health and Human Services; *WIC*, Special Supplemental Nutrition Program for Women, Infants, and Children.

*Level of prevention rationale: Programs that provide food only are regarded as primary; programs that provide food, nutrients at a mandated level of recommended dietary allowances or an educational component are regarded as secondary; and programs that used health screening measures on enrollment were regarded as tertiary.

TABLE 10-2

Common Foodborne Illnesses

Illness	Signs and Symptoms	Onset and Duration	Causes and Prevention	Comments
Bacillus cereus	Watery diarrhea, abdominal cramping, vomiting	6-15 hours after consumption of contaminated food; duration 24 hours in most instances	Meats, milk, vegetables, and fish have been associated with the diarrheal type; vomiting-type outbreaks have generally been associated with rice products; potato, pasta and cheese products; food mixtures such as sauces, puddings, soups, casseroles, pastries, and salads may also be a source.	*B. cereus* is a gram-positive, aerobic spore former.
Campylobacter jejuni	Diarrhea (often bloody), fever, and abdominal cramping	2-5 days after exposure; duration 2-10 days	Drinking raw milk or eating raw or undercooked meat, shellfish, or poultry; to prevent exposure, avoid raw milk and cook all meats and poultry thoroughly; it is safest to drink only pasteurized milk; the bacteria may also be found in tofu or raw vegetables. Hand-washing is important for prevention; wash hands with soap before handling raw foods of animal origin, after handling raw foods of animal origin, and before touching anything else; prevent cross-contamination in the kitchen; proper refrigeration and sanitation are also essential.	Top source of foodborne illness; some people develop antibodies to it, but others do not. In persons with compromised immune systems, it may spread to the bloodstream and cause sepsis; may lead to arthritis or to GBS; 40% of GBS in the United States is caused by campylobacteriosis and affects the nerves of the body, beginning several weeks after the diarrheal illness; can lead to paralysis that lasts several weeks and usually requires intensive care.
Clostridium botulinum	Muscle paralysis caused by the bacterial toxin: double or blurred vision, drooping eyelids, slurred speech, difficulty swallowing, dry mouth, and muscle weakness; infants with botulism appear lethargic, feed poorly, are constipated, and have a weak cry and poor muscle tone	In foodborne botulism symptoms generally begin 18-36 hours after eating contaminated food; can occur as early as 6 hours or as late as 10 days; duration days or months	Home-canned foods with low acid content such as asparagus, green beans, beets, and corn; outbreaks have occurred from more unusual sources such as chopped garlic in oil, hot peppers, tomatoes, improperly handled baked potatoes wrapped in aluminum foil, and home-canned or fermented fish. Persons who home-can should follow strict hygienic procedures to reduce contamination of foods; oils infused with garlic or herbs should be refrigerated; potatoes that have been baked while wrapped in aluminum foil should be kept hot until served or refrigerated; because high temperatures destroy the botulism toxin, persons who eat home-canned foods should boil the food for 10 minutes before eating.	If untreated, these symptoms may progress to cause paralysis of the arms, legs, trunk, and respiratory muscles; long-term ventilator support may be needed. Throw out bulging, leaking, or dented cans and jars that are leaking; safe home-canning instructions can be obtained from county extension services or from the U.S. Department of Agriculture; honey can contain spores of *C. botulinum* and has been a source of infection for infants; children younger than 12 months old should not be fed honey.

Clostridium perfringens	Nausea with vomiting, diarrhea, and signs of acute gastroenteritis lasting 1 day	Within 6-24 hours from the ingestion	Ingestion of canned meats or contaminated dried mixes, gravy, stews, refried beans, meat products, and unwashed vegetables. Cook foods thoroughly; leftovers must be reheated properly or discarded.	
Cryptosporidium parvum	Watery stools, diarrhea, nausea, vomiting, slight fever, and stomach cramps	2-10 days after being infected	Contaminated food from poor handling. Hand washing is important.	Protozoa causes diarrhea among immune-compromised patients.
Enterotoxigenic Escherichia coli (ETEC)	Watery diarrhea, abdominal cramps, low-grade fever, nausea and malaise	With high infective dose, diarrhea can be induced within 24 hours	Contamination of water with human sewage may lead to contamination of foods; infected food handlers may also contaminate foods; dairy products such as semisoft cheeses may cause problems, but this is rare.	More common with travel to other countries; in infants or debilitated elderly persons, electrolyte replacement therapy may be necessary.
Escherichia coli O157:H7 Enterohemorrhagic *E. coli* (EHEC)	Hemorrhagic colitis (painful, bloody diarrhea)	Onset is slow, usually approximately 3-8 days after ingestion Duration 5-10 days	Undercooked ground beef and meats, from unprocessed apple cider, or from unwashed fruits and vegetables; sometimes water sources; alfalfa sprouts, unpasteurized fruit juices, dry-cured salami, lettuce, spinach, game meat, and cheese curds Cook meats thoroughly, use only pasteurized milk, and wash all produce well.	Antibiotics are not used because they spread the toxin further; the condition may progress to hemolytic anemia, thrombocytopenia, and acute renal failure, requiring dialysis and transfusions; HUS can be fatal, especially in young children; there are several outbreaks each year, particularly from catering operations, church events, and family picnics; *E. coli* O157:H7 can survive in refrigerated acid foods for weeks (Mayerhauser, 2001).
Listeria monocytogenes (LM)	Mild fever, headache, vomiting, and severe illness in pregnancy; sepsis in the immuno-compromised patient; meningoencephalitis in infants; and febrile gastroenteritis in adults	Onset 2-30 days Duration variable	Processed, ready-to-eat products such as undercooked hot dogs, deli or lunchmeats, and unpasteurized dairy products; postpasteurization contamination of soft cheeses such as feta or Brie, milk, and commercial coleslaw; cross-contamination between food surfaces has also been a problem. Use pasteurized milk and cheeses; wash produce before use; reheat foods to proper temperatures; wash hands with hot, soapy water after handling these ready-to-eat foods; discard foods by their expiration dates.	May be fatal. Caution must be used by pregnant women, who may pass the infection on to their unborn child.

Continued

TABLE 10-2

Common Foodborne Illnesses—cont'd

Illness	Signs and Symptoms	Onset and Duration	Causes and Prevention	Comments
Norovirus	Gastroenteritis with nausea, vomiting, and/or diarrhea accompanied by abdominal cramps; headache, fever/chills, and muscle aches may also be present.	24 to 48 hours after ingestion of the virus, but can appear as early as 12 hours after exposure	Foods can be contaminated either by direct contact with contaminated hands or work surfaces that are contaminated with stool or vomit or by tiny droplets from nearby vomit that can travel through air to land on food; although the virus cannot multiply outside of human bodies, once on food or in water, it can cause illness; most cases occur on cruise ships.	Symptoms are usually brief and last only 1 or 2 days; however, during that brief period, people can feel very ill and vomit, often violently and without warning, many times a day; drink liquids to prevent dehydration.
Salmonella	Diarrhea, fever, and abdominal cramps	12-72 hours after infection Duration usually 4-7 days	Ingestion of raw or undercooked meat, poultry, fish, eggs, unpasteurized dairy products; unwashed fruits and raw vegetables (melons and sprouts) Prevent by thorough cooking, proper sanitation, and hygiene.	There are many different kinds of *Salmonella* bacteria; *S. typhimurium* and *S. enteritidis* are the most common in the United States. Most people recover without treatment, but some have diarrhea that is so severe that the patient needs to be hospitalized; this patient must be treated promptly with antibiotics; the elderly, infants, and those with impaired immune systems are more likely to have a severe illness.
Shigellosis	Bloody diarrhea, fever, and stomach cramps	24-48 hours after exposure Duration 4-7 days	Milk and dairy products; cold mixed salads such as egg, tuna, chicken, potato, and meat salads Proper cooking, reheating, and maintenance of holding temperatures should aid in prevention; careful hand washing is essential.	This is caused by a group of bacteria called *Shigella;* it may be severe in young children and the elderly; severe infection with high fever may be associated with seizures in children younger than 2 years old.
Staphylococcus aureus	Nausea, vomiting, retching, abdominal cramping, and prostration	Within 1-6 hours; rarely fatal Duration 1-2 days	Meat, pork, eggs, poultry, tuna salad, prepared salads, gravy, stuffing, cream-filled pastries Cooking does not destroy the toxin; proper handling and hygiene are crucial for prevention.	Refrigerate foods promptly during preparation and after meal service.

Streptococcus pyogenes	Sore and red throat, pain on swallowing; tonsillitis, high fever, headache, nausea, vomiting, malaise, rhinorrhea; occasionally a rash occurs	Onset 1-3 days	Milk, ice cream, eggs, steamed lobster, ground ham, potato salad, egg salad, custard, rice pudding, and shrimp salad; in almost all cases, the foodstuffs were allowed to stand at room temperature for several hours between preparation and consumption.	Entrance into the food is the result of poor hygiene, ill food handlers, or the use of unpasteurized milk. Complications are rare; treated with antibiotics.
Vibrio vulnificus	Vomiting, diarrhea, or both; illness is mild	Gastroenteritis occurs about 16 hours after eating contaminated food. Duration about 48 hours	Seafood, especially raw clams and oysters, that has been contaminated with human pathogens; although oysters can only be harvested legally from waters free from fecal contamination, even these can be contaminated with *V. vulnificus* because the bacterium is naturally present.	This is a bacterium in the same family as those that cause cholera; it yields a *Norovirus*; it may be fatal in immunocompromised individuals.
Yersinia enterocolitica	Common symptoms in children are fever, abdominal pain, and diarrhea, which is often bloody; in older children and adults, right-sided abdominal pain and fever may be predominant symptom and may be confused with appendicitis.	1-2 days after exposure Duration 1-3 weeks or longer	Contaminated food, especially raw or undercooked pork products; postpasteurization contamination of chocolate milk, reconstituted dry milk, pasteurized milk, and tofu are also high-risk foods; cold storage does not kill the bacteria. Cook meats thoroughly; use only pasteurized milk; proper hand washing is also important.	Infectious disease caused by the bacterium *Yersinia;* in the United States most human illness is caused by *Y. enterocolitica;* it most often occurs in young children. In a small proportion of cases, complications such as skin rash, joint pains, or spread of bacteria to the bloodstream can occur.

Adapted with permission from Escott-Stump S: Nutrition and diagnosis-related care, ed 7, Baltimore, 2011, Lippincott Williams & Wilkins. Other sources: http://www.cdc.gov/health/diseases; http://www.cfsan.fda.gov/~mow/intro.html, accessed April 23, 2010.

GBS, Guillian-Barré Syndrome; *HUS*, hemolytic uremic syndrome.

CLINICAL INSIGHT

Global Food Safety

The United States imports produce, meat, and seafood from other countries to meet the consumer demands for foods that are not readily available in the country. Global importation creates potential danger to the public. Our current food supply is becoming much harder to trace back to a single source, and because of this, it is imperative that safety concerns be addressed globally, as well as in the United States. Leadership from food growers, producers, distributors and those involved in food preparation is essential to ensure a safe food supply. Protecting the food supply chain requires several safety management systems such as hazard analysis, critical control points, good manufacturing practice, and good hygiene practice (Aruoma, 2006). Food safety also includes attention to issues such as the use of toxins and pesticides in countries where standards and enforcement may be variable, as well as the importance of clean water. Finally, the effect of global warming on food production is an increasing concern.

of global food safety issues (see *Clinical Insight:* Global Food Safety).

Hazard Analysis Critical Control Points

An integral strategy to reduce foodborne illness is risk assessment and management. **Risk assessment** entails hazard identification, characterization, and exposure. **Risk management** covers risk evaluation, option assessment and implementation, monitoring and review of progress. One formal program, organized in 1996, is the **Hazard Analysis Critical Control Points (HACCP)**, a systematic approach to the identification, evaluation, and control of food safety hazards. HACCP involves identifying any biologic, chemical, or physical agent that is likely to cause illness or injury in the absence of its control as it pertains to food production. It also involves identifying points at which control can be applied, thus preventing or eliminating the food safety hazard or reducing it to an acceptable level. Restaurants and health care facilities are obligated to use HACCP procedures in their food handling practices.

There is an increased risk to health care professionals with direct patient contact, as well as those involved in community education. Those who serve populations at the greatest risk for foodborne illness have a special need to be involved in the network of food safety education and to communicate this information to their clients. Adoption of the HACCP regulations, food quality assurance programs, handling of fresh produce guidelines, technologic advances designed to reduce contamination, increased food supply regulations, and a greater emphasis on food safety education has contributed to a substantial decline in foodborne illness. Figure 10-1 shows a graphic used to explain HACCP to those who are cooking meals in large quantity.

FOOD AND WATER SAFETY

Although individual educational efforts are effective in raising awareness of food safety issues, food and water safety must be examined on a national, systems-based level (ADA, 2009). Several federal health initiatives include objectives relating to food and water safety, pesticide and allergen exposure, food-handling practices, reducing disease incidence associated with water, and reducing food- and water-related exposure to environmental pollutants. Related agencies can be found in Table 10-3.

Contamination

Controls and precautions in the area of limiting potential contaminants in the water supply are of continuing importance. Water contamination with arsenic, lead, pesticides, mercury, chlorine, herbicides, and *Escherichia coli* has been repeatedly highlighted by the media. It has been estimated that many public water systems, built using early twentieth-century technology, will need to invest more than $138 billion during the next 20 years to ensure continued safe drinking water (ADA, 2009). The effect on the potential safety of foods that have contact with these contaminants is an ongoing issue being monitored by advocacy and professional groups and governmental agencies.

Of interest to many is the issue of the potential hazards of ingestion of seafood that has been in contact with methyl mercury present naturally in the environment and released into the air from industrial pollution. Mercury has accumulated in bodies of water (i.e., streams, rivers, lakes, and oceans) and in the flesh of seafood in these waters (U.S. Food and Drug Administration and Environmental Protection Agency, 2009). The body of knowledge on issues such as this is constantly being updated, and there are now recommendations to restrict the consumption of certain fish such as shark, mackerel, tilefish, tuna, and swordfish by pregnant women (Center for Food Safety and Applied Nutrition, 2009). (See Chapter 16 for further discussion.) Other contaminants in fish, polychlorinated biphenyls, and dioxin are also of concern (Mozaffarian and Rimm, 2006).

There are precautions in place at the federal, state, and local levels that need to be addressed by dietetics professionals whose roles include advocacy, communication, and education. Both members of the public and local health officials must understand the risks and the importance of carrying out measures for food and water safety and protection. Both the EPA and the Center for Food Safety and Applied Nutrition (CFSAN) provide ongoing monitoring and guidance. In addition, food and water safety and foodborne illness issues are monitored by state and local health departments.

Organic Foods and Pesticide Use

The use of pesticides and contaminants from the water supply affect produce quality. The debate continues about

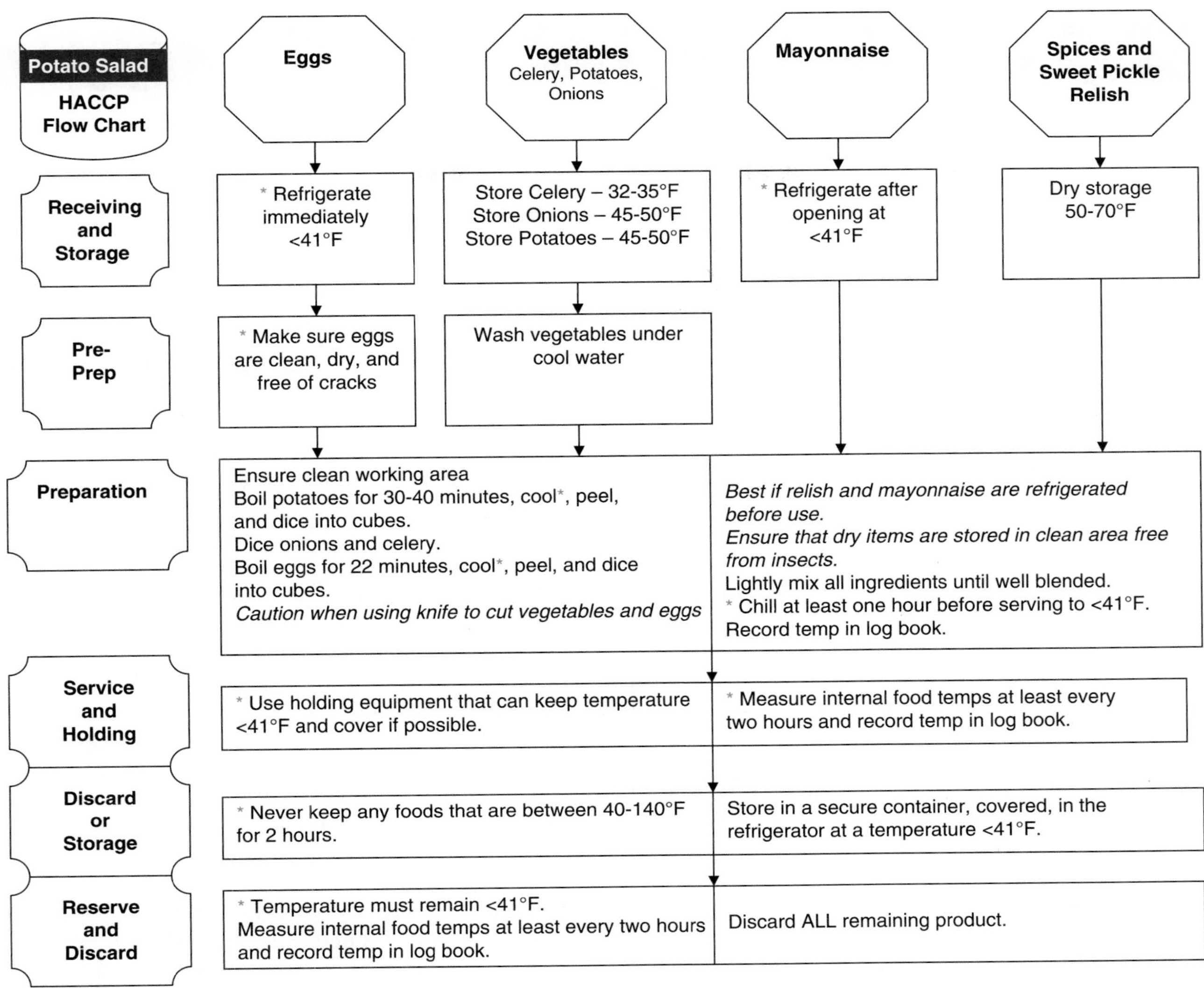

FIGURE 10-1 The Seven Steps of HACCP and a Sample Flow Chart
1. Hazard analysis-what can go wrong?
2. Determine the critical control points (CCPs).
3. Establish critical limits.
4. Establish a system to monitor CCPs.
5. Decide upon a corrective action.
6. Verify that HACCP is working properly.
7. Document and demonstrate it works.

*Critical Control Point in food handling.

whether or not organic foods are worth the extra cost. However, the beneficial effects of organic farming also need to be considered. Most experts agree that fruit such as apples may be healthier if chosen in the organic aisle. Otherwise, fruits with a thick skin, such as banana, are acceptable in either form. See *Clinical Insight:* Is Organic Produce Healthier?

Bioterrorism and Food-Water Safety

Bioterrorism is the deliberate use of microorganisms or toxins from living organisms to induce death or disease. Threats to the nation's food and water supplies have made food **biosecurity**, or precautions to minimize risk, an issue when addressing preparedness planning. The CDC has identified seven foodborne pathogens as having the potential to be used by bioterrorists to attack the food supply: tularemia, brucellosis, *Clostridium botulinum* toxin, epsilon toxin of *Clostridium perfringens*, *Salmonella*, *E. coli*, and *Shigella*. These pathogens, along with potential water contaminants, such as mycobacteria, *Legionella*, *Giardia*, viruses, arsenic, lead, copper, methyl butyl ether, uranium, and radon, are the targets of federal systems put in place to monitor the safety of the food and water supply. Current surveillance systems are designed to detect foodborne illness outbreaks resulting from food spoilage, poor food handling practices, or other unintentional sources, but they were not designed to identify an intentional attack.

Consequences of a compromised food and water supply would be physical, psychological, political, and economic. Compromise could occur with food being the primary agent such as a vector to deliver a biologic or chemical weapon or with food being a secondary target, leaving an inadequate

CLINICAL INSIGHT

Is Organic Produce Healthier?

By Christine McCullum-Gómez, PhD, RD, Food and Nutrition Consultant, Houston, TX

There are a variety of reasons why organic foods facilitate the creation of a healthful, sustainable food system (McCullum-Gómez and Scott, 2009). First, some organic fruits, vegetables, and juices may contain more antioxidants and polyphenols compared with their conventionally grown counterparts (Dani et al., 2008; Mitchell et al., 2007; Olsson et al., 2006), although this is an ongoing debate (Benbrook et al., 2009; Dangour et al., 2009a; Dangour et al., 2009b; Lairon, 2009). Second, organic meat may reduce the development of human antibiotic resistance and lessen air and water pollution (American Medical Association, 2009). Third, consumption of organic versus conventional dairy products may yield a lower risk of eczema during the first two years of life, possibly from higher intake of ω-3 fatty acids or conjugated linoleic acids (Kummeling et al., 2008).

Fortunately, **organic foods** are becoming more available in the marketplace. A 2009 survey showed sales of organic food in the United States grew by almost 16 percent in 2008 over 2007, totaling $22.9 billion in 2008 sales; 3.5 percent of all food sales (Organic Trade Association, 2009). These foods are produced following practices described in the United States Department of Agriculture (USDA) National Organic Program (NOP), a marketing program with a certification process throughout the production and manufacturing chain, required for labeling a product "organic" (U.S. Department of Agriculture, 2009). Organic foods that are certified through the USDA NOP must meet the same State and Federal food safety requirements as non-organic foods (National Organic Program, 2009; Riddle, 2009).

Although it has been suggested that organically grown fruits and vegetables may have a greater risk of pathogenic contamination than their counterparts, very few studies have confirmed these risks (Mukherjee et al., 2006). In a longitudinal survey of fresh produce grown by U.S. farmers in the upper Midwest, preharvest microbiological quality of produce from three farm types (organic, semiorganic, and conventional) was very similar during two seasons. Produce type (leafy greens, lettuces and cabbages) influences *Escherichia coli* contamination more than the type of farm (Mukherjee et al., 2006). Indeed, the way manure is treated and stored has a large impact on *E. coli* levels. When manure is composted before it is spread on soil, it generates heat that can kill most of the *E. coli* (Semenova et al., 2009). In organic farming, raw animal manure must be composted (§205.203), unless it is applied to land used for a crop not intended for consumption or incorporated into the soil not less than 120 days prior to the harvest (Electronic Code of Federal Regulations, Title 7: Agriculture. Part 205—National Organic Program, 2010).

The Food, Conservation and Energy Act of the Farm Bill helps to fund organic certification costs and to enhance data collection on organic agriculture. Organic agriculture offers numerous opportunities to reduce exposure to detrimental pesticides from the food and water supply (Greene et al., 2009; Lu et al., 2006; Lu et al., 2008), which is particularly important for high-risk groups including pregnant women, infants, young children, and farm workers (Arcury et al., 2007; Huen et al., 2009). Organically cultivated foods can also promote a more sustainable food system by reducing soil erosion; rehabilitating poor soils; and sequestering carbon in soil, which may reduce carbon levels in the atmosphere (Greene et al., 2009; Niggli et al., 2009). Organic agriculture reduces energy requirements for production by 25 to 50 percent (Niggli et al., 2009). These lower energy inputs decrease greenhouse gas emissions (Ziesemer, 2007). In addition, biodiversity is enhanced and farms are more resilient to unpredictable weather patterns and pest outbreaks that are predicted with climate change (Niggli et al., 2009; Worldwatch Institute, 2008). Public investment in organic agriculture facilitates wider access to organic food for consumers, helps farmers capture high-value markets, and conserves natural resources, including soil and water (Greene et al., 2009).

food supply to feed a region or the nation. Intentional use of a foodborne pathogen as the primary agent might be mistaken as a routine outbreak of foodborne illness. Distinguishing normal illness fluctuation from an intentional attack depends on having in place a system for preparedness planning, rapid communication, and central analysis.

Experience with the series of hurricanes in 2005 emphasizes the need to provide access to a safe food and water supply after emergencies and disasters. Access to food and water may be limited, which, in the case of bioterrorism, results in social disruption and self-imposed quarantine. These situations require a response different from the traditional approach to disaster relief, during which it is assumed that hungry people will seek assistance and have confidence in the safety of the food that is offered (Bruemmer, 2003). In the event of a disaster, dietetics professionals can play a key role by being aware of their environment, knowing available community and state food and nutrition resources, and participating in coordination and delivery of relief to victims of the disaster.

TABLE 10-3

Food and Water Safety Resources

American Egg Board	http://www.aeb.org
American Dietetic Association	http://www.eatright.org/
American Meat Institute	http://www.meatami.com
CFSAN	http://www.cfsan.fda.gov
CFSCAN—Food and Water Safety—Disasters	http://www.cfsan.fda.gov/~dms/fsdisas.html
CDC	http://www.cdc.gov
CDC Disaster	http://www.bt.cdc.gov/disasters/
FEMA	http://www.fema.gov
Food Chemical News	http://www.foodchemicalnews.com
Food Marketing Institute	http://www.fmi.org
Food Marketing Institute—Bird Flu	http://www.fmi.org/foodsafety/avian_flubrochure.htm
FoodNet	http://www.cdc.gov/foodnet/
Food Preservation and Safety, Iowa State University	http://www.foodpres.com
Foundation for Food Irradiation Education	http://www.food-irradiation.com
Grocery Manufacturers of America	http://www.gmabrands.org
International Food Information Council	http://ific.org/food
National Broiler Council	http://www.eatchicken.com
National Cattleman's Beef Association	http://www.beef.org/
National Institutes of Health	http://www.nih.gov
National Food Safety Database	http://www.foodsafety.gov
National Restaurant Association Educational Foundation	http://www.edfound.org
The Partnership for Food Safety Education	http://www.fightbac.org
Produce Marketing Association	http://www.pma.com
PulseNet	http://www.cdc.gov/pulsenet/whatis.html
U.S. Department of Agriculture	http://www.usda.gov
U.S. Department of Agriculture Food Safety and Inspection Service	http://www.fsis.usda.gov
U.S. Department of Education	http://www.ed.gov
U.S. Department of Health and Human Services	http://os.dhhs.gov
U.S. EPA—Office of Ground and Drinking Water	http://www.epa.gov/safewater
U.S. EPA Seafood Safety	http://www.epa.gov/ost/fish
U.S. Food and Drug Administration	http://www.fda.gov
U.S. Poultry and Egg Association	http://www.poultryegg.org

NOTE: Specific websites often change because of updating. Go to the home website and use a search to find the desired resources.

CDC, Centers for Disease Control and Prevention; *CFSAN*, Center for Food Safety and Applied Nutrition; *EPA*, Environmental Protection Agency; *FEMA*, Federal Emergency Management Agency.

DISASTER PLANNING

Dietetics and health professionals working in food service are expected to plan for the distribution of safe food and water in any emergency situation. This may include choosing food preparation and distribution sites, establishing temporary kitchens, preparing foods with limited resources, and keeping prepared food safe to eat through HACCP procedures (Puckett and Norton, 2009). To prepare for such planning, several federal agencies share the responsibility for food and water safety.

Planning, surveillance, detection, response, and recovery are the key components of public health disaster preparedness. The key agencies are the USDA, the **Department of Homeland Security (DHS)** and the Federal Emergency Management Agency (FEMA), the CDC, and the FDA. In conjunction with DHS, USDA operates Protection of the Food Supply and Agricultural Production (PFSAP). PFSAP handles issues related to food production, processing, storage, and distribution. It addresses threats against the agricultural sector and border surveillance. PFSAP conducts food safety activities concerning meat, poultry, and egg inspection and provides laboratory support, research, and education on outbreaks of foodborne illness.

Ready.gov (www.ready.gov) is an education tool informing the public on how to prepare for a national emergency, including possible terrorist attacks. In addition, the USDA FSIS operates the Food Threat Preparedness Network (PrepNet) and the Food Biosecurity Action Team (F-Bat). PrepNet ensures effective coordination of food security efforts, focusing on preventive activities to protect the food supply. F-Bat assesses potential vulnerabilities along the farm-to-table continuum, provides guidelines to industry on food security and increased plant security, strengthens FSIS's coordination and cooperation with law enforcement agencies, and enhances security features of FSIS laboratories (Bruemmer, 2003).

CDC has three operations relating to food security and disaster planning: PulseNet, FoodNet, and the Centers for Public Health Preparedness. PulseNet is a national network of public health laboratories that performs deoxyribonucleic acid fingerprinting on foodborne bacteria, assists in detecting foodborne illness outbreaks and tracing them back to their source, and provides linkages among sporadic cases. FoodNet is the Foodborne Diseases Active Surveillance Network, which functions as the principle foodborne disease component of the CDC's Emerging Infections Program, providing active laboratory-based surveillance. The Centers for Public Health Preparedness funds academic centers linking schools of public health with state, local, and regional bioterrorism preparedness and public health infrastructure needs (Bruemmer, 2003).

CFSAN in the FDA is concerned with regulatory issues such as seafood HACCP, safety of food and color additives, safety of foods developed through biotechnology, food labeling, dietary supplements, food industry compliance, and regulatory programs to address health risks associated with foodborne chemical and biologic contaminants. CFSAN also runs cooperative programs with state and local governments.

The **Federal Emergency Management Agency (FEMA)**, under the DHS, provides emergency support functions after a disaster or emergency. FEMA identifies food and water needs, arranges delivery, and provides assistance with temporary housing and other emergency services. Agencies that assist FEMA include the USDA, the Department of Defense, the USDHHS, the EPA, and the General Services Administration. Major players include voluntary agencies such as the American Red Cross, the Salvation Army, and community-based agencies and organizations. Disaster management is evolving as it is tested by both manufactured and natural disasters.

CLINICAL SCENARIO

Dietitians and nutritionists play an important role in emergency preparedness. The role of qualified nutrition professionals will vary with the type of emergency of disaster (e.g., hurricane, flood, foodborne illness outbreak, ice storm). As an emerging nutrition professional, you can play a role within your own family and community by helping them to prepare safe and adequate food for an emergency.

Your family is composed of seven members: two parents, one infant on infant formula, one school-age child, one teenager, and two grandparents. The grandparents are on moderate food restrictions that reduce sugar and sodium. Review information on emergency preparedness information from the American Red Cross (www.redcross.org) and the Department of Home Land Security (www.dhs.gov.org) and propose an emergency food package for your family that includes food and water and supplies, including menus for 7 days.

Nutrition Diagnostic Statement

Lack of access to safe foods and water related to no planning as evidenced by insufficient preparation and food and water supplies for emergencies.

Nutrition Care Questions

1. What steps can you take to design a plan?
2. How many days of food and water should be available?
3. How concerned are you about expiration dates?

USEFUL WEBSITES

American Dietetic Association
http://www.eatright.org/

American Heart Association
http://www.americanheart.org

Centers for Disease Control
http://www.cdc.gov/

Dietary Guidance
http://fnic.nal.usda.gov/nal_display/index.php?info_center=4&tax_level=1&tax_subject=256

Dietary Guidelines for Americans
http://www.cnpp.usda.gov/dietaryguidelines.htm

Environmental Protection Agency (Fish)
http://www.epa.gov/ost/fish

Federal Emergency Management Agency
http://www.fema.gov/

Homeland Security
http://www.dhs.gov/dhspublic

Food Safety
http://www.foodsafety.gov/

Hazard Analysis Critical Control Points
http://www.fda.gov/Food/FoodSafety/HazardAnalysisCriticalControlPointsHACCP/HACCPPrinciplesApplicationGuidelines/default.htm

Head Start
http://www.acf.hhs.gov/programs/ohs/legislation/index.html

Healthy People 2010 and 2020
http://www.healthypeople.gov/

MyPlate
http://www.chooseMyPlate.gov

National Academy Press—Dietary Reference Intakes
http://www.nap.edu/topics.php?topic=380

National Center for Health Statistics
http://www.cdc.gov/nchs/

National Health and Nutrition Examination Study
http://www.cdc.gov/nchs/nhanes.htm

U.S. Department of Agriculture Farm to School Initiative
http://www.fns.usda.gov/cnd/F2S/Default.htm
U.S. Department of Agriculture Nutrient Database
http://www.ars.usda.gov/nutrientdata
U.S. Department of Agriculture Nutrition Assistance Programs
http://www.fns.usda.gov/fns/
What We Eat in America
www.ars.usda.gov/ba/bhnrc/fsrg

REFERENCES

American Dietetic Association (ADA): Position of the American Dietetic Association: food and water safety, *J Am Diet Assoc* 109:1449, 2009.

American Dietetic Association: the role of registered dietitians and dietetic technicians, registered in health promotion and disease prevention programs, *J Am Diet Assoc* 106:1875, 2006.

American Medical Association: *Report of the Council on Science and Public Health*. (CSAPH). *CSAPH Report 8-A-09. Sustainable Food, Resolution* 405: A-08.2008. Accessed 20 June 2009 from http://www.ama-assn.org/ama1/pub/upload/mm/443/csaph-rep8-a09.pdf.

Arcury T, et al: Pesticide urinary metabolite levels of children in Eastern North Carolina farmworker households, *Environ Health Perspect* 115:1254, 2007.

Aruoma OI: The impact of food regulation on the food supply chain, *Toxicology* 221:119, 2006.

Benbrook C, et al: Methodologic flaws in selecting studies and comparing nutrient concentrations led Dangour to miss the emerging forest amid the trees, *Am J Clin Nutr* 90: 1700, 2009.

Bruemmer B: Food biosecurity, *J Am Diet Assoc* 103:687, 2003.

Center for Food Safety and Applied Nutrition (CFSAN), U.S. Department of Health and Human Services, Food and Drug Administration: Food. Accessed 27 December 2009 from http://www.fda.gov/food/default.htm.

Clark MA, Fox MK: Nutritional quality of the diets of US public school children and the role of the school meal programs, *J Am Diet Assoc* 109:S44, 2009.

Condon EM, et al: School meals: types of foods offered to and consumed by children at lunch and breakfast, *J Am Diet Assoc* 109:S67, 2009.

Dangour AD, et al: Nutritional quality of organic foods: a systematic review, *Am J Clin Nutr* 90:680, 2009a.

Dangour AD, et al: Reply to DL Gibbon and C Benbrook et al, *Am J Clin Nutr* 90:1701, 2009b.

Dani C, et al: Intake of purple grape juice as a hepatoprotective agent in Wistar rats, *J Med Food* 11:127, 2008.

Edelstein S, et al: Reaching out to those at highest nutritional risk. In *Nutrition in public health*, ed 2, Sudbury, MA, 2010, Jones and Bartlett, p 122. (In press.)

Electronic Code of Federal Regulations (e-CFR): Title 7: Agriculture. Part 205—National Organic Program. Accessed 4 January 2010 from.http://ecfr.gpoaccess.gov/cgi/t/text/text-idx?c=ecfr&sid=49c75b1e28f8cd145546869235346e46&rgn=div5&view=text&node=7:3.1.1.9.32&idno=7

Greene C, et al: *Emerging issues in the US organic industry, Economic Information Bulletin Number EIB-55*, Washington DC, June 2009, United States Department of Agriculture, Economic Research Service.

Healthy People 2000: *National health promotion and disease prevention objectives*, Washington, DC, 1990, U.S. Department of Health and Human Services.

Healthy People 2010: *National health promotion and disease prevention objectives*, Washington, DC, 2000, U.S. Department of Health and Human Services.

Healthy People 2020: *National health promotion and disease prevention objectives*, Washington, DC, 2010, U.S. Department of Health and Human Services.

Huen K, et al: Developmental changes in PON1 enzyme activity in young children and effects on PON1 polymorphisms, *Environ Health Perspect* 117:1632, 2009.

Kummeling I, et al: Consumption of organic food and risk of atopic disease during the first 2 years of life in the Netherlands, *Br J Nutr* 99:598, 2008.

Lairon D: Nutritional quality and safety of organic food: a review, *Agron Sustain Dev* 2009; doi: 10.10151/agro/2009019.

Lu C, et al: Dietary intake and its contribution to longitudinal pesticide exposure in urban/suburban children, *Environ Health Perspect* 116:537, 2008.

Lu C, et al: Organic diets significantly lower children's dietary exposure to organophosphorus pesticides, *Environ Health Perspect* 114:260, 2006.

Mayerhauser CM: Survival of enterhemorrhagic Escherichia coli 0157: H7 in retail mustard, *J Food Prot* 64:783, 2001.

McCullum-Gómez C, Scott AM: Hot topic: perspective on the benefit of organic foods, September 2009. Accessed 2 December 2009 from http://www.eatright.org/About/Content.aspx?id=10614.

Mendoza JA, et al: Change in dietary energy density after implementation of the Texas Public School Nutrition Policy, *J Am Diet Assoc* 110:434, 2010.

Mitchell AE, et al: Ten year comparison of the influence of organic and conventional crop management on the content of flavonoids in tomatoes, *J Agric Food Chem* 55:6154, 2007.

Mozaffarian D, Rimm EB: Fish intake, contaminants, and human health: evaluating the risks and the benefits, *JAMA* 296:1885, 2006.

Mukherjee A, et al: Longitudinal microbiological survey of fresh produce grown by farmers in the upper Midwest, *J Food Prot* 69:1928, 2006.

National Organic Program (NOP): *Organic production and handling standards*, Washington, DC, United States Department of Agriculture (USDA), Agricultural Marketing Service. Accessed 25 July 2009 from http://www.ams.usda.gov/AMSv1.0/getfile?dDocName=STELDEV3004445&acct=nopgeninfo.

Niggli U, et al: *Low greenhouse gas agriculture: mitigation and adaptation potential of sustainable farming systems*, Rome, Italy, 2009, Food and Agriculture Organization (FAO) of the United Nations, Accessed 29 June 2009 from ftp://ftp.fao.org/docrep/fao/010/ai781e/ai781e00.pdf.

Olsson ME, et al: Antioxidant levels and inhibition of cancer cell proliferation in vitro by extracts from organically and conventionally cultivated strawberries, *J Agri Food Chem* 54:1248, 2006.

Organic Trade Association: *Organic Trade Association's 2009 organic industry survey*, Greenfield, Ma, 2009, Organic Trade Association. Accessed 1 July 2009 from http://www.ota.com.

Puckett R, Norton C: Are you prepared? Developing a disaster plan for your facility, *ADA Times*, November-December 2005. Accessed 27 December 2009 from http://www.eatright.org.

Riddle JA: *Organic food safety—regulatory requirements*, College of Food, Agricultural and Natural Resource Sciences, University of Minnesota, Organic Ecology Research and Outreach

Program. Accessed 30 November 2009 from www.organic ecology.umn.edu.

Rose D, et al: The importance of a multi-dimensional approach for studying the links between food access and consumption, *J Nutr* 2010. [Epub ahead of print.]

Sallis JF, Glanz K: Physical activity and food environments: solutions to the obesity epidemic, *Milbank Q* 87:123, 2009.

Semenova AV, et al: COLIWAVE: a simulation model for survival of *E. coli* 0157:H7 in dairy manure and manure-amended soil, *Ecol Model* 2009; doi: 10.1016/j.ecolmodel.2009.10.028.

U.S. Department of Agriculture (USDA): Country of origin labeling, Washington, DC. Accessed 27 December 2009 from http://www.ams.usda.gov/nop/AMSv1.0/Cool.

U.S. Department of Agriculture (USDA), Agricultural Research Service (ARS): *What we eat in America (WWEIA), NHANES, Overview*, Beltsville, Md, USDA. Accessed 27 December 2009 from http://www.ars.usda.gov/Services/docs.htm?docid=13793.

U.S. Department of Health and Human Services (USDHHS) Institutes of Health: 5 a day, 2005. Accessed 27 December 2009 from http://www.5aday.gov.

U.S. Food and Drug Administration (FDA) and U.S. Environmental Protection Agency (EPA): Mercury and fish. Accessed 27 December 2009 from http://www.epa.gov/ost/fish.

Winslow CEA: The untilled field of public health, *Mod Med* 2:183, 1920.

Worldwatch Institute: *Questions and answers about global warming and abrupt climate change*, Washington, DC, 2008, Worldwatch Institute. Accessed 26 July 2009 from http://www.worldwatch.org/node/3949.

Ziesemer J: *Energy use in organic food systems*. Natural Resources Management and Environment Department, Food and Agriculture Organization of the United Nations (FAO), Rome, Italy, 2007, FAO. Accessed 3 July 2009 from http://www.fao.org/docs/eims/upload/233069/energy-use-oa.pdf.

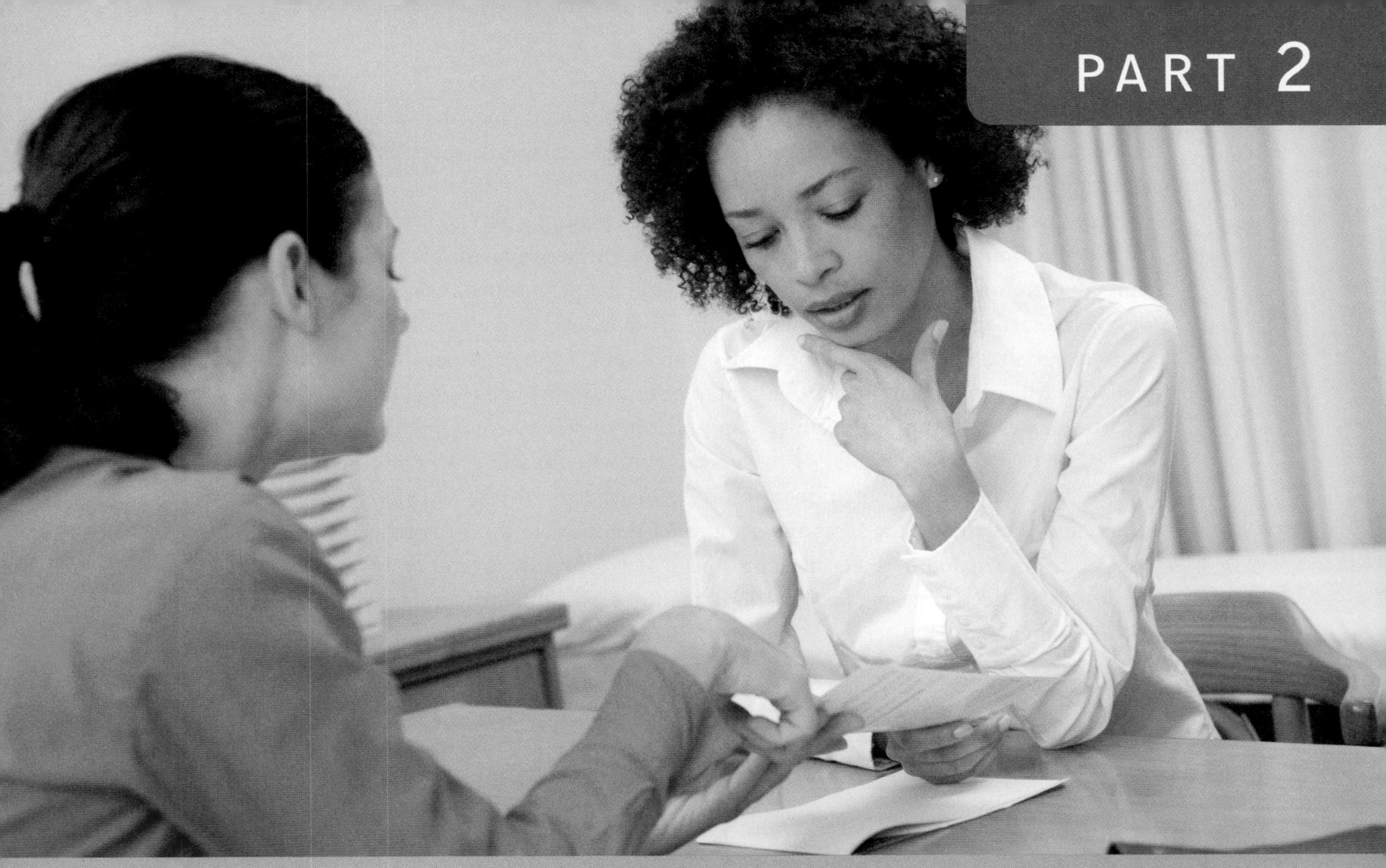

PART 2

Nutrition Diagnosis and Intervention

The type of nutrition care provided for an individual varies depending on the findings of the assessment process. The environment, surgery or trauma, food allergies, inadequate access to safe or sufficient food, stages of growth and development, harmful beliefs, lack of knowledge, and socioeconomic issues can all affect the intake of an adequate diet. In the healthy individual, omission of a specific food group or intake of high-energy, nutrient-poor foods does not lead to failed nutritional status overnight. It is the prolonged intake of such imbalances or a dramatic and acute insufficiency that leads to undesirable nutritional consequences. Indeed, inadequacy of the types or amounts of macro- or micronutrients, fluid, or even physical activity may cause a decline in health status or immunity.

The establishment of nutrition diagnoses and a standardized language helps to define and promote effective care according to specific nutrition problems. Such problems may be found in an individual, a group (such as persons who have diabetes or celiac disease), or even a community (such as sites where local produce is grown in mineral-depleted soil.) Thus step two of the nutrition care process involves identifying the appropriate diagnosis or diagnoses. It includes an analysis of the factors affecting adequacy of the current nutritional intake and overall nutritional status. In most cases, institutions use standards of care or national practice guidelines that describe recommended actions in the nutrition care process. These standards serve as the basis for assessing quality of care provided.

Step three of the nutrition care process requires planning and goal-setting, followed by the selection of interventions that fit the cause of the problem. For example, nutrition education is an appropriate intervention for the person who has little knowledge of how to manage his or her gluten-free diet. Educating individuals about their "total diet" is a viable approach, but any other nutrition diagnoses should be addressed as well. Coordination of care may be helpful to refer the individual to available cookbooks, health services, and support groups. Manipulation of dietary components, provision of enteral or parenteral nutrition, or in-depth nutrition counseling may also be needed.

The final step of the nutrition care process is specific to the individual patient or client, and is related to the signs and symptoms identified in the assessment. A separate chapter is not written here because this fourth step (monitoring and evaluation) would be developed according to the nutrition diagnoses, assessment factors, and outcomes for the individual being served.

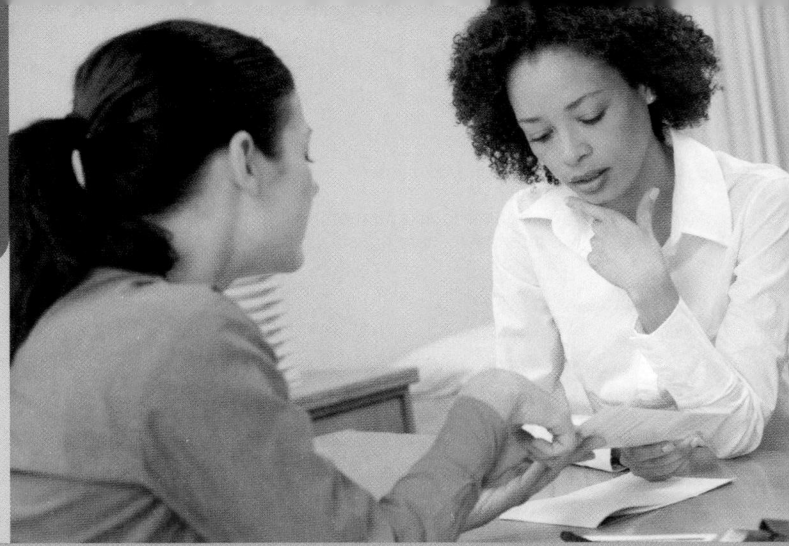

CHAPTER 11

Pamela Charney, PhD, RD
Sylvia Escott-Stump, MA, RD, LDN

Overview of Nutrition Diagnosis and Intervention

KEY TERMS

assessment, diagnosis, interventions, monitoring, evaluation (ADIME) format
advance directives
case management
Centers for Medicare and Medicaid Services (CMS)
critical pathways
discharge planning
disease management
electronic health record (EHR)
electronic medical record (EMR)
evidence-based guidelines (EBGs)
Health Insurance Portability and Accountability Act (HIPAA)
managed-care organizations (MCOs)
nutrition care process (NCP)
nutrition diagnosis
nutrition prescription
palliative care
patient-centered medical home (PCMH)
patient-focused care
personal health record (PHR)
preferred-provider organization (PPO)
problem, etiology, signs and symptoms (PES) statement
process improvement (PI)
protected health information (PHI)
room service
sentinel events
standards of care
Standards of Professional Performance (SOPPs)
subjective, objective, assessment, plan (SOAP) note format
The Joint Commission (TJC)
utilization management

Nutrition care is an organized group of activities allowing identification of nutritional needs and provision of care to meet these needs. Comprehensive service may involve different health care providers—the physician, registered dietitian (RD), nurse, pharmacist, physical or occupational therapist, social worker, speech therapist, and case manager—who are integral in achieving desired outcomes, regardless of the care setting. A collaborative approach helps to ensure that care is coordinated and that team members and the patient are aware of all goals and priorities. Team conferences, formal or informal, are useful in all settings—a clinic, a hospital, the home, the community, a long-term care facility, or any other site where nutrition problems may be identified. Coordinating the activities of health care professionals also requires documentation of the process and regular discussions to offer complete nutritional care.

THE NUTRITION CARE PROCESS

The **nutrition care process (NCP)** was established by the American Dietetic Association (ADA) as a standardized process for the provision of nutrition care. The patient or client is the central focus of the NCP (Figure 11-1), and benefits from the critical thinking of the RD and effective, interdisciplinary decision-making. The NCP includes four steps to be completed by the RD: (1) nutrition assessment,

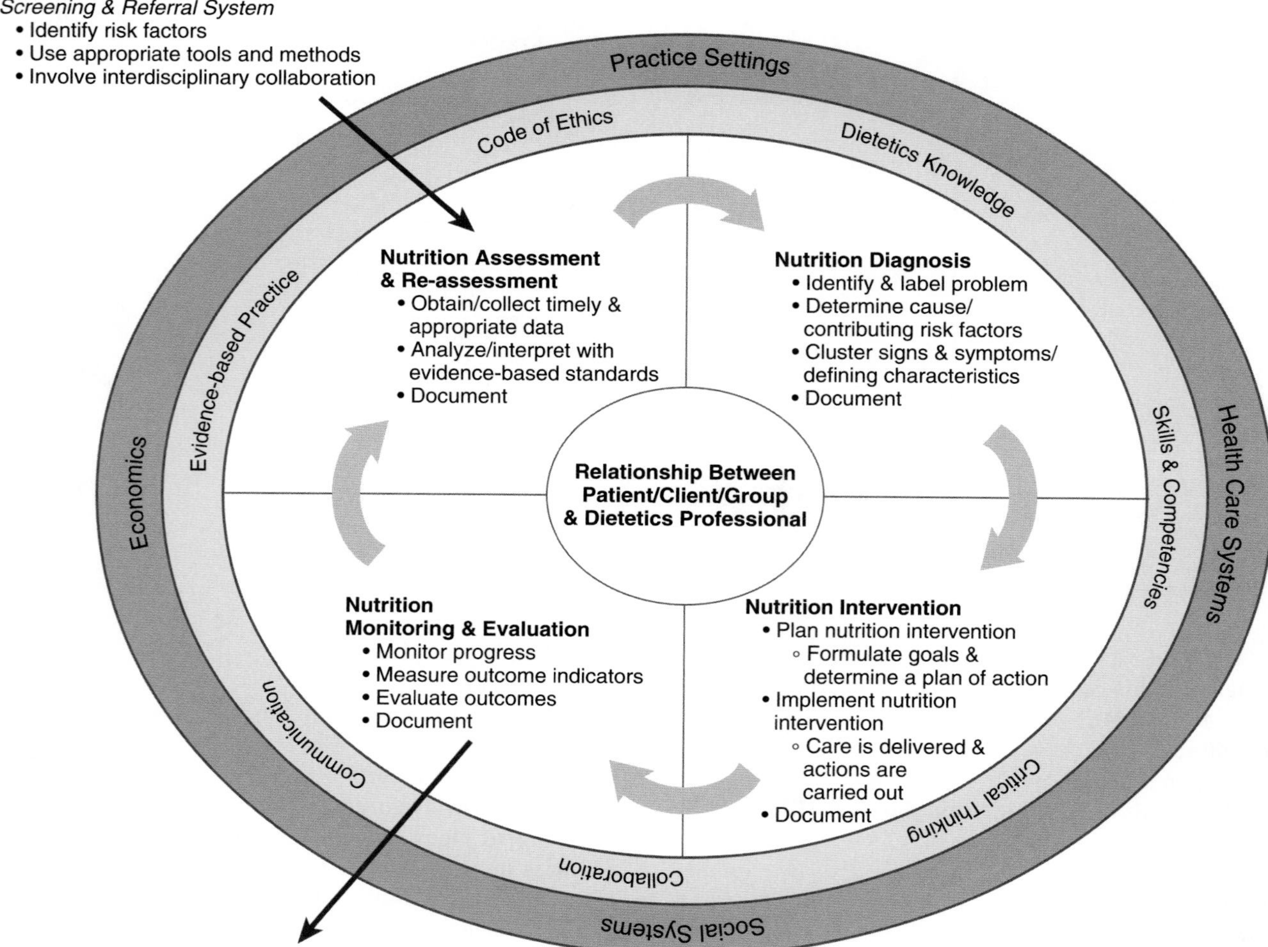

FIGURE 11-1 The nutrition care process. *(©2011 American Dietetic Association. Reprinted with permission.)*

(2) nutrition diagnosis, (3) nutrition intervention, and (4) monitoring and evaluation (American Dietetic Association [ADA], 2010).

Nutrition Screening and Assessment

Nutrition screening provides a mechanism to identify patients or clients who would benefit from nutrition assessment. Most health care facilities have developed a multidisciplinary admission screening process that is completed by nursing staff during admission to the facility. One efficient mechanism for completing the nutrition screen is to incorporate the screen into this admission assessment. The nutrition risk screen should be quick, easy to administer, and cost-effective while maintaining accuracy. Patients identified as "at risk" during the admission screen should be referred to the RD for nutrition assessment. Table 11-1 lists information that is frequently included in a nutrition screen.

When the ADA's Evidence Analysis Library (EAL) team conducted a systematic review of acute care screening tools, they determined that the Malnutrition Screening Tool had acceptable reliability and validity (ADA, 2010). Rescreening should occur at regular intervals during the admission. In hospitalized patients, there may be a relationship between length of stay and worsening nutrition status. Policies for nutrition rescreening should take into account the average length of time a patient will stay at the facility. Nutrition assessment is needed when the screening highlights potential areas of concern (see Chapter 4 for methods and tools).

Nutrition Diagnosis

After assessment of nutrition status using all of the available data, **nutrition diagnoses** (problems or needs) are identified, prioritized, and documented in the medical record. Selection of an accurate nutrition diagnosis is guided by critical

TABLE 11-1

Nutrition Risk Screening

Responsible Party	Action	Documentation
Admitting health care professional	Assess weight status—Has the patient lost weight without trying before admission?	Check yes or no on admission screen.
Admitting health care professional	Assess GI symptoms—Has the patient had GI symptoms preventing usual intake over the past 2 weeks?	Check yes or no on admission screen.
Admitting health care professional	Determine need to consult RD.	If either screening criterion is "yes," consult RD for nutrition assessment.

GI, Gastrointestinal; *RD*, registered dietitian.

evaluation of each component of the assessment, combined with critical judgment and decision-making skills. Patients with nutrition diagnoses may be at higher risk for nutrition-related complications such as increased morbidity, increased length of hospital stay, and infectious complications. Nutrition-related complications can lead to a significant increase in costs associated with hospitalization, lending support to the early diagnosis of nutrition problems followed by prompt intervention.

Many facilities use standardized formats to facilitate communication of information gathered in the nutrition assessment and nutrition diagnosis phase. A nutrition diagnosis includes documentation of the **problem, etiology, signs and symptoms (PES)** in a simple, clear statement. Methods used for documenting nutrition care in the medical record are determined at the facility level. RDs in private practice should also develop a systematic method for documenting care provided. Box 11-1 lists the nutrition diagnoses currently in use by the ADA.

Nutrition Intervention

Nutrition interventions are the actions taken intended to address the nutrition problem. Because the intervention must be an action taken by the RD, assessment of the problem must focus on any nutrition-related causes of the problem rather than the medical diagnosis. Nutrition

BOX 11-1

Nutrition Diagnoses and Sample Codes

Intake — NI

Defined as "actual problems related to intake of energy, nutrients, fluids, bioactive substances through oral diet or nutrition support"

Caloric Energy Balance (1)

Defined as "actual or estimated changes in energy (kcal)"

- ☐ Not in use — NI-1.1
- ☐ Increased energy expenditure — NI-1.2
- ☐ Not in use — NI-1.3
- ☐ Inadequate energy intake — NI-1.4
- ☐ Excessive energy intake — NI-1.5

Oral or Nutrition Support Intake (2)

Defined as "actual or estimated food and beverage intake from oral diet or nutrition support compared with patient goal"

- ☐ Inadequate oral food or beverage intake — NI-2.1
- ☐ Excessive oral food or beverage intake — NI-2.2
- ☐ Inadequate intake from enteral or parenteral nutrition infusion — NI-2.3
- ☐ Excessive intake from enteral or parenteral nutrition — NI-2.4
- ☐ Inappropriate infusion of enteral or parenteral nutrition (use with caution) — NI-2.5

Fluid Intake (3)

Defined as "actual or estimated fluid intake compared against patient goal"

- ☐ Inadequate fluid intake — NI-3.1
- ☐ Excessive fluid intake — NI-3.2

Continued

BOX 11-1

Nutrition Diagnoses and Sample Codes—cont'd

Intake	NI
Bioactive Substances (4)	
Defined as "actual or observed intake of bioactive substances, including single or multiple functional food components, ingredients, dietary supplements, alcohol"	
☐ Inadequate bioactive substance intake	NI-4.1
☐ Excessive bioactive substance intake	NI-4.2
☐ Excessive alcohol intake	NI-4.3
Nutrient (5)	
Defined as "actual or estimated intake of specific nutrient groups or single nutrients as compared with desired levels"	
☐ Increased nutrient needs (specify)	NI-5.1
☐ Malnutrition	NI-5.2
☐ Inadequate protein-energy intake	NI-5.3
☐ Decreased nutrient needs (specify)	NI-5.4
☐ Imbalance of nutrients	NI-5.5
Fat and Cholesterol (51)	
☐ Inadequate fat intake	NI-51.1
☐ Excessive fat intake	NI-51.2
☐ Inappropriate intake of food fats *(specify)* ______	NI-51.3
Protein (52)	
☐ Inadequate protein intake	NI-52.1
☐ Excessive protein intake	NI-52.2
☐ Inappropriate intake of amino acids *(specify)* ______	NI-52.3
Carbohydrate and Fiber Intake (53)	
☐ Inadequate carbohydrate intake	NI-53.1
☐ Excessive carbohydrate intake	NI-53.2
☐ Inappropriate intake of types of carbohydrate *(specify)* ______	NI-53.3
☐ Inconsistent carbohydrate intake	NI-53.4
☐ Inadequate fiber intake	NI-53.5
☐ Excessive fiber intake	NI-53.6
Vitamin Intake (54)	
☐ Inadequate vitamin intake *(specify)* ______	NI-54.1
☐ Excessive vitamin intake *(specify)* ______	NI-54.2
☐ A ☐ C	
☐ Thiamin ☐ D	
☐ Riboflavin ☐ E	
☐ Niacin ☐ K	
☐ Folate ☐ Other ______	
Mineral Intake (55)	
☐ Inadequate mineral intake *(specify)*	NI-55.1
☐ Calcium ☐ Iron	
☐ Potassium ☐ Zinc	
☐ Other ______	
☐ Excessive mineral intake (specify)	NI-55.2
☐ Calcium ☐ Iron	
☐ Potassium ☐ Zinc	
Other ______	

BOX 11-1

Nutrition Diagnoses and Sample Codes—cont'd

Clinical	**NC**
Defined as "nutritional findings or problems identified as related to medical or physical conditions"	
Functional (1)	
Defined as "change in physical or mechanical functioning that interferes with or prevents desired nutritional consequences"	
☐ Swallowing difficulty	NC-1.1
☐ Chewing (masticatory) difficulty	NC-1.2
☐ Breastfeeding difficulty	NC-1.3
☐ Altered gastrointestinal function	NC-1.4
Biochemical (2)	
Defined as "change in capacity to metabolize nutrients as a result of medications, surgery, or as indicated by altered lab values"	
☐ Impaired nutrient utilization	NC-2.1
☐ Altered nutrition-related laboratory values	NC-2.2
☐ Food medication interaction	NC-2.3
Weight (3)	
Defined as "chronic weight or changed weight status when compared with usual or desired body weight"	
☐ Underweight	NC-3.1
☐ Involuntary weight loss	NC-3.2
☐ Overweight or obesity	NC-3.3
☐ Involuntary weight gain	NC-3.4
Behavioral-Environmental	**NB**
Defined as "nutritional findings or problems identified as related to knowledge, attitudes or beliefs, physical environment, or food supply and safety"	
Knowledge and Beliefs (1)	
Defined as "actual knowledge and beliefs as observed or documented"	
☐ Food and nutrition-related knowledge deficit	NB-1.1
☐ Harmful beliefs or attitudes about food or nutrition-related topics (use with caution)	NB-1.2
☐ Not ready for diet or lifestyle change	NB-1.3
☐ Self-monitoring deficit	NB-1.4
☐ Disordered eating pattern	NB-1.5
☐ Limited adherence to nutrition-related recommendations	NB-1.6
☐ Undesirable food choices	NB-1.7
Physical Activity and Function (2)	
Defined as "actual physical activity, self-care, and quality of life problems as reported, observed or documented"	
☐ Physical inactivity	NB-2.1
☐ Excessive exercise	NB-2.2
☐ Inability or lack of desire to manage self-care	NB-2.3
☐ Impaired ability to prepare foods/meals	NB-2.4
☐ Poor nutrition quality of life	NB-2.5
☐ Self-feeding difficulty	NB-2.6
Food Safety and Access (3)	
Defined as "actual problems with food access or food safety"	
☐ Intake of unsafe food	NB-3.1
☐ Limited access to food	NB-3.2

intervention involves two steps: planning and implementation. During the planning phase of the nutrition intervention, the RD, patient or client, and others as needed collaborate to identify goals and objectives that will signify success of the intervention. Patient-centered goals and objectives are set, and then implementation begins. Interventions may include food and nutrition therapies, nutrition education, counseling, or coordination of care such as providing referral for financial or food resources. Because the care process is continuous, the initial plan may change as the condition of the patient changes, as new needs are identified, or if the interventions are unsuccessful.

Interventions should be specific; they are the "what, where, when, and how" of the care plan (ADA, 2010). For example, in a patient with "inadequate oral food or beverage intake," an objective might be to increase portion sizes at two meals per day. This could be implemented through provision of portions that are initially 5% larger with a gradual increase to 25% larger portion sizes. Plans should be communicated to the health care team and the patient to ensure understanding of the plan and its rationale. Thorough communication by the RD increases the likelihood of adherence to the plan. Box 11-2 presents the NCP applied to a sample patient, JW.

Monitoring and Evaluation of Nutrition Care

The fourth step in the NCP involves monitoring and evaluation of the effect of nutrition interventions. This clarifies the effect that the RD has in the specific setting, whether health care, education, consulting, food services, or research. During this step, the RD first determines indicators that should be monitored. These indicators should match the signs and symptoms identified during the assessment process. For example, if excessive sodium intake was identified during the assessment, then an evaluation of the sodium intake is needed at a designated time for follow-up.

In the clinical setting the goal of nutrition care is to meet the nutritional needs of the patient or client; thus the interventions must be monitored and the meeting of the objectives evaluated frequently. This ensures that unmet objectives are addressed and that care is evaluated and modified in a timely manner. Monitoring and evaluation are not unique to nutrition practice. Evaluation of the monitored indicators provides objective data to demonstrate effectiveness of nutrition interventions, regardless of the setting or focus. If objectives are written in measurable, behavioral terms, evaluation is relatively easy because new behavior is being measured against a behavior that has already been defined.

An example in clinical practice is the sample case in Box 11-2. Here, monitoring and evaluation include weekly reviews of his nutritional intake, including an estimation of energy intake. If intake was less than the goal of 1800 kcal, the evaluation might be: "JW was not able to increase his calorie intake to 1800 kcal because of his inability to cook and prepare meals for himself." A revision in the care plan at this point might include the following: "JW will be provided a referral to local agencies (Meals on Wheels) that can provide meals at home." This new intervention is then implemented with continued monitoring and evaluation to determine whether the new objective can be met.

When evaluation reveals that objectives are not being met or that new needs have arisen, the process begins again with reassessment, identification of new nutrition diagnoses, and formulation of a new NCP. For example, in JW's case, during his hospitalization, high-calorie snacks were provided. However, monitoring reveals that JW's usual eating pattern does not include snacks, and thus he was not consuming them. The evaluation showed these snacks to be an ineffective intervention. JW agrees to a new intervention—the addition of one more food to his meals. Further monitoring and evaluation will be needed to ascertain if this new intervention improves his intake.

Evidence-Based Guidelines

Evidence-based practice is use of current "best evidence" in making decisions about the care of individual patients. "Best evidence" includes high-quality research, systematic reviews of the literature, and metaanalysis to support decisions made in practice. Comprehensive use of **evidence-based guidelines (EBGs)** leads to improved quality of care. The guides may also create new research questions.

In the 1990s, the ADA began developing nutrition practice guidelines and evaluating how their use affected clinical outcomes; diabetes management was among the first (Franz et al., 2008). These evidence-based nutrition practice guidelines are disease- and condition-specific recommendations with toolkits. Medical nutrition therapy (MNT) evidence-based guides are available to assist dietetic practitioners in providing nutrition care, especially for diabetes and prerenal failure. MNT provided by a Medicare Part B licensed provider can be reimbursed when the EBGs are used and all procedural forms are properly documented and coded (White et al., 2008).

To define professional practice by the RD, the ADA has published a Scope of Dietetics Practice Framework, a Code of Ethics, and the **Standards of Professional Performance (SOPPs)**. Specialized standards for knowledge, skills, and competencies required to provide care at the generalist, specialist, and advanced practice level for a variety of populations are now complete for many areas of practice. Benefits of nutrition therapy can be communicated to physicians, insurance companies, administrators, or other health care providers using evidence provided from these guidelines. The EBGs include major recommendations, background information, and a reference list.

Overall, the ADA's EAL provides the best available evidence to answer questions that arise during provision of nutrition care. Use of this library is essential to protect the practitioner and the public from the consequences of ineffective care. These guidelines are extremely valuable for staff orientation, competence verification, and training of RDs anywhere in the world.

Accreditation and Surveys

Accreditation by **The Joint Commission (TJC)**, formerly the Joint Commission on Accreditation of Healthcare

BOX 11-2

Applying the Nutrition Care Process for Patient JW

JW is a 70-year-old white man admitted for cardiac bypass surgery. JW lives alone in his own home. He lost his wife 3 months ago, and for the past 6 months he rarely has sat down to a cooked meal. The nutrition risk screen reveals that he has lost weight without trying and has been eating poorly for several weeks before admission, leading to referral to the RD for nutrition assessment (Step 1 of the nutrition care process).

Assessment: Chart review and patient interview reveals the following data:

Laboratory Data and Medications

Glucose and electrolytes: WNL
Albumin: 3.8 g/dL
Cholesterol/triglycerides: WNL
Medications: Inderal

Anthropometric Data

Height: 70″
Weight: 130 lb (15 lb weight loss over 3 months)

Nutrition Interview Findings

Caloric intake: 1200 kcal/day (less than energy requirements as stated in the recommended dietary allowances)
Meals: irregular throughout the day; drinks coffee frequently

Medical History

History of hypertension, thyroid dysfunction, asthma, prostate surgery

Psychosocial Data

New widower; indicates depression and loneliness without his wife

Nutrition Diagnosis: JW has been consuming fewer calories than he requires and has little interest in eating. RD determines his nutrition diagnosis and establish objectives for his care.

Nutrition Diagnostic (PES Statement): Involuntary weight loss related to depression and poor oral food and beverage intake as evidenced by 15-lb loss in 3 months.

Interventions: Identification of the nutrition diagnosis allows the RD to focus the nutrition intervention on treatment of the cause of the problem (in this case the missing meals). Goal setting is the first step, and short-term and long-term plans are established. In the education process the client and the RD must jointly establish achievable goals. Objectives should be expressed in behavioral terms and stated in terms of what the patient will do or achieve when the objectives are met. Objectives should reflect the educational level and the economic and social resources available to the patient and the family.

Short-Term Objectives

During the hospitalization, JW will maintain his current weight; following discharge he will begin to slowly gain weight up to a target weight of 145 lb.

While in the hospital, JW will include nutrient-dense foods in his diet, especially if his appetite is limited.

Long-Term Objectives

JW will modify his diet to include adequate calories and protein through the use of nutrient-dense foods to prevent further weight loss and eventually promote weight gain.

Following discharge, JW will attend a local senior center for lunch on a daily basis to help improve his socialization and caloric intake.

Monitoring and Evaluation: Choosing the means for monitoring if the interventions, and nutritional care activities have met the objectives or goals is important. Evaluation of the monitoring criteria will provide the RD with information on outcomes, and this should occur over time. Finally, documentation is important for each step of the process to ensure communication between all parties.

For JW, weekly weight measurements and nutrient intake analyses are required while he is in the hospital and biweekly weight measurements at the senior center or clinic when he is back at home. If nutrition status is not improving, which in this case would be evidenced by JW's weight records, and the goals are not being met, it is important to reassess JW and perhaps develop new goals and definitely create plans for new interventions.

PES, Problem, etiology, and signs and symptoms; *RD*, registered dietitian; *WNL*, within normal limits.

Organizations, involves a peer review process. TJC survey teams evaluate health care institutions to evaluate their compliance with established minimum standards. TJC requires that nutrition screening be completed within 24 hours of admission to acute care, but does not mandate a method to accomplish screening.

TJC focuses on the facility's actual performance of important governance, managerial, clinical, and support functions. It also focuses on the continual **process improvement (PI)** in an organization's performance of these functions. Standards are provided in the *Accreditation Manual for Hospitals* document, which is updated and revised on a yearly basis. This document consists of three sections: (1) patient-focused functions; (2) organization-focused functions; and (3) structures with functions, which provides descriptions of the various departments and their roles. Its approach is a functional one, and all departments and disciplines must be familiar with relevant issues found in applicable chapters. Most chapters contain standards that affect the care provided by a dietitian.

The "Care of the Patient" section contains standards that apply specifically to medication use, rehabilitation, anesthesia, operative and other invasive procedures, and special treatments, as well as nutrition care standards. The focus of the nutrition care standards is provision of appropriate nutrition care in a timely and effective manner using an interdisciplinary approach. Appropriate care requires screening of patients for nutrition needs, assessing and reassessing patient needs, developing an NCP, ordering and communicating the diet order, preparing and distributing the diet order, monitoring the process, and continually reassessing and improving the NCP. A facility can define who, when, where, and how the process is accomplished; but TJC specifies that a qualified dietitian must be involved in establishing this process. A plan for the delivery of nutrition care may be as simple as providing a regular diet for a patient who is not at nutritional risk or as complex as managing tube feedings in a ventilator-dependent patient, which involves the collaboration of multiple disciplines.

The accreditation process typically involves an on-site survey that lasts for several days. During this survey adherence to standards is ascertained through interviews, review of documents (including patient medical records), and visits to patient care and other areas. In addition, a tracer method is now being used, which identifies an issue that surveyors can follow throughout the care of a specific patient.

RDs are actively involved in the survey process. Standards set by TJC play a large role in influencing the standards of care delivered to patients in all health care disciplines. For more information, see the TJC website at www.jointcommission.org.

Dietitians are also involved with surveys from other regulatory bodies, such as a state or local health department, a department of social services, or licensing organizations. **Sentinel events** are unintended events that are unanticipated and often unwelcome (Ash, 2007). These events must be prevented. When or if they do occur, the outcomes must be documented in the medical record. Regardless of the source of the survey, it is imperative to follow all regulations and guidelines at all times and not just when a survey is due.

DOCUMENTATION IN THE NUTRITION CARE RECORD

MNT and other nutrition care provided must be documented in the health or medical record. The medical record is a legal document; if interventions are not recorded, it is assumed that they have not occurred. Documentation affords the following advantages:

- It ensures that nutrition care will be relevant, thorough, and effective by providing a record that identifies the problems and sets criteria for evaluating the care.
- It allows the entire health care team to understand the rationale for nutrition care, the means by which it will be provided, and the role each team member must play to reinforce the plan and ensure its success.

The medical record serves as a tool for communication among members of the health care team. Beginning in 2014, health care facilities must use electronic health records (EHRs) to document patient care, store and manage laboratory and test results, communicate with other entities, and maintain all information related to an individual's health. During the transition period, those using paper documentation maintain paper charts that typically include sections for physician orders, medical history and physical examinations, laboratory test results, consults, and progress reports. Although the format of the medical record varies depending on facility policies and procedures, in most settings all professionals document care in the medical record. The RD must ensure that all aspects of nutrition care are summarized succinctly in the medical record.

Medical Record Charting

Problem-oriented medical records (POMRs) are used in many facilities. The POMR is organized according to the patient's primary problems. Entries into the medical record can be done in many styles. One of the most common forms is the **subjective, objective, assessment, plan (SOAP) note format** (Table 11-2).

The **assessment, diagnosis, interventions, monitoring, evaluation (ADIME) format** is used by many nutrition departments to reflect the steps of the NCP (Box 11-3; Table 11-3). See Table 11-4 for common nutrition diagnostic (PES) statements.

The important factor is the content of the documentation, not necessarily the style. All entries made by the dietitian should address the issues of nutrition status and needs. Notes must be accurate and concise, and they must be able to convey important information to the physician and other health care team members so that they might take action. In a paper-based system, the following are general guidelines for documentation in the hospital setting:

- All entries should be written in black pen or typewritten.
- Documentation should be complete, clear, concise, objective, legible, and accurate.
- Entries should include date, time, and service. Each page should include the patient's name and hospital number.
- Entries should be in chronologic order and be consecutive.
- The first word of every statement should be capitalized, with periods placed at the end of each thought. Complete sentences are not necessary, but grammar and spelling should be correct.
- All entries should be consistent and noncontradictory.

Text continued on p. 266

TABLE 11-2

Evaluation of a Note in SOAP Format

	Outstanding 2 Points	Above Expectations 1 Point	Below Expectations 0 Points	Score
DATE & TIME		Present	Not present	
S (SUBJECTIVE) Tolerance of current diet Reports of wt loss or appetite decrease Chewing or swallowing difficulties Previously unreported food allergies Pertinent diet hx information	Pertinent components documented. Captures essence of pt's perception of medical problem.	Accurately summarizes most of the pertinent information.	One or more pertinent elements missing.	
O (OBJECTIVE) Diet order √ Pt dx Ht, wt, DBW, %DBW √ UBW, % UBW Pertinent laboratory values √ Diet-related meds Estimated nutrient needs (EER & protein)	All necessary elements documented accurately.	Necessary elements documented. No more than one item missing or irrelevant data documented.	One or more pertinent elements omitted and irrelevant data documented.	
A (ASSESSMENT) S + O = A Nutritional status assessed Appropriateness of current diet order noted Interpretation of abnormal laboratory values (to assess nutritional status) Comments on diet hx (if appropriate) Comments of tolerance of diet (if appropriate) Rationale for suggested changes (if appropriate)	Sophisticated assessment drawn from items documented in S & O. Appropriate conclusions drawn.	Appropriate, effective assessment, but not based on documentation in S & O.	Unacceptable assessment or no assessment. Disease pathophysiologic findings documented as assessment of nutritional status.	
P (PLAN) Dx (if appropriate) Request more labs or calorie count Rx (if appropriate) Suggestions for changing diet Suggestions for adding supplements TF/TPN recs Recs for vitamin supplements Suggestions for referrals F/U Plans for future care Follow-up prn vs. continue to monitor nutritional status Monitor tolerance of TF/TPN (if approp.) Encourage PO (if appropriate)	Appropriate nutritional care plan documented reflecting pt's nutritional status.	Vague nutritional care plan documented reflecting pt's nutritional status. Minor errors in care plan. At least one necessary element missing.	MD's orders documented as nutritional care plan. More than one necessary element missing. Unacceptable and/or inappropriate care plan documented.	
SIGNATURE & CREDENTIALS		Present	Not present	

Courtesy Sara Long, PhD, RD.

DBW, Desired body weight; *Dx*, diagnosis; *EER*, estimated energy requirements; *F/U*, follow up; *ht*, height; *hx*, history; *PO*, by mouth; *PRN*, as necessary; *pt*, patient; *Rx*, prescription; *SOAP*, subjective, objective, assessment, plan; *TF*, tube feeding; *TPN*, total parenteral nutrition; *UBW*, usual body weight; *wt*, weight.

TABLE 11-3

Evaluation of a Note in ADIME Format

	Outstanding 2 Points	Above Expectations 1 Point	Below Expectations 0 Points	Score
DATE & TIME		Present	Not present	
A (ASSESSMENT) Reports of wt loss or appetite decrease Chewing or swallowing difficulties Previously unreported food allergies Pertinent diet hx information Estimated nutrient needs (EER & protein) Diet order √ Pt dx Ht, wt, DBW, %DBW √ UBW, % UBW if appropriate Pertinent laboratory values √ Diet-related meds	Pertinent components documented. Captures essence of pt's perception of medical problem.	Accurately summarizes most of the pertinent information.	One or more pertinent elements missing or irrelevant data documented.	
D (NUTRITION DIAGNOSIS) Written in PES statement(s) using standardized language for the nutrition care process	Necessary PES statement(s) stated accurately & prioritized.	No more than one item missing.	Not written in PES statement format or standardized. language not used. Medical dx listed as nutrition dx.	
I (INTERVENTION) Aimed at cause of nutr dx; can be directed at reducing effects of signs & symptoms Planning: prioritize nutr dx, jointly establish goals w/ pt, define nutrition Rx, identify specific nutr interventions Implementation: action phase, includes carrying out & communicating plan of care, continuing data collection & revising nutr intervention as warranted based on pt's response	Appropriate & specific plan(s) AND implementation to remedy nutr dx documented.	Plans or implementation missing. Vague plans or intervention documented.	MD's orders documented as intervention, or inappropriate plan or intervention documented.	
M (MONITORING) & E (EVALUATION) Determines progress made by pt & if goals are being met Tracks pt outcomes relevant to nutr dx Can be organized into one or more of following: Nutr-Related Behavioral & Environmental Outcomes Food & Nutrient Intake Outcomes Nutr-Related Physical Sign & Symptom Outcome Nutr-Related Pt-Centered Outcome	Appropriate nutr care outcomes relevant to nutr dx & intervention plans & goals documented. Nutr care outcomes defined, specific indicators (can be measured & compared to established criteria) identified.	No more than one item missing.	Nutr care outcome not relevant to nutr dx, intervention, or plans/goals. Nutr care outcomes cannot be measured or compared with established criteria.	
SIGNATURE & CREDENTIALS		Present	Not present	

Courtesy Sara Long, PhD, RD.

ADIME, Assessment, diagnosis, intervention, monitoring, evaluation; *DBW*, desirable body weight; *dx*, diagnosis; *EER*, estimated energy requirement; *ht*, height; *hx*, history; *MD*, medical doctor; *meds*, medications; *nutr*, nutrition; *PES*, problem, etiology, signs and symptoms; *pt*, patient; *Rx*, prescription; *UBW*, usual body weight; *w/*, with; *wt*, weight.

BOX 11-3

Chart Note Using ADIME

Nutrition Assessment

- Pt is 66-year-old woman admitted with abdominal pain: Ht: 62 cm; Wt: 56 kg; IBW: 52-58 kg
- Laboratory values noted: Na 134, calcium 8, total protein 5.8, albumin 3
- EEN: 1568-1680 calories (28-30 cal/kg) and 56-73 g protein (1-1.3 g/kg)
- Current diet is low residue with pt consuming 25% of meals recorded
- Consult for education received

Nutrition Diagnosis

- Food- and nutrition-related knowledge deficit related to lack of prior exposure to information as evidenced by client having no prior knowledge of need for low-residue diet (NB-1.1).

Nutrition Intervention

- Education: Will provide pt with written and verbal instruction on low-residue diet.
- Goals: Pt will be able to develop 1-day menu using dietary restrictions.
- Pt will be able to identify good sources of calcium and protein from list of foods appropriate for low-residue diet.
- Pt will ask appropriate questions and verbalize understanding of dietary modifications.

Monitoring and Evaluation

- Follow up with pt regarding questions about diet indicated no further questions; good comprehension.
- Evaluation: anticipate no problems following diet at home. Gave business card/phone contact.

J Wilson, MS, RD 1/2/11 @ 10:15 AM

EEN, Early enteral nutrition; *ht*, height; *IBW*, ideal body weight; *Na*, sodium; *pt*, patient; *wt*, weight.

TABLE 11-4

Types of Consults and Sample PES Statements

Type of Consult	Nutrition Diagnosis Problem (P)	Related to Etiology (E)	As Evidenced by Signs and Symptoms (S)
Weight loss	Inadequate energy intake	Calorie intake not meeting caloric needs	X-lb weight loss in Y days Weight below IBW range
	Inadequate protein/energy intake	Protein/calorie intake < bodily needs	BMI <19 Decreased oral intake (X%), infection
	Inadequate oral food/ beverage intake	Calorie intake < calorie expenditure	
	Involuntary weight loss	Increased caloric needs	
	Inadequate energy intake	Intake < calculated bodily needs	Oral intake ≤25% X-lb weight loss in Y days Weight < IBWR
	Inadequate oral food/ beverage intake	Oral intake < recommended/ calculated	X-lb weight loss in Y days Oral intake ≤50% Low total protein Low albumin Stage X pressure ulcer on ____________
	Involuntary weight loss	Weight loss > expected or desired	Weight loss >5% in 30 days 7.5% in 90 days 10% in 180 days
	Disordered eating pattern	Attitudes related to food, eating, or weight management	Refusal to eat Y meal(s) per day X-lb weight loss in Y days
	Self-feeding difficulty	Impaired ability to place food in mouth	X-lb weight loss in Y days Rapid weight loss Advanced stages of Parkinson disease or MS Excessive shaking of hands

Continued

TABLE 11-4

Types of Consults and Sample PES Statements—cont'd

Type of Consult	Nutrition Diagnosis Problem (P)	Related to Etiology (E)	As Evidenced by Signs and Symptoms (S)
Pressure ulcer w/ poor PPO intake and weight loss	Inadequate protein/energy intake Inadequate oral food/ beverage intake	Protein/calorie intake < calculated needs Protein/calorie intake < protein/calorie needs Increased expenditure/protein needs	X-lb weight loss in Y days Weight below IBWR BMI <19 Stage X pressure ulcer on ________ Reported X% intake
Pressure ulcer-eating well	Inadequate protein intake	Increased protein needs Oral intake not meeting needs	Stage X pressure ulcer on ________
Pressure ulcer	Increased nutrient needs	Increased demand for energy and protein	Loss of skin integrity Stage X pressure ulcer on ________
	Increased protein needs	Increased demand for protein intake	Low albumin Low total protein Stage X pressure ulcer on ________
Overweight/obesity	Excessive oral food/beverage intake Excessive energy intake Overweight/obesity	Calorie intake > caloric expenditure	Weight > IBWR X-lb weight gain in Y month(s) Elevated BMI Decreased mobility
	Excessive energy intake	Calorie intake exceeds calculated needs	X-lb rapid weight gain in Y days Overweight Obesity Morbid obesity
Weight gain	Excessive energy intake Involuntary weight gain	Calorie intake > caloric expenditure Increased fluid intake	X-lb weight gain in Y month(s) X-lb weight gain in Y days
	Involuntary weight gain	Weight gain > expected or desired	Weight gain >5% in 30 days 7.5% in 90 days 10% in 180 days
	Physical inactivity	Calorie intake > calorie expenditure	X-lb weight gain in Y month(s) refuses activity, bed bound X-lb gradual weight gain in Y days refuses physical therapy
Low HgB/Hct	Inadequate mineral intake (iron)	Increased needs Iron intake not meeting needs Lower iron containing foods or substances than meets needs	Low HgB Low Hct Low RBC Anemia
Low albumin, HgB/Hct	Inadequate oral food/ beverage intake Increased nutrient needs (protein, iron)	Intake not meeting needs Increase nutrient demand for acute phase proteins	Low albumin Low HgB/Hct Low RBC Stress, trauma, inflammation, wound healing

TABLE 11-4

Types of Consults and Sample PES Statements—cont'd

Type of Consult	Nutrition Diagnosis Problem (P)	Related to Etiology (E)	As Evidenced by Signs and Symptoms (S)
Abnormal laboratory values	Altered nutrition-related laboratory values	Change in ability to eliminate the byproducts of metabolism Change in ability to metabolize, absorb, or excrete specific nutrients	Low albumin Low albumin (edema) Low albumin (high CRP)
	Altered nutrition-related laboratory values	Chang in ability to eliminate by-product of metabolism	Elevated BUN, creatinine Elevated calculated osmolality Elevated Chol., TG, LDL Elevated CO_2 Elevated glucose
	Impaired nutrient use	Change in ability to absorb, metabolize, or excrete specific nutrients	Elevated glucose X-lb weight loss in Y days Low albumin Low total protein Low iron
Diabetes	Excessive carbohydrate intake Inadequate carbohydrate intake	Intake > needs Intake < needs	Elevated glucose Low glucose
	Inconsistent Carbohydrate intake	Inappropriate pattern of carbohydrate intake throughout the day	Uncontrolled glucose levels Need for no concentrated sweets diet
Tube feeding	Inadequate intake from enteral/parenteral nutrition infusion Excessive intake from enteral/parenteral nutrition Inadequate fluid intake Excessive fluid intake	Intake < caloric needs Diet and TF do not meet needs Intake > caloric needs Diet and TF exceed needs Intake < calculated needs Intake > calculated needs	X-lb weight loss in Y days X-lb weight gain in Y days Elevated BUN, calc. osmo. Low calc. osmol.
	Inadequate intake from enteral nutrition infusion	Lower calorie and nutrient intake than meets bodily needs	Low infusion rate X-lb weight loss in Y days
Dehydration	Inadequate fluid intake	Fluid intake < bodily needs	Elevated BUN Elevated calculated osmolality Elevated BUN/creatinine ratio Elevated Na^+/K^+
Edema/fluid overload	Involuntary weight gain Excessive oral food/beverage intake Excessive fluid intake	Fluid intake > needs Fluid intake > body's ability to excrete fluid	X-lb weight gain in Y days Low Na^+ Low HgB/Hct Elevated BUN (in CHF)
Dysphagia	Swallowing difficulty Inadequate oral food/beverage intake	Impaired movement of food/liquid from mouth to stomach Inability to consume regular consistency food and/or fluids Intake < calculated needs	Choking, coughing, gurgling during meals Need for mechanically altered diet
GERD	Altered GI function	Inability to tolerate certain foods	Reflux, sharp GI pain while eating

Continued

TABLE 11-4

Types of Consults and Sample PES Statements—cont'd

Type of Consult	Nutrition Diagnosis Problem (P)	Related to Etiology (E)	As Evidenced by Signs and Symptoms (S)
Constipation	Inadequate fiber intake	Low intake of fiber containing foods/substances	Constipation
SIADH	Excessive fluid intake	Intake > body's ability to excrete excess fluid	Low Na^+
Medications (example: calcitonin salmon [Miacalcin] spray)	Inadequate mineral intake (calcium)	Low calcium intake	Use of calcitonin salmon spray without a calcium supplement Low oral intake of high calcium foods
Hospice	Increased energy needs Decreased energy needs	RMR > calculated requirements	Cancer Head trauma
End-stage disease	Increased energy needs	Increased RMR	End stage disease process Weight loss expected
Financial constraints	Limited access to food	Inability to acquire food	Homeless resident X-lb weight loss in Y days Malnutrition No income/no job

BMI, Body mass index; *BUN*, blood urea nitrogen; *calc. osmol.*, calculation of osmolity; *CHF*, congestive heart failure; *CO_2*, carbon dioxide; *Chol*, cholesterol; *CRP*, C-reactive protein; *Hct*, hematocrit; *HgB*, hemoglobin; *IBW*, ideal body weight; *IBWR*, ideal body weight range; *K^+*, potassium; *LDL*, low-density lipoprotein; *MS*, multiple sclerosis; *Na^+*, sodium; *PES*, problem, etiology, and signs and symptoms; *PO*, by mouth; *RBC*, red blood cell; *TF*, tube feeding; *G*, triglyceride; *w/*, with.

- All entries must be signed at the end and should include credentials (e.g., *J. Wilson, RD*). No one should ever chart or sign the medical record for another individual.
- Personal opinions and comments criticizing or casting doubt on the professionalism of others should never be included.
- Documentation must be done at the time of the actual procedure or service.
- Late entries should be identified as such, including the actual date and time of the entry and the date and time it should have been recorded. *Never* add notes after the fact without accurately authenticating, dating, and referencing the original entry.
- Paper medical record entries should always be legible. When correcting an error draw a single line through the error and initial. *Never* use correction fluid, correction tape, self-adhesive labels, or thick marker strokes. *Never* remove an original and replace it with a copy.
- If information is accidentally omitted, write "see addendum" by the original entry, add the date and initial, and write the content in the medical record, identified as an addendum with the date and time of the original entry.

Electronic Health Records and Nutrition Informatics

Prior to the early 1990s, technology advances did not meet the needs of clinicians in practice. Since then, costs for memory space have decreased, hardware has become more portable, and system science has sufficiently advanced to make EHRs a permanent fixture in health care. Additional impetus to change standard practice came with publication of several Institute of Medicine reports that brought to light a high rate of preventable medical errors along with the recommendation to use technology as a tool to improve health care quality and safety.

Clinical information systems used in health care are known by different names; although some use electronic medical record (EMR), EHR, and personal health record (PHR) interchangeably, there are important differences. **Electronic health record (EHR)** describes information systems that contain all the health information for an individual. Another term that might be seen includes an **electronic medical record (EMR)**, which typically describes a clinical information system used by a health care organization to document patient care. Both the EHR and EMR are maintained by health care providers. In contrast, the **personal health record (PHR)** is a system that is used by the consumer to maintain health information. A PHR can be web-based, free-standing, or integrated to a facility's EMR.

EHRs include all of the information typically found in a paper-based documentation system along with tools such as clinical decision support, electronic medication records, and alert systems that will support clinicians in making decisions regarding patient care. By 2014, all health care providers will use EHRs to enter, store, retrieve, and manage information related to patient care. Dietitians must have at least a basic understanding of technology and health information management to ensure a smooth transition from paper to EHR. Such transition will include the development of nutrition screens for patient admission, documentation, information sharing, decision support tools, and order entry. Customization capabilities vary depending on vendor contracts; RDs managing nutrition services must be involved in EHR system decisions at the very beginning, prior to communication of a request for proposals to potential vendors.

In both paper and electronic formats, medical records and the information contained are vital conduits for communicating patient care to others, providing information for quality evaluation and improvement, and as a legal document. RD documentation includes information related to NCPs. Documentation must follow the facility policy and be brief and concise while accurately describing actions taken to those authorized to view the record. Figure 11-2 shows how a computerized medical record might look when using the ADIME method.

Federal requirements mandate that provider systems be "interoperable," meaning that information can be safely and securely exchanged between providers and facilities. Although this concept seems simple on the surface, problems with interoperability will be very difficult and expensive to overcome. The transition from paper to electronic documentation can be facilitated by thorough planning, training, and support. Many RDs in practice have little experience with technology; they may not fully understand the practice improvement that can be realized with proper implementation and use of technology. Others may resist any change in the workplace that interrupts their current workflow. Change is never easy (Schifalacqua, 2009).

Clinical system vendors might convince administrators that the transition will be simple and that time savings will be realized immediately following implementation. Quite often this is not the case, leading to unsatisfied clinicians and an expensive tool that is not properly used (Demiris, 2007). RDs participating in implementation of EHRs in health care must be aware of possible resistance or "human issues," ensuring that all involved are properly trained.

INFLUENCES ON NUTRITION AND HEALTH CARE

The health care environment has undergone considerable change related to the provision of care and reimbursement in the last decade. Governmental influences, cost containment issues, changing demographics, and the changing role of the patient as a "consumer" have influenced the health care arena. The United States currently spends more on health care than any other nation, yet health care outcomes lag far behind those seen in other developed nations. Exponential increases in health care costs in the United States have been a major impetus for drives to reform how health care is provided and paid for in the United States (Ross, 2009).

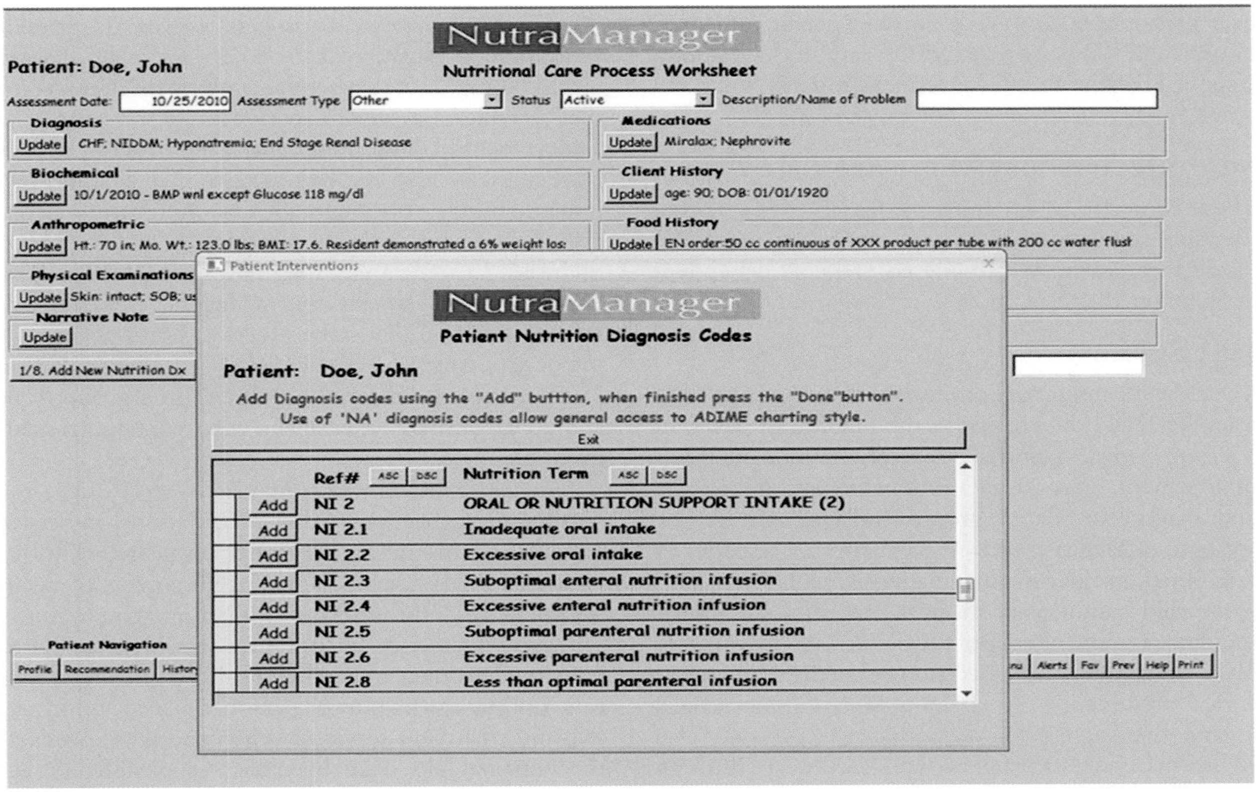

FIGURE 11-2 Example of electronic chart note using drop-down boxes on computer. *(Courtesy Maggie Gilligan, RD, owner of NUTRA-MANAGER, 2010.)*

Affordable Health Care for America: Reconciliation Bill

All Americans will have access to quality, affordable health care under a final package of health insurance reforms signed into law in March 2010. The law will protect Americans from insurance industry practices, offer the uninsured and small businesses the opportunity to obtain affordable health care plans, cover 32 million uninsured Americans, and reduce the deficit by $143 billion over the next decade.

Confidentiality and the Health Insurance Portability and Accountability Act

Privacy and security of personal information is of concern in all health care settings. In 1996 Congress passed the **Health Insurance Portability and Accountability Act (HIPAA)** (Centers for Medicare and Medicaid Services, 2010). The initial intent of HIPAA was to ensure that health insurance eligibility was maintained when people changed or lost jobs. The Administrative Simplification provisions of HIPAA require development of national standards that maintain privacy of **protected health information (PHI)**. HIPAA requires that health care facilities and providers (covered entities) take steps to safeguard PHI. Although HIPAA does not prevent sharing of patient data required for an incident of care, patients must be notified if their medical information is to be shared outside of the care process or if protected information (e.g., address, e-mail, income) is to be shared. RDs must use common sense when working with PHI; it is never appropriate to look at another person's medical record unless the RD is involved in the care of that patient. Violations of HIPAA rules have resulted in large fines and loss of jobs.

Patient Protection and Affordable Care Act

The Patient Protection and Affordable Care Act was written in 2010. Final regulations require group health plans and health insurance issuers to provide coverage of dependent children younger than age 26.

Payment Systems

One of the largest influences on health care delivery in the last decade has been the change in the method of payment for services provided. There are several common methods of reimbursement: cost-based reimbursement, negotiated bids, and diagnostic-related groups (DRGs). Under the DRG system, a facility receives payment for a patient's admission based on the principal diagnosis, secondary diagnosis (comorbid conditions), surgical procedure (if appropriate), and the age and gender of the patient. Approximately 500 DRGs cover the entire spectrum of medical diagnoses and surgical treatments. **Preferred-provider organizations (PPOs)** and **managed-care organizations (MCOs)** also changed health care. MCOs finance and deliver care through a contracted network of providers in exchange for a monthly premium, changing reimbursement from a fee-for-service system to one in which fiscal risk is borne by health care organizations and physicians. New legislation will likely change the face of reimbursement even more.

Quality Management

To contain health care costs while providing efficient and effective care that is of consistently high quality, practice guidelines or **standards of care** are used. These sets of recommendations serve as a guide for defining appropriate care for a patient with a specific diagnosis or medical problem. They help to ensure consistency and quality for both providers and clients in a health care system and, as such, are specific to an institution or health care organization. **Critical pathways**, or care maps, identify essential elements that should occur in the patient's care and define a timeframe in which each activity should occur to maximize patient outcomes. They often use an algorithm or flowchart to indicate the necessary steps required to achieve the desired outcomes. **Disease management** is designed to prevent a specific disease progression or exacerbation, and to reduce the frequency and severity of symptoms and complications. Education and other strategies maximize compliance with disease treatment. Educating a patient with type 1 diabetes regarding control of blood glucose levels would be an example of a disease management strategy aimed at decreasing the complications (nephropathy, neuropathy, and retinopathy) and the frequency with which the client needs to access the care provider. Decreasing the number of emergency room visits related to hypoglycemic episodes is a sample goal.

Patient-Centered Care and Case Management

The **case management** process strives to promote the achievement of patient care goals in a cost-effective, efficient manner. It is an essential component in delivering care that provides a positive experience for the patient, ensures achievement of clinical outcomes, and uses resources wisely. Case management involves assessing, evaluating, planning, implementing, coordinating, and monitoring care, especially in patients with chronic disease or those who are at high risk. In some areas, dietitians have added skill sets that enable them to serve as case managers. **Utilization management** is a system that strives for cost efficiency by eliminating or reducing unnecessary tests, procedures, and services. Here, a manager is usually assigned to a group of patients and is responsible for ensuring adherence to preestablished criteria.

The **patient-centered medical home (PCMH)** is a new development that focuses on the relationship between the patient and his or her personal physician. The personal physician takes responsibility for all aspects of health care for the patient and acts to coordinate and communicate with other providers as needed. Other providers such as nurses, health educators, and allied health professionals may be called on by the patient or personal physician for preventative and treatment services. When specialty care is needed, the personal physician becomes responsible for ensuring that care is seamless and that transitions between care sites go smoothly (Backer, 2007; Ornstein 2008). The RD should be considered part of the medical home treatment plan.

Regardless of model, the facility must manage patient care prudently. Nutrition screening can be very important in identifying patients who are nutritionally compromised. Early identification of these factors allows for timely intervention and helps prevent the comorbidities often seen with malnutrition, which may cause the length of stay and costs to increase. The **Centers for Medicare and Medicaid Services (CMS)** has identified several conditions, such as heart failure, for which no additional reimbursement will be received if a patient is readmitted to acute care within 30 days of a prior admission. Although many view this rule as punitive, it does provide an opportunity for RDs to demonstrate how nutrition services, including patient education, can save money through decreased readmissions.

Other recent developments include "never events." Never events are those occurrences that should never happen in a facility that provides high-quality, safe, **patient-focused care**. RDs must pay attention to new or worsening pressure ulcers and central line infections as potential "never events."

Staffing and Nutrition Coding

Staffing also affects the success of nutrition care. Clinical dietitians may be centralized (all are part of a core nutrition department) or decentralized (individual dietitians are part of a unit or service that provides care to patients), depending on the model adopted by a specific institution. Certain departments such as food service, accounting, and human resources remain centralized in most models because some of the functions for which these departments are responsible are not directly related to patient care. Dietitians should be involved in the planning for any redesign of patient care. Regardless of where dietitians work, they need to implement the NCP, use the standardized terminology of the profession, and code their services accurately (see *Focus On:* Nutrition Standardized Language and Coding Practices).

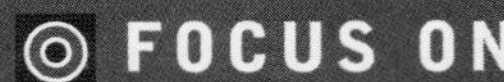

FOCUS ON

Nutrition Standardized Language and Coding Practices

ICD codes were developed in the late 1800s as a mechanism to monitor and track mortality rates in medical practice. The ICD coding system has been revised and updated several times and is used by most countries. Medical records departments review medical records and assign codes to the medical diagnoses as well as complicating factors ("comorbidities") to determine reimbursement rates. Commonly, pulmonary, gastrointestinal, endocrine, mental disorders, and cancer can lead to malnutrition* as a comorbid factor. Thus coordinated nutrition care and coding for malnutrition are important elements in patient services.

Use of the nutrition codes and evidence-based guides established by the ADA should improve client outcomes and reimbursement. A study by White et al (2008) found that self-employed RDs are more likely to be reimbursed by private or commercial payers, and RDs working in clinic settings are more likely to be reimbursed by Medicare. RDs must know and be accountable for both the business and clinical side of their nutrition practices (White et al., 2008). Several members of the ADA are active on medical committees where coding and reimbursement issues are being evaluated and updated.

Using correct codes and following payers' claims processing policies and procedures are essential. For example, an NPI is a 10-digit number that is required on claims. To apply for an NPI, registered dietitians can complete the online application at the NPPES website at https://nppes.cms.hhs.gov/NPPES/Welcome.do.

ADA, American Dietetic Association; *ICD*, International Classification of Disease; *NPI*, National Provider Identifier; *NPPES*, National Plan and Provider Enumeration System; *RD*, registered dietitian.

*For the malnutrition identified during the nutrition care process, Code 261 is "evident malnutrition."

NUTRITION INTERVENTIONS

The RD is the only licensed provider who can reliably offer food and nutrition services that are credible and highly individualized. The RD expert is able to inform, educate, and inspire his or her clients. This guidance is health-enhancing and, often, life-changing. The profession offers stringent guidelines for practice, with science-based information that is not compromised by market forces. The RD must complete continuing education and rigorous reviews of competency every 5 years to maintain that credential. In addition, there are a myriad of position papers and journal articles that keep members up to date to support the "total diet approach" to good nutritional intake.

The evaluation of general and modified diets requires in-depth knowledge of the nutrients contained in different foods. In particular, it is essential to be aware of the nutrient-dense foods that contribute to dietary adequacy. Balance and judgment are needed. Sometimes a vitamin-mineral supplement is necessary to meet the patient's needs when the intake is limited. Chapter 3 and Appendixes 46-58 provide detailed information on specific minerals and vitamins and the foods that contain them.

Interventions: Food and Nutrient Delivery

The **nutrition prescription** designates the type, amount, and frequency of nutrition based on the individual's disease process and disease management goals. The prescription may specify a caloric level or other restriction to be implemented. It may also limit or increase various components of the diet, such as carbohydrate, protein, fat, alcohol, fiber, water, specific vitamins or minerals, bioactive substances such as phytonutrients (see Chapter 3). RDs write the nutrition prescription following diagnosis of nutrition problems.

Note that a diet order differs from a nutrition prescription. In most states, only a licensed independent health care provider can enter diet orders into a patient's medical record. Typically, physicians, physician assistants, and advanced practice nurses are considered to be licensed independent providers. In some facilities, RDs have been granted order-writing privileges. It should be remembered that the ability to enter orders does not absolve the RD of the need to communicate and coordinate care with the provider who is ultimately responsible for all aspects of patient care.

Therapeutic or modified diets are based on a general, adequate diet that has been altered to provide for individual requirements, such as digestive and absorptive capacity, alleviation or arrest of a disease process, and psychosocial factors. In general, the therapeutic diet should vary as little as possible from the individual's normal diet. Personal eating patterns and food preferences should be recognized, along with socioeconomic conditions, religious practices, and any environmental factors that influence food intake, such as where the meals are eaten and who prepares them (see "Cultural Aspects of Dietary Planning" in Chapter 12).

A nutritious and adequate diet can be planned in many ways. One foundation of such a diet is the MyPlate Food Guidance System (see Fig. 12-1). This is a basic plan; additional foods or more of the foods listed are included to provide additional energy and increase the intake of required nutrients for the individual. The Dietary Guidelines for Americans are also used in meal planning and to promote wellness. The dietary reference intakes (DRIs) and specific nutrient recommended dietary allowances are formulated for healthy persons, but they are also used as a basis for evaluating the adequacy of therapeutic diets. Nutrient requirements specific to a particular person's genetic makeup, disease state, or disorder must always be kept in mind during diet planning.

Modifications of the Normal Diet

Normal nutrition is the foundation on which therapeutic diet modifications are based. Regardless of the type of diet prescribed, the purpose of the diet is to supply needed nutrients to the body in a form that it can handle. Adjustment of the diet may take any of the following forms:

- Change in consistency of foods (liquid diet, pureed diet, low-fiber diet, high-fiber diet)
- Increase or decrease in energy value of diet (weight-reduction diet, high-calorie diet)
- Increase or decrease in the type of food or nutrient consumed (sodium-restricted diet, lactose-restricted diet, fiber-enhanced diet, high-potassium diet)
- Elimination of specific foods (allergy diet, gluten-free diet)
- Adjustment in the level, ratio, or balance of protein, fat, and carbohydrate (diet for diabetes, ketogenic diet, renal diet, cholesterol-lowering diet)
- Rearrangement of the number and frequency of meals (diet for diabetes, postgastrectomy diet)
- Change in route of delivery of nutrients (enteral or parenteral nutrition)

Diet Modifications in Hospitalized Patients

Food is an important part of nutrition care. Attempts should be made to honor patient preferences during illness and recovery from surgery. Imagination and ingenuity in menu planning are essential when planning meals acceptable to a varied patient population. Attention to color, texture, composition, and temperature of the foods, coupled with a sound knowledge of therapeutic diets, is required for menu planning. However, to the patient, good taste and attractive presentation are most important. When possible, patient choices of food are most likely be consumed. The ability to make food selections gives the patient an option in an otherwise limiting environment.

Hospitals have to adopt a diet manual that serves as the reference for that facility. The ADA has an online manual that can be purchased for several users per facility. All hospitals or health care institutions have basic, routine diets designed for uniformity and convenience of service. These standard diets are based on the foundation of an adequate diet pattern with nutrient levels as derived from the DRIs. Types of standard diets vary but can generally be classified as general or regular or modified consistency. The diets should be realistic and meet the nutritional requirements of the patients. The most important consideration of the type of diet offered is providing foods that the patient is willing and able to eat and that fit in with any required dietary restrictions. Shortened lengths of stay in many health care settings result in the need to optimize intake of calories and protein and this often translates into a liberal approach to therapeutic diets. This is especially true when the therapeutic restrictions might compromise intake and subsequent recovery from surgery, stress, or illness.

Regular or General Diet

"Regular" or "general diets are used routinely and serve as a foundation for more diversified therapeutic diets. In some institutions a diet that has no restrictions is referred to as the *regular* or *house* diet. It is used when the patient's medical condition does not warrant any limitations. This is a basic, adequate, general diet of approximately 1600 to 2200 kcal; it usually contains 60 to 80 g of protein, 80 to 100 g of fat, and 180 to 300 g of carbohydrate. Although there are no particular food restrictions, some facilities have instituted regular diets that are low in fat, saturated fat, cholesterol, sugar, and salt to follow the dietary recommendations for the general population. In other facilities the diet focuses on providing foods the patient is willing and able to eat, with less focus on restriction of nutrients. Many institutions have a selective menu that allows the patient certain choices; the adequacy of the diet varies based on the patient's selections.

Consistency Modifications

Modifications in consistency may be needed for patients who have limited chewing or swallowing ability. Chopping, mashing, pureeing, or grinding food modifies its texture. See Chapter 41 and Appendix 35 for more information on consistency modifications and for neurologic changes in particular.

Clear liquid diets include some electrolytes and small amounts of energy from tea, broth, carbonated beverages, clear fruit juices, and gelatin. Milk and liquids prepared with milk are omitted, as are fruit juices that contain pulp. Fluids and electrolytes are often replaced intravenously until the diet can be advanced to a more nutritionally adequate one.

There is little scientific evidence supporting the use of clear liquid diets as transition diets after surgery (Jeffery et al., 1996). The average clear liquid diet contains only 500 to 600 kcal, 5 to 10 g of protein, minimum fat, 120 to 130 g of carbohydrate, and small amounts of sodium and potassium. It is inadequate in calories, fiber, and all other essential nutrients and should be used only for short periods. In addition, full liquid diets are also not recommended for a prolonged time. If needed, oral supplements may be used to provide more protein and calories.

Food Intake

Food served does not necessarily represent the actual intake of the patient. Prevention of malnutrition in the health care setting requires observation and monitoring of the adequacy of patient intake. If food intake is inadequate, measures should be taken to provide foods or supplements that may be better accepted or tolerated. Regardless of the type of diet prescribed, both the food served and the amount actually eaten must be considered to obtain an accurate determination of the patient's energy and nutrient intake. Nourishments and calorie-containing beverages consumed between meals are also considered in the overall intake. It is important that the RD maintain communication with nursing and food service personnel to determine adequacy of intake. Although calorie counts are often inaccurate and incomplete, they are sometimes used to justify the need for enteral or parenteral nutrition.

Acceptance and Psychological Factors

Meals and between-meal nourishments are often highlights of the day and are anticipated with pleasure by the patient. Mealtime should be as positive an experience as possible. Whatever setting the patient is eating in should be comfortable for the patient. Food intake is encouraged in a pleasant room with the patient in a comfortable eating position in bed or sitting in a chair located away from unpleasant sights or odors. Eating with others often promotes better intake.

Arrangement of the tray should reflect consideration of the patient's needs. Dishes and utensils should be in a convenient location. Independence should be encouraged in those who require assistance in eating. The caregiver can accomplish this by asking patients to specify the sequence of foods to be eaten and having them participate in eating, if only by holding their bread. Even visually impaired persons can eat unassisted if they are told where to find foods on the tray. Patients who require feeding assistance should be fed when the foods are still at an optimal temperature. The feeding process requires about 20 minutes as a general rule.

Poor acceptance of foods and meals may be caused by unfamiliar foods, a change in eating schedule, improper food temperatures, the patient's medical condition, or the effects of medical therapy. Food acceptance is improved when personal selection of menus is encouraged. There is a revolution occurring in hospital food service. Most hospitals have a **room service**–style menu or are actively working to implement one to solve the problems related to dissatisfaction and poor intake.

Patients should be given the opportunity to share concerns regarding meals, which may improve acceptance and intake. In encouraging acceptance of a therapeutic diet, the attitude of the caregiver is important. The nurse who understands that the diet contributes to the restoration of the patient's health will communicate this conviction by actions, facial expressions, and conversation. Patients who understand that the diet is important to the success of their recovery usually accept it more willingly. When the patient must adhere to a therapeutic dietary program indefinitely, an interdisciplinary approach will help him or her achieve nutritional goals. Because they have frequent contact with patients, nurses play an important role in a patient's acceptance of nutrition care. Ensuring that the nursing staff is aware of the NCP can greatly improve the probability of success.

Interventions: Nutrition Education and Counseling

Nutrition education is an important part of the MNT provided to many patients. The goal of nutrition education is to help the patient acquire the knowledge and skills needed to make changes, including modifying behavior to facilitate sustained change. Nutrition education and dietary changes can result in many benefits, including control of the disease or symptoms, improved health status, enhanced quality of life, and decreased health care costs.

As the average length of hospital stays has decreased, the role of the in-patient dietitian in educating inpatients has changed to providing brief education or "survival skills." This education includes the types of foods to limit, timing of meals, and portion sizes. Follow-up outpatient counseling should be encouraged to reinforce the basic counseling given during hospitalization. See Chapter 14 for managing nutrition support and Chapter 15 for counseling skills.

Intervention: Coordination of Care

Nutrition care is part of **discharge planning**. Education, counseling, and mobilization of resources to provide home care and nutrition support are included in discharge procedures. Completing a discharge nutritional summary for the next caregiver is imperative for optimal care. Appropriate discharge documentation includes a summary of nutrition therapies and outcomes; pertinent information such as weights, laboratory values, and dietary intake; potential drug-nutrient interactions; expected progress or prognosis; and recommendations for follow-up services. Types of therapy attempted and failed can be very useful information.

The amount and type of instruction given, the patient's comprehension, and the expected degree of adherence to the prescribed diet are included. An effective discharge plan increases the likelihood of a positive outcome for the patient.

Regardless of the setting to which the patient is discharged, effective coordination of care begins on day 1 of a hospital or nursing home stay and continues throughout the institutionalization. The patient should be included in every step of the planning process whenever possible to ensure that decisions made by the health care team reflect the desires of the patient.

When needed, the RD refers the patient or client to other caregivers, agencies, or programs for follow-up care or services. For example, use of the home-delivered meal program of the Older Americans Act Nutrition Program has traditionally served frail, homebound, older adults, yet studies show that older adults who have recently been discharged from the hospital may be at high nutritional risk but not referred to this service (Sahyoun et al., 2010). Thus the RD plays an essential role in making the referral and coordinating the necessary follow-up.

NUTRITION FOR THE TERMINALLY ILL OR HOSPICE PATIENT

Maintenance of comfort and quality of life are most typically the goals of nutrition care for the terminally ill patient. Dietary restrictions are rarely appropriate. Nutrition care should be mindful of strategies that facilitate symptom and pain control. Recognition of the various phases of dying—denial, anger, bargaining, depression, and acceptance—will help the health care practitioner understand the patient's response to food and nutrition support.

The decision as to when life support should be terminated often involves the issue of whether to continue enteral or parenteral nutrition. With **advance directives**, the patient can advise family and health care team members of his or her individual preferences with regard to end-of-life issues. Food and hydration issues may be discussed, such as whether tube feeding should be initiated or discontinued and under what circumstances. Nutrition support should be continued as long as the patient is competent to make this choice (or if specified in the patient's advance directives).

In advanced dementia, the inability to eat orally can lead to weight loss. One clear goal-oriented alternative to tube feeding may be the order for "comfort feeding only" to ensure an individualized feeding plan (Palecek et al., 2010). **Palliative care** encourages the alleviation of physical symptoms, anxiety, and fear while attempting to maintain the patient's ability to function independently.

Hospice home care programs allow terminally ill patients to stay at home and delay or avoid hospital admission. Quality of life is the critical component. Indeed, individuals have the right to request or refuse nutrition and hydration as medical treatment (ADA, 2008). RD intervention may benefit the patient and family as they adjust to issues related to the approaching death. Families who might be accustomed to a modified diet should be reassured if they are uncomfortable about easing dietary restrictions. Ongoing communication and explanations to the family are important and helpful. RDs should work collaboratively to make recommendations on providing, withdrawing, or withholding nutrition and hydration in individual cases and serve as active members of institutional ethics committees (ADA, 2008). The RD, as a member of the health care team, has a responsibility to promote use of advanced directives of the individual patient and to identify their nutritional and hydration needs.

CLINICAL SCENARIO

Mr. B, a 47-year-old man, 6 ft 2 in tall and weighing 200 lb, is admitted to the hospital with chest pain. Three days after admission, at patient care rounds, it is discovered that Mr. B has gained 30 pounds over the last 2 years. Review of the medical record reveals the following laboratory data: LDL: 240 (desirable 130), HDL 30 (desirable >50), triglyceride 350 (desirable <200). Blood pressure is 120/85. Current medications: multivitamin/mineral daily. Cardiac catheterization is scheduled for tomorrow. Diet is poor; skips meals and eats very large dinner meals.

Nutrition Diagnostic Statement

Altered nutrition-related laboratory values related to undesirable food choices as evidenced by elevated LDL and low HDL.

Nutrition Care Questions

1. What other information do you need to develop a nutrition care plan?
2. Was nutrition screening completed in a timely manner? Discuss the implications of timing of screening versus implementing care.
3. Develop a chart note, using ADIME format, based on this information and the interview you conduct with the patient.
4. What nutrition care goals would you develop for this patient during his hospital stay?
5. What goals would you develop for this patient after discharge? Discuss how the type of health care insurance coverage the patient has might influence this plan.

HDL, High-density lipoprotein; *LDL*, low-density lipoprotein.

USEFUL WEBSITES

American Dietetic Association
www.eatright.org

Centers for Medicare and Medicaid Services
www.cms.hhs.gov

The Joint Commission
www.jointcommission.org

REFERENCES

American Dietetic Association (ADA): *Evidence analysis library*. Accessed 5 May 2010 from http://www.adaevidencelibrary.com.

American Dietetic Association (ADA): *International nutrition and diagnostic terminology*, ed 3, Chicago, Il, 2010, American Dietetic Association.

American Dietetic Association (ADA): Position of the American Dietetic Association: Ethical and legal issues in nutrition, hydration and feeding, *J Am Diet Assoc* 108:873, 2008.

Ash J et al: The extent and importance of unintended consequences related to computerized provider order entry, *J Am Med Inform Assoc* 14:415, 2007.

Backer LA: The medical home. An idea whose time has come … again, *Fam Pract Manag* 14:38, 2007.

Centers for Medicare and Medicaid Services. Accessed 1 November 2010 at https://www.cms.gov/hipaageninfo/.

Demiris G, et al: Current status and perceived needs of information technology in Critical Access Hospitals, *Informatics in Primary Care* 15:45, 2007.

Franz MJ, et al: Evidence-based nutrition practice guidelines for diabetes and scope and standards of practice, *J Am Diet Assoc* 108:S52, 2008.

Jeffery KM, et al: The clear liquid diet is no longer necessary in the routine postoperative management of surgical patients, *Am J Surg* 62:167, 1996.

Ornstein S, et al: Improving the translation of research into primary care practice: results of a national quality improvement demonstration project, *Jt Comm J Qual Patient Saf* 34:379, 2008.

Palecek EJ, et al: Comfort feeding only: a proposal to bring clarity to decision-making regarding difficulty with eating for persons with advanced dementia, *J Am Geriatr Soc* 58:580, 2010.

Ross JS: Health reform redux: learning from experience and politics, *Am J Public Health* 99:779, 2009.

Sahyoun NR, et al: Recently hospital-discharged older adults are vulnerable and may be underserved by the Older Americans Act nutrition program, *J Nutr Elder* 29:227, 2010.

Schifalacqua M, et al: Roadmap for planned change, part I: change leadership and project management, *Nurse Leader* 7:26, 2009.

White JB, et al: Registered dietitians' coding practices and patterns of code use, *J Am Diet Assoc* 108:1242, 2008.

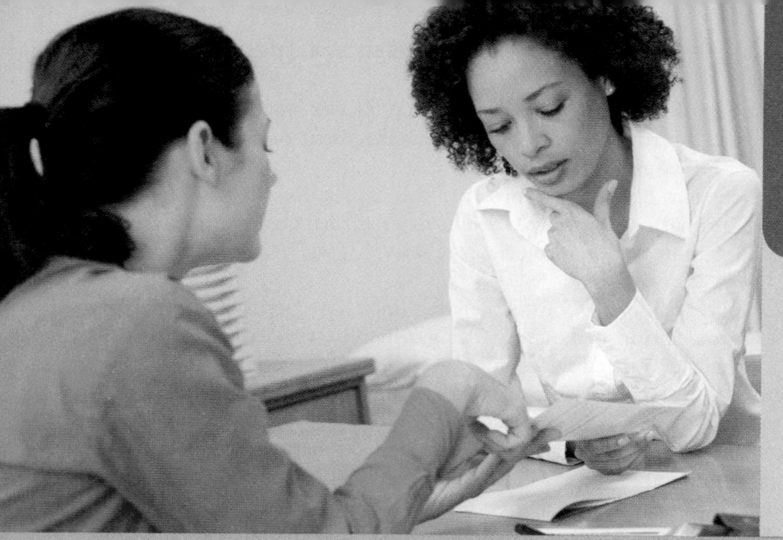

CHAPTER 12

Deborah H. Murray, MS, RD, LD
David H. Holben, PhD, RD, LD
Janice L. Raymond, MS, RD, CD

Food and Nutrient Delivery: Planning the Diet with Cultural Competency

KEY TERMS

adequate intake (AI)
daily reference intake (DRI)
daily reference values (DRVs)
daily value (DV)
Dietary Guidelines for Americans (DGA)
dietary reference intake (DRI)
estimated average requirement (EAR)
estimated safe and adequate daily dietary intake (ESADDI)
flexitarian
food insecurity
functional food
health claim
Healthy Eating Index (HEI)
locovore
MyPlate Food Guidance System
nutrition facts label
phytochemicals
recommended dietary allowance (RDA)
reference daily intakes (RDIs)
tolerable upper intake level (UL)
vegan

An appropriate diet is adequate and balanced and considers the individual's characteristics such as age and stage of development, taste preferences, and food habits. It also reflects the availability of foods, socioeconomic conditions, cultural practices and family traditions, storage and preparation facilities, and cooking skills. An adequate and balanced diet meets all the nutritional needs of an individual for maintenance, repair, living processes, growth, and development. It includes energy and all nutrients in proper amounts and in proportion to each other. The presence or absence of one essential nutrient may affect the availability, absorption, metabolism, or dietary need for others. The recognition of nutrient interrelationships provides further support for the principle of maintaining food variety to provide the most complete diet.

Dietitians translate food, nutrition, and health information into food choices and diet patterns for groups and individuals. With increasing knowledge of how diet influences diseases that lead to premature disability and mortality among Americans, an appropriate diet helps reduce the risk of developing chronic diseases and conditions. In this era of vastly expanding scientific knowledge, food intake messages for health promotion and disease prevention change rapidly. The public often hears references to functional food ingredients, which provide more benefits than just basic nutrition.

DETERMINING NUTRIENT NEEDS

According to the Food and Nutrition Board, choosing a variety of foods should provide adequate amounts of nutrients. A varied diet may also ensure that a person is consuming sufficient amounts of **functional food** constituents that, although not defined as nutrients, have biologic effects and may influence health and susceptibility to disease. Examples include foods containing dietary fiber and carotenoids, as well as lesser known **phytochemicals** (components of plants that have protective or disease-preventive properties) such as isothiocyanates in broccoli or other cruciferous vegetables and lycopene in tomato products (see Chapter 20).

WORLDWIDE GUIDELINES

Numerous standards serve as guides for planning and evaluating diets and food supplies for individuals and population groups. The Food and Agriculture Organization and the World Health Organization of the United Nations have established international standards in many areas of food quality and safety, as well as dietary and nutrient recommendations. In the United States the Food and Nutrition Board (FNB) of the Institute of Medicine (IOM) has led the development of nutrient recommendations since the 1940s. Since the mid-1990s, nutrient recommendations developed by the FNB have been used by the United States and Canada.

The U.S. Department of Agriculture (USDA) and U.S. Department Health and Human Services (USDHHS) have a shared responsibility for issuing dietary recommendations, collecting and analyzing food composition data, and formulating regulations for nutrition information on food products. Health Canada is the agency responsible for Canadian dietary recommendations; in Australia, the guidelines are available through the National Health and Medical Research Council. The Japan Dietetic Association updates their guidelines every four years, the latest designed as the "Spinning Top" from the Ministry of Health, Labor and Welfare. Indeed, many countries have issued guidelines appropriate for the circumstances and needs of their populations.

Dietary Reference Intakes

American standards for nutrient requirements have been the recommended dietary allowances (RDAs) established by the FNB of the IOM. They were first published in 1941 and most recently revised between 1997 and 2002. Each revision incorporates the most recent research findings. In 1993 the FNB developed a framework for the development of nutrient recommendations, called **dietary reference intakes (DRI)**. Nutrition and health professionals should always use updated food composition databases and tables and inquire whether data used in computerized nutrient analysis programs have been revised to include the most up-to-date information. An interactive DRI calculator is available at http://fnic.nal.usda.gov/interactiveDRI/.

Estimated Safe and Adequate Daily Dietary Intakes

Numerous nutrients are known to be essential for life and health, but data for some are insufficient to establish a recommended intake. Intakes for these nutrients are **estimated safe and adequate daily dietary intakes (ESADDIs)**. Most intakes are shown as ranges to indicate that not only are specific recommendations not known, but also at least the upper and lower limits of safety should be observed.

DRI Components

The DRI model expands the previous RDA, which focused only on levels of nutrients for healthy populations to prevent deficiency diseases. To respond to scientific advances in diet and health throughout the life cycle, the DRI model now includes four reference points: adequate intake (AI), estimated average intake (EAR), RDA, and tolerable upper intake level (UL).

The **adequate intake (AI)** is a nutrient recommendation based on observed or experimentally determined approximation of nutrient intake by a group (or groups) of healthy people when sufficient scientific evidence is not available to calculate an RDA or an EAR. Some key nutrients are expressed as an AI, including calcium (see Chapter 3). The **estimated average requirement (EAR)** is the average requirement of a nutrient for healthy individuals; a functional or clinical assessment has been conducted, and measures of adequacy have been determined. An EAR is the amount of a nutrient with which approximately one half of individuals would have their needs met and one half would not. The EAR should be used for assessing the nutrient adequacy of populations, but not for individuals.

The **recommended dietary allowance (RDA)** presents the amount of a nutrient needed to meet the requirements of almost all (97% to 98%) of the healthy population of individuals for whom it was developed. An RDA for a nutrient should serve as a goal for intake for individuals, not as a benchmark for adequacy of diets of populations. Finally the **tolerable upper intake level (UL)** was established for many nutrients to reduce the risk of adverse or toxic effects from consumption of nutrients in concentrated forms—either alone or combined with others (not in food)—or from enrichment and fortification. A UL is the highest level of daily nutrient intake that is unlikely to have any adverse health effects on almost all individuals in the general population. The DRIs for the macronutrients, vitamins and minerals, including the ULs are presented on the inside front cover and opening page of this text. The acceptable macronutrient distribution ranges are based on energy intake by age and sex. See Table 12-1 and the DRI tables on the inside front cover of this text.

Target Population

Each of the nutrient recommendation categories in the DRI system is used for specific purposes among individuals or populations. The EAR is used for evaluating the nutrient intake of populations. The AI and RDA can be used for individuals. Nutrient intakes between the RDA and the UL may further define intakes that may promote health or prevent disease in the individual.

Age and Gender Groups

Because nutrient needs are highly individualized depending on age, sexual development, and the reproductive status of females, the DRI framework has 10 age groupings, including age-group categories for children, men and women 51 to 70 years of age, and those older than 70 years of age. It separates three age-group categories each for pregnancy and lactation—younger than 18 years, 19 to 30 years, and 31 to 50 years of age.

Reference Men and Women

The requirement for many nutrients is based on body weight, according to reference men and women of

TABLE 12-1

Acceptable Macronutrient Distribution Ranges

Nutrient	AMDR (Percentage of Daily Energy Intake) 1-3 Years	4-18 Years	>19 Years	AMDR Sample Diet Adult, 2000-kcal/day Diet % Reference*	g/Day
Protein†	5-20	10-30	10-30	10	50
Carbohydrate	45-65	45-65	45-65	60	300
Fat	30-40	25-35	20-35	30	67
α-Linolenic acid (*ω-3)‡	0.6-1.2	0.6-1.2	0.6-1.2	0.8	1.8
Linolenic acid (ω-6)	5-10	5-10	5-10	7	16
Added sugars§	≤25% of total calories			500	125

Modified from Food and Nutrition Board, Institute of Medicine: Dietary reference intakes for energy, carbohydrate, fiber, fat, fatty acids, cholesterol, protein, and amino acids, Washington DC, 2002, National Academies Press.

AMDR, Acceptable macronutrient distribution range; *DHA*, docosahexaenoic acid; *DRI*, dietary reference intake; *EPA*, eicosapentaenoic acid.

*Suggested maximum.

†Higher number in protein AMDR is set to complement AMDRs for carbohydrate and fat, not because it is a recommended upper limit in the range of calories from protein.

‡Up to 10% of the AMDR for α-linolenic acid can be consumed as EPA, DHA, or both (0.06%-0.12% of calories).

§Reference percentages chosen based on average DRI for protein for adult men and women, then calculated back to percentage of calories. Carbohydrate and fat percentages chosen based on difference from protein and balanced with other federal dietary recommendations.

designated height and weight. These values for age-sex groups of individuals older than 19 years of age are based on actual medians obtained for the American population by the third National Health and Nutrition Examination Survey, 1988 to 1994. Although this does not necessarily imply that these weight-for-height values are ideal, at least they make it possible to define recommended allowances appropriate for the largest number of people.

NUTRITIONAL STATUS OF AMERICANS

Food and Nutrient Intake Data

Information about the diet and nutritional status of Americans and the relationship between diet and health is collected by 22 federal agencies. This effort is coordinated by the USDA and USDHHS through the National Nutrition Monitoring and Related Research Program, (See Chapter 10). Overall, analysis of the American diet shows that the population is slowly changing eating patterns and adopting more healthy diets. Intake of total fat, saturated fatty acids, and cholesterol has decreased in some segments of the population; servings of fruits and vegetables have risen to four per day. Hospitals have even taken on the challenge for healthier food intake (see *Focus On:* The "Healthy Food In Health Care" Pledge).

Unfortunately, gaps still exist between actual consumption and government recommendations in certain population subgroups. Nutrition-related health measurements indicate that overweight and obesity are increasing from lack of physical activity. Hypertension remains a major public health problem in middle-age and older adults and in non-Hispanic blacks in whom it increases the risk of stroke and coronary heart disease. Osteoporosis develops more often among non-Hispanic whites than non-Hispanic blacks. Finally, in spite of available choices, many Americans experience **food insecurity**, meaning that they lack access to adequate and safe food for an active, healthy life. Table 12-2 provides a list of food components and public health concerns related to those components.

Healthy Eating Index

The Center for Nutrition Policy and Promotion of the USDA releases the **Healthy Eating Index (HEI)** to measure how well people's diets conform to recommended healthy eating patterns. The index provides a picture of foods people are eating, the amount of variety in their diets, and compliance with specific recommendations in the Dietary Guidelines for Americans (DGA). The HEI is designed to assess and monitor the dietary status of Americans by evaluating 10 components, each representing different aspects of a healthy diet. The dietary components used in the evaluation include grains, vegetables, fruits, milk, meat, total fat, saturated fat, cholesterol, sodium, and variety. Data from the HEI over time show that Americans are reducing total and saturated fat and eating a wider variety of foods. The 2005 report suggests that milk intake is still low (Guenther et al., 2008). The overall HEI score ranges from 0 to 100. Interestingly, women generally have scores higher than men, and toddlers have the highest scores.

Nutrition Monitoring Report

At the request of the USDHHS and USDA, the Expert Panel on Nutrition Monitoring was established by the Life Sciences Research Office of the Federation of American

FOCUS ON

The "Healthy Food in Health Care" Pledge

Health care facilities across the nation have recognized that their systems of purchasing, producing and distributing food are misaligned with the U.S. dietary guidelines and have joined a movement to change their practices. The organization promoting this plan is called "Health Care Without Harm." In 2009, The American Medical Association (AMA) approved a new policy resolution in support of practices and policies within health care systems that promote and model a healthy and ecologically sustainable food system. The resolution also calls on the AMA to work with health care and public health organizations to educate the health care community and the public about the importance of healthy and ecologically sustainable food systems. Hospitals are using the online pledge form to commit to these eight steps:

1. Work to source locally (see *Focus On:* What is a Locovore?).
2. Encourage vendors to supply foods without harmful chemicals and antibiotics and to support the health of farmers and the environment.
3. Implement a program to adopt sustainable food procurement.
4. Communicate to group purchasing organizations a desire to source locally and to source foods that do not contain harmful chemicals.
5. Educate patients and the community about nutritious, socially just, and ecologically sustainable food practices and procedures.
6. Minimize or beneficially reuse food waste and support the use of food packaging that is ecologically protective.
7. Develop a program to promote and source from producers and processors that uphold the dignity of family, farmers, and their communities, and support humane and sustainable agriculture systems.
8. Report annually.

Modified from Health Care without Harm. Accessed 24 May 2010 from http://www.noharm.org.

Societies for Experimental Biology to review the dietary and nutritional status of the American population. In general, the committee concluded that the food supply in the United States is abundant, although some people may not receive enough nutrients for various reasons. Nutrient intakes are most likely to be low in persons living below the poverty level. Intakes of nutrients reported to be low in the general population are even lower in the poverty group. Chapter 10 describes this report more fully.

NATIONAL GUIDELINES FOR DIET PLANNING

Eating can be one of life's greatest pleasures. People eat for enjoyment and to obtain energy and nutrients. Although many genetic, environmental, behavioral, and cultural factors affect health, diet is equally important for promoting health and preventing disease. Yet within the past 40 years, attention has been focused increasingly on the relationship of nutrition to chronic diseases and conditions. Although this interest derives somewhat from the rapid increase in number of older adults and their longevity, it is also prompted by the desire to prevent premature deaths from diseases such as coronary heart disease, diabetes mellitus, and cancer. Approximately two thirds of deaths in the United States are caused by chronic disease.

Current Dietary Guidance

In 1969 President Nixon convened the White House Conference on Nutrition and Health (AJCN, 1969). Increased attention was being given to prevention of hunger and disease. The development of dietary guidelines in the United States is discussed in Chapter 10. Guidelines directed toward prevention of a particular disease, such as those from the National Cancer Institute; the American Diabetes Association; the American Heart Association; and the National Heart, Lung, and Blood Institute's cholesterol education guidelines, contain recommendations unique to particular conditions. The American Dietetic Association supports a total diet approach, in which the overall pattern of food eaten, consumed in moderation with appropriate portion sizes and combined with regular physical activity, is key. Various guidelines that can be used by health counselors throughout the developed world are summarized in Box 12-1.

Implementing the Guidelines

The task of planning nutritious meals centers on including the essential nutrients in sufficient amounts as outlined in the newest DRIs, in addition to appropriate amounts of energy, protein, carbohydrate (including fiber and sugars), fat (especially saturated and *trans*-fats), cholesterol, and salt. Suggestions are included to help people meet the specifics of the recommendations. When specific numeric recommendations differ, they are presented as ranges.

To help people select an eating pattern that achieves specific health promotion or disease prevention objectives, nutritionists should assist individuals in making food choices (e.g., to reduce fat, to increase fiber). Although numerous federal agencies are involved in the issuance of dietary guidance, the USDA and USDHHS lead the effort. The **Dietary Guidelines for Americans (DGA)** were first published in 1980 and are revised every five years; the most recent guidelines were released in 2010 (Box 12-2). The DGA are designed to motivate consumers to change their eating and activity patterns by providing them with positive, simple messages. Using consumer research, the DGA develop messages that expand the influence of the dietary guidelines to encourage

TABLE 12-2

Food Components and Public Health Concerns

Food Component	Relevance to Public Health
Energy	The high prevalence of overweight indicates that an energy imbalance exists among Americans because of physical inactivity and underreporting of energy intake or food consumption in national surveys.
Total fat, saturated fat, and cholesterol	Intakes of fat, saturated fatty acids, and cholesterol among all age groups older than 2 years of age are above recommended levels. Cholesterol intakes are generally within the recommended range of 300 mg/dL or less.
Alcohol	Intake of alcohol is a public health concern because it displaces food sources of nutrients and has potential health consequences.
Iron and calcium	Low intakes of iron and calcium continue to be a public health concern, particularly among infants and females of childbearing age. Prevalence of iron deficiency anemia is higher among these groups than among other age and sex groups. Low calcium intake is a particular concern among adolescent girls and adult women in most racial and ethnic groups.
Sodium*	Sodium intake exceeds government recommendations of 2300 mg/day in most age and sex groups. Strategies to lower intake can be found at the Institute of Medicine website at http://www.iom.edu/Reports/2010/Strategies-to-Reduce-Sodium-Intake-in-the-United-States.aspx
Other nutrients at potential risk	Some population or age groups may consume insufficient amounts of total carbohydrate and carbohydrate constituents such as dietary fiber; protein; vitamin A; carotenoids; antioxidant vitamins C and E; folate, vitamins B_6. and B_{12}; magnesium, potassium, zinc, copper, selenium, phosphorus, and fluoride. Studies also suggest that vitamin D deficiency is very common.
Unbalanced Nutrients	Intakes of polyunsaturated and monounsaturated fatty acids, *trans*-fatty acids, and fat substitutes are often excessive.

*Recommended intake of 1500 mg or less in at-risk populations defined as African-Americans, people with hypertension, and anyone 40 years or older (IOM, 2004).

BOX 12-1

Universal Prescription for Health and Nutritional Fitness

- Adjust energy intake and exercise level to achieve and maintain appropriate body weight.
- Eat a wide variety of foods to ensure nutrient adequacy.
- Increase total carbohydrate intake, especially complex carbohydrates.
- Eat less total fat and less saturated fat.
- Eat more fiber-rich foods, including whole grains, fruits, and vegetables.
- Eat fewer high cholesterol foods.
- Limit or omit high-sodium foods.
- Reduce intake of concentrated sugars.
- Drink alcohol in moderation or not at all.
- Meet the recommendations for calcium, especially important for adolescents and women.
- Meet the recommendation for iron, especially for children, adolescents, and women of childbearing age.
- Limit protein to no more than twice the recommended dietary allowance.
- If using a daily multivitamin, choose dietary supplements that do not exceed the dietary reference intake.
- Drink fluoridated water.

consumers to adopt them and ultimately change their behaviors. The messages reach out to consumers' motivations, individual needs, and life goals, and can be used in education, counseling, and communications initiatives (USDA, 2005).

The **MyPlate Food Guidance System**, shown in Figure 12-1, replaces the MyPyramid and offers a guide for daily food choices and portions. Consumers can use chooseMyPlate.gov as a resource.

For comparison, see the Eating Well with Canada's Food Guide as shown in *Clinical Insight:* Nutrition Recommendations for Canadians and Figure 12-2.

FOOD AND NUTRIENT LABELING

To help consumers make choices between similar types of food products that can be incorporated into a healthy diet, the Food and Drug Administration (FDA) established a voluntary system of providing selected nutrient information on food labels. The regulatory framework for nutrition information on food labels was revised and updated by the USDA (which regulates meat and poultry products and eggs) and the FDA (which regulates all other foods) with enactment of the Nutrition Labeling and Education Act (NLEA) in 1990. The labels became mandatory in 1994.

Mandatory Nutrition Labeling

As a result of the NLEA, nutrition labels must appear on most foods except products that provide few nutrients (such as coffee and spices), restaurant foods, and ready-to-eat

BOX 12-2

The 2010 Dietary Guidelines for Americans—Focal Points

Unlike previous Dietary Guidelines, reduction of calories in general, and reduction of dietary components that most contribute these excess calories, such as solid fats, added sugars, and refined grains, is the underlying message.

The emphasis is placed more on dietary patterns instead of individual nutrients and food groups to enable diverse approaches to complying with the Dietary Guidelines.

Whenever possible, the goal should be to encourage consumption of whole, minimally processed foods as the source of nutrients. The following concepts form the basis of the 2010 Dietary Guidelines for Americans Committee report:

- Reduce calorie consumption.
- Shift food intake patterns to a more plant-based diet that emphasizes vegetables, cooked dry beans and peas, fruits, whole grains, and nuts and seeds.
- Reduce intake of foods containing added sugars, solid fats, refined grains, and sodium.
- Meet the Physical Activity Guidelines for Americans by reducing sedentary behavior and screen time, and increasing physical activity at school, work, and community.
- Prevent excessive maternal weight gain and obesity in young children through attention to breastfeeding, early advice to parents, changes in school food offerings and physical activity, and preventive measures from the White House Task Force on Obesity.

Accessed 24 May 2010 from http://www.healthierus.gov/dietaryguidelines.

foods prepared on site, such as supermarket bakery and deli items. Providing nutrition information on many raw foods is voluntary. However, the FDA and USDA have called for a voluntary point-of-purchase program in which nutrition information is available in most supermarkets. Nutrition information is provided through brochures or point-of-purchase posters for the 20 most popular fruits, vegetables, and fresh fish and the 45 major cuts of fresh meat and poultry.

Nutrition information for foods purchased in restaurants is widely available at the point of purchase or from Internet sites or toll-free numbers. New legislation may require chains with 20 or more locations to disclose on their menus or menu board the number of calories per menu item, with additional nutrition information including total calories and calories from fat, and amounts of fat, saturated fat, cholesterol, sodium, total carbohydrates, complex carbohydrates, sugars, dietary fiber, and protein available upon request.

Ready-to-eat unpackaged foods in delicatessens or supermarkets may provide nutrition information voluntarily. However, if nutrition claims are made, nutrition labeling is required at the point of purchase. If a food makes the claim of being organic, it also must meet certain criteria and labeling requirements.

CLINICAL INSIGHT

Nutrition Recommendations for Canadians

The revision to Canada's Food Guide to Healthy Eating was released in 2007 and developed age- and gender-specific food intake patterns. These age- and gender-specific suggestions include 4 to 7 servings of vegetables and fruits, 3 to 7 servings of grain products, 2 to 3 servings of milk or milk alternatives, and 1 to 3 servings of meat or meat alternatives. Canada's Eating Well with Canada's Food Guide contains four food groupings presented in a rainbow shape (Health Canada, 2007).

Tips include:

- Consume no more than 400-450 mg of caffeine per day.
- Eat at least one dark green and one orange vegetable each day.
- Make at least half of grain products consumed each day whole grain.
- Compare the Nutrition Facts table on food labels to choose products that contain less fat, saturated fat, *trans* fat, sugar, and sodium.
- Drink skim, 1% or 2% milk, or fortified soy beverages each day. Check the food label to see if the soy beverage is fortified with calcium and vitamin D.
- Include a small amount (30-45 mL [2-3 Tbsp]) of unsaturated fat each day to get the fat needed.
- Limit the intake of soft drinks, sports drinks, energy drinks, fruit drinks, punches, sweetened hot and cold beverages, and alcohol.
- Eat at least two Food Guide Servings of fish each week.
- Build 30-60 minutes of moderate physical activity into daily life for adults and at least 90 minutes a day for children and youth.

The Canadian Food Guide recognizes the cultural, spiritual, and physical importance of traditional Aboriginal foods as well as the role of nontraditional foods in contemporary diets, with a First Nations, Inuit, and Métis guide available. The guide is available in 12 languages.

Data from Health Canada: Eating well with Canada's food guide, Her Majesty the Queen in Right of Canada, represented by the Minister of Healthy Canada, 2007. Accessed 17 January 2010 from http://www.hc-sc.gc.ca/fn-an/food-gu.

Standardized Serving Sizes on Food Label

Serving sizes of products are set by the government based on reference amounts commonly consumed. For example, a serving of milk is 8 oz, and a serving of salad dressing is

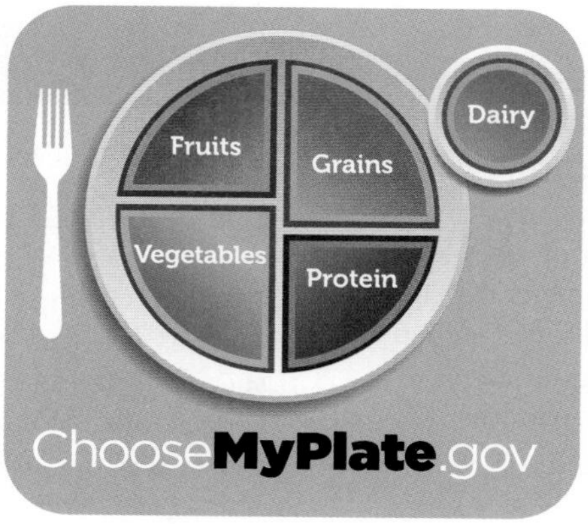

Balancing Calories

- Enjoy your food, but eat less.
- Avoid oversized portions.

Foods to Increase

- Make half your plate fruits and vegetables.
- Make at least half your grains whole grains.
- Switch to fat-free or low-fat (1%) milk.

Foods to Reduce

- Compare sodium in foods like soup, bread, and frozen meals – and choose the foods with lower numbers.
- Drink water instead of sugary drinks.

FIGURE 12-1 MyPlate showing the five essential food groups. *(From the United States Department of Agriculture (USDA). Accessed June 10, 2011 from http://www.chooseMyPlate.gov/.)*

2 tbsp. Standardized serving sizes make it easier for consumers to compare the nutrient contents of similar products (Figure 12-3).

Nutrition Facts Label

The **nutrition facts label** on a food product provides information on its per-serving calories and calories from fat. The label must list the amount (in grams) of total fat, saturated fat, trans fat, cholesterol, sodium, total carbohydrate, dietary fiber, sugar, and protein. For most of these nutrients the label also shows the percentage of the **daily value (DV)** supplied by a serving, showing how a product fits into an overall diet by comparing its nutrient content with recommended intakes of those nutrients. DVs are not recommended intakes for individuals; they are simply reference points to provide some perspective on daily nutrient needs. DVs are based on a 2000-kcal diet. For example, individuals who consume diets supplying more or fewer calories can still use the DVs as a rough guide to ensure that they are getting adequate amounts of vitamin C but not too much saturated fat.

The DVs exist for nutrients for which RDAs already exist (in which case they are known as **reference daily intakes [RDIs]**) (Table 12-3) and for which no RDAs exist (in which case they are known as **daily reference values [DRVs]** [Table 12-4]). However, food labels use only the term *daily value*. RDIs provide a large margin of safety; in general, the RDI for a nutrient is greater than the RDA for a specific age-group. The term *RDI* replaces the term *U.S. RDAs* used on previous food labels. The previously mentioned nutrients must be listed on the food label.

As new DRIs are developed in various categories, labeling laws are updated. Figure 12-4 shows a sample nutrition facts label, and Box 12-3 provides tips for reading and understanding food labels. The FDA has a helpful website to assist consumers with reading labels (http://www.fda.gov/Food/LabelingNutrition/ConsumerInformation/UCM078889.htm).

Nutrient Content Claims

Nutrient content terms such as *reduced sodium*, *fat free*, *low calorie*, and *healthy* must now meet government definitions that apply to all foods (Box 12-4). For example, *lean* refers to a serving of meat, poultry, seafood, or game meat with less than 10 g of fat, less than 4 g of saturated fat, and less than 95 mg of cholesterol per serving or per 100 g. Extra

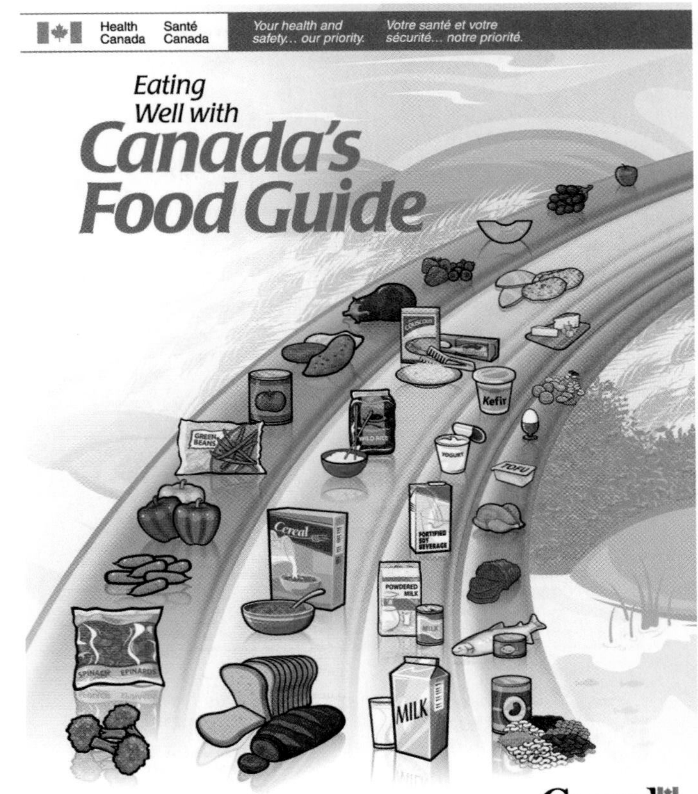

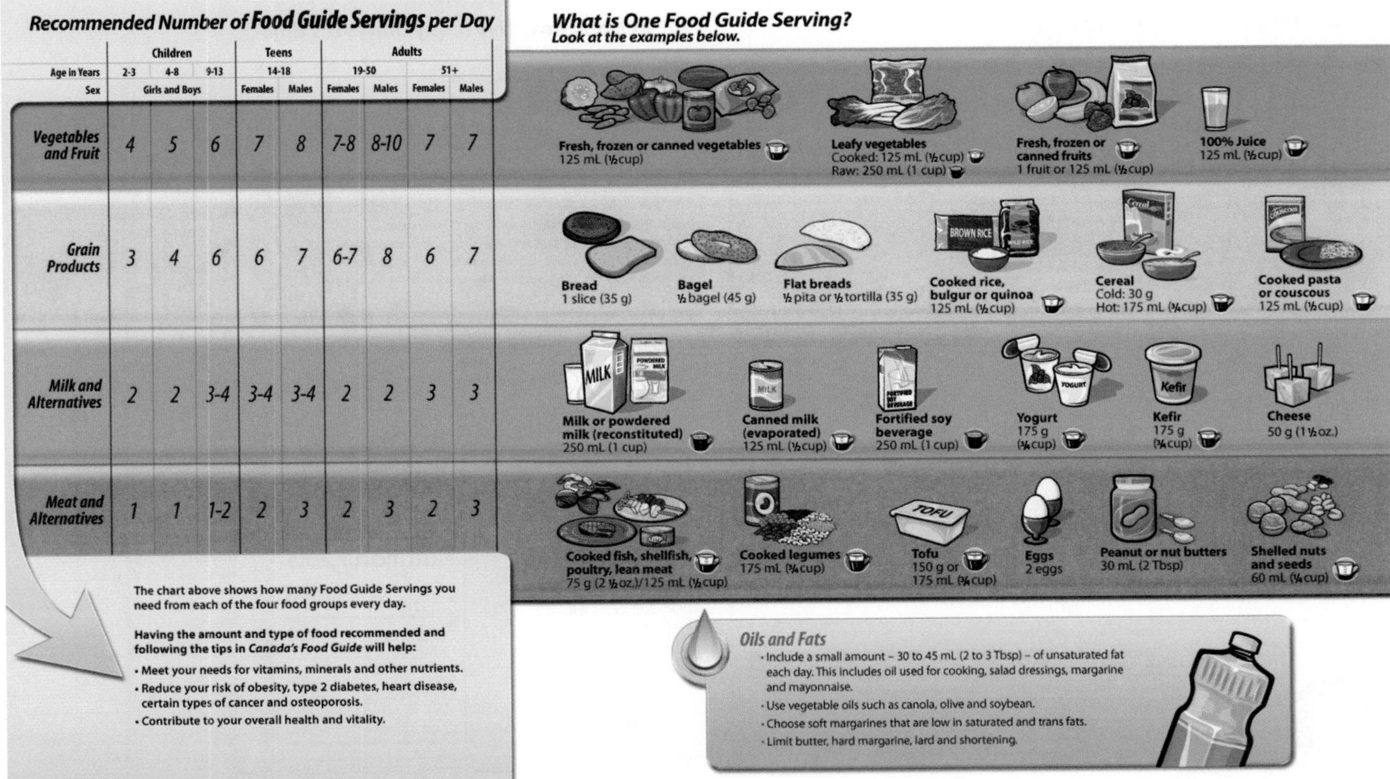

Recommended Number of Food Guide Servings per Day

	Children			Teens		Adults			
Age in Years	2-3	4-8	9-13	14-18		19-50		51+	
Sex	Girls and Boys			Females	Males	Females	Males	Females	Males
Vegetables and Fruit	4	5	6	7	8	7-8	8-10	7	7
Grain Products	3	4	6	6	7	6-7	8	6	7
Milk and Alternatives	2	2	3-4	3-4	3-4	2	2	3	3
Meat and Alternatives	1	1	1-2	2	3	2	3	2	3

FIGURE 12-2 Eating well with Canada's food guide. *(Reprinted with permission from Health Canada. Data from Health Canada: Eating well with Canada's food guide, Her Majesty the Queen in Right of Canada, represented by the Minister of Healthy Canada, 2007. Accessed 22 May 2010 from www.hc-sc.gc.ca/fn-an/food-guide-aliment.*

Make each Food Guide Serving count...
wherever you are – at home, at school, at work or when eating out!

- **Eat at least one dark green and one orange vegetable each day.**
  - Go for dark green vegetables such as broccoli, romaine lettuce and spinach.
  - Go for orange vegetables such as carrots, sweet potatoes and winter squash.
- **Choose vegetables and fruit prepared with little or no added fat, sugar or salt.**
  - Enjoy vegetables steamed, baked or stir-fried instead of deep-fried.
- **Have vegetables and fruit more often than juice.**

- **Make at least half of your grain products whole grain each day.**
  - Eat a variety of whole grains such as barley, brown rice, oats, quinoa and wild rice.
  - Enjoy whole grain breads, oatmeal or whole wheat pasta.
- **Choose grain products that are lower in fat, sugar or salt.**
  - Compare the Nutrition Facts table on labels to make wise choices.
  - Enjoy the true taste of grain products. When adding sauces or spreads, use small amounts.

- **Drink skim, 1%, or 2% milk each day.**
  - Have 500 mL (2 cups) of milk every day for adequate vitamin D.
  - Drink fortified soy beverages if you do not drink milk.
- **Select lower fat milk alternatives.**
  - Compare the Nutrition Facts table on yogurts or cheeses to make wise choices.

- **Have meat alternatives such as beans, lentils and tofu often.**
- **Eat at least two Food Guide Servings of fish each week.***
  - Choose fish such as char, herring, mackerel, salmon, sardines and trout.
- **Select lean meat and alternatives prepared with little or no added fat or salt.**
  - Trim the visible fat from meats. Remove the skin on poultry.
  - Use cooking methods such as roasting, baking or poaching that require little or no added fat.
  - If you eat luncheon meats, sausages or prepackaged meats, choose those lower in salt (sodium) and fat.

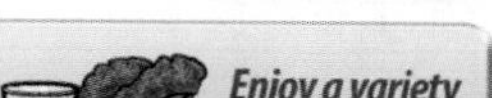

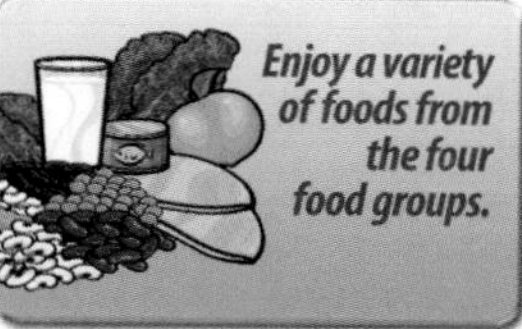

Enjoy a variety of foods from the four food groups.

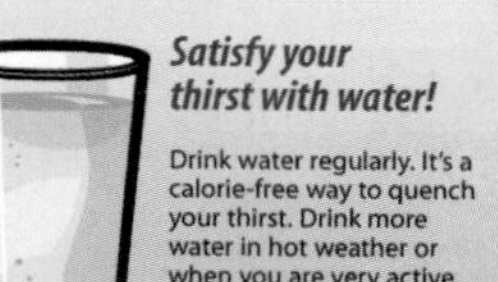

Satisfy your thirst with water!

Drink water regularly. It's a calorie-free way to quench your thirst. Drink more water in hot weather or when you are very active.

* Health Canada provides advice for limiting exposure to mercury from certain types of fish. Refer to www.healthcanada.gc.ca for the latest information.

Advice for different ages and stages...

Children

Following *Canada's Food Guide* helps children grow and thrive.

Young children have small appetites and need calories for growth and development.

- Serve small nutritious meals and snacks each day.
- Do not restrict nutritious foods because of their fat content. Offer a variety of foods from the four food groups.
- Most of all... be a good role model.

Women of childbearing age

All women who could become pregnant and those who are pregnant or breastfeeding need a multivitamin containing **folic acid** every day. Pregnant women need to ensure that their multivitamin also contains **iron**. A health care professional can help you find the multivitamin that's right for you.

Pregnant and breastfeeding women need more calories. Include an extra 2 to 3 Food Guide Servings each day.

Here are two examples:
- Have fruit and yogurt for a snack, or
- Have an extra slice of toast at breakfast and an extra glass of milk at supper.

Men and women over 50

The need for **vitamin D** increases after the age of 50.

In addition to following *Canada's Food Guide*, everyone over the age of 50 should take a daily vitamin D supplement of 10 μg (400 IU).

How do I count Food Guide Servings in a meal?

Here is an example:

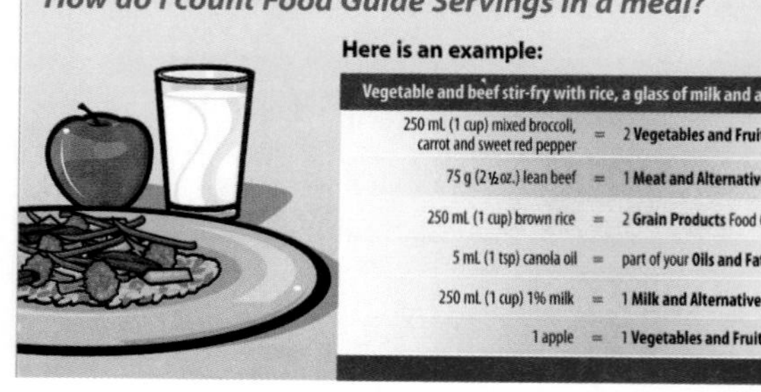

Vegetable and beef stir-fry with rice, a glass of milk and an apple for dessert		
250 mL (1 cup) mixed broccoli, carrot and sweet red pepper	=	2 **Vegetables and Fruit** Food Guide Servings
75 g (2 ½ oz.) lean beef	=	1 **Meat and Alternatives** Food Guide Serving
250 mL (1 cup) brown rice	=	2 **Grain Products** Food Guide Servings
5 mL (1 tsp) canola oil	=	part of your **Oils and Fats** intake for the day
250 mL (1 cup) 1% milk	=	1 **Milk and Alternatives** Food Guide Serving
1 apple	=	1 **Vegetables and Fruit** Food Guide Serving

Eat well and be active today and every day!

The benefits of eating well and being active include:

- Better overall health.
- Lower risk of disease.
- A healthy body weight.
- Feeling and looking better.
- More energy.
- Stronger muscles and bones.

Be active

To be active every day is a step towards better health and a healthy body weight.

Canada's Physical Activity Guide recommends building 30 to 60 minutes of moderate physical activity into daily life for adults and at least 90 minutes a day for children and youth. You don't have to do it all at once. Add it up in periods of at least 10 minutes at a time for adults and five minutes at a time for children and youth.

Start slowly and build up.

Eat well

Another important step towards better health and a healthy body weight is to follow *Canada's Food Guide* by:

- Eating the recommended amount and type of food each day.
- Limiting foods and beverages high in calories, fat, sugar or salt (sodium) such as cakes and pastries, chocolate and candies, cookies and granola bars, doughnuts and muffins, ice cream and frozen desserts, french fries, potato chips, nachos and other salty snacks, alcohol, fruit flavoured drinks, soft drinks, sports and energy drinks, and sweetened hot or cold drinks.

Read the label

- Compare the Nutrition Facts table on food labels to choose products that contain less fat, saturated fat, trans fat, sugar and sodium.
- Keep in mind that the calories and nutrients listed are for the amount of food found at the top of the Nutrition Facts table.

Nutrition Facts
Per 0 mL (0 g)

Amount	% Daily Value
Calories 0	
Fat 0 g	0 %
Saturates 0 g + Trans 0 g	0 %
Cholesterol 0 mg	
Sodium 0 mg	0 %
Carbohydrate 0 g	0 %
Fibre 0 g	0 %
Sugars 0 g	
Protein 0 g	
Vitamin A 0 %	Vitamin C 0 %
Calcium 0 %	Iron 0 %

Limit trans fat

When a Nutrition Facts table is not available, ask for nutrition information to choose foods lower in trans and saturated fats.

Take a step today...

- ✓ Have breakfast every day. It may help control your hunger later in the day.
- ✓ Walk wherever you can – get off the bus early, use the stairs.
- ✓ Benefit from eating vegetables and fruit at all meals and as snacks.
- ✓ Spend less time being inactive such as watching TV or playing computer games.
- ✓ Request nutrition information about menu items when eating out to help you make healthier choices.
- ✓ Enjoy eating with family and friends!
- ✓ Take time to eat and savour every bite!

For more information, interactive tools, or additional copies visit Canada's Food Guide on-line at:
www.healthcanada.gc.ca/foodguide

or contact:

Publications
Health Canada
Ottawa, Ontario K1A 0K9
E-Mail: publications@hc-sc.gc.ca
Tel.: 1-866-225-0709
Fax: (613) 941-5366
TTY: 1-800-267-1245

Également disponible en français sous le titre : Bien manger avec le Guide alimentaire canadien

This publication can be made available on request on diskette, large print, audio-cassette and braille.

FIGURE 12-2, cont'd

Nutrition Facts

Serving Size:About (20g)
Servings Per Container:16

	Amount Per Serving	%Daily Value*
Total Calories	60	
Calories From Fat	15	
Total Fat	2 g	3%
Saturated Fat	1 g	4%
Trans Fat	0 g	
Cholesterol	0 mg	0%
Sodium	45 mg	2%
Total Carbohydrates	15 g	5%
Dietary Fiber	4 g	17%
Sugars	4 g	
Sugar Alcohols (Polyols)	3 g	
Protein	2 g	
Vitamin A		0%
Vitamin C		0%
Calcium		2%
Iron		2%

*Percent Daily Values are based on a 2,000 calorie diet.
Ingredients: Wheat flour,unsweetened chocolate, erythritol, inulin, oat flour, cocoa power, evaporated cane juice, whey protein concencrate, corn starch (low glycemic), natural flavors, salt, baking soda, wheat gluten, guar gurn

FIGURE 12-3 Standard food label showing serving size.

Nutrition Facts

Serving Size 1 cup (228g)
Servings Per Container 2 — Start here

Amount Per Serving	
Calories 250	Calories from Fat 110
	% Daily Value*
Total Fat 12g	18%
Saturated Fat 3g	15%
Trans Fat 3g	
Cholesterol 30mg	10%
Sodium 470mg	20%
Potassium 700mg	20%
Total Carbohydrate 31g	10%
Dietary Fiber 0g	0%
Sugars 5g	
Protein 5g	
Vitamin A	4%
Vitamin C	2%
Calcium	20%
Iron	4%

Check calories

Quick guide to % DV: 5% or less is low; 20% or more is high

Limit these

Get enough of these

Footnote

* Percent Daily Values are based on a 2,000 calorie diet. Your Daily Values may be higher or lower depending on your calorie needs.

	Calories:	2,000	2,500
Total Fat	Less than	65g	80g
Sat Fat	Less than	20g	25g
Cholesterol	Less than	300mg	300mg
Sodium	Less than	2,400mg	2,400mg
Total Carbohydrate		300g	375g
Dietary Fiber		25g	30g

FIGURE 12-4 Nutrition facts label information. *(Source: U.S. Food and Drug Administration. Accessed 22 May 2010 from http://www.health.gov/dietaryguidelines/dga2005/healthieryou/html/tips_food_label.html.)*

TABLE 12-3

Reference Daily Intakes

Nutrient	Amount
Vitamin A	5000 IU
Vitamin C	60 mg
Thiamin	1.5 mg
Riboflavin	1.7 mg
Niacin	20 mg
Calcium	1 g
Iron	18 mg
Vitamin D	400 IU
Vitamin E	30 IU
Vitamin B_6	2 mg
Folic acid	0.4
Vitamin B_{12}	6 mcg
Phosphorus	1 g
Iodine	150 mcg
Magnesium	400 mg
Zinc	15 mg
Copper	2 mg
Biotin	0.3 mg
Pantothenic acid	10 mg
Selenium	70 mcg

From Center for Food Safety & Applied Nutrition: A food labeling guide, College Park, Md, 1994, U.S. Department of Agriculture, revised 1999.

TABLE 12-4

Daily Reference Values

Food Component	DRV	Calculation
Fat	65 g	30% of kcal
Saturated fat	20 g	10% of kcal
Cholesterol	300 mg	Same regardless of kcal
Carbohydrates (total)	300 g	60% of calories
Fiber	25 g	11.5 g per 1000 kcal
Protein	50 g	10% of kcal
Sodium	2400 mg	Same regardless of kcal
Potassium	3500 mg	Same regardless of kcal

DRV, Daily reference value.

NOTE: The DRVs were established for adults and children over 4 years old. The values for energy yielding nutrients below are based on 2,000 calories per day.

BOX 12-3

Tips for Reading and Understanding Food Labels

Interpret the Percent Daily Value.

Nutrients with %DV of 5 or less are considered low.

Nutrients with %DV of 10-19 or less are considered moderate or "good sources."

Nutrients with %DV of 20 or more are considered high or "rich sources."

Prioritize nutrient needs and compare %DV levels accordingly. For example, if a consumer wishes to lower osteoporosis risk versus limiting sodium, a packaged food containing 25%DV calcium and 15%DV sodium may be considered a sensible food selection.

Note the calories per serving and the servings per container. Consider how the energy value of a specific food fits into the total energy intake "equation." Be conscious of the portion size that is consumed and "do the math" as to how many servings per container that portion would be.

Be aware of specific nutrient content claims. As shown in Box 12-4, there are many nutrient content claims, but only specific ones may relate to personal health priorities. For example, if there is a positive family history for heart disease, the "low fat" nutrient claim of 3 grams or less per serving may serve as a useful guide during food selection.

Review the ingredient list. Ingredients are listed in order of prominence. Pay particular attention to the top five items listed. Ingredients that contain sugar often end in *-ose*. The term *hydrogenated* signals that processed, trans, or saturated fats may have been incorporated. Sodium-containing additives may be present in multiple forms. In an effort to lower the amount of heavily processed food consumed, look for ingredient lists containing more nutrient-dense food items and fewer additives.

BOX 12-4

Nutrient Content Claims

Free: *Free* means that a product contains no amount of, or only trivial or "physiologically inconsequential" amounts of, one or more of these components: fat, saturated fat, cholesterol, sodium, sugar, or calories. For example, *calorie-free* means the product contains fewer than 5 calories per serving, and *sugar-free* and *fat-free* both mean the product contains less than 0.5 g per serving. Synonyms for *free* include *without, no,* and *zero.* A synonym for fat-free milk is *skim.*

Low: *Low* can be used on foods that can be eaten frequently without exceeding dietary guidelines for one or more of these components: fat, saturated fat, cholesterol, sodium, and calories. Synonyms for low include *little, few, low source of,* and *contains a small amount of.*

- **Low fat:** 3 g or less per serving
- **Low saturated fat:** 1 g or less per serving
- **Low sodium:** 140 mg or less per serving
- **Very low sodium:** 35 mg or less per serving
- **Low cholesterol:** 20 mg or less and 2 g or less of saturated fat per serving
- **Low calorie:** 40 calories or less per serving

Lean and extra lean: *Lean* and *extra lean* can be used to describe the fat content of meat, poultry, seafood, and game meats.

Lean: less than 10 g fat, 4.5 g or less saturated fat, and less than 95 mg cholesterol per serving and per 100 g

Extra lean: less than 5 g fat, less than 2 g saturated fat, and less than 95 mg cholesterol per serving and per 100 g

Reduced: *Reduced* means that a nutritionally altered product contains at least 25% less of a nutrient or of calories than the regular, or reference, product. However, a *reduced* claim cannot be made on a product if its reference food already meets the requirement for a "low" claim.

Less: *Less* means that a food, whether altered or not, contains 25% less of a nutrient or of calories than the reference food. For example, pretzels that have 25% less fat than potato chips could carry a *less* claim. *Fewer* is an acceptable synonym.

Light: *Light* can mean two things:

- First, that a nutritionally altered product contains one-third fewer calories or half the fat of the reference food. If the food derives 50% or more of its calories from fat, the reduction must be 50% of the fat.
- Second, that the sodium content of a low-calorie, low-fat food has been reduced by 50%. In addition, *light in sodium* may be used on food in which the sodium content has been reduced by at least 50%.

The term *light* still can be used to describe such properties as texture and color, as long as the label explains the intent (e.g., *light brown sugar* and *light and fluffy*).

High: *High* can be used if the food contains 20% or more of the daily value for a particular nutrient in a serving.

Good source: *Good source* means that one serving of a food contains 10% to 19% of the daily value for a particular nutrient.

More: *More* means that a serving of food, whether altered or not, contains a nutrient that is at least 10% of the daily value more than the reference food. The 10% of daily value also applies to *fortified, enriched, added, extra,* and *plus* claims, but in these cases the food must be altered.

Data from Food and Drug Administration. Accessed 18 January 2010 from http://www.fda.gov/Food/GuidanceComplianceRegulatoryInformation/GuidanceDocuments/FoodLabelingNutrition/FoodLabelingGuide/default.htm.

lean meat or poultry contains less than 5 g of fat, less than 2 g of saturated fat, and the same cholesterol content as lean, per serving, or per 100 g of product.

Health Claims

A **health claim** is allowed only on appropriate food products that meet specified standards. The government requires that health claims be worded in ways that are not misleading (e.g., the claim cannot imply that the food product itself helps prevent disease). Health claims cannot appear on foods that supply more than 20% of the DV for fat, saturated fat, cholesterol, and sodium. The following is an example of a health claim for dietary fiber and cancer: "Low-fat diets rich in fiber-containing grain products, fruits, and vegetables may reduce the risk of some types of cancer, a disease associated with many factors." Box 12-5 lists health claims that manufacturers can use to describe food-disease relationships.

DIETARY PATTERNS AND COUNSELING TIPS

Vegetarian Diet Patterns

Vegetarian diets are popular. Those who choose them may be motivated by philosophic, religious, or ecologic concerns, or by a desire to have a healthier lifestyle. Considerable evidence attests to the health benefits of a vegetarian diet. Studies of Seventh-Day Adventists indicate that the diet results in lower rates of type 2 diabetes, breast and colon cancer, and cardiovascular and gallbladder disease.

Of the millions of Americans who call themselves vegetarians, many eliminate "red" meats but eat fish, poultry, and dairy products. A lactovegetarian does not eat meat, fish, poultry, or eggs, but does consume milk, cheese, and other dairy products. A lactoovovegetarian also consumes eggs. A **vegan** does not eat any food of animal origin. The vegan diet is the only vegetarian diet that has any real risk of providing inadequate nutrition, but this risk can be avoided by careful planning (American Dietetic Association [ADA], 2009). A new type of semivegetarian is known as a **flexitarian.** Flexitarians generally adhere to a vegetarian diet for the purpose of good health and do not follow a specific ideology. They view an occasional meat meal as acceptable.

Vegetarian diets tend to be lower in iron than omnivorous diets, although the nonheme iron in fruits, vegetables, and unrefined cereals is usually accompanied either in the food or in the meal by large amounts of ascorbic acid that aids in iron assimilation. Vegetarians do not have a greater risk of iron deficiency than those who are not vegetarians (ADA, 2009). Vegetarians who consume no dairy products may have low calcium intakes, and vitamin D intakes may be inadequate among those in northern latitudes where there is less exposure to sunshine. The calcium in some vegetables is inactivated by the presence of oxalates. Although phytates in unrefined cereals also can inactivate calcium, this is not a problem for Western vegetarians, whose diets tend to be based more on fruits and vegetables than on the unrefined cereals of Middle Eastern cultures. Long-term vegans may develop megaloblastic anemia because of a deficiency of vitamin B_{12}, found only in foods of animal origin. The high levels of folate in vegan diets may mask the neurologic damage of a vitamin B_{12} deficiency. Vegans should have a reliable source of vitamin B_{12} such as fortified breakfast cereals, soy beverages, or a supplement. Although most vegetarians meet or exceed the requirements for protein, their diets tend to be lower in protein than those of omnivores. This lower intake may help vegetarians retain more calcium from their diets. Furthermore, lower protein intake usually results in lower dietary fat because many high-protein animal products are also rich in fat (ADA, 2009).

Well-planned vegetarian diets are safe for infants, children, and adolescents and can meet all of their nutritional requirements for growth. They are also adequate for pregnant and lactating females. The key is that the diets be well planned. Vegetarians should pay special attention to ensure that they get adequate calcium, iron, zinc, and vitamins B_{12} and D. Calculated combinations of complementary protein sources is not necessary, especially if protein sources are reasonably varied. Table 12-5 highlights many of the phytochemicals and functional components rich in many vegetable-based diets. A useful website on vegetarian meal planning is available at http://www.eatright.org/ through the American Dietetic Association. See also *Focus On:* The "Healthy Food In Health Care" Pledge earlier in the chapter.

CULTURAL ASPECTS OF DIETARY PLANNING

To plan diets for individuals or groups that are appropriate from a health and nutrition perspective, it is important that registered dietitians and health providers use resources that are targeted to the specific client or group. Numerous population subgroups in the United States and throughout the world have specific cultural, ethnic, or religious beliefs and practices to consider. These groups have their own set of dietary practices or beliefs, which are important when considering dietary planning (Diabetes Care and Education Dietetic Practice Group, 2010). The IOM report entitled *Unequal Treatment* recommends that all health care professionals receive training in cross-cultural communication to reduce ethnic and racial disparities in health care; indeed, cultural competence is central to professionalism and quality (Betancourt and Green, 2010).

Attitudes, rituals, and practices surrounding food are part of every culture in the world and there are so many cultures in the world that it defies enumeration. Many world cultures have influenced American cultures as a result of immigration and intermarriage. This makes planning a menu that embraces cultural diversity and is sensitive to the needs of a specific group of people a major challenge. It is tempting to simplify the role of culture by attempting to categorize dietary patterns by race, ethnicity, or religion. However, this type of generalizing can lead to inappropriate labeling and misunderstanding.

BOX 12-5

Health Claims for Diet-Disease Relationships

(Approved Claim [Model Claim, Statements and Claim Requirements])

Calcium and Osteoporosis (Regular exercise and a healthy diet with enough calcium helps teens and young adult white and Asian women maintain good bone health and may reduce their high risk of osteoporosis later in life.)

Sodium and Hypertension (Diets low in sodium may reduce the risk of high blood pressure, a disease associated with many factors.)

Sodium and Hypertension (Diets low in sodium may reduce the risk of high blood pressure, a disease associated with many factors.)

Dietary Fat and Cancer (Development of cancer depends on many factors. A diet low in total fat may reduce the risk of some cancers.)

Dietary Saturated Fat and Cholesterol and Risk of Coronary Heart Disease (Although many factors affect heart disease, diets low in saturated fat and cholesterol may reduce the risk of this disease.)

Fiber-Containing Grain Products, Fruits, and Vegetables and Cancer (Low-fat diets rich in fiber-containing grain products, fruits, and vegetables may reduce the risk of some types of cancer, a disease associated with many factors.)

Fruits, Vegetables and Grain Products that contain Fiber, particularly Soluble Fiber, and Risk of Coronary Heart Disease (Diets low in saturated fat and cholesterol and rich in fruits, vegetables, and grain products that contain some types of dietary fiber, particularly soluble fiber, may reduce the risk of heart disease, a disease associated with many factors.)

Fruits and Vegetables and Cancer (Low-fat diets rich in fruits and vegetables [*foods that are low in fat and may contain dietary fiber, vitamin A, or vitamin C*] may reduce the risk of some types of cancer, a disease associated with many factors. Broccoli is high in vitamin A and C, and it is a good source of dietary fiber.)

Folate and Neural Tube Defects (Healthful diets with adequate folate may reduce a woman's risk of having a child with a brain or spinal cord defect.)

Dietary Noncariogenic Carbohydrate Sweeteners and Dental Caries (Full claim: Frequent between-meal consumption of foods high in sugars and starches promotes tooth decay. The sugar alcohols in [*name of food*] do not promote tooth decay; Shortened claim on small packages only: Does not promote tooth decay.)

Soluble Fiber from Certain Foods and Risk of Coronary Heart Disease (Soluble fiber from foods such as [*name of soluble fiber source, and, if desired, name of food product*], as part of a diet low in saturated fat and cholesterol, may reduce the risk of heart disease. A serving of [*name of food product*] supplies __ grams of the [*necessary daily dietary intake for the benefit*] soluble fiber from [*name of soluble fiber source*] necessary per day to have this effect.)

Soy Protein and Risk of Coronary Heart Disease (1. 25 grams of soy protein a day, as part of a diet low in saturated fat and cholesterol, may reduce the risk of heart disease. A serving of [*name of food*] supplies __ grams of soy protein. 2. Diets low in saturated fat and cholesterol that include 25 grams of soy protein a day may reduce the risk of heart disease. One serving of [*name of food*] provides __ grams of soy protein.)

Plant Sterol and Stanol Esters and Risk of Coronary Heart Disease (1. Foods containing at least 0.65 gram per of vegetable oil sterol esters, eaten twice a day with meals for a daily total intake of least 1.3 grams, as part of a diet low in saturated fat and cholesterol, may reduce the risk of heart disease. A serving of [*name of food*] supplies __ grams of vegetable oil sterol esters. 2. Diets low in saturated fat and cholesterol that include two servings of foods that provide a daily total of at least 3.4 grams of plant stanol esters in two meals may reduce the risk of heart disease. A serving of [*name of food*] supplies __ grams of plant stanol esters.)

Whole Grain Foods and Risk of Heart Disease and Certain Cancers ("Diets rich in whole grain foods and other plant foods and low in total fat, saturated fat, and cholesterol may reduce the risk of heart disease and some cancers.")

Potassium and the Risk of High Blood Pressure and Stroke ("Diets containing foods that are a good source of potassium and that are low in sodium may reduce the risk of high blood pressure and stroke.")

Fluoridated Water and Reduced Risk of Dental Carries ("Drinking fluoridated water may reduce the risk of [*dental caries or tooth decay*].")

Saturated Fat, Cholesterol, and *Trans* Fat, and Reduced Risk of Heart Disease ("Diets low in saturated fat and cholesterol, and as low as possible in *trans* fat, may reduce the risk of heart disease.")

Data from Food and Drug Administration. Accessed 18 January 2010 from http://www.fda.gov/Food/GuidanceComplianceRegulatoryInformation/GuidanceDocuments/FoodLabelingNutrition/FoodLabelingGuide/ucm064919.htm.

FOCUS ON

What is a Locovore?

There is a growing movement in the United States fueled by books like the Omnivore's Dilemma (Pollan et al., 2006). One component of this movement is a collaborative effort to build a more locally based, self-reliant food economy—one in which sustainable food production, processing, distribution, and consumption are integrated to enhance the economic, environmental, and social health of a particular place. **Locovores** are those who eat food grown or produced locally or within a certain radius. The locovore movement encourages consumers to buy from farmers' markets or even to produce their own food. They argue that locally produced food is fresher and more nutritious and uses less fossil fuel to grow and transport. Another component of this movement is the condemnation of the factory farming method of grain feeding animals. These operations are known as concentrated animal feeding operations. There is a growing demand for meat that is grass or range fed and not transported long distances.

To illustrate this point, consider the case of Native Americans. There are more than 500 different tribes spread across all 50 states. The food and customs of the tribes in the Southwest are drastically different than those of the Northwest. When discussing traditional foods among Native Americans, the situation is further complicated by the fact that many tribes were removed from their traditional lands by the U.S. government. Thus a Montana tribe that once depended on hunting bison and gathering local roots and berries may now be living in Oklahoma.

Another example of the complexity of diet and culture in the United State is that of African Americans. "Soul food" is commonly identified with African Americans from the South. Traditional food choices include grits, collard greens prepared with ham hocks and lard, with a side of corn bread. But this by no means represents the diet of all African Americans. African Americans may be eating the foods of their homeland. An Ethiopian meal might consist of a vegetable stew served atop bread known as *injera*, whereas someone eating the food of Ghana would probably be eating a stew atop rice or yams.

When faced with planning a diet to meet the needs of an unfamiliar culture, it is important to avoid forming opinions that are based on inaccurate information or stereotyping

TABLE 12-5

Phytochemicals and Functional Components in Foods

Compound	Function	Food Sources
Carotenoids		
β-carotene	May neutralize free radicals that damage cells, boost antioxidant defenses	Carrots, dark orange fruits, butternut squash, cantaloupe
Lutein	Much discovered about its role in protecting the eyes from oxidation; also being investigated for potentially reducing the risk of colon, breast, lung, and skin cancer (www.luteininfo.com)	Deep green vegetables, kale, spinach, collards, corn, eggs, citrus
Lycopene	Protects prostrate health by reducing risk of prostate cancer; may also aid in preserving bone health	Processed tomato products, guava, pink grapefruit, watermelon
Diallyl sulfides	Along with promoting heart health, boosts production of enzymes that benefit the immune system	Onions, garlic, scallions, leeks, chives
Ellagic acid	May block body's production of enzymes needed for tumor growth; causes cancer cell death in the test tube; functions as antioxidant; possible antiviral and antibacterial activities	Strawberries, raspberries, pomegranates, cranberries, walnuts
Flavonoids		
Anthocyanins	Most studied; may neutralize free radicals, bolster antioxidant defenses, especially at the DNA level; contributes to heart health and vision and brain function by reducing oxidation of LDL cholesterol	Berries, (especially dark-colored), cherries, red grapes
Lignans	Acting as phytoestrogens, may boost immune function and contribute to maintaining heart health; may also help block some hormone related cancers	Flax seed, rye, some vegetables

Continued

TABLE 12-5

Phytochemicals and Functional Components in Foods—cont'd

Compound	Function	Food Sources
Limonene	Boosts levels of naturally occurring liver enzymes involved in detoxification of carcinogens	Essential oils of citrus fruits and other plants
Phytic acid	May suppress oxidation reactions in the colon that produce free radicals; reduces rate of starch digestion and thus blood glycemic response; converted to related compounds in body involved in cellular communication; may be effective in slowing tumor growth	Wheat bran, flax seed, sesame seeds, beans and other high-fiber foods
Proanthocyanidins (condensed tannins or procyanidins)	The active component of cranberries that contributes to urinary tract health but may also have a role in heart health	Cranberries, cocoa, cinnamon, peanuts, wine, grapes, strawberries, peanut skins
Phenols	May boost antioxidant defense while maintaining healthy vision	Apples, pears, citrus fruits, parsley, carrots, broccoli, cabbage, cucumbers, squash, yams, tomatoes
Phytoestrogens	Genistein and daidzein; may contribute to healthy bones, brain function, and immune function; relationship of phytoestrogens and cancers is still being debated	Soybeans, soybean products
Plant stanols and sterols	May help bolster the benefits of a heart-healthy diet with exercise, thus reducing the risk of heart disease	Corn, soy, wheat, fortified foods, beverages, fortified table spreads, fortified chocolate, peanut oil
Prebiotics		
	Nondigestible food ingredients such as dietary fibers that provide food for gut bacteria to grow on; may improve gastrointestinal health and immune function; insulin and oligofructose are the most commonly studied prebiotics	Whole grains (especially oatmeal), flax and barley; greens; berries, bananas, and other fruits; legumes; onions, garlic, honey, leeks
Probiotics		
	Beneficial bacteria that improve gastrointestinal health and may improve calcium absorption	Yogurt (with active, live culture), kefir, buttermilk and other fermented dairy products; fermented vegetables such as kim chi and sauerkraut; and fermented soy products such as miso and tempeh
Organosulfuric compounds	Believed to fight cancer cell growth; may be useful in treating arthritic joints	Garlic, onions, chives, citrus fruits, broccoli, cabbage, cauliflower, Brussels sprouts

From Center for Food Safety & Applied Nutrition: A Food Labeling Guide, College Park, Md, 1994, U.S. Dept of Agriculture, revised 1999.
DNA, Deoxyribonucleic acid; *LDL*, low-density lipoprotein.

(see Chapter 15). Some cultural food guides have even been developed for specific populations (Figure 12-5) for helping to manage disease conditions.

Religion and Food

Dietary practices have been a component of religious practice for all of recorded history. Some religions forbid the eating of certain foods and beverages; others restrict foods and drinks during holy days. Specific dietary rituals may be assigned to members with designated authority or with special spiritual power (e.g., medicine men, priests). Sometimes dietary rituals or restrictions are observed based on gender. Dietary and food preparation practices (e.g., halal and kosher meat preparation) can be associated with rituals of faith.

Fasting is practiced by many religions. It has been identified as a mechanism that allows one to improve one's body, to earn approval (as with Allah or Buddha), or to understand and appreciate the sufferings of others. Attention to specific eating behaviors such as overeating, use of alcoholic or stimulant-containing beverages, and vegetarianism are also considered by some religions. Before planning menus for members of any religious group, it is important to gain an understanding of some traditions or dietary practices (Table 12-6). In all cases, discussing the personal dietary preferences of an individual is imperative (Kittler and Sucher, 2008).

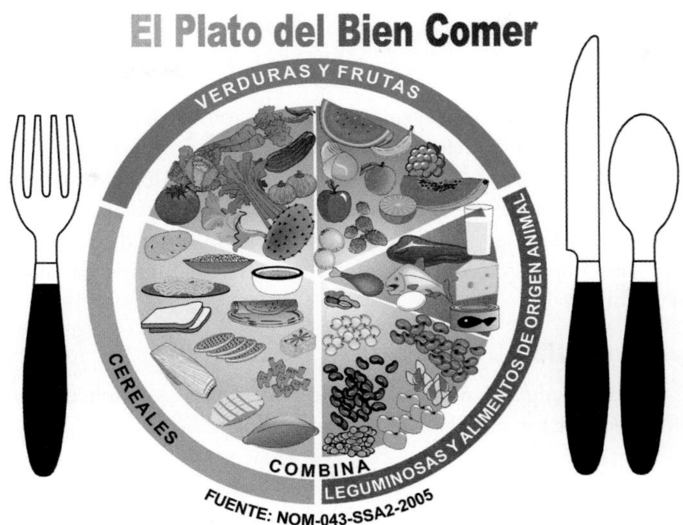

FIGURE 12-5 El Plato del Bien Comer. (The Plate of Good Eating.) *(Norma Oficial Mexicana NOM-043-SSA2-2005. Servicios básicos de salud. Promoción y educación para la salud en materia alimentaria. Criterios para brindar orientación. México, DF. Diario Oficial de la Federación, 23 de enero de 2006. Official Mexican Standard NOM-043-SSA2-2005. Basic health services. Promotion and health education with regard to food. Criteria for counseling. Government Gazzette. Mexico, January 23, 2006.)*

TABLE 12-6

Some Religious Dietary Practices

	Buddhist	Hindu	Jewish (Orthodox)	Muslim	Christian Roman Catholic	Christian Eastern Orthodox	Christian Mormon	Christian Seventh Day Adventist
Beef	A	X						A
Pork	A	A	X	X				X
Meats, all	A	A	R	R	R	R		A
Eggs/dairy	O	O	R			R		O
Fish	A	R	R			R		A
Shellfish	A	R	X			O		X
Alcohol		A		X			X	X
Coffee/tea				A			X	X
Meat/dairy at same meal			X					
Leavened foods			R					
Ritual slaughter of meats			+	+				
Moderation	+			+				+
Fasting*	+	+	+	+	+	+	+	

Modified from Kittler PG, Sucher KP: *Food and culture*, ed 5, Belmont, Ca, 2008, Wadsworth/Cengage Learning.

Escott-Stump S: Nutrition and diagnosis-related care, ed 7, Baltimore, Md, 2011, Lippincott Williams & Wilkins.

+, Practiced; *A*, avoided by the most devout; *O*, permitted, but may be avoided at some observances; *R*, some restrictions regarding types of foods or when a food may be eaten; *X*, prohibited or strongly discouraged.

*Fasting varies from partial (abstention from certain foods or meals) to complete (no food or drink).

CLINICAL SCENARIO

Marty is a 45-year-old Jewish male who emigrated from Israel to the United States 3 years ago. He follows a strict kosher diet. In addition, he does not drink milk but does consume other dairy products. He has a body mass index of 32 and a family history of heart disease. He has come to you for advice on increasing his calcium intake.

Nutrition Diagnostic Statement

Knowledge deficit related to calcium as evidenced by request for nutrient and dietary information.

Nutrition Care Questions

1. What type of dietary guidance would you offer Marty?
2. What type of dietary plan following strict kosher protocols would meet his daily dietary needs and promote weight loss?
3. What suggestions would you offer him about dietary choices for a healthy heart?
4. Which special steps should Marty take to meet calcium requirements without using supplements?
5. How can food labeling information be used to help Marty meet his weight loss and nutrient goals and incorporate his religious dietary concerns?

USEFUL WEBSITES

American Dietetic Association
http://www.eatright.org

Center for Nutrition Policy and Promotion, U.S. Department of Agriculture
http://www.usda.gov/cnpp/

Centers for Disease Control—Health Literacy
http://www.cdc.gov/healthmarketing/healthliteracy/training/page5711.html

Cost of Food at Home
http://www.cnpp.usda.gov/USDAFoodCost-Home.htm

Dietary Guidelines for Americans
http://www.health.gov/DietaryGuidelines

Eat Smart, Play Hard
http://www.fns.usda.gov/eatsmartplayhardkids/

Ethnic Food Guides
http://fnic.nal.usda.gov/nal_display/index.php?info_center=4&tax_level=3&_tax_subject=256&topic_id=1348&level3_id=5732

Food and Drug Administration, Center for Food Safety and Applied Nutrition
http://www.cfsan.fda.gov

Food and Nutrition Information Center, National Agricultural Library, U.S. Department of Agriculture
http://www.nal.usda.gov/fnic/

Health Canada
http://www.hc-sc.gc.ca/fn-an/index_e.html

Healthy Eating Index
http://www.cnpp.usda.gov/HealthyEatingIndex.htm

Institute of Medicine, National Academy of Sciences
http://www.iom.edu/

International Food Information Council
http://ific.org

MyPlate Food Guidance System
http://www.chooseMyPlate.gov/

National Center for Health Statistics
http://www.cdc.gov/nchs/nhanes.htm

Nutrition.gov (U.S. government nutrition site)
http://www.nutrition.gov

U.S. Department of Agriculture
http://www.usda.gov

REFERENCES

American Dietetic Association (ADA): Position of the American Dietetic Association: vegetarian diets, *J Am Diet Assoc* 109:1266, 2009.

American Journal of Clinical Nutrition: White House Conference on Food, Nutrition and Health, *AJCN* 11:1543, 1969.

Betancourt JR, Green AR: Commentary: linking cultural competence training to improved health outcomes: perspectives from the field, *Acad Med* 85:583, 2010.

Diabetes Care and Education Dietetic Practice Group, Goody CM, Drago L, editors: *Cultural food practices*, Chicago, 2010, American Dietetic Association.

Guenther P et al: Healthy eating index, *J Am Diet Assoc* 108:1854-1864, 2008.

Health Canada: *Eating well with Canada's food guide*, Her Majesty the Queen in Right of Canada, represented by the Minister of Healthy Canada, 2007. Accessed 18 January 2010 from www.hc-sc.gc.ca/fn-an/food-guide-aliment.

Institute of Medicine (IOM), Food and Nutrition Board, Consensus Report: Dietary reference intakes: water, potassium, sodium, chloride, and sulfate. Accessed 11 March, 2011 at http://www.iom.edu/reports/2004/dietary-reference-intakes-water-potassium-sodium-chloride-and-sulfate.aspx.

Kittler PG, Sucher KP: *Food and culture*, ed 5, Belmont, CA, 2008, Wadsworth/Cengage Learning.

Pollan M: *The omnivore's dilemma: a natural history of four meals*, New York, 2006, Penguin.

U.S. Department of Agriculture, Center for Nutrition Policy and Promotion: *Healthy eating index 2005*. Accessed 16 April 2007 from www.cnpp.usda.gov.

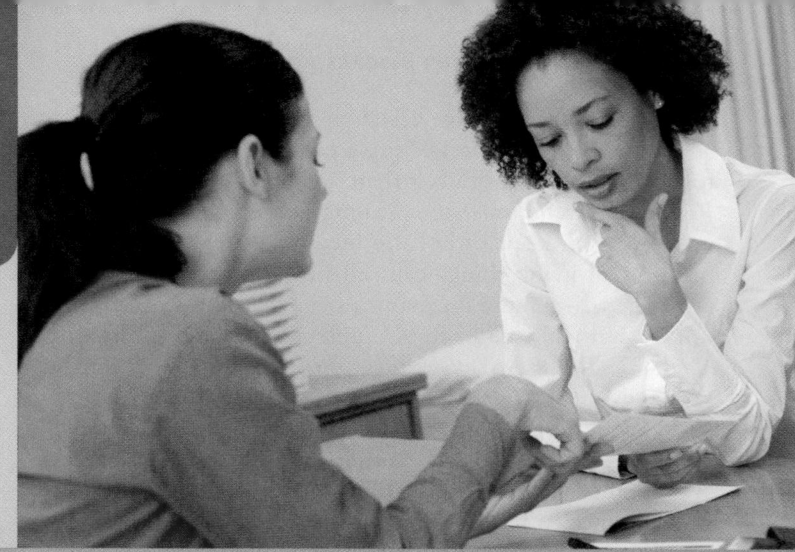

CHAPTER 13

Cynthia A. Thomson, PhD, RD

Food and Nutrient Delivery: Bioactive Substances and Integrative Care

KEY TERMS

adverse events (AEs)
acupuncture
botanicals
chi (Qi)
chiropractic
Codex Alimentarius Commission (Codex)
Commission E Monographs
complementary and alternative medicine (CAM)
dietary supplement
Dietary Supplement Health and Education Act (DSHEA)
functional medicine
functional nutrition assessment
health claim
holistic therapies
homeopathy
integrative medicine
meridians
moxibustion
naturopathy
pharmacognosy
phytotherapy
qualified health claim
structure-function claim
subluxation
traditional Oriental medicine

INTEGRATIVE MEDICINE

Integrative medicine focuses on healing-oriented medicine that considers the whole person (body, mind, spirit) and all aspects of lifestyle. Emphasis is placed on the therapeutic relationship and appropriate therapies, both conventional and alternative. A multidisciplinary approach that moves beyond conventional medicine practitioners is needed; here, patients and health care providers are partners in promoting wellness. The scope of care includes wellness and prevention, and, when illness does occur, a reliance on less invasive approaches is emphasized. Yet integrative care is evidence-based by critically evaluating all medical and healing approaches.

Complementary and alternative medicine (CAM) refers to those practices that are not a customary part of conventional medicine. This includes such treatment methodologies as acupuncture, meditation, naturopathy, and chiropractic care. **Integrative medicine** is slightly different than CAM in that it is focused on the combined use of conventional and CAM approaches, and is defined as the comprehensive integration of appropriate complementary approaches along with conventional medical approaches into the care of the whole person, with the goal of achieving optimal health outcomes (Kiefer, 2009).

CAM and integrative therapies are not new. In fact, their roots can be traced to early Greek and Chinese cultures. Although natural therapies are often described as being "cutting edge," they are actually much older than conventional Western medical interventions. Experts estimate that herbal remedies and ayurveda, the traditional medicine of India, are more than 5000 years old. CAM therapies are **holistic therapies**, derived from the Greek word *holos*, meaning *whole.* They are based on the theory that health is a vital dynamic state, reflecting a profound will and wisdom to maintain wellness rather than just the absence of disease. *Vis mediatrix naturae*, the healing force of nature, is the underlying precept of holistic medicine. According to this precept, all living things can self-heal, and organisms have inherent self-defense mechanisms against illness. According to the National Center for Complementary and Alternative Medicine (NCCAM) classification scheme, CAM can be grouped as (1) alternative medical systems such as naturopathy, traditional Chinese Medicine, ayurveda, and homeopathy; (2) mind-body therapies such as meditation, prayer, art or music therapy, and cognitive behavior therapy; (3) biologically based therapies such as the use of herbs, whole-foods diets, and nutrient supplementation; (4) manipulative therapies such as massage, chiropractic medicine, osteopathy, and yoga; and (5) and medical systems based on energy therapies such as qi gong, magnetic therapy, or reiki.

Functional medicine has some components of CAM therapy, but shifts the disease-centered focus of traditional medical practice to a more patient-centered approach (Institute of Functional Medicine, 2011). The goal is to evaluate the whole person rather than individual symptoms, and to consider care in relation to prevention as well as long-term support for health. Diet, nutrition, and exercise are considered central to "best medical practice" in the delivery of functional medicine. The philosophy also embraces biochemical individuality, hormonal and neurotransmitter imbalance, oxidative stress and detoxification, immune enhancement, and the overall dynamic balance of internal and external factors important to health and longevity.

Increasingly, health care practitioners, including dietetics professionals, are involved in the provision of care based on an integrative approach. For example, **functional nutrition assessment** (as defined in *New Directions:* Functional Nutrition Assessment in Chapter 6) is being included more frequently as part of a complete health evaluation. As the cost of health care escalates, providers are actively seeking integrative care as a plausible approach to reducing costs and enhancing client satisfaction (Maizes, 2009; Ullman, 2009). Diet therapy and dietary supplementation are modalities commonly practiced in the context of CAM and integrative and functional medicine. Several diet-based therapies are listed as CAM modalities, including the Ornish, Zone, Atkins, and Pritikin diets, as well as macrobiotic and vegetarian diets. See Table 13-1 for descriptions of modalities identified as within the scope of CAM.

Use of Complementary and Alternative Therapies

The use of CAM therapies to enhance conventional medical practices has increased in the United States since the 1960s. A significant number of Americans use some form of CAM therapy even more frequently than they see a primary care physician. Figure 13-1 shows the frequency of use of CAM therapies.

Data from the Alternative Health/Complementary and Alternative Medicine supplement to the 2007 National Health Interview Survey (NHIS), administered by the Centers for Disease Control and Prevention, showed that among the 29,266 American households and 75,764 people surveyed, 38.3% of adults and one in nine children reported use of CAM within the previous 12 months (Barnes et al., 2008). Use has been shown to be greatest among women, people ages 30-69, people with higher education, those residing in the western United States, and people who were hospitalized in the previous 12 months (National Center for Complementary and Alternative Medicine, 2005). By race

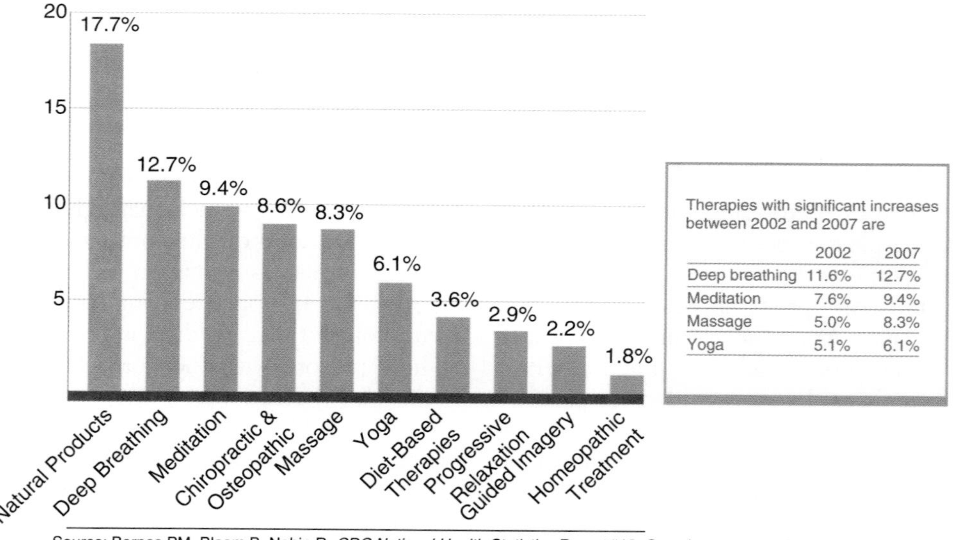

	2002	2007
Deep breathing	11.6%	12.7%
Meditation	7.6%	9.4%
Massage	5.0%	8.3%
Yoga	5.1%	6.1%

Source: Barnes PM, Bloom B, Nahin R. *CDC National Health Statistics Report* #12. Complementary and Alternative Medicine Use Among Adults and Children: United States, 2007. December 2008.

FIGURE 13-1 The ten most common complementary and alternative medicine therapies used by adults. *(Source: http://nccam.nih.gov/news/camstats/2007/graphics.htm. Accessed 24 May 2010.)*

TABLE 13-1

Description of Commonly Used Complementary and Alternative Medicine Therapies

	Description
Naturopathy (natural medicine)	Based on the concept of the healing force of nature that emphasizes the prevention of disease and the maintenance of health. Derived from the Hippocratic precept, "First do no harm." Naturopathic physicians avoid therapies that weaken the body's innate ability to self-heal or that take over a function of the body; instead, naturopathic practice emphasizes the concepts of wellness, prevention, and the role of the health care provider as a teacher. Diagnosis and treatment based on natural laws. May prescribe medications. Licensure required in most states. Training includes pathology, microbiology, histology, and physical and clinical diagnosis; **pharmacognosy** (clinical training in botanical medicine), hydrotherapy, physiotherapy, therapeutic nutrition, and homeopathy. Modalities include phytotherapy (treatment with plant-based preparations), electrotherapy, physiotherapy, minor surgery, mechanotherapy, and therapeutic manipulation. Nutrition and dietary supplementation routinely used.
Chiropractic	Embraces many of the same principles as naturopathy, particularly the belief that the body has the ability to heal itself and that the practitioner's role is to assist the body in doing so; like naturopathy, chiropractic focuses on wellness and prevention and favors noninvasive treatments. Chiropractors do not prescribe drugs or perform surgery. Focus on locating and removing interferences to the body's natural ability to maintain health, called **subluxations** (specifically musculoskeletal problems that lead to interference with the proper function of the nervous system). The central approach is the manual manipulation of the body, such as spinal adjustment and muscle work, with support from physiologic approaches to healing such as lifestyle modification. Two fundamental precepts: (1) the structure and condition of the body influence how well the body functions, and (2) the mind-body relationship is important in maintaining health and in promoting healing. Licensed and regulated in all 50 states and in some 30 countries. Must complete a 4-year program from a federally accredited college of chiropractic and, like other licensed practitioners, successfully pass an examination administered by a national certifying body.
Homeopathy	The root words of *homeopathy* are derived from the Greek *homios*, meaning *like* and *pathos*, meaning *suffering*. Homeopathy is a medical theory and practice advanced to counter the conventional medical practices of 200 years ago. It endeavors to help the body heal itself by treating like with like, commonly known as the "law of similars"; the law of similars is based on the theory that, if a large amount of a substance causes symptoms in a healthy person, a smaller amount of the same substance can be used to treat an ill person • Samuel Hahnemann, an 18th-century German physician, is credited with founding homeopathy. • The amounts of the remedies used in homeopathic medicines are extremely diluted; according to homeopathic principles, remedies are potentized (i.e., they become more powerful through shaking). • A tincture is made directly from the source material. One drop of the tincture is then mixed with 99 drops of water or alcohol to make the first potency. The mixture is vigorously shaken more than 100 times, a process called *succussion.* • The minimum-dose principle means that many homeopathic remedies are so dilute that no actual molecules of the healing substance can be detected by chemical tests. • The goal of homeopathy is to select a remedy that will bring about a sense of well-being on all levels—physical, mental, and emotional—and that will alleviate physical symptoms and restore the patient to a state of wellness and creative energy. • Clinical evidence on the efficacy of homeopathy is highly contradictory.

Continued

TABLE 13-1

Description of Commonly Used Complementary and Alternative Medicine Therapies—cont'd

	Description
Traditional Oriental medicine	Based on the concept that energy, also termed **chi (Qi)** or life-force energy, is the center of body functions. Chi is the intangible force that animates life and enlivens all activity. Wellness is a function of the balanced and harmonious flow of chi, whereas illness or disease results from disturbances in its flow; wellness also requires preserving equilibrium between the contrasting states of yin and yang (the dual nature of all things). The underlying principle is preventive in nature, and the body is viewed as a reflection of the natural world. Four substances—blood, jing (essence, substance of all life), shen (spirit), and fluids (body fluids other than blood)—constitute the fundamentals. The nutritional modality has several components: food as a means of obtaining nutrition, food as a tonic or medicine, and the abstention from food (fasting); foods are classified according to taste (sour, bitter, sweet, spicy, and salty) and property (cool, cold, warm, hot, and plain) to regulate yin, yang, chi, and blood. The **meridians** are channels that carry chi and blood throughout the body; these are not channels per se, but rather they are invisible vertical networks that act as energy circuits, unifying all parts of the body and connecting the inner and the outer body; organs are not viewed as anatomic concepts but as energetic fields.
Acupuncture	Acupuncture is the use of thin needles, inserted into points on the meridians, to stimulate the body's chi, or vital energy. **Moxibustion**, the application of heat along meridian acupuncture points for the purpose of affecting chi and blood so as to balance substances and organs, is related to acupuncture. This therapy is used to treat disharmony in the body, which leads to disease. Disharmony, or loss of balance, is caused by a weakening of the yin force in the body, which preserves and nurtures life, or a weakening of the yang force, which generates and activates life. The concept of yin and yang expresses the dual nature of all things, the opposing but complementary forces that are interdependent on each other and must exist in equilibrium.
Massage therapy/ body work	The philosophy behind massage therapy and body work is that there is a healing that occurs through the action of touching. Massage therapy became a profession in the United States in the 1940s and has grown in use over the last several decades. The key principles of body work are the importance of increasing blood circulation, moving lymphatic tissue to remove waste and release toxins, calming of the spirit, enhancing physiologic functions of body systems, and improving musculoskeletal function. This therapy has also been widely used to reduce stress and increase energy.

or ethnicity, Native Americans (50.3%) and Hawaiians and Pacific Islanders (43.2%) report the highest use of CAM, followed by non-Hispanic whites (43.1%). Factors associated with greater CAM use among children include adolescence, college-educated parents, concurrent prescription medication use, and reported anxiety or stress, as well as dermatologic conditions, sinusitis, and musculoskeletal conditions (Birdee, 2010).

Between 2002 and 2007, use of CAM therapies acupuncture, deep breathing, massage therapy, meditation, naturopathy, and yoga increased. Vegetarian diets were most commonly used (3.5% of adults), followed by the Atkins Diet (1.7%), macrobiotic (0.2%), and Zone diets (0.2%). Megavitamin therapy was reportedly used by 2.8% of the adult population surveyed (Barnes et al., 2008).

Those who use these therapies believe that these options are beneficial to their overall health and are more congruent with their values about health than conventional therapies. Frequently, there is an increased reliance on CAM therapies when conventional medicine has little to offer in terms of effective treatment, or when the current conventional approach has significant risks and side effects that motivate patients to explore alternatives. CAM therapies are also often considered when conventional therapies or diagnostic workups are not deemed effective by the patient (as in insomnia, pain, anxiety), when CAM approaches have been shown to be effective (chiropractic medicine for back pain, acupuncture for pain relief, select dietary supplementation for joint pain associated with osteoarthritis), and when CAM approaches are supported by significant historical evidence of efficacy. The recent NHIS survey also suggested that CAM use increases when conventional treatments are too costly. Figure 13-2 shows the frequency of CAM use by medical diagnosis.

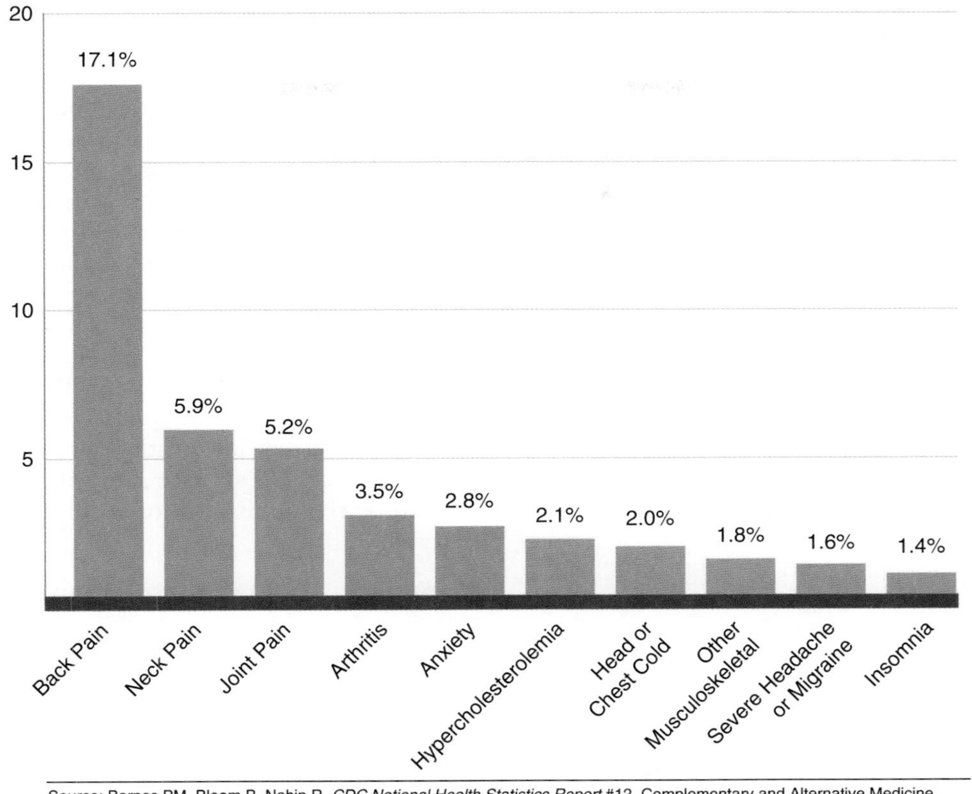

FIGURE 13-2 Diseases for which complementary and alternative medicine therapies are most often used by adults. *(Source: http://nccam.nih.gov/news/camstats/2007/graphics.htm. Accessed 24 May 2010.)*

As a result of the increased interest in these therapies, the Office of Alternative Medicine of the National Institutes of Health (NIH) was created in 1992 to evaluate their effectiveness. This office became the 27th institute or center within the NIH in 1998. Renamed NCCAM, the Center explores complementary and alternative healing practices scientifically, using research, training, outreach, and integration. (Ahn et al, 2010) In addition to research funding, there has been an increased awareness of expanding training needs as well as medical reimbursement for provision of CAM therapies in the context of conventional medical systems. Increasingly, nursing and medical curricula include CAM training.

DIETARY SUPPLEMENTATION

Dietary supplementation is common practice among Americans, particularly among those at risk or diagnosed with clinical conditions such as cancer, cardiovascular disease, diabetes, or hypertension. Consumers and health professionals should be aware that there is limited information on the effects of dietary supplements taken concurrently with prescription and other over-the-counter medications (Farmer Miller et al., 2008).

Historically, dietetics professionals focused their assessment, care plan, and counseling on diet or food-related recommendations. The 2007 NHIS survey of CAM use indicated that nonvitamin, nonmineral, natural products are the most common form of CAM. The demand for information in this area from dietetics professionals remains high. In fact, the 2009 Position Paper of the American Dietetic Association on nutrient supplementation calls on registered dietitians to be the "first source" of information on nutrient supplementation (Marra et al., 2009).

Dietary supplements have been officially defined under the **Dietary Supplement Health and Education Act (DSHEA)** of 1994 as products intended to supplement the diet that contain one or more of the following ingredients: a vitamin, mineral, herb or other botanical, amino acid, concentrate, metabolite, constituent, extract, or combinations of these ingredients. Dietary supplements are intended for ingestion in pill, capsule, tablet, or liquid form and are not to be represented for use as a conventional food or as the sole item of a meal or diet. They should be labeled as a *dietary supplement* and carry the dietary supplement facts label (Figure 13-3). Dietary supplements must be differentiated from drugs, cosmetics, and foods; see Figure 13-4.

Botanicals, plants (including their leaves, flowers, stems, rhizomes, or roots) that are used for medicinal purposes, are formulated in a wide variety of forms, including teas, infusions, and decoctions (concentrated beverage made from boiling plant root), as well as extracts (including tinctures, alcohol solvent, and glycerite-glycerol solvent) and pill forms (capsules, tablets, lozenges, soft gels) (see Botanical Formulations in Box 13-1). Topical application of botanicals or nutrients in the form of creams or essential oils such as are used in aromatherapy are not classified as dietary supplements under the current regulatory definition. Created in Germany, the **Commission E Monographs** on phytomedicines were developed by an expert commission of scientists and health care professionals as references for practice of **phytotherapy**, the science of using plant-based medicines to prevent or treat illness.

In recent years the Office of Dietary Supplements has worked collaboratively with several organizations and experts to develop a database of dietary supplements used in the United States. Because the database provides specific information on the nutrient, herbal, or other constituents contained in a supplement, it allows clinicians to more accurately assess the appropriate use of select supplements by their patients. The database includes dietary supplement label information for more than 4000 supplements, including the structure and function claims. The information is linked to PubMed, allowing clinicians access to peer-reviewed information on use in human trials, **adverse events (AEs)** associated with use, and information regarding the mechanism of action (National Institutes of Health, 2010).

Supplement Facts

Serving Size 1 Capsule

Amount Per Capsule	% Daily Value
Calories 20	
Calories from Fat 20	
Total Fat 2 g	3%*
Saturated Fat 0.5 g	3%*
Polyunsaturated Fat 1 g	†
Monounsaturated Fat 0.5 g	†
Vitamin A 4250 IU	85%
Vitamin D 425 IU	106%
Omega-3 fatty acids 0.5 g	†

* Percent Daily Values are based on a 2,000 calorie diet.
† Daily Value not established.

Ingredients: Cod liver oil, gelatin, water, and glycerin.

FIGURE 13-3 A dietary supplement facts label per Food and Drug Administration regulation as defined under the Dietary Supplement Health Education Act. *(Source: http://www.fda.gov/Food/DietarySupplements/ConsumerInformation/ucm110493.htm. Accessed 24 May 2010.)*

Trends in Dietary Supplement Use

Dietary supplement use is common among adults in the United States and is growing among children as well. About one third of adults use a multivitamin and mineral supplement regularly (American Dietetic Association, 2009). The NHIS CAM survey showed the most common nonvitamin, nonmineral supplements consumed were fish oils, glucosamine, echinacea, flaxseed, and ginseng (Barnes et al., 2008). Children commonly consume the same dietary supplements taken by adults. Use of dietary supplements has been shown to increase with advancing age, white race, and female gender. Reports find that use of dietary supplements is highest among those in the best state of health; most frequently supplements are taken by those with a body mass index less than 25 kg/m^2 who are nonsmokers, are physically active, report good health, adhere to a healthy diet, and use food labels in making food choices, as well as among those with high incomes and education (Archer, 2005).

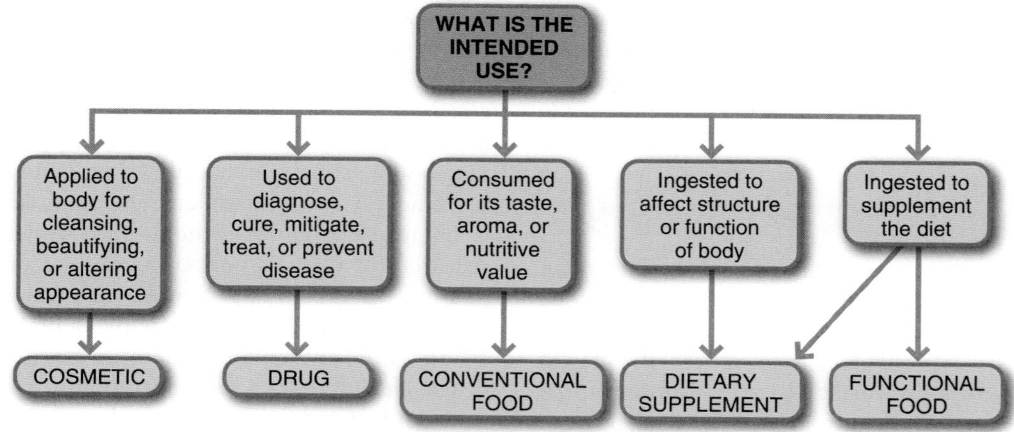

FIGURE 13-4 Use of dietary supplementation in clinical practice requires use of a credible resource for evaluation and application. *(From Thomson CA, Newton T: Dietary supplements: evaluation and application in clinical practice, Topics Clin Nutr 20(1):32, 2005. Reprinted with permission.)*

BOX 13-1

Botanical Formulations

Type	Form
Bulk Herbs	
	Sold loose to be used as teas, in cooking, and to prepare capsules; rapidly lose potency; should be stored in opaque containers, away from heat and light
Beverages	
Teas	Beverage weak in concentration; steep fresh or dried herbs in a cup of hot water for a few minutes, strain, and drink
Infusions	More concentrated than teas; steep fresh or dried herbs for approximately 15 min to allow more of the active ingredients to be extracted than for teas
Decoctions	Most concentrated of the beverages, made by boiling the root, rhizome, bark or berries for 30-60 min to extract the active ingredients
Extracts	
	Herbs are extracted with an organic solvent to dissolve the active components; forms a concentrated form of the active ingredients
Tinctures	Extract in which the solvent is alcohol
Glycerites	Extract in which the solvent is glycerol or a mixture of glycerol, propylene glycol, and water; more appropriate for children than a tincture
Pill Forms	
	Pills should be taken with at least 4-8 oz of water to avoid leaving residue in the esophagus
Capsules	Herbal material is enclosed in a hard shell made from animal-derived gelatin or plant-derived cellulose
Tablets	Herbal material is mixed with filler material to form the hard tablet; may be uncoated or coated with films
Lozenges	Also called *troches*; method of preparation allows the active components to be readily released in the mouth when chewed or sucked
Soft gels	Soft capsule used to encase liquid extracts such as ω-3 fatty acids or vitamin E
Essential oils	Fragrant, volatile plant oils; used for aromatherapy, bathing; concentrated form and not to be used internally unless specifically directed (such as enteric-coated peppermint oil)

Use of herbal products has been more difficult to evaluate; products are often taken intermittently to treat specific health care problems, and use can be quite variable. Some herbal products commonly consumed include St. John's wort, echinacea, garlic, saw palmetto and ginkgo biloba, ginseng, soy, valerian, cranberry, and black cohosh (Ernst, 2005). For several dietary supplements enough evidence has accumulated to justify an evidence assessment report by multidisciplinary teams of scientific experts under the Agency for Healthcare Research and Quality or the preparation of a Cochrane Database Review (CDR). A CDR is published as a summation of efficacy and safety of the use of a select supplement in specific medical conditions. Table 13-2 presents commonly used dietary supplements and related information regarding clinical efficacy in the form of CDR.

Potentially At-Risk Populations

Although dietary supplementation is most common among those who are likely to be at lowest risk for nutrient deficiency, select groups within the population are more likely to require dietary supplementation. For example, dietary intake inadequacies have been reported among the elderly (Chernoff, 2005), those of lower socioeconomic status (Karp et al., 2005), and those on energy- or fat-restricted diets (Dwyer et al., 2005). In addition, select physiologic states such as pregnancy and lactation increase requirements for select nutrients (e.g., iron, calcium, folate) that are sometimes difficult to meet through dietary changes alone. Furthermore, chronic illness may result in either increased requirements for certain nutrients (e.g., malabsorptive disorders and general supplementation, osteoporosis and bone-related nutrients, elevated serum homocysteine levels in cardiac disease, and increased B vitamin requirements). Finally, lifestyle choices may increase nutrient needs (e.g., increased vitamin C requirement in smokers, increased folate requirement in alcohol users, and increased iron requirements in iron-deficient athletes). Thus clinicians should be aware of these at-risk subgroups and complete a nutrition assessment to determine the need for supplementation on an individual basis. See Chapters 6 and 8.

TABLE 13-2

Select Cochrane Database Reviews of Nutrient and Botanical Supplementation Efficacy

Dietary Supplement	Use	Sufficient Evidence of Therapeutic Benefit?	Reference
Nutrients			
Antioxidant supplements (mixed)	Gastrointestinal cancer prevention	NO	Bjelakovic G et al: *Cochrane Database Syst Rev* 18(4):CD004183, 2008.
	Macular degeneration	YES with antioxidant mixture plus zinc	Evans JR: *Cochrane Database Syst Rev* (2):CD000254, 2009.
	Preeclampsia	NO	Rumbold et al: *Cochrane Database Syst Rev* CD004227, 2008.
	Mortality	NO	Bjelakovic G et al: *Cochrane Database Syst Rev* CD007176, 2008.
Calcium	Colorectal cancer and polyps	YES, for recurrent adenomatous polyps, not CRC specifically	Weingarten MA et al: *Cochrane Database Syst Rev* (1):CD003548, 2008.
	Hypertension	YES, with pregnancy; 50% reduction in preeclampsia	Hofmeyr GT et al: *Cochrane Database Syst Rev* (1):CD001059, 2010.
		NO, adults with HTN	Dickinson HO et al: *Cochrane Database Syst Rev* (2):CD004639, 2009.
DHEA	Cognitive function in healthy elderly	NO	Evans JG: *Cochrane Database Syst Rev* (2):CD006221, 2006.
Folic acid	Cognition and dementia	NO, with or without B_{12}, possible in people with elevated homocysteine	Malouf R et al: *Cochrane Database Syst Rev* (4):CD004514, 2008.
Omega-3 fatty acids	Cardiovascular disease treatment and prevention	NO, inconclusive	Hooper L et al: *Cochrane Database Syst Rev* 142(3):CD003177, 2009.
	Crohn disease	NO	Turner D et al: *Cochrane Database Syst Rev* CD006320, 2009.
	Intermittent claudication	NO	Sommerfield T, et al: *Cochrane Database Syst Rev* (3):CD003833, 2007.
Probiotics	Infectious diarrhea	YES	Allen SJ et al: *Cochrane Database Syst Rev* (2):CD003048, 2009.
Selenium	Critical illness (adult)	NO	Avenell et al: *Cochrane Database Syst Rev* 18(4):CD003703, 2007.
	Asthma	Somewhat	Allam MF, Lucane RA: *Cochrane Database Syst Rev* (2):CD003538, 2005.
Vitamin C	Asthma	NO	Ram et al: *Cochrane Database Syst Rev* (4):CD000993, 2004.
	Common cold	NO, maybe with severe physical exercise or cold environment	Hemila H et al: *Cochrane Database Syst Rev* 18(3):CD000980, 2007.
	Pneumonia	NO, general population YES, those with low plasma concentrations	Hemila H, Louhiala P: *Cochrane Database Syst Rev* 24(1):CD005532, 2007.
Vitamin D	Fractures w/ osteoporosis	NO, possibly with calcium, likely in deficient people	Avenell A et al: *Cochrane Database Syst Rev* (1):CD000227, 2009.
Botanicals			
Cranberry	Urinary tract infections	YES, in women with recurrent UTIs	Jepson RG and Craig JC: *Cochrane Database Syst Rev* (2):CD001321, 2008.
Echinacea	Common cold	YES, with *Echinacea purpurea*	Linde K et al: *Cochrane Database Syst Rev* (2):CD000530, 2006.
Ginkgo biloba	Ischemic stroke recovery	NO	Zeng X et al: *Cochrane Database Syst Rev* 19(4):CD003691, 2005.

TABLE 13-2

Select Cochrane Database Reviews of Nutrient and Botanical Supplementation Efficacy—cont'd

Dietary Supplement	Use	Sufficient Evidence of Therapeutic Benefit?	Reference
	Dementia/cognition	NO, not convincing	Birks J, Evans JG: *Cochrane Database Syst Rev* (4):CD003120, 2009.
Garlic	Peripheral arterial occlusive disease	NO	Jepson RG et al: *Cochrane Database Syst Rev* (2):CD000095, 2008.
Kava	Anxiety	YES	Pittler MH, Ernst E: *Cochrane Database Syst Rev* (1):CD003383, 2009.
Milk thistle	Alcoholic liver disease or hepatitis B and C	Somewhat; trials needed	Rambaldi A et al: *Cochrane Database Syst Rev* (2):CD003620, 2007.
Saw palmetto	Benign prostatic hyperplasia	NO; trials needed	Tacklind J et al: *Cochrane Database Syst Rev* (3):CD001423, 2009.
St. John's wort	Depression	YES, with hypericum	Linde K et al: *Cochrane Database Syst Rev* (2):CD000448, 2008.

Cochrane Database reviews can be found online at: www.cochrane.org/reviews and are also listed in MedLine and PubMed peer-review citation indexes.

CRC, Colorectal cancer; *DHEA,* dehydroepiandrosterone; *HTN,* hypertension; *UTI,* urinary tract infection.

Routine use of multivitamin-mineral supplements may be an appropriate recommendation to ensure dietary adequacy. Because many American adults do not meet even the estimated average requirement for vitamin C, D, and E or minerals such as calcium, many suggest that adults in the United States should regularly take a multivitamin-mineral supplement. To further address this issue, the NIH convened a Conference on Multivitamin/Mineral Supplements and Chronic Disease Prevention in 2006 to develop a consensus statement. Even though the panel report states that there is insufficient evidence to show that multivitamin-mineral supplements will reduce the risk for certain chronic diseases (see full report at http://ods.od.nih.gov/news/Results_of_MultivitaminMineral_Supplements_2006.aspx; Neuhouser, 2009), many nutrition practitioners and health care providers continue to recommend a daily multivitamin-mineral supplement to their patients on a routine basis. In some instances supplementation is considered standard of practice. An example is the recommendation that all women of childbearing age take a multivitamin with 400 mcg of folic acid to reduce the risk for neural tube defects in unborn children.

In the area of botanical supplementation there is less evidence of the existence of at-risk populations who require supplementation. Rather, botanical supplements are more generally used to alleviate symptoms of illness or disease. There can be wide variability in response, and routine recommendations for all patients may not be appropriate For example, although there is some support for the use of garlic to reduce serum cholesterol levels, routine supplementation with garlic for all patients with hypercholesterolemia is not appropriate. The patient may be taking prescription medications to treat the elevated cholesterol, may be at risk for increased bleeding time with long-term garlic use, or may be intolerant of the potential gastrointestinal discomfort of supplemental garlic.

In addition to reviewing the available evidence, an assessment of each patient's clinical situation is important. If the therapy is both effective and safety has been demonstrated, recommending a dietary supplement or a CAM therapy may make sense. Unfortunately, either the evidence for CAM therapy is not clear and consistent (especially in regard to general lack of studies) or safety is a concern. These gray areas are challenging for clinicians when making specific recommendations. Certainly the use of a CAM or dietary supplement that has not been shown to be effective and carries a safety risk should be discouraged.

DIETARY SUPPLEMENT REGULATION

Botanical products are regulated in the United States as dietary supplements. The DSHEA of 1994 clarifies marketing regulations for botanicals and reclassifies them as dietary supplements, distinct from food or drugs. A variety of potential labeling approaches are used by the dietary supplement industry to market supplements. These include qualified health claims; unqualified health claims; claims based on an authoritative statement; nutrient content claims; dietary guidance statements; and structure-function claims, which is the most commonly used approach.

A **health claim** is a written claim on the dietary supplement label that has two essential components: (1) a *substance* and (2) a *disease* or health-related condition. It describes the relationship between these two components; a statement lacking either of these components does not meet the regulatory definition of a health claim. Furthermore, it must meet the significant scientific agreement standard and requires prenotification of the Food and Drug Administration (FDA). Although it does require approval by the FDA, a general health claim does not require the level of scientific evidence of a qualified health claim.

A **qualified health claim** is a label health claim based on emerging scientific evidence that, on review of this evidence by the FDA, is approved for use on a food or dietary supplement label, given sufficient evidence exists to make the requested label claim (see Chapter 12 for more details). Remember that qualified health claims must be petitioned for by a body outside the FDA such as the supplement manufacturer; thus, although evidence may exist for use of select dietary supplements for select health symptoms, unless a request is formally made to FDA, such a claim will not be developed. Other types of health claims are the *authoritative statement* (FDA Modernization Act of 1997) and *dietary guidance statements*, which are based on published statements from authoritative organizations and agencies, as well as statements found within the body of the dietary guidelines.

Of greatest concern is the set of **structure-function claims**. Under DSHEA, the physiologic effects of a product can be noted, but no claims about prevention or cure of specific conditions can be made. A product manufacturer cannot claim that a dietary supplement "prevents heart disease," but it can state that the product "helps increase blood flow to the heart." Such subtle differences are unlikely to be discerned by the average consumer, leading to misinterpretation and potentially inappropriate use of the products. Furthermore, these claims do not require FDA prenotification, and the manufacturer assumes responsibility for ensuring the accuracy and truthfulness of the statement. All products must display the following disclaimer: "This statement has not been evaluated by the Food and Drug Administration. This product is not intended to diagnose, treat, cure, or prevent any disease." However, there is no research as to the awareness or interpretation of this statement by consumers. Consumers must educate themselves about the appropriate application of each dietary supplement they choose to use and about selection of quality products.

A report from the International Food Information Council (IFIC) suggests that consumers cannot clearly distinguish qualified from unqualified health claims and that they prefer structure-function claims for their positive focus and brevity. Among the more common problems that have been reported since the passage of DSHEA are misrepresentation of product contents; variable potency and recommended dosages among products; inadequate information about how a company's herbs are grown and processed; and poor standards of quality, product safety, or activity of ingredients. Although rare, herb contamination and misidentification do occur. Governmental and industry entities have developed high-quality manufacturing guidelines (good manufacturing practices [GMPs]) for all dietary supplements, including botanical products. Under the GMP rule manufacturers are required to establish and meet specifications for identity, purity, quality, strength and composition of dietary supplements (Food and Drug Administration, 2007)

In December 2006 the Dietary Supplement and Nonprescription Drug Consumer Protection Act was signed into law, setting requirements for both labeling and mandatory (rather than voluntary) AE reporting related to dietary supplement and over-the-counter (OTC) medication interactions (Frankos, 2009).

Another agency has international significance. The **Codex Alimentarius Commission (Codex)** was created in 1963 by two U.N. organizations, the Food and Agriculture Organization and the World Health Organization, to protect the health of consumers and to ensure fair practices in international food trade (Food and Drug Administration, 2010). Codex participants work on the development of food standards, codes of practice, and guidelines for products such as dietary supplements. Codex standards and guidelines are developed by committees from 180 member countries, where they voluntarily review and provide comments on standards at several stages in the development process (Crane et al., 2010).

ASSESSMENT OF DIETARY SUPPLEMENT USE

Popular interest in the use of dietary supplements for health applications is widespread in the United States. Health care professionals should be aware that, although nutrient supplementation is generally recommended to enhance the relative adequacy of the diet or to meet increased requirements associated with illness or disease, the therapeutic action of many botanical products is similar to that of drugs; so the potential for harmful interactions exists. Consumers may not be well informed about the safety and efficacy of supplements and some have difficulty interpreting product labels (American Dietetic Association, 2009).

Health care professionals should also be aware that their patients typically do not inform them of their use of botanicals or other dietary supplements; practitioners must inquire about the use of supplements by their patients. To facilitate obtaining information, health care providers should approach patients in an open, nonjudgmental manner. Key items and issues to be inquired about are summarized in Box 13-2. Not only should all dietary supplements be reviewed, but it is recommended that patients bring all supplements into the clinic to be evaluated. In this way the health care provider can review dose, dosage form, additive sources of the same nutrient or botanical, frequency of use, rationale for use, any identified side effects, and the patient-perceived efficacy of each supplement. This should be done on a regular basis. It is particularly important

BOX 13-2

Evaluating Dietary Supplement Use: The Patient–Health Care Provider Information Exchange

Ask

- What dietary supplements are you taking (type: vitamin, mineral, botanical, amino acid, fiber)?
- What antacids or other OTC medications or food products are you taking that provide supplemental nutrients, herbals, fiber, etc.?
- Why are you taking these dietary supplements? Include review of patient's medical diagnosis and symptoms for reasons why he or she may be taking supplements (e.g., osteoarthritis, heart disease, high blood pressure, night sweats, loss of memory, fatigue).
- How long have you been taking these dietary supplements?
- What dose or how much are you taking? For each, include chemical form and review and photocopy labels.
- With what frequency are you taking each supplement?
- What are the sources of the supplements (e.g., OTC or prescribed, Internet, health care provider) and manufacturers of the supplements?
- Is it touted as being preventive or to have treatment effects? What does the label claim? Supplemental brochures or materials?
- Who recommended the supplement (e.g., media, physician, nurse, dietitian, alternative medicine practitioner, friend, family)?

Evaluate

- Dietary intake (including intake of fortified foods, energy or sports bars, or beverages)
- Health status and health history—include lifestyle habits (e.g., smoking, alcohol, exercise)
- Biochemical profile, laboratory data
- Prescribed and OTC medications
- Clinical response
- Adverse events, symptoms

Educate

- Scientific evidence of benefit and effectiveness
- Potential interaction with foods, nutrients, and medications or other dietary supplements
- Appropriate dose, brand, and chemical form; duration of supplementation; appropriate follow-up
- Quality of products, manufacturers, good manufacturing practices (USP, Consumer Labs)
- Mechanism of action of the primary active ingredient
- Appropriate storage of the dietary supplement
- Administration instructions: with food? Without food? Potential food-supplement interactions?
- Awareness and reporting of any side effects or adverse events, symptoms
- Recommend necessary dietary changes
- Remind that a nutritional *supplement* should supplement the diet

Document

- List specific supplements and brand names of each supplement being taken.
- Record batch number from bottle in case of an adverse event.
- Record patient perception and expected level of compliance.
- Monitor efficacy and safety, including health outcomes and adverse effects.
- Record medication-supplement or supplement-supplement interactions.
- Plan for follow-up.

From Practice Paper of the American Dietetic Association: Dietary supplements, J Am Diet Assoc 105(3):466, 2005. Reprinted with permission.

OTC, Over the counter.

that dietary supplement use be reviewed before surgery because some dietary supplements and botanicals alter the rate of blood coagulation. Table 13-3 provides specific recommendations regarding the discontinuation of dietary supplements before surgery to avoid complications associated with prolonged bleeding time.

Although a listing of efficacy and safety issues of select supplements is provided in the form of Cochrane database reviews in this chapter (see Table 13-3), the list is somewhat limited. A more extensive list is not provided because it is imperative that practitioners seek current data sources for this information, which is expanding rapidly. Practitioners should use the most up-to-date information when formulating recommendations for their patients. See Box 13-3 for a listing of reliable and comprehensive data sources.

Intake and follow-up information about these therapies provides important pharmacologic and treatment information for the health care provider. In particular, dietary supplements that have similar actions to prescription and OTC medications should generally not be combined, because the effects can be additive and cause harm (DeBusk, 2000). Conversely, dietary supplements that counter the effects of prescription and OTC medications should not be

BOX 13-3

Evidence-Based Dietary Supplement Resources

Websites

Agency for Healthcare Research Quality, USDHHS: http://www.ahrq.gov
American Botanical Council: www.herbalgram.org
American Dietetic Association, Complementary Care Dietetic Practice Group: www.complementarynutrition.org
American Herbal Products Association: http://www.ahpa.org
Consumer Laboratories: www.consumerlab.com
Computer-assisted research on dietary supplements (CARDS): http://ods.od.nih.gov/Research/CARDS_Database.aspx
Dietary supplements database (IBIDS): www.dietary-supplements.info.nih.gov
Federal Trade Commission: http://www.ftc.gov/bcp/menus/consumer/health/drugs.shtm
Food and Drug Administration (FDA): http://www.fda.gov/Food/DietarySupplements/default.htm
Herb Research Foundation: www.herbs.org
International bibliographic information on dietary supplements database: http://dietary-supplements.info.nih.gov/Health_Information/IBIDS_Overview.aspx
Mayo Clinic: http://www.mayoclinic.com/health/nutrition-and-healthy-eating/MY00431/DSECTION=nutritional-supplements
National Center for Complementary and Alternative Medicine: http://nccam.nih.gov
NHANES online analysis of dietary supplements (NOADS), 2006: http://ods.od.nih.gov/index.aspx
Natural Standard: http://www.naturalstandard.com
Office of Dietary Supplements: http://ods.od.nih.gov
Pharmacist's letter/natural medicine database: www.naturaldatabase.com
Supplement watch: www.supplementwatch.com
United States Pharmacopoeia: www.usp.org

Text/Print

Blumenthal M, editor: *The ABC clinical guide to herbs*, Silver Springs, Md, 2003, American Botanical Council.
Brunton L et al: *Goodman and Gilman's manual of pharmacology and therapeutics*, New York, 2008, McGraw-Hill.
Gruenwald J: *PDR for herbal medicines*, ed 3, Montvale, N.J., 2004, Medical Economics.
Sarubin-Fragakis A: *The health professionals guide to dietary supplements*, ed 3, Chicago, Ill, 2007, American Dietetic Association.

TABLE 13-3

Recommended Times for Preoperative Discontinuation of Select Common Dietary Supplements

Dietary Supplement	Recommended Discontinuation Time Before Surgery
Echinacea	Insufficient data
Garlic	7 days
Gingko	36 hours
Ginseng	7 days
Kava	24 hours
St. John's wort	5 days
Valerian	Insufficient data
Vitamin E	7 days

Data from Ang-Lee MK et al: Herbal medicines and perioperative care, JAMA 286:208, 2001.

combined, such as taking a blood pressure–lowering medication along with a botanical that can raise blood pressure. Funding studies that evaluate botanical-drug interactions is a priority of the NCCAM.

Beyond evaluating the efficacy of dietary supplements, safety must also be addressed. Although select safety issues have been identified, some may go unreported and use of that supplement discontinued, with no formal report of the AE being filed. As an example, more than 4 million Americans are taking antithrombotic therapy. Approximately 180 dietary supplements have been identified as having anticoagulation, antiplatelet, antagonistic, or drug-metabolizing activity. AEs should be reported to the health care institutions, poison control centers, and MedWatch. Manufacturers of dietary supplements should also maintain their own reporting system for AEs (Talati and Gurnani, 2009).

AEs should be reported to MedWatch. Reports can be filed by the individual, health care provider, or industry. AE reports are forwarded to the Center for Food Safety and Applied Nutrition where they are further evaluated by qualified reviewers. In 2008 a total of 1,080 reports were filed—the majority from mandatory rather than voluntary sources. The majority were related to use of vitamins or mixed-nutrient products (Frankos, 2009).

Many health care professionals remain uncomfortable recommending dietary supplements. Guidelines for recommending and selling dietary supplements and a clinical practice paper have been previously published (Thomson et al., 2005). Internet resources are listed at the end of this chapter. An algorithm for assessing and recommending dietary supplements is presented. Practitioners must take the initiative to develop the appropriate knowledge, skills, and resources to provide optimal care in the area of dietary supplementation.

GUIDELINES FOR COUNSELING

The goal of CAM counseling is to determine which supplements clients are using and the health goals they hope to achieve through the use of these products. People typically do not divulge their use of dietary supplements or CAM use to their health care practitioners. This is especially true for minority racial and ethnic groups. It is imperative that the practitioner establish rapport with the client to enhance disclosure of CAM use (Chao, 2008). Being nonjudgmental of the client's practices fosters a constructive dialogue. The health care practitioner's role is as a coach who helps clients assess the need for supplements and helps them to become more knowledgeable about their options (see Box 13-2).

For discussion of dietary supplement use, clients should bring with them all prescriptions, OTC medications, and dietary supplements they are using. In addition, a dietary supplement intake assessment form should be completed by each patient or client and reviewed in detail by the health care provider. Note that, in addition to a listing of specific supplements, nutrients, and botanicals, the form also identifies the health conditions that motivated the use of supplements. In the case of calcium, it is also imperative to collect information about antacid use because this is a major source of calcium supplementation.

Each supplement should be discussed individually in terms of what the client hopes to achieve by using that supplement, whether the preparation is appropriate for the client's health goals, and whether the dosage being taken and the length of time for supplementation is supported by published clinical trials. How to recognize a quality preparation for each supplement (in particular if the manufacturer is compliant with GMPs), any known safety concerns and contraindications, and any known or potential interactions between each supplement and prescription or OTC medications and other dietary supplements or foods should also be reviewed (see Chapter 9).

The client should be instructed to use the dosage commonly recommended for that specific botanical. A low starting dose, even less than the recommended dose, should be encouraged and the response monitored to minimize the chances of an adverse reaction. Dietary supplement use by clients provides an excellent platform for teaching consumers analytic skills that will serve them well in their pursuit of increased self-management of their health.

The Office of Dietary Supplements has developed facts sheets for an extensive list of dietary supplements that can be used by health care professionals to educate patients. The FDA has published tips for the dietary supplement user in making informed choices regarding which supplements to consider taking. Tips include advice regarding (1) assessment of present diet, (2) informing health care providers of dietary supplement use, (3) potential medication–dietary supplement interactions, (4) reporting of AEs, and (5) assessment of the validity of information. See Box 13-4 for issues to consider when choosing a botanical.

Resources for Clinicians

As awareness of dietary supplement use expands within the health care community, the number of evidence-based resources available to clinicians is also growing considerably. It is advisable that clinicians have access to at least one online resource that is updated at regular intervals. Resources that provide reference to the original research are preferable. In addition, accessing available medical literature is advised, given that there are a growing number of studies being published in peer-reviewed literature. Finally, contacting health care providers and researchers who are actively working in this area can be invaluable in terms of increasing awareness of safety issues, understanding mechanisms of biologic activity, and assessing the level of evidence for clinical efficacy.

CLINICAL SCENARIO

Ellen is 66 years old and has been diagnosed as having hypertension, hypercholesterolemia, and type 2 diabetes. She has been referred by her physician for nutritional counseling, with a specific request from the referring physician that you evaluate any herbal preparations she is taking. At the initial consult, Ellen tells you she is taking the following dietary supplements: garlic pills, ginseng, ginkgo, and St. John's wort, along with the following medications: warfarin, a tricyclic antidepressant, and blood pressure–lowering medication.

Nutrition Diagnostic Statement

Bioactive substance intake related to daily intake of multiple supplements as evidenced by intake of supplements that conflict with medications (warfarin, garlic, St. John's wort).

Nutrition Care Questions

1. What recommendations would you make about Ellen's diet?
2. What additional questions would you ask regarding Ellen's supplements?
3. List potential adverse interactions between the botanicals and the prescription drugs.
4. How would you counsel Ellen?

BOX 13-4

Guidelines for Choosing Botanical Products

1. Be sure the choice of a botanical is appropriate to the health care goals and compatible with any prescription and over-the-counter medications or other dietary supplements. Information is available at www.consumerlab.com for validation of specific product brands on the market.
2. Investigate the quality of the manufacturer whose product is being considered. At a minimum, it is important to know that the retail suppliers carry only manufacturers that adhere to high-quality standards or that the health care professional recommending a product is knowledgeable about the quality of dietary supplements. Some of the questions to ask are how herbs are grown, selected, stored, and processed to ensure absence of microbial contamination, proper identification, and potency.
3. Investigate the potential for pesticide contamination, which can be minimized by choosing organically grown herbs whenever possible.
4. Investigate the claims being made about the products and avoid products with exaggerated claims associated with them.
5. Use the dietary supplement label to obtain important information, including:
   - The complete botanical name of the product to confirm that this is the appropriate botanical
   - The part of the plant used to prepare the product, confirming that it is the part that contains the active components
   - The concentration of the botanical or nutrient and whether the concentration is appropriate for obtaining the reported benefits of the product (i.e., neither too weak nor too strong)
   - The daily dosage needed to obtain the desired effect
   - A lot number, which is helpful if problems arise because it allows the product to be tracked through each stage of the manufacturing process
   - An expiration date
   - A recognized seal of approval that indicates good manufacturing practices have been used in the production of the product and that the product has passed independent analyses confirming that the label accurately represents the product
   - A toll-free number for contacting the manufacturer in the event of adverse reactions
6. After determining that a manufacturer and its product meet these standards, compare prices among products of similar quality. Prices can vary widely.

Adapted from DeBusk RM: A practical guide to herbal supplements for nutrition practitioners, Topics Clin Nutr 16:53, 2001.

USEFUL WEBSITES

Agency for Healthcare Research and Quality
http://www.ahrq.org

Arthritis Foundation Supplement Guide
http://www.arthritistoday.org/treatments/supplement-guide/conditions.php

CAM on PubMed
http://nccam.nih.gov/camonpubmed/

Computer Access to Research on Dietary Supplements
http://dietary-supplements.info.nih.gov/Research/CARDS_Database.aspx

Dietary Supplements Labels Database
http://dietarysupplements.nlm.nih.gov/dietary

Consumer Lab
http://www.consumerlab.com/

Cochrane Database Review
http://www2.Cochrane.org/reviews/

Food and Drug Administration—Dietary supplement advice
http://www.fda.gov/ForConsumers/ConsumerUpdates/ucm153239.htm

Institute for Functional Medicine
http://www.functionalmedicine.org

MedWatch
http://www.fda.gov/medwatch/

Memorial Sloan Kettering Cancer Center's About Herbs, Botanicals & Other Products
www.mskcc.org/AboutHerbs

National Center for Complementary and Alternative Medicine
http://nccam.nih.gov/

Office of Dietary Supplements
http://ods.od.nih.gov/Health_Information/Health_Information.aspx

REFERENCES

Ahn AC, et al: Applying principles from complex systems to studying the efficacy of CAM therapies, *J Altern Complement Med* 16:1015, 2010.

Allam MF, Lucane RA: Selenium supplementation for asthma, *Cochrane Database Syst Rev* CD003538, 2005.

Allen SJ, et al: Probiotics for treating infectious diarrhea, *Cochrane Database Syst Rev* CD003048, 2009.

American Dietetic Association: Position of the American Dietetic Association: nutrient supplementation, *Am Diet Assoc* 109:2073, 2009.

Ang-Lee MK, et al: Herbal medicines and perioperative care, *JAMA* 286:208, 2001.

Archer SL: Association of dietary supplement use with specific micronutrient intakes among middle-aged American men and women: the INTERMAP Study, *J Am Diet Assoc* 105:1106, 2005.

Avenell A, et al: Selenium supplementation for critically ill adults, *Cochrane Database Syst Rev* CD003703 October 18, 2007.

Avenell A, et al: *Cochrane Database Syst Rev* (1):CD000227, 2009.

Barnes P, et al: Complementary and alternative medicine use among adults and children: United States, 2007, *Natl Health Stat Report* 10(12):1, 2008.

Birdee GS, et al: Factors associated with pediatric use of complementary and alternative medicine, *Pediatrics* 125:249, 2010.

Birks J, Evans JG: Ginkgo biloba for cognitive impairment and dementia, *Cochrane Database Syst Rev* CD003120, 2009.

Bjelakovic G, et al: Antioxidant supplements for preventing gastrointestinal cancers, *Cochrane Database Syst Rev* 18(4):CD004183, 2008.

Bjelakovic G, et al: Antioxidant supplements for prevention of mortality in healthy participants and patients with diseases, *Cochrane Database Syst Rev* 16(2):CD007176, 2008.

Chao MT, et al: Disclosure of complementary and alternative medicine to conventional medical providers: variation by race/ethnicity and type of CAM, *J Natl Med Assoc* 100:1341, 2008.

Chernoff R: Micronutrient requirements in older women, *Am J Clin Nutr* 81:1204S, 2005.

Crane NT, et al: The role and relevance of Codex in Nutrition Standards, *Am Diet Assoc* 110:672, 2010.

DeBusk RM: *Herbs as medicine: what you should know*, Tallahassee, FL, 2000, PR Treadwell.

Dickinson HO, et al: Calcium supplementation for the management of primary hypertension in adults, *Cochrane Database Syst Rev* CD004639, 2009.

Dwyer JT, et al: Dietary supplements in weight reduction, *J Am Diet Assoc* 105:80S, 2005.

Ernst E: The efficacy of herbal medicine-an overview, *Fundamental Clin Pharmacol* 19:405, 2005.

Evans JG: Dehydroepiandrosterone (DHEA) supplementation for cognitive function, *Cochrane Database Syst Rev* CD006221, 2006.

Evans JR: Antioxidant vitamin and mineral supplements for age-related macular degeneration, *Cochrane Database Syst Rev* CD000254, 2009.

Farmer Miller N, et al: Dietary supplement use in individuals living with cancer and other chronic conditions: a population-based study, *J Am Diet Assoc* 108:483, 2008.

Food and Drug Administration: Current good manufacturing practice in manufacturing, packaging, labeling, or holding operations for dietary supplements. Final rule, *Fed Regist* 72:34751, 2007.

Food and Drug Administration (FDA): *What is Codex?* Accessed 24 May 2010 from http://www.fda.gov/Food/DietarySupplements/GuidanceComplianceRegulatoryInformation/ucm113860.htm#what.

Frankos VH, et al: FDA regulation of dietary supplements and requirements regarding adverse event reporting, *Clin Pharmacol Ther* 87:239, 2010.

Hemila H, et al: Vitamin C for preventing and treating the common cold, *Cochrane Database Syst Rev* 18(3):CD000993, 2007.

Hemila H, Louhiala P: Vitamin C for preventing and treating pneumonia, *Cochrane Database Syst Rev* 24(1):CD005532, 2007.

Hofmeyr GT, Atallah AN, Duley L: Calcium supplementation during pregnancy for preventing hypertensive disorders and related problems, *Cochrane Database Syst Rev* (1):CD001059, 2010.

Hooper L, et al: ω 3 fatty acids for prevention and treatment of cardiovascular disease, *Cochrane Database Syst Rev* CD003177, 2009.

Institute of Functional Medicine. Website http://www.functionalmedicine.org/about/whatis.asp accessed 1/16/2011.

Jepson RG, Craig JC: Cranberries for preventing urinary tract infections, *Cochrane Database Syst Rev* CD001321, 2008.

Jepson RG, et al: *Cochrane Database Syst Rev* (2):CD000095, 2008.

Karp RJ, et al: The appearance of discretionary income: influence on the prevalence of under and over nutrition, *Int J Equity Health* 28:4, 2005.

Kiefer D, et al: An overview of CAM: components and clinical uses, *Nutr in Clin Pract* 24:549, 2009.

Linde K, et al: Echinacea for preventing and treating the common cold, *Cochrane Database Syst Rev* CD000530, 2006.

Linde K, et al: St John's wort for depression, *Cochrane Database Syst Rev* CD000448, 2008.

Maizes VM, et al: Integrative medicine and patient-centered care, *Explore (NY)* 5(5):277, 2009.

Malouf R, et al: Folic acid with or without vitamin B_{12} for cognition and dementia, *Cochrane Database Syst Rev* CD004514, 2008.

Marra MV, et al: Position of the American Dietetic Association: nutrient supplementation, *JADA* 190:2073, 2009.

National Center for Complementary and Alternative Medicine (NCCAM): *NCCAM funding: appropriations history*. Accessed 8 December 2005 from www.nccam.nih.gov/news/camsurvey.htm.

National Institutes of Health (NIH): *Dietary supplements labels database*. Accessed 20 May 2010 from http://dietarysupplements.nlm.nih.gov/dietary/.

Neuhouser ML, et al: Multivitamin use and risk of cancer and cardiovascular disease in the Women's Health Initiative cohorts, *Arch Intern Med* 169:294, 2009.

Pittler MH, Ernst E: Kava extract for treating anxiety, *Cochrane Database Syst Rev* CD003383, 2009.

Rambaldi A, et al: Milk thistle for alcoholic and/or hepatitis B or C virus liver diseases, *Cochrane Database Syst Rev* CD003620, 2007.

Rumbold A, et al: Antioxidants for preventing pre-eclampsia. *Cochrane Database Syst Rev* D004227, 2008.

Sommerfield T, et al: ω-3 fatty acids for intermittent claudication, *Cochrane Database Syst Rev* CD003833, 2007.

Tacklind J, et al: Serenoa repens for benign prostatic hyperplasia, *Cochrane Database Syst Rev* CD001423, 2009.

Talati AR, Gurnani AK: Dietary supplements adverse event reports: review and analysis, *Food & Drug Law J* 64:503, 2009.

Thomson CA, et al: Practice Paper of the American Dietetic Association: dietary supplements, *J Am Diet Assoc* 105:460, 2005.

Turner D, et al: ω 3 fatty acids (fish oil) for maintenance of remission in Crohn's disease. *Cochrane Database Syst Rev* CD006320, 2009.

Ullman D: A review of a historical summit on integrative medicine, *eCAM Advance Access* 31 August 2009. doi:10.1093/ecam/nep128.

Weingarten MA, et al: Dietary calcium supplementation for preventing colorectal cancer and adenomatous polyps, *Cochrane Database Syst Rev* CD003548, 2008.

Zeng X, et al: Ginkgo biloba for acute ischaemic stroke, *Cochrane Database Syst Rev* 19(4):CD003691, 2005.

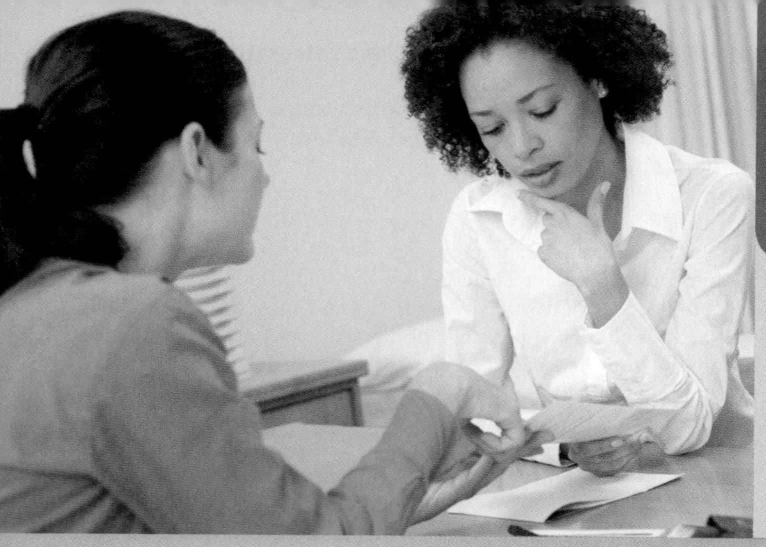

CHAPTER 14

Janice L. Raymond, MS, RD, CD
Carol S. Ireton-Jones, PhD, RD, LD, CNSD, FACN

Food and Nutrient Delivery: Nutrition Support Methods

KEY TERMS

advance directives
bolus feeding
catheter
central parenteral nutrition (CPN)
closed enteral system
computerized prescriber order entry (CPOE)
continuous drip infusion
durable medical equipment (DME) provider
enteral nutrition (EN)
essential fatty acid deficiency (EFAD)
extended dwell catheter
french size
gastrointestinal decompression
gastrojejunostomy
hang time
hemodynamic stability
home enteral nutrition (HEN) support
home parenteral nutrition (HPN)
intermittent drip feeding
lumen
modular enteral feeding
multiple lumen tubes
nasoduodenal tube (NDT)
nasogastric tube (NGT)
nasojejunal tube (NJT)
open enteral system
osmolality
osmolarity
parenteral nutrition (PN)
percutaneous endoscopic gastrostomy (PEG)
percutaneous endoscopic jejunostomy (PEJ)
peripheral parenteral nutrition (PPN)
peripherally inserted central catheter (PICC or PIC)
polymeric formula
rebound hypoglycemia
refeeding syndrome
sentinel event
total nutrient admixture (3-in-1)
transitional feeding

Nutrition support is the delivery of formulated enteral or parenteral nutrients for the purpose of maintaining or restoring nutritional status. **Enteral nutrition (EN)** refers to the provision of nutrients into the gastrointestinal tract (GIT) through a tube or **catheter**. In certain instances EN may include the use of formulas as oral supplements or meal replacements. **Parenteral nutrition (PN)** is the provision of nutrients intravenously.

Sections of this chapter were written by Charles Mueller, PhD, RD, CNSD, CDN and Abby S. Bloch, PhD, Rd, FADA for the previous edition of this text.

RATIONALE AND CRITERIA FOR APPROPRIATE NUTRITION SUPPORT

When patients are unable to eat enough to support their nutritional needs for more than a few days, nutrition support should be considered. EN should be the first consideration. Using the gut for nutrition versus using only PN is preferable for preserving the mucosal barrier function and integrity. The act of feeding the GIT has been shown to attenuate the catabolic response and preserve immunologic function (ASPEN, 2010). EN decreases the incidence of hyperglycemia when compared with PN. At this time, there is insufficient evidence to draw conclusions about the effect of EN versus PN on length of stay and mortality (American Dietetic Association, 2010).

Criteria must be applied to select appropriate candidates for nutrition support (Table 14-1). PN should be used in patients who are or will become malnourished and who do not have sufficient gastrointestinal function to

TABLE 14-1

Conditions That Often Require Nutrition Support

Recommended Route of Feeding	Condition	Typical Disorders
Enteral nutrition	Inability to eat	Neurologic disorders (dysphagia) Facial trauma Oral or esophageal trauma Congenital anomalies Respiratory failure (on a ventilator) Traumatic brain injury Comatose state GI surgery (e.g., esophagectomy)
	Inability to eat enough	Hypermetabolic states such as with burns Cancer Heart failure Congenital heart disease Impaired intake after orofacial surgery or injury Anorexia nervosa HIV/AIDS Failure to thrive Cystic fibrosis
	Impaired digestion, absorption, metabolism	Severe gastroparesis Inborn errors of metabolism Crohn disease Short bowel syndrome with minimum resection Pancreatitis
Parenteral nutrition	Gastrointestinal incompetency	Short bowel syndrome—major resection Severe acute pancreatitis with intolerance to enteral feeding Severe inflammatory bowel disease Small bowel ischemia Intestinal atresia Severe liver failure Persistent postoperative ileus Intractable vomiting/diarrhea refractory to medical management Distal high-output fistulas Severe GI Bleeding
	Critical illness with poor enteral tolerance or accessibility	Multiorgan system failure Major trauma or burns Bone marrow transplantation Acute respiratory failure with ventilator dependency and gastrointestinal malfunction Severe wasting in renal failure with dialysis Small bowel transplantation, immediate after surgery

McClave SA et al: Guidelines for the provision and assessment of nutrition support therapy in the adult critically ill patient, JPEN J Parenter Enteral Nutr 33: 277, 2009.

AIDS, Acquired immune deficiency syndrome; *GI*, gastrointestinal; *HIV*, human immunodeficiency virus.

be able to restore or maintain optimal nutritional status (McClave et al., 2009). Figure 14-1 presents an algorithm for selecting EN and PN routes. Although these guidelines can assist with the selection of the best type of nutrition, the choice is not always easy. For example, access methods are not universally available in every health care setting. Therefore, if a specific type of small bowel access is not available for EN, PN may be the only realistic option. Often PN is used temporarily until adequate gastrointestinal function can support either EN or oral intake. In this situation a combination of feeding methods is used (see "Transitional Feeding" later in the chapter).

In a **computerized prescriber order entry (CPOE)**, the prescriber enters orders directly into a computer system, usually aided by decision-support technology (Bankhead et al., 2009). Although methods of nutrition support can be standardized for the course of certain disease states or treatments, every patient presents an individual challenge. Nutrition support must often be adapted to unanticipated developments or complications. The optimal treatment plan requires interdisciplinary collaboration that is closely aligned with the overall patient care plan. In a few instances nutrition support may be warranted but physically impossible to implement within the overall care plan.

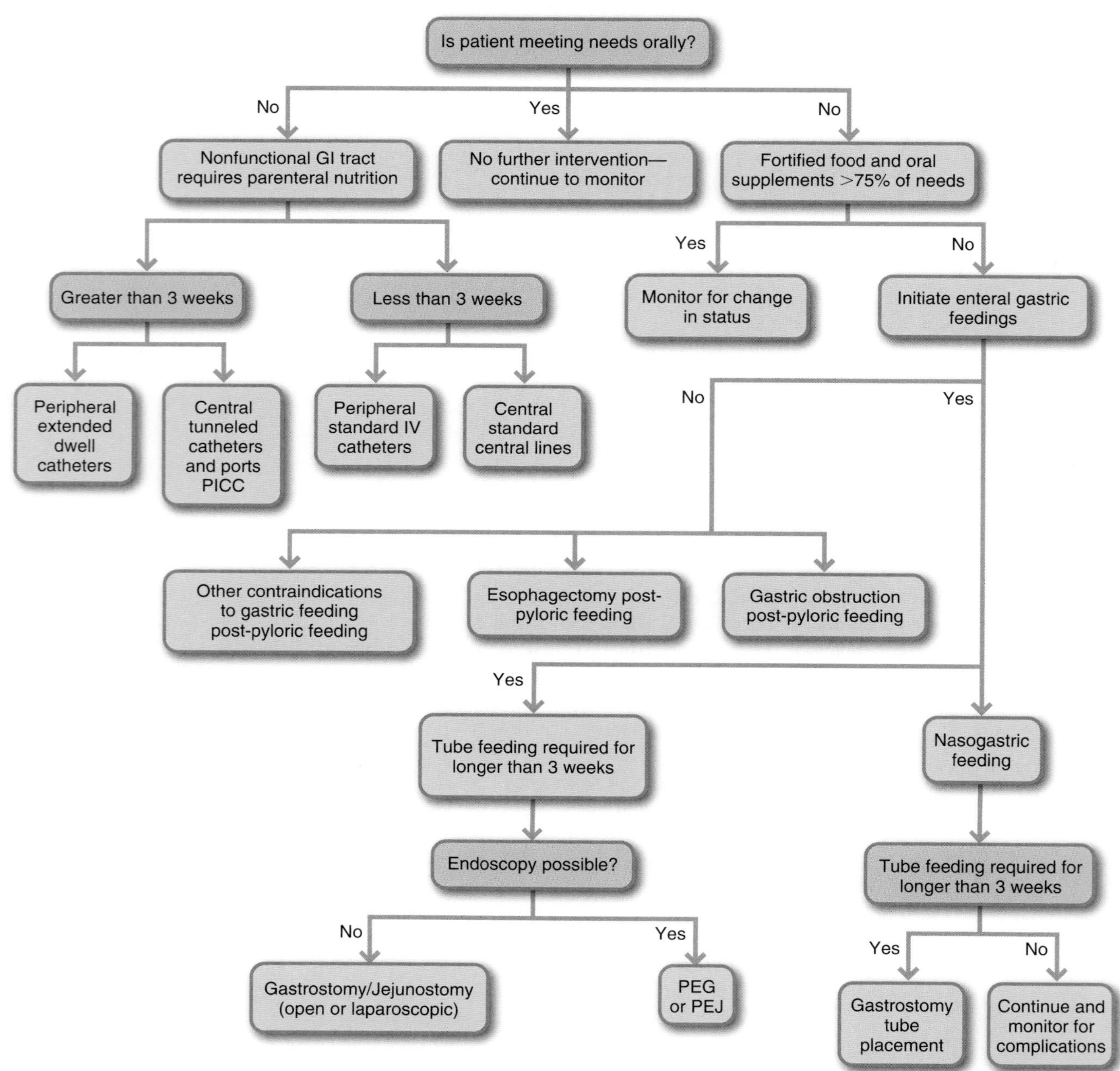

FIGURE 14-1 Algorithm for route selection for nutrition support.

Conversely, nutrition support may be achievable but not warranted because of the prognosis, unacceptable risk, or the patient's right to self-determination. In all cases, it is important to prevent errors in ordering, delivery, and monitoring of nutrition support to prevent undesirable risks or outcomes (**sentinel events**) such as an unexpected death, serious physical injury with loss of limb or function, or psychological injury (Joint Commission, 2010).

ENTERAL NUTRITION

By definition, *enteral* implies using the GIT, primarily via "tube feeding." When a patient has been determined to be a candidate for EN, the location of nutrient administration and type of enteral access device is selected. Enteral access selection depends on the (1) anticipated length of time enteral feeding will be required, (2) degree of risk for aspiration or tube displacement, (3) patient's clinical status, (4) presence or absence of normal digestion and absorption, (5) patient's anatomy (e.g., feeding tube placement is not possible in some very obese patients), and (6) whether a surgical intervention is planned.

In a **closed enteral system** the container or bag is prefilled with sterile liquid formula by the manufacturer, and is ready to administer. In an **open enteral system**, the person administering the feeding must open and pour the feeding into the container or bag. Both systems are effective when sanitation is a priority. **Hang time** is the length of time an enteral formula is considered safe for delivery to the patient; most facilities allow a 4 hour hang time before the product is changed for open systems and 24-48 hours for closed systems.

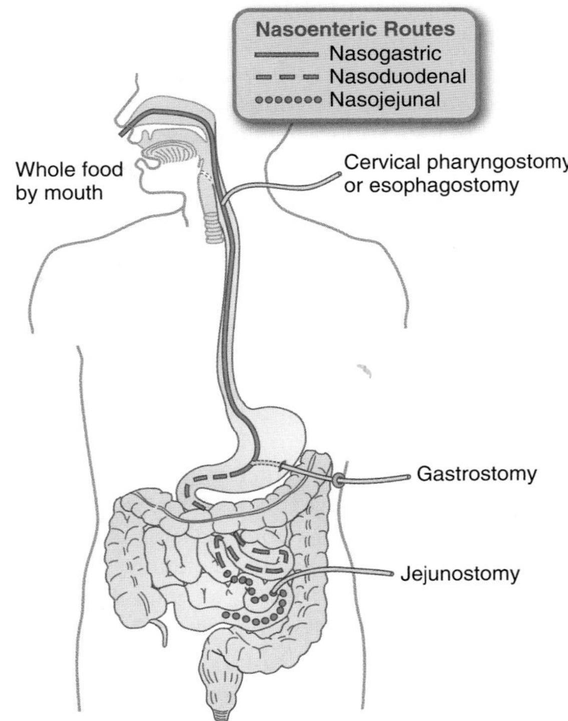

FIGURE 14-2 Diagram of enteral tube placement.

Short-Term Enteral Access

Nasogastric Route

Nasogastric tubes (NGTs) are the most common way to access the GIT. They are generally appropriate only for those requiring short-term EN, which is defined as 3 or 4 weeks. Typically, the tube is inserted at the bedside by a nurse or dietitian. The tube is passed through the nose into the stomach (Figure 14-2). Patients with normal gastrointestinal function tolerate this method, which takes advantage of normal digestive, hormonal, and bactericidal processes in the stomach. Rarely, complications can occur (Box 14-1).

NG feedings can be administered by bolus injection or by intermittent or continuous infusions (see "Administration" later in this chapter). Soft, flexible, and well-tolerated polyurethane or silicone tubes of various diameters, lengths, and design features may be used, depending on formula characteristics and feeding requirements. Tube placement is verified by aspirating gastric contents in combination with auscultation of air insufflation into the stomach or by radiographic confirmation of the tube tip location. Techniques for placing a tube are described by Metheny and Meert (2004).

BOX 14-1

Potential Complications of Nasoenteric Tubes

Esophageal strictures
Gastroesophageal reflux resulting in aspiration pneumonia
Incorrect position of the tube leading to pulmonary injury
Mucosal damage at the insertion site
Nasal irritation and erosion
Pharyngeal or vocal cord paralysis
Rhinorrhea, sinusitis
Ruptured gastroesophageal varices in hepatic disease
Ulcerations or perforations of the upper gastrointestinal tract and airway

Adapted from McClave SA et al: Guidelines for the provision and assessment of nutrition support therapy in the adult critically ill patient, JPEN J Parenter Enteral Nutr 33: 277, 2009.

Gastric versus Small-Bowel Feeding

The decision to use a small-bowel feeding tube versus a gastric tube is multifaceted. It is much easier to place tubes into the stomach; therefore gastric feedings generally result in a patient being fed sooner. However, ease of access is only one consideration. Gastric feedings may not be well tolerated, especially in critically ill patients (see Chapter 39).

Signs and symptoms of intolerance to gastric feeding include abdominal distention and discomfort; vomiting; and persistent, high gastric residuals (defined as more than 400 mL). Patients receiving gastric feedings are often thought to be at higher risk of aspiration pneumonia, but this is debatable (Bankhead et al., 2009).

Nasoduodenal or Nasojejunal Route

For those patients unable to tolerate gastric feedings who require relatively short-term nutrition support, a **nasoduodenal tube (NDT)** or a **nasojejunal tube (NJT)** is indicated. This requires that the tip of the tube pass through the pylorus and into the duodenum or pass all the way through the duodenum and into the jejunum. Positioning of these tubes requires one of the following techniques: (1) intraoperative placement (generally not just for the purpose of placing a feeding tube), (2) endoscopic or fluoroscopic guidance, (3) spontaneous placement that depends on a gastric tube migrating into the duodenum by peristalsis, or (4) bedside placement using a computer guidance system (Figure 14-3). Spontaneous migration of a gastric tube cannot be used for an NJT. Confirmation that the tube has migrated to the correct position can take several days and requires x-ray confirmation. This can result in delayed feedings

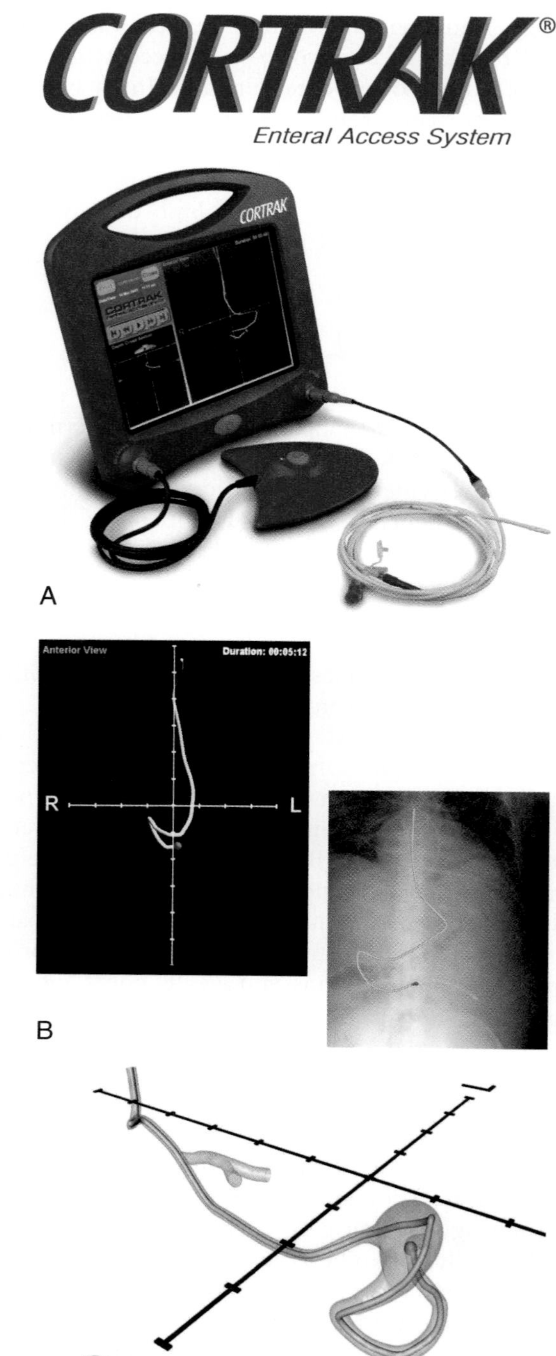

FIGURE 14-3 Computerized Cortrak tube feeding placement system. **A,** CORTRAK System; **B,** CORTRAK Anterior View compared to abdominal radiograph; **C,** 3-Dimensional graphic representation of a CORTRAK feeding tube in post pyloric position. *(Used with permission from CORPAK MedSystems.)*

Long-Term Enteral Access

Gastrostomy or Jejunostomy

When enteral feedings are necessary for more than 3-4 weeks, gastrostomy or jejunostomy should be considered to prevent some of the complications related to nasal and upper GIT irritation (see Box 14-1) and for the general comfort of the patient (Figure 14-4). These procedures can be done surgically and this may be the most efficient method if the patient is otherwise undergoing surgery (e.g., patients undergoing esophagectomies commonly have jejunal feeding tubes placed at the time of surgery). Nonoperative procedures are now far more common.

The **percutaneous endoscopic gastrostomy (PEG)** is a nonsurgical technique for placing a tube directly into the stomach through the abdominal wall; the technique is performed using an endoscope, with the patient under local anesthesia. Tubes are endoscopically guided from the mouth into the stomach or the jejunum and then brought out through the abdominal wall. The short procedural time required for insertion, limited need for anesthesia, and minimum wound complications also make it preferable for the physician and others caring for the patient.

PEG tubes used are generally large bore (feeding tubes are measured as **french size**), making clogging less likely. It is possible to convert a PEG to a **gastrojejunostomy** by threading a small-bore tube through the PEG tube into the jejunum using either fluoroscopy or endoscopy. PEGs may have a short piece of tubing that can be used to inject feedings with a syringe or to connect to a feeding bag. PEGs that are "low profile" are flush to the skin. These feeding tubes, also known as "buttons", are a good choice

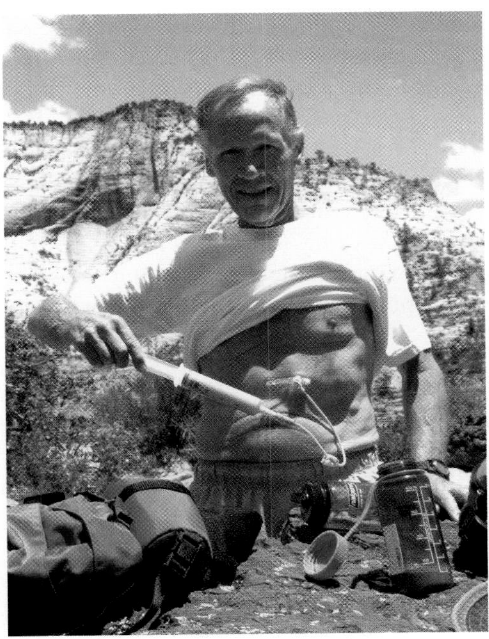

FIGURE 14-4 A man with a gastrostomy tube out hiking. *(From Oley Foundation, Albany NY www.oley.org.)*

for those patients prone to pulling on their tubes (e.g., children, older adults with dementia). They are also beneficial for those who are active and want to avoid the bulkiness of a feeding tube under their clothing.

Other Minimally Invasive Techniques

High-resolution video cameras have made percutaneous radiologic and laparoscopic gastrostomy and jejunostomy enteral access an option for patients in whom endoscopic procedures are contraindicated. Using fluoroscopy, a radiologic technique, tubes can be guided visually into the stomach or the jejunum and then brought out through the abdominal wall to provide the access route for enteral feedings. Laparoscopic or fluoroscopic techniques are used in some facilities and offer alternative options for enteral access (Nikolaidis, 2005).

Multiple Lumen Tubes

Gastrojejunal dual tubes are available for either endoscopic or surgical placement. These tubes are designed for patients in whom prolonged **gastrointestinal decompression** is anticipated. The **multiple lumen tube** has one **lumen** for decompression and one to feed into the small bowel. These tubes are used for early postoperative feeding.

Formula Content and Selection

A wide variety of enteral feeding products are commercially available. A **modular enteral feeding** is created by combining separate nutrient sources or by modifying existing formulas. For the most sterile product, it is best to use standardized commercial products and to avoid using multiple additives or drugs. The less the products are handled, the safer they are for the patient.

Enteral formulas can be classified as (1) standard **polymeric formula**; (2) elemental, predigested, or chemically defined; or 3) specialized. Many formulas are available within each of these categories. Hospitals and other health care institutions generally have a product formulary that determines which products can be used in that facility. The suitability of an enteral formula for a specific patient should be based on the functionality of the GIT, the clinical status of the patient, and the patient's nutrient needs. In some situations the cost of the formula is a major factor. In the past, **osmolality** was considered key to patient tolerance and the goal was to provide feedings that were the same osmolality as body fluids (290 mOsm/kg). However, studies done in the mid-1980s showed that patients can tolerate feedings with a wide variance of osmolarity.

Formulas are classified in a variety of ways, usually based on protein or overall macronutrient composition. Most patients with a variety of clinical conditions tolerate standard formulas intended to meet the nutritional requirements of general patient populations. The formulas are lactose-free, contain 1 to 1.2 kcal/mL, and are used as over-the-counter oral supplements and tube-feeding formulas. Some standard formulas are more concentrated to provide 1.5 to 2 kcal/mL when fluid restriction is required for patients with cardiopulmonary, renal, and hepatic failure, or for patients who have trouble tolerating high-volume feedings. Formulas intended for use as supplements to oral diets are flavored and contain simple sugars for palatability. See Appendix 32.

The Food and Drug Administration states that enteral formulas are a food; thus they are not under regulatory control. Manufacturers do not need to register their products with FDA nor get FDA approval before producing or selling them. Products are often introduced with little scientific evidence to support claims that are made. Evaluation of the suitability and efficacy of products, whether for individual or institutional use, is increasingly complex. A product making claims of pharmacologic effects must be evaluated using clinical evidence before a decision is made to use it (Box 14-2).

Protein

The amount of protein in enteral formulas varies from 6% to 25% of total kilocalories. The protein is typically derived from casein, whey, or soy protein isolate. Standard formulas provide intact protein, whereas elemental or predigested formulas have protein as di- and tripeptides and amino acids. The latter require less digestion. Specialized formulas may have the protein as crystalline amino acids for conditions such as renal or hepatic failure. These truly elemental formulas may also be used in the case of severe allergies. (Gottschlich 2006), In some cases specific amino acids have been added to enteral formulas. For example, arginine is added to renal products and critical care products because it is considered to be a conditionally essential amino acid in those clinical situations. See Chapter 39 for further discussion.

BOX 14-2

Factors to Consider When Choosing an Enteral Formula

Ability of the formula to meet the patient's nutritional requirements
Caloric and protein density of the formula (i.e., kcal/mL, g protein/mL, kcal : nitrogen ratio)
Gastrointestinal function of the patient
Presence of lactose, which may not be tolerated
Sodium, potassium, magnesium, and phosphorus content of the formula, especially in cardiopulmonary, renal, or hepatic failure
Type of protein, fat, carbohydrate, and fiber in the formula tolerable for the patient's digestive and absorptive capacity
Viscosity of the formula related to tube size and method of feeding

Carbohydrate

The percentage of total calories provided as carbohydrates in enteral formulas varies from 30% to 85% of kilocalories. Corn syrup solids are usually the carbohydrate found in standard formulas. Sucrose is added to flavored formulas that are meant for oral consumption. Hydrolyzed formulas have carbohydrate from cornstarch or maltodextrin. A recent innovation in the carbohydrate component of enteral formulas is fructooligosaccharides (FOS). These oligosaccharides are fermented to short-chain fatty acids and used as fuel by colonocytes (Charney, 2006).

Formulas are lactose-free. Lactose is not used as a carbohydrate source in most formulas because lactase deficiency is common in acutely ill patients. Fiber or carbohydrate that cannot be digested by human enzymes, although digested by colonic microflora into short-chain fatty acids, is frequently added to enteral formulas. Fibers are classified as water soluble (pectins and gums) or water insoluble (cellulose or hemicellulose) (see Chapters 1 and 3). The effectiveness of different fibers in enteral formulas used to treat gastrointestinal symptoms in acutely ill patients is controversial (see Chapter 39).

Lipid

Lipid varies from 1.5% to 55% of the total kilocalories in enteral formulas; between 15% and 30% of the total kilocalories of standard formulas are provided by lipids, usually from corn, soy, sunflower, safflower, or canola oils. Elemental formulas usually have minimum amounts of long-chain fat. Approximately 2% to 4% of daily energy intake from linoleic and linolenic acid is necessary to prevent **essential fatty acid deficiency (EFAD)**. The remainder of the fat in enteral formulas is in the form of long-chain and medium-chain triglycerides (MCTs). Formulas contain a combination of ω-3 fatty acids and ω-6 fatty acids. The ω-3 fatty acids include eicosapentaenoic acid and docosahexanoic acid. These are considered advantageous compared with ω-6 fatty acids because of their antiinflammatory effect; see Chapter 6.

MCTs can be added to enteral formulas because they do not require bile salts or pancreatic lipase for digestion and are absorbed directly into the portal circulation. Most formulas provide 0% to 85% of fat as MCTs. MCTs do not provide the essential linoleic or linolenic acids; they must therefore be provided in combination with long-chain triglycerides.

Vitamins, Minerals, and Electrolytes

Most, but not all available formulas are designed to meet the dietary reference intakes (DRIs) for vitamins and minerals if a sufficient volume is taken. However, DRIs are intended for healthy populations, not for acute or chronically ill people. Formulas intended for use in renal and hepatic failure are intentionally low in specific vitamins, minerals, and electrolytes. In contrast, disease-specific formulas often are supplemented with antioxidant vitamins and minerals with the intention of improving immune function and accelerating wound healing. Electrolytes are provided in relatively modest amounts compared with the oral diet and may require supplementation when diarrhea or drainage losses occur.

Fluid

Fluid needs for adults can be estimated at 1 mL of water per kilocalorie consumed, or 30 to 35 mL/kg of usual body weight (see Chapter 7). Without an additional source of fluid, tube-fed patients may not get enough free water to meet their needs, particularly when concentrated formulas are used. Standard (1 kcal/mL) formulas contain approximately 85% water by volume, but concentrated (2 kcal/mL) formulas contain only approximately 70% water by volume. All sources of fluid being given to a patient receiving EN, including feeding tube flushes, medications, and intravenous fluids, should be considered when determining and calculating a patient's intake. Additional water can be provided through the feeding tube as needed.

Administration

The three common methods of tube-feeding administration are (1) bolus feeding, (2) intermittent drip, and (3) continuous drip. Method selection is based on the patient's clinical status, living situation, and quality-of-life considerations. One method can serve as a transition to another method as the patient's status changes.

Bolus

The feeding modality of choice when patients are clinically stable with a functional stomach is the syringe bolus method (see Figure 14-4). Syringe **bolus feedings** administered in 5 to 20 minutes are more convenient and less expensive than pump or gravity bolus feedings, and should be encouraged when tolerated. A 60-mL syringe is used to infuse the formula. If bloating or abdominal discomfort develops, the patient is encouraged to wait 10 to 15 minutes before proceeding with the remainder of formula allocated for that feeding. Patients with normal gastric function can usually tolerate 500 mL of formula at each feeding. People receiving home EN may tolerate greater volumes of formula over time. Three or four bolus feedings per day can provide the daily nutritional requirements for most patients. Feedings should be at room temperature because cold formula can cause gastric discomfort.

Intermittent Drip

Quality-of-life issues are often the reason for the initiation of **intermittent drip feeding** regimens, which allow mobile patients more free time and autonomy compared with continuous drip infusions. These feedings can be given by pump or gravity drip. Gravity feeding is done by pouring formula into a feeding bag with a roller clamp. The clamp is adjusted to the desired drips per minute. A schedule is based on four to six feedings per day administered for 20 to 60 minutes. Formula administration is initiated at 100 to 150 mL per feeding and increased incrementally as tolerated. Success with this method of feeding depends largely on the degree of mobility, alertness, and motivation of the patient to tolerate the regimen.

Continuous Drip

Continuous drip infusion of formula requires a pump. This method is appropriate for patients who do not tolerate large-volume infusions during a given feeding such as those occurring with bolus or intermittent methods. Patients with compromised gastrointestinal function because of disease, surgery, cancer therapy, or other physiologic impediments are candidates for continuous drip infusion. Patients that are being fed into the small intestine should be fed only by continuous drip infusion. The feeding rate goal, in milliliters per hour, is set by dividing the total daily volume by the number of hours per day of administration (usually 18 to 24 hours). Feeding is started at one quarter to one half of the goal rate and is advanced every 8 to 12 hours to the final volume.

Formulas can generally be started at full strength; however, high osmolality formulas may require more time to achieve tolerance and should be advanced conservatively. Dilution of formulas is not necessary and can lead to underfeeding.

Modern enteral pumps are small and easy to handle. Many pumps are battery operated for up to 8 hours in addition to being electrically powered, allowing flexibility and mobility for the patient. Most pumps have a complete delivery system available, including bags and tubing compatible with proper pump operation.

Monitoring and Evaluation

Monitoring for Complications

Abdominal leakage of gastric contents from a gastrostomy site can cause skin erosion and skin breakdown, leading to infection and peritonitis; however, fewer than 10% of patients experience serious complications. Other complications can be prevented or managed with careful patient monitoring. Box 14-3 provides a comprehensive list of complications associated with EN.

Aspiration is a concern for patients receiving EN and is also a controversial topic because many experts believe

BOX 14-3

Complications of Enteral Nutrition

Access Problems

Leakage from ostomy/stoma site
Pressure necrosis/ulceration/stenosis
Tissue erosion
Tube displacement/migration
Tube obstruction

Administration Problems

Microbial contamination
Misplacement of tube, causing infection or aspiration pneumonia or peritonitis
Regurgitation

Gastrointestinal Complications

Constipation
Delayed gastric emptying
Diarrhea
- Osmotic diarrhea, especially if sorbitol is given in liquid drug preparations
- Secretory

Distention/bloating/cramping
Formula choice/rate of administration
High gastric residuals
Intolerance of nutrient components
Maldigestion/malabsorption
Medications
Nausea/vomiting
Treatment/therapies

Metabolic Complications

Drug-nutrient interactions
Glucose intolerance/hyperglycemia
Hydration status—dehydration/overhydration
Hypoalbuminemia
Hyponatremia
Hypoglycemia
Hyperkalemia/hypokalemia
Hyperphosphatemia/hypophosphatemia
Micronutrient deficiencies
Refeeding syndrome

Data from Hamaoui E, Kodsi R: Complications of enteral feeding and their prevention. In Rombeau JL, Rolandelli RH, editors: Clinical nutrition: enteral tube feeding, Philadelphia, 1997, Saunders; Merck Manual online. Accessed 29 May 2010 from http://www.merckmanuals.com/professional/sec01/ch003/ch003b.html.

the issue is not aspiration of formula into the airway, but aspiration of throat contents and saliva. To minimize the risk of aspiration, patients should be positioned with their heads and shoulders above their chests during and immediately after feeding (ASPEN, 2010, Bankhead et al., 2009).

There is confusion in the literature as to the efficacy of checking gastric residuals, because procedures are not standardized and the practice of checking residuals does not protect the patient from aspiration. Stable patients, especially those who have been fed by tube for long periods, do not need residuals checked regularly. Also, it is difficult to aspirate the stomach contents, and the residuals may contain more secretions and gastric fluids than formula. In critically ill patients the best methods for decreasing the risk of aspiration are elevating the head of the bed, continuous subglottic suctioning, and oral decontamination (American Dietetic Association, 2010; Bankhead et al., 2009).

Diarrhea is a common complication, often from colonic bacterial overgrowth, antibiotic therapy, and gastrointestinal motility disorders associated with acute and critical illness. Hyperosmolar medications such as magnesium-containing antacids, sorbitol-containing elixirs, and electrolyte supplements can also contribute to diarrhea. Adjustment of medications or administration methods can frequently correct the diarrhea. The addition of FOS, pectin, and other fibers, bulking agents, and antidiarrheal medications can also be beneficial. Use of a predigested formula can also be considered when managing diarrhea in a tube-fed patient.

Among stable patients receiving EN, constipation can become a problem. Fiber-containing formulas or stool-bulking medication may be helpful, and adequate fluid must be provided. Again, medications should be reviewed. Narcotic pain relievers have the side effect of slowing GIT activity. Gastrointestinal motility should be assessed because diarrhea can coexist with constipation, usually when there is also a fecal impaction.

Monitoring for Tolerance and Nutritional Intake Goals

Monitoring the patient's actual intake and tolerance is necessary to ensure that nutrition goals are achieved and maintained. Monitoring of metabolic and gastrointestinal tolerance, hydration status, and nutritional status is extremely important (Box 14-4). It is important to avoid use of blue dye to evaluate the contents of aspirate; the risks outweigh any perceived benefit (American Dietetic Association, 2010). Another concern is gastroparesis or high gastric residuals. In these cases, a promotility drug may be beneficial to increase gastrointestinal transit, improve EN delivery, and improve feeding tolerance (American Dietetic Association, 2010). The development and use of practice guidelines, institutional protocols, and standardized ordering procedures are helpful to ensure optimal, safe monitoring of EN (ASPEN, 2010).

It is important to monitor actual intake compared with prescribed intake. During routine patient care, feeding time is commonly lost from the prescribed feeding schedule as a result of (1) a dislodged tube, (2) gastrointestinal intolerance, (3) medical procedures requiring discontinuation of feeding, and (4) difficulties with the feeding tube position. When feedings must be turned off for long periods of time the result can be inadequate nutrition and adjustment in the tube feeding regimen should be made. For example, if tube feedings are being turned off for 2 hours every afternoon for physical therapy, the rate on the feeding should be turned up and the length of feeding time decreased to accommodate the therapy schedule.

BOX 14-4

Monitoring the Patient Receiving Enteral Nutrition

Abdominal distention and discomfort
Fluid intake and output (daily)
Gastric residuals (every 4 hr) if appropriate
Signs and symptoms of edema or dehydration (daily)
Stool output and consistency (daily)
Weight (at least 3 times/wk)
Nutritional intake adequacy (at least 2 times/wk)
Serum electrolytes, blood urea nitrogen, creatinine, (2-3 times/wk)
Serum glucose, calcium, magnesium, phosphorus, (weekly or as ordered)

Adapted from McClave SA et al: Guidelines for the provision and assessment of nutrition support therapy in the adult critically ill patient, JPEN J Parenter Enteral Nutr 33: 277, 2009.

PARENTERAL NUTRITION

PN provides nutrients directly into the bloodstream intravenously. PN is indicated when the patient requires nutrition support but is unable or unwilling to take adequate nutrients orally or enterally. PN may be used as an adjunct to oral or EN to meet nutrient needs. Alternatively, PN may be the sole source of nutrition during recovery from illness or injury, or may be a life-sustaining therapy for patients who have lost the function of their intestine for nutrient absorption. The practitioner must choose between central and peripheral access. *Central access* refers to catheter tip placement in a large, high-blood-flow vein such as the superior vena cava; this is **central parenteral nutrition (CPN)**. **Peripheral parenteral nutrition (PPN)** refers to catheter tip placement in a small vein, typically in the hand or forearm.

The osmolarity of the PN solution dictates the location of the catheter; central catheter placement allows for the higher caloric PN formulation and therefore greater osmolarity (Table 14-2). The use of PPN is limited in that it is short-term therapy with a minimum effect on nutritional status; the type and amount of fluids that can be provided peripherally do not fully meet nutrition requirements.

TABLE 14-2

Osmolarity of Nutrients in PN Solutions

Nutrient	Osmolarity (mOsm/mL)	Sample Calculations
Dextrose 5%	0.25	500 mL = 125 mOsm
Dextrose 10%	0.505	500 mL = 252 mOsm
Dextrose 50%	2.52	500 mL = 1260 mOsm
Dextrose 70%	3.53	500 mL = 1765 mOsm
Amino Acids 8.5%	0.81	1000 mL = 810 mOsm
Amino Acids 10%	0.998	1000 mL = 998 mOsm
Lipids 10%	0.6	500 mL = 300 mOsm
Lipids 20%	0.7	500 mL = 350 mOsm
Electrolytes	Varies by additive	
Multitrace elements	0.36	5 mL = 1.8 mOsm
Multivitamin concentrate	4.11	10 mL = 41 mOsm

Data from RxKinetics: Calculating osmolarity of an IV admixture. Accessed 29 May 2010 from http://www.rxkinetics.com/iv_osmolarity.html.

Volume-sensitive patients such as those with cardiopulmonary, renal, or hepatic failure are not good candidates for PPN. PPN may be appropriate when used as a supplemental feeding or in transition to enteral or oral feeding, or as a temporary method to begin feeding when central access has not been initiated. Calculation of the osmolarity of a parenteral solution is important to ensure venous tolerance (Kumpf et al., 2005). **Osmolarity**, or mOsm/mL is used to calculate IV fluids rather than osmolality which is used for body fluids.

Access

Peripheral Access

Nutrient solutions not exceeding osmolalities of 800 to 900 mOsm/kg of solvent can be infused through a routine peripheral intravenous angiocatheter placed in a vein in good condition (Matarese and Steiger, 2006). Protocols for dressing changes and rotation of the site are used to prevent thrombophlebitis, the principal complication of peripheral catheters.

A beneficial development in peripheral catheter technology is the **extended dwell catheter**. These catheters are sometimes called *midline* or *midclavicular catheters*, depending on their position. Extended dwell catheters require a vein large enough to advance the catheter 5 to 7 inches into the vein. These catheters can remain at the original site for 3 to 6 weeks and make PPN a more feasible option in patients with veins large enough to tolerate the catheter (Krzywda et al., 2005).

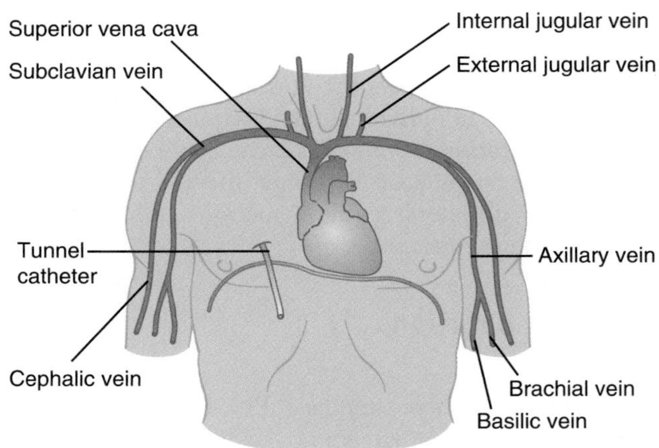

FIGURE 14-5 Venous sites from which the superior vena cava may be accessed.

Short-Term Central Access

Catheters used for CPN ideally consist of a single lumen. If central access is needed for other reasons, such as hemodynamic monitoring, drawing blood samples, or giving medications, multiple-lumen catheters are available. To reduce the risk of infection, the catheter lumen used to infuse CPN should be reserved for that purpose only. Catheters are most commonly inserted into the subclavian vein and advanced until the catheter tip is in the superior vena cava, using strict aseptic technique. Alternatively, an internal or external jugular vein catheter can be used with the same catheter tip placement. However, the motion of the neck makes this site much more difficult for maintaining the sterility of a dressing. Radiologic verification of the tip site is necessary before infusion of nutrients can begin. Strict infection control protocols should be used for catheter placement and maintenance (Krzywda et al., 2005). Figure 14-5 shows alternative venous access sites for CPN; femoral placement is also possible.

A **peripherally inserted central catheter (PICC or PIC)** may be used for short- or moderate-term infusion in the hospital or in the home. This catheter is inserted into a vein in the antecubital area of the arm and threaded into the subclavian vein with the catheter tip placed in the superior vena cava. Trained nonphysicians can insert a PICC, whereas placement of a tunneled catheter is a surgical procedure (Krzywda et al., 2005). All catheters must have radiologic confirmation of the placement of the catheter tip prior to initiating any infusion.

Long-Term Central Access

A commonly used long-term catheter is a "tunneled" catheter. This single- or multiple-lumen catheter is placed in the cephalic, subclavian, or internal jugular vein and fed into the superior vena cava. A subcutaneous tunnel is created so that the catheter exits the skin several inches from its venous entry site. This allows the patient to care for the catheter more easily as is necessary for long-term infusion. Another type of long-term catheter is a surgically implanted port under the skin where the catheter would normally exit at the end of the subcutaneous tunnel. A special needle must access the entrance port. Ports can be single or double; an individual port is equivalent to a lumen. Both tunneled catheters and PICCs can be used for extended therapy in the hospital or for home infusion therapy. Care of long-term catheters requires specialized handling and extensive patient education.

Parenteral Solutions

Protein

Commercially available standard PN solutions are composed of all the essential amino acids and only some of the nonessential crystalline amino acids. Nonessential nitrogen is provided principally by the amino acids alanine and glycine, usually without aspartate, glutamate, cysteine, and taurine. Specialized solutions with adjusted amino acid content that contain taurine are available for infants, for whom taurine is thought to be conditionally essential.

The concentration of amino acids in PN solutions ranges from 3% to 20% by volume. Thus a 10% solution of amino acids supplies 100 g of protein per liter (1000 mL). The percentage of a solution is usually expressed at its final concentration after dilution with other nutrient solutions. The caloric content of amino acid solutions is approximately 4 kcal/g of protein provided. Approximately 15% to 20% of total energy intake should come from protein (Kumpf et al., 2005).

Specialized solutions for patients with renal or liver disease are available, but are used infrequently because of their expense and the lack of conclusive research data supporting their efficacy. Recently, the amino acid glutamine has been suggested as an additive for patients requiring PN in the critical care setting (Martindale, 2009). Glutamine is not yet readily available in a commercial form and is therefore not routinely added to PN formulations.

Carbohydrates

Carbohydrates are supplied as dextrose monohydrate in concentrations ranging from 5% to 70% by volume. The dextrose monohydrate yields 3.4 calories per gram. As with amino acids, a 10% solution yields 100 g of carbohydrates per liter of solution. The use of carbohydrates (100 g daily for a 70-kg person) ensures that protein is not catabolized for energy during conditions of normal metabolism.

Maximum rates of carbohydrate administration should not exceed 5 to 6 mg/kg/min in critically ill patients. When PN solutions provide 15% to 20% of total calories as protein, 20% to 30% of total calories as lipid, and the balance from carbohydrate (dextrose), infusion of dextrose should not exceed this amount. Excessive administration can lead to hyperglycemia, hepatic abnormalities, or increased ventilatory drive (see Chapter 35).

Lipid

Lipid emulsions, available in 10%, 20%, and 30% concentrations, are composed of aqueous suspensions of soybean or safflower oil, with egg yolk phospholipid as the emulsifier. Lipid emulsions should not be used when a patient has an egg allergy. The three-carbon molecule, glycerol, which is water soluble, is added to the emulsion. Glycerol is oxidized and yields 4.3 kcal/g.

Dietitians may be asked to calculate what the patient is receiving. A 10% emulsion provides 1.1 kcal/mL, a 20% emulsion provides 2 kcal/mL, and 30% emulsion provides 2.9 kcal/mL. Providing 20% to 30% of total calories as lipid emulsion should result in a daily dosage of approximately 1 g of fat per kilogram of body weight. Administration should not exceed 2.5 g of lipid emulsion per kilogram of body weight per day. In the hospital lipid is infused during 24 hours when mixed with the dextrose and amino acids. Alternatively, lipids can be provided separately by infusion via an infusion pump. For adult patients receiving PN at home, the PN will most often be infused during 10-12 hours per day with the lipid as part of the PN solution.

Approximately 10% of calories per day from fat emulsions provide the 2% to 4% of calories from linoleic acid required to prevent EFAD. Soybean and safflower oils are rich sources of linoleic acid, providing approximately 40%. Linoleic acid alters prostaglandin metabolism, thereby producing both proinflammatory and immunosuppressive effects, particularly at high doses and at faster infusion rates (Mizock and DeMichele, 2004). Therefore it is important not to use high doses of linoleic acid in the solutions.

Electrolytes, Vitamins, Trace Elements

General guidelines for daily requirements for electrolytes are given in Table 14-3, for vitamins in Table 14-4, and for trace elements in Table 14-5. Parenteral solutions also represent a significant portion of total daily fluid and electrolyte intake. Once a solution is prescribed and initiated, adjustments for proper fluid and electrolyte balance may be necessary, depending on the stability of the patient. The choice of the salt form of electrolytes (e.g., chloride, acetate) affects acid-base balance.

TABLE 14-3

Daily Electrolyte Requirements During Total Parenteral Nutrition—Adults

Electrolyte	Standard Intake/Day
Calcium	10-15 mEq
Magnesium	8-20 mEq
Phosphate	20-40 mmol
Sodium	1-2 mEq/kg + replacement
Potassium	1-2 mEq/kg
Acetate	As needed to maintain acid-base balance
Chloride	As needed to maintain acid-base balance

From McClave SA et al: Guidelines for the provision and assessment of nutrition support therapy in the adult critically ill patient, JPEN J Parenter Enteral Nutr 33:277, 2009.

TABLE 14-4

Adult Parenteral Multivitamins: Comparison of Guidelines and Products

Vitamin	NAG-AMA Guidelines	FDA Requirements	MVI-12	MVI-13 (Infuvite) Baxter
A (retinol)	3300 units (1 mg)	3300 units (1 mg)	3300 units (1 mg)	3300 units (1 mg)
D (ergocalciferol cholecalciferol))	200 units (5 mcg)	200 units (5 mcg)	200 units (5 mcg)	200 units (5 mcg)
E (mcg-tocopherol)	10 units (10 mg)	10 units (10 mg)	10 units (10 mg)	10 units (10 mg)
B_1 (thiamin)	3 mg	6 mg	3 mg	6 mg
B_2 (riboflavin)	3.6 mg	3.6 mg	3.6 mg	3.6 mg
B_3 (niacinamide)	40 mg	40 mg	40 mg	40 mg
B_5 (dexpanthenol)	15 mg	15 mg	15 mg	15 mg
B_6 (pyridoxine)	4 mg	6 mg	4 mg	6 mg
B_{12} (cyanocobalamin)	5 mcg	5 mcg	5 mcg	5 mcg
C (ascorbic acid)	100 mg	200 mg	100 mg	200 mg
Biotin	60 mcg	60 mcg	60 mcg	60 mcg
Folic acid	400 mcg	600 mcg	400 mcg	600 mcg
K		150 mcg	0	150 mcg

From Fed Reg 66(77), 2000.

AMA, American Medical Association; *FDA,* U.S. Food and Drug Administration; *MVI-12* and *MVI-13,* multivitamin supplements; *NAG,* National Advisory Group.

TABLE 14-5

Daily Trace Element Supplementation for Adult Parenteral Formulations

Trace Element	Intake
Chromium	10-15 mcg
Copper	0.3-0.5 mg
Manganese	60-100 mcg
Zinc	2.5-5.0 mg
Selenium	20-60 mcg

Because parenterally administered vitamins and trace elements do not go through the digestive and absorptive processes, these recommendations are lower than the DRIs. Recently a review of the micronutrient needs of patients receiving PN, especially those receiving long-term home parenteral nutrition (HPN), has raised awareness of the need for careful review of patient requirements compared with the content of current trace element formulations. Monitoring of manganese and chromium status is recommended for patients receiving PN for longer than 6 months (Buchman, 2009). Iron is not normally part of parenteral infusions because it is not compatible with lipids and may enhance certain bacterial growth. Additionally, care must be taken to ensure that a patient can tolerate the separate iron infusion. When patients receive iron on an outpatient basis, the first dose should be done in a controlled setting (such as an outpatient infusion suite) to observe for any reactions that the patient might experience.

Fluid

Fluid needs for PN or EN are calculated similarly. Maximum volumes of CPN rarely exceed 3 L, with typical prescriptions of 1.5 to 3 L daily. In critically ill patients volumes of prescribed CPN should be closely coordinated with their overall care plan. The administration of other medical therapies requiring fluid administration, such as intravenous medications and blood products, necessitates careful monitoring. Patients with cardiopulmonary, renal, and hepatic failure are especially sensitive to fluid administration. For HPN, higher volumes may be best provided in separate infusions. For example, if additional fluid is required as a result of high output by the patient, then a liter bag of intravenous fluid containing minimal electrolytes may be infused during a short time during the day if the PN is infused over night. See Appendix 32 on calculating PN prescriptions.

Compounding Methods

PN prescriptions have historically required preparation or compounding by competent pharmacy personnel under laminar airflow hoods using aseptic techniques. Hospitals may have their own compounding pharmacy or may purchase PN solutions that have been compounded outside the hospital in a central location, and then returned to the hospital for distribution to individual patients. A third method of providing PN solutions is to utilize multichamber bag technology whereby solutions are manufactured in a quality-controlled environment using good manufacturing processes. These PN solutions are standardized but are available in multiple formulas with varying amounts of dextrose and amino acids, making them suitable for CPN or

PPN infusion. They contain conservative amounts of electrolytes or may be electrolyte free. These products have a shelf life of 2 years and do not need to be refrigerated unless the product covering has been opened to reveal the infusion bag (Figure 14-6). Institutions frequently use standardized solutions, which are compounded in batches, thus saving labor and lowering costs; however, flexibility for individualized compounding should be available when warranted (Kumpf et al., 2005).

Prescriptions for PN are compounded in two general ways. One method compounds all components except the fat emulsion, which is infused separately. Solutions are usually mixed in one bag at a 1:1 dextrose-to-amino acid volume ratio. The second method combines the lipid emulsion with the dextrose and amino acid solution and is referred to as a **total nutrient admixture** or **3-in-1** solution. The PN Safe Practices Guidelines provide practitioners with information on many techniques and procedures that enhance safety and prevent mistakes in the preparation of PN (Seres, 2006).

A number of medications, including antibiotics, vasopressors, narcotics, diuretics, and many other commonly administered drugs, can be compounded with PN solutions. In practice this occurs infrequently because it requires specialized knowledge of physical compatibility or incompatibility of the solution contents. The most common drug additives are insulin for persistent hyperglycemia and histamine-2 antagonists to avoid gastroduodenal stress ulceration (Kumpf et al., 2005). One other consideration is that the PN usually is ordered 24 hours prior to its administration, and patient status may have changed.

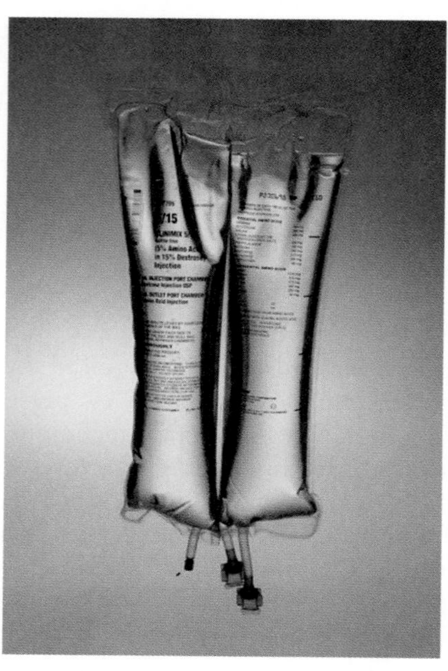

FIGURE 14-6 Baxter Clinimix Compounding System. *(Image provided by Baxter Healthcare Corporation. CLINIMIX is a trademark of Baxter International Inc.)*

Administration

The methods used to administer PN are addressed after the goal infusion rate, based on calculations, has been established. PN calculations and orders are inherently complex and protocols for ordering PN vary considerably among institutions. Nevertheless, general considerations as listed in Box 14-5 can be applied to almost any protocol.

Continuous Infusion

Parenteral solutions are usually initiated below the goal infusion rate via a volumetric pump and then increased incrementally over a 2- or 3-day period to attain the goal infusion rate. Some practitioners start PN based on the amount of dextrose, with initial prescriptions containing 100 to 200 g daily and advancing over a 2- or 3-day period to a final goal. With high dextrose concentrations, abrupt cessation of CPN should be avoided, particularly if the patient's glucose tolerance is abnormal. If CPN is to be stopped, it is prudent to taper the rate of infusion in an unstable patient to prevent **rebound hypoglycemia**, low blood sugar levels resulting from abrupt cessation. For most stable patients this is not necessary.

Cyclic Infusion

Individuals who require PN at home will benefit from a cyclic infusion; this entails infusion of PN for 8- to 12-hour periods, usually at night. This allows the person to have a free period of 12 to 16 hours each day, which may improve quality of life. The goal cycle for infusion time is established incrementally when a higher rate of infusion or a more concentrated solution is required. Cycled infusions should not be attempted if glucose intolerance or fluid tolerance is a problem. The pumps used for home infusion of PN are small and convenient, allowing mobility during daytime infusions. Administration time may be decreased because of patient ambulation and bathing, tests or other treatments, intravenous administration of medications, or other therapies.

Monitoring and Evaluation

As with enteral feeding, routine monitoring of PN is necessary more frequently for the patient receiving PN in the hospital. For patients receiving HPN, initial monitoring is done on a weekly basis or less frequently as the patient becomes more stable on PN. Monitoring is done not only to evaluate response to therapy, but to ensure compliance with the treatment plan.

The primary complication associated with PN is infection (Box 14-6). Therefore strict adherence to protocols and monitoring for signs of infection such as chills, fever, tachycardia, sudden hyperglycemia, or elevated white blood cell count are necessary. Monitoring of metabolic tolerance is also critical. Electrolytes, acid-base balance, glucose tolerance, renal function, and cardiopulmonary and **hemodynamic stability** (maintenance of adequate blood pressure) can be affected by PN and should be monitored

BOX 14-5

Nutrition Care Process for Enteral and Parenteral Nutrition

Assessment

1. Clinical status, including medications
2. Fluid requirement
3. Route of administration
4. Energy (kcal) requirement
5. Protein requirement
6. Carbohydrate/lipid considerations
7. Micronutrient considerations
8. Formula selection or PN solution considerations
   - A. Concentration (osmolarity)
   - B. Protein content
   - C. Carbohydrate/lipid content
   - D. Micronutrient content
   - E. Special formula considerations
9. Calculations
   - A. Energy: use kcal/mL formula
   - B. Protein: use g/1000 mL
   - C. Fat and micronutrient considerations: units/1000 mL
   - D. Fluid considerations: extra water, IV fluids (including medications)

Nutrition Diagnosis

1. Identify the problems affecting oral nutritional intake.
2. Identify problems related to access or administration of tube feedings.
3. Write PES statements. These may include inadequate or excess infusion of enteral or parenteral nutrition, or other nutrition diagnoses.

Intervention

1. Each problem should have an intervention and a way to evaluate it.
2. Recommend what method and how to begin feedings.
3. Recommend how to advance feedings.
4. Determine how fluids will be given in adequate amounts.
5. Calculate final feeding prescription.

Monitoring and Evaluation

1. Describe clinical signs and symptoms to monitor for feeding tolerance.
2. List laboratory values and other measurements to be monitored.
3. Determine how feeding outcomes will be evaluated.

IV, Intravenous; *PES*, problem, etiology, and signs and symptoms; *PN*, parenteral nutrition.

BOX 14-6

Parenteral Nutrition Complications

Mechanical Complications

Air embolism
Arteriovenous fistula
Brachial plexus injury
Catheter fragment embolism
Catheter misplacement
Cardiac perforation
Central vein thrombophlebitis
Endocarditis
Hemothorax
Hydromediastinum
Hydrothorax
Pneumothorax or tension pneumothorax
Subcutaneous emphysema
Subclavian artery injury
Subclavian hematoma
Thoracic duct injury

Infection and Sepsis

Catheter entrance site
Catheter seeding from bloodborne or distant infection
Contamination during insertion
Long-term catheter placement
Solution contamination

Metabolic Complications

Dehydration from osmotic diuresis
Electrolyte imbalance
Essential fatty acid deficiency
Hyperosmolar, nonketotic, hyperglycemic coma
Hyperammonemia
Hypercalcemia
Hyperchloremic metabolic acidosis
Hyperlipidemia
Hyperphosphatemia
Hypocalcemia
Hypomagnesemia
Hypophosphatemia
Rebound hypoglycemia on sudden cessation of PN in patient with unstable glucose levels
Uremia
Trace mineral deficiencies

Gastrointestinal Complications

Cholestasis
Gastrointestinal villous atrophy
Hepatic abnormalities

Adapted from McClave SA et al: Guidelines for the provision and assessment of nutrition support therapy in the adult critically ill patient, JPEN J Parenter Enteral Nutr 33: 277, 2009.

PN, Parenteral nutrition.

TABLE 14-6

Inpatient Parenteral Nutrition Monitoring

Variable to Be Monitored	Suggested Frequency	
	Initial Period*	**Later Period***
Weight	Daily	Weekly
Serum electrolytes	Daily	1-2/wk
Blood urea nitrogen	3-wk	Weekly
Serum total calcium or ionized Ca^+, inorganic phosphorus, magnesium	3-wk	Weekly
Serum glucose	Daily	3-wk
Serum triglycerides	Weekly	Weekly
Liver function enzymes	3-wk	Weekly
Hemoglobin, hematocrit	Weekly	Weekly
Platelets	Weekly	Weekly
WBC count	As indicated	As indicated
Clinical status	Daily	Daily
Catheter site	Daily	Daily
Temperature	Daily	Daily
I&O	Daily	Daily

McClave SA et al: Guidelines for the provision and assessment of nutrition support therapy in the adult critically ill patient, JPEN J Parenter Enteral Nutr 33:277, 2009.

I&O, Intake and output; *WBC,* white blood cell.

*Initial period is that period in which a full glucose intake is being achieved. Later period implies that the patient had achieved a steady metabolic state. In the presence of metabolic instability, the more intensive monitoring outlined under initial period should be followed.

I&O refers to all fluids going into the patient: oral, intravenous, medication; and all fluid coming out: urine, surgical drains, exudates.

carefully. Table 14-6 lists parameters that should be monitored routinely.

The CPN catheter site is a potential source for introduction of microorganisms into a major vein. Protocols to prevent infection vary and should follow Centers for Disease Control Prevention guidelines (Centers for Disease Control and Prevention [CDC] and O'Grady, 2002). Catheter care and prevention of catheter-related bloodstream infections are of utmost importance in both the hospital and alternate settings. These infections are not only costly but may be life-threatening. Catheter care is dictated by the site of the catheter and the setting in which the patient receives care.

REFEEDING SYNDROME

Patients who require enteral or PN therapies may have been eating poorly prior to initiating therapy because of the disease process and may be moderately to severely malnourished. Aggressive administration of nutrition, particularly via the intravenous route, can precipitate **refeeding syndrome** with severe, potentially lethal electrolyte fluctuations involving metabolic, hemodynamic, and neuromuscular problems. Refeeding syndrome occurs when energy substrates, particularly carbohydrate, are introduced into the plasma of anabolic patients (Parrish, 2009).

Proliferation of new tissue requires increased amounts of glucose, potassium, phosphorus, magnesium, and other nutrients essential for tissue growth. If intracellular electrolytes are not supplied in sufficient quantity to keep up with tissue growth, low serum levels of potassium, phosphorus, and magnesium develop. Low levels of these electrolytes are the hallmark of refeeding syndrome, especially hypokalemia. Carbohydrate metabolism by cells also causes a shift of electrolytes to the intracellular space as glucose moves into cells for oxidation. Rapid infusion of carbohydrate stimulates insulin release, which reduces salt and water excretion and increases the chance of cardiac and pulmonary complications from fluid overload.

Patients starting on PN who have received minimal nutrition for a significant period should be monitored closely for electrolyte fluctuation and fluid overload. A review of baseline laboratory values, including glucose, magnesium, potassium, and phosphorus should be completed and any abnormalities corrected prior to initiating nutrition support, particularly PN. Conservative amounts of carbohydrate and adequate amounts of intracellular electrolytes should be provided. The initial PN formulation should usually contain 25% to 50% of goal dextrose concentration and be increased slowly to avoid the consequences of hypophosphatemia, hypokalemia, and hypomagnesemia. PN compatibilities must be assessed when very low levels of dextrose are provided with higher levels of amino acids and electrolytes. The syndrome also occurs in enterally fed patients, but less often because of the effects of the digestive process.

In managing the nutrition care process, refeeding syndrome is an undesirable outcome that requires monitoring and evaluation. Most often, the nutrition diagnosis may be "excessive carbohydrate intake" or "excessive infusion from enteral or parenteral nutrition" in the undernourished patient. Thus, in the early phase of refeeding, nutrient prescriptions should be moderate in carbohydrate and supplemented with phosphorus, potassium, and magnesium (Kraft et al., 2005).

TRANSITIONAL FEEDING

All nutrition support care plans strive to use the GIT when possible, either with EN or by a total or partial return to oral intake. Therefore patient care plans frequently involve **transitional feeding**, moving from one type of feeding to another, with several feeding methods used simultaneously while continuously administering estimated nutrient requirements. This requires careful monitoring of patient tolerance and quantification of intake from parenteral, enteral, and oral routes. Most experts advise that initial oral diets be low in simple carbohydrates and fat, as well as lactose free. These provisions make digestion easier and minimize the possibility of osmotic diarrhea. Attention to individual tolerance and food preferences also helps maximize intake.

Parenteral to Enteral Feeding

To begin the transition from PN to EN, introduce a minimal amount of enteral feeding at a low rate of 30 to 40 mL/hr to establish gastrointestinal tolerance. When there is severe gastrointestinal compromise, predigested formula to initiate enteral feedings may be better tolerated. Once formula has been given during a period of hours, the parenteral rate can be decreased to keep the nutrient levels at the same prescribed amount. As the enteral rate is increased by 25 to 30 mL/hr increments every 8 to 24 hours, the parenteral prescription is reduced accordingly. Once the patient is tolerating about 75% of nutrient needs by the enteral route, the PN solution can be discontinued. This process ideally takes 2 to 3 days; however, it may become more complicated, depending on the degree of gastrointestinal function. At times the weaning process may not be practical, and PN can be stopped sooner, depending on overall treatment decisions and likelihood for tolerance of enteral feeding.

Parenteral to Oral Feeding

The transition from parenteral to oral feeding is ideally accomplished by monitoring oral intake and concomitantly decreasing the PN to maintain a stable nutrient intake. Approximately 75% of nutrient needs should be met consistently by oral intake before the PN is discontinued. The process is less predictable than the transition to enteral feeding. Variations include the patient's appetite, motivation, and general well being. It is important to continue monitoring the patient for adequate oral intake once PN has been stopped and to initiate alternate nutrition support if necessary. Generally patients are transitioned from clear liquids to a diet that is low in fiber and fat and is lactose free. It takes several days for the GIT to regain function; during that time, the diet should be composed of easily digested foods.

Special nutrient needs may be employed, especially when transitioning a patient with gastrointestinal disorders such as short bowel syndrome. Specialized nutrients, optimized drug therapy, and nutrition counseling should be comprehensive to improve outcome. Some PN patients may not be able to fully discontinue PN, but may be able to use PN less than 7 days per week, necessitating careful attention to nutrient intake. A skilled registered dietitian (RD) can coordinate diet and PN needs for this type of patient (Matarese and Steiger, 2006).

Enteral to Oral Feeding

A stepwise decrease is also used to transition from EN to oral feeding. It is effective to move from continuous feeding to a 12- and then an 8-hour formula administration cycle during the night; this reestablishes hunger and satiety cues for oral intake during daytime. In practice, oral diets are often tried after inadvertent or deliberate removal of a nasoenteric tube. This type of interrupted transition should be monitored closely for adequate oral intake. Patients receiving EN who desire to eat and for whom it is not contraindicated can be encouraged to do so. A transition from liquids to easy-to-digest foods may be necessary during a period of days. Patients who cannot meet their needs by the oral route can be maintained by a combination of EN and oral intake.

Oral Supplements

The most common types of oral supplements are commercial formulas meant primarily to augment the intake of solid foods. They often provide approximately 250 kcal/8-oz or 240-mL portion and approximately 8 to 14 g of intact protein. Some products have 360 or 500 or as much as 575 kcal in a can. There are different types of products for different disease states.

Fat sources are often long-chain triglycerides, although some supplements contain MCTs. More concentrated and thus more nutrient-dense formulas are also available. A variety of flavors, consistencies, and modifications of nutrients are appropriate for various disease states. Some oral supplements provide a nutritionally complete diet if taken in sufficient volume.

The form of carbohydrate is a key factor to patient acceptance and tolerance. Supplements with appreciable amounts of simple carbohydrate taste sweeter and have higher osmolalities, which may contribute to gastrointestinal intolerance. Individual taste preferences vary widely, and normal taste is altered by certain drug therapies, especially chemotherapy. Concentrated formulas or large volumes can contribute to taste fatigue and early satiety. Thus both oral dietary intake and the actual intake of prescribed supplements should be monitored.

Oral supplements that contain hydrolyzed protein and free amino acids such as those developed for patients with renal, liver, and malabsorptive diseases tend to be mildly to markedly unpalatable, and acceptance by the patient depends on motivation. Some of these formulas also lack sufficient vitamins and minerals and are not nutritionally complete.

Although commercially available supplements are most commonly used for convenience, modules of protein, carbohydrate, or fat or commonly available food items can produce highly palatable additions to a diet. As examples, liquid or powdered milk, yogurt, tofu, or protein powders can be used to enrich cereals, casseroles, soups, or milk shakes. Thickening agents are now used to add variety, texture, and aesthetics to pureed foods, which are used when swallowing ability is limited (see Chapter 41). Imagination and individual tailoring can increase oral intake, avoiding the necessity for more complex forms of nutrition support.

NUTRITION SUPPORT IN LONG-TERM AND HOME CARE

Long-Term Care

Long-term care (LTC) generally refers to a skilled nursing facility. Health care provided in this environment focuses on quality of life, self-determination, and management of acute and chronic disease. Indications for EN and PN are generally the same for older patients as for younger adults, and varies according to the age, gender, and disease state of the individual. PN and EN are often provided to these facilities by offsite pharmacies that specialize in LTC. These providers may employ dietitians and specially trained nurses to assist the facilities with education and training on PEN.

Advance directives are legal documents that residents use to state their preferences about aspects of care, including those regarding the use of nutrition support. These directives may be written in any setting, including acute or home care, but are especially useful in LTC to guide interventions on behalf of long-term care residents when they are no longer able to make decisions.

Differentiation between the effects of advanced age versus malnutrition is an assessment challenge for dietitians working in long-term care (Raymond, 2006). This is an area of active research, as is the influence that nutrition support has on the quality of life among long-term care residents. Studies generally show that use of nutrition support in older adults is beneficial, especially when used in conjunction with physical activity. However, when there is a terminal illness or condition, starting nutrition support may have no advantage and may prolong suffering in some cases. It is prudent for dietitians to be involved in ethical decisions according to the policies of their institutions.

Home Care

Home enteral nutrition (HEN) or **home parenteral nutrition (HPN)** support usually entails the provision of nutrients or formulas, supplies, equipment, and professional clinical services. Resources and technology for safe and effective management of long-term enteral or parenteral therapy are widely available for the home-care setting. Although home nutrition support has been available for more than 20 years, few outcome data have been generated. Because mandatory reporting requirements do not exist in the United States for patients receiving home nutrition support, the exact number of patients receiving this support is unknown.

The elements needed to implement home nutrition successfully include identification of appropriate candidates and a feasible home environment with responsive caregivers, a choice of a suitable nutrition support regimen, training of the patient and family, and a plan for medical and nutritional follow-up by the physician as well as by the home infusion provider (Box 14-7). These objectives are best achieved through coordinated efforts of an interdisciplinary team (see *Clinical Insight:* Home Tube Feeding—Key Considerations).

Patients receiving HEN may receive supplies only, or formula and supplies with or without clinical oversight by the provider. Many enteral patients receive services from a **durable medical equipment (DME) provider** that may or may not provide clinical services. A home infusion provider provides intravenous therapies, including home PN, intravenous antibiotics, and other therapies. Home nursing agencies may be associated with a DME company or a home infusion agency to provide nursing services to home EN or PN patients. Often the patient's reimbursement source for home therapy plays a major role in determining the type of home infusion provider. In fact, reimbursement is a key component of a patient's ability to receive home therapy of any kind and should be evaluated early in the care plan so that appropriate decisions can be made prior to discharge or initiating a therapy (Wojtylak, 2007).

Companies that provide home infusion services for EN or PN may be private or affiliated with acute care facilities. Criteria for selecting a home-care company to provide nutrition support should be based on the company's ability

BOX 14-7

Considerations When Deciding on Home Nutrition Support

Sanitation of the home environment to preserve the patient's health and reduce risk of infection

Potential for improvement in quality of life and nutritional status

The financial and time commitment needed by patient or family; potential loss of income outside the home in some cases

Ability to understand the techniques for administration of the product and safe use of all equipment and supplies

Any physical limitations that prevent the implementation of HEN or HPN therapy

Capacity for patient or caregiver to contact medical services when needed

HEN, Home enteral nutrition; *HPN*, home parenteral nutrition.

CLINICAL INSIGHT

Home Tube Feeding—Key Considerations

What Is the Best Kind of Tube?

In general, nasal tubes should be avoided because they are more difficult to manage, clog easily, are easily dislodged, and over time can cause tissue irritation and even erosion. PEG tubes are now the most common and preferred method for home tube feedings. They can be either low-profile (flat to the abdomen), button-type tubes, or they can have a short piece of tubing attached through the abdomen and into the stomach. The button tubes require some manual dexterity to access and can be difficult to use for patients who are very obese. **Percutaneous endoscopic jejunostomy (PEJ)** tubes are best for patients who require postpyloric feedings as a result of intolerance of gastric feeding, but PEJ feedings require a pump, which severely limits mobility of the patient.

What Is the Best Method of Administration?

Bolus feeding is the easiest administration method and should generally be tried first. It should be started slowly at half of an 8-oz can four to six times a day. If bolus feeding is not tolerated, gravity feeding is a second option. It does require a bag and pole, but can be accomplished fairly quickly and requires less manual dexterity than bolus feeding.

Pump feeding is sometimes necessary when a patient requires small amounts of formula delivered slowly. Although it is well tolerated, it has major implications for a patient at home because even the simplest pump is often viewed as "high tech." Its use greatly limits mobility, and, like any piece of equipment, it can break and interrupt feeding schedules.

What is the Best Way to Educate the Patient and Caregiver?

Directions should be written in common measurements such as cups, tablespoons, and cans rather than milliliters.

The enteral nutrition regimen should be as simple as possible; use whole cans of formula rather than partial cans.

Additives to the feedings should be minimized to avoid confusion and clogging of the feedings tubes.

Provide clear directions for gradually increasing to the goal feeding rate.

Provide clear directions for water flushing of the tube and for additional water requirements to prevent dehydration.

Discuss common problems that may come up and provide guidance for resolving them.

Make sure that the patient or caregiver can demonstrate understanding of the feeding process by either explaining it or by doing it.

to provide ongoing monitoring, patient education, and coordination of care. When a patient is receiving home EN or PN, it is important to determine if the provider has an RD on staff or access to the services of a RD. The RD is uniquely qualified not only to provide oversight and monitoring for the patient while receiving EN or PN, but also to provide the appropriate nutrition counseling and food suggestions when the patient transitions between therapies (Fuhrman, 2009).

ETHICAL ISSUES

Whether to provide or withhold nutrition support is often a central issue in "end-of-life" decision making. For patients who are terminally ill or in a persistent vegetative state, nutrition support can extend life to the point that issues of quality of life and the patient's right to self-determination come into play. Often surrogate decision makers are involved in treatment decisions. The nutrition support practitioner has a responsibility to know whether documentation, such as a living will regarding the patient's wishes for nutrition support, is in the medical record and whether counseling and support resources for legal and ethical aspects of patient care are available to the patient and his or her significant others.

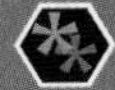 CLINICAL SCENARIO

A 24-year-old has newly diagnosed type 1 diabetes mellitus and Crohn's disease. She recently had surgery for removal of one third of her ileum. She is 75% of her usual weight, which is 125 lb; she is 65 inches tall. She requires specialized nutrition support for several months until her body adapts to the shortened bowel.

Nutrition Diagnostic Statements

- Involuntary weight loss related to poor intake, surgery, and pain during flare-up of Crohn's disease as evidenced by 25% weight loss.
- Inadequate oral food and beverage intake related to recent ileal resection as evidenced by 75% of usual weight and need for artificial nutrition.

Nutrition Care Questions

1. What immediate nutrition support method would be recommended?
2. What long-term nutrition support plan is likely to be designed?
3. What specialty products, if any, might be beneficial?
4. What parameters would you monitor to determine tolerance and response to the nutrition plan?

USEFUL WEBSITES

American Dietetic Association—Evidence Analysis Library
http://www.adaevidencelibrary.com/topic.cfm?cat=3016
American Society for Parenteral and Enteral Nutrition
http://www.nutritioncare.org/
Infusion Nurses Society
http://www.ins1.org
Medscape—Integrated Med Information
http://www.medscape.com/
Oley Foundation
http://www.oley.org/

REFERENCES

American Dietetic Association: *Evidence analysis library*, 2010. Accessed 29 May 2010 from http://www.adaevidencelibrary.com/topic.cfm?cat=3016&library=EBG.

American Society for Parenteral and Enteral Nutrition Board of Directors and American College of Critical Care Medicine: Nutrition guidelines for the provision and assessment of nutrition support therapy in the adult critically ill patient, *JPEN J Parenter Enteral Nutr* 33:3, 2010.

Bankhead R, et al: ASPEN: enteral nutrition practice recommendations, *JPEN J Parenter Enteral Nutr* 33:122, 2009.

Buchman AL, et al: Micronutrients in parenteral nutrition: too little or too much? The past, present, and recommendations for the future, *Gastroenterology* 137:1S, 2009.

Centers for Disease Control and Prevention, O'Grady NP, et al: *Guidelines for the prevention of intravascular catheter-related infections*, 9 August 2002. Accessed January 2006 from http://www.cdc.gov/mmwr/preview/mmwrhtml/rr5110a1.htm.

Charney P, Malone A: *ADA pocket guide to enteral nutrition*, Chicago, 2006, American Dietetic Association.

Fuhrman MP, et al: Home care opportunities for food and nutrition professionals, *JADA J Am Diet Assoc* 109:1092, 2009.

Gottschlich MM: Adult enteral nutrition: formulas and supplements. In Buchman A, editor: *Clinical nutrition in gastrointestinal disease*, Thoroughfare, N.J., 2006, Slack Inc.

Joint Commission on Accreditation of Healthcare Organizations: *Sentinel Event Policy and Procedures*, July 2007. Accessed 29 May 2010 from http://www.jointcommission.org/SentinelEvents/PolicyandProcedures/.

Kraft MD, et al: Review of the refeeding syndrome, *Nutr Clin Pract* 20:625, 2005.

Krzywda EA, et al: Parenteral nutrition access and infusion equipment. In Merritt R, editor: *The ASPEN nutrition support practice manual*, ed 2, Silver Spring, MD, 2005, American Society for Parenteral and Enteral Nutrition.

Kumpf VJ, et al: Parenteral nutrition formulations: preparation and ordering. In Merritt R, editor: *The ASPEN Nutrition support practice manual*, ed 2, Silver Spring, MD, 2005, American Society for Parenteral and Enteral Nutrition.

Martindale RD, et al: Guidelines for the provision and assessment of nutrition support therapy in the adult critically ill patient: Society of Critical Care Medicine and the American Society for Parenteral and Enteral Nutrition: executive summary, *Crit Care Med* 37:1757, 2009.

Matarese LE, Steiger E: Dietary and medical management of short bowel syndrome in adult patients, *J Clin Gastroenterol Suppl* 2:S85, 2006.

McClave SA, et al: Guidelines for the provision and assessment of nutrition support therapy in the adult critically ill patient, *JPEN J Parenter Enteral Nutr* 33:277, 2009.

Metheny NA, Meert KL: Monitoring tube feeding placement, *Nutr Clin Pract* 19:487, 2004.

Mizock BA, DeMichele SJ: The acute respiratory distress syndrome: role of nutritional modulation of inflammation through dietary lipids, *Nutr Clin Pract* 19:563, 2004.

Nikolaidis P, et al: Practice patterns of nonvascular interventional radiology procedures at academic centers in the United States? *Acad Radiol* 12:1475, 2005.

Parrish CR: The refeeding syndrome in 2009: prevention is the key to treatment, *J Support Oncol* 7:20, 2009

Raymond J: Long-term care. In Lysen L, editor: *Quick reference to clinical dietetics*, ed 2, Sudbury, Mass, 2006, Jones and Bartlett.

Seres D, et al: Parenteral nutrition safe practices: results of the 2003 American Society for Parenteral and Enteral Nutrition survey, *JPEN J Parenter Enteral Nutr* 30:259, 2006.

Wojtylak F, Hamilton: Reimbursement for home nutrition support. In Ireton-Jones C, DeLegge M, editors: *Handbook of home nutrition support*, Sudbury, MA, 2007, Jones and Bartlett.

CHAPTER 15

Karen Chapman-Novakofski, PhD, RD, LDN

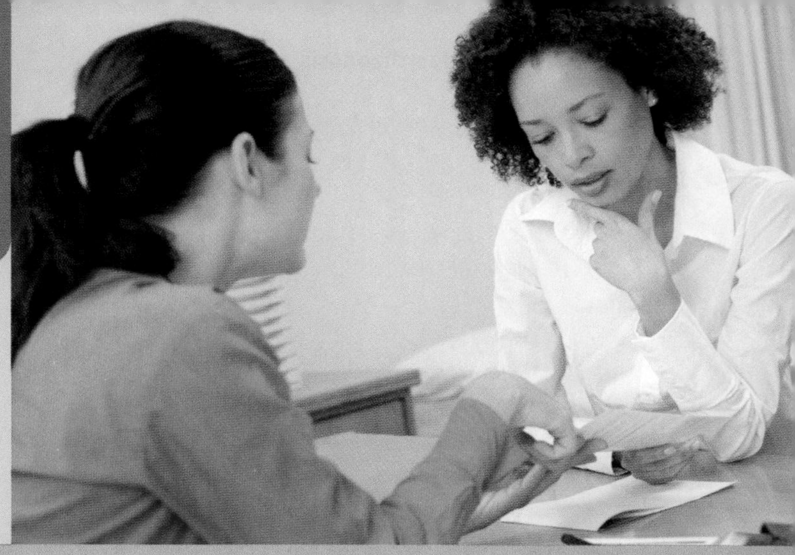

Education and Counseling: Behavioral Change

KEY TERMS

alignment
ambivalence
behavior change
behavior modification
cognitive behavioral therapy (CBT)
cultural competency
discrepancy
double-sided reflection
empathy
health belief model (HBM)
health literacy
maleficence
motivational interviewing (MI)
negotiation
normalization
peer educator
reflective listening
reframing
self-efficacy
self-management
self-monitoring
social cognitive theory (SCT)
stages of change
theory of planned behavior (TPB)
transtheoretical model (TTM)

Key factors in changing nutrition behavior are the person's awareness that a change is needed and the motivation to change. Nutrition education and nutrition counseling both provide information and motivation, but they do differ. *Nutrition education* can be individualized or delivered in a group setting; it is usually more preventive than therapeutic, and there is a transmission of knowledge. *Counseling* is most often used during medical nutrition therapy, one on one. In the one-on-one setting, the nutritionist sets up a transient support system to prepare the client to handle social and personal demands more effectively while identifying favorable conditions for change. The goal of nutrition counseling is to help individuals make meaningful changes in their dietary behaviors.

Sections of this chapter were written by Linda Snetselaar, PhD, RD for the previous edition of this text

BEHAVIOR CHANGE

Although there are differences between education and counseling as intervention techniques, the distinctions are not as important as the desired outcome, behavior change. **Behavior change** requires a focus on the broad range of activities and approaches that affect the individual choosing food and beverages in his or her community and home environment. **Behavior modification** implies the use of techniques to alter a person's behavior or reactions to environmental cues through positive and negative reinforcement, and extinction of maladaptive behaviors. In the context of nutrition, both education and counseling can assist the individual in achieving short-term or long-term health goals. Education provides the knowledge and skills needed to change; counseling is aimed at the other steps shown in Figure 15-1.

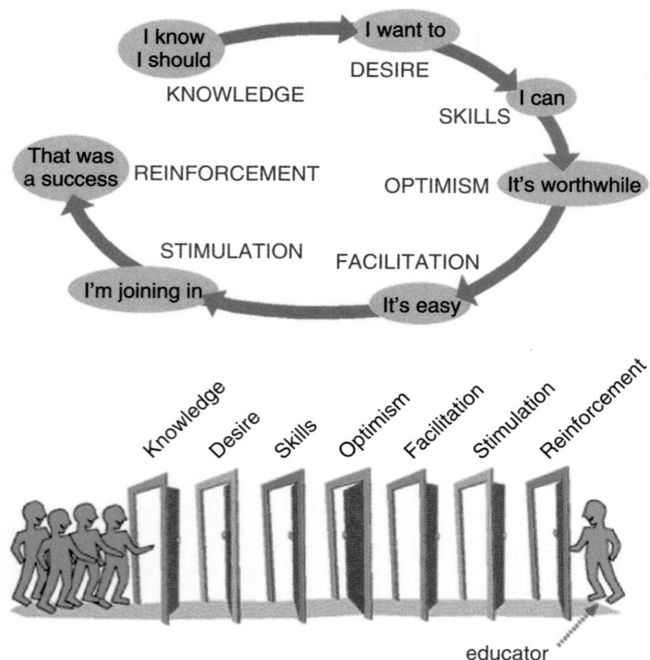

FIGURE 15-1 Seven steps to behavior change. *(Accessed 31 May 2010 from http://www.comminit.com/en/node/201090.)*

Factors Affecting the Ability to Change

Multiple factors affect a person's ability to change, the educator's ability to teach new information, and the counselor's ability to stimulate and support small changes. Inability to afford nutrition counseling, unstable living environments, inadequate family or social support, expensive food costs, insufficient transportation, and low literacy are some of the socioeconomic factors that may be barriers for obtaining and maintaining a healthy diet. With a population that is culturally diverse, it is imperative to appreciate the differences in beliefs or understanding that may lead to the inability to change.

Physical and emotional factors also make it hard to change, especially for seniors. Older adults need education and counseling programs that address low vision, poor hearing, limited mobility, decreased dexterity, and memory problems or cognitive impairments (Kamp et al., 2010).

Trust and respect are essential for all helping relationships. The quality of the provider-patient relationship can have either a positive or a negative effect on the outcome of the sessions. If a treatment plan is complex and not understood, decreased adherence is likely. When uncertain of comprehension, asking a few questions can be quite helpful to identify gaps in the patient's knowledge, understanding, or motivation.

Cultural Competency

The health care community was the first to promote **cultural competency** and, although there is no agreement on its exact definition, it is fair to say it involves cultural sensitivity or awareness. It requires respecting and understanding the attitudes, values, and beliefs of others; willingness to use cultural knowledge while interacting with clients; and consideration of culture during discussions and recommendations (Ulrey and Amason, 2001). Culture encompasses more than race, religion, or ethnicity; it includes community perspectives and perceptions. Care must be taken not to label people with a stereotype (Stein, 2009).

Gregg et al. (2006) define the following five tenets as the basis for cultural competency:

- Understanding the role of culture. Learning the skills to elicit patients' individual beliefs and interpretations and to negotiate conflicting beliefs is important to good patient care, regardless of the social, ethnic, or racial backgrounds of the patient.
- Learning about culture and becoming "culturally competent" is not a panacea for health disparities.
- *Culture*, *race*, and *ethnicity* are distinct concepts. Just learning about the culture will not eliminate racism.
- Culture is mutable and multiple; any understanding of a particular cultural context is always incompletely true, always somewhat out of date, and partial.
- Context is critical. Because culture is so complex, so shape-shifting, and so ultimately inseparable from its social and economic context, it is impossible to consider it as an isolated or static phenomenon.

Multicultural awareness is the first step toward establishing rapport and becoming a competent nutrition educator or counselor. It is important to evaluate one's own beliefs and attitudes and become comfortable with differences among racial, ethnic, or religious beliefs, culture, and food practices (*Clinical Insight:* The Counselor Looks Within). Heightening awareness of personal biases and increasing sensitivity allows the counselor to be more effective in understanding what the client may need to move forward.

Implementation of a cultural competency in interactions with patients or clients may seem like a very time-consuming challenge, without readily available resources in some cases. However, having this skill will in the end result in a more thorough communication with the patient or client and ultimately a better outcome. The Joint Commission continues to strengthen guidelines related to communication and cultural competency with guidelines and roadmaps for hospitals (The Joint Commission, 2010). Cultural competency is expected to be added as a Joint Commission standard in the future (Stein, 2009).

Communication

One of the most essential competencies in the delivery of health care is effective multicultural communication. The United States will continue to become more diverse. By the year 2050, it is estimated that almost 25% of the total U.S. population will be Hispanic. Of those who are non-Hispanic, projections for 2050 reflect a population that is 72.1% white, 14.6% black, and 8% Asian (Shrestha, 2010). Each culture has values, ideas, assumptions, and beliefs about life and a common system of encoding and decoding verbal and nonverbal messages (Ulrey and Amason, 2001).

Language is always important in communication. Although knowing several languages can be an asset, many will rely on translators. Unofficial translators, such as family or friends, are not usually a good choice because of a lack of understanding of nutrition and health. Using professional translators is also not without limitations in that the educator needs to understand not only the client but also the interpreter. The educator should maintain contact with the client and explain the role of the interpreter (Mossavar-Rahmani, 2007). When working with clients who have limited ability to speak and understand English, always use common terms, avoiding slang and words with multiple meanings. Always speak directly to the client, even when using a translator, and watch the client for nonverbal responses during the translation.

Communication not only encompasses language but also the context in which words are interpreted, including posture, gestures, concepts of time, spatial relationships, the role of the individual within a group, status and hierarchy of persons, and the setting (Satia-About et al., 2002). Nonverbal messages convey information about relationships. The way in which cultures combine verbal and nonverbal messages to transmit a message determines the context of the communication (Kittler and Sucher, 2007). Spatial relationships vary among cultures and among individuals. Movements such as gestures, facial expressions, and postures are often the cause of confusion and misinterpretations in intercultural communication. Good posture is an important sign of respect in nearly all cultures. Rules regarding eye contact are usually complex and vary according to issues such as gender, distance apart, and social status (*Clinical Insight:* Body Language and Communication Skills).

All counselors should be empathetic, genuine, and respectful. A good way to begin communication is by finding out how the client prefers to be addressed. Although in America it is common to call strangers and acquaintances by their given names, nearly all other cultures expect a more respectful approach. Listening sensitively, sharing control, accepting differences, demonstrating sincere concern, respecting other cultures, seeking feedback, and being natural and honest are strategies important to achieving client compliance and satisfaction (Patterson, 2004). Use of these techniques helps make the counseling sessions more effective and satisfying for both parties.

CLINICAL INSIGHT

The Counselor Looks Within

Before entering a counseling relationship and after reflecting on the session, the nutritionist should look inward and consider any factors that affect his or her own thinking and how they might affect the client. The nutritionist should reflect on ethical issues, such as the autonomy of the client, and beneficence versus **maleficence** (harm). An example may be when a female client decides not to set goals for her blood glucose levels and not to learn the amounts of carbohydrates in foods (autonomy). These choices serve as barriers to the benefit the counselor would make in teaching these **self-management** tools (beneficence) and the need for nonmaleficence (do no harm). Whenever clients decide a behavior change is not right for them, the counselor's role is not to force the issue but to encourage its future consideration.

CLINICAL INSIGHT

Body Language and Communication Skills

Active listening forms the basis for effective nutrition counseling. There are two aspects to effective listening: nonverbal and verbal. Nonverbal listening skills consist of varied eye contact, attentive body language, a respectful but close space, adequate silence, and encouragers. Eye contact is direct yet varied. Lack of eye contact implies that the counselor is too busy to spend time with the client. When the counselor leans forward slightly and has a relaxed posture and avoids fidgeting and gesturing, the client will be more at ease. Silence can give the client time to think and provide time for the counselor to contemplate what the client has said. Shaking one's head in agreement can be a positive encourager, leading to more conversation. Moving forward slightly toward the client is an encourager that allows for more positive interaction.

Verbal components of listening include keeping the focus on the client by demonstrating a willingness to listen. Often the nutritionist feels obligated to solve a problem or give advice. These two desires can decrease the time left for active listening. Emphasize questions that are open to detailed descriptions. Use questions that begin with "what," "how," "why," and "could."

Two types of encouragers are important in counseling: paraphrasing and summarizing. Paraphrasing is a brief repeat of the essence of what the speaker has said, using fresh and concise wording. It is not parroting or word swapping. Paraphrasing is not easy and requires careful listening and caring. Summarizing is lengthier than paraphrasing because it uses more information and summarizes what has been said during a longer period. In general, it is important to establish the interactive relationship before beginning the actual process of nutrition counseling.

Message Framing

The way in which a message is framed can influence its persuasiveness and effectiveness. Framing a message in a positive way focuses on the positive aspects of change; framing it with a negative spin highlights what could be lost without the change. By observing the community in which one practices, the counselor can adjust his or her comments accordingly. Visiting a grocery store, restaurants in the neighborhood, schools, or social centers will help the nutritionist understand the client's perspective. For example, knowing that fresh produce is not readily available from the local grocery store, the counselor may discuss the benefits of using canned or frozen vegetables instead of praising only the benefits of raw vegetables.

Messages and materials must be available for various educational levels, English language proficiencies, geographic locations, sexual orientation (lesbian, gay, bisexual, transgender), and folk customs and beliefs. Instructional information should be simple, clear, and free from bias in content and use of graphics or pictures.

Health Literacy

Low **health literacy** is common among older adults, minorities, and those who are medically underserved or have a low socioeconomic status (Health Resources and Services Administration, 2010). This problem can lead to poor management of chronic health conditions, as well as low adherence to recommendations. The counselor should be careful to avoid jargon and to use language or examples that have relevance to the client. Although there are many guidelines for writing health materials at lower literacy levels, oral communication requires interactive dialogue for assessment of the client's understanding and ability to absorb potentially complex concepts. Relying on the client's educational attainment provides some guidance, but asking the client to repeat explanations in his or her own words can also help the nutrition educator evaluate the client's level of understanding. Useful resources from the Agency on Healthcare Research and Quality are *Rapid Estimate of Adult Health Literacy in Medicine (REALM)* and *Short Assessment of Health Literacy for Spanish Adults (SAHLSA-50)* (Agency on Healthcare Research and Quality, 2010).

Models for Behavior Change

Changing behavior is the ultimate goal for nutrition counseling and education. Simply providing a pamphlet or a list of foods usually does not change eating behavior. Because so many different factors influence what someone eats, nutritionists have been learning from behavioral scientists to identify and intervene based on mediators of people's eating behavior. Health professionals can support individuals in deciding what and when to change by using a variety of health behavior theories. Some of the most common theories for behavior change are listed in Table 15-1, with examples described in the following paragraphs.

TABLE 15-1

Overview of Behavior Theories Used in Nutrition Education and Counseling

Health Belief Model (HBM)	Perceived susceptibility: an individual's belief regarding the chance that he or she may get a condition or disease
	Perceived severity: an individual's belief of how serious a condition and its consequences are
	Perceived benefits: an individual's belief in the positive effects of the advised action in the reducing risk or the seriousness of a condition
	Perceived barriers: an individual's belief about the tangible and psychological costs of the advised action
	Self-efficacy: an individual's belief that he or she is capable of performing the desired action
	Cues to action: strategies to activate one's readiness to change a behavior
Social Cognitive Theory (SCT)	Personal factors: outcome expectations, self-efficacy, reinforcements, impediments, goals and intentions, relapse prevention
	Behavioral factors: knowledge and skills, self-regulation and control, and goal setting
	Environmental factors: include imposed, selected, and created environments
Theory of Planned Behavior (TPB)	Subjective norms: the people who may influence the patient
	Attitudes: what the patient thinks about the behavior
	Perceived control: how much control the patient has to change things that affect the behavior
	Behavioral intention: whether the patient plans to perform the behavior
Transtheoretical Model (TM), or Stages of Change Model	Precontemplation: The individual has not thought about making a change.
	Contemplation: The individual has thought about making a change but has done no more than think about it.
	Preparation: The individual has taken some steps to begin to make the desired change.
	Action: The individual has made the change and continues it for less than 6 months.
	Maintenance: The individual has continued the behavior for longer than 6 months.
	Termination: The individual no longer thinks about the change; it has become a habit.

Health Belief Model

The **health belief model (HBM)** focuses on a disease or condition, and factors that may influence behavior related to that disease (Contento, 2007). The HBM has been used most with behaviors related to diabetes and osteoporosis, focusing on barriers to and benefits of changing behaviors (Sedlak et al., 2007; Tussing and Chapman-Novakofski, 2005).

Social Cognitive Theory

Social cognitive theory (SCT) represents the reciprocal interaction among personal, behavioral, and environmental factors (Bandura, 1977, 1986). This theory is quite extensive and includes many variables; some of the most important to counseling include self-efficacy, goal setting, and relapse prevention.

Transtheoretical Model of Change

The **transtheoretical model (TTM)**, or **stages of change** model, has been used for many years to alter addictive behaviors. TTM describes behavior change as a process in which individuals progress through a series of six distinct stages of change, as shown in Table 15-1 (Prochaska et al., 1992; Prochaska and DiClemente, 1982; Sigman-Grant, 1996). The value of the TTM is in determining the individual's current stage, then using change processes matched to that stage (Resnicow et al., 2006). Recently, however, the effectiveness of the TTM has been questioned (Salmela et al., 2009).

Theory of Planned Behavior

The **theory of planned behavior (TPB)** is based on the concept that intentions predict behavior (Ajzen, 1991). Intentions are predicted by attitudes, subjective norms (important others), and perceived control. This theory is most successful when a discrete behavior is targeted (e.g. milk consumption), but has also been used for healthy diet consumption (Brewer et al., 1999; Pawlak et al., 2009).

COUNSELING STRATEGY: COGNITIVE BEHAVIORAL THERAPY

Cognitive behavior therapy (CBT) can be used to help individuals develop skills to achieve healthier eating habits. Instead of helping to decide *what* to change, it helps to identify *how* to change thinking, behavior, and communication. Lifestyle modification can be time-consuming and skill-intensive, but new methods include use of the Internet and cognitive therapy to alter distorted thinking. CBT can be used for obesity treatment to promote and encourage self-care among patients, or for managing chronic diseases such as diabetes or cardiovascular disease.

Many textbooks describe the CBT process. For example, for a textbook on eating disorders describes steps such as shaping concerns and mindsets, managing dietary restraint and rules, and handling events and moods related to eating (Fairburn et al., 2003). CBT counselors can help clients explore troubling themes, strengthen their coping skills, and focus on their well being. The CBT process is practical, action-oriented, and goal-directed. CBT training is available from many universities or centers for cognitive therapy (National Alliance on Mental Illness, 2010).

COUNSELING STRATEGY: MOTIVATIONAL INTERVIEWING

Motivational interviewing (MI) has been used to encourage clients to identify discrepancies between how they would like to behave and how they are behaving, and then motivate them to change (Miller and Rollnick, 2002). Studies point to the positive influence of MI on changes in dietary behavior, either alone or in combination with other strategies. These include increases in self-efficacy in relation to dietary changes, increased fruit and vegetable intake, and decreased body mass index. As with any strategy, better outcomes were associated with longer interventions and increased number of counseling session (Martins and McNeil, 2009). The following are principles used in MI to enhance behavior change.

Expressing Empathy

Empathy, nutrition counselor acceptance of what a client feels in times of turmoil, can often result in change. Acceptance facilitates change. Beyond this acceptance is a skillful form of **reflective listening**, which allows the client to describe thoughts and feelings, while the nutritionist reflects back understanding. Many clients have no one with whom to discuss problems in their lives. This opportunity to have someone listen and understand the emotions behind the words is crucial to eventual dietary change.

As clients review situations in their lives and lack of time for dietary changes, the nutrition counselor will hear **ambivalence**. On the one hand, clients want to make changes; on the other hand, they want to pretend that change is not important. Ambivalence is normal.

Client: I feel totally worthless. On one hand, I want to follow this new eating pattern, and on the other, I want to eat spontaneously, not worrying about decreasing my fat intake.

Nutrition Counselor: Your feelings are normal. You are having a difficult time merging new and old habits. This happens to many people.

Developing Discrepancy

An awareness of consequences is important. Identifying the advantages and disadvantages of modifying a behavior, or developing **discrepancy**, is a crucial process in making changes.

Client: I want to follow the new eating pattern, but I just can't afford it.

Nutrition Counselor: Let's look at your diet record and discuss some healthy, low-cost changes.

Rolling with Resistance (Legitimation, Affirmation)

Invite new perspectives without imposing them. The client is a valuable resource in finding solutions to problems. Perceptions can be shifted, and the nutrition counselor's role is to help with this process. For example, a client who is wary of describing why she is not ready to change may become much more open to change if she sees openness to her resistive behaviors. When it becomes okay to discuss resistance, the rationale for its original existence may seem less important.

Client: I just feel that my level of enthusiasm for following the diet is low. It all seems like too much effort.
Nutrition Counselor: I appreciate your concerns. At this point in following a new diet, many people feel the same way. Tell me more about your concerns and feelings.

Supporting Self-Efficacy

Belief in one's own capability to change is an important motivator. The client is responsible for choosing and carrying out personal change. However, the nutrition counselor can support **self-efficacy** by having the client try behaviors or activities while the counselor is there.

Client: I just don't know what to buy once I get to the grocery store. I end up with hamburger and potato chips.
Nutrition Counselor: Let's think of one day's meals right now. Then we can make a grocery list from that.

First Session

The first session of a one-on-one educational intervention establishes the counseling relationship. The environment should be conducive to privacy, and there should be a plan for reduction of interruptions (e.g., no telephone calls). The counselor should be seated in a manner that reflects interest in the client, such as sitting directly across from one another in chairs without a desk as a barrier. In this first session, it is most important to establish rapport and invite input from the client.

Establishing Rapport

To build rapport, one begins by asking how the client prefers to be addressed.

"Good afternoon Mrs. Jones. My name is Ms. Kathy Smith. Please call me Kathy. Do you prefer I use Mrs. Jones, or your first name as we talk?"

It is acceptable to ask one or two questions that are relevant to important aspects of the client's life or conversational to allow the client to adjust.

"I see you live in _________. Have you always lived there?"

"The traffic has been really bad with all the road repair. Did you have a difficult time getting here?"

Some clients may choose very little conversation, while others are quite talkative. At some point, the nutrition counselor needs to move the conversation to the point of the visit.

"We have about _________ minutes to meet today. I thought we might talk about how you're doing with your dietary changes. How does this sound to you?"

In an initial visit, the counselor introduces the subject of the session and invites the client to contribute. The following are sample conversations:

"The purpose of this visit is to see how you are doing in covering your dietary carbohydrate intake with insulin." (SCT, self-efficacy)
"In looking at your monitoring tools, it seems that you have had excellent progress at some times and at other times it may have been more difficult. Is there an area in particular that you'd like to work on?"
"Could we talk about your diet records to identify problems we could solve?" (HBM, perceived barriers)

Although not every first session lends itself to an assessment of the client's readiness to change, at some point after the topic has been agreed upon, the counselor must assess if the client is ready to change. To identify in which of these three stages a client is, see Figure 15-2.

It may be difficult to build rapport with some clients. Someone who appears hostile, unusually quiet, or dismissive may have more success with either a different nutritionist or with someone with whom he or she has background in common. In those cases, working with a peer educator may be most effective. The **peer educator** should ideally share similarities with the target population in terms of age or ethnicity, and have primary experience in the nutrition topic (e.g., has breastfed her infant) (Pérez-Escamilla et al., 2008). Peer educators are usually community health workers or paraprofessionals. The Expanded Food and Nutrition Education Program (EFNEP) has demonstrated the effectiveness and cost efficiency of peer educators (Dollahite et al., 2008). In prenatal or WIC clinics, breastfeeding peer counselors are often highly effective in helping new mothers with their questions and concerns.

Assessment Results: Choosing Focus Areas

The purpose of assessment is to identify the client's stage of change and to provide appropriate help in facilitating change. The assessment should be completed in the first visit if possible. If conversation extends beyond the designated time for the session, the assessment steps should be completed at the next session. The nutritional assessment requires gathering the appropriate anthropometric, biochemical, clinical, dietary, and economic data relating to the

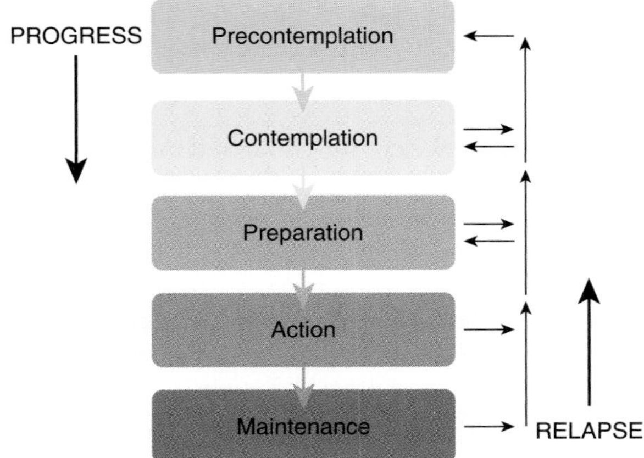

FIGURE 15-2 A model of the stages of change. In changing, a person progresses down these steps to maintenance. If relapse occurs, he or she gets back on the steps at some point and works down them again.

client's condition. The nutritional diagnosis then focuses on any problems related to food or nutrient intake.

Determining present eating habits provides ideas on how to change in the future. It is important to review the client's eating behavior, to identify areas needing change, and to help the client select goals that will have the most effect on health conditions. For instance, if the nutrition diagnosis includes excessive fat intake (nutrient intake [NI]-5102), inappropriate intake of food fats (NI-51.3), excessive energy intake (NI-1.5), inadequate potassium intake (NI-55.1), food- and nutrition-related knowledge deficit (nutrition behavior [NB]-1.1), and impaired ability to prepare foods or meals (NB-2.4), the counselor may need to focus on the last diagnosis before the others. If all other diagnoses are present except impaired ability to prepare foods or meals (NB-2.4), the nutritionist may want to have a discussion about whether excessive fat intake, inappropriate intake of types of food fats, or excessive energy intake are more appealing or possible for the client to focus on first.

Assessment of Readiness to Change

Once the nutrition diagnosis is selected for intervention, it is important to assess readiness for changes. Using a ruler that allows the client to select his or her level of intention to change is one method of allowing client participation in the discussion. The counselor asks the client, "On a scale of 1 to 12, how ready are you right now to make any new changes to eat less fat? (1 = not ready to change; 12 = very ready to change)." The nutritionist may use this method with each nutrition diagnosis to help the client decide where to focus first.

Three possibilities for readiness exist: (1) not ready to change; (2) unsure about change; (3) ready to change. These three concepts of readiness have condensed the six distinct stages of change described in this chapter to assist the counselor in determining the level of client readiness. There are many concepts to remember, and readiness to change may fluctuate during the course of the discussion. The counselor must be ready to move back and forth between the phase-specific strategies. If the client seems confused, detached, or resistant during the discussion, the counselor should return and ask about readiness to change. If readiness has lessened, tailoring the intervention is necessary. Not every counseling session has to end with the client's agreement to change; even the decision to think about change can be a useful conclusion.

NOT-READY-TO-CHANGE COUNSELING SESSIONS

In approaching the "not-ready-to-change" stage of intervention, there are three goals: (1) facilitate the client's ability to consider change, (2) identify and reduce the client's resistance and barriers to change, and (3) identify behavioral steps toward change that are tailored to each client's needs. At this stage identifying barriers (HBM), the influence of subjective norms and attitudes (TPB), or personal and environmental factors (SCT) that may have negative influences on the intention to change can be helpful. To achieve these goals, several communication skills are important to master: asking open-ended questions, listening reflectively, affirming the patient's statements, summarizing the patient's statements, and eliciting self-motivational statements.

Asking Open-Ended Questions

Open-ended questions allow the client to express a wider range of ideas, whereas closed questions can help in targeting concepts and eliminating tangential discussions. For the person who is not ready to change, targeted discussions around difficult topics can help focus the session. The nutritionist asks questions that must be answered by explaining and discussing, not by one-word answers. This is particularly important for someone who is not ready to change, because it opens the discussion to problem areas that keep the client from being ready. The following statements and questions are examples that create an atmosphere for discussion:

- "We are here to talk about your dietary change experiences to this point. Could you start at the beginning and tell me how it has been for you?" *(SCT, personal factors)*
- "What are some things you would like to discuss about your dietary changes so far? What do you like about them? What don't you like about them?" *(TPB, attitudes)*

Reflective Listening

Nutrition counselors not only listen but also try to tag the feelings that surface as a client is describing difficulties with an eating pattern. Listening is not simply hearing the words spoken by the client and paraphrasing them back. Figure 15-3 shows a nutrition counselor listening reflectively to her client.

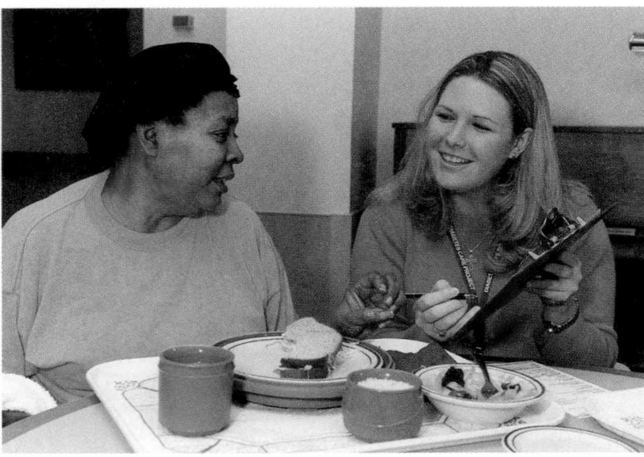

FIGURE 15-3 This nutrition counselor is using reflective listening techniques with her client.

Reflective listening involves a guess at what the person feels and is phrased as a statement, not a question. By stating a feeling, the nutrition counselor communicates understanding. The following are three examples of listening reflectively:

Client: "I really do try, but I am retired and my husband always wants to eat out. How can I stay on the right path when that happens?"
Nutrition Counselor: "You feel frustrated because you want to follow the diet, but at the same time you want to be spontaneous with your husband. Is this correct?" (reflective listening; TPB, subjective norms; HBM, barriers; SCT, personal factors)
Client: "I feel like I let you down every time I come in to see you. We always discuss plans and I never follow them. I almost hate to come in."
Nutrition Counselor: "You are feeling like giving up. You haven't been able to modify your diet, and it is difficult for you to come into our visits when you haven't met the goals we set. Is this how you are feeling?"(reflective listening) Can you think of a specific time when you feel that you had an opportunity to achieve your plan, but didn't?" (HBM, barriers)
Client: "Some days I just give up. It is on those days that I do very badly in following my diet."
Nutrition Counselor: "You just lose the desire to try to eat well on some days and that is very depressing for you. Do I have that right?"(rephrasing) "Are those days when something in particular has happened? (HBM, barriers)

Affirming

Counselors often understand the idea of supporting a client's efforts at following a new eating style but do not put those thoughts into words. When the counselor affirms someone, there is alignment and normalization of the client's issues. In **alignment** the counselor tells the client that he or she understands these difficult times. **Normalization** means telling the client that he or she is perfectly within reason and that it is very normal to have such reactions and feelings. The following statements indicate affirmation:

- "I know that it is hard for you to tell me this. But thank you."
- "You have had amazing competing priorities. I feel that you have done extremely well, given your circumstances."
- "Many people I talk with express the same problems. I can understand why you are having difficulty."

Summarizing

The nutrition counselor periodically summarizes the content of what the client has said by covering all the key points. Simple and straightforward statements are most effective, even if they involve negative feelings. If conflicting ideas arise, the counselor can use the strategy exemplified by the statement, "On the one hand you want to change, but love those old eating patterns." This helps the client recognize the dichotomy in thinking that often prevents behavior change.

Eliciting Self-Motivational Statements

The four communication strategies (asking open-ended questions, listening reflectively, affirming, and summarizing) are important when eliciting self-motivational statements. The goal here is for the client to realize that a problem exists, that concern results, and that positive steps in the future can be taken to correct the problem. The goal is to use these realizations to set the stage for later efforts at dietary change. Examples of questions to use in eliciting self-motivational feeling statements follow.

Problem Recognition

- "What things make you think that eating out is a problem?"
- "In what ways has following your diet been a problem?"

Concern

- "How do you feel when you can't follow your diet?"
- "In what ways does not being able to follow your diet concern you?"
- "What do you think will happen if you don't make a change?"

Intention to Change

- "The fact that you're here indicates that at least a part of you thinks it's time to do something. What are the reasons you see for making a change?"
- "If you were 100% successful and things worked out exactly as you would like, what would be different?"
- "What things make you think that you should keep on eating the way you have been?" And in the opposite direction, "What makes you think it is time for a change?"

Optimism

- "What encourages you that you can change if you want to?"
- "What do you think would work for you if you decided to change?"

Clients in this "not-ready-to-change" category have already told the counselor they are not doing well at making changes. Usually if a tentative approach is used by asking permission to discuss the problem, the client will not refuse. One asks permission by saying, "Would you be willing to continue our discussion and talk about the possibility of change?" At this point, it is helpful to discuss thoughts and feelings about the current status of dietary change by asking open-ended questions:

- "Tell me why you picked ________ on the ruler." (Refer to previous discussion on the use of a ruler.)
- "What would have to happen for you to move from a ________ to a ________ (referring to a number on the ruler)? How could I help get you there?"
- "If you did start to think about changing, what would be your main concern?"

To show real understanding about what the client is saying, it is beneficial to summarize the statements about his or her progress, difficulties, possible reasons for change, and what needs to be different to move forward. This paraphrasing allows the client to rethink his or her reasoning about readiness to change. The mental processing provides new ideas that can promote actual change.

Ending the Session

Counselors often expect a decision and at least a goal-setting session when working with a client. However, it is important in this stage to realize that traditional goal setting will result in feelings of failure on both the part of the client and the nutritionist. If the client is not ready to change, respectful acknowledgment of this decision is important. The counselor might say, "I can understand why making a change right now would be very hard for you. The fact that you are able to indicate this as a problem is very important, and I respect your decision. Our lives do change, and, if you feel differently later on, I will always be available to talk with you. I know that, when the time is right for you to make a change, you will find a way to do it." When the session ends, the counselor will let the client know that the issues will be revisited after he or she has time to think. Expression of hope and confidence in the client's ability to make changes in the future, when the time is right, will be beneficial. Arrangements for follow-up contact can be made at this time.

With a client who is not ready to change it is easy to become defensive and authoritarian. At this point, it is important to avoid pushing, persuading, confronting, coaxing, or telling the client what to do. It is reassuring to a nutritionist to know that change at this level will often occur outside the office. The client is not expected to be ready to do something during the visit (see *New Directions:* Dietitian Counselor as Life Coach).

NEW DIRECTIONS

Dietitian Counselor as Life Coach

By Marjorie Geiser, RD, NSCA-CPT

More and more registered dietitian (RD) nutrition counselors are turning to life coaching to enhance nutrition counseling skills and increase client success. Coaching moves the focus away from the RD as the expert who tells the client what to do, to realizing that clients do know how they want to accomplish their goals. Many clients already know the information the RD provides, but the RD can be most valuable by helping them apply that information. Life coaching involves asking questions to help clients look within to answer the questions they didn't think of. It is not therapy; it is simply asking questions without an agenda. It is taking the client from where he or she is currently to where he or she wants to be. It is helping the client accomplish more sooner.

UNSURE-ABOUT-CHANGE COUNSELING SESSIONS

The only goal in the "unsure-about-change" session is to build readiness to change. This is the point at which changes in eating behavior can escalate. This "unsure" stage is a transition from not being ready to deal with a problem eating behavior to preparing to continue the change. It involves summarizing the client's perceptions of the barriers to a healthy eating style and how they can be eliminated or circumvented to achieve change. Heightened self-efficacy may provide confidence that goals can be achieved. A restatement of the client's self-motivational statements assists in setting the stage for success. The client's ambivalence is discussed, listing the positive and negative aspects of change. The nutritionist can restate any statements that the client has made about intentions or plans to change or to do better in the future.

One crucial aspect of this stage is the process of discussing thoughts and feelings about current status. Use of open-ended questions encourages the client to discuss dietary change progress and difficulties. Change is promoted through discussions focused on possible reasons for change. The counselor might ask the question: "What would need to be different to move forward?"

This stage is characterized by feelings of ambivalence. The counselor should encourage the client to explore ambivalence to change by thinking about "pros" and "cons." Some questions to ask are:

- "What are some of the things you like about your current eating habits?"
- "What are some of the good things about making a new or additional change?"
- "What are some of the things that are not so good about making a new or additional change?"

By trying to look into the future, the nutrition counselor can help a client see new and often positive scenarios. As a change facilitator, the counselor helps to tip the balance away from being ambivalent about change toward considering change by guiding the client to talk about what life might be like after a change, anticipating the difficulties as well as the advantages. An example of an opening to generate discussion with the client might be: "I can see why you're unsure about making new or additional changes in your eating habits. Imagine that you decided to change. What would that be like? What would you want to do?" The counselor then summarizes the client's statements about the "pros" and "cons" of making a change and includes any statements about wanting, intending, or planning to change.

The next step is to negotiate a change. There are three parts to the **negotiation** process. The first is setting goals. Set broad goals at first and hold more specific nutritional goals until later. "How would you like things to be different from the way they are?" and "What is it that you would like to change?"

The second step in negotiation is to consider options. The counselor asks about alternative strategies and options and then asks the client to choose from among them. This is effective because, if the first strategy does not work, the client has other choices. The third step is to arrive at a plan, one that has been devised by the client. The counselor touches on the key points and the problems and then asks the client to write down the plan.

To end the session the counselor asks about the next step, allowing the client to describe what might occur next in the process of change. The following questions provide some ideas for questions that might promote discussion:

- "Where do you think you will go from here?"
- "What do you plan to do between now and the next visit?"

RESISTANCE BEHAVIORS AND STRATEGIES TO MODIFY THEM

Resistance to change is the most consistent emotion or state when dealing with clients who have difficulty with dietary change. Examples of resistance behaviors on the part of the client include contesting the accuracy, expertise, or integrity of the nutrition counselor; or directly challenging the accuracy of the information provided (e.g., the accuracy of the nutrition content). The nutrition counselor may even be confronted with a hostile client. Resistance may also surface as interrupting, when the client breaks in during a conversation in a defensive manner. In this case, the client may speak while the nutrition counselor is still talking without waiting for an appropriate pause or silence. In another, more obvious manner, the client may break in with words intended to cut off the nutrition counselor's discussion.

When clients express an unwillingness to recognize problems, cooperate, accept responsibility, or take advice, they may be denying a problem. Some clients blame other people for their problems (e.g., a wife may blame her husband for her inability to follow a diet). Other clients may disagree with the nutrition counselor when a suggestion is offered, but they frequently provide no constructive alternative. The familiar "Yes, but …" explains what is wrong with the suggestion but offers no alternative solution.

Clients try to excuse their behavior. A client may say, "I want to do better, but my life is in a turmoil since my husband died 3 years ago." An excuse that was once acceptable is reused even when it is no longer a factor in the client's life.

Some clients make pessimistic statements about themselves or others. This is done to dismiss an inability to follow an eating pattern by excusing poor compliance as just a given resulting from past behaviors. Examples are "My husband will never help me" or "I have never been good at sticking with a goal. I'm sure I won't do well with it now."

In some cases, clients are reluctant to accept options that may have worked for others in the past. They express reservations about information or advice given. "I just don't think that will work for me." Some clients will express a lack of willingness to change or an intention not to change. They make it very clear that they want to stop the dietary regimen.

Often clients show evidence that they are not following the nutrition counselor's advice. Clues that this is happening include using a response that does not answer the question, providing no response to a question, or changing the direction of the conversation.

These types of behavior can occur within a counseling session as clients move from one stage to another. They are not necessarily stage-specific, although most are connected with either the "not ready" or "unsure-about-change" stages. A variety of strategies are available to assist the nutrition counselor in dealing with these difficult counseling situations. These strategies include reflecting, double-sided reflection, shifting focus, agreeing with a twist, emphasizing personal choice, and reframing. Each of these options is described in the following paragraphs.

Reflecting

In reflecting, the counselor identifies the client's emotion or feeling and reflects it back. This allows the client to stop and reflect on what was said. An example of this type of counseling is, "You seem to be very frustrated by what your husband says about your food choices."

Double-Sided Reflection

In **double-sided reflection**, the counselor uses ideas that the client has expressed previously to show the discrepancy between the client's current words and the previous ones. For example:

Client: "I am doing the best I can." (Previously this client stated that she sometimes just gives up and doesn't care about following the diet.)
Nutrition Counselor: "On the one hand you say you are doing your best, but on the other hand I recall that you said you just felt like giving up and didn't care about following the diet. Do you remember that? How was that point in time different than now?"

Shifting Focus

Clients may hold onto an idea that they think is getting in the way of their progress. The counselor might question the feasibility of continuing to focus on this barrier to change when other barriers may be more appropriate targets. For example:

Client: "I will never be able to follow a low–saturated fat diet as long as my grandchildren come to my house and want snacks."
Nutrition Counselor: "Are you sure that this is really the problem? Is part of the problem that you like those same snacks?"
Client: "Oh, you are right. I love them."
Nutrition Counselor: "Could you compromise? Could you ask your grandchildren which of this long list of low–saturated fat snacks they like and then buy them?"

Agreeing with a Twist

This strategy involves offering agreement, then moving the discussion in a different direction. The counselor agrees with a piece of what the client says but then offers another perspective on his or her problems. This allows the opportunity to agree with the statement and the feeling, but then to redirect the conversation onto a key topic. For example:

Client: "I really like eating out, but I always eat too much, and my blood sugars go sky high."
Nutrition Counselor: "Most people do like eating out. Now that you are retired it is easier to eat out than to cook. I can understand that. What can we do to make you feel great about eating out so that you can still follow your eating plan and keep your blood glucose values in the normal range?"

Reframing

With **reframing** the counselor changes the client's interpretation of the basic data by offering a new perspective. The counselor repeats the basic observation that the client has provided and then offers a new hypothesis for interpreting the data. For example:

Client: "I gave up trying to meet my dietary goals because I was having some difficulties when my husband died, and I have decided now that I just cannot meet those strict goals."
Nutrition Counselor: "I remember how devastated you were when he died and how just cooking meals was an effort. Do you think that this happened as a kind of immediate response to his death and that you might have just decided that all of the goals were too strict at that time?" (Pause)
Client: "Well, you are probably right."
Nutrition Counselor: "Could we look at where you are now and try to find things that will work for you now to help you in following the goals we have set?"

These strategies help by offering tools to ensure that nutrition counseling is not ended without appropriate attempts to turn difficult counseling situations in a more positive direction.

Self-Efficacy and Self-Management

Counselors should always emphasize that any future action belongs to the client, that the advice can be taken or disregarded. This emphasis on personal choice (autonomy) helps clients avoid feeling trapped or confined by the discussion. Belief in the ability to change through his or her own decisions is an essential and worthy goal. A sense of self-efficacy reflects the belief about being capable of influencing events and choices in life. These beliefs determine how individuals think, feel, and behave. If people doubt their capabilities, they will have weak commitments to their goals. Success breeds success, and failure breeds a sense of failure. Having resilience, positive role models, and effective coaching can make a significant difference.

READY-TO-CHANGE COUNSELING SESSIONS

The major goal in the "ready-to-change" session is to collaborate with the client to set goals that include a plan of action. The nutrition counselor provides the client with the tools to use in meeting nutrition goals. This is the stage of change that is most often assumed when a counseling session begins. To erroneously assume this stage means that inappropriate counseling strategies set the stage for failure. Misaligned assumptions often result in lack of adherence on the part of the client and discouragement on the part of the nutritionist. Therefore it is important to discuss the client's thoughts and feelings about where he or she stands relative to the current change status. Use of open-ended questions helps the client confirm and justify the decision to make a change and in which area. The following questions may elicit information about feelings toward change:

- "Tell me why you picked _____ on the ruler."
- "Why did you pick (nutrition diagnosis 1) instead of (other nutrition diagnoses)?"

In this stage, goal setting is extremely important. Here the counselor helps the client set a realistic and achievable short-term goal: "Let's do things gradually. What is a reasonable first step? What might be your first goal?"

Action Plan

Following goal setting, an action plan is set to assist the client in mapping out the specifics of goal achievement. Identifying a network to support dietary change is important. What can others do to help?

Early identification of barriers to adherence is also important. If barriers are identified, plans can be formed to help eliminate these roadblocks to adherence.

Many clients fail to notice when their plan is working. Clients can be asked to summarize their plans and identify markers of success. The counselor then documents the plan for discussion at future sessions and ensures that the clients also have their plans in writing. The session should be closed with an encouraging statement and reflection about how the client identified this plan personally. Indicate that each person is the expert about his or her own behavior. Compliment the client on carrying out the plan. Ways to express these ideas to clients are:

- "You are working very hard at this, and it's clear that you're the expert about what is best for you. You can do this!"
- "Keep in mind that change is gradual and takes time. If this plan doesn't work, there will be other plans to try."

The key point for this stage is to avoid telling the client what to do. Clinicians often want to provide advice. However, it is critical that the client express ideas of what will work best: "There are a number of things you could do, but what do you think will work best for you?" The next contact may be in person, online, or by phone.

Following up with clients by phone or online has become a popular counseling method for many nutritionists. When behavior and counseling theories are combined with phone counseling, the results have been effective in managing weight, type 2 diabetes, and hypertension (Eakin et al., 2009; Kim et al., 2009). Online weight reduction programs have also been successful, especially when the websites are interactive and communication with counselors is available (Krukowski et al., 2009).

EVALUATION OF EFFECTIVENESS

Clinicians need to evaluate their services. Just completing the process does not mean that outcomes will match the goals. The sessions must be confidential, empowering, and personalized. When the American Dietetic Association Evidence Analysis Library Nutrition Counseling Workgroup conducted a review of literature related to behavior change theories and strategies used in nutrition counseling, they found the following (Spahn et al., 2010):

1. Strong evidence supports the use of a CBT in facilitating modification of targeted dietary habits, weight, and cardiovascular and diabetes risk factors.
2. MI is a highly effective counseling strategy, particularly when combined with CBT.
3. Few studies have assessed the application of the TTM or SCT on nutrition-related behavior change.
4. **Self-monitoring**, meal replacements, and structured meal plans are effective; financial reward strategies are not.
5. Goal setting, problem solving, and social support are effective strategies.
6. Research is needed in more diverse populations to determine the most effective counseling techniques and strategies.

CLINICAL SCENARIO

Mrs. Lee is originally from mainland China. She has been living in your area for several years and has numerous health problems, including high blood pressure and glaucoma. You have been asked to counsel her about making changes in her diet. Because her vision is poor, she will not be able to use printed materials that you have in your office that have been translated into Chinese.

Nutrition Diagnostic Statement

Impaired ability to prepare food and meals related to inability to see as evidenced by client report and history of glaucoma

Nutrition Care Questions

1. What steps should you take to make her comfortable with this session?
2. Should you invite family members to attend the counseling session? Why or why not?
3. What tools might be useful to help Mrs. Lee understand portions or types of food that she should select?
4. Would a supermarket tour be useful? Why or why not?
5. What other types of information will be needed to help Mrs. Lee?

USEFUL WEBSITES

American Counseling Association
http://www.counseling.org/

American Dietetic Association—Nutrition Diagnosis and Intervention
http://eatright.org/

Counseling Relationships—Code of Ethics
http://www.counseling.org/Resources/CodeOfEthics/TP/Home/CT2.aspx

Cultural Competency
http://www.thinkculturalhealth.org/
Cultural Competency Resources
http://www.thinkculturalhealth.org/online_resources.asp
Cultural Competency with Adolescents
http://www.ama-assn.org/ama1/pub/upload/mm/39/culturallyeffective.pdf
International Coaching Federation
http://www.coachfederation.org/
Journal of Counseling Psychology
http://www.apa.org/pubs/journals/cou/
Office of Minority Health
http://minorityhealth.hhs.gov/
Society for Nutrition Education
http://www.sne.org/

REFERENCES

Agency on Healthcare Research and Quality (AHRQ): *Health literacy measurement tools*. Accessed 31 May 2010 from http://www.ahrq.gov/populations/sahlsatool.htm.

Ajzen I: The theory of planned behavior, *Organ Behav Hum Decis Process* 50:179, 1991.

Bandura A: *Social foundations of thought and action*, Englewood Cliffs, N.J., 1986, Prentice-Hall.

Bandura A: *Social learning theory*, New York, 1977, General Learning Press.

Brewer JL, et al: Theory of reasoned action predicts milk consumption in women, *J Am Diet Assoc* 99:39, 1999.

Contento I: *Nutrition education: linking research, theory and practice*, Sudbury, Mass, 2007, Jones and Bartlett.

Dollahite J, et al: An economic evaluation of the expanded food and nutrition education program, *J Nutr Educ Behav* 40:134, 2008.

Eakin E, et al: Telephone counseling for physical activity and diet in primary care patients, *Am J Prev Med* 36:142, 2009.

Fairburn CG, et al: *Enhanced cognitive behavior therapy for eating disorders: the core protocol*, St Louis, 2003, Elsevier.

Gregg J, et al: Losing culture on the way to competence: the use and misuse of culture in medical curriculum, *Acad Med* 81:542, 2006.

Health Resources and Services Administration (HRSA): *Health literacy*. Accessed 31 May 2010 from http://www.hrsa.gov/healthliteracy/.

Kamp B, et al: Position of the American Dietetic Association, American Society for Nutrition, and Society for Nutrition Education: food and nutrition programs for community-residing older adults, *J Nutr Educ Behav* 42:72, 2010.

Kim Y, et al: Telephone intervention promoting weight-related health behaviors, *Prev Med* 16 December 2009. [Epub ahead of print.]

Kittler PG, Sucher KP: *Food and culture*, ed 5, Belmont, Calif, 2007, Wadsworth- Thomson Learning.

Krukowski RA, et al: Recent advances in internet-delivered, evidence-based weight control programs for adults, *J Diabetes Sci Technol* 3:184, 2009.

Martins RK, McNeil DW: Review of motivational interviewing in promoting health behaviors, *Clin Psychol Rev* 29:283, 2009.

Miller W, Rollnick S: *Motivational interviewing: preparing people for change*, ed 2, New York, 2002, Guilford.

Mossavar-Rahmani Y: Applying motivational enhancement to diverse populations, *J Am Diet Assoc* 107:918, 2007.

National Alliance on Mental Illness (NAMI): *Cognitive-behavioral therapy*. Accessed 31 May 2010 from http://www.nami.org/Template.cfm?Section=About_Treatments_and_Supports&template=/ContentManagement/ContentDisplay.cfm&ContentID=7952.

Patterson CH: Do we need multicultural counseling competencies? *J Mental Health Couns* 26:67, 2004.

Pawlak R, et al: Predicting intentions to eat a healthful diet by college baseball players: applying the theory of planned behavior, *J Nutr Educ Behav* 41:334, 2009.

Pérez-Escamilla R, et al: Impact of peer nutrition education on dietary behaviors and health outcomes among Latinos: a systematic literature review, *J Nutr Educ Behav* 40:208, 2008.

Prochaska JO, DiClemente CC: Transtheoretical therapy: toward a more integrative model of change, *Psychother Theory Res Pract* 20:276, 1982.

Prochaska JO, et al: In search of how people change, *Am Psychol* 47:1102, 1992.

Resnicow K, et al: Motivational interviewing for pediatric obesity: conceptual issues and evidence review, *J Am Diet Assoc* 106:2024, 2006.

Salmela S, et al: Transtheoretical model-based dietary interventions in primary care: a review of the evidence in diabetes, *Health Educ Res* 24:237, 2009.

Satia-Abouta J, et al: Dietary acculturation: applications to nutrition research and dietetics, *J Am Diet Assoc* 102:1105, 2002.

Sedlak CA, et al: DXA, health beliefs, and osteoporosis prevention behaviors, *J Aging Health* 19:742, 2007.

Shrestha LB: The changing demographic profile of the United States, *Congressional Research Service Report for Congress*. Accessed 30 January 2010 from http://www.fas.org/sgp/crs/misc/index.html.

Sigman-Grant M: Stages of change: a framework for nutrition interventions, *Nutr Today* 31:162, 1996.

Spahn JM, et al: State of the evidence regarding behavior change theories and strategies in nutrition counseling to facilitate health and food behavior change, *J Am Diet Assoc* 110:879, 2010.

Stein K: Navigating cultural competency: in preparation for an expected standard in 2010, *J Am Diet Assoc* 109:1676, 2009.

The Joint Commission: *Advancing Effective Communication, Cultural Competence, and Patient- and Family-Centered Care: A Roadmap for Hospitals*, Oakbrook Terrace, IL, 2010, The Joint Commission.

Tussing L, Chapman-Novakofski K: Osteoporosis prevention education: behavior theories and calcium intake, *J Am Diet Assoc* 105:92, 2005.

Ulrey KL, Amason P: Intercultural communication between patients and health care providers: an exploration of intercultural communication effectiveness, cultural sensitivity, stress and anxiety, *Health Comm* 13:449, 2001.

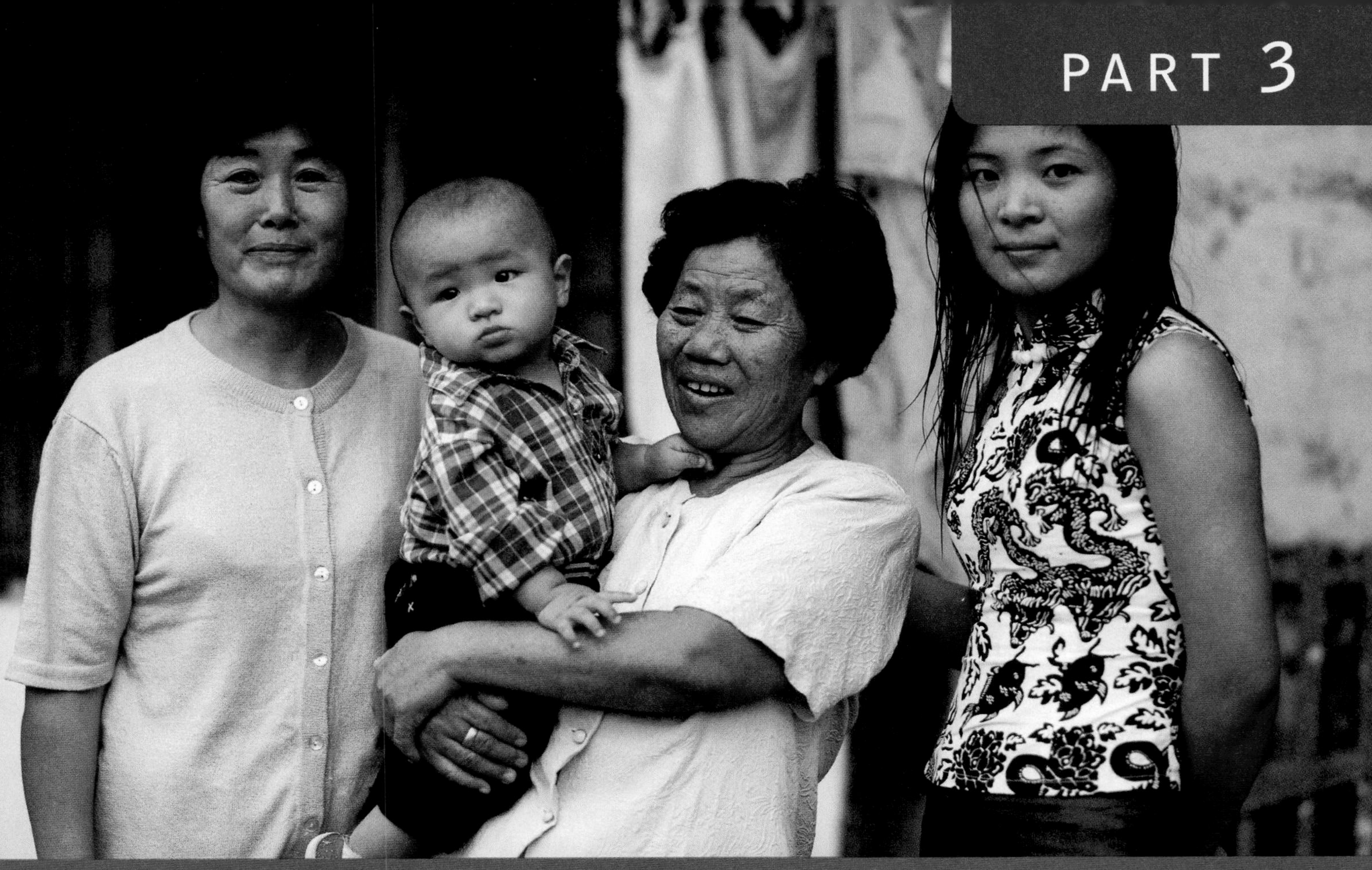

PART 3

Nutrition in the Life Cycle

The importance of nutrition throughout the life cycle cannot be refuted. However, the significance of nutrition during specific times of growth, development, and aging is becoming increasingly appreciated.

Health professionals have recognized for quite some time the effects of proper nutrition during pregnancy on the health of the infant and mother, even after her childbearing years. Maternal nutrition and possibly even paternal nutrition before conception affect the health of the newborn. "Fetal origin" has far more lifelong effects than originally thought.

Establishing good dietary habits during childhood lessens the possibility of inappropriate eating behavior later in life. Although the influence of proper nutrition on morbidity and mortality usually remains unacknowledged until adulthood, dietary practices aimed at preventing the degenerative diseases that develop later in life should be instituted in childhood.

During early adulthood many changes begin that lead to the development of diseases of aging years later. Many of these changes can be accelerated or slowed over the years, depending on the quality of the individual's nutritional intake, the health of the gut, and the function of the immune system.

With the rapid growth of the population of older adults has evolved a need to expand the limited nutrition data currently available for these individuals. Although it is known that energy needs decrease with aging, little is known about whether requirements for specific nutrients increase or decrease. Identifying the unique nutritional differences among the various stages of aging is becoming even more important.

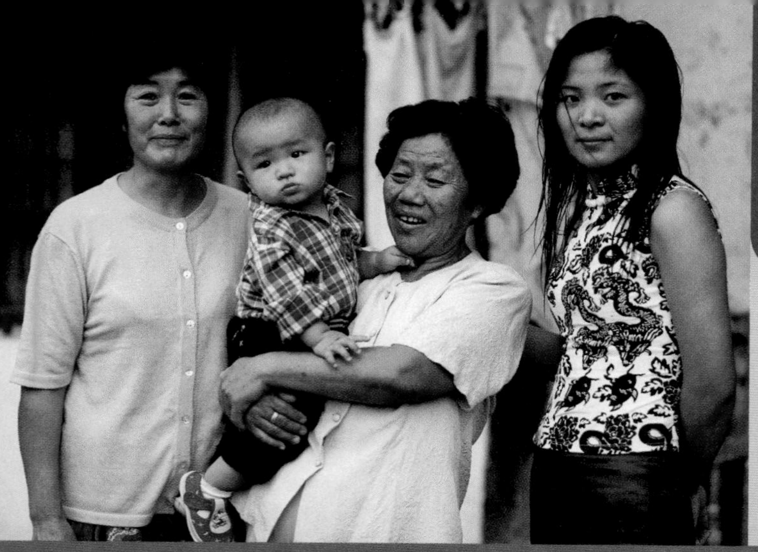

CHAPTER 16

Miriam Erick, MS, RD, CDE, LDN

Nutrition in Pregnancy and Lactation

KEY TERMS

amenorrhea
amylophagia
assisted reproductive technology (ART)
colostrum
congenital anomalies
eclampsia
epigenetic effects
failure to thrive (FTT)
fetal alcohol syndrome (FAS)
fetal origins of disease
geophagia
gestational diabetes mellitus (GDM)
gestational hypertension
gravida
hyperemesis gravidarum (HG)
intrauterine fetal demise (IUFD)
intrauterine growth restriction (IUGR)
lactation
let-down
macrosomia
nausea and vomiting in pregnancy (NVP)
neural tube defect (NTD)
oxytocin
perinatal mortality
pica
pre-eclamptic toxemia (PET)
pregnancy-induced hypertension (PIH)
pregorexia
prolactin
ptyalism
teratogenicity

Optimal preconceptual nutrition supports successful conception when it includes adequate amounts of all of the required vitamins, minerals, and energy-providing macronutrients. Because the developing fetus depends solely on the transfer of substrates from its host, there is simply no other means to acquire nutrition in utero. The cliché that the "fetus is the perfect parasite" implies the fetus takes entirely what it requires at the expense of the host. However, at some point nutritional deficiency can result in premature labor, relieving the host of an ongoing nutritional debt. After birth, quality nutrition during **lactation** continues the process of providing nutritional building blocks for maximal cerebral development, and growth of all body organs in the neonate.

This time period in the human experience—creating a new human being—sets the stage for the health of future generations. The quality and quantity of in-utero nourishment on the developing zygote, then fetus, then neonate, then adult emerges as one explanation for diseases that manifest in adulthood. This concept is known as **fetal origins of disease** or *developmental origins of health and disease* (Niljand, 2008; Solomons, 2009).

PRECONCEPTION AND FERTILITY

Traditional pregnancy partners were usually "man and wife," or mother and father. Advances in **assisted reproductive**

technology (ART) mean that "parents" may be egg or sperm donors. ART can involve in vitro fertilization (IVF), cryo embryo transfer, IVF with donor oocytes, intracytoplasmic sperm injection, a gestational carrier, or surrogate mother.

Reproductive Readiness and Fertility

Preconceptual guidance is based on findings that many women enter pregnancy with suboptimal nutrition intake. One study of 249 pregnant women who reported for their first prenatal visit found low dietary intakes of vitamin E, folate, iron, and magnesium in the preconceptual period and during pregnancy (Pinto et al., 2009). Although current public health recommendations promote mostly folate supplementation, there is some evidence that other nutrients also reduce the risk of congenital defects, such as vitamins B_{12}, B_6, and niacin, iron, and magnesium (Gaber et al., 2007). Thus a preconceptual multinutrient supplement confers more benefit than single supplements for a pregnant woman, or **gravida**.

Causes of infertility can be male factor (25% to 40%), ovulation defect (20% to 30%), fallopian tube defect (20% to 30%), unexplained causes (10% to 20%), endometriosis (5% to 10%), and other causes (4%). Infertility may also be due to extremes in body mass index (BMI) in either partner. Women with less than 17% body fat often do not menstruate, and those with less than 22% often do not ovulate. Women at risk include those with excessive exercise regimens, eating disorders, or both.

Dietary changes have been shown to decrease ovulatory disorders and improve fertility. Vitamin D deficiency in both men and women can be associated with infertility (Ozkan et al., 2009). Calcium has been shown to be important in males for spermatogenesis, sperm motility, hyperactivation, and acrosome (area of the sperm that contains digestive enzymes to break down the outer layers of the ovum) reactions. Recommendations include eating a lower glycemic diet (including high-fat dairy products, but reducing *trans*-fats), obtaining iron from plant sources, consuming a multivitamin daily, and being moderately physically active (Chavarro et al., 2007).

Toxins

Exposure to environmental chemicals such as dioxins, polybrominated biphenyls, phthalate esters, and other industrial products (endocrine disruptors) and heavy metals are known to damage sperm health (Meeker et al., 2008). Healthier sperm counts are associated with avoidance of tobacco and alcohol as well as an optimal diet with zinc, folic acid, and antioxidants (Gaur et al., 2010).

Screening is critical in women for occupational toxin exposure as well as for alcohol, tobacco, and intravenous and recreational drug use (Hannigan et al., 2009). Women with high fish consumption are at risk for entering pregnancy with toxic levels of mercury. Mercury levels decline once fish consumption is reduced. Unfortunately, even when a medical university in Taiwan advised women that fish containing high levels of mercury might be harmful to the brains of their developing fetuses, more than two thirds of the women indicated they would not change their fish intake (Chien et al., 2010).

Maternal caffeine intake and infertility relationships are often debated (Cochrane Update, 2009). A few studies have associated caffeine with increased rates of miscarriage or adverse pregnancy outcome (Jahanfar and Sharifah, 2009). However, caffeinated beverages are not considered to be of high nutritional quality and moderation is encouraged to ensure consumption of fluids with better nutrients, such as soy milk, low-fat dairy, and 100% fruit juices.

Obesity, Endocrine Conditions, and Oxidative Stress

Obesity is often correlated with poor prepregnancy health care, inaccurate self-categorization of weight, unsuccessful weight loss attempts, and insufficient advice regarding the importance of prepregnancy weight loss (Callaway et al., 2009a). In men elevated BMI is associated with lower testosterone levels (Chavarro et al., 2007). Obese women have a higher likelihood of prediabetes, undiagnosed diabetes preconceptually, or prolonged hyperglycemia; they also often have higher rates of fetal **congenital anomalies** (Selvaraj et al., 2008). Thus reducing obesity preconceptually may lower the risk of birth defects (American Dietetic Association, 2009; Biggio, 2010; Dheen, 2009).

Polycystic ovary syndrome (PCOS) affects 5% to 10% of women of reproductive age. These ovarian cysts alter the testosterone-estrogen balance, which results in insulin resistance and infertility. PCOS is often treated successfully with metformin (Grassi, 2008). See Chapter 32.

Hypothyroidism is also associated with reduced fertility (Hoy-Rosas, 2009). The thyroid hormone requirement increases 20% to 40% during gestation (Yassa et al., 2010). Pregnant women with treated hypothyroidism must increase their T4 levels to prevent transient hypothyroxinemia, associated with preterm birth or low birth weight (LBW) (Yassa et al., 2010). See Chapter 32.

Finally, oxidative stress depletes nutrient stores and contributes to a host of pregnancy complications. A healthy, antioxidant-rich diet and an exercise program help women prepare for an optimal pregnancy outcome. Box 16-1 lists some risk factors for birth defects.

CONCEPTION

Conception involves a complex series of endocrine events in which a healthy sperm fertilizes a healthy ovum (egg) within 24 hours of ovulation (see Table 16-1). An optimal environment is needed, including adequate nutrition and the absence of hostile factors. Conception itself does not guarantee successful pregnancy outcome. Low levels of copper and zinc adversely affect the development of the oocyte. Cloning experiments have shown that once the oocyte is fertilized, there is no further genetic material that is incorporated into the genetic sequence of that embryo. Exposures of the embryo or fetus to specific maternal nutrients can turn on or off the imprinting genes that control growth and development.

BOX 16-1

Potential Risk Factors for Development of Birth Defects

Assisted reproductive technologies
Birth trauma
Bacterial or viral infection during pregnancy
Genetic alterations
Gene-environmental interactions, such as maternal smoking
Hormonal conditions (hypothyroidism, PCOS)
Hyperglycemia
Hypoxia during pregnancy
In utero exposure to toxins (lawn chemicals, formaldehyde, endocrine disruptors, agricultural products, pesticides, carbon monoxide)
Maternal alcohol ingestion
Maternal medication or substance exposure (phenytoin, antihypertensive medications, aspirin), illicit recreational substances
Mother born in a different country
Nutrient deficits during pregnancy, such as iodine, vitamin B_{12}, vitamin D, vitamin A, vitamin K, copper, zinc, folic acid, choline
Obesity
Older mother
Oxidative stress
Premature birth
Radiation exposure

Adapted from Erick M: Gestational malnutrition. Lecture at Brigham and Women's Hospital, Boston, Mass,. December 2008.

PCOS, Polycystic ovary syndrome.

PREGNANCY

The eventual infant from a gestational carrier's womb will not be the same as one that had been carried by the biologic mother, even though the genes themselves are the same (Wilkins-Haug, 2009). This phenomenon reflects the effects of deoxyribonucleic acid (DNA) methylation from the maternal diet, known as epigenetics. **Epigenetic effects** involve the mechanisms by which DNA transcription is altered in various tissues and at different times without changing the underlying gene sequence. Unfortunately, the biologic changes of early pregnancy are difficult to visualize without sophisticated equipment.

Physiologic Changes of Pregnancy

Blood Volume and Composition

Blood volume expands approximately 50% by the end of pregnancy. This results in decreased levels of hemoglobin, serum albumin, other serum proteins, and water-soluble vitamins. The decline in serum albumin may be the result of fluid accumulation. The decrease in water-soluble vitamin concentrations makes determination of an inadequate intake or a deficient nutrient state difficult. In contrast, serum concentrations of fat-soluble vitamins and other lipid fractions such as triglycerides, cholesterol, and free fatty acids increase.

Cardiovascular and Pulmonary Function

Increased cardiac output accompanies pregnancy, and cardiac size increases by 12%. Diastolic blood pressure decreases during the first two trimesters because of peripheral vasodilatation, but returns to prepregnancy values in the third trimester. Mild lower extremity edema is a normal condition of pregnancy resulting from the pressure of the expanding uterus on the inferior vena cava. Blood return to the heart decreases, leading to decreased cardiac output, a fall in blood pressure, and lower-extremity edema. Mild physiologic lower extremity edema is associated with slightly larger babies and a lower rate of prematurity.

Maternal oxygen requirements increase and the threshold for carbon dioxide lowers, making the pregnant woman feel dyspneic. Adding to this feeling of dyspnea is the growing uterus pushing the diaphragm upward. Compensation results from more efficient pulmonary gas exchange.

Gastrointestinal Function

During pregnancy the function of the gastrointestinal (GI) tract changes in several ways that affect nutritional status. In the first trimester nausea and vomiting may occur, followed by a return of appetite that may be ravenous (see "Nausea, Vomiting, and Hyperemesis Gravidarium"). Cravings for and aversions to foods are common. Increased progesterone concentrations relax the uterine muscle to allow for fetal growth while also decreasing GI motility with increased reabsorption of water. This often results in constipation. In addition, a relaxed lower esophageal sphincter and pressure on the stomach from the growing uterus can cause regurgitation and gastric reflux (see "Heartburn").

Gallbladder emptying becomes less efficient because of the effect of progesterone on muscle contractility. Constipation, dehydration, a low-calorie diet, or poor intake are risk factors for gallstone development. During the second and third trimesters, the volume of the gallbladder doubles and its ability to empty efficiently is reduced. Gallbladder disease affects approximately 3.5% of pregnant women.

Celiac disease affects approximately 1 in 333 people, more than previously thought. It adversely affects fertility and absorption of nutrients. Women with celiac disease are at high risk of spontaneous abortion and premature deliveries. Some prenatal supplements may contain gluten or wheat binders and should be avoided. See Chapter 29.

Placenta

The placenta produces several hormones responsible for regulating fetal growth and development of maternal support tissues. It is the conduit for exchange of nutrients, oxygen, and waste products. Placental insults compromise the ability to nourish the fetus, regardless of how well nourished the

Text continued on p. 349

TABLE 16-1

The Carnegie Criteria

Carnegie Stage	Time Postovulation	Structure Size	Major Events	Other Events
Stage 1 Oocyte (egg) is fertilized.	1 day	0.1-0.15 mm—Approximately the size of a pencil point	Fertilization begins when the sperm penetrates the oocyte. This requires the sperm, which can survive up to 48 hours, to travel 10 hours up the female reproductive track. Then the sperm must successfully penetrate the zona pellucida, a tough membrane surrounding the egg. This process takes approximately 20 minutes. Once the fertilization is successful, the structure now becomes a zygote. This is the end of the fertilization process.	**Optimal amounts of folate** are needed for cell division and formation of DNA.
Stage 2 Cleavage First Cell Division	1.5-3 days	0.1-0.2 mm	Zygote begins to divide. Division begins to occur approximately every 24 hours. When cell division generates a mass of approximately 16 cells, the zygote now becomes a morula. (This structure is mulberry shaped.)	The newly created morula (formerly a zygote, which is less than 16 cells) leaves the fallopian tube and enters the uterine cavity 3-4 days after fertilization.
Stage 3 Early Blastocyst	4 days	0.1-0.2 mm	The morula enters the uterus and cell division continues. A cavity (hole) forms in the middle of the morula. This structure is now called a blastocele. Cells are flattening and compacting inside the cavity. The zona pellucida remains the same size as it was after fertilization of the egg by the sperm, with the cavity (hole) in the center.	The presence of the blastocele indicates two cell types are being formed: embryoblasts (which are on the *inside* of the blastocele) and trophoblasts, which are on the outside portion of the blastocele.
Stage 4 Implantation Begins HCG levels rise	5-6 days	0.1-0.2 mm	Pressure from the blastocele expanding in the middle of the blastocyte against the rigid wall of the zona pellucida creates a "hatching" of the blastocyte from this zona pellucida. Separation of these two elements is complete. Corpus Luteum: The yellow glandular mass in the ovary formed by an ovarian follicle that has matured and discharged its ovum.	The outer layers of the trophoblast cells secrete an enzyme that erodes the epithelial lining of the uterine cavity so the blastocyte can implant. Trophoblast cells secrete HCG. HCG stimulates the corpus luteum to continue progesterone production. Progesterone is a C21 steroid secreted by the corpus luteum and in the placenta; important intermediate in steroid biosynthesis to support the pregnancy. Progesterone has a short half-life and is metabolized by the liver.

Continued

TABLE 16-1

The Carnegie Criteria—cont'd

Carnegie Stage	Time Postovulation	Structure Size	Major Events	Other Events
Stage 5 Implantation Complete	7-12 days	0.1-0.2 mm	Trophoblast cells continue to engulf and destroy cells of the uterine lining, creating blood pools and stimulating new capillaries to grow. This begins the growth of the placenta. Ectopic pregnancies are those that do not implant in the uterus at this time and can develop up until 16 weeks before eventually becoming a life-threatening problem.	Blastocyst layer: forming two inner cell masses, which differentiate into two layers: epiblast: top layer of cells, which becomes the embryo and the amniotic cavity hypoblast: lower layer of cells, which become the yolk sac
Stage 6 Primitive Streak	13 days	0.2 mm	Placental formation: Chorionic villi "fingers" form in the placenta, anchoring the embryo to the uterus. Blood vessels begin appearing first in the placenta surrounding the embryo. Stalk Formation: The embryo is attached to the developing placenta by a stalk, which later becomes part of the umbilical cord. Gastrulation: A narrow line of cells appear on the surface of the formerly two-layered embryonic disc, which is called the *primitive streak*, which marks the bilateral symmetry in the embryo. Cells now migrate from the outer edges of the disc into the primitive streak and down, creating a new third layer. These three layers (see right column) are the ectoderm, mesoderm and the endoderm.	Ectoderm: Top layer of the embryonic disc will later form skin, hair, lenses of the eye, lining of the internal and external ear, nose, sinuses, mouth, anus, tooth enamel (Vello et al., 2009), pituitary and mammary glands, and all parts of the nervous system. Mesoderm: Middle cell layer of the embryonic disc and precursor to the muscles, bones, lymphatic tissue, spleen, blood cells, heart, lungs, reproductive, and excretory systems. Endoderm: Inner cell layer of the embryonic disc, which will eventually form the lining of the lungs, the tongue, tonsils, urethra and associated glands, the bladder, and the digestive tract. **Consider vitamins A, E, C.**
Stage 7 Neurulation	16 days	0.4 mm	Formation of a new cell layer—the ectoderm, which changes the two-layer disc into a three-layer disc.	Neural crest cells originate at the top of the neural tube and mitigate extensively, differentiating into many cell types such as neurons, glial cells, pigmented cells of the epidermis, epinephrine producing cells of the adrenal glands, and various skeletal (Wai-Man See et al., 2008) and connective tissues of the head.

			Rho B and Slug protein are the proteins now present in stage 7, which promote migration. The loss of N-cadherin, a protein required for left-right symmetry, also helps to initiate the migration of the neural crest cells.	Crest cells are important because they travel along to many areas of the developing embryo and give rise to multiple parts of the mature body, including sensory ganglia and melanocytes. These cells migrate from the neural plate, to the forebrain and mandibular and hyoid arches. They travel around the developing eye in three main pathways, forming the maxillary, mandibular, median, and lateral nasal processes. These cells develop into a variety of tissues, such as connective tissue, cartilage, and bone.
Stage 8	17-19 days	1-1.5 mm	Primitive pit, notochordal canal, and neuroenteric canals. The embryonic area is now shaped like a pear and the head region is broader than the tail region. By stage 8, the blood cells are already developed and begin to form channels alongside the epithelial cells, which form at the same time. *Sonic hedgehog (SHH)* is the name of a series of three genes that are forming and look like a hedgehog. These genes encode for signaling molecules that are involved in patterning processes during embryogenesis. SHH are secreted from the notochord. Various levels of SHH result in different types of cells formed in the developing fetus.	The ectoderm has thickened to form the neural plate, which then flattens out to form the neural groove. This groove is the precursor of the embryo's nervous system and it is one of the first organs to develop. **Consider vitamin B_{12}, ω-3 fatty acids, folate, and choline.** Some roles of SHH: purkinje neuron development involved in separation of the single eye filed into two bilateral fields implicated in hair development important in limb development
Stage 9 Appearance of Somites	19-21 days postovulation	1.5-2.1 mm	Embryo looks like a peanut with a larger head end compared with the tail end. One to three pairs of somites are present in stage 9. Every ridge, bump, and recess now indicates cellular differentiation.	Somites, which look like "bumps," are forming on this comma-shaped structure. Somites are composed of tissue and are considered the mesoderm and appear on either side of the neural groove. A head ridge rises on either side of the primitive streak, which is now ¼ to ⅓ the length of the embryo.

Continued

TABLE 16-1

The Carnegie Criteria—cont'd

Carnegie Stage	Time Postovulation	Structure Size	Major Events	Other Events
			Secondary blood vessels now appear in the chorion and placenta. Hematopoietic cells appear on the yolk sac simultaneously with endothelial cells, which evolve to form blood vessels for the newly emerging blood cells.	Endocardial (muscle) cells begin to fuse and form into the early embryo's two heart tubes.
Stage 10	21-23 days postovulation	1.5-3 mm	Neural folds and heart folds begin to fuse. On each side of the neutral tube, between 4 and 12 pairs of somites can exist by the end of stage 10. The cells, which will become eyes, appear as thickened circles just off the neural folds. Other newly differentiated cells will become the ears. At this time, the embryo looks like an old fashioned key-hole with a big oval top, with an ear of corn in the bottom ⅔ of the structure.	Rapid cellular growth and changes elongate the embryo and expand the yolk sac. The neural folds are rising and fusing at several points along the neural tube, as the budding somites appear to "zip" the neural tube closed. Failure of the neural tube to close results in spina bifida, which varies in severity. Neural crest cells eventually contribute to the skull and face of the embryo. The two endocardial tubes, formed during stage 9, now fuse in stage 10. Together they form one single tube generated from the cells in the "roof" of the neural tube. The heart tube takes on an S shape, establishing the asymmetry of the heart.
Stage 11	23-25 days postovulation	2.5-3 mm	Major event: two pharyngeal arches appear.	A primitive S-shaped heart is beating and peristaltic muscle contractions begin. This is *not* true circulation because blood vessel development is incomplete. **Consider Vitamin A.**
Stage 12			Beginning cells of the liver are forming.	Upper limb buds appear.
Stage 13	26-30 days postovulation	4-6 mm; size of the head of a pencil eraser	First thin surface layer of skin appears to cover the embryo.	
Stage 14	31-35 days postovulation	5-7 mm	Esophagus is forming.	
Stage 15			Future cerebral hemispheres are distinct.	

Stage 16		9-11 mm	Future lower jaw now visible.	Hind brain begins to develop.
Stage 17			Heart separates into four distinct chambers.	
Stage 18			Kidneys begin to produce urine.	
Stage 19			Semicircular canals are forming in the inner ear.	Gonads are forming.
Stage 20			Spontaneous movement begins.	
Stage 21			Intestines begin to recede into the abdominal cavity. Failure to recede results in a condition known as *gastroschisis.*	
Stage 22			Limbs begin to ossify.	**Consider the bone nutrients.**
Stage 23 First Trimester End of Embryonic Period	56-60 days postovulation	23-26 mm	In the head and neck, the head is erect and round. External ear is completely developed. Eyes are closed but retina is fully pigmented. Eyelids begin to unite and are half-closed.	Taste buds begin to form on the surface of the tongue. Primary teeth are at cap stage. Bones of the palate begin to fuse. **For bone, consider vitamins A, D, and K.** **For eyes, consider vitamin A and ω-3 fatty acids.**
			Intestines begin to migrate from the umbilical cord into the body cavity.	Upper and lower limbs are well formed. Fingers get bigger and toes are no longer webbed. All digits are separate and distinct.
			Layers of rather flattened cells—the precursor of the layer of skin—replaces the thin ectoderm.	The "tail" has disappeared.
Second Trimester	61-68 days postovulation	31-42 mm	In the head and neck, the basic brain structure is complete and the brain mass is rapidly dividing. Sockets for all 20 teeth are formed in the gum line. Face has human appearance.	The brain from weeks 12-23 has a smooth surface, with two to three layers differentiated in the cerebral cortex. **For the brain, consider folate, iodine, choline, ω-3 fatty acid, vitamin D.** **For the face, consider various B vitamins.**
			In the abdomen, the intestines have migrated into the abdomen from the umbilical cord. Digestive tract muscles are functional and practice contractions. Liver begins to secrete bile, bile pigments, cholesterol and inorganic salts. Bile is stored in the gallbladder. The development of the thyroid and pancreas are complete. Insulin begins to be secreted.	Genitals begin to show sex-specific characteristics. Fingernails begin to grow from nail buds. Skin develops reflexes and is reportedly very sensitive. **For the thyroid, consider iodine.**

Continued

TABLE 16-1

The Carnegie Criteria—cont'd

Carnegie Stage	Time Postovulation	Structure Size	Major Events	Other Events
Second Trimester: Approximately 14 Weeks		Length: crown-rump 2.5 inches (61 mm). Length is a better measure at this time. Weight: 0.3-0.5 oz or 8 to 14 g.	In the head and neck, the fetal head is 50% of the structure. Sucking muscles of mouth fill out cheeks. Tooth buds continue to develop and salivary glands start functioning. Hair pattern starting to be discernible.	In the thorax, heart tones can be detected with sensitive equipment. The lungs start to develop further as the fetus inhales and exhales amniotic fluid essential for proper lung development. **Consider vitamin A.**
			Able to identify gender. Sweat glands begin to develop.	In the abdomen, the spleen now assumes removal of old red blood cells and production of antibodies begins.
Second Trimester: 16 weeks postovulation		Length: 4.3-4.6 inches (108-111 mm) Weight: approximately 2.3 oz (80 g)	Mother has approximately 7.5 oz or 250 mL of amniotic fluid surrounding the conceptus.	Fingerprints and toe prints begin. Eyes now straight-forward in final position and start blinking. Ears move into final places at side of head.
			In the blood and nervous system, circulation is functionally complete. Placenta is now almost same size as fetus. Nerves are beginning to be coated in myelin, which is a fatty substance that surrounds nerve fibers to speed nerve cell transmission and insulates them for uninterrupted impulses.	In the abdomen, meconium begins to develop in the fetal bowels. Meconium is the product of cell loss, digestive secretions, and swallowed amniotic fluid. **For myelin, consider iron.** **For kidneys, consider vitamin A.**

Adapted from The Visible Embryo. Accessed 18 June 2010 from www.visembryo.com.

DNA, Deoxyribonucleic acid; *HCG*, human chorionic gonadotropin; *SHH*, sonic hedgehog.

mother. Placental insults can be the result of poor placentation from early pregnancy or small infarcts associated with preeclampsia (PET) or hypertension disorders. Placental size can be 15% to 20% lower than normal in fetuses with **intrauterine growth restriction (IUGR)**. A small placenta has a smaller surface area of placental villi, with a reduced functional capacity. Important research about the role of imprinting and epigenetics in placental function is underway (Wilkins-Haug, 2009).

Renal Function

The glomerular filtration rate (GFR) increases by 50% during pregnancy, although the volume of urine excreted each day is not increased. The blood volume increases because of the increased GFR with lower serum creatinine and blood urea nitrogen concentrations. Renal tubular resorption is less efficient than in the nonpregnant state, and glucosuria may occur, along with increased excretion of water-soluble vitamins. Small amounts of glucosuria increase the risk for urinary tract infections. Pregnant women who present with acute pyelonephritis are hospitalized for aggressive antibiotic treatment, as this infection can easily affect the respiratory system.

Uterine Environment

A less than ideal intrauterine environment resulting from maternal infection, stressful events, poor nutrition, or excess saturated fat intake can negatively influence the development of different cell types and organs (Tamashiro and Moran, 2010). Nonetheless, the goal is to support a healthy environment through a proper balance of nutrients and the avoidance of teratogens.

A system depicting embryonic changes was compiled by scientists and embryologists in 1913. This system is known as the "Carnegie criteria," with 23 stages of developmental milestones. For example, multiple nutrients are involved in the creation of bone (see Box 16-2). Specific nutrients are involved at the different Carnegie stages, see *The Visible Embryo* from www.visembryo.com

Optimizing outcomes includes adequate prenatal care, minimizing stress, and ensuring a healthy pregnancy diet (Rifas-Shiman et al., 2009). Fortunately, women with poor socioeconomic status can improve their diet quality with nutrition education. Women with preexisting depression are at risk for poor pregnancy outcome and postpartum depression, which not only puts the mother at risk but also the newborn. Inadequate nutrient intake (such as ω-3 fatty acids), poor self-care, or a combination of both, are complex causes but are important to distinguish (Leung et al., 2009).

The effect of poor maternal nutrition follows both infant and mother for decades (Cox and Phelan, 2008). Maternal nutritional status has been evaluated primarily for infant birth weight, risk of **neural tube defects (NTDs)**, and fetal alcohol syndrome (FAS), a major cause of mental retardation and learning disorders. Birth weight is highly correlated with infant mortality and morbidity. Infants born small for gestational age are known to have major organs that are

BOX 16-2
Bone Nutrients

Protein

Forms organic matrix, for collagen, production of hormones, growth factors.

Minerals

Boron: Considered to have minor role in bone function.
Calcium: Main bone-forming mineral; 99% in skeleton.
Copper: Functions in lysyl oxidase, an enzyme essential for cross-linking of collagen fibrils.
Fluoride: Can replace hydroxyl groups in hydroxyapatite to form less soluble fluoroapatite..
Iron: Cofactor in enzyme involved in collagen bone matrix synthesis, cofactor in 25-hydroxycholecalciferol hydroxylase.
Magnesium: 60% of this mineral is in bone; it has an indirect role in ATP metabolism.
Manganese: For biosynthesis of mucopolysaccharides in bone matrix, cofactor for several enzymes in bone tissue.
Phosphorous: Essential bone-forming mineral.
Zinc: For osteoblastic activity, collagen synthesis, alkaline phosphatase activity.

Fat-Soluble Vitamins

Vitamin A: Essential in bone remodeling process: osteoblasts and osteoclasts have receptors for retinoic acid.
Vitamin D: Maintains calcium levels.
Vitamin K: Cofactor for gamma carboxylation of glutamic acid residues, including osteocalcin, the noncollagenous protein of bone.

Water-Soluble Vitamins

Folic acid: Coenzyme mediating variety of reactions critical to nucleic and amino acid metabolism critical to bone development.
Riboflavin: Needed to convert vitamin B_6 and folate into active forms.
Vitamin B_6: Essential Cofactor for enzyme ornithine decarboxylase; osteoblast NADPH concentrations, essential for Vitamin K.
Vitamin B_{12}: Osteoblast function; cofactor for osteoblast-related proteins (bone alkaline phosphatase and osteocalcin); iron formation.
Vitamin C: Hydroxylation of lysine, proline; cross-linking of collagen fibril; stimulates alkaline phosphatase for osteoblast formation.

ATP, Adenosine triphosphate; *NADPH*, nicotinamide adenine dinucleotide phosphate.

Adapted from Palacios C: The role of nutrients in bone health, from A to Z. *Crit Rev Food Sci Nutr* 46(8):621, 2006.

small; they are at increased risk for hypertension, obesity, learning disorders, behavioral problems, glucose intolerance, and cardiovascular disease (see Chapter 43). Intrauterine food restriction or hyperglycemia may reprogram leptin levels and neuropeptide Y, possibly contributing to metabolic conditions later in life (Page et al., 2009). Infants born large for gestational age (LGA) often have hyperglycemia at birth.

Preconceptual vitamin D status is thought to influence 3% of the human genome, including bone health throughout life. Indeed, maternal vitamin D status may program neonatal skeletal development. A study in Finland found that, although the total vitamin D intake met the current recommendations for this nutrient, 71% of women and 15% of newborns were vitamin D–deficient (Viljakainen et al., 2010). A dose of vitamin D that provides for 25-hydroxyvitamin D (25[OH]D) sufficiency in the mother during pregnancy should provide for normal cord blood concentrations of 25(OH)D for the infant.

Effects of Nutritional Status on Pregnancy Outcome

Any adverse maternal condition puts the fetus at risk for being delivered prematurely. Prematurity has significant inherent health risks. One theory for prematurity is the pregnancy is not obtaining adequate nutrients to continue growth and development of the fetus or the placenta. For example, Table 16-2 presents the roles of specific nutrients for neonatal brain development.

Researchers speculate that maternal starvation causes alterations in DNA, regulated by various nutrients very early in pregnancy or at the time of conception. In the early 1900s women with poor nutritional status had adverse pregnancy outcomes with hemorrhage at delivery, prolonged labor, and LBW infants. During World War II, the effects of severe food deprivation on previously well-nourished populations were explored. Higher rates of spontaneous abortion, stillbirths, neonatal deaths, and congenital malformations were noted in offspring born to women who conceived during the famine; surviving infants were smaller. Likewise, results from the Chinese famine of 1959 to 1961 showed similar results in the offspring conceived during this period of maternal malnutrition (Zammit et al., 2007). Smaller organs are found in offspring of mothers who were malnourished during pregnancy (Kyle and Picard, 2006).

Even today, subclinical malnutrition may lead to poor reproductive performance. Women experiencing anorexia

CLINICAL INSIGHT

High-Risk Pregnancies

The majority of pregnancies proceed without major risk to either mother or fetus. Approximately 10% of all pregnancies are considered "high risk," meaning there is a maternal preexisting complication or a situation that antedates pregnancy or presents in current gestation that puts the mother or the fetus at risk for a poor outcome. Women who present with the following issues need increased medical surveillance and nutrition assessment to ensure the most favorable outcomes, controlled medical costs, and the fewest complications.

Anemias: microcytic or macrocytic
Cardiovascular issues: hypertension and preeclampsia, deep-vein thrombosis, maternal cardiac structural defects
Endocrine issues: polycystic ovary syndrome, thyroid disease, gestational diabetes, type 1 diabetes
Functional alterations: deafness, blindness, paralysis, paraplegia, quadriplegia
Gastrointestinal issues: food allergies, celiac disease, gastric bypass, Crohn's disease, ulcerative colitis
Hyperemesis gravidarum or nausea and vomiting of pregnancy
Infections: HIV and AIDS, malaria, chicken pox, rubella, measles, mumps, West Nile virus, parvovirus, Lyme disease, dental disease
Maternal genetic diseases or mental retardation
Medical problems: lupus, myasthenia gravis, cystic fibrosis, pancreatitis, PKU, cancer, obesity, sickle cell disease
Obesity: BMI >30
Organ transplants: heart, kidneys, liver, lung, stem-cell, liver-intestinal
PROM: early rupture of the chorion (outer layer) and the amnion (inner layer) of the amniotic sac
Placenta previa—complete or marginal: abnormal presentation of the placenta with placenta presenting and obstructing the cervix; cannot deliver fetus through placenta
Psychiatric: eating disorders, depression, bipolar disorders, Munchausen syndrome, suicidal ideation, substance abuse
Reproductive issues: incompetent cervix, uterine anomalies, fibroids; multiple gestations; ovarian hyperstimulation syndrome
Respiratory issues: asthma, tuberculosis, adult respiratory distress disorder, SARS
Surgeries: gastric bypass, cancers, emergency appendicitis

AIDS, Acquired immune deficiency syndrome; *HIV*, human immunodeficiency virus; *PKU*, phenylketonuria; *PROM*, premature rupture of the membranes; *SARS*, sudden acute respiratory syndrome.

TABLE 16-2

Key Nutrients for Fetal and Neonatal Brain Development

Nutrient	Function in Brain	Effect of Deficiency
Energy: protein, carbohydrate, fat	Cell proliferation and differentiation, synaptogenesis, growth factor synthesis	Global effect including cortex, hippocampus, white matter.
Iron	Myelin, monoamine synthesis, neuronal and glial energy metabolism.	White matter-striatal-frontal; hippocampus-frontal
Zinc	DNA synthesis, neurotransmitter release	Autonomic nervous system, hippocampus, cerebellum
Copper	Neurotransmitter synthesis, neuronal and glial energy metabolism, antioxidant activity	Cerebellum
Long-chain polyunsaturated fatty acids	Myelin formation, synaptogenesis	Cortex of the brain, the eye
Choline	Neurotransmitter synthesis, DNA methylation, myelin synthesis	Hippocampus, white matter

Adapted from Georgieff MK: Nutrition and the developing brain: nutrient priorities and measurement, Am J Clin Nutr 85:1S, 2007.
DNA, Deoxyribonucleic acid.

nervosa and bulimia nervosa can have **amenorrhea**, infertility, and reduced rates of pregnancy. Women with a history of eating disorders should therefore be carefully monitored. This includes looking for **pregorexia**, a form of increased calorie expenditure and caloric restraint during pregnancy (Mathieu, 2009). See *Clinical Insight:* High-Risk Pregnancies.

The developing fetus may be unable to obtain optimal nutrients from a host who is compromised nutritionally. Compromises in structural or cognitive potential may not be evident when an infant is born, but may manifest later in life when various stages of growth are arrested or altered. Attention deficit disorder in some children may be related to suboptimal gestational iodine or low vitamin D transfer in a depleted mother (Cui et al., 2007).

LBW (<2500 g) and especially very low birth weight (<1500 g) are major factors for **perinatal mortality** (infant deaths occurring between 28 weeks' gestation and 4 weeks' postpartum). These deaths may occur from necrotizing enterocolitis, respiratory distress syndrome, intraventricular hemorrhage, cerebral palsy, or retinopathy of prematurity. Maternal obesity in the African American population has been associated with a 40% higher incidence of stillbirths compared with women with normal BMI status (Salihu et al., 2007).

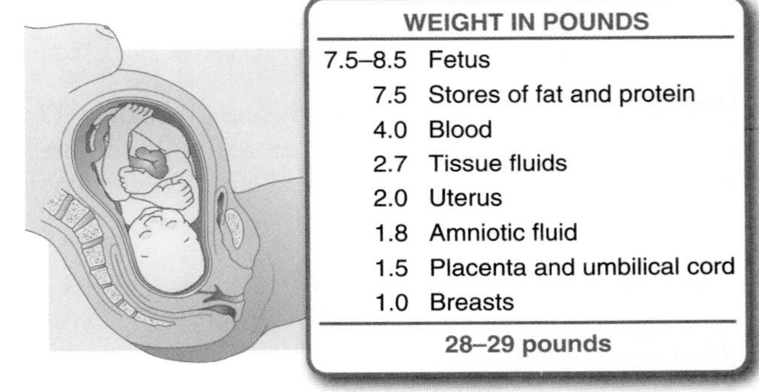

FIGURE 16-1 Distribution of weight gain during pregnancy.

Maternal Weight Gain

With a singleton gestation, less than half of the total weight gain of a normal-weight pregnant woman resides in the fetus, placenta, and amniotic fluid. The remainder is in maternal reproductive tissues (breast tissues and uterus), interstitial fluid, blood volume, and maternal adipose tissue. Gradually, increased subcutaneous fat in the abdomen, back, and upper thigh serves as an energy reserve for pregnancy and lactation. The normal distribution of weight gain is illustrated in Figure 16-1. Although this chart implies the fetus at term constitutes approximately 27% of the total pregnancy weight gain, this may not be true for all pregnancies.

In normal-weight women living in healthy environments, a gestational weight gain of 25 to 35 lb is associated with a favorable outcome at term. Guidelines issued by the Institute of Medicine (IOM) recommend a weight gain of 25 to 35 lb for women of normal weight (pregravid BMI 18.5 to 24.9), 28 to 40 lb for underweight women (BMI <18.5), and 15 to 25 lb for overweight women (BMI 25 to 29.9) (Rasmussen and Yaktine, 2009; Figure 16-2).

Weight loss during pregnancy should be discouraged. As adipose tissue is mobilized, there is concern for the release of semivolatile organic compounds, which can have an effect on the developing fetal brain that is not clear.

Obesity

Pregravid obesity is described as class I (BMI 30-34.9), class II (BMI 35-39.9), and class III (BMI more than 40); optimal gestational gains for these groups are not yet known. Studies indicate that 50% of high-BMI women gain more

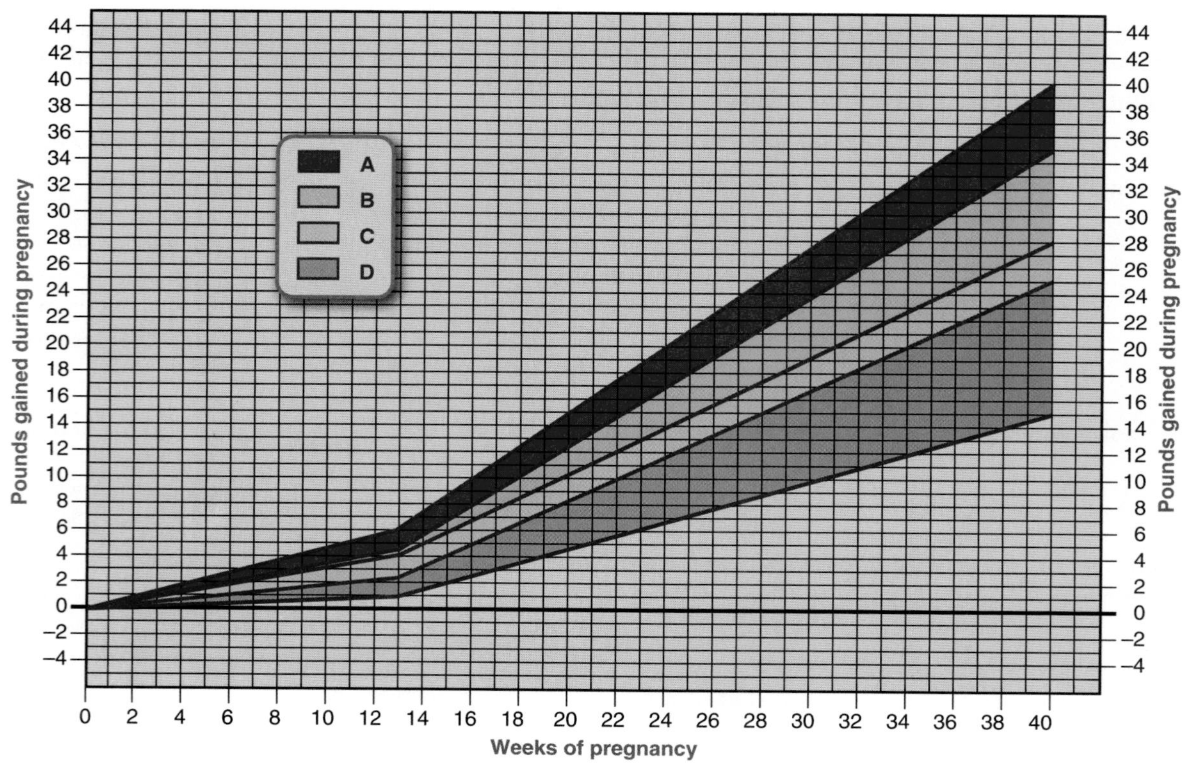

FIGURE 16-2 Desirable weight gain during pregnancy. Females who are of normal weight before their pregnancy should aim for a weight gain in the B to C range (25-35 lb) during pregnancy. Underweight females should gain in the A to B range (28-40 lb). Females who are overweight before pregnancy should gain in the D range (11-20 lb).

than the target weight recommendations, thus reflecting the increasing prevalence of obesity among U.S. women (Stotland et al., 2005).

Overweight and obese women are at increased risk for **intrauterine fetal demise (IUFD)** or miscarriage. The risks for **gestational diabetes mellitus (GDM)**, pregnancy-induced hypertension (PIH), and cesarean section increase in this same group (American Congress of Obstetricians and Gynecologists [ACOG], 2005). When ultrasound studies examined the lean to fat mass in fetuses of women with GDM, their fetuses showed an accelerated rate of growth (de Santis et al., 2010). The risk for delivery of a very preterm (<32 weeks) infant or an infant with a cardiac defect, NTD, or **macrosomia** (birthweight > 4000 g) increases in women who are obese (Artal et al., 2010). Obesity is associated with a high risk of hypertensive disorders (Callaway et al., 2009b).

An association between maternal obesity and increased incidence of NTDs has not been explained, but obesity itself is an inflammatory state. Low grade systemic inflammation is associated with higher levels of C-reactive protein, interleukin-6, and leptin. A sustained state of hyperglycemia or hyperinsulinism may be related to NTDs as well (Yazdy et al., 2010). Folate intake of 600 mcg/day is less protective against NTDs in obese women than in normal-weight pregnant women; obese women may need more (Scialli and Public Affairs Committee, 2006). There is speculation that the increased body size may require additional supplementation. Since vitamin B12 is a cofactor for methionine synthase, an enzyme that plays a key role in folate metabolism, it may also be required in larger amounts to prevent NTDs. In addition, there is a suggestion that nutrients such as iron, magnesium and niacin may play a role in NDTs (Groenen, 2004). Inadequate choline may be implicated in NDTs since, like folate, it functions as a methyl donor (Zeisel, 2009). A proactive nutritional goal is to choose foods of high antioxidant quality. Indeed, the benefits of prepregnancy maternal weight loss include improved plasma lipids, glucose, and uric acid, which may also reduce pregnancy risk factors.

Postbariatric Surgery. The prevalence of obesity has resulted in more gastric bypass operations for weight reduction, which has tremendous implications for pregnancy. Although prepregnancy weight loss may improve fertility, it has the potential to provide a suboptimal uterine environment for the developing fetus. Pregnancy should be delayed for at least 1 year after this surgery, and adequate nutrient supplementation is essential.

Operative complications are not uncommon, such as intestinal hernias. Deficiencies in iron, vitamins A, D, B_{12}, K, and folate, and calcium can result in maternal complications (severe anemia) or fetal complications, such as congenital abnormalities, smaller kidneys, neonatal rickets, IUGR and **failure to thrive (FTT)** (Faintuch et al., 2009; Guelinckx et al., 2009). An optimum nutrient prescription and caloric requirement for pregnant women following

BOX 16-3

Risk Factors for Poor Pregnancy Outcome in Teenagers

Young maternal age, especially younger than age 16
Pregnancy less than 2 years after onset of menarche
Poor nutrition and low prepregnancy weight
Poor weight gain
Infection
Sexually transmitted disease or infection
Preexisting anemia
Substance abuse: smoking, drinking, and drugs
Poverty
Lack of social support
Low educational level
Rapid repeat pregnancies
Lack of access to age-appropriate prenatal care
Late entry into the health system
Unmarried status
Unstable housing, shelter living, homelessness

bariatric surgery has not been determined and thus must be individualized. Low intakes of calcium, vitamin B_{12}, and iron have been noted in this population (Faintuch et al., 2009).

Adolescent Pregnancy

Public health initiatives have helped reduce the incidence of teen pregnancies; however, teenage pregnancy continues as a major public health problem in the United States and is associated with significant medical and nutritional risks. Approximately 1 million U.S. adolescents become pregnant every year, accounting for 25% of U.S. pregnancies. Teens have a higher incidence of delivering a LBW infant. Risk factors for poor outcome in pregnant adolescents are listed in Box 16-3.

Poor outcomes are especially common in obese teens who become pregnant. Excess body fat, particularly of visceral distribution, has been linked with proinflammatory cytokines, chronic low-grade inflammation, low total-body iron metabolism, increased fatigue, and reduced physical activity (Tussing-Humphreys et al., 2009). Many other teens enter pregnancy with suboptimal nutritional status, especially for iron, calcium, and folic acid. Young maternal age is a significant risk factor for developmental defects, such as inadequate neonatal tooth enamel formation (Vello et al., 2009).

Improved dietary practices can be one of the most important factors for the pregnant teen or young mother. In counseling teen mothers, the nutrition professional must be aware of the teen's psychosocial, cultural, and literacy level; economic status and dependencies; and any educational frameworks that influence her food choices. Benefits of nutritional counseling for pregnant adolescents are presented in Figure 16-3.

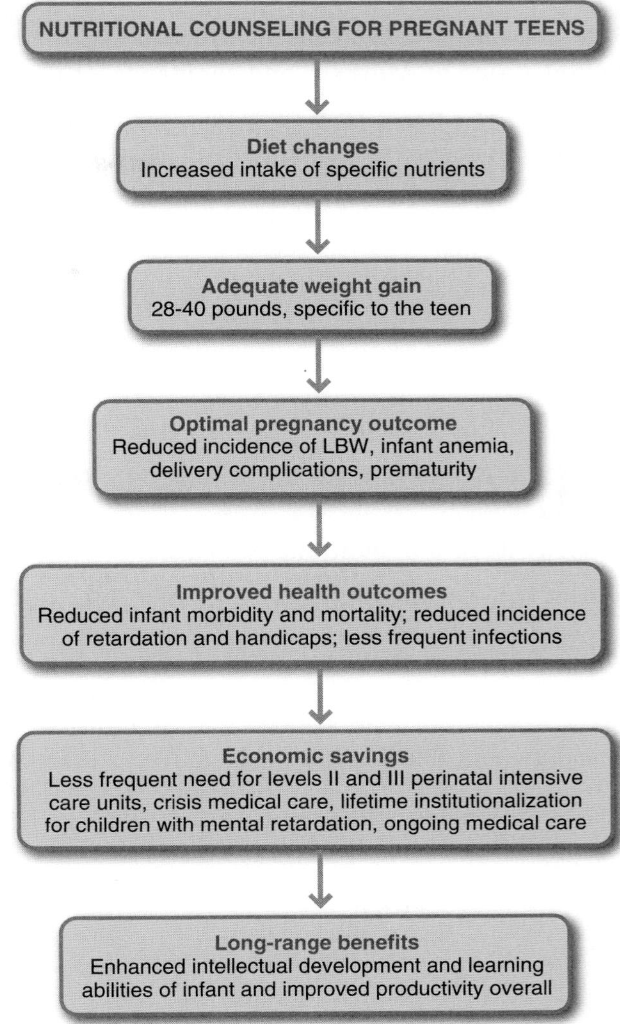

FIGURE 16-3 Benefits of nutritional counseling for pregnant adolescents.

Multiple Births

The incidence of multiple births in the United States is rising in part because of the increased use of fertility drugs and ART. Infants of multiple-birth pregnancies have a greater risk of premature delivery with accompanying IUGR or LBW than do singletons. Adequate maternal weight gain has been shown to be particularly important in these higher-risk pregnancies.

Multifetal gestations undergo significant maternal physiological adaptations beyond the usual pregnancy changes, including increased plasma volume, metabolic rate, and increased insulin resistance (Goodnight and Newman, 2009). Optimal weight gain and infant gestational ages for this population are presented in Table 16-3.

The optimal nutritional requirements for twins and higher-order multiples are not yet known. One nutritional plan is summarized in Table 16-4. Although this plan has not included iodine specifically, it is imperative to meet at least the singleton recommendation of 220 mcg/day, with

TABLE 16-3

Weight Gains of Mothers and Incidence of Low Birth Weights in Multiple-Birth Pregnancies

Plurality	Live-Born Infants	LBW (%) (Less Than 2500 g)	VLBW (%) (Less Than 1500 g)	Maternal Weight Gain by 24 Wk (lb)	Weight Gain Total (lb)	Weeks Gestation	Mean Birth Weight (g)
Singletons	3.8M	6	1	12	25-35	38-41	3700-4000
Twins	96,445	50	10	24	40-45	36-37	2500-2800
Triplets	4168	90	32	36	50-60	34-35	1900-2200

From Luke B: Managing maternal nutrition: prenatal and postpartum, Perinat Nutr Rep 3:2, 1997; Heron et al: Annual summary of vital statistics, 125:4, 2007.

LBW, Low birth weight; *VLBW*, very low birth weight.

TABLE 16-4

Nutrient Recommendations for Twins

Nutrient	Twins	Comments
Calories	40-45 kcal/kg normal weight BMI	Weight is not specified—pregravid, ideal or current?
Protein	14.4%-18.1% of total calories	Depending on calorie requirements, could be as high as 175 g/day.
Carbohydrate	350 g/day for normal weight gravid	Encourage low glycemic choices.
Fat	156 g/day for normal weight gravid	Encourage healthy fats.
Vitamin D	1000 IU/day	Assessment of maternal levels should be considered in first and early third trimester to allow alterations in the supplemental dose.
Vitamin C	500-1000 mg/day	This is half of the UL of 1800-2000 mg/day.
Vitamin E	400 mg/day	This is half of the UL of 800-1000 mg/day.
Zinc	15 mg/day (T1); 45 mg/day (T2-3)	Diet alone may not be enough. Supplementation may be required.
Iron	30 mg/day	For nonanemic twins. Rosello-Soberon (2005) reported an estimated 869 mg/day iron requirement for twins compared with 476 mg for a singleton pregnancy.
Folic acid	1000 mcg/day	
Calcium	1500 mg/day (T1); 2500 mg (T2-3)	UL: 2500 mg/day
Magnesium	400 mg/day (T1); 800 mg/day (T2-3)	
DHA/EPA	300-500 mg/day	

Adapted from Goodnight W, Newman R: Optimal nutrition for improved twin pregnancy outcome, Obstet Gynecol 114:1121, 2009.

BMI, Body mass index; *DHA*, docosahexaenoic acid; *EPA*, eicosapentaenoic acid; *T*, trimester; *UL*, tolerable upper limit.

the upper limit for singleton gestation at 900 mcg for mothers younger than 18 years old and 1100 mcg for those 19 years and older. The dietary reference intakes (DRIs) for choline for the singleton gestation are important as well; include 450 mg/day with a tolerable upper limit of 3 g/day for women younger than 18 and 3.5 grams for women older than 19.

Nutritional Supplementation During Pregnancy

Supplementation of a mother's diet during pregnancy may take the form of additional energy, protein, vitamins, or minerals that exceed her routine daily intake. The more compromised the nutritional status of the woman, the greater is the benefit for pregnancy outcome with improved diet and nutritional supplementation. Judicious use of supplements is needed in high-risk pregnancies and in undernourished women, women with substance abuse, teenage mothers, women with a short interval between pregnancies, women with a history of delivering an LBW infant, and women with a multiple gestation pregnancy.

Under the auspices of the U.S. Department of Agriculture (USDA), pregnant women at nutritional risk are encouraged to enroll in the Special Supplemental Nutrition

Program for Women, Infants and Children (WIC). For U.S. citizens, the WIC program serves eligible pregnant women, postpartum women until 6 months' postpartum, breastfeeding women until 1 year postpartum, and infants and children up to the age of 5 years (see Chapter 10). "Nutritional risk" criteria may include anemia, poor gestational weight gain, inadequate diet, or FTT in the infant or child. Outcome studies show higher mean birth weights and higher mean gestational ages in infants born to WIC participants.

Many pregnant women and some providers have limited knowledge regarding the nutrients in the supplements they have been prescribed or have been advised to purchase over the counter. There is great variability in the composition of supplements as demonstrated in Table 16-5, and formulations change frequently. It is important to read the label

TABLE 16-5

Comparison of Some Prenatal Supplements

Nutrient	Example #1 (3 caps per day)	Example #2 (2 caps per day)	Example #3 (2 tabs per day)	Example #4 (1 tab per day)	Children's chewable Multivitamin-mineral (1 per day for adults)
Vitamin A IU	5000 (2000 IU retinyl palmitate and 3000 IU as mixed carotenoids)	8000 (100% as mixed carotenoids)	8000 (4800 IU retinyl palmitate and 3200 IU beta carotene)	4000 (100% as beta carotene)	3000
Vitamin D IU	1,000	400	400	400	400
Vitamin E IU	50	18.2	60	30	30
Vitamin K mcg	100		—	—	—
Vitamin B_1 (thiamine) mg	4	1.6	3.0	1.8	1.5
Vitamin B_2 (riboflavin) mg	3.6	1.7	3.4	1.7	1.7
Vitamin B_3 (niacin) mg	30	20	40	20	15
Pantothenic acid mg	16	6	20	—	10
Vitamin B_6 mg	10	2.2	4	2.6	2
Vitamin B_{12} mcg	200	2.6	12	8	6
Folic acid mcg	1000 (500 mcg as calcium folate and 500 mcg as 5-MTHF)	1000	800	800	400
Vitamin C mg	150	110	120	—	60
Choline mg			10	—	38
Biotin mcg	50	300	600	—	40
Calcium mg	200	200	400	200	100
Copper mcg	2	2	2		2
Iron mg	45	27	20	28	18
Chromium mcg	100	120	—		—
Iodine mcg	150	150	—	—	150
Magnesium mg	100	80	300	—	20
Zinc mg	25	15	20	25	12
Selenium mcg	50	70	—		—
Manganese mg	5	2	2		—
Phosphorous mg	—	—	—	—	100
Sodium mg	—	—	—	—	10

DHA, Docosahexaenoic acid; *5-MTHF*, 5-methyltetrahydrofolate.

of prenatal supplements—some are much more complete than others and some are little more than a children's chewable multivitamin mineral with extra folic acid and iron. Approximately 60% of prenatal supplements include the recommended dietary allowance (RDA) for iodine, but an analysis found that the actual amount of iodine differed from the amount listed on the label (Leung, 2009). Women often need advice on local, suitable choices for themselves or their children.

Nutrition Requirements

Fetal growth demands additional nutrients and these requirements are defined in the DRIs, which include RDAs and adequate intakes (AIs). These DRIs are found on the inside front cover.

Energy

Additional energy is required during pregnancy to support the metabolic demands of pregnancy and fetal growth. Metabolism increases by 15% in the singleton pregnancy. The 2002 DRIs for energy for the pregnant female are the same as for the nonpregnant female in the first trimester, then increase by 340 to 360 kcal/day during the second trimester and by another 112 kcal/day in the third trimester (Institute of Medicine [IOM], 2002). If maternal weight gain is within the desirable limits, the range of acceptable energy intakes varies widely, given individual differences in energy output and basal metabolic rate.

Exercise. Energy expended in voluntary physical activity is the largest variable in overall energy expenditure. Physical activity increases energy expenditure proportional to body weight. However, most pregnant women compensate for increased weight gain by slowing their work pace; thus total daily energy expenditure may not be substantially greater than before pregnancy.

Excessive exercise, combined with inadequate energy intake, may lead to suboptimal maternal weight gain and poor fetal growth. Therefore a pregnant woman should always discuss exercise with her primary health practitioner. Exercising during pregnancy at high altitudes may compromise fetal oxygen delivery, especially for women who are not acclimatized to higher elevations. Resting uterine blood flow is lower in residents residing at 3100 m than at 1600 m, and blood flow is likely to decrease further during exercise in proportion to the intensity and duration.

Consequences of Energy Restriction. A once-popular concept held that the fetus develops at the expense of the mother during nutritional deprivation. However, evidence from famines clearly contradicts this assumption. It is now accepted that a malnourished mother is proportionately less affected than her fetus. One consequence of severe energy restriction is increased ketone production. Although the fetus has a limited ability to metabolize ketone bodies, the short- and long-term effects of maternal ketonemia are unclear. Both animal and human data indicate that ketone bodies are normally presented to the fetal brain at various times during pregnancy. After an overnight fast, maternal blood ketone body concentrations are greater in pregnant than in nonpregnant women, and even ketonuria can be detected. When ketonuria is present, it indicates a lack of energy-providing macronutrients, which also reduces vitamin and mineral intake. Box 16-4 describes some of the causes of fetal malnutrition.

BOX 16-4

Causes of Fetal Malnutrition

Acute change in maternal condition, such as a stroke
GI disease cancers of the intestinal tract, gastric bypass
Hyperemesis gravidarum
Infections
Parasite infestation
Lack of food due to war, famine, natural disasters (e.g., earthquake, tsunami)
Maternal gallbladder disease causing malabsorption
Mother with active eating disorder, such as anorexia nervosa
Multiple gestations
Pica
Placental compromise: placenta previa, hypertensive disorders, abruptions
Poverty

GI, Gastrointestinal.

Protein

There is an additional protein requirement for pregnancy to support the synthesis of maternal and fetal tissues, but the magnitude of this increase is uncertain. Protein requirement increases throughout gestation and is maximized during the third trimester. The current RDA of 0.8 g/kg/day of protein for pregnant women is the same as that for the nonpregnant women in the first half of pregnancy. Needs increase in the second half to 71 g/day, based on 1.1 gm/kg/day of prepregnant weight (IOM, 2002). For each additional fetus, another 25 g/day of protein is recommended; this may be as much as 175 g/day for the normal-weight woman carrying a twin gestation who is consuming 3500 kcal/day (Goodnight and Newman, 2009).

Protein deficiency during pregnancy has adverse consequences. Limited intakes of protein and energy usually occur together, making it difficult to separate the effects of energy deficiency from those of protein deficiency.

Carbohydrates

DRIs for carbohydrates in pregnancy are estimated average requirements (EARs) at 135 g/day; the RDA is 175 g/day (IOM, 2002). This 135 to 175 g/day is recommended to provide enough calories in the diet to prevent ketosis and maintain appropriate blood glucose during pregnancy. With an average 2000 calorie/day regimen, 175 g translates to 700 calories, or 35%. The amount may be greater in women consuming more calories, but careful carbohydrate choices are needed to include all the daily nutrients for pregnancy.

Fiber

Daily consumption of whole-grain breads and cereals, leafy green and yellow vegetables, and fresh and dried fruits should be encouraged to provide additional minerals, vitamins, and fiber. The DRI for fiber during pregnancy is 28 g/day (IOM, 2002) and if met, will help a great deal in managing the constipation that often accompanies pregnancy.

Lipids

There is no DRI for lipids during pregnancy. The amount of fat in the diet should depend on energy requirements for proper weight gain. However, there is a recommendation (an AI of 13 g/day) for the amount of ω-6 polyunsaturated fatty acids (linoleic acid) and an AI of 1.4 g/day for the amount of ω-3 polyunsaturated fatty acids (α-linolenic acid) in the diet (IOM, 2002). The recommendation for docosahexaenoic acid is 300 mg/day. Essential fatty acid requirements can usually be met by one to two portions of fish per week (Simpson et al., 2010b). See *Focus On:* Omega-3 Fatty Acids in Pregnancy and Lactation.

Vitamins

All vitamins are needed for optimal pregnancy outcome. In some instances the provision of these specific vitamins may be met through diet, and for others a supplement is necessary. Periconceptional multivitamin supplementation has been documented to reduce the risk of heart defects in infants if started very early in pregnancy. Most vitamin and mineral recommendations increase approximately 15% from nonpregnant values. Refer to the DRI tables on the inside cover.

Folic Acid. For nonpregnant adult women, the recommended intake is 400 mcg/day for dietary folate equivalent. Folic acid requirements increase during pregnancy for maternal erythropoiesis, DNA synthesis, and fetal and placental growth. The Centers for Disease Control and Prevention recommends that all women of childbearing age increase their intake of folic acid; obese women even more so. More than half of all U.S. pregnancies are unplanned and the neural tube closes by 28 days of gestation, before most women realize they are pregnant (Goldberg et al., 2006; see Table 16-1). Because the average amount of folic acid received through food fortification (grains) in the United States is only 128 mcg/day, there is a need for the additional 400 mcg/day of synthetic folic acid from supplements or fortified foods (Simpson et al., 2010a).

Folic acid deficiency is marked by a reduced rate of DNA synthesis and mitotic activity in individual cells. White cell morphologic and biochemical changes signaling deficiency precede overt megaloblastic anemia, the latest stage of folate deficiency, which may not present until the third trimester (see Chapter 33). Maternal folate deficiency is associated with an increased incidence of congenital malformations, including cleft lip and palate and NTDs. Indeed, approximately 2500 new cases of NTDs occur in the United States each year; the NTD recurrence rate may be as high as 2% to 10%. Red blood cell folate concentrations exceeding 906 mmol/L (400 ng/mL) are associated with the fewest NTDs.

FOCUS ON

Omega-3 Fatty Acids in Pregnancy and Lactation

Our ancestors consumed a diet with equal amounts of ω-3 and ω-6 fatty acids with a ratio of 1 : 1. American diets are currently estimated to contain a ratio of ω-3 to ω-6 fatty acids of 1 : 10. This dramatic decrease in the consumption of ω-3 fatty acids over many centuries is thought to affect overall disease prevalence, as well as pregnancy outcome.

Fatty acids are found in all cell membranes. They compose 60% of the dry weight of fetal brain, half of which is as ω-6 and the other half as ω-3 (arachidonic acid) and docosahexaenoic acid [DHA], respectively). Because DHA is important for the growth and development of the fetal central nervous system and the retina, the prenatal diet should include adequate amounts of preformed DHA. 300 mg during pregnancy and during lactation is recommended (Institute of Medicine, 2002). The main food source of DHA is fatty, cold-water fish; and two to three fish meals per week of low-mercury fish during pregnancy appear to provide adequate amounts of DHA. An example of a low-mercury fish high in DHA is sardines. The consumer is advised to follow "safe-fish" guidelines by monitoring information that is found on www.seaturtles.org/gotmercury.htm.

Other options to increase the DHA content in the diet of pregnant and lactating women include the consumption of ω-3–enriched eggs and the use of DHA supplements. Vegetable sources of ω-3 fats include flax seeds and nuts, especially walnuts and walnut oil, although they are less efficient in being converted to DHA. Any pregnant woman allergic to fish should seek an algae source of supplemental DHA (Arterburn et al., 2008). Women should be asked if a supplement has DHA or cod-liver oil; the latter has high amounts of vitamin A (retinoic acid) that can be of concern.

The breast-fed infant obtains DHA through maternal milk when the mother eats sufficient quantities of foods containing DHA. If the mother is not consuming fish or DHA supplements, a DHA liquid supplement can be given to the infant. Most infant formulas are fortified with DHA.

Women who smoke, consume alcohol moderately or heavily, or use recreational drugs are at risk for marginal folate status, as are those with malabsorption syndromes or genetic differences related to methylation and metabolic use of dietary folate. See Chapters 5 and 8. Malformations can occur in infants of women using the anticonvulsant medications phenytoin, carbamazepine, diphenylhydantoin; oral contraceptives; the diuretic triamterene; and trimethoprim. Women using antiseizure medications must be closely monitored when starting folic acid because folic acid supplementation can reduce seizure threshold.

Vitamin B_6. Vitamin B_6 functions as a cofactor in approximately 50 decarboxylase and transaminase enzymes, especially in amino acid metabolism. Although this vitamin catalyzes a number of reactions involving neurotransmitter production, it is not known whether this function is involved in the relief of nausea or vomiting. Because meat, fish, and poultry are good dietary sources, deficiency is not common and routine prenatal vitamins are sufficient (Simpson et al., 2010a). Megadoses such as 25 mg three times per day has questionable efficacy.

Vitamin B_{12}. Cobalamin is required for enzyme reactions and for generation of methionine and tetrahydrofolate. B_{12} is found almost exclusively in foods of animal origin (meats, dairy products); therefore vegetarians are at greatest risk for dietary vitamin B_{12} deficiency and should be supplemented (Simpson et al., 2010a). Deficiencies in both folate and vitamin B_{12} have been related to depression in adults. There is concern regarding inadequate amounts of these nutrients during fetal brain development affecting infant cognitive and motor development (Black, 2008).

Choline. Choline is an essential nutrient because it cannot be synthesized in sufficient quantities to meet metabolic demands. It is needed for structural integrity of cell membranes, cell signaling, and nerve impulse transmission, and is a major source of methyl groups. Choline has been shown to support adequate neurogenesis in folic-acid deficient mice whose mothers were supplemented (Craciunescu et al., 2010). The IOM recommends choline at 450 mg/day during pregnancy, 25 mg more than for the nonpregnant woman. Choline-rich foods are beef liver, pork, chicken, turkey, fish, egg yolks, soy lecithin, and wheat germ. Pregnant women who are not eating these foods may need supplementation. The prenatal supplement should be evaluated for its choline content; many popular brands do not contain choline.

Vitamin C. Ascorbic acid is involved in collagen synthesis and functions as an antioxidant. Daily consumption of food sources high in this nutrient should be encouraged. At this time there are no recommendations to suggest supplemental vitamin C for the prevention of premature ruptured membranes and pre-eclamptic toxemia (PET).

Vitamin A. Vitamin A deficiency is teratogenic, as noted by xerophthalmia in developing countries. In human cord blood, vitamin A concentrations correlate with birth weight, head circumference, length, and gestation duration. Low maternal vitamin A concentration can result in reduced kidney size in newborns (Goodyer et al., 2007). Infants born prematurely have low vitamin A stores and poor lung function (Darlow and Graham, 2009).

Prenatal vitamin A supplementation is usually not warranted, and in developing countries should not exceed 3000 mcg (10,000 IU)/day (Simpson et al., 2010b). Very high doses of vitamin A (>30,000 IU) may increase the risk for a neural crest defect (Neural Crest and Associated Disorders, 2009). Women who take isotretinoin (Accutane) for acne should stop before they become pregnant. It is a vitamin A analog. As such, the infants of women who become pregnant while on isotretinoin are at extremely high risk for fetal anomalies (NICHD, 2001).

Vitamin D. Vitamin D and its metabolites cross the placenta and appear in fetal blood in the same concentration as in maternal circulation. Vitamin D enhances immune function and brain development (Feron et al., 2005). Vitamin D may have a role in cytokine (Th_1 and Th_2) regulation, multiple sclerosis, diabetes, and autism. Low vitamin D levels during pregnancy predispose to PET, a hypertensive condition of pregnancy affecting up to 8% of pregnant women (Duley, 2009). Maternal vitamin D deficiency is associated with neonatal hypocalcemia, which can manifest in inadequate fetal bone mineralization, hypoplasia of tooth enamel, or convulsions (Cambadoo et al., 2007).

Vitamin D blood concentrations are often low in infants born to vitamin D–deficient mothers. Vitamin D deficiency is increasingly recognized in dark-skinned and veiled women in the northern latitudes where sun exposure is low (Simpson et al., 2010b). Women who are at risk of entering pregnancy with low vitamin D levels include those with BMI greater than 30 and those with a high use of sunscreen, along with poor dietary intake. Poor muscular performance is associated with vitamin D deficiency. The rate of cesarean section deliveries is found to be inversely related to vitamin D status (Merewood et al., 2009). Vitamin D supplementation may be needed to reach desired serum concentrations of more than 20 ng/ml (50 nmol/L) (Simpson et al., 2010b). Use caution not to overdose; excessive amounts of vitamin D are undesirable.

Vitamin E. Vitamin E requirements are increased during pregnancy. Although deficiency during pregnancy is speculated to cause miscarriage, preterm birth, PET, and IUGR (Gagne et al., 2009), vitamin E deficiency specifically has not yet been reported in human pregnancy. Vitamin E is an important lipophilic antioxidant. Of the many tocopherols and tocotrienols, alpha tocopherol is the most biologically active form and is found in all lipoproteins. See Chapter 3.

Vitamin K. Usual diets do not provide adequate amounts of vitamin K as most food sources are dark leafy green vegetables, and are not consumed in recommended quantities. Vitamin K has an important role in bone health as well as in coagulation homeostasis, so adequate amounts during pregnancy are vital. Vitamin K deficiency has been reported in women who have had hyperemesis gravidarum (HG), Crohn's disease, and gastric bypass (Brunnetti-Pierri et al., 2007).

Minerals

Calcium. Hormonal factors strongly influence calcium metabolism in pregnancy. Human chorionic somatomammotropin from the placenta increases the rate of maternal bone turnover. Estrogen inhibits bone resorption, provokes a compensatory release of parathyroid hormone, and maintains maternal serum calcium while enhancing maternal absorption of calcium across the gut. The net effect of these changes is the promotion of progressive calcium retention to meet progressively increasing fetal skeletal demands for mineralization. Fetal hypercalcemia and subsequent endocrine adjustments ultimately stimulate the mineralization process.

Approximately 30 g of calcium is accumulated during pregnancy, almost all of it in the fetal skeleton (25 g). The remainder is stored in the maternal skeleton, held in reserve for the calcium demands of lactation. Most fetal accretion occurs during the last trimester of pregnancy, an average of 300 mg/day.

The upper limit for calcium intake during pregnancy is 2500 mg/day. Overconsumption of calcium in food form is not common; however, elevated serum level of calcium can be the result of excess antacid ingestion for heartburn or gastroesophageal reflux disease.

Copper. Diets of pregnant women are often marginal in copper. Copper deficiency alters embryo development and induced-copper deficiency has been shown to be teratogenic. Not only are there genetic mutations, as in Menkes disease, but also secondary deficiencies from excessive zinc or iron intake, certain drugs, and bariatric surgery (Uriu-Adams et al., 2010). These inadequacies cause decreased activity of cuproenzymes, increased oxidative stress, altered iron metabolism, abnormal protein crosslinking, decreased angiogenesis and altered cell signaling (Uriu-Adams et al., 2010). See Chapter 3

Fluoride. The role of fluoride in prenatal development is controversial. Development of primary dentition begins at 10 to 12 weeks' gestation. From the sixth to the ninth month, the first four permanent molars and eight of the permanent incisors are forming. Thus 32 teeth are developing during gestation. Controversy involves the extent to which fluoride is transported across the placenta and its value in-utero in the development of caries-resistant permanent teeth (see Chapter 26).

Iodine. Iodine is part of the thyroxine molecule, with a critical role in the metabolism of macronutrients. Adequate gestational iodine is associated with a higher intelligence quotient in the child and attention deficit may be associated with milder iodine deficiency (Hoy-Rosas, 2009). In instances in which preconception iodine intake cannot be ensured, supplementation before the end of the second trimester protects the fetal brain from the effects of deficiency (see Chapter 3). To ensure adequate iodine, food is often fortified with iodized salt. Yet many people worldwide are at risk for iodine deficiency caused by low intake of sea products and fish, produce grown in iodine-deficient soils, or food industry use of noniodized salt. Women who emigrate from other countries may have low iodine status because of the low iodine content of their agricultural soil. If urinary iodine levels are low, supplementation is needed (Simpson et al., 2010b). See Table 16-6.

Iron. A marked increase in the maternal blood supply during pregnancy greatly increases the demand for iron. Normal erythrocyte volume increases by 20% to 30% in pregnancy. A pregnant woman must consume an additional 700 to 800 mg of iron throughout her pregnancy—500 mg for hematopoiesis, and 250 to 300 mg for fetal and placental tissues. Most accretion occurs after the 20th week of gestation when maternal and fetal demands are greatest.

A first trimester ferritin level should be assessed before prescribing iron. Foods containing ascorbic acid enhance absorption. If anemia is not improved with iron therapy, it is advised to check vitamin B_6 status. (Hisano et al., 2010). Because many women do not enter pregnancy with sufficient iron stores to cover the physiologic needs of pregnancy, iron supplementation (usually a ferrous salt) is often necessary. Supplementation may be necessary in the

TABLE 16-6

Assessing Iodine Nutrition

Urinary iodine Excretion (mcg/L)	Corresponding iodine intake (mcg/day)	Classification and Implication
<20	<30	Insufficient: severe deficiency
20-49	30-47	Insufficient: moderate deficiency
50-99	75-149	Insufficient: mild deficiency
100-199	150-299	Adequate: optimal nutritional status
200-299	300-499	More than adequate: risk of iodine-induced hyperthyroidism within 5-10 years in susceptible groups
>300	>449	Risk of adverse health consequences such as iodine-induced hyperthyroidism, autoimmune thyroid disease

World Health Organization, United Nations Children's Fund, Assessment of iodine deficiency disorders and monitoring their elimination, pg 33, ISBN 978 92 4 159582 7, 2007.

third trimester, earlier in pregnancy, or in nonpregnant states if serum ferritin is less than 20 mcg/L, hematocrit is less than 32%, or hemoglobin is less than 10.9 g/dL (Simpson et al., 2010b). Inadequate iron consumption may lead to poor hemoglobin production, followed by compromised delivery of oxygen to the uterus, placenta, and developing fetus. The added workload of the heart from maternal anemia with increased cardiac output can lead to preterm delivery, fetal growth retardation, LBW, or inferior neonatal health.

Although the implications of excessive iron intake for women and their infants are not yet clearly defined, some studies suggest a relationship with GDM (Chen et al., 2009).

Magnesium. The full-term fetus accumulates 1 g of magnesium during gestation. The IOM reports that magnesium supplementation during pregnancy reduces the incidence of PET and IUGR; see "Edema and Leg Cramps."

Phosphorus. Phosphorus is found in a wide variety of foods and deficiency is rare when one is eating. Low phosphorous levels, indicative of "refeeding syndrome" have been found in women experiencing severe vomiting or other situations resulting in starvation. Hypophosphatemia can be life threatening because phosphorous is important in energy metabolism as a component of adenosine triphosphate (ATP) and must be promptly replenished, as with intravenous phosphorous (Stanza et al., 2008).

Sodium. The hormonal milieu of pregnancy affects sodium metabolism. Increased maternal blood volume leads to increased glomerular filtration of sodium of 5,000 to 10,000 mEq/day. Compensatory mechanisms maintain fluid and electrolyte balance.

Restriction of dietary sodium or the use of diuretics in pregnant women with edema is not recommended. Rigorous sodium restriction stresses the renin-angiotensin-aldosterone system, resulting in water intoxication and renal and adrenal tissue necrosis. Although moderation in the use of salt and other sodium-rich foods is appropriate for everyone, aggressive restriction is usually unwarranted in pregnancy. Consumption of sodium should remain above 2 to 3 g/day. Use of iodized salt should be encouraged.

Zinc. A zinc-deficient diet does not result in the effective mobilization of zinc stored in the maternal skeleton; therefore a compromised zinc status develops rapidly. Zinc deficiency is highly teratogenic and leads to congenital malformations, abnormal brain development in the fetus, and abnormal behavior in the newborn. A low zinc level also adversely affects vitamin A status. Women with low plasma zinc concentrations are at 2.5 times greater risk for delivering an infant weighing less than 2000 g; women younger than 19 years old have an even higher risk (Rwebembera et al., 2005; Scheplyagina, 2005). Evaluating nutritional status using plasma zinc requires caution because homeostatic mechanisms can maintain plasma concentrations for weeks despite inadequate intake (Charney and Malone, 2009). Zinc is available in red meat, seafood, including oysters, and unrefined grains. Extra supplementation is usually not required (Simpson et al., 2010b).

Guide for Eating During Pregnancy

Recommended Food Intake

The increased requirements of pregnancy can be met by following the Daily Food Guide (Table 16-7). Box 16-5 provides a summary of nutritional care.

Calcium Intake

Milk is one choice for a calcium source for the pregnant woman to meet her increased calcium requirements. A number of milk choices are available: whole milk, low fat milk, skim milk, nonfat powdered milk, buttermilk, acidophilus milk, Lactaid-treated milk, evaporated milk, enriched soy milk, enriched rice and other grain milks, enriched nut milks, and yogurt. Goat milk is also available, but usually has low folate content. Approximately ⅓ cup of dried skim milk is equivalent to 1 cup of fluid milk. Milk can be made richer in calcium, protein, and calories by adding 2 tablespoons of dried nonfat milk to a glass of fluid milk.

Not all milk products are fortified with vitamin D_3, a derivative from an animal source. Some soy milks are fortified with vitamin D_2; because this is a nonanimal source, it may be preferred by vegans. Vitamin D_2 potency is less than one third that of vitamin D_3.

There are many other calcium-containing foods such as spinach, kale, and other dark green leafy vegetables, tofu, canned salmon, almonds, and calcium-fortified drinks and juices. See Table 3-25 in Chapter 3. Many women, primarily non–white women, are less able to digest the disaccharide lactose present in milk, unless it is taken in small amounts or milk is in a cooked product. If necessary, calcium

BOX 16-5

Summary of Nutritional Care During Pregnancy

1. Energy intake to meet nutritional needs and allow for approximately a 0.4-kg (14-oz) weight gain per week during the last 30 weeks of pregnancy
2. Protein intake to meet nutritional needs, approximately an additional 25 g/day; additional 25 g/day/fetus if more than one fetus; 20% of energy intake from protein
3. IODIZED sodium intake that is not excessive, but no less than 2-3 g/day
4. Mineral and vitamin intakes to meet the recommended daily allowances (folic acid and possibly iron supplementation is required)
5. Alcohol omitted
6. Omission of toxins and nonnutritive substances from food, water, and environment as much as possible

TABLE 16-7

Daily Food Guide for Females

Food Group	Minimum Number of Servings		
	Nonpregnant 11- to 24-Year-Olds	Nonpregnant 25- to 50-Year-Olds	Pregnant or Lactating
Protein, foods	5*	5*	7†
Milk products	3	2	3
Breads, grains	7	6	7
Whole-grain	4	4	4
Enriched	3	3	3
Fruits, vegetables	5	5	5
Vitamin C rich	1	1	1
β-carotene rich	1	1	1
Folate rich	1	1	1
Other	2	2	2
Unsaturated fats	3	3	3

Modified from Nutrition during pregnancy and the postpartum period: a manual for health care professionals, 1990, California Department of Health Services, Maternal Child Health Branch.

*Equivalent in protein to 5 oz of animal protein; at least three servings per week should be from the vegetable proteins.

†Equivalent in protein to 7 oz of animal protein; at least one of these servings should be a vegetable protein

supplements such as calcium lactate or calcium carbonate may be prescribed (see Chapter 25).

Fluids

Drinking 8 to 10 glasses of quality fluid daily, mainly water, is encouraged. Although the 2004 report by the National Academies set the AI at 1.5 L/day, with an upper limit of 2.3 L/day, evaluation of a woman's body size as well as climatic conditions are important considerations. Adequate hydration improves the overall sense of well being. Frequent urination is often a complaint from pregnant women; however, optimal hydration reduces risks for urinary tract infections, kidney stones, and constipation.

Alcohol

Abundant evidence from both animal studies and human experience associates maternal alcohol consumption with **teratogenicity** and a specific pattern of abnormalities in the neonate. Features of **fetal alcohol syndrome (FAS)** include prenatal and postnatal growth failure, developmental delay, microcephaly, eye changes (including involvement of the epicanthal fold), facial abnormalities, and skeletal joint abnormalities (Figure 16-4). However, many children adversely affected by maternal drinking during pregnancy cannot be identified early in life using current diagnostic criteria for fetal alcohol spectrum disorder. Alcohol has been shown to alter gene expression. Changes involve proteins associated with central nervous system development; organ morphogenesis; immunologic responses; endocrine function; ion homeostasis; and skeletal, cardiovascular, and cartilage development.

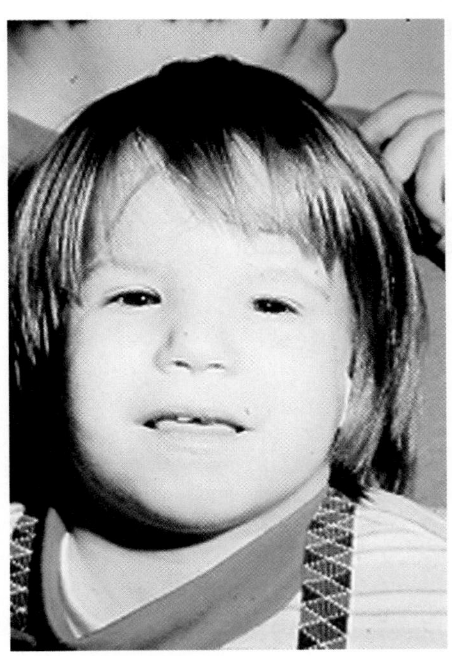

FIGURE 16-4 One-year-old child with fetal alcohol syndrome. *(From Streissguth AP et al: Teratogenic effects of alcohol in humans and laboratory animals, Science 209:353, 1980.)*

Use of alcohol during pregnancy has been associated with an increased rate of spontaneous abortion, placenta abruptio, LBW deliveries, mental retardation, and cognitive compromise. The American Congress of Obstetricians and Gynecologists (ACOG), as well as the March of Dimes and other professional organizations, recommend that alcohol not be used during pregnancy. Reduced-alcohol wines and beers do contain small amounts of alcohol and are also contraindicated. Despite the multiple warnings of fetal injury caused by alcohol, it has been shown that some women continue to consume alcohol in pregnancy (Crozier et al., 2009; Hannigan et al., 2009).

Nonnutritive Substances in Foods

Artificial Sweeteners. The artificial sweeteners sold in the United States have chemical names of *saccharin*, *acesulfame-K*, *sucralose*, and *aspartame*; brand names are *Sweet 'n' Low*, *Sunette* (or *Sweet One*), *Splenda*, *Equal*, or *NutraSweet*, respectively.

Saccharin is a weak carcinogenic in rats in very high doses. However, its consumption in pregnancy has not been restricted. Acesulfame-K consumption by pregnant women is classified as safe, even without long-term studies during human pregnancy. Both saccharin and acesulfame-K cross the placenta and appear in breast milk, but have no known adverse effect on the fetus or infant. Sucralose, a carbohydrate derived from sucrose, was approved for general use in all foods by the Food and Drug Administration (FDA) in 1998. It has not been found to be mutagenic or teratogenic in high doses in animals.

Aspartame is unsafe for women with phenylketonuria (PKU), regardless of whether they are pregnant. Aspartame is metabolized to phenylalanine and aspartic acid. Women with PKU are advised to follow a lifelong low-protein diet and should always be followed by qualified nutrition specialists, especially if they become pregnant. High circulating concentrations of phenylalanine are known to damage the fetal brain (see Chapter 44).

The plant derived sweetener stevia, has not been found to affect fetal development.

Bisphenol-A. Bisphenol-A, or BPA, an endocrine disruptor, may affect thyroid function in humans, especially in the fetus. It may also decrease the serum T_4 half-life by activating hepatic enzymes (Pearce and Braverman, 2009). It should be eliminated if possible from the diet of the pregnant woman, and has been eliminated from plastic bottles and dishes used in feeding the newborn in the US and many other countries (Kubwabo et al., 2009).

Lead and Other Contaminants. Contaminants in food are the exception rather than the rule in the United States, but they do occur. In high concentrations, they can pass across the placenta to the fetus (Figure 16-5). Poorly glazed dishware and leaded crystal decanters often contain high amounts of lead. Old cookware coated with polytetrafluoroethylene (Teflon) are sources of contamination and need to be avoided. Pregnant women should be advised against using dolomite as a calcium supplement because it comes from seashells or sea coral, which have been shown to contain heavy metals, such as lead, the result of dumping industrial wastes in the oceans.

Listeria Monocytogenes. *Listeria monocytogenes* infects 2500 Americans each year; 500 of those infected die. Pregnant women are 20 times more likely than other healthy adults to become infected with *Listeria*. It is a known cause of spontaneous abortion and meningitis of the fetus and newborn. *Listeria* is a soilborne organism; infection results from eating contaminated foods of animal origin and raw vegetables. Raw milk, smoked seafood, frankfurters, pâté, soft cheeses, cold cuts from the deli counter, and uncooked meats are likely sources. Produce irrigated with wastewater needs to be carefully washed with potable water before ingestion.

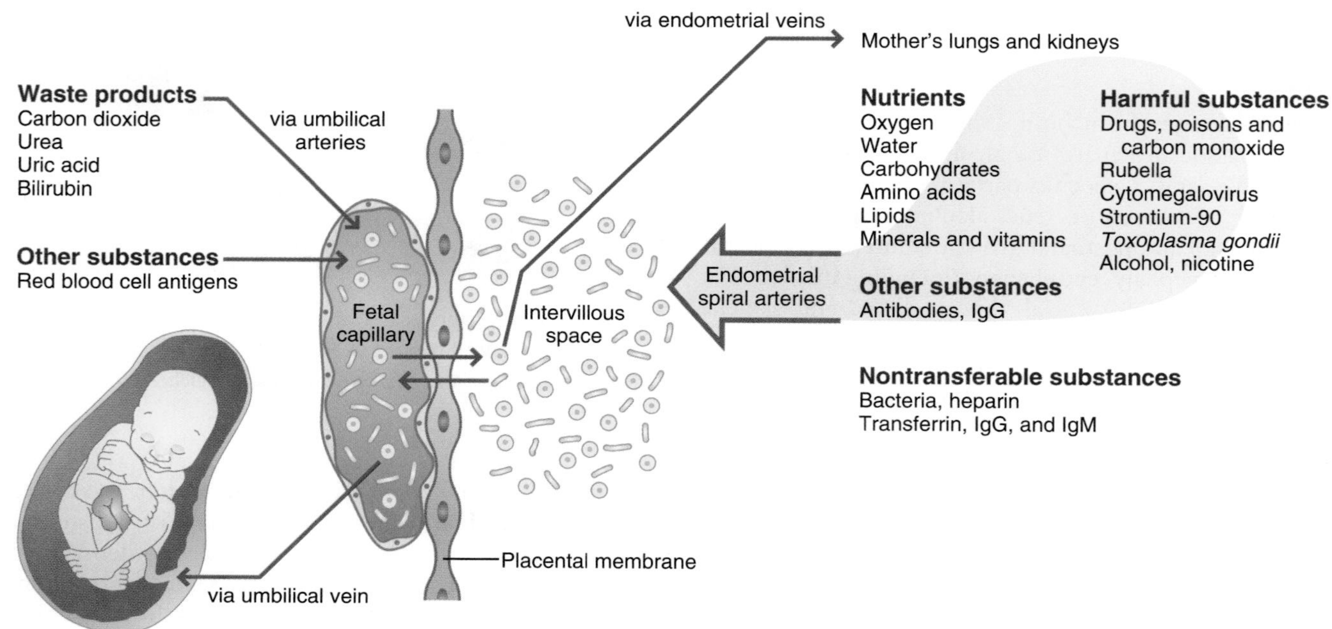

FIGURE 16-5 Transfer of substances across the placental membrane. *Ig*, Immunoglobulin.

Melamine. Melamine is a chemical additive that was criminally added to infant formula from China to increase the nitrogen content; this was discovered when analyzed by modern technology. It is a toxic substance and leads to renal damage or death in infants who ingest it. (Wen et al., 2010).

Mercury. In January 2001 the USDA and the FDA issued a warning for pregnant and lactating women and women of childbearing age to limit consumption of shark, mackerel, tilefish, tuna, and swordfish to no more than two times a week in 4-oz portions. Traces of methyl mercury are found in most fish, but concentrations may be higher in fish from waters close to areas of industrial mercury pollution. The usual concentration of methyl mercury in most fish ranges from less than 0.01 ppm to 0.5 ppm. Few species of fish reach the FDA limit for human consumption of 1 ppm except shark, swordfish, large tuna (the type used to make sushi or fresh steaks), tilefish, and king mackerel. Seafoods (canned tuna, shrimp, pollock, salmon, cod, catfish, clams, flatfish, crabs, and scallops) are continually at risk of mercury contamination and women are advised to regularly check the latest advisories. Farm-raised fish are subject to mercury contamination via acid rain.

Polychlorinated Biphenyls. More than 1.2 billion pounds of polychlorinated biphenyls (PCBs) were produced in the United States before 1976, and half still remain in the water systems. Although PCBs can be absorbed through the skin and lungs, they primarily enter the body from ingestion of contaminated fatty fish such as salmon, lake trout, and carp. They readily pass through the placenta and breast milk; thus pregnant and nursing women and women of childbearing age should avoid eating fish from water known to be contaminated with PCBs. Questions regarding mercury, PCBs, and other contaminants can be directed to state land and natural resource departments.

Cravings and Harmful Beliefs, Avoidances, and Aversions

Most women change their diets during their pregnancies. Change may be due to medical advice, cultural beliefs, or a change in food preference and appetite. Food avoidances may not reflect a mother's conscious choice to eliminate certain foods during her pregnancy. Some reasons for food avoidance may include smell adversity caused by enhanced perception of aromas, a heightened gag response, getting ill while eating or smelling a particular food, or altered gastric comfort.

Cravings and Aversions. Cravings and aversions are powerful urges toward or away from foods, including foods about which women experience no unusual attitudes when not pregnant. The most commonly craved foods are sweets and dairy products or foods that are quick to eat. The most common aversions reported are to alcohol, coffee, other caffeinated drinks, and meats. However, cravings and aversions are not limited to any particular food or food groups.

Pica. Consumption of nonfood substances (**pica**) during pregnancy most often involves **geophagia** (consumption of dirt or clay) or **amylophagia** (consumption of starch such as laundry starch). Other substances include ice, paper, burnt matches, stones or gravel, charcoal, soot, cigarette ashes, antacid tablets, milk of magnesia, baking soda, and coffee grounds.

The incidence of pica is not limited to any one geographic area, race, sex, culture, or social status; nor is it limited to pregnancy. Its cause in pregnancy is poorly understood. One theory suggests that pica relieves nausea and vomiting. It has also been hypothesized that a deficiency of an essential nutrient such as calcium or iron results in the eating of nonfood substances that contain these nutrients. Malnutrition can be a consequence when nonfood substances displace essential nutrients in the diet. Starch in excessive amounts can contribute to obesity and can be deleterious in managing diabetes mellitus. Some substances contain toxic compounds or heavy metals; others interfere with the absorption of iron or other minerals. Excessive intake of starch and clay can lead to intestinal obstruction.

Complications and Nutritional Implications

Constipation and Hemorrhoids

Pregnant women become constipated if they fail to consume adequate water and fiber. Women who are treated with ondansetron (Zofran) for nausea and vomiting often experience severe constipation. Straining during stooling (*val salva*) increases the risk for hemorrhoids. Increased consumption of fluids, fiber-rich foods (see Appendix 41), and dried fruits (especially prunes and apricots), and nuts usually controls these problems. Some women may also require a bulking type of stool softener.

Diabetes Mellitus

The Hyperglycemia Adverse Pregnancy Outcome (HAPO) trial recently defined *GDM* as having one positive glucose reading after a 75-g glucose challenge (Table 16-8). Glucose intolerance may be associated with obesity. Women with

TABLE 16-8

Recommendations for the Diagnosis of GDM

Time	HAPO* Recommendations	Current Standards
Fasting	<92 mg/dL	<95 mg/dL
1 hour	<180 mg/dL	<180 mg/dL
2 hour	<153 mg/dL	<155 mg/dL
3 hour	Not performed	<140 mg/dL

References:

Hadar E et al: Towards new diagnostic criteria for diagnosing GDM: the HAPO study, J Perinat Med 37:447, 2009.

Metzger B et al: Hyperglycemia and adverse pregnancy outcomes, N Engl J Med 358:1991, 2008.

GDM, Gestational diabetes mellitus; *HAPO*, Hyperglycemia Adverse Pregnancy Outcome trial.

(*The challenge is proposed to by 75 grams of glucola)

recurrent preterm births are often treated with 17 α-hydroxyprogesterone caproate, which increases insulin resistance and the rate of GDM (Waters et al., 2009). Women diagnosed with GDM are at risk for future type 2 diabetes mellitus and cardiovascular disease. Although low serum 25(OH)D concentrations correlate with impaired glucose intolerance (von Hurst et al., 2009), no recommendations for nutrient supplementation have been made.

Fetuses of mothers with type 1 or type 2 diabetes are at risk for cardiac defects, such as transposition of the great vessels, double outlet of the right ventricle, tetralogy of Fallot, and mitral and pulmonary atresia (Corrigan et al., 2009). Fetuses of women with GDM are at risk for hypoglycemia at birth, a neonatal intensive care stay, macrosomia, or shoulder dystocia (HAPO Study Cooperative Research Group, 2010). These infants may have lower levels of potassium, zinc, manganese, and chromium (Afridi et al., 2009).

Approaches to reduce the incidence of GDM include providing women with supplemental probiotics before and during pregnancy. Probiotics appear to alter maternal microbiota, change the immune response (Luoto, 2010), and support better glucose tolerance and lower body weight (Laitinen et al., 2009). Women with GDM or elevated first-trimester uric acid concentrations may benefit from a low glycemic prenatal diet (Laughton et al., 2009). See Chapter 31.

Edema and Leg Cramps

Mild, physiologic edema is usually present in the extremities in the third trimester and should not be confused with the pathologic, generalized edema associated with PIH. Normal edema in the lower extremities in pregnancy is caused by the pressure of the enlarging uterus on the vena cava, obstructing the return of blood flow to the heart. When a woman reclines on her side, the mechanical effect is removed, and extravascular fluid is mobilized and eventually eliminated by increased urine output. No dietary intervention is required. Magnesium supplementation has been recommended to reduce leg cramps in pregnancy; however, it may not be effective for every pregnant woman (Nygaard et al., 2008; Sohrabvand et al., 2006).

Heartburn

Gastric esophageal reflux is common during the latter part of pregnancy, and often occurs at night. In most cases this is an effect of pressure of the enlarged uterus on the intestines and stomach, which, in combination with the relaxation of the esophageal sphincter, may result in regurgitation of stomach contents into the esophagus. Relief may occur by suggesting that the pregnant woman eat frequent small meals and stay upright for at least 3 hours after a meal and before lying down. Smaller plates can be used to remind a woman about reduced gastric volume. See Chapter 28.

Nausea, Vomiting, and Hyperemesis Gravidarum

Morning sickness, **nausea and vomiting in pregnancy (NVP)**, affects 50% to 90% of all pregnant women during the first trimester and usually resolves at approximately 17 weeks gestation. Motion, loud noises, bright lights, and adverse climate conditions may trigger the nausea (Erick, 2004). Fortunately, most women with NVP are functional, able to work, do not lose weight, and are helped by simple dietary measures. Small, frequent snacks of carbohydrate foods reduce nausea for some, whereas protein foods may help others. Diets high in ginger and protein can reduce symptoms of nausea (Levine et al., 2008). Ginger reduces symptoms of NVP better than vitamin B_6 (Chittumma et al., 2007; Ensiyeh and Sakineh, 2009). Other therapies suggested include crackers or potato chips, elastic wrist bands, electronic wrist bands ("Relief Bands"), special lollipops ("Preggie Pops"), red raspberry leaf tea, noise reduction, acupuncture, and hypnosis. Some even try "Morning Sickness Magic," a tonic containing peach, ginger, raspberry leaf, vitamin B_6, and folate.

Some women do not tolerate the odors from hot foods, and room-temperature foods may be preferred. Smelling lemons may help block noxious odors (Erick, 2004). Unfortunately, there is no cure-all. Women suffering with nausea should eat whatever reduces the sensation of nausea and avoid odors that trigger nausea.

When early pregnancy is characterized by excessive vomiting and weight loss, fluid and electrolyte imbalances can occur. Here, "morning sickness" becomes **hyperemesis gravidarum (HG)**; this occurs in approximately 1% to 2% of pregnancies. Hospitalization for nutrition support and hydration is usually indicated. Appropriate weight gain for pregnancy; correction of fluid and electrolyte deficits; avoidance of ketosis; control of HG symptoms; and achievement of nitrogen, vitamin, and mineral balance are the goals in management (Austin, 2010).

Complications of HG vary, but may include global subluxation (Zeller, 2007), chondrodysplasia punctata, splenic avulsion (Nguyen et al., 1995), ruptured esophagus, and gestational malnutrition (Fejzo et al., 2009). A nuisance factor is **ptyalism** gravidarum, or excess saliva. Salivary output can be substantial and can be a source of lost electrolytes. Output of 500-1000 mL/day is not uncommon. Another difficult to identify but serious complication may be Wernicke encephalopathy with at least 49 cases being reported worldwide by 2006 (Chiossi et al., 2006) (see Chapter 3). Here intravenous administration of 100-mg thiamin for several days may be required (Austin, 2010).

In HG, enteral nutrition has variable effectiveness. Part of the challenge is that many obstetricians lack knowledge in tube placement, and women with severe emesis and retching have often dislodged tubes and are sometimes reluctant for replacement. If tubes are placed during a hospitalization, frequent nursing checks during the night disrupt sleep and add to sleep deprivation issues, which have not been widely recognized. Parenteral nutrition is used if the GI tract is not accessible, or if enteral nutrition is not tolerated (Austin, 2010). Because pregnancy is a condition of accelerated starvation, refeeding syndrome is often seen (Majumdar and Dada, 2010). Electrolytes such as phosphorous, magnesium, and potassium must be evaluated daily because low levels may result in cardiac irregularities and respiratory failure (Stanza et al., 2008). See Chapter 14.

Pregnancy-Induced Hypertension

Pregnancy-induced hypertension (PIH) includes gestational hypertension, PET, and eclampsia. **Gestational hypertension** is a maternal blood pressure equal to or greater than 140/90 with no proteinuria that develops after mid-pregnancy. These women may develop **pre-eclamptic toxemia (PET)**, defined as a systolic blood pressure of 140 or more, or a diastolic blood pressure of more than 90, plus urinary protein of more than 300 mg from a 24-hour urine sample. Severe PET is defined as a systolic blood pressure of more than 160 or a diastolic blood pressure of more than 110, plus more than 5 g of protein in a 24-hour urine sample. PET is associated with decreased uterine blood flow from vasospasm, leading to reduced placental size, compromised fetal nourishment, and an IUGR fetus.

The cause of PET is unknown; however, the disease complicates 5% to 8% of pregnancies (Getahun et al., 2007). Theories regarding causes are varied and include vascular injury to the placental blood vessels, high BMI, nulliparity, advanced maternal age, multifetal gestation, non-white race, renal disease, high pregnancy weight gain, and low levels of vitamin D (Getahun et al., 2007). Very young women with first pregnancies are also known to have higher incidences of PET. The incidence of PET is also increased in women with autoimmune diseases such as type 1 diabetes and rheumatoid arthritis.

PET is more common in dark-skinned women living in northern latitudes and others with a high prevalence of hypovitaminosis D. Low levels of vitamin D produce elevated cytokines. There is a reduction in the levels of circulating $1,25(OH)2D_3$ in preeclamptic patients (Spinnato, 2007) ; this may be caused by a disturbance in 1β-hydroxylation within the placenta.

Eclampsia is PIH resulting in grand mal seizures. Symptoms that precede seizure are dizziness, headache, visual disturbances, facial edema, right-sided epigastric pain, anorexia, nausea, and vomiting. Fetal death often results in women who develop eclampsia. A small percent of cases of eclampsia present in the postpartum period. Eclampsia can be fatal to the mother if not treated promptly. Intravenous magnesium supplementation may be used.

LACTATION

Exclusive breast-feeding is unequivocally the preferred method of infant feeding for the first 4 to 6 months of life. Both the American Dietetic Association and the American Academy of Pediatrics (AAP) have issued position statements in support of breast-feeding (James and Lessen, 2009). Other supporters include Healthy People 2010, The WIC program, and the U.S. Breastfeeding Committee.

Benefits

Breast-feeding can reduce the incidence of both types 1 and 2 diabetes (Gunderson et al., 2007; Malcova et al., 2006). An excellent way to promote breast-feeding is to discuss its benefits, as shown in Box 16-6.

In 1991 the World Health Organization and the United Nations Children's Fund adopted the Baby-Friendly Hospital Initiative, a global effort to increase the incidence and duration of breast-feeding. To become "baby friendly," a hospital must show to an outside review board that it implements the "Ten Steps to Successful Breast-feeding," a guideline for mother-baby management in the hospital; see *Clinical Insight:* Baby-Friendly Hospital Initiative: Ten Steps to Successful Breast-Feeding.

Contraindications

Breast-feeding is contraindicated for infants with galactosemia and for mothers who have active untreated tuberculosis or are positive for human T-cell lymphotropic virus type 1 or 2, who use drugs of abuse, have human immunodeficiency virus (in the United States), or who take certain medications (i.e., antimetabolites and chemotherapeutic agents). The use of radioactive isotopes requires temporary cessation of breast-feeding (Lawrence and Lawrence, 2005).

Physiology of Lactation

Mammary gland growth during menarche and pregnancy prepares the woman for lactation. Hormonal changes

CLINICAL INSIGHT

Baby-Friendly Hospital Initiative: Ten Steps to Successful Breast-Feeding

1. Have a written breast-feeding policy that is routinely communicated to all health care staff.
2. Train all health care staff in the skills necessary to implement this policy.
3. Inform all pregnant women about the benefits and management of breast-feeding.
4. Help the mother initiate breast-feeding within a half-hour of birth.
5. Show mothers how to breast-feed and how to maintain lactation, even if they are separated from their infants.
6. Give newborn infants no food or drink other than breast milk unless medically indicated.
7. Practice rooming-in; allow mothers and infants to remain together 24 hours a day.
8. Encourage breast-feeding on demand.
9. Give no artificial teats or pacifiers (also called dummies or soothers) to breast-feeding infants.
10. Foster the establishment of breast-feeding support groups and refer mothers to them on discharge from the hospital or clinic.

From Ebrahim GJ: The baby-friendly hospital initiative, J Trop Pediatr 39:2, 1993, by permission of Oxford University Press.

BOX 16-6

Benefits of Breast-Feeding

For Infant

Decreases Incidence and Severity of Infectious Diseases

- Bacterial meningitis
- Bacteremia
- Diarrhea
- Late-onset sepsis in preterm infants
- Necrotizing enterocolitis
- Otitis media
- Respiratory tract infection
- Urinary tract infection

Decreases Rates of

- Asthma
- Food allergies
- Hodgkin disease
- Hypercholesterolemia
- Leukemia
- Lymphoma
- Overweight and obesity
- Sudden infant death syndrome
- Types 1 and 2 diabetes

Promotes

- Analgesia during painful procedures (heel stick for newborns)
- Enhanced performance on cognitive development tests
- Mother-child bonding

For Mother

- Decreases menstrual blood loss
- Decreases postpartum bleeding
- Decreases risk of hormonal (breast and ovarian) cancers
- Promotes earlier return to prepregnancy weight
- Increases child spacing
- Promotes rapid uterine involution
- Decreases risk of postmenopausal hip fracture and osteoporosis

Adapted from American Academy of Pediatrics: Breastfeeding and the use of human milk, Pediatrics 115:496, 2005.

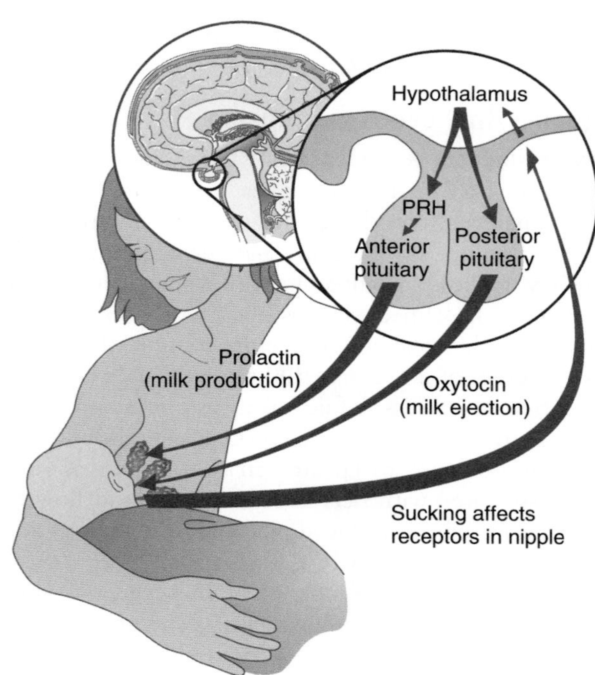

FIGURE 16-6 Physiology of milk production and the let-down reflex. *PRH,* Pituitary-releasing hormone.

markedly increase breast, areola, and nipple size. In pregnancy, hormones significantly increase ducts and alveoli and influence mammary growth. Late in pregnancy the lobules of the alveolar system are maximally developed, and small amounts of colostrum may be released for several weeks before term and for a few days after delivery. After birth there is a rapid drop in circulating levels of estrogen and progesterone accompanied by a rapid increase in prolactin secretion, setting the stage for a copious milk supply.

The usual stimulus for milk production and secretion is suckling. Subcutaneous nerves of the areola send a message via the spinal cord to the hypothalamus, which in turn transmits a message to the pituitary gland, where both the anterior and posterior areas are stimulated. **Prolactin** from the anterior pituitary stimulates alveolar cell milk production, as shown in Figure 16-6.

Oxytocin from the posterior pituitary stimulates the myoepithelial cells of the mammary gland to contract, causing movement of milk through the ducts and lactiferous sinuses, a process referred to as **let-down**. "Let-down" is highly sensitive. Oxytocin may be released by visual, tactile, olfactory, and auditory stimuli; and even by thinking about the infant. Oxytocin secretion can also be inhibited by pain, emotional and physical stress, fatigue, and anxiety. Women who have diabetes, who are obese, who are stressed during delivery, or who have retained placental fragments in the uterus are at risk for delayed milk production, when signs of lactogenesis are absent 72 hours after birth (Lawrence and Lawrence, 2005).

Nutritional Requirements of Lactation

Lactation is nutritionally demanding, especially for the woman who nurses her infant exclusively for a number of months. Increased intake of most nutrients is advised. The nutritional status of lactating women who have previously undergone gastric bypass surgery needs close attention because suboptimal levels of iron, vitamin A, vitamin D, vitamin K, folate, and calcium have been reported (Guelinckx et al., 2009).

Milk production is most affected by the frequency of suckling and maternal hydration. However, milk composition varies according to the mother's diet. For example, the fatty acid composition of a mother's milk reflects her dietary intake. In addition, milk concentrations of selenium, iodine, and some of the water-soluble B vitamins reflect the maternal diet. Breast milk of malnourished mothers has been shown to have lower levels of various nutrients, reflecting the foods she has available to eat.

Energy

Milk production is 80% efficient: production of 100 mL of milk (approximately 75 kcal) requires an 85-kcal expenditure (Lawrence and Lawrence, 2005). During the first 6 months of lactation, average milk production is 750 mL/day, with a range of 550 to more than 1200 mL/day. Because production is a function of the frequency, duration, and intensity of infant suckling, infants who feed well are likely to stimulate the production of larger volumes of milk.

The DRI for energy during lactation is 330 kcal greater during the first 6 months of lactation and 400 kcal greater during the second 6 months of lactation over that for a nonpregnant woman. It is the same as the DRI during the second trimester of pregnancy (IOM, 2002). The obese and overweight woman may not require the full 330 to 400 extra kcal/day. Maternal fat stores accumulated during pregnancy provide approximately 100 to 150 kcal per day to support the early months of lactation. When the reserve fat stores have been depleted, dietary energy support for lactation must be increased if the mother intends to provide all or most of her infant's nutrition through breast milk alone. During the second 6 months of lactation, production generally drops to an average of 600 mL/day or approximately 20 oz/day.

Healthy breast-feeding women can lose as much as 1 pound per week and still supply adequate milk to maintain their infants' growth. Breast-feeding women should be reminded of the energy expenditure required to produce milk: approximately 0.67 kcal per 1 cc of breast milk output. Milk production decreases in mothers whose intakes are suboptimal; less than 1800 calories/day, and breast milk will reflect the nutrient profile of the maternal diet. Appropriate fluid intake (such as drinking for thirst) and adequate rest are also needed.

Protein

The DRI suggests an additional 25 g of protein a day for lactation, or 71 g of protein a day. This is based on an RDA of 1.1 gm/kg/day of prepregnancy weight. Clinical judgment is necessary with protein recommendations because 71 g/day may be too low in an overweight woman and too high for the woman with a lower BMI. Women with surgical delivery and women who enter pregnancy in poor nutritional shape may need additional protein. The average protein requirement for lactation is estimated from milk composition data and the mean daily volume of 750 mL, assuming 70% efficiency in the conversion of dietary protein to milk protein.

Breast milk has a whey/casein ratio of 90:10 early in lactation, which changes to 80:20 as an average, and to 60:40 as the baby gets older. It is speculated that this ratio makes breast milk more digestible. In contrast, the whey/casein ratio of cow's milk protein is 18:82.

Carbohydrates

The RDA for carbohydrate is 210 g/day (IOM, 2002). This 210 g/day is the recommended amount to provide enough calories in the diet for adequate volumes of milk and to maintain an adequate energy level during lactation. This may need to be adjusted depending on activity of the mother and the amount of breast-feeding. The woman with a poor gestation weight gain may require more carbohydrates.

Lipid

The amount and type of fat in breast milk directly reflects the maternal diet. The "fore" milk or first milk in a feeding is lower in fat than the "hind" milk at the end of a feeding. Dietary fat choices by the mother can increase or decrease specific fatty acids in her milk. Severe restriction of energy intake results in mobilization of body fat, and the milk produced has a fatty acid composition resembling that of the mother's body fat.

There is no DRI for total lipids during lactation because it depends on the amount of energy required by the mother to maintain milk production. DRIs state a recommended amount of specific long-chain polyunsaturated fatty acids in human milk because their presence in the maternal diet is crucial for fetal and infant brain development. The AI for ω-6 polyunsaturated fatty acids is 13 g/day, and the AI for ω-3 polyunsaturated fatty acids is 1.3 g/day (IOM, 2002). *Trans* fats should be avoided completely by the nursing mother so that the potential for their appearance in her breast milk is reduced.

Human milk contains 10 to 20 mg/dL of cholesterol, resulting in an approximate consumption of 100 mg/day by the infant. The amount of cholesterol in milk does not reflect the mother's diet; however, the cholesterol content of the milk decreases over time as lactation progresses.

Vitamins and Minerals

The vitamin D content of milk is related to maternal vitamin D intake and the degree of sun exposure. Numerous case reports document marginal or significant vitamin D deficiency in pregnant women and in infants of lactating women who are veiled, dark skinned, with BMI of more than 30, who use sunscreens heavily, or who live in northern latitudes with decreased sun exposure. Women with lactose intolerance who do not drink vitamin D–fortified milk or take a vitamin supplement may be at higher risk for vitamin D deficiency. Because of reports of clinical rickets, the AAP recommends that all breast-fed infants receive an additional 200 IU (5 mcg) of vitamin D daily beginning at 2 months of age (Lawrence and Lawrence, 2005). During lactation, supplements administered directly to the infant allow the infant to easily achieve vitamin D sufficiency; the mother may need much higher doses (100 mcg or 4000 IU per day) to achieve adult-normal 25(OH)D concentrations and vitamin D adequacy in her exclusively breast-fed infant.

The calcium content of breast milk is not related to maternal intake, and there is no convincing evidence that maternal change in bone mineral density is influenced by calcium intake across a broad range of intakes up to 1600 mg/day. In a community study of 210 Sri Lankan women, prolonged lactation was not shown to have detrimental effects on bone density mass (Lenora et al., 2009).

The amount of iodine in breast milk may not always reflect maternal intake. See "Iodine" earlier in this chapter. In the US the presence of the industrial pollutant, perchlorate, has been shown to inhibit iodine uptake. Perchlorate has been found in mothers' milk as well as in the water supply (Dasgupta et al., 2008). This may explain why iodine levels in some individuals are low, despite what appears to be an adequate amount of iodine in the diet.

The requirements for zinc during lactation are greater than those during pregnancy. In the process of normal lactation the zinc content of breast milk drops dramatically during the first few months from 2 to 3 mg/day to 1 mg/day by the third month after birth.

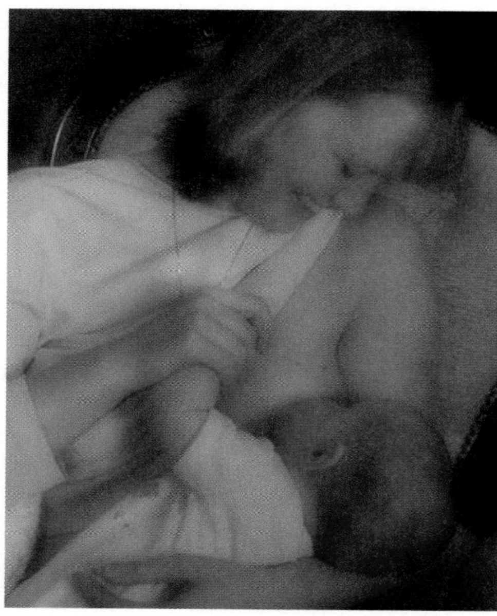

FIGURE 16-7 A nursing mother and her infant enjoy the close physical and psychologic contact that accompanies breast-feeding. *(Courtesy Kelly Carlson Atlec, Fairbanks, Alaska.)*

Breast-Feeding an Infant

Preparation

The advantages of breast-feeding should be presented throughout the childbearing years (Figure 16-7). During the last months of pregnancy, counseling on the process of lactation should be made available to women who have decided to breast-feed. Fathers or partners should be encouraged to participate in counseling sessions because the emotional support they provide contributes to the success of lactation.

Colostrum

Colostrum is the thin, yellow, milky fluid that is the first milk available after birth. It is higher in protein and lower in fat and carbohydrate than mature milk. Colostrum provides approximately 20 kcal/oz and is a rich source of antibodies (Lawrence and Lawrence, 2005). The unique properties of colostrum include that it is lower in lactose than mature milk, facilitates the passage of meconium (first stool of neonate), is high in antioxidants, and is lower in water-soluble vitamins than mature milk. Colostrum is also higher in fat-soluble vitamins, protein, sodium, potassium, chloride, zinc, and immunoglobulins than mature milk.

The Technique

Breast-feeding is a learned skill for both mother and her infant. The baby should be put to breast soon after birth and remain in direct skin-to-skin contact until the first feed is accomplished (American Academy of Pediatrics, 2005). Lactating women may experience a tingling sensation in the breast signaling the let-down reflex. Practice, patience, and perseverance are necessary. Within 48 to 96 hours after birth the breasts become fuller and firmer as the milk volumes increase. Women should be encouraged to pump and store breast milk in the likelihood of needing to be away from the infant for a feeding or two. Use of a breast pump facilitates breast milk expression; pump rentals may be covered by insurance.

Women who have insulin-dependent diabetes may experience "lactation hypoglycemia" as they increase their breast-feeding sessions. Those who have had cesarean deliveries or those who are taking pain medication may have difficulty with discerning let-down from low glucose levels. Frequent glucose monitoring needs to be emphasized to ensure safety for both mother and baby.

There is no need to offer breast-fed babies additional water because 87% of breast milk is water. However, cases of hypernatremic dehydration caused by suboptimal breast-feeding do occur. Most cases involve young and first-time mothers who may feel intimidated and overwhelmed at delivery, lack breast-feeding education, and are unaware of the consequences of dehydration. Extreme heat or hot weather may also contribute to this problem. The consequence of hypernatremic dehydration can be permanent brain damage or death. Therefore it is vital to evaluate the breast-feeding in the clinic at followup. Problems identified can then be addressed, and a plan of care can be implemented.

All breast-fed newborns should be seen within 3 to 5 days of birth by an experienced health care professional (AAP, 2005).

Exclusive breast-feeding is recommended for the first 6 months, but may continue for the first year or as long as it is mutually desired by mother and child (AAP, 2005).

Exercise and Breast-Feeding

The breast-feeding mother should be encouraged to get back to exercise a few weeks after delivery, after lactation is well established. Aerobic exercise at 60% to 70% of maximum heart rate has no adverse effect on lactation; infants gain weight at the same rate, and the mother's cardiovascular fitness improves. Exercise also improves plasma lipids and insulin response in lactating women.

Transfer of Drugs into Human Milk

Almost all drugs taken by the mother appear in her milk to some degree. The amount that usually transfers is quite small. Many factors influence how medications transfer into human milk: milk/plasma ratio, molecular weight of the drug, and the protein binding and lipid solubility of the drug.

It is estimated that more than 500,000 pregnancies in the United States each year involve women who have psychiatric illnesses that either antedate the pregnancy or emerge during pregnancy and an estimated one third of them require a psychotropic medication (ACOG 2009; Voyer and Moretti, 2009). The need for medication must be balanced against the risk of an untreated illness. Websites that can provide more information include the AAP, www.aap.org, and the National Institutes of Health, http://www.nimh.nih.gov/health/publications/mental-health-medications/complete-index.shtml.

Failure to Thrive in the Breast-Fed Infant

Insufficient milk supply is rarely a problem for the well-fed, well-rested, and unstressed mother. Sucking stimulates the flow of milk; thus feeding on demand should supply ample amounts of milk to the infant. If the baby continues to gain weight and length steadily, has at least six to eight wet diapers daily, and has frequent stools, the milk supply is probably adequate.

Occasionally, however, an infant fails to thrive while seeming to nurse properly. Figure 16-8 illustrates potential problems in the mother or the infant that should be investigated during the course of evaluation. If the cause of the problem cannot be identified or the defined problem cannot be corrected, it may be necessary to encourage the mother to use commercial infant formula for at least partial nutritional support of the infant. A thorough assessment of the maternal diet and health habits is always necessary. Women who consume diets low in vitamins D or B_{12} or iodine produce milk with low levels; the result is FTT in the breast-fed infant.

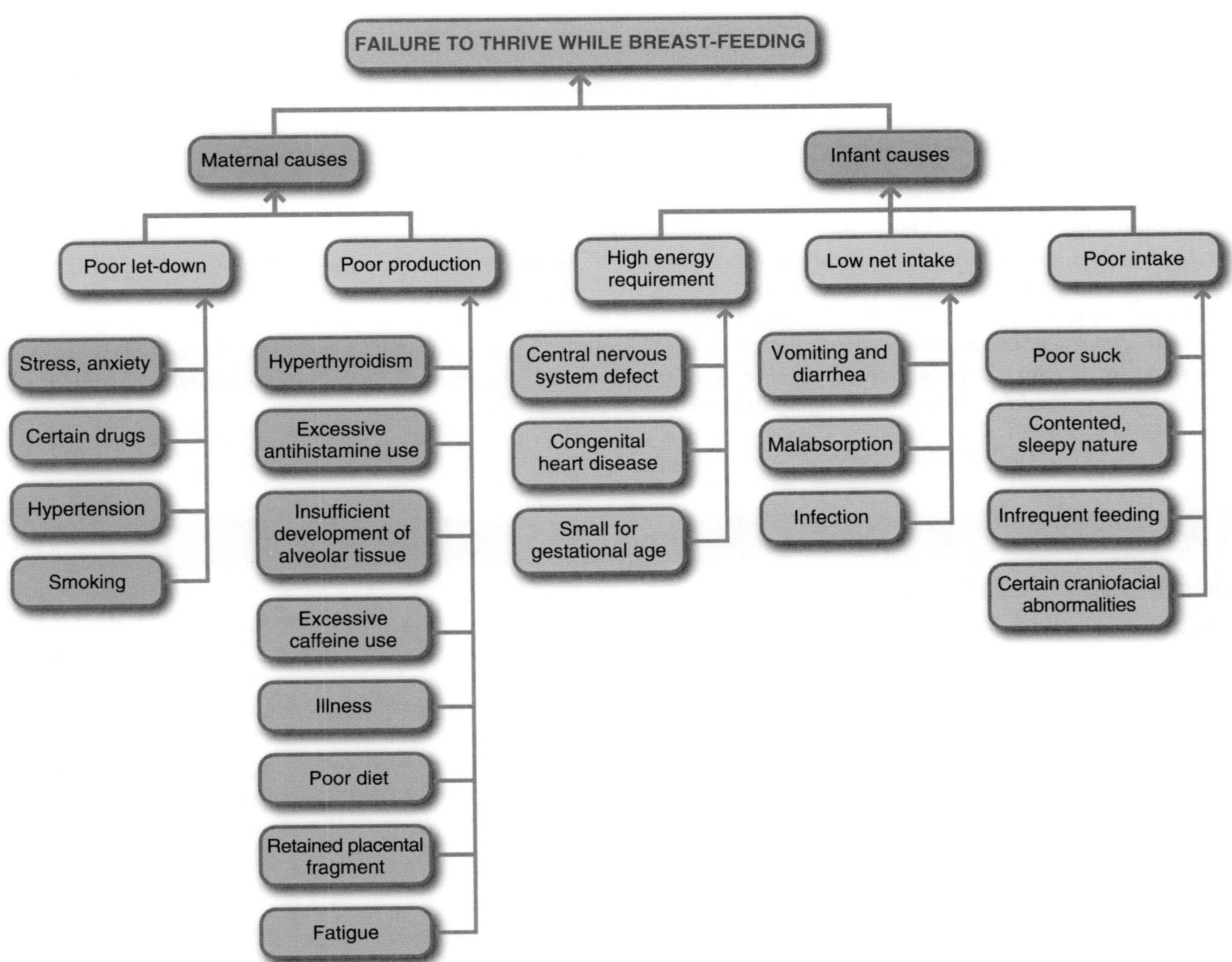

FIGURE 16-8 Diagnostic flow chart for failure to thrive in the breast-feeding infant.

Three cases of dilated cardiomyopathy in male neonates caused by low vitamin D intakes in the lactating mothers have been reported. Two cases from the United Arab Emirates found congestive cardiac failure in two 9-month-old babies who were also noted to have rickets (Amirlak et al., 2008). Both mothers were also diagnosed with vitamin D deficiencies, being heavily clothed. Dilated cardiomyopathy associated with hypocalcemic rickets has been reported in the United States in breast-fed black infants (Brown et al., 2009).

Sometimes the infant may become intolerant or allergic to something the mother has ingested. Cow's milk protein, notably casein, has been implicated, as have peanuts. At this time, the amount or the frequency has not been conclusively determined (Sicherer SH et al., 2010; DesRoches A et al., 2010; Lopez-Exposito I et al., 2009). When suspicious foods are removed from the mother's diet, it is important to assess the nutritional quality of her diet and supplement her appropriately (see Chapter 27).

Other Problems of Breast-Feeding

Overweight lactating women can restrict their energy intake by 500 kcal per day by decreasing consumption of foods high in fat and simple sugars, but they must increase their intake of foods high in calcium, vitamin D, vitamin A, vitamin C, and ω-3 fats to provide key nutrients for their milk supply.

Breast augmentation, a procedure in which an implant is inserted into the breast to enlarge it, is a common elective breast procedure. Periareolar and transareolar incisions can cause lactation insufficiency. These mothers should be encouraged to breast-feed, and their infants monitored for appropriate weight gain.

Reduction mammoplasty is often recommended for women with extremely large breasts who suffer from back, shoulder, or neck pain or poor body image. There are wide variations in milk production, from a little to full production, depending on the amount of tissue removed and the type of surgical incision. These mothers should also be encouraged to breast-feed and be given anticipatory guidance and support; their infants should be monitored closely for appropriate weight gain.

There can be a number of other hurdles to overcome to breast-feed successfully. These problems and their solutions are discussed in Table 16-9.

CLINICAL SCENARIO 1

Jean is a 34-year-old woman who is pregnant for the first time. She has a sister who has spina bifida and an older brother who had a stroke when he was 14. Jean has been tested and found to have a genetic defect known as C>T in the methylene-tetrahydrofolate receptor (MTHFR), which is a concern for her. She is worried about using the traditional prenatal vitamin-mineral supplement because she has been cautioned that she is unable to metabolize folic acid from diet and supplements. She is asking for your advice for a successful pregnancy.

Nutrition Diagnostic Statement

Altered nutrient (folic acid) metabolism related to a genetic alteration as evidenced by positive results for C>T in the MTHFR gene and family history of spina bifida and stroke.

Nutrition Care Questions

1. What advice would you give Jean about any special dietary changes?
2. Jean knows that there is a special prenatal vitamin-mineral supplement available but does not know how to obtain it. How will you help Jean find this supplement?
3. What are the risks for a successful pregnancy outcome if Jean cannot find this special prenatal supplement?

TABLE 16-9

Management of Breast-Feeding Difficulties

Problem	Approaches to Management
Retracted nipples	Before feeding the infant, roll the nipple gently between the fingers until erect.
Baby's mouth not open wide enough	Before feeding, depress the infant's lower jaw with one finger as the nipple is guided into the mouth.
Baby sucks poorly	Stimulate sucking motions by pressing upward under the baby's chin. Expression of colostrums often occurs, and the taste may stimulate sucking.
Baby demonstrates rooting but does not grasp the nipple; eventually cries in frustration	Interrupt the feeding, comfort the infant; the mother should take time to relax before trying again.
Baby falls asleep while nursing	If the infant falls asleep early in the feeding, the mother should awaken the infant by holding him or her upright, rubbing his or her back, talking to him or her, or providing similar quiet stimuli; another effort at feeding can then be made. If the baby falls asleep again, the feeding should be postponed.

CLINICAL SCENARIO 2

Elena is a 23-year-old woman who has a 2-year-old child and a 10-day-old infant via cesarean delivery; she has a history of postpartum depression. She has come to the Women, Infants, and Children clinic for certification as a breast-feeding mother. She is breast-feeding her infant every 3 hours, but is concerned that he may not be getting enough milk. While with the nutritionist in the clinic, she begins to cry and talk about her sore nipples, profound fatigue, and worry. A 24-hour recall of foods eaten the day before reveals that Elena skipped breakfast and ate some microwave meals for lunch and dinner.

The nutritionist asks permission to watch Elena nurse her infant. Because she is not supporting the infant's back and buttocks firmly, the infant tugs at the nipple and causes the soreness. The nutritionist then weighs the infant and finds that he has already regained his birth weight.

Nutrition Diagnostic Statement

Difficulty breast-feeding related to poor infant positioning as evidenced by mom's reports of fatigue and sore nipples.

Nutrition Care Questions

1. What would you say to Elena regarding her concern that her son may not be getting enough milk?
2. What would you recommend to improve the infant's position during nursing? How would this improve the nursing experience?
3. What advice would you give Elena about her fatigue?
4. How would you design an eating plan that Elena could follow?

Other Common Nutrition Diagnostic Statements in Pregnant or Lactating Women

Harmful beliefs related to nutritional requirements during pregnancy as evidenced by pica with consumption of laundry starch two times daily with lunch and dinner meals

Limited access to food related to low income and misunderstanding of the use of WIC vouchers as evidenced by other family members using the WIC foods in the household

Obesity related to frequent meals and snacking during pregnancy as evidenced by weight gain of 30 pounds in second trimester

Intake of unsafe foods related to storing fresh milk on the counter as evidenced by home visit by social worker and discussions with client

Inconsistent carbohydrate intake related to management of gestational diabetes as evidenced by nutritional history of skipping breakfast and sometimes lunch

Abnormal gastrointestinal function related to heartburn as evidenced by complaints of reflux after every meal and excessive use of antacids

Inadequate food and beverage intake related to irregular income as evidenced by discussion about migrant status and the challenges during pregnancy

Breast-feeding difficulty related to frequent nipple soreness as evidenced by mother's hesitancy to continue nursing her 6-month-old

USEFUL WEBSITES

Agency for Toxic Substances and Disease Registry, Polychlorinated Biphenyls
http://www.atsdr.cdc.gov/tfacts17.html

Breastfeeding After Breast Reduction
www.bfar.org

Centers for Disease Control, Listeriosis
http://www.cdc.gov/nczved/divisions/dfbmd/diseases/listeriosis/

Mercury
www.gotmercury.org

Women's Health—Breastfeeding
http://www.womenshealth.gov/breastfeeding/

REFERENCES

Afridi HI, et al: Status of essential trace metals in biological samples of diabetic mothers and their neonates, *Arch Gynecol Obstet* 280:415, 2009.

Amirlak I, et al: Dilated cardiomyopathy secondary to nutritional rickets, *Ann Trop Paediatr* 93:227, 2008.

American Dietetic Association: Position of the American Dietetic Association and American Society for Nutrition: obesity, reproduction and pregnancy outcome, *J Am Diet Assoc* 109:918, 2009.

American Academy of Pediatrics: breastfeeding and the use of human milk, *Pediatrics* 115:496, 2005.

American College of Obstetricians and Gynecologists: ACOG Committee Opinion number 315, Sept 2005. Obesity in pregnancy, *Obstet Gynecol* 106(3):671, 2005.

American Congress of Obstetricians and Gynecologists (ACOG): ACOG Practice Bulletin. Use of psychiatric medications during pregnancy and lactation, *Obstet Gynecol* 111:1001, 2009.

Artal R, et al: Weight gain recommendations in pregnancy and the obesity epidemic, *Obstet Gynecol* 115:152, 2010.

Arterburn LM, et al: Algal-oil capsules and cooked salmon: nutritionally equivalent sources of docosahexaenoic acid, *J Am Diet Assoc* 108:1204, 2008.

Austin T: Nutrition management of the hyperemesis gravidarum patient, *Nutrition Support Line* 32(2):16, 2010.

Biggio JR, et al: Fetal anomalies in obese women: the contribution of diabetes, *Ob Gyn* 115:290, 2010.

Black MM: Effect of vitamin B_{12} and folate deficiency on brain development in children, *Food Nutr Bull* 29:S126, 2008.

Brown J, et al: Hypocalcemic rickets and dilated cardiomyopathy: case reports and review of the literature, *Pediatric Cardiol* 30:6, 2009.

Brunetti-Pierri N, et al: Gray matter heterotopias and brachytelephalangic chondrodysplasia punctata: a complication of hyperemesis gravidarum induced vitamin K deficiency? *Am J Gen Med* Part A:143:200, 2007.

Callaway LK, et al: Barriers to addressing overweight and obesity before conception, *Med J Aust* 191:425, 2009a.

Callaway LK, et al: Obesity and the hypertensive disorders of pregnancy, *Hypertens Preg* 28:473, 2009b.

Cambadoo L, et al: Maternal vitamin D deficiency associated with neonatal hypocalcaemic convulsions, *Nutr J* 6:23, 2007.

Charney P, Malone AM: *ADA pocket guide to nutrition assessment*, ed 2, Chicago, 2009, American Dietetic Association.

Chen KK, et al: Iron supplementation in pregnancy and development of gestational diabetes—a randomized placebo-controlled trial, *BJOG* 116:389, 2009.

Chavarro JE, et al: Diet and lifestyle in the prevention of ovulatory disorder infertility, *Obstet Gynecol* 110:1050, 2007.

Chien LC, et al: Hair mercury concentration and fish consumption: risk and perception of risk among women of childbearing age, *Environ Res* 110:123, 2010.

Chiossi G, et al. Hyperemesis gravidarum complicated by Wernicke's encephalopathy: background, case report and review of the literature, *Obstet Gynecol Surv* 61(4):255, 2006.

Chittumma P, et al: Comparison of the effectiveness of ginger and vitamin B_6 for the treatment of nausea and vomiting in early pregnancy: a randomized double-blind controlled trial, *J Med Assoc Thai* 90:15, 2007.

Cochrane Update: Effects of restricted caffeine intake by mother on fetal, neonatal and pregnancy outcome, *Obstet Gynecol* 14:161, 2009.

Corrigan N, et al: Fetal cardiac effects of maternal hyperglycemia during pregnancy, *Birth Defects Res A Clin Mol Teratol* 85:523, 2009.

Craciunescu CN, et al: Dietary choline reverses some, but not all, effects of folate deficiency on neurogenesis and apoptosis in fetal mouse brain, *J Nutr* 140:1162, 2010.

Crozier SR, et al: Do women change their health behaviours in pregnancy? Findings from the Southampon Women's Survey, *Paediatric Perinatal Epidemiol* 23:446, 2009.

Cui X, et al: Maternal vitamin D depletion alters neurogenesis in the developing rat brain, *Int J Dev Neurosci* 25:227, 2007.

Cox JT, Phelan ST: Nutrition during pregnancy, *Obstet Gynecol Clin North Am* 35:369, 2008.

Darlow BA, Graham P: Vitamin A supplementation to prevent mortality and short term and long term morbidity in very low birthweight infants (review), *The Cochrane Collaborative*, *The Cochrane Library* 4, 2008. Accessed from http://www.thecochranelibrary.com.

Dasgupta PK, et al: Intake of iodine and perchlorate and excretion in human milk, *Environ Sci Technol* 42:81, 2008.

Dheen ST, et al: Recent studies on neural tube defects in embryos of diabetic pregnancy: an overview, *Curr Med Chem* 16:2345, 2009.

De Santis MS, et al: Growth of fetal lean and fat mass in gestational diabetes, *Ultrasound Obst Gynecol* 36:328, 2010.

DesRoches A, Infante-Rivard C, et al: Peanut allergy: is maternal transmission of antigen during pregnancy and breastfeeding a risk factor? *J Investig Allergol Clin Immunol* 20(4):289, 2010.

Duley L: The global impact of pre-eclampsia and eclampsia, *Semin Perinatol* 33:130, 2009.

Ensiyeh J, Sakineh MA: Comparing ginger and vitamin B_6 for the treatment of nausea and vomiting in pregnancy: a randomized controlled trial, *Midwifery* 25:649, 2009.

Erick M: *Managing morning sickness: a survival guide for pregnant women*, Boulder, Colo, 2004, Bull Publishing.

Faintuch J, et al: Pregnancy nutritional indices and birth weight after Roux-en-Y gastric bypass, *Obes Surg* 19:583, 2009.

Fejzo MS, et al: Symptoms and pregnancy outcomes associated with extreme weight loss among women with hyperemesis gravidarum, *J Women's Health* 18:1981, 2009.

Feron F, et al: Developmental vitamin D_3 deficiency alters the adult brain, *Brain Res Bull* 65:14, 2005.

Gaber KR, et al: Maternal vitamin B_{12} and risk of neural tube defects in Egyptian patients, *Clin Lab* 53:69, 2007.

Gagne A, et al: Absorption, transport, and bioavailability of vitamin E and its role in pregnant women, *J Obstet Gynaecol Can* 210, 2009.

Gaur DS, et al: Alcohol intake and cigarette smoking: impact of two major lifestyle factors on male infertility, *Indian J Pathol Microbiol* 53:35, 2010.

Georgieff MK: Nutrition and the developing brain: nutrient priorities and measurement, *Am J Clin Nutr* 85:1S, 2007.

Getahun D, et al: Primary preeclampsia in the second pregnancy: effect of changes in prepregnancy body mass index between pregnancies, *Ob Gyn* 110:1319, 2007.

Goldberg BB, et al: Prevalence of periconceptual folic acid use and perceived barriers to postgestational continuance of supplemental folic acid: survey from a Teratogen Information Service, *Birth Defects Res A Clin Mol Teratol* 76:193, 2006.

Goodnight W, Newman R: Optimal nutrition for improved twin pregnancy outcome, *Obstet Gynecol* 114:1121, 2009.

Goodyer P, et al: Effects of maternal vitamin A status on kidney development: a pilot study, *Pediatr Nephrol* 22:209, 2007.

Grassi A: Recognition and treatment approaches for polycystic ovary syndrome. In *Women's health report*, Chicago, Ill, Summer 2008, American Dietetic Association, Women's Health Dietetic Practice Group.

Groenen PM, et al: Low maternal dietary intakes of iron, magnesium and niacin are associated with spina bifida in the offspring, *J Nutr* 134:1516, 2004.

Guelinckx I, et al: Reproductive outcome after bariatric surgery: a critical review, *Hum Reprod Update* 15:189, 2009.

Gunderson EP, et al: Lactation and changes in maternal metabolic risk factors, *Obstet Gynecol* 109:729, 2007.

Hadar E, et al: Towards new diagnostic criteria for diagnosing GDM: the HAPO study, *J Perinat Med* 37:447, 2009.

HAPO Study Cooperative Research Group, Hyperglycemia and Adverse Pregnancy Outcome (HAPO) Study: associations with maternal body mass index, *Am J Ostet Gynecol* 202:255, 2010.

Hannigan JH, et al: A 14-year retrospective maternal report of alcohol consumption in pregnancy predicts pregnancy and teen outcomes, *Alcohol* 44:583, 2009.

Hisano M, et al: Vitamin B_6 deficiency and anemia in pregnancy, *Eur J Clin Nutr* 64:221, 2010.

Hoy-Rosas J: Iodine and reproductive nutrition. In *Women's health report*, Chicago, Ill, Spring 2009, American Dietetic Association, Women's Health Dietetic Practice Group.

Institute of Medicine (IOM), Food and Nutrition Board: *Dietary reference intakes for energy, macronutrients, carbohydrates, fiber, fat and fatty acids*, Washington, DC, 2002, National Academies Press.

Jahanfar S, Sharifah H: Effects of restricted caffeine intake by mother on fetal, neonatal and pregnancy outcome, *Cochrane Database of Systemic Reviews*. 2:CD006965, 2009.

James J, Lessen R: Position of the American Dietetic Association: promoting and supporting breastfeeding, *J Am Diet Assoc*, 109:1926, 2009.

Kubwabo C, et al: Migration of bisphenol A from plastic baby bottles, baby bottle liners and reusable polycarbonate drinking bottles, *Food Addit Contam Part A Chem Anal Control Expo Risk Assess* 26:928, 2009.

Kyle UG, Picard C: The Dutch Famine of 1944-45: a pathological model of long-term consequences of wasting disease, *Curr Opin Clin Nutr Metab Care* 9:388, 2006.

Laitinen K, et al: Probiotics and dietary counseling contribute to glucose regulation during and after pregnancy: a randomized controlled trial, *Br J Nutr* 101:1679, 2009.

Laughton SK: Elevated first trimester uric acid concentrations are associated with the development of gestational diabetes, *Am J Ob Gyn* 201:402, 2009.

Lawrence RA, Lawrence RM: *Breastfeeding: a guide for the medical profession*, Philadelphia, 2005, Mosby.

Lenora J, et al: Effects of multiparity and prolonged breast-feeding on maternal bone density: a community-based cross-sectional study, *BMC Women's Health* 9:19, 2009.

Levine ME, et al: Protein and ginger for the treatment of chemo-induced delayed nausea, *J Alter Complement Med* 14:545, 2008.

Leung AM, et al: Iodine content of prenatal multivitamins in the United States, *N Engl J Med* 360:939, 2009.

Leung BMT, Kaplan BJ: Perinatal depression: prevalence, risks and the nutrition link—A review of the literature, *J Am Diet Assoc* 109:1566, 2009.

Lopez-Exposito I, Song Y, et al. Maternal peanut exposure during pregnancy and lactation reduces peanut allergy risk in offspring, *J Allergy Clin Immunol* 124:1039, 2009 Nov.

Luoto R, et al: Impact of maternal probiotic-supplemented dietary couselling on pregnancy outcome and prenatal and postnatal growth: a double-blind, placebo-controlled study, *Br J Nutr* 103(12):1792, 2010.

Majumdar S, Dada B: Refeeding syndrome: a serious and potentially life-threatening complication of severe hyperemesis gravidarum, *J Obstet Gynaecol* 30:416, 2010.

Malcova H, et al: Absence of breast-feeding is associated with the risk of type I diabetes: a case-control study in a population with rapidly increasing incidence, *Eur J Pediatr* 165:114, 2006.

Mathieu J: What is pregorexia? *J Am Dent Assoc* 109:976, 2009.

Meeker JD, et al: Cadmium, lead and other metals in relation to semen quality: human evidence for molybdenum as a male reproductive toxicant, *Environ Health Perspect* 116:1473, 2008.

Merewood A, et al: Association between vitamin D deficiency and primary cesarean section, *J Clin Endocrin Metab* 94:940, 2009.

Metzger B, et al: Hyperglycemia and adverse pregnancy outcomes, *N Engl J Med* 358:1991, 2008.

National Institute for Child Health and Human Development (NICHD), National Institutes of Health: *Moderate doses of vitamin A do not pose risk of birth defects*, 2001. Accessed 1 December 2006 from http://www.nichd.nih.gov//new/releases/vitama.cfm.

Neural Crest and Associated Disorders: Vertebrate embryology. Accessed 11 November 2009 from http://www.brown.edu/Courses/BI0032/neurcrst/migrate.htm.

Niljand MJ: Prenatal origins of adult disease, *Curr Opin Ob Gyn* 20:132, 2008.

Nguyen N, et al: Splenic avulsion in a pregnant patient with vomiting, *Can J Surg* 38:464, 1995.

Nygaard IH, et al: Does oral magnesium substitution relieve pregnancy-induced leg cramps? *Eur J Obstet Gynecol Reprod Biol* 141:23, 2008.

Ozkan S, et al: Replete vitamin D stores predict reproductive success following in vitro fertilization, *Fertil Steril* 7 July 2009. [Epub ahead of print.]

Palacios C. The role of nutrients in bone health, from A to Z. *Crit Rev Food Sci Nutr* 46(8):621, 2006.

Page KC, et al: Maternal and postweaning diet interaction alters hypothalamic gene expression and modulates response to a high-fat diet in male offspring, *Am J Physiol Regul Integr Comp Physiol* 297:1049, 2009.

Pearce EN, Braverman LE: Environmental pollutants and the thyroid, *Best Pract Res Clin Endocrinol Metab* 23:801, 2009.

Pinto E, et al: Dietary intake and nutritional adequacy prior to conception and during pregnancy: a follow-up study in the north of Portgal, *Publ Health Nutr* 12:922, 2009.

Rasmussen KM, Yaktine AL, editors: *Weight gain during pregnancy: re-examining the recommendations*, Washington, DC, 2009, The National Academies Press.

Rifas-Shiman SL, et al: Dietary quality during pregnancy varies by maternal characteristics in project VIVA: a US cohort, *J Am Diet Assoc* 109:1004, 2009.

Rosello-Soberon ME, et al: Twin pregnancies: eating for three? Maternal nutrition update, *Nutr Rev* 63(9):95-302, 2005.

Rwebembera AA, et al: Relationship between infant birth weight <2000 g and maternal zinc levels at Muhimbili National Hospital, Dar Es Salamm, Tanzania, *J Trop Pediatr* 52:118, 2005.

Salihu HM, et al: Extreme obesity and risk of stillbirth among black and white gravidas, *Obstet Gynecol* 110:552, 2007.

Scheplyagina LA: Impact of the mother's zinc deficiency on the woman's and newborn's health status, *J Trace Elem Med Biol* 19:29, 2005.

Scialli AR, Public Affairs Committee of the Teratology Society: Teratology public affairs committee position paper: maternal obesity and pregnancy, *Birth Defects Res A Clin Mol Teratol* 76:73, 2006.

Selvaraj N, et al: Oxidative stress: does it play a role in the genesis of early glycated proteins? *Med Hypotheses* 70:265, 2008.

Sicherer SH, Wood RA et al. Maternal consumption of peanuts during pregnancy is associated with peanut sensitization in atopic infants, *J Allergy Clin Immunol* 126:1191, 2010.

Simpson JL, et al: Micronutrients and women of reproductive potential: required dietary intake and consequences of dietary deficiency or excess. Part I—folate, vitamin B_{12} and vitamin B_6, *J Matern Fetal Neonatal Med* 23:1323, 2010.

Simpson JL, et al: Micronutrients and women of reproductive potential: required dietary intake and consequences of dietary deficiency or excess. Part II—vitamin D, vitamin A, iron, zinc, iodine, essential fatty acids, *J Matern Fetal Neonatal Med* 24:1, 2011.

Sohrabvand F, et al: Vitamin B supplementation for leg cramps during pregnancy, *Intl J Gynaecol Obstet* 95:48, 2006.

Solomons NW: Developmental origins of health and disease: concepts, caveats and consequences for public health nutrition, *Nutr Rev* 67:S12, 2009.

Spinnato JA II, et al: Antioxidant therapy to prevent preeclampsia: a randomized controlled trial, *Obstet Gynecol* 110:1311, 2007.

Stanza Z, et al: Nutrition in clinical practice—the refeeding syndrome: illustrative cases and guidelines for prevention and treatment, *Eur J Clin Nutr* 62:687, 2008.

Stotland N, et al: Body mass index, provider advice and target gestational weight gain, *Obstet Gynecol* 105:633, 2005.

Tamashiro KL, Moran TH: Perinatal environment and its influences on metabolic programming of offspring, *Physiol Behav* 100:560, 2010.

Tussing-Humphreys LM, et al: Excess adiposity, inflammation and iron-deficiency in female adolescents, *J Am Diet Assoc* 109:297, 2009.

Uriu-Adams JY, et al: Influence of copper on early development: prenatal and postnatal considerations, *Biofactors* 36:136, 2010.

Vello M, et al: Prenatal and neonatal risk factors for the development of enamel defects in low birth weight children, *Oral Dis* 2009.

Viljakainen HT, et al: Maternal vitamin D status determines bone variables in the newborn, *J Clin Endocrinol Metab* 95:1749, 2010.

Von Hurst PR, et al: Vitamin D supplementation reduces insulin resistance in South Asian women living in New Zealand who are insulin resistant and vitamin D deficit: a randomized, placebo controlled trial, *Br J Nutr* 28:1, 2009.

Voyer Lavigne S, Moretti M: Medication in pregnancy and lactation, *Obstet Gynecol* 114:166, 2009.

Wai-Man See A, et al: A nutritional model of late embryonic vitamin A deficiency produces defects in organogenesis at a high penetrance and reveals new roles for the vitamin in skeletal development, *Dev Biol* 316:171, 2008.

Waters TP, et al: Effect of 17 a-hydroxyprogesterone caproate on glucose intolerance in pregnancy, *Obstet Gynecol* 14:45, 2009.

Wen JG, et al: Melamine related bilateral renal calculi in 50 children: single center experience in diagnosis and treatment, *J Urol* 183:1533, 2010.

Wilkins-Haug L: Epigenetics and assisted reproduction, *Curr Opin Obstet Gynecol* 21:201, 2009.

Yassa L, et al: Thyroid Hormone Early Adjustment in Pregnancy (The THERAPY) Trial, *J Clin Endocrinol Metab* 12 May 2010. [Epub ahead of print.]

Yazdy MM, et al: Maternal dietary glycemic intake and the risk of neural tube defects, *Am J Epidemiol* 171:407, 2010.

Zammit S et al. Schizophrenia and neural tube defects: comparisons from an epidemiological perspective, *Schizophr Bull* 33(4):853-858, 2007.

Zeisel SH, daCosta K: Choline: an essential nutrient for public health, *Nutrition Reviews* 67:615, 2009.

Zeller J, et al: Spontaneous globe subluxation in a patient with hyperemesis gravidarum: a case report and review of the literature, *J Emerg Med* 32:285, 2007.

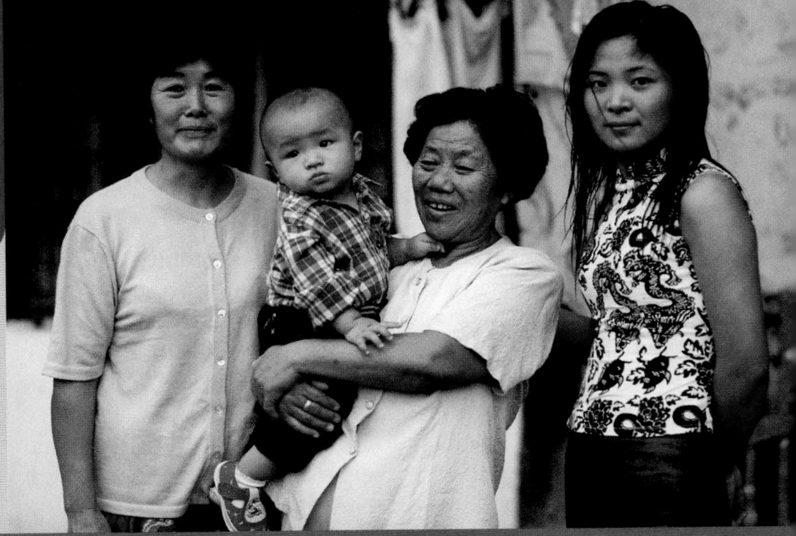

CHAPTER 17

Cristine M. Trahms, MS, RD, CD, FADA
Kelly N. McKean, MS, RD, CD

Nutrition in Infancy

KEY TERMS

arachidonic acid (ARA)
casein
casein hydrolysate
catch-up growth
colostrum
docosahexaenoic acid (DHA)
growth channel
electrolytically reduced iron
lactalbumin
lactoferrin
lag-down growth
palmar grasp
pincer grasp
renal solute load
secretory immunoglobin A (sIgA)
whey proteins

During the first 2 years of life, which are characterized by rapid physical and social growth and development, many changes occur that affect feeding and nutrient intake. The adequacy of infants' nutrient intakes affects their interaction with their environment. Healthy, well-nourished infants have the energy to respond to and learn from the stimuli in their environment and to interact with their parents and caregivers in a manner that encourages bonding and attachment.

PHYSIOLOGIC DEVELOPMENT

The length of gestation, the mother's prepregnancy weight, and the mother's weight gain during gestation determine an infant's birth weight. After birth, the growth of an infant is influenced by genetics and nourishment. Most infants who are genetically determined to be larger reach their **growth channel**, a curve of weight and length or height gain throughout the period of growth, at between 3 and 6 months of age. However, many infants born at or below the tenth percentile for length may not reach their genetically appropriate growth channel until 1 year of age; this is called **catch-up growth**. Infants who are larger at birth and who are genetically determined to be smaller grow at their fetal rate for several months and often do not reach their growth channel until 13 months of age. This phenomenon during the first year of life is called **lag-down growth**.

Infants lose approximately 6% of their body weight during the first few days of life, but their birth weight is usually regained by the seventh to tenth day. Growth thereafter proceeds at a rapid but decelerating rate. Infants usually double their birth weight by 4 to 6 months of age and triple it by the age of 1 year. The amount of weight gained by the infant during the second year approximates the birth weight. Infants increase their length by 50% during the first year of life and double it by 4 years. Total body fat increases rapidly during the first 9 months, after which the rate of fat gain tapers off throughout the rest of childhood. Total body water decreases throughout infancy from 70% at birth to 60% at 1 year. The decrease is almost all in extracellular water, which declines from 42% at birth to 32% at 1 year of age.

The stomach capacity of infants increases from a range of 10 to 20 mL at birth to 200 mL by 1 year, enabling infants to consume more food at a given time and at less frequent intervals as they grow older. During the first weeks of life, gastric acidity decreases and for the first few months remains lower than that of older infants and adults. The rate of emptying is relatively slow, depending on the size and composition of the meal.

Fat absorption varies in the neonate. Human milk fat is well absorbed, but butterfat is poorly absorbed, with fecal excretions of 20% to 48%. The fat combinations in commercially prepared infant formula are well absorbed. The infant's lingual and gastric lipases hydrolyze short- and medium-chain fatty acids in the stomach. Gastric lipase also hydrolyzes long-chain fatty acids and is important in initiating the digestion of triglycerides in the stomach. Most long-chain triglycerides pass unhydrolyzed into the small intestine, where they are broken down by pancreatic lipase. The bile salt–stimulated lipase present in human milk is stimulated by the infant's bile salts and hydrolyzes the triglycerides in the small intestine into free fatty acids and glycerol. Bile salts, which are effective emulsifiers when combined with monoglycerides, fatty acids, and lecithin, aid in the intestinal digestion of fat.

The activities of the enzymes responsible for the digestion of disaccharides—maltase, isomaltase, and sucrase—reach adult levels by 28 to 32 weeks' gestation. Lactase activity (responsible for digesting the disaccharide in milk) reaches adult levels by birth. Pancreatic amylase, which digests starch, continues to remain low during the first 6 months after birth. If the infant consumes starch before this time, increased activity of salivary amylase and digestion in the colon usually compensate.

The neonate has functional but physiologically immature kidneys that increase in size and concentrating capacity in the early weeks of life. The kidneys double in weight by 6 months and triple in weight by 1 year of age. The last renal tubule is estimated to form between the eighth fetal month and the end of the first postnatal month. The glomerular tuft is covered by a much thicker layer of cells throughout neonatal life than at any later time, which may explain why the glomerular filtration rate is lower during the first 9 months of life than it is in later childhood and adulthood. In the neonatal period the ability to form acid, urine, and concentrate solutes is often limited. The renal concentrating capacity at birth may be limited to as little as 700 mOsm/L in some infants. Others have the concentrating capacity of adults (1200 to 1400 mOsm/L). By 6 weeks, most infants can concentrate urine at adult levels. Renal function in a normal newborn infant is rarely a concern; however, difficulties may arise in infants with diarrhea or those who are fed formula that is too concentrated (Butte et al., 2004).

NUTRIENT REQUIREMENTS

Nutrient needs of infants reflect rates of growth, energy expended in activity, basal metabolic needs, and the interaction of the nutrients consumed. Balance studies have defined minimum acceptable levels of intakes for a few nutrients, but for most nutrients the suggested intakes have been extrapolated from the intakes of normal, thriving infants consuming human milk. The dietary reference intakes (DRIs) for infants are shown in the inside front cover.

Energy

Full-term infants who are breast-fed to satiety and infants who are fed a standard 20-kcal/oz formula generally adjust their intake to meet their energy needs when caregivers are sensitive to the infants' hunger and satiety cues. An effective method for determining the adequacy of an infant's energy intake is to carefully monitor gains in weight, length, head circumference, and weight-for-length for age and plot these data on the World Health Organization (WHO) growth charts shown in Appendix Tables 9, 10, 13, and 14. It is important to recognize that during the first year a catch-up or lag-down period in growth may occur.

If infants begin to experience a decrease in their rate of weight gain, do not gain weight, or lose weight, their energy and nutrient intake should be monitored carefully. If the rate of growth in length decreases or ceases, potential malnutrition, an undetected disease, or both should be investigated thoroughly. If the weight gain proceeds at a much more rapid rate than growth in length, the energy concentration of the formula, the quantity of formula consumed, and the amount and type of semisolid and table foods offered should be evaluated. The activity level of the infant should also be assessed. Infants who are at the highest end of the growth charts for weight-for-length, or who grow rapidly in infancy, tend to be at greater risk for obesity later in life.

Protein

Protein is needed for tissue replacement, deposition of lean body mass, and growth (Rodriguez, 2005). Protein requirements during the rapid growth of infancy are higher per kilogram of weight than those for older children or adults. Recommendations for protein intake are based on the composition of human milk, and it is assumed that the efficiency of human milk use is 100%.

Infants require a larger percentage of total amino acids as essential amino acids than do adults. Histidine seems to be an essential amino acid for infants, but not for adults. Tyrosine, cystine, and taurine may be essential for premature infants.

Human milk or infant formula provides the major portion of protein during the first year of life. The amount of protein in human milk is adequate for the first 6 months of life, even though the amount of protein in human milk is considerably less than in infant formula. From 6 to 12 months of age the diet should be supplemented with additional sources of high-quality protein such as yogurt, strained meats, or cereal mixed with formula or human milk.

Infants may not receive adequate protein if their formula is excessively diluted for a prolonged period, as may be done to treat diarrhea after an enteric illness, or they have multiple food allergies causing their intake to be restricted (see Chapter 27).

Lipids

The current recommendation for infants younger than 1 year of age is to consume a minimum of 30 g of fat per day. This quantity is present in human milk and all infant formulas. Significantly lower fat intakes (e.g., with skim-milk feedings) may result in an inadequate total energy intake. An infant may try to correct the energy deficit by increasing the volume of milk ingested but usually cannot make up the entire deficit this way.

Human milk contains a generous amount of the essential fatty acids linoleic acid and α-linolenic acid, as well as the longer-chain derivatives **arachidonic acid (ARA)** (C20:4ω-6) and **docosahexaenoic acid (DHA)** (C22:6ω-3). Infant formulas are supplemented with linoleic acid and α-linolenic acid, from which ARA and DHA are derived. Increasingly, many formulas are also supplemented with ARA and DHA.

Linoleic acid, which is essential for growth and dermal integrity, should provide 3% of the infant's total energy intake, or 4.4 g/day for infants younger than 6 months of age and 4.6 g/day for infants 7 months to 1 year of age. In human milk 5% of the kilocalories and 10% in most infant formulas are derived from linoleic acid. Smaller amounts of α-linolenic acid, a precursor of the ω-3 fatty acids DHA and eicosapentaenoic acid (EPA), should be included. The current recommendation is 0.5 g/day during the first year of life.

Because DHA can be formed by desaturation of α-linolenic acid, the importance of dietary DHA intake is uncertain. The concentration of DHA in human milk varies, depending on the amount of DHA in the mother's diet. DHA and ARA are the major ω-3 and ω-6 long-chain polyunsaturated fatty acids (LCPUFAs) of neural tissues, and DHA is the major fatty acid of the photoreceptor membranes of the retina. Some studies suggest that supplementation of DHA and ARA positively affects visual acuity and psychomotor development, especially in premature infants. However, other studies have shown no differences in development. The American Academy of Pediatrics (AAP) has not taken an official stand on the addition of LCPUFAs to infant formula; however, they are now added to most infant formulas.

Carbohydrates

Carbohydrates should supply 30% to 60% of the energy intake during infancy. Approximately 40% of the energy in human milk and 40% to 50% of the energy in infant formulas is derived from lactose or other carbohydrates. Although rare, some infants cannot tolerate lactose and require a modified formula in their diet (see Chapters 29 and 44).

Botulism in infancy is caused by the ingestion of *Clostridium botulinum* spores, which germinate and produce toxin in the bowel lumen. The carbohydrates honey and corn syrup, occasionally used in home-prepared foods, have been identified as the only food sources of these spores in infants' diets. The spores are extremely resistant to heat treatment and are not destroyed by current methods of processing. Thus honey and corn syrup should not be fed to infants younger than 1 year of age because they have not yet developed the immunity required to resist botulism spore development.

Water

The water requirement for infants is determined by the amount lost from the skin and lungs and in the feces and urine, in addition to a small amount needed for growth. The recommended total water intake for infants, based on the DRIs, is 0.7 L/day for infants up to 6 months and 0.8 L/day for infants 7 to 12 months of age. Note that total water includes all water contained in food, beverages, and drinking water. Water requirements per kilogram of body weight are shown in Table 17-1.

Because the renal concentrating capacity of young infants may be less than that of older children and adults, they may be vulnerable to developing a water imbalance. Under ordinary conditions, human milk and formula that is properly prepared supply adequate amounts of water. However, when formula is boiled, the water evaporates and the solutes become concentrated; therefore boiled milk or formula is inappropriate for infants. In very hot, humid environments, infants may require additional water. When losses of water are high (e.g., vomiting and diarrhea), infants should be monitored carefully for fluid and electrolyte imbalances.

Water deficits result in hypernatremic dehydration and its associated neurologic consequences (e.g., seizures, vascular damage). Hypernatremic dehydration has been reported in breast-fed infants who lose greater than 10% of their birth weight in the first few days of life (Leven and Macdonald, 2008). Because of the potential for hypernatremic dehydration, careful monitoring of volume of intake, daily weights, and hydration status (e.g., number of wet diapers) in all newborns is warranted.

Water intoxication results in hyponatremia, restlessness, nausea, vomiting, diarrhea, and polyuria or oliguria; seizures can also result. This condition may occur when water

TABLE 17-1

Water Requirements of Infants and Children

Age	Water Requirement (mL/kg/day)
10 days	125-150
3 mo	140-160
6 mo	130-155
1 yr	120-135
2 yr	115-125
6 yr	90-100
10 yr	70-85
14 yr	50-60

From Barness LA: Nutrition and nutritional disorders. In Behrman RE, Kliegman RM: Nelson textbook of pediatrics, ed 17, Philadelphia, 2003, Saunders.

is provided as a replacement for milk, the formula is excessively diluted, or bottled water is used instead of an electrolyte solution in the treatment of diarrhea.

Minerals

Calcium

Breast-fed infants retain approximately two thirds of their calcium intake. The recommended adequate intake (AI), the mean intake, is based on calcium intakes in healthy breast-fed infants. The AI for infants 0 to 6 months of age is 200 mg/day; for infants 7 to 12 months of age the AI is 260 mg/day; formulas are enhanced accordingly.

Fluoride

The importance of fluoride in preventing dental caries has been well documented. However, excessive fluoride may cause dental fluorosis, ranging from fine white lines to entirely chalky teeth (see Chapter 26). To prevent fluorosis, the tolerable upper intake level for fluoride has been set at 0.7 mg/day for infants up to 6 months and 0.9 mg/day for infants 7 to 12 months of age.

Human milk is very low in fluoride. Commercially prepared infant cereals, wet pack cereals, and fruit juice produced with fluoridated water are significant sources of fluoride in infancy. Fluoride supplementation is not recommended for infants younger than 6 months of age. After tooth eruption it is recommended that fluoridated water be offered several times per day to breast-fed infants, those who receive cow's milk, and those fed formulas made with water that contains less than 0.3 mg of fluoride/L (American Academy of Pediatrics [AAP], 2009).

Iron

Full-term infants are considered to have adequate stores of iron for growth up to a doubling of their birth weight. This occurs at approximately 4 months of age in full-term infants and much earlier in prematurely born infants. Recommended intakes of iron increase according to age, growth rate, and iron stores. At 4 to 6 months of age, infants who are fed only human milk are at risk for developing a negative iron balance and may deplete their reserves by 6 to 9 months. Iron in human milk is highly bioavailable; however, breast-fed infants should receive an additional source of iron by 4 to 6 months of age (AAP, 2005). Iron-fortified cereals and infant formula are common food sources. Cow's milk is a poor source of iron and should not be given before 12 months of age. The AAP recommends iron supplementation of 1 mg/kg/day starting at 4 months of age and continuing until appropriate complementary foods have been introduced (Baker and Greer, 2010).

Iron deficiency and iron deficiency anemia are common health concerns for the older infant. The prevalence of iron deficiency in children 9 months to 3 years of age who are living in the United States and the United Kingdom and are primarily among low socioeconomic and minority groups is higher than the 10% in the general population, and has been estimated at 30% (Eden, 2005).

Monitoring iron status is important because of the long-term cognitive effects of iron deficiency in infancy (Eden, 2005). Low hemoglobin concentrations at 8 months of age correlate with impaired motor development at 18 months of age (Sherriff et al., 2001). In addition, children with chronic iron deficiency in infancy demonstrate long-term developmental deficits and behavioral issues in early adolescence.

Zinc

Newborn infants are immediately dependent on a dietary source of zinc. Zinc is better absorbed from human milk than from infant formula. Human milk and infant formulas provide adequate zinc (0.3 to 0.5 mg/100 kcal) for the first year of life. Other foods (e.g., meats, cereals) should provide most of the zinc required during the second year. Infants who are zinc-deficient can exhibit growth retardation (Cole and Lifshitz, 2008).

Vitamins

Vitamin B_{12}

Milk from lactating mothers who follow a strict vegan diet may be deficient in vitamin B_{12}, especially if the mother followed the regimen for a long time before and during her pregnancy. Vitamin B_{12} deficiency has also been diagnosed in infants breast-fed by mothers with pernicious anemia (Weiss et al., 2004) (see Chapter 32).

Vitamin D

Human milk derived from an adequately fed, lactating mother supplies all the vitamins the term infant needs except for vitamin D; human milk contains approximately only 20 international units (IU)/L (0.5 mcg cholecalciferol) of vitamin D. For the prevention of rickets and vitamin D deficiency, the AAP recommends a minimum vitamin D intake of 400 IU per day shortly after birth for all infants. All breast-fed infants need a vitamin D supplement of 400 IU per day. Formula-fed infants who consume less than 1000 mL of formula per day also need supplementation (Wagner and Greer, 2008). There appears to be a higher risk of rickets among young, breast-fed infants and children with dark skin (Weisberg et al., 2004). Because a variety of environmental and family lifestyle factors can affect both sunlight exposure and absorption of vitamin D, the AAP recommendations to provide supplemental vitamin D are appropriate for all infants. Supplementation up to 800 IU of vitamin D per day may be needed for infants at higher risk, such as premature infants, dark-skinned infants and children, and those who reside in northern latitudes or at higher altitudes (Misra et el., 2008).

The Food and Drug Administration (FDA) states that some droppers that come with liquid vitamin D supplements could hold more than the 400 IU per day recommended by the AAP. Thus it is important that parents or caregivers provide only the recommended amount. Excessive vitamin D can cause nausea and vomiting, loss of appetite, excessive thirst, frequent urination, constipation, abdominal pain, muscle weakness, muscle and joint aches, confusion, fatigue or damage to kidneys.

Vitamin K

The vitamin K requirements of the neonate need special attention. Deficiency may result in bleeding or hemorrhagic disease of the newborn. This condition is more common in breast-fed infants than in other infants because human milk contains only 2.5 mcg/L of vitamin K, whereas cow's milk–based formulas contain approximately 20 times this amount. All infant formulas contain a minimum of 4 mcg of vitamin K per 100 kcal of formula. The AI for infants is 2 mcg/day during the first 6 months and 2.5 mcg/day during the second 6 months of life. This can be supplied by mature breast milk, although perhaps not during the first week of life. For breast-fed infants vitamin K supplementation is necessary during that time to considerably decrease the risk for hemorrhagic disease. Most hospitals require that infants receive an injection of vitamin K as a prophylactic measure shortly after birth.

Supplementation

Vitamin and mineral supplements should be prescribed only after careful evaluation of the infant's intake. Commercially prepared infant formulas are fortified with all necessary vitamins and minerals; therefore formula-fed infants rarely need supplements. Breast-fed infants need additional vitamin D supplementation shortly after birth and iron by 4 to 6 months of age (see *Focus On:* Vitamin and Mineral Supplementation Recommendations for Full-Term Infants). Chapter 43 discusses the feeding of premature or high-risk infants and their special needs.

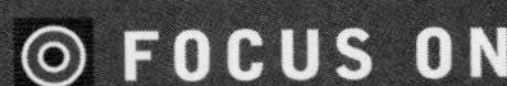

FOCUS ON

Vitamin and Mineral Supplementation Recommendations for Full-Term Infants

Vitamin D

Supplementation shortly after birth of 400 IU/day for all breast-fed infants and infants consuming less than 1000 mL of vitamin D–fortified formula each day

Vitamin K

Supplementation soon after birth to prevent hemorrhagic disease of the newborn

Fluoride

Supplement of 0.25 mg/day after 6 months of age if fluoride concentration of water is less than 0.3 ppm

Iron

Breast-Fed Infants

Approximately 1 mg/kg/day by 4 to 6 months of age, preferably from supplemental foods, and only iron-fortified formulas for weaning or supplementing breast milk

Formula-Fed Infants

Only iron-fortified formula during the first year of life

Modified from American Academy of Pediatrics, Committee on Nutrition: Pediatric nutrition handbook, ed 6, Elk Grove Village, Ill, 2009, American Academy of Pediatrics.

MILK

Human Milk

Human milk is unquestionably the food of choice for the infant. Its composition is designed to provide the necessary energy and nutrients in appropriate amounts. It contains specific and nonspecific immune factors that support and strengthen the immature immune system of the newborn and thus protect the body against infections. Human milk also helps prevent diarrhea and otitis media (AAP, 2005). Allergic reactions to human milk protein are rare. Moreover, the closeness of the mother and infant during breast-feeding facilitates attachment and bonding (see Chapter 16) and breast milk provides nutritional benefits (e.g., optimal nourishment in an easily digestible and bioavailable form), decreases infant morbidity, provides maternal health benefits (e.g., lactation amenorrhea, maternal weight loss, some cancer protection), and has economic and environmental benefits (American Dietetic Association [ADA], 2009).

During the first few days of life, a breast-feeding infant receives **colostrum**, a yellow, transparent fluid that meets the infant's needs during the first week. It contains less fat and carbohydrate but more protein and greater concentrations of sodium, potassium, and chloride than mature milk. It is also an excellent source of immunologic substances.

Note that breast feeding may not be appropriate for mothers with certain infections or those who are taking medications that may have untoward effects on the infant. For example, a mother who is infected with human immunodeficiency virus can transmit the infection to the infant and a mother using psychotropic drugs or other pharmacologic drugs may pass the medication to the infant through her breast milk (AAP, 2005). See Chapter 16.

The American Dietetic Association (ADA) and the AAP support exclusive breast feeding (EBF) for the first 6 months of life and then breast feeding supplemented by complementary foods until at least 12 months (AAP, 2005; ADA, 2009). It is important to note the ages of the infants in these recommendations; adding other foods at too young of an age decreases breast-milk intake and increases early weaning. Healthy Children 2020 objectives propose to support breast-feeding among mothers of newborn infants (see *Focus On:* Healthy Children 2020 Objectives: Nourishment of Infants).

FOCUS ON

Healthy Children 2020 Objectives: Nourishment of Infants

Healthy People 2020 is a comprehensive set of health objectives for the United States to achieve during the second decade of the 21st century. Healthy People 2020 identifies a wide range of public health priorities and specific, measurable objectives. The objectives have 42 focus areas, one of which is Maternal, Infant, and Child Health. The objectives related to nourishment of infants are as follows:

GOAL: Improve the health and well being of women, infants, children, and families.

Objective: Increase the proportion of infants who are breastfed to 81.9% in the early postpartum period, to 60.6% at 6 months, and to 34.1% at 1 year of age. Increase the proportion of infants that are exclusively breastfed to 46.2% through 3 months of age and 25.5% through 6 months of age.

Objective: Reduce the proportion of breastfed newborns who receive formula supplementation within the first 2 days of life to 14.2%.

GOAL: Promote health and reduce chronic disease risk through the consumption of healthful diets and achievement and maintenance of healthy body weights.

Objective: Eliminate very low food security among children. Objective: Reduce iron deficiency among children ages 1 to 2 years to less than 14.3%.

GOAL: Prevent and control oral and craniofacial diseases, conditions, and injuries and improve access to preventive services and dental care.

Objective: Reduce the proportion of young children with dental caries in their primary teeth.

The complete text of the Healthy People 2020 Objectives can be found at www.healthypeople.gov/2020/topics objectives2020/default.aspx

Composition of Human and Cow's Milk

The composition of human milk is different from that of cow's milk; for this reason, unmodified cow's milk is not recommended for infants until at least 1 year of age. Both provide 20 kcal/oz; however, the nutrient sources of the energy are different. Protein provides 6% to 7% of the energy in human milk and 20% of the energy in cow's milk. Human milk is 60% **whey proteins** (mainly lactalbumins) and 40% casein; by contrast, cow's milk is 20% whey proteins and 80% casein. **Casein** forms a tough, hard-to-digest curd in the infant's stomach, whereas **lactalbumin** in human milk forms soft, flocculent, easy-to-digest curds. Taurine and cystine are present in higher concentrations in human milk than in cow's milk; these amino acids may be essential for premature infants. Lactose provides 42% of the energy in human milk and only 30% of the energy in cow's milk.

Lipids provide 50% of the energy in human and whole cow's milk. Linoleic acid, an essential fatty acid, provides 4% of the energy in human milk and only 1% in cow's milk. The cholesterol content of human milk is 10 to 20 mg/dL compared with 10 to 15 mg/dL in whole cow's milk. Less fat is absorbed from cow's milk than from human milk; a lipase in human milk is stimulated by bile salts and contributes significantly to the hydrolysis of milk triglycerides.

All of the water-soluble vitamins in human milk reflect maternal intake. Cow's milk contains adequate quantities of the B-complex vitamins, but little vitamin C. Human milk and supplemented cow's milk provide sufficient vitamin A. Human milk is a richer source of vitamin E than cow's milk.

The quantity of iron in human and cow's milk is small (0.3 mg/L). Approximately 50% of the iron in human milk is absorbed, whereas less than 1% of the iron in cow's milk is absorbed. The bioavailability of zinc in human milk is higher than in cow's milk. Cow's milk contains three times as much calcium and six times as much phosphorus as human milk, and its fluoride concentration is twice that of human milk.

The much higher protein and ash content of cow's milk results in a higher **renal solute load**, or amount of nitrogenous waste and minerals that must be excreted by the kidney. The sodium and potassium concentrations in human milk are about one third those in cow's milk, contributing to the lower renal solute load of human milk. The osmolality of human milk averages 300 mOsm/kg, whereas that of cow's milk is 400 mOsm/kg.

Antiinfective Factors

Human milk and colostrum contain antibodies and antiinfective factors that are not present in infant formulas. **Secretory immunoglobulin A (sIgA)**, the predominant immunoglobulin in human milk, plays a role in protecting the infant's immature gut from infection. Breast feeding should be maintained until the infant is at least 3 months of age to obtain this benefit.

The iron-binding protein **lactoferrin** in human milk deprives bacteria of iron and thus slows their growth. Lysozymes, which are bacteriolytic enzymes found in human milk, destroy the cell membranes of bacteria after the peroxides and ascorbic acid that are also present in human milk have inactivated them. Human milk enhances the growth of the bacterium *Lactobacillus bifidus*, which produces an acidic gastrointestinal (GI) environment that interferes with the growth of certain pathogenic organisms. Because of these antiinfective factors, the incidence of infections is lower in breast-fed infants than in formula-fed infants.

Colonization with nonpathogenic microbiota is important for infant health and may affect health in later life. By the time a mother weans her infant, the baby's GI tract has established its normal flora. This ecosystem in early life is influenced by such factors as mode of birth, environment, diet, and use of antibiotics (Marques et al., 2010). The role and safety of supplemental probiotic use is under study.

Formulas

Infants that are not breastfed are usually fed a formula based on cow's milk or a soy product. Many mothers may also choose to offer a combination of breast milk and formula feedings. Those infants who have special requirements receive specially designed products.

Commercial formulas made from heat-treated nonfat milk or a soy product and supplemented with vegetables fats, vitamins, and minerals are formulated to approximate, as closely as possible, the composition of human milk. They provide the necessary nutrients in an easily absorbed form. The manufacture of infant formulas is regulated by the FDA through the Infant Formula Act (Nutrient Requirements for Infant Formulas, 1985). By law, infant formulas are required to have a nutrient level that is consistent with these guidelines (Table 17-2). Refer to individual manufacturers' websites to obtain the most accurate information and compare the composition of various infant formulas and feeding products.

Formulas are also available for older infants and toddlers. However, typically "older infant" formulas are unnecessary unless toddlers are not receiving adequate amounts of infant or table foods.

Efforts are ongoing to manufacture infant formulas that closely approximate human milk. Recent additions to infant formulas include ARA, DHA, prebiotics, and probiotics. No current documentation shows that the growth or development of formula-fed infants is compromised when they consume formulas without these additives. The declining prevalence of anemia in infants is credited to the use of iron-fortified formula. The AAP recommends iron-fortified formulas for all formula-fed infants. The widespread theory that iron-fortified formula may cause constipation, loose stools, colic (severe abdominal pain), and spitting up has not been confirmed by clinical studies (AAP, 1999).

Various products are available for infants who cannot tolerate the protein in cow's milk–based formulas. Soy-based infant formulas are recommended for (1) infants in vegetarian families, and (2) infants with galactosemia or hereditary primary lactase deficiency. Soy formulas are not recommended for children known to have protein allergies because many infants who are allergic to cow's milk protein also develop allergies to soy protein (Bhatia and Greer, 2008) (see Chapter 27).

Infants who cannot tolerate cow's milk–based or soy products can be fed formulas made from a **casein hydrolysate**, which is casein that has been split into smaller components by treatment with acid, alkali, or enzymes. These formulas do not contain lactose. For infants who have severe food protein intolerances and cannot tolerate hydrolysate formulas, free amino acid–based formulas are available. Other formulas are available for children with problems such as malabsorption or metabolic disorders (e.g., phenylketonuria) (see Chapters 18 and 44).

Soy-based formulas are under regular scrutiny. Full-term infants ingesting soy formulas grow and absorb minerals as well as infants fed cow's milk–based formulas, but they are exposed to several thousand times higher levels of phytoestrogens and isoflavones. The biologic effect of these elevated isoflavone levels on long-term infant development is not yet clear (National Toxicology Program, 2010). Soy-based formulas are not recommended for preterm infants

TABLE 17-2

Nutrient Levels in Infant Formulas As Specified by the Infant Formula Act

Specified Nutrient Component	Minimum Level Required (per 100 kcal of energy)
Protein (g)	1.8
Fat (g)	3.3
Percentage of calories	30
Linoleic acid (mg)	300
Percentage of calories	2.7
Vitamin A (IU)	250
Vitamin E (IU)	0.7
Vitamin D (IU)	40
Vitamin K (mcg)	4
Thiamin (mcg)	40
Riboflavin (mcg)	60
Niacin (mcg)	250
Ascorbic acid (mg)	8
Pyridoxine (mcg)	35
Vitamin B_{12} (mcg)	0.15
Folic acid (mcg)	4
Biotin (mcg) (non-milk–based formulas only)	1.5
Pantothenic acid (mcg)	300
Choline (mg) (non-milk–based formulas only)	7
Inositol (mg) (non-milk–based formulas only)	4
Calcium (mg)	60
Phosphorus (mg)	30
Iron (mg)	0.15
Zinc (mg)	0.5
Magnesium (mg)	6
Manganese (mcg)	5
Sodium (mg)	20
Potassium (mg)	80
Iodine (mcg)	5
Chloride (mg)	55
Copper (mcg)	60

From Nutrient requirements for infant formulas, Final Rule (21 CFR 107), Fed Reg 50:45106, 1985.

because of the increased risk for osteopenia (Bhatia and Greer, 2008).

The protein in soy infant formula is soy protein isolate supplemented with L-methionine, L-carnitine, and taurine. Contaminants include phytates, which bind minerals and niacin; and protease inhibitors, which have antitrypsin, antichymotrypsin, and antielastin properties. Aluminum from mineral salts is found in soy infant formulas at concentrations of 600-1300 ng/mL, levels that exceed aluminum concentrations in human milk of 4-65 ng/mL (Bhatia and Greer, 2008).

Whole Cow's Milk

Some parents may choose to transition their infant from formula to fresh cow's milk before 1 year of age. However, the AAP Committee on Nutrition has concluded that infants should not be fed whole cow's milk during the first year of life (AAP, 2009). Infants who are fed whole cow's milk have been found to have lower intakes of iron, linoleic acid, and vitamin E, and excessive intakes of sodium, potassium, and protein. Cow's milk may cause a small amount of GI blood loss.

Low-fat (1% to 2%) and nonfat milk are also inappropriate for infants during the first 12 months of life. The infants may ingest excessive amounts of protein in large volumes of milk in an effort to meet their energy needs, and the decreased amount of essential fatty acids may be insufficient for preventing deficiency (AAP, 2009). In addition, substitute or imitation milks such as rice, oat, or nut milks are inappropriate and should not be fed to infants unless they are properly supplemented.

Formula Preparation

Commercial infant formulas are available in ready-to-feed forms that require no preparation, as concentrates prepared by mixing with equal parts of water, and in powder form that is designed to be mixed with 2 oz of water per level scoop of powder.

Infant formulas should be prepared in a clean environment. All equipment, including bottles, nipples, mixers, and the top of the can of formula, should be washed thoroughly. Formula may be prepared for up to a 24-hour period and refrigerated. Formula for each feeding should be warmed in a hot water bath. Microwave heating is not recommended because of the risk of burns from formula that is too hot or unevenly heated. Any formula warmed and not consumed at that feeding should be discarded.

FOOD

Dry infant cereals are fortified with **electrolytically reduced iron**, which is iron that has been fractionated into small particles for improved absorption. Four level tablespoons of cereal provide approximately 5 mg of iron or approximately half the amount the infant requires. Therefore infant cereal is usually the first food added to the infant's diet.

Strained and "junior" vegetables and fruits provide carbohydrates and vitamins A and C. Vitamin C is added to numerous jarred fruits and all fruit juices. In addition, tapioca is added to several of the jarred fruits. Milk is added to the creamed vegetables, and wheat is incorporated into the mixed vegetables.

Most strained and junior meats are prepared with water. Strained meats, which have the highest energy density of any of the commercial baby foods, are an excellent source of high-quality protein and heme iron.

Numerous dessert items are also available such as puddings and fruit desserts. The nutrient composition of these products varies, but all contain excess energy in the form of sugar and modified cornstarch or tapioca starch. Most infants do not need this excess energy.

Various commercially prepared foods and organically grown products are available for infants. See Chapter 10 for a discussion of organic foods. These products vary widely in their nutrient value. Foods for infants should be thoughtfully selected to meet their nutritional and developmental needs.

Mothers who would like to make their own infant food can easily do so by following the directions in Box 17-1. Home-prepared foods are generally more concentrated in nutrients than commercially prepared foods because less water is used. Salt and sugar should not be added to foods prepared for infants.

BOX 17-1

Directions for Home Preparation of Infant Foods

1. Select fresh, high-quality fruits, vegetables, or meats.
2. Be sure that all utensils, including cutting boards, grinder, knives, and other items, are thoroughly cleaned.
3. Wash hands before preparing the food.
4. Clean, wash, and trim the food in as little water as possible.
5. Cook the foods until tender in as little water as possible. Avoid overcooking, which may destroy heat-sensitive nutrients.
6. Do not add salt or sugar. Do not add honey to food intended for infants younger than 1 year of age.*
7. Add enough water for the food to be easily puréed.
8. Strain or purée the food using an electric blender, a food mill, a baby food grinder, or a kitchen strainer.
9. Pour purée into an ice cube tray and freeze.
10. When the food is frozen hard, remove the cubes and store in freezer bags.
11. When ready to serve, defrost and heat in a serving container the amount of food that will be consumed at a single feeding.

*Clostridium botulinum spores, which cause botulism, have been reported in honey; young infants do not have the immune capacity to resist this infection.

FEEDING

Early Feeding Patterns

Because milk from a mother with an adequate diet is uniquely designed to meet the needs of the human infant, breast feeding for the first 6 months of life is strongly recommended. Most chronic medical conditions do not contraindicate breast-feeding.

A mother should be encouraged to nurse her infant immediately after birth. Those who care for and counsel parents during the first postpartum days should acquaint themselves with ways in which they can be supportive of breast-feeding. Ideally, counseling and preparation for breast feeding starts in the last few months or weeks of pregnancy (see Chapter 16).

Regardless of whether infants are breast-fed or formula fed, they should be held and cuddled during feedings. Once a feeding rhythm has been established, infants become fussy or cry to indicate they are hungry, whereas they often smile and fall asleep when they are satisfied (Table 17-3). Infants, not adults, should establish the feeding schedules. Initially, most infants feed every 2 to 3 hours; by 2 months of age most feed every 4 hours. By 3 to 4 months of age infants have usually matured enough to allow the mother to omit night feedings.

Bisphenol A (BPA) is a chemical present in many hard plastic bottles, such as baby bottles and reusable cups, and metal food and beverage containers, including canned liquid infant formula. Concern has been raised about the potential effects of BPA on the brain, behavior, and prostate gland in fetuses, infants, and young children. Studies are ongoing; however, in the interim the FDA recommends taking reasonable steps to reduce human exposure to BPA. The major U.S. manufacturers have stopped producing BPA-containing bottles and infant feeding cups for the U.S. market. The FDA is facilitating the development of alternatives to BPA for the linings of infant formula cans and supporting efforts to replace or minimize BPA in other food can linings (Food and Drug Administration [FDA], 2010).

TABLE 17-3

Satiety Behaviors in Infants

Age (Weeks)	Behavior
4-12	Draws head away from the nipple Falls asleep When nipple is reinserted, closes lips tightly Bites nipple, purses lips, or smiles and lets go
16-24	Releases nipple and withdraws head Fusses or cries Obstructs mouth with hands Pays more attention to surroundings Bites nipple
28-36	Changes posture Keeps mouth tightly closed Shakes head as if to say "no" Plays with utensils Uses hands more actively Throws utensils
40-52	See behaviors listed for previous age range Sputters with tongue and lips Hands bottle or cup to mother

From Pipes PL: Health care professionals. In Garwood G, Fewell R, editors: Educating handicapped infants, Rockville, Md, 1982, Aspen Systems.

Development of Feeding Skills

At birth, infants coordinate sucking, swallowing, and breathing, and are prepared to suckle liquids from the breast or bottle, but are not able to handle foods with texture. During the first year, typical infants develop head control, the ability to move into and sustain a sitting posture, and the ability to grasp, first with a **palmar grasp** and then with a refined **pincer grasp** (Figure 17-1). They develop mature sucking and rotary chewing abilities and progress from being fed to feeding themselves using their fingers. In the second year, they learn to feed themselves independently with a spoon (Figure 17-2).

Addition of Semisolid Foods

Developmental readiness and nutrient needs are the criteria that determine appropriate times for the addition of various foods. During the first 4 months of life, the infant attains head and neck control, and oral motor patterns progress from a suck to a suckling to the beginnings of a mature sucking pattern. Puréed foods introduced during this phase are consumed in the same manner as are liquids, with each suckle being followed by a tongue-thrust swallow. Table 17-4 lists developmental landmarks and their indications for semisolid and table food introduction.

Between 4 and 6 months of age, when the mature sucking movement is refined and munching movements (up-and-down chopping motions) begin, the introduction of strained foods is appropriate. Infant cereal is usually introduced first. To support developmental progress, cereal is offered to the infant from a spoon, not combined with formula in a bottle. Thereafter various commercially or home-prepared foods may be offered. The sequence in which these foods are introduced is not important; however, it is important that one single ingredient food (e.g., peaches, not peach cobbler, which has many ingredients) be introduced at a time. Introducing a single new food at a time at 2- to 7-day intervals enables parents to identify any allergic responses or food intolerances (Butte et al., 2004). Introducing vegetables before fruits may increase vegetable acceptance.

Infants demonstrate their acceptance of new foods by slowly increasing the variety and quantity of solids they accept. Breast-fed infants seem to accept greater quantities than do formula-fed infants. Parents who thoughtfully offer a variety of nourishing foods are more likely to provide a well-balanced diet and help their children learn to accept more flavors.

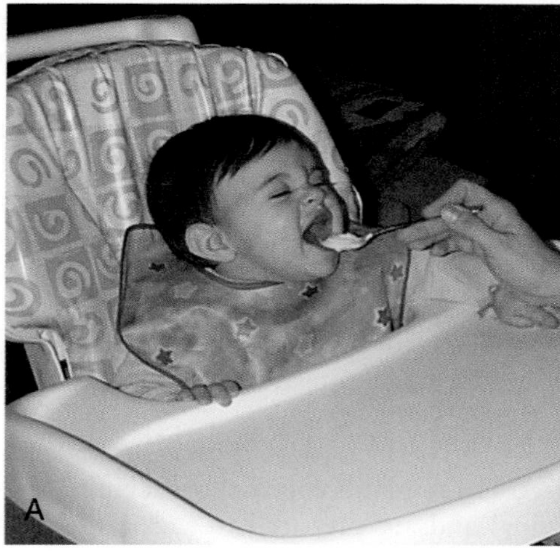

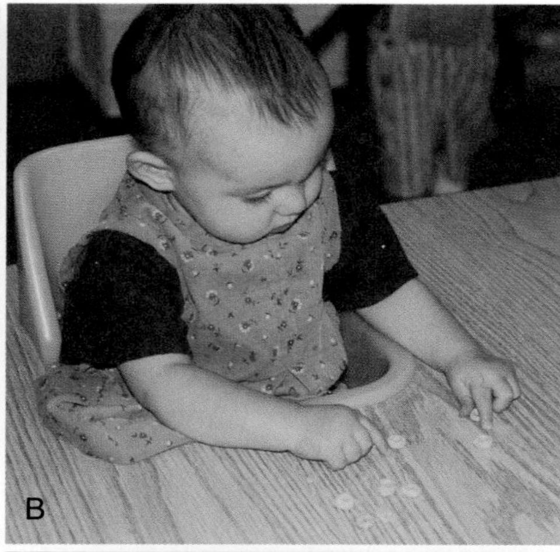

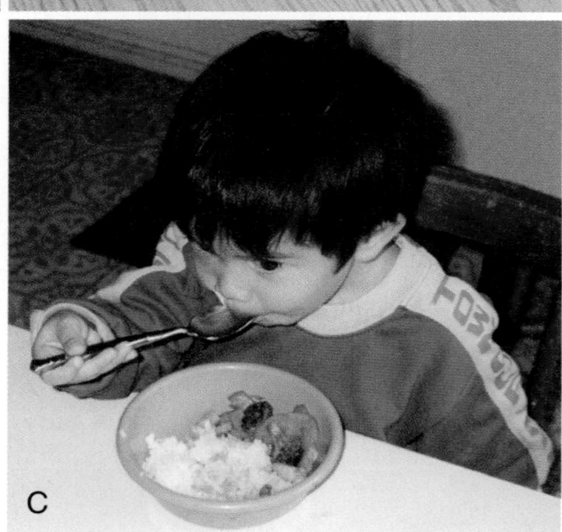

FIGURE 17-1 Development of feeding skills in infants and toddlers. **A,** This 7-month-old child shows the beginnings of involvement with feeding by anticipating the spoon. **B,** This 9-month-old girl is using a refined pincer grasp to pick up her food. **C,** This 19-month-old boy is beginning to use his spoon independently, although he is not yet able to rotate his wrist to keep food on it.

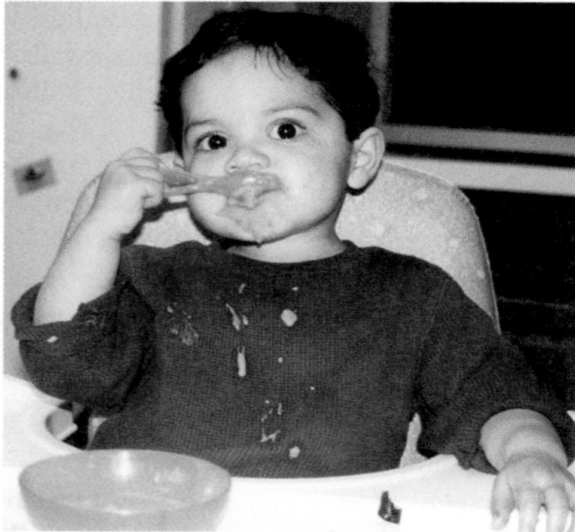

FIGURE 17-2 This 2-year-old is skilled at self-feeding because he has the ability to rotate his wrist and elevate his elbow to keep food on the spoon.

As oral-motor maturation proceeds, an infant's rotary chewing ability develops, indicating a readiness for more textured foods such as well-cooked mashed vegetables, casseroles, and pasta from the family menu. Learning to grasp—with the palmar grasp, then with an inferior pincer grasp, and finally with the refined pincer grasp—indicates a readiness for finger foods such as oven-dried toast, arrowroot biscuits, or cheese sticks (see Figure 17-1). Table 17-5 presents recommendations for adding foods to an infant's diet. Foods with skins or rinds and foods that stick to the roof of the mouth (e.g., hot dogs, grapes, bread with peanut butter) may cause choking and should not be offered to young infants.

During the last quarter of the first year, infants can approximate their lips to the rim of the cup and can drink if the cup is held for them. During the second year they gain the ability to rotate their wrists and elevate their elbows, thus allowing them to hold the cup themselves and manage a spoon. They are very messy eaters at first, but by 2 years of age most typical children skillfully feed themselves (see Figure 17-2).

Weaning from Breast or Bottle to Cup

The introduction of solids into an infant's diet begins the weaning process in which the infant transitions from a diet of only breast milk or formula to a more varied one. Weaning should proceed gradually and be based on the infant's rate of growth and developmental skills. Weaning foods should be carefully chosen to complement the nutrient needs of the infant, promote appropriate nutrient intake, and maintain growth.

TABLE 17-4

Feeding Behaviors: Developmental Landmarks During the First 2 Years of Life

Developmental Landmarks	Change Indicated	Examples of Appropriate Foods
Tongue laterally transfers food in the mouth Shows voluntary and independent movements of the tongue and lips Sitting posture can be sustained Shows beginning of chewing movements (up and down movements of the jaw)	Introduction of soft, mashed table food	Tuna fish; mashed potatoes; well-cooked, mashed vegetables; ground meats in gravy and sauces; soft, diced fruit such as bananas, peaches, and pears; flavored yogurt
Reaches for and grasps objects with palmar grasp Brings hand to mouth	Finger feeding (large pieces of food)	Oven-dried toast, teething biscuits; cheese sticks (should be soluble in the mouth to prevent choking)
Voluntarily releases food (refined digital [pincer] grasp)	Finger feeding (small pieces of food)	Bits of cottage cheese, dry cereal, peas, and other bite-size vegetables; small pieces of meat
Shows rotary chewing pattern	Introduction of food of varied textures from family menu	Well-cooked, chopped meats and casseroles; cooked vegetables and canned fruit (not mashed); toast; potatoes; macaroni, spaghetti; peeled ripe fruit
Approximates lips to rim of the cup	Introduction of cup for sipping liquids	
Understands relationship of container and its contents	Beginning of self-feeding (though messiness should be expected)	Food that when scooped adheres to the spoon, such as applesauce, cooked cereal, mashed potatoes, cottage cheese, yogurt
Shows increased movements of the jaw Shows development of ulnar deviation of the wrist	More skilled at cup and spoon feeding	Chopped fibrous meats, such as roast and steak; raw vegetables and fruit (introduced gradually)
Walks alone	May seek food and obtain food independently	Foods of high nutritional value
Names food, expresses preferences; prefers unmixed foods Goes on food jags Appetite appears to decrease		Balanced food choices, with child permitted to develop food preferences (parents should not be concerned that these preferences will last forever)

Modified from Trahms CM, Pipes P: Nutrition in infancy and childhood, ed 6, New York, 1997, McGraw-Hill.

TABLE 17-5

Suggested Ages for the Introduction of Juice, Semisolid Foods, and Table Foods

	Age (mo)		
Food	**4-6**	**6-8**	**9-12**
Iron-fortified cereals for infants	Add		
Vegetables		Add strained.	Gradually eliminate strained foods and introduce table foods.
Fruits		Add strained.	Gradually eliminate strained foods; introduce chopped, well-cooked, or canned foods.
Meats		Add strained or finely chopped table meats.	Decrease the use of strained meats; increase the varieties of table meats offered.
Finger foods, such as arrowroot biscuits, oven-dried toast		Add foods that can be secured with a palmar grasp.	Increase the use of small finger foods as the pincer grasp develops.
Well-cooked mashed or chopped table foods prepared without added salt or sugar			Add and introduce use of spoon.
Juice or formula by cup			Add

Modified from Trahms CM, Pipes P: Nutrition in infancy and childhood, ed 6, New York, 1997, McGraw-Hill.

Many infants begin the process of weaning with the introduction of the cup at approximately 6 to 9 months of age and complete the process when they are able to ingest an adequate amount of milk or formula from a cup at 18 to 24 months of age. Parents of infants who are breast-fed may choose to transition the infant directly to a cup or have an intermittent transition to a bottle before the cup is introduced.

Early Childhood Caries

Early childhood caries (ECC), or "baby bottle tooth decay," is the most common chronic disease of childhood. ECC is a pattern of tooth decay that involves the upper anterior and sometimes lower posterior teeth. ECC is common among infants and children who are allowed to bathe their teeth in sugar (sucrose or lactose) throughout the day and night. If infants are given sugar-sweetened beverages or fruit juice in a bottle during the day or at bedtime after teeth have erupted, the risk of dental caries increases (see Chapter 26).

To promote dental health, infants should be fed and burped and then put to bed without milk, juice, or food. Juice should not be introduced into the diet before 6 months of age. Juice should be limited to 4 to 6 oz/day for infants and young children and offered to children only from a cup (AAP, 2007). Parents and caregivers can be taught effective oral health practices for infants, not only by dentists but by other paraprofessionals (MacIntosh et al., 2010).

Feeding Older Infants

As maturation proceeds and the rate of growth slows down, infants' interest in and approach to food changes. Between 9 and 18 months of age most reduce their breast-milk or formula intake. They can become finicky about what and how much they eat.

In the weaning stage infants have to learn many manipulative skills, including the ability to chew and swallow solid food and use utensils. They learn to tolerate various textures and flavors of food, eat with their fingers, and then feed themselves with a utensil. Very young children should be encouraged to feed themselves. See *Clinical Insight:* A New Look at the Food Practices of Infants and Toddlers.

At the beginning of a meal, children are hungry and should be allowed to feed themselves; when they become tired, they can be helped quietly. Emphasis on table manners and the fine points of eating should be delayed until they have the necessary maturity and developmental readiness for such training.

The food should be in a form that is easy to handle and eat. Meat should be cut into bite-size pieces. Potatoes and vegetables should be mashed so that they can be eaten easily with a spoon. Raw fruits and vegetables should be in sizes that can be picked up easily. In addition, the utensils should be small and manageable. Cups should be easy to hold, and dishes should be designed so that they do not tip over easily.

Type of Food

In general, children prefer simple, uncomplicated foods. Food from the family meal can be adapted for the child and served in child-size portions. Children younger than 6 years of age usually prefer mild-flavored foods. Because a young child's stomach is small, a snack may be required between meals. Fruit, cheese, crackers, dry cereal, fruit juices, and milk contribute nutrients and energy. Children ages 2 to 6 years often prefer raw instead of cooked vegetables and fruits.

CLINICAL INSIGHT

A New Look at the Food Practices of Infants and Toddlers

The Feeding Infants and Toddlers Study was a national random sample of more than 2500 infants and toddlers from 4 to 24 months of age and their mothers.

- Assuming that a variety of nutritious foods are offered to infants and toddlers, parents and caregivers should encourage self-feeding without concern for compromising energy intake and nutrient adequacy (Carruth et al., 2004a).
- Parents and caregivers should offer a variety of fruits and vegetables daily; sweets, desserts, sweetened beverages, and salty snacks should be offered only occasionally. Because family food choices influence the foods offered to infants, family-based approaches to healthy eating habits should be encouraged (Fox et al., 2004).
- By 24 months of age, 50% of toddlers were described as picky eaters. When offering a new food, caregivers need to be willing to provide 8 to 15 repeated exposures to enhance acceptance of that food (Carruth et al., 2004b).
- Infants and toddlers have an innate ability to regulate energy intake. Parents and caregivers should understand the cues of hunger and satiety and recognize that coercive admonitions about eating more or less food can interfere with the infant's or toddler's innate ability to regulate energy intake (Fox et al., 2006).
- On average, infants and toddlers were fed seven times per day, and the percentage of children reported to be eating snacks increased with age. Snack choices for infants and toddlers could be improved by delaying the introduction of and limiting foods that have a low nutrient content and are energy dense (Skinner et al., 2004).

Infants should be offered foods that vary in texture and flavor. Infants who are accustomed to many kinds of foods are less likely to limit their variety of food choices later. To add variety to an infant's diet, vegetables and fruits can be added to cereal feedings. It is important to offer various foods and not allow the infant to continue consuming a diet consisting of one or two favorite foods. Older infants generally reject unfamiliar foods the first time they are offered. When parents continue to offer small portions of these foods without comment, infants become familiar with them and often accept them. It is important that fruit juice does not replace more nutrient-dense foods. If excessive amounts of juice are consumed, children may fail to thrive.

Serving Size

The size of a serving of food offered to a child is very important. At 1 year of age infants eat one third to one half the amount an adult normally consumes. This proportion increases to one half an adult portion by the time the child reaches 3 years of age and increases to about two thirds by 6 years of age. Young children should not be served a large plateful of food; the size of the plate and the amount should be in proportion to their age. A tablespoon (not a heaping tablespoon) of each food for each year of age is a good guide to follow. Serving less food than parents think or hope will be eaten helps children eat successfully and happily. They will ask for more food if their appetite is not satisfied.

Forced Feeding

Children should not be forced to eat; instead, the cause for the unwillingness to eat should be determined. A typical, healthy child eats without coaxing. Children may refuse food because they are too inactive to be hungry or too active and overtired. To avoid both overfeeding and underfeeding, parents should be responsive to the cues for hunger and satiety offered by the infant. A child who is fed snacks or given a bottle too close to mealtime (within 90 minutes) is not hungry for the meal and may refuse it (Butte et al., 2004).

Parents who support the development of self-feeding skills respond to the infant's need for assistance and offer encouragement for self-feeding; they also allow the infant to initiate and guide feeding interactions without excessive pressure on the infant for neatness in self-feeding or amount of food consumed. If a child refuses to eat, the family meal should be completed without comment, and the plate should be removed. This procedure is usually harder on the parent than on the child. At the next mealtime, the child will be hungry enough to enjoy the food presented.

Eating Environment

Young children should eat their meals at the family table; it gives them an opportunity to learn table manners while enjoying meals with a family group. Sharing the family fare strengthens ties and makes mealtime pleasant. However, if the family meal is delayed, the children should receive their meal at the usual time. When children eat with the family, everyone must be careful not to make unfavorable comments about any food. Children are great imitators of the people they admire; thus, if the father or older siblings make disparaging remarks about squash, for example, young children are likely to do the same.

The Bright Futures materials and guidelines (www.brightfutures.org/nutrition/) provide information and support to families as they guide their children to healthy eating habits and nourishment.

CLINICAL SCENARIO

Lela is a 12-week-old girl who was born by cesarean section at 42 weeks' gestation to an 18-year-old single mother. Her mother gained 70 lb during the pregnancy. Lela's weight-for-length is plotted at the 95th percentile, and her length and weight continue in the same channels as at birth.

Lela's mother chose to feed Lela infant formula rather than breast-feed. Lela is offered Similac Advance formula that is prepared with 1 scoop of powder mixed in 2 oz of water. Lela consumes approximately six 8-oz bottles per day and is fed on demand. She usually sleeps during the night, but if she is fussy, her mother gives her small amounts of commercially prepared infant cereal, vegetables, and fruit.

Nutrition Diagnostic Statement

Excessive oral food and beverage intake related to using foods to soothe baby as evidenced by weight for height greater than the 95th percentile for age.

Nutrition Care Questions

1. What additional information is needed to get an accurate assessment of this infant's intake?
2. When you assess Lela's growth, what are your expectations for her growth rate? Do you have concerns about her rate of growth?
3. What is Lela's estimated energy intake? Is this appropriate?
4. The American Academy of Pediatrics recommendations suggest that the addition of complimentary foods be delayed until after 4 months of age. How would you assess Lela's readiness for semisolid foods? Which infant skills would you assess in a feeding evaluation?

Other Common Nutrition Diagnostic Statements in Infants:

Inadequate energy intake related to poor sucking reflex as evidenced by growth retardation and small head circumference

Underweight related to inadequate prenatal growth and prematurity as evidenced by weight of 2100 grams at birth

Harmful beliefs related to nutritional requirements for infants as evidenced by mother's comments about diluting formula to save money

USEFUL WEBSITES

American Academy of Pediatrics
www.aap.org/

Bright Futures: Nutrition in Practice
www.brightfutures.org/nutrition/

CDC and WHO Growth Charts
www.cdc.gov/growthcharts/

Healthy People 2020: Objectives for Improving Health
www.healthypeople.gov/

University of Washington Assuring Pediatric Nutrition in the Hospital and Community
http://depts.washington.edu/nutrpeds/

REFERENCES

American Academy of Pediatrics (AAP), Committee on Nutrition: Iron fortification of infant formulas, *Pediatrics* 104:119, 1999.

American Academy of Pediatrics (AAP), Committee on Nutrition: The use and misuse of fruit juice in pediatrics, *Pediatrics* 107:1210, 2001 (reaffirmed Feb 2007).

American Academy of Pediatrics (AAP), Committee on Nutrition: *Pediatric nutrition handbook*, ed 6, Elk Grove Village, IL, 2009, The Academy.

American Academy of Pediatrics (AAP), Section on Breastfeeding: breastfeeding and the use of human milk, *Pediatrics* 115:496, 2005.

American Dietetic Association: Position of the American Dietetic Association: promoting and supporting breastfeeding, *J Am Diet Assoc* 109:1926, 2009.

Baker RD, Greer FR; American Academy of Pediatrics, Committee on Nutrition: diagnosis and prevention of iron-deficiency anemia in infants and young children (0-3 years of age), *Pediatrics* 126;1040, 2010.

Bhatia J, Greer F; American Academy of Pediatrics, Committee on Nutrition: use of soy protein–based formulas in infant feeding, *Pediatrics* 121:1062, 2008.

Butte N, et al: The Start Healthy feeding guidelines for infants and toddlers, *J Am Diet Assoc* 104:442, 2004.

Carruth BR, et al: Developmental milestones and self-feeding behaviors in infants and toddlers, *J Am Diet Assoc* 104:S51, 2004a.

Carruth BR, et al: Prevalence of picky eaters among infants and toddlers and their caregivers' decisions about offering a new food, *J Am Diet Assoc* 104:S57, 2004b.

Cole CR, Lifshitz F: Zinc nutrition and growth retardation, *Pediatr Endocrinol Rev* 5:889, 2008.

Eden AN: Iron deficiency and impaired cognition in toddlers: an underestimated and undertreated problem, *Pediatr Drugs* 7:347, 2005.

Food and Drug Administration (FDA): Update on bisphenol A for use in food contact applications, 2010. Accessed from http://www.fda.gov/NewsEvents/%20PublicHealthFocus/ucm197739.htm.

Fox MK, et al: Feeding infants and toddlers study: what foods are infants and toddlers eating? *J Am Diet Assoc* 104:S22, 2004.

Fox MK, et al: Relationship between portion size and energy intake among infants and toddlers: evidence of self-regulation, *J Am Diet Assoc* 106:S77, 2006.

Leven LV, MacDonald PD: Reducing the incidence of neonatal hypernatraemic dehydration, *Arch Dis Child* 93:811, 2008.

Marques TM, et al: Programming infant gut microbiota: influence of dietary and environmental factors, *Curr Opin Biotechnol* 21(2):149, 2010.

MacIntosh AC, et al: The impact of community workshops on improving early childhood oral health knowledge, *Pediatric Dent* 32:110, 2010.

Misra M, et al: Vitamin D deficiency in children and its management: review of current knowledge and recommendations, *Pediatrics* 122:398, 2008.

National Toxicology Program (NTP): *Draft NTP brief on soy infant formula*, Washington, DC, 16 March 2010, US Department of Health and Human Services.

Nutrient Requirements for Infant Formulas, Final Rule (21 CFR 107), *Fed Reg* 50:45106, 1985.

Rodriguez NR: Optimal quantity and composition of protein for growing children, *J Am Coll Nutr* 24:150S, 2005.

Sherriff A, et al: Should infants be screened for anemia? A prospective study investigating the ratio between hemoglobin at 8, 12, and 18 months and development at 18 months, *Arch Dis Child* 84:480, 2001.

Skinner JD, et al: Meal and snack patterns of infants and toddlers, *J Am Diet Assoc* 104:S65, 2004.

Wagner CL, Greer FR; American Academy of Pediatrics, Section on Breastfeeding; American Academy of Pediatrics, Committee on Nutrition: prevention of rickets and vitamin D deficiency in infants, children, and adolescents, *Pediatrics* 122:1142, 2008.

Weisberg P, et al: Nutritional rickets among children in the United States: review of cases reported between 1986 and 2003, *Am J Clin Nutr* 80:1697S, 2004.

Weiss R, et al: Severe vitamin B_{12} deficiency in an infant associated with a maternal deficiency and a strict vegetarian diet, *J Pediatr Hematol Oncol* 26:270, 2004.

CHAPTER 18

Betty L. Lucas, MPH, RD, CD
Sharon A. Feucht, MA, RD, CD
Beth N. Ogata, MS, RD, CD, CSP

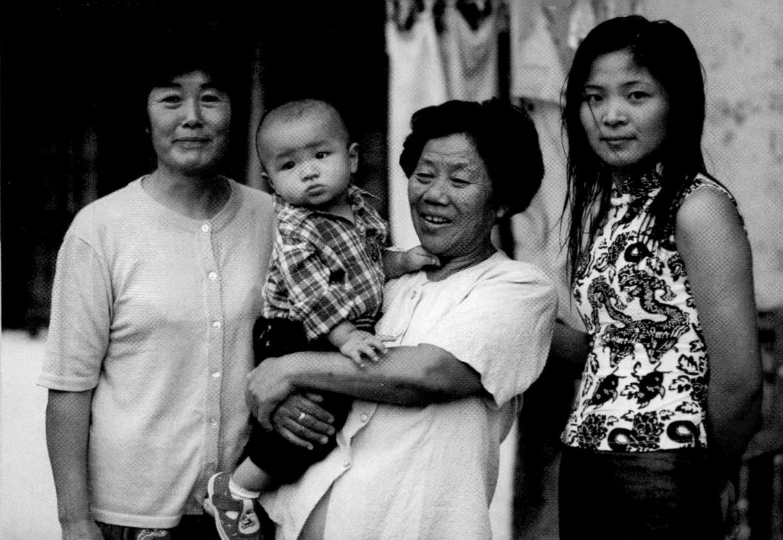

Nutrition in Childhood

KEY TERMS
adiposity rebound
catch-up growth
failure to thrive (FTT)
food jags
growth channels
primarily wasted
stunted growth

The period that begins after infancy and lasts until puberty is often referred to as the *latent* or *quiescent* period of growth—a contrast to the dramatic changes that occur during infancy and adolescence. Although physical growth may be less remarkable and proceed at a steadier pace than it did during the first year, these preschool and elementary school years are a time of significant growth in the social, cognitive, and emotional areas.

GROWTH AND DEVELOPMENT

Growth Patterns

The rate of growth slows considerably after the first year of life. In contrast to the usual tripling of birth weight that occurs in the first 12 months, another year passes before the birth weight quadruples. Likewise, birth length increases by 50% in the first year but does not double until approximately the age of 4 years. Increments of change are small compared with those of infancy and adolescence; weight typically increases an average of 2 to 3 kg (4½ to 6½ lb) per year until the child is 9 or 10 years old. Then the rate increases, signaling the approach of puberty. Height increase increments average 6 to 8 cm (2½ to 3½ inches) per year from 2 years of age until puberty.

Growth is generally steady and slow during the preschool and school age years, but it can be erratic in individual children, with periods of no growth followed by growth spurts. These patterns usually parallel similar changes in appetite and food intake. For parents, periods of slow growth and poor appetite can cause anxiety, leading to mealtime struggles.

Body proportions of young children change significantly after the first year. Head growth is minimal, trunk growth slows substantially, and limbs lengthen considerably, all of which create more mature body proportions. Walking and increased physical activity of the now erect child lead to the legs straightening and increased muscle strength in the abdomen and back.

The body composition of preschool and school age children remains relatively constant. Fat gradually decreases during the early childhood years, reaching a minimum between 4 and 6 years of age. Children then experience the **adiposity rebound**, or increase in body fatness in preparation for the pubertal growth spurt. Earlier adiposity rebound has been associated with increased adult body mass index (BMI) (Williams, 2009). A BMI at an "end" of the charts (e.g., less than 3rd or greater than 97th percentiles) requires careful evaluation to describe the degree of underweight or obesity (Flegal, 2009). Sex differences in body composition become increasingly apparent—boys have more lean body mass per centimeter of height than girls. Girls have a higher percentage of weight as fat than boys, even in the preschool years, but these differences in lean body mass and fat do not become significant until adolescence.

Assessing Growth

A complete nutritional assessment includes the collection of anthropometric data. This includes length or stature, weight, and weight-for-length or BMI, all of which are plotted on the Centers for Disease Control and Prevention (CDC) growth charts (see Appendixes 9 through 16). Other measurements that are less commonly used but that provide estimates of body composition include upper-arm circumference and triceps or subscapular skin folds. Care should be taken to use standardized equipment and techniques for obtaining and plotting growth measurements. Charts designed for birth to 36 months of age are based on length measurements and nude weights, whereas charts used for 2- to 20-year-olds are based on stature (standing height) and weight with light clothing and without shoes (see Chapter 6).

The proportion of weight to length or height is a critical element of growth assessment. This parameter is determined by plotting the weight-for-length on the WHO birth- to 24-month growth charts or calculating BMI and plotting it on the 2- to 20-year-old CDC growth charts. Growth measurements obtained at regular intervals provide information about an individual's growth pattern. One-time measurements do not allow for interpretation of growth status. Growth channels are not well established until after 2 years of age. Children generally maintain their heights and weights in the same **growth channels** during the preschool and childhood years, although rates of growth can vary within a selected period.

Regular monitoring of growth enables problematic trends to be identified early and intervention initiated so that long-term growth is not compromised. Weight that increases rapidly and crosses growth channels suggests the development of obesity. Lack of weight gain or loss of weight over a period of months may be a result of undernutrition, an acute illness, an undiagnosed chronic disease, or significant emotional or family problems. However, many children are evaluated by health care professionals only when they are ill, so growth evaluation and development may not be a focus of care. Figure 18-1 demonstrates the changes that can occur in growth parameters.

Catch-Up Growth

A child who is recovering from an illness or undernutrition and whose growth has slowed or ceased experiences a greater than expected rate of recovery. This recovery is referred to as **catch-up growth**, a period during which the body strives to return to the child's normal growth channel. The degree of growth suppression is influenced by the timing, severity, and duration of the precipitating cause, such as a severe illness or prolonged nutritional deprivation.

Initial studies supported the thesis that malnourished infants who did not experience immediate catch-up growth would have permanent growth retardation. However, studies of malnourished children from developing countries who subsequently received adequate nourishment, as well as reports of children who were malnourished because of chronic disease such as celiac disease or cystic fibrosis, have shown that these children caught up to their normal growth channels after the first year or two of life.

The nutritional requirements for catch-up growth depend on whether the child has overall **stunted growth** (both height and weight are proportionally low) and is chronically malnourished, or is **primarily wasted**, meaning that the weight deficit exceeds the height deficit. A chronically malnourished child may not be expected to gain more than 2-3 g/kg/day, whereas as a child who is primarily wasted may gain as much as 20 g/kg/day.

Nutrient requirements, especially for energy and protein, depend on the rate and stage of catch-up growth. For instance, more protein and energy are needed during the initial period of very rapid weight gain and for those in whom lean tissue is the major component of the weight gain. In addition to energy, other nutrients are important, including vitamin A, iron, and zinc.

Current growth parameters are used to evaluate the child's weight in relation to age and stature, and to estimate a "desirable" or goal weight. Formulas are then used to estimate the minimum and maximum energy needed for catch-up growth. After a child who is wasted catches up in weight, dietary management must change to slow the weight gain velocity and avoid excessive gain. The catch-up in linear growth peaks approximately 1 to 3 months after treatment starts, whereas weight gain begins immediately.

NUTRIENT REQUIREMENTS

Because children are growing and developing bones, teeth, muscles, and blood, they need more nutritious food in proportion to their size than do adults. They may be at risk for malnutrition when they have a poor appetite for a long period, eat a limited number of foods, or dilute their diets significantly with nutrient-poor foods.

The dietary reference intakes (DRIs) are based on current knowledge of nutrient intakes needed for optimal health (Institute of Medicine [IOM], 2006). See inside front cover. Most data for preschool and school age children are values interpolated from data on infants and adults. The DRIs are meant to improve the long-term health of the population by reducing the risk of chronic disease and preventing nutritional deficiencies. Thus, when intakes are less than the recommended level, it cannot be assumed that a particular child is inadequately nourished.

Energy

The energy needs of healthy children are determined by basal metabolism, rate of growth, and energy expenditure of activity. Dietary energy must be sufficient to ensure growth and spare protein from being used for energy, but not allow

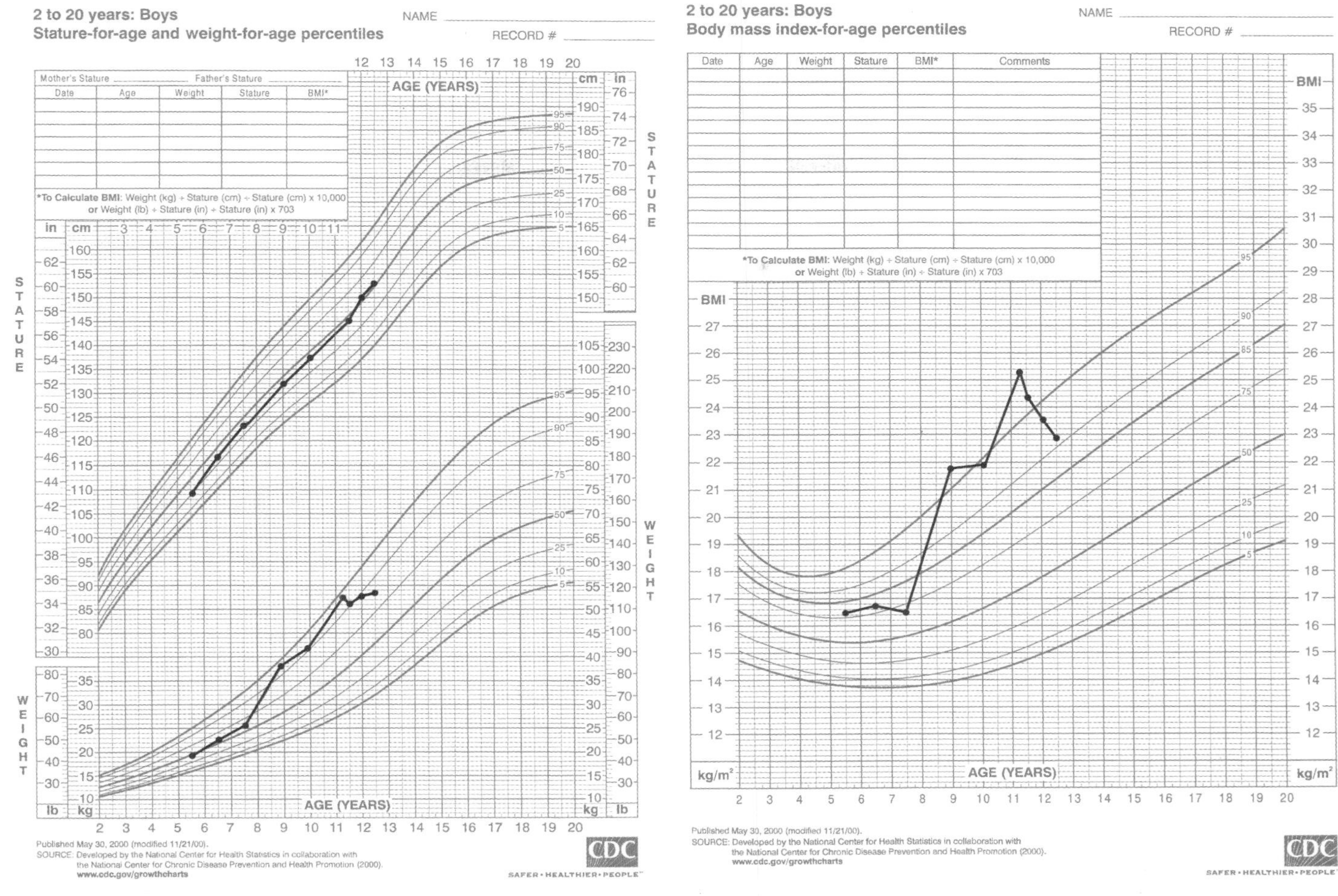

FIGURE 18-1 A, Growth chart and BMI chart for an 8-year-old boy who gained excessive weight after having leg surgery and being immobilized in a body cast for 2 months. The surgery and immobilization were followed by a long period of stress caused by family problems. At the age of 11 years, he became involved in a weight management program.

excess weight gain. Suggested intake proportions of energy are 45% to 65% as carbohydrate, 30% to 40% as fat, and 5% to 20% as protein for 1- to 3-year-olds, with carbohydrates the same for 4- to 18-year-olds, 25% to 35% as fat, and 10% to 30% as protein (IOM, 2006).

The DRIs for estimated energy requirement (EER) are average energy requirements based on life-stage groupings for healthy individuals of normal weight. Toddlers 13 through 35 months are grouped together; for older children the EERs are divided by sex and age (3-8 years and 9-18 years.) The EER includes the total energy expenditure plus energy needed for growth (see Chapter 2). The DRIs are applied to child nutrition programs and other guidelines (IOM, 2006). See Box 18-1 for examples of determining EER for two children. On an individual basis, it can be useful to estimate energy requirements using kilocalories per kilogram of weight or per centimeter of height.

Protein

The need for protein decreases from approximately 1.1 g/kg in early childhood to 0.95 g/kg in late childhood (Table 18-1). Protein intake can range from 5% to 30% of total energy depending on age. Protein deficiency is uncommon in American children, partly because of the cultural emphasis on protein foods. National surveys show that less than 3% of children fail to meet the recommended dietary allowance (Moshfegh et al., 2005). Children who are most at risk for inadequate protein intake are those on strict vegan diets; those with multiple food allergies; or who have limited food selections because of fad diets, behavioral problems, or inadequate access to food.

Minerals and Vitamins

Minerals and vitamins are necessary for normal growth and development. Insufficient intake can cause impaired growth and result in deficiency diseases. See Chapter 3. The DRIs are listed inside the front cover.

Iron

Children between 1 and 3 years of age are at high risk for iron-deficiency anemia. The rapid growth period of infancy is marked by an increase in hemoglobin and total iron mass. National Health and Nutrition Examination Survey (NHANES) data indicate that children with prolonged

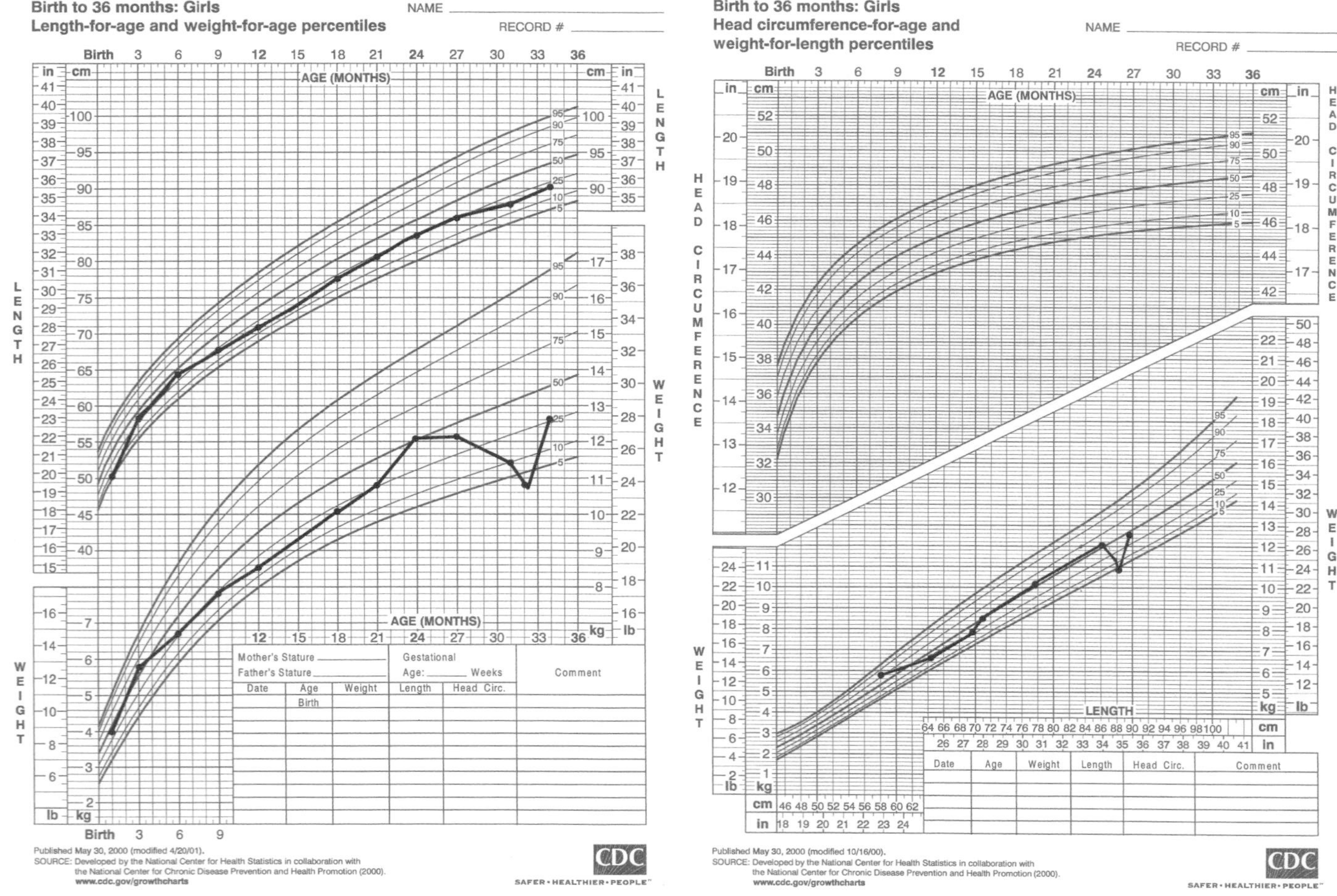

FIGURE 18-1, cont'd B, Growth charts for a 2-year-old girl who experienced significant weight loss during a prolonged period of diarrhea and feeding problems. After being diagnosed with celiac disease, she began following a gluten-free diet and entered a period of catch-up growth. *(Source of growth charts only: The National Center for Health Statistics in collaboration with the National Center for Chronic Disease Prevention and Health Promotion, 2000.)*

TABLE 18-1

Protein Dietary Reference Intakes (DRIs) for Children through Age 13 Years

		Protein
Age	**Grams/Day***	**Grams/Kilogram/Day**
1-3 yr	13 g/day	1.10 g/kg/day
4-8 yr	19 g/day	0.95 g/kg/day
9-13 yr	34 g/day	0.95 g/kg/day

Adapted from Feucht S: Dietary reference intakes (DRI) review: case studies illustrating energy and protein for children and adolescents with special needs, Nutr Focus Newsletter 20:1, 2005.

*Recommended dietary allowance for reference individual (g/day).

bottle feeding and those of Mexican-American descent are at highest risk for iron deficiency. The reason for the association between iron deficiency and ethnicity is not clear (Brotanek et al., 2005). Recommended intakes must factor in the absorption rate and quantity of iron in foods, especially those of plant origin.

Calcium

Calcium is needed for adequate mineralization and maintenance of growing bone in children. The RDA for calcium for children 1 to 3 years old is 700 mg/day, for children 4 to 8 years it is 1000 mg/day, and for those 9 to 18 years it is 1300 mg per day (Ross et al., 2011). Actual need depends on individual absorption rates and dietary factors such as quantities of protein, vitamin D, and phosphorus. Because milk and other dairy products are primary sources of calcium, children who consume limited amounts of these foods are at risk for poor bone mineralization (Figure 18-2). Other calcium-fortified foods such as soy and rice milks and fruit juices are also good sources (see Table 3-25).

BOX 18-1

Determining Estimated Energy Requirements

(Examples using data from Box 2-1, Chapter 2)

1. For 13- to 35-month-old children:

$$\text{EER (kcal)} = (89 \times \text{wt [kg]} - 100) + 20$$

An 18-month-old boy has a length of 84 cm and weighs 12.5 kg

$$\text{EER (kcal)} = (89 \times 12.5 - 100) + 20$$

$$\text{EER (kcal)} = (1113 - 100) + 20$$

$$\text{EER (kcal)} = 1033$$

2. For girls 3 through 8 years:

$$\text{EER (kcal)} = 135.3 - (30.8 \times \text{age [y]}) + \text{PA} \times (10 \times \text{wt [kg]} + 934 \times \text{ht [m]}) + 20$$

A 6½-year-old girl is 112 cm tall, weighs 20.8 kg, and has moderate activity (PA coefficient of 1.31)

$$\text{EER (kcal)} = 135.3 - 30.8 \times 6.5 + 1.31 \times (10 \times 20.8 + 934 \times 1.12) + 20$$

$$\text{EER (kcal)} = 135.3 - 200.2 + 1.31 \times (208 + 1046.1) + 20$$

$$\text{EER (kcal)} = 135.3 - 200.2 + 1642.9 + 20$$

$$\text{EER (kcal)} = 1598$$

EER, Estimated energy requirement; *PA*, physical activity.

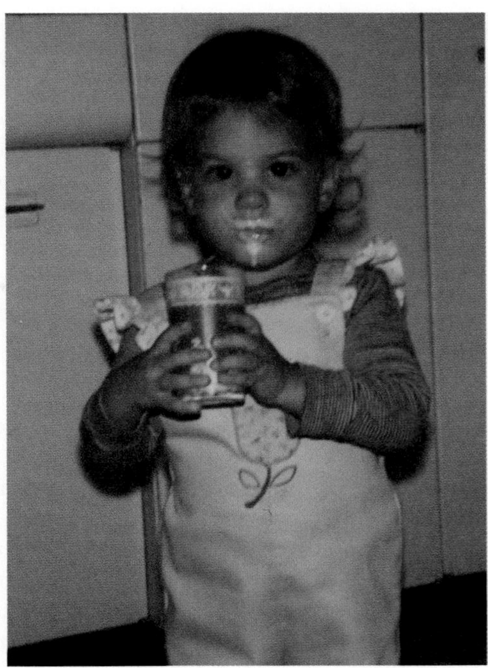

FIGURE 18-2 Milk and other dairy products supply preschool children with the calcium and vitamin D needed for growing bones.

Zinc

Zinc is essential for growth; a deficiency results in growth failure, poor appetite, decreased taste acuity, and poor wound healing. Because the best sources of zinc are meat and seafood, some children may regularly have low intakes. Marginal zinc deficiency has been reported in preschool and school age children. Diagnosis may be difficult because laboratory parameters, including plasma, serum erythrocyte, hair, and urine, are of limited value in determining zinc deficiency. There is a positive influence of zinc supplementation on growth and serum zinc concentrations. Improving zinc nutrition status by food and supplementation programs has shown efficacy (see Chapter 3).

Vitamin D

Vitamin D is needed for calcium absorption and deposition of calcium in the bones, as well as prevention of cancer, autoimmune disorders, cardiovascular disease, and infectious disease. Because this nutrient is also formed from sunlight exposure on the skin, the amount required from dietary sources depends on factors such as geographic location and time spent outside.

The new DRI for vitamin D for infants is 400 IU (10 mcg) per day and for children is 600 IU (15 mcg) per day (Ross et al., 2011). Vitamin D–fortified milk is the primary source of this nutrient, and breakfast cereals and nondairy milks are often fortified with vitamin D. Dairy products such as cheese and yogurt, however, are not always made from fortified milk. It is becoming more common to measure serum 25(OH) vitamin D 25-hydroxy in children; however, there is some controversy regarding what constitutes optimal levels.

Vitamin-Mineral Supplements

Almost 40% of preschool children are given a multivitamin-mineral supplement, but this percentage usually decreases with older children (Picciano et al., 2007). Families with more education, health insurance coverage, and higher incomes generally have higher rates of supplement use, although these may not be the families who are at greatest risk for having inadequate diets. Supplements do not necessarily fulfill specific nutrient needs. For instance, although many children consume less than the recommended amount of calcium, children's vitamin-mineral supplements typically do not contain significant amounts of calcium. Careful evaluation of each pediatric supplement is suggested because many types are available but incomplete.

Evidence shows that fluoride can help prevent dental caries. If a community's water supply is not fluoridated, fluoride supplements are recommended from 6 months until 16 years of age. However, individual family practices should be assessed, including the child's primary source of fluids (e.g., drinking water, juices, or other beverages) and fluoride sources from child care, school, toothpaste and mouthwash.

The AAP does not support giving healthy children routine supplements of any vitamins or minerals other than fluoride. However, children at risk for inadequate nutrition who may benefit from supplementation include those (1) with anorexia, inadequate appetite, or who consume fad diets; (2) with chronic disease (e.g., cystic fibrosis, inflammatory bowel disease, hepatic disease); (3) from deprived families or those who are abused or neglected; (4) using a dietary program to manage obesity; (5) who do not consume adequate amounts of dairy products; and (6) with failure to thrive (FTT) (American Academy of Pediatrics [AAP], 2009).

Children who routinely take a multiple vitamin or a vitamin-mineral supplement usually do not experience negative effects if the supplement contains nutrients in amounts that do not exceed the DRIs, especially the tolerable upper intake level. However, children should not take megadoses, particularly of the fat-soluble vitamins because large amounts can result in toxicity (see Chapter 3). Because many vitamin-mineral supplements look and taste like candy, parents should keep them out of reach of children to avoid excessive intake of nutrients such as iron.

Complementary nutrition therapies or herbal product use is becoming more common for children, especially those with special needs such as children with Down syndrome, autism spectrum disorder (ASD), or cystic fibrosis (Harris, 2005). Practitioners should inquire as to the use of these products and therapies in nutrition assessments, be knowledgeable about their efficacy and safety, and help families determine whether they are beneficial and how to use them (see Chapter 13).

PROVIDING AN ADEQUATE DIET

The development of feeding skills, food habits, and nutrition knowledge parallels the cognitive development that takes place in a series of stages, each laying the groundwork for the next. Table 18-2 outlines the development of feeding skills in terms of Piaget's theory of child psychology and development.

Intake Patterns

Children are most likely to consume inadequate amounts of calcium, vitamin D, vitamin E, magnesium, and vitamin A (Moshfegh, 2009; Moshfegh et al., 2005). However, clinical signs of malnutrition in American children are rare.

Children's food patterns have changed over the years. Although they drink less milk, more of it is low-fat or nonfat milk. The total fat as a percent of energy intake has decreased, but remains above recommendations. More energy comes from snacks, and portion sizes have increased. In addition, more food is consumed in environments other than the home (American Dietetic Association [ADA], 2008). Foods with low nutrient density (soft drinks, baked and dairy desserts, sweeteners, and salty snacks) often displace nutrient-dense foods (ADA, 2008). National food intake studies of children and adolescents indicate that most of their diets do not meet the national recommendations for food groups (ADA, 2008). Most children ages 2 to 3 years have high-quality diets; as they grow older, diet quality declines.

Like physical growth patterns, food intake patterns are not smooth and consistent. Although subjective, appetites usually follow the rate of growth and nutrient needs. By a child's first birthday, milk consumption begins to decline. In the next year vegetable intake decreases; intakes of cereals, grain products, and sweets increase. Young children often prefer softer protein sources instead of meats that are harder to chew.

Changes in food consumption are reflected in nutrient intakes. The early preschool years show a decrease in calcium, phosphorus, riboflavin, iron, and vitamin A compared to infancy. Intakes of most other key nutrients remain relatively stable. During the early school years, a pattern of consistent and steadily increased intakes of most nutrients is seen until adolescence. In healthy children a wide variability of nutrient intake is seen at any age.

Factors Influencing Food Intake

Numerous influences, some obvious and others subtle, determine the food intake and habits of children. Habits, likes, and dislikes are established in the early years and carried through to adulthood. The major influences on food intake in the developing years include family environment, societal trends, the media, peer pressure, and illness or disease.

Family Environment

For toddlers and preschool children the family is the primary influence in the development of food habits. In young children's immediate environment, parents and older siblings are significant models. Food attitudes of parents can be strong predictors of food likes and dislikes and diet complexity in children of primary school age. Similarities between children's and their parents' food preferences are likely to reflect genetic and environmental influences (Savage, 2007).

Contrary to common belief, young children do not have the innate ability to choose a balanced, nutritious diet; they can choose one only when presented with nutritious foods. A positive feeding relationship includes a division of responsibility between parents and children. The parents and other adults are to provide safe, nutritious, developmentally appropriate food as regular meals and snacks. The children decide how much, if any, they eat (Satter, 2000).

Eating together at family meals is becoming less common, partly because of family schedules, more time eating in front of the television, and the decreasing amount of time devoted to planning and preparing family meals. School age children and adolescents who eat more dinners with their families consume more fruits and vegetables, less soda, and fewer fried foods than those who rarely eat dinner with their families (Larson, 2007).

TABLE 18-2

Feeding, Nutrition, and Piaget's Theory of Cognitive Development

Developmental Period	Cognitive Characteristics	Relationships to Feeding and Nutrition
Sensorimotor (birth-2 yr)	Neonate progresses from automatic reflexes to a child with intentional interaction with the environment and the beginning use of symbols.	Progression involves advancing from sucking and rooting reflexes to the acquisition of self-feeding skills. Food is used primarily to satisfy hunger, as a medium to explore the environment, and as an opportunity to practice fine motor skills.
Preoperational (2-7 yr)	Thought processes become internalized; they are unsystematic and intuitive. Use of symbols increases.	Eating becomes less the center of attention and is secondary to social, language, and cognitive growth. Food is described by color, shape, and quantity, but the child has only a limited ability to classify food into "groups."
	Reasoning is based on appearances and happenstance. The child's approach to classification is functional and unsystematic. The child's world is viewed egocentrically.	Foods tend to be categorized into "like" and "don't like." Foods can be identified as "good for you," but reasons why they are healthy are unknown or mistaken.
Concrete operational (7-11 yr)	The child can focus on several aspects of a situation simultaneously.	The child begins to realize that nutritious food has a positive effect on growth and health but has a limited understanding of how or why.
	Cause-and-effect reasoning becomes more rational and systematic. The ability to classify, reclassify, and generalize emerges. A decrease in egocentrism permits the child to take another's view.	Mealtimes take on a social significance. The expanding environment increases the opportunities for influences on food selection; for example, peer influence increases.
Formal operational (11 yr and beyond)	Hypothetical and abstract thought expand.	The concept of nutrients from food functioning at physiologic and biochemical levels can be understood.
	The child's understanding of scientific and theoretical processes deepens.	Conflicts in making food choices may be realized (i.e., knowledge of the nutritious value of foods may conflict with preferences and nonnutritive influences).

The atmosphere around food and mealtime also influences attitudes toward food and eating. Unrealistic expectations for a child's mealtime manners, arguments, and other emotional stress can have a negative effect. Meals that are rushed create a hectic atmosphere and reinforce the tendency to eat too fast. A positive environment is one in which sufficient time is set aside to eat, occasional spills are tolerated, and conversation that includes all family members is encouraged (Figure 18-3).

Societal Trends

Because almost three fourths of women with school age children are employed outside the home, children may eat one or more meals at a child care center or school. In these settings all children should have access to nutritious meals served in a safe and sanitary environment that promotes healthy growth and development (ADA, 2005, 2006). Because of time constraints, family meals may include more convenience or fast foods. However, having a mother who is employed outside the home does not seem to affect children's dietary intakes negatively. Food service in group settings such as child care centers, Head Start programs, preschool programs, and in elementary schools is regulated by federal or state guidelines. Many facilities and some in-home child care centers may participate in the U.S. Department of Agriculture (USDA) Child and Adult Care Food Program. However, the quality of meals and snacks can vary greatly; parents should investigate food service when considering child care options. In addition to providing children with optimal nutrients, a program should offer food that is appealing, safely prepared, and appropriate, incorporating cultural and developmental patterns (ADA, 2005).

Approximately one in five American children lives in a family with an income below the poverty line; these children constitute 35% of all the poor in the United States (DeNavas-Walt et al., 2009). The increasing numbers of single-parent households predominantly headed by women have lower incomes and less money for all expenses, including food, than households headed by men. This phenomenon makes these families increasingly vulnerable to multiple stressors such as marginal health and nutritional status partly because of lack of jobs, child care, adequate housing, and health insurance.

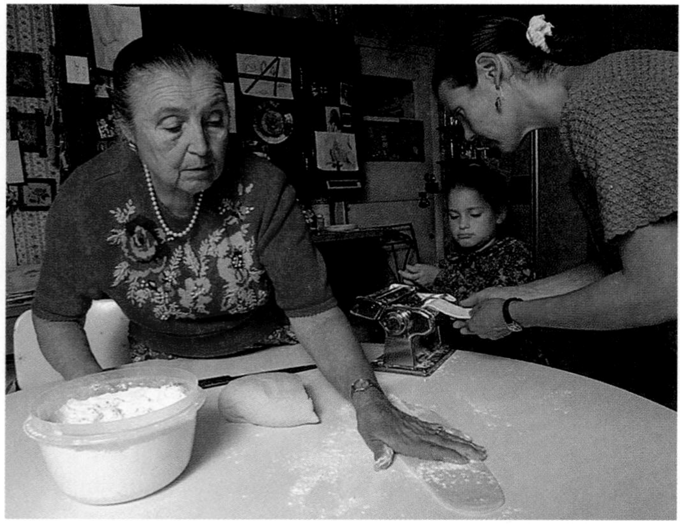

FIGURE 18-3 Three generations of Italian Americans make a pasta dinner. The custom of eating authentically prepared foods gives meals a place of prominence in this home—meals that will not be replaced with fast foods eaten on the run. *(From Leahy J, Kisilay P: Foundations of nursing practice: a nursing process approach, Philadelphia, 1998, Saunders.)*

In 2008, 16% of households with children in the United States experienced food insecurity. Federal food and nutrition assistance programs (including National School Lunch, Food Stamp Program, and Special Supplemental Nutrition Program for Women, Infants and Children (WIC)) provided benefits to four out of five food-insecure households' children (ADA, 2010; Nord, 2009). See Chapter 10. The food stamp allotment for families, based on the USDA Thrifty Food Plan, does not provide adequate funds to purchase food based on the government's nutrition guidelines, especially when labor is considered (Davis and You, 2010). Food insecurity also increases the risk for children younger than age 3 years to be iron-deficient with anemia (Skalicky et al., 2005). Studies suggest that intermittent hunger in American children is associated with increased developmental risk (Rose-Jacobs et al., 2008) (see *Focus On:* Childhood Hunger and Its Effect on Behavior and Emotions).

Media Messages

Food is marketed to children using a variety of techniques, including television advertising, in-school marketing, sponsorship, product placement, Internet marketing, and sales promotion. Television advertising and in-school marketing are regulated to some degree. By the time the average American child graduates from high school, he or she has

FOCUS ON

Childhood Hunger and Its Effect on Behavior and Emotions

It is well accepted that malnourished children are less responsive, less inquisitive, and participate in less exploratory behavior than well-nourished infants. Specific nutrient deficiencies such as iron deficiency anemia can also result in a decreased ability to pay attention and poorer problem-solving skills. Less clear is the effect of periodic hunger or food insecurity on a child's behavior and functioning. With recent federal welfare reform legislation and economic downturns, an increasing number of children from low-income families are at risk for limited food resources (American Dietetic Association, 2010).

In the 1990s the Community Childhood Hunger Identification Project conducted surveys using standardized questions and large, rigorously selected samples to categorize families as "hungry," "at risk for hunger," or "not hungry" (Kleinman et al., 1998). It was estimated that each year 8% of children younger than 12 years of age in the United States experience prolonged periods in which they have insufficient food. Data from 2008 indicated that 16.2 million children (22.5% of all children) live in food-insecure households (Food Research and Action Center, 2009). The number of children in food-insecure households continues to increase. A longitudinal study following approximately 21,000 children from kindergarten through third grade found that persistent food insecurity was predictive of impaired academic outcomes, poorer social skills, and a tendency to increased body mass index (Jyoti et al., 2005).

Although these studies have limitations because of other factors that may affect a child's functioning (e.g., stress, family dysfunction, or substance abuse), a correlation exists between children's lack of sufficient food and their behavioral and academic functioning. As future studies provide more evidence of this relationship, it will be clear that social policies need to ensure the provision of children's basic needs for optimal growth and development.

watched 15,000 hours of television and spent 11,000 hours in the classroom. In a random sample of television advertising to children, 20% of commercials were for food. Of these, 70% were for items high in sugar or fat, and more than 25% were for fast-food restaurants (Bell, 2009).

Screen time can also be detrimental to growth and development because it encourages inactivity and passive use of leisure time. Indeed, television viewing and its multiple media cues to eat have been suggested as a factor contributing to excessive weight gain in school-age children and adolescents (Laurson, 2008). In addition, the types of food eaten during television viewing can contribute to increased dental caries resulting from the continued exposure of the teeth to dense carbohydrate- and sugar-laden foods (Palmer, 2005).

Preschool children are generally unable to distinguish commercial messages from regular programs. In fact, they often pay more attention to the commercials. As children get older, they gain knowledge about the purpose of commercial advertising and become more critical of its validity, but are still susceptible to the commercial message. Media literacy education programs teach children and adolescents about the intent of advertising and media messages and how to evaluate and interpret their obvious and subtle influences.

Fortunately, some media messages are beneficial. For example, public health messages about eating fish versus the risks of acquiring mercury are important. See *Focus On:* Childhood Methylmercury Exposure and Toxicity: Media Messaging.

Peer Influence

As children grow, their world expands and their social contacts become more important. Peer influence increases with age and affects food attitudes and choices. This may result in a sudden refusal of a food or a request for a currently popular food. Decisions about whether to participate in school meals may be made more on the basis of friends' choices than on the menu. Such behaviors are developmentally typical. Positive behaviors such as a willingness to try new foods can be reinforced. Parents need to set limits on undesirable influences but also need to be realistic; struggles over food are self-defeating.

FOCUS ON

Childhood Methylmercury Exposure and Toxicity: Media Messaging

Mercury toxicity can cause neurologic problems, which can lead to cognitive and motor deficits. Toxicity related to prenatal exposure is well documented, and there is evidence that postnatal exposure is dangerous as well (Myers et al., 2009; Oken and Bellinger, 2008). Exposure to mercury can occur through environmental contact and eating contaminated foods. Methylmercury, the most toxic form of mercury accumulates in fish.

Public health agencies have looked at balancing the benefits of minimizing exposure to this neurotoxin with the risk of limiting intake of docosahexaenoic acid (DHA) and eicosapentaenoic acid (EPA) as well as a source of high biologic value protein. DHA and EPA are essential ω-3 fatty acids and have received much attention because of their importance in cognitive and vision development and their cardiovascular benefits (Mahaffey et al., 2008). In addition, fish advisories are available in certain states. The U.S. Environmental Protection Agency's (EPA) reference dose for methylmercury is based on body weight: 0.1 mcg/kg/day. For a 20-kg child, this is approximately 14 mcg/week (US EPA, 2010). The methylmercury content of 3 ounces of albacore tuna is approximately 29.7 mcg, canned light tuna approximately 10 mcg, and fresh or frozen salmon approximately 1.2 mcg. The Food and Drug Administration (FDA) and EPA have made recommendations for fish intake by young children:

Do not eat shark, swordfish, king mackerel, or tilefish because they contain high levels of mercury.

Eat up to 12 oz (two average meals) a week of a variety of fish and shellfish that are lower in mercury.

Five of the most commonly eaten fish that are low in mercury are shrimp, canned light tuna, salmon, pollock, and catfish.

Another commonly eaten fish, albacore ("white") tuna has more mercury than canned light tuna. So, when choosing two meals of fish and shellfish, eat up to 6 ounces (one average meal) of albacore tuna per week, but only 3 ounces for a child.

Check local advisories about the safety of fish caught by family and friends in local lakes, rivers, and coastal areas. If no advice is available, eat up to 6 ounces (3 oz for a child) per week of fish caught from local waters, but don't consume any other fish during that week.

Follow these same recommendations when feeding fish and shellfish to young children, but serve smaller portions.

Resources:

EPA: http://www.epa.gov/waterscience/fish/advice/index.html

FDA: http://www.fda.gov/Food/FoodSafety/Product-specificInformation/Seafood/FoodbornePathogensContaminants/Methylmercury/default.htm

Illness or Disease

Children who are ill usually have a decreased appetite and limited food intake. Acute viral or bacterial illnesses are often short-lived but may require an increase in fluids, protein, or other nutrients. Chronic conditions such as asthma, cystic fibrosis, or chronic renal disease may make it difficult to obtain sufficient nutrients for optimal growth. Children with these types of conditions are more likely to have behavior problems relating to food. Children requiring special diets (e.g., those who have diabetes or phenylketonuria) not only have to adjust to the limits of foods allowed, but also have to address issues of independence and peer acceptance as they grow older. Some rebellion against the prescribed diet is typical, especially as children approach puberty.

Feeding Preschool Children

From 1 to 6 years of age children experience vast developmental progress and acquisition of skills. One-year-old children primarily use fingers to eat and may need assistance with a cup. By 2 years of age, they can hold a cup in one hand and use a spoon well (see Figure 17-2, but may prefer to use their hands at times. Six-year-old children have refined skills and are beginning to use a knife for cutting and spreading.

As the growth rate slows after the first year of life, appetite decreases, which often concerns parents. Children have less interest in food and an increased interest in the world around them. They can develop **food jags** which can be periods when foods that were previously liked are refused, or there are repeated requests to eat the same food meal after meal. This behavior may be attributable to boredom with the usual foods or may be a means of asserting newly discovered independence. Parents may have concerns with their child's seemingly irrational food behavior. Struggles over control of the eating situation are fruitless; no child can be forced to eat. This period is developmental and temporary.

A positive feeding relationship includes a division of responsibility between parents and children. Young children can choose a balanced nutritious diet if presented with nutritious foods. The parents and other adults provide safe, nutritious, developmentally appropriate food as regular meals and snacks; and the children decide how much, if any, they eat (Satter, 2000). Parents maintain control over what foods are offered and have the opportunity to set limits on inappropriate behaviors. Neither rigid control nor a laissez-faire approach is likely to succeed. Parents and other care providers should continue to offer a variety of foods, including the child's favorites, and not make substitutions a routine.

With smaller stomach capacities and variable appetites, preschool children should be offered small servings of food four to six times a day. Snacks are as important as meals in contributing to the total daily nutrient intake. Carefully chosen snacks are those dense in nutrients and least likely to promote dental caries. A general rule of thumb is to offer 1 tablespoon of each food for every year of age and to serve more food according to the child's appetite. Table 18-3 is a guide for food and portion size.

Senses other than taste play an important part in food acceptance by young children. They tend to avoid food with extreme temperatures, and some foods are rejected because of odor rather than taste. A sense of order in the food presentation is often required; many children will not accept foods that touch each other on the plate, and mixed dishes or casseroles with unidentifiable foods are not popular. Broken crackers may go uneaten or a sandwich may be refused because it is "cut the wrong way."

The physical setting for meals is important. Children's feet should be supported, and chair height should allow a comfortable reach to the table at chest height. Sturdy, child-size tables and chairs are ideal, or a high chair or booster seat should be used. Dishes and cups should be unbreakable and heavy enough to resist tipping. For very young children, a shallow bowl is often better than a plate for scooping. Thick, short-handled spoons and forks allow for an easier grasp.

Young children do not eat well if they are tired; this should be considered when meal and play times are scheduled. A quiet activity or rest immediately before eating is conducive to a relaxed, enjoyable meal. However, children also need active, large-motor activities and time in the fresh air to stimulate a good appetite.

Fruit juices and juice drinks are a common beverage for young children; they frequently replace water and milk in children's diets. In addition to altering the diet's nutrient content, excessive intake of fruit juice can result in carbohydrate malabsorption and chronic, nonspecific diarrhea (AAP, 2001). This suggests that juices, especially apple and pear, should be avoided when using liquids to treat acute diarrhea. For children with chronic diarrhea, a trial of restricting fruit juices may be warranted before more costly diagnostic tests are done.

When children aged 2 to 11 years consume 100% juice, their intakes have significantly higher intakes of energy, carbohydrates, vitamins C and B_6, potassium, riboflavin, magnesium, iron, and folate, and significantly lower intakes of total fat, saturated fatty acids, discretionary fat, and added sugar; this 100% juice intake does not correlate with overweight later (Nicklas et al., 2008). However, excess juice intake (12 to 30 oz/day) by young children may decrease a child's appetite, resulting in decreased food intake and poor growth. Here, a reduction in juice intake results in improved growth (AAP, 2001). Fruit juice intake should be limited to 4-6 oz/day for children 1 through 6 years of age and 8-12 oz/day (in two servings) for older children and adolescents (AAP, 2009).

Large volumes of sweetened beverages, combined with other dietary and activity factors, may contribute to overweight in a child. High intake of fructose, especially from sucrose and high-fructose corn syrup in processed foods and beverages, may lead to increased plasma triglycerides and insulin resistance (Vos et al., 2008). In several studies, low calcium intake and obesity have been correlated with high intake of sugar-sweetened beverages in preschool children

TABLE 18-3

Suggested Portion Sizes for Children*

These suggestions are not necessarily appropriate for all children (and may be inappropriate for some children with medical conditions that greatly affect nutrient needs). They are intended to serve as a general framework that can be individualized based on a child's condition and growth pattern.

	1- to 3-Year-Olds	4- to 6-Year-Olds	7- to 12-Year-Olds	Comments
Grain Products	Bread: ½ to 1 slice Rice, pasta, potatoes: ¼ to ½ cup Cooked cereal: ¼ to ½ cup Ready-to-eat cereal: ¼ to ½ cup Tortilla: ½ to 1	Bread: 1 slice Rice, pasta, potatoes: ½ cup Cooked cereal: ½ cup Ready-to-eat cereal: ¾ to 1 cup Tortilla: 1	Bread: 1 slice Rice, pasta, potatoes: ½ cup Cooked cereal: ½ cup Ready-to-eat cereal: 1 cup Tortilla: 1	Include whole grain foods and enriched grain products.
Vegetables	Cooked or pureed: 2 to 4 Tablespoons Raw: few pieces, if child can chew well	Cooked or pureed: 3 to 4 Tablespoons Raw: few pieces	Cooked or pureed: ½ cup Raw: ½ to 1 cup	Include one green leafy or yellow vegetable for vitamin A, such as spinach, carrots, broccoli, or winter squash.
Fruit	Raw (apple, banana, etc.): ½ to 1 small, if child can chew well Canned: 2 to 4 Tablespoons Juice: 3 to 4 ounces	Raw (apple, banana, etc.): ½ to 1 small, if child can chew well Canned: 4 to 8 Tablespoons Juice: 4 ounces	Raw (apple, banana, etc.): 1 small Canned: ¾ cup Juice: 5 ounces	Include one vitamin C–rich fruit, vegetable, or juice, such as citrus juices, an orange, grapefruit sections, strawberries, melon in season, a tomato, or broccoli.
Milk and Dairy Products	Milk, yogurt, pudding: 2 to 4 ounces Cheese: ¾ ounce	Milk, yogurt, pudding: ½ to ¾ cup Cheese: 1 ounce	Milk, yogurt, pudding: 1 cup Cheese: 1½ ounces	
Meat, Poultry, Fish, Other Protein	Meat, poultry, fish: 1 to 2 ounces Eggs: ½ to 1 Peanut butter: 1 Tablespoon Cooked dried beans: 4 to 5 Tablespoons	Meat, poultry, fish: 1 to 2 ounces Eggs: 1 to 2 Peanut butter: 2 Tablespoons Cooked dried beans: 4 to 8 Tablespoons	Meat, poultry, fish: 2 ounces Eggs: 2 Peanut butter: 3 Tablespoons Cooked dried beans: 1 cup	

Modified from Lowenberg ME: Development of food patterns in young children. In Trahms CM, Pipes P: Nutrition in infancy and childhood, ed 6, St Louis, 1997, WCB/McGraw-Hill and Harris AB, et al: *Nutrition strategies for children with special needs*, 1999, USC University Affiliated Program, Los Angeles.

*This is a guide to a basic diet. Fats, oils, sauces, desserts, and snack foods provide additional kilocalories to meet the needs of a growing child. Foods can be selected from this pattern for meals and snacks.

(Dubois et al., 2007; Keller et al., 2009; Lim et al., 2009). High milk and low sweetened-beverage intake is associated with improved nutrient intake, including calcium, potassium, magnesium, and vitamin A (O'Neil et al., 2009). Children should be offered milk, water, and healthy snacks throughout the day instead of sugar-sweetened choices.

Excess sodium is another concern. An increase in sodium or salt intake results in an increase in systolic blood pressure and diastolic blood pressure (ADA, 2010). A reduction in the use of processed foods may be warranted for children with elevated blood pressure. The Dietary Approaches to Stop Hypertension diet is useful for all age groups because it increases potassium, magnesium, and calcium in relation to sodium intake. See Chapter 34.

Meal time in group settings is an ideal opportunity for nutrition education programs focused on various learning activities around food (Figure 18-4). Experiencing new foods, participating in simple food preparation, and planting a garden are activities that develop and enhance positive food habits and attitudes.

Feeding School-Age Children

Growth from ages 6 to 12 years is slow but steady, paralleled by a constant increase in food intake. Children are in school a greater part of the day; and they begin to participate in clubs, organized sports, and recreational programs. The influence of peers and significant adults such as teachers, coaches, or sports idols increases. Except for severe issues, most behavioral problems connected with food have been resolved by this age, and children enjoy eating to alleviate hunger and obtain social satisfaction.

School-age children may participate in the school lunch program or bring a lunch from home. The National School Lunch Program, established in 1946, is administered by the USDA. Children from low-income families are eligible for free or reduced-price meals. In addition, the School Breakfast Program, begun in 1966, is offered in approximately 85% of the public schools that participate in the lunch program. The USDA also offers the Afterschool Snacks and Summer Food Service for organized programs, the Fresh Fruit and Vegetable Program in selected schools, and the Special Milk program for children not participating in school lunch (see Chapter 10).

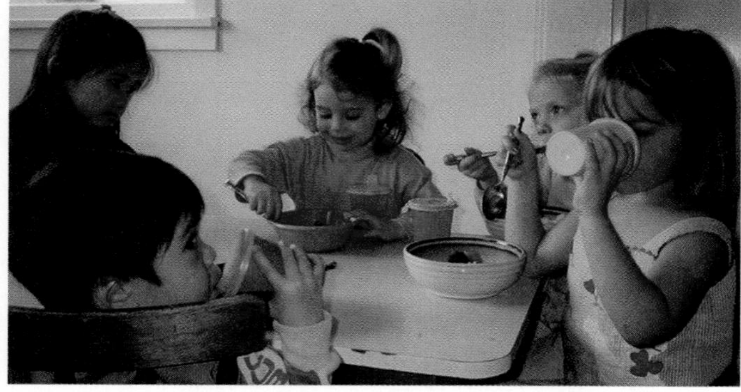

FIGURE 18-4 Children who eat with each other in an appropriate environment often eat more nutritiously and try a wider variety of foods than when eating alone.

More than 70% of schools met USDA standards for current target nutrients but less than one third of schools met standards for fat in lunch; levels of sodium remain high, whereas fiber is low relative to the DRI (Crepinsek, 2009). Of schools studied, 42% did not offer any fresh fruit or raw vegetables in the reimbursable school lunch on a daily basis (Gordon et al., 2007). New criteria for a broader number of specific nutrient targets and recommendations for menu planning using a food-based approach consistent with the DRI have been published (IOM, 2010). Efforts have been made to decrease food waste by altering menus to accommodate student preferences, allowing students to decline one or two menu items and offering salad bars. Efforts to increase participation in school lunch require consistent messages that support healthful eating.

School wellness policies were required by the school year 2006-2007 in institutions participating in school lunch and school breakfast programs. A survey indicated that many parents, although supportive of snack food restrictions and desirous of more physical education, were unaware of the required school wellness policies (Action for Healthy Kids, 2005). A survey of school food services directors revealed that 97% of school districts have policies that address nutrition standards for National School Lunch Program meals; in those districts, more than 92% have implemented activities including nutrition education, physical activity, and nutrition guidelines (School Nutrition Association, 2007). The school, including the administration, teachers, students, and food service personnel together with families and the community, are encouraged to work together to support nutrition integrity in the educational setting (ADA, 2006).

Consumption of school meals is also affected by the daily school schedule and the amount of time allotted for children to eat. When recess is scheduled before lunch rather than after, intake is better. A Montana "Recess Before Lunch" pilot study documented improvement in the mealtime atmosphere and students' behavior. Discipline problems on the playground, in the lunchroom, and in the classroom decreased (Montana Office of Public Instruction, 2010).

Children who require a special diet because of certain medical conditions such as diabetes, hyperlipidemia, or documented food allergy are eligible for modified school meals. Children with developmental disabilities are eligible to attend public school from ages 3 to 21 years, and some of them need modified school meals (e.g., meals that are texture modified, or with increased or decreased energy density). To receive modified meals, families must submit written documentation by a medical professional of the diagnosis, meal modification, and rationale. For children receiving special education services, the documentation for meals and feeding can be incorporated as objectives in a child's individual education plan (IEP) (see Chapter 45).

Studies of lunches packed at home indicate that they usually provide fewer nutrients but less fat than school lunch meals. Favorite foods tend to be packed, so children have less variety. Food choices are limited to those that travel well and require no heating or refrigeration. A typical well-balanced lunch brought from home could include a sandwich with whole-grain bread and a protein-rich filling; fresh vegetables, fruit, or both; low-fat milk; and possibly a cookie, a graham cracker, or another simple dessert. Food safety measures (e.g., keeping perishable foods well chilled) must be observed when packing lunches for school.

Today many school age children are responsible for preparing their own breakfasts. It is not uncommon for children to skip this meal altogether, even children in the primary grades. Children who skip breakfast tend to consume less calories and nutrients than those who eat breakfast (Wilson, 2006). Reviews of the effects of breakfast on cognition and school performance suggest that children who go to school without breakfast are more likely to experience performance deficits than those who eat breakfast (Rampersaud et al., 2005). See *Focus On:* Breakfast: Does It Affect Learning?

Snacks are commonly eaten by school age children, primarily after school and in the evening. As children grow older and have money to spend, they tend to consume more snacks from vending machines, fast-food restaurants, and neighborhood grocery stores. Families should continue to offer wholesome snacks at home and support nutrition education efforts in the school. In most cases, good eating habits established in the first few years help children through this period of decision making and responsibility. Developing and supporting programs and policies that ensure access to better-quality food, larger quantities of food, and better living conditions for low-income children help to reduce health disparities where present (Yoo et al., 2009).

Nutrition Education

As children grow, they acquire knowledge and assimilate concepts. The early years are ideal for providing nutrition information and promoting positive attitudes about all foods. This education can be informal and take place in the home with parents as models and a diet with a wide variety of foods. Food can be used in daily experiences for the toddler and preschooler and to promote the development of language, cognition, and self-help behaviors (i.e., labeling; describing size, shape, and color; sorting; assisting in preparation; and tasting).

More formal nutrition education is provided in preschools, Head Start programs, and public schools. Some programs such as Head Start have federal guidance and standards that incorporate healthy eating and nutrition education for the families involved. Nutrition education in schools is less standard and frequently has minimum or no requirements for inclusion in the curriculum or the training of teachers. Recent recommendations include policies in schools promoting coordination between nutrition education; access to and promotion of child nutrition programs; and cooperation with families, the community, and health services (ADA, 2006).

FOCUS ON

Breakfast: Does It Affect Learning?

The educational benefits of school meal programs and especially the role of breakfast in better school performance have been debated and discussed for decades. Studies of healthy 9- to 11-year-old children have shown that those who skipped breakfast and were then given a variety of tests made more errors, had slower stimulus discrimination, and had slower memory recall (Pollitt et al., 1998). Similar studies in other countries with children who were at nutritional risk (i.e., had wasted and stunted growth) and skipped breakfast demonstrated even poorer performance on the learning tasks (Rampersaud et al., 2005). Recent school-based breakfast experiments in 9- to 11-year-old and 6- to 8-year-old children found similar positive results with breakfast consumption (i.e., enhanced short-term memory, better spatial memory, and improved processing of complex visual stimuli) (Mahoney et al., 2005), but other reports are less supportive (Rampersaud et al., 2005). These studies suggest that brain functioning is sensitive to short-term variations in nutrient availability. A short fast may impose greater stress on young children than on adults, resulting in metabolic alterations as various homeostatic mechanisms work to maintain circulating glucose concentrations.

School breakfast programs result in better academic performance, achievement test scores, and attendance (Rampersaud et al., 2005). In addition, breakfast contributes significantly to the child's overall nutrient intake. These studies underscore the potential benefits—not only for low-income and at-risk children but also for all school children—of a breakfast at home or school meal programs that include breakfast. Based on a study of the most recent data available from 2002-2003, nearly 50% of children eligible participate in a school breakfast program, which is up from almost 29% participation in the 1992-93 school year (Dahl and Scholz, 2011).

Teachers attempting to teach children nutrition concepts and information should take into account the children's developmental level. The play approach, based on Piaget's theory of learning, is one method for teaching nutrition and fitness to school-age children (Rickard et al., 1995). Activities and information that focus on real-world relationships with food are most likely to have positive results. Meals, snacks, and food preparation activities provide children opportunities to practice and reinforce their nutrition knowledge and demonstrate their cognitive understanding. Involving parents in nutrition education projects can produce positive outcomes that are also beneficial in the home. Many written and electronic resources on nutrition education for children exist, such as at the National Center for Education in Maternal and Child Health.

NUTRITIONAL CONCERNS

Overweight and Obesity

The increasing prevalence of overweight children is a significant and alarming public health problem. The most recent NHANES reported an obesity (BMI higher than the 95th percentile) prevalence of 16.9% in children ages 2 to 19 years, and high BMI (BMI higher than the 85th percentile) prevalence of 31.7% (Ogden et al., 2010). For children 2 to 5 years of age, the prevalence is 10.4% for obese and 21.1% for high BMI (Ogden et al., 2010). This prevalence has remained relatively constant (except for an increase among the heaviest 6-19 year old boys) between 1999-2000 and 2007-2008.

Terminology for BMI categories related to overweight and obesity continues to change. The most recent Expert Committee report suggests the following terms to describe risk based on BMI: *obesity* as BMI at or above the 95th percentile and *overweight* as BMI between the 85th and 94th percentiles (Barlow et al., 2007). Determining whether growing children are obese is difficult. Some excess weight may be gained at either end of the childhood spectrum; the 1-year-old toddler and the prepubescent child may weigh more for developmental and physiologic reasons, but this extra weight is often not permanent. BMI, a useful clinical tool for screening for overweight, has limitations in determining obesity because of variability related to sex, race, body composition, and maturation stage.

The CDC growth charts allow tracking of BMI from age 2 into adulthood; thus children can be monitored periodically, and intervention provided when the rate of BMI change is excessive. The BMI charts show the adiposity rebound, which normally occurs in children between 4 and 6 years of age. Children whose adiposity rebound occurs before 5½ years of age are more likely to weigh more as adults than those whose adiposity rebound occurs after 7 years of age. The timing of the adiposity rebound and excess fatness in adolescence are two critical factors in the development of obesity in childhood, with the latter being the most predictive of adult obesity and related morbidity (Williams, 2009).

Although genetic predisposition is an important factor in obesity development, the increases in the prevalence of overweight children cannot be explained by genetics alone. Factors contributing to excess energy intake for the pediatric population include ready access to eating and food establishments, eating tied to sedentary leisure activities, children making more food and eating decisions, larger portion sizes, and decreased physical activity. In addition, American children snack three times a day, with chips, candy, and other low-nutrient foods providing more than 27% of their daily energy intake; this contributes 168 kcals/day (Piernas and Popkin, 2010).

Inactivity plays a major role in obesity development, whether it results from screen time, limited opportunities for physical activity, or safety concerns that prevent children from enjoying free play outdoors. Although increased television viewing and computer and handheld game use has been associated with childhood overweight, a review suggests that the greater risk of overweight is related to television viewing plus a low activity level (Ritchie et al., 2005). The need to use automobiles for short trips limits children's opportunities to walk to local destinations, a phenomenon particularly relevant to children in the suburbs.

Obesity in childhood is not a benign condition, despite the popular belief that overweight children will outgrow their condition. The longer a child has been overweight, the more likely the child is to be overweight or obese during adolescence and adulthood. Consequences of overweight in childhood include psychosocial difficulties such as discrimination from others, a negative self-image, depression, and decreased socialization. Many overweight children have one or more cardiovascular risk factors such as hyperlipidemia, hypertension, or hyperinsulinemia (Daniels, 2009). An even more dramatic health consequence of overweight is the rapid increase in the incidence of type 2 diabetes in children and adolescents, which has a serious effect on adult health, development of other chronic diseases, and health care costs (see Chapter 31).

The AAP has developed guidelines for overweight screening and assessment for children from age 2 through adolescence (Barlow et al., 2007). In addition to growth parameters, other important information includes dietary intake and patterns, previous growth patterns, family history, physical activity, and family interactions. The U.S. Preventive Services Task Force (USPSTF) recommends obesity screening for 6- to 18-year olds and referral to treatment programs, if appropriate (USPSTF, 2010).

A 2010 paper described a lower prevalence of obesity among children who were exposed to the following routines: regularly eating the evening meal as a family, obtaining adequate night-time sleep, and having limited screen-viewing time (Anderson, 2010). Interventions for obesity in children have had limited effect on the childhood obesity problem, especially for black, Hispanic, and Native American populations. Success is most likely to result from programs that include comprehensive behavioral components such as family involvement, dietary modifications, nutrition information, physical activity, and behavioral strategies (Barlow et al., 2007). Incorporating behavioral intervention in obesity treatment improves outcomes and is most effective with a team approach. Depending on the child, goals for weight change may include a decrease in the rate of weight gain, maintenance of weight, or, in severe cases, gradual weight loss (see Chapter 22). An individualized approach should be tailored to each child, with minimum use of highly restrictive diets or medication, except if there are other significant diseases and no other options. (Barlow et al., 2007).

Intervention strategies require family involvement and support. Incorporating motivational interviewing and stages of change theory into the comprehensive program will likely be more successful (Kirk et al., 2005) (see Chapter 15). Changes to address overweight should include the child's input, with choices and plans that modify the family's food and activity environment, not just the child's. Adequate energy and nutrients are needed to ensure maintenance of height velocity and nutrient stores. The hazards of treating overweight children too aggressively include alternate periods of undereating and overeating, feelings of failure in meeting external expectations, ignoring internal cues for appetite and satiation, feelings of deprivation and isolation, an increased risk for eating disorders, and a poor or an increasingly poor self-image.

Some children with special health care needs, such as those with Down syndrome, Prader-Willi syndrome, short stature, and limited mobility, are at increased risk for being overweight. Their size, level of activity, and developmental status need to be considered when estimating energy intake and providing dietary guidance to their families (see Chapter 45).

Prevention of childhood obesity is an important public health priority in the United States. The Institute of Medicine (IOM) has published recommendations that target families, health care professionals, industry, schools, and communities (IOM, 2005; Kirk et al., 2005). The recommendations include schools (improved nutritional quality of food sold and served, increased physical activity, wellness education), industry (improved nutrition information for consumers clear media messages), health care professionals (tracking BMI, providing counseling for children and families), and communities and government (better access to healthy foods, improved physical activity opportunities). Schools are a natural environment for obesity prevention, which can include nutrition and health curricula, opportunities for physical education and activity, and appropriate school meals. Recent efforts have resulted in school nutrition policies that limit the kinds of products sold in vending machines and food and beverages sold for fundraising. More research is also needed to develop effective prevention strategies that incorporate cultural competency for high-risk populations.

Families are essential for modeling food choices, healthy eating, and leisure activities for their children. Parents influence children's environment by choosing nutrient-rich foods, having family meals (including breakfast), offering regular snacks, and spending time together in physical activity, all of which can be critical in overweight prevention. Reducing sedentary behaviors can increase energy expenditure and reduce prompts to eat; the AAP recommends limiting television and video time to no more than 2 hours per day (AAP, 2003; Epstein et al., 2008). Parents exerting too much control over their child's food intake or promoting a restrictive diet may cause children to be less able to self-regulate and more likely to overeat when the opportunity is available (Ritchie et al., 2005). Health professionals should support positive parenting within the child's developmental level (Satter, 2005).

Underweight and Failure to Thrive

Weight loss, lack of weight gain, or **failure to thrive (FTT)** can be caused by an acute or chronic illness, a restricted diet, a poor appetite (resulting from constipation, medication, or other issues), feeding problems, neglect, or a simple lack of food. Some experts prefer the terms *pediatric undernutrition* or *growth deficiency*. Infants and toddlers are most at risk for poor growth, often as a result of prematurity, medical conditions, developmental delays, inadequate parenting, or all of these. Dietary practices can also contribute to poor growth, including food restrictions in preschool children stemming from parents' concerns about obesity, atherosclerosis, or other potential health problems.

A careful assessment is critical and must include the social and emotional environment of the child and any physical findings. If neglect is documented to be a contributing factor, health professionals are obligated to report the case to the local child protective services (Block and Krebs, 2005). Because of the complexity of growth failure, an interdisciplinary team is ideal for assessments and interventions.

The provision of adequate energy and nutrients and nutrition education should be one part of an overall interdisciplinary plan to assist children and their families. Attempts should be made to increase children's appetites and modify the environment to ensure optimal intake. Frequent, small meals and snacks should be offered at regular times, using developmentally appropriate, nutrient-dense foods. This optimizes the smaller stomach capacity of the young child and provides structure and predictability for the eating environment. Families should receive support for positive parent-child interactions, with respect for the division of responsibility in feeding and avoidance of any pressure or coercion on the child's eating. Severe malnutrition may require carefully planned interventions and close monitoring to prevent refeeding syndrome.

Chronic constipation can result in poor appetite, diminished intake, and FTT. Adding legumes and fruits (especially dried fruits), vegetables, high fiber breakfast cereals, bran muffins, or all of these to the diet can help relieve constipation, improve appetite, and eventually promote weight gain. Because the fiber intake of children is often low, especially in children who are picky eaters, fiber intake should always be addressed in the evaluation.

Iron Deficiency

Iron deficiency is one of the most common nutrient disorders of childhood. The highest prevalence of anemia in children occurs in those younger than 2 years of age. Iron deficiency is less of a problem among older preschool and school-age children.

Infants with iron deficiency, with or without anemia, tend to score lower on standardized tests of mental development and pay less attention to relevant information needed for problem solving. Poorer cognitive performance and delayed psychomotor development have been reported in infants and preschool children with iron deficiency. Deficiency can have long-term consequences, as demonstrated by poorer performance on developmental tests in late childhood and early adolescence (Lozoff, 2006, 2007). Iron intake should be considered during assessments of individual diets and in policy decisions intended to address the nutrition needs of low-income, high-risk children.

In addition to growth and the increased physiologic need for iron, dietary factors also play a role. For example, a

1-year-old child who continues to consume a large quantity of milk and excludes other foods may develop anemia. Many young preschool children do not like meat, so most of their iron is consumed in the nonheme form from fortified cereals, which is absorbed less efficiently (see Chapter 33).

Dental Caries

Nutrition and eating habits are important factors affecting oral health. An optimal nutrient intake is needed to produce strong teeth and healthy gums. The composition of the diet and an individual's eating habits (e.g., dietary carbohydrate intake, eating frequency) are significant factors in the development of dental caries (see Chapter 26).

Allergies

Food allergies usually present during infancy and childhood and are more likely when a child has a family history of allergies. Allergic symptoms are most often seen as respiratory or gastrointestinal responses or involve the skin, but may include fatigue, lethargy, and behavior changes. Controversy exists over the definition of *food allergy*, *food intolerance*, and *food sensitivity*, and some tests for food allergies are unspecific and equivocal (see Chapter 27).

Attention Deficit Hyperactivity Disorder

Attention deficit hyperactivity disorder is a clinical diagnosis based on specific criteria: excessive motor activity, impulsiveness, a short attention span, a low tolerance for frustration, and an onset before 7 years of age. Various dietary factors have been suggested as a cause of this disorder, including artificial flavors and colors, sugar, altered fatty acid metabolism, and allergies. Over the years, dietary treatments have been promoted such as the Feingold diet, the omission of sugar, allergy elimination diets, and supplements of vitamins and essential fatty acids (see Chapter 45).

Autism Spectrum Disorders (ASDs)

ASDs affect 1 in 110 children and are diagnosed by impairments in three behavioral categories: social interactions, verbal and nonverbal communication, and restricted or repetitive behaviors. These impairments can affect nutrient intake and eating behaviors if a child accepts only specific foods, refuses new or unfamiliar foods, or has increased hypersensitivities (e.g., to texture, temperature, color, and smell) or difficulty making transitions. Children with an ASD often refuse fruits and vegetables and may eat only a few foods from the other food groups. Although most children have normal growth parameters, their restricted diets make them at risk for marginal or inadequate nutrient intake. They are often very resistant to taking a vitamin-mineral supplement, even though they could benefit from one.

Popular nutrition advice for children with ASDs include elimination diets (e.g., gluten-free or casein-free), essential fatty acid supplements, large doses of vitamins, and other alternative therapies. Despite anecdotal reports of benefits, few well-designed controlled studies have been done to test the effectiveness of these interventions, and currently there is no strong evidence of benefits (Milward et al., 2008). Behavioral nutrition interventions may increase the types of food accepted at home and school. If families want to try alternative dietary therapies, nutrition professionals can help them ensure that the child's diet is adequate and any supplements are safe (see Chapter 45).

PREVENTING CHRONIC DISEASE

The roots of chronic adult diseases such as heart disease, cancer, diabetes, and obesity are often based in childhood—a phenomenon that is particularly relevant to the increasing rate of obesity related diseases such as type 2 diabetes. To help decrease the prevalence of chronic conditions in Americans, government and nonprofit agencies have been promoting healthy eating habits for children. Their recommendations include the Dietary Guidelines for Americans, the USDA MyPlate, the National Cholesterol Education Program (NCEP), and the National Cancer Institute Dietary Guidelines (see Chapter 12).

Dietary Fat and Cardiovascular Health

Compared with their counterparts in many other countries, American children and adolescents have higher blood cholesterol levels and higher intakes of saturated fatty acids and cholesterol. Autopsy studies demonstrate that early coronary atherosclerosis begins in childhood and adolescence and is related to high serum total cholesterol, low-density lipoprotein (LDL) cholesterol, and very-low-density lipoprotein cholesterol levels, and low high-density lipoprotein levels (AAP, 2009).

The AAP recommendations for lipid screening and prevention of cardiovascular disease in children are similar to recommendations published for adults (Daniels, 2008; Lichtenstein, 2006). For children older than 2 years of age, nutrition recommendations are the same as those for adults: (1) no more than 30% of energy from fat (10% or less from saturated fat); and (2) 200-300 mg/day of cholesterol. Cholesterol screening is also recommended for children with risk factors—family history of dyslipidemia or premature cardiovascular disease (Daniels, 2008) (see Chapter 33).

Dietary trends have demonstrated a decrease in total fat, saturated fat, and percentage of energy from fat in children's diets; but at the same time overweight has increased with increased risk of cardiovascular disease (Gidding et al., 2005). Recommendations include a balanced energy intake; sufficient physical activity to maintain a healthy weight; increased intake of fruits, vegetables, fish, and whole grains; and use of low-fat dairy products (Daniels, 2008). Reports have shown that from age 4 to adolescence, children can consume diets that comply with the NCEP guidelines without compromising energy or nutrient intake (Gidding et al., 2005). A long-term dietary intervention study demonstrated improved lipid levels and improved eating habits in children with elevated LDL cholesterol levels (Van Horn et al., 2005). Health practitioners should assess each child individually regarding total fat intake and excessive consumption of low-fat and nonfat foods especially by preschool children (see Chapter 33).

Calcium and Bone Health

Osteoporosis prevention begins early by maximizing calcium retention and bone density during childhood and adolescence, when bones are growing rapidly and are most sensitive to diet and physical activity (see Chapter 25). To reach the maximum calcium balance during puberty, children may need to consume more than the recommended amount. However, mean dietary intakes of calcium are lower than the AI, with 20% to 30% of pubertal girls having intakes less than 500 mg/day. Although calcium supplementation coupled with an average calcium dietary intake in pubertal children has been shown to increase bone mineral density significantly, it is less certain whether this benefit is long term (Matkovic et al., 2005). One longitudinal study of white children from infancy to 8 years of age found that bone mineral content was positively correlated with intake of protein and several minerals, suggesting that many nutrients are related to bone health in children (Bounds et al., 2005). Because food consumption surveys show that children are drinking more soft drinks and noncitrus juices and less milk, education is needed to encourage young people to consume an appropriate amount of calcium from food sources and possibly supplements.

Fiber

Education about dietary fiber and disease prevention has mainly been focused on adults, and only limited information is available on the dietary fiber intake of children. Dietary fiber is needed for health and normal laxation in children. National survey data indicate that preschool children consume a mean of 9.5 g/day of dietary fiber; school age children consume approximately 11.6 g/day (Moshfegh, 2005). This is lower than the DRI for children, which is based on the same 14 g/1000 kcal as adults because of lack of scientific evidence for the pediatric population (IOM, 2006). Generally, higher fiber intakes are associated with more nutrient-dense diets in young children (Kranz et al., 2005).

Physical Activity

A decreased level of physical activity in children has been noted for several decades. Participation in school physical education programs has declined over time and generally decreases with increasing age (ADA, 2008). Regular physical activity not only helps control excess weight gain, but also improves strength and endurance, enhances self-esteem, and reduces anxiety and stress. Activity, combined with an optimal calcium intake, is associated with increased bone mineral density in children and adolescents. Current physical activity recommendations for those ages 6 through 17 years of age are 60 minutes or more of physical activity every day with the majority at a moderate or vigorous aerobic intensity. Children and adolescents should do vigorous intensity activity on at least 3 days per week and include muscle-strengthening and bone-strengthening activity on at least 3 days per week. Information regarding activities that will meet these recommendations and are appropriate for children is available (U.S. Department of Health and Human Services, 2010). The Kid's MyActivity Pyramid promotes substituting sedentary activities for more physically active choices (Figure 18-5). The Dietary Guidelines for Americans and MyPlate have also been applied to children and their parents (www.chooseMyPlate.gov/kids).

CLINICAL SCENARIO

Brian is a 7-year, 4-month-old boy who gained 15 lb during the past school year. His height is 50½ inches and his weight is 70 pounds. Brian moved to a new home and began a new school a year ago after his parents' divorce. After-school care has been provided by an older neighbor, who loves to bake for Brian. Because he has no friends in the neighborhood, his main leisure activities have been watching television and playing video games. His mother reports that they have been relying more on take-out and fast-food meals because of the time constraints of her full-time job, and she has gained weight herself. However, she has recently started an aerobics class with a friend and is interested in developing healthier eating habits.

After joint sessions with Brian and his mother, the following goals were identified by the family: (1) explore after-school care at the local community center, which has sports activities; (2) alter shopping and food preparation to emphasize the MyPlate and low-fat choices; (3) begin weekend swimming or bicycling for the family; and (4) limit television and video games to no more than 2 hours daily.

After 4 months, most of the changes have been made, except for participating in the weekend family activity and watching less television on the weekends. However, Brian is now playing soccer, has lost 4 pounds, and is taller. He is 51 inches tall and weighs 66 lb.

Nutrition Diagnostic Statement

Overweight/obesity as evidenced by BMI-for-age at 95th percentile or more related to physical inactivity and excess energy intake.

Nutrition Care Questions

1. What recommendations should be made to prevent Brian and his mother from resuming their old habits?
2. Calculate and plot Brian's BMI over time. Discuss the changes.
3. What other activities can Brian try to help him avoid or reduce the tendency to eat when he is not hungry?
4. What would you suggest to promote a positive feeding relationship between Brian and his mother, considering his age and level of development?
5. How can Brian's mother alter some of his favorite recipes to lower the fat content? For example, his favorite meal is fried chicken with gravy, mashed potatoes, and ice cream.
6. Are there any nutrient-related concerns because Brian is using diet to help with weight management?

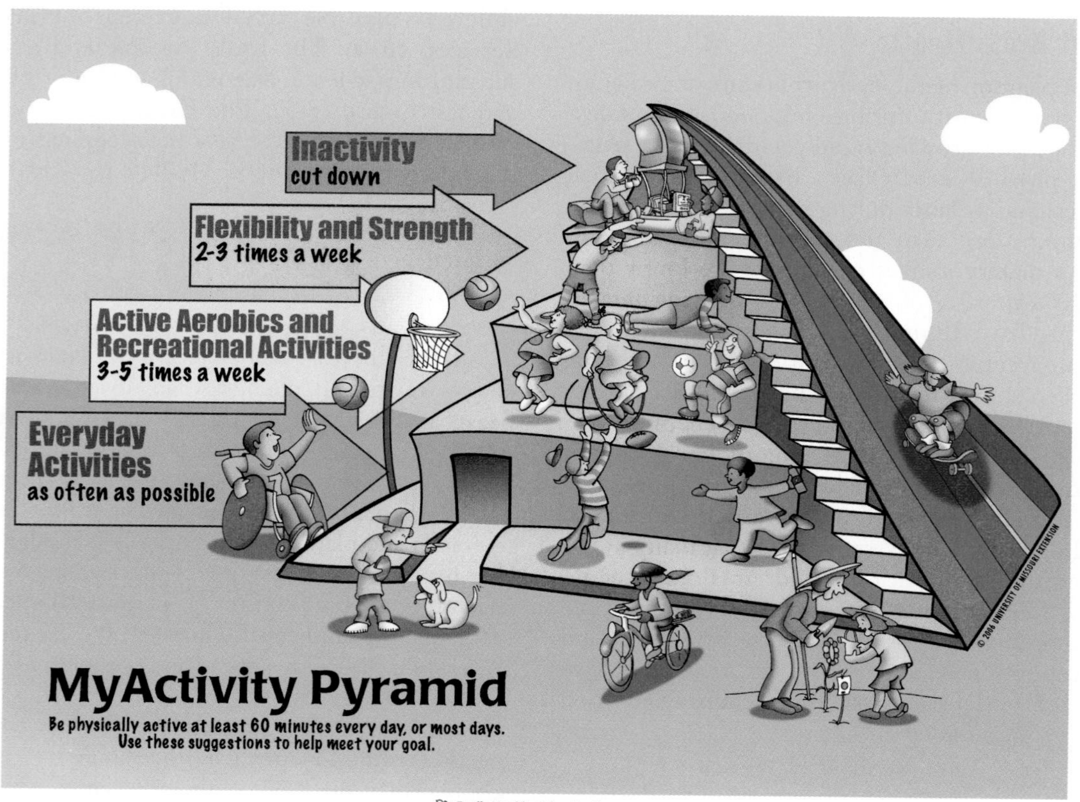

Family Nutrition Education Programs

MyActivity Pyramid

Be physically active at least 60 minutes every day, or most days.
Use these suggestions to help meet your goal:

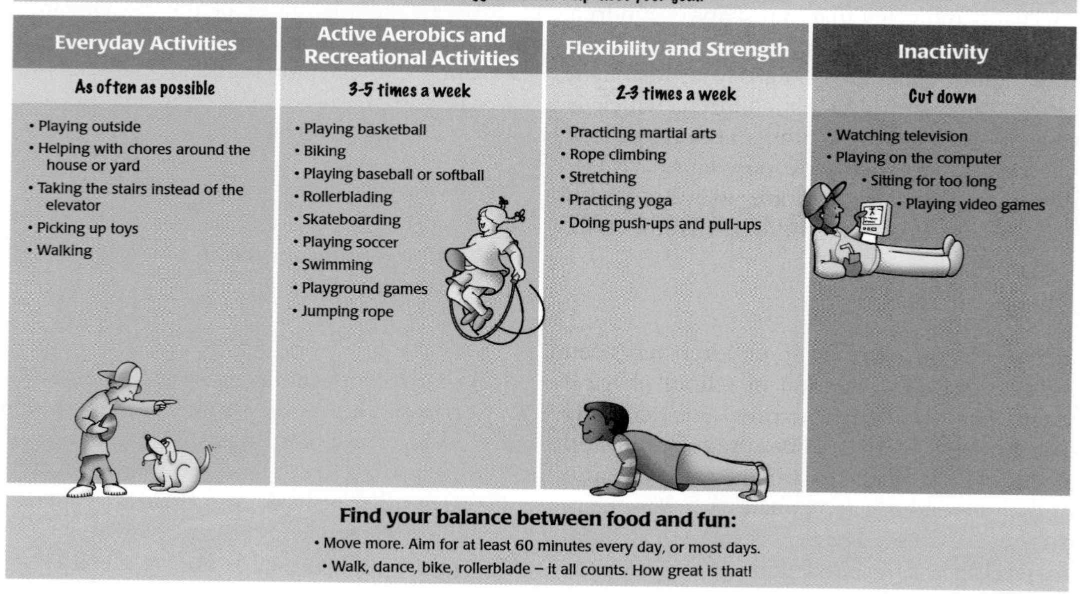

Everyday Activities	Active Aerobics and Recreational Activities	Flexibility and Strength	Inactivity
As often as possible	3-5 times a week	2-3 times a week	Cut down
• Playing outside • Helping with chores around the house or yard • Taking the stairs instead of the elevator • Picking up toys • Walking	• Playing basketball • Biking • Playing baseball or softball • Rollerblading • Skateboarding • Playing soccer • Swimming • Playground games • Jumping rope	• Practicing martial arts • Rope climbing • Stretching • Practicing yoga • Doing push-ups and pull-ups	• Watching television • Playing on the computer • Sitting for too long • Playing video games

Find your balance between food and fun:

- Move more. Aim for at least 60 minutes every day, or most days.
- Walk, dance, bike, rollerblade – it all counts. How great is that!

This publication is adapted from USDA's MyPyramid and was funded in part by USDA's Food Stamp Program.

UNIVERSITY OF MISSOURI Extension ■ Issued in furtherance of Cooperative Extension Work Acts of May 8 and June 30, 1914, in cooperation with the United States Department of Agriculture. L. Jo Turner, Interim Director, Cooperative Extension, University of Missouri, Columbia, MO 65211. ■ University of Missouri Extension does not discriminate on the basis of race, color, national origin, sex, sexual orientation, religion, age, disability or status as a Vietnam-era veteran in employment or programs. ■ If you have special needs as addressed by the Americans with Disabilities Act and need this publication in an alternative format, write: ADA Officer, Extension and Agricultural Information, 1-98 Agriculture Building, Columbia, MO 65211, or call (573) 882-7216. Reasonable efforts will be made to accommodate your special needs.

N 386

Revised 7/06/100M

FIGURE 18-5 MyActivity Pyramid. *(This publication is adapted from the U.S. Department of Agriculture's (USDA's) MyPyramid and was funded in part by the USDA's Food Stamp Program. Issued in furtherance of Cooperative Extension Work Acts of May 8 and June 30, 1914, in cooperation with the United States Department of Agriculture. L. Jo Turner, Interim Director, Cooperative Extension, University of Missouri, Columbia, MO, July, 2006.)*

USEFUL WEBSITES

Bright Futures in Practice: Nutrition
www.brightfutures.org/nutrition/
Eat Well, Play Hard
http://counties.cce.cornell.edu/erie/ewph.html
Growth Charts
www.cdc.gov/growthcharts/
Guidelines for Physical Activity
www.health.gov/paguidelines/guidelines
MyPlate Food Guidance System
www.chooseMyPlate.gov
National Center for Education in Maternal and Child Health
www.ncemch.org
www.mchlibrary.info/KnowledgePaths/kp_childnutr.html
Nutrition and Physical Activity
www.cdc.gov/nccdphp/dnpa/
Pediatric Nutrition Practice Group—American Dietetic Assn.
www.pnpg.org/
USDA Food and Nutrition Service—School Meals
www.fns.usda.gov/cnd

REFERENCES

Action for Healthy Kids: *Parents' views on school wellness practices*, September 2005. Accessed 16 March 2010 from www.actionforhealthykids.org.

American Academy of Pediatrics (AAP), Committee on Nutrition: The use and misuse of fruit juice in pediatrics, *Pediatrics* 107:1210, 2001. (Reaffirmed October 2006.)

American Academy of Pediatrics (AAP), Committee on Nutrition: prevention of pediatric overweight and obesity, *Pediatrics* 112:424, 2003. (Reaffirmed February 2007.)

American Academy of Pediatrics (AAP): *Pediatric nutrition handbook*, ed 6, Elk Grove Village, IL, 2009, AAP.

American Dietetic Association (ADA): Position of the American Dietetic Association: local support for nutrition integrity in schools, *J Am Diet Assoc* 106:122, 2006.

American Dietetic Association (ADA): Position of the American Dietetic Association: child and adolescent nutrition assistance programs, *J Am Diet Assoc* 110:791, 2010.

American Dietetic Association (ADA): Position of the American Dietetic Association: nutrition guidance for healthy children aged 2 to 11 years, *J Am Diet Assoc* 108:1038, 2008.

American Dietetic Association (ADA): Position of the American Dietetic Association: benchmarks for nutrition programs in child care settings, *J Am Diet Assoc* 105:979, 2005.

Anderson SE, Whitaker RC: Household routines and obesity in US preschool-aged children, *Pediatrics* 8 February 2010. [Epub ahead of print.]

Barlow SE, et al: Expert Committee recommendations regarding the prevention, assessment, and treatment of child and adolescent overweight and obesity: summary report, *Pediatrics* 120:S164, 2007.

Bell RA, et al: Frequency and types of foods advertised on Saturday morning and weekday afternoon English- and Spanish-language American television programs, *J Nutr Educ Behav* 41:406, 2009.

Block RW, Krebs NF, American Academy of Pediatrics, Committee on Child Abuse and Neglect, Committee on Nutrition: failure to thrive as a manifestation of child neglect, *Pediatrics* 116:1234, 2005.

Bounds W, et al: The relationship of dietary and lifestyle factors to bone mineral indexes in children, *J Am Diet Assoc* 105:735, 2005.

Brotanek JM, et al: Iron deficiency, prolonged bottle-feeding, and racial/ethnic disparities in young children, *Arch Pediatr Adolesc* 159:1038, 2005.

Crepinsek MK, et al: Meals offered and served in US public schools: do they meet nutrient standards? *J Am Diet Assoc*, 109:S31, 2009.

Dahl MW, Scholz JK: *The National School Lunch Program and School Breakfast Program: evidence on participation and noncompliance*, Congressional Budget Office, U.S. Congress and Dept. of Economics, Institute of Research on Poverty, and NBER, University of Wisconsin, Madison, WI. Accessed 12 April 2011 from http://www.ssc.wisc.edu/~scholz/Research/Lunch.pdf.

Davis GC, You W: The thrifty food plan is not thrifty when labor cost is considered, *J Nutr* 140:854, 2010.

Daniels SR: Complications of obesity in children and adolescents, *Int J Obes* 33:S60, 2009.

Daniels SR, Greer FR, Committee on Nutrition: lipid screening and cardiovascular health in childhood, *Pediatrics* 122:198, 2008.

DeNavas-Walt C, et al: *U.S. Census Bureau, current population reports, P60-236, income, poverty, and health insurance coverage in the United States: 2008*, Washington, DC, 2009, U.S. Government Printing Office.

Dubois L, et al: Regular sugar-sweetened beverage consumption between meals increases risk of overweight among preschool-aged children, *J Am Diet Assoc* 107:924, 2007.

Epstein LH, et al: A randomized trial of the effects of reducing television viewing and computer use on body mass index in young children, *Arch Pediatr Adolesc Med* 162:239, 2008.

Flegal KM, et al: Characterizing extreme values of body mass index-for-age by using the 2000 Centers for Disease Control and Prevention growth charts, *Am J Clin Nutr* 90:1314, 2009.

Food Research and Action Center: *Hunger and food insecurity in the United States*, 2009. Accessed 16 March 2010 from http://www.frac.org/html/hunger_in_the_us/hunger_index.html.

Gidding SS, et al: Dietary recommendations for children and adolescents: a guide for practitioners: consensus statement from the American Heart Association, *Circulation* 112:2061, 2005.

Gordon A, et al: *School nutrition dietary assessment study-III: volume II: student participation and dietary intakes*, Princeton, N.J., 2007, Mathematical Policy Research, Inc.

Harris AB: Evidence of increasing dietary supplement use in children with special health care needs: strategies for improving parent and professional communication, *J Am Diet Assoc* 105:34, 2005.

Institute of Medicine (IOM), Food and Nutrition Board, Committee on Prevention of Obesity in Children and Youth, Koplan JP, Liverman CT, Kraak VA, editors: *Preventing childhood obesity: health in the balance*, Washington, DC, 2005, National Academies Press.

Institute of Medicine (IOM), Food and Nutrition Board: *Dietary reference intakes: the essential guide to nutrient requirements*, Washington, DC, 2006, National Academies Press.

Institute of Medicine (IOM): *School meals: building blocks for healthy children*, Washington DC, 2010, National Academies Press.

Jyoti DF, et al: Food insecurity affects school children's academic performance, weight gain, and social skills, *J Nutr* 135:2831, 2005.

Keller KL, et al: Increased sweetened beverage intake is associated with reduced milk and calcium intake in 3- to 7-year-old children at multi-item laboratory lunches, *J Am Diet Assoc* 109:497, 2009.

Kirk S, et al: Pediatric obesity epidemic: treatment options, *J Am Diet Assoc* 105:S44, 2005.

Kleinman RE, et al: Hunger in children in the United States; potential behavioral and emotional correlates, *Pediatrics* 101:e3, 1998.

Kranz S, et al: Dietary fiber intake by American preschoolers is associated with more nutrient-dense diets, *J Am Diet Assoc* 105:221, 2005.

Larson NI, et al: Family meals during adolescence are associated with higher diet quality and healthful meal patterns during young adulthood, *J Am Diet Assoc* 107:1502, 2007.

Laurson KR, et al: Combined influence of physical activity and screen time recommendations on childhood overweight, *Pediatrics* 153:209, 2008.

Lichtenstein AH, et al: Diet and lifestyle recommendations revision 2006: a scientific statement from the American Heart Association Nutrition Committee, *Circulation* 114:82, 2006.

Lim S, et al: Obesity and sugar-sweetened beverages in African-American preschool children: a longitudinal study, *Obesity* 17:1262, 2009.

Lozoff B, et al: Long-lasting neural and behavioral affects of iron deficiency in infants, *Nutrition Revises* 64(5):S34, 2006.

Lozoff B, et al: Preschool-aged children with iron deficiency anemia show altered affect and behavior, *J Nutr* 137:683, 2007.

Mahaffey KR, et al: Methylmercury and ω-3 fatty acids: co-occurrence of dietary sources with emphasis on fish and shellfish, *Environ Res* 107:20, 2008.

Mahoney CR, et al: Effect of breakfast composition on cognitive processes in elementary school children, *Physiol Behav* 85:635, 2005.

Matkovic V, et al: Calcium supplementation and bone mineral density in females from childhood to young adulthood: a randomized controlled trial, *Am J Clin Nutr* 81:175, 2005.

Milward C, et al: Gluten- and casein-free diets for autistic spectrum disorder, *Cochrane Database Syst Rev* 2008, issue 2. Art. No.: CD003498. DOI: 10.1002/146518583.CD003498.pub3.

Montana Office of Public Instruction: *The Montana Office of Public Instruction School nutrition programs pilot project—a recess before lunch policy in four Montana schools*. Accessed 6 May 2010 from http://opi.mt.gov/pdf/schoolfood/rbl/RBL Pilot.pdf.

Moshfegh A, et al: *What we eat in America, NHANES 2001-2002: usual nutrient intakes from food compared to dietary reference intakes*, Washington, DC, 2005, U.S. Department of Agriculture, Agricultural Research Service.

Moshfegh A, et al: *What we eat in America, NHANES 2005-2006: usual nutrient intakes from food and water compared to 1997 dietary reference intakes for vitamin D, calcium, phosphorus, and magnesium*, Washington, DC, 2009, U.S. Department of Agriculture, Agricultural Research Service.

Myers GH, et al: Postnatal exposure to methyl mercury from fish consumption: a review and new data from the Seychelles Child Development Study, *NeuroToxicity* 30:338, 2009.

Nicklas TA, et al: Association between 100% juice consumption and nutrient intake and weight of children aged 2 to 11 years, *Arch Pediatr Adolesc Med* 162:557, 2008.

Nord M: *Food insecurity in households with children: prevalence, severity, and household characteristics*, USDA Econ Res Serv; September 2009. Accessed 10 May 2010 from http://www.ers.usda.gov/Publications/EIB56/.

Ogden CL, et al: Prevalence of high body mass index in US children and adolescents, 2007-2008, *JAMA* 303:242, 2010.

Oken E, Bellinger DC: Fish consumption, methylmercury and child neurodevelopment, *Curr Opin Pediatr* 20:178, 2008.

O'Neil CE, et al: Impact of dairy and sweetened beverage consumption on diet and weight of a multiethnic population of head start mothers, *J Am Diet Assoc* 109:874, 2009.

Palmer CA: Dental caries and obesity in children: different problems, related causes, *Quintessence Int* 36:457, 2005.

Picciano MF, et al: Dietary supplement use among infants, children, and adolescents in the United States, 1999-2002, *Arch Pediatr Adolesc Med* 161:978, 2007.

Piernas C, Popkin BM: Trends in snacking among U.S. children, *Health Affairs J* 29:398, 2010.

Pollitt E, et al: Fasting and cognition in well- and undernourished school children: a review of three experimental studies, *Am J Clin Nutr* 67(Suppl):779,1998.

Rampersaud GC, et al: Breakfast habits, nutritional status, body weight, and academic performance in children and adolescents, *J Am Diet Assoc* 105:743, 2005.

Rickard KA, et al: The play approach to learning in the context of families and schools: an alternative paradigm for nutrition and fitness education in the 21st century, *J Am Diet Assoc* 95:1121, 1995.

Ritchie LD, et al: Family environment and pediatric overweight: What is a parent to do? *J Am Diet Assoc* 105:S70, 2005.

Rose-Jacobs R, et al: Household food insecurity: associations with at-risk infant and toddler development, *Pediatrics* 121:65, 2008.

Ross, CA, et al, editors, *Institute of Medicine (IOM): Dietary Reference Intakes for Calcium and Vitamin D*, Washington, DC, 2011, The National Academies Press. Accessed at www.nap.edu.

Satter E: *Child of mine—feeding with love and good sense*, Palo Alto, Calif, 2000, Bull Publishing Co.

Satter E: *Your child's weight: helping without harming*, Madison, Wisc, 2005, Kelcy Press.

Savage JS, et al: Parental influence on eating behavior: conception to adolescence, *J Law Med Ethics* 35:22-34, 2007.

School Nutrition Association: From cupcakes to carrots: local wellness policies one year later. September, 2007, School Nutrition Association, National Harbor, MD.

Skalicky A, et al: Child food security and iron deficiency anemia in low-income infants and toddlers in the United States, *Matern Child Health J* 19 November 2005:1-9. [Epub ahead of print.] Accessed 5 May 2010 from http://www.cdc.gov/pcd/issues/2010/mar/08_0257.htm.

U.S. Department of Health and Human Services: *2008 physical activity guidelines for Americans*. Accessed 6 May 2010 from http://www.health.gov/paguidelines/guidelines.

U.S. Environmental Protection Agency: *What you need to know about mercury in fish and shellfish*. Accessed 16 March

2010 from http://www.epa.gov/waterscience/fish/advice/index.html.

U.S. Preventive Services Task Force, Agency for Healthcare Research and Quality: *Screening for obesity in children and adolescents*, Rockville, Md, 2010. Accessed 6 May 2010 from http://www.uspreventiveservicestaskforce.org/uspstf/uspschobes.htm.

Van Horn L, et al: Children's adaptations to a fat-reduced diet: the intervention study in children (DISC), *Pediatrics* 115:1723, 2005.

Vos MB, et al: Dietary fructose consumption among US children and adults: the Third National Health and Nutrition Examination Survey, *Medscape J Med* 10:160, 2008.

Williams SM, Goulding A: Patterns of growth associated with timing of adiposity rebound, *Obesity* 17:335, 2009.

Wilson NC, et al: Eating breakfast and its impact on children's daily diet, *Nutrition & Dietetics* 63:15, 2006.

Yoo JP, et al: Material hardship and the physical health of school-aged children in low-income households, *Am J Public Health* 99:829, 2009.

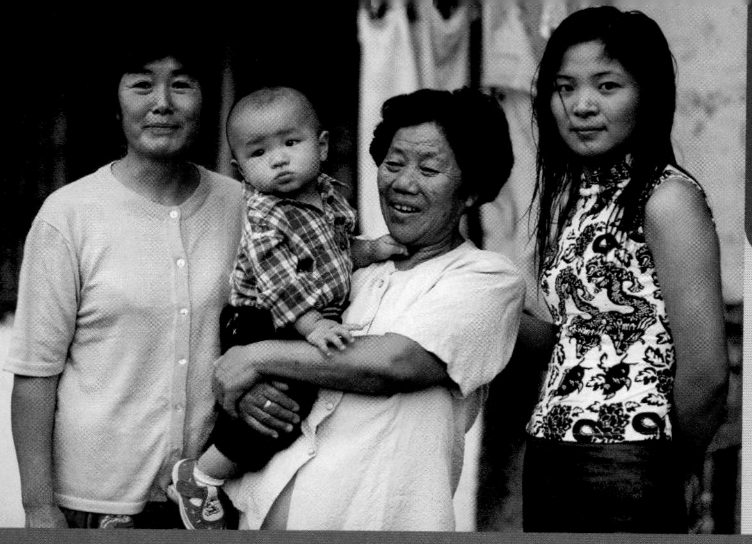

CHAPTER 19

Jamie S. Stang, PhD, MPH, RD, LN
Nicole Larson, PhD, MPH, RD

Nutrition in Adolescence

KEY TERMS

adolescence
body image
disordered eating
growth spurt
gynecologic age
menarche
peak height gain velocity
physiologic anemia of growth
pubarche
puberty
sexual maturity rating (SMR)
Tanner stage
thelarche

Adolescence is one of the most exciting yet challenging periods in human development. Generally thought of as the period of life that occurs between 12 and 21 years of age, adolescence is a period of tremendous physiologic, psychologic, and cognitive transformation during which a child becomes a young adult. The gradual growth pattern that characterizes early childhood changes to one of rapid growth and development, affecting both physical and psychosocial aspects of health. Changes in cognitive and emotional functioning allow teens to become more independent as they mature. Peer influence and acceptance may become more important than family values, creating periods of conflict between teens and parents. Because all of these changes have a direct effect on the nutrient needs and dietary behaviors of adolescents, it is important that health care providers develop a full understanding of how these developmental changes of adolescence can affect nutritional status.

GROWTH AND DEVELOPMENT

Puberty is the period of rapid growth and development during which a child physically develops into an adult and becomes capable of sexual reproduction. It is initiated by the increased production of reproductive hormones such as estrogen, progesterone, and testosterone and is characterized by the outward appearance of secondary sexual characteristics such as breast development in females and the appearance of facial hair in males (Table 19-1).

Psychological Changes

Adolescence is often depicted as a time of irrational behavior. The physical growth of puberty transforms the teen body into an adultlike form, leading adults to believe that adolescent development is complete. However, the social and emotional development of adolescence lags behind. The mismatch between how teens look and how they act may lead adults to deduce that the adolescent is "not acting his or her age." The rebellion that is associated with the teen years is actually the manifestation of their search for independence and a sense of autonomy. Food can be, and often is, used as a means of exerting autonomy. Adolescents may choose to become vegetarian as a way to differentiate themselves from their meat-eating parents or to express their moral and ethical concerns over animal welfare

TABLE 19-1

Ratings of Sexual Maturation*

	Pubic Hair	Genitalia	Corresponding Changes
Males			
Stage 1	None	Prepubertal	
Stage 2	Small amount at outer edges of pubis, slight darkening	Beginning penile enlargement Testes enlarged to 5-mL volume Scrotum reddened and changed in texture	Increased sweat gland activity
Stage 3	Covers pubis	Penis longer Testes enlarged to 8-10 mL Scrotum enlarged	Voice changes Faint mustache and facial hair Axillary hair Beginning of peak height gain velocity (growth spurt of 6-8 inches)
Stage 4	Adult type, does not extend to thighs	Penis wider and longer Testes enlarged to 12 mL Scrotal skin darker	End of peak height gain velocity More facial hair Darker hair on legs Voice deeper Possibly severe acne
Stage 5	Adult type, spreads to thighs	Adult penis Testes enlarged to 15 mL	Significantly increased muscle mass
Females			
Stage 1	None	No change from childhood	
Stage 2	Small amount, downy, on medial labia	Breast buds	Increased sweat gland activity Beginning of peak height gain velocity (growth spurt of 3-5 inches)
Stage 3	Increased, darker, curly	Larger, but no separation of the nipple and the areola	End of peak height gain velocity Beginning of acne Axillary hair
Stage 4	More abundant, coarse texture	Larger Areola and nipple form secondary mound	Possibly severe acne Menarche begins
Stage 5	Adult, spreads to medial thighs	Adult distribution of breast tissue, continuous outline	Increased fat and muscle mass

Modified from Tanner JM: Growth at adolescence, ed 2, Oxford, 1962, Blackwell Scientific Publications.
*See Appendixes 17 and 18.

or the environment. Eating fast food becomes a strong social factor for adolescents that differentiates them from their parents and older generations. In their minds, asking teens to stop eating fast food is equivalent to asking them to stop being adolescents.

Cognitive and emotional development is best understood when it is divided into three periods: early, middle, and late adolescence (Ingersoll, 1992). Each period has unique features in terms of the ability to synthesize information and apply health concepts, and this has a direct bearing on methods used when providing nutritional counseling and designing educational programs.

Early adolescence, occurring between the ages of 13 and 15, is characterized by the following:

- Preoccupation with body size and shape, and **body image** (the mental self-concept and perception of personal body size) as a result of the rapid growth and development that has occurred
- Continuation of trust and respect for adults as authority figures; however, this diminishes during this phase of psychosocial development
- Strong influence of peers, especially around areas of body image and appearance, with peer pressure peaking at approximately 14 years of age
- Desire for autonomy but still wanting parental approval for major decisions and still seeking parental security when experiencing stress
- Expanded cognitive ability, including abstract reasoning
- Increased spending money resulting in more independent purchasing power, including for snacks and meals

Middle adolescence, occurring between the ages of 15 and 17, is characterized by the following:

- Persistence of peer group influence; however, teens are influenced by fewer individuals with whom they closely bond
- Decreased trust in adult authority and wisdom
- Less pronounced body image issues as the adolescent becomes more comfortable in his or her adultlike body shape and size
- More pronounced social, emotional, and financial independence, leading to increased independent decision making related to food and beverage intake
- Significant cognitive development as abstract reasoning is nearly complete and egocentrism decreases

Late adolescence, occurring between the ages of 18 and 21, is characterized by the following:

- Fully developed abstract reasoning; however, teens may still revert to less complex thinking patterns when they are stressed
- Developed future orientation, which is required to understand the link between current behavior and chronic health risks
- Development of social, emotional, financial, and physical independence from family as teens leave home to attend college or seek full-time employment
- Development of a core set of values and beliefs that guides moral, ethical, and health decisions

The psychosocial development of adolescents has a direct bearing on the foods and beverages they choose. Teens in early to mid-adolescence are at risk for restricting calories as a means of dieting because of body image concerns. Because abstract reasoning ability is not yet fully developed, teens of this age are generally unable to see the relationship between their current behaviors and their future health risk. Nutrition education and counseling methods that focus on how adolescents look, such as improving skin appearance or promoting hair growth, are most likely to be effective with young teens.

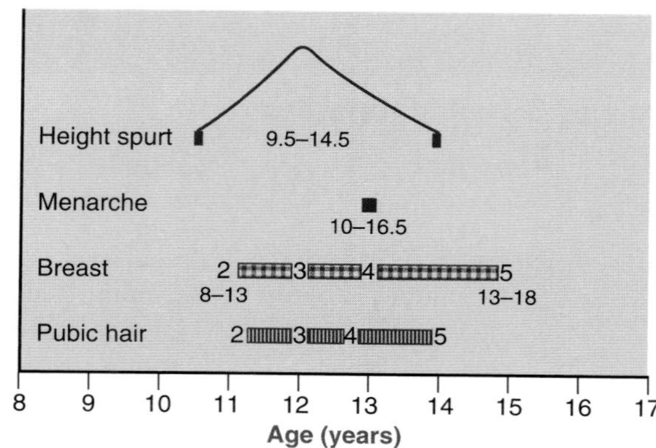

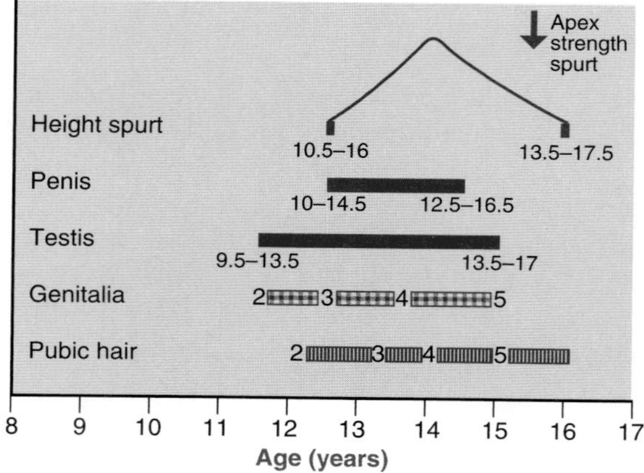

FIGURE 19-1 Sequence of events during puberty in females *(upper chart)* and males *(lower chart)*. Breast, genitalia, and pubic hair development are numbered 2 to 5 based on the Tanner developmental stages. *(From Marshall WA, Tanner JM: Variations in the pattern of pubertal changes in males, Arch Dis Child 45:13, 1970.)*

Sexual Maturity

Sexual maturity rating (SMR), also known as **Tanner stage**, is used to clinically assess the degree of sexual maturation during puberty (Tanner, 1962). Among males SMR is based on genital and pubic hair development (see Figure 19-1 and Table 19-1). Among females SMR is assessed by breast and pubic hair development. SMR is measured through a series of five stages, with stage 1 marking prepubertal development and stage 5 marking the completion of physical growth and development. See Appendix Tables 17 and 18. The five stages of SMR correlate highly with other markers of growth and development during puberty such as alterations in height, weight, body composition, and endocrine functioning. A thorough understanding of the relationship between physical growth and development and SMR enables health care professionals to assess an adolescent's potential for future growth.

In general, females enter puberty earlier than males. An example of ethnic variation in female development is shown in data from the National Health and Nutrition Examination Study III (NHANES III). It suggests that most non-Hispanic black and Mexican American females reach breast development stage 2 (**thelarche**) at 9.6 years of age, 8 months earlier than non-Hispanic white females (Rosenfield, 2009). Racial and ethnic differences in maturation are also seen for pubic hair stage 3 (**pubarche**), which occurs earlier among most non-Hispanic black females (10.6 years) compared with Mexican American and white females (11.6 years). Most females enter puberty at least 2.5 years earlier than their male counterparts, with Mexican American youth showing the greatest gender variance in age at pubarche.

Data from NHANES III also suggest variation in the timing of pubarche among males of different racial and ethnic backgrounds (Rosenfield, 2009). The median age among non-Hispanic white and black males (12.3 and 12.5 years) is approximately 6 months earlier than among Mexican American males (13.2 years).

Adolescent females with a body mass index (BMI) in the 85th percentile or higher are four times more likely to have

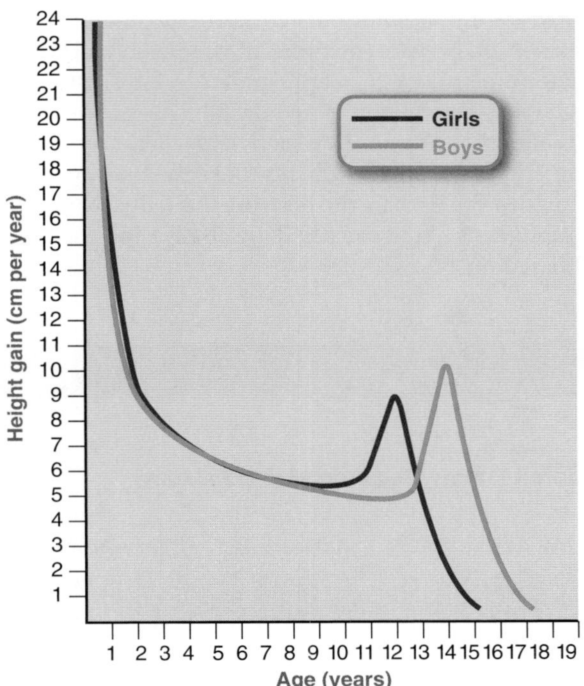

FIGURE 19-2 Typical individual velocity curves for supine length or height in males and females. Curves represent the growth velocity of the typical boy and girl at any given age.

reached thelarche by age 8 and twice as likely by 9.6 years of age than normal weight females (Rosenfeld, 2009). Excessive body weight among young females plays a larger role in the timing and duration of puberty among females than among males.

Menarche, the onset of menses or menstruation, is often considered the hallmark of puberty among females (at 12.5 years in the average girl). However, the onset of menses can occur anywhere between the ages of 8 and 17 years (Rosenfeld, 2009; Tanner, 1962). The median age of menarche is 12.1 years for black, 12.3 years for Mexican American, and 12.6 years for white females (Rosenfeld, 2009).

Excessive body weight among females was associated with both earlier onset of puberty as well as earlier menses among females of all racial and ethnic groups. Females with a BMI in the 85th percentile or higher are four times as likely to have experienced menses by age 10.6 years of age.

In summary, puberty may begin earlier but last longer for nonwhite females (Rosenfeld, 2009). Although racial and ethnic differences in the age of pubarche were noted for males, the differences were not as pronounced. No significant relationship between weight status and pubarche was found among males.

Linear Growth

The velocity of physical growth during adolescence is much higher than that of early childhood (Figure 19-2). On average, adolescents gain approximately 20% of their adult height during puberty. There is a great deal of variability in the timing and duration of growth among adolescents, illustrated in Figure 19-3 by a group of 13-year-old males.

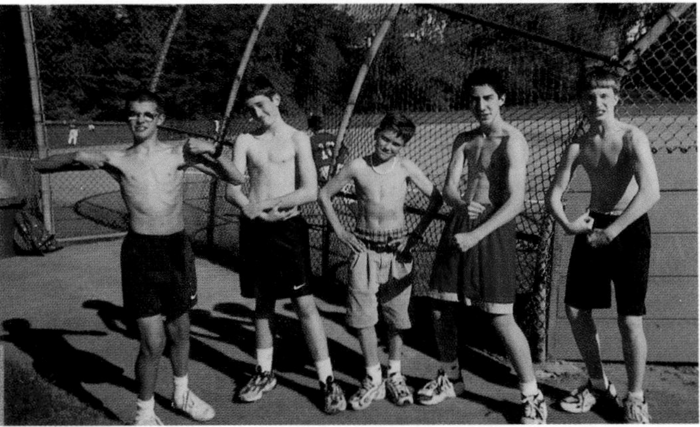

FIGURE 19-3 These males are all 13 years old, but their energy needs vary according to their individual growth rates.

Linear growth occurs throughout the 4 to 7 years of pubertal development in most teens; however, the largest percentage of height is gained during an 18- to 24-month period commonly referred to as the **growth spurt**. The fastest rate of growth during the growth spurt is labeled the **peak height gain velocity**. Although growth slows after the achievement of sexual maturity, linear growth and weight acquisition continue into the late teens for females and early 20s for males and young men. Most females gain no more than 2 to 3 inches after menarche, although females who have early menarche tend to grow more after its onset than do those having later menarche.

Increases in height are accompanied by increases in weight during puberty. Teens gain 40% to 50% of adult body weight during adolescence. The majority of weight gain coincides with increases in linear height. However, it should be noted that teens may gain more than 15 pounds after linear growth has ceased. Changes in body composition accompany changes in weight and height. Males gain twice as much lean tissue as females, resulting in differentiation in percent body fat and lean body mass. Body fat levels increase from prepuberty averages of 15% for males and 19% for females to 15% to 18% in males and 22% to 26% in females. Differences in lean body mass and body fat mass affect energy and nutrient needs throughout adolescence and differentiate the needs of females from those of males.

NUTRIENT REQUIREMENTS

The dietary reference intakes (DRIs) for adolescents are listed by chronologic age and gender. Although the DRIs provide an estimate of the energy and nutrient needs for an individual adolescent, actual need varies greatly between teens as a result of differences in body composition, degree of physical maturation, and level of physical activity. Therefore health professionals should use the DRIs as a guideline during nutritional assessment, but should rely on clinical judgment and indicators of growth and physical maturation to make a final determination of an individual's nutrient and energy requirements.

Energy

Estimated energy requirements (EERs) vary greatly among males and females because of variations in growth rate, body composition, and physical activity level (PAL). EERs are calculated using an adolescent's gender, age, height, weight, and PAL, with an additional 25 kcal/day added for energy deposition or growth (Institute of Medicine [IOM], 2006). To determine adequate energy intake (in kilocalories), physical activity assessment is required. The energy requirements allow for four levels of activity (sedentary, low active, active, and very active), which reflect the energy expended in activities other than the activities of daily living. Tables 19-2 and 19-3 show the EER (kcal/day) for each activity level based on PALs.

TABLE 19-2

Estimated Energy Requirements for Adolescent Males

			Estimated Energy Requirements (kcal/day)			
Age	Reference Weight (kg [lb])	Reference Height (m [in])	Sedentary PAL*	Low Active PAL*	Active PAL*	Very Active PAL*
9	28.6 (63.0)	1.34 (52.8)	1505	1762	2018	2334
10	31.9 (70.3)	1.39 (54.7)	1601	1875	2149	2486
11	35.9 (79.1)	1.44 (56.7)	1691	1985	2279	2640
12	40.5 (89.2)	1.49 (58.7)	1798	2113	2428	2817
13	45.6 (100.4)	1.56 (61.4)	1935	2276	2618	3038
14	51.0 (112.3)	1.64 (64.6)	2090	2459	2829	3283
15	56.3 (124)	1.70 (66.9)	2223	2618	3013	3499
16	60.9 (134.1)	1.74 (68.5)	2320	2736	3152	3663
17	64.6 (142.3)	1.75 (68.9)	2366	2796	3226	3754
18	67.2 (148)	1.76 (69.3)	2383	2823	3263	3804

Data from Institute of Medicine, Food and Nutrition Board: Dietary reference intakes for energy, carbohydrate, fiber, fat, fatty acids, cholesterol, protein, and amino acids, Washington, DC, 2002, National Academies Press.

PAL, Physical activity level.

*PAL categories, which are based on walking per day at 2-4 mph, are as follows: sedentary, no additional activity; low active, 1.5-2.9 miles/day; active, 3-5.8 miles/day; and very active, 7.5-14 miles/day (see Table 2-3).

TABLE 19-3

Estimated Energy Requirements for Adolescent Females

			Estimated Energy Requirements (kcal/day)			
Age	Reference Weight (kg [lb])	Reference Height (m [in])	Sedentary PAL*	Low Active PAL*	Active PAL*	Very Active PAL*
9	29.0 (63.9)	1.33 (52.4)	1390	1635	1865	2248
10	32.9 (72.5)	1.38 (54.3)	1470	1729	1972	2376
11	37.2 (81.9)	1.44 (56.7)	1538	1813	2071	2500
12	40.5 (89.2)	1.49 (58.7)	1798	2113	2428	2817
13	44.6 (91.6)	1.51 (59.4)	1617	1909	2183	3640
14	49.4 (108.8)	1.60 (63)	1718	2036	2334	3831
15	52.0 (114.5)	1.62 (63.8)	1731	2057	2362	2870
16	53.9 (118.7)	1.63 (64.2)	1729	2059	2368	2883
17	55.1 (121.4)	1.63 (64.2)	1710	2042	2353	2871
18	56.2 (123.8)	1.63 (64.2)	1690	2024	2336	2858

Data from Institute of Medicine, Food and Nutrition Board: Washington, DC, 2002, National Academies Press.

PAL, Physical activity level.

*PAL categories, which are based on walking per day at 2-4 mph are as follows: sedentary, no additional activity; low active, 1.5-2.9 miles/day; active, 3-5.8 miles/day; and very active, 7.5-14 miles/day (see Table 2-3).

Adequacy of energy intake for adolescents is best assessed by monitoring weight and BMI. Excessive weight gain indicates that energy intake is exceeding energy needs, whereas weight loss or a drop in BMI below an established percentile curve suggests that energy intake is inadequate to support the body's needs. Groups of adolescents who are at elevated risk for inadequate energy intake include teens who "diet" or frequently restrict caloric intake to reduce body weight; individuals living in food-insecure households, temporary housing, or on the street; adolescents who frequently use alcohol or illicit drugs, which may reduce appetite or replace food intake; and teens with chronic health conditions such as cystic fibrosis, Crohn disease, or muscular dystrophy.

Recent concerns about excessive energy intake among youths have centered on the intakes of added fats and sugars in their diets. The mean daily intake of added sugars by 9- to 13-year-old males is 29.2 tsp, among 14- to 18-year-old males is 34.4 tsp, among 9- to 13-year-old females is 23.2 tsp, and among 14- to 18-year-old females is 25.2 tsp (National Cancer Institute, 2010). When one considers that a cup of sugar is approximately 48 tsp, it is apparent that adolescents consume a great deal of energy through added sugars. Soft drinks provide 37% of added sugars in the U.S. diet (Bachman et al., 2008). NHANES data revealed that 9- to 13-year-olds consume 1.5 servings of soft drinks daily, whereas 14- to 18-year-olds consume 2.7 servings, the highest intake of any age group (Frazao, 2005). Added fats are consumed by adolescents largely through snack foods, baked goods, and fast food (Bachman et al., 2008). Corn, potato, and other chips have been shown to provide 16% of added fats in the U.S. diet, and half of all potatoes were fried potatoes or chips (Bachman et al., 2008). Counseling related to excessive energy intakes among adolescents should focus on intake of discretionary calories, especially those from added sweeteners consumed through soft drinks and candy and from added fats consumed through snack foods and fried food.

Protein

During adolescence protein requirements vary with degree of physical maturation. The DRIs for protein intake are estimated to allow for adequate pubertal growth and positive nitrogen balance (IOM, 2006). Table 19-4 illustrates the protein requirements for adolescents. Actual protein needs are best determined based on a per kilogram of body weight method during puberty to account for differences in rates of growth and development among teens.

Insufficient protein intake is uncommon in the U.S. adolescent population. However, as with energy intake, food security issues, chronic illness, frequent dieting, and substance use may compromise protein intakes among adolescents. Teens who follow vegan or macrobiotic diets are also at elevated risk for inadequate protein intake.

When protein intake is inadequate, alterations in growth and development are seen. In the still-growing adolescent, insufficient protein intake results in delayed or stunted increases in height and weight. In the physically mature teen, inadequate protein intake can result in weight loss, loss of lean body mass, and alterations in body composition. Impaired immune response and susceptibility to infection may also be seen.

TABLE 19-4

Protein: Estimated Average Requirements and Recommended Dietary Allowances for Adolescents

Age (yr)		EAR (g/kg/day)	RDA (g/kg/day)
9-13		0.76	0.95 or 34 g/day*
14-18	Males	0.73	0.85 or 52 g/day*
14-18	Females	0.71	0.85 or 46 g/day*

Data from Institute of Medicine, Food and Nutrition Board: Dietary reference intakes for energy, carbohydrate, fiber, fat, fatty acids, cholesterol, protein, and amino acids, Washington, DC, 2002, National Academies Press.

EAR, Estimated average requirement; *RDA*, recommended dietary allowance.

*Based on average weight for age.

Carbohydrates and Fiber

Carbohydrate requirements of adolescents are estimated to be 130 g/day (IOM, 2006). The requirements for carbohydrates, as for most nutrients, are extrapolated from adult needs and should be used as a starting point for the determination of an individual adolescent's actual need. Teens who are very active or are actively growing need additional carbohydrates to maintain adequate energy intake, whereas teenagers who are inactive or have a chronic condition that limits mobility may require fewer carbohydrates. Whole grains are the preferred source of carbohydrates because these foods provide vitamins, minerals, and fiber. Intake of carbohydrates is adequate in most teens, with less than 3% of adolescents in the United States reporting intakes less than the recommended dietary allowance value (Moshfegh et al., 2005).

Fiber intakes of youth are low, however, because of poor intake of whole grains, fruits, and vegetables. The adequate intake (AI) values for fiber intake among adolescents are 31 g/day for males 9 to 13 years old, 38 g/day for males 14 to 18 years old, and 26 g/day for 9- to 18-year-old females (IOM, 2006). These values are derived from calculations that suggest that an intake of 14 g/1000 calories provides optimal protection against cardiovascular disease (CVD) and cancer (IOM, 2006). Adolescents who require less energy intake because of activity restrictions may have needs that are lower than the AI values.

Data from the 2005-2006 What We Eat in America survey, a component of the NHANES, suggest that median intakes of fiber are 15.2 g/day for teenage males and 12.3 g/day for females (U.S. Department of Agriculture [USDA], 2008). The disparities between fiber recommendations and actual intakes suggest that more emphasis needs to be placed on educating adolescents about optimal sources of carbohydrates, including whole grains, fruits, vegetables, and legumes.

Fat

DRI values for absolute fat intake have not been established for adolescents. Instead it is recommended that fat intakes not exceed 30% to 35% of total caloric intake, with no more than 10% of calories coming from saturated fatty acids. However, specific recommendations for intakes of ω-6 and ω-3 fatty acids have been set in an attempt to ensure that teens consume adequate essential fatty acids to support growth and development, as well as to reduce chronic disease risk later in life. The AI for ω-6 polyunsaturated fatty acids (linoleic acid) are 12 g/day for 9- to 13-year-old males, 10 g/day for 9- to 13-year-old females, 16 g/day for 14- to 18-year-old males and 11 g/day for 14- to 18-year-old females (IOM, 2006). Estimated requirements for ω-3 polyunsaturated fatty acids (α-linolenic acid) among teens are 1.2 g/day for 9- to 13-year-old males, 1 g/day for 9- to 13-year-old females, 1.6 g/day for 14- to 18-year-old males, and 1.1 g/day for 14- to 18-year-old females (IOM, 2006).

Minerals and Vitamins

Micronutrient needs of youth are elevated during adolescence to support physical growth and development. However, micronutrients involved in the synthesis of lean body mass, bone, and red blood cells are especially important during adolescence. Vitamins and minerals involved in protein, ribonucleic acid, and deoxyribonucleic acid synthesis are needed in greatest amounts during the growth spurt. Needs decline after physical maturation is complete. However, the requirements for vitamins and minerals involved in bone formation are elevated throughout adolescence and into adulthood, because bone density acquisition is not completed by the end of puberty.

In general, adolescent males require greater amounts of most micronutrients during puberty, with the exception of iron. Micronutrient intakes during adolescence are inadequate among some subgroups of teens, especially among females. Tables 19-5 and 19-6 based on the 2005-2006 What We Eat in America survey, illustrates the adequacy of micronutrient intakes among U.S. adolescents compared with DRI recommendations. These data suggest that in all age and gender categories the intakes of vitamin E, calcium, and fiber are too low. Teenage females between the ages of 14 and 18 years old are most likely to consume inadequate intakes of the most vitamins and minerals, and benefit the most from nutrition intervention.

TABLE 19-5

Mean Intakes of Select Nutrients Compared to DRIs: Adolescent Males

	Mean Intake	9-13 year old RDA/AI	14-18 year old RDA/AI
Vitamin A (mcg RAE)	651	600	700
Vitamin E (mg)	7.3	11	15
Thiamin (mg)	2.05	0.9	1.2
Riboflavin (mg)	2.65	0.9	1.3
Niacin (mg)	31.1	12	16
Vitamin B_6 (mg)	2.34	1	1.3
Folate (Ug DEF)	658	300	400
Vitamin B_{12} (mcg)	7.31	1.8	2.4
Vitamin C (mg)	96.9	45	75
Phosphorus (mg)	1586	1250	1250
Magnesium (mg)	287	240	410
Iron (mg)	19.6	8	11
Zinc (mg)	14.7	8	11
Calcium (mg)	1186	1300	1300
Sodium (mg)	4266	1500	1500
Fiber (g)	15.2	31	38

Data sources: U.S. Department of Agriculture, Agricultural Research Service. 2008. Nutrient Intakes from Food: Mean Amounts Consumed per Individual, One Day, 2005-2006. Available: www.ars.usda.gov/ba/bhnrc/fsrg. Accessed Jan 29, 2010.

AI, Adequate intake; *DRI*, dietary reference intake; *NA*, not available; *RDA*, recommended dietary allowance.

TABLE 19-6

Mean Intakes of Select Nutrients Compared to DRIs: Adolescent Females

	Mean Intake	9- to 13-Year Old Female RDA/AI	14 to 18-year-old females RDA/AI
Vitamin A (mcg RAE)	474	600	700
Vitamin E (mg)	6.1	11	15
Thiamin (mg)	1.38	0.9	1
Riboflavin (mg)	1.75	0.9	1
Niacin (mg)	19.3	12	14
Vitamin B_6 (mg)	1.52	1	1.2
Folate (Ug DEF)	482	300	400
Vitamin B_{12} (mcg)	3.96	1.8	2.4
Vitamin C (mg)	75.2	45	65
Phosphorus (mg)	1077	1250	1250
Magnesium (mg)	216	240	360
Iron (mg)	13.3	8	15
Zinc (mg)	9.6	8	9
Calcium (mg)	849	1300	1300
Sodium (mg)	2950	1500	1500
Fiber (g)	12.3	26	26

Data sources: U.S. Department of Agriculture, Agricultural Research Service. 2008. Nutrient Intakes from Food: Mean Amounts Consumed per Individual, One Day, 2005-2006. Available: www.ars.usda.gov/ba/bhnrc/fsrg. Accessed Jan 29, 2010.

AI, Adequate intake; *DRI*, dietary reference intake; *NA*, not available; *RDA*, recommended dietary allowance.

Calcium

Because of accelerated muscular, skeletal, and endocrine development, calcium needs are greater during puberty and adolescence than during childhood or adult years. Bone mass is acquired at much higher rates during puberty than any other time of life; rates of bone accretion during adolescence may be four times as high as rates during early childhood or adulthood (Stransky and Rysava, 2009). In fact, females accrue approximately 92% of their bone mass by the age of 18 years, making adolescence a crucial time for osteoporosis prevention (IOM, 2006; Word Health Organization, 2003).

The AI for calcium is 1300 mg for all adolescents with an upper level intake of 3000 mg/day. Calcium intake declines with age during adolescence, especially among females. Research suggests that high soft drink consumption in the adolescent population contributes to low calcium intake by displacing milk consumption. Increasing intakes of sweetened soft drinks are found to be related to decreasing numbers of servings of dairy foods and a decrease in the adequacy of calcium intake among children and adolescents (Rajeshwari et al., 2005). Interventions to promote calcium consumption among youth should focus not only on increasing dairy product intake, but also on decreasing intakes of soft drinks and increasing intakes of calcium-fortified foods such as orange juice, bread, dark-green vegetables, nuts, and ready-to-eat cereals.

Iron

Iron requirements are increased during adolescence for the deposition of lean body mass, increase in red blood cell volume, and to support iron lost during menses among females. Iron needs are highest during periods of active growth among all teens, and are especially elevated after the onset of menses in adolescent females. The DRI for iron among females increases from 8 mg/day before age 13 (or before the onset of menses) to 15 mg/day after the onset of menses. Among adolescent males recommended intakes increase from 8 to 11 mg/day, with higher levels required during the growth spurt. Iron needs remain elevated for women after age 18, but fall back to prepubescent levels in men once growth and development are completed.

Median intakes of iron among adolescents less than desirable. Increased needs for iron, combined with low intakes of dietary iron, place adolescent females at risk for iron deficiency and anemia. It is estimated that 9% of adolescent females 12 to 15 years old and 11% to 16% of females 16 to 19 years old are iron deficient, with 2% to 3% classified as having iron-deficiency anemia (Centers for Disease Control and Prevention [CDC], 1998).

Rapid growth may temporarily decrease circulating iron levels, resulting in **physiologic anemia of growth**. Other risk factors for iron-deficiency anemia are listed in Box 19-1. Recent data suggest that overweight adolescents are almost three times more likely to experience iron deficiency than their normal-weight peers despite having similar dietary intakes of iron and vitamin C (Tussing-Humphreys et al., 2009). During adolescence, iron deficiency anemia may impair the immune response, decrease resistance to infection, and decrease cognitive functioning and short-term memory.

BOX 19-1

Risk Factors for Iron Deficiency

Inadequate Iron Intake/Absorption/Stores

- Vegetarian eating styles, especially vegan diets
- Macrobiotic diet
- Low intakes of meat, fish, poultry, or iron-fortified foods
- Low intake of foods rich in ascorbic acid
- Frequent dieting or restricted eating
- Chronic or significant weight loss
- Meal skipping
- Substance abuse
- History of iron-deficiency anemia
- Recent immigration from developing country
- Special health care needs

Increased Iron Requirements and Losses

- Heavy or lengthy menstrual periods
- Rapid growth
- Pregnancy (recent or current)
- Inflammatory bowel disease
- Chronic use of aspirin, nonsteroidal antiinflammatory drugs (e.g., ibuprofen), or corticosteroids
- Participation in endurance sports (e.g., long-distance running, swimming, cycling)
- Intensive physical training
- Frequent blood donations
- Parasitic infection

Reprinted with permission from Stang J, Story M, editors: Guidelines for adolescent nutrition services, Minneapolis, 2005, Center for Leadership Education and Training in Maternal and Child Nutrition, Division of Epidemiology and Community Health, School of Public Health, University of Minnesota.

Folic Acid

The DRI for folate intake among teens is 300 mcg/day for 9- to 13-year-old males and females, increasing to 400 mcg/day for 14- to 18-year-olds (IOM, 2006). The need for folate increases during later adolescence to support accretion of lean body mass and to provide AI among females of reproductive age as a preventive measure against neural tube defects. Food sources of folate should include both naturally occurring folate, found in dark green leafy vegetables and citrus fruit, as well as folic acid found in fortified grain products.

Median intakes of folate reported in the 2005-2006 What We Eat in America survey suggest that adolescent females are at greater risk for inadequate intake of folate than are males (USDA, 2008). This is cause for concern among adolescent females who have achieved menses and are sexually active, as having adequate folic acid status prior to conception is important for the prevention of birth defects.

Vitamin D

Vitamin D plays an important role in facilitating calcium and phosphorus absorption and metabolism, which has important implications for bone development during adolescence (IOM, 2010). Vitamin D can be synthesized by the exposure of skin to sunlight; however, many individuals live in latitudes that prevent them from synthesizing vitamin D for 6 or more months each year (Ginde et al., 2009). Individuals with darkly pigmented skin may also have a limited capacity for vitamin D production by the body (McDowell et al., 2008). The current RDA for vitamin D requirements among adolescents is 600 IU/day (IOM 2010).

NHANES data collected during the preceding few decades has established that serum 25 (OH) vitamin D levels decreased among adolescents over time (Ginde et al., 2009). The reductions were especially obvious among black participants. Greater declines in serum vitamin D status were found among females than males. The reduction in vitamin D status is troubling for adolescent females because of their poor intake of calcium and elevated lifetime risk for osteoporosis.

A criteria of less than 10 ng/mL for deficiency and 30 ng/mL or more for sufficiency has been suggested; however, this is an area of current debate. Using this definition, less than 1% of white adolescents are vitamin D–deficient and 39% of females and 29% of males are not vitamin D–sufficient (Ginde et al., 2009). Mexican American females have a vitamin D deficiency prevalence of 2%, whereas less than 1% of their male peers are deficient. More than half (59%) of Mexican American teen males and 76% of females are thought to be vitamin D–insufficient. Black teens appear to have the highest rates of vitamin D deficiency and insufficiency, probably because of their dark pigmentation, with 4% of adolescent black males and 10% of adolescent black females deficient; 75% of black males and 92% of black females are vitamin D–insufficient.

Thus low vitamin D intake is a potential health risk for adolescents and deserves greater attention during nutrition assessment, education, and intervention. Vitamin D intake and adequacy should be assessed for all adolescents who live in northern climates, who have limited sun exposure, who have lactose intolerance or milk allergy, who have developmental disabilities that may limit outdoor activities, or who have darkly pigmented skin.

Supplement Use by Adolescents

The consumption of moderate portions of a wide variety of foods is preferred to nutrient supplementation as a method for obtaining adequate nutrient intake. Despite this recommendation, studies show that adolescents do not consume nutrient-dense foods and usually have inadequate intakes of many vitamins and minerals; thus supplements may be beneficial for many teens. National surveys show that 30% to 40% of adolescents report using vitamin or mineral supplements (Shaikh et al., 2009). The adolescents most likely to use supplements are those with a higher household income, a high degree of food security, and health insurance. Supplement users usually meet national guidelines for physical activity, dietary intake, and screen time.

The use of herbal and botanical supplements is not well documented. It is estimated that 29% of adolescents consume nonnutritional supplements, including herbal weight loss products (Yussman et al., 2006). Surveys suggest that herbal weight loss products are most commonly used, with up to 18% of youth reporting their use (Calfee and Fadale, 2006). Creatine, guarana, energizers (e.g., bee pollen), L-carnitine, and coenzyme Q_{10} are other products that are commonly reported by adolescents. The short- and long-term effects of nonnutritional supplement use by children and adolescents are not known. Health professionals should screen adolescents for supplement use and should counsel them accordingly.

FOOD HABITS AND EATING BEHAVIORS

Food habits that are seen more frequently among teens than other age groups include irregular consumption of meals, excessive snacking, eating away from home (especially at fast-food restaurants), dieting, and meal skipping. Many factors contribute to these behaviors, including decreasing influence of family, increasing influence of peers, exposure to media, employment outside the home, greater discretionary spending capacity, and increasing responsibilities that leave less time for teens to eat meals with their families. Socioeconomic status, family meal frequency, and home availability of healthy foods have been positively associated with vegetable, fruit and starchy food patterns (Cutler et al., 2011). Most adolescents are aware of the importance of nutrition and the components of a healthy diet; however, they may have many barriers to overcome.

Teens perceive taste preferences, hectic schedules, the accessibility of different foods at home and school, and social support from family and friends to be key factors that affect their food and beverage choices (Goh et al., 2009; Powers et al., 2010). For example, parents may positively influence the food and beverage choices of teens by modeling healthy eating habits, selecting healthy foods for family meals, encouraging healthy eating, and setting limits on the consumption of unhealthy snack foods. Friends influence each other through modeling and shared activities, such as eating out at fast-food restaurants and purchasing snacks at convenience stores near school.

Developmentally, many teens lack the ability to associate current eating habits with future disease risk. Teens are often more focused on "fitting in" with their peers. They adopt health behaviors that demonstrate their quest for autonomy and make them feel more like adults such as drinking alcohol, smoking, and engaging in sexual activity. Nutrition education and counseling should focus on short-term benefits, such as improving school performance, looking good, and having more energy. Messages should be positive, developmentally appropriate, and concrete. Specific skills such as choosing water or milk over sugar-sweetened drinks, ordering broiled rather than fried meats, and choosing baked rather than fried snack chips are key concepts to include.

Irregular Meals and Snacking

Meal skipping is a common behavior among adolescents. Meal skipping increases throughout adolescence as teens try to sleep longer, try to lose weight through calorie restriction, and try to manage their busy lives. Breakfast is the most commonly skipped meal. National data suggest that 30% of adolescents (12-19 years) skip breakfast on a given day (Moshfegh, 2005). Adolescent males are more likely than females (38% vs. 27%) to report having breakfast daily, whereas females are more likely than males (16% vs. 13%) to report never eating breakfast (Timlin et al., 2008). Breakfast skipping has been associated with poor health outcomes including higher BMI; poorer concentration and school performance; and increased risk of inadequate nutrient intake, especially of calcium and fiber (Rampersaud et al., 2005).

Teens who skip meals often snack in response to hunger instead of eating a meal. Most teens (89%) consume at least one snack per day and the majority of teens who report snacking consume two or more snacks per day (Sebastian et al., 2008). On a given day, more than one third of all fruit servings, approximately one fourth of all grain and milk servings, and approximately 15% of vegetable servings are consumed at snacking occasions. However, snacks also provide more than one third of discretionary calories and added sugars, and approximately one fourth of solid fats (Sebastian et al., 2008). Snack foods consumed by teens are often high in added fats, sweeteners, and sodium. Soft drinks and other sugar-sweetened beverages are commonly consumed, accounting for 13% of daily caloric intake among teens (Wang et al., 2008). Because snacks are prevalent and often consumed in place of meals, teens should be encouraged to make healthy choices when choosing these snack foods and beverages. Box 19-2 provides ideas for healthy snacks or meal alternatives for teens.

BOX 19-2

Teen-Friendly Healthy Snacks

Pudding made with skim milk
A glass of skim milk sweetened with a teaspoon of chocolate or strawberry syrup
Soft pretzels warmed in the microwave and topped with mustard or salsa
Sliced apples dipped in peanut butter or fat-free caramel dip
English muffin mini-pizzas (topped with tomato or pizza sauce and mozzarella cheese)
Air-popped popcorn
Peeled and sectioned oranges
Hummus and pita bread
Mozzarella or string cheese
Baked tortilla chips with bean dip or salsa
Baked potato (microwaved) topped with salsa, yogurt, or fat-free sour cream
Graham crackers, animal crackers containing no *trans* fat
Frozen yogurt or juice bars
Fruit drink spritzer (half cranberry juice and half seltzer water)
Trail mix (dried fruit with nuts and seeds)
Baby carrots and low-fat ranch dressing
Low fat granola bars
Mini-rice cakes or popcorn cakes
Sandwich wraps with slices of turkey, cheese, and tomato

Adapted with permission from Stang J, Story M, editors: Guidelines for adolescent nutrition services, Minneapolis, 2005, Center for Leadership Education and Training in Maternal and Child Nutrition, Division of Epidemiology and Community Health, School of Public Health, University of Minnesota.

Fast Foods and Convenience Foods

Convenience foods include foods and beverages from vending machines, canteens, school stores, fast-food restaurants, and convenience stores. As adolescents spend considerable amounts of time in and around schools, convenience foods available at school and in the surrounding neighborhood may have a great influence on their eating patterns. National data indicate vending machines are available in 62% of middle schools and 86% of high schools (O'Toole et al., 2007). One third of middle schools and half of all high schools have a school store or canteen where students can purchase food or beverages (O'Toole et al., 2007). In addition, one third of U.S. middle schools and high schools have at least one fast-food restaurant or convenience store within walking distance (Zenk and Powell, 2008). Fast-food restaurants and convenience stores are socially acceptable places for teens to work and spend time with their friends.

Convenience foods tend to be low in vitamins, minerals, and fiber, but high in calories, added fat, sweeteners, and sodium (Gordon et al., 2007). National data suggest that 59% of adolescents (12-19 years) consume at least one item from a fast-food restaurant and 44% to 55% consume at least one convenience food item at school on a given day (Fox et al., 2009; Sebastian et al., 2009). Few teens are willing to stop purchasing convenience foods; the low price, convenient access, and taste appeal to them (Figure 19-4). Health professionals should refrain from asking teenagers to not eat these foods and should instead counsel them on how to make wise and healthy choices. Concrete guidelines, such as choosing snacks or vending and fast-food options with fewer than 5 g of fat per serving, are easy for adolescents to remember. Teens can also be encouraged to check labels to determine if foods are made from whole grains or are high in added sweeteners or sodium.

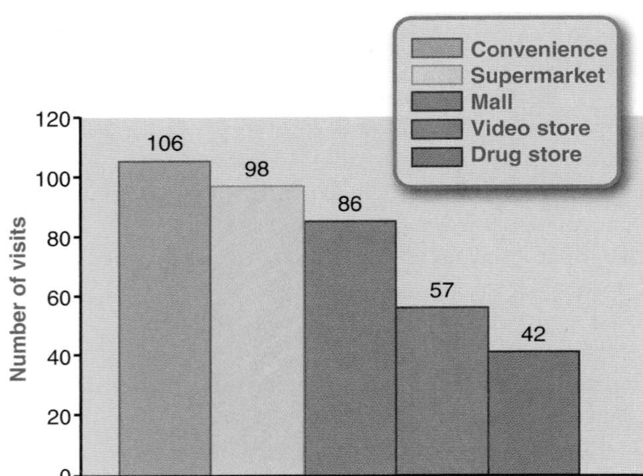

FIGURE 19-4 Store visits by teenagers in a 30-day period. *(Data from Channel One Network, New York, 2000.)*

Family Meals

The frequency with which adolescents eat meals with their families decreases with age (National Center on Addiction and Substance Abuse, 2007). Half of 12-year-olds eat dinner with their families every day in a typical week compared with just 27% of 17-year-olds. Adolescents who eat meals with their families have been found to have better academic performance and to be less likely to engage in risky behaviors such as drinking alcohol and smoking compared with peers who do not frequently engage in family meals (Neumark-Sztainer et al., 2010).

Developing healthful eating patterns at family meals during adolescence may improve the likelihood that individuals will choose to consume nutritious foods in adulthood (Larson et al., 2007). Family meals not only allow for more communication between teens and their parents, but they also provide an ideal environment during which parents can model healthy food and beverage choices and attitudes toward eating. Teens who eat at home more frequently have been found to consume fewer soft drinks and more calcium-rich foods, fruit, and vegetables (see *Focus On:* Family Meals and Nutritional Benefits for Teens).

Media and Advertising

Marketing to teenagers has become a multibillion-dollar business. It is estimated that the nation's largest food and beverage companies spend $1.6 billion per year to market their products to youth (Federal Trade Commission, 2008). Food and beverage companies promote their products to youth using a number of different techniques (e.g., contests, product placements, sponsorships, celebrity endorsements, viral marketing) and multiple platforms.

American youth spend 7.5 hours per day with media and, given the amount of time they spend using more than one medium at a time, they are exposed to more than 10.5 hours of media content (Rideout et al., 2010). Outside of school work, on an average day, youth spend 4.5 hours watching television and movies, 2.5 hours listening to radio or recorded music, 1.5 hours using a computer, 1.2 hours playing video games, and 38 minutes reading magazines or books. The majority of youth (71%) have a television and 33% have Internet access in their bedroom. As the time that youth spend with media has increased over time (Rideout et al., 2010), so has the ability for advertisers to influence their eating behaviors. It is estimated that teenagers (13-17 years) view more than 28,000 television advertisements per year or more than 217 hours of advertising (Gantz et al., 2007). More than 20% of television advertisements viewed by teens are for food products (Gantz et al., 2007), and most viewed food advertisements (89%) are for products high in fat, sugar, or sodium (Powell et al., 2007). In addition, more than two thirds of the nation's largest food and beverage companies market their products to youth online (Federal Trade Commission, 2008). Media literacy education can and should be taught to teens to assist them in determining the accuracy and validity of media and advertising messages.

Dieting and Body Image

Body image concerns are common during adolescence. Many teens describe themselves as being overweight despite being of normal weight, signifying a disturbance in their

FOCUS ON

Family Meals and Nutritional Benefits for Teens

When teens regularly share mealtimes with their families, they are more likely to have diets of higher nutritional quality (Neumark-Sztainer et al., 2010). One study examined whether this relationship may hold true not only for the general population, but also for racially diverse teens at risk for academic failure (Fulkerson et al., 2009). Students at six alternative high schools in the Minneapolis-St. Paul metropolitan area of Minnesota were surveyed about their dietary practices and other aspects of health. More than half (60%) of students at these schools qualified for free or reduced-price school meals. Among these students, 50% reported eating family dinners five to seven times per week, 24% reported eating family dinners one to four times per week, and 26% reported not eating family dinners in the past week. The results showed that family dinner frequency was related to higher daily fruit consumption and lower rates of overweight. However, in contrast to other studies, family dinner frequency was not related to vegetable consumption, high-fat food intake, regular soda consumption, or use of weight-loss practices. Health professionals should be aware that intervention programs to promote family meals may be beneficial, but such programs need to direct attention to the specific needs of at-risk teens, including the affordability of healthful foods for families.

body image. Data from the Youth Risk Behavior Survey (YRBS) found that 16% of U.S. high school students described themselves as being overweight despite being of normal weight (Talamayan et al., 2006). Females were more likely to report this misperception than males (25% vs. 7%).

Poor body image can lead to weight control issues and dieting. Data from the 2007 YRBS show that 45% of U.S. high school students were attempting to lose weight. White and Hispanic females had the highest prevalence of dieting at 62%, followed by black females (49%), Hispanic males (38%), white males (29%), and black males (25%) (Eaton et al., 2008). The prevalence of dieting increased with age among females, but decreased with age among males.

Approximately half (53%) of females and 28% of males reported eating fewer calories or less fat in the previous month to either lose weight or prevent weight gain (Eaton et al., 2008). Additionally, 67% of females and 55% of males had exercised in the previous month to lose weight or prevent weight gain. These behaviors can be viewed as healthy weight loss behaviors when used in moderation, and can be a starting point for nutrition education and counseling to improve eating behaviors.

Not all dieting behaviors have the potential to improve health, however. High-risk dieting practices are used by many teens and carry with them the risk of poor nutritional status and increased risk for **disordered eating** (see Chapter 23). Fasting, or refraining from eating for more than 24 hours, was practiced by 16% of female and 7% of male U.S. high school students in the past month as a means of dieting (Eaton et al., 2008). Seven percent of females and four percent of males had used diet pills to lose weight; the prevalence of this behavior was higher among white and Hispanic students and increased with age. The use of purging methods, including vomiting and laxative or diuretic use, was reported by 6% of females and 2% of males. White and Hispanic females were more likely to report purging behaviors than black females. In contrast, black and Hispanic males were more likely to report purging behaviors than white males.

NUTRITION SCREENING, ASSESSMENT, AND COUNSELING

The Guidelines for Adolescent Preventive Services recommend that adolescents have an annual health screening to determine risk factors for acute and chronic disease, with screening for nutrition risk (American Medical Association, 2006). Nutrition screening should include the assessment of height, weight, and BMI to determine weight status; detection of potentially high-risk dietary habits such as calorie restriction, vegetarianism, and dealing with food allergies; and the evaluation of the presence of iron-deficiency anemia (females only). See Chapters 6-9.

Weight, height, and BMI should be plotted using the Centers for Disease Control and Prevention National Center for Health Statistics BMI tables to determine appropriateness of weight for height. Although BMI is not a direct measure of body fatness and thus cannot be used to clinically assess obesity, it is highly correlated with body fatness and is the recommended screening method for weight status among youth (Freedman and Sherry, 2009). A BMI below the fifth percentile may signal the presence of chronic or metabolic disease, growth failure, or an eating disorder. A BMI at or above the 85th percentile, but below the 95th percentile, indicates that an adolescent is at risk for overweight, whereas a BMI at or above the 95th percentile indicates the presence of overweight. All BMI values that indicate the presence of overweight risk should be corroborated with a direct measure of body fat to determine that excessive fat, or obesity, is truly indicated.

When nutrition screening indicates the presence of nutritional risk, a full assessment should be conducted. Components of a full nutrition assessment are listed in Table 19-7. Nutrition assessment should include a complete evaluation of food intake through a 24-hour recall, dietary records, or brief food frequency questionnaire (see Chapter 6). The adequacy of energy, fiber, macronutrients, and micronutrients should be determined, as well as excessive intake of any dietary components such as sodium or sweeteners.

Nutritional assessments also should include an evaluation of the nutritional environment, including parental, peer, school, cultural, and personal lifestyle factors. The attitude of the adolescent toward food and nutrition is also important; helping them overcome their perceived barriers to eating well is an essential component of nutrition counseling,

Teens who live in food-insecure households, temporary housing, or shelters, or who have run away from home are at especially high nutritional risk, as are adolescents who use alcohol and street drugs. It is important that health professionals working with high-risk teens develop partnerships with community-based food assistance programs to ensure that youths have access to a steady, nutritious food supply. Homeless teens, as well as those living in temporary shelters, benefit from nutrition counseling focusing on lightweight, low-cost, prepackaged foods that do not require refrigeration or cooking facilities. Dried fruit, nuts, granola bars, cereal bars, tuna in pouches, and meat jerky are foods that should be available for runaway or homeless teens.

Education and counseling should be tailored to meet any specific nutrition diagnoses identified during the assessment. A teen who has been found to be overweight with type 2 diabetes requires a different type and intensity of counseling than a teen who has been diagnosed with iron-deficiency anemia. Knowledge, attitude, and behavior must be addressed when guiding adolescents toward acquiring healthful food habits. For a plan to succeed, the adolescent must be willing to change; therefore an assessment of a teenager's desire to change is essential. Encouraging the desire to change usually requires much attention (see Chapter 15).

Information can be provided in various settings ranging from the classroom to the hospital. The clinician must understand the change process and how to meaningfully

TABLE 19-7

Elements of a Nutritional Screening and Assessment for Adolescents

	Medical and Psychosocial History	Growth and Development	Diet and Physical Activity	Routine Screenings and Laboratory Tests
Components of an initial nutrition screening	Medical history Psychosocial history Socioeconomic status and history	BMI SMR	Meal and snacking patterns Nutrient and nonnutrient supplement use Food security Food allergies and intolerances Special dietary practices Alcohol consumption Physical activity and competitive sports	Hemoglobin (females) Serum cholesterol or blood lipids Blood pressure
Indications for an in-depth nutritional assessment	Chronic disease Substance use Poverty or homelessness Depression or dysthymia Disordered eating Eating disorders Body image disorders Pregnancy or lactation	Underweight Overweight At risk for overweight Delayed sexual maturation Short stature or stunting	Food insecurity Meal skipping Inadequate micronutrient intake Excessive intake of total or saturated fat Food allergy or intolerance Vegetarian diet Use of nonnutritional or herbal supplements Competition in competitive sports Chronic dieting Fasting Alcohol consumption	Hypertension Hyperlipidemia Iron deficiency anemia Hyperglycemia

Reprinted with permission from Stang J, Story M, editors: Guidelines for adolescent nutrition services, Minneapolis, 2005, Center for Leadership Education and Training in Maternal and Child Nutrition, Division of Epidemiology and Community Health, School of Public Health, University of Minnesota.

BMI, Body mass index; *SMR,* sexual maturity rating.

communicate this process. Parents may be included in the process and are encouraged to be supportive. Recommended eating plans based on recommended energy intakes for adolescents are shown in Table 19-8.

SPECIAL CONCERNS

Vegetarian Dietary Patterns

As adolescents mature they begin to develop autonomous social, moral, and ethical values. These values may lead to vegetarian eating practices because of concerns about animal welfare, the environment, or personal health. Concerns about body weight also motivate some adolescents to adopt a vegetarian diet because it is a socially acceptable way to reduce dietary fat. Recent data confirm that adolescents who consume vegetarian diets are less likely to be overweight or obese than their omnivorous peers (Robinson-O'Brien et al., 2009). Well-planned vegetarian diets that include a variety of legumes, nuts, and whole grains can provide adequate nutrients for teens who have completed the majority of their growth and development (Figure 19-5).

Vegetarian diets that become increasingly more restrictive should be viewed with caution, however, because this may signal the development of disordered eating, with the vegetarian diet used as a means to hide a restriction of food intake (Robinson-O'Brien et al., 2009). Both teen males and females who adopt vegetarian dietary patterns have been found to use more high-risk weight control behaviors, especially vomiting, to lose weight (Robinson-O'Brien et al., 2009). This increased risk for unhealthy weight control behaviors seems to persist even after the vegetarian eating style is discontinued, suggesting that although the issues are related, vegetarian diets likely do not cause disordered eating and instead may serve as an early symptom.

Vegetarian adolescents often have high intakes of iron, vitamin A, and fiber and low intakes of dietary cholesterol. Vegetarian diets that include eggs or dairy products are consistent with the Dietary Guidelines for Americans and can meet the DRIs for all nutrients. A sample eating plan to assist vegetarian teens in achieving adequate energy and nutrient intakes is listed in Table 19-9. Vegan and macrobiotic diets, which do not include animal products of any kind, do not provide natural sources of vitamin B_{12} and may be deficient in calcium, vitamin D, zinc, and iron (Kirby &

TABLE 19-8

Recommended Number of Servings for Adolescents Ages 13 and 16 Years Based on Activity Level

	Grains (ounce)	Vegetables (cup)	Fruit (cup)	Milk (cup)	Meat or Beans (ounce)	Whole Grains (ounce)*
Males						
13 Years						
≤30 min physical activity/day	6	2.5	2	3	5.5	3
30-60 min physical activity/day	7	3	2	3	6	3.5
≥60 min physical activity/day	9	3.5	2	3	6.5	4.5
16 Years						
≤30 min physical activity/day	8	3	2	3	6.5	4
30-60 min physical activity/day	10	3.5	2.5	3	7	5
≥60 min physical activity/day	10	4	2.5	3	7	4
Females						
13 Years						
≤30 min physical activity/day	5	2	1.5	3	5	3
30-60 min physical activity/day	6	2.5	2	3	5.5	3
≥60 min physical activity/day	7	3	2	3	6	3.5
16 Years						
≤30 min physical activity/day	6	2.5	1.5	3	5	3
30-60 min physical activity/day	6	2.5	2	3	5.5	3
≥60 min physical activity/day	8	3	2	3	6.5	4

*Number of servings of whole grains are not in addition to but are included in the number of servings of grains.

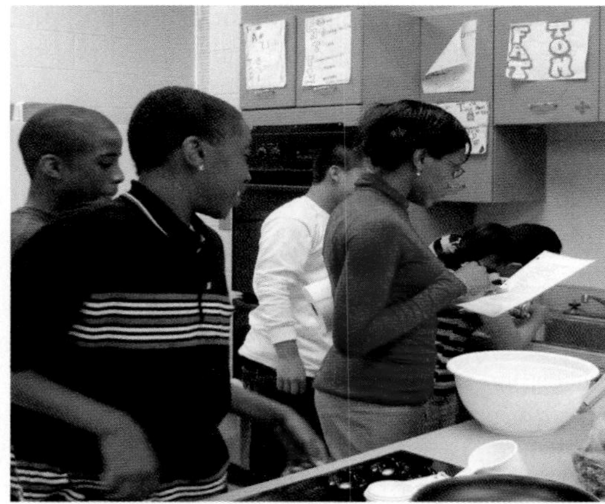

FIGURE 19-5 Teenagers who help to prepare safe, nutritious meals become engaged in the healthy eating process.

TABLE 19-9

Suggested Daily Food Intake Guide for Vegetarian Adolescents

Food Group	Servings/Day*
Bread, grains, cereal	9-11
Legumes	2-3
Vegetables	4-5
Fruits	4
Nuts, seeds	1
Milk, yogurt, cheese	3
Eggs (limit three/week)	½
Fats, oils (added)	4-6
Sugar (added teaspoons)	6-9

Modified from Story M, Holt K, Sofka D, editors: Bright futures in practice: nutrition, ed 2, Arlington, Va, 2002, National Center for Education in Maternal and Child Health.

*Age 11 years or older; 2200-2800 kcal.

Danner, 2009). Therefore it is imperative that vegan adolescents choose foods that are fortified with these nutrients or take a daily multivitamin-mineral supplement. Adolescents and their caregivers should be instructed on the planning of well-balanced vegetarian diets and fortified foods that can prevent potential nutrient deficiencies.

Disordered Eating and Eating Disorders

It is estimated that 10% to 20% of teens engage in disordered eating behaviors, such as binge-purge behavior, compensatory exercise, laxative and diuretic abuse, and binge eating (CDC 2008). These behaviors do not occur with enough regularity or frequency to be diagnosed as an eating disorder, but may still have significant health implications for teens. Symptoms that may signal the presence of disordered eating behaviors include recurring gastrointestinal complaints, amenorrhea, or unexplained weight loss. Overweight females have been found to be twice as likely to engage in disordered eating behaviors. A screening for disordered eating can easily be done and should include questions about body dissatisfaction, fear of becoming obese, frequency of dieting and fasting, use of laxatives and diuretics, use of diet pills, fear of certain foods (e.g., foods containing fat or sugar), vomiting, bingeing, and compensatory exercise (see Chapter 23).

Eating disorders are the third most common chronic illness in adolescent females, with an incidence of from 1.5% to 5%. In general, anorexia nervosa is characterized by a dangerously low body weight, preoccupation with thinness, and restrictive dietary behaviors. Bulimia nervosa is characterized by a body weight that is close to normal, episodes of uncontrollable eating (bingeing), and efforts to eliminate calories or food from the body (purging). Binge eating disorder is characterized by frequent, recurrent episodes of binge eating and loss of control over eating.

Diagnostic criteria for eating disorders provided by the *Diagnostic and Statistical Manual of Mental Disorders*, 4th edition, need to be used judiciously with adolescents because of issues surrounding normal growth and development. The wide variability in the rate, timing, and velocity of height and weight gain during normal puberty; the absence of menstrual periods in early puberty combined with the unpredictability of menses soon after menarche; and the cognitive inability to understand abstract concepts limit the application of the diagnostic criteria to adolescents (American Dietetic Association, 2006). Adolescents are particularly vulnerable to the complications of eating disorders. The effect of malnutrition on linear growth, brain development, and bone acquisition can be persistent and irreversible. Yet with early and aggressive treatment, adolescents have the potential for a better outcome than adults who have had the disease longer (Steinhausen, 2008).

Obesity

Adolescent obesity has both short- and long-term health consequences. Adolescents who are overweight are at higher risk for hyperlipidemia, hypertension, insulin resistance, and type 2 diabetes compared with normal weight peers (Cali and Carpior, 2008; Daniels et al., 2005). Data from NHANES suggest that the prevalence of metabolic syndrome is increasing among adolescents, from a rate of 9.2% in the 1988-1994 survey to 12.7% in the 1999-2000 survey (de Ferranti et al., 2006). Epidemiologic studies of obesity and disease risk demonstrate an increased risk of morbidity from coronary heart disease, arteriosclerosis, specific types of cancer, gout, and arthritis among individuals who were overweight or obese during adolescence (van Dam et al., 2006).

Adolescent weight status is evaluated based on BMI (weight/height^2 [kg/m^2]) as shown in Appendixes 12 and 16. Among 12- to 19-year-olds in the United States, the prevalence of overweight, characterized by a BMI higher than the 85th percentile, is 34.2% (Ogden et al., 2010). The prevalence of obesity (BMI ≥95th percentile) is 18.1%. Obesity is a complex, multifactorial health issue that is influenced by genetics, metabolic efficiency, PAL, dietary intake, and environmental and psychosocial factors. Adolescents who are found to be overweight should have a fasting lipid profile completed and should be assessed for additional risk factors for chronic disease, such as personal history of hypertension, hyperlipidemia, and tobacco use, and family history of hypertension, early cardiovascular death, stroke, hyperlipidemia, and type 2 diabetes mellitus (Krebs et al., 2007). If risk factors are noted, aspartate aminotransferase and alanine aminotransferase measurements to assess liver function should be obtained as well.

A fasting glucose level should be drawn on any overweight adolescent with two or more risk factors for CVD or with a family history of diabetes. Obese teens should undergo the same laboratory assessments as overweight children, with the addition of microalbumin/creatinine or microalbumin/creatinine ratio. Additional assessments for conditions such as sleep apnea, orthopedic disorders, polycystic ovary disease, and hormonal abnormalities should be performed based on presenting symptoms.

Recent guidelines for adolescent overweight and obesity suggest a staged care treatment process based on a teen's BMI, age, motivation, and the presence of comorbid conditions (Spear et al., 2007). Four stages are recommended, with progress through the stages based on age, biological development, level of motivation, weight status, and success with previous stages of treatment. Each of the stages is briefly described in the following text.

Overweight adolescents start out in Stage 1 if they do not display comorbid conditions or have not completed the adolescent growth spurt. Stage 1 consists of general nutrition and physical activity advice to promote health and prevent disease. Educational components for this stage of treatment include consuming 5 or more servings of fruits and vegetables per day, reducing consumption of sweetened beverages, participating in at least 60 minutes of physical activity each day, and limiting screen time (movies, Internet, television, and computer and video games) to no more than 2 hours per day. Nutrition topics that are particularly important to discuss with overweight adolescents during Stage 1 include the importance of breakfast consumption, limiting food eaten outside the home or school (including fast food), eating meals with their family at least five times per week, and appropriate portion size. This stage of obesity treatment can be provided by a single health care provider, including physicians, nurses, and dietitians who have training in pediatric weight management.

Stage 2 builds on the same concepts as Stage 1, but in a more structured way. A key component of Stage 2 is the monitoring of food and beverage intake by adolescents or their parents, usually done through daily food and exercise journals or record books. Screen time is more limited in Stage 2 to less than 1 hour per day and a meal plan is introduced to provide further guidance for dietary intake. Successful lifestyle changes should be reinforced through the use of age-appropriate, nonfood rewards such as tickets to a local event or museum, jewelry, clothing, or music. Stage 2 can be provided by a single health care provider with training in motivational counseling. Referrals for additional services such as physical therapy or counseling may be necessary for some adolescents during Stage 2. Monthly follow-up and assessment of progress is suggested for both Stages 1 and 2.

Stage 3 is more structured than Stage 2 and is provided by a multidisciplinary team consisting of a physician or pediatric nurse practitioner, a counselor (psychologist or social worker), a registered dietitian, and an exercise physiology or physical therapist. This treatment stage recommends 8-12 weeks of weekly appointments with the adolescent and their family, followed by monthly or bimonthly follow-up appointments. A highly structured meal plan and physical activity schedule are implemented, along with a formal behavior modification program.

Stage 4 treatment is reserved for severely obese adolescents or those who have significant comorbidities that require concerted intervention. This treatment stage is available only in clinical settings that employ a full range of health professionals who are specifically trained in the behavioral and medical management of pediatric obesity. Intensive dietary regimens such as meal replacement, protein-sparing modified fasts, oral medication, and bariatric surgery may be used in this stage.

Concern has been expressed regarding the use of bariatric surgery in adolescents. Recommendations for bariatric surgery suggest that it is only appropriate in severely overweight teens (BMI >40) with severe comorbid medical conditions or those with a BMI of more than 50 who have completed most of their physical growth and development (Pratt et al., 2009). Difficulty in complying with dietary restrictions following surgery may lead to complications such as dumping syndrome following high carbohydrate intake, voluntary excessive food intake, meat impacted in a gastrojejunal anastomosis, and B vitamin deficiency caused by poor compliance with vitamin-mineral supplementation

Hyperlipidemia and Hypertension

Hyperlipidemia and hypertension, both risk factors for CVD, are apparent in adolescence and have been shown to be predictive of CVD risk in later life (Celermajer and Ayer, 2006; Gidding, 2007). Table 19-10 lists the classification criteria for the diagnosis of hyperlipidemia among youth. National data suggest that one in five adolescents 12-19 years old has elevated blood lipid levels (CDC, 2010). The prevalence of hyperlipidemia among adolescents was not consistent, however. The prevalence of hyperlipidemia was 14% among normal weight, 22% among overweight, and 43% among obese teens. The prevalence of low high-density lipoprotein (HDL) cholesterol and high triglyceride levels appeared to increase with age. Adolescent males were almost three times more likely to have low HDL cholesterol levels compared with females at any age. These youth are considered candidates for therapeutic lifestyle counseling with emphasis on nutrition and physical activity intervention.

It is important to consider secondary causes of hyperlipidemia when determining dietary treatment options (Table 19-11). Nutrition intervention for elevated blood lipids focuses on reducing the intake of total, saturated, and trans fat and limiting dietary cholesterol intakes. Promoting healthy lifestyle behaviors to reduce CVD risk should include a discussion of the benefits of regular physical activity in addition to dietary recommendations.

National screening criteria for blood pressure levels among adolescents are listed in Tables 19-12 and 19-13.

TABLE 19-10

Classification of LDL and Total Cholesterol Levels in Adolescents*

	Acceptable	Borderline	High
Total cholesterol (mg/dL)	≤170	170-199	≥200
LDL cholesterol (mg/dL)	<110	110-129	≥130
HDL cholesterol (mg/dL)	≥35	Not applicable	Not applicable
Triglycerides (mg/dL)	≤150	Not applicable	Not applicable

Data from National Cholesterol Education Program (U.S.): Report of the expert panel on blood cholesterol levels in children and adolescents, NIH publication no. 91-2732, Bethesda, Md, 1991, National Institutes of Health, National Heart, Lung, and Blood Institute; National Cholesterol Education Program: Cholesterol in childhood (RE9805) policy statement, Am Acad Pediatr 101(1):141, 1998. Accessed 10 November 2006 from http://www.aappolicy.aappublications.org/.

*Based on the average of two measurements.

HDL, High-density lipoprotein; *LDL*, low-density lipoprotein.

TABLE 19-11

Secondary Causes of Hyperlipidemia

Lipid Abnormality			
Anabolic steroid use	↑ LDL	↓ HDL	
Anorexia nervosa	↑ LDL		
Cigarette smoking		↓ HDL	
Diabetes	↑ LDL	↑ TG	↓ HDL
Hypothyroidism		↑TG	
Liver disease, obstructive	↑ LDL		
Medications: corticosteroids, bile acid–binding resins, anticonvulsants, certain oral contraceptives, isotretinoin (Accutane), medroxyprogesterone (Depo Provera)	Varies		
Overweight or obesity	↑ LDL	↑ TG	↓ HDL
Renal disease	Varies		
Therapeutic diet: ketogenic; high carbohydrate	↑ LDL	↑ TG	
Transplant (bone marrow, heart, kidney, or liver)		↑ TG	↓ HDL

Reprinted with permission from Stang J, Story M, editors: Guidelines for adolescent nutrition services, Minneapolis, 2005, Center for Leadership Education and Training in Maternal and Child Nutrition, Division of Epidemiology and Community Health, School of Public Health, University of Minnesota.

HDL, High-density lipoprotein; *LDL*, low-density lipoprotein; *TG*, triglyceride.

TABLE 19-12

90th and 95th Percentiles for Blood Pressure for Adolescent Males by Height Percentiles

	Height Percentiles*	Systolic BP (mm Hg)							Diastolic BP (mm Hg)						
Age	BP†	5%	10%	25%	50%	75%	90%	95%	5%	10%	25%	50%	75%	90%	95%
10	90th	111	112	114	115	117	119	119	73	73	74	75	76	77	78
	95th	115	116	117	119	121	122	123	77	78	79	80	81	81	82
11	90th	113	114	115	117	119	120	121	74	74	75	76	77	78	78
	95th	117	118	119	121	123	124	125	78	78	79	80	81	82	82
12	90th	115	116	118	120	121	123	123	74	75	75	76	77	78	79
	95th	119	120	122	123	125	127	127	78	79	80	81	82	82	83
13	90th	117	118	120	122	124	125	126	75	75	76	77	78	79	79
	95th	121	122	124	126	128	129	130	79	79	80	81	82	83	83
14	90th	120	121	123	125	126	128	128	75	76	77	78	79	79	80
	95th	124	125	127	128	130	132	132	80	80	81	82	83	84	84
15	90th	122	124	125	127	129	130	131	76	77	78	79	80	80	81
	95th	126	127	129	131	133	134	135	81	81	82	83	84	85	85
16	90th	125	126	128	130	131	133	134	78	78	79	80	81	82	82
	95th	129	130	132	134	135	137	137	82	83	83	84	85	86	87
17	90th	127	128	130	132	134	135	136	80	80	81	82	83	84	84
	95th	131	132	134	136	138	139	140	84	85	86	87	87	88	89

From National High Blood Pressure Education Program Working Group on High Blood Pressure in Children and Adolescents: Fourth report on the diagnosis, evaluation, and treatment of high blood pressure in children and adolescents, Pediatrics 114(2):555-576, 2004. This supplement is a work of the U.S. government, published in the public domain by the American Academy of Pediatrics. Available at http://www.pediatrics.org/cgi/content/full/114/2/S2/555.

BP, Blood pressure.

*Height percentile determined by standard growth curves.

†Blood pressure percentile determined by a single measurement.

TABLE 19-13

90th and 95th Percentiles for Blood Pressure for Adolescent Females by Height Percentiles

	Height Percentiles*	Systolic BP (mm Hg)							Diastolic BP (mm Hg)						
Age	BP†	5%	10%	25%	50%	75%	90%	95%	5%	10%	25%	50%	75%	90%	95%
10	90th	112	112	114	115	116	118	118	73	73	73	74	75	76	76
	95th	116	116	117	119	120	121	122	77	77	77	78	79	80	80
11	90th	114	114	116	117	118	119	120	74	74	74	75	76	77	77
	95th	118	118	119	121	122	123	124	78	78	78	79	80	81	81
12	90th	116	116	117	119	120	121	122	75	75	75	76	77	78	78
	95th	119	120	121	123	124	125	126	79	79	79	80	81	82	82
13	90th	117	118	119	121	122	123	124	76	76	76	77	78	79	79
	95th	121	122	123	124	126	127	128	80	80	80	81	82	83	83
14	90th	119	120	121	122	124	125	125	77	77	77	78	79	80	81
	95th	123	124	125	126	127	129	129	81	81	81	82	83	84	84
15	90th	120	121	122	123	125	126	127	78	78	78	79	80	81	81
	95th	124	125	126	127	129	130	131	82	82	82	83	84	85	86
16	90th	121	122	123	124	126	127	128	78	78	79	80	81	81	82
	95th	125	126	127	128	130	131	132	82	82	83	84	85	85	86
17	90th	122	122	123	125	126	127	128	78	79	79	80	81	81	82
	95th	125	126	127	129	130	131	132	82	83	83	84	85	85	86

From National High Blood Pressure Education Program Working Group on High Blood Pressure in Children and Adolescents: Fourth report on the diagnosis, evaluation, and treatment of high blood pressure in children and adolescents, Pediatrics 114(2):555-576, 2004. This supplement is a work of the U.S. government, published in the public domain by the American Academy of Pediatrics. Available at http://www.pediatrics.org/cgi/content/full/114/2/S2/555.

BP, Blood pressure.

*Height percentile determined by standard growth curves.

†Blood pressure percentile determined by a single measurement.

Teenagers 17 years of age and younger are determined to have prehypertension if their average blood pressure readings fall between the 90th and 94th percentiles. Hypertension is diagnosed when the average of three blood pressure measurements exceed the 95th percentile for age, gender, and height.

Dietary counseling and weight management are integral components of hypertension treatment. The Dietary Approaches to Stop Hypertension (DASH) eating pattern has been shown to be effective in reducing blood pressure in many individuals (see Chapter 34 and Appendix 33). In addition to the DASH diet, teens with elevated blood pressure should be counseled to reduce sodium intake to less than 2000 mg/day and to achieve and maintain a healthy body weight.

Physical Activity

National recommendations for physical activity suggest that all youth should be active at least 60 minutes each day, including participating in vigorous activity at least 3 days each week (U.S. Department of Health and Human Service, 2008). In addition, muscle-strengthening and bone-strengthening activities should each be included in the 60 minutes of physical activity at least three times a week. However, many youths do not meet these recommendations. Only 35% of U.S. students report being physically active for 5 days or more per week, with males nearly twice as likely to meet recommendations as females (CDC, 2008).

Teenage athletes have unique nutrient needs. Adequate fluid intake to prevent dehydration is especially critical for young athletes. Young adolescents are at higher risk for dehydration because they produce more heat during exercise but have less ability to transfer heat from the muscles to the skin. They also sweat less, which decreases their capacity to dissipate heat through the evaporation of the sweat (see Chapter 24).

Athletes who participate in sports that use competitive weight categories or emphasize body weight are at elevated risk for the development of disordered eating behaviors. A concern among female athletes is the female athlete triad relationship, a constellation of low body weight and inadequate body fat levels, amenorrhea, and osteoporosis (see Chapter 23). Female athlete triad may lead to premature bone loss, decreased bone density, increased risk of stress fractures, and eventual infertility (Gottschlich and Young, 2008). Nutrition assessment and education for teenaged athletes should focus on obtaining adequate energy and macro- and micronutrients to meet the needs for growth and development and to maintain a healthy body weight. The use of anabolic agents (such as steroids or insulin) and other ergogenic supplements should also be included in nutrition screening. Survey data suggest that up to 8% of high school students use creatine, 5% use steroids, and 4% use androstenedione (Castillo and Comstock, 2007; CDC, 2008).

Pregnancy

Adolescent females who become pregnant are at particularly high risk for nutritional deficiencies because of elevated nutrient needs. Pregnant adolescents with a **gynecologic age** (the number of years between the onset of menses and current age) of less than 4 and those who are undernourished at the time of conception have the greatest nutritional needs. As with adult women, pregnant teens require additional folic acid, iron, zinc, calcium, and other micronutrients to support fetal growth (see Chapter 16). Pregnant teens should have a full nutrition assessment done early in pregnancy to determine any nutrient deficiencies and to promote adequate weight gain. Weight gain recommendations for pregnancy are listed in Chapter 16. Referral to appropriate food assistance programs such as the Special Supplemental Food Program for Women, Infants and Children is an important part of prenatal nutrition education.

USEFUL WEBSITES

American Academy of Pediatrics Media Matters Program
www.aap.org/advocacy/mmcamp.htm

American Alliance for Health, Physical Education, Recreation and Dance
www.aahperd.org

American School Health Association
www.ashaweb.org

Bright Futures
www.brightfutures.org

Centers for Disease Control and Prevention
www.cdc.gov

Empowered Parents
www.empoweredparents.com

National Collegiate Athletics Association
www.ncaa.org

National Eating Disorder Association
www.nationaleatingdisorders.org

School Nutrition Association
www.schoolnutrition.org

Vegetarian Resource Group
www.vrg.org

CLINICAL SCENARIO

Shawna is a 17-year-old girl who is being seen at the pediatric clinic today for a preemployment physical. The physician has recommended that she talk with you, the nutritionist, about her eating habits because her hemoglobin level was low. When you question Shawna about her eating habits, she reveals that she skips breakfast each day because she doesn't have time to eat in the morning, but she does have a cup of coffee on her way to school at 7:15 am. Shawna's first food intake is usually a snack from the vending machine at 10:30 am, which consists of a candy bar or a bag of chips and a soft drink. Occasionally she purchases ala carte lunches of tacos or a burger, but generally she skips lunch. Shawna gets out of school at 2 pm and goes to work at the mall. She has a half-hour break in the late afternoon, so she goes to the food court for dinner. The evening meal usually consists of one to two slices of pizza, two tacos, or one to two pieces of chicken with a soft drink. About half of the time she also orders fries or chips. When Shawna gets home from work at 9 pm, she usually has a snack of ice cream, tortilla chips, spicy cheese puffs, or microwave popcorn. She usually has a large glass of juice or lemonade with her snack.

When you suggest to Shawna that she might benefit from eating meals rather than snacks, she says she doesn't have time to cook meals, especially in the morning. She also tells you that there are no other food choices besides fast foods at the mall where she works.

Nutrition Diagnostic Statements

1. Undesirable food choices related to perceived limitations of work and school as evidenced by daily intake of high-fat, high-sugar foods.
2. Inadequate iron intake related to low intake of iron-containing foods as evidenced by diet history reflecting 70% of dietary reference intake for iron.

Nutrition Care Questions

1. What types of foods might you suggest to Shawna to have for breakfast? Why would you choose these foods?
2. What is the recommended iron intake for a girl of Shawna's age? Does it appear that she is getting adequate iron intake from her diet? What food choices would you recommend for Shawn to increase her hemoglobin level?
3. How much calcium does a 17-year-old teen girl need? What suggestions could you make to increase Shawna's calcium intake based on the foods she likes and the places she eats?
4. What types of foods might you suggest that Shawna choose at the mall fast food court to improve her nutrient intake and to help treat her anemia?

REFERENCES

American Dietetic Association: Position of the American Dietetic Association: nutrition intervention in the treatment of anorexia nervosa, bulimia nervosa, and eating disorders not otherwise specified (EDNOS), *J Am Diet Assoc* 106:2073, 2006.

American Medical Association: Guidelines for adolescent preventive services recommendations monograph, 2006. Accessed 12 December 2006 from www.ama-assn.org/ama/upload/mm/39/gapsmono.pdf.

Bachman JL, et al: Sources of food group intakes among the US populations, 2001-2002, *J Am Diet Assoc* 108:804, 2008.

Calfee R, Fadale P: Popular ergogenic drugs and supplements in young athletes, *Pediatrics* 117:e577, 2006.

Cali AMG, Caprio S: Obesity in children and adolescents, *J Clin Endocrinol Metab* 93:S31, 2008.

Castillo EM, Comstock RD: Prevalence of performance-enhancing substances among United States adolescents, *Pediatr Clin N Am* 54:663, 2007.

Celermajer DS, Ayer JG: Childhood risk factors for adult cardiovascular disease and primary prevention in childhood, *Heart* 92:1701, 2006.

Centers for Disease Control and Prevention: Recommendations to prevent and control iron deficiency in the United States. *MMWR* 47(RR-3):1-29, 1998. Available online at http://www.cdc.gov/mmwr/preview/mmwrhtml/00051880.htm through http://www.cdc.gov. Accessed Jan 11, 2011.

Centers for Disease Control and Prevention (CDC): Youth risk behavior surveillance—United States 2007, *MMWR Morb Mortal Wkly Rep* 57(SS-4), 2008.

Centers for Disease Control and Prevention (CDC): Prevalence of abnormal lipid levels among youths—United States, 1999-2006, *MMWR Morb Mortal Wkly Rep* 59(2):29, 2010.

Cutler GJ, et al: Multiple Sociodemographic and Socioenvironmental Characteristics Are Correlated with Major Patterns of Dietary Intake in Adolescents. *J Am Diet Assoc* 111:230, 2011.

Daniels SR, et al: Overweight in children and adolescents: pathophysiology, consequences, prevention, and treatment, *Circulation* 111:1999, 2005.

De Ferranti SD, et al: Inflammation and changes in metabolic syndrome abnormalities in US adolescents: findings from the 1988-1994 and 1999-2000 National Health and Nutrition Examination surveys, *Clin Chem* 52:1325, 2006.

Eaton DK, et al: Youth risk behavior surveillance—United States, 2007, *MMWR Surveill Summ* 57(4):1, 2008.

Federal Trade Commission: *Marketing food to children and adolescents: a review of industry expenditures, activities, and self-regulation*, Washington, DC, 2008, Federal Trade Commission.

Fox C, et al: Availability and consumption of competitive foods in US public schools, *J Am Diet Assoc* 109:S57, 2009.

Frazao E: Meal patterns, milk and soft drink consumption and supplement use, *Agriculture Information Bulletin 796-804*, February 2005, USDA Economic Research Service. Accessed from http://www.ers.usda.gov/publications/aib796/aib796-4/aib796-4.pdf

Freedman DS, Sherry B. The Validity of BMI as an Indicator of Body Fatness and Risk Among Children. PEDIATRICS Vol. 124 Supplement September 2009, pp. S23-S34.

Fulkerson J, et al: Are there nutritional and other benefits associated with family meals among at-risk youth? *J Adolesc Health* 45:389, 2009.

Gantz W, et al: *Food for thought: television food advertising to children in the United States*, Menlo Park, Calif, 2007, Kaiser Family Foundation.

Gidding SS: Physical activity, physical fitness and cardiovascular risk factors in childhood, *Am J Lifestyle Med* 1:499, 2007.

Ginde AA, et al: Demographic differences and trends of vitamin D insufficiency in the US population, 1988-2004, *Arch Intern Med* 169:626, 2009.

Goh YY, et al: Using community-based participatory research to identify potential interventions to overcome barriers to adolescents' healthy eating and physical activity, *J Behav Med* 32:491, 2009.

Gordon A, et al: *School Nutrition Dietary Assessment Study-III: volume I: school foodservice, school food environment, and meals offered and served*, Princeton, N.J., 2007, Mathematica Policy Research, Inc.

Gottschlich LM, Young CC: Female athlete triad, eMedicine specialties, 30 May 2008. Accessed 1 March 2010 from http://emedicine.medscape.com/article/89260-overview.

Ingersoll GM: Psychological and social development. In McAnarney ER, Kreipe RE, editors: *Textbook of adolescent medicine*, Philadelphia, 1992, Saunders.

Institute of Institute of Medicine (IOM) Food and Nutrition Board: *Dietary Reference Intakes for Calcium and Vitamin D.* Washington, DC, 2010, National Academies Press.

Institute of Medicine (IOM), et al: *Dietary reference intakes: the essential guide to nutrient requirements*, Washington, DC, 2006, National Academies Press.

Kirby M, Danner E: Nutritional deficiencies in children on restricted diets, *Pediatr Clin N Am* 56:1085, 2009.

Krebs NF, et al: Assessment of child and adolescent overweight and obesity, *Pediatrics* 120:S193, 2007.

Larson xxx, et al: Family meals during adolescence are associated with higher diet quality and healthful meal patterns during young adulthood, *J Am Diet Assoc* 107:1502, 2007.

McDowell MA, et al: Blood folate levels: the latest NHANES results, *NCHS Data Brief* 6:1, 2008. Accessed 30 June 2008 from http://www.cdc.gov/nchs/data/databriefs/db06.htm.

Moshfegh A, et al: What we eat in America, NHANES 2001-2002: usual nutrient intakes from food compared to dietary reference intakes, 2005. Accessed 6 December 2005 from http://www.ars.usda.gov/Services/docs.htm?docid=9098.

National Cancer Institute: Risk factor monitoring and methods, 2010. Accessed 8 February 2010 from http://riskfactor.cancer.gov/diet/usualintakes/pop/t35.html.

National Center on Addiction and Substance Abuse: The importance of family dinners IV, September 2007. Accessed 10 February 2010 from http://casafamilyday.org/familyday/files/themes/familyday/pdf/Family-Dinners-IV.pdf.

Neumark-Sztainer D, et al: Family meals and adolescents: what have we learned from Project EAT (Eating Among Teens), *Public Health Nutr* 13:1113, 2010.

O'Toole T, et al: Nutrition services and foods and beverages available at school: results from the School Health Policies and Programs Study 2006, *J Sch Health* 77:500, 2007.

Ogden CL, et al: Prevalence of high body mass index in US children and adolescents, 2007-2008, *JAMA* 303:242, 2010.

Powell L, et al: Nutritional content of television food advertisements seen by children and adolescents in the United States, *Pediatrics* 120:576, 2007.

Powers TG, et al: Obesity prevention in early adolescence: student, parent, and teacher views, *J Sch Health* 80:13, 2010.

Pratt JSA, et al: Best practice updates for pediatric/adolescent weight loss surgery, *Obesity* 17:901, 2009.

Rajeshwari R, et al: Secular trends in children's sweetened beverage consumption (1973 to 1994): The Bogalusa Heart Study, *J Am Diet Assoc* 105:208, 2005.

Rampersaud GC, et al: Breakfast habits, nutritional status, body weight, and academic performance in children and adolescents, *J Am Diet Assoc* 105(5):743, 2005.

Rideout VJ, et al: *Generation M^2: media in the lives of 8- to 18-year-olds*, Menlo Park, Calif, 2010, Kaiser Family Foundation.

Robinson-O'Brien R, et al: Adolescent and young adult vegetarianism: better dietary intake and weight outcomes but increased risk of disordered eating behaviors, *J Am Diet Assoc* 109:648, 2009.

Rosenfield RL, et al: Thelarche, pubarche and menarche attainment in children with normal and elevated body mass index, *Pediatrics* 123(1):84, 2009.

Sebastian RS, et al: Effect of snacking frequency on adolescents' dietary intakes and meeting national recommendations, *J Adolesc Health* 42:503, 2008.

Sebastian RS, et al: US adolescents and MyPyramid: Associations between fast-food consumption and lower likelihood of meeting recommendations, *J Am Diet Assoc* 109:226, 2009.

Shaikh U, et al: Vitamin and mineral supplement use by children and adolescents in the 1999-2004 National Health and Nutrition Examination Survey, *Arch Pediatr Adolesc Med* 163:150, 2009.

Spear BA, et al: Recommendations for treatment of child and adolescent overweight and obesity, *Pediatrics* 120:S254, 2007.

Steinhausen HC: Outcome of eating disorders, *Child Adolesc Adol Psych* 18:225, 2008.

Stransky M, Rysava L: Nutrition as prevention and treatment of osteoporosis, *Physiolog Res* 58:S7, 2009.

Talamayan KS, et al: Prevalence of overweight misperception and weight control behaviors among normal weight adolescents in the United States, *ScientificWorldJournal* 6:365, 2006.

Tanner J: *Growth at adolescence*, Oxford, 1962, Blackwell Scientific Publications.

Timlin MT, et al: Breakfast eating and weight change in a 5-year prospective analysis of adolescents: Project EAT (Eating Among Teens), *Pediatrics* 121:e638, 2008.

Tussing-Humphreys LM: Excess adiposity, inflammation and iron-deficiency in female adolescents, *J Am Diet Assoc* 109:297, 2009.

U.S. Department of Agriculture, Agricultural Research Service: Nutrient intakes from food: mean amounts consumed per individual, one day, 2005-2006, 2008. Accessed 29 January 2010 from www.ars.usda.gov/ba/bhnrc/fsrg.

U.S. Department of Health and Human Services, Physical Activity Guidelines Steering Committee: 2008 physical activity guidelines for Americans, 2008. Available at: *www.health.gov/paguidelines*. Accessed Jan 14, 2011.

Van Dam RM, et al: The relationship between overweight in adolescence and premature death in women, *Ann Intern Med* 145:91, 2006.

Wang YC, et al: Increasing caloric contribution from sugar-sweetened beverages and 100% fruit juices among US children and adolescents, 1988-2004, *Pediatrics* 121:e1604, 2008.

World Health Organization: *Prevention and management of osteoporosis*. Report of a Scientific Group, WHO Technical Report Series no. 921, Geneva, 2003, World Health Organization.

Yussman SM, et al: Herbal products and their association with substance use in adolescents, *J Adolescent Health* 38:395, 2006.

Zenk S, Powell L: U.S. secondary schools and food outlets, *Health Place* 14:336, 2008.

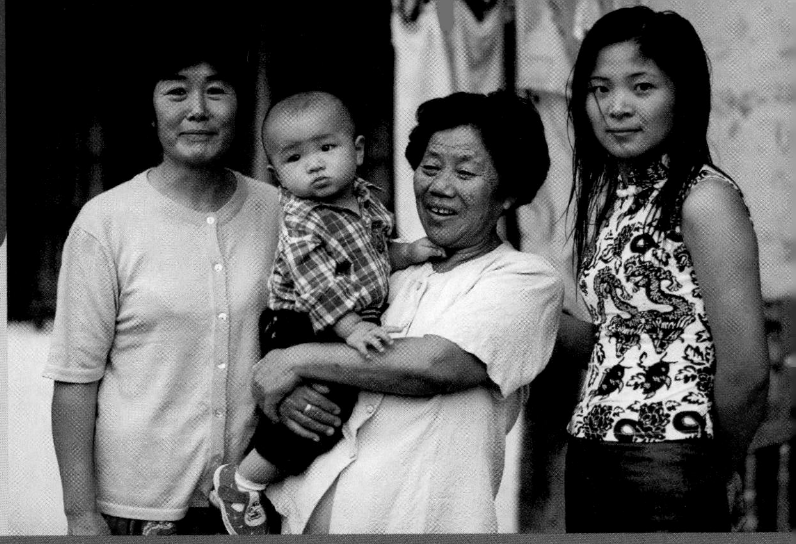

CHAPTER 20

Judith L. Dodd, MS, RD, LDN, FADA

Nutrition in the Adult Years

KEY TERMS

consumer price index (CPI)
food security
functional foods
health-related quality of life (HRQOL)
isoflavones
metabolic syndrome
phytochemicals
phytoestrogens
phytonutrients
prebiotics
premenstrual syndrome (PMS)
probiotics
wellness

This chapter emphasizes the background and tools for encouraging adults to set nutrition-related lifestyle goals that promote positive health and reduce risk factors. Other chapters of this text provide in-depth information about the major chronic diseases and conditions that affect food and nutrition choices in the adult years, including cardiovascular disease (CVD), diabetes, cancer, weight control, and osteoporosis. The focus here is on achieving and maintaining positive health, and in making lifestyle choices to achieve the goals for Healthy People 2020 (see Chapter 10).

SETTING THE STAGE: NUTRITION IN THE ADULT YEARS

This chapter focuses on nutrition- and food-related behaviors for the years following adolescence but before one is deemed an "older adult," often defined as age 65. Admittedly this is a large age span, and, like all population groups, it is heterogeneous. The dietary reference intakes (DRIs) on the inside cover of this text provide an overview of the nutrient recommendations for age groups under the DRI umbrella. Nutrient needs are similar but, as in all life stages, are affected by gender, state of health, medications, and lifestyle choices such as eating behaviors, smoking, and activity. These are markers, determined through assessment, that the nutrition and health professional can use to determine this population's needs. Other markers are less evident and include the adult's perceptions of quality of life and motivation in the areas of nutrition and health. When the objectives are prevention and behavior change, such markers become critical.

A first step for dietetics and health professionals is to recognize that many adults are prime targets for nutrition and health information that offers positive guidance. As with any group, adults need to be approached with strategies and guidance that fit their health and education needs. The American Dietetic Association (ADA) Trends surveys offer some insights. These surveys include a representative sampling of adult Americans with a focus on food, nutrition, and activity messages and consumers' reactions to these messages. Because this survey was conducted every 2 years for 12 years and was repeated in 2008, Trends provides a snapshot of attitudes about the importance of nutrition, activity, and sources of information. In 2002, 38% of Americans believed they had made significant adjustments in achieving a healthful and nutritious diet. Trends 2008 continued to show positive gains in that 43% of the respondents noted they were making positive steps (ADA, 2008).

Eating Habits of American Adults

Surveys such as ADA Trends support the idea that an increasing number of adults, more women than men, are seeking nutrition information and using it to make positive lifestyle changes. In a recent survey almost 70% of 30,000 U.S. adults said that they are trying to eat healthier foods; half are looking for nutrition value and have an ongoing concern about controlling calories (Dornblaser, 2006). According to the ADA's survey three in five consumers said diet, nutrition, and physical activity are "very important" to them personally, women more so than men. Younger adults were less likely than older adults to rate diet and nutrition as "very important," whereas exercise and physical activity were very important across the life cycle. Of relevance is the fact that reasons for not adjusting their diet or exercise patterns more were most likely to be satisfaction with their current health and nutrition status (79%) and concerns for not having to give up foods they like (73%). For those interested in changing their beliefs and behaviors, time limitations, lack of practical information, and unclear guidelines were noted (ADA, 2008)

A review of the health and nutrition information in magazines and on television reinforces the idea that nutrition and health information is "in." However, consumers are selective about their personal concerns. The International Food Information Council (IFIC) Foundation Food and Health Survey found that half of Americans are trying to lose weight, two thirds report making changes in the types and amounts of food eaten, and 70% express concerns with their weight (IFIC, 2009). Messages regarding the potential benefits and risks of certain foods and nutrients are being heard by consumers. Messages such as the negative effect of saturated fat, *trans*-fatty acids, and sodium are acknowledged; two in five adults said they were planning to eat more whole grains during the year they were surveyed (Harris Interactive Poll, 2006). This has driven the marketing of "healthful foods" as well as the demand for creating and marketing foods that fit this image (Sloan, 2006).

Where consumers get their information is another factor to consider. Both the source and the message affect the scientific value, but to the adult consumer the promise of specific benefit is more important than the standard "it's good for you" message. Both television and magazines are major sources of food and nutrition information for adults, and the Internet has surpassed newspapers. When it comes to credible sources, 78% of survey respondents rate registered dietitians as credible, followed by doctors and nurses (ADA, 2008.)

Consumers are using the labels on foods and beverages, including both the Nutrition Facts Panel and other label information, to get health information. Although 84% of the population is aware of MyPyramid which has recently been updated to MyPlate, only 25% report customizing their diets using these guidance systems (IFIC, 2009). Consumers will continue to need help in using the new website, www.chooseMyPlate.gov to improve their diets.

Nutrition Information and Education for Adults

Frequently, mainstream adults are ignored as a unique segment of the population needing a positive message. Preventive strategies are likely to be targeted to address the formative years of prenatal, infancy, childhood, adolescence, and young adulthood. The older adult group is likely to be targeted with health intervention strategies and quality-of-life messages. But the population group in the middle of the continuum, the adult age 25 to approximately 65, is likely to be segmented in reference to a disease state, a life event, or a lifestyle choice. For example, adults are targeted as having or being at risk for diabetes or heart disease, in need of a medication, being pregnant, or being an athlete.

The adult who is not pregnant, an athlete, or "sick," but who seeks guidance on normal nutrition or prevention of disease may be directed toward diets for chronic disease or weight loss. Such information may be a good fit when the information is based on science. Fortunately, the guidance provided by such groups as the American Heart Association (AHA), the ADA, the American Diabetes Association, and the American Cancer Society (ACS) mirror the Dietary Guidelines for Americans 2010 (DGA) (USDHHS, 2010). The AHA released guidelines in 2006 defining new goals with a focus on improving overall health and achieving improved cardiovascular health of all Americans by 20% by 2020 (Lloyd-Jones, 2010).

Adults are prime targets for information on chronic disease prevention and weight management; however, the messages may appear to be conflicting or less sensational than advice promising quick solutions. In spite of this, health education and public health programs, along with improved research and care, have contributed to changes in morbidity and mortality of the adult population (Centers for Disease Control and Prevention [CDC], 2009a). U.S. adults are on a path to positive change, moving from knowledge to action (National Center for Health Statistics [NCHS], 2009).

Adults in the awareness and action stages are likely to be looking for answers, often short-term fixes or reversals of a health problem. For example, adults might want to know where carbohydrates fit into the total diet and whether there are "better carbs." What's the message on fat now that *trans*-fats have been almost banned? Are there "good fats?" What is a "healthy" or "unhealthy" food or diet? Should I be buying organically grown or locally grown foods? What should I do about sodium? How can I practice food safety?

Guidance based on science generally addresses total diet and lifestyle rather than single nutrients or foods. The concepts of *healthful eating*, *nutrient density*, and *nutritious food* are being debated by food and nutrition professionals. The idea of expressing nutrient density using food labels is a major discussion point. Unfortunately, food and nutrition debates are fodder for media coverage, adding to the confusion and perception of mixed messages. There is ongoing effort to sort out information on food labels, particularly front-of-package systems meant to help consumers understand what is in their food (Institute of Medicine [IOM], 2010; Thompson, 2010).

But adults are a population group with both the interest and the ability to seek out their own resources and answers. A search for information on choosing foods for health can result in evidence-based information such as the DGA, as well as questionable guidance based on single studies or product promotion. The combination of marketing and electronic media makes it easier to mix science with speculation and outright untruths. Adults with an interest in improving the nutritional quality of their diet may end up with noncredible advice pointing to supplements as quick-fix solutions.

Consider the adult years as a time for health promotion, health maintenance, and disease prevention, along with the interventions that accompany the progression of chronic disease that can come with aging. It is a time for adults to take responsibility and control. The Food and Health Survey and the ADA Trends study are examples of benchmark studies that provide a snapshot of consumer attitudes on food and health. Such studies provide the dietetic and health professional the information on "hot buttons" issues of importance to consumers. Examining these and other surveys targeting adults is critical to presenting relevant information and also initiating and reinforcing positive nutrition and health behaviors.

THE WELLNESS YEARS

The adult years are a broad span chronologically and are complicated by physiologic, developmental, and social factors. Along with their genetic and social history, adults have accumulated the results of behaviors and risks from environmental factors. These factors shape the heterogeneity of the adult years. Nonetheless, the adult years are an ideal time for positive health promotion and disease prevention messages. In the transitions from early to middle adulthood, health and wellness may take on a new importance. This may be the result of a life event or education (an epiphany) which triggers an awareness that being well and staying well are important. Examples include learning the results of a screening for blood pressure, cholesterol, or diabetes; facing the reality of death; the self-reflection that occurs when personal health or that of a peer or family member is in crisis; or realizing that clothes don't fit as well as they should. Regardless of the reason, the concept of wellness takes on a new meaning and these events are teachable moments.

The Wellness Councils of America (WELCOA) describes **wellness** as a process that involves being aware of better health and actively working toward that goal (WELCOA, 2009). With this mindset, a state of wellness can exist at any age and can start at any point in a person's life course. Wellness is more than physical health and well-being. A state of well-being includes mental and spiritual health and encompasses the ability of a person to move through Maslow's Hierarchy of Needs (Maslow, 1970).

The ability to address nutrition needs requires **food security** (i.e., access to a safe, acceptable, and adequate source of food). The current economic climate has put added emphasis on food security. Hispanic and black Americans in all age groups are more likely to live in poverty than white and Asian Americans (CDC, 2009a). Indeed, the highest levels of food insecurity are in black and Hispanic households (CDC, 2006a).

In 2008, it was estimated that 85% of U.S. households were food secure throughout the entire year and 15% were food insecure at least some time during the year, an increase of 11.1% over 2007 (U.S. Department of Agriculture [USDA] and Economic Research Service [ERS], 2010). Hunger and poverty statistics released by Feeding America, formerly Second Harvest, note that in 2008 39.8 million people were living in poverty (Food Research and Action Center, 2010).

Participation in the Supplemental Nutrition Assistance Program (SNAP), previously "Food Stamps," is a marker of food insecurity. Slightly more than half of all Americans between the ages of 20 and 65 will at some point receive food stamps, an indicator of the risk for food insecurity in the adult years (Sandoval et al., 2009). Although most SNAP recipients are children or older adults, working-age women represent 28% of those enrolled in the program and working-age men represented 14% (USDA and ERS, 2010). Access to affordable food is a basic requirement for wellness and nutrition in the adult years.

One's perceptions of personal health (both mental and physical) relate to views on wellness and perceptions of quality of life. **Health-related quality of life (HRQOL)** is a concept used to measure the effects of current health conditions on a person's day-to-day life. To capture this and create a tool for professionals, the CDC measures population HRQOL perceptions, including the perception of "feeling healthy." Using HRQOL, one can learn about how adults relate their health to their daily performance. Americans report feeling "unhealthy" approximately 6 days a month and "healthy" or "full of energy" approximately 19 days a month; adults with the lowest income levels and more chronic diseases report more "unhealthy" days (CDC, 2006a).

The adult years offer unique opportunities to evaluate health status, build on positive factors, and change the negative factors that affect quality of life. See Fig. 20-1. Because adults are teachers, coaches, parents, caregivers, and work-site leaders, targeting the wellness-related attitudes and behaviors of adults can potentially have a multiplier effect. A positive wellness focus may influence not only the health of the adult, but also those in his or her sphere of influence.

LIFESTYLE AND HEALTH RISK FACTORS

Lifestyle choices, including activity, lay the framework for health and wellness. The health of people living in the

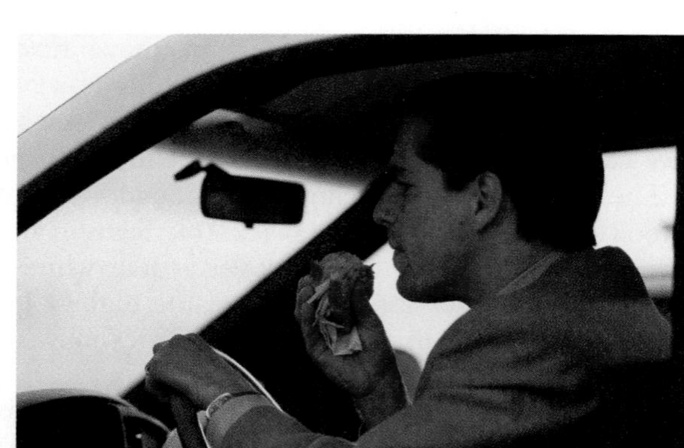

FIGURE 20-1 Eating quickly without attention, when stressed or when multi-tasking often results in poor nutritional intake in the adult years. *(© 2011 Photos.com a division of Getty Images. All rights reserved.)*

United States has continued to improve during the previous 55 years in part because of education that has led to lifestyle changes. Life expectancy has continued to increase (projected at 77.9 years), and the morbidity and mortality rate from heart disease, cancer, and stroke has dropped. Overall mortality was 25% higher for black Americans that white Americans in 2007; this has only slightly improved since 1990 when the gap was 37% (CDC, 2009a). This is an area for increased emphasis on prevention and intervention initiatives.

Even when the emphasis is on wellness, there is a strong link to risk factors that influence morbidity and mortality. In the United States the leading causes of death and debilitation among adults include (1) heart disease, (2) cancer, (3) cerebrovascular disease, (4) chronic lower respiratory disease, (5) accidents (unintentional injuries), and (6) diabetes (CDC, 2009b). Chronic diseases, including heart disease, stroke, cancer, and diabetes, are among the most costly and preventable of all health problems and account for one third of the years of potential life lost before age 65 and for 75% of the nation's medical care costs (CDC, 2009b). Four of these chronic diseases have links to diet and lifestyle, including CVD, diabetes, certain cancers, and osteoporosis.

Overweight and obesity is either a precursor or complication in all of these diseases. The prevalence of overweight, as measured by a body mass index (BMI) of 25 or more, has increased at all ages, but appears to be holding steady. It is important when looking at the overall health of adults to consider elevated BMI as a major risk factor. Hypertension, hyperlipidemia, and elevated blood glucose are often seen together with or without obesity, known as the **metabolic syndrome**.

Obesity and overweight directly link with calorie imbalance. It is estimated that less than half of U.S. adults participate in regular physical activity, with one fourth reporting no activity. Many health risks in the adult years, including coronary artery disease, certain types of cancer, hypertension, type 2 diabetes, depression, anxiety, and osteoporosis have a relationship with lack of participation in regular physical activity and poor eating behaviors. One cannot achieve positive health without a combination of physical activity and food choices that fit personal needs for energy balance and nutrition.

On the other end of the weight spectrum is chronic underweight, frequently accompanied by undernutrition. Anorexia nervosa is the extreme condition, found in both genders across the age span. An unhealthy weight or unhealthy concern about body weight not only affects overall health but in women can also affect fertility and the ability to conceive.

HEALTH DISPARITIES

Implementation of Healthy People goals are based in part on eliminating disparities that increase the health risks for affected populations. Such disparities are related to inadequate access to a safe and affordable food supply and health care based on race, ethnicity, gender, education, income level, and geographic location. Inadequate access to care is a disparity that has a major effect on a person's wellness. Men of working age are nearly twice as likely as women to have no usual source of health care (NCHS, 2009). Chronic diseases and obesity have been shown to be more of a burden to racial minorities and women (CDC, 2009a, 2010). There is a higher incidence of heart disease, diabetes, and obesity or overweight in low-income, black, and Hispanic populations (AHA and American Stroke Association, 2005). These same population groups have limited access to preventive care, nutrition education, and guidance (U.S. Department of Health and Human Services [USDHHS], 2010).

Food insecurity and limited access to healthful foods are also disparities. It is often more expensive to eat healthy foods than less healthy, high-calorie foods. Limited skills in the areas of wise food purchasing and food preparation coupled with limited food and equipment resources further complicate a person's ability to follow advice for a healthy lifestyle. This emphasizes the need for adult consumer education in basic food skills.

The problems associated with chronic diseases are similar in other countries (World Health Organization [WHO], 2009). Human immunodeficiency virus, acquired immune deficiency syndrome, tuberculosis, and tropical diseases are barriers to global achievement of positive health status. Indeed, the eight United Nations millennium development goals seek to reduce the number of people who suffer from hunger and increase access to safe water and sanitation (WHO, 2009).

Emphasis: Women's Health

The reproductive years constitute a significant stage of a woman's life. Many issues that affect the health of women are related to the monthly hormonal shifts associated with menses. Osteoporosis, heart disease, and some cancers are disease states that are affected by specific hormones. Pregnancy and breast-feeding have an effect on a woman's health (see Chapter 16). Breast-feeding helps control weight, lower the risk for diabetes, and improves bone health (Stuebe et al., 2005). Therefore encouraging women to breast-feed is a potential prevention strategy for the future health of both the mother and her infant.

Shifts of estrogen and progesterone hormones trigger the female reproductive cycle and affect health. Associated with menses is a complex set of physical and psychologic symptoms known as **premenstrual syndrome (PMS)**. Reported symptoms vary, but are described as general discomfort, anxiety, depression, fatigue, breast pain, and cramping. Such symptoms are reported to occur approximately 1 week to 10 days before the onset of menses and increase in severity into menses. Currently, there is no single cause or intervention identified for PMS. Hormone imbalance, neurotransmitter synthesis defects, and low levels of certain nutrients (i.e., vitamin B_6 and calcium) have been implicated (National Institutes of Health [NIH] and Office of Dietary Supplements [ODS], 2007). A diet high in sodium and refined carbohydrates has been implicated, but the evidence is not complete enough to make recommendations (NIH and ODS, 2007). A greater emphasis on a plant-based diet of whole grains, fruits, vegetables, lean or low-fat protein sources, and low-fat dairy or soy beverages is a reasonable intervention and may cause relief in some women. Exercise and relaxation techniques have been reported as lessening the symptoms.

When menses end, either because of age or surgical removal of reproductive organs, women have unique health and nutrition concerns. Perimenopause and menopause generally begin in the late forties. However, genetics, general health, and the age that menses began can alter the timing of this marker. Typically, estrogen production decreases around age 50, when endogenous estrogen circulation decreases approximately 60%. The effects include a cessation of menses and the loss of the healthful benefits of estrogen. Even after the ovaries cease production, a weaker form of estrogen continues to be produced by the adrenal glands, and some is stored in adipose tissue (Barrett-Connor et al., 2005).

As estrogen decreases, symptoms associated with menopause may occur. Both the onset of menopause and the reported side effects vary. Some women experience a gradual decline in the frequency and duration of menses, whereas others experience an abrupt cessation. The symptoms most often reported include low energy levels and vasomotor symptoms (hot flashes). Bone, heart, and brain health are affected. The decrease in circulating estrogen limits the body's ability to remodel bones, resulting in a decrease of bone mass. Lower levels of circulating estrogen also affect blood lipid levels, increasing both total cholesterol and low-density lipoprotein cholesterol levels, and decreasing high-density lipoprotein (HDL) levels. Brain function, particularly memory, is also affected; negative changes may be somewhat alleviated with hormone therapy (MacLennan et al., 2006).

Managing menopause promotes emphasis on plant-based foods for the benefits of phytoestrogens, soluble fiber, and other components. Having sufficient calcium, vitamin D, vitamin K, and magnesium, and using the DRI as the guideline, is important for protecting bone health. Although soy (isoflavones) continues to be suggested by the popular press as a way to control hot flashes, current research does not support these suggestions for all women.

Heart disease, cancer, and stroke continue to be the leading causes of death in women (CDC, 2006b). As reported earlier, weight is a risk factor for heart disease and some cancers. Weight gain is an issue for women, with the 35% prevalence of obesity in American women aged 20-74 years as compared with 33% in the same aged men. One-half of non-Hispanic black women and two fifths of Hispanic women are obese, compared with one third of non-Hispanic white women (CDC, 2009a). Physical activity with aerobic endeavors and resistance and weight-bearing exercise is protective for bone, cardiovascular, and emotional health. The key nutrition message is one of balanced food intake with nutrient dense foods that are low in fat.

Emphasis: Men's Health

The leading causes of death among American men include heart disease, prostate and lung cancers, and unintentional injuries (CDC, 2006c). For the adult man, a diet that supports reducing the risk for heart disease is especially important because men develop heart disease at a younger age than women. Regular exercise and activity are important. Along with contributing to cardiovascular health, weight-bearing exercise has a positive effect on bone health.

Another issue in adult men is iron intake. Unless adult men are diagnosed with iron-deficiency anemia and require additional iron, they should not get additional iron from multivitamin or mineral supplements, enriched sports drinks, or energy bars. Excessive iron intake is problematic because it is an oxidant in the body; men and postmenopausal women do not have menstruation, pregnancy, or lactation to get rid of excess iron. A certain percentage of men carry the genetic variant for hemochromatosis and iron overload, and in this situation iron is particularly dangerous. See Chapter 33.

INTERVENTIONS: NUTRITION AND PREVENTION

Adults are in the ideal life-cycle phase for health promotion and disease prevention nutrition advice because of the combination of life experience and influence. This group has the potential to shape personal lifestyle choices and influence others. The tools are in place, including the DGA, MyPlate, and the Nutrition Facts panel on food labels. Alternative patterns exist to support those who choose to be vegetarian or vegan (Craig et al., 2009).

Implementation of positive choices and moving people along the continuum of a healthy lifestyle are other issues. Many consumers are aware of the concerns associated with lifestyle and diet (IFIC, 2009). They are also aware of the implied promises for good health that come with messages from the media, friends, and health professionals. However, they are unlikely to move from awareness to action without motivation stronger than another promise. Consumers often do not want to give up the foods they like for fear that healthy foods would not taste good (ADA, 2008). A total diet approach of making gradual changes of food and lifestyle choices may help. The Small Step Program available through the U.S. Department of Health and Human Services is an example of such an approach in a simple, Internet-based program (USDHHS, 2006). "America on the Move" is another program that puts emphasis on achievable goals while maintaining calorie balance through small changes.

However, the steps to prevention and health promotion, even when small, are personal responsibilities that cannot be legislated. Americans have many choices: what and where they eat, where they receive their information, and what they include or remove from their lifestyle. Adults in our culture value choice; it is a right, even if it leads to poor health, chronic disease, or death. Some messages are directed at reaching adults where they live and work. Adults in developed countries are mobile, and for the working adult populations, much of the day is tied to a work site. There are increasing efforts in both the private and public sectors to promote positive work site nutrition-related behaviors and programs.

FOOD TRENDS AND PATTERNS

Where one eats, who prepares it, and how much is consumed are all patterns of behavior and choice. There is no stereotypic "adult" when it comes to lifestyles. Adults may be single or partnered, with or without children, working outside the home or at home. The sit-down family meals at home have given way to eating on the run, take-out, and drive-through. Too little time for planning or preparation and limited cooking skills can lead to reliance on processed foods, speed-scratch cooking (combining processed with fresh ingredients), or more food prepared out of the home. Today's economic climate and changing dietary recommendations present new challenges. The nutrient-dense approach is essential (Miller et al., 2009). Reaching both men and women with an understandable and relevant message, especially heads of households or gatekeepers, is critical.

According to the **consumer price index (CPI)** it is estimated that Americans spend up to 48.5% of their food dollars away from home. The CPI for food measures the average change over time in the prices paid by urban consumers, using a representative market basket of consumer goods and services. The Economic Research Service (ERS) of the USDA follows these expenditures and manages the data set. This is a valuable resource for monitoring expenditures and planning for meaningful interventions.

Changing food patterns and the use of more processed and purchased foods result in an increase of foods higher in sodium with added fat and sweeteners, and a decrease in use of basic foods such as fruits, vegetables, and whole grains. Portion sizes (either the amount presented or the amount eaten) replace serving sizes (what is recommended as a serving by the DGA or other source), as others determine what is considered a "meal" or "snack." Portions have continued to increase in size, as evidenced from using the tool "Portion Distortion" available at http://hp2010.nhlbihin.net/portion/keep.htm.

Dietary changes have affected nutrition and are already reflected in the current concerns for weight and nutrient imbalances. The DGA 2010 and MyPlate can be viewed as attempts to put more emphasis on basic foods that are nutrient-dense rather than calorie-dense, and on total amounts of foods per day rather than numbers of servings. The most current information is reflected in the information used to shape the 2010 DGAs (USDHHS, 2010).

Current adult diets are likely to be higher in total fat than the 30% of total calories recommended in the 2010 DGA and include a predominance of carbohydrates as added sugar and refined grains. Fruit and vegetable guidelines are not being met. Although chicken and fish servings have increased, animal sources outweigh plant-based protein sources. Health guidelines continue to move in the direction of increasing plant based foods. Key nutrients that may be in short supply are calcium, magnesium, and potassium; the antioxidants vitamins A, C, and E; and vitamin D (USDHHS, 2010).

NUTRITIONAL SUPPLEMENTATION

The position of the ADA that the best nutritional strategy for promoting optimal health and reducing the risk of chronic disease is to wisely choose a wide variety of nutrient-rich foods. Additional nutrients from fortified foods and supplements can help some people meet their nutritional needs as specified by science-based nutrition standards such as the DRI (Hasler et al., 2009). In making this statement, the ADA puts food first but leaves the door open for those with specific nutrient needs, identified through assessment by a dietetic or health professional, to be nutritionally supplemented.

Traditionally, one thinks of vitamins and minerals, fiber, and protein as nutrient supplements, generally in a pill, capsule, or liquid form. The DRIs are the standards used with most adults. However, food fortification is another form of nutrient supplementation. The level of fortified foods (such as "energy bars" or "sports drinks") in the marketplace puts another layer of potential nutrient sources in the mix with traditional supplements. Less traditional supplements such as herbals and other natural dietary "enhancers" are also added to the array of supplements available to consumers.

Americans frequently do not meet the dietary recommendations for promoting optimal health. Several segments of the adult population fall into high-risk groups who are unlikely to meet their nutrient needs because of life stage (e.g., pregnancy), alcohol or drug dependency, food insecurity, chronic illness, recovery from illness, or choosing a nutritionally restrictive diet or lifestyle (ADA, 2008). Other persons with special needs include those with food allergies or intolerances that eliminate major food groups, persons using prescription drugs or therapies that change the way the body uses nutrients, those with disabilities that limit their ability to enjoy a varied diet, and those who are just unable or unwilling because of time or energy to prepare or consume a nutritionally adequate diet. These adults potentially need a nutritional supplement. See Chapter 13.

FUNCTIONAL FOODS

Adults interested in attaining and maintaining wellness are frequently interested in altering dietary patterns or choosing foods for added health benefits. The desire for fewer calories and multiple health benefits, especially when children are in the home, is driving the growth in the U.S. functional foods market. Examples of **functional foods** are fruits and vegetables (especially dark colored ones), flax seeds, whole grains, the oils of fish, certain spices, yogurt, nuts, soy, and legumes that are believed to have benefits beyond their usual nutrient value (IFIC, 2010). Functional foods can include whole foods and fortified, enriched, or enhanced foods. The potential benefit for health is when these foods are consumed as part of a varied diet on a regular basis (Marra and Boyar, 2009).

Providing this information to the segment of the adult population that is looking for ways to enhance its health not only gains the adults' attention but also takes nutrition guidance to a higher level. Research continues to provide information on dietary patterns and components of foods that may have added benefits for health. Helping to lower blood cholesterol or control blood sugar, serving as an antioxidant or scavenger against harmful components, promoting a healthy gastrointestinal tract, or stimulating activity of detoxification enzyme systems in the liver are examples of benefits being reported and researched for validity. See *Focus On:* Eating to Detoxify.

Adults who have no major health problems that would restrict food choices can benefit from guidance on meeting the recommendations of MyPlate and the DGA as a first step. This guidance is based on increasing the intake of fruits, vegetables (including legumes), grains (with emphasis on whole grains), and seeds and nuts—some of the same foods known to have components that go beyond the benefits associated with major nutrients. Most of these components that are considered dietary enhancers are associated with plant foods.

Phytochemicals or **phytonutrients** (from the Greek word *phyto* for *plant*) are biologically active and naturally occurring chemical components in plant foods. In plants phytochemicals act as natural defense systems for their host and offer protection against microbial invasions or infections. They also provide color, aroma, and flavor, with more than 2000 plant pigments identified (see Figure 20-2). These include flavonoids, anthocyanins, and carotenoids (see Chapter 4). There is even interest in resveratrol from grape juice and red wines. See *Focus On:* Alcohol: A Functional Food? As part of human consumption phytonutrients can have an anti-oxidant, detoxification, and anti-inflammatory functions in the body.

Soy is another example of a food with value beyond quality protein. The health benefits of soy products or components of soy include reducing the risk for heart disease and certain types of cancer and reducing vasomotor symptoms (hot flashes) in menopausal females. Note that soy itself, as a plant, has no cholesterol and is a source of **isoflavones**, a **phytoestrogen** or plant estrogen. In 1999 the Food and Drug Administration (FDA) approved a food label claim for soy, addressing its potential role in reducing the risk of heart disease (Food and Drug Administration, 1999). To qualify, the food needs to have 6.25 g of soy protein in one serving; be low in fat (less than 3 g); be low in saturated fat (1 g or less) and cholesterol (less than 20 mg); and have no more than 480 mg of sodium for an individual food, 720 mg if an entrée, and 960 mg if a meal. In January 2006 the AHA released the results of a review of 22 randomized trials on the effect of soy protein with isoflavones on serum cholesterol (Sacks et al., 2006). The committee found that soy

FOCUS ON

Alcohol: A Functional Food?

There are some benefits to moderate intake of alcohol for specific population groups. The extent to which these benefits are related to lifestyle are unclear. There is evidence that increasing alcoholic beverage consumption is associated with a decline in total diet quality (Breslow, 2010). However, light to moderate intake of alcohol is associated with a lower risk for cardiovascular disease (CVD); these benefits appear to be independent of other CVD risk factors, including age, sex, smoking habits, and BMI. Women age 55 and older and men age 45 and older at risk for heart disease were in the groups most likely to benefit (USDHHS, 2006). In younger adults, the benefits may be offset by the increases in alcohol-related accidents.

Polyphenols in red wine (especially Pinot Noir) have protective effects. The question of energy intake by those who enjoy wine is a factor, and lifestyles are being explored. For example, in a Danish study of 3.5 million supermarket purchases, those who bought wine were also more likely to buy fruits, vegetables, olives, and low-fat cheeses than those who bought beer (Johansen et al., 2006). The high wine intake by the French, the "French paradox" and with Mediterranean diets has also shown benefits.

Based on the literature, the best advice may be to proceed cautiously. One should be the legal age to use alcohol; drink responsibly; enjoy it with a healthful meal; and be medically able to use alcohol based on health, life stage (no alcohol while pregnant or breast-feeding), and medications. *Moderation* is defined as one drink a day for women and up to two drinks per day for men. A *drink* is defined as 12 oz of regular beer, 5 oz of wine, or 1.5 oz of 80-proof distilled liquor.

FOCUS ON

Eating To Detoxify

L. Kathleen Mahan, RD, CDE, and Sheila Dean, DSc, RD, CDE

Current thinking on eating to detoxify for optimal health is based on a system of choosing foods to protect, maintain, and renew the body. The body is protected from xenobiotics (compounds foreign to the body) by natural barriers, including the gastrointestinal system, the lungs, and the skin. When compounds that are potentially harmful or unknown cross these barriers, the body's detoxification systems, which are series of metabolic reactions, go into play, with the result of decreasing the negative effect of the xenobiotics, drugs, or toxins.

Toxins may be of external origin (also referred to as *xenobiotics* or *exogenous toxins*), such as chemicals and pollutants in the air or water, food additives, or drugs. They may also be generated internally (referred to as *endogenous toxins*), as the end-products from the metabolism of hormones, bacterial byproducts, and other complex molecules. The prolonged presence of these molecules can have damaging effects on tissues or lead to undesirable imbalances.

The detoxification process occurs in two classical steps, named *Phase 1* and *Phase 2*, each involving a battery of enzymes of broad specificity. Specifically, Phase 1 reactions are catalyzed by the cytochrome P450 (CYP450) supergene family of isoenzymes, which have very broad substrate specificity. The products generated from Phase 1 reactions are often reactive intermediate metabolites or reactive oxygen species, which may cause tissue damage. The reactions in Phase 2 generally involve conversion or conjugation of the intermediate metabolites of Phase 1 by the addition of a water-soluble group to the reactive site into the final products that are eliminated. In some cases, a toxin may be directly converted via Phase 1 or Phase 2. Although both phases have different characteristics, it is essential that they function in balance with one another to minimize the presence of intermediate metabolites and carry through an effective detoxification.

Although as much as 75% of detoxification activity occurs in the liver, much of the remainder takes place in the intestinal mucosa wall. An additional small percentage occurs in other tissues. Although the liver is thought of as the detoxification site, it makes sense that the intestine also plays an important role in detoxification, because the gastrointestinal lining provides the initial physical barrier to the largest load of xenobiotics.

The potential power of these systems to protect the body is demonstrated by a closer look at the major barrier, the gut. More than half the body's lymphoid tissue surrounds the digestive tract. Gut-associated lymphoid tissue (GALT) generates almost 70% of the body's antibodies and contains the greatest number of lymphocytes in the body. It is the GALT immunoglobulins that prevent absorption of bacteria and viruses. Secretory immunoglobin A is a part of the major immune system of the gut and has been reported to directly deactivate enzymes and toxins from bacteria such as *Escherichia coli.*

The mechanisms for the food and nutrient link to detoxification are being explored, but it is suggested that phytochemicals are involved, along with more traditional nutrients that build and support the enzyme systems. Isothiocyanates such as sulforaphanes found in cruciferous vegetables; organosulfuric compounds in garlic, onions, and other members of the allium family; and the components present in **prebiotics** (nondigestible food products that stimulate the growth of bacteria already present in the colon); and the bacteria of **probiotics** are examples of food choices that can affect detoxification in both prevention and healing.

Foods with phytochemicals that boost detoxification include:

- At least 1 cup of cruciferous vegetables (cabbage, broccoli, collards, kale, Brussels sprouts) daily for their Phase 2 enzyme promoting effect
- A few cloves of garlic, which also promote Phase 2 enzymes
- Decaffeinated green tea in the morning.
- Fresh vegetable juices including carrots, celery, cilantro, beets, parsley, and ginger
- Herbal teas containing a mixture of burdock root, dandelion root, ginger root, licorice root, sarsaparilla root, cardamom seed, cinnamon bark and other herbs
- High-quality, sulfur-containing foods—eggs or whey protein, garlic, onions
- Limonene in citrus peels, caraway, and dill oil
- Bioflavonoids in grapes, berries, and citrus fruits that promote Phase 1 enzymes
- Dandelion greens to help liver detoxification, improve the flow of bile, and increase urine flow
- Celery to increase the flow of urine and aid in detoxification
- Cilantro, which may help remove heavy metals
- Rosemary, which has carnosol, a potent booster of detoxification enzymes
- Curcuminoids (turmeric and curry) for their antioxidant and antiinflammatory action
- Chlorophyll in dark green leafy vegetables and in wheat grass

Hyman M: Systems biology, toxins, obesity, and functional medicine in managing biotransformation: the metabolic, genomic, and detoxification balance points, The Proceedings from the 13th International Symposium of The Institute for Functional Medicine, Gig Harbor, Wash, 2006, Institute of Functional Medicine.

Lyon M et al: Clinical approaches to detoxification and biotransformation. In Jones DS, editor: Textbook of functional medicine, Institute for Functional Medicine, Gig Harbor, Washington, 2006.

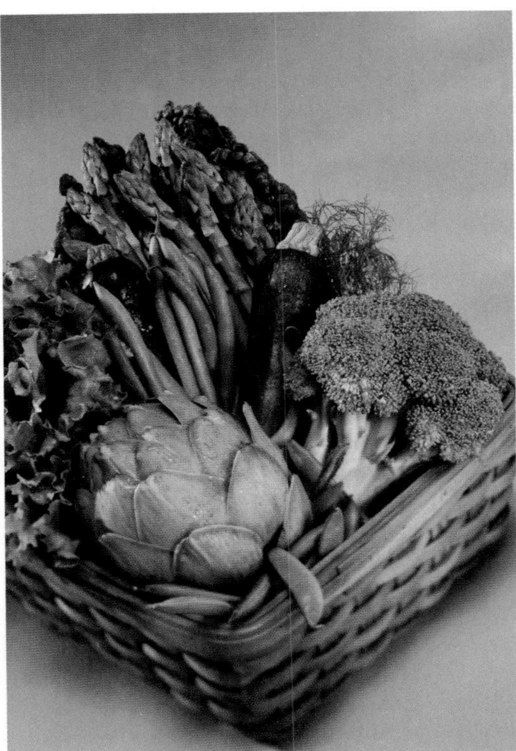

FIGURE 20-2 Phytochemicals in vegetables can have powerful anti-oxidant, detoxification, and anti-inflammatory functions in the body. (*© 2011 Photos.com a division of Getty Images. All rights reserved.*)

protein and isoflavones have not been shown to lessen vasomotor symptoms of menopause and show no significant effects on HDL cholesterol or triglyceride levels. This controversy illustrates the questions that arise when studying the use of food or food components at levels beyond what are consumed in a traditional diet (Maskarinec, 2005).

Foods that fit the FDA label claim for soy protein have a positive nutrition profile by virtue of the label requirements, and moderate amounts of soy foods can be part of a balanced diet even for cancer survivors (Maskarinec, 2005). The ACS concludes that cancer survivors may safely consume up to three servings daily (American Cancer Society, 2010). Soy can be used to displace animal protein and help lower intake of saturated fat, but soy is not recommended as a therapy to reduce LDL cholesterol or other cardiovascular risk factors (Lichtenstein et al., 2006). Whole soy foods continue to be a reasonable part of a diet with a role in both disease prevention and health promotion. (Messina, 2009).

One cannot address dietary guidance without considering the issues of both functional components and functional foods. Rather than isolating and promoting food components, current thinking supports the emphasis on food as a package and as a first source for nutrients and potential enhancers (Figure 20-2). In the big picture it is the person's health status, lifestyle choices, and genetics that form his or her potential for wellness, but dietary enhancement is a tool that gains attention and helps the person move forward on the wellness continuum.

CLINICAL SCENARIO

Lee is a 35-year-old woman who lives in an urban neighborhood with her husband and 12-year-old daughter. She is 5 ft, 10 in tall and currently weighs 165 pounds. In the past 2 years she has gained 10 pounds. At a recent neighborhood health fair Lee's blood glucose and blood pressure screening results were higher than they had been a year ago but were still in a good range. She has a family history of heart disease and diabetes and recognizes that her weight gain is an issue. Her grandmother recently died of colon cancer. Both she and her husband work full time, and blending their schedules with that of their daughter is hectic. Lee does all the cooking and shopping, although they eat out (fast food or take out) for most lunches and at least two dinners a week. They have no regular activity or exercise. They have minimum health insurance that requires a large copayment; thus they don't have an ongoing health care routine.

Lee made an appointment with her health care source. She asked for some dietary counseling and was asked to bring a 1-day food recall for the registered dietitian. She reported the following: breakfast: egg and sausage on a bagel, coffee; mid-morning: low-fat snack bar from vending machine with coffee; lunch: double burger with cheese on a bun and large fries, diet soda; dinner: chicken and rice casserole, corn, lettuce salad with diet ranch dressing; evening: dish of ice cream.

Nutrition Diagnostic Statements

1. Physical inactivity related to lifestyle issues as evidenced by no regular physical activity and a 10-lb weight gain.
2. Undesirable food choices related to high fat and low fruit and vegetable intake as evidenced by diet history revealing high-fat foods at every meal and an average of one fruit or vegetable each day.

Nutrition Care Questions

1. What lifestyle factors and nutrition triggers are likely to be identified by the dietitian?
2. What foods should Lee consider including in her diet to build a prevention-related meal plan?
3. Plan a meal pattern and two sample meals that illustrate your recommendations, including at least one at-home and away-from-home breakfast, lunch, and dinner.

USEFUL WEBSITES

America on the Move
https://aom3.americaonthemove.org/default.aspx

American Dietetic Association
http://www.eatright.org/

Centers for Disease Control and Prevention Health
http://www.cdc.gov/women/
http://www.cdc.gov/men/
http://www.cdc.gov/nchs/hdi.htm
Dietary Guidelines for Americans
http://www.dietaryguidelines.gov
Food and Agriculture Organization
http://www.fao.org/
Healthy People 2010
http://www.healthypeople.gov/hp2020/Objectives/TopicAreas.aspx
Institute of Medicine
http://www.iom.edu/
Flax Council of Canada
http://www.flaxcouncil.ca/
U.S. Department of Agriculture: Agricultural Research Service
http://www.ars.usda.gov/
U.S. Department of Agriculture: MyPlate
http://www.chooseMyPlate.gov/
U.S. Department of Health and Human Services: Small Steps
http://www.smallstep.gov/
Wellness Councils of America
http://www.welcoa.org/

REFERENCES

American Cancer Society. Accessed March 2010 from www.cancer.org.

American Dietetic Association (ADA): *Nutrition and you: trends 2008*, Chicago, 2008, American Dietetic Association.

American Heart Association, American Stroke Association: *A nation at risk: obesity in the United States*, Stanford, Calif, 2005, Robert Wood Johnson Foundation.

Barrett-Connor E, Laughlin GA: Hormone therapy and coronary artery calcification in asymptomatic postmenopausal women: the Rancho Bernardo Study, *Menopause* 1(1):40, 2005

Breslow RA, et al: Alcoholic beverage consumption, nutrient intakes and diet quality in the US adult population, 1999-2006, *J Am Diet Assoc* 110:561, 2010.

Centers for Disease Control and Prevention (CDC): *Chronic disease prevention and health promotion*, 2010. Accessed 20 January 2010 from http://www.cdc.gov/nccdphp/overview.htm.

Centers for Disease Control and Prevention (CDC): *Data 2010: The Healthy People 2010 database*, 2006a. Accessed 1 April 2010.

Centers for Disease Control and Prevention (CDC): *Health data interactive*, 2009a. Accessed March 2010 from http://www.cdc.gov/nchs/hdi.htm.

Centers for Disease Control and Prevention (CDC): *Leading causes of death in females: United States*, 2006b. Accessed March 2010 from http://www.cdc.gov/women/lcod/.

Centers for Disease Control and Prevention (CDC): *Leading causes of death in males: United States*, 2006c. Accessed March 2010 from http://www.cdc.gov/men/lcod/index.htm.

Centers for Disease Control and Prevention (CDC): *National vital statistics report: deaths: final data for 2006*, 2009b. Accessed March 2010 from http://www.cdc.gov/nchs.

Craig WJ, et al: Position of the American Dietetic Association: vegetarian diets, *J Am Diet Assoc* 109:1266, 2009.

Dornblaser L: *Trends in the food industry*, Chicago, 2006, Food Marketing Institute (FMI) Trade Show.

Food Research and Action Center (FRAC): *Hunger and poverty statistics: hunger in America*. Accessed March 2010 from http://feedingamerica.org.

Food and Drug Administration (FDA): *Qualified health claims: withdrawn soy protein and cancer*, 1999. Accessed 7 October 2005 from http://www.cfsan.fda.gov/~dms/lab-qhc.html.

Harris Interactive Poll, Gullo K, editor: *Healthcare news: Healthy eating messages appear to be resonating with consumers, according to new Harris interactive survey*, Rochester, N.Y., 2006, Harris Interactive. Accessed 15 May 2007 from http://www.harrisinteractive.com/news/allnewsbydate.asp?NewsID51039.

Hasler CM, et al: Position of the American Dietetic Association: functional foods, *J Am Diet Assoc* 109:739, 2009.

Institute of Medicine (IOM): *Examination of front-of-package nutrition rating systems and symbols*. Accessed March 2010 from http://www.iom.edu/Activities/Nutrition/NutritionSymbols.aspx.

Institute of Medicine (IOM), National Academy of Sciences (NAS): *Dietary reference intake (DRI) series*, Washington, DC, 1998-2004, National Academies Press.

International Food Information Council (IFIC): *Background on functional foods, IFIC Foundations*. Accessed 12 June 2010 from http://www.foodinsight.org/Resources/Detail.aspx?topic=Background_on_Functional_Foods.

International Food Information Council (IFIC): *Food & health survey: consumer attitudes toward food, nutrition & health: a benchmark survey 2009*, Washington, DC, 2009. Accessed March 2010 from http://www.foodinsight.org/.

Johansen D, et al: Food buying habits of people who buy wine or beer: cross sectional study, *Br Med J* 332:519, 2006.

Lichtenstein AH, et al: Diet and lifestyle recommendations revision 2006: a scientific statement from the American Heart Association Nutrition Committee, *Circulation* 114:82, 2006.

Lloyd-Jones DM, et al: Defining and setting national goals for cardiovascular health promotion and disease reduction, *Circulation* 121:586, 2010.

MacLennan AH, et al: Hormone therapy, timing of initiation, and cognition in women older than 60 years: the REMEMBER pilot study, *Menopause* 13:28, 2006.

Marra MV, Boyar AP: Position of the American Dietetic Association: nutrient supplementation, *J Am Diet Assoc* 109:2073, 2009.

Maskarinec G: Commentary: soy foods for breast cancer survivors and women at high risk for breast cancer, *J Am Diet Assoc* 105:10, 1524, 2005.

Maslow A: *Motivation and personality*, ed 2, New York, 1970, Harper.

Messina M, et al: Report on the 8th International Symposium on the Role of Soy in Health Promotion and Chronic Disease Prevention and Treatment, *J Nutr* 139:796S, 2009.

Miller GD, et al: It is time for a positive approach to dietary guidance using nutrient density as a basic principle, *J Nutr* 139:1198, 2009.

National Center for Health Statistics (NCHS): *Health, United States, 2004 with chart book on trends in the health of Americans*, Hyattsville, Md, 2009, NCHS.

National Institutes of Health (NIH), Office of Dietary Supplements (ODS): *Dietary supplement fact sheet: B6*, 24 August 2007. Accessed May 2010 from http://ods.od.nih.gov/factsheets/vitaminb6.asp.

Sacks F, et al: Soy protein, isoflavones, and cardiovascular health: an American Heart Association Science Advisory for Professionals from the Nutrition Committee, *Circulation* 113:1034,

2006. Accessed 15 May 2006 from http://www.circulationaha.org.

Sandoval DA, et al: The increasing risk of poverty across the American life course, *Demography* 46:717, 2009.

Sloan AE: Top 10 functional food trends, *Food Technol* 60(4):22, 2006. Accessed 15 May 2006 from www.ift.org.

Stuebe AM, et al: Duration of lactation and incidence of type 2 Diabetes, *JAMA* 294:2601, 2005.

Thompson A: *FDA working to replace misleading food labels*, Live Science. Accessed March 2010 from http://www.livescience.com/health/food-labels-100314html.

U.S. Department of Agriculture (USDA), Economic Research Service (ERS): *Food CPI and expenditures*. Accessed March 2010 from http://www.ers.usda.gov/Briefing//CPIFoodANDEspenditures/, http://www.ersusda.gov/Briefing//CPIFoodAndExtpenditures/overview.htm.

U.S. Department of Health and Human Services (USDHHS): *Healthy People 2010*. Accessed March 2010 from http://www.healthypeople.com.

U.S. Department of Health and Human Services (USDHHS): *Small steps: a web-based wellness program*, April 2006. Accessed 1 April 2006 from http://www.smallstep.gov.

U.S. Department of Health and Human Services (USDHHS): *Dietary Guidelines for Americans, 2010*. ed 7, Washington, DC, December 2010, U.S. Government Printing Office.

Wellness Councils of America (WELCOA): *The 7 benchmarks of success*, Omaha, Nebr, 2009, WELCOA. Accessed March 2010 from http://www.welcoa.org/.

World Health Organization (WHO): *Progress on health-related millennium development goals (MDGs)*, Copenhagen, May 2009, WHO. http://www.who.int/whosis/whostat/2009/en/index.html, accessed March, 2010.

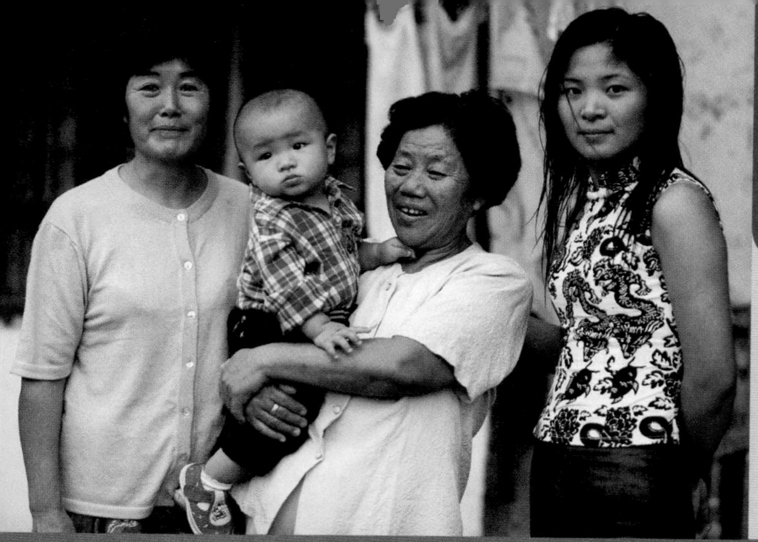

CHAPTER 21

Nancy S. Wellman, PhD, RD, FADA
Barbara J. Kamp, MS, RD

Nutrition in Aging

KEY TERMS

achlorhydria
activities of daily living (ADLs)
age-related macular degeneration (AMD)
assisted living communities (ALCs)
baby boomer
cataract
diabetic retinopathy
dysgeusia
dysphagia
functionality
geriatrics
gerontology
glaucoma
home- and community-based services (HCBS)
hyposmia
instrumental activities of daily living (IADLs)
Minimum Data Set (MDS)
Omnibus Reconciliation Act (OBRA)
one percent rule
polypharmacy
pressure ulcers
presbycusis
quality of life
Resident Assessment Instrument (RAI)
sarcopenia
sarcopenic obesity
sedentary death syndrome (SeDS)
senescence
skilled nursing facility (SNF)
supercentenarians
xerostomia

THE OLDER POPULATION

Older adults in the United States are living longer, healthier, and more functionally fit lives than ever before. Life expectancy increased by 30 years in the twentieth century. Those born today can expect to live an average of 77.9 years. Women who reach age 65 can expect to live an additional 19.9 years, and men, 17.2 years. By the year 2020 the population older than age 65 will grow from approximately 40 million to 55 million, increasing from 13% to 20% of the population. The fastest-growing segment is those older than age 85, currently almost 6 million and increasing to almost 7 million in 2020. Members of minority groups will also increase from 20% to 24% of the older population (U.S. Administration on Aging [USAoA], 2010). See Figures 21-1 and 21-2.

By 2030 the number of older adults will exceed the number of school-age children in 10 states—Florida, Pennsylvania, Vermont, Wyoming, North Dakota, Delaware, New Mexico, Montana, Massachusetts, and West Virginia. A few years ago no state had more people older than age 65 than those younger than 18. Twenty-six states will double their older-than-65 population by 2030, when the oldest of the **baby boomer** generation enter their 80s. Growth in the older-than-65 population will equal 3.5 times the U.S. growth as a whole. This demographic shift has enormous social, economic, and political implications (He, 2005).

Women live longer than men. The older-than-65 female/male ratio is 136:100; it increases to 216:100 among those older than age 85. More than 72% of older men are married, whereas only 42% of older women are married. Half of women over age 75 live alone; thus more men die married and most women die unmarried.

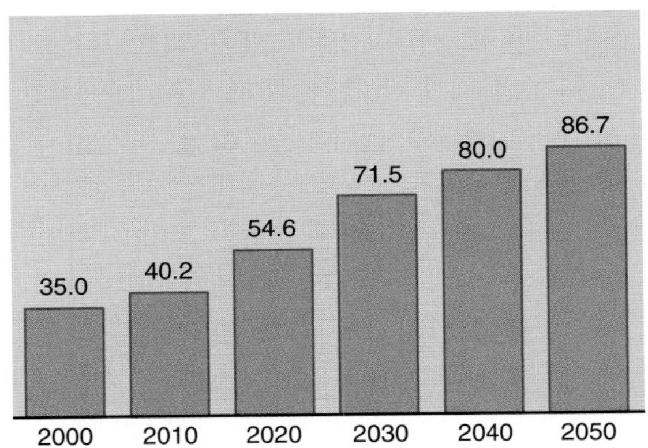

FIGURE 21-1 Population ages 65 and older: 2000 to 2050. *(Data from He W et al:* U.S. Census Bureau, current population reports, P23-209, 65+ in the United States: 2005, *Washington, DC, 2005, U.S. Government Printing Office.)*

Classification

Everyone knows people older than themselves, but those considered "old" depends a lot on one's own age. Youngsters consider their 20- or 30-something parents old. Today gray hair color, wrinkles, retirement, or age 65 no longer defines *old.* Yet qualifying as an "older adult" is based on the minimum eligibility age of 65 in many federal programs. The U.S. Census Bureau uses a stratified system to define this generation-spanning age-group; those aged 65 to 74 are the *young old;* 75 to 84, *old;* and 85 or older, *oldest old.* Some consider today's *new old* to be those in their 90s. The more than 100,000 centenarians alive today are no longer considered unique and many of them still live independently. See *Focus On:* Centenarians...Life in the Blue Zone.

GERONTOLOGY + GERIATRICS = THE SPECTRUM OF AGING

Gerontology is the study of normal aging, including factors in biology, psychology, and sociology. **Geriatrics** is the study of the chronic diseases frequently associated with aging, including diagnosis and treatment. Although medical nutrition therapy has commonly been practiced in hospitals, nutrition services have moved out of hospitals and into

FOCUS ON

Centenarians...Life in the Blue Zone

By Janice M. Raymond, RD, MS

Centenarians are the fastest growing segment of older adults in the United Stated and in developed nations, including Japan. The worldwide estimate of centenarians is 450,000. The U.S. Census Bureau estimates for 2009 there are about 65,000 centenarians and more than 1 million by 2050. As with the aging population as a whole, women represent 85% of the long-lived. A new group of individuals older than age 110, **supercentenarians**, have sufficient numbers to merit dedicated research.

What is known about extremely long-lived individuals? Centenarians generally have delays in functional decline. They also tend to either never develop a chronic disease or develop one late in life. Much has been written about longevity in the southern Japanese prefecture of Okinawa. The ongoing Okinawa Centenarian Study suggests that low caloric intake may produce fewer destructive free radicals. This intake plus an active lifestyle, natural ability to combat the stresses of life, and a genetic predisposition favor a healthy, functional, longer life.

Buettner and colleagues (2008) worked with the National Institute on Aging to identify communities around the world where people are living longer and living measurably better. They called these areas, where people reach the age of 100 at rates 10 times greater than in the United States, the *Blue Zones.* One such community was Okinawa. Others included the Nicoya Peninsula in Costa Rica and Sardinia in Italy. Residents of Loma Linda in California boast the longest life spans in America. They found that these groups had common characteristics related to food: very little animal protein and four to six servings of fruits, vegetables, legumes, and nuts. But eating wisely is only part of what seems to be a prescription for long life. The people of these communities don't smoke and make regular low-intensity exercise part of their daily routine (e.g., gardening, walking). They are people who can articulate their purpose in life, are spiritually fulfilled, and have strong social networks.

In the New England Centenarian Study, independent function to at least age 90 is a predominant feature. Other important factors are that few centenarians are obese, they rarely smoke, and they consume little or no alcohol. At least 50% of centenarians have first-degree relatives or grandparents who also achieved very old age, and many have exceptionally old siblings (Boston University School of Medicine, 2010).

FIGURE 21-2 Percent of people ages 65 and older in poverty by sex, race, and Hispanic origin. Note: The term *non-Hispanic white alone* is used to refer to people who reported being white and no other race and who are not Hispanic. The term *black alone* is used to refer to people who reported being black or African American and no other race, and the term *Asian alone* is used to refer to people who reported only Asian as their race. Reference population: These data refer to the resident population. *(U.S. Census Bureau: Population estimates and projections, 2000.)*

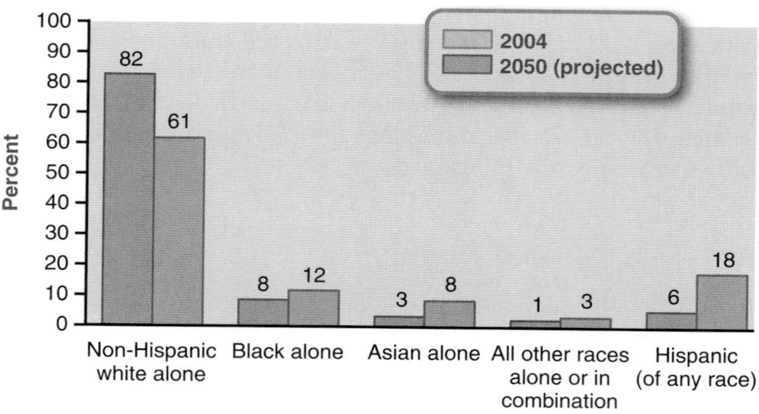

homes and communities where the focus is on health promotion, risk reduction, and disease prevention.

NUTRITION IN HEALTH PROMOTION AND DISEASE PREVENTION

In aging nutrition care is not only disease management or medical nutrition therapy; it has broadened with a stronger focus on healthy lifestyles and disease prevention. Without increased emphasis on better diets and more physical activity at all ages, health care expenditures will rise exorbitantly as the population ages. Thus it is never too late to emphasize nutrition for health promotion and disease prevention. Older Americans, more than any other age group, want health and nutrition information and are willing to make changes to maintain their independence and quality of life. They often need help in improving self-care behaviors. They want to know how to eat healthier, exercise safely, and stay motivated.

Nutrition may include three types of preventive services. In *primary prevention*, the emphasis is on nutrition in health promotion and disease prevention. Pairing healthy eating with physical activity is equally important.

Secondary prevention involves risk reduction and slowing the progression of chronic nutrition-related diseases to maintain functionality and quality of life. *Functionality* is perceived as a positive way to discuss fitness versus disability and dependence, because the term *exercise* is not appealing. Many community dining centers funded through the Older Americans Act (OAA) Nutrition Programs attract participants through new fitness programs

In *tertiary prevention*, case management and discharge planning often involve chewing and appetite problems, modified diets, and functional limitations. Complicated cases are often influenced by nutrition issues; case managers can benefit from consulting with dietitians (see *New Directions:* Providing Health Care for Older Americans Means Jobs).

THEORIES ON AGING

Gerontologists study aging and have diverse theories about why the body ages. No single theory can fully explain the complex processes of aging. A good theory should integrate knowledge and tell how and why phenomena are related. Broadly, theories can be grouped into two categories: predetermined and accumulated damage. A loss of efficiency comes about as some cells wear out, die, or are not replaced. This is sometimes referred to as the **one percent rule**; most organ systems lose approximately 1% of their functioning each year, starting at age 30. A recent theory is that the cause of age-related health decline is malfactioning telomeres. So far the studies are in mice (Sahin et al., 2011). Most likely several theories explain the heterogeneity in older populations. See Table 21-1.

PHYSIOLOGIC CHANGES

Aging is a normal biologic process. However, it involves some decline in physiologic function. Organs change with age. The rates of change differ among individuals and within organ systems. It is important to distinguish between normal changes of aging and changes caused by chronic disease such as atherosclerosis.

The human growth period draws to a close at approximately age 30, when senescence begins. **Senescence** is the organic process of growing older and displaying the effects of increased age. Disease and impaired function are not inevitable parts of aging. Nevertheless, there are certain systemic changes that occur as part of growing older. These changes result in varying degrees of efficiency and functional decline. Factors such as genetics, illnesses, socioeconomics, and lifestyle all determine how aging progresses for each person. Indeed, one's outward expression of age may or may not reflect one's chronologic age and there is a need to eliminate ageist stereotypes. See Figure 21-3.

Body Composition

Body composition changes with aging. Fat mass and visceral fat increase, whereas lean muscle mass decreases. **Sarcopenia**, the loss of muscle mass, strength, and function,

NEW DIRECTIONS

Providing Health Care for Older Americans Means Jobs

Registered dietitians (RDs) were identified by the Institute of Medicine in 2000 as "the single group with the standardized education and clinical training necessary to be directly reimbursed through Medicare as providers of nutrition therapy." The projected growth for dietitians is 15% overall, but a remarkable 70% in home and residential care. The Centers for Medicare and Medicaid Services is contracting with chronic care improvement programs for individuals with nutrition-related conditions, including heart failure, diabetes, and chronic obstructive pulmonary disease. RDs have more opportunities because of the major expansion of medical nutrition therapy under the Medicare Reform/Prescription Drug Law.

There are few college nutrition courses on healthy aging, but many on maternal and child health. Nutrition textbooks have focused on geriatric illnesses and malnutrition (O'Neill et al., 2005). There is a need to better prepare future RDs for these new opportunities. Nutrition students are encouraged to work with older adults because jobs are growing rapidly and financial incentives are strong.

Improving knowledge and attitudes about aging takes exposure to positive RD role models and older adults in a wide variety of settings. There are opportunities in service projects, internship placements, and summer externships at community dining centers, retirement centers, and assisted living and continuous-care facilities. Volunteering at food banks on days when older adults are scheduled to pick up groceries, teaming up with volunteers who deliver meals to the frail homebound, and participating in mealtime assistance for nursing home residents who cannot eat independently are good opportunities. Student associations can sponsor activities that foster interactions across the spectrum of aging, from the well active to the frail needy.

Full-time RDs have been shown to improve the quality of nursing home care because their expertise is essential to prevent unintended weight loss, dehydration, and pressure ulcers. Assisted living facilities and continuous-care communities present job opportunities as they expand and serve more at-risk persons. Positive experiences are sure to reduce ageist stereotypes, increase interest, and develop the skills needed to ride America's age wave.

TABLE 21-1

Theories on Aging

Category	Theory	Description
Predetermination: A built-in mechanism determines when aging begins and time of death	Pacemaker theory	"Biologic clock" is set at birth, runs for a specified time, winds down with aging, and ends at death.
	Genetic theory	Life span is determined by heredity.
	Rate of living theory	Each living creature has a finite amount of a "vital substance," and, when it is exhausted, the result is aging and death.
	Oxygen metabolism theory	Animals with the highest metabolisms are likely to have the shortest life spans.
	Immune system theory	Cells undergo a finite number of cell divisions that eventually cause deregulation of immune function, excessive inflammation, aging, and death.
Accumulated damage: Systemic breakdown over time	Crosslink theory	With time proteins, DNA and other structural molecules in the body make inappropriate attachments, or crosslinks, to each other, leading to decreased mobility, elasticity, and cell permeability.
	Wear-and-tear theory	Years of damage to cells, tissues, and organs eventually take their toll, wearing them out and ultimately causing death.
	Free radical theory	Accumulated, random damage caused by oxygen radicals slowly cause cells, tissues, and organs to stop functioning.
	Somatic mutation theory	Genetic mutations caused by oxidizing radiations and other factors accumulate with age, causing cells to deteriorate and malfunction.

DNA, Deoxyribonucleic acid.

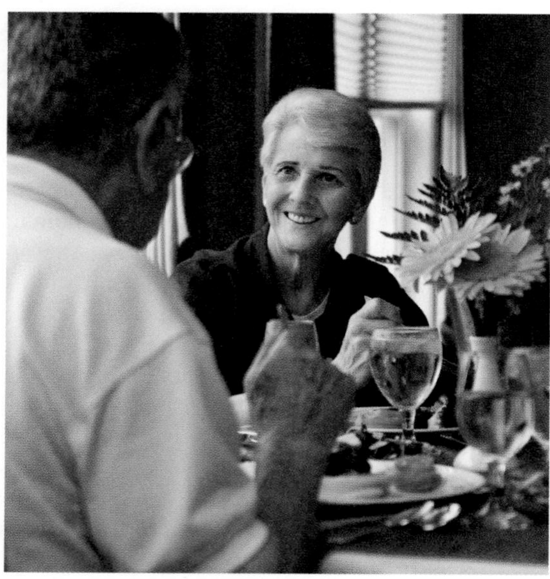

FIGURE 21-3 Enjoying a meal together, these older people are interested in knowing how good nutrition can keep them vigorous and healthy. *(© 2011 Photos.com a division of Getty Images. All rights reserved.)*

can be age-related, and can significantly affect an older adult's quality of life by decreasing mobility, increasing risk for falls, and altering metabolic rates (Janssen, 2009; Thomas, 2010). Sarcopenia accelerates with a decrease in physical activity, but weight-bearing exercise can slow its pace. Although inactive persons have faster and greater losses of muscle mass, sarcopenia is also found in active older individuals, to a lesser degree. Currently no specified degree of lean body mass loss determines the diagnosis of sarcopenia. All losses are important because of the close connection between muscle mass and strength. By the fourth decade of life evidence of sarcopenia is detectable, and the process accelerates after approximately age 75.

Sarcopenic obesity is the loss of lean muscle mass in older persons with excess adipose tissue. Together the excess weight and decreased muscle mass exponentially compound to further decrease physical activity, which in turn accelerates sarcopenia. An extremely sedentary lifestyle in obese persons is a major detractor from quality of life.

Sedentary lifestyle choices can lead to **sedentary death syndrome (SeDS)**, a phrase coined by The President's Council on Physical Fitness. It describes the life-threatening health problems caused by a sedentary lifestyle. *Sedentary lifestyle* can be defined as a level of inactivity below the threshold of the beneficial health effects of regular physical activity or, more simply, burning fewer than 200 calories in physical activity per day. *The Surgeon General's Vision for a Healthy and Fit Nation 2010* emphasizes health consequences of inactivity as greater risk for cardiovascular disease (CVD), hypertension, diabetes, dyslipidemia, obesity, overweight, and even death (U.S. Department of Health and Human Services, 2010).

Few older adults achieve the minimum recommended 30 or more minutes of moderate physical activity on 5 or more days per week. Only 22% of adults older than age 65 report engaging in regular leisure time physical activity (Centers for Disease Control and Prevention, 2006). Inactivity is more common in older people than younger people; women often report no leisure-time activity. The American College of Sports Medicine position emphasizes that all older adults should engage in regular physical activity and avoid an inactive lifestyle (American College of Sports Medicine, 2009). The Centers for Disease Control and Prevention (2010) quantifies the amount of exercise older adults need and the National Institute on Aging (2010) has a guide for physical activity.

Taste and Smell

Sensory losses affect people to varying degrees, at varying rates, and at different ages (Benelam, 2009; Schiffman, 2009). Genetics, environment, and lifestyle are all part of the decline in sensory competence. Age-related alterations to the sense of taste, smell, and touch can lead to poor appetite, inappropriate food choices, and lower nutrient intake. Although some **dysgeusia** (altered taste), loss of taste, or **hyposmia** (decreased sense of smell) are attributable to aging, many changes are due to medications. Other causes include conditions such as Bell's palsy; head injury; diabetes; liver or kidney disease; hypertension; neurologic conditions, including Alzheimer's disease and Parkinson's disease; and zinc or niacin deficiency. Untreated mouth sores, tooth decay, poor dental or nasal hygiene, and cigarette smoking also can decrease these senses.

Because taste and smell sensation thresholds are higher, older adults may be tempted to over-season foods, especially to add more salt, which may have a negative effect in many older adults. Because taste and smell stimulate metabolic changes such as salivary, gastric acid, and pancreatic secretions and increases in plasma levels of insulin, decreased sensory stimulation may impair these metabolic processes as well.

Hearing and Eyesight

In the United States 30% to 35% of adults ages 65 to 75 and 50% of those older than age 75 have some degree of hearing loss (National Institute on Deafness, 2006). Approximately one in four older adults who need a hearing aid actually use one. The most common type of hearing loss is **presbycusis**. This loss is usually greater in the high-pitched tonal range (e.g., telephone ring). The cumulative effect of exposure to daily noises such as traffic, construction, loud music, noisy office, and machines causes a change to the inner ear complex. The change occurs slowly over time, and sufferers may not be aware of the loss.

Some vitamins may play a part in hearing loss. Vitamin B_{12}, a nutrient often found to be deficient in the diets of older adults, has been associated with increased ringing in the ears, presbycusis, and reduced auditory brainstem response. Vitamin D may have an effect on hearing loss because of the role it plays in calcium metabolism, fluid and nerve transmission, and bone structure.

Vision loss is not a part of normal aging. However, everyone's vision changes with age. For most the changes are small and correctable with glasses, improved lighting, or large print. Reading glasses often become necessary in the fourth decade of life.

Immunocompetence

As immunocompetence declines with age, immune response is slower and less efficient. Changes occur at all levels of the immune system, from chemical alterations within the cells to differences in the kinds of proteins found on the cell surface and even to mutations to entire organs. The progressive decline in T-lymphocyte function and cell-mediated immunity contributes to the increased infection and cancer rates seen in aging populations. The mechanisms of age-related changes in immune function are not fully understood but likely depend on environmental factors and lifestyle choices that affect overall immune function. Maintaining good nutritional status promotes good immune function.

Oral

Diet and nutrition can be compromised by poor oral health. Tooth loss, use of dentures, and **xerostomia** (dry mouth) can lead to difficulties in chewing and swallowing. Decreases in taste sensation and saliva production make eating less pleasurable and more difficult. Oral diseases and conditions are common among Americans who grew up without the benefit of community water fluoridation and other fluoride products. Missing, loose, or rotten teeth or poor-fitting, painful dentures make it difficult to eat some foods. People with these mouth problems often prefer soft, easily chewed foods and avoid some nutritionally dense options such as whole grains, fresh fruits and vegetables, and meats.

The nutrition-related consequences of taking five or more medications or over-the-counter drugs daily (**polypharmacy**) are significant. More than 400 commonly used medications can cause dry mouth. See Chapter 9. Preparing foods that are moisture-rich such as hearty soups and stews, adding sauces, and pureeing and chopping foods can all make meals easier to eat. In addition, those with poor oral health may benefit from fortified foods with increased nutrient density. Although 30% of today's adults 65 years and older no longer have any natural teeth, tooth loss is no longer part of normal aging.

Gastrointestinal

Some gastrointestinal (GI) changes may be age-related. Rather than ascribing any of these disorders to aging, the true clinical cause should be determined. GI changes can negatively affect a person's nutrient intake, starting in the mouth. **Dysphagia**, a dysfunction in swallowing, is commonly associated with neurologic diseases and senility. It increases the risk for aspiration pneumonia, an infection caused by food or fluids entering the lungs. Thickened liquids and texture-modified foods can help people with dysphagia eat safely. The National Dysphagia Diet is in Appendix 35 and appropriate levels of texture modification are also defined in Chapter 41.

Gastric changes can also occur. Decreased gastric mucosal function leads to an inability to resist damage such as ulcers, cancer, and infections. Gastritis causes inflammation and pain, delayed gastric emptying, and discomfort. These all affect the bioavailability of nutrients such as calcium and zinc and increase the risk of developing a chronic deficiency disease such as osteoporosis.

Achlorhydria is the insufficient production of stomach acid. Approximately 30% of those older than age 50 have achlorhydria. Sufficient stomach acid and intrinsic factor are required for the absorption of vitamin B_{12}. Although substantial amounts are stored in the liver, B_{12} deficiency does occur. Symptoms, often misdiagnosed because they mimic Alzheimer's disease or other chronic conditions, include extreme fatigue, dementia, confusion, and tingling and weakness in the arms and legs (see Chapters 3, 33 and 41).

The incidence of diverticulosis increases with age. Half of the population older than age 60 develop it, but only 20% of them have clinical manifestations. The most common problems with diverticular disease are lower abdominal pain and diarrhea (see Chapter 29).

Constipation is defined as having fewer bowel movements than usual, having difficulty or excessive straining at stool, painful bowel movements, hard stool, or incomplete emptying of the bowel. Older adults are more likely than younger adults to become constipated. Primary causes include insufficient fluids, lack of physical activity, and low intake of dietary fiber. Constipation is also caused by delayed transit time in the gut and some medications like narcotics. (See Chapter 9).

Cardiovascular

CVD includes heart disease and stroke. Although the effects of CVD are often measured by deaths in later life, it is not a disease of aging. This nutrition-related disease has its roots in unhealthy food choices made throughout one's lifetime (Neidert, 2005). CVD is the leading cause of deaths in both genders in the United States, in all racial and ethnic groups. CVD age-related changes are extremely variable and are affected by environmental influences such as smoking, exercise, and diet. Changes include decreased arterial wall compliance, decreased maximum heart rate, decreased responsiveness to *b*-adrenergic stimuli, increased left ventricle muscle mass, and slowed ventricular relaxation. Often the end result of hypertension and artery disease is chronic heart failure. A low sodium diet and fluid restriction is integral to the treatment of this condition. These necessary diet restrictions in conjunction with other side effects of heart failure often lead to decreased nutrient consumption. See Chapter 34 for discussion of the multifaceted approach required to manage CVD in the elderly.

Renal

Age-related changes in renal function vary tremendously. Some older adults experience little change, whereas others can have devastating, life-threatening change. On average glomerular filtration rate, measured in creatinine clearance rates, declines by approximately 8 to 10 $mL/min/1.73m^2$/decade after age 30 to 35. The resulting increase in serum creatinine concentrations should be considered when determining medication dosages. The progressive decline in renal function can lead to an inability to excrete concentrated or dilute urine, a delayed response to sodium deprivation or a sodium load, and delayed response to an acid load. Renal function is also affected by dehydration, diuretic use, and medications, especially antibiotics.

Neurologic

There can be significant age-related declines in neurologic processes. Cognition, steadiness, reactions, coordination, gait, sensations, and daily living tasks can decline as much as 90% or as little as 10%. On average, the brain loses 5% to 10% of its weight between the ages of 20 and 90, but most if not all neurons are functional until death unless a specific pathologic condition is present.

It is important to make the distinction between normal, age-related decline and impairment from conditions such as dementia, a disease process. Memory difficulties do not necessarily indicate dementia, Alzheimer's disease, Parkinson's disease, or any mental disorder (see Chapter 41). Many changes in memory can be attributed to environmental factors, including stress, chemical exposure, and poor diet rather than to physiologic processes. However, even mild cognitive impairment that affects approximately 20% of those older than age 70 may affect eating, chewing, and swallowing, thus increasing the risk of malnutrition.

COMMON HEALTH PROBLEMS

Eye Disease

Age-related macular degeneration (AMD) is the leading cause of blindness in people older than age 65 in the United States; it may also be linked to an increased risk for stroke (Wong, 2006). AMD occurs when the macula, the center part of the retina, degrades. The result is central vision loss. The macular pigment is composed of two chemicals, lutein and zeaxanthin. A diet rich in fruits and vegetables may help delay or prevent the development of AMD. Zinc has also been shown to decrease the risk of developing AMD. Finally, correcting obesity and smoking are modifiable factors that can reduce progression of AMD (Clemons, 2006).

Glaucoma is damage to the optic nerve resulting from high pressure in the eye. It is the second most common cause of vision loss in the United States and affects approximately 3 million Americans. Hypertension, diabetes, and CVD all increase the risk of glaucoma.

A **cataract** is a clouding of the lens of the eye. Approximately half of Americans 65 and older have some degree of clouding of the lens. The most common treatment is surgery; the clouded lens is removed and replaced with a permanent prosthetic lens. A diet high in antioxidants such as beta-carotene, selenium, resveratrol, and vitamins C and E may delay cataract development. Studies show that a high sodium intake may increase risk of cataract development. Ultraviolet (UV) radiation exposure is directly related to 5% of worldwide cataracts. When the UV index is 3 and above, protective sunglasses are recommended (World Health Organization, 2009).

Diabetic retinopathy is a complication of diabetes (see Chapter 31). It occurs when blood vessels of the retina leak and produce spotty hemorrhages. Not all persons with diabetes develop retinopathy; blood glucose control can help protect the retina from damage.

All forms of vision loss can negatively affect nutritional status. Those with moderate-to-severe vision loss may have difficulty shopping for, identifying, and preparing foods and self-feeding.

Depression

Psychological changes often manifest as depression and its extent can vary widely from person to person. Among older persons depression is often caused by other conditions such as heart disease, stroke, diabetes, cancer, grief, or stress. Depression in older people is frequently undiagnosed or misdiagnosed because symptoms are confused with other medical illnesses. Untreated depression can have serious side effects for older adults. It diminishes the pleasures of living, including eating; it can exacerbate other medical conditions; and it can compromise immune function. It is associated with decreased appetite, weight loss, and fatigue. Nutritional care plays an important role in addressing this condition (see Chapter 42). Providing nutrient- and calorie-dense foods, additional beverages, texture-modified foods, and favorite foods at times when people are most likely to eat the greatest quantity can be very effective. In that comorbidities lead to polypharmacy and concern regarding drug-drug interactions, providers may choose to omit antidepressants, which leaves the depression untreated.

Pressure Ulcers

Pressure ulcers, formerly called *bedsores* or *decubitus ulcers*, develop from continuous pressure that impedes capillary blood flow to skin and underlying tissue. Several factors contribute to the formation of pressure ulcers, but impaired mobility and urinary incontinence are key. Older adults with neurologic problems, those heavily sedated, and those with dementia are often unable to shift positions to alleviate pressure. Paralysis, incontinence, sensory losses, and rigidity can all contribute to the problem. Notably malnutrition (inadequate protein) and undernutrition (inadequate energy intake) set the stage for its development and can delay wound healing. The escalating chronic nature of pressure ulcers in bed-ridden or sedentary elderly requires vigilant attention to nutrition.

Several classification systems exist to describe pressure ulcers. The four stages of pressure ulcers, based on the depth of the sore and level of tissue involvement, are described in Table 21-2. Thomas (2009) suggests that wound nutrition equals whole-body nutrition, and coordinated efforts of a multidisciplinary treatment team are important. Nutrition recommendations for the treatment of pressure ulcers are as follows (Doley, 2010; Thomas, 2009):

- Optimize protein intake with a goal of 1.25 to 2 g/kg/day.
- Meet calorie requirements at 30-40 kcal/kg/day.
- Assess the effect of medications on wound healing and supplement if indicated.
- Replace micronutrients if depleted—routine supplementation is not warranted.

Frailty and Failure to Thrive

The four syndromes known to be predictive of adverse outcomes in older adults that are prevalent in patients with frailty or "geriatric failure to thrive" include impaired physical functioning, malnutrition, depression, and cognitive impairment. Symptoms include weight loss, decreased appetite, poor nutrition, dehydration, inactivity, and impaired immune function. Interventions should be directed at easily remediable contributors in the hope of improving overall functional status. Nutrition interventions, especially those rectifying protein-energy malnutrition (PEM), are essential.

QUALITY OF LIFE

Quality of life is a general sense of happiness and satisfaction with one's life and environment. Health-related quality of life is the personal sense of physical and mental health and the ability to react to factors in the physical and social environments. To assess health-related quality of life, common measures and scales, either general or disease-specific, can be used. Because older age is often associated with health problems and decrease in functionality, quality-of-life issues become relevant.

Food and nutrition contribute to one's physiologic, psychological, and social quality of life. A measure of nutrition-related quality of life has been proposed to document quality-of-life outcomes for individuals receiving medical nutrition therapy. Effective strategies to improve eating and thereby improve nursing home residents' quality of life are well established but could be more widely implemented (Kamp et al., 2010; Neidert, 2005).

Functionality

Functionality and *functional status* are terms used to describe physical abilities and limitations in, for example, ambulation. **Functionality**, the ability to perform self-care, self-maintenance, and physical activities, correlates with independence and quality of life. Disability rates among older adults are declining, but the actual number considered disabled is increasing as the size of the aging population grows. Limitations in **activities of daily living (ADLs)** (toileting, bathing, eating, dressing) and **instrumental activities of daily living (IADLs)** such as managing money, shopping, telephone use, travel in community, housekeeping, preparing meals, taking medications correctly, and other individual self-performance skills needed in everyday life, are used to monitor physical function.

Many nutrition-related diseases affect functional status in older individuals. Inadequate nutrient intake may hasten loss of muscle mass and strength, which can have a negative effect on performing ADLs. Among the older adults who have one or more nutrition-related chronic diseases, impaired physical function may cause greater disability, with increased morbidity, nursing home admissions or death.

Weight Maintenance

Obesity

The prevalence of obesity in all ages has increased during the past 25 years in the United States; older adults are no exception. Obesity rates are greater among those ages 65 to 74 than among those age 75 and older. Obesity is associated with increased mortality and contributes to many chronic diseases: type 2 diabetes, heart disease, hypertension, arthritis, dyslipidemia, and cancer. Obesity causes a progressive decline in physical function, which may lead to increased frailty. Overweight and obesity can lead to a decline in IADLs.

Current data demonstrate that weight-loss therapy improves physical function, quality of life, and reduces the medical complications associated with obesity in older persons (Villareal, 2005). Accordingly, weight loss therapies that maintain muscle and bone mass are recommended for obese older adults. Lifestyle changes that include diet, physical activity, and behavior modification techniques are the most effective. The goals of weight loss and management for adults are the same for the general population, and should include prevention of further weight gain, or reduction of body weight, and maintenance of long-term weight loss.

Weight loss of 10% of total body weight over 6 months should be the initial goal. After that, strategies for maintenance should be implemented. Dietary changes include an energy deficit of 500-1000 kcal/day. Usual caloric goals range from 1200-1800 kcal/day but should not be less than 800 kcal/day. It is critical for the older adult on a calorie-restricted diet to meet nutrient requirements. This may necessitate the use of a multivitamin or mineral supplement as well as nutrition education.

Underweight and Malnutrition

The actual prevalence of underweight among older adults is quite low; older women older than age 65 are three times as likely as their male counterparts to be underweight (Federal Interagency Forum, 2008). However, many older adults are at risk for undernutrition and malnutrition. Among those hospitalized, 40% to 60% are malnourished or at risk for malnutrition, 40% to 85% of nursing home residents have malnutrition, and 20% to 60% of home care

TABLE 21-2

Pressure Ulcer Stages and Nutritional Recommendations

Suspected Deep Tissue Injury Purple or maroon localized area of discolored intact skin or blood-filled blister caused by damage of underlying soft tissue from pressure or shear. The area may be preceded by tissue that is painful, firm, mushy, boggy, warmer, or cooler as compared with adjacent tissue. Deep tissue injury may be difficult to detect in individuals with dark skin tones. Evolution may include a thin blister over a dark wound bed. The wound may further evolve and become covered by thin eschar. Evolution may be rapid, exposing additional layers of tissue even with optimal treatment.	Energy: 30 calories/kg BW Normal protein requirements in healthy adults are approximately 0.8 g/kg of body weight and 1 g/kg BW in the elderly.
Stage I Intact skin with nonblanchable redness of a localized area, usually over a bony prominence. Darkly pigmented skin may not have visible blanching; its color may differ from the surrounding area. The area may be painful, firm, soft, warmer, or cooler as compared with adjacent tissue. Stage I may be difficult to detect in individuals with dark skin tones. May indicate "at-risk" persons (a heralding sign of risk).	Energy: 30 to 35 calories/kg BW Protein: 1.25 to 1.5 grams/kg BW Fluid: 30 to 33 cc/kg BW; possibly less fluid for patients with severe renal disease or congestive heart failure.
Stage II Partial thickness loss of dermis presenting as a shallow open ulcer with a red pink wound bed without slough. May also present as an intact or open or ruptured serum-filled blister. Presents as a shiny or dry, shallow ulcer without slough or bruising. This stage should not be used to describe skin tears, tape burns, perineal dermatitis, maceration, or excoriation. Bruising indicates suspected deep tissue injury.	Energy: 30 to 35 calories/kg BW Protein: 1.25 to 1.5 grams/kg BW Fluid: 30 to 33 cc/kg BW; possibly less fluid for patients with severe renal disease or congestive heart failure.
Stage III Full-thickness tissue loss. Subcutaneous fat may be visible but bone, tendon, or muscle are not exposed. Slough may be present but does not obscure the depth of tissue loss. May include undermining and tunneling. The depth of a stage III pressure ulcer varies by anatomic location. The bridge of the nose, ear, occiput, and malleolus do not have subcutaneous tissue, and stage III ulcers can be shallow. In contrast, areas of significant adiposity can develop extremely deep stage III pressure ulcers. Bone and tendon are not visible or directly palpable.	Energy: 35 to 40 calories/kg BW Protein: 1.5 to 1.75 g/kg BW (Note: Assessment of protein needs should be determined after an assessment of visceral protein status has been completed, keeping in mind that stressed patients with protein depletion usually cannot metabolize more than 2 g/kg BW per day.) Fluid: 30 to 33 cc/kg BW; possibly less fluid for patients with severe renal disease or congestive heart failure. Additional fluids are needed for patients with draining wounds, fever, and other fluid losses. Patients on air-fluidized beds may become dehydrated because of increased evaporative water loss; extra 10 to 15 mL/kg BW may be needed. A multivitamin with 15 mg of zinc will be adequate for most patients.

TABLE 21-2

Pressure Ulcer Stages and Nutritional Recommendations—cont'd

Stage IV Full-thickness tissue loss with exposed bone, tendon, or muscle. Slough or eschar may be present on some parts of the wound bed. Often include undermining and tunneling. The depth of a stage IV pressure ulcer varies by anatomic location. The bridge of the nose, ear, occiput, and malleolus do not have subcutaneous tissue, and these ulcers can be shallow. Stage IV ulcers can extend into muscle and supporting structures (e.g., fascia, tendon, or joint capsule), making osteomyelitis possible. Exposed bone or tendon is visible or directly palpable.	Energy: 35 to 40 calories/kg BW Protein: 1.75 to 2 g/kg BW (Note: Assessment of protein needs should be determined after an assessment of visceral protein status has been completed, keeping in mind that stressed patients with protein depletion usually cannot metabolize more than 2 g/kg of body weight each day.) Fluid: 30 to 33 cc/kg BW; possibly less fluid for patients with severe renal disease or congestive heart failure. Additional fluids are needed for patients with draining wounds, fever, and other fluid losses. Patients on air-fluidized beds may become dehydrated because of increased evaporative water loss; extra 10 to 15 mL/kg body weight may be needed. A multivitamin with 15 mg of zinc/day may be adequate for most patients; some may require more zinc.
Unstageable Full-thickness tissue loss in which the base of the ulcer is covered by slough (yellow, tan, gray, green, or brown) or eschar (tan, brown, or black) in the wound bed. Until enough slough or eschar is removed to expose the base of the wound, the true depth, and therefore stage, cannot be determined. Stable (dry, adherent, intact without erythema or fluctuance) eschar on the heels serves as "the body's natural (biologic) cover" and should not be removed.	Often treated as a stage IV.

Sources: National Pressure Ulcer Advisory Panel, 2007; reprinted with permission. American Dietetic Association. Consultant Dietitians in Health Care Facilities. Pocket Resource for Nutrition Assessment. 2005 Revision; 69-73.

BW, Body weight.

patients are malnourished. Many community-residing older persons consume fewer than 1000 kcal/day, an amount not adequate to maintain good nutrition. Some causes of undernutrition include medications, depression, decreased sense of taste or smell, poor oral health, chronic diseases, dysphagia, and other physical problems that make eating difficult. Social causes may include living alone, inadequate income, lack of transportation, and limitations in shopping for and preparing food.

Health care professionals frequently overlook PEM. The physiologic changes of aging, as well as changes in living conditions and income, all contribute to the problem. Symptoms of PEM are often attributed to other conditions, leading to misdiagnosis. Some common symptoms are confusion, fatigue, and weakness. Older adults with low incomes, who have difficulty chewing and swallowing meat, who smoke, or engage in little or no physical activity are at increased risk of developing PEM.

Strategies to decrease PEM include increased caloric and protein intake. In a clinical setting nutritional oral supplements and enteral feedings may be used. Frailty is often related to micronutrient deficiencies, especially in women (Michelon, 2006). Older malnourished adults are at risk of refeeding syndrome when they begin to receive nutrition support, and this should be assessed (see Chapter 14).

In a community setting older adults should be encouraged to eat energy-dense and high-protein foods. Diet restrictions should be liberalized to offer more choices. Adding gravies and creams can increase calories and soften foods for easier chewing (Joshipura, 2009). Federal food and nutrition services are also available for older adults.

NUTRITION SCREENING AND ASSESSMENT

The Mini Nutritional Assessment (MNA) (Bauer, 2008) includes two sections: screening and assessment. The Short Form is the most widely used screening method to identify malnutrition in noninstitutionalized older adults. It includes six questions and a body mass index (BMI) evaluation, or a calf circumference, if a BMI is not possible. The MNA

Short Form has been validated (Kaiser, 2009). For a complete nutrition assessment, the full MNA is used. It is the most commonly used assessment tool in long-term care (see Figs 4-4 and 4-5.).

Some assessment measures are not necessarily accurate or feasible to use with older adults (Morley, 2009). Physical and metabolic changes of aging can yield inaccurate results. An illustration of this is anthropometric measurements such as height and weight, and BMI. With aging, fat mass increases and height decreases as a result of vertebral compression (Villareal, 2005). An accurate height measure may be difficult in those unable to stand up straight, the bed bound, those with spinal deformations such as a dowager's hump, and those with osteoporosis. Measuring arm span or knee height may give more accurate measurements. See Appendix 20. BMIs based on questionable heights are inaccurate. Clinical judgment is needed for accuracy.

Body composition measures may also be ineffective. Skin-fold thickness and mid-arm circumference used to detect changes in body fat are limited in their ability to distinguish between changes in fat and muscle mass, because of decreased elasticity and increased compressibility of older skin. Mid-arm muscle circumference measures may be more accurate and sensitive to weight change than overall body composition measurements.

NUTRITION NEEDS

Many older adults have special nutrient requirements because aging affects absorption, use, and excretion of nutrients (Kuczmarski and Weddle, 2005). The dietary reference intakes (DRIs) separate the cohort of people age 50 and older into two groups, ages 50-70 and 71 and older. Based on the Healthy Eating Index, older Americans need to increase their intakes of whole grains, dark green and orange vegetables, legumes, and milk; choose more nutrient-dense forms of foods, that is, foods low in solid fats and free of added sugars; and lower their intake of sodium and saturated fat (Juan, 2008). Other studies show that older persons have low intakes of calories, total fat, fiber, calcium, magnesium, zinc, copper, folate, and vitamins B_{12}, C, E, and D (Box 21-1).

The Mifflin-St. Jeor energy equation can be used to assess calorie needs in older adults (see Chapter 2). DRI tables (Table 21-3; see inside cover) can also be used. Here, DRIs for energy suggest 3067 kcal/day for men and 2403/day for women 18 years; subtract 10 kcal/day for men and 7 kcal/day for women for each year of age older than 19 years.

The DRIs are not specific for protein in older adults. After age 65, the minimum protein requirement is 1 g protein/kg of body weight (Chernoff, 2004). New evidence

BOX 21-1

Dietary Guidelines for Americans

KEY RECOMMENDATIONS FOR OLDER ADULTS

- **Maintain calorie balance over the lifetime to achieve and sustain a healthy weight.** Healthy eating patterns limit intake of sodium, solid fats, added sugars, and refined grains. Increased physical activity and reduced time spent in sedentary behaviors are also desired.
- **Focus on consuming nutrient-dense foods and beverages.** A healthy eating pattern emphasizes nutrient-dense foods and beverages. Select fat-free or low-fat milk and milk products, seafood, lean meats and poultry, eggs, beans and peas, and nuts and seeds. Choose vegetables, fruits, whole grains, and milk and milk products for more potassium, dietary fiber, calcium, and vitamin D as nutrients of concern. Eat a variety of vegetables, especially dark-green and red and orange vegetables, beans and peas. Consume at least half of all grains as whole grains.
- **Nutrient needs should be met primarily through consuming foods.** When needed, fortified foods and dietary supplements may be useful in providing one or more nutrients that otherwise might be consumed in less than recommended amounts. Consume foods fortified with vitamin B12, such as fortified cereals, or dietary supplements. Two eating patterns that are beneficial are Vegetarian adaptations and the DASH (Dietary Approaches to Stop Hypertension) Eating Plan.
- **A healthy eating pattern should prevent foodborne illness.** Four basic food safety principles (Clean, Separate, Cook, and Chill) work together to reduce the risk of foodborne illnesses. In addition, some foods (such as milks, cheeses, and juices that have not been pasteurized, and undercooked animal foods) pose high risk for foodborne illness and should be avoided.
- **Use alcohol in moderation.** If alcohol is consumed, it should be consumed in moderation—up to one drink per day for women and two drinks per day for men—and only by adults of legal drinking age.
- Individuals should meet the following recommendations as part of a healthy eating pattern while staying within their calorie needs.
- Information on the type and strength of evidence supporting the Dietary Guidelines recommendations can be found at http://www.nutritionevidencelibrary.gov.

Source: U.S. Department of Health and Human Services, U.S. Department of Agriculture: Dietary Guidelines for Americans, 2010, ed 7, Washington, DC, 2010, U.S. Government Printing Office.

supports 1 g/kg, even up to 1.2 gm/kg. In those individuals with impaired renal function or long-standing diabetes, .8g/kg to 1.0 g/kg may be more appropriate. Even protein distribution throughout the day with no single serving exceeding 30 g (Symons et al., 2009) should be a goal.

MEDICARE BENEFITS

The Social Security Act of 1965 created the Medicare program to cover most of the health care costs of those 65 and older and persons with disabilities. However, this federally funded health insurance program does not cover the entire cost of long-term care (LTC). A portion of payroll taxes and monthly premiums deducted from Social Security payments finance Medicare.

Medicare benefits are provided in four parts. *Part A* covers inpatient hospital care, some skilled nursing care, hospice care, and some home health care costs for limited periods of time. It is premium-free for most citizens. *Part B* has a monthly premium that helps pay for doctors, outpatient hospital care, and some other care not covered by Part A (physical and occupational therapy, for example). *Part C* allows private insurers, including health maintenance organizations (HMOs) and referred provider organizations (PPOs), to offer health insurance plans to Medicare beneficiaries. These must provide the same benefits the original Medicare plan provides under Parts A and B. Part C HMOs and PPOs may also offer additional benefits, such as dental and vision care. *Part D* provides prescription drug benefits through private insurance companies.

The 2010 health care reform legislation changed Medicare to include an annual wellness visit and a personalized prevention assessment and plan with no copayment or deductible. Prevention services include referrals to education and preventive counseling or community-based interventions to address risk factors. The new law mandates the creation of the Independence at Home Demonstration Project, a demonstration program to begin by 2012. It will enroll chronically ill Medicare beneficiaries to test a payment incentive and service delivery system that uses physician- and nurse practitioner–directed home-based primary care teams aimed at reducing costs and improving health outcomes. The 2010 law expands medical nutrition therapy reimbursement for registered dietitians to cover therapy considered reasonable and necessary for the prevention of an illness or disability.

The Home and Community-Based Services (HCBS) Waivers, Section 1915 (c), provide service to nursing home–appropriate older adults to help prevent or decrease nursing home or LTC institutionalization. States may offer an unlimited variety of services under this waiver. These waiver programs may provide both traditional medical services (dental, skilled nursing) and nonmedical services (meal delivery, case management, environmental modifications). States have the discretion to choose the number of older persons served. Forty-eight states (Michigan and Utah are the exceptions) and the District of Columbia offer services through HCBS waivers; currently there are approximately 287 active programs.

NUTRITION SUPPORT SERVICES

U.S. Department of Health and Human Services Older Americans Act Nutrition Program (OAA)

The OAA Nutrition Program is the largest, most visible, federally funded community-based nutrition program for older persons. Primarily a state-run program, it has few federal regulations and considerable variation in state-to-state policies and procedures. This nutrition program provides congregate and home-delivered meals (usually 5 days/week), nutrition screening, education, and counseling, as well as an array of other supportive and health services. Although frequently called *meals on wheels*, that term accurately refers *only* to the home-delivered meals. Participants are poorer, older, sicker, frailer, more likely to live alone, be members of minority groups, and live in rural areas (USAoA, 2008). The OAA Nutrition Program, available to persons age 60 and older, successfully targets those in greatest economic and social need, with particular attention to low-income minorities and rural individuals. More than half of the OAA annual budget supports the Nutrition Program, which provides approximately 240 million congregate and home-delivered meals to 2.6 million older adults annually. Home-delivered meals have grown to more than 60% of all meals served; almost half of the programs have waiting lists. To receive home-delivered meals, an individual must be assessed to be homebound or otherwise isolated. Home-delivered meal recipients are especially frail; half are at high nutrition risk or are malnourished and approximately one-third qualify as nursing-home appropriate.

At congregate sites, the Nutrition Program provides access and linkages to other community-based services. It is the primary source of food and nutrients for many program participants and presents opportunities for active social engagement and meaningful volunteer roles. Participants have higher daily intakes of key nutrients than similar non-participants. The meals are nutritionally dense per calorie and each meal supplies more than 33% of the recommended dietary allowances (an OAA requirement) and provides 40% to 50% of daily intakes of most nutrients (USAoA, 2008). Otherwise, inadequate nutrient intake affects approximately 37% to 40% of community-dwelling individuals 65 years of age and older (Federal Interagency Forum, 2008).

The OAA Nutrition Program has neither received the research or evaluation attention that a program its size deserves, nor the growth in federal funding to keep pace with inflation and the growing numbers of older adults (Wellman, 2010). The program reaches fewer than 5% of older Americans, and those served average fewer than three meals per week. The OAA Nutrition Program is closely linked to **home- and community-based services (HCBS)** through cross-referrals through the Aging Network. Because older adults are being discharged earlier from hospitals and

TABLE 21-3

Nutrient Needs Change With Aging

Nutrient	Changes with Aging	Practical Solutions
Energy	Basal metabolic rate decreases with age because of changes in body composition. Energy needs decrease ~3% per decade in adults.	Encourage nutrient-dense foods in amounts appropriate for caloric needs.
Protein 0.8 g/kg minimum	Minimal change with age but research is not conclusive. Requirements vary with chronic disease, decreased absorption, and synthesis.	Protein intake should not be routinely increased; excess protein could unnecessarily stress aging kidneys.
Carbohydrates 45%-65% of total calories Men 30 g fiber Women 21 g fiber	Constipation may be a serious concern for many.	Emphasize complex carbohydrates: legumes, vegetables, whole grains, fruits to provide fiber, essential vitamins, minerals. Increase dietary fiber to improve laxation especially in older adults.
Lipids 20%-35% total calories	Heart disease is a common diagnosis.	Overly severe restriction of dietary fats alters taste, texture, and enjoyment of food; can negatively affect overall diet, weight, and quality of life. Emphasize healthy fats rather restricting fat.
Vitamins and Minerals	Understanding vitamin and mineral requirements, absorption, use, and excretion with aging has increased but much remains unknown.	Encourage nutrient-dense foods in amounts appropriate for caloric needs. Oxidative and inflammatory processes affecting aging reinforce the central role of micronutrients, especially antioxidants.
Vitamin B_{12} 2.4 mg	Risk of deficiency increases because of low intakes of vitamin B_{12}, and decline in gastric acid, which facilitates B12 absorption.	Those 50 and older should eat foods fortified with the crystalline form of vitamin B_{12} such as in fortified cereals or supplements.

Vitamin D 800-1,000 IU	Risk of deficiency increases as synthesis is less efficient; skin responsiveness as well as exposure to sunlight decline; kidneys are less able to convert D3 to active hormone form. As many as 30%-40% of those with hip fractures are vitamin D insufficient.	Supplementation may be necessary. This supplement is inexpensive, whereas testing for vitamin D deficiency is costly and the laboratory methods are not completely assured at this point. A supplement is indicated in virtually all institutionalized older adults.
Folate 400 µg	May lower homocysteine levels; possible risk marker for atherothrombosis, Alzheimer disease, and Parkinson disease.	Fortification of grain products has improved folate status. When supplementing with folate, must monitor B_{12} levels.
Calcium 1200 mg	Dietary requirement may increase because of decreased absorption; only 4% of women and 10% of men age 60 and older meet daily recommendation.	Recommend naturally occurring and fortified foods. Supplementation may be necessary.
Potassium 4700 mg	Potassium-rich diet can blunt the effect of sodium on blood pressure.	Recommend meeting potassium recommendation with food, especially fruits and vegetables.
Sodium 1500 mg	Risk of hypernatremia caused by dietary excess and dehydration. Risk of hyponatremia caused by fluid retention.	Recommend consuming 1500 to no more than 2300 mg/d.
Zinc Men 11 mg Women 8 mg	Low intake associated with impaired immune function, anorexia, loss of sense of taste, delayed wound healing, and pressure ulcer development.	Encourage food sources: lean meats, oysters, dairy products, beans, peanuts, tree nuts and seeds.
Water	Hydration status can easily be problematic. Dehydration causes decreased fluid intake, decreased kidney function, increased losses caused by increased urine output from medications (laxatives, diuretics). Symptoms: electrolyte imbalance, altered drug effects, headache, constipation, blood pressure change, dizziness, confusion, dry mouth and nose.	Encourage fluid intake of at least 1500 mL/day or 1 mL per calorie consumed. Risk increases because of impaired sense of thirst, fear of incontinence, and dependence on others to get beverages. Dehydration is often unrecognized; it can present as falls, confusion, change in level of consciousness, weakness or change in functional status, or fatigue.

nursing homes, many require a care plan that includes home-delivered meals and other nutrition services (e.g., nutrition screening, assessment, education, counseling, and care planning). Many states are creating programs to provide necessary medical, social, and supportive HCBS, including home-delivered meals, nutrition education, and counseling services (Kuczmarski and Weddle, 2005).

USDA Food Assistance Programs

Several U.S. Department of Agriculture (USDA) food and nutrition assistance programs (www.fns.usda.gov/fns/default.htm) are available to older adults. All USDA programs are means tested (i.e., recipients must meet income criteria). These programs are discussed further in Chapter 10.

Supplemental Nutrition Assistance Program

The Supplemental Nutrition Assistance Program (SNAP) program (formerly Food Stamps) is designed to end hunger and improve nutrition and health of low-income Americans. Beneficiaries use electronic benefit transfer (EBT) cards to purchase certain foods at authorized retail food stores. The program is operated by state and local welfare offices under USDA guidance. Currently SNAP serves less than one third of eligible older adults—the lowest participation rate of all demographic groups. Reasons for the low participation rate include the myth that only a $10 monthly benefit is provided, feeling stigmatized as a welfare recipient, feeling the application process is overly intrusive, eligibility confusion, mistrusting the EBT cards, and lack of outreach.

The goal of SNAP nutrition education is to make healthy choices within a limited budget and choose active lifestyles consistent with the current Dietary Guidelines for Americans and MyPlate. State cooperative extension offices, nutrition education networks, public health departments, welfare agencies, and university centers generally provide the nutrition education. Unfortunately, little outreach specific to older adults is offered.

Commodity Supplemental Food Program

The Commodity Supplemental Food Program (CSFP) strives to improve the health of low-income Americans by supplementing their diets with nutritious USDA commodity foods. It provides food and administrative funds to states, but not all are enrolled. In states, CSFP administration may be located in diverse sites such as public health, nutrition services, or agriculture departments. Eligible populations include adults age 60 and older with incomes less than 130% of the poverty level. Local CSFP agencies determine eligibility, distribute the foods, and provide nutrition education. The food packages do not provide a complete diet, but may be good sources of nutrients frequently lacking in low-income diets.

Seniors' Farmers Market Nutrition Program

The Seniors' Farmers Market Nutrition Program (SFMNP) is administered by state departments of agriculture, aging and disability services, health and human service, markets, public health, state units on aging, or state food and nutrition services. SFMNP provides coupons to low-income older individuals to purchase fresh, unprepared foods at farmers' markets, roadside stands, and community-supported agriculture programs. It provides eligible older adults with local, seasonal access to fresh fruits, vegetables, and herbs.

Medicaid and Nutrition Services

The Social Security Act suggests seven core HCBS waiver program services: case management, homemaker services, home health aide services, personal care services, adult day health, rehabilitation, and respite care. Note that nutrition service is not a core Medicaid service. Older persons who are eligible for nursing home placement are not usually able to shop for food, store food safely, or plan and prepare nutritionally appropriate meals. Thus a strong argument can be made to fund all or some meals and nutrition services based on health and nutrition risk criteria. Yet only 38 states include meals or nutrition services among the specified benefits available through Medicaid waivers. Approved nutrition services include home-delivered meals, nutrition risk reduction counseling, and nutritional supplements as appropriate.

ASSISTED LIVING AND SKILLED CARE FACILITIES

Several million older adults live in senior housing of various types, (assisted living or residential care communities, skilled senior apartments, continuing care communities, independent retirement living). Some sites have supportive services available to their residents, including meals and services through the older adult nutrition program.

Assisted living communities (ALCs) generally serve the fastest growing population segment—those ages 85 and older. The estimated 33,000 licensed ALCs are home to approximately 1 million persons. They combine housing and personalized supportive and health care for those who need help with ADLs. Often residents move to ALCs when they can no longer safely live alone, have some cognitive impairment, and require supervision and "cueing" about their daily routine. ALCs usually involve the resident's family, neighbors, and friends. Care is provided in ways that promote maximum independence and dignity. Assisted living residences cost less than nursing home care. Residents are encouraged to maintain active social lives with planned activities, exercise classes, religious and social functions, and field trips directed by the facilities. These facilities are not required to provide therapeutic diets and can be a problem for patients with special requirements, such as those with heart failure.

Comprehensive state regulations for food and nutrition services in ALCs are rare, but there is early consensus of what should be regulated (Chao, 2009). Emphasizing that food and nutrition matter at every age, it is essential that support for nutrition and quality of life extend beyond food availability and safety. Dietitian expertise is needed for nutrition assessment and care planning to meet special needs such as type and amounts of macronutrients and micronutrients, texture modifications, and quality of food choices and presentation.

Surprisingly, fewer than 4% or 1.4 million seniors live in the approximately 15,730 **skilled nursing facilities (SNFs)** or LTC facilities (Centers for Medicare and Medicaid Services, 2010). The percentage of the population that lives in institutional settings, including nursing homes, increases dramatically with age, especially for those older than age 85. These percentages have declined since 1990, likely because of healthier aging, the federal cost-containment policy to rebalance LTC away from nursing homes to HCBS, and increased availability of hospice (He, 2005).

Skilled nursing facilities are federally regulated under the auspices of the Centers for Medicare and Medicaid Services; ALCs are subject to individual state regulations. More residents are there for short-stay, postacute care; thus more comprehensive medical nutrition therapy is needed. Nutritional care within long-term living facilities must be directed toward identifying and responding to changing physiologic and psychological needs over time that protect against avoidable decline. Attractive and palatable food served in an atmosphere that encourages eating independence, or assistance with eating provided when necessary, helps to promote nutritional well-being. For older adults, overall health goals may not warrant implementation of strict therapeutic diets that are often unpalatable and lessen quality of life. In terminal care for hospice patients, interventions include providing comfort foods and emotional support for family and friends.

In 1987 Congress approved reform legislation as a part of the **Omnibus Reconciliation Act (OBRA)** to improve quality of care in SNFs by strengthening standards that must be met for Medicare and Medicaid reimbursement. SNFs are required to conduct periodic assessments to determine the residents' needs; to provide services that ensure residents maintain the highest practical physical, mental and psychological well being; and to ensure that no harm is inflicted. This is accomplished using the **Minimum Data Set (MDS)**, which is part of the federally mandated process for clinical assessment of residents of LTC facilities licensed under Medicare or Medicaid. Section K of the MDS is specific to nutrition and is generally the responsibility of the dietitian to complete, but can be done by nursing staff (Figure 21-4). This form documents "triggers" that may place a resident at nutrition risk and therefore requires an intervention. This assessment must be done at admission and if there is a significant change in the resident's condition such as weight loss or skin breakdown. Reassessment is required quarterly and annually. The entire process is known as the **Resident Assessment Instrument (RAI)**. It provides the individual assessment of each resident's functional capabilities and helps identify problems and develop a care plan.

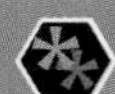

CLINICAL SCENARIO

MF is an 84-year-old white woman resident in a skilled nursing facility with unintentional weight loss. She was admitted 3 months ago from the hospital after a hip fracture. She had been residing in an independent living facility for several years. She reports she has been eating poorly because of difficulty moving around, being generally uncomfortable, and states, "If I am not active I don't need to eat so much." Intake is less than 50% of regular diet. No problems chewing or swallowing are noted after a speech language pathologist's evaluation. Admission weight was 112 pounds; current weight is 95 pounds. Self-reported height is 5′3″; albumin, 3.2; Hgb/Hct, normal; total cholesterol, 135; and Mini Nutrition Assessment score, 3. Hip scans show slow fracture healing and no improvement in bone density; currently being supplemented with calcium 1000 mg/d and vitamin D 400 IU/d. Blood pressure, 128/80 with furosemide (Lasix); other medications are lorazepam (Ativan), oxycodone, senna (Senokot-S), docusate (Colace), and megestrol acetate (Megace).

Nutrition Diagnostic Statement

Unintentional weight loss related to intake of less than 50% at meals with limited physical activity as evidenced by weight loss of 17 lb.

Nutrition Care Questions

1. Comment on the appropriateness of and use for each medication. Would you suggest any changes or additional medications?
2. What strategies could you use to help improve this resident's food and fluid intake?
3. What suggestions are appropriate to promote fracture healing and increase bone density?
4. Do you suspect that this client is constipated? What would you recommend in terms of food choices to deal with this?

USEFUL WEBSITES

Administration on Aging
http://www.aoa.gov

American Association of Homes and Services for the Aging
http://www.aahsa.org

American Association of Retired Persons
http://www.aarp.org

American Geriatrics Society
http://www.americangeriatrics.org

Centers for Medicare and Medicaid Services
http://www.cms.hhs.gov/

International Longevity Center
http://www.ilcusa.org/

Section K	Swallowing/Nutritional Status
K0100. Swallowing Disorder Signs and symptoms of possible swallowing disorder	
↓ **Check all that apply**	
☐	**A. Loss of liquids/solids from mouth when eating or drinking**
☐	**B. Holding food in mouth/cheeks or residual food in mouth after meals**
☐	**C. Coughing or choking during meals or when swallowing medications**
☐	**D. Complaints of difficulty or pain with swallowing**
☐	**Z. None of the above**
K0200. Height and Weight - While measuring, if the number is X.1 - X.4 round down; X.5 or greater round up	
☐☐ inches	**A. Height** (in inches). Record most recent height measure since admission
☐☐☐ pounds	**B. Weight** (in pounds). Base weight on most recent measure in last 30 days; measure weight consistently, according to standard facility practice (e.g., in a.m. after voiding, before meal, with shoes off, etc.)
K0300. Weight Loss	
Enter Code ☐	**Loss of 5% or more in the last month or loss of 10% or more in last 6 months** 0. **No** or unknown 1. **Yes, on** physician-prescribed weight-loss regimen 2. **Yes, not on** physician-prescribed weight-loss regimen
K0500. Nutritional Approaches	
↓ **Check all that apply**	
☐	**A. Parenteral/IV feeding**
☐	**B. Feeding tube** - nasogastric or abdominal (PEG)
☐	**C. Mechanically altered diet** - require change in texture of food or liquids (e.g., pureed food, thickened liquids)
☐	**D. Therapeutic diet** (e.g., low salt, diabetic, low cholesterol)
☐	**Z. None of the above**
K0700. Percent Intake by Artificial Route - Complete K0700 only if K0500A or K0500B is checked	
Enter Code ☐	**A. Proportion of total calories the resident received through parenteral or tube feeding** 1. **25% or less** 2. **26-50%** 3. **51% or more**
Enter Code ☐	**B. Average fluid intake per day by IV or tube feeding** 1. **500 cc/day or less** 2. **501 cc/day or more**

FIGURE 21-4 The Minimum Data Set, Section K version 3.0. *(From the Centers for Medicare & Medicaid Services, Baltimore, MD.)*

Minimum Data Set
http://www.cms.gov/IdentifiableDataFiles/10_LongTermCareMinimumDataSetMDS.asp

Meals on Wheels Association of America
http://www.mowaa.org/

Mini Nutritional Assessment
http://www.mna-elderly.com/default.html

National Association of Area Agencies on Aging
http://www.n4a.org/

National Association of Nutrition and Aging Services Programs
http://www.nanasp.org

National Citizen's Coalition for Nursing Home Reform
http://www.nccnhr.org/

National Institute on Aging
http://www.nih.gov/nia

National Institutes of Health Senior Health
http://nihseniorhealth.gov/

Older Americans Act Nutrition Program
http://www.aoa.gov/AoARoot/AoA_Programs/HCLTC/Nutrition_Services/index.aspx

Okinawa Centenarian Study
http://www.okicent.org/

U.S. Food and Drug Administration: To Your Health—Food Safety for Seniors
http://www.fda.gov/Food/ResourcesForYou/Consumers/Seniors/default.htm

REFERENCES

American College of Sports Medicine: Position stand: exercise and physical activity for older adults, *Med Sci Sports Exerc* 41:1510, 2009. Accessed 1 June 2010 from http://journals.lww.com/acsmmsse/Fulltext/2009/07000/Exercise_and_Physical_Activity_for_Older_Adults.20.aspx.

Bauer JM, et al: The Mini Nutritional Assessment—its history, today's practice, and future perspectives, *Nutr Clin Pract* 23:388, 2008.

Benelam B: Satiety and the anorexia of ageing: review, *Br J Comm Nurs* 14:332, 2009.

Boston University School of Medicine: *Why study centenarians? An overview*, 2010. Accessed 3 July 2010 from http://www.bumc.bu.edu/centenarian/overview/.

Buettner D: *The blue zones*, Washington, DC, 2008, The National Geographic Society.

Centers for Disease Control and Prevention: *How much physical activity do older adults need?* U.S. Department of Health and Human Services, 2006. Accessed 1 June 2010 from http://www.cdc.gov/physicalactivity/everyone/guidelines/olderadults.html.

Centers for Medicare and Medicaid Services: http://www.cms.hhs.gov/. Accessed 12/12/10.

Chao SY, et al: What food and nutrition services should be regulated in assisted-living facilities for older adults? *J Am Diet Assoc* 109:1048, 2009.

Chernoff R: Protein and older adults, *J Am Coll Nutr* 23:627S-630S, 2004.

Clemons TE, et al: Cognitive impairment in the age-related eye disease study: AREDS report no. 16, *Arch Ophthalmol* 124:537, 2006.

Doley J: Nutrition management of pressure ulcers, *Nutr Clin Prac* 25:50, 2010.

Federal Interagency Forum on Aging-Related Statistics: *Older Americans 2008: key indicators of well-being*, Washington, DC, 2008, U.S. Government Printing Office. Accessed 1 June 2010 from http://www.agingstats.gov/.

He W, et al: *U.S. Census Bureau, Current Population Reports, P23-209, 65+ in the United States: 2005*, Washington, DC, 2005, U.S. Government Printing Office. Accessed 1 June 2010 from http://www.census.gov/prod/2006pubs/p23-209.pdf.

Institute of Medicine, Committee on Nutrition Services for Medicare Beneficiaries: *The role of nutrition in maintaining health in the nation's elderly*, Washington, DC, 2000, National Academies Press.

Janssen I: Sarcopenia. In Bales CW, Ritchie CS, editors: *Handbook of clinical nutrition and aging*, ed 2, Totowa, N.J., 2009, Humana Press.

Joshipura K, Dietrich T: Nutrition and oral health: a two-way relationship. In Bales CW, Ritchie CS, editors: *Handbook of clinical nutrition and aging*, ed 2, Totowa, N.J., 2009, Humana Press.

Juan WY, et al: *Diet quality of older Americans in 1994-96 and 2001-02 as measured by the healthy eating index-2005, Nutrition Insight 41*, Washington, DC, 2008, U.S. Department of Agriculture, Center for Nutrition Policy and Promotion. Accessed 1 June 2010 from http://www.cnpp.usda.gov/Publications/NutritionInsights/Insight41.pdf.

Kaiser MJ, et al: Validation of the mini nutritional assessment short-form (MNA®-SF): a practical tool for identification of nutritional status, *J Nutr Health Aging* 13:782, 2009.

Kamp B, et al: Position statement of the American Dietetic Association, American Society for Nutrition, and Society for Nutrition Education: food and nutrition programs for community-residing older adults, *J Am Diet Assoc* 110:463, 2010.

Kuczmarski MF, Weddle DO: American Dietetic Association position statement: nutrition across the spectrum of aging, *J Am Diet Assoc* 105:616, 2005. Accessed 1 June 2010 from http://www.eatright.org/About/Content.aspx?id=8374.

Michelon E, et al: Vitamin and carotenoid status in older women: associations with the frailty syndrome, *J Gerontol A: Biol Sci Med Sci* 61:600, 2006.

Morley JE: Update on nutritional assessment strategies. In Bales CW, Ritchie CS, editors: *Handbook of Clinical Nutrition and Aging*, ed 2, Totowa, N.J., 2009, Humana Press.

National Institute on Aging: *Exercise and physical activity for older adults guide*, 20 January 2010. Accessed 1 June 2010 from http://nihseniorhealth.gov/exerciseforolderadults/toc.html.

National Institute on Deafness and Other Communicative Disorders, National Institutes of Health: What is presbycusis? 2006. Accessed 1 June 2010 from http://www.nidcd.nih.gov/health/hearing/presbycusis.htm#what.

Neidert KC: American Dietetic Association position statement: liberalization of the diet prescription improves quality of life for older adults in long-term care, *J Am Diet Assoc* 105:1955, 2005.

O'Neill PS, et al: Aging in community nutrition, diet therapy, and nutrition and aging textbooks, *Gerontol Geriatr Educ* 25:65, 2005.

Sahin E, et al: Telomere dysfunction induces metabolic and mitochondrial compromise, *Nature* 470:359, 2011.

Schiffman S: Sensory impairment: taste and smell impairments with aging. In Bales CW, Ritchie CS, editors: *Handbook of clinical nutrition and aging*, ed 2, Totowa, N.J., 2009, Humana Press.

Symons TB, et al: A moderate serving of high-quality protein maximally stimulates skeletal muscle protein synthesis in young and elderly subjects, *J Am Diet Assoc* 109:1582, 2009.

Thomas DR: The relationship of nutrition and pressure ulcers. In Bales CW, Ritchie CS, editors: *Handbook of clinical nutrition and aging*, ed 2, Totowa, N.J., 2009, Humana Press.

Thomas DR: Sarcopenia, *Clin Geriatr Med* 26(2):331, 2010.

U.S. Administration on Aging: National survey of OAA participants, 2008, Aging Integrated Database. Accessed 1 June 2010 from http://www.agidnet.org/.

U.S. Administration on Aging (USAoA): *Profile of older Americans 2010*. Accessed 1 June 2010 from http://www.aoa.gov/AoARoot/Aging_Statistics/Profile/index.aspx.

U.S. Department of Health and Human Services (USDHHS): *2010 Surgeon General's vision for a healthy and fit nation*, Rockville, Md, 2010, U.S. Department of Health and Human Services, Office of the Surgeon General. Accessed 1 June 2010 from http://www.surgeongeneral.gov/.

U.S. Department of Health and Human Services (USDHHS), U.S. Department of Agriculture (USDA): *Dietary Guidelines for Americans, 2010*, ed 7, Washington, DC, 2010, U.S. Government Printing Office. Accessed 1 June 2010 from http://www.healthierus.gov/dietaryguidelines/.

Villareal DT, et al: Obesity in older adults: position statement of the American Society for Nutrition and The Obesity Society, *Am J Clin Nutr* 82:923, 2005.

Wellman NS: Aging at home: more research on nutrition and independence, please, *Am J Clin Nutr* 91:1151, 2010.

World Health Organization (WHO): *Fact sheet No 305: ultraviolet radiation and human health*, December 2009. Accessed 1 June 2010 from http://www.who.int/mediacentre/factsheets/fs305/en/.

Wong TY, et al: Age-related macular degeneration and risk for stroke, *Ann Intern Med* 145:98, 2006.

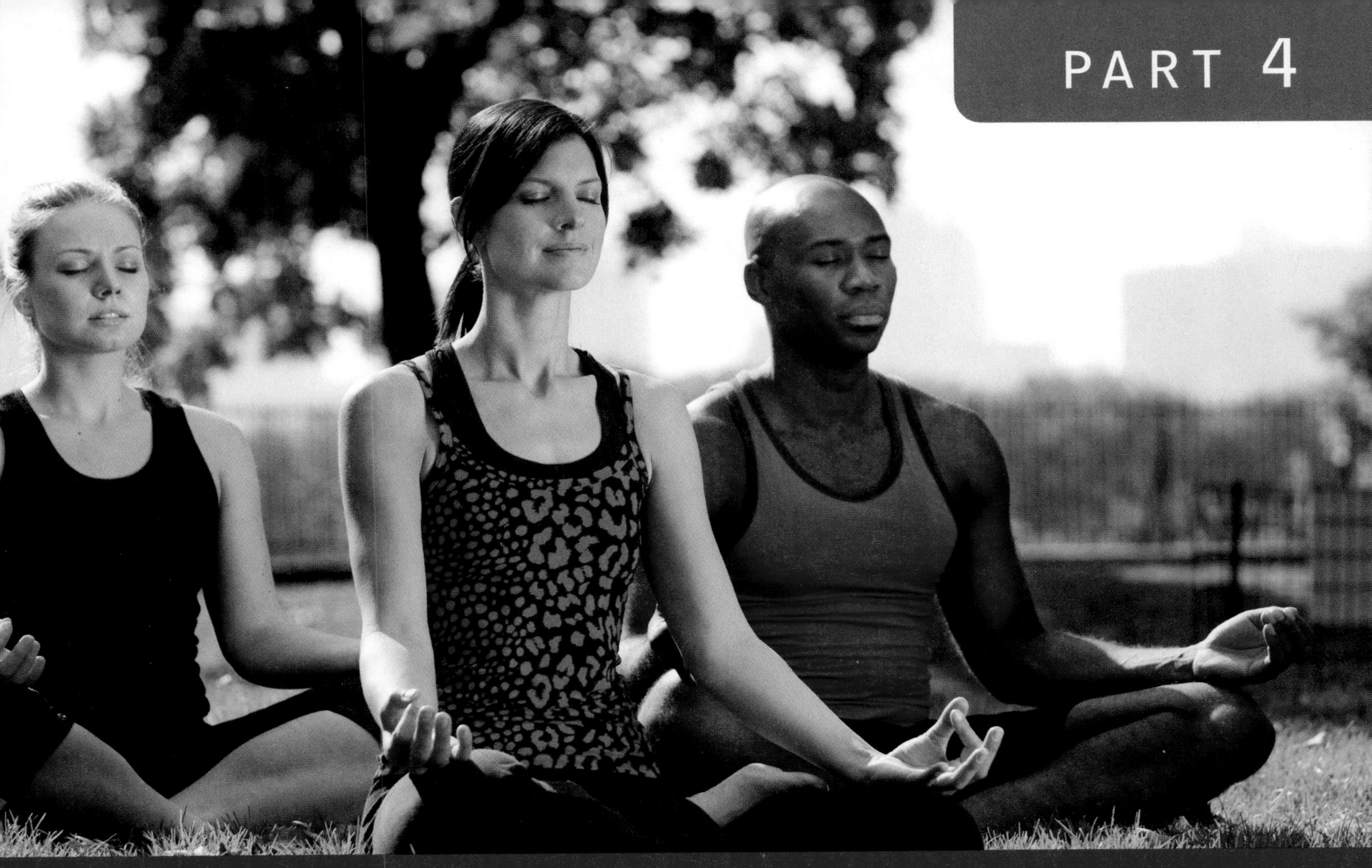

PART 4

Nutrition for Health and Fitness

The chapters in this section reflect the evolution of nutritional science, from the identification of nutrient requirements and the practical application of this knowledge to the concepts that relate nutrition to the prevention of chronic and degenerative diseases and optimization of health and performance.

The relationship between nutrition and dental disease has long been recognized. In more recent decades the possibility of reducing the incidence of osteoporosis by emphasizing appropriate nutrition has accumulated supportive evidence. Medical research now shows the role of nutrition on gene expression; dietary intake can turn on or turn off the inflammatory process, a key factor in disease onset and management.

Weight management and exercise form the basis for a great deal of nutrition in health, fitness, and disease prevention. Understanding the role of nutrition in sports and in optimizing performance has led to dietary and exercise practices generally applicable to a rewarding, healthy lifestyle.

The opportunities for members of an affluent society to choose from a great variety of foods has led to an overabundant intake of energy for many individuals. Efforts to reduce body weight, widely pursued with varying degrees of enthusiasm and diligence, are often disheartening, making the knowledge presented here so important. Frustration with dieting and stress often lead to eating disorders, which are increasing in frequency and require attention and understanding from the nutrition professional.

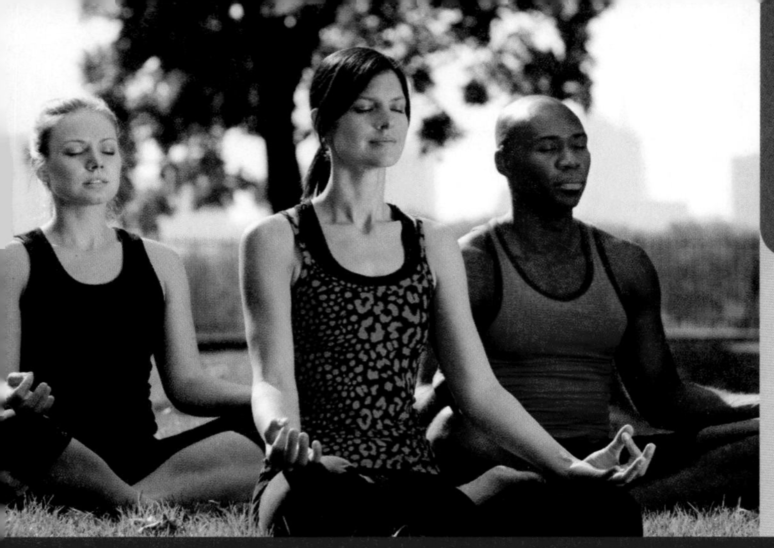

CHAPTER 22

Lucinda K. Lysen, RD, RN, BSN
Donna A. Israel, PhD, RD, LD, LPC, FADA

Nutrition in Weight Management

KEY TERM

activity thermogenesis (AT)
adipocyte
adipocytokines
adiponectin
adiposity rebound
android fat distribution
bariatric surgery
body mass index (BMI)
brown adipose tissue (BAT)
catecholaminergic
comorbidities
essential fat
fat mass
fat-free mass (FFM)
gastric banding
gastric bypass
gastroplasty
ghrelin
gynoid fat distribution
hormone-sensitive lipase (HSL)
hyperphagia
hyperplasia
hypertrophy
hypophagia
incretin
insulin
lean body mass (LBM)
leptin
lifestyle modification
lipogenesis
lipoprotein lipase (LPL)
liposuction
metabolic syndrome (MetS)
morbid obesity
night-eating syndrome (NES)
nonalcoholic fatty liver disease (NAFLD)
nonexercise activity thermogenesis (NEAT)
obesity
obesogen
orlistat
overweight
sensory-specific satiety
sibutramine
storage fat
semivolatile organic compounds (SVOCs)
underweight
vagus nerve
very-low-calorie diet (VLCD)
visceral adipose tissue (VAT)
white adipose tissue (WAT)
yo-yo effect

Sections of this chapter were written by Molly Gee, MED, RD for the previous edition of this text.

Body weight is the sum of bone, muscle, organs, body fluids, and adipose tissue. Some or all of these components are subject to normal change as a reflection of growth, reproductive status, variation in physical activity, and the effects of aging. Consistent body weight is orchestrated by neural, hormonal, and chemical mechanisms as well as individual genetic polymorphisms that balance energy intake and expenditure within fairly precise limits (de Luis et al., 2006). Abnormalities of these complex mechanisms can result in weight fluctuations, most commonly overweight and obesity.

On the other end of the weight spectrum is underweight. Although the inability to gain weight can also be a primary problem, low body weight is usually secondary to a disease state, an eating disorder, or a psychological problem (see Chapter 23). In the elderly or in children, unintentional weight loss can be especially detrimental and should be addressed early to prevent malnutrition or other undesirable consequences.

BODY WEIGHT COMPONENTS

Body weight is often described in terms of its composition, and different models have been advanced to estimate body fat. Body composition is discussed in detail in Chapter 6. Traditionally, a two-compartment model divides the body into **fat mass**, the fat from all body sources including the brain, skeleton, and adipose tissue, and **fat-free mass (FFM)**, which includes water, protein, and mineral components (Figure 22-1). The proportions of FFM are relatively constant from person to person.

Although *FFM* is often used interchangeably with the term *lean body mass*, it is not exactly the same. **Lean body mass (LBM)** is muscle. LBM is higher in men than in women, increases with exercise, and is lower in older adults. It is the major determinant of the resting metabolic rate (RMR). It follows that a decrease in LBM could hinder the progress of weight loss. Therefore, to achieve long-term weight-loss, the loss of fat mass while maintaining FFM and RMR is desirable (Stiegler and Cunliffe, 2006). Water, which makes up 60% to 65% of body weight, is the most variable component of LBM, and the state of hydration can induce fluctuations of several pounds.

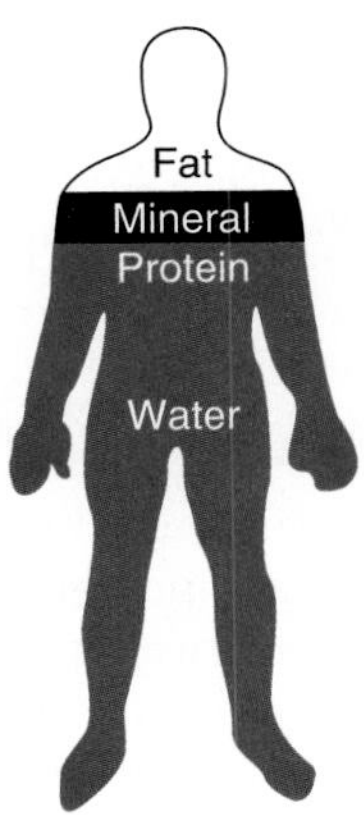

FIGURE 22-1 The components of fat-free mass in the body.

Body Fat

Total body fat is the combination of "essential" and "storage" fats, usually expressed as a percentage of total body weight that is associated with optimum health. Muscle and even skeletal mass adjust to some extent to support the burden of adipose tissue.

Essential fat, necessary for normal physiologic functioning, is stored in small amounts in the bone marrow, heart, lung, liver, spleen, kidneys, muscles, and the nervous system. In men, approximately 3% of body fat is essential. In women, essential fat is higher (12%) because it includes body fat in the breasts, pelvic regions, and thighs that support the reproductive process.

Storage fat is the energy reserve, primarily as triglycerides (TGs) in adipose tissue. This fat accumulates under the skin and around the internal organs to protect them from trauma. Most storage fat is "expendable." The fat stores in adipocytes are capable of extensive variation. This allows for the changing requirements of growth, reproduction, aging, environmental and physiologic circumstances, the availability of food, and the demands of physical activity. Total body fat (essential fat plus storage fat) as a percentage of body weight that is associated with optimal health is 10% to 25% in men and 18% to 30% in women, although professional and elite athletes have body fat levels much lower than those of the average person, with an average for optimal fitness of 12% to 18% for men and 16% to 25% for women (Wilmore et al., 1986).

Adipose Tissue Composition

Adipose tissue exerts a profound influence on whole-body homeostasis. Adipose tissue is located primarily under the skin, in the mesenteries and omentum, and behind the peritoneum. Although it is primarily fat, it also contains small amounts of protein and water. **White adipose tissue (WAT)** stores energy as a repository for TGs, serves as a cushion to protect abdominal organs, and insulates the body to preserve heat. Carotene gives it a slight yellow color. **Brown adipose tissue (BAT)** is a rapid source of energy for infants, found primarily in the scapular and subscapular areas as 5% of their body weight. The brown color is due to extensive vascularization for energy and heat production. Its function in humans remains poorly understood, and by adulthood BAT is no longer available (Hansen and Kristiansen, 2006).

Adipocyte Size and Number

The mature fat cell (**adipocyte**) consists of a large central lipid droplet surrounded by a thin rim of cytoplasm, which contains the nucleus and the mitochondria. These cells can store fat equal to 80% to 95% of their volume. Gains in weight and adipose tissue occur by increasing the number of cells, the size of cells as lipid is added, or a combination of the two.

Hyperplasia (increased number of cells) occurs as a normal growth process during infancy and adolescence. Cell number increases in both lean and obese children into adolescence, but the number increases faster in obese children. In teens and adults, increases in fat cell size are more common, but hyperplasia can also occur after the fat content of existing cells has reached capacity.

During normal growth, the greatest percentage of body fat (approximately 25%) is set by 6 months of age. In lean children, fat cell size then decreases; this decrease does not occur in obese children. At the age of 6 years in lean children, **adiposity rebound** occurs, especially in girls, with an increase in body fat. An early adiposity rebound occurring before 5.5 years is predictive of a higher level of adiposity at 16 years of age and in adulthood; a period of later rebound is correlated with normal adult weight (Rolland-Cachera, 2005).

With **hypertrophy** (increased cell size), fat depots can expand as much as 1000 times at any age as long as space is available. With weight loss as a result of trauma, illness, or starvation, fat cell size decreases but cell numbers remain the same (Bjorntorp and Sjostrom, 1971). Although weight loss of any amount in severely obese individuals improves basic adipocyte physiology, a weight loss of at least 5% is required to decrease fat cell size (de Luis et al., 2006; Varady et al., 2009).

Fat Storage

Most depot fat comes directly from dietary TGs. The fatty acid composition of adipose tissue mirrors the fatty acid composition of the diet. Even excess dietary carbohydrate and protein are converted to fatty acids in the liver by the comparatively inefficient process of **lipogenesis**. Under normal conditions, little dietary carbohydrate is used to produce adipose tissue; it requires three times more energy to convert excess energy from carbohydrate to fat storage as that from dietary fat. Recommendations simply to reduce dietary fat are ineffective; total reduction of calories is needed for weight loss to occur.

Semivolatile organic compounds (SVOCs) accumulate in adipose tissues from exposure to toxins, chemicals, and pesticides.

When adipose tissue is mobilized during weight loss, SVOCs are released. See *Clinical Insight:* What's in That Fat When You Lose It? Obese women should lose weight before becoming pregnant because the effect of SVOCs on the developing fetal brain is not yet known (see Chapter 16).

Lipoprotein Lipase

Dietary TG is transported to the liver by chylomicrons. Endogenous TGs, synthesized in the liver from free fatty acids, travel as part of very-low-density lipoprotein particles. The enzyme **lipoprotein lipase (LPL)** moves lipid from the blood into the adipose cell where it hydrolyzes TG into free fatty acids and glycerol. Glycerol proceeds to the liver; fatty acids enter the adipocyte and are reesterified into TGs. When needed by other cells, TGs are hydrolyzed once again to fatty acids and glycerol by **hormone-sensitive lipase (HSL)** within the adipose cell; they are then released into the circulation.

Hormones affect LPL activity in different adipose tissue regions. Estrogens stimulate LPL activity in the gluteofemoral adipocytes and thus promote fat storage in this area for childbearing and lactation. In the presence of sex steroid hormones, a normal distribution of body fat exists. With a decrease in sex steroid hormones, as occurs with menopause or gonadectomy, there is a tendency to increase central obesity.

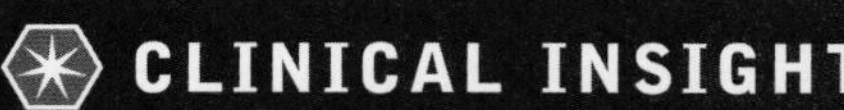

What's in That Fat When You Lose It?

Sheila Dean, DSc, RD, LD, CCN, CDE

The role of toxins in obesity development and later fat loss is becoming of increasing concern as the emerging evidence forms a plausible link between toxins and obesity. Exposure to toxins comes from two main sources: the environment (external toxins) and the gut (breakdown products of our metabolism) or internal toxins. Both can overload the body's endogenous detoxification mechanisms. When this happens these toxins are stored in the body's depot fat. This can necessitate the deposition of more fat and obesity development, or, in the case of weight or fat loss, the release of these toxins can interfere with the body's functioning and even its ability to continue to lose more fat (Barouki, 2010; Imbeault et al., 2002; Tremblay et al., 2004).

Toxins alter metabolism, disrupt endocrine function, damage the mitochondria, increase inflammation and oxidative stress, lower thyroid hormones, and alter circadian rhythms and the autonomic nervous system. These all interfere with key weight control mechanisms in the body. Using a comprehensive approach to obesity, including the assessment and treatment of toxin-mediated effects can result in more effective body fat and weight management. Simple lifestyle choices, as well as medical detoxification, can reduce exposure to toxins and enhance mobilization and elimination of stored and external toxins (Hyman, 2006).

REGULATION OF BODY WEIGHT

Regulatory systems such as neurochemicals, body-fat stores, protein mass, hormones, and postingestion factors all play a role in regulating intake and weight. Regulation takes place on both a short- and a long-term basis. Short-term regulation governs consumption of food from meal to meal; long-term regulation is controlled by the availability of adipose stores and hormone responses.

Metabolic Rate and Voluntary Activity

The RMR explains 60% to 70% of total energy expenditure. RMR declines with age or with restriction of energy intake. When the body is suddenly deprived of adequate energy from involuntary or deliberate starvation, the RMR conserves energy by dropping rapidly, by as much as 15% in 2 weeks.

Activity thermogenesis (AT) is the energy expended in voluntary activity, the most variable component of energy expenditure. Under normal circumstances physical activity accounts for 15% to 30% of total energy expenditure. Yet all activity counts. **Nonexercise activity thermogenesis (NEAT)** is the energy expended for everything that is not sleeping, eating, or sportslike exercise. It includes going to work, typing, doing yard work, toe-tapping, even fidgeting (see Chapter 2). NEAT and a sedentary lifestyle may have profound importance in weight management. NEAT varies as much as 2000 kcal/day between individuals (Levine et al., 2007). To reverse obesity, individual strategies should promote standing and ambulating for 2.5 hours per day and should also reengineer work, school, and home environments to support a more active lifestyle (Levine, 2007).

Short- and Long-Term Regulation

Short-term controls are concerned primarily with factors governing hunger, appetite, and satiety. Satiety is associated with the postprandial state when excess food is being stored. Hunger is associated with the postabsorptive state when those stores are being mobilized. Physical triggers for hunger are much stronger than those for satiety, and it is easier to override the signals for satiety.

When either overfeeding or underfeeding occurs, younger individuals exhibit spontaneous **hypophagia** (undereating) or **hyperphagia** (overeating) accordingly. Older individuals do not have the same responsiveness; they are more vulnerable to unexplained weight losses or gains because they are unable to control spontaneous, short-term changes in food intake.

Long-term regulation seems to involve a feedback mechanism in which a signal from the adipose mass is released when "normal" body composition is disturbed, as when weight loss occurs. **Adipocytokines** are proteins released by the adipose cell into the bloodstream that act as signaling molecules. Younger persons have more responsiveness to this feedback than do older adults. See Table 22-1 and *Focus On:* Signals from a Host of Hormones.

Set Point Theory

Fat storage in nonobese adults appears to be regulated in a manner that preserves a specific body weight. In both animals and humans, deliberate efforts to starve or overfeed are followed by a rapid return to the original body weight, a "set point." Body weight remains remarkably stable from internal regulatory mechanisms that are genetically determined. Some studies suggest that body weight can be displaced only temporarily and that RMR lowers, resulting in a regain of lost weight; other studies have not shown this adaptive metabolic response.

FOCUS ON

Signals from a Host of Hormones

A host of hormones—insulin, leptin, adiponectin, and ghrelin, among others—communicate with the hypothalamus to control a person's intake and weight. These regulatory hormones govern feeding in response to signals originated in affected body tissues.

Insulin controls the amount of glucose in the blood by moving it into the cells for energy. **Leptin**, which is produced mainly by fat cells, contributes to long-term fullness by sensing the body's overall energy stores. **Adiponectin** is also made by fat cells and apparently helps the body respond better to insulin by boosting metabolism. **Ghrelin**, the hunger hormone, tells the brain when the stomach is empty, prompting hunger pangs and a drop in metabolism.

The stomach communicates with the brain via the **vagus nerve**, part of the autonomic nervous system that travels from the brain to the stomach. When filled with food or liquid, the stomach's stretch receptors send a message to the brain indicating satiety. Gastric bypass surgery reduces the stomach to the size of an egg, and triggers a sharp drop in ghrelin levels, which lessens hunger and oral intake (Blackburn, 2008). Unfortunately, traditional dieting tends to boost ghrelin levels.

WEIGHT IMBALANCE: OVERWEIGHT AND OBESITY

Overweight occurs as a result of an imbalance between food consumed and physical activity. Obesity is a complex issue related to lifestyle, environment, and genes. Environmental and genetic factors have a complex interaction with psychological, cultural, and physiologic influences. Over the years, many hypotheses have evolved to explain why some people become fat and others remain lean, and why it is so difficult for reduced-obese persons to maintain weight loss. No single theory can completely explain all manifestations of obesity or apply consistently to all persons.

Prevalence

The United States has the highest prevalence of obesity among the developed nations. However, increases in the prevalence of overweight and obesity have been observed throughout the world. The international trend is often called "globesity."

The estimates of overweight and obesity among children and adults are based on measured weights and heights from the National Health and Nutrition Examination Survey

TABLE 22-1

Regulatory Factors Involved in Feeding and Weight Management

Brain Neurotransmitters	Characteristics and Function
Norepinephrine and dopamine	Released by the SNS in response to dietary intake; mediate the activity of areas in the hypothalamus that govern feeding behavior. Fasting and semistarvation lead to decreased SNS activity and increased adrenal medullary activity with a consequent increase in epinephrine, which fosters substrate mobilization. Dopaminergic pathways in the brain play a role in the reinforcement properties of food.
Serotonin, neuropeptide Y, and endorphins	Decreases in serotonin and increases in neuropeptide Y have been associated with an increase in carbohydrate appetite. Neuropeptide Y increases during food deprivation; it may be a factor leading to an increase in appetite after dieting. Preferences and cravings for sweet, high-fat foods observed among obese and bulimic patients involve the endorphin system.
CRF	Involved in controlling adrenocorticotropic hormone release from the pituitary gland, CRF is a potent anorexic agent and weakens the feeding response produced by norepinephrine and neuropeptide Y. CRF is released during exercise.
Gut Hormones	
Incretins	Gastrointestinal peptides increase the amount of insulin released from the beta cells of the pancreas after eating, even before blood glucose levels become elevated. They also slow the rate of absorption by reducing gastric emptying and may directly reduce food intake. Incretins also inhibit glucagon release from the alpha cells of the pancreas. (See GLP-1 and GIP.)
CCK	Released by the intestinal tract when fats and proteins reach the small intestine, receptors for CCK have been found in the gastrointestinal tract and the brain. CCK causes the gallbladder to contract and stimulates the pancreas to release enzymes. At the brain level, CCK inhibits food intake.
Bombesin	Released by enteric neurons; reduces food intake and enhances the release of CCK.
Enterostatin	A portion of pancreatic lipase involved specifically with satiety following the consumption of fat.
Adiponectin	An adipocytokine secreted by the adipose tissue that modulates glucose regulation and fatty acid catabolism. Levels of this hormone are inversely correlated with BMI. The hormone plays a role in metabolic disorders such as type 2 diabetes, obesity, and atherosclerosis. Levels drop after gastric bypass surgery for up to 6 months (Couce et al., 2006).
Glucagon	Increased secretion of glucagon is caused by hypoglycemia, increased levels of norepinephrine and epinephrine, increased plasma amino acids, and cholecystokinin. Decreased secretion of glucagon occurs when insulin or somatostatin is released.
Apolipoprotein A-IV	Synthesized and secreted by the intestine during lymphatic secretion of chylomicrons. After entering the circulation, a small portion of apolipoprotein A-IV enters the CNS and suppresses food consumption.
Fatty acids	Free fatty acids, triglycerides, and glycerol are factors that also affect uptake of glucose by peripheral tissues.
GLP-1 and GIP	Released by intestinal mucosa in presence of meals rich in glucose and fat; stimulate insulin synthesis and release; GLP-1 decreases glucagon secretion, delays gastric emptying time, and may promote satiety; examples of incretin hormones.
Insulin	Acts in the CNS and the periphery nervous system to regulate food intake. Insulin is involved in the synthesis and storage of fat. Impaired insulin activity may lead to impaired thermogenesis. It is possible that obese persons with insulin resistance or deficiency have a defective glucose disposal system and a depressed level of thermogenesis. The greater the insulin resistance, the lower the thermic effect of food. Fasting insulin levels increase proportionately with the degree of obesity; however, many obese persons demonstrate insulin resistance because of a lack of response by insulin receptors, impaired glucose tolerance, and associated hyperlipidemia. These sequelae can usually be corrected with weight loss.
Leptin	An adipocytokine secreted by the adipose tissue, correlated with percent of body fat. Primary signal from energy stores; in obesity loses the ability to inhibit energy intake or to increase energy expenditure (Enriori et al., 2006). Compared with men, women have significantly higher concentrations of serum leptin.

TABLE 22-1

Regulatory Factors Involved in Feeding and Weight Management—cont'd

Brain Neurotransmitters	Characteristics and Function
Resistin	An adipocytokine expressed primarily in adipocytes; antagonizes insulin action (Goldstein and Scalia, 2007).
Ghrelin	Produced primarily by the stomach; acts on the hypothalamus to stimulate hunger and feeding. Ghrelin levels are highest in lean individuals and lowest in the obese. Increased levels are seen in people who are dieting, and suppressed levels are noted after gastric bypass, possibly counteracted by adiponectin (Couce et al., 2006).
PYY_{3-36}	Secreted by endocrine cells lining the small bowel and colon in response to food; a "middle man" in appetite management. PYY seems to work opposite from ghrelin; it induces satiety.
IL-6 and TNF-α	Both are gut hormones. Cytokines secreted by adipose tissue and participate in metabolic events. Impair insulin signals in muscle and liver. Levels are proportional to body fat mass (Thomas et al., 2010).
Other Hormones	
Thyroid hormones	Modulate the tissue responsiveness to the catecholamines secreted by the SNS. A decrease in triiodothyronine lowers the response to SNS activity and diminishes adaptive thermogenesis. Women should be tested for hypothyroidism, particularly after menopause. Weight regain after weight loss may be a function of a hypometabolic state; energy restriction produces a transient, hypothyroid, hypometabolic state.
Visfatin	An adipocytokine protein secreted by visceral adipose tissue that has an insulin-like effect; plasma levels increase with increasing adiposity and insulin resistance (Stevens and Vidal-Puig, 2006).
Adrenomedullin	A new regulatory peptide secreted by adipocytes as a result of inflammatory processes.

BMI, Body mass index; *CCK,* cholecystokinin; *CNS,* central nervous system; *CRF,* corticotropin-releasing factor; *GIP,* glucose-dependent insulinotropic peptide; *GLP-1,* glucagon-like peptide 1; *IL-6,* interleukin-6; PYY_{3-36}, peptide YY_{3-36}; *SNS,* sympathetic nervous system; *TNF-α,* tumor necrosis factor–α.

(NHANES), conducted by the National Center for Health Statistics (Centers for Disease Control and Prevention [CDC], 2007). An estimated 66% of U.S. adults are overweight, and 32% are obese. In Canada 36% of adults are overweight and another 23% are obese (Statistics Canada, 2010). In Europe between 15% and 25% of adults are obese. In the United States, prevalence of obesity is higher in black and Hispanic populations, especially among Mexican-American women (CDC, 2007; Figure 22-2).

Unfortunately, children are not immune to the epidemic. Obesity is now the most common pediatric nutritional problem in the United States. Nearly 1/3 of children and adolescents between ages 2 and 19 years are overweight. See *New Directions*: Organizing to Solve the Childhood Obesity Problem "Within a Generation."

Causes of Overweight and Obesity

Heredity and Nutrigenomics

Many hormonal and neural factors involved in weight regulation are determined genetically. These include the short- and long-term signals that determine satiety and feeding activity. Small defects in their expression or interaction could contribute significantly to weight gain.

The number and size of fat cells, regional distribution of body fat, and RMR are also influenced by genes. Studies of twins confirm that genes determine 50% to 70% of the predisposition to obesity (Prentice, 2005). Although numerous genes are involved, several have received much attention—the Ob gene, the adiponectin (ADIPOQ) gene, the FTO gene, and the β3-adrenoreceptor gene. The Ob gene produces leptin. Mutations in the Ob gene, leptin receptor (LEPR), or ADIPOQ genes can result in obesity or metabolic syndrome (MetS), especially if diet provides too much saturated fat (Ferguson et al., 2010). The β3-adrenoreceptor gene, located primarily in the adipose tissue, is thought to regulate RMR and fat oxidation in humans. The FTO gene predisposes to diabetes by its effect on body mass (Frayling et al., 2007).

Nutritional or lifestyle choices can activate or deactivate those obesity-triggering genes. Thus the answer to successful long-term weight management is likely to include behavioral application of individual genetics. One day soon, specific deoxyribonucleic acid tests may give accurate predictions about an individual's response to a low-fat diet, a low-carbohydrate diet, or a balanced diet (Ashley et al., 2010). Nutritional counseling can truly be personalized (see Chapter 5).

Inadequate Physical Activity

Lack of exercise and a generally sedentary lifestyle, compounded by chronic overeating, are also causes of weight

NEW DIRECTIONS

Organizing to Solve the Childhood Obesity Problem "Within a Generation"

Because the number of obese children in the US has tripled since 1980, and obesity now rivals smoking as the largest cause of preventable death and disease (Ogden et al., 2002 and Ogden et al., 2010), a new foundation was launched in the spring of 2010 to address this serious epidemic of childhood obesity. This foundation—***Partnership for a Healthier America*** has as its mission, the simple concept that children should have good, nutritious food to eat and the chance to be physically active every day in order to become healthy adults.

The objectives of the partnership are to support the national goal of solving the childhood obesity challenge "within a generation" set by First Lady Michelle Obama who also serves as Honorary Chair of the new organization. The Partnership brings together the public and private sectors, organizations, business and thought leaders, the media, and states and local communities to make meaningful and measurable commitments for fighting childhood obesity. The plan has four pillars:

- Offering parents the tools and information they need to make healthy choices for their children
- Getting healthier food into the nation's schools
- Ensuring that all families have access to healthy, affordable food in their communities
- Increasing opportunities for children to be physically active, both in and out of school.

The partnership will support, unite and inspire families from every corner of the United States to implement and sustain the 4 pillar plan. The initiative was started with the *Let's Move!* Campaign. www.letsmove.gov/

The White House Task Force on Childhood Obesity—Report to the President "Solving the Problem of Childhood Obesity within a Generation" (Task Force, 2010) can be accessed at www.nj.gov/health/fhs/shapingnj/pdf/wh_obesity_report.pdf

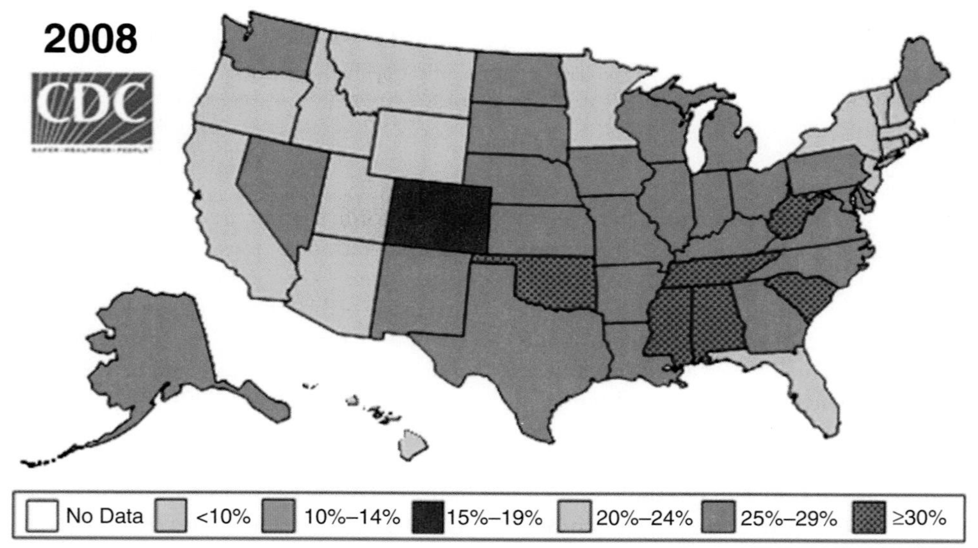

FIGURE 22-2 Prevalence of obesity among U.S. adults in 2008. *(Centers for Disease Control and Prevention (CDC) Behavioral Risk Factor Surveillance System Survey, June 13, 2010.)*

gain. The sedentary nature of society is a factor in the growing problem of obesity. Fewer people are exercising, and more time is being spent in low-energy, screen-watching activities such as watching television or movies, using the computer, playing video games, and sitting in cars driving to work or events.

Inflammation

Adipose tissue actively secretes a wide range of pro- and antiinflammatory cytokines that are influenced by single-nucleotide polymorphisms in the cytokine genes; effects include insulin insensitivity, hyperlipidemia, muscle protein loss, and oxidant stress (Grimble, 2010). Scientists have found a direct relationship between obesity and inflammatory diseases such as cardiovascular disorders, some cancers, and type 2 diabetes.

Metabolic signals are triggered in the hypothalamus of obese individuals, laying the groundwork for chronic inflammation and tissue damage during a prolonged period. In mice fed a high-fat diet, the "master switch" of inflammation turns on the hypothalamus. In humans, chronic overeating "flips on" the inflammation switch, leading to weight gain and insulin resistance. In insulin-resistant individuals on a weight-loss diet, ezetimibe (Zetia) reduces hepatic steatosis and inflammatory markers (Chan et al., 2010).

A combined approach of diet and drug is likely to improve health outcomes. Simple diet and lifestyle changes can alter obesity-related inflammation. Foods such as oranges are antiinflammatory, whereas cream may be proinflammatory and red wine is neutral. Genotypic factors influence the effectiveness of immunonutrients; antioxidants and ω-3 polyunsaturated fatty acid decrease the intensity of the inflammatory process (Grimble, 2010). For further information on inflammation, see Chapter 6.

Sleep, Stress, and Circadian Rhythms

Shortened sleep alters the endocrine regulation of hunger and appetite. Hormones that affect appetite take over and may promote excessive energy intake. Thus recurrent sleep deprivation can modify the amount, composition, and distribution of food intake and may contribute to the obesity epidemic. It is estimated that more than 50 million Americans suffer from sleep deprivation. Others may have shift work or exposure to bright light at night, increasing the disruption of circadian rhythms and enhancing the prevalence of adiposity (Garaulet et al., 2010).

There is also a relationship between sleep, disrupted circadian rhythm, genes, and the metabolic syndrome. The cellular lipid membrane content of monounsaturated fatty acids from the diet may be protective against development of metabolic syndrome (Garaulet et al., 2009). Stress is another factor. Cortisol is released under stress; it stimulates insulin release to maintain blood glucose levels in the "fight-or-flight" response. Thus an increase in appetite occurs. Cortisol levels are typically high in the early morning and low around midnight. Individuals with **night-eating syndrome (NES)** have a delayed circadian rhythm of meal intake as a result of genetically programmed neuroendocrine factors, including altered cortisol levels (Stunkard and Lu, 2010).

Taste, Satiety, and Portion Sizes

Food and its taste elements evoke pleasure responses. The endless variety of food available at any time at a reasonable cost can contribute to higher calorie intake; people eat more when offered a variety of choices than when a single food is available. Normally, as foods are consumed, they become less desirable; this phenomenon is known as **sensory-specific satiety**. Overriding this principle is the "all-you-can-eat buffet" in which the diner reaches satiety for one food but has many choices for the "next course." Although sensory-specific satiety can promote the intake of a varied or nutritionally balanced diet, it can also lead to overconsumption of energy.

Active overeating is partly the result of excessive portion sizes that are now accepted as normal. The portions and calories that restaurants and fast-food outlets offer in one meal often exceed a person's energy needs for the entire day. High intake of energy-dense food can also be problematic.

Obesogens

Obesogens are chemical compounds foreign to the body that act to disrupt the normal metabolism of lipids, ultimately resulting in over fatness and obesity (Grun and Blumberg, 2006). Obesogens can be called "endocrine disruptors" in that they alter lipid homeostasis and fat storage, change metabolic set points, disrupt energy balance, or modify the regulation of satiety and appetite to promote accumulation of fat and obesity. Examples of suspected obesogens in the environment and food supply are bisphenol A and phthalates which are found in many plastics used in food packaging and which migrate into foods processed or stored in them (Grun, 2010). See *Clinical Insight:* What's in That Fat When You Lose It?

Viruses and Pathogens

In the last two decades, at least ten adipogenic pathogens have been identified, including viruses, scrapie agents (spongiform encephalopathies from sheep or goats), bacteria, and gut microflora (Pasarica and Dhurandhar, 2007). Whether or not "infectobesity" is a relevant contributor to the obesity epidemic remains to be determined. A human adenovirus, adenovirus-36, is capable of inducing adiposity in experimentally infected animals by increasing the replication, differentiation, lipid accumulation, and insulin sensitivity in fat cells and reduces leptin secretion and expression (van Ginnekin et al., 2009).

Assessment

Overweight is a state in which the weight exceeds a standard based on height. **Obesity** is a condition of excessive fatness, either generalized or localized. Overweight and obesity usually parallel each other, but it is possible to be overweight according to standards, but not be overfat or obese. It is also possible to have excessive fatness, and yet not be overweight.

It is important to assess body fatness or adiposity to determine the health risks as explained in detail in Chapter 6. Clinically practical assessment tools are: 1) the **body mass index (BMI)** or W/H^2, in which W= weight in kg and H = height in meters, 2) the waist circumference, 3) the waist-to-hip ratio, and 4) the Deurenberg equation which predicts body fat percentage (Deurenberg and Deurenberg-Yap, 2003).

The NIH guidelines classify individuals with a BMI of 25 as overweight and those with a BMI of 30 or more as obese (Table 22-2). Optimal BMI for longevity varies with race, gender, and age. BMI that increases over time have a substantial effect on health outcomes (Newby et al., 2006). See Chapter 6 and Appendix 23.

Waist circumference of more than 40 inches in men and more than 35 inches in women signifies increased risk, equivalent to a BMI of 25 to 34. When waist circumference and percentage of fat are both high, they are significant predictors of heart failure and other risks associated with obesity (Nicklas et al., 2007). Waist circumference is a strong correlate of insulin sensitivity index in older adults; measurement of waist circumference is helpful to assess disease risk (Racette et al., 2006). Waist/hip ratio (WHR) is a measurement in which a ratio of more than 0.8 for women and 1 for men is also associated with high risk for cardiovascular events.

TABLE 22-2

Classification of Overweight and Obesity

Classification	Body Mass Index (kg/m^2)
Underweight	<18.5
Normal	18.5-24.9
Overweight	25.0-29.9
Obesity, class I	30.0-34.9
Obesity, class II	35.0-39.9
Extreme obesity, class III	>40

From National Institutes of Health, National Heart, Lung, and Blood Institute: Clinical guidelines on the identification, evaluation, and treatment of overweight and obesity in adults—the evidence report, NIH Publication No. 98-4083, 1998.

The Deurenberg equation using the BMI, age, and gender of an individual to determine body fatness is as follows (Deurenberg and Deurenberg-Yap, 2003):

$$\%\text{ body fat} = (1.2 \times \text{BMI}) + (0.23 \times \text{age in yrs}) - (10.8 \times \text{G}) - 5.4$$

$$\text{G} = 1 \text{ for male; G} = 0 \text{ for female}$$

For example if BMI = 28, age = 21 and G = female:

$$\begin{aligned}\%\text{ body fat} &= (1.2 \times 28) + (0.23 \times 21) - (10.8 \times 0) - 5.4 \\ &= 33.6 + 4.83 - 0 - 5.4 \\ &= 33\%\end{aligned}$$

A body fat percentage of 20% to 25% or more in a male and 25% to 32% or more in a female is usually considered to be excessive and associated with the metabolic and health risks of obesity.

Health Risks and Longevity

In general, obesity can be viewed as metabolically unhealthy. Chronic diseases such as heart disease, type 2 diabetes, hypertension, stroke, gallbladder disease, infertility, sleep apnea, hormonal cancers, and osteoarthritis tend to worsen as the degree of obesity increases (Figure 22-3).

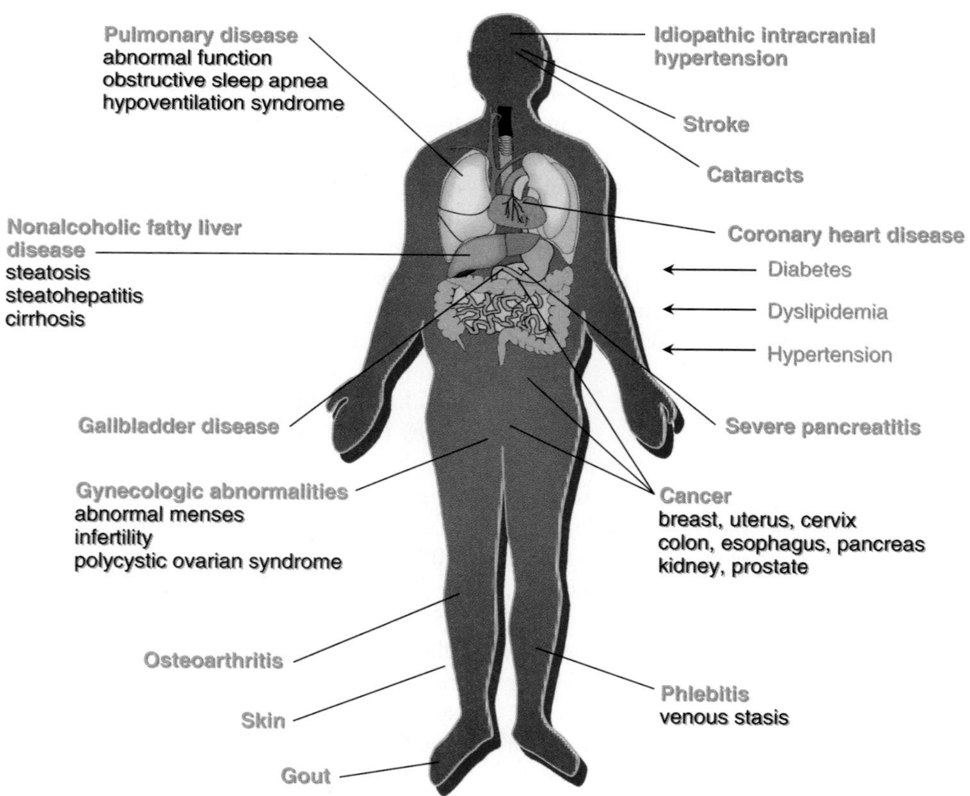

FIGURE 22-3 The medical complications of obesity are extensive. *(Reprinted with permission from Delichatsios HK: Obesity assessment in the primary care office, Harvard Medical School. 23rd Annual International Conference-Practical approaches to the treatment of obesity, Boston, June 18-20 2009, GL Blackburn, course director.)*

A subset of obese persons who are metabolically normal seems to exist. This subgroup has uncomplicated, early-onset obesity, hyperplastic adipocytes, and normal quantities of visceral fat. However, they are the exception and not the rule. Estimates using mortality data from the NHANES surveys show that thousands of deaths are related to obesity. Moderately high BMI in adolescence is correlated with premature death in younger and middle-age women (van Dam et al., 2006). Increased adiposity and reduced physical activity are strong independent risk factors for death in women.

A huge study of more than 100,000 U.S. men and women age 50 and older who took part in a 9-year Cancer Prevention Study II Nutrition Cohort found that obesity is linked to death. Those individuals with very large waists (at least 47 inches in men and 43 inches in women) had twice the risk of mortality compared with those with small waists (35 inches or less for men and 30 inches or less for women). This was true at all BMIs, but was strongest in women of normal weight, indicating the danger of waistline, abdominal, or visceral fat (Jacobs et al., 2010).

Several large studies have determined that the optimal BMI with the least risk for mortality is a BMI of 23 to 24.9. BMI above or below this range seems to increase mortality risk (Adams et al., 2006; Jee et al., 2006). The optimal range for longevity appears to be within the range of 20.5 to 24.9.

Nonalcoholic fatty liver disease (NAFLD) is associated with obesity and may progress to end-stage liver disease. Obesity is also a risk factor for cancer, infertility, poor wound healing, and poor antibody response to hepatitis B vaccine. Thus the costs of obesity are staggering. Health economists estimate costs of overweight and obesity to account for nearly 10% of total annual U.S. medical expenditures. The Internal Revenue Service issued a rule in 2002 qualifying obesity as a disease, allowing taxpayers to claim weight loss expenses as a medical deduction if undertaken to treat an existing disease.

The U.S. government recognizes the immense effect of obesity on the health and financial well-being of its citizens. Healthy People 2020 objectives also identify the implications of overweight and obesity (see Chapter 12). The objectives include targets to increase the proportion of adults who are at a healthy weight and to reduce the proportion of adults, children, and adolescents who are obese. Overweight adolescents often become obese adults; obese individuals are at increased risk for **comorbidities** of type 2 diabetes, hypertension, stroke, certain cancers, infertility, and other conditions.

Fat Deposition and the Metabolic Syndrome

Regional patterns of fat deposit are controlled genetically and differ between and among men and women. Two major types of fat deposition are currently recognized: excess subcutaneous truncal-abdominal fat (the apple-shaped **android fat distribution**) and excess gluteofemoral fat in thighs and buttocks (the pear-shaped **gynoid fat distribution**). The android shape is more common among men. The fat deposits support the demands of pregnancy and lactation. Women with the gynoid type of obesity do not develop the impairments of glucose metabolism in those with an android deposition. Postmenopausal women more closely follow the male pattern of abdominal fat stores.

Visceral obesity, or excessive **visceral adipose tissue (VAT)** under the peritoneum and in the intraabdominal cavity, is highly correlated with insulin resistance. Individuals diagnosed with the **metabolic syndrome (MetS)** have three or more of the following abnormalities: waist circumference of more than 102 cm (40 in) in men and more than 88 cm (35 in) in women, serum TGs of at least 150 mg/dL, high-density lipoprotein (HDL) level less than 40 mg/dL in men and less than 50 mg/dL in women, blood pressure 135/85 mm Hg or higher, or fasting glucose 100 mg/dL or higher. Increased visceral fat is a risk factor for coronary artery disease, dyslipidemia, hypertension, stroke, type 2 diabetes, and MetS (Goodpaster, 2005; Gower et al., 2006). By the same token, both VAT and low cardiorespiratory fitness (CRF) levels are associated with a deteriorated cardiometabolic risk profile. Achieving a low level of VAT and a high level of CRF are important targets for cardiometabolic health (Rheaume, 2011).

Calorie Restriction and Longevity

Balancing energy intake and energy expenditure is the basis of weight management throughout life. **Lifestyle modification**, becoming aware of eating behavior triggers to manage them more effectively, is vital for permanent change to occur. A key recommendation is to prevent gradual weight gain over time by making small decreases in overall calories and increasing physical activity. Patterns of healthful eating and regular physical activity should begin in childhood and continue throughout adulthood. The aging process with a lower RMR introduces special challenges. Energy balance must be maintained by adjusting or reducing caloric intake and increasing physical activity to prevent weight gain.

Prolonged calorie restriction (CR) increases life span and slows aging in animals. The apparent generality of the longevity-increasing effects of CR has prompted speculation that similar results could be obtained in humans. Two biomarkers of longevity (fasting insulin level and body temperature) are decreased by prolonged CR in humans (Heilbronn et al., 2006). Proponents of CR for antiaging believe that cutting calorie intake reduces aging and chronic disease development. In rodents with Alzheimer disease, heart disease, and stroke, decreased deterioration of nerves and increased nerve creation was also demonstrated (Mayo Clinic, 2010). Whether CR can slow the aging process, however, remains an important question (Fontana, 2009; Phelan, 2006). The Calorie Restriction (CR) Society International (www.crsociety.org) supports the efforts of people who practice CR for current health, future longevity, or other benefits; those curious about or interested in understanding the effects of the diet; and those interested in the development of related, science-based health-enhancing and life-extension technologies.

Weight Discrimination

Widespread bias and discrimination based on weight have been documented in education, employment, and health care. Like other forms of prejudice, this stems from a lack of understanding of the chronic disease of obesity and its medical consequences. Despite laws designed to prevent discrimination based on appearance, unfavorable attitudes and practices still persist. Overweight children experience adverse social, educational, and psychological consequences as a result of weight bias (Latner et al., 2005). There are automatic negative associations for obese people among health professionals, exercise science students, and obese individuals themselves (Brown, 2006; Carr and Friedman, 2005). It is essential to break down the barriers caused by ignorance and indifference. Patient support groups help to correct the negative effect of this type of discrimination.

MANAGEMENT OF OBESITY IN ADULTS

The management of obesity has evolved over the years. Initially, clinicians focused entirely on weight loss, and little was known about weight maintenance. It soon became clear that focusing on weight loss without attention to weight maintenance was inappropriate, unfair, and possibly harmful to anyone trying to manage his or her weight.

Treatment has also evolved. Years ago, an energy-restricted diet was the only treatment. Eventually, lifestyle modifications were added. The importance of physical activity was recognized as an essential ingredient for weight maintenance after weight loss. Today, a chronic disease-prevention model incorporates both lifestyle interventions and interdisciplinary therapies from physicians, dietitians, exercise specialists, and behavior therapists. Weight-reduction programs with the most promise of success integrate healthier food choices, exercise, and lifestyle modification. Pharmacologic treatment and surgical intervention are appropriate in some circumstances but are not a substitute for the necessary changes in eating and physical activity pattern. The American Dietetic Association (ADA) Evidence Analysis Library (EAL) provides reliable treatment guidelines (Figure 22-4).

Goals of Treatment

The goal of obesity treatment should focus on weight management, attaining the best weight possible in the context of overall health. Achieving an "ideal" body weight or percentage of body fat is not always realistic; under some circumstances, it may not be appropriate at all. Depending on the type and severity of the obesity and the age and lifestyle of the individual, successfully reducing body weight varies from a being relatively simple to being virtually impossible.

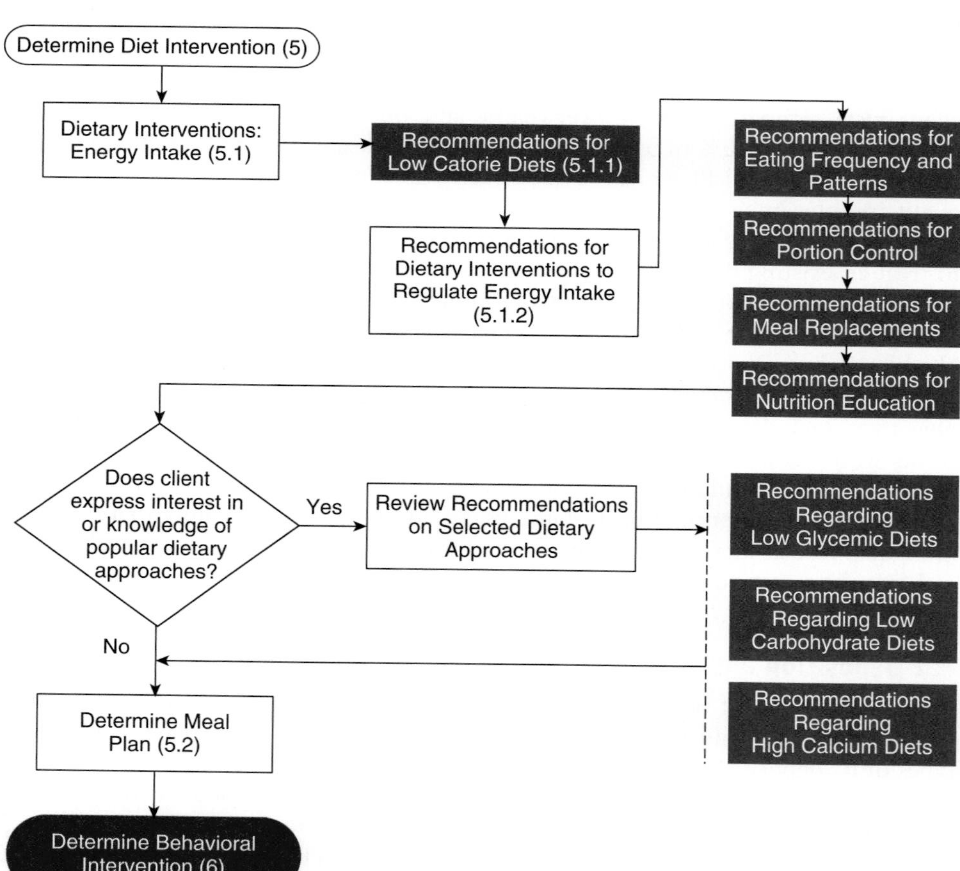

FIGURE 22-4 Algorithm for managing obesity using nutrition care process intervention terms. *(© American Dietetic Association. Reprinted with permission.)*

Maintaining present body weight or achieving a moderate loss is beneficial. Obese persons who lose even small amounts of weight (5% to 10% of initial body weight) are likely to improve blood glucose, blood pressure, and cholesterol levels.

Despite the recognition that modest weight loss is beneficial and may be more achievable, obese persons usually have self-defined goal weights that differ considerably from the goals suggested by professionals. Therefore health professionals must help their patients accept more modest, realistic weight-loss goals.

Rate and Extent of Weight Loss

Reduction of body weight involves the loss of both protein and fat, in amounts determined to some degree by the rate of weight reduction. A drastic reduction in calories resulting in a high rate of weight loss can mimic the starvation response. Tissue response to starvation is one of adaptation to an anticipated period of deprivation. The classic starvation studies done by Keys (1950) found that during the first 10 days of a fast and after use of glycogen stores, approximately 8% to 12% of the energy expenditure is from protein and the balance is from fat. As starvation progresses, up to 97% of energy expenditure is from stored TG. Metabolic aberrations during starvation include bradycardia, hypotension, dry skin and hair, easy fatigue, constipation, nervous system abnormalities, depression, and even death.

Mobilizing fat, with more than twice the kilocalories of protein, is more efficient and also spares vital LBM. Steady weight loss over a longer period favors reduction of fat stores, limits the loss of vital protein tissues, and avoids the sharp decline in RMR that accompanies rapid weight reduction. Calorie deficits that result in a loss of approximately 0.5 to 1 lb per week for persons with a BMI of 27 to 35, and 1 to 2 lb per week for those with BMIs greater than 35, should continue for approximately 6 months for a reduction of 10% of body weight (American Dietetic Association [ADA], 2010). For the next 6 months the focus changes from weight loss to weight maintenance. Following this phase, further weight loss may be considered.

Even with the same caloric intake, rates of weight reduction vary. Men reduce weight faster than women of similar size because of their higher LBM and RMR. The heavier person expends more energy than one who is less obese, and loses faster on a given calorie intake than a lighter person. Many obese persons who fail to lose weight on a diet actually consume more energy than they report and overestimate their physical activity levels.

Weight goals should be individualized and realistic, with reduction of body fat as the focus. For example, neither the morbidly obese nor the gynoid types will be able to maintain a large weight loss. Female models of dress sizes 6 to 10 and male models with 30-inch to 34-inch waists are not appropriate role models for the obese population; even BMIs of 25 are unreasonable goals for many dieters. See *Focus On:* The Influence of Fashion on Societal Food Patterns.

FOCUS ON

The Influence of Fashion on Societal Food Patterns

Contributed by Mousavi Jazayeri, PhD

The media can influence attitudes toward appearance and the body. Historically, the meaning of art and beauty has differed across cultures (Barber, 1995). The international reach of today's media, which features images of slim models and athletes, has shifted norms of beauty and changed attitudes about attractiveness. In most of the world, being thin and slim has become a symbol of beauty. Fashion models, celebrities, gymnasts, runners, skaters, divers and dancers are often underweight when compared with the recommended guidelines for a healthy body mass index. Susceptibility to the media's thin ideal and body dissatisfaction leads to restraint or emotional eating behaviors (Anschultz et al., 2008). Images of ultrathin models may exert strong pressure on young girls to lose weight. For young women who wish to bear children, maintaining a sufficient amount of body fat is necessary. Thus a more sensible perception of an attractive body image may help to change attitudes (Bonafini and Pozzilli, 2010). The need for "normal-weight" role models is highlighted by a series of weight loss–related deaths of young models. Models and athletes who maintain a healthy weight could help to reduce the ill effects of the media on body image and health outcomes.

Lifestyle Modification

Behavior modification is the cornerstone of lifestyle intervention. It focuses on restructuring a patient's environment, nutritional intake, and physical activity by using goal setting, stimulus control, problem solving, cognitive restructuring, self-monitoring, and relapse prevention (Berkel et al., 2005). It also provides feedback on progress and places the responsibility for change and accomplishment on the patient.

In goal setting, most behavioral programs try to achieve a 0.5- to 1-lb weight loss per week by providing calorie, fat grams, and physical activity targets. It is important to identify goals that support a client's sense of self-efficacy.

Stimulus control involves modification of (1) the settings or the chain of events that precede eating, (2) the kinds of foods consumed when eating does occur, and (3) the consequences of eating. Patients are taught to slow their rate of eating to become mindful of satiety cues and reduce food intake. Strategies such as putting down the utensils between bites, pausing during meals, and chewing for a minimum number of times are some ways to slow the eating process.

Problem solving is the process of defining the intake problem, generating possible solutions, evaluating and choosing the best solution, implementing the new behavior,

BOX 22-1

Lifestyle Modification Strategies

Setting Easy-To-Achieve Short-Term Goals

Increase number of minutes of walking on weekends.
Include one fruit at lunch.
Trim regular food portions.

Self-Monitoring

Use a food and activity log.
Use a daily planner.
Perform a regular weigh-in (i.e., daily or weekly).

Stimulus Control

Shop when not hungry and with a grocery list.
Make eating a singular activity (e.g., turn off the television).

Confronting Barriers

Practice problem-solving steps.
Plan ahead (e.g., keep healthful snacks on hand).

Sleep and Stress Management

Increase sleep and rest.
Practice a daily exercise routine.
Practice daily meditation or yoga.
Practice progressive relaxation and visual imagery exercises.

Social Support

Attend organized commercial support meetings or classes.
Use family, friends, and co-workers as support systems.

Contracting

Make realistic, simple, and achievable healthful goals.
Useful for short-term change.

Modified from Foreyt JP: Need for lifestyle intervention: how to begin, Am J Cardiovasc 96:11E, 2005.

evaluating outcomes, and reevaluating alternative solutions if needed.

Cognitive restructuring teaches patients to identify, challenge, and correct the negative thoughts that frequently undermine their efforts (see Chapter 15). Some lifestyle modification strategies are listed in Box 22-1.

Self-monitoring with daily records of place and time of food intake, as well as accompanying thoughts and feelings, helps identify the physical and emotional settings in which eating occurs. Physical activity is typically recorded in minutes or calories expended. Self-monitoring also gives clues to the occurrence of relapses and consequent guilt and how they can be prevented.

A comprehensive program of lifestyle modification produces a loss of approximately 10% of initial weight in 16 to 26 weeks, as revealed by a review of recent randomized controlled trials (RCTs), including the Diabetes Prevention Program. Long-term weight control is facilitated by continued patient-therapist contact, whether provided in person or by telephone, mail, or e-mail. Multiple strategies for behavioral therapy are often needed (ADA, 2010).

Technology shows promise as a delivery mechanism. Both e-mail and phone consults appear to be viable methods for contact and support as part of structured behavioral weight loss programs. Future treatment methods may include augmenting behavioral interventions with specific stimulus controls, self-monitoring with pharmacotherapy, targeted interventions available from the Internet, meal replacements, and telephone interventions. Nontraditional behavioral interventions for children and culturally sensitive interventions for racial and ethnic minority populations are needed (Berkel et al., 2005).

Dietary Modification Recommendations

Weight-loss programs with any degree of success integrate food-choice changes with exercise, behavior modification, nutrition education, and psychological support. When these approaches fail to bring about the desired reduction in body fat, medication may be added. For **morbid obesity** (BMI of 40 or greater), surgical intervention may be required.

Weight-loss programs should combine a nutritionally balanced dietary regimen with exercise and lifestyle modification at the least possible expense. Selecting the appropriate treatment strategy depends on the goals and health risks of the patient. Treatment options include:

- A low-calorie diet, increased physical activity, and lifestyle modification
- The preceding plus pharmacotherapy
- Surgery plus an individually prescribed dietary regimen, physical activity, and lifestyle modification program
- Prevention of weight regain through energy balance.

Restricted-Energy Diets

A balanced, restricted-energy diet is the most widely prescribed method of weight reduction. The diet should be nutritionally adequate except for energy, which is decreased to the point at which fat stores must be mobilized to meet daily energy needs. A caloric deficit of 500 to 1000 kcal daily usually meets this goal. The energy level varies with the individual's size and activities, usually ranging from 1200 to 1800 kcal daily. Regardless of the level of CR, healthful eating should be taught and recommendations for increasing physical activity should be included.

The low-calorie diet should be individualized for carbohydrates (50% to 55% of total kilocalories), using sources such as vegetables, fruits, beans, and whole grains. Generous protein, approximately 15% to 25% of kilocalories, is needed to prevent conversion of dietary protein to energy. Fat content should not exceed 30% of total calories. Extra fiber is recommended to reduce caloric density, to promote satiety by delaying stomach-emptying time, and to decrease to a small degree the efficiency of intestinal absorption. New food products made from oats and beverages with coconut oil may promise to enhance satiety by intake before a meal, with the expectation of reduced overall caloric intake. There are no current studies that suggest that coconut oil is effective for weight loss and it may contribute to weight gain with its 120 kcal and 13 g of fat per tablespoon. Otherwise, by combining oats with other fiber-rich foods, satiety may be increased.

Calculating fat as a percentage of calories is useful. A simple rule is to divide ideal calorie level by 4 for a 25% fat intake (e.g., an 1800-kcal intake needs 450 kcal from fat, or, at approximately 9 kcal/g, approximately 50 g of fat). Giving the person license to distribute fat grams throughout the day makes the approach more appealing, involves the person in the process, and decreases energy intake without hunger. Total calories must also be considered.

Alcohol and foods high in sugar should be limited to small amounts for palatability. Alcohol makes up 10% of the diet for many regular drinkers and contributes 7 kcal/g. Heavy drinkers who consume 50% or more of daily calories from alcohol may have a depressed appetite, whereas moderate users tend to gain weight with the added alcohol calories. Habitual use of alcohol may result in lipid storage, weight gain, or obesity.

Artificial sweeteners and fat substitutes improve the acceptability of limited food intakes for some people. There is no evidence that using artificial sweeteners reduces food intake or results in weight loss.

Vitamin and mineral supplements that meet age-related requirements are usually recommended with less than 1200 kcal for women or 1800 kcal for men. It is difficult to choose foods to maintain this calorie level and meet all nutritional requirements every day.

Formula Diets and Meal Replacement Programs

Formula diets are commercially prepared, ready-to-use, portion-controlled meal replacements. These meal replacements can be found over the counter (OTC) in drug stores, supermarkets, and franchised weight loss centers or in a clinical setting as drinks, prepackaged meals (entrees), or meal bars. The goal is to provide structure and replace other higher calorie foods. Per serving, most meal replacements include 0 to 5 g of fiber, 10 to 14 g of protein, various amounts of carbohydrate, 0 to 10 g of fat, and 25% to 30% of recommended dietary allowances for vitamins and minerals. Usually shakes are milk or soy based and are high in calcium with 150 to 250 kcal/8 oz. Some shakes are prepared using a blender at home and are made with a purchased powder. People who have difficulty with self-selection or portion control may use meal replacements as part of a comprehensive weight management program. Substituting one or two daily meals or snacks with meal replacements is a successful weight loss and weight maintenance strategy (ADA, 2010).

Commercial Programs

Millions of Americans turn to commercial weight-loss or self-help programs in search of permanent weight loss. The more caloric-restricted programs are usually medically supervised in a health care setting. As Table 22-3 illustrates, the programs vary considerably. Some require the use of proprietary prepackaged low-fat meals. Prepackaged diets appeal to some people because they allow them to avoid making choices about food. Some provide classes on self-introspection, behavior modification, and nutrition.

Use of the Internet has spawned a new generation of commercial programs. The importance of a tailored approach was the conclusion of an RCT comparing an Internet-based tailored weight management program with an information-only Internet weight management program based in an integrated health care setting (Rothert, 2006).

With the exception of Weight Watchers, the evidence to support the use of the major commercial and self-help weight loss programs is suboptimal. The reported results are probably a best-case scenario because many studies do not control for high attrition rates. More controlled trials are needed to assess the efficacy and cost-effectiveness of commercial programs. Thus it is important to evaluate all weight loss programs for sound nutritional practices. Consumers are savvy, and many programs have begun to report data on dropout or success rates, as well as weight maintenance.

Extreme Energy Restriction and Fasting

Extreme energy-restricted diets provide fewer than 800 kcal per day, and starvation or fasting diets provide fewer than 200 kcal per day. Fasting is seldom prescribed as a treatment; however, it is frequently invoked as a part of religious or protest regimen or in a personal effort to lose weight. Under these circumstances it is seldom continued long enough to produce the serious neurologic, hormonal, and other side effects that accompany prolonged starvation. More than 50% of the rapid weight reduction is fluid, which often leads to serious hypotension. Accumulation of uric acid can precipitate episodes of gout; gallstones can also occur. Also, as fat stores diminish, molecules are released that can affect further weight loss. See *Clinical Insight:* What's in That Fat When You Lose It? Sometimes what starts as extreme energy restriction to lose weight leads to more disordered eating patterns (see Chapter 23).

Very-Low-Calorie Diets

Diets providing 200 to 800 kcal are classified as **very-low-calorie diets (VLCDs)**. Little evidence suggests that intakes of fewer than 800 calories daily are of any advantage. Most VLCDs are hypocaloric but relatively rich in protein (0.8-1.5 g/kg IBW per day). They are designed to include a full complement of vitamins, minerals, electrolytes, and essential fatty acids, but not calories; they are given in a form that completely replaces usual food intake; and they are usually given for a period of 12 to 16 weeks. Their major advantage is rapid weight loss. Because of potential side effects, prescription of these diets is reserved for persons with a BMI of more than 30 for whom other diet programs with psychotherapy have been unsuccessful. Occasionally VLCDs may be indicated for persons with a BMI of 27 to 30 who have comorbidities or other risk factors.

The VLCD that first became popular in the early 1970s resulted in several deaths; however, improved protein formulations have increased acceptability and safety for

TABLE 22-3

Popular Commercial Diet Programs

Name	Foods or Products	Education	Teachers/ Counselors	Maintenance
VLCD Programs				
Medifast www.medifast.net	Special drink; physician supervised	Weekly individual sessions Weekly group meetings	Supervised by MDs	Weekly meetings for 5 mo
Optifast www.optifast.com	Special drink; physician supervised	Weekly individual sessions with MD 1½-hr weekly group meetings One meeting with RD	MDs, RNs, RDs, and psychologists at most locations	No time limit, begins at 20th week
Diet Programs				
Diet Center www.dietcenter.com	Regular food	Daily individual sessions	Trained staff	Weekly meetings for the first 3 mo; biweekly for months 4-6; monthly for months 6-12
Jenny Craig www.jennycraig.com	Prepackaged foods	14 1-hr video group classes; weekly individual sessions	RDs and psychologists	Monthly meetings for 6 mo or 1 yr
Nutrisystem www.nutrisystem.com	Prepackaged foods	30-min weekly group meetings; 10-min weekly individual sessions	College graduates	1-yr transition diet; program and regular foods
Weight Watchers www.weightwatchers.com	Regular food	45-min weekly group meetings	Program graduates	Weekly meetings for 6 wk; free meetings if maintain goal weight
The Solution www.shapedown.com	Regular food	Weekly 2-hr group meetings	RDs and psychologists certified by the program	Monthly meetings for 6 mo-1 yr; weekly meetings as necessary; no time limit
Internet-Based Diets				
Cyberdiet www.dietwatch.com www.cyberdiet.com	Regular food	Personal and professional e-counseling provide weekly meal plans and nutrition and fitness report cards; Professional e-counseling provides biweekly chats with an RD in chat rooms, bulletin boards; e-newsletter	RDs; physiologists; fitness trainers, chefs, MDs, and psychologists	Maintenance program once personal goals are met
eDiets www.ediets.com	Regular food	Weekly meal plan and exercise routines Chat rooms, bulletin boards, e-newsletter	RDs, RNs, fitness trainers, counselors, psychologists	Maintenance meal plans
Nutrio www.nutrio.com	Regular food	Daily and weekly meal plans; exercise and nutrition logs, community message boards, and e-newsletter	RDs, exercise physiologists, and psychologists	Maintenance meal plans
Set Point Health www.setpointhealth.com	Regular food and pre-packaged food	Customized eating plans; one-to-one online sessions with lifestyle coaches	MD directed; RDs and chefs	Maintenance program available

MD, Medical doctor; *RD*, registered dietitian; *VLCD*, very-low-calorie diet.

those with morbid obesity. The VLCDs can lead to an increase of urinary ketones that interfere with the renal clearance of uric acid, resulting in increased serum uric acid levels or gout. Higher serum cholesterol levels resulting from mobilization of adipose stores pose a risk of gallstones. Additional adverse reactions include cold intolerance, fatigue, light-headedness, nervousness, euphoria, constipation or diarrhea, dry skin, anemia, and menstrual irregularities; some of these are related to triiodothyronine (thyroid) deficiency.

Even though there are significantly greater weight losses with VLCDs in the short term, there are no significant differences in the weight losses in the long term (Gilden and Wadden, 2006). Thus there does not seem to be reason to recommend these VLCDs over more moderate CR except rarely. For those who have lost weight on a VLCD, limiting dietary fat intake and maintaining physical activity are both important factors for the prevention of weight regain. To promote better weight loss, patients should limit their fat intake to less than 30% of calories and increase activity levels.

Popular Diets and Practices

Each year, new approaches to weight loss find their way to the consumer through the popular press and media. Some of the programs are sensible and appropriate, whereas others emphasize fast results with minimum effort. Some of the proposed diets would lead to nutritional deficiencies over an extended period; however, the potential health risks are seldom realized because the diets are usually abandoned after a few weeks. Diets that emphasize fast results with minimum effort encourage unrealistic expectations, setting the dieter up for failure, subsequent guilt, and feelings of helplessness at ever managing the weight problem.

The low-carbohydrate, high-fat diet restricts carbohydrates to less than 20% of calories (and often less than 10% in the beginning), and fat constitutes 55% to 65% of calories, with protein making up the balance. Protein obtained from animal sources means that fat, saturated fat, and cholesterol intakes are high. Although these diets feature high ketone production, they suppress appetite to only a minor degree. The initial rapid weight loss from diuresis is secondary to the carbohydrate restriction. Examples of severe carbohydrate-restricted diets include *Dr. Atkins' New Diet Revolution* and *The Carbohydrate Addict's Diet*. The *Zone* and the *South Beach Diet* both restrict carbohydrates to no more than 40% of total calories, with fat and protein providing 30% of calories each. This diet composition is claimed to keep insulin in check, which is blamed for fat storage. The diet includes generous amounts of fiber and fresh fruits and vegetables. There is attention to the kind of fat, with emphasis on monounsaturated and polyunsaturated fat and limitation of saturated fat. Weight loss ensues not because insulin is kept in a narrow range, but because calories are restricted.

The EAL examined 14 studies on the effectiveness of the low-carbohydrate diets (Atkins, South Beach). Consumption of ad libitum low-carbohydrate diets (only limiting carbohydrate) and reduced-calorie diets both lower total caloric intake. However, ad libitum low-carbohydrate diets often result in greater body weight loss and fat loss in the first 6 months. After 1 year the differences are no longer significant (ADA, 2010).

Very-low-fat diets contain less than 10% of calories from fat, such as *Dr. Dean Ornish's Program for Reversing Heart Disease* and *The Pritikin Program*. These diets produce rapid weight loss and are very restrictive. A more popular variation limits fat to 20% of total energy intake. Because fat provides more than two times the energy per gram as protein or carbohydrate (9 kcal versus 4 kcal), an effective diet can be one that includes extensive controls on this nutrient.

Moderate-fat, balanced-nutrient reduction diets contain 20% to 30% of calories from fat, 15% to 20% of calories from protein, and 55% to 60% of calories from carbohydrate. *Volumetrics*, a program in this category, focuses on the energy density of foods (Rolls et al., 2005). Foods high in water content have a low energy density. These include fruits, vegetables, low-fat milk, cooked grains, lean meats, poultry, fish, and beans. Low–water containing foods that are energy dense such as potato chips, crackers, and fat-free cookies are restricted.

The U.S. Department of Agriculture (USDA) supported a scientific review of popular diets to assess their efficacy for weight loss and weight maintenance, as well as their effect on metabolic parameters, psychological well being, and reduction of chronic disease. A summary is shown in Table 22-4.

Physical Activity

Physical activity is the most variable component of energy expenditure. Increases in energy expenditure through exercise and other forms of physical activity are important components of interventions for weight loss and its maintenance. By increasing LBM in proportion to fat, physical activity helps to balance the loss of LBM and reduction of RMR that inevitably accompany intentional weight reduction. Other positive side effects of increased activity include strengthening cardiovascular integrity, increasing sensitivity to insulin, and expending additional energy and therefore calories.

Adequate levels of physical activity appear to be 60 to 90 minutes daily, as recommended by the USDA. This is also the amount of activity reported by those in the National Weight Control Registry (NWCR) who have kept off at least 10% of their weight for at least a year. Overweight and obese adults should gradually increase to these levels of physical activity. There is evidence that, even if an overweight or obese adult is unable to achieve this level of activity, significant health benefits can be realized by participating in at least 30 minutes of daily activity of moderate intensity (ADA, 2010). Therefore it is important to target these levels of physical activity to improve health-related outcomes and to facilitate long-term weight control (Jakicic, 2006).

Both aerobic and resistance training should be recommended. Resistance training increases LBM, adding to

TABLE 22-4

Results of U.S. Department of Agriculture Scientific Review of Popular Diets

Area	Finding
Weight loss	Diets that reduce caloric intake result in weight loss; all popular diets result in short-term weight loss if followed.
Body composition	All low-calorie diets result in a loss of body fat. In the short term, high-fat, low-carbohydrate ketogenic diets cause a greater loss of body water than body fat.
Nutritional adequacy	• High-fat, low-carbohydrate diets are low in vitamins E and A; thiamin; B_6; and folate; and the minerals calcium, magnesium, iron, and potassium. They are also low in dietary fiber. • Very-low-fat diets are low in vitamins E and B_{12} and the mineral zinc. • With proper food choices, a moderate-fat, balanced nutrient–reduction diet is nutritionally adequate.
Metabolic parameters	• Low-carbohydrate diets cause ketosis and may significantly increase blood uric acid concentrations. • Blood lipid levels decline as body weight decreases. • Energy restriction improves glycemic control. • As body weight declines, blood insulin and plasma leptin levels decrease. • As body weight declines, blood pressure decreases.
Hunger and compliance	No diet was optimal for reducing hunger.
Effect on weight maintenance	Controlled clinical trials of high-fat, low-carbohydrate, low-fat, and very-low-fat diets are lacking; therefore no data are available on weight maintenance after weight loss or long-term health benefits or risk.

From Freedman M et al: Popular diets: a scientific review, Obes Res 9:1S, 2001.

the RMR and the ability to use more of the energy intake, and it increases bone mineral density, especially for women (see Chapter 24). Aerobic exercise is important for cardiovascular health through elevated RMR, calorie expenditure, energy deficit and loss of fat. In addition to the physiologic benefits of exercise are relief of boredom, increased sense of control, and improved sense of well-being. The whole family can get involved in pleasurable activities (Figure 22-5).

Consistency is the key to realizing the health and weight-management benefits of exercise. Previous exercise recommendations for health called for 20 to 60 minutes of moderate- to high-intensity endurance exercise performed three or more times weekly. It now appears that most health benefits can be gained by physical activity of moderate intensity (enough to expend 200 kcal daily) accumulated in intermittent short bouts, such as 20 to 30 minutes of high-intensity activity 4 to 7 days per week (Institute of Medicine, 2002). High-intensity activity is not required. Contrary to popular belief, spot reduction (i.e., reducing fat in one area of the body) is not possible with exercise; fat is burned from the largest concentrations of adipose tissue.

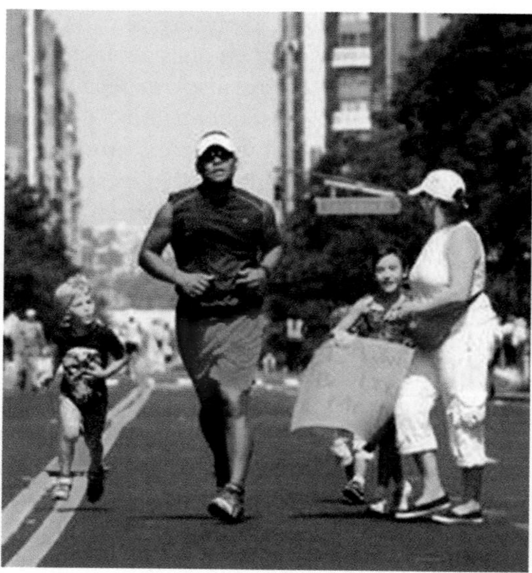

FIGURE 22-5 Jogging is an excellent aerobic activity for the whole family. *(Photo printed with permission from Dr. David Rivera, 2010.)*

Pharmaceutical Management

Appropriate pharmacotherapy can augment diet, physical activity, and behavior therapy as treatment for patients with a BMI of 30 or higher or patients with 27 or higher who also have significant risk factors or disease. These agents can decrease appetite, reduce absorption of fat, or increase energy expenditure. As with any drug treatment, physician monitoring for efficacy and safety is necessary. Pharmacotherapy is not a "magic pill"; dietitians should collaborate with other health professionals regarding the use of Food and Drug Administration (FDA)–approved pharmacotherapy. Not all individuals respond, but for patients who do respond, clinical trials suggest that a weight loss of approximately 2 to 20 kg can be expected usually during the first 6 months of treatment. Medication without lifestyle modification is less effective.

Medications currently available can be categorized as central nervous system (CNS)–acting agents and non–CNS-acting agents. The CNS-acting agents fall into the categories of catecholaminergic agents, serotoninergic agents, and combination catecholaminergic-serotoninergic agents. Common side effects of CNS-acting agents are dry mouth, headache, insomnia, and constipation. Only sibutramine (Meridia) and orlistat are approved by the FDA for long-term use in the treatment of obesity (Food and Drug Administration, 2009).

Catecholaminergic drugs act on the brain, increasing the availability of norepinephrine. Drug Enforcement Agency Schedule II anorexic agents such as amphetamines have a high potential for abuse and are not recommended for obesity treatment.

Serotoninergic agents act by increasing serotonin levels in the brain. Two drugs in this category, fenfluramine (commonly used in combination with phentermine, known as "fen-phen") and dexfenfluramine, were removed from the market in 1997 after concerns were raised regarding the possible side effects of cardiac valvulopathy, regurgitation, and primary pulmonary hypertension.

Sibutramine is a combination of catecholaminergic and serotoninergic agents, which inhibit the reuptake of serotonin and norepinephrine in the CNS to increase satiety, reduce hunger, and lessen the drop in metabolic rate that often occurs with weight loss. Because it stimulates the sympathetic nervous system, patients taking sibutramine may experience cardiovascular side effects; it is not appropriate for patients with a history of cardiovascular disorders. Sibutramine should not be used in combination with certain antidepressant agents such as monoamine oxidase inhibitors, selective serotonin reuptake inhibitors or other central-acting agents such as pseudoephedrine (Ephedra). The interaction may cause a hypertensive crisis.

Orlistat inhibits gastrointestinal lipase, which reduces approximately one third the amount of fat that is absorbed from food. Depending on the fat content of a person's diet, this lowered absorption can represent 150 to 200 kcal/day. With lowered fat-soluble vitamin absorption, supplements are typically recommended, separated by 2 hours or more. Weight loss of 3 to 5 kg in orlistat-treated patients is common. Side effects are gastrointestinal: oily spotting, fecal urgency, and flatus with discharge. Health benefits include reduced low-density lipoprotein (LDL) cholesterol and elevated HDL cholesterol, improved glycemic control, and reduced blood pressure.

Other drugs targeting weight loss and obesity through the CNS pathways or peripheral adiposity signals are in early-phase clinical trials. Currently, the only FDA-approved OTC weight-loss product is Alli, which contains 50% of the prescription dose of orlistat. OTC and natural weight-loss products hold varying degrees of efficacy (Table 22-5).

Other Nonsurgical Approaches

The "non-diet" paradigm maintains that the body will attain its natural weight if the individual eats healthfully, becomes attuned to hunger and satiety cues, and incorporates physical activity. This approach focuses on achieving health rather than attaining a certain weight. Advocates for this approach promote size acceptance and respect for the diversity of body shapes and sizes. Given the evidence that a 5% to 10% loss of initial weight can result in health benefits, that many persons set weight-loss goals that are unrealistic, and that fat discrimination continues to plague society, this approach may help some persons to develop a better relationship with food and a healthier perspective about their bodies.

Bariatric Surgery

Bariatric surgery is an accepted form of treatment for extreme or class III obesity with a BMI of 40 or greater, or a BMI of 35 or greater with comorbidities. Gastroplasty procedures are restrictive because they decrease the amount of food entering the gastrointestinal tract. Other surgical procedures, such as Roux-en-Y, are restrictive and cause malabsorption because they also prevent food from being absorbed from the gastrointestinal tract.

Before any extremely obese person is considered for surgery, failure of a comprehensive program that includes CR, exercise, lifestyle modification, psychological counseling, and family involvement must be demonstrated. *Failure* is defined as an inability of the patient to reduce body weight by one third and body fat by one half and an inability to maintain any weight loss achieved. Such patients have intractable morbid obesity and should be considered for surgery.

If surgery is chosen, the patient is evaluated extensively with respect to physiologic and medical complications, psychological problems such as depression or poor self-esteem, and motivation. Counseling sharply improves the outcomes for dieting and drug therapy in this population (Wadden and Sarwer, 2006). Postoperative follow-up requires evaluation at regular intervals by the surgical team and a registered dietitian. In addition, behavioral or psychological support is necessary. Generally, bariatric surgery improves self-image and may alleviate depression.

Gastric Bypass, Gastroplasty, and Gastric Banding

Both gastroplasty and gastric bypass procedures reduce the amount of food that can be eaten at one time and produce early satiety (Figure 22-6). The new stomach capacity may be as small as 1 oz (20 to 30 mL) or approximately 2 tablespoons. After surgery the patient's diet progresses from clear liquid, to full liquid, to puree, soft, and finally to a regular diet as tolerated, with emphasis on protein intake (Table 22-6). The results of gastric surgery are more favorable than those from the intestinal bypass surgery practiced during the 1970s. On average the reduction of excess body weight after

TABLE 22-5

Nonprescription Weight Loss Products

Product	Claim	Effectiveness	Safety
Alli: OTC version of prescription drug orlistat (Xenical)	Decreases absorption of dietary fat	Effective; weight-loss amounts typically less for OTC versus prescription	FDA investigating reports of liver injury, pancreatitis
Bitter orange	Increases calories burned	Insufficient reliable evidence to rate	Possibly unsafe
Chitosan	Blocks absorption of dietary fat	Insufficient reliable evidence to rate	Possibly safe
Chromium	Increases calories burned, decreases appetite, and builds muscle	Insufficient reliable evidence to rate	Likely safe
CLA	Reduces body fat and builds muscle	Possibly effective	Possibly safe
Country mallow (heartleaf)	Decreases appetite and increases calories burned	Insufficient reliable evidence to rate	Likely unsafe and banned by FDA
Ephedra (Ma Huang)	Decreases appetite	Possibly effective	Likely unsafe and banned by FDA
Green tea extract	Increases calorie and fat metabolism and decreases appetite	Insufficient reliable evidence to rate	Possibly safe
Guar gum	Blocks absorption of dietary fat and increases feeling of fullness	Possibly ineffective	Likely safe
Hoodia	Decreases appetite	Insufficient reliable evidence to rate	Insufficient information
Senna	Cathartic; causes diarrhea	Insufficient reliable evidence	Likely unsafe

Data from Natural Medicines in the Clinical Management of Obesity, Natural Medicines Comprehensive Database, http://naturaldatabase.therapeuticresearch.com:80/ce/ceCourse.aspx?s=ND&cs=&pc=09%2D32&cec=1&pm=5, Accessed on April 19, 2011.

CLA, Conjugated linoleic acid; *FDA*, Food and Drug Administration; *OTC*, over the counter.

TABLE 22-6

Diet Progression After Gastric Bypass

Phases of Diet	Total Quantity	Typical Progression after Surgery	Sample Food Items
Liquid diet	No more than ½ cup total	1-2 days	Plain and flavored waters, broth, unsweetened juices, diet gelatin, noncarbonated diet drinks, strained cream soups
Semisolids and pureed diet	Gradually increase from ½ cup to no more than ¾ cup total	Day 3 to 3 weeks	Blenderized or pureed soft meats, fish, chicken, turkey. Pureed fruits and tender vegetables. Hot cereals cooked in milk. Yogurt.
Soft foods	Meals should be from ¾ cup to no more than 1 cup total	3 to 6 weeks	Foods that can be mashed with a fork, such as ground or finely diced meats, canned or soft, fresh fruit, and cooked vegetables.
Regular small meals and snacks	No more than 1 cup total; meat should be no more than 2 oz	6 weeks and beyond	Firmer foods without being pureed. Avoid popcorn, nuts, meats with gristle, dried fruits, vegetables and fruits that are stringy or coarse, sodas, bread, granola.

Adapted from Mayo Clinic, Gastric bypass diet. Accessed 11 July 2010 from http://www.mayoclinic.com/health/gastric-bypass-diet/my00827.

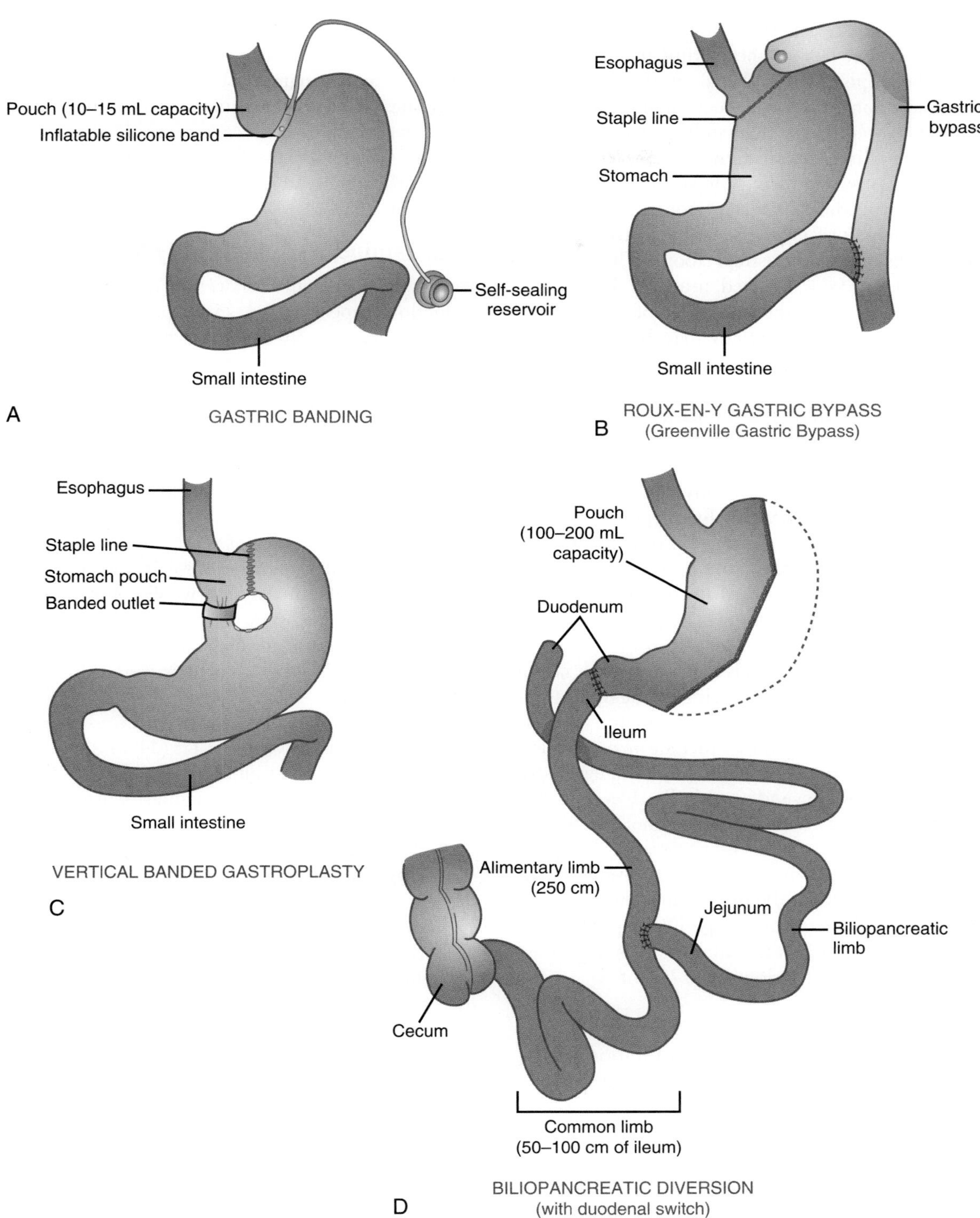

FIGURE 22-6 Bariatric surgeries.

gastric restriction surgery correlates to approximately 30% to 40% of initial body weight. In addition to the greater absolute weight loss observed, the gastric bypass tends to have sustainable results with significant resolution of hypertension, type 2 diabetes mellitus, osteoarthritis, back pain, dyslipidemia, cardiomyopathy, nonalcoholic steatohepatitis, and sleep apnea. However, late complications may be seen, such as vitamin deficiency, electrolyte problems or even intestinal failure.

Gastroplasty reduces the size of the stomach by applying rows of stainless-steel staples to partition the stomach and create a small gastric pouch, leaving only a small opening (0.8-1 cm) into the distal stomach. This opening may be banded by a piece of mesh to prevent it from enlarging during the years after surgery. Vertical-banded gastroplasty is the most popular surgery. In the lap-band procedure, also called **gastric banding**, the band creating the reduced stomach pouch can be adjusted so that the opening to the rest of the stomach can be made smaller or enlarged. The band, filled with saline, has a tube exiting from it to the surface of the belly just under the skin; this allows for the injection of additional fluid or reduction of fluid into the lap band. Patients who undergo the banding procedures will not require folic acid, iron, or vitamin B_{12} replacements

Gastric bypass involves reducing the size of the stomach with the stapling procedure, but then connecting a small opening in the upper portion of the stomach to the small intestine by means of an intestinal loop. The original operation in the late 1960s evolved into the Roux-en-Y gastric bypass. Because use of the lower part of the stomach is omitted, the gastric bypass patient may have dumping syndrome as food empties quickly into the duodenum (see Chapter 28). The tachycardia, sweating, and abdominal pain are so negative that they motivate the patient to make the appropriate behavioral changes and refrain from overeating. However, patients tend to choose liquids; weight loss can be deterred by drinking too much calorically dense liquid such as milk shakes and soft drinks. Eventually the pouch expands to accommodate 4 to 5 oz at a time. Frequently, gastric bypass surgery leads to bloating of the pouch, nausea, and vomiting. A postsurgical food record noting the tolerance for specific foods in particular amounts helps in devising a program to avoid these episodes.

Completion of bypass surgery leads to malnutrition, which requires lifelong follow-up and monitoring by the multidisciplinary team. Nutritional status should be evaluated periodically by a dietitian. Monitoring should include an assessment of total body-fat loss, potential anemia, and deficiencies of potassium, magnesium, folate, and vitamin B_{12}. Ice-cube pica and iron deficiency anemia are possible (Kushner and Shanta Retelny, 2005). Supplementation is necessary. An adult vitamin-mineral supplement (one liquid or chewable tablet twice daily) containing 1200-1500 mg calcium citrate,1000-2000 IU vitamin D, 500 mcg vitamin B_{12}, 400 mcg folic acid, and 65-80 mg elemental iron with vitamin C is suggested (Kuluck et al., 2010; Snyder-Marlow et al., 2010.)

Liposuction

Liposuction (or liposculpture) involves aspiration of fat deposits by means of a 1- to 2-cm incision through which a tube is fanned out into the adipose tissue. The most successful operations are performed on younger persons with only small amounts of fat to be removed, where the elastic properties of the skin are able to allow tightening over the aspirated areas. It is not usually a weight-reduction technique but rather a cosmetic surgery because usually only approximately 5 lb of fat are removed at a time. Deaths, severe infections, cellulitis, and hemorrhage have occurred.

COMMON PROBLEMS IN OBESITY TREATMENT

Prognosis for maintaining reduced weight is typically poor. Continued dieting, with repeated ups and downs, leads gradually to a net increase in body fat and thus to a health risk for hyperlipidemia, hypertension, diabetes, and even osteoarthritis. Women having bariatric surgery had lower serum 25-hydroxyvitamin D (s25D) and higher parathyroid hormone (sPTH). The major determinant of s25D and sPTH was weight. Hyperparathyroidism in obesity did not indicate vitamin D insufficiency. Low s25D was not associated with comorbid conditions, apart from osteoarthritis (Grethen, 2011).

Maintaining Reduced Body Weight

Energy requirements for weight maintenance after weight reduction appear to be 25% lower than at the original weight. The net effect is that reduced-obese persons are faced with the necessity of maintaining a reduced energy intake even after the desired weight has been lost. Whether this reduced intake must be maintained indefinitely is not known.

The NWCR consists of more than 5000 individuals who have been successful in long-term weight loss maintenance. The purpose of establishing the NWCR is to identify the common characteristics of those who succeed in long-term weight loss maintenance. There is very little similarity in how these individuals lost weight but there are some common behaviors they all have for keeping their weight off. Lifestyle modification and a sense of self-efficacy appear to be essential. To maintain their weight loss, NWCR participants report:

1. Eating a relatively low-fat (24%) diet
2. Eating breakfast almost every day
3. Weighing themselves regularly, usually once per day to once per week
4. Engaging in high levels (60 to 90 minutes/day) of physical activity

Weight loss maintenance may get easier over time; after individuals have successfully maintained their weight loss for 2 to 5 years, the chance of longer-term success greatly increases (Wing and Phelan, 2005). Support groups are valuable for reduced-obese persons who are maintaining a new lower weight; they help individuals facing similar problems. Two self-help support groups are Overeaters Anonymous and Take Off Pounds Sensibly. These groups are inexpensive, continuous, include a "buddy system," and encourage participation on a regular basis or as often as needed. Weight Watcher programs offer free lifelong maintenance classes for those who have reached and are maintaining their goal weights.

Interestingly, boring and monotonous diets can be a management strategy. Diets that are repetitious without change from meal to meal are one consideration because people tend to overeat when they have many mealtime choices. Overall, a common sense approach is needed. Some phrases can be shared with individuals who are trying to maintain their weight loss, including:

1. The best diet is "don't buy it."
2. "Easy does it"—use moderation at all meals.

3. "Don't drink your calories."
4. Keep the "extras" to no more than 200 kcal per day.

Plateau Effect

A common experience for the person in a weight-reduction program is arrival at a weight plateau, when weight remains at the same level for a long period. Eventually weight loss halts completely. One theory is that interim plateaus reflect a reduction of lipid in individual adipocytes to some level that signals metabolic adjustment and weight maintenance. Another theory is that there is a release of toxins from adipose tissue that act as endocrine disruptors and inflammatory agents and affect subsequent weight loss. See *Clinical Insight:* What's in That Fat When You Lose It? To move out of this phase usually requires increasing the activity level.

Any weight loss, whether fast or slow, results in a loss of the extra muscle that has developed to support the excess adipose tissue. Because this extra LBM has contributed to an increased metabolic rate, RMR decreases as LBM is lost. The fact that RMR decreases rapidly at the onset of a weight-reduction diet, by as much as 15% within 2 weeks, indicates that other adaptations to the lower weight and the threat of deprivation are taking place.

Other factors join to decrease RMR and limit effectiveness of the restricted energy intake. A decrease in the total kilocalories ingested results in a decrease in total energy expenditure. Because a body that weighs less requires less energy expenditure to move around, the cost of physical activity is also less. A state of equilibrium is eventually reached at which the energy intake is equal to energy expenditure. Unless a change is made in either nutritional intake or physical activity, weight loss stops at this point.

Weight Cycling

Repeated bouts of weight loss and regain, known as weight cycling or the **yo-yo effect**, occurs in men and women and is common in both overweight and nonoverweight individuals. The effect of weight cycling appears to result in increased body fatness and weight with the end of each cycle. There are metabolic and psychological effects that are undesirable.

WEIGHT MANAGEMENT IN CHILDREN

Almost 32% of US children ages 2-19 are overweight or obese (Ogden et al, 2010). Obese children are often the targets of discrimination. Childhood obesity increases the risk of obesity in adulthood. For the child who is obese after 6 years of age, the probability of obesity in adulthood is significantly greater if either the mother or the father is obese.

The BMI tables for determining childhood obesity are available for use by health care practitioners (see Appendixes 12 and 16). Children whose BMI is greater than the 85th percentile are six times more likely to be overweight later (Nadir et al., 2006). In addition, children who have growth failure and undernutrition in utero or in the early years of life tend to become overweight in later childhood with subsequent risks of elevated blood pressure, lipid, and glucose levels (Stein et al., 2005). Obesity that begins in childhood tends to lead to hypertension, elevated LDL cholesterol, and TGs in adults (Thompson et al., 2007).

Children with a body mass index (BMI) in the 85th percentile or higher with complications of obesity, or with a BMI in the 95th percentile or higher with or without complications, should be carefully assessed for genetic, endocrinologic, and psychologic conditions, and secondary complications such as hypertension, dyslipidemias, sleep apnea, and orthopedic problems. If the complications cause serious morbidity and require rapid weight loss, referral to a pediatric obesity specialist may be necessary. Otherwise, parent and child readiness to make changes should be evaluated and eating and activity patterns carefully assessed.

Once assessment is complete, treatment can begin. The primary goal of treatment is to achieve healthy eating and activity, not to achieve an IBW. For children 7 years of age and younger the goal is prolonged weight maintenance or slowing of the rate of weight gain, which allows for a gradual decline in BMI as children grow in height. This is an appropriate goal in the absence of any secondary complications of obesity. However, if secondary complications are present, children in this age group may benefit from weight loss if their BMI is at the 95th percentile or higher. For children older than 7 years, prolonged weight maintenance is appropriate if their BMI is between the 85th and 95th percentile and if they have no secondary complications. If a secondary complication is present or if BMI is at the 95th percentile or above, weight loss (about 1 lb per month) is advised. If the weight appropriate for the child's anticipated adult height has already been reached, maintenance at that weight should be the lifetime goal. The child who already exceeds an optimal adult weight can safely experience a slow weight loss of 10 to 12 lb per year until the optimal adult weight is reached. Balanced micronutrient intake for children includes 45% to 60% of kcal from carbohydrate, 25% to 40% from fat, and 10% to 35% from protein.

The child who needs to reduce weight is going to require more attention from family and health professionals. This attention should be directed to all the areas mentioned previously, with family modification of eating habits and increased physical activity. The program should be long term over the entire growth period and perhaps longer.

Inactivity is often coupled with sedentary hobbies, excessive TV watching, or prolonged sitting in front of a computer or game screen. However, there is a new theory that physical inactivity appears to be the result of fatness rather than its cause (Metcalf et al., 2010). This requires further research, but does suggest that factors other than inactivity may be more important in obesity development in children. See New Directions—Organizing to Solve the Childhood Obesity Problem "Within a Generation."

WEIGHT IMBALANCE: EXCESSIVE LEANNESS OR UNINTENTIONAL WEIGHT LOSS

Almost eclipsed by the attention focused on obesity is the need for some people to gain weight. The term **underweight** is applicable to those who are 15% to 20% or more below accepted weight standards. Because underweight is often a symptom of disease, it should be assessed medically. A low BMI (<18.5) is associated with greater mortality risk than that of individuals with optimal BMI (18.5-24.9), especially with aging and in the elderly. Undernutrition may lead to underfunction of the pituitary, thyroid, gonads, and adrenals. Other risk factors include loss of energy and susceptibility to injury and infection, as well as a distorted body image and other psychological problems (see Chapter 21).

Cause

Underweight or unintentional weight loss can be caused by (1) inadequate oral food and beverage intake, with insufficient quantities to match activity; (2) excessive physical activity, as in the case of compulsive athletic training; (3) inadequate capacity for absorption and metabolism of foods consumed; (4) a wasting disease that increases the metabolic rate and energy needs, as in cancer, acquired immune deficiency syndrome (AIDS), or hyperthyroidism; or (5) excess energy expenditure during psychological or emotional stress (see Chapter 23).

Assessment

Assessing the cause and extent of underweight before starting a treatment program is important. A thorough history and pertinent medical tests usually determine whether underlying disorders are causing the underweight. From anthropometric data such as arm muscle and fat areas, it is possible to determine whether health-endangering underweight really exists. Assessment of body fatness is useful, especially in dealing with the patient who has an eating disorder (see Chapter 23). Biochemical measurements will indicate whether malnutrition accompanies the underweight (see Chapter 8). Use of an eating inventory questionnaire can identify persons at risk of unintentional weight loss (Hays et al., 2006).

Management

Any underlying cause of unintentional weight loss or low BMI must be the first priority. A wasting disease or malabsorption requires treatment. Nutrition support and dietary changes are effective along with treatment of the underlying disorder (Table 22-7).

If the cause of the underweight is inadequate oral food and beverage intake, activity should be modified and psychological counseling started if necessary.

Appetite Enhancers

The FDA has approved orexigenic agents that include corticosteroids, cyproheptadine, loxiglumide (cholecystokinin antagonist), megestrol acetate, mirtazapine, dronabinol, oxoglutarate, anabolic agents (testosterone or Anadrol), oxandrin, and growth hormone. Use of orexigenic agents for weight loss in seniors is saved for those whose conditions are refractory to usual treatments. One third of older adults, especially women, exhibit weight loss in combination with depression. Mirtazapine is an effective antidepressant that is well tolerated and increases appetite. Dronabinol is used for

TABLE 22-7

Nutrition Management of Unintentional Weight Loss

Concern	Tips
Anxiety, stress, depression	Antidepressants can help; monitor choice to be sure they do not contribute to weight loss.
Cancer	Gastrointestinal cancers are especially detrimental. Some treatments and medications can cause loss of appetite, as can the cancer itself.
Celiac disease	Ensure that all gluten-containing foods and ingredients are eliminated from the diet.
Changes in activity level or dietary preparation methods	Avoid skipping meals; prepare foods with high energy density.
Diabetes, new onset	See a physician; monitor medications and meals accordingly.
Dysphagia or chewing difficulties	Alter food and liquid textures accordingly to improve chewing and swallowing capability.
Hyperthyroidism	Too much thyroxine can cause weight loss.
Inflammatory bowel disease	Check medications and treatments to determine if new choices are in order.
Intestinal ischemia	See a physician.
Medications	Some medications can cause weight loss; check with the physician; add snacks or enhanced meals if needed.
Nausea and vomiting	Infections, other illnesses, hormonal changes, and some medications cause nausea and vomiting; small, frequent meals are useful; serve liquids between meals instead of with meals to reduce fullness.
Pancreatitis and cystic fibrosis	Monitor for sufficiency of pancreatic enzyme replacement.

chemotherapy-induced nausea and vomiting in cancer and AIDS patients; it has been shown to induce weight gain in patients with dementia.

High-Energy Diets

A careful history may reveal inadequacies in dietary habits and nutritional intakes. Meals should be scheduled and relaxed instead of hastily planned or quickly eaten. The underweight person frequently must be encouraged to eat, even if not hungry. The secret is to individualize the program with readily available foods that the individual really enjoys, with a plan for regular eating times throughout the day. In addition to meals, snacks are usually necessary to adequately increase the energy intake. Often a liquid supplement taken with meals or between meals is effective; it is nutritious as well as easy to prepare and consume.

The energy distribution of the diet should be approximately 30% of the kilocalories from fat, with the majority from monounsaturated or polyunsaturated sources and at least 12% to 15% of the kilocalories from protein. A basic vitamin and mineral supplement may be encouraged. In addition to an intake according to estimated energy requirements for the present weight, 500 to 1000 extra kilocalories per day should be planned. If 2400 kcal maintains the current weight, 2900 to 3400 kcal would be required for weight gain. The intake should be increased gradually to avoid gastric discomfort, discouragement, electrolyte imbalances, and heart dysfunction. Step-up plans are outlined in Table 22-8.

In underweight children, nonnutritional factors, insufficient caloric intake, excessive nutrient losses, and abnormal energy metabolism may contribute to growth failure and morbidity. Thus adequate nutritional support should be an integral part of the management plan. Lipid-based nutrient

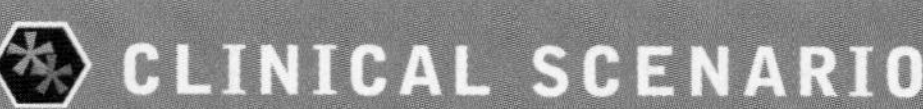

Maria is a 45-year-old Latina woman who has tried numerous weight-loss programs. She has followed strict diets and has never exercised in previous weight-loss attempts. She takes several cardiac medications, none of which she can remember. Her blood pressure is 160/90, she is 5 ft 4 in, and she weighs 195 lb. Her lowest body weight was 130 lb at age 30, maintained for 2 years. Maria mentioned that she tried numerous diets while a teenager, when she weighed 170 lb for 3 years. What guidelines would you offer to Maria at this time?

Nutrition Diagnostic Statements

1. Limited adherence to nutrition-related recommendations related to multiple failed weight-loss attempts as evidenced by no change in weight
2. Overweight and obesity related to excessive energy intake as evidenced by weight 70 lbs over desirable weight

Nutrition Care Questions

1. How would you address the concern about medications?
2. What types of exercise would you be likely to discuss?
3. Which macro- and micronutrients would you discuss with Maria (e.g., total fat, saturated fat, sodium, potassium, calcium)?
4. How would you bring up exercise and what would you recommend for Maria?
5. What would be the goals of her treatment?

TABLE 22-8

Suggestions for Increasing Energy Intake

Additional Foods	kcal	Protein (g)
Plus 500 kcal (Served Between Meals)		
1. 1 c dry cereal	110	2
1 banana	80	
1 c whole milk	159	8
1 slice toast	60	2
1 T peanut butter	86	4
	495	16
2. 8 saltine crackers	99	3
1 oz cheese	113	7
1 c ice cream	290	6
	502	16
3. 6 graham cracker squares	165	3
2 T peanut butter	172	8
1 c orange juice	122	
2 T raisins	52	
	511	11

Continued

TABLE 22-8

Suggestions for Increasing Energy Intake—cont'd

Additional Foods	kcal	Protein (g)
Plus 1000 kcal (Served Between Meals)		
1. 8 oz fruit flavored whole milk yogurt	240	9
1 slice bread	60	2
2 oz cheese	226	14
1 apple	87	
¼ of 14-inch cheese pizza	306	16
1 small banana	81	1
	1000	42
2. Instant Breakfast with whole milk	280	15
1 c cottage cheese	239	31
½ c pineapple	95	
1 c apple juice	117	3
6 graham cracker squares	165	
1 pear	100	1
	996	50
Plus 1500 kcal (Served Between Meals)		
1. 2 slices bread	120	4
2 T peanut butter	172	8
1 T jam	110	
4 graham cracker squares	110	2
8 oz fruit-flavored whole milk yogurt	240	9
¾ c roasted peanuts	628	28
1 c apricot nectar	143	1
	1523	52
2. 1 baked custard	285	13
Instant Breakfast with whole milk	280	15
1 c dry cereal	110	2
1 banana	80	
1 c dry cereal	110	2
1 c whole milk	159	8
1 c orange juice	122	
4 T raisins	104	
1 bagel	165	6
2 T cream cheese	199	
2 T jam	110	
	1514	46

supplements are fortified products that are often ready-to-use therapeutic foods or highly concentrated supplements that can be administered at "point of service" or emergency settings (Chaparro and Dewey, 2010).

USEFUL WEBSITES

American Obesity Association
http://www.obesity.org/

America on the Move
http://www.americaonthemove.org

American Society of Bariatric Surgery
http://www.asmbs.org/

Calorie Restriction Society International
www.crsociety.org

Centers for Disease Control and Prevention (CDC)
http://www.cdc.gov/

International Association for the Study of Obesity
http://www.iaso.org/

International Obesity Task Force
http://www.iotf.org

Let's Move!
www.letsmove.gov/

National Heart, Lung, and Blood Institute: Identification, Evaluation, and Treatment of Overweight and Obesity in Adults

http://www.nhlbi.nih.gov/guidelines/obesity/ob_home.htm

The Obesity Society

http://www.naaso.org

Shape Up America!

http://www.shapeup.org/

Weight Control Network: National Institute of Diabetes and Digestive and Kidney Disease

http://win.niddk.nih.gov/

REFERENCES

Adams KF, et al: Overweight, obesity, and mortality in a large prospective cohort of persons 50 to 71 years old, *N Engl J Med* 355:763, 2006.

American Dietetic Association: *Evidence-based nutrition practice guideline on adult weight management, dietary intervention algorithm*, published on May 2006 at www.adaevidencelibrary.com/topic.cfm?cat=2849 and copyrighted by the American Dietetic Association. Accessed 10 July 2010.

Anschultz DJ, et al: Susceptibility for thin ideal media and eating styles, *Body Image* 5:70, 2008.

Ashley EA, et al: Clinical assessment incorporating a personal genome, *Lancet* 375:1497, 2010.

Barber N: The evolutionary psychology of physical attractiveness: sexual selection and human morphology, *Evol Hum Behav* 16:395, 1995.

Barouki R: Linking long-term toxicity of xeno-chemicals with short-term biological adaptation, *Biochimi* 99:1222, 2010.

Bonafini BA, Pozzilli P: Body weight and beauty: the changing face of the ideal female body weight, *Obes Rev* 19 May 2010. [Epub ahead of print.]

Berkel LA, et al: Behavioral interventions for obesity, *J Am Diet Assoc* 105:S35, 2005.

Bjorntorp P, Sjostrom L: Number and size of adipose fat cells in relation to metabolism in human obesity, *Metabolism* 20:703, 1971.

Blackburn GL: *Break through your set point*, New York, 2008 Harper-Collins.

Brown I: Nurses' attitudes toward adult patients who are obese: literature review, *J Adv Nurs* 55:265, 2006.

Carr D, Friedman MA: Is obesity stigmatizing? Body weight, perceived discrimination, and psychological well-being in the United States, *J Health Soc Behav* 46:264, 2005.

Centers for Disease Control and Prevention (CDC): *Overweight and obesity trends*, 2007. Accessed 12 May 2010 from www.cdc.gov/nccdphp/obesity/trend/index.htm.

Chan DC, et al: Effect of ezetimibe on hepatic fat, inflammatory markers, and apolipoprotein B-100 kinetics in insulin-resistant obese subjects on a weight loss diet, *Diab Care* 33:1134, 2010.

Chaparro CM, Dewey KG: Use of lipid-based nutrient supplements (LNS) to improve the nutrient adequacy of general food distribution rations for vulnerable sub-groups in emergency settings, *Matern Child Nutr* 6:1S, 2010.

Couce ME, et al: Is ghrelin the culprit for weight loss after gastric bypass surgery? A negative answer, *Obes Surg* 16:870, 2006.

De Luis DA, et al: Influence of ALA54THR polymorphism of fatty acid binding protein 2 on lifestyle modification response in obese subjects, *Ann Nutr Metab* 50:354-360, 2006

Deurenberg P, Deurenberg-Yap M: Validity of body composition methods across ethnic population groups, *Acta Diabetol* 40:2465, 2003.

Enriori JP, et al: Leptin resistance and obesity, *Obesity* 14:254s, 2006.

Food and Drug Administration (FDA): *FDA approves orlistat for over-the-counter use*, 2009. Accessed 11 July 2010 from http://www.fda.gov/NewsEvents/Newsroom/PressAnnouncements/2007/ucm108839.htm.

Ferguson JF, et al: Gene-nutrient interactions in the metabolic syndrome: single nucleotide polymorphisms in ADIPOQ and ADIPOR1 interact with plasma saturated fatty acids to modulate insulin resistance, *Am J Clin Nutr* 91:794, 2010.

Fontana L: *Calorie restriction, endurance exercise, and successful aging.* 62nd Annual Scientific Meeting of the Gerontological Society of America, Atlanta, Ga, 21-22 November 2009.

Frayling TM, et al: A common variant in the FTO gene is associated with body mass index and predisposes to childhood and adult obesity, *Science* 316:389, 2007.

Garaulet M, et al: CLOCK genetic variation and metabolic syndrome risk: modulation by monounsaturated fatty acids, *Am J Clin Nutr* 90:1466, 2009.

Garaulet M, et al: The chronobiology, etiology and pathophysiology of obesity, *Int J Obes (Lond)* 22 June 2010. [Epub ahead of print.]

Gilden TA, Wadden TA: The evolution of very-low-calorie diets: an update and meta-analysis, *Obesity* 14:1283, 2006.

Goldstein BJ, Scalia R: Adipokines and vascular disease in diabetes, *Curr Diab Rep* 7:25, 2007.

Goodpaster BH, et al: Obesity, regional fat distribution, and the metabolic syndrome in older men and women, *Arch Int Med* 165:777, 2005.

Gower BA, et al: Changes in intra-abdominal fat in early postmenopausal women: effects of hormone use, *Obesity* 14:1046, 2006.

Grethen E, McClintock R, Gupta CE, Jones R, Cacucci BM, Diaz D, Fulford AD, Perkins SM, Considine RV, Peacock M: Vitamin D and Hyperparathyroidism in Obesity, *Clin Endocrinol Metab* 2011 Feb 16.

Grimble RF: The true cost of in-patient obesity: impact of obesity on inflammatory stress and morbidity, *Proc Nutr Soc* 69:511, 2010.

Grun F: Obesogens, *Curr Opin Endocrinal Diabetes Obes* 17:453, 2010.

Grun F, Blumberg B: Environmental obesogens: organotins and endocrine disruption via nuclear receptor signaling, *Endocrinology* 147:s50, 2006.

Hansen JB, Kristiansen K: Regulatory circuits controlling white versus brown adipocyte differentiation, *Biochem J* 398:153, 2006.

Hays NP, et al: Eating behavior and weight change in healthy postmenopausal women: results of a 4-year longitudinal study, *J Gerontol A Biol Sci Med Sci* 61:608, 2006.

Heilbronn LK, et al: Effect of 6-month calorie restriction on biomarkers of longevity, metabolic adaptation, and oxidative stress in overweight individuals: a randomized, controlled trial, *JAMA* 295:1539, 2006.

Hyman M: *Systems biology, toxins, obesity, and functional medicine.* The Proceedings From the 13th International Symposium of The Institute for Functional Medicine, 2006.

Imbeault P, et al: Weight loss-induced rise in plasma pollutant is associated with reduced skeletal muscle oxidative capacity, *Am J Physiol Endocrinol Metab* 282:E574, 2002.

Institute of Medicine, Food and Nutrition Board: *Dietary reference intakes for energy, carbohydrate, fiber, fat, fatty acids, cholesterol, protein, and amino acids*, Washington, DC, 2002, National Academies Press.

Jacobs EJ, et al: Waist circumference and all-cause mortality in a large US cohort, *Arch Intern Med* 170:1293, 2010

Jakicic JM: Treatment and prevention of obesity: what is the role of exercise? *Nutr Rev* 64:S57, 2006.

Jee SH, et al: Body-mass index and mortality in Korean men and women, *N Engl J Med* 355:779, 2006.

Keys A: *The biology of human starvation*, Minneapolis, 1950, University of Minnesota Press.

Kuluck D, et al: The bariatric surgery patient: a growing role for registered dietitians, *J Am Diet Assoc* 110:593, 2010.

Kushner RF, Shanta Retelny V: Emergence of pica (ingestion of non-food substances) accompanying iron deficiency anemia after gastric bypass surgery, *Obes Surg* 15:1491, 2005.

Latner JD, et al: Stigmatized students: age, sex, and ethnicity effects in the stigmatization of obesity, *Obes Res* 13:1226, 2005.

Levine JA: Nonexercise activity thermogenesis—liberating the life-force, *J Intern Med* 262:273, 2007.

Mayo Clinic: Calorie restriction for anti-aging. Accessed 16 April 2010 from http://www.mayoclinic.com/.

Metcalf BS, et al: Fatness leads to inactivity, but inactivity does not lead to fatness: a longitudinal study in children (EarlyBird 45), *Arch Dis Child* 23 June 2010. [Epub ahead of print.]

Nadir PR, et al: Identifying risk for obesity in early childhood, *Pediatrics* 118:e594, 2006.

Newby PK, et al: Longitudinal changes in food patterns predict changes in weight and body mass index and the effects are greatest in obese women, *J Nutr* 136:2580, 2006.

Nicklas B: Polymorphisms of angiotensinogen and angiotensin-converting enzyme associated with lower extremity arterial disease in the health, aging and body composition study, *J Hum Hypertens* 1(8):673, 2007

Ogden CL, et al: Prevalence of high body mass index in US children and adolescents, 2007-2008, *JAMA*, 303:242, 2010.

Ogden CL, et al: Prevalence and trends in overweight among US children and adolescents, 1999-2000, *JAMA* 288:1728, 2002.

Pasarica M, Dhurandhar NV: Infectobesity: obesity of infectious origin, *Adv Food Nutr Res* 52:61, 2007.

Phelan JP, Rose, MR: Calorie restriction increases longevity substantially only when the reaction norm is steep, *Biogerontology* 7:161, 2006.

Prentice AM: Early influences on human energy regulation: thrifty genotypes and thrifty phenotypes, *Physiol Behav* 86:640, 2005.

Racette SB, et al: Abdominal adiposity is a stronger predictor of insulin resistance than fitness among 50-95 year olds, *Diabetes Care* 29:673, 2006

Rhéaume C, Arsenault BJ, Dumas MP, Pérusse L, Tremblay A, Bouchard C, Poirier P, Després JP: Contributions of Cardiorespiratory Fitness and Visceral Adiposity to Six-Year Changes in Cardiometabolic Risk Markers in Apparently Healthy Men and Women, *Clin Endocrinol Metab* 2011 Feb 16.

Rolland-Cachera MF: Rate of growth in early life: a predictor of later health? *Adv Exp Med Biol* 569:35, 2005.

Rolls BJ, et al: Provision of foods differing in energy density affects long-term weight loss, *Obes Res* 13:1052, 2005.

Rothert K, et al: Web-based weight management programs in an integrated health care setting: a randomized controlled trial, *Obesity* 14:266, 2006.

Snyder-Marlow G, et al: Nutrition care for patients undergoing laparoscopic sleeve gastrectomy for weight loss, *J Am Diet Assoc* 110:6000, 2010.

Statistics Canada: Accessed 7 July 2010 from http://www.statcan.gc.ca/pub/82-620-m/2005001/pdf/4224906-eng.pdf.

Stein AD, et al: Childhood growth and chronic disease: evidence from countries undergoing nutrition transition, *Matern Child Nutr* 1:177, 2005.

Stevens JM, Vidal-Puig AJ: An update on visfatin/pre-B cell colony-enhancing factor, an ubiquitously expressed, illusive cytokine that is regulated in obesity, *Curr Opin Lipidol* 17:128, 2006.

Stiegler P, Cunliffe A: The role of diet and exercise for the maintenance of fat-free mass and resting metabolic rate during weight loss, *Sports Med* 36:239, 2006.

Stunkard A, Lu XY: Rapid changes in night eating: considering mechanisms, *Eat Weight Disord* 15:e2, 2010.

Task Force on Childhood Obesity, Domestic Policy Council: Solving the Problem of Childhood Obesity Within a Generation—White House Task Force on Childhood Obesity —Report to the President, May, 2010.

Thomas S, et al: Bariatric surgery and the gut hormone response, *Nutr Clin Pract* 25:2, 2010.

Thompson DR, et al: Childhood overweight and cardiovascular disease risks: the National Heart, Lung and Blood Institute Growth and Health Study, *J Pediatr* 150:18, 2007.

Tremblay A, et al: Thermogenesis and weight loss in obese individuals: a primary association with organochlorine pollution, *Int J Obes Relat Metab Disord* 228:936, 2004.

Van Dam RM, et al: The relationship between overweight in adolescence and premature death in women, *Ann Intern Med* 145:91, 2006.

Van Ginnekin V, et al: Infectobesity: viral infections (especially with human adenovirus-36: Ad-36) may be a cause of obesity, *Med Hypotheses* 72:383, 2009.

Varady KA, et al: Degree of weight loss required to improve adipokine concentrations and decrease fat cell size in severely obese women, *Metabolism* 58:1096, 2009.

Wadden T, Sarwer DB: Behavioral assessment of candidates for bariatric surgery: a patient-oriented approach, *Surg Obes Relat Dis* 2:171, 2006.

Wilmore JH, et al: Body composition: a round table, *The Physician and Sportsmedicine* 14(3):144, 1986.

Wing RR, Phelan S: Long-term weight loss maintenance, *Am J Clin Nutr* 82:222S, 2005.

CHAPTER 23

Janet E. Schebendach, PhD, RD

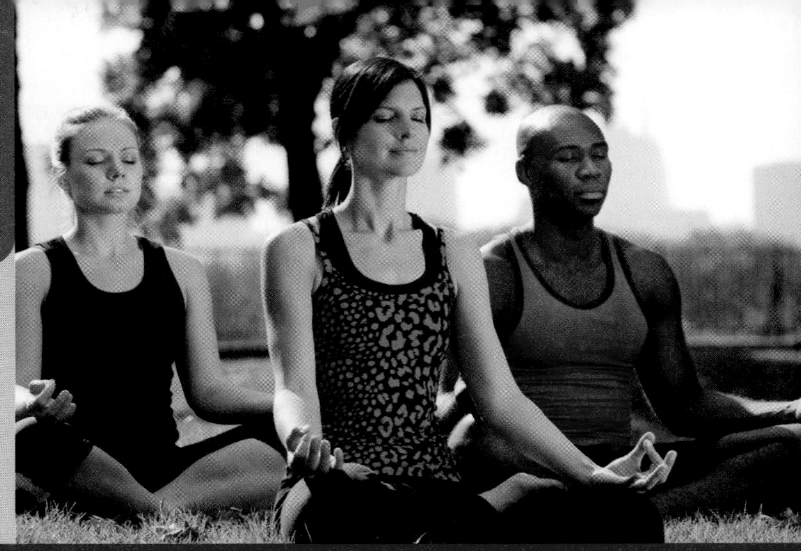

Nutrition in Eating Disorders

KEY TERMS
amenorrhea
anorexia nervosa (AN)
binge
binge eating disorder (BED)
body image distortion
bulimia nervosa (BN)
cognitive behavioral therapy (CBT)
Diagnostic and Statistical Manual of Mental Disorders, IV, TR (DSM-IV-TR)
eating disorder not otherwise specified (EDNOS)
hypercarotenemia
lanugo
low T3 syndrome
purging
Russell sign

Eating disorders (EDs) are debilitating psychiatric illnesses characterized by a persistent disturbance of eating habits or weight control behaviors that result in significantly impaired physical health and psychosocial functioning. American Psychiatric Association (APA) diagnostic criteria are available for anorexia nervosa (AN), bulimia nervosa (BN), eating disorder not otherwise specified (EDNOS), and binge eating disorder (BED). Childhood eating disturbances and the female athlete triad are also characterized by disordered eating and weight control behaviors (see Chapters 22 and 24).

DIAGNOSTIC CRITERIA

Diagnostic criteria for EDs have been established by the APA and are currently published in the **Diagnostic and Statistical Manual of Mental Disorders IV, TR (DSM-IV-TR)**; however, these criteria are currently under revision. For an update on the status of proposed revisions, the reader is referred to the following APA website: http://www.dsm5.org.

Anorexia Nervosa

A core clinical feature of **anorexia nervosa (AN)** is voluntary self-starvation resulting in emaciation. The reported lifetime prevalence of AN in women is 0.3% to 3.7%, depending on how strictly diagnostic criteria are defined (American Psychiatric Association [APA], 2006). Among men, lifetime prevalence has recently been estimated at 0.3% (Treasure et al., 2010). AN is more prevalent in Westernized, postindustrialized societies; however, more global distribution of EDs (Becker, 2004), including third world countries is expected. Genetic, biologic, and psychosocial factors contribute to the pathogenesis of this disorder (Treasure et al., 2010).

Initial presentation of AN typically occurs during adolescence or young adulthood; however, later onset (i.e., initial onset at age 25 or older) may develop in response to adverse life events. Incidence rates for AN among middle-age women (older than age 50) account for less than 1% of newly diagnosed AN patients (APA, 2006).

BOX 23-1

American Psychiatric Association (DSM-IV) Criteria

Anorexia Nervosa

A. Refusal to maintain body weight at or above a minimally normal weight for age and height (e.g., weight loss leading to maintenance of body weight less than 85% of that expected; or failure to make expected weight gain during period of growth, leading to body weight less than 85% of that expected)

B. Intense fear of gaining weight or becoming fat, even though underweight

C. Disturbance in the way in which one's body weight or shape is experienced, undue influence of body weight or shape on self-evaluation, or denial of the seriousness of the current low body weight

D. In postmenarcheal females, amenorrhea (i.e., the absence of at least three consecutive menstrual cycles)

1. Restricting type: During the current episode of AN, not regularly engaged in binge eating or purging behavior
2. Binge eating–purging type: During the current episode of AN, regularly engaged in binge eating and purging behavior

Bulimia Nervosa

A. Recurrent episodes of binge eating. An episode of binge eating is characterized by both of the following:

1. Eating, in a discrete period (e.g., within any 2-hour period), an amount of food that is definitely larger than most people would eat during a similar period of time and under similar circumstances
2. A sense of lack of control over eating during the episode (e.g., a feeling that one cannot stop eating or control what or how much one is eating)

B. Recurrent inappropriate compensatory behavior to prevent weight gain, such as self-induced vomiting; misuse of laxatives, diuretics, enemas, or other medications; fasting; or excessive exercise

C. Binge eating and inappropriate compensatory behaviors both occurring, on average, at least twice a week for 3 months

D. Self-evaluation unduly influenced by body shape and weight

E. Disturbance not exclusively occurring during episodes of AN

1. Purging type: During the current episode of BN, regularly engaged in self-induced vomiting or the misuse of laxatives, diuretics, or enemas
2. Nonpurging type: During the current episode of BN, use of other inappropriate compensatory behaviors such as fasting or excessive exercise but not regularly engaged in self-induced vomiting or the misuse of laxatives, diuretics, or enemas

Eating Disorder Not Otherwise Specified

EDNOS is for disorders of eating that do not meet criteria for any specific eating disorder. For example:

1. For females, all of the criteria for AN are met except that the individual has regular menses.
2. All of the criteria for AN are met except that, despite significant weight loss, the individual's current weight is in the normal range.
3. All of the criteria for BN are met except that the binge eating and inappropriate compensatory mechanisms occur at a frequency of less than twice a week or for a duration of less than 3 months.
4. An individual of normal body weight regularly uses inappropriate compensatory behavior after eating small amounts of food.
5. An individual repeatedly chews and spits out, but does not swallow, large amounts of food.

Binge Eating Disorder

A. Recurrent episodes of binge eating in the absence of the regular use of inappropriate compensatory behaviors characteristic of BN

B. Binge episodes occurring at least 2 days per week for a period of 6 months

From American Psychiatric Association: Diagnostic and statistical manual of mental disorders, *DSM-IV-TR*, ed 4, text revision, Washington, DC, 2000, American Psychiatric Association. Changes in these diagnostic criteria are expected in the 5th revision of the DSM.

AN, Anorexia nervosa, *BN*, bulimia nervosa, *EDNOS*, eating disorder not otherwise specified.

Criteria for the establishment of a diagnosis of AN were first published in 1972 by Feighner and associates. The APA first published criteria for the diagnosis of AN in 1980; however, it was not until 1987 that the APA recognized AN and BN as two separate and distinct clinical entities. See Box 23-1 for the current diagnostic criteria for AN.

The DSM-IV-TR defines AN "refusal to maintain a body weight at or above a minimally normal weight for age and height (e.g., body weight less than 85% of that expected)" (APA, 2000). The weight deficit may occur secondary to purposeful weight loss or manifest as failure to gain weight during periods of linear growth in children and adolescents. The DSM-5 is likely to eliminate the 85% cutoff point for body weight deficit.

Determination of "minimally normal weight" is problematic. Metropolitan Life Insurance Company weight standards are often used; however, recommended weight for height differs between the 1959 and 1983 tables. Dietitians often calculate desirable body weight using the Hamwi method.* This is not recommended in patients with an ED because it calculates a "normal" body weight much lower than other standards. Use of BMI has become increasingly accepted in the management of AN patients. Although a body mass index (BMI) of 19-25 kg/m^2 is considered normal for most healthy individuals, a BMI of 19-20 kg/m^2 represents a low-normal target body weight for AN patients (Royal College of Psychiatrists, 2005).

In children and adolescents, growth records should be obtained to determine if linear growth has deviated from premorbid height curves. If stunting has occurred, calculation of the weight deficit should be based on the premorbid height percentile. In 11- to 17-year-olds a normal body weight can be derived from the National Center for Health Statistics (NCHS) weight and height tables (see Appendixes 11 and 15).

BMI norms (see Appendixes 12 and 16) vary with age; therefore assessment of BMI in children and adolescents should be related to BMI percentiles (Royal College of Psychiatrists, 2005). Once again, if growth retardation is suspected, assessment of BMI should be based on expected rather than actual height. A BMI in the range of the 14th to 39th percentile can be used to assign an initial treatment goal weight, with adjustments made for prior weight, stage of pubertal development, and anticipated growth (Golden et al., 2008).

Patients with AN have **body image distortion**, causing them to feel fat despite their often cachectic state. Some individuals feel overweight all over, whereas others are overly concerned about the fatness of a specific body part such as the abdomen, buttocks, or thighs.

Amenorrhea, defined as the absence of at least three consecutive menstrual cycles in postmenarcheal women, is a problematic diagnostic criterion because some patients continue to menstruate regardless of a low body weight (Attia and Roberto, 2009); this criterion will most likely be eliminated from DSM-5 to be released soon. Development of AN during prepubescence may result in arrested sexual maturation and delayed menarche (primary amenorrhea). Young adolescent males with AN may have estrogen and testosterone deficiency and arrested growth and sexual development.

AN is categorized into two diagnostic subtypes: restricting and binge eating and purging. The restricting type is characterized by food restriction without binge eating or purging (self-induced vomiting or misuse of laxatives, enemas, or diuretics). Binge eating and purging is characterized by regular episodes of binge eating or purging behavior. Patients may initially present with the restricting subtype but migrate to the binge-and-purge subtype as the duration of their illness progresses.

*Hamwi Method for women: 100 lb for the first 5 feet of height plus 5 lb per inch for every inch over 5 feet plus 10% for a large frame and minus 10% for a small frame. For men: 106 lb for the first 5 feet of height plus 6 lb per inch for every inch over 5 feet plus 10% for a large frame and minus 10% for a small frame.

Psychological features associated with AN include perfectionism, compulsivity, harm avoidance, feelings of ineffectiveness, inflexible thinking, overly restrained emotional expression, and limited social spontaneity. Several psychiatric conditions may also coexist with AN, and these include depression, anxiety disorders, obsessive-compulsive disorder (OCD), personality disorders, and substance abuse.

Lifetime comorbid depression has been reported in 50% to 75% of AN patients; however, symptoms may remit during the course of nutrition rehabilitation and weight restoration. Because the rate of suicide is greater among individuals with AN than in the general population, ongoing psychiatric assessment is critical More than 40% of AN patients also have OCD. Onset of OCD frequently predates AN, and many patients remain symptomatic despite weight restoration (APA, 2006).

Crude mortality rates range from 0% to 8% across studies, with a cumulative mortality rate of 2.8% (Keel, 2010). Malnutrition, dehydration, and electrolyte abnormalities may precipitate death by inducing heart failure or fatal arrhythmias (McCallum et al., 2006). Overall, approximately 50% of deaths are attributed to medical complications directly related to AN (Steinhausen, 2002).

Bulimia Nervosa

Bulimia nervosa (BN) is a disorder characterized by recurrent episodes of binge eating followed by one or more inappropriate compensatory behaviors to prevent weight gain. These behaviors include self-induced vomiting, laxative misuse, diuretic misuse, compulsive exercise, or fasting. The lifetime prevalence of BN among young adult women in the United States is estimated to be 1% to 3%. The rate of occurrence in men is approximately one tenth that in women.

Unlike AN patients with binge-and-purge subtype, patients with BN are typically within the normal weight range. Like their AN counterparts, these individuals place considerable importance on body shape and size, and they are often frustrated by their inability to attain an underweight state.

It is commonly thought that vomiting is the predominant feature of BN; however, it is the binge eating behavior that is central to the diagnosis. A **binge** is consumption of an unusually large amount of food in a discrete period (usually approximately 2 hours). There is a sense of lack of control over the eating episode. Although the amount of food and caloric content of a binge vary, binges are often in the range of 1000 to 2000 calories (Fairburn and Harrison, 2003). Although BN patients typically binge on energy-dense foods like desserts and savory snacks, binges can also include lower-calorie foods like fruit and salad. Patients may report a binge episode when the amount of food consumed is clearly not excessive. Although these "subjective binges" may not support a diagnosis of BN, these individuals have feelings about their eating behavior that merit further exploration.

BN patients engage in compensatory behaviors intended to offset food binges. The choice of compensatory behaviors further classifies BN into purging and nonpurging subtypes. Patients with **purging** type BN regularly engage in self-induced vomiting or the misuse of laxatives, enemas, or diuretics. Those with nonpurging-type BN do not regularly engage in purging behaviors but rather fast or excessively exercise to compensate for their binge. To meet full DSM-IV-TR criteria for BN bingeing, both binge eating and recurrent inappropriate compensatory behaviors must occur, on average, at least twice a week for 3 months; the frequency at which these behaviors are required to occur are likely to decrease in the upcoming DSM-5. Current APA diagnostic criteria for BN are listed in Box 23-1.

Adverse emotional states such as labile mood, frustration, anxiety, and impulsivity are often found in patients with BN. Psychiatric comorbidities, including depression, anxiety disorders, personality disorders, substance abuse, and self-injurious behaviors, are also common in BN. Compared with AN, BN patients are usually embarrassed and distressed by their symptoms, making it easier to engage them in treatment.

Causal factors proposed for the development of BN include addictive, family, sociocultural, cognitive-behavioral, and psychodynamic models (APA, 2006). BN, with or without comorbid psychiatric illness, should be treated and monitored by a mental health professional.

Mortality rates for BN are lower than those for AN. Crude mortality rates range from 0% to 2% across studies, with a cumulative mortality rate of 0.4% (Keel and Brown, 2010).

Eating Disorder Not Otherwise Specified

Under DSM-IV, approximately half of the individuals with EDs fall into the **eating disorder not otherwise specified (EDNOS)** diagnostic group. Essentially these individuals meet most, but not all, of the criteria for AN or BN (e.g., a woman might meet all diagnostic criteria for AN except amenorrhea; a previously obese patient who, despite extreme weight loss, pathologic eating behavior, and amenorrhea fails to meet the AN criterion of body weight less than 85% of expected; a person who binges and purges, but with less frequency or for a shorter duration, than is specified for BN; or the individual who does not binge but vomits after eating a normal-size meal or snack). Clinically the EDNOS patient should receive treatment consistent with reasonable and customary care for either AN or BN. Inadequate treatment may lead to the development of full criteria AN or BN. In addition, patients who meet criteria for BED, a diagnostic group for research purposes only, are clinically diagnosed with EDNOS. See Box 23-1 for APA diagnostic criteria for EDNOS. Proposed revisions to the diagnostic criteria (DSM-V) are likely to result in a greater number of patients meeting criteria for AN and BN, and fewer meeting criteria for a subclinical ED (i.e., EDNOS).

Binge Eating Disorder

Research criteria for **binge eating disorder (BED)** are listed in Box 23-1. Binge eating, similar to that seen in BN, is characteristic of BED; however, there are no inappropriate compensatory behaviors after the binge. Binge episodes must occur at least 2 days per week for a period of 6 months.

Persons with BED experience a feeling of powerlessness over their eating, similar to that felt by BN patients. Significant emotional distress characterized by feelings of disgust, guilt, and depression occurs after a binge. Onset of BED generally occurs in late adolescence or in the early twenties, with women being 1.5 times more likely to develop this disorder than men.

Most patients with this disorder are overweight, with 15% to 50% prevalence among participants in weight-control programs. Patients with BED may have a higher lifetime prevalence of major depression, substance abuse, and personality disorders.

Eating Disorders in Childhood

Onset of EDs most typically occurs during adolescence and young adulthood. When an ED is suspected in a child or young teen, use of DSM criteria may be problematic because clinical presentation often differs from that seen in older adolescents and young adults. Complaints of nausea, abdominal pain, and difficulty in swallowing may coexist with concerns about weight, shape, and body fatness. Food avoidance, self-induced vomiting, and excessive exercise may occur, but laxative misuse is uncommon.

Any child or adolescent practicing unhealthy weight-control practices or thinking obsessively about food, body weight or shape, or exercise may be at risk for an ED. Other obsessive behaviors and depression may coexist in these children as well. Early-onset AN may result in delayed or stunted growth, osteopenia, and osteoporosis. AN has been reported in children as young as 7 years of age. The boy/girl ratio may be higher in this younger age group, and it appears in many different cultures and ethnic groups. BN in children is rare (APA, 2006).

The relationship between problematic childhood eating behaviors and subsequent development of EDs in later life is of concern. A longitudinal study of 800 children found that eating conflicts, food struggles, and unpleasant meals were risk factors for the later development of an ED (Kotler et al., 2001).

Childhood eating disturbances described by Bryant-Waugh (2007) include AN and, rarely, BN, as well as food avoidance emotional disorder, selective eating, restrictive eating, food refusal, functional dysphagia, and pervasive refusal syndrome (Table 23-1). Changes in the diagnostic criteria for childhood EDs have also been proposed for DSM-5 and are being developed (Bryant-Waugh et al., 2010).

TREATMENT APPROACH

Treatment of EDs requires a multidisciplinary approach that includes psychiatric, psychological, medical, and nutrition interventions. Treatment, provided at several levels of care depending on severity of illness, includes inpatient hospitalization, residential treatment, day hospitalization, intensive outpatient treatment, and outpatient treatment.

TABLE 23-1

Eating Disorders in Children Aged 8 to 14 Years

Eating Disturbance	Characteristics
Anorexia nervosa	Determined weight loss (e.g. through food avoidance, self-induced vomiting, excessive exercising, abuse of laxatives) Abnormal cognitions regarding weight and/or shape Morbid preoccupation with weight and/or shape, food, and/or eating
Bulimia nervosa	Recurrent binges and purges and/or food restriction Sense of lack of control Abnormal cognitions regarding weight and/or shape

From Bryant-Waugh R, and Lask, R: Overview of the eating disorders. In Lask B, Bryant-Waugh R, editors: Eating disorders in childhood and adolescence, 3rd Ed., East Sussex, UK, 2007, Routledge.

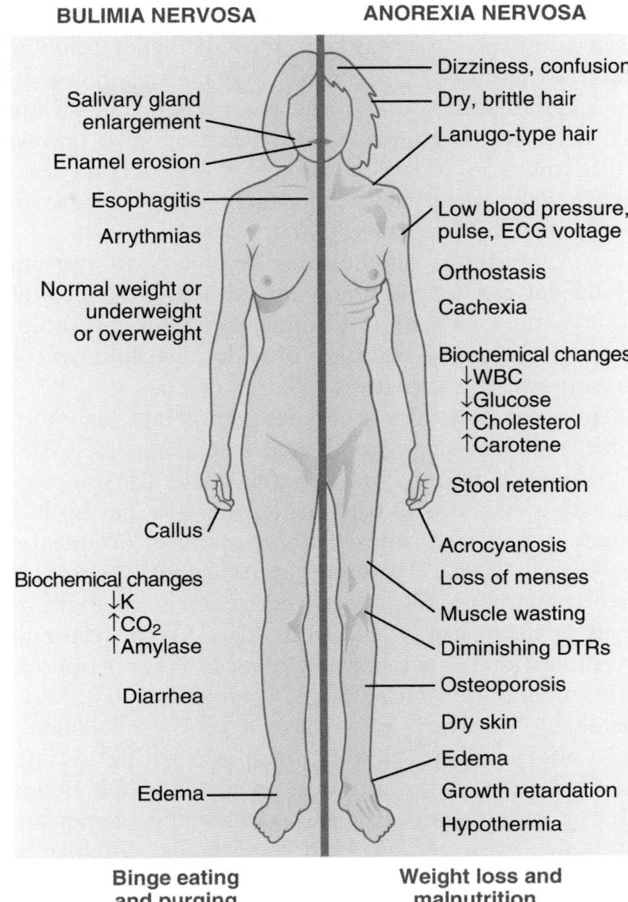

FIGURE 23-1 Physical and clinical signs and symptoms of bulimia nervosa and anorexia nervosa. *DTRs*, Deep tendon reflexes; *ECG*, electrocardiogram; *WBC*, white blood cell.

Inpatient treatment can be provided on a psychiatric or medical unit; a behavioral protocol developed specifically for the management of eating-disordered patients is highly recommended. Residential treatment programs also provide 24-hour care, but they are not usually equipped to handle the medically or psychiatrically unstable patient. Day hospital programs are also available. In this setting, patients initially receive 6 to 8 hours of specialized multidisciplinary treatment for 5 to 7 days per week. As treatment progresses, required attendance tapers off. The least intensive form of treatment is outpatient care; however, this still requires the ongoing, coordinated effort of physicians, psychotherapists, and nutritionists. Intensive outpatient treatment programs are also available. In this setting, patients receive several hours of multidisciplinary care each week. This may be scheduled in the late afternoon or early evening so the patient can attend after school or work.

The *Practice Guideline for the Treatment of Patients with Eating Disorders* (APA, 2006) provides comprehensive guidelines for the formulation and implementation of treatment plans in patients with AN, BN, EDNOS, and BED. These guidelines provide specific treatment recommendations (e.g., nutritional rehabilitation, medical management, psychological interventions, medication management) and level-of-care guidelines for patients with EDs. In addition, the Society for Adolescent Medicine (SAM, 2003), the American Academy of Pediatrics (2003), Committee on Adolescence (Rosen et al., 2010) and the American Dietetic Association (ADA, 2006) have published policy statements and positions regarding guidelines for effective treatment of EDs.

CLINICAL CHARACTERISTICS AND MEDICAL COMPLICATIONS

Although EDs are classified as psychiatric illnesses, they are associated with significant medical complications, morbidity, and mortality. Numerous physiologic changes result from the weight-control habits of patients with AN and BN. Some are minor changes that occur secondary to reduced energy intake, some are pathologic alterations that may have long-term consequences, and a few represent potentially life-threatening conditions.

Anorexia Nervosa

Patients with AN have a typical and distinctive appearance (Figure 23-1). Their cachectic and prepubescent body habitus often makes them look younger than their age. Common physical findings include **lanugo**, soft, downy hair growth, dry and brittle hair, hypercarotenemia, cold intolerance, and cyanosis of the extremities.

Protein-energy malnutrition with resultant loss of lean body mass is associated with reduced left ventricular mass and systolic dysfunction in AN. Cardiovascular complications include bradycardia, orthostatic hypotension, and cardiac arrhythmias. Protein-calorie malnutrition and deficiencies of thiamin, phosphorus, magnesium, and selenium have been associated with heart failure in AN; however, cardiac function is largely reversible with correction of dietary deficiencies and adequate weight restoration (Birmingham and Gritzner, 2007).

Gastrointestinal complications secondary to starvation include delayed gastric emptying, decreased small bowel motility, and constipation. Complaints of abdominal bloating and a prolonged sensation of abdominal fullness complicate the refeeding process.

Significant bone loss occurs frequently and early in the course of illness among both males and females, with an estimated 92% having bone mineral density (BMD) consistent with a diagnosis of osteopenia, and 40% having BMD consistent with a diagnosis of osteoporosis (Mehler and MacKenzie, 2009). Hormone replacement therapy and treatment with bisphosphonates have been found to be ineffective or inadequately studied in AN. Weight restoration is recommended as the first line of treatment for improved BMD in adolescent girls with AN (Golden, 2005). Unfortunately, AN patients often have a protracted course of illness associated with frequent relapse resulting in weight loss. Under these circumstances, reversibility of bone mineralization may be difficult and some studies demonstrate that bone density is not fully recoverable (Mehler and MacKenzie, 2009).

Children and adolescents with AN develop unique medical complications that affect normal growth and development such as growth retardation, reduction in peak bone mass, and structural abnormalities in the brain (SAM, 2003).

Bulimia Nervosa

Clinical signs and symptoms of BN are more difficult to detect because patients are usually of normal weight and secretive in behavior. When vomiting occurs, there may be clinical evidence such as (1) scarring of the dorsum of the hand used to stimulate the gag reflex, known as **Russell sign**; (2) parotid gland enlargement; and (3) erosion of dental enamel with increased dental caries resulting from the frequent presence of gastric acid in the mouth.

Chronic vomiting can result in dehydration, alkalosis, and hypokalemia. Common clinical manifestations include sore throat, esophagitis, mild hematemesis (vomiting of blood), abdominal pain, and subconjunctival hemorrhage. More serious gastrointestinal complications include Mallory-Weiss esophageal tears, rare occurrence of esophageal rupture, and acute gastric dilation or rupture. Ipecac, used to induce vomiting, may cause irreversible myocardial damage and sudden death.

Laxative abuse may lead to dehydration, elevation of serum aldosterone and vasopressin levels, rectal bleeding, intestinal atony, and abdominal cramps. Diuretic abuse may lead to dehydration and hypokalemia. Cardiac arrhythmias can occur secondary to electrolyte and acid-base imbalance caused by vomiting, laxative, and diuretic abuse. Although the profound amenorrhea associated with AN is uncommon in BN, menstrual irregularities may occur (see Figure 23-1).

PSYCHOLOGICAL MANAGEMENT

EDs are complex psychiatric illnesses that require psychological assessment and ongoing treatment. Evaluation of the patient's cognitive and psychological stage of development, family history, family dynamics, and psychopathologic condition is essential for the development of a comprehensive psychosocial treatment program.

The long-term goals of psychosocial interventions in AN are (1) to help patients understand and cooperate with their nutritional and physical rehabilitation, (2) to help patients understand and change behaviors and dysfunctional attitudes related to their EDs, (3) to improve interpersonal and social functioning, and (4) to address psychopathologic and psychological conflicts that reinforce or maintain eating-disordered behaviors.

In the acute stage of illness, malnourished AN patients are typically negativistic and obsessional, making it difficult to conduct formal psychotherapy. At this stage of treatment, psychological management is often focused on positive behavioral reinforcement of weight restoration. This includes praise for positive efforts, reassurance, coaching, and encouragement. Inpatient behavioral management typically uses reinforcers that link attainment of privileges such as physical activity (versus bed rest), off-unit passes, and visitation privileges with attainment of targeted weight gain and improved eating behaviors.

Once acute malnutrition has been corrected and weight restoration is underway, the AN patient is more likely to benefit from psychotherapy. Psychotherapy can help the patient understand and change core dysfunctional thoughts, attitudes, motives, conflicts, and feelings related to his or her ED. Associated psychiatric conditions, including deficits in mood, impulse control, and self-esteem, as well as relapse prevention, should be addressed in the psychotherapeutic treatment plan. Several years of ongoing psychotherapy may be necessary for recovery.

Cognitive behavioral therapy (CBT) is a highly effective intervention for treatment of the acute symptoms of BN (Fairburn, 2008). Nevertheless, clinicians may combine elements of several types of psychotherapy during treatment. In some cases, adjunctive family and marital therapy may also be beneficial.

Several validated psychological instruments and questionnaires are available for the assessment of patients with EDs self-report measures may be used for screening purposes, whereas structured interviews are often used to confirm the diagnosis. Representative instruments include the Eating Attitudes Test, Eating Disorder Inventory, Eating Disorder Examination, Eating Disorders Questionnaire, and the Yale-Brown-Cornell Eating Disorder Scale (APA, 2006).

NUTRITION REHABILITATION AND COUNSELING

Nutrition rehabilitation includes nutrition assessment, medical nutrition therapy (MNT), nutrition counseling, and nutrition education. Although the EDs are distinct illnesses, similarities exist in nutritional consequences and nutritional management.

Nutrition Assessment

Nutrition assessment routinely includes a diet history and the assessment of biochemical, metabolic, and anthropometric indices of nutrition status.

Diet History

Guidelines should include assessment of energy intake, macronutrient, micronutrient, and fluid consumption, as well as eating attitudes, and eating behaviors (see Chapter 4).

Anorexia Nervosa

Patients with restricting subtype AN generally consume less than 1000 kcal/day. Assessment of typical energy intake prevents overfeeding or underfeeding at the inception of nutritional rehabilitation and opens a dialogue regarding caloric requirements during the refeeding and weight-maintenance phases of nutritional rehabilitation. Inadequate energy intake results in decreased consumption of carbohydrate, protein, and fat. Patients with AN were historically described as *carbohydrate restrictors*, but at present there is a tendency to avoid fat-containing foods. Observed food intake in 30 patients revealed that patients with AN consumed significantly less fat (15% to 20% of calories) than healthy controls. Percent of calories contributed by protein may be in the average to above-average range, but the adequacy of intake is relative to total caloric consumption. For example, the percentage of calories may remain the same, but as the calorie intake continues to drop, the actual amount of protein falls also. Patients with binge-purge subtype AN have more chaotic diet patterns, and energy consumption should be assessed across the spectrum of restriction and binge eating (Burd et al., 2009).

Vegetarianism is common among AN patients. The nutritionist should determine if adoption of the vegetarian diet predated the development of AN. A vegetarian diet adopted during the course of AN is a covert means of limiting food choice that may justifiably be considered as part of the psychopathologic findings of the disorder (Royal College of Psychiatrists, 2005). Many treatment programs prohibit vegetarian diets during the weight restoration phase of treatment; others allow it. The relationship of social, cultural, and family influences, as well as religious beliefs relative to the patient's vegetarian status must also be explored. If an AN patient is permitted to follow a vegan or vegetarian diet during weight restoration, care must be taken to provide adequate phosphate for prevention of hypophosphatemia, particularly during the initial stage of refeeding (Royal College of Psychiatrists, 2005).

Inadequate caloric intake, limited variety in the diet, and poor food group representation result in inadequate vitamin and mineral consumption in AN. In general, micronutrient intake parallels macronutrient intake; thus AN patients who consistently restrict dietary fat are at greater risk for inadequate essential fatty acid intake and fat-soluble vitamin intake. Based on a 30-day diet history, Hadigan and colleagues (2000) found that more than 50% of 30 AN patients failed to meet dietary reference intake requirements for vitamin D, calcium, folate, vitamin B_{12}, magnesium, copper, and zinc.

When obtaining a diet history, typical fluid intake should also be determined because abnormalities in fluid balance are prevalent in this population. Some patients severely restrict intake because they are intolerant of feeling full after fluid ingestion, whereas others drink excessive amounts, attempting to stave off hunger. Extremes in fluid restriction or ingestion may require monitoring of urine specific gravity and serum electrolytes.

Many AN patients consume excessive amounts of artificial sweeteners and artificially sweetened beverages (Marino et al., 2009). Use of these products should be addressed during the course of nutrition rehabilitation.

Bulimia Nervosa

Chaotic eating, ranging from restriction to normal eating to binge eating, is a hallmark feature of bulimia nervosa Energy intake in BN can be unpredictable. The caloric content of a binge, the degree of caloric absorption after a purge, and the extent of calorie restriction between binge episodes make assessment of total energy intake challenging. Bulimic patients assume that vomiting is an efficient mechanism for eliminating calories consumed during binge episodes; however, this is a common misconception. In a study of the caloric content of foods ingested and purged in a feeding laboratory, it was determined that, as a group, BN subjects consumed a mean of 2131 kcal during a binge and vomited only 979 kcal afterward (Kaye et al., 1993). As a rule of thumb, patients should be advised that approximately 50% of energy consumed during a binge is retained.

Because of day-to-day variability, a 24-hour recall is not a particularly useful assessment tool. To assess energy intake, it is helpful to estimate daily food consumption over the course of a week. First determine the number of non-binge days (which may include restrictive and normal intake days) and approximate their caloric content; then determine the number of binge days and approximate caloric content, and deduct 50% of the caloric content of binges that are purged (vomited); finally, average the caloric intake over the 7-day period. Determination of this average energy intake, as well as the range of intake, will be useful information for the counseling process.

Nutrient intake in patients with BN varies with the cycle of binge eating and restriction, and it is likely that overall diet quality and micronutrient intake is inadequate. A 14-day dietary intake study of 50 BN patients revealed that at least

BOX 23-2

Assessment of Eating Attitudes, Behaviors, and Habits

1. Eating attitudes
   A. Food aversions
   B. Safe, risky, forbidden foods
   C. Magical thinking
   D. Binge trigger foods
   E. Ideas on appropriate amounts of food
2. Eating behaviors
   A. Ritualistic behaviors
   B. Unusual food combinations
   C. Atypical seasoning of food
   D. Excessive and atypical use of non-caloric sweeteners
   E. Atypical use of eating utensils
3. Eating habits
   A. Intake pattern
      (1) Number of meals and snacks
      (2) Time of day
      (3) Duration of meals and snacks
      (4) Eating environment—where and with whom
      (5) How consumed—sitting or standing
   B. Avoidance of specific food groups, particularly those with higher energy density
   C. Evidence of diet variety
   D. Fluid intake—restricted or excessive

Adapted from: Schebendach J, Nussbaum M: Nutrition management in adolescents with eating disorders, Adolesc Med: State of the Art Rev 3(3):545, 1992.

50% of participants consumed less than two thirds of the recommended dietary allowance (RDA) for calcium, iron, and zinc on nonbinge days. Furthermore, 25% of participants still had inadequate intakes of zinc and iron when overall intake (i.e., binge and non-binge days) was assessed (Gendall, 1997). It is important to note that even when the diet appears adequate, nutrient loss will occur secondary to purging, thus making it difficult to assess true adequacy of nutrient intake. Use of vitamin and mineral supplements should also be determined but, once again, retention after purging must be considered.

Eating Behavior

Characteristic attitudes, behaviors, and eating habits seen in AN and BN are shown in Box 23-2. Food aversions, common in this population, include red meat, baked goods, desserts, full-fat dairy products, added fats, fried foods, and caloric beverages. Patients with EDs often regard specific foods or groups of foods as absolutely "good" or absolutely "bad." Irrational beliefs and dichotomous thinking about food choices should be identified and challenged throughout the treatment process.

In the assessment it is important to determine unusual or ritualistic behaviors, which may include ingestion of food in an atypical manner or with nontraditional utensils; unusual food combinations; or the excessive use of spices, vinegar, lemon juice, and artificial sweeteners. Meal spacing and length of time allocated for a meal should also be determined. Many patients save their self-allotted food ration until late in the day; others are fearful of eating past a certain time of day.

Many AN patients eat in an excessively slow manner, often playing with their food and cutting it into small pieces. This is sometimes regarded as a tactic to avoid food intake, but it may also be an effect of starvation (Keys et al., 1950). Time limits for meal and snack consumption are frequently incorporated into behavioral treatment plans.

Many BN patients eat quickly, reflecting their difficulties with satiety cues. In addition, BN patients may identify foods they fear will trigger a binge episode. The patient may have an all-or-nothing approach to "trigger" foods. Although the patient may prefer avoidance, assistance with reintroduction of controlled amounts of these foods at regular times and intervals is helpful.

Biochemical Assessment

The marked cachexia of AN may lead one to expect biochemical indices of malnutrition (see Chapter 8), but this is rarely the case. Compensatory mechanisms are remarkable, and laboratory abnormalities may not be observed until the illness is far advanced.

Significant alterations in visceral protein status are uncommon in AN. Indeed, adaptive phenomena that occur in chronic starvation are aimed at the maintenance of visceral protein metabolism at the expense of the somatic compartment. Serum albumin levels are generally within normal limits, but may be masked by dehydration in early treatment (Swenne, 2004).

Despite consumption of a typically low-fat, low-cholesterol diet, a high total cholesterol level is commonly found in malnourished AN patients (Rigaud et al., 2009). Despite hyperlipidemia, a fat- and cholesterol-restricted diet is not warranted during nutritional rehabilitation. If hyperlipidemia predated the development of AN, or if a strong family history of hyperlipidemia is identified, the patient should be reassessed after weight restoration and a period of weight stabilization.

Patients with BN may also have abnormal lipid levels. Patients with BN are prone to eating low-fat, low-energy foods during the restriction phase and high-fat, high-sugar foods during binge episodes. Premature prescription of a low-fat, low-cholesterol diet may only reinforce this dichotomous approach to eating. Care must be taken to balance extremes in the types and amounts of foods consumed. An accurate lipid profile can be obtained only after a period of dietary stabilization. Patients with BN may also have difficulty complying with the fast required for an accurate lipid profile.

Low serum glucose results from a deficit of precursors needed for gluconeogenesis and glucose production.

Thyroid hormone production tends to be normal, but the peripheral deiodination of thyroxine favors formation of the less metabolically active reduced triiodothyronine (rT3) rather than triiodothyronine (T3) resulting in **low T3 syndrome** (Figure 32-2). This metabolic state is characteristic of AN and typically resolves with weight restoration. Thyroid hormone replacement is not recommended (APA, 2006).

Vitamin and Mineral Deficiencies

Hypercarotenemia is a common finding in AN, attributed to mobilization of lipid stores, catabolic changes caused by weight loss, and metabolic stress. Excessive dietary intake of carotenoids is less common. Normalization of serum carotene occurs during the course of nutrition rehabilitation.

Despite obviously deficient diets, reports of clinical and biochemical findings of true deficiency diseases are uncommon. The decreased need for micronutrients in a catabolic state, use of vitamin supplements, and selection of micronutrient-rich foods may be protective. Documented cases of riboflavin, vitamin B_6, thiamin, niacin, folate, and vitamin E deficiencies have been reported in lower-weight and more chronically ill patients with AN (Altinyazar et al., 2009; Castro, 2004; Jagielska et al., 2007; Prousky, 2003). Patients avoiding animal foods may also be at risk for B_{12} deficiency (Royal College of Psychiatrists, 2005).

Iron requirements in AN are decreased secondary to amenorrhea and the overall catabolic state. At treatment onset, the hemoglobin level may be falsely elevated as a result of dehydration resulting in hemoconcentration. Malnourished patients may also have fluid retention, and associated hemodilution may falsely lower the hemoglobin level. In severely malnourished AN patients, iron use may be blocked. Loss of lean tissue results in decreased red blood cell mass. Iron released from red cell mass is bound to ferritin and stored. Saturated ferritin-bound iron stores increase the risk of unbound iron that may result in cell damage, and use of iron supplements should be avoided at this phase of treatment (Royal College of Psychiatrists, 2005). During nutrition rehabilitation and weight restoration, ferritin-bound iron is taken out of storage; this is generally adequate to meet the need for cellular repair and increased red blood cell mass. Patients should, however, be periodically reassessed for depletion of their reserve and the possible need for supplemental iron later in treatment. Hutter and colleagues (2009) presents a comprehensive review of hematological changes that occur in AN.

Zinc deficiency may occur secondary to inadequate energy intake, avoidance of red meat, and the adoption of vegetarian food choices. Although zinc deficiency may be associated with altered taste perception and weight loss, there is no evidence that deficiency causes or perpetuates symptoms of AN. Although supplemental zinc is purported to enhance food intake and weight gain in AN patients, there is poor evidence to support this claim (Lock and Fitzpatrick, 2009).

Although the high prevalence of osteopenia and osteoporosis in AN is largely due to hormone imbalance and weight loss, concurrent dietary deficiencies of calcium, magnesium, and vitamin D likely contribute to the overall pathogenesis. Dual x-ray absorptiometry to determine the degree of impaired bone mineralization is recommended (see Chapter 25).

Fluid and Electrolyte Balance

Vomiting and laxative and diuretic use can result in significant fluid and electrolyte imbalances in patients with EDs. Laxative use may result in hypokalemia, and diuretic use can also cause hypokalemia and dehydration. Vomiting may result in dehydration, hypokalemia, and alkalosis with hypochloremia. Hyponatremia is another serious complication, but is seen less frequently.

Urine concentration is decreased, and urine output is increased in semistarvation. Edema may occur in response to malnutrition and refeeding. Depletion of glycogen and lean tissue is accompanied by obligatory water loss that reflects characteristic hydration ratios. For example, the obligatory water loss associated with glycogen depletion may be in the range of 600-800 mL. Varying degrees of fluid intake, ranging from restricted to excessive, may affect electrolyte values in AN patients (see Chapter 7).

Energy Expenditure

Resting energy expenditure (REE) is characteristically low in malnourished AN patients (de Zwaan et al., 2002). Weight loss, decreased lean body mass, energy restriction, and decreased leptin levels have been implicated in the pathogenesis of this hypometabolic state. Refeeding increases and normalizes REE in AN patients. An exaggerated diet-induced thermogenesis (DIT) has also been reported in AN during the course of refeeding (de Zwann et al., 2002). This may pose metabolic resistance to weight gain during the course of nutritional rehabilitation in patients with AN (see Chapter 2).

Patients with BN can have unpredictable metabolic rates. Dietary restraint between episodes of binge eating may place bulimic patients in a state of semistarvation (resulting in a hypometabolic rate). However, binge eating followed by purging can increase the metabolic rate secondary to a preabsorptive release of insulin, which activates the sympathetic nervous system (de Zwann et al., 2002).

Baseline and follow-up assessment of REE may be clinically useful throughout the course of nutritional rehabilitation (Dragani et al., 2006; Schebendach, 2003); however, access to standard indirect calorimetry is typically limited to research settings. Although portable, handheld devices like the MedGem have been increasingly popular in the general population, a recent study of AN patients found poor agreement between MedGem and a standard indirect calorimeter measurements of REE (Hlynsky et al., 2005).

Anthropometric Assessment

Patients with AN have protein-energy malnutrition characterized by significantly depleted adipose and somatic protein stores, but a relatively intact visceral protein compartment. These patients meet the criteria for a diagnosis of severe protein-energy malnutrition. A goal of nutritional rehabilitation is restoration of body fat and fat-free mass. Although these compartments do regenerate, the extent and rate vary.

Percent body fat can be estimated from the sum of four skinfold measurements (triceps, biceps, subscapular, and suprailiac crest) (see Figures 6-4, 6-5, and 6-6) using the calculations of Durnin and colleagues (Durnin and Rahaman, 1967; Durnin and Womersley, 1974) (see Appendix 24). This method has been validated against underwater weighing to assess percentage of body fat in adolescent girls with AN (Probst, 2001). A more accurate measurement of percentage of body fat can be obtained from underwater weighing or from a dual-energy x-ray absorptiometry (DEXA) scan (see Figure 6-10) equipped with body composition software; however, these methods are not generally available in an office or clinic setting (see Chapter 6 on Physical Assessment).

Bioelectrical impedance analysis (BIA) is more readily available, but shifts in intracellular and extracellular fluid compartments in patients with severe EDs may affect the accuracy of body fat measurement. To improve the validity of BIA measurement in AN patients (see Figure 6-9), the measurement should be done in the morning before ingestion of all food and liquid, using a reclining chair that is always reclined to the same position to prevent differential pooling of fluids (Sunday and Halmi, 2003). A comparison of body composition measurements assessed by several impedance methods, as well as DEXA, has been reported in AN patients and healthy controls (Moreno et al., 2008).

For practical purposes the midarm muscle circumference, derived from midarm circumference and triceps skinfold measurements (see Figure 6-7), can be easily obtained and compared with sex- and age-matched population standards (see Appendixes 25 and 26). Baseline and follow-up measurements can be easily obtained during nutritional rehabilitation.

Body weight is assessed and routinely monitored in patients with EDs. In AN weight gain is necessary. In BN the short-term goal should be weight maintenance. Although weight loss may be warranted, this cannot be addressed until chaotic eating patterns are stabilized.

Rate of weight gain in AN may be affected by hydration status, glycogen stores, metabolic factors, and changes in body composition (Box 23-3). Rehydration and replenished glycogen stores contribute to weight gain during the first few days of refeeding. Thereafter weight gain results from increased lean and fat stores. It is generalized that one needs to increase or decrease caloric intake by 3500 kcal to cause a 1-lb change in body weight, but the true energy cost depends on the type of tissue gained. More energy is required to gain fat versus lean tissue, but weight gain may be a mix of fat and lean tissue.

In adult women with AN, short-term weight restoration has been associated with a significant increase in truncal fat with central adiposity (Grinspoon, 2001; Mayer, 2005; Mayer et al., 2009); however, this abnormal distribution appears to normalize within 1 year of weight maintenance (Mayer et al., 2009). In adolescent girls with AN, short-term weight restoration is associated with normalization of body fat without increased central adiposity (de Alvaro et al., 2007; Misra, 2003).

BOX 23-3

Factors Affecting Rate of Weight Gain in Anorexia Nervosa

1. Fluid balance
   - A. Polyuria seen in semistarvation
   - B. Edema
     - (1) Starvation
     - (2) Refeeding
   - C. Hydration ratios in tissues
     - (1) Glycogen: 3-4:1
     - (2) Protein: 3-4:1
2. Metabolic rate
   - A. Resting energy expenditure
   - B. Postprandial energy expenditure
   - C. Respiratory quotient
3. Energy cost of tissue gained
   - A. Adipose tissue
   - B. Lean body mass
4. Previous obesity
5. Physical activity

Adapted from Schebendach J, Nussbaum M: Nutrition management in adolescents with eating disorders, Adolesc Med: State of the Art Rev 3(3):545, 1992.

The anthropometric status of patients with EDs should be assessed and monitored regularly (see Chapter 6). The patient's goal weight can be determined by various methods, none of which is perfect. The height, weight, and BMI percentile tables of the NCHS should be used to assess boys and girls up to 20 years of age (see Appendixes 11 and 12 and 15 and 16). A bone age can be obtained in adolescents with stunted height to determine catch-up growth potential.

If a patient is hospitalized, a daily preprandial, early-morning weight should be obtained. On an outpatient basis a gowned weight should be obtained on the same scale, at approximately the same time of day, at least once a week in early treatment. Before weigh-in the patient should void, and urine specific gravity should be checked for dehydration or fluid loading. If the patient claims to be unable to provide a urine specimen, the physician should examine the patient to see whether the bladder is full. Patients may resort to deceptive tactics (water loading, hiding heavy objects on their person, and withholding urine and bowel movements) to make a mandated weight goal.

MEDICAL NUTRITION THERAPY AND COUNSELING

Treatment of an ED may begin at one of four levels of care: outpatient, intensive outpatient, day treatment, inpatient. The registered dietitian (RD) is an essential part of the treatment team at all levels of care.

In AN the chosen level of care is determined by the severity of malnutrition, degree of medical and psychiatric instability, duration of illness, and growth failure. In some instances, treatment begins on an inpatient unit but is stepped down to a less intensive level of care as weight restoration progresses. In other instances, treatment begins on an outpatient basis; however, if the rate of weight gain is inadequate, care is stepped up to a more intensive level.

In BN treatment typically begins and continues on an outpatient basis. On occasion a BN patient may be directly admitted to an intensive outpatient or day treatment program. However, inpatient hospitalization is relatively uncommon and generally is of short duration and for the specific purpose of fluid and electrolyte stabilization.

Anorexia Nervosa

Guidelines for MNT in AN are summarized in Box 23-4. Goals for nutrition rehabilitation include restoration of body weight and normalization of eating patterns and behaviors. Although MNT is an essential component of treatment, guidelines are largely based on clinical experience rather than scientific evidence.

Weight restoration is essential for recovery. The medically unstable, severely malnourished, or growth-retarded patient typically requires supervised weight gain in a specialized hospital unit or residential ED treatment program. In these settings, the energy prescription and desired rate of weight gain are usually determined by the medical doctor or the treatment team. Treatment programs often have three phases to the weight restoration process: weight stabilization and prevention of further weight loss, weight gain, and weight maintenance. Although the duration of these phases vary, the weight restoration process is typically the longest and is obviously influenced by patient's state of malnutrition.

Treatment plans typically include a targeted rate of expected rate of weight gain. Gains of 2 to 3 lb/week for the hospitalized patient and 0.5 to 1 lb/week for the outpatient are reasonable and attainable goals. Although the initial calorie prescription may be in the range of 1000 to 1600 kcal/day (30 to 40 kcal/kg of body weight per day), progressive increases in energy intake will be needed to promote a consistent and targeted rate of weight gain. To accomplish this, the caloric prescription is often increased in 100 to 200 calorie increments every 2 to 3 days. In some treatment programs, however, the prescription is increased in larger increments (e.g., in 500-calorie increments) (Yager and Andersen, 2005).

Aggressive refeeding of severely malnourished AN patients (i.e., those weighing less than 70% standard body weight) may precipitate life-threatening complications of the refeeding syndrome during the first week of oral, nasogastric, or intravenous refeeding. Manifestations of the syndrome are fluid and electrolyte imbalance; cardiac, neurologic, and hematologic complications; and sudden death. High-risk patients need to be carefully monitored with daily measurements of serum phosphorus, magnesium,

BOX 23-4

Guidelines for Medical Nutrition Therapy of Anorexia Nervosa

1. Caloric prescription:
- **A.** Initial weight gain
  - **(1)** Initial prescription: 30 to 40 kcal/kg/day (approximately 1000 to 1600 kcal/day)
  - **(2)** Assess risk for refeeding syndrome
- **B.** Controlled weight gain phase
  - **(1)** Increase calories in small, progressive increments (i.e., 100 kcal) to promote expected rate of controlled weight gain (e.g., 2-3 lb/week for inpatients, 0.5 to 1 lb/week for outpatients)
  - **(2)** Late treatment: 70 to 100 kcal/kg/day
Females: 3000 to 4000 kcal/day
Males: 4000 to 4500 kcal/day
  - **(3)** If patient requires a higher kcal prescription, evaluate for vomiting, discarding food, increased exercise, increased resting energy expenditure and/or induced thermogenesis
- **C.** Weight maintenance phase
  - **(1)** Adults: 40 to 60 kcal/kg/day
  - **(2)** Ongoing growth and development in children and adolescents: 40-60 kcal/kg/day

2. Macronutrients
- **A.** Protein
  - **(1)** Minimum intake = RDA in g/kg ideal body weight
  - **(2)** 15% to 20% kcal
  - **(3)** High biologic value sources
- **B.** Carbohydrate
  - **(1)** 50% to 55% kcal
  - **(2)** Provide sources of insoluble fiber for treatment of constipation
- **C.** Fat
  - **(1)** 30% kcal, including sources of essential fatty acids
  - **(2)** Encourage small increases in fat intake until goal can be attained

3. Micronutrients
- **A.** 100% RDA multivitamin with minerals supplement with the exception of iron
- **B.** Avoid supplemental iron during initial phase of weight restoration; reassess need during late treatment
- **C.** Determine need for supplemental thiamin during course of weight restoration

Adapted from: Luder E, Schebendach J: Nutrition management of eating disorders, Top Clin Nutr 8:48, 1993.

RDA, Recommended dietary allowance.

potassium, and calcium for the first 5 days of refeeding and every other day for several weeks thereafter. Supplemental phosphorus, magnesium, and potassium may be given orally or intravenously. Children and adolescents with AN may be at increased risk for refeeding syndrome and care must be taken not to over-prescribe calories in this age group (O'Connor and Goldin, 2010) (see Chapter 14).

Caloric prescriptions in the range of 3000 to 4000 kcal/day (70 to 100 kcal/kg of body weight per day) may ultimately be needed later in the course of weight restoration, and male AN patients may require even more—4000 to 4500 kcal/day (APA, 2006). Changes in REE, DIT, and the type of tissue gained are all factors. In addition, the energy cost of physical activity must be considered because many AN patients expend significant amounts of energy in physical activity or fidgeting behavior (de Zwann et al., 2002).

Patients who require extraordinarily high energy intakes should be questioned or observed for discarding of food, vomiting, exercising, and excessive physical activity, including fidgeting. After the goal weight is attained, the caloric prescription may be slowly decreased to promote weight maintenance. However, caloric prescriptions may remain at higher levels in adolescents with the potential for continued growth and development.

AN patients receiving care in less structured treatment settings such as outpatient treatment programs may be particularly resistant to formalized meal plans. A practical approach may be the addition of 200 to 300 calories per day to the patient's typical (baseline) energy intake. However, the nutritionist must carefully query and assess intake as these patients may overestimate their food and energy consumption.

Once the caloric prescription is calculated, a reasonable distribution of macronutrients must be determined. Patients may express multiple food aversions. Extreme avoidance of dietary fat is common, but continued omission will make it difficult to provide concentrated sources of energy needed for weight restoration. A dietary fat intake of approximately 30% of calories is recommended. This can be accomplished easily when AN patients are treated on inpatient units or in day hospital programs. However, on an outpatient basis small, progressive increases in dietary fat intake rather than a set optimal amount right away may be met with less resistance. Although some patients will accept small amounts of added fat (such as salad dressing, mayonnaise, or butter), many do better when the fat content is less obvious (as in cheese, peanut butter, granola, and snack foods). Encouraging the gradual change from fat-free products (fat-free milk) to low-fat products (1% or 2% milk) and finally to full-fat items (whole milk) is also acceptable to some patients.

A protein intake in the range of 15% to 20% of total calories is recommended. To ensure adequacy the minimum protein prescription should equal the RDA for age and sex in grams per kilogram of ideal body weight (see inside front cover). Vegetarian diets are often requested but should be discouraged during weight restoration.

Carbohydrate intake in the range of 50% to 55% of calories is well tolerated. Sources of insoluble fiber should be included for optimal health, but also to relieve the constipation frequently seen in this population.

Although vitamin and mineral supplements are not universally prescribed, the potential for increased needs during the later stages of weight gain must be considered. Prophylactic prescription of a vitamin and mineral supplement providing 100% of the RDA may be reasonable, but iron supplementation may be contraindicated early in treatment. During weight restoration, prophylactic thiamin supplementation, at a dose of 25 mg/day, may also be warranted; and higher doses may be required if thiamin deficiency is biochemically confirmed (Royal College of Psychiatrists, 2005). Owing to the increased risk of low BMD, liberal amounts of calcium and vitamin D–rich foods must be encouraged. There is, however, no clear consensus on the use of calcium and vitamin D supplements in this population., however vitamin D status should be assessed. See Chapter 8.

Delayed gastric emptying with complaints of abdominal distention and discomfort after eating are common in AN. In early treatment intake is generally low and can be tolerated in three meals per day. However, as the caloric prescription increases, between-meal feedings become essential. The addition of an afternoon or evening snack may relieve the physical discomfort associated with larger meals, but some patients express feelings of guilt for "indulging" between meals. Commercially available, defined-formula liquid supplements containing 30 to 45 calories per fluid ounce are often prescribed once or twice daily. Patients are fearful that they will become accustomed to the large amount of food required to meet increased caloric requirements; thus use of a liquid supplement is appealing because it can easily be discontinued when the goal weight is attained.

Institutions vary with respect to their menu-planning protocol. In some institutions the meal plan and food choices are initially fixed without patient input. As treatment progresses and weight is restored, the patient generally assumes more responsibility for menu planning. In other inpatient programs the patient participates in menu planning from the beginning of treatment. Some institutions have established guidelines that the patient must comply with to maintain the "privilege" of menu planning. Guidelines may require a certain type of milk (e.g., whole versus low fat), and the inclusion of specific types of foods such as added fats, animal proteins, desserts, and snacks. A certain number of servings from the different food groups may be prescribed at different calorie levels. Meal-planning systems also vary among treatment programs. Some design their own, others use food group exchanges or the MyPlate system, and some formulate an individualized meal plan for each patient.

There are no outcome studies to suggest that one method of meal planning is superior to another, and treatment programs tend to have their own philosophy about menu planning. Despite differences in protocol, AN patients consistently find it difficult to make food choices. The RD can be extremely helpful in providing a structured meal plan and guidance in the selection of nutritionally adequate meals. In a study of recently weight-restored, hospitalized AN patients, those who selected more energy-dense foods and a diet with greater variety had better treatment outcomes during the 1-year period immediately following hospital discharge, and this effect was independent of total caloric intake (Schebendach et al., 2008).

In an outpatient setting the treatment team obviously has less control over the AN patient's food choices, energy intake, and energy distribution. Under these circumstances the RD must use counseling skills to begin the process of developing a plan for nutritional rehabilitation. AN patients are typically precontemplative and, at best, ambivalent about making changes in eating behavior, diet, and body weight; some are defiant and hostile on initial presentation. At this point the nutrition counselor's use of motivational interviewing techniques may help the AN patient resolve ambivalence toward the idea of change and move beyond the precontemplative stage (see Figure 15-3). Use of cognitive behavior therapy may be useful in the nutrition counseling of AN patients (ADA, 2006); the reader is referred to Fairburn (2008) for a thorough review of these techniques.

Effective nutritional rehabilitation and counseling must ultimately result in weight gain and improved eating attitudes and behaviors. A comprehensive review of nutrition counseling techniques can be found in Chapter 15 and in Herrin (2003) and Stellefson Myers (2006).

Bulimia Nervosa

Guidelines for MNT in BN are summarized in Box 23-5. BN is described as a state of dietary chaos, characterized by periods of uncontrolled, poorly structured eating, which are often followed by a periods of restrained food intake. The nutritionist's role is to help develop a reasonable plan of controlled eating while assessing the patient's tolerance for structure. Because BN patients are hospitalized infrequently, nutrition counseling will most likely begin in an outpatient treatment setting.

In BN much of the patient's eating and purging behavior is aimed at weight loss. Although weight reduction may be a reasonable long-term goal, immediate goals must be interruption of the binge-and-purge cycle, restoration of normal eating behavior, and stabilization of body weight. Attempts at dietary restraint for the purpose of weight loss typically exacerbate binge-purge behavior in BN patients.

Patients with BN have varying degrees of metabolic efficiency, which must be taken into account when prescribing the baseline diet. Assessment of REE along with clinical signs of a hypometabolic state such as a low T3 level and cold intolerance are useful in determining the caloric prescription. If a low metabolism is suspected, a caloric prescription of 1500 to 1600 calories daily is a reasonable place to start. Another technique that is helpful in establishing an initial caloric prescription is to base it on the patient's present intake by using the following method:

BOX 23-5

Guidelines for Medical Nutrition Therapy of Bulimia Nervosa

1. Caloric prescription for weight maintenance
   - **A.** If there is evidence of a hypometabolic rate provide 1500 to 1600 kcal/day diet if patient is hypometabolic.
   - **B.** If metabolic rate appears to be normal, provide DRI for energy if metabolic rate is normal.
   - **C.** Monitor body weight and adjust caloric prescription for weight maintenance.
   - **D.** Avoid weight reduction diets until eating patterns and body weight are stabilized.
2. Macronutrients
   - **A.** Protein
     - **(1)** Minimum intake is RDA in g/kg of ideal body weight.
     - **(2)** Provide 15% to 20% kcal.
     - **(3)** Provide high biologic–value sources.
   - **B.** Carbohydrate
     - **(1)** Provide 50% to 55% kcal.
     - **(2)** Encourage insoluble fiber for treatment of constipation.
   - **C.** Fat
     - **(1)** Provide approximately 30% kcal.
     - **(2)** Provide source of essential fatty acids.
3. Micronutrients
   - **A.** Provide 100% RDA multivitamin with minerals supplement.
   - **B.** Note that iron-containing preparation may aggravate constipation.

Adapted from: Luder E, Schebendach J: Nutrition management of eating disorders, Top Clin Nutr 8:48, 1993.

DRI, Dietary reference intake; RDA, recommended dietary allowance.

1. For a typical week ask the patient to estimate the number of binge-purge days, binge-nonpurge days, moderate-intake days, and restrained-intake days.
2. Have the patient describe a typical food intake on a binge-purge day, a binge-nonpurge day, a moderate-intake day, and a restrained-intake day.
3. Estimate 50% of the caloric intake on the binge-purge days and 100% of caloric intake on the binge-nonpurge days, moderate-intake days, and restrained-intake days.
4. Calculate the total caloric intake during the 7-day period.
5. Calculate an average daily intake. The RD can then formulate an initial eating and meal plan based on this estimated average daily intake.

Body weight should be monitored with a goal of stabilization. If the patient's weight is stabilized on a lower-than-average caloric intake, small but consistent increases in the caloric intake should be prescribed every 1 to 2 weeks. This will induce incremental increases in the metabolic rate (Schebendach, 2003).

BN patients need a great deal of encouragement to follow weight-maintenance versus weight-loss diets. They must be reminded that attempts to restrict caloric intake may only increase the risk of binge eating and that their pattern of restrained intake followed by binge eating has not facilitated weight loss in the past.

A balanced macronutrient intake is essential for the provision of a regular meal pattern. This should include sufficient carbohydrates to prevent craving and adequate protein and fat to promote satiety. In general, a balanced diet providing 50% to 55% of the calories from carbohydrate, 15% to 20% from protein, and 25% to 30% from fat is reasonable. Small amounts of dietary fat should be encouraged at each meal. As is the case with AN, this may be better tolerated when provided in a less obvious manner, such as in peanut butter, cheese, or whole milk.

Adequacy of micronutrient intake relative to the caloric prescription and variety of intake should be assessed. A multivitamin and mineral preparation may be prescribed to ensure adequacy, particularly in the initial phase of treatment.

Bingeing, purging, and restrained intake often impair recognition of hunger and satiety cues. The cessation of purging behavior coupled with a reasonable daily distribution of calories at three meals and prescribed snacks can be instrumental in strengthening these biologic cues. Many patients with BN are afraid to eat earlier in the day because they are fearful that these calories will contribute to caloric excess if they binge later. They may also digress from their meal plans after a binge, attempting to restrict intake to balance out the binge calories. Patience and support are essential in this process of making positive changes in their eating habits.

CBT, a highly structured psychotherapeutic method used to alter attitudes and problem behaviors by identifying and replacing negative, inaccurate thoughts and changing the rewards of the behavior, is the treatment of choice in BN (APA, 2006). When applied to an ED, CBT is typically a 20-week intervention that consists of three distinct and systematic phases of treatment: (1) establishing a regular eating pattern, (2) evaluating and changing beliefs about shape and weight, and (3) preventing relapse.

When the BN patient is receiving CBT, the RD can be instrumental in helping the patient establish a regular meal pattern (phase 1). However, the RD and the psychotherapist must maintain active communication to avoid overlap in the counseling sessions. If the BN patient is engaged in a type of psychotherapy other than CBT, the RD should incorporate more CBT skills into the nutrition counseling sessions (Herrin, 2003). See Fairburn (2008) for guidance on CBT techniques.

Patients with BN are typically more receptive to nutrition counseling than AN patients and less likely to present in the precontemplation stage of change. Suggested strategies for nutrition counseling at the precontemplation, contemplation, preparation, action, and maintenance stages are given in Table 23-2 (see Chapter 15).

TABLE 23-2

Counseling Strategies Using the Stages of Change Model in Eating Disorders

Stage of Change	Counseling Strategies
Precontemplation	• Establish rapport. • Assess nutrition knowledge, beliefs, attitudes. • Conduct thorough review of food likes and dislikes, safe and risky foods, forbidden foods (assess reason), binge and purge foods. • Assess physical, anthropometric, metabolic status. • Assess level of motivation. • Use motivational interviewing techniques. • Decisional balance: weigh costs and benefits of maintaining current status versus costs and benefits of change.
Contemplation	• Identify behaviors to change; prioritize. • Identify barriers to change. • Identify coping mechanisms. • Identify support systems. • Discuss self-monitoring tools: food and eating behavior records. • Continue motivational interviewing technique.
Preparation	• Implement nutrition-focused CBT • Implement self-monitoring tools: food and eating behavior records. • Determine list of alternative behaviors to bingeing and purging.
Action	• Develop a plan of healthy eating. • Reinforce positive decision making, self-confidence, and self-efficacy. • Promote positive self-rewarding behaviors. • Develop strategies for handling impulsive behaviors, high-risk situations, and "slips." • Continue CBT. • Continue self-monitoring.
Maintenance and relapse	• Identify strategies; manage high-risk situations. • Continue positive self-rewarding behaviors. • Reinforce coping skills and impulse-control techniques. • Reinforce relapse prevention strategies. • Determine and schedule follow-up sessions needed for maintenance and reinforcement of positive changes in eating behavior and nutrition status.

Modified from Stellefson Myers E: Winning the war within: nutrition therapy for clients with anorexia or bulimia nervosa, Dallas, TX, 1999, Helm Publishing.

CBT, Cognitive behavioral therapy.

Binge Eating Disorder

Strategies for treatment of BED include nutrition counseling and dietary management, individual and group psychotherapy, and medication. Some treatment programs focus primarily on nutrition counseling and weight loss. Although successful weight loss and decreased frequency of binge eating episodes may result, relapse occurs often. Other treatment programs focus primarily on reduction of binge episodes rather than weight loss. Self-acceptance, improved body image, increased physical activity, and better overall nutrition are also goals of treatment in BED. Several self-help manuals are available for the treatment of BED (Sysko and Walsh, 2008), and these approaches can be augmented with guidance from psychotherapists and nutritionists.

Monitoring Nutritional Rehabilitation

Guidelines for patient monitoring are indicated in Box 23-6. The health professional, patient, and family must be realistic

BOX 23-6
Patient Monitoring

1. Body weight
   - A. Establish goal weight.
   - B. Determine:
     - (1) Acceptable rate of weight gain in AN
     - (2) Maintenance weight range in BN
   - C. Monitor weight:
     - (1) Inpatient
       - a. Daily, or every other day
       - b. Gowned
       - c. Preprandial
       - d. Postvoid
       - e. Urine specific gravity measured
       - f. Additional, random, afternoon, or evening weight if fluid loading is suspected
     - (2) Day treatment:
       - a. Variable, depending on diagnosis, age of patient, and treatment setting (i.e., daily, several times per week, once per week)
       - b. Gowned
       - c. Postvoid
       - d. Same time of day
       - e. Same scale
       - f. Urine specific gravity measured
     - (3) Outpatient:
       - a. Once every 1-2 week in early treatment, less frequently in mid- to late treatment
       - b. Gowned
       - c. Postvoid
       - d. Same time of day
       - e. Same scale
       - f. Urine specific gravity measured
2. Height
   - A. Obtain baseline (NCHS percentile for children and adolescents).
   - B. Monitor every 1-2 months in patients with growth potential.
3. Anthropometric measurements (optional)
   - A. Obtain baseline:
     - (1) Skinfolds; triceps, biceps, subscapula, suprailiac
     - (2) Midarm circumference
     - (3) Midarm muscle circumference
   - B. Monitor
     - (1) Inpatient: as medically indicated
     - (2) Outpatient: as medically indicated
4. Resting and postprandial energy expenditure (optional)
   - A. Obtain baseline
   - B. Monitor
     - (1) Inpatient: as medically indicated
     - (2) Outpatient: as medically indicated
5. Outpatient diet monitoring
   - A. Anorexia nervosa
     Daily food record to include:
     - (1) Food
     - (2) Fluid: caloric, noncaloric, alcohol
     - (3) Artificial sweeteners
     - (4) Eating behavior: time, place, how eaten, with whom
     - (5) Exercise
   - B. Bulimia nervosa
     Daily food record to include:
     - (1) Food
     - (2) Fluid: caloric, non-caloric, alcohol
     - (3) Artificial sweeteners
     - (4) Eating behavior: time, place, how eaten, with whom
     - (5) Emotions and feelings when eating
     - (6) Foods eaten at a binge
     - (7) Time and method of purge
     - (8) Exercise

Adapted from: Luder E, Schebendach J: Nutrition management of eating disorders, Top Clin Nutr 8:48, 1993.

AN, Anorexia nervosa; *BN*, bulimia nervosa; *NCHS*, National Center for Health Statistics.

BOX 23-7

Topics for Nutrition Education

1. Guidelines for healthy eating: energy, macronutrients, vitamins, minerals, fluids and electrolytes
2. Impact of malnutrition on adolescent growth and development
3. Impact of malnutrition on behavior
4. Set-point theory and the determination of a healthy body weight goal
5. Impact of dieting on metabolism
6. Restrained eating and disinhibition
7. Causes of bingeing and purging, and techniques to break the cycle
8. Changes in body composition that occur during weight restoration
9. Exercise and energy balance
10. Ineffectiveness of vomiting, laxatives, and diuretics in long-term weight control
11. Portion control
12. Social and holiday dining
13. Hunger and satiety cues
14. Interpreting food labels

Adapted from: Schebendach J, Nussbaum MP: Nutrition management in adolescents with eating disorders, Adolesc Med State Art Rev 3(3):545, 1992.

about treatment, which is often a long-term process. Although outcomes may be favorable, the course of treatment is rarely smooth, and clinicians must be prepared to monitor progress carefully.

Nutrition Education

Patients with EDs may appear quite knowledgeable about food and nutrition. Despite this, nutrition education is an essential component of their treatment plan. Indeed, some patients spend significant amounts of time reading nutrition-related information, but their sources may be unreliable, and their interpretation potentially distorted by their illness. Malnutrition may impair the patient's ability to assimilate and process new information. Early- and mid-adolescent development is characterized by the transition from concrete to abstract operations in problem solving and directed thinking, and normal developmental issues must be considered when teaching adolescents with EDs (see Chapter 19).

Nutrition education materials must be thoroughly assessed to determine if language and subject matter are bias free and appropriate for AN and BN patients. For example, literature provided by many health organizations promotes a low-fat diet and low-calorie lifestyle for the prevention and treatment of chronic disease. This material is in direct conflict with a treatment plan that encourages increased caloric and fat intake for the purpose of nutritional rehabilitation and weight restoration.

Although the interactive process of a group setting may have advantages, these topics can also be effectively incorporated into individual counseling sessions. Topics for nutrition education are suggested in Box 23-7.

Prognosis

Relapse rates after weight restoration in AN are high, with as many as 50% of patients requiring rehospitalization within 1 year of inpatient treatment (Walsh et al., 2006). Follow-up studies suggest that two thirds of AN patients have enduring morbid food and weight preoccupation (APA, 2006). In general, adolescents have better outcomes than adults, and younger adolescents have better outcomes than older adolescents. Outcomes studies in treated BN patients suggest a short-term success rate of 50% to 70%; however, relapse rates in the range of 30% to 85% have also been reported (APA, 2006).

USEFUL WEBSITES

Academy for Eating Disorders: For Professionals Working in the Area of Eating Disorders
http://www.aedweb.org

National Association of Anorexia Nervosa and Associated Disorders
http://www.anad.org

National Eating Disorders Association
http://www.nationaleatingdisorders.org

American Psychiatric Association
Proposed revisions to eating disorders diagnostic criteria: http://www.dsm5.org/ProposedRevisions

CLINICAL SCENARIO

Jennifer is a 19-year-old woman. Her height is 65″ and her weight is 138 lb. Laboratory data: glucose, 82 mg/dL; albumin, 4.2 g/dL; cholesterol, 180 mg/dL; potassium, 2.7 mmol/L; serum CO_2, 31 mmol/L. Anthropometric status: Skin folds: triceps, 20 mm; biceps, 7 mm; subscapular, 10 mm; suprailiac, 13 mm; midarm circumference, 26.7 cm; midarm muscle circumference, 20.4 cm.

Jennifer has always been unhappy with her weight. She went on every fad diet throughout high school and lost some weight but always regained it. About 1 year ago, Jennifer began binge eating. Binge episodes now occur three to four times per week. During these binges Jennifer consumes about 1500 to 2000 kcal in a 2-hour period. Binge foods include ice cream, cookies, potato chips, and other foods. Jennifer describes them as "fattening and unhealthy." After binge eating Jennifer feels extremely guilty, and vomiting is immediately self-induced. Jennifer always tries to eat as little as possible the next day, sometimes consuming only 700 or 800 kcal. Three months ago Jennifer started to overdose on laxatives about three times a week. She occasionally uses over-the-counter diet pills, but they never really help. Jennifer feels fat in her abdomen, buttocks, and thighs. Her physical activity includes 100 sit-ups and 100 leg lifts three or four times per week.

Nutrition Diagnostic Statement

Disordered eating pattern related to binging and purging as evidenced by self-induced vomiting following binge episodes accompanied by guilt and restricted eating

Nutrition Care Questions

1. What are some possible medical complications that Jennifer may develop secondary to binge eating and her compensatory behaviors?
2. Discuss her laboratory values and what you might expect to happen to these indices during rehabilitation.
3. Determine Jennifer's ideal body weight and goal weight for short-term and long-term treatment.
4. Calculate Jennifer's initial caloric prescription and discuss how you arrived at this.
5. Plan a sample menu.
6. Discuss how you would handle foods that Jennifer considers binge "trigger" foods.
7. What would you suggest for Jennifer to help control her episodes of vomiting, laxative use, and diet pill use?

REFERENCES

Altinyazar V, et al: Anorexia nervosa and Wernicke Korsakoff's syndrome: atypical presentation by acute psychosis, *Int J Eat Disord* 2009. [Epub ahead of print.]

American Academy of Pediatrics: Policy statement: identifying and treating eating disorders, *Pediatrics* 111:204, 2003.

American Dietetic Association: Nutrition intervention in the treatment of anorexia nervosa, bulimia nervosa, and other eating disorders, *J Am Diet Assoc* 106:2073, 2006.

American Psychiatric Association: *Diagnostic and statistical manual for mental disorders*, ed 4, text revision, Washington, DC, 2000, APA Press.

American Psychiatric Association: *Practice guidelines for the treatment of patients with eating disorders*, ed 3, *Am J Psychiatry* 2006. Accessed 1 October 2006 from www.Psych.org/edu/cme/pgeatingdisorders3rdedition.cfm.

Attia E, Roberto CA: Should amenorrhea be a diagnostic criterion for anorexia nervosa, *Int J Eat Disord* 42:581, 2009.

Becker AE: New global perspectives on eating disorders, *Cult Med Psychiatry* 28:433, 2004.

Birmingham CL, Gritzner S: Heart failure in anorexia nervosa: case report and review of the literature, *Eating Weight Disord* 12:e7, 2007.

Bryant-Waugh R: Overview of the eating disorders. In Lask B, Bryant-Waugh R, editors: *Eating disorders in childhood and adolescence*, ed 3, East Sussex, UK, 2007, Routledge.

Bryant-Waugh R: Feeding and eating disorders in childhood, *Int J Eat Disord* 43:98, 2010.

Burd C, et al: An assessment of daily food intake in participants with anorexia nervosa in the natural environment, *Int J Eat Disord* 42:371, 2009.

Castro J, et al: Persistence of nutritional deficiencies after short-term weight recovery in adolescents with anorexia nervosa, *Int J Eat Disord* 35:169, 2004.

de Alvaro M, et al: Regional fat distribution in adolescents with anorexia nervosa: effect of duration of malnutrition and weight recovery, *Eur J Clin Nutr* 157:473, 2007.

de Zwann M, et al: Research on energy expenditure in individuals with eating disorders: a review, *Int J Eating Disord* 31:361, 2002.

Dragani B, et al: Dynamic monitoring of restricted eating disorders by indirect calorimetry: a useful cognitive model, *Eating Weight Disord* 11:e9, 2006.

Durnin JVGA, Rahaman MM: The assessment of the amount of body fat in the human body from measurements of skinfold thickness, *Br J Nutr* 21:681, 1967.

Durnin JVGA, Womersley J: Body fat assessed from total body density and its estimation from skinfolds thickness: measurements of 481 men and women aged from 16 to 72 years, *Br J Nutr* 32:77, 1974.

Fairburn CG: *Cognitive behavior therapy and eating disorders*, New York, 2008, Guilford Press.

Fairburn CG, Harrison PJ: Eating disorders, *Lancet* 361:407, 2003.

Feighner JP, et al: Diagnostic criteria for use in psychiatric research, *Arch Gen Psychiatry* 26:57, 1972.

Gendall KA, et al: The nutrient intake of women with bulimia nervosa, *Int J Eat Disord* 21:115, 1997.

Golden NH, et al: Alendronate for the treatment of osteopenia in anorexia nervosa: a randomized, double-blind, placebo-controlled trial, *J Clin Endocrinol Metabol* 90:3179, 2005.

Golden NH, et al: Treatment goal weight in adolescents with anorexia nervosa, *Int J Eat Disord* 41:301, 2008.

Grinspoon S, et al: Changes in regional fat distribution and the effects of estrogen during spontaneous weight gain in women with anorexia nervosa, *Am J Clin Nutr* 73:865, 2001.

Hadigan CM, et al: Assessment of macronutrient and micronutrient intake in women with anorexia nervosa, *Int J Eating Disord* 28(3):284, 2000.

Herrin M: *Nutrition counseling in the treatment of eating disorders*, New York, 2003, Brunner-Routledge.

Hlynsky J, et al: The agreement between the MedGem indirect calorimeter and a standard indirect calorimeter, *Eating Weight Disord* 10:e83, 2005.

Hutter G, et al: The hematology of anorexia nervosa, *Int J Eat Disord* 42:293, 2009.

Jagielska G, et al: Pellagra: a rare complication of anorexia nervosa, *Eur Child Adolesc Psychiatry* 16:417, 2007.

Kaye WH, et al: Amounts of calories retained after binge eating and vomiting, *Am J Psychiatry* 150:969, 1993.

Keys A, et al: *The biology of human starvation*, vols 1 and 2, Minneapolis, 1950, University of Minnesota Press.

Keel PK, Brown TA: Update on course and outcome in eating disorders, *Int J Eat Disord* 43:195, 2010.

Kotler LA, et al: Longitudinal relationships between childhood, adolescent, and adult eating disorders, *J Am Acad Child Adolesc Psychiatry* 40:1434, 2001.

Lock JD, Fitzpatrick KK: Anorexia nervosa, *Clin Evid* Mar 10:1001, 2009.

Marino JM, et al: Caffeine, artificial sweetener, and fluid intake in anorexia nervosa, *Int J Eat Disord* 42:540, 2009.

Mayer L, et al: Body fat redistribution after weight gain in women with anorexia nervosa, *Am J Clin Nutr* 81:1286, 2005.

Mayer ES, et al: Adipose tissue redistribution after weight restoration and weight maintenance in women with anorexia nervosa, *Am J Clin Nutr* 90:1132, 2009.

McCallum K, et al: How should the clinician evaluate and manage the cardiovascular complications of anorexia nervosa? *Eating Disord* 14(1):73, 2006.

Mehler PS, MacKenzie TD: Treatment of osteopenia and osteoporosis in anorexia nervosa: a systematic review of the literature, *Int J Eat Disord* 42:195, 2009.

Misra S, et al: Regional body composition in adolescents with anorexia nervosa and changes with weight recovery, *Am J Clin Nutr* 77:1361, 2003.

Moreno MV, et al: Assessment of body composition in adolescent subjects with anorexia nervosa by bioimpedance, *Med Eng Phys* 30:783, 2008.

O'Connor GO, Goldin J: The refeeding syndrome and glucose load, *Int J Eat Disord* 2010. [Epub ahead of print.]

Probst M, et al: Body composition of anorexia nervosa patients assessed by underwater weighing and skin-fold thickness measurements before and after weight gain, *Am J Clin Nutr* 73:190, 2001.

Prousky JE: Pellagra may be a rare secondary complication of anorexia nervosa: a systematic review of the literature, *Alternative Med Rev* 8:180, 2003.

Rigaud D, et al: Hypercholesterolaemia in anorexia nervosa: frequency and changes during refeeding, *Diabetes Metab* 35:57, 2009.

Rosen DS and the Committee on Adolescence. Identification and management of eating disorders in children and adolescents. *Pediatrics* 126:1240, 2010.

Royal College of Psychiatrists: *Guidelines for the nutritional management of anorexia nervosa*, Council Report CR130, July 2005.

Schebendach J: The use of indirect calorimetry in the clinical management of adolescents with nutritional disorders, *Adoles Med* 14:77, 2003.

Schebendach J, et al: Dietary energy density and diet variety as predictors of outcome in anorexia nervosa, *Am J Clin Nutr* 87:810, 2008.

Society for Adolescent Medicine: Position paper: eating disorders in adolescents, *J Adolesc Health* 33:96, 2003.

Steinhausen HC: The outcome of anorexia nervosa in the 20th century, *Am J Psychiatry* 159:1284, 2002.

Stellefson Myers E: *Winning the war within: nutrition therapy for clients with eating disorders*, ed 2, Dallas, Tex, 2006, Helm Publishing.

Sunday SR, Halmi KA: Energy intake and body composition in anorexia and bulimia nervosa, *Phys Behav* 78:11, 2003.

Swenne I: The significance of routine laboratory analyses in the assessment of teenage girls with eating disorders and weight loss, *Eating Weight Disord* 9:269, 2004.

Sysko R, Walsh BT: A critical evaluation of the efficacy of self-help interventions for the treatment of bulimia nervosa and binge-eating disorder, *Int J Eat Disord* 41:97, 2008.

Treasure J, et al: Eating disorders, *Lancet* 375:583, 2010.

Walsh BT, et al: Fluoxetine after weight restoration in anorexia nervosa: a randomized controlled trial, *JAMA* 295(22):2605, 2006.

Yager J, Andersen AE: Anorexia nervosa, *N Engl J Med* 353:1481, 2005.

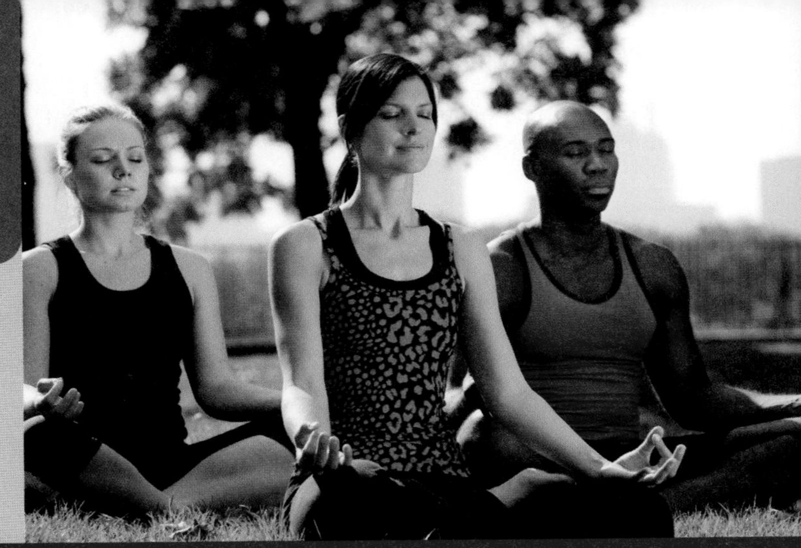

CHAPTER 24

Lisa Dorfman, MS, RD, CSSD, LMHC

Nutrition in Exercise and Sports Performance

KEY TERMS

actomyosin
adenosine diphosphate (ADP)
adenosine triphosphate (ATP)
aerobic metabolism
anabolic effects
anaerobic metabolism
androgenic effects
creatine phosphate (CP)
dehydroepiandrosterone (DHEA)
ergogenic aid
female athlete triad
glycemic index
glycogen
glycogen loading (glycogen supercompensation)
glycogenolysis
glycolysis
high-intensity interval training (HIIT)
hypohydration
human growth hormone (HGH)
lactic acid
mitochondria
myoglobin
preexercise sports drinks (PRXs)
respiratory exchange ratio (RER)
reactive oxygen species (ROS)
sports anemia
thermoregulation
Vo_2max

Successful athletic performance is a combination of favorable genetics, desire, proper training, and a sensible approach to nutrition. Whether an athlete is recreational or elite, young or mature, the importance of nutrition as a contributing factor to success in training and competition has been recognized for decades. Athletes attempting to gain a competitive edge will try almost any dietary regimen or artificial means, including nutritional supplements and oral or injectable medications, in the hope of reaching a new level of wellness or physical performance. Unfortunately, there is a plethora of misinformation on the topic of sports nutrition. Among college athletes, men are more likely than women to rely on strength coaches for supplement information. Athletes rely on trainers (71%), coaches (60%), and physicians (41%); they also refer to the Internet (79%), magazines (68%), and television (52%) for guidance (Malinauskas et al., 2007). Athletes can benefit from nutrition education and intervention by nutrition experts—increasing knowledge, self-efficacy, and dietary improvement.

ENERGY PRODUCTION

The human body must be supplied continuously with energy to perform its many complex functions. As a person's energy demands increase with exercise, the body must provide additional energy, or the exercise will cease. Two metabolic systems supply energy for the body: one dependent on oxygen (**aerobic metabolism**), and the other independent of oxygen (**anaerobic metabolism**). The use of one system over the other depends on the duration, intensity, and type of physical activity.

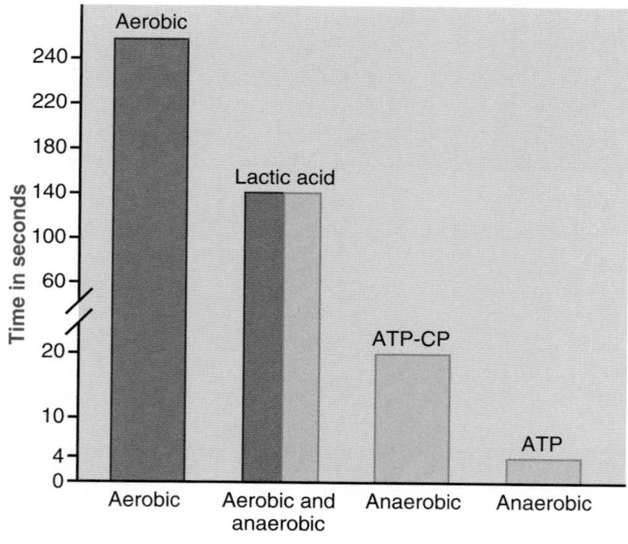

FIGURE 24-1 Classification of activities based on duration of performance and the predominant pathways of energy production. One can see that the duration of activity can continue much longer when energy is produced by aerobic metabolism.

Adenosine Triphosphate

The body obtains its continuous supply of fuel through **adenosine triphosphate (ATP)**, found within the cells of the body. ATP is the energy currency of the cell. The energy produced from the breakdown of ATP provides the fuel that activates muscle contraction. The energy from ATP is transferred to the contractile filaments (myosin and actin) in the muscle, which form an attachment of actin to the cross-bridges on the myosin molecule, thus forming **actomyosin**. Once activated the myofibrils slide past each other and cause the muscle to contract.

Resynthesizing Adenosine Triphosphate

Although ATP is the main currency for energy in the body, it is stored in limited amounts. In fact, only approximately 3 oz of ATP is stored in the body at any one time. This provides only enough energy for several seconds of exercise. ATP must continually be resynthesized to provide a constant energy source during exercise. When ATP loses a phosphate, thus releasing energy, the resulting **adenosine diphosphate (ADP)** is enzymatically combined with another high-energy phosphate from **creatine phosphate (CP)** to resynthesize ATP. The concentration of high-energy CP in the muscle is five times that of ATP.

Creatine kinase is the enzyme that catalyzes the reaction of CP with ADP and inorganic phosphate. It is the fastest and most immediate means of replenishing ATP, and it does so without the use of oxygen (anaerobic). Although this system has great power, it is time-limited because of the concentration of CP found in the muscles (see "Creatine" later in the chapter).

The energy released from this ATP-CP system will only support an all-out exercise effort of a few seconds, such as in a power lift, tennis serve, or sprint. If the all-out effort continues for longer than 8 seconds or if moderate exercise is to proceed for longer periods, an additional source of energy must be provided for the resynthesis of ATP (Figure 24-1). The production of ATP carries on within the muscle cells through either the anaerobic or aerobic pathways.

Anaerobic or Lactic Acid Pathway

The next energy pathway for supplying ATP for more than 8 seconds of physical activity is the process of anaerobic **glycolysis**. In this pathway the energy in glucose is released without the presence of oxygen. **Lactic acid** is the end product of anaerobic glycolysis. Without the production of lactic acid, glycolysis would shut down. The coenzyme called nicotinic acid dehydrogenase (NAD) is in limited supply in this pathway. When NAD is limited, the glycolytic pathway cannot provide constant energy. By converting pyruvic acid to lactic acid, NAD is freed to participate in further ATP synthesis. The amount of ATP furnished is relatively small (the process is only 30% efficient). This pathway contributes energy during an all-out effort lasting up to 60 to 120 seconds. Examples are a 440-yard sprint and many sprint-swimming events.

Although this process provides immediate protection from the consequences of insufficient oxygen, it cannot continue indefinitely. When exercise continues at intensities beyond the body's ability to supply oxygen and convert lactic acid to fuel, lactic acid accumulates in the blood, lowers the pH to a level that interferes with enzymatic action, and causes fatigue. Lactic acid can be removed from the muscle; transported into the bloodstream; and converted to energy in muscle, liver, or brain. Otherwise, it is converted to glycogen. Conversion to **glycogen** occurs in the liver and to some extent in muscle, particularly among trained athletes.

The amount of ATP produced through glycolysis is small compared with that available through aerobic pathways. Substrate for this reaction is limited to glucose from blood sugar or the glycogen stored in the muscle. Liver glycogen contributes but is limited.

Aerobic Pathway

Production of ATP in amounts sufficient to support continued muscle activity for longer than 90 to 120 seconds requires oxygen. If sufficient oxygen is not present to combine with hydrogen in the electron transport chain, no further ATP is made. Thus the oxygen furnished through respiration is of vital importance. Here, glucose can be broken down far more efficiently for energy, producing 18 to 19 times more ATP. In the presence of oxygen, pyruvate is converted to acetyl coenzyme A (CoA), which enters the **mitochondria**. In the mitochondria acetyl CoA goes through

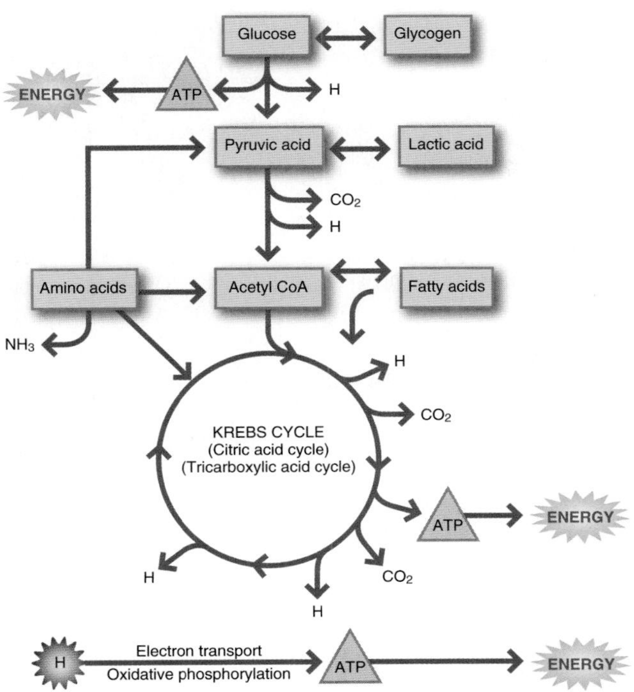

FIGURE 24-2 Pathways of energy production. *ATP*, Adenosine triphosphate; *CoA*, coenzyme A; *H*, hydrogen atoms.

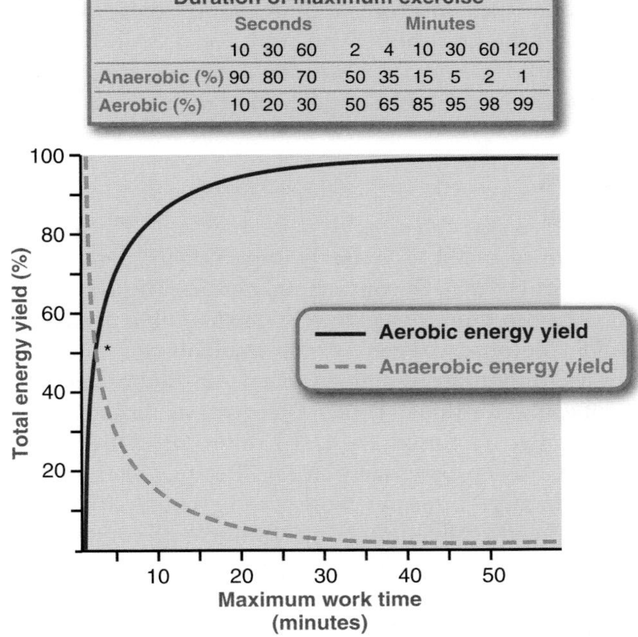

FIGURE 24-3 Relative contribution of aerobic and anaerobic energy during maximum physical activity of various durations. Note that 90 to 120 seconds of maximum effort requires 50% of the energy from each of the aerobic and anaerobic processes. This is also the point at which the lactic acid pathway for energy production is at its maximum.

the Krebs cycle, which generates 36 to 38 ATP per molecule of glucose (Figure 24-2).

Aerobic metabolism is limited by the availability of substrate, a continuous and adequate supply of oxygen, and the availability of coenzymes. At the onset of exercise and with the increase in exercise intensity, the capability of the cardiovascular system to supply adequate oxygen is a limiting factor, and this is largely due to the level of conditioning. The aerobic pathway can also provide ATP by metabolizing fats and proteins. A large amount of acetyl CoA, which enters the Krebs cycle and provides enormous amounts of ATP, is provided by β-oxidation of fatty acids. Proteins may be catabolized into acetyl CoA or Krebs cycle intermediates, or they may be directly oxidized as another source of ATP.

Energy Continuum

A person who is exercising may use one or more energy pathways. For example, at the beginning of any physical activity, ATP is produced anaerobically. As exercise continues, the lactic acid system produces ATP for exercise. If the person continues to exercise and does so at a moderate intensity for a prolonged period, the aerobic pathway will become the dominant pathway for fuel. On the other hand, the anaerobic pathway provides most of the energy for short-duration, high-intensity exercise such as sprinting; the 200-meter swim; or high-power, high-intensity moves in basketball, football, or soccer.

The production of ATP for exercise is on a continuum that depends on the availability of oxygen. Other factors that influence oxygen capabilities, and thus energy pathways, are the capacity for intense exercise and its duration. These two factors are inversely related. For example, an athlete cannot perform high-power, high-intensity moves over a prolonged period. To do this, he or she would have to decrease the intensity of the exercise to increase its duration (Figure 24-3).

The aerobic pathway cannot tolerate the same level of intensity as duration increases because of the decreased availability of oxygen and accumulation of lactic acid. As the duration of exercise increases, power output decreases. The contribution of energy-yielding nutrients must be considered also. As the duration of exercise lengthens, fats contribute more as an energy source. The opposite is true for high-intensity exercise; when intensity increases, the body relies increasingly on carbohydrates as substrate.

FUELS FOR CONTRACTING MUSCLES

Sources of Fuel

Protein, fat, and carbohydrate are all possible sources of fuel for muscle contraction. The glycolytic pathway is restricted to glucose, which can originate in dietary carbohydrates or stored glycogen, or it can be synthesized from the carbon skeletons of certain amino acids through the process of gluconeogenesis. The Krebs cycle is fueled by three-carbon fragments of glucose; two-carbon fragments of fatty acids; and carbon skeletons of specific amino acids, primarily alanine and the branched-chain amino acids. All these substrates can be used during exercise; however, the intensity and duration of the exercise determine the relative rates of substrate use.

Intensity

The intensity of the exercise is important in determining what fuel will be used by contracting muscles. High-intensity, short-duration exercise has to rely on anaerobic production of ATP. Because oxygen is not available for anaerobic pathways, only glucose and glycogen can be broken down anaerobically for fuel. When glycogen is broken down anaerobically, it is used 18 to 19 times faster than when glucose is broken down aerobically. Persons who are performing in high-intensity workouts or competitive races may run the risk of running out of muscle glycogen before the event or exercise is done as a result of its high use.

Sports that use both the anaerobic and aerobic pathways also have a higher glycogen use rate and, like anaerobic athletes, athletes in these sports also run the risk of running out of fuel before the race or exercise is finished. Sports such as basketball, football, soccer, and swimming are good examples; glycogen usage is high because of the intermittent bursts of high-intensity sprints and running drills. In moderate-intensity sports or exercise such as jogging, hiking, aerobic dance, gymnastics, cycling, and recreational swimming, approximately half of the energy for these activities comes from the aerobic breakdown of muscle glycogen, whereas the other half comes from circulating blood glucose and fatty acids.

Moderate- to low-intensity exercise such as walking is fueled entirely by the aerobic pathway; thus a greater proportion of fat can be used to create ATP for energy. Fatty acids cannot supply ATP during high-intensity exercise because fat cannot be broken down fast enough to provide the energy. Also, fat provides less energy per liter of oxygen consumed than does glucose (4.65 kcal/L of O_2 versus 5.01 kcal/L of O_2). Therefore when less oxygen is available in high-intensity activities, there is a definite advantage for the muscles to be able to use glycogen because less oxygen is required (Figure 24-4).

In general, both glucose and fatty acids provide fuel for exercise in proportions depending on the intensity and duration of the exercise and the fitness of the athlete. Exertion of extremely high intensity and short duration draws primarily on reserves of ATP and CP. High-intensity exercise that continues for more than a few seconds depends on anaerobic glycolysis. During exercise of low-to-moderate intensity (60% of maximum oxygen uptake [Vo_2max]), energy is derived mainly from fatty acids. Carbohydrate becomes a larger fraction of the energy source as intensity increases until, at an intensity level of 85% to 90% Vo_2max, carbohydrates from glycogen is the principal energy source, and the duration of activity is limited (Figure 24-5).

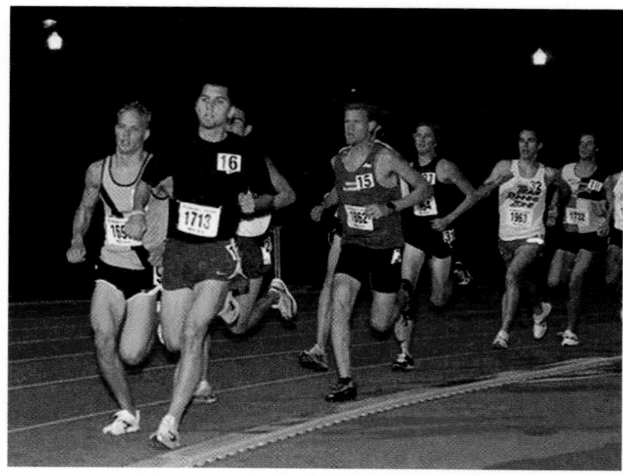

FIGURE 24-4 Running is a high-intensity exercise in which both carbohydrates and fat are used as fuels, depending on the speed and length of the event. *(Courtesy Richard Andrews, Titusville, Fl.)*

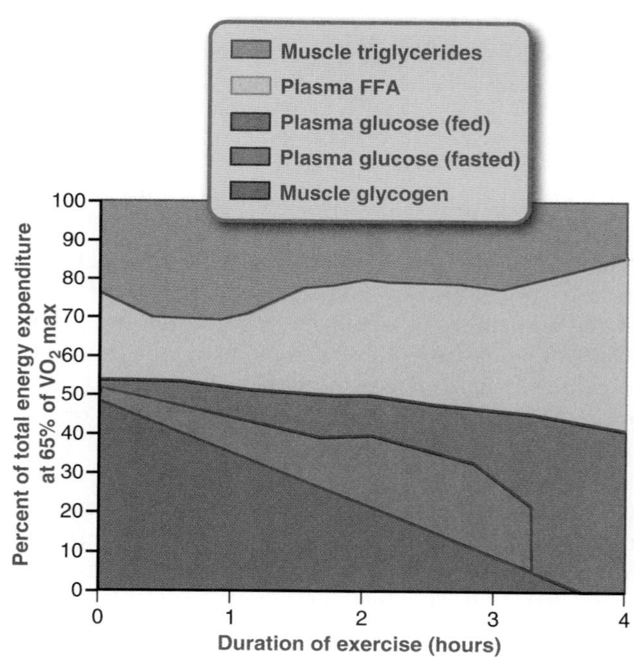

FIGURE 24-5 Sources of energy during 4 hours of exercise. *FFA*, Free fatty acid.

Duration

The duration of a training session determines the substrate used during the exercise bout. For example, the longer the time spent exercising, the greater the contribution of fat as the fuel. Fat can supply up to 60% to 70% of the energy needed for ultra-endurance events lasting 6 to 10 hours. As the duration of exercise increases, the reliance on aerobic metabolism becomes greater, and a greater amount of ATP can be produced from fatty acids. However, fat cannot be metabolized unless a continuous stream of some carbohydrates is also available through the energy pathways. Therefore muscle glycogen and blood glucose are the limiting factors in human performance of any type of intensity or duration.

Effect of Training

The length of time an athlete can oxidize fatty acids as a fuel source is related to the athlete's conditioning, as well as the exercise intensity. In addition to improving cardiovascular systems involved in oxygen delivery, training increases the number of mitochondria and the levels of enzymes involved in the aerobic synthesis of ATP, thus increasing the capacity for fatty acid metabolism. Increases in mitochondria with aerobic training are seen mainly in the type IIA (intermediate fast-twitch) muscle fibers. These fibers however quickly lose their aerobic capacity with the cessation of aerobic training, reverting to the genetic baseline.

These changes from training result in a lower **respiratory exchange ratio (RER)**, the amount of CO_2 produced divided by the amount of O_2 consumed, lower blood lactate and catecholamine levels, and a lower net muscle glycogen breakdown at a specific power output. These metabolic adaptations enhance the ability of muscle to oxidize all fuels, especially fat.

NUTRITIONAL REQUIREMENTS OF EXERCISE

Energy

The most important component of successful sport training and performance is to ensure adequate calorie intake to support energy expenditure and maintain strength, endurance, muscle mass and overall health. Energy and nutrient requirements vary with weight, height, age, sex, and metabolic rate (see Chapter 2) as well as the type, frequency, intensity, and duration of training and performance.

Individuals who participate in an overall fitness program (i.e., 30 to 40 min/day, three times per week) can generally meet their daily nutritional needs by following a normal diet providing 25 to 35 kcal/kg/day or roughly 1800 to 2400 calories a day. However, the 50-kg athlete engaging in more intense training of 2 to 3 hours/day five to six times a week or high-volume training of 3 to 6 hours in one to two workouts per day 5 to 6 days a week may expend up to an additional 600 to 1200 calories a day, thus requiring 50 to 80 kcal/kg/day or roughly 2500 to 4000 kcal/day. For elite athletes or heavier athletes, daily calorie needs can reach 150 to 200 kcal/kg, or roughly 7500 to 10,000 calories a day, depending on the volume and intensity of different training phases.

Meeting caloric needs for many fitness-minded and or elite, intensely training individuals can be a challenge. For working individuals, balancing daily training schedules with work and family responsibilities can compromise the quantity, quality, and timing of meals, which can greatly affect energy, strength levels, and overall health. In the elite athlete, consuming enough food at regular intervals without compromising performance is challenging, particularly for the collegiate athlete. School schedules, budgets, cafeteria schedules, travel requirements, and a varying appetite can further complicate the situation.

TABLE 24-1

Comparison of the Electrolyte Content between Standard Sport Drinks and Endurance-Specific Sport Drinks

Electrolyte	Sweat Loss mg/L	Standard Sport Drink mg/L	Endurance Specific Sport Drink mg/L
Sodium	900-2600	200-450	800-1110
Potassium	100-200	80-125	390-650
Magnesium	60-260	0	10-615
Chloride	900-1900	0	390-1550
Calcium	50-100	0	250-500

Source: First endurance. Accessed 14 July 2010 from http://blog.firstendurance.com/tag/electrolytes/.

Meeting the daily energy needs and the appropriate macronutrient distribution for active individuals may necessitate the use of sports bars, drinks, and convenience foods and snacks in addition to whole foods and meals. Dietitians need to be flexible in accommodating lifestyles and eating behaviors when designing meal plans for maximum sport performance.

Sports Supplements

Sports supplements include the easy-to-carry, easy-to-consume, and easy-to-digest meal-replacement powders, ready-to-drink supplements, energy bars, and energy gels. This group represents 50% to 70% of the industry's sales. These products are typically fortified with 33% to 100% of the recommended dietary allowances (RDAs) for vitamins and minerals; provide varying amounts and types of carbohydrates, protein, and fat; and are ideal for athletes on the run. They provide a portable, easy-to-consume food that can be used pericompetitively; while traveling; at work; in the car; or throughout the day at a multievent meet such as in track and field, swimming, diving, or gymnastics.

Many fitness-minded and athletic individuals use these products as a convenient way to enhance their current diet. These products are generally regarded as safe. However, if they are substituted in the place of whole foods on a regular basis, they can deprive the athlete of a well-balanced diet. They may also contain excesses of sugars, fats, and protein and banned substances such as caffeine, Ephedra, and other botanicals. See Table 24-1.

WEIGHT MANAGEMENT

In efforts to maximize performance, many athletes alter normal energy intake to either gain or lose weight. Although such efforts are sometimes appropriate, weight-reduction programs may involve elements of risk. For some young athletes achievement of an unrealistically light weight can jeopardize growth and development. Chronic dieting by female athletes can lead to eating disorders, delayed menarche, amenorrhea, and potential osteoporosis (see Chapters 23 and 25).

The goal weight of an athlete should be based on body fatness. Adequate time should be allowed for a slow, steady weight loss of approximately 1 to 2 lb each week over several weeks. Weight loss should be achieved before the competitive season begins to ensure maximum strength. In addition, the exercise should be of moderate intensity because at this level a greater proportion of energy is derived from fat than carbohydrate and the exercise can be sustained longer. When planned school-based activity programs are in effect, up to a 50% reduction in the incidence of overweight is feasible (Foster et al., 2008). Appropriate programs for weight management are discussed in Chapter 22.

Weight gain should be achieved through a gradual increase in energy intake combined with a strength training program to maximize muscle weight gain over fat gain. A realistic goal is ½ to 1 lb weekly. Fat intake should not exceed 30% of kilocalories from fat, and protein should be 1 to 1.5 g/kg of body weight. The professional working with an elite athlete must remember the tremendous motivation that comes from a desire to perform well in the sport.

MACRONUTRIENTS

Individuals engaging in a general fitness program can typically meet their macronutrient needs by consuming a normal diet of 45% to 55% of calories from carbohydrates (3 to 5 g/kg/day), 10% to 15% from protein (0.8 to 1 g/kg/day) and 25% to 35% from fat (0.5 to 1.5 g/kg/day). Athletes involved in moderate- to high-volume training need greater amounts of carbohydrates and protein to meet macronutrient needs. An intake of at 60% to 70% of total calories (5 to 8 g/kg/day or 250 to 1200 g/day for 50- to 150-kg athletes) should be met by carbohydrates. The remaining calories should be obtained from protein and fat. These percentages are only guidelines for estimating macronutrient requirements

Specific macronutrient recommendations should be used when counseling an active individual or athlete. When energy intake is high (more than 4500 calories/day), even a diet containing only 50% of the calories from carbohydrates would provide 500 g of carbohydrates, which is sufficient to maintain muscle glycogen stores. Similarly, if protein intake in this high-calorie diet were low, at 10% of calories, absolute protein intake would still exceed the recommendation for a 70-kg athlete. Thus specific recommendations should be based on an individual's body size, body composition, sport, and gender. Calories and nutrients should come from a wide variety of foods on a daily basis.

CARBOHYDRATE

The first source of glucose for the exercising muscle is its own glycogen store. When this is depleted, **glycogenolysis** and then gluconeogenesis (both in the liver) maintain the glucose supply (see Chapter 3). During endurance exercise that exceeds 90 minutes, such as marathon running, muscle glycogen stores become progressively lower. When they drop to critically low levels, high-intensity exercise cannot be maintained. In practical terms the athlete is exhausted and must either stop exercising or drastically reduce the pace. Athletes often refer to this as "hitting the wall."

Glycogen depletion may also be a gradual process, occurring over repeated days of heavy training, in which muscle glycogen breakdown exceeds its replacement, as well as during high-intensity exercise that is repeated several times during competition or training. For example, a distance runner who averages 10 miles per day but does not take the time to consume enough carbohydrates in his or her diet, or the swimmer who completes several interval sets at maximum oxygen consumption within hours can deplete glycogen stores rapidly. A high-carbohydrate or **glycogen loading (glycogen supercompensation)** diet can help athletes maximize glycogen stores and be able to continue endurance performance.

The amount of carbohydrate required depends on the athlete's total daily energy expenditure, type of sport, gender, and environmental conditions. Recommendations should provide for daily carbohydrate intake in grams relative to body mass, and allow flexibility for the athlete to meet these targets within the context of their energy needs and other dietary goals. Carbohydrate intake of 5 to 7 g/kg/day can meet general training needs, and 7 to 10 g/kg/day will suffice for endurance athletes. For example, a 70-kg (154-lb) athlete would consume 350 to 700 g of carbohydrate daily (see Table 24-1).

Types of Carbohydrate

Even though the effects of different sugars on performance, substrate use, and recovery has been studied extensively, the optimal type of carbohydrate for the athlete is debatable. The **glycemic index** represents the ratio of the area under the blood glucose curve resulting from the ingestion of a given quantity of carbohydrate and the area under the glucose curve resulting from the ingestion of the same quantity of white bread or glucose (see Chapter 31 and Appendix 43). Studies concerning whether the glycemic index of carbohydrate in the preexercise meal affects performance are inconclusive (Lin-Wu and Williams, 2006; Wong et al., 2009).

Carbohydrate Intake Before Exercise

The preevent or pretraining meal serves two purposes: (1) it keeps the athlete from feeling hungry before and during the exercise and (2) it maintains optimal levels of blood glucose for the exercising muscles. A preexercise meal can improve performance compared with exercising in a fasted state. Athletes who train early in the morning before eating or drinking risk developing low liver glycogen stores that can impair performance, particularly if the exercise regimen involves endurance training. **Preexercise sports drinks (PRXs)** are commonly used in athletic competitions requiring aerobic power. PRX (containing 14 g/serving of fructose, medium-chain triglycerides, and amino acids mixed with 8 oz of water) given 30 minutes prior to performing enhances indices of aerobic performance, specifically Vo_2max, time to exhaustion, and percentage of nonprotein fat substrate use (Byars et al., 2010).

Carbohydrate feedings before exercise can enhance liver glycogen stores. Although allowing for personal preferences and psychological factors, the preevent meal should be high in carbohydrates, nongreasy, and readily digested. Fat should be limited because it delays gastric emptying time and takes longer to digest. A meal eaten 3.5 to 4 hours before competition should be limited to 25% of the kilocalories from fat. Closer to the event, the fat content should be less than 25% (Box 24-1).

Exercising with a full stomach may cause indigestion, nausea, and vomiting. Thus the pregame meal should be eaten 3 to 4 hours before an event and should provide 200 to 350 g of carbohydrates (4 g/kg). Allowing time for partial digestion and absorption provides a final addition to muscle glycogen, additional blood sugar, and also relatively complete emptying of the stomach. To avoid gastrointestinal (GI) distress, the carbohydrate content of the meal should be reduced when the meal is close to the exercise time. For example, 4 hours before the event it is suggested that the athlete consume 4 g of carbohydrate per kilogram of body weight, whereas 1 hour before the competition the athlete would consume 1 g of carbohydrate per kilogram of body weight.

Commercial liquid formulas providing an easily digested high-carbohydrate fluid are popular with athletes and probably leave the stomach faster. Foods high in fiber, fat, and lactose will cause GI distress for some (e.g., bloating, gas, or diarrhea) and should be avoided before competition. Athletes should always use what works best for them by experimenting with foods and beverages during practice sessions and planning ahead to ensure that they have these foods available when they compete.

Carbohydrate Intake During Exercise

Carbohydrate consumed during endurance exercise lasting longer than 1 hour ensures the availability of sufficient amounts of energy during the later stages of exercise, improves performance, and enhances feeling of pleasure during and following exercise (Backhouse et al., 2005). Carbohydrate feeding does not prevent fatigue; rather, it simply delays it. During the final minutes of exercise, when muscle glycogen is low and athletes rely heavily on blood glucose for energy, their muscles feel heavy, and they must concentrate to maintain exercise at intensities that are ordinarily not stressful when muscle glycogen stores are full. Glucose ingestion during exercise has also been shown to spare endogenous protein and carbohydrates in fed cyclists without glycogen depletion (van Hamont et al., 2005). Thus consuming an exogenous carbohydrate during endurance exercise helps to maintain blood glucose and improve performance.

The form of carbohydrate does not seem to matter physiologically. Some athletes prefer to use a sports drink,

BOX 24-1

Examples of Pre-event Meals

For athletes who compete in events such as track or swimming meets or soccer, basketball, volleyball, and wrestling tournaments, nutritious, easy-to-digest food and fluid choices require attention. The athlete should consider the amount of time between eating and performance when choosing foods during these all-day events. Suggested precompetition menus include the following:

1 Hour or Less Before Competition—Approximately 100 kcal

One of these choices:

Fresh fruit such as a banana or orange slices
Half of a sports energy bar
½ plain bagel or English muffin
Crackers such as saltines or low-fiber cracker
Small box of low-fiber cereal
8-12 oz of a sports drink or endurance sports drink

2 to 3 Hours Before Competition—Approximately 300-400 kcal

One of these choices:

½ of turkey sandwich on white bread with baked chips
½ bagel with low sugar jelly and 1 banana
2 pancakes with lite or sugar-free syrup and berries
32 fluid oz of a sports drink or 32-oz endurance drink with protein
1 low-sugar smoothie with berries, banana, and 1 scoop soy or whey protein
1 sports energy bar, 1 cup sports drink, 1 cup water

3 to 4 Hours Before Competition—Approximately 700 kcal

One of these selections:

Scrambled egg whites with white toast with low-sugar jam and banana
1 bagel with fat-free or low-fat cream cheese and low-sugar jelly and 1 banana
1 6-in turkey sub on Italian bread with lettuce, tomato, and mustard
1 3-oz grilled chicken breast with small baked potato, roll, and water
2 cups plain pasta with 1 plain roll
1 can of low fat sport shake with no more than 25 g protein, 1 sports bar, 1 banana, water

whereas others prefer to eat a solid or gel and consume water. If a sports drink with carbohydrates is consumed during exercise, the rate of carbohydrate ingestion should be approximately 26 to 30 g every 30 minutes, an amount equivalent to 1 cup of a 6% to 8% carbohydrate solution taken every 15 to 20 minutes. This ensures that 1 g of carbohydrate will be delivered to the tissues per minute at the time fatigue sets in. It is unlikely that a carbohydrate concentration of less than 5% is enough to help performance, but solutions with a concentration greater than 10% are often associated with abdominal cramps, nausea, and diarrhea.

Combining protein and carbohydrates in a sport fluid or snack may also improve performance, muscle protein synthesis and net balance, and recovery. A small amount of amino acids ingested in small amounts alone or in conjunction with carbohydrates before or after exercise appears to improve net protein balance and may stimulate protein synthesis and improve net protein balance at rest during exercise and postexercise recovery (Millard-Stafford et al., 2005).

Carbohydrate Intake After Exercise

On average, only 5% of the muscle glycogen used during exercise is resynthesized each hour following exercise. Accordingly, at least 20 hours will be required for complete restoration after exhaustive exercise, provided approximately 600 g of carbohydrates are consumed. The highest muscle glycogen synthesis rates have been reported when large amounts of carbohydrates—1 to 1.85 g/kg/hr—are consumed immediately after exercise and at 15- to 60-minute intervals thereafter for up to 5 hours after exercise. Delaying carbohydrate intake for too long after exercise reduces muscle glycogen resynthesis.

It also appears that the consumption of carbohydrates with a high glycemic index results in higher muscle glycogen levels 24 hours after exercise compared with the same amount of carbohydrates provided as foods with a low glycemic index (Wilson M et al., 2009). Adding approximately 5 to 9 g of protein with every 100 g of carbohydrate eaten after exercise may further increase glycogen resynthesis rate, provide amino acids for muscle repair and promote a more anabolic hormonal profile (Millard-Stafford et al., 2005).

Many athletes find it difficult to consume food immediately after exercise. Usually when body or core temperature is elevated, appetite is depressed, and it is difficult to consume carbohydrate-rich foods. Many athletes find it easier and simpler to drink their carbohydrate or to consume easy-to-eat, carbohydrate-rich foods such as fruit pops, bananas, oranges, melon, or apple slices.

PROTEIN

There has been considerable debate regarding the protein needs of athletes. The current RDA is 0.8 g/kg bodyweight and the acceptable macronutrient distribution range for protein for 18 years and older is 10% to 35% of total calories. Factors affecting the protein needs of athletes include age, gender, mass, fitness level, regimen, and phase of training. Nitrogen balance studies in endurance athletes suggest a range of 1.2 g/kg to 1.4 g/kg/day, and for strength athletes 1.2 to 1.7 g/kg/day with the higher end of the range recommended in early season (Rodriguez et al., 2009).

Reports of food intake in athletes and nonathletes consistently indicate that protein represents from 12% to 20% of total energy intake or 1.2 to 2 g of protein per kilogram of body weight daily. The exception to the rule is small, active women who may consume a low-energy intake in conjunction with an exercise or training program. Although these women may consume close to the RDA for protein in conjunction with the restricted energy intake, it may be inadequate to maintain lean body mass.

Intermittent bouts of **high-intensity interval training (HIIT)** depletes energy substrates and allows for metabolite accumulation. Studies suggest that supplementation with beta-alanine may improve endurance performance as well as lean body mass (Smith et al., 2009). However, the need for protein during exercise is just slightly elevated above that for sedentary persons. Consuming more protein than the body can use is not necessary and should be avoided.

When athletes consume diets that are high in protein, they compromise their carbohydrate status, which may affect their ability to train and compete at peak levels. High protein intakes can also result in diuresis and potential dehydration. Protein foods are often also high in fat, and consumption of excess protein can create difficulty in maintaining a low-fat diet.

Protein Needs for Resistance Exercise

Protein needs for resistance exercise involve maintenance (minimum protein required to accomplish nitrogen equilibrium), and the need for increasing lean tissue (positive nitrogen balance). For bodybuilders or persons interested in increasing body mass, the mythology of increased protein need is rampant. Strategies to increase the concentration and availability of amino acids after resistance exercise such as timing of snacks and meals have become an area of interest. See *Clinical Insight:* How Does Type, Timing, and Amount of Protein Affect Muscle Hypertrophy?

FAT

Even though maximum performance is impossible without muscle glycogen, fat also provides energy for exercise. Fat is the most concentrated source of food energy, supplying 9 kcal/g. Essential fatty acids are necessary for cell membranes, skin, hormones, and transport of fat-soluble vitamins. The body has total glycogen stores (both muscle and liver) equaling approximately 2600 calories, whereas each pound of body fat supplies 3500 calories. This means that an athlete weighing 74 kg (163 lb) with 10% body fat has 16.3 lb of fat, which equals 57,000 calories.

Fat is the major, if not most important, fuel for light- to moderate-intensity exercise. Although fat is a valuable metabolic fuel for muscle activity during longer aerobic exercise and performs many important functions in the body, more

CLINICAL INSIGHT

How Does Type, Timing, and Amount of Protein Affect Muscle Hypertrophy?

Although many factors appear to contribute to overall muscle hypertrophy, nutritional factors that control protein synthesis during exercise are not well understood, leaving experts in discord about the type, amount, and timing of meals to enhance protein synthesis and muscle hypertrophy (Pennings, 2010). Resistance training and diet consistently appear to play a role in postworkout muscle protein synthesis. Many studies support supplementation of free-form amino acids or whole protein to enhance training. A 2005 study with resistance-trained participants for 14 weeks demonstrated that the administration of a protein supplement resulted in greater increases in cross-sectional muscle size of types I and II fibers and greater increase in squat height (Anderson et al., 2005). In another study, a postexercise trial, including a mixture of carbohydrate and whey protein consumed 1 hour after exercise resulted in a more immediate and overall greater protein synthesis response, whereas the addition of free essential amino acids before and after exercise also was shown to cause a rapid increase in protein synthesis and balance (Kerksick and Leutholtz, 2005). This higher rate of protein synthesis after exercise has been shown to occur in both young and elderly men (Pennings, 2010).

Although the optimal amount of amino acids to ingest for maximum protein synthesis is not known, a study examined the effect of 25 g of whey and casein protein solution before and after a strength-training session (STS). When consumed 30 minutes before an STS, there were significant increases in growth hormone, testosterone, free fatty acids, and serum insulin, and significantly increased postexercise oxygen consumption and respiratory exchange ratio during the 2 hours after exercise; hence there was a more anabolic environment for muscle growth (Hulmi et al., 2005).

For athletes interested in muscle hypertrophy, it appears that the neither the type nor the amount of protein matters if the day's total amount is within the recommended range for resistance-training athletes of 1.2 to 2 g of protein per kilogram of body weight per day. Sports nutrition professionals can use these data to construct pre- and postworkout formulas to enhance the resistance training sessions of their clients.

than the usual recommended amount of fat is not indicated. In addition, athletes who consume a high-fat diet typically consume fewer calories from carbohydrate.

The diet content also determines which substrate is used during an exercise bout. If an athlete is consuming a high-carbohydrate diet, he or she will use more glycogen as fuel for the exercise. If the diet is high in fat, more fat will be oxidized as a fuel source. Fat oxidation rates decline after the ingestion of high-fat diets, partly because of adaptations at the muscle level and decreased glycogen stores. Fasting longer than 6 hours optimizes fat oxidation; however, the ingestion of carbohydrates in the hours before or at the beginning of an exercise session augments the rate of fat oxidation significantly when compared with fasting (Achten and Jeukendrup, 2004).

Exercise intensity and duration are important determinants of fat oxidation. Fat oxidation rates decrease when exercise intensity becomes high. A high-fat diet has been shown to compromise high-intensity performance even when a high-fat diet regimen is followed by carbohydrate loading before high-intensity performance (Havemann et al., 2005). The mode and duration of exercise can also affect fat oxidation; running increases fat oxidation more than cycling (Achten and Jeukendrup, 2004).

Fats, Inflammation and Sports Injury

When players get injured, they want to heal and get back on the field as soon as possible. Specific foods at the right time can help to provide energy for rehabilitation, rebuild strength, and ensure a complete, healthy, and faster recovery.

Stress to muscle leads to inflammation, bruising and tissue breakdown. Failure to decrease inflammation can lead to scar tissue, poor mobility, and delayed recovery times. The inflammatory stage is impacted by foods, especially the types of dietary fat consumed. A diet high in trans fats, saturated fats, and some ω-6 vegetable oils has been shown to promote inflammation while a diet high in monounsaturated fat and essential ω-3 fats has been shown to be anti-inflammatory. Monounsaturated fats like olive, peanut, canola, and sesame oils as well as avocado also inhibit and reduce inflammation by interfering with pro-inflammatory compounds such as leukotrienes, which are produced naturally by the body. Diets high in ω-3s have been shown to increase collagen deposition and promote healing. New research also suggests that ω-3s may impact healing from concussions.

Supplemental ω-3 fat has been recommended during the inflammation stage especially when the diet is deficient. However, there are also concerns regarding the usual source of ω-3 fats and fish oils since some have been found to be contaminated with mercury and polychlorinated biphenyls (PCBs), toxins dangerous to humans.

Fruits and vegetables are also good sources of alpha linolenic acid, an ω-3. See Appendix 40. However, the conversion to the more active forms of ω-3s, DHA and EPA, in the body is very low. Plant-based foods rich in ALA include: kidney beans, navy beans, tofu, winter and summer squash, certain berries such as raspberries and strawberries, broccoli, cauliflower, green beans, romaine lettuce, and collard greens. Wheat germ and free-range beef and poultry are also good sources of ω-3 fats since they are fed with ω-3 rich food.

VITAMINS AND MINERALS

Unless an individual is deficient in a given nutrient, supplementation with that nutrient does not have a major effect on performance. Several nutrients are of concern for athletes. A daily intake of less than one third of the RDA for thiamin, riboflavin, B_6, and vitamin C, even when other vitamins are supplemented, may lead to a significant decrease in Vo_2max and the anaerobic threshold in less than 4 weeks. Iron and calcium are the two minerals most likely to be low in the diet of young athletes.

Training and work schedules, low-nutrient snacks, infrequent nutrient-dense meals, and overall low calorie intakes may cause inadequate intakes of vitamins and minerals. Because many women athletes are also vegetarians, zinc, iron, and vitamin B_{12} may be of concern. In one study, female athletes failed to meet the estimated average requirement for folate in 48% of cases, calcium (24%), magnesium (19%), and iron (4%) (Heaney et al., 2010).

When limited to 100% of the dietary reference intakes (DRIs), vitamin supplementation is generally regarded as safe. Excess amounts may contribute to health problems; athletes need to understand that more is not always better. The DRIs for vitamins and minerals are the guide for determining nutritional needs, and upper levels have been established (see Chapter 12 and inside front cover).

B Vitamins

Increased energy metabolism creates a need for more of the B vitamins that serve as part of coenzymes involved in the energy cycles. Studies have shown that athletes can become depleted in some B vitamins, and in these athletes dietary change or supplementation improves exercise performance. For some athletes such as wrestlers, gymnasts, or rowers who consume low-calorie diets for long periods, a B-vitamin supplement to meet the RDA may be appropriate. There is no evidence that supplementing the well-nourished athlete with more B vitamins will increase performance

A deficiency of vitamin B_{12} could develop in a vegetarian athlete after several years of a strict vegan intake; thus a vitamin B_{12} supplement is warranted. There is a possibility of altered B_{12} metabolism based on serum homocysteine concentrations. The intake of folic acid is marginal for a large portion of the U.S. population and could be low in an athlete whose consumption of whole fruits and vegetables is low. A folate supplement to meet the RDA plus wheat, grain, and fortified products can be suggested to boost dietary intake of folate.

Antioxidants

Antioxidants have been studied individually and collectively for their potential to enhance exercise performance or to prevent exercise-induced muscle tissue damage. Cells continuously produce free radicals and **reactive oxygen species (ROS)** as a part of metabolic processes. The rate of whole-body oxygen consumption during exercise may increase 10- to 15-fold, or as much as 100-fold in active peripheral skeletal muscles. Oxidative stress increases the generation of lipid peroxides and free radicals. The magnitude of stress depends on the ability of the body's tissues to detoxify ROS.

Free radicals are neutralized by antioxidant defense systems that protect the cell membrane from oxidative damage. These systems include catalase; superoxide dismutase; glutathione peroxidase; antioxidant vitamins A, E, and C; selenium; and phytonutrients such as carotenoids (see *Focus On:* Eating to Detoxify in Chapter 20).

Whether exercise increases the need for additional antioxidants in the diet is unclear. Watson and colleagues (2005) compared antioxidant-restricted diets and high-antioxidant diets of trained athletes running for 40 minutes (acute high-intensity exercise); they found an increased rate of perceived exertion, significantly higher levels of oxidative stress markers, and up to 1 hour of recovery in those with antioxidant-deficient diets. In a more recent study, for the first time the antioxidant status of athletes was changed by live-high-train-low (LHTL) conditioning or acute hypoxic exposure, and remained impaired after 14 days of recovery (Pialoux et al., 2010).

Vitamins with antioxidant activity neutralize free radicals. The question is whether they enhance recovery from exercise. Susceptibility to oxidative stress appears to vary from person to person and the effect varies by diet, lifestyle, environmental factors, and training (Pialoux et al., 2009). Antioxidant nutrients may enhance recovery from exercise, maintaining optimal immune response, and lowering lipid peroxidation after exercise.

Evidence suggests that the antioxidant compounds found in tart cherry juice can help to reduce inflammation, muscle damage and oxidative stress following marathon running. An unexpected effect of tart cherry juice is that it may also have beneficial effect on sleep which has been attributed to the high melatonin content of tart cherries and its impact on sleep quality (Howatson et al., 2010; Kuehl et al., 2010; Pigeon et al., 2010). A diet rich in fruits and vegetables can ensure an adequate intake of antioxidants and prudent use of an antioxidant supplement may provide insurance against a suboptimal diet and the increased stress from exercise.

Vitamin C

Vitamin C is involved in a number of important biochemical pathways that are important to exercise metabolism and the health of athletes. The effect of vitamin C supplementation on performance has received considerable attention, mainly because athletes consume vitamin C in large quantities, generally because of the volume of food they consume. In studies in which athletes were deficient in vitamin C, supplementation improved physical performance, but a thorough analysis of these studies supports the general conclusion that vitamin C supplementation does not increase physical performance capacity in subjects with normal body levels of vitamin C. On the other hand, because exercise is a stressor to the body, some nutritionists recommend that the active individual may need more vitamin C than the DRI.

Vitamin E

Vitamin E is used widely as a supplement by athletes who hope to improve performance. Vitamin E may protect against exercise-induced oxidative injury and acute immune response changes. Over the course of an exercise season with intense workouts and competition, vitamin E supplementation of 200 to 450 IU daily may prevent oxidative injury; further studies are recommended.

Vitamin D

Research has shown that up to 77% of athletes who live in northern climates with little winter sunlight may be affected by deficiencies of vitamin D (Cannell et al., 2009).

Athletes who are at risk for Vitamin D deficiency include those who:

are lactose intolerant and avoid milk and dairy

don't consume fish

live in colder, less sunny climates

have darker skin, like African-Americans, even if they live and train in sunny climates

use sun block on exposed areas or wear extensive clothing (Cannell et al., 2009; Larson-Meyer and Willis, 2010)

Blood tests can determine deficiency states. A measurement of 25-(OH) vitamin D levels of 50 ng/mL or less may be cause for concern. The most improvement with supplementation will be for those with a value of 15 to 30 ng/mL, followed by those with 30 to 50 ng/mL (Cannell et al., 2009).

Although the specific amount of vitamin D needed to reverse deficiency states has not been determined, partly because it is dependent on the extent of deficiency, athletes should be tested and guided by a health professional if diagnosed with a deficiency. The RDA for males and females under age 70 is 600 IU and for those 70 and over, 800 IU/day. The tolerable upper intake level (UL) is 4000 IU/day for all individuals age 9 and older (IOM, 2011).

Iron

Iron is critical for sport performance. As a component of hemoglobin, it is instrumental in transporting oxygen from the lungs to the tissues. It performs a similar role in **myoglobin**, which acts within the muscle as an oxygen acceptor to hold a supply of oxygen readily available for use by the mitochondria. Iron is also a vital component of the cytochrome enzymes involved in the production of ATP. Thus it follows that iron-deficiency anemia limits aerobic endurance and the capacity for work. Even partial depletion of iron stores in the liver, spleen, and bone marrow, as evidenced by low serum ferritin levels, can have a detrimental effect on exercise performance, even when anemia is not present (see Chapters 8 and 33).

Although iron-deficiency anemia is not frequent in athletes, suboptimal serum ferritin levels are relatively common (Sinclair and Hinton, 2005). Athletes at risk are the rapidly growing male adolescent; the female athlete with heavy menstrual losses; the athlete with an energy-restricted diet; distance runners who may have increased GI iron loss, hematuria, hemolysis caused by foot impact, and myoglobin leakage; and those training heavily in hot climates with heavy sweating. All athletes, especially female long-distance runners and vegetarians, should be screened periodically to assess their iron status.

Heavy training can also cause a transient decrease in serum ferritin and hemoglobin that may be experienced by some athletes. This was once called **sports anemia**, but erythrocyte morphology remains normal, and performance does not appear to deteriorate. These decreases in serum ferritin and hemoglobin are a result of an increase in plasma volume, which causes a hemodilution and appears to have no effect on performance (see Chapter 33).

Some athletes, especially long-distance runners, experience GI bleeding. Iron loss through GI bleeding can be detected by fecal hemoglobin assays. GI bleeding is related to the intensity and duration of the exercise, the ability of the athlete to stay hydrated, how well the athlete is trained, and whether he or she has taken ibuprofen before the competition.

The iron concentration in sweat is lower in a hot environment. Iron supplementation can be beneficial in improving iron stores of athletes who are iron depleted, but the effects on aerobic performance of nonanemic athletes are equivocal. Because large doses of iron (75 mg/day) may be toxic in persons with the genetic disorder hemochromatosis (see Chapter 33), such supplements should be used only by those diagnosed as iron depleted or anemic.

If true iron depletion is present, iron supplementation along with vitamin C to enhance its absorption is appropriate. Oral iron therapy is effective and maintains performance in runners who are deficient in iron but not anemic (see Chapter 33). Some athletes experience iron deficiency without anemia, a condition with normal hemoglobin levels but reduced levels of serum ferritin (20 to 30 ng/mL; see Chapter 8). Iron supplementation may restore serum ferritin to normal; it may not have an effect on performance (Williams, 2005).

Calcium

Osteoporosis is a major health concern, especially for women. Although the disease has been regarded as a problem of older women, young women, especially those who have had interrupted menstrual function, may be at risk for decreased bone mass.

The **female athlete triad** is a disturbing pattern in women's athletics (see Chapter 23). Strategies to promote the resumption of menses include estrogen replacement therapy, weight gain, and reduced training. Regardless of menstrual history, most female athletes need to increase their calcium and vitamin D_3 intake, as well as magnesium. Low-fat and nonfat dairy products, calcium-fortified fruit juices, calcium-fortified soy milk, and tofu made with calcium sulfate are all good sources.

FLUID

Maintaining fluid balance requires the constant integration of input from hypothalamic osmoreceptors and vascular baroreceptors so that fluid intake matches or modestly exceeds fluid loss (Murray, 2006). Proper fluid balance maintains blood volume, which in turn supplies blood to the skin for body temperature regulation. Because exercise produces heat, which must be eliminated from the body to maintain appropriate temperatures, regular fluid intake is essential. Any fluid deficit that is incurred during an exercise session can potentially compromise the subsequent exercise bout.

The body maintains appropriate temperatures by **thermoregulation**. As heat is generated in the muscles during exercise, it is transferred via the blood to the body's core. Increased core temperature results in increased blood flow to the skin; in cool to moderate ambient temperatures, heat is then transferred to the environment by convection, radiation, and evaporation.

Environmental conditions have a large effect on thermoregulation. When ambient temperatures range from warm to hot, the body must dissipate the heat generated from exercise, as well as the heat absorbed from the environment. When this occurs, the body relies solely on the evaporation of sweat to maintain appropriate body temperatures. Thus maintaining hydration becomes crucial when ambient temperatures reach or exceed 36° C (96.8° F). The hotter the temperature, the more important sweating is for body-heat dissipation. Exercise in the heat also affects blood flow and alters the stress response, with modest changes in circulating leukocytes and cytokines. A critical threshold for elevation of body temperature is 6° F (3.5° C), above which the systemic inflammatory response leads to heatstroke (Peake, 2010).

Humidity affects the body's ability to dissipate heat to a greater extent than air temperatures. As humidity increases, the rate at which sweat evaporates decreases, which means more sweat drips off the body without transferring heat from the body to the environment. Combining the effects of a hot, humid environment with a large metabolic heat load produced during exercise taxes the thermoregulatory system to its maximum. Ensuring proper and adequate fluid intake is key to reducing the risk of heat stress.

Fluid Balance

Body fluid balance is regulated by mechanisms that reduce urinary water and sodium excretion, stimulate thirst, and control the intake and output of both water and electrolytes. In response to dehydration, antidiuretic hormone (ADH or vasopressin) and the renin-angiotensin II–aldosterone system increase water and sodium retention by the kidneys and provoke an increase in thirst. These hormones maintain the osmolality, sodium content, and volume of extracellular fluids and play a major role in the regulation of fluid balance (see Chapter 7).

Water losses throughout the course of the day include those from sweat and the respiratory tract, plus losses from the kidneys and GI tract. When fluid is lost from the body in the form of sweat, plasma volume decreases and plasma osmolality increases. The kidneys, under hormonal control, regulate water and solute excretion in excess of the obligatory urine loss. However, when the body is subjected to hot environments, hormonal adjustments occur to maintain body function. Some of these adjustments include the body's conservation of water and sodium and the release of ADH by the pituitary gland to increase water absorption from the kidneys. These changes cause the urine to become more concentrated, thus conserving fluid and making the urine a dark gold color. This feedback process helps to conserve body water and blood volume.

At the same time, aldosterone is released from the adrenal cortex and acts on the renal tubules to increase the resorption of sodium, which helps maintain the correct osmotic pressure. These reactions also activate thirst mechanisms in the body. However, in situations in which water losses are increased acutely such as in athletic workouts or competition, the thirst response can be delayed, making it difficult for athletes to trust their thirst to ingest enough fluid to offset the volume of fluid lost during training and competition. A loss of 1.5 to 2 L of fluid is necessary before the thirst mechanism kicks in, and this level of water loss already has a serious effect on temperature control. Athletes need to rehydrate on a timed basis rather than as a reaction to thirst, and it should be enough to maintain the preexercise weight.

Daily Fluid Needs

Daily fluid intake recommendations for sedentary individuals vary greatly because of the wide disparity in daily fluid needs created by body size, physical activity, and environmental conditions. The DRI for water and electrolytes identify the adequate intake for water to be 3.7 L/day in men (130 oz/day, 16 cups of fluid/day) and 2.7 L/day for women (95 oz/day, approximately 12 cups/day) (Institute of Medicine, 2004). Approximately 20% of the daily water need comes from water found in fruits and vegetables; the remaining 80% is provided by beverages, including water, juice, milk, coffee, tea, soup, sports drinks, and soft drinks.

When individuals work, train, and compete in warm environments, their fluid needs can increase to more than 10 L/day. The water required to excrete the urea from protein metabolism and excess electrolyte intake adds to the daily needs. However, for active individuals this volume is relatively small (130 mL/1000 kcal) and inconsequential because usually they are consuming more than 2 L each day (Murray, 2006).

Fluid Replacement

Several opinions are published by a variety of professional organizations that address fluid and electrolyte replacement before, during, and after exercise. A summary of these recommendations can be found in Box 24-2. The groups that developed these statements include the American College of Sports Medicine, the National Athletic Trainers Association, the American Academy of Pediatrics, the American Dietetic Association and the Dietitians of Canada, the International Marathon Directors Association, the Inter-Association Task Force on External Heat Illnesses, and USA Track and Field.

When possible, fluid should be consumed at rates that closely match sweating rate. It appears that plain water is not the best beverage to consume following exercise to replace the water lost as sweat (Murray, 2006). Although specific recommendations differ slightly, the intent is to keep athletes well hydrated.

Electrolytes

The replacement of electrolytes as well as water is essential for complete rehydration (see Table 24-1).

Sodium

It is important to include sodium in fluid-replacement solutions, especially with excessive intake of plain water (Hew, 2005; Noakes et al., 2005). For events lasting more than 2 hours, sodium should be added to the fluid to replace losses and to prevent hyponatremia. Rehydration with water alone dilutes the blood rapidly, increases its volume, and stimulates urine output. Blood dilution lowers both sodium and the volume-dependent part of the thirst drive, thus removing much of the drive to drink and replace fluid losses.

The potential benefits of temporary hyperhydration with sodium salts is important. Sodium losses can contribute to heat cramping, especially among football players (Stofan et al., 2005). Besides individual variations, the intensity and duration of workouts appear to play a role in the amount of sodium lost.

Water-soluble electrolytes such as sodium can move rapidly across the proximal intestines. During prolonged exercise lasting more than 4 to 5 hours, including sodium in replacement fluids increases palatability and facilitates fluid uptake in the intestines. Both sodium and carbohydrate are actively transported from the lumen to the bloodstream.

Water replacement in the absence of supplemental sodium can lead to decreased plasma sodium concentrations. As plasma sodium levels fall below 130 mEq/L, symptoms can include lethargy, confusion, seizures, or loss of consciousness. Exercise-induced hyponatremia may result from fluid overloading during prolonged exercise over 4 hours. Hyponatremia is associated with individuals who drink plain water in excess of their sweat losses or who are less physically conditioned and produce a saltier sweat.

BOX 24-2

Summary of Guidelines for Proper Hydration

General Guidelines

Monitor fluid losses: Weigh in before and after practice, especially during hot weather and the conditioning phase of the season.

Do not restrict fluids before, during, or after the event.

Do not rely on thirst as an indicator of fluid losses.

Drink early and at regular intervals throughout the activity.

Do not consume alcohol before, during, or after exercise because it may act as a diuretic and prevent adequate fluid replenishment.

Discourage caffeinated beverages a few hours before and after physical activity because of their diuretic effect.

Before Exercise

Drink approximately 400 to 600 mL (14 to 22 oz) of water or sports drink (approximately 17 oz) 2 to 3 hr before the start of exercise.

During Exercise

Drink 150 to 350 mL (6 to 12 oz) of fluid every 15 to 20 min, depending on race speed, environmental conditions, and tolerance; no more than 1 C (8 to 10 oz) every 15 to 20 min, although individualized recommendations must be followed.

After Exercise

Drink 25% to 50% more than existing weight loss to ensure hydration 4-6 hours after exercise.

Drink 450 to 675 mL (16 to 24 oz) of fluid for every pound of body weight lost during exercise.

If an athlete is participating in multiple workouts in 1 day, then 80% of fluid loss must be replaced before the next workout.

Electrolyte Replacement

Sodium: 0.5 to 0.7 g/L in activity longer than 1 hour to enhance palatability and the drive to drink and to reduce the risk of hyponatremia and minimize risk of muscle cramps.

Data from Murray R: Fluid, electrolytes, and exercise. In Danford M, editor: Sports nutrition: a practice manual for professionals, ed 4, Washington, DC, 2006, American Dietetic Association.

Potassium

As the major electrolyte inside the body's cells, potassium works in close association with sodium and chloride in maintaining body fluids, as well as generating electrical impulses in the nerves, muscles, and heart. Potassium balance is regulated by aldosterone and regulation is precise. Although aldosterone acts on sweat glands to increase the resorption of sodium, potassium secretion is unaffected. Loss of potassium from skeletal muscle has been implicated in fatigue during athletic events. There is little loss of potassium through sweat; loss of 32 to 48 mEq/day does not appear to be significant and is easily replaced by diet.

Fluid Absorption

The speed at which fluid is absorbed depends on a number of different factors, including the amount, type, temperature, and osmolality of the fluid consumed and the rate of gastric emptying. Because glucose is actively absorbed in the intestines, it can markedly increase both sodium and water absorption. A carbohydrate-electrolyte solution enhances exercise capacity by elevating blood sugar, maintaining high rates of carbohydrate oxidation, preventing central fatigue, and reducing perceived exertion (Byrne et al., 2005).

Early studies indicate that water absorption is maximized when luminal glucose concentrations range from 1% to 3% (55 to 140 mM); however, most sports drinks contain two to three times this quantity without causing adverse GI symptoms. To determine the concentration of carbohydrate in a sports drink, the grams of carbohydrate or sugar in a serving are divided by the weight of a serving of the drink, which is usually 240 g, the approximate weight of 1 cup of water. A 6% carbohydrate drink contains 14 to 16 g of carbohydrate per 8 oz (1 cup).

Cold water is preferable to warm water because it attenuates changes in core temperature and peripheral blood flow, decreases sweat rate, speeds up gastric emptying, and is absorbed more quickly.

Children

Because young children are likely to participate in physical activities less than 60 minutes in duration there is often little attention to their hydration. Children do not drink enough when offered fluids freely during exercise in hot and humid climates. But children differ from adults in that, for any given level of dehydration, their core temperatures rise faster than those of adults, putting them at far greater risk for heat stress. Children who participate in sports activities must be taught to prevent dehydration by drinking above and beyond thirst and at frequent intervals, such as every 20 minutes.

A rule of thumb is that a child 10 years of age or younger should drink until he or she does not feel thirsty and then should drink an additional half a glass (⅓ to ½ cup). Older children and adolescents should follow the same guidelines; however, they should consume an additional cup of fluid (8 oz). When relevant, regulations for competition should be modified to allow children to leave the playing field periodically to drink. One of the hurdles to getting children to consume fluids is to provide fluids they like. Providing a sports drink that will maintain the drive to drink and rehydrate them is the key.

Older Athletes

Older, mature, or masters-level athletes are also at risk for dehydration and need to take precautions when exercising or staying fit. **Hypohydration** (water loss exceeding water intake with a body water deficit) in older individuals can affect circulatory and thermoregulatory function to a greater extent and may be caused by the lower skin blood flow, causing core temperature to rise. Because the thirst drive is reduced in older adults, they need to drink adequately before exercise, well before they become thirsty. Women athletes need to drink more than men during interval exercise in the heat. Fluid balance is maintained better when palatable carbohydrate and electrolyte solutions are offered (Baker et al., 2005).

Hydration at High Altitudes

Unacclimated individuals undergo a plasma volume contraction when acutely exposed to moderately high altitude. This is the result of increased renal sodium and water excretion and decreased voluntary sodium and water intake. Respiratory losses are increased by high ventilatory rates and typically dry air. The result is an increase in serum hematocrit and hemoglobin, which increases the oxygen-carrying capacity of the blood, but at the cost of reduced blood volume, stroke volume, and cardiac output. Fluid requirements increase as a result. With acclimation, red blood cell production increases and plasma and blood volume return to pre–high altitude levels.

OTHER CONSIDERATIONS

Alcohol

Alcohol is a central nervous system depressant. Pure alcohol supplies 7 kcal/g and is a source of energy that is metabolized more like fat. For alcohol to be used by muscle, it must first be metabolized in the liver. Alcohol consumption immediately before or during exercise has a detrimental effect on athletic performance, even though, by reducing feelings of insecurity, tension, and discomfort, it may cause the athlete to believe that he or she is performing better. Some athletes incorrectly believe that because alcohol contains carbohydrates, they can load up on beer to improve their performance. Perceptual motor performance, gross motor skills, balance, and coordination are affected by alcohol consumption.

Alcohol may cause reduced glucose secretion from the liver, which may lead to hypoglycemia and early fatigue during endurance exercise. Alcohol may also be a contributing factor to hypothermia if consumed during exercise in cold weather. Alcohol should not be used to replace fluids immediately after exercise because of its diuretic effect and adverse effects on blood glucose and glycogen levels. Chronic alcohol use causes the loss of many nutrients important for performance and health, including thiamin, vitamin B_6, and calcium.

Caffeine

Caffeine contributes to endurance performance, apparently because of its ability to enhance mobilization of fatty acids and thus conserve glycogen stores. Caffeine may also directly affect muscle contractility, possibly by facilitating calcium transport. It could reduce fatigue as well by reducing plasma potassium accumulation, which contributes to fatigue. Probably some ergogenic effects occur at doses of 6.5 mg/kg of body weight when taken before endurance exercise, however, caffeine does not seem to offer any benefits before high-intensity exercise.

Because of this potential ergogenic effect, caffeine is banned by the International Olympic Committee (IOC), although the banned level is much higher than that needed to enhance performance. An energy-enhancing effect is seen with only 1.5 to 3 mg of caffeine per pound (3.3 to 6.6 mg/kg). For a 150-lb man this is equivalent to only one 10-oz cup of coffee. As fluid-replacement beverages, tea, iced tea, coffee, cola, caffeinated water, and some of the new caffeine-containing energy drinks are poor choices because of their diuretic effect and variable carbohydrate content. The diuretic action of caffeine could have negative consequences for athletes with excessive water needs or for those participating in long-distance events who do not want to have to urinate during the event. As a restricted drug by the IOC, caffeine is considered a doping agent if the intake results in urine caffeine concentrations of more than 12 mg/L.

ERGOGENIC AIDS

Ergogenic aids include any training technique, mechanical device, nutrition practice, pharmacologic method, or physiologic technique that can improve exercise performance capacity and training adaptations. The use of ergogenic aids in the form of dietary supplements is widespread in all sports. Many athletes, whether recreational, elite, or professional, use some form of dietary supplementation (e.g., substances obtainable by prescription or by illegal means or others marked as supplements, vitamins, or minerals) to improve athletic performance or to assist with weight loss (Dhar et al., 2005). Research suggests that 50% to 98.6% of university athletes use some form of supplements as ergogenic aids (Kristiansen et al., 2005; Neiper, 2005).

Reasons for supplement use differ between genders. Women athletes reported taking supplements for their health or to overcome an inadequate diet, whereas men may take supplements to improve speed, agility, strength, and power. Health reasons (45%), immune system enhancement (40%), and performance improvement (25%) have also been cited as reasons for supplement use (Neiper, 2005). Performance enhancement supplements are pills, drinks, bars, or gels that improve speed, strength, or performance, or minimize or delay fatigue (Bishop, 2010). Supplements used to help build body mass and reduce weight or excess body fat may also enhance exercise performance. The most common supplements used by athletes are described in Tables 24-2 and 24-3.

Athletes are bombarded with advertisements and testimonials from other athletes and coaches about the effects of dietary supplements on performance. The Dietary Supplement Health and Education Act (DSHEA) protects dietary supplements from being required to demonstrate proof of efficacy or safety (see Chapter 13). Under this act the Food and Drug Administration no longer has regulatory control of supplements and they are now classified as foods. Manufacturers are allowed to publish limited information about the benefits of dietary supplements in the form of statements of support, as well as so-called structure and function claims. This results in a great deal of printed material that can be confusing to athletes at the point of sale of nutritional products.

Research suggests that the Internet, family members, friends, physicians, or pharmacists guide supplement choices for women athletes; whereas the store nutritionist, fellow athletes, friends, or coaches, advise on supplement decisions for men athletes (Kristiansen et al., 2005). Many believe that ergogenic aids will improve their performance and assist in recovery. As in the past and probably in the future, many of these ergogenic aids are not supported by scientific studies. In fact, many act only as placebos (Figure 24-6).

Many of these supplements confer no performance or health benefit, and some may actually be detrimental to both performance and health when taken for prolonged periods. They may contain excessive doses of potentially toxic ingredients or contain significant amounts of ingredients not approved by the IOC, the World Anti-Doping Agency, the National Collegiate Athletic Association (NCAA), Major League Baseball, and the National Football League (NFL) (Maughan, 2005).

Sports nutritionists need to know how to evaluate the scientific merit of articles and advertisements about exercise and nutrition products so they can separate marketing hype from scientifically based training and nutrition practices. Performance-enhancing substances such as anabolic-androgenic steroids, tetrahydrogestrinone, and androstenedione (andro); stimulants such as ephedra; and nonsteroidal agents such as recombinant human erythropoietin (EPO), human growth hormone (HGH), creatine, and β-hydroxy-β-methylbutyrate (HMB) may cause serious side effects, including adverse cardiovascular changes and sudden death (Dhar et al., 2005).

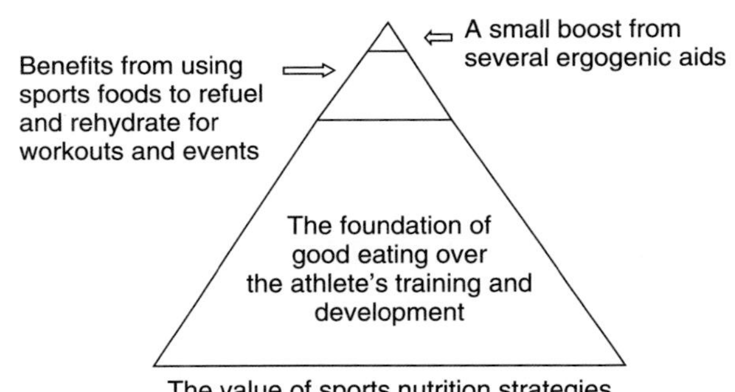

FIGURE 24-6 The value of sports nutrition strategies versus sports drinks and ergogenic aids. *(From Australia Sports. Accessed 14 July 2010 at http://fulltext.ausport.gov.au/fulltext/2001/ascpub/images/FactSupp2.gif.)*

TABLE 24-2

Recommendations for Use of Sport Foods and Drinks

Sport Food	Characteristics	Guidelines for Consumption in Exercise		
		Before	During	After
Sports drink	CHO: 5%-7% by volume (approximately 14 g/8 oz) Sodium: 20-30 mEq/L (110-165 mg/8 oz) Multiple carbohydrates with high glycemic indices	0.5 L (16 oz) 1 hr before exercise	150-300 mL every 15-20 min (20-40 oz/hr)	24 oz/lb of body weight lost
High CHO energy drink	CHO: >13% by volume (more than 50 g/8 oz) Optional B vitamins: thiamin, niacin, and riboflavin at 10%-40% of RDA	0.5 L (16 oz) 2-5 hr before exercise	Typically not advised for use during the event	Immediately after and at 1-hr intervals to deliver 1 g CHO/kg of body weight
Sports bar	CHO: >70% of total kcal High glycemic index Fat: low (1-2 g/bar) or absent Vitamins and minerals not critical component	One bar 2 hr before exercise	Usually not advised except for those desiring solid foods during long-duration events	One to two bars immediately after exercise and with daily meals as desired
Sports shake	CHO: >65% of total kcal (>18 g/100 mL) High glycemic index Fat: not to exceed 25% of total kcal Protein: 15%-20% of total kcal Vitamins and minerals: optional at low levels (10%-40% of RDA)	0.5 L (16 oz) 2-5 hr before exercise	Not recommended	Immediately after exercise to deliver 1 g CHO/kg body weight and as a supplement to daily meals
Energy gel	CHO: >50% by volume (>50 g/100 mL or 15 g/oz) Vitamins and minerals: trace or absent Avoid those with herbs	1 packet before exercise; consume adequate fluid to promote absorption	If overall fluid intake is adequate, enough to supply 30-60 g CHO/hr	Immediately after exercise and at 1-hr intervals to deliver 1 g CHO/kg body weight
Shot bloks	Organic electrolyte chew Gelatin consistency CHO: 24 g/1 oz 3 bloks = 100 cal plus electrolytes	Not applicable	3-6 bloks every hour with water	Not applicable
Sports beans	CHO: 25 g/1 oz 14 beans = 100 cal 10% DV of vitamins B_1, B_2, B_3 20% DV of vitamins C and E	Not applicable	Up to 14 pieces per hour for energy	Not applicable

Modified from Gatorade Sports Science Institute.

CHO, Carbohydrate; *DV*, daily value; *RDA*, recommended dietary allowance.

Muscle-Building Supplements

Muscle-building supplements include amino acids, HMB, creatine, prohormones, glutamine, protein, high-calorie powders, protein-fortified beverages and bars, and other compounds listed in Table 24-2.

Amino Acids

Protein or amino acid supplementation in the form of powders or pills is not necessary and should be discouraged. Taking large amounts of protein or amino acid supplements can lead to dehydration, hypercalciuria, weight gain, and stress on the kidney and liver. Taking single amino acids or in combination, such as arginine and lysine, may interfere with the absorption of certain other essential amino acids. An additional concern is that substituting amino acid supplements for food may cause deficiencies of other nutrients found in protein-rich foods such as iron, zinc, niacin, and thiamin. Athletes and coaches need to realize that amino

TABLE 24-3

Ergogenic Aids

Ergogenic Aid	Reported Action/Claim	Research on Ergogenic Effects	Side Effects	Legality
α-Ketoglutarate	Intermediate in Krebs cycle.	Some evidence as anticatabolic after surgery; unclear in training.	None	Legal
ALA	Enzyme found in mitochondria involved in energy production.	No studies of use in humans for sport; used in Europe with persons with diabetes to treat insulin resistance and neuropathy.	None	Legal
Amino Acids				
Arginine	Protein synthesis; precursor to creatine and potential to increase GH; precursor to NO.	Little evidence; some rationale for athletic improvement may be the result of role as precursor to NO; some improvement in cardiac patients on protocol of 1.5 g/10 kg of body weight for 7 days.	None	Legal
Branched-chain amino acids	Decreases mental fatigue. Decreases exercise-induced protein degradation and muscle enzyme release.	Some evidence that decreased fatigue may occur at higher altitudes.	Mild	Legal
EAAs		Limited; suggests 3-6 g of EAAs before exercise; stimulates protein synthesis.	Same as protein	Legal
Glutamine	Boosts immunity; stimulates protein and glycogen synthesis.	May boost immunity with branched-chain amino acids and enriched whey.	None	Legal
HMB	Anticatabolic; enhances recovery by stimulating protein and glycogen synthesis.	Minimum gains in strength and lean body mass in untrained athletes and the elderly; possibly catabolic with prolonged exercise; mixed reports in trained subjects.	None with short-term use	Legal
Chokeberry juice	Enhances endogenous antioxidant defense system.	Limits exercise-induced oxidative damage to red blood cells.	None reported	Legal
Chitosan	Inhibits fat absorption; lowers cholesterol.	No evidence in humans.	None reported	Legal
Citrus aurantium, bitter orange, synephrine	Increases metabolism.	No evidence of weight-reducing properties.	None reported	Legal
Ciwujia aka Siberian ginseng ES	Improves CF, FAM, and EP.	Mixed; limited research shows improvement in CF, FAM, EP, although studies flawed	None reported	Legal
Chondroitin sulfate	Builds and grows cartilage.	No studies that it is effective in treating arthritis or joint damage or helps torn ligaments or cartilage.	None	Legal

Continued

TABLE 24-3

Ergogenic Aids—cont'd

Ergogenic Aid	Reported Action/Claim	Research on Ergogenic Effects	Side Effects	Legality
Ephedrine, other sympathomimetics Pseudoephedrine, ma huang	Stimulates central nervous system; increases energy.	With caffeine, increases energy, time to exhaustion; increases metabolism without exercise; without caffeine, no benefits.	Restlessness, nervousness, tachycardia, arrhythmias, hypertension, death	Banned by NFL, NCAA, and IOC
Glucosamine	Serves as nonsteroidal antiinflammatory drug alternative.	Readily absorbed; benefit in reducing pain and need for medication.	None reported	Legal
Green tea extract	Antioxidant; increases energy expenditure.	Limited; may increase energy expenditure.	Same as caffeine	Legal
Human growth hormone	Anabolic effect on muscle growth; increases fat metabolism.	Limited ergogenic benefits.	Significant and dangerous	Illegal
MSM	Metabolite of dimethylsulfoxide, a solvent used topically for analgesic and antiinflammatory properties.	Little evidence of effectiveness for pain control in humans.	None	Legal
NO	Promotes a "muscle pump," signals muscle growth and speeds recovery.	No evidence that NO promotes muscle growth synthesis or improves muscle strength.	None	Legal
Ornithine-α-ketoglutarate	Anabolic/catabolic	Limited; may improve protein balance, gains in bench press, but no significant gains in muscle mass, GH, squat strength, or training capacity.	None reported	Legal
Oxygenated beverages	Increases aerobic metabolism, decreases lactic acid, improves endurance.	Performance hydration and blood oxygenation unaffected by oxygenated water.	None	Legal
Ribose	3-Carbon carbohydrate; involved in synthesis of adenosine triphosphate.	Limited; can increase exercise capacity in heart patients; no effect on exercise capacity in trained or untrained subjects.	None reported	Legal
Sodium bicarbonate	Buffers lactic acid production; delays fatigue.	Increases body's ability to buffer lactic acid during sub max exercise for events lasting 1-7 min.	Stomach distress: bloating, diarrhea; dangerous in high doses; alkalosis	Legal
Sodium phosphate	Buffer	Some; increases Vo_2max and anaerobic threshold by 5%-10%; improves endurance.	Stomach distress	Legal
Tribulus terrestris	Increases endogenous steroid production; promotes skeletal hypertrophy.	Mixed; no effect on strength or change in body composition.	Potentially dangerous at high doses	Legal
Vanadyl sulfate (Vanadium)	Trace mineral; may affect protein and glucose metabolism.	No effect on strength training or muscle mass during training.	None reported	Legal

For additional information go to http://gssiweb.org/Article_Detail.aspx?articleid=704&level=3&topic=9.

ALA, α-Lipoic acid; *CF*, cardiorespiratory fitness; *EAA*, essential amino acid; *EP*, endurance performance; *ES*, *Eleutherococcus senticosus;* *FAM*, fat metabolism; *GH*, growth hormone; *HMB*, β-hydroxy-β-methylbutyrate; *IOC*, International Olympic Committee; *MSM*, methylsulfonylmethane; *NCAA*, National Collegiate Athletic Association; *NFL*, National Football League; *NO*, nitric oxide.

acid supplements taken in large doses have not been tested in human subjects, and no margin of safety is available. It is important for the health professional to develop a strategy to approach and discuss this supplement use effectively with both athletes and coaches.

Branched-chain amino acids

The BCAAs include leucine, isoleucine, and valine and they make up 35% to 40% of the essential amino acids (EAAs) in the body's protein and 14% of the total AAs in muscle. In order to get energy, the body can break down muscle to get the BCAAs. During times of stress, BCAAs are required more than any other EAA.

BCAAs consumed before and after training have been shown to increase protein synthesis and muscle gains beyond normal adaptation. They have been reported to decrease exercise-induced protein breakdown and muscle enzyme release, which is a sign of muscle damage. Some research suggests that 14 grams of BCAAs during eight weeks of weight training can produce a significantly greater weight gain in lean mass.

Dairy products and red meat contain the greatest amounts of BCAAs. Whey protein and egg protein supplements are also good sources.

Branched-chain amino acid	Food sources
Leucine	meats, dairy, nuts, beans, brown rice, soy, and whole wheat
Isoleucine	meats, chicken, eggs, fish, almonds, chickpeas, soy protein, and most seeds
Valine	meat, dairy, soy protein, grains, peanuts, and mushrooms

Leucine is the most readily oxidized BCAA and is most effective at causing insulin secretion from the pancreas. It lowers elevated blood sugar levels and aids in growth hormone production. Leucine works in conjunction with isoleucine and valine to protect muscle and act as fuel for the body. Doses of up to 2 grams (2000 mg) post workout have been suggested by some experts for accelerating muscle repair and recovery.

β-Hydroxy-β-Methylbutyrate

HMB is an important compound made in the body and a metabolite of the essential amino acid leucine. In humans oral administration of HMB has been associated with increased body mass across the young, elderly, untrained, trained, and clinically cachexic (Wilson JM et al., 2009). The effects of HMB supplementation in trained athletes is not clear, with most studies reporting nonsignificant gains in muscle mass (Palisin and Stacy, 2005). Regarding HMB supplementation and exercise recovery, several studies have found that subjects supplemented with HMB may have less stress-induced muscle protein breakdown. Recent research suggests that both acute and chronic administration of HMB are associated with less exercise-induced muscle damage and soreness (Wilson JM et al., 2009), Additional research is necessary to determine the effectiveness of this supplement both as an ergogenic and recovery aid for athletes.

Creatine

Creatine is an amino acid normally produced in the body from arginine, glycine, and methionine. Most dietary creatine comes from meat, but half is manufactured in the liver and kidneys. For meat eaters, dietary intake of creatine is approximately 1 g daily. The body also synthesizes approximately 1 g of creatine per day, for a total production of approximately 2 g daily.

In normal healthy persons approximately 40% of muscle creatine exists as free creatine; the remainder combines with phosphate to form CP. Approximately 2% of the body's creatine is broken down daily to creatinine before excretion by the kidneys. The normal daily excretion of creatinine is approximately 2 g for most persons. Those with lower levels of intramuscular creatine such as vegetarians may respond to creatine supplementation (Williams, 2006).

Creatine is one of the most researched and popular sports supplements. It supplies most of the energy for short-term, maximum exercise such as weight lifting, running a 100-m sprint, swinging a bat, or punting a football. Supplementation elevates muscle creatine levels and facilitates the regeneration of CP, which helps to regenerate ATP. When creatine stores in the muscles are depleted, ATP synthesis is prevented and energy can no longer be supplied at the rate required by the working muscle. Improved athletic performance has been attributed to this ATP resynthesis.

Creatine supplementation increases body mass or muscle mass during training; short-term gains may be primarily water, whereas long-term gains along with resistance training are muscle mass (Williams, 2006). Studies suggest that creatine does not enhance exercise and events lasting more than 90 seconds (Astorino et al., 2005). However, creatine supplementation may improve submaximal exercise performance for HIIT, which promotes fitness similar to endurance training (Graef et al., 2009).

Creatine absorption appears to be stimulated by insulin. Therefore ingesting creatine supplements in combination with carbohydrate, amino acid, or protein can increase muscle creatine concentrations (Buford TW, 2007). Once creatine is taken up by the muscles, it is trapped within the muscle tissue. It is estimated that muscle creatine stores decline slowly and will still be elevated 2 to 3 months after ingestion of 20 g of creatine for 5 days.

Current thought is to consume creatine at a dose of 2 to 5 g daily. Human muscle appears to have an upper limit of creatine storage; thus excess creatine presumably will be of little benefit. Few data exist on the long-term benefits and risks of creatine supplementation. There have been anecdotal descriptions of athletes who have had muscle strains and tears, dehydration, and kidney damage (Rodriquez et al., 2009). Thus the American College of

Sports Medicine advises against taking creatine for youth 18 years old and younger.

Peptide Hormones

Erythropoietin. EPO is commonly used to keep up the body's production of red blood cells in patients with bone marrow suppression such as patients with leukemia, those who are receiving chemotherapy, or those with renal failure (see Chapter 36). In athletes, injections increase the serum hematocrit and oxygen-carrying capacity of the blood and thus enhance Vo_2max and endurance. EPO use as an ergogenic aid is difficult to detect because it is a hormone produced by the kidneys, although newer blood tests can detect its use. Typically, athletes with elevated hematocrit have been banned from endurance sports for suspected EPO misuse; however, despite its ban by the IOC, it is still commonly abused. Drastically high hematocrit combined with exercise-induced dehydration can lead to thick or viscous blood, which can lead to coronary or cerebral vascular occlusions, heart attack, or stroke. EPO can also cause elevated blood pressure or elevated potassium levels.

Human growth hormone (HGH) has many functions in the body, and it is produced naturally throughout life. It stimulates protein synthesis, enhances carbohydrate and fat metabolism, helps to maintain sodium balance, and stimulates bone and connective tissue turnover. HGH production decreases with age after the peak growth years. The amount secreted is affected by diet, stress, exercise, nutrition, and medications. HGH is banned by the IOC; however, it continues to be abused by athletes. Potential side effects can include skin changes, darkening of moles, an adverse effect on glucose metabolism and on the lipid profile, and growth of bones as evidenced by a protruding jaw and boxy forehead.

Prohormones and Steroids

Prohormones are popular among bodybuilders, many of whom believe that these prohormones are natural boosters of anabolic hormones. Androstenedione, 4-androstenediol, 19-nor-4-androstenedione, 19-nor-4-androstenediol, 7-keto dehydroepiandrosterone (DHEA) and 7-keto DHEA are naturally derived precursors to testosterone and other anabolic steroids. Androstenedione is an anabolic androgenic steroid used to increase blood testosterone levels for the purpose of increasing strength and lean body mass, although there is no research that it has that effect in humans. Although theoretically prohormones may increase testosterone levels, there is no evidence that these compounds affect training adaptations in younger men with normal hormone levels. They may even increase estrogen levels and low-density lipoprotein cholesterol levels and reduce high-density lipoprotein (HDL) cholesterol.

Androstenedione. Androstenedione (andro) is a prehormone, an inactive precursor to both female estrogen and male testosterone. It has about one seventh of the activity of testosterone and is a precursor that directly converts to testosterone by a single reaction. It is naturally produced in the body from either DHEA or 17-α-hydroxyprogesterone. Some researchers have found that taking andro elevates testosterone more than DHEA does; however, the induced increase lasts only several hours and remains at peak levels for just a few minutes. Acute or long-term administration of testosterone precursors does not effectively increase serum testosterone levels and fails to produce any significant changes in lean body mass, muscle strength, or performance improvement (Smurawa and Congeni, 2007).

Adverse reactions occur in male and female athletes, including muscle tightness and cramps, increased body weight, acne, GI problems, changes in libido, amenorrhea, liver damage, and stunted growth in adolescents. Consumption of a prohormone supplement can alter a patient's hypothalamic-pituitary-gonadal axis. Andro-related hormones may abnormally elevate estrogen-related hormones and alter elevations of serum estrogen, which is thought to increase the risk for developing prostate or pancreatic cancers. A significant decline in HDLs occur, leading to an increased cardiovascular disease risk (Dhar et al., 2005). Therefore taking androstenedione may be irresponsible because of the potential risks associated with long-term use. Until there is scientific support for its use, andro should not be sold under the assumption that it is either an effective or a safe athletic ergogenic aid. Clearly adolescents and women of childbearing age should not use it. In 1998 andro was added to the list of banned substances by the IOC and several amateur and professional organizations, including the NFL and the NCAA.

Dehydroepiandrosterone (DHEA) is a weak androgen and product of dehydroandrosterone-3-sulfate (DHEA-S) and is used to elevate testosterone levels. It is a precursor to more potent testosterone and dihydrotestosterone. Although DHEA-S is the most abundant circulating adrenal hormone in humans, its physiologic role is poorly understood. DHEA has been labeled the "fountain of youth" hormone because its levels peak during early adulthood. The decline with aging has been associated with increased fat accumulation and risk of heart disease. Several studies have suggested a positive correlation between increased plasma levels of DHEA and improved vigor, health, and well-being in persons who range in age from 40 to 80 years. By decreasing cortisol output from the liver by 50%, DHEA could have an anabolic effect. If this were to occur in muscle tissue as well, the anabolic effect would be comparable to that of anabolic steroids; however, no proof of this currently exists.

DHEA supplementation does not increase testosterone levels or increase strength in men, but it may increase testosterone levels in women with a virilizing effect. Because DHEA can take several different hormonal pathways, the one that it follows depends on several factors, including existing levels of other hormones. It can take several routes in the body and interact with certain enzymes along the sex-steroid pathway. Thus it can turn into less desirable byproducts of testosterone, including dihydrotestosterone, which is associated with male-pattern baldness, prostate enlargement, and acne.

Until recently DHEA was a prescription drug, but it is now sold over the counter. Analysis of DHEA products on the market shows a dramatic difference between the amount stated on the label and the actual amount in the product.

The benefits of taking DHEA for sports performance have not been clearly established, and the effects of chronic DHEA ingestion are not known. Long-term safety has not been established, and there are concerns that chronic use in men may worsen prostate hyperplasia or even promote prostate cancer. DHEA is not recommended for athletic use because it can alter the testosterone-epitestosterone ratio so that it exceeds the 6:1 limit set by the IOC, the U.S. Olympic Committee, the NFL, and the NCAA.

Steroids. Androgenic-anabolic steroids (AASs) categorize all male sex steroid hormones, their synthetic derivatives, and their active metabolites used to enhance athletic performance and appearance (DiLuigi et al., 2005). AAS use was reported in the 1950 Olympics and was banned in 1976. Steroids may be used in oral or intramuscular preparations.

The legal and illegal use of these drugs is increasing as a result of society's preoccupation with increasing muscle strength, size, and libido. Originally designed for therapeutic uses to provide enhanced anabolic potency, nontherapeutic use of AAS is increasing among adolescents and females (DiLuigi et al., 2005). Anecdotal evidence suggests widespread use of anabolic steroids among athletes (20% to 90%), especially at the professional and elite amateur levels. Use among high school boys is approximately 5% to 10%; rates among college athletes are slightly higher. Use of multiple steroids simultaneously in excess of therapeutic doses by 10-fold to 100-fold is known as "stacking" (Trenton and Currier, 2005). See Box 24-3 for a list of commonly abused steroids.

Short-term administration of these drugs by athletes can increase strength and body weight. **Anabolic effects** include increased muscle mass; increased bone mineral density; increased blood cell production; decreased body fat; increased heart, liver, and kidney size; vocal cord changes; and increased libido. Anabolic steroids increase protein synthesis in skeletal muscles and reverse catabolic processes; however, increased muscle mass and strength are observed only in athletes who maintain a high-protein, high-calorie diet during steroid administration. **Androgenic effects** are the development of secondary sexual characteristics in men, changes in genital size and function, and growth of auxiliary pubic and facial hair (Trenton and Currier, 2005). Some adverse effects associated with steroid use are irreversible, especially in women (Table 24-4).

BOX 24-3

Commonly Abused Steroids

Oral

oxymetholone (Anadrol)
oxandrolone (Oxandrin)
methandrostenolone (Dianabol)
stanozolol (Winstrol)

Injectable Steroids

stanozolol (Sanobolic)
nandroline decanoate (Deca Durabolin)
nandrolone phenylpropionate (Durabolin)
testosterone cypionate (Depo-Testosterone)
boldenone undecylenate (Equipoise)

TABLE 24-4

Effects of Androgenic Anabolic Steroids in Athletes

Children	Premature closing of growth plates
Males	Increase sex drive, acne vulgaris, enlarged breasts, testicular hypotrophy, infertility
Females	Clitoris enlargement, excessive body hair
Athletic performance	Increased strength and lean body mass; no increase in endurance performance
Cardiovascular system	Increased blood pressure, depression of HDL, HDL2, and HDL3 cholesterol
Hormonal changes	Disturbance in endocrine and immune function
Hepatic system	Peliosis (purpura), hepatitis, increased liver enzymes, jaundice, cancer
Immune compromised—those with HIV, AIDS, hepatitis	Infections from injectable forms
Mental health	Increase in aggressive behavior, mood disturbances (e.g., depression, hypomania, psychosis, homicidal rage, mania, delusions)
Metabolic changes	Changes in hemostatic system and urogenital tract, altered glucose metabolism, immune system suppression, low thyroid hormone levels
Physical	Short stature, tendon rupture
Skin	Acne, cysts, oily scalp

AIDS, Acquired immune deficiency syndrome; *HDL*, high-density lipoprotein; *HIV*, human immunodeficiency virus.

CLINICAL SCENARIO

Ben is a 21-year-old active college student who is interested in building muscle mass and losing body fat. His height is 5 ft 8 in, and his weight is 160 lb. Ben says that, although he is very disciplined, he has weekend splurges of a pizza and a six-pack of beer, as well as chips, ribs, and nuts during football, basketball, and baseball season. He does not work out on the weekends. He cannot understand why he is not losing body fat because he works out twice a day, includes resistance training and cardiovascular exercise, and eats the following:

Before Breakfast

1 protein bar with 45 g of protein and 300 calories

After Workout

1 protein drink with 30 g of protein

Breakfast

1 protein smoothie with berries and 60 g of protein
1 oatmeal with 1 whey protein scoop (25 g of protein)

Snack

3 oz bologna or ham

Lunch

1 turkey sandwich with 6-9 oz of protein, lettuce, and tomato

Before Afternoon Workout

1 protein bar with 60 g of protein

After Workout

Protein drink with 45 g of protein

Dinner

½ chicken, string beans, and a lettuce salad with olive oil

Nutrition Diagnostic Statement

Excessive protein intake related to frequent intake of protein bars and supplemental beverages, as evidenced by an intake of 265 g of protein per day from these products compared with a recommended dietary allowance (RDA) of 55 to 75 g/day for normal growth and development.

Nutrition Care Questions

1. How many grams of protein is Ben consuming? What is his protein per kilogram of body weight consumption? Can this be a contributing factor to his difficulty with losing body fat?
2. What level of protein intake would you recommend for him? Is this different from the RDA for normal growth and development? Are there healthier sources of protein that he can consume?
3. What is the calorie cost of his weekend splurges? Are they in excess of his calorie needs? And if so, by how much? What type of recovery beverages and protein dosages may be more suitable for Ben to consume? What additional questions would you ask Ben about his bars and supplements?
4. What nutrients are in deficient amounts in Ben's diet? Including what foods in his diet would be beneficial?
5. What are other changes Ben can make on the weekends? What foods and exercise will help him reduce his body fat and manage his weight better?

USEFUL WEBSITES

American College of Sports Medicine
www.acsm.org

American Council on Exercise
www.acefitness.org

American Sport Education Program
www.americanrunning.org

Australian Institute of Sport
www.ausport.gov.au

Drug Free Sport
http://www.drugfreesport.com

Gatorade Sports Science Institute
www.gssiweb.com

Informed-choice
www.informed-choice.org

International Society of Sports Nutrition
www.theissn.org

Sports and Cardiovascular and Wellness Dietitians Dietetic Practice Group of the American Dietetic Association
www.scandpg.org

Sport Science
www.sportsci.org

REFERENCES

Achten J, Jeukendrup AE: Optimizing fat oxidation through exercise and diet, *Nutrition* 20:716, 2004.

Anderson LL, et al: Effect of resistance training and combined with timed ingestion of protein muscle fiber size and muscle strength, *Metabolism* 54:151, 2005.

Astorino T, et al: Is running performance enhanced with creatine serum ingestion? *J Strength Cond Res* 19:730, 2005.

Backhouse SH, et al: Effect of carbohydrate and prolonged exercise on affect and perceived exertion, *Med Sci Sports Exerc* 37:1768, 2005.

Baker LB, et al: Sex differences in voluntary fluid intake by older adults during exercise, *Med Sci Sports Exerc* 37:789, 2005.

Bishop D: Dietary supplements and team-sport performance, *Sports Med* 40:995, 2010.

Buford TW, et al: International Society of Sports Nutrition position stand: creatine supplementation and exercise. *Int Soc Sports Nutr* 30:4, 2007

Byars A, et al: The influence of a pre-exercise sports drink (PRX) on factors related to maximal aerobic performance, *J Int Soc Sports Nutr* 7:12, 2010.

Byrne C, et al: Water versus carbohydrate electrolyte replacement during loaded marching under heat stress, *Mil Med* 170:715, 2005.

Cannell JJ, et al: Athletic performance and vitamin D, *Med Sci Sports Exerc* 41:1102, 2009.

Dhar R, et al: Cardiovascular toxicities of performance-enhancing substances in sports, *Mayo Clin Proc* 80:1307, 2005.

DiLuigi L, et al: Androgenic-anabolic steroids abuse in males, *J Endocrinol Invest* 28:81S, 2005.

Foster GD, et al: A policy-based school intervention to prevent overweight and obesity, *Pediatrics* 121:e794, 2008.

Graef JL, et al: The effects of four weeks of creatine supplementation and high-intensity interval training on cardiorespiratory fitness: a randomized controlled trial, *J Int Soc Sports Nutr* 6:18, 2009.

Havemann L, et al: Fat adaptation followed by carbohydrate loading compromises high intensity sprint performance, *J Appl Physiol* 100:194, 2005.

Heaney S, et al: Comparison of strategies for assessing nutritional adequacy in elite female athletes' dietary intake, *Int J Sport Nutr Exerc Metab* 20:245, 2010.

Hew TD: Women hydrate more during a marathon race: hyponatremia in the Houston Marathon: a report on 60 cases, *Clin J Sport Med* 15:148, 2005.

Howatson G, et al: Influence of tart cherry juice on indices of recovery following marathon running, *Scand J Med Sci Sports* 37:843, 2010

Hulmi JJ, et al: Protein ingestion prior to strength exercise affects blood hormones and metabolism, *Med Sci Sports Exerc* 37:1990, 2005.

Institute of Medicine (IOM), Food and Nutrition Board: *Dietary reference intakes (DRIs) for water, potassium, sodium and chloride and sulfate*, Washington, DC, 2004, National Academies Press.

Institute of Medicine (IOM), Food and Nutrition Board: *Dietary Reference Intakes for Calcium and Vitamin D*, Washington, DC, 2011, National Academies Press.

Kerksick C, Leutholz B: Nutrient administration and resistance training, *J Int Soc Sports Nutr* 2:50, 2005.

Kristiansen M, et al: Dietary supplement use by university athletes at a Canadian university, *Int J Sports Nutr Exerc Metab* 15:195, 2005.

Kuehl KS, Perrier ET, Elliot DL, Chesnutt JC: Efficacy of tart cherry juice in reducing muscle pain during running a randomized controlled trial, *J Int Soc Sports Nutr* 7:17, 2010.

Larson-Meyer DE, Willis KS: Vitamin D and athletes, *Curr Sports Med Rep*, 9:220, 2010

Lin-Wu CL, Williams C: A low glycemic index meal before exercise improves endurance running capacity in men, *Int J Sport Nutr Exerc Metab* 16:510, 2006.

Malinauskas BM, et al: Supplements of interest for sport-related injury and sources of supplement information among college athletes, *Adv Med Sci* 52:50, 2007.

Maughan RJ: Contamination of dietary supplements and positive drug tests in sport, *J Sports Sci* 23:883, 2005.

Millard-Stafford M, et al: Recovery from run training: efficacy of a carbohydrate-protein beverage? *Int J Sport Nutr Exerc Metab* 15:610, 2005.

Murray R: Fluids, electrolytes, and exercise. In Danford M, editor: *Sports nutrition: a practice manual for professionals*, ed 4, Washington, DC, 2006, American Dietetic Association.

Neiper A: Nutritional supplement practices in UK junior national track and field athletes, *Br J Sports Med* 39:645, 2005.

Noakes TD, et al: Three independent biological mechanisms cause exercise-associated hyponatremia: evidence from 2,135 weighed competitive performances, *Proc Natl Acad Sci* 102:18550, 2005.

Palisin T, Stacy JJ: Beta-hydroxy-methylbutyrate and its use in athletics, *Curr Sports Med Rep* 4:220, 2005.

Peake J: Heat, athletes and immunity, *Am J Lifestyle Med* 4:320, 2010.

Pennings B, et al: Exercising before protein intake allows for greater use of dietary protein—derived amino acids for de novo muscle protein synthesis in both young and elderly men, *Am J Clin Nutr* 93(2)322, 2010.

Pialoux V, et al: Effects of acute hypoxic exposure on prooxidant/antioxidant balance in elite endurance athletes, *Int J Sports Med* 30:87, 2009.

Pialoux V, et al: Antioxidant status of elite athletes remains impaired 2 weeks after a simulated altitude training camp, *Eur J Nutr* 49:285, 2010.

Pigeon WR, et al: Effects of a tart cherry juice beverage on the sleep of older adults with insomnia: a pilot study, *J Med Food* 13:579, 2010.

Rodriguez NR, et al: Position of the American Dietetic Association, Dietitians of Canada, and the American College of Sports Medicine: nutrition and athletic performance, *J Am Diet Assoc* 109:509, 2009.

Sinclair L, Hinton P: Prevalence of iron deficiency with and without anemia in recreationally active men and women, *J Am Diet Assoc* 105:975, 2005.

Smith AE, et al: Effects of beta-alanine supplementation and high-intensity interval training on endurance performance and body composition in men: a double-blind trial, *J Int Soc Sports Nutr* 6:5, 2009.

Smurawa TM, Congeni JA: Testosterone precursors: use and abuse in pediatric athletes, *Pediatr Clin North Am* 54:787, 2007.

Stofan J, et al: Sweat and sodium losses in NCAA football players: a precursor to heat cramps? *J Sport Nutr Exerc Metabol* 15:641, 2005.

Trenton AJ, Currier GW: Behavioral manifestations of anabolic steroid use, *CNS Drugs* 19:571, 2005.

Van Hamont D, et al: Reduction in muscle glycogen and protein utilization with glucose feeding during exercise, *Int J Sport Nutr Exerc Metabol* 15:350, 2005.

Watson TA, et al: Antioxidant restriction and oxidative stress in short-duration exhaustive exercise, *Med Sci Sports Exerc* 37:63, 2005.

Williams M: Dietary supplements and sports performance: metabolites, constituents, and extracts, *J Int Soc Sports Nutr* 3:1, 2006.

Williams M: Dietary supplements and sport performance: minerals, *J Int Soc Sports Nutr* 2(1):43, 2005.

Wilson JM, et al: Acute and timing effects of beta-hydroxy-beta-methylbutyrate (HMB) on indirect markers of skeletal muscle damage, *Nutr Metab* 6:6, 2009.

Wilson M, et al: Effect of glycemic index meals on recovery and subsequent endurance capacity, *Int J Sports Med* 30:898, 2009.

Wong SH, et al: Effect of preexercise glycemic-index meal on running when CHO-electrolyte solution is consumed during exercise. *Int J Sport Nutr Exerc Metab* 19:222, 2009.

CHAPTER 25

Karen Chapman-Novakofski, PhD, RD, LDN

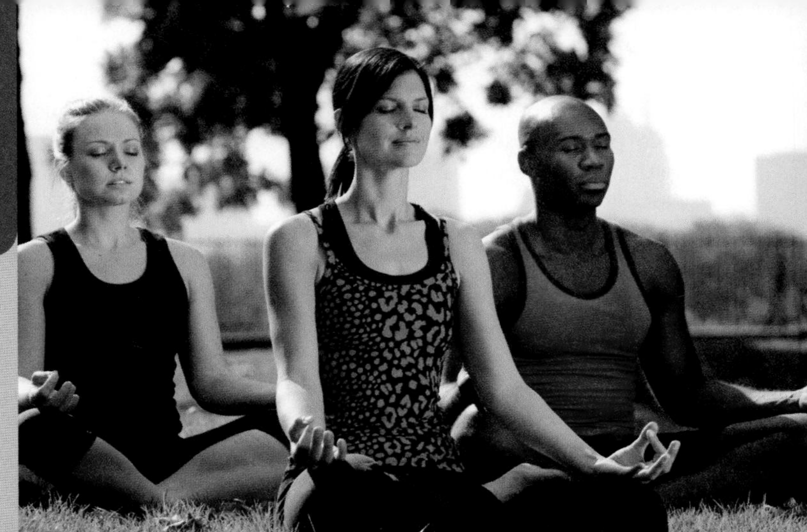

Nutrition and Bone Health

KEY TERMS

25-hydroxy vitamin D (calcidiol)
1,25-dihydroxy vitamin D_3 (calcitriol)
age-related primary osteoporosis
bisphosphonates
bone densitometry
bone mineral content (BMC)
bone mineral density (BMD)
bone modeling
bone remodeling
calcium homeostasis
calcitonin
cancellous bone
cortical bone
estrogen-androgen deficient osteoporosis
estrogen receptor (ER)
estrogen replacement therapy (ERT)
hydroxyapatite
intermittent parathyroid hormone (PTH) therapy
osteoid
osteoblast
osteocalcin
osteoclast
osteocyte
osteomalacia
osteopenia
osteoporosis
parathyroid hormone (PTH)
peak bone mass (PBM)
secondary osteoporosis
selective estrogen receptor modulator (SERM)
trabecular bone

Adequate nutrition is essential for the development and maintenance of the skeleton (i.e., bone health). Although diseases of the bone such as osteoporosis and **osteomalacia** (a condition of impaired mineralization caused by vitamin D and calcium deficiency) have complex causes, the development of these diseases can be minimized by providing adequate amounts of nutrients throughout the life cycle. Of these diseases, osteoporosis is the most common and destructive of productivity and quality of life.

The number of people older than 65 years in the United States is projected to reach almost 25% of the population by 2020. The average life expectancy in the United States is almost 81 years for women and 74 for men. As a result of the increasing numbers of older adults, osteoporosis with resulting hip fractures has become more significant in cost, morbidity, and mortality in the United States. Although the use of bone-building nutrients is necessary after the onset of osteoporosis, the benefits of adequate intakes (AIs) of bone-building nutrients during adolescence and adulthood are significant.

Sections of this chapter were written by John J.B. Anderson, PhD for the previous edition of this text.

BONE STRUCTURE AND BONE PHYSIOLOGY

Bone is a term used to mean both an organ, such as the femur, and a tissue, such as trabecular bone tissue. Each bone contains bone tissues of two major types, trabecular and cortical. These tissues undergo bone modeling during growth (height gain) and bone remodeling after growth ceases.

Composition of Bone

Bone consists of an organic matrix or **osteoid**, primarily collagen fibers, in which salts of calcium and phosphate are deposited in combination with hydroxyl ions in crystals of **hydroxyapatite**. The cablelike tensile strength of collagen and the hardness of hydroxyapatite combine to give bone its great strength. Other components of the bone matrix include osteocalcin, osteopontin, and several other matrix proteins.

Types of Bone Tissue

Approximately 80% of the skeleton consists of compact or cortical bone tissue. Shafts of the long bones contain primarily **cortical bone**, which consists of osteons or Haversian systems that undergo continuous but slow remodeling, and both contain an outer periosteal layer of compact circumferential lamellae and an inner endosteal layer of trabecular tissue. The remaining 20% of the skeleton is **trabecular** or **cancellous bone** tissue, which exists in the knobby ends of the long bones, the iliac crest of the pelvis, the wrists, scapulas, vertebrae, and the regions of bones that line the marrow. Trabecular bone is less dense than cortical bone as a result of an open structure of interconnecting bony spicules that resemble a sponge in appearance; thus trabecular bone is also called *spongy bone* or *spongiosa.*

The elaborate interconnecting components (columns and struts) of trabecular bone tissue add support to the cortical bone shell of the long bones and provide a large surface area that is exposed to circulating fluids from the marrow, and is lined by a disproportionately larger number of cells than cortical bone tissue. Therefore trabecular bone tissue is much more responsive to estrogens or the lack of estrogens than cortical bone tissue (Figure 25-1). The loss of trabecular bone tissue late in life is largely responsible for the occurrence of fractures, especially those of the spine.

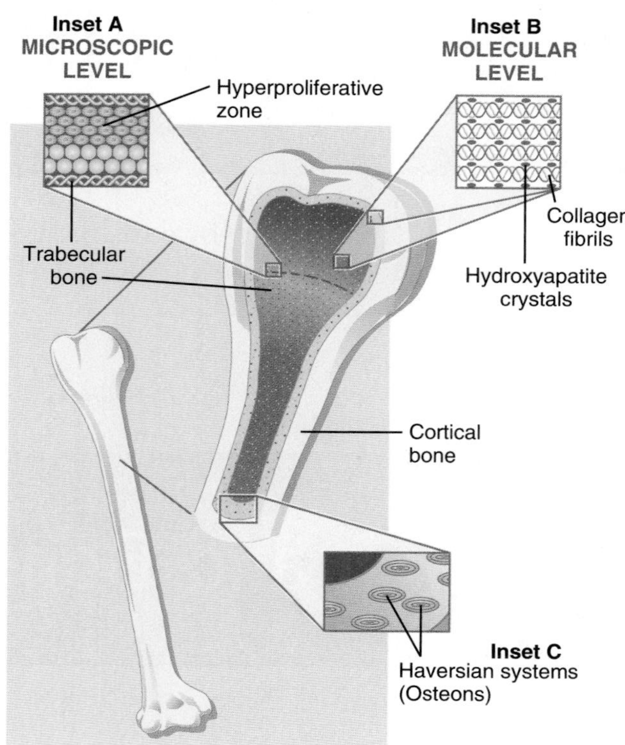

FIGURE 25-1 Schematic diagram of the structure of a long bone (hemisection of a long bone, such as the tibia). The ends of the long bones contain high percentages of trabecular (cancellous) bone tissue, whereas the shaft contains predominately cortical bone tissue. *Inset A* includes an enlarged section (approximately 100-fold) of the growth plate (epiphysis) and the subjacent hyperproliferative zone containing cartilage cells stacked like coins. *Inset B* includes a section of collagen molecules (triple helices) surrounded by mineralized deposits (dark spheroids) at a magnification of approximately 1,000,000-fold. These collagen-mineral complexes exist in both trabecular and cortical bone tissues. *Inset C* shows the cross-section of half of the mid-shaft of a long bone (magnification 10-fold). This section of cortical bone tissue contains vertical Haversian systems (osteons) that run parallel with the shaft axis; many are required to extend this system from one end of the shaft to the other. At the center of each osteon is a canal that contains an artery that supplies bone tissues with nutrients and oxygen, a vein for removing wastes, and a nerve for returning afferent relays to the brain. *(Copyright John J. B. Anderson and Sanford C. Garner.)*

Bone Cells

Osteoblasts are responsible for the formation or production of bone tissue, and **osteoclasts** govern the resorption or breakdown of bone (also see "Bone Modeling and Bone Remodeling" later in this chapter). The functions of these two cell types are listed in Table 25-1.

Two other important cell types also exist in bone tissue, **osteocytes** and bone-lining cells (inactive osteoblasts), both of which are derived from osteoblasts. The origin of the osteoblasts and osteoclasts is from primitive precursor cells found in bone marrow, now known to be stimulated by hormones and growth factors as part of their differentiation to become mature, functional bone cells.

Cartilage

In the embryo, cartilage forms the first temporary skeleton, until it develops into a mature bone matrix. In the adult, cartilage is found as flexible supports in areas such as the nose and ear. Cartilage is not bone, and is neither vascularized nor calcified.

Calcium Homeostasis

Bone tissue serves as a reservoir of calcium and other minerals that are used by other tissues of the body. **Calcium homeostasis** is the process of maintenance of a constant serum calcium concentration. The body is almost totally

TABLE 25-1

Functions of Osteoblasts and Osteoclasts

Osteoblasts	Osteoclasts
Bone Formation	**Bone Resorption**
Synthesis of matrix proteins: Collagen type 1 (90%); Osteocalcin and others (10%) Mineralization	Degradation of bone tissue via enzymes and acid (H^+) secretion
Communication: Secretion of cytokines that act on osteoblasts	Communication: Secretion of enzymes that act on osteoclasts

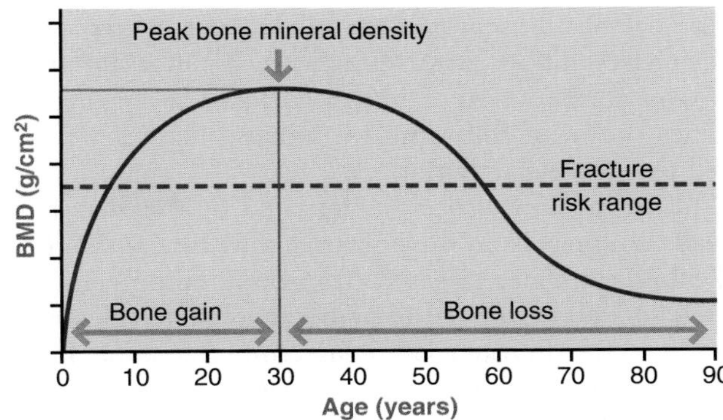

FIGURE 25-2 The early gain and later loss of bone in females. Peak bone mineral density (BMD) is typically achieved by age 30. Menopause occurs at approximately age 50 or within a few years. Postmenopausal women typically enter the fracture risk range after age 60. Men have a more gradual decline in BMD, which starts at 50 years. *(Copyright John J. B. Anderson and Sanford C. Garner.)*

reliant on this bone tissue source of calcium when the diet is inadequate. Bone tissue is also dynamic, because it undergoes bone turnover via both modeling early in life and remodeling after skeletal growth (height gain) ceases.

Although 99% of the body calcium is found in the skeleton, the remaining 1% is critical to a great variety of indispensable life processes. The concentration of calcium in blood and other extracellular fluids is regulated by complex mechanisms that balance calcium intake and excretion with bodily needs. When calcium intake is not adequate, homeostasis is maintained by drawing on mineral from the bone to keep the serum calcium ion concentration at its set level (approximately 10 mg/dL). Depending on the amount of calcium required, homeostasis can be accomplished by drawing from two major skeletal sources: readily mobilizable calcium ions in the bone fluid, or through osteoclastic resorption from the bone tissue itself. The daily turnover of skeletal calcium ions (transfers in and out of bone) is surprisingly high, which supports the dynamic activity of bone tissue in calcium homeostasis.

Blood calcium concentration is regulated by two calcium-regulating hormones -**parathyroid hormone (PTH)** and **1,25 dihydroxy vitamin D_3 (calcitriol)**. Through direct actions on the skeleton and kidney and indirect actions in the gut, PTH contributes to overall calcium homeostasis. **Intermittent parathyroid hormone (PTH) therapy** contributes to bone formation by prolonging the life of osteoblasts. However, high continuous levels of PTH contribute to bone loss (Kousteni and Bilezikian, 2008).

Active vitamin D, as calcitriol, also plays a role by increasing the efficiency of intestinal calcium absorption in the upper half of the small bowel. Vitamin D works in concert with PTH, enhancing bone release of calcium to maintain blood values. Vitamin D primarily is obtained from sunlight's interaction with precursors in the skin and secondarily from the diet. Calcitriol also has a direct effect on osteoblasts to increase the formation of several bone matrix proteins and other local factors needed for new bone formation and the suppression of bone degradation. The optimal intake and blood values for vitamin D remain under study. (see Chapter 3 and Chapter 8).

Bone Modeling

Bone modeling is the term applied to the growth of the skeleton until mature height is achieved. For example, during bone modeling long bones elongate and widen by undergoing great internal changes as well as external expansions in their structures. In modeling, the formation of new bone tissue occurs first and is followed by the resorption of old tissue. In long bones growth occurs both at terminal epiphyses (growth plates that undergo hyperproliferation) and circumferentially in lamellae; at each location cells undergo division and contribute to the formation of new bone tissue (see Figure 25-1).

Bone modeling is typically completed in females by ages 16 to 18 and in males by ages 18 to 20. After growth (height gain) ceases, gains in bone tissue may continue by the process known as *bone consolidation.* The major event of the skeleton in early life is growth, whereas there is an inevitable decline of bone mass in later stages of life (Figure 25-2).

Bone Remodeling

After skeletal growth is completed, bone continuously undergoes change in response to strains on the skeleton. Bone adapts to changes in lifestyle factors and dietary intakes, maintains calcium concentration in extracellular fluids, and repairs microscopic fractures that occur over time. **Bone remodeling** is a process in which bone is continuously resorbed through the action of the osteoclasts and reformed through the action of the osteoblasts. A greater proportion occurs in the trabecular bone, especially at those sites located in areas subject to the greatest weight-bearing strains. In normal young adults the resorption and formation phases are tightly coupled, and bone mass is maintained at zero balance. In seniors bone loss involves an uncoupling of the phases of bone remodeling with an increase of resorption over formation and thus bone loss. Trabecular bone declines the most following menopause because of unopposed osteoclastic activity.

The remodeling process is initiated by the *activation* of preosteoclastic cells in the bone marrow. Interleukin (IL)-1 and other cytokines released from bone-lining cells act as the triggers in the activation of precursor stem cells in bone marrow. The preosteoclast cells from the bone marrow migrate to the surfaces of bone while differentiating into mature osteoclasts. The osteoclasts then cover a specific area of trabecular or cortical bone tissue. Acids and proteolytic enzymes released by the osteoclasts form small cavities on bone surfaces and *resorb* both bone mineral and matrix on the surface of trabecular bone or cortical bone. The resorptive process is rapid, and it is completed within a few days, whereas the refilling of these cavities by osteoblasts is slow (i.e., on the order of 3 to 6 months or even as long as a year or more in older adults).

The *rebuilding* or *formation* stage involves secretion of collagen and other matrix proteins by the osteoblasts, also derived from precursor stem cells in bone marrow. Collagen polymerizes to form mature triple-stranded fibers, and other matrix proteins are secreted. Within a few days salts of calcium and phosphate begin to precipitate on the collagen fibers, developing into crystals of hydroxyapatite. Approximately 4% of the total bone surface is involved in remodeling at any given time as new bone is renewed continually throughout the skeleton. Even in the mature skeleton, bone remains a dynamic tissue. Normal bone turnover is illustrated in Figure 25-3.

When the resorption and formation phases are in balance, the same amount of bone tissue exists at the completion of the formation phase as at the beginning of the resorption phase. The benefit to the skeleton of this remodeling is the renewal of bone without any microfractures. However, when dietary calcium is low, osteoclastic resorption becomes relatively greater than formation by osteoblasts because of a persistently elevated PTH concentration in blood (Figure 25-4). Then large amounts of bone tissue are removed and typically not fully replaced. The net result is a decrease in both bone mineral content (BMC) and bone mineral density (BMD).

The action of PTH in promoting activity of the osteoclasts is countered by estrogen, which reduces the response of osteoblasts to PTH. PTH acts directly on osteoblasts, which increase the production of IL-6 and other cytokines that in turn stimulate osteoclasts to resorb bone. Estrogen helps to block the production of PTH-stimulated cytokines. See Fig. 25-5. **Calcitonin**, a vestigial hormone, may directly inhibit osteoclast activity (resorption), but the significance of its physiologic role in human subjects is not clear.

Osteocalcin and Bone Markers

Osteocalcin is a protein derived from osteoblasts. In bone matrix, osteocalcin assists in the mineralization process, perhaps acting to stop the formation of crystals and to prevent overmineralization. Interpretation of its level in blood is complicated by the fact that it is involved in both formation and resorption, which typically occur simultaneously at several different skeletal sites. There is difficulty in using it as a marker for predicting future fracture risk. Some osteocalcin is secreted by osteoblasts directly into the circulating blood, with a reciprocal relationship between bones and energy metabolism. Leptin influences osteoblast functions and, in turn, osteocalcin influences energy metabolism through increased insulin secretion and sensitivity, increased energy expenditure, and fat mass reduction (Hinoi et al., 2009).

Bone markers are used for research and for monitoring the effectiveness of medication on bone turnover. Plasma

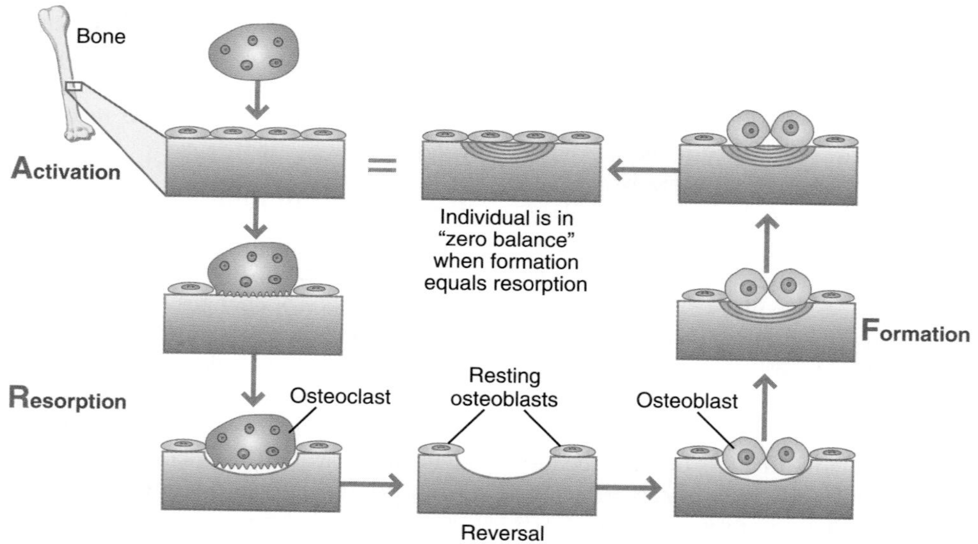

FIGURE 25-3 Normal bone turnover in healthy adults. *(Copyright John J. B. Anderson and Sanford C. Garner.)*

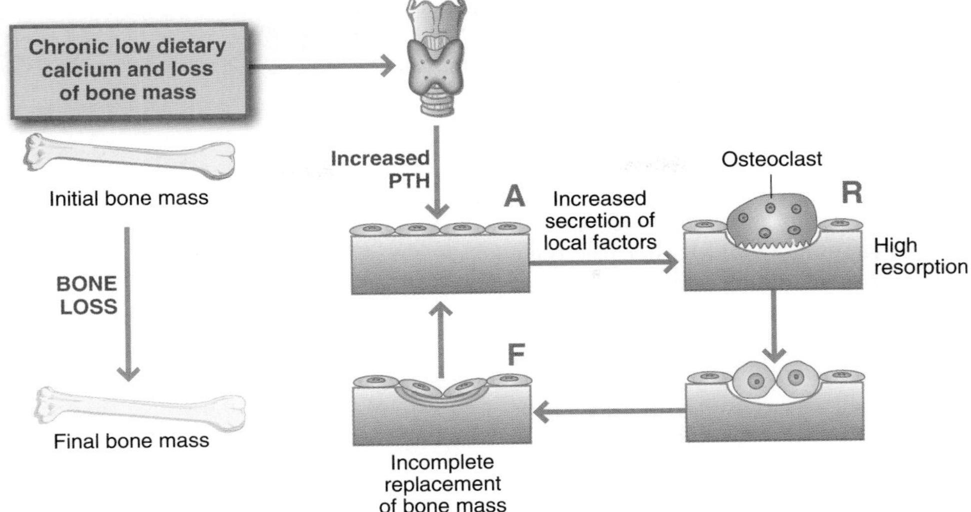

FIGURE 25-4 Effects of persistently elevated serum concentration of parathyroid hormone (PTH) on bone mass; this incorporates the effect of estradiol, counteracting the effect of PTH. *(Copyright John J. B. Anderson and Sanford C. Garner.)*

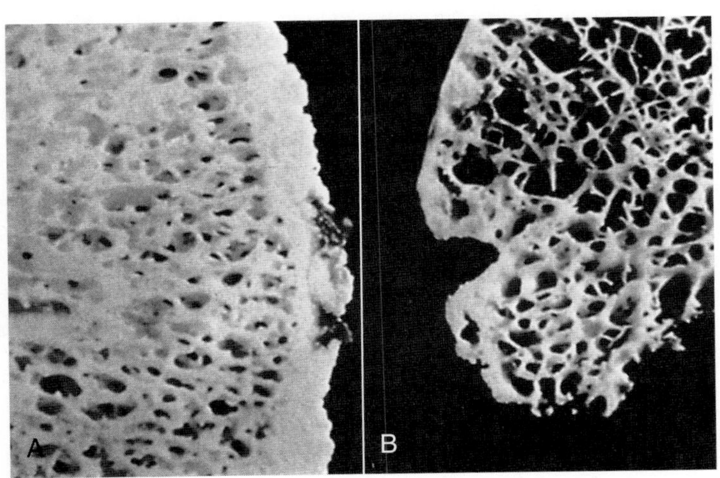

FIGURE 25-5 Difference between normal bone **(A)** and osteoporotic bone **(B)**. *(From Maher AB et al: Orthopaedic nursing, Philadelphia, 1994, Saunders.)*

bone-specific alkaline phosphatase is a marker of bone formation, although total plasma alkaline phosphatase may also be used. Other markers of bone resorption include plasma crosslinked collagen telopeptides, urinary N-telopeptides, and plasma tartrate-resistant acid phosphatase.

BONE MASS

Bone mass is a generic term that refers to BMC but not to BMD. **Bone mineral content (BMC)** is more appropriately used in assessing the amount of bone accumulated before the cessation of growth (height gain), whereas **bone mineral density (BMD)** is better used to describe bone after the developmental period is completed. These measurements are often used interchangeably, but BMD is more useful for monitoring bone changes in adults. However, neither BMC nor BMD provides information on the microarchitectural (three-dimensional) structural quality of bone tissue (i.e., index of risk of fracture).

Accumulation of Bone Mass

During the growth periods of childhood, puberty, and early adulthood, formation exceeds the resorption of bone. **Peak bone mass (PBM)** is reached by 30 years of age or so (see Figure 25-2). The long bones stop growing in length by approximately age 18 in females and age 20 in males, but bone mass continues to accumulate for a few more years by a process known as consolidation (i.e., filling-in of osteons in the shafts of long bones). The age when BMD acquisition ceases varies, depending not only on diet but also on physical activity.

Peak Bone Mass

PBM is greater in men than in women because of men's larger frame size. BMC, but not necessarily BMD, is typically lower in women. Both the lean and fat components of body composition contribute to these differences in bone mass. BMD is also greater in blacks and Hispanics than in whites and Asians, related to larger muscle mass, differences in body weight, lifestyle factors, and dietary intake (Pothiwala et al., 2006). Hereditary factors also contribute to the extent of accumulation of PBM.

PBM is related to appropriate intake of calories, protein, calcium, phosphorus, and vitamins D and K. Because bone formation begins in the embryo, more attention is being focused on maternal nutrition and health as a predictor of the child's future PBM (Prentice et al., 2011). Physical activity also plays a role. Children's activities should include ground-force reactions, such as running, skipping, or jumping, as these activities are site-specific to the bone. The importance of strengthening exercise continues to be investigated. The optimal time to begin physical activity to enhance PBM is not exact.

Body weight is positively associated with BMD, probably attributable to both adipose and lean mass (Reid, 2008). PBM is diminished in cases of anorexia nervosa (Misra and Klibanski, 2006), as well as in chronic diseases.

Loss of Bone Mass

Age is an important determinant of BMD. At approximately age 40, BMD begins to diminish gradually in both sexes, but bone loss increases greatly in women after age 50 or after menopause. A continuous loss thereafter in postmenopausal women occurs at rate of 1% to 2% per year during the next decade. Men continue to have bone loss, but at a much lower rate than women of the same age until age 70, when the loss rates are about the same for both genders. Loss of bone mass is the result of changes in the hormone-directed mechanisms that govern bone remodeling.

Cortical bone tissue and trabecular bone tissue undergo different patterns of aging. Loss of cortical bone eventually plateaus and may even cease late in life. Trabecular bone loss begins in both sexes as early as 40 years of age. Premenopausal loss of trabecular bone in women is much greater than that of cortical bone. Loss of both kinds of bone accelerates in women after menopause, although trabecular bone is also lost at a much higher rate than cortical bone. Differences between normal and osteoporotic bone—both trabecular and cortical tissues—are shown in Figure 25-6.

The accelerated bone loss rate of 2% to 3% per year continues for between 5 and 10 years after menopause, and then the rate declines gradually to 0.5% to 1% per year thereafter. Some postmenopausal women lose bone at an even faster rate (Figure 25-7). If the age of a woman is known, her vertebral bone mass may be predicted (see *Clinical Insight:* Postmenopausal Women at High Risk for Hip Fracture).

The normal bone loss that occurs with aging in both sexes is related to the decline of osteoblastic function such as the reduced production of collagen, osteocalcin, osteopontin, and other matrix proteins. As a result of the uncoupling of the remodeling process, osteoclastic resorption

CLINICAL INSIGHT

Postmenopausal Women at High Risk for Hip Fracture

It is important to identify women who are at risk of developing osteoporosis as early as possible so that measures can be taken to monitor bone status and to prevent further bone loss. Because low bone mineral density (BMD) is a major risk factor for osteoporosis, its assessment is clinically useful. Assessment of bone status based on the existence of one or more risk factors such as age, height, weight, smoking status, alcohol consumption, drug use, calcium intake, exercise, frame size, and selected bone markers is not sufficiently accurate. BMD as measured by bone densitometry is more clinically useful. Typically total body BMD and the regional sites such as the proximal femur and lumbar vertebrae are measured by dual-energy x-ray absorptiometry.

A BMD measurement of an at-risk woman entering menopause (before becoming estrogen deficient) serves as a baseline for subsequent measurements as the individual becomes increasingly estrogen deficient and loses bone mass. This information helps physicians and patients make decisions about the need for and use of drug therapy such as bisphosphonates, parathyroid hormone drugs, and selective estrogen receptor modulators. For men or women on long-term glucocorticosteroid therapy, a BMD measurement may indicate the need for treatment with a bone-preserving medication or calcitonin.

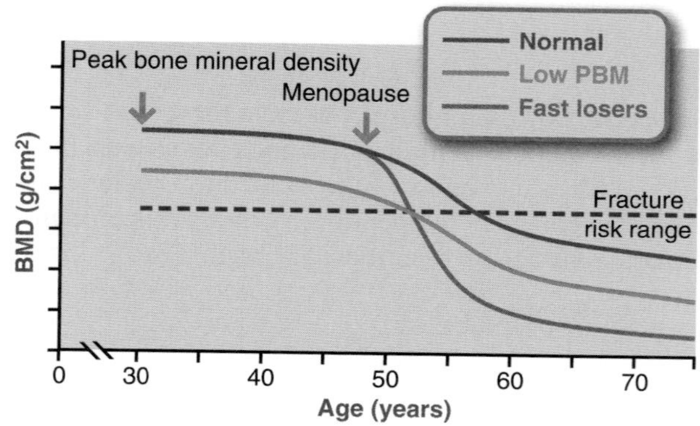

FIGURE 25-6 Variable patterns of bone loss of women following the onset of menopause at approximately 50 years of age. The rapid loss of bone mineral density (BMD) in some women referred to as *fast losers* is contrasted to the loss of *slow losers.* Women who develop low peak BMD have less bone mass than women with normal BMD, but they also can lose BMD either as slow or fast losers. *(Copyright John J. B. Anderson and Sanford C. Garner.)*

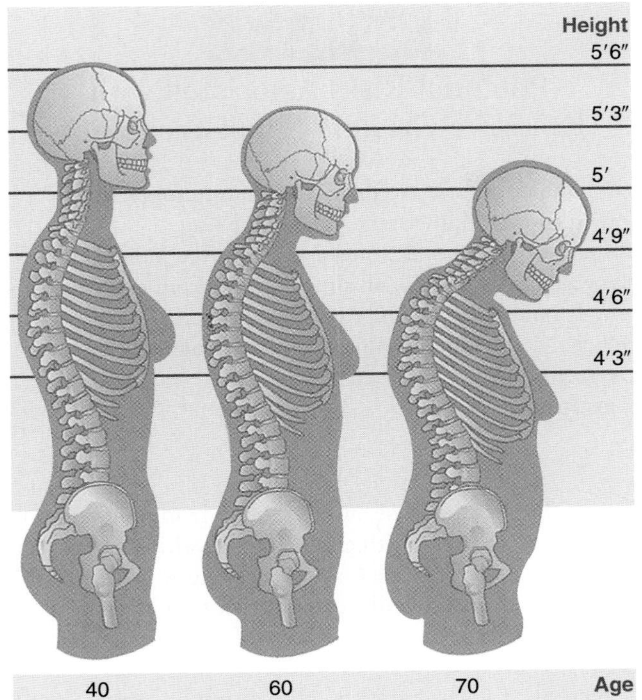

FIGURE 25-7 Normal spine at age 40 and osteoporotic changes at ages 60 and 70. These changes can cause a loss of as much as 6 to 9 inches in height and result in the dowager's hump *(far right)* in the upper thoracic vertebrae. *(From Ignatavicius D, Workman M: Medical-surgical nursing: critical thinking for collaborative care, ed 5, Philadelphia, 2006, Saunders.)*

exceeds formation with an increasing differential. Bone loss in men accelerates in later years, typically in ages 60 through 79. The reason for bone loss in men is very similar to that in women, being either age-related, idiopathic, or secondary to an underlying disease or medication. The prevalence of low bone mass and osteoporosis in men is increasing as more men are being screened or diagnosed using dual-energy x-ray absorptiometry (DEXA). It has been estimated that 39% of osteoporotic fractures are in men (Khosla, 2010.)

Measurement of Bone Mineral Content and Bone Mineral Density

Bone densitometry measures bone mass on the basis of tissue absorption of photons produced by one or two monoenergetic x-ray tubes. DEXA (see Chapter 6 and Fig. 6-10) is available in most hospitals and many clinics for the measurement of the total body and regional skeletal sites such as the lumbar vertebrae and the proximal femur (hip). Results of DEXA measurements are commonly expressed as T-scores.

Ultrasound Measurements of Bone

Quantitative ultrasound measurements of the heel bone (calcaneus) and the kneecap are becoming popular. Ultrasound instruments measure the velocity of sound waves transmitted through bone and broadband ultrasound attenuation (BUA). Measurements at the calcaneus correlate well with BMD measurements at this same skeletal site, meaning that low values by DEXA are typically mirrored by low values of BUA. However, ultrasound measurements are considered screening tools, whereas DEXA measurements are considered diagnostic.

Fracture Risk Assessment

The World Health Organization (WHO) developed an algorithm to predict fracture by using femoral head BMD and clinical indicators of low bone mass. This uses economic modeling to guide the most cost-effective instances to begin medications. Vertebral fractures that are confirmed by x-rays are a strong predictor of future vertebral fractures, as well as fractures at other sites (National Osteoporosis Foundation [NOF], 2010). DEXA scans can also identify vertebral fractures.

NUTRITION AND BONE

Calcium, phosphate, and vitamin D are essential for normal bone structure and function. Protein, calories, and other micronutrients also help develop and maintain bone (Tucker, 2009).

Protein

Both protein and calcium are important components of PBM, especially before puberty (Rizzoli, 2008). Adequate protein intake, with adequate calcium intake, is needed for optimal bone health. A meta-analysis of studies concerned with protein intake and indicators of bone health found a slight positive effect on BMD, but it did not influence the risk of fracture over the long-term for total protein, animal protein, or vegetable protein (Darling et al., 2009;) unfortunately, this analysis did not consider calcium intake.

The negative effects of either too high or too low an intake of protein is more pronounced with inadequate calcium intake, especially in seniors (Tucker, 2009). The theory that higher protein intakes produce a higher acidic load, which increases calcium urinary excretion, has not been verified.

Very low protein intake may theoretically negatively affect bone turnover and development. In cases of negative nitrogen balance, such as with fracture or surgery, higher protein intake may be advised.

Minerals

Calcium from Foods

Calcium intake in the primary prevention of osteoporosis has received much attention. The Institute of Medicine Dietary Reference Intakes (DRIs) for calcium and vitamin D, are given as RDAs. The RDA for calcium from preadolescence (age 9 years) through adolescence (up to 19 years) was increased to 1300 mg/day for both genders (IOM, 2011). The RDAs for calcium adults, pregnant and lactating women and children, are listed on the inside front cover).

People older than 11 years, particularly females, typically do not receive the recommended amount of calcium. According to the National Health and Nutrition Examination Survey (2007), teen and adult women consume considerably less than the current RDAs. Males are more likely to consume somewhat greater amounts than females, but after 50 years of age they also do not meet the recommended levels. These deficits translate, on average, into the need for an additional 500 mg/day for teenage girls and adult women.

Food sources are recommended first for supplying calcium needs because of the coingestion of other essential nutrients. In the United States, the primary source of calcium is dairy foods, and this intake is higher in white than in black women (Plawecki et al., 2009). However, calcium fortification of nondairy foods such as nondairy milks and other beverages, juices, breakfast cereals, bread, and some crackers is common.

Calcium bioavailability from foods is generally good, and the amount of calcium in the food is more important than its bioavailability. However, the order of concern relative to calcium absorption efficiency is first the individual's need for calcium, second the amount consumed because absorption efficiency is inversely related to amount consumed, and third the intake of absorption enhancers or inhibitors. For example, absorption from foods high in oxalic and phytic acid (certain vegetables and legumes) is lower than from dairy products.

The amount of calcium in foods varies with the brand, serving size, and whether it has been fortified. Read the Nutrition Facts label to determine the amount of calcium per serving. Multiply the daily value (DV) percentage by 10 to determine the milligrams of calcium. For example, a 20% DV equals 200 mg of calcium (see Chapter 12). Labeling for "excellent" (>200 mg/serving) and "good" (100-200 mg/serving) sources of calcium are regulated by the Food and Drug Administration (FDA).

Calcium from Supplements

Reaching RDA levels of calcium from foods should be the first goal, but if insufficient amounts of calcium from foods are consumed, supplements of calcium should then be ingested to reach the age-specific RDA. The upper limit of safety for calcium intake is 2500 mg for everyone older than 1 year except for youth age 9-18 years and pregnant or lactating women when it is 3000 mg/day. Box 25-1 lists the potential risks associated with excessive calcium intake.

An increasing percentage of the population is taking calcium supplements. Persons who should take supplements include those not meeting the RDA on most days, those taking corticosteroids, those with low bone mass or osteoporosis, women who are perimenopausal or postmenopausal, and those who are lactose intolerant. Calcium carbonate is the most common form of calcium supplement. It should be taken with food because an acidic environment enhances absorption. For those with achlorhydria, which often occurs in seniors, calcium citrate may be more appropriate because it does not require an acidic environment for absorption and does not further reduce the acidity of the stomach (Straub, 2007).

Calcium supplementation absorption is optimal when taken as individual doses of 500 mg or less. Many formulations include vitamin D, because the likelihood of needing vitamin D is high if calcium supplementation is needed. Choosing a supplement that has the United States Pharmacopeia designation increases the likelihood that the supplement quantity is consistent with the label, and that good manufacturing practices are used.

BOX 25-1

Potential Risks Associated with Excessive Calcium Supplementation

Contamination of bone meal or dolomite supplements with cadmium, mercury, arsenic, or lead
Urinary tract or renal stones in susceptible individuals
Hypercalcemia or milk alkali syndrome from extremely high intakes (>4000 mg/day)
Deficiency of iron and other mineral divalent cations resulting from decreased absorption
Constipation

Phosphate

Phosphate salts are available in practically all foods either naturally or because of processing. In healthy adults, the urinary phosphorus excretion approximately equals intake.. The regulation of phosphorus levels in the blood is tightly controlled by an interaction between vitamin D from the kidney, PTH from the parathyroid glands, and fibroblast growth factor 23 from bone. Both calcium and phosphate ions in a ratio of approximately 1:1 are needed for the mineralization of bone.

Excessive phosphorus intake as phosphates can greatly alter the calcium/phosphate ratio, especially if calcium intakes are low. Too much phosphate compared with calcium lowers the serum calcium ion concentration, which then stimulates PTH; if this pattern of intake becomes chronic, bone loss is thought to follow.

Soft drinks are poor in nutrient value but high in phosphate content. However, studies have found that the soft drink primarily displaces milk as a beverage, so the negative effect is from lower calcium intake rather than higher phosphate intake. Some studies have found a negative correlation between soft drink intake and BMD in women but not in men. Those at high risk and those who have osteoporosis may want to avoid these beverages because an effect is theoretically possible (Tucker, 2009).

Magnesium

Magnesium dietary deficits seem to have little effect on bone tissue, but one report suggests that meeting the RDIs for magnesium improve BMD (Ryder et al., 2005). However, diets deficient in magnesium are likely deficient in other nutrients that are needed for healthy bone growth and maintenance. Nevertheless, magnesium deficiency may affect the quality of bone by decreasing bone formation, preventing the optimal crystal formation, and having a negative effect on PTH (Rude et al., 2009).

Trace Minerals

Few studies are available about the effects of trace elements on bone. Iron, zinc, copper, manganese, and boron may function in bone cells, but their specific roles in preventing bone loss are not well established. In one study, supplementation of copper, fluoride, manganese, and zinc along with calcium for 1 year resulted in a reduced loss of lumbar BMD compared with the greater loss in a group receiving only calcium supplementation (Nieves, 2005).

Boron

Boron is used by osteoblasts for bone formation. It is required to convert estrogen to its most active form, 17-beta-estradiol, and estrogen is involved in bone metabolism. However, it is not known whether, or how much boron is required for optimal bone health. (Hakki et al., 2010; Nielsen, 2008).

Copper

Copper is needed for the enzyme that increases the crosslinking of collagen and elastin molecules, and it may have roles in other enzymes of bone cells. Because of the changes induced in the two matrix proteins by low copper intakes, bone mineralization may also be reduced, especially in seniors.

Fluoride

Fluoride ions enter the hydroxyapatite crystals of bone as substitutes for hydroxyl ions. Water containing 1 ppm of fluoride does not help bone in the same way that it helps tooth surfaces. Within narrow limits of safety (less than 2 ppm), fluoride ions have little effect on increasing the hardness of bone mineral. At intakes of 2 ppm or greater, fluoride may produce bone that is subject to increased microfractures because of the change in the properties of the hydroxyapatite crystals.

Iron

Iron serves as a catalytic cofactor for the vitamin C–dependent hydroxylations of proline and lysine in collagen maturation. Iron also has other roles in osteoblasts and osteoclasts in mitochondrial oxidative-phosphorylation, as well as in other heme- and nonheme-containing enzymes, similar to the needs of other cells in the body.

Manganese

Manganese is required for the biosynthesis of mucopolysaccharides in bone matrix formation, and it also acts as a cofactor in energy-generating reactions.

Zinc

Zinc is essential for several critical enzymes in osteoblasts that are essential for collagen synthesis and other products. In addition, alkaline phosphatase requires zinc for its activity in the osteoblasts.

Vitamins

Vitamin D

An individual's vitamin D status depends mostly on sunlight exposure, and secondarily on dietary intake of vitamin D. The synthesis of vitamin D by skin exposed to sunlight varies considerably as a result of many factors, including skin tone, sunscreen use, environmental latitude, and age (McCarty, 2008). The skin of older individuals is less efficient at producing vitamin D following exposure to ultraviolet (UV) light because the skin is thinner and it contains fewer cells that can synthesize vitamin D. In addition, older adults living in nursing homes and similar institutions typically have little exposure to sunlight. Those who live at northern latitudes in the United States and Canada are at increased risk of osteoporosis because of limited UV light during winter months.

The few foods that naturally contain vitamin D are egg yolks, fatty fish such as salmon, mackerel, catfish, tuna, and sardines, cod liver oil, and mushrooms (see Appendix 51). The vitamin D content of fish varies, as does the content in UV-exposed mushrooms. Fluid milk in the United States is fortified with vitamin D at a standardized level of 400 IU per quart, whereas other foods, including juices, cereals, yogurt, and margarines, may be fortified in varying amounts. The RDAs for vitamin D across the life cycle are shown inside the front cover. The upper limit is 100 μg (4000 IU) for everyone older than 8 years, and lower levels for younger children (see inside front cover). From any source, vitamin D must be hydroxylated in the kidney before becoming the physiologically active calcitriol.

To prevent rickets, the American Academy of Pediatrics recommends that all infants who are exclusively breastfed be supplemented with 400 IU of vitamin D. Infants who are both formula and breastfed should also be supplemented until they are consistently taking 1 liter (1 quart) of formula a day. They further recommend continuing the supplementation until 1 year of age, when children begin drinking vitamin D–fortified milk (Wagner and Greer, 2008).

The older adult is at increased risk for vitamin D deficiency. Risks are from decreased synthesis of vitamin D by the skin because of changes in the skin and decreased exposure to sunlight; increased body fat; decreased renal function that decreases the hydroxylation of vitamin D to its active form; and decreased levels of insulin-like growth factor 1, calcitonin, and estrogen, which affect hydroxylase activity. In general, seniors may benefit from daily vitamin D supplementation of 10-20 mg (400 IU-800 IU) to reach serum **25-hydroxy vitamin D (calcidiol)** levels of at least 30 ng/mL (75 nmol/L). Older adults who are frail or institutionalized may need up to 50 mcg (2000 IU)/day. Mobility, skin tone, body weight, and dietary habits may modify these recommendations (Oudshoorn et al., 2009). The most common blood test for vitamin D status is serum 25-hydroxyvitamin D level, although other tests may also be used.

Vitamin K

Vitamin K is an essential micronutrient for bone health. Its role in posttranslational modification of several matrix proteins, including osteocalcin, is well established. Following bone resorption, osteocalcin is released and enters the blood. In this way, osteocalcin serves as a serum bone marker for predicting the risk of a fracture (see Appendix 30). Many older adults have inadequate intakes of vitamin K, primarily because their consumption of dark-green leafy vegetables is so low. Most of the vitamin K intake in the United States is from green leafy vegetables, with about one third from fats and oils. Although menaquinones, a form of vitamin K, are formed in the gut by bacteria, the influence of this source on vitamin K status appears to be weak. It is important to consider the vitamin K intake in older persons who may also be taking blood-thinning medications (vitamin K antagonists). Rather than having these patients avoid vitamin K in foods and thus jeopardize their bone status, it is better to have the vitamin K daily intake be consistent and regulate the vitamin K antagonist medication. In fact, it has been shown that therapeutic international normalized ratio (INR) ranges from blood thinning medication can be achieved with vitamin K in low-dose supplementation, and when fluctuations are few (Ford and Moll, 2008).

Vitamin A (Retinol)

Vitamin A consumption is generally considered to be beneficial to bone growth and maintenance. Lycopene may be protective against oxidative stress; more research is suggested (MacKinnon et al, 2011).

Excessive retinol intake (but not carotenoids) may contribute to risk for hip fractures. However, there is not complete understanding, and many still question the effect on bone of excessive retinol intake (Ribaya-Mercado and Blumberg, 2007). Nevertheless, concern remains that the combined intakes of supplemental vitamin A and vitamin A from fortified foods may be too high in the United States, especially in health-conscious postmenopausal white women. The window of safe consumption of vitamin A is fairly narrow, but it may be even narrower for seniors.

Other Dietary Components

Several other dietary factors have been associated with bone health but their relative quantitative importance is not clear.

Alcohol

Moderate consumption of wine and beer may be beneficial to bone in men and postmenopausal women. Nonalcoholic constituents, such as silicon in beer, need further investigation.

In men, high liquor intakes (>2 drinks/d) are associated with significantly lower BMD (Kanis et al., 2005; Tucker et al, 2009). Heavy alcohol consumption also may be accompanied by poor dietary intake, cigarette smoking, poor balance, and an increased risk of falls.

Caffeine and Soft Drinks

The relationship of moderate consumption of caffeine to osteoporosis has not been clearly established. *Excessive* caffeine intake may have a deleterious effect on BMD (Ruffing et al., 2006). Intake of colas is also associated with lower BMD. Although the primary issue may be displacement of dairy beverages, there is also a potential direct effect (Tucker, 2009). Rapid metabolizers of caffeine may be a high risk group for bone loss (Hallström et al, 2010.)

Dietary Fiber

Excessive dietary fiber intake may interfere with calcium absorption, but any interference is considered extremely small in the typical low-fiber diet. Vegans who may consume as much as 50 g of fiber a day are most likely to have a significant depression in intestinal calcium absorption, but this is often offset by adequate calcium intake.

Isoflavones

The isoflavones in soybeans function both as estrogen agonists and antioxidants in bone cells. They inhibit bone resorption in female animal models without ovaries, but not in young adult females with normal estrogen status. Some but not all studies show modest skeletal benefits.

Potassium bicarbonate

The skeleton serves as a buffer to help regulate acid-base balance, and a high-acid diet may contribute to the progressive decline in bone mass and osteoporosis (Sebastian, 2005).

In postmenopausal women, an oral dose of potassium bicarbonate sufficient to neutralize endogenous acid improves calcium balance and bone. Decreased bone resorption and an increased rate of bone formation can result. See *Clinical Insight:* Urine pH—How Does Diet Affect It? in Chapter 36.

Sodium

A high sodium intake may contribute to osteoporosis because of increased calcium excretion (Massey, 2005). While the calciuric effect of sodium has been speculated, there seem to be no adverse effects with adequate calcium and vitamin D intake (Ilich et al, 2010).

Vegetarian Diets

Though research is inconclusive, vegetarian diets may be more beneficial for bone than animal-based diets. They may provide less calcium than animal diets but animal proteins contribute to urine acidity. In general, fruits and vegetables in the diet promote an alkaline urine and less need for neutralizing calcium. In addition they are high in potassium, which is considered a bone-protective nutrient. See *Clinical Insight:* Urine pH—How Does Diet Affect It? in Chapter 36. Polyphenols and other antioxidants in plant foods support optimal functioning and health of bone cells and provide many bone-healthy nutrients.

OSTEOPENIA AND OSTEOPOROSIS

Osteoporosis may have its origin in early life during the period of skeletal growth and PBM accumulation. The WHO defines osteoporosis in terms of decline in BMD.

Definitions

When BMD falls sufficiently below healthy values (1 standard deviation [SD] according to WHO standards) low bone mass or **osteopenia** exists. **Osteoporosis** occurs when the BMD becomes so low (greater than 2.5 SDs below healthy values) that the skeleton is unable to sustain ordinary strains. However, the National Osteoporosis Foundation (2010) states that the WHO BMD diagnostic classification should not be applied to premenopausal women, men younger than 50 years of age, or children. Clinical assessment and ethnically adjusted Z-scores are thought to be more reflective of the norms in other groups.

Prevalence

It is estimated that 8 million women and 2 million men in the United States are classified as osteoporotic. More than 2 million osteoporotic fractures were estimated to occur in 2005, which represents a cost of billions of dollars in health care and rehabilitation services. One fourth of these osteoporosis-related fractures involve the vertebrae; 297,000 are fractures of the hip, which typically result in incapacitation, long-term nursing care, and significant mortality.

Types of Osteoporosis

Osteoporosis is considered to have a broad spectrum of variant forms. There are two types of primary osteoporosis, distinguished in general by sex, the age at which fractures occur, and the kinds of bone involved. **Secondary osteoporosis** results when an identifiable drug or disease process causes loss of bone tissue (Box 25-2).

Estrogen-androgen deficient osteoporosis occurs in women within a few years of menopause from loss of trabecular bone tissue and cessation of ovarian production of estrogens. BMC and BMD measurements of the lumbar spine of women with postmenopausal osteoporosis may be as much as 25% to 40% lower than in age-matched nonosteoporotic control women of the same age range. Other bone sites with a preponderance of trabecular bone such as the pelvis, ribs, and proximal femur also display low BMD. Rarely, men may develop androgen-deficient osteoporosis if they have a significant decline in androgen production. This osteoporosis is characterized by fractures of the distal radius (Colles fractures) and "crush" fractures of the lumbar vertebrae that are often painful and deforming.

Age-related primary osteoporosis occurs at approximately age 70 and beyond. Both cortical and trabecular bone tissues undergo remodeling, but more remodeling occurs in trabecular tissue. In seniors, the processes of bone resorption and bone formation become uncoupled. Many women lose several inches in height between 50 and 80 years of age. Although age-associated osteoporosis affects both sexes, women are more severely affected because they have a smaller skeletal mass than men and they live longer.

Fractures may occur during ordinary activities, such as lifting a sack of groceries or stepping over a shower opening, but more hip fractures result from a fall. Hip fractures affect nearly 20% of postmenopausal women up to age 80 and almost 50% of those beyond that age, and the hip fracture numbers are steadily increasing in men. A dramatic increase in hip fractures occurs late in life, and almost all women beyond 80 years of age are at risk of hip fracture. Although fractures of the hips characterize this osteoporosis, vertebral fractures also increase with age. Wedge fractures of vertebrae typically lead to back pain, loss of height, spinal deformity, and kyphosis or "dowager's hump."

Causes and Risk Factors

Osteoporosis is a complex heterogeneous disorder and many risk factors contribute during a lifetime. Low BMD is common to all types of osteoporosis, but an imbalance between bone resorption and formation results from an array of factors characteristic of each form of this disease. Loss of bone mass to a degree that produces fractures can result from (1) an excessive acceleration of resorption, especially after menopause; or (2) a suboptimal peak bone mass that results in bone after menopause (or later in life in men) that becomes fragile and susceptible to fracture. Risk factors for osteoporosis include age, race, gender, and factors noted in Box 25-3.

BOX 25-2

Medical Conditions That Deplete Calcium and Promote Risk of Osteoporosis

Chronic diarrhea or intestinal malabsorption
Chronic obstructive lung disease
Chronic renal disease
Diabetes
Hemiplegia
Hyperparathyroid disease
Hyperthyroidism
Scurvy
Subtotal gastrectomy

BOX 25-3

Risk Factors for Developing Osteoporosis

Age, especially older than age 60
Amenorrhea in women as a result of excessive exercise
Androgen depletion with hypogonadism in men
Cigarette smoking
Estrogen depletion from menopause or early oophorectomy
Ethnicity: white or Asian
Excessive intake of alcohol, caffeine, fiber
Female gender
Family history of osteoporosis
Inadequate calcium or vitamin D intake
Lack of exercise
Prolonged use of certain medications (see Box 25-4)
Sarcopenia
Underweight, low body mass index, low body fatness

Alcohol and Cigarettes

Cigarette smoking and excessive alcohol consumption are risk factors for developing osteoporosis, probably because of toxic effects on osteoblasts. Moderate alcohol intake has no detrimental effect on bone, and some studies show a modest positive effect in postmenopausal women. Three or more drinks per day is associated with increased risk of falling and may pose other threats to bone health. The risk appears significant even after adjusting for BMD when comparing smokers versus nonsmokers (North America Menopause Society, 2010). Excessive consumption (more than three drinks a day) for an extended period may result in bone loss. The combination of smoking and alcohol, common among young women and men, places them at increased risk for osteoporosis.

Body Weight

Body weight is a principal determinant of bone density and fracture risk; adipose tissue mass is a major contributor (Reid, 2010). The greater the body mass, the greater the BMD. Fat and bone are linked by pathways involving adiponectin; insulin, amylin, and preptin; and leptin and adipocytic estrogens, which ultimately serve the function of providing a skeleton appropriate to the mass of adipose tissue it is carrying (Reid, 2010).

The lower the body mass, the lower the BMD. Young girls who are typically premenarcheal may incur fractures with minimum trauma because of low BMC and BMD related to rapid growth in height that is not accompanied with a proportionate increase in weight (Goulding et al., 2005). Young, overweight males with low bone mass may also suffer fractures (Goulding et al., 2005). Weight loss from dieting, bariatric surgery, or sarcopenia are also associated with bone loss. Thus being overweight is protective against osteoporosis and underweight is a risk factor for fractures (Reid, 2010).

Ethnicity

Whites and Asians suffer more osteoporotic fractures than blacks and Hispanics, who usually have a greater bone density. However, hypovitaminosis D with secondary hyperparathyroidism occurs more often in the black population. Thin women, particularly of northern European ancestry, have the highest risk of osteoporosis.

Lactation

A striking but transient bone loss occurs in women who breast-feed for 6 months or longer, especially from the femoral neck and lumbar spine. Sufficient calcium and vitamin D intake are essential during this time for the mother to replete her own serum and storage levels, but repletion typically does not occur until several months after peak lactation. Several successive pregnancies and lactations over a relatively few years may contribute to significant bone loss by the end of the period of childbearing if nutrition is inadequate.

Limited Weight-Bearing Exercise

Maintenance of healthy bone requires exposure to weight-bearing pressures. A good diet plus exercise from roughly ages 10 to 20 years is particularly important for skeletal growth, accrual of bone mass, and increased femoral bone dimensions (Iuliano-Burns et al., 2005). Physical activity, especially upper body activities, is thought to contribute to an increase in bone mass or density (Chubak et al., 2006). Lack of exercise and a sedentary mode of living may also contribute to bone loss, although the most important influence is probably an inadequate accumulation of bone mass.

Exercise is beneficial for reducing skeletal inflammatory markers in frail older individuals (Lambert et al., 2008). Stresses from muscle contraction and maintaining the body in an upright position against the pull of gravity stimulate osteoblast function. Bones not subjected to normal use rapidly lose mass.

Immobility in varying degrees is well recognized as a cause of bone loss. Invalids confined to bed or persons unable to move freely are commonly affected. Astronauts living in conditions of zero gravity for only a few days experience bone loss, especially in the lower extremities; appropriate exercise is a feature of their daily routines.

Loss of Menses

Loss of menses at any age is a major determinant of osteoporosis risk in women. Acceleration of bone loss coincides with menopause, either natural or surgical, at which time the ovaries stop producing estrogen. Estrogen replacement therapies have been shown to conserve BMD and reduce fracture risk within the first few years following menopause, at least in short-term studies.

Any interruption of menstruation for an extended period results in bone loss. The amenorrhea that accompanies excessive weight loss seen in patients with anorexia nervosa or in individuals who participate in high-intensity sports, dance, or other forms of exercise has the same adverse effect on bones as menopause. BMD in amenorrheic athletes has been measured at levels 25% to 40% below normal. Young women with the "female athlete triad" of disordered eating, amenorrhea, and low BMD are at increased risk for having fractures. These young women may benefit from the use of oral contraceptive agents plus calcium and vitamin D supplements.

Nutrients

Many nutrients and several nonnutrients have been implicated as causal risk factors for osteoporosis and have been discussed in previous paragraphs. Frank vitamin D deficiency has been widely reported at northerly latitudes in North America and Europe. Vitamin D insufficiency is now considered more common at latitudes closer to the equator than previously thought because of reduced exposure to sunlight during the year (Hypponen and Power, 2007).

Medications

A number of medications contribute adversely to osteoporosis, either by interfering with calcium absorption or by actively promoting calcium loss from bone (Box 25-4). For example, corticosteroids affect vitamin D metabolism and can lead to bone loss. Excessive amounts of exogenous thyroid hormone can promote loss of bone mass over time.

Prevention of Osteoporosis and Fractures

The increasing longevity of the population emphasizes the need for prevention of osteoporosis. Universal guidelines apply to everyone. Consuming adequate amounts of calcium and vitamin D, lifelong muscle strengthening and weight-bearing exercise, avoidance of tobacco, moderate or no intake of alcohol, and steps to avoid falls are all part of the holistic approach to a lifestyle that promotes bone health (NAMS, 2010).

BOX 25-4

Medications That Increase Calcium Loss and Promote Risk of Osteoporosis

- Aluminum-containing antacids
- Corticosteroids
- Cyclosporine
- Heparin
- Lasix and thiazide diuretics
- Lithium
- Methotrexate
- Phenobarbital
- Phenothiazine derivatives
- Phenytoin (Dilantin)
- Thyroid hormone
- Tetracycline

Exercise

To preserve bone health through adulthood, the American Academy of Sports Medicine recommends weight-bearing activity three to five times per week and resistance exercise two to three times per week with moderate to high bone-loading force for a combination of 30 to 60 minutes per week. Regular walking and swimming appear to have minor benefits in older individuals. More active participation (such as weight-bearing exercises and intensive walking) has positive effects on BMD.

Medical Nutrition Therapy

Calcium (1000 mg/day) and vitamin D (800 to 1000 units/day) are typically recommended as supplements for patients being treated with one of the bone drugs, either antiresorptive or anabolic. These amounts are considered both safe and sufficient for bone formation. The efficacy of calcium or calcium plus vitamin D supplementation continues to be investigated. Several studies report a reduction in fracture risk for postmenopausal women when supplements with calcium and vitamin D are used (Stránský and Rysavá, 2009). In a meta-analysis of 15 publications of nursing home residents, supplementation with calcium (1200 mg) and vitamin D (800 IU) reduced fracture risk and improved BMD (Parikh et al., 2009). Several studies also report the efficacy of calcium and vitamin D supplementation in older adults who live at home.

Interventions with children also show the benefits of calcium supplementation on PBM (Lanham-New, 2008). Reports are not consistent, however, possibly because of the variation in calcium and vitamin D status or environmental factors. Thus, because of the range of nutrients involved in bone health, a healthy diet emphasizing the key nutrients seems most promising in achieving an intake for optimal bone health (Tucker, 2009).

FDA-Approved Drug Treatments

Estrogen replacement therapy (ERT) is hormone-replacement therapy approved by the FDA as treatment for the prevention of osteoporosis. Because of potential side effects, nonestrogen treatment for prevention is recommended, especially if menopausal symptom relief is not a goal.

Bisphosphonates act as antiresorbers on osteoclasts to reduce their bone-degradative activities. They have been shown to be effective in reducing the incidence of new fractures (Epstein, 2006). The bisphosphonates act by inhibiting osteoclast-mediated bone resorption. Examples include alendronate, risedronate, ibandronate, and zoledronic acid. Side effects include gastrointestinal problems and rare cases of jaw necrosis.

Calcitonin, the hormone, is used to inhibit osteoclastic bone resorption by blocking the stimulatory effects of PTH on these cells. Calcitonin can be administered by nasal spray. It improves BMD, especially of the lumbar spine, and it may reduce the recurrence of fractures in patients with osteoporosis. Calcitonin is approved by the FDA for postmenopausal treatment of osteoporosis, but it is recommended that the women be at least five years' postmenopausal.

PTH therapy is approved by the FDA for the treatment of postmenopausal women and men at high risk for fracture, and for those on long-term glucocorticoid therapy. PTH works by increasing osteoblast number and function (Kousteni and Bilezikian, 2008). PTH increases spine, hip, and total body BMD. PTH is often prescribed first, followed by bisphosphonates, so that an increase in bone mass is followed by antiresorptive therapy (Cosman, 2008).

Selective estrogen receptor modulators (SERMs) are able to stimulate **estrogen receptors (ER)** in bone tissue and yet have very little effect on the ERs of the breast or uterus. Another term for SERMs is *estrogen agonist* or *antagonist* because they act as weak estrogen agonists at times and as weak estrogen antagonists at others. Two examples of these drugs are tamoxifen and raloxifene. The most common side effect is hot flashes.

Drug Treatments Not Yet Approved By the FDA

Calcitriol is 1,25-dihyroxy vitamin D3, and has had little use in the treatment of osteoporosis because of its potential toxicity. Calcium plus calcitriol may be useful, however, in patients who are taking high-dose corticosteroid therapy, during which vertebral fractures are common.

Growth hormone and insulin-like growth factors may improve bone through anabolic effects, but more research is needed.

Osteoprotegerin (OPG) is a natural cytokine secreted by osteoblasts as well as other cell types. OPG can be detected in human serum and inactivates another cytokine that affects osteoclasts, thereby inhibiting osteoclast activation and bone resorption. Final results from clinical trials are anticipated.

PTH 1-84 is an intact human recombinant form of PTH undergoing clinical trials.

Sodium fluoride treatment increases bone mass, especially in trabecular bone. However, the quality of the bone typically is not normal. Fluoride ions become incorporated at the surfaces of hydroxyapatite crystals; the size and structure of the crystals become so altered that the mechanical competence of the bone declines. Fluoride therapy is not likely ever to be approved by the FDA.

Strontium ranelate is the mechanism supporting the reduction in spine and nonspine fractures; yet, the use of strontium is not clear.

Prevention of Falls

Fractures of the humerus, wrist, pelvis, and hip are often age related, resulting from a combination of osteoporosis and falling. Although only a small percentage of falls result in fractures, preventing falls through education and attention to the living environment of older adults is an important measure. Wearing girdles with built-in pads to protect the hips during a fall has been demonstrated in some, but not all, studies to significantly reduce the rate of fractures in a well-controlled investigation. A physical therapist can often evaluate the home to provide advice on reducing the likelihood of falls.

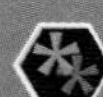

CLINICAL SCENARIO

Annie B., a 70-year-old white woman of Northern European ancestry, developed lactose intolerance during her early 50s when she had a serious gastrointestinal infection. She currently is retired, lives alone, and stays indoors most of each day watching television. Approximately 3 years ago at age 67, she had dual-energy x-ray absorptiometry (DEXA) measurements that showed that she had low bone mineral density (BMD) values of her proximal femur and lumbar vertebrae (both values are classified as osteoporotic according to World Health Organization definitions). Her physician recommended that she start taking supplements of calcium (1000 mg/day) and vitamin D (800 units/day) because of her lactose intolerance and her lack of consumption of all dairy products.

Annie took the supplements regularly for a year when a second set of DEXA measurements revealed that she had practically maintained her BMD values of 1 year earlier, with only a small decline in BMD. However, her continuing low measurements concerned her physician, and he ordered laboratory tests of calcium-regulatory hormones to see if she had any hormonal complications. These tests showed that her parathyroid hormone and 25-hydroxy vitamin D concentrations fell in the upper half of the normal range for each variable. Other routine measurements such as serum calcium and phosphate were normal. After discussion of her high risk of an osteoporotic fracture, her physician decided to place Annie on a bisphosphonate drug in addition to calcium and vitamin D.

After 1 year on the new therapy and continuation of the calcium and vitamin D, her BMD values (her third set of DEXA measurements) actually increased a few percentage points, even though they remained within the classification of osteoporosis. She was then instructed by her physician to continue indefinitely on this therapeutic regimen.

Nutrition Diagnostic Statement

Inadequate calcium and vitamin D intake related to avoidance of dairy products as evidenced by diet history revealing less

CLINICAL SCENARIO—cont'd

than 20% of estimated requirements. Note: This may be resolved once she starts taking supplements.

Nutrition Care Questions

1. How would you classify Annie's calcium intake at the initial visit with her physician (who did not take a diet history or estimate her calcium intake)? Her vitamin D intake? Her exposure to sunlight?
2. What would you have recommended to improve her calcium intake from foods so that she could reduce her supplemental calcium to 500 mg/day? Why would you recommend foods to provide calcium rather than supplements? Could you make similar recommendations for improving her intake of vitamin D from foods?
3. Design a set (3 days minimum) of daily menus that provide approximately 800 mg of calcium from foods alone, which, coupled with a 500-mg supplement, would provide a total of 1300 mg, the current adequate intake for calcium. Similarly, design these same meals to include 400 units of vitamin D, with another 400 units coming from supplements.

USEFUL WEBSITES

Center for Disease Control and Prevention
http://www.cdc.gov/nutrition/everyone/basics/vitamins/calcium.html

Menopause
http://www.menopause.org/

National Institutes of Health—Bone Health
http://www.nichd.nih.gov/health/topics/bone_health.cfm

National Osteoporosis Foundation
http://www.nof.org/

REFERENCES

Chubak J, et al: Effect of exercise on bone mineral density and lean mass in postmenopausal women, *Med Sci Sports Exerc* 38:1236, 2006.

Cosman F: Parathyroid hormone treatment for osteoporosis, *Cur Opin Endocrin Diab Obes* 15:495, 2008.

Darling AL, et al: Dietary protein and bone health: a systematic review and meta-analysis, *Am J Clin Nutr* 90:1674, 2009.

Epstein S: Update of current therapeutic options for the treatment of postmenopausal osteoporosis, *Clin Ther* 28:151, 2006.

Ford SK, Moll S: Vitamin K supplementation to decrease variability of international normalized ratio in patients on vitamin K antagonists: a literature review, *Curr Opin Hematol* 15(5):504, 2008.

Goulding A, et al: Bone and body composition of children and adolescents with repeated forearm fractures, *J Bone Miner Res* 20:2090, 2005.

Hakki SS, et al: Boron regulates mineralized tissue-associated proteins in osteoblasts (MC3T3-E1), *J Trace Elem Med Biol* 24(4):243, 2010.

Hallström H, et al: Coffee consumption and CYP1A2 genotype in relation to bone mineral density of the proximal femur in elderly men and women: a cohort study. *Nutr Metab (Lond)* 7:12, 2010.

Hinoi E, et al: An osteoblast-dependent mechanism contributes to the leptin regulation of insulin secretion, *Ann N Y Acad Sci* 1173:E20, 2009.

Hypponen E, Power C: Hypovitaminosis D in British adults at age 45 y: nationwide cohort study of dietary and lifestyle predictors, *Am J Clin Nutr* 85:860, 2007.

Ilich JZ, et al: Higher habitual sodium intake is not detrimental for bones in older women with adequate calcium intake, *Eur J Appl Physiol* 109:745, 2010.

Institute of Medicine (IOM): *Standing Committee on the Scientific Evaluation of Dietary Reference Intakes, Food and Nutrition Board: Dietary reference intakes for calcium and vitamin D*, Washington, DC, 2011, National Academy Press. Accessed at www.nap.edu.

Iuliano-Burns S, et al: Diet and exercise during growth have site-specific skeletal effects: a co-twin study, *Osteoporos Int* 16:1225, 2005.

Kanis JA, et al: Alcohol intake as a risk factor for fracture, *Osteopros Int* 16:737, 2005.

Khosla S: Update in male osteoporosis, *J Clin Endocrinol Metab* 95:3, 2010.

Kousteni S, Bilezikian JP: The cell biology of parathyroid hormone in osteoblasts, *Curr Osteoporos Rep* 6:72, 2008.

Lambert CP, et al: Exercise but not diet-induced weight loss decreases skeletal muscle inflammatory gene expression in frail obese elderly persons, *J Appl Physiol* 105:473, 2008.

Lanham-New SA: Importance of calcium, vitamin D and vitamin K for osteoporosis prevention and treatment, *Proc Nutr Soc* 67:163, 2008.

MacKinnon AS, et al: Dietary restriction of lycopene for a period of one month resulted in significantly increased biomarkers of oxidative stress and bone resorption in postmenopausal women. *J Nutr Health Aging* 15:133, 2011.

Massey LK: Effect of dietary salt intake on circadian calcium metabolism, bone turnover, and calcium oxalate kidney stone risk in postmenopausal women, *Nutr Res* 25:891, 2005.

McCarty CA: Sunlight exposure assessment: can we accurately assess vitamin D exposure from sunlight questionnaires? *Am J Clin Nutr* 87:1097, 2008.

Misra M, Klibanski A: Anorexia nervosa and osteoporosis, *Rev Endocr Metab Disord* 7:91, 2006.

National Health and Nutrition Examination Survey (NHANES): NHANES home. Accessed 2 April 2010 from www.cdc.gov/nchs/nhanes.htm.

National Osteoporosis Foundation [NOF.] Website http://www.nof.org/. Accessed 7/13/10.

Nielsen FH: Is boron nutritionally relevant? *Nutr Rev* 66:183, 2008.

Nieves JW: Osteoporosis: the role of micronutrients, *Am J Clin Nutr* 81:1232S, 2005.

North America Menopause Society (NAMS): Management of osteoporosis in post-menopausal women: 2010 position statement of the North America Menopause Society, *Menopause* 17:25, 2010.

Oudshoorn C, et al: Ageing and vitamin D deficiency: effects on calcium homeostasis and considerations for vitamin D supplementation, *Br J Nutr* 101:1597, 2009.

Parikh S, et al: Pharmacological management of osteoporosis in nursing home populations: a systematic review, *J Am Geriatr Soc* 57:327, 2009.

Plawecki KL, et al: Assessing calcium intake in postmenopausal women, *Prev Chronic Dis* 6:124, 2009.

Pothiwala P, et al: Ethnic variation in risk for osteoporosis among women: a review of biological and behavioral factors, *J Womens Health* 15:709, 2006.

Prentice A: Milk intake, calcium and vitamin d in pregnancy and lactation: effects on maternal, fetal and infant bone in low- and high-income countries, *Nestle Nutr Workshop Ser Pediatr Program* 67:1, 2011.

Reid IR: Fat and bone, *Arch Biochem Biophys* 503(1):20, 2010.

Reid IR: Relationships between fat and bone, *Osteoporos Int* 19:595, 2008.

Ribaya-Mercado JD, Blumberg JB: Vitamin A: is it a risk factor for osteoporosis and bone fracture? *Nutr Rev* 65:425, 2007.

Rizzoli R: Nutrition: its role in bone health, *Best Pract Res Clin Endocrinol Metab* 22:813, 2008.

Rude RK, et al: Skeletal and hormonal effects of magnesium deficiency, *J Am Coll Nutr* 28:131, 2009.

Ruffing J, et al: Determinants of bone mass and bone size in a large cohort of physically active young adult men, *Nutr Metabol* 3:14, 2006.

Ryder KM, et al: Magnesium intake from food and supplements is associated with bone mineral density in healthy older white subjects, *J Am Geriatr Soc* 53:1875, 2005.

Sebastian A: Dietary protein content and the diet's net acid load: opposing effects on bone health, *Am J Clin Nutr* 82:921, 2005.

Stránský M, Rysavá L: Nutrition as prevention and treatment of osteoporosis, *Physiol Res* 58:S7, 2009.

Straub DA: Calcium supplementation in clinical practice: a review of forms, doses, and indications, *Nutr Clin Pract* 22:286, 2007.

Tucker KL: Osteoporosis prevention and nutrition, *Curr Osteoporos Rep* 7:111, 2009.

Tucker KL, et al: Effects of beer, wine, and liquor intakes on bone mineral density in older men and women, *Am J Clin Nutr* 89:1188, 2009.

Wagner CL, Greer FR: American Academy of Pediatrics Section on Breastfeeding, American Academy of Pediatrics Committee on Nutrition: Prevention of rickets and vitamin D deficiency in infants, children, and adolescents, *Pediatrics* 122:1142, 2008.

CHAPTER 26

Diane Rigassio Radler, PhD, RD

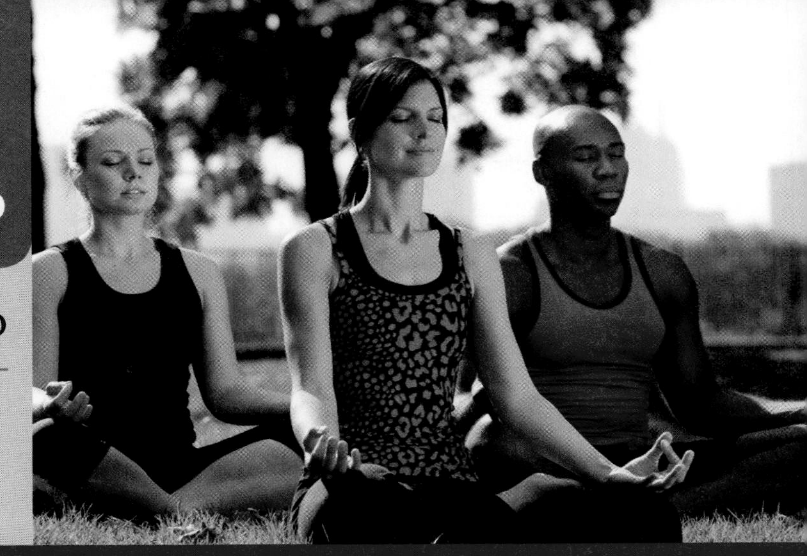

Nutrition for Oral and Dental Health

KEY TERMS

anticariogenic
calculus
candidiasis
cariogenic
cariogenicity
cariostatic
demineralization
dental caries
dental erosion
dentin
early childhood caries (ECC)
edentulism
enamel
fermentable carbohydrate
fluoroapatite
fluorosis
gingiva
gingival sulcus
hydroxyapatite
lingual caries
periodontal disease
plaque
remineralization
root caries
stomatitis
Streptococcus mutans
xerostomia

Diet and nutrition play key roles in tooth development, integrity of the **gingiva** (gums) and mucosa, bone strength, and the prevention and management of diseases of the oral cavity. Diet has a local effect on tooth integrity; the type, form, and frequency of foods and beverages consumed have a direct effect on the oral pH and microbial activity, which may promote dental decay. Nutrition systemically affects the development, maintenance, and repair of teeth and oral tissues.

Nutrition and diet affect the oral cavity, but the reverse is also true; that is, the status of the oral cavity may affect one's ability to consume an adequate diet and achieve nutritional balance. Indeed, there is a lifelong synergy between nutrition and the integrity of the oral cavity in health and disease related to the known roles of diet and nutrients in the growth, development, and maintenance of the oral cavity structure, bones, and tissues (Touger-Decker et al., 2007).

Sections of this chapter were written by Riva Touger-Decker, PhD, RD, FADA for the previous edition of this text.

NUTRITION FOR TOOTH DEVELOPMENT

Primary tooth development begins at 2 to 3 months' gestation. Mineralization begins at approximately 4 months' gestation and continues through the preteen years. Therefore maternal nutrition must supply the preeruptive teeth with the appropriate building materials. Inadequate maternal nutrition consequently affects tooth development.

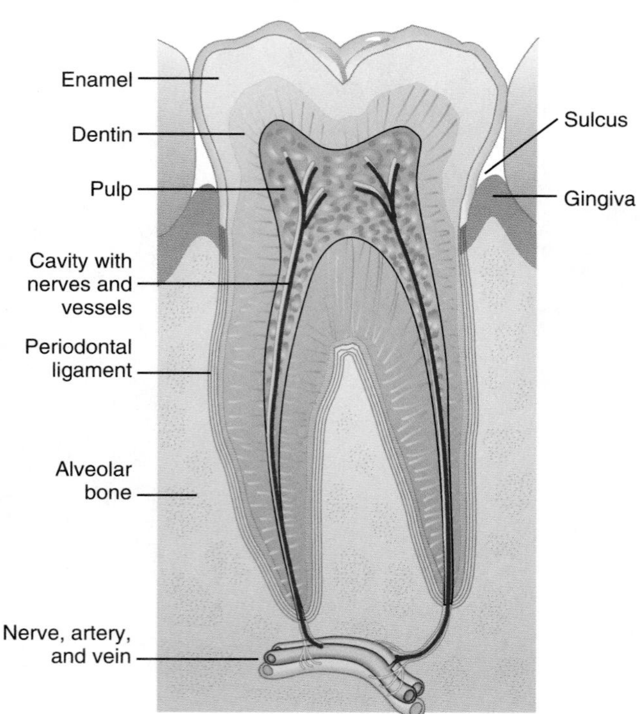

FIGURE 26-1 Anatomy of a tooth.

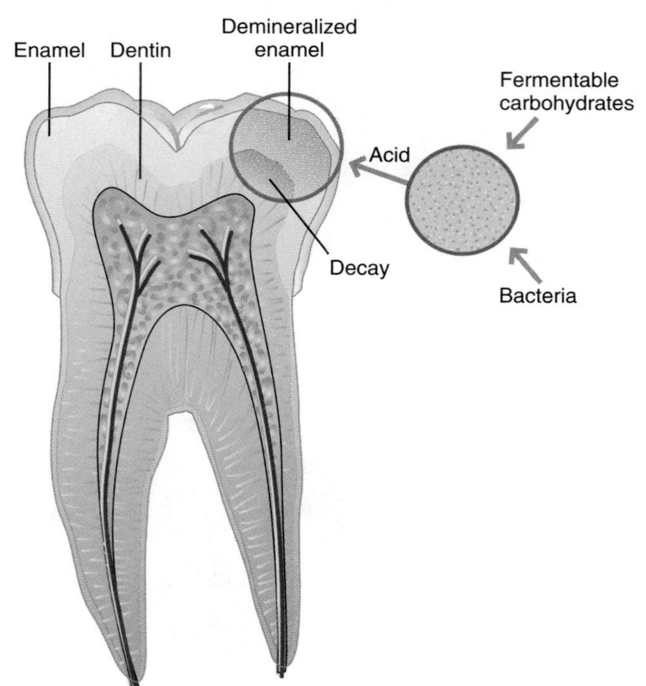

FIGURE 26-2 Formation of dental caries.

Teeth are formed by the mineralization of a protein matrix. In **dentin**, protein is present as collagen, which depends on vitamin C for normal synthesis. Vitamin D is essential to the process by which calcium and phosphorus are deposited in crystals of **hydroxyapatite**, a naturally occurring form of calcium and phosphorus that is the mineral component of **enamel** and dentin. Fluoride added to the hydroxyapatite provides unique caries-resistant properties to teeth in both prenatal and postnatal developmental periods.

Diet and nutrition are important in all phases of tooth development, eruption, and maintenance (Figure 26-1). Posteruption, diet and nutrient intake continue to affect tooth development and mineralization, enamel development and strength, and eruption patterns of the remaining teeth. The local effects of diet, particularly fermentable carbohydrates and eating frequency, affect the production of organic acids by oral bacteria and the rate of tooth decay as described later in this chapter.

DENTAL CARIES

Dental caries is one of the most common infectious diseases. According to a Surgeon General's report on oral health in 2000, dental caries is seven times more common than hay fever and five times more common than asthma. Unfortunately, differences are evident in caries prevalence; approximately 20% to 25% of U.S. children have 80% of the dental caries. Trends in dental caries have demonstrated that children who come from homes in which parents have at least a college education have fewer caries than children from homes in which parents have less than a college education (Centers for Disease Control and Prevention [CDC], 2010). These differences, or health disparities, may happen as a result of lack of access to care, cost of care not reimbursed by third-party payors (e.g., insurance, Medicaid), lack of knowledge of preventive dental care, or a combination of factors.

Pathophysiology

Dental caries is an oral infectious disease in which organic acid metabolites lead to gradual **demineralization** of tooth enamel, followed by rapid proteolytic destruction of the tooth structure. Caries can occur on any tooth surface. The cause of dental caries involves many factors. Four factors must be present simultaneously: (1) a susceptible host or tooth surface; (2) microorganisms such as *Streptococcus* or *Lactobacillus* in the dental plaque or oral cavity; (3) fermentable carbohydrates in the diet, which serve as the substrate for bacteria; and (4) time (duration) in the mouth for bacteria to metabolize the fermentable carbohydrates, produce acids, and cause a drop in salivary pH to less than 5.5. Once the pH is acidic, which can occur within minutes, oral bacteria can initiate the demineralization process. Figure 26-2 shows the formation of dental caries.

Susceptible Tooth

The development of dental caries requires the presence of a tooth that is vulnerable to attack. The composition of enamel and dentin, the location of teeth, the quality and quantity of saliva, and the presence and extent of pits and fissures in the tooth crown are some of the factors that

BOX 26-1

Factors Affecting Cariogenicity of Foods

Frequency of consumption
Food form (liquid or solid, slowly dissolving)
Sequence of eating certain foods and beverages
Combination of foods
Nutrient composition of foods and beverages
Duration of exposure of teeth

govern susceptibility. Alkaline saliva may have a protective effect, whereas acidic saliva increases susceptibility to decay.

Microorganisms

Bacteria are an essential part of the decay process. **Streptococcus mutans** is the most prevalent, followed by *Lactobacillus casein* and *Streptococcus sanguis*. All three contribute to the process because they metabolize carbohydrates in the mouth, producing acid as a byproduct, which is sufficient to cause decay. Genetic variations of the type and quantity of bacteria present in the oral cavity may put someone at an increased risk for caries and periodontal disease, but the quantity and quality of oral hygiene contributes directly to the risk of oral infectious disease.

Substrate

Fermentable carbohydrates, those carbohydrates susceptible to the actions of salivary amylase, are the ideal substrate for bacterial metabolism. The acids produced by their metabolism cause a drop in salivary pH to less than 5.5, creating the environment for decay. Bacteria are always present and begin to reduce pH when they have exposure to fermentable carbohydrates.

Although both the Dietary Guidelines for Americans and the MyPlate Food Guidance system support a diet high in carbohydrates, it is important to be aware of the cariogenicity of foods. **Cariogenicity** refers to the caries-promoting properties of a diet or food. The cariogenicity of a food varies, depending on the form in which it occurs, its nutrient composition, when it is eaten in relation to other foods and fluids, the duration of its exposure to the tooth, and the frequency with which it is eaten (Box 26-1).

Individuals should be aware of the form of food consumed and the frequency of intake to integrate positive diet and oral hygiene habits to reduce risk of oral disease.

Fermentable carbohydrates are found in three of the five MyPlate food groups: (1) grains, (2) fruits, and (3) dairy. Although some vegetables may contain fermentable carbohydrates, little has been reported about the cariogenicity, or caries-promoting properties, of vegetables. Examples of grains and starches that are cariogenic by nature of their fermentable carbohydrate composition include crackers, chips, pretzels, hot and cold cereals, and breads.

All fruits (fresh, dried, and canned) and fruit juices may be cariogenic. Fruits with high water content, such as melons, have a lower cariogenicity than others such as bananas and dried fruits. Fruit drinks, sodas, ice teas, and other sugar-sweetened beverages; desserts; cookies; candies; and cake products may be cariogenic. Dairy products sweetened with fructose, sucrose, or other sugars can also be cariogenic because of the added sugars; however, dairy products are rich in calcium, and their alkaline nature may have a positive influence, reducing the cariogenic potential of the food.

Like other sugars (glucose, fructose, maltose, and lactose), sucrose stimulates bacterial activity. The causal relationship between sucrose and dental caries has been established (Marshall, 2007; Moynihan, 2005). All dietary forms of sugar, including honey, molasses, brown sugar, and corn syrup solids, have cariogenic potential and can be used by bacteria to produce organic acid.

Caries Promotion by Individual Foods

It is important to differentiate between cariogenic, cariostatic, and anticariogenic foods. **Cariogenic** foods are those that contain fermentable carbohydrates, which, when in contact with microorganisms in the mouth, can cause a drop in salivary pH to 5.5 or less and stimulate the caries process.

Cariostatic foods do not contribute to decay, are not metabolized by microorganisms, and do not cause a drop in salivary pH to 5.5 or less within 30 minutes. Examples of cariostatic foods are protein foods such as eggs, fish, meat, and poultry; most vegetables; fats; and sugarless gums. Sugarless gum may help to reduce decay potential because of its ability to increase saliva flow and because it uses noncarbohydrate sweeteners (Deshpande, 2008; Splieth, 2009).

Anticariogenic foods are those that, when eaten before an acidogenic food, prevent plaque from recognizing the acidogenic food. Examples are aged cheddar, Monterey Jack, and Swiss because of the casein, calcium, and phosphate in the cheese. The five-carbon sugar alcohol, xylitol, is considered anticariogenic because bacteria cannot metabolize five-carbon sugars in the same way as six-carbon sugars like glucose, sucrose, and fructose. It is not broken down by salivary amylase and is not subject to bacterial degradation. Salivary stimulation leads to increased buffering activity of the saliva and subsequent increased clearance of fermentable carbohydrates from tooth surfaces. Another anticariogenic mechanism of xylitol gum is that it replaces fermentable carbohydrates in the diet. *S. mutans* cannot metabolize xylitol and is inhibited by it. Both the antimicrobial activity against *S. mutans* and the effect of gum chewing on salivary stimulation are protective. Brands of chewing gum that include xylitol are Arm and Hammer Advance White, Dentyne Ice, Spry, and Trident.

Remineralization is mineral restoration of the hydroxyapatite in dental enamel. Casein phosphopeptide-amorphous calcium phosphate (CPP-ACP; Recaldent) is a substance that promotes remineralization of enamel surfaces. It is currently available as an ingredient in Trident White brand chewing gums (Ramalingam, 2005). CPP-ACP has also exhibited anticariogenic activity in randomized, controlled clinical trials of sugar-free gum and a tooth cream (Walker et al., 2010). Its use for that purpose is not suggested at this time.

Factors Affecting Cariogenicity of Food

Cariogenicity also is influenced by the volume and quality of saliva; the sequence, consistency, and nutrient composition of the foods eaten; dental plaque buildup; and the genetic predisposition of the host to decay.

Form and Consistency

The form and consistency of a food have a significant effect on its cariogenic potential and pH-reducing or buffering capacity. Food form determines the duration of exposure or retention time of a food in the mouth, which, in turn, affects how long the decrease in pH or the acid-producing activity will last. Liquids are rapidly cleared from the mouth and have low adherence (or retentiveness) capabilities. Solid foods such as crackers, chips, pretzels, dry cereals, and cookies can stick between the teeth (referred to as the *interproximal spaces*) and have high adherence (or retention) capability.

Consistency also affects adherence. Chewy foods such as gum drops and marshmallows, although high in sugar content, stimulate saliva production and have a lower adherence potential than solid, sticky foods such as pretzels, bagels, or bananas. High-fiber foods with few or no fermentable carbohydrates, such as popcorn and raw vegetables, are cariostatic.

Exposure

The duration of exposure may be best explained with starchy foods, which are fermentable carbohydrates subject to the action of salivary amylase. The longer starches are retained in the mouth, the greater their cariogenicity (Fontana, 2006). Given sufficient time, such as when food particles become lodged between the teeth, salivary amylase makes additional substrate available as it hydrolyzes starch to simple sugars. Processing techniques, either by partial hydrolysis or by reducing particle size, make some starches rapidly fermentable by increasing their availability for enzyme action.

Sugar-containing candies rapidly increase the amount of sugar available in the oral cavity to be hydrolyzed by bacteria. Sucking on hard candies such as lollipops or sugared breath mints results in prolonged sugar exposure in the mouth. Simple carbohydrate-based snacks and dessert foods (e.g., potato chips, pretzels, cookies, cakes, and doughnuts) provide gradually increasing oral sugar concentrations for a longer duration because these foods often adhere to the tooth surfaces and are retained for longer periods than candies (Fontana, 2006).

Nutrient Composition

Nutrient composition contributes to the ability of a substrate to produce acid and to the duration of acid exposure. Dairy products, by virtue of their calcium- and phosphorus-buffering potential, are considered to have low cariogenic potential. Evidence suggests that cheese and milk, when consumed with cariogenic foods, help to buffer the acid pH produced by the cariogenic foods. Because of the anticariogenic properties of cheese, eating cheese with a fermentable carbohydrate, such as dessert at the end of a meal, may decrease the cariogenicity of the meal and dessert (Moynihan, 2005).

Nuts, which do not contain a significant amount of fermentable carbohydrates and are high in fat and dietary fiber, are cariostatic. Protein foods such as seafood, meats, eggs, and poultry, along with other fats such as oils, margarine, butter, and seeds, are also cariostatic.

Sequence and Frequency of Eating

Eating sequence and combination of foods also affect the caries potential of the substrate. Bananas, which are cariogenic because of their fermentable carbohydrate content and adherence capability, have less potential to contribute to decay when eaten with cereal and milk than when eaten alone as a snack. Milk, as a liquid, reduces the adherence capability of the fruit. Crackers eaten with cheese are less cariogenic than when eaten alone.

The frequency with which a cariogenic food or beverage is consumed determines the number of opportunities for acid production. Every time a fermentable carbohydrate is consumed, a decline in pH is initiated within 5 to 15 minutes, causing caries-promoting activity. Small, frequent meals and snacks, often high in fermentable carbohydrate, increase the cariogenicity of a diet more than a diet consisting of three meals and minimal snacks. Eating several cookies at once, followed by brushing the teeth or rinsing the mouth with water, is less cariogenic than eating a cookie several times throughout a day. Table 26-1 lists messages that can be given to children to prevent caries.

The Decay Process

The carious process begins with the production of acids as a by-product of bacterial metabolism taking place in the dental plaque. Decalcification of the surface enamel continues until the buffering action of the saliva is able to raise the pH above the critical level. See Box 26-2 for prevention guidelines.

Plaque is a sticky, colorless mass of microorganisms and polysaccharides that forms around the tooth and adheres to teeth and gums. It harbors acid-forming bacteria and keeps the organic products of their metabolism in close contact with the enamel surface. As a cavity develops, the plaque blocks the tooth, to some extent, from the buffering and remineralization action of the saliva. In time the plaque combines with calcium and hardens to form **calculus**.

An acidic pH is also required for plaque formation. Soft drinks (diet and regular), sports beverages, citrus juices and "ades," and vitamin C supplements have high acid content. Research using National Health and Nutrition Examination Survey III data reported significantly more dental caries in children (ages 2 to 10 years) who consumed large amounts of carbonated soft drinks or juices when compared with children who had high consumption of water or milk (Sohn, 2006). Other beverages and foods contribute to **dental erosion**, a loss of minerals from tooth surfaces by a chemical process in the presence of acid (Wongkhantee, 2006).

TABLE 26-1

Nutrition Messages Related to Oral Health for 3- to 10-Year-Old Children and Their Caregivers

Message	Rationale
Starchy, sticky, or sugary foods should be eaten with nonsugary foods.	The pH will rise if a nonsugary item that stimulates saliva is eaten immediately before, during, or after a challenge.
Combine dairy products with a meal or snack.	Dairy products (nonfat milk, yogurt) enhance remineralization and contain calcium.
Combine chewy foods such as fresh fruits and vegetables with fermentable carbohydrates.	Chewy, fibrous foods induce saliva production and buffering capacity.
Space eating occasions at least 2 hours apart and limit snack time to 15-30 minutes.	Fermentable carbohydrates eaten sequentially one after another promote demineralization.
Limit bedtime snacks.	Saliva production declines during sleep.
Limit consumption of acidic foods such as sports drinks, juices, and sodas.	Acidic foods promote tooth erosion that increases risk for caries.
Combine proteins with carbohydrates in snacks: Examples: tuna and crackers, apples and cheese	Proteins act as buffers and are cariostatic.
Combine raw and cooked or processed foods in a snack.	Raw foods encourage mastication and saliva production, whereas cooked or processed foods may be more available for bacterial metabolism if eaten alone.
Encourage use of xylitol- or sorbitol-based chewing gum and candies immediately following a meal or snack.*	Five minutes of exposure is effective in increasing saliva production and dental plaque pH.
Sugar-free chewable vitamin and mineral supplements and syrup-based medication should be recommended.	Sugar-free varieties are available and should be suggested for high–caries risk groups.
Encourage children with pediatric GERD to adhere to dietary guidelines.	GERD increases risk for dental erosion and thus increases risk for caries.

Modified from Mobley C: Frequent dietary intake and oral health in children 3 to 10 years of age, Building Blocks 25(1):17-20, 2001.

GERD, Gastroesophageal reflux disease.

*Gum is not recommended for children younger than 6 years old.

BOX 26-2

Caries Prevention Guidelines

- Brush at least twice daily, preferably after meals.
- Rinse mouth after meals and snacks.
- Chew sugarless gum for 15 to 20 min after meals and snacks.
- Floss twice daily.
- Use fluoridated toothpastes.
- Pair cariogenic foods with cariostatic foods.
- Snack on cariostatic and anticariogenic foods such as cheese, nuts, popcorn, and vegetables.
- Limit between-meal eating and drinking of fermentable carbohydrates.

For example, diet soft drinks, which may not contain sugar, also are acidic by nature and therefore cause a drop in pH. Chewable vitamin C supplements provide an acidic substance that directly contacts tooth surfaces and causes a drop in pH of the oral cavity, making teeth susceptible to erosion.

Roles of Saliva

Salivary flow clears food from around the teeth. By means of the bicarbonate-carbonic acid and phosphate buffer system, it also provides buffering action to neutralize bacterial acid metabolism. Chewing promotes saliva production and may account for the reduced cariogenicity of fermentable carbohydrates consumed with a meal.

Saliva is supersaturated with calcium and phosphorus. Once buffering action has restored pH above the critical point, remineralization can occur. If fluoride is present in the saliva, the minerals are deposited in the form of **fluoroapatite**, which is resistant to erosion. It should be noted that salivary production decreases as a result of diseases affecting salivary gland function (e.g., Sjögren's syndrome); as a side-effect of fasting; as a result of radiation therapy to the head and neck involving the parotid gland; normally during sleep; with the use of medications associated with reduced salivary flow; or with **xerostomia**, dry mouth caused by inadequate saliva production. There are estimates that between 400 and 500 medications currently available by prescription or over the counter may cause dry mouth. The degree of xerostomia may vary but may be caused by medications such as those to treat depression, hypertension, anxiety, human immunodeficiency virus (HIV), and allergies, to name a few.

Caries Patterns

Caries patterns describe the location and surfaces of the teeth affected. Coronal caries affect the crown of the tooth, the part of the tooth visible above the gum line, and may occur on any tooth surface. Although the overall incidence of decay in the United States has declined, as many as 17% of children between 2 and 4 years of age have tooth decay. According to the National Oral Health Surveillance System, many states report 40% to 70% of children having some decay by age 8.

Root caries, occurring on the root surfaces of teeth secondary to gingival recession, affect a large portion of the older population. Root caries is a dental infection that is increasing in older adults, partly because this population is retaining their natural teeth longer. The gums recede in older age, exposing the root surface. Other factors related to the increased incidence of this decay pattern are lack of fluoridated water, poor oral hygiene practices, decreased saliva, frequent eating of fermentable carbohydrates, and dementia (Chalmers, 2008;). Management of root caries includes dental restoration and nutrition counseling. Poor oral health from caries, pain, or edentulism may adversely affect dietary intake and nutritional status in the older adult (Quandt, 2009).

Lingual caries, or caries on the lingual side (surface next to or toward the tongue) of the anterior teeth, are seen in persons with gastrointestinal reflux, bulimia, or anorexia-bulimia (see Chapter 23). Frequent intake of fermentable carbohydrates, combined with regurgitation or induced vomiting of acidic stomach contents, results in a constant influx of acid into the oral cavity. The caries are the end result of tooth erosion characterized by erosion of the palatal and buccal surfaces of the maxillary anterior teeth and the lingual surfaces of the palatal surface of the maxillary posterior teeth (Holbrook, 2009).

Fluoride

Fluoride is a primary anticaries agent. Used systemically and locally, it is a safe, effective public health measure to reduce the incidence and prevalence of dental caries (Palmer and Wolfe, 2005). Water fluoridation began in 1940; by 1999 the Centers for Disease Control and Prevention listed water fluoridation as one of the top 10 greatest public health achievements of the 20th century because of its influence on decreasing the rate of dental caries (CDC, 2006). The effect of fluoride on caries prevention continues with water fluoridation, fluoridated toothpastes, oral rinses, and dentifrices, as well as beverages made with fluoridated water. Optimal water fluoridation concentrations (0.7 to 1.2 ppm) can provide protection against caries development without causing tooth staining (Palmer and Wolfe, 2005). See *Focus On:* Water Fluoridation.

Mechanism of Action

There are four primary mechanisms of fluoride action on teeth: (1) when incorporated into enamel and dentin along with calcium and phosphorus, it forms fluoroapatite, a compound more resistant to acid challenge than hydroxyapatite; (2) it promotes repair and remineralization of tooth surfaces with early signs of decay (incipient carious lesions); (3) it helps to reverse the decay process while promoting the development of a tooth surface that has increased resistance to decay; and (4) helps to deter the harmful effects of bacteria in the oral cavity by interfering with the formation and function of microorganisms.

FOCUS ON

Water Fluoridation

Fluoride supplementation has been endorsed as a public health measure by the American Dental Association and American Dietetic Association (American Dental Association, 2005; Palmer and Wolfe, 2005). The American Academy of Pediatrics, American Dental Association, and the American Academy of Pediatric Dentistry have developed a dosing schedule for fluoride supplementation that is aimed at providing adequate fluoride while preventing fluorosis.

1. All possible sources of fluoride must be taken into account. These include:
    - Knowing the fluoride content of the child's primary drinking water source and all other sources of water for the child (eg, other home, child care, school, relative or caregiver's house, bottled water).
    - Other sources of fluoride, such as prescriptions from the dentist, fluoride mouthrinse in school, or fluoride varnish.
2. If it is determined that fluoride access is limited, then supplementation should be written.
3. No child younger than 6 months of age and no child older than 16 years of age should be supplemented.
4. No child who has adequate access to (and is drinking) appropriately fluoridated community water should be supplemented.

The American Dental Association published a new guideline in 2010, recommending fluoride supplements be prescribed only to children determined to be high risk for the development of caries.

http://www.aap.org/oralhealth/pact/ch6_sect3b.cfm accessed 11 Mar 2011

Food Sources

Most foods, unless prepared with fluoridated water, contain minimal amounts of fluoride, except for brewed tea, which has approximately 1.4 ppm (Morin, 2006). Fluoride may be unintentionally added to the diet in a number of ways, including through the use of fluoridated water in the processing of foods and beverages. Fruit juices and drinks, particularly white grape juice produced in cities with fluoridated water, may have increased fluoride content; however, because of the wide variation in fluoride content, it is difficult to estimate amounts consumed.

Supplementation

It is prudent for health professionals to consider a child's fluid intake as well as food sources and the availability of fluoridated water in the community before prescribing fluoride supplements. Because bones are repositories of fluoride, bone meal, fish meal, and gelatin made from bones are potent sources of the mineral. In communities without fluoridated water, dietary fluoride supplements may be recommended for children ages 6 months to 16 years.

Fluoride can be used topically and systemically. When consumed in food and drink, it enters the systemic circulation and is deposited in bones and teeth. Systemic sources have a topical benefit as well by providing fluoride to the saliva. A small amount of fluoride enters the soft tissues; the remainder is excreted. The primary source of systemic fluoride is fluoridated water; food and beverages supply a smaller amount. Table 26-2 contains a schedule of fluoride supplementation for the public through age 16.

Fluoride supplements are not recommended for formula-fed infants or for breast-fed infants living in fluoridated communities if these infants receive drinking water between feedings. If the infant does not drink water between feedings or drinks bottled water when on a diet of only breast milk, he or she should be supplemented according to the fluoride supplement guidelines. Fluoride supplements must be prescribed by the child's doctor; they are not available as over-the-counter supplements (American Dental Association, 2005).

TABLE 26-2

Dietary Fluoride Supplement Schedule

	Fluoride Ion Level In Drinking Water (ppm)*		
Age	**<0.3 ppm**	**0.3-0.6 ppm**	**>0.6 ppm**
Birth-6 mo	None	None	None
6 mo-3 yr	0.25 mg/day[†]	None	None
3-6 yr	0.50 mg/day	0.25 mg/day	None
6-16 yr	1.0 mg/day	0.50 mg/day	None

Approved by The American Dental Association, The American Academy of Pediatrics, and The American Academy of Pediatric Dentistry, 1994.

*1 ppm = 1 mg/L.

[†]2.2 mg of sodium fluoride contains 1 mg of fluoride ion.

Topical fluoride sources include toothpastes, gels, and rinses used by consumers daily, along with more concentrated forms applied by dental professionals in the form of gels, foams, and rinses. Frequent fluoride exposure via topical fluorides, fluoridated toothpastes, rinses, and fluoridated water is important in maintaining an optimal concentration of fluoride, but excess intake should be avoided. (See Chapter 3.)

Excess Fluoride

Fluorosis occurs when too much fluoride is provided during tooth development and can range from mild to severe and present on teeth from unnoticeable to very apparent dark spots on teeth (Alvarez, 2009). Causes of mild fluorosis from excessive fluoride intake include misuse of dietary fluoride supplements, ingestion of fluoridated toothpastes and rinses, or excessive fluoride intake secondary to fluoride in foods and beverages processed in fluoridated areas and transported to other areas (Palmer and Wolfe, 2005). Topical fluorides, available as fluoridated toothpaste and mouthwashes, are effective sources of fluoride that can be used in the home, school, or dental office. Caries prevention efforts in preschool children include diet modification, water fluoridation or supplements in nonfluoridated areas, and supervised toothbrushing with fluoridated toothpaste (Alvarez, 2009).

Children younger than 6 years of age should not use fluoridated mouthwashes, and older children should be instructed to rinse, but not swallow, mouthwash. No more than a pea-size amount of toothpaste should be placed on a child's toothbrush to reduce the risk of accidental fluoride ingestion. Topical fluorides may be administered in the dental office.

Fluoride gels often are prescribed for adults and older adults. Such gels are effective in reducing the risk of coronal and root decay and tooth loss (Weintraub, 2006). Fluoride is most effective when given from birth through ages 12 to 13, the period when mineralization of unerupted permanent teeth occurs.

EARLY CHILDHOOD CARIES

Early childhood caries (ECC), often called "baby-bottle tooth decay," describes a caries pattern in the maxillary anterior teeth of infants and young children. Characteristics include rapidly developing carious lesions in the primary anterior teeth and the presence of lesions on tooth surfaces not usually associated with a high caries risk. Because tooth decay remains a common oral disease of childhood, caries are a primary marker for a child's oral health. Good behavioral habits and child nutrition patterns must be encouraged, beginning in infancy.

Pathophysiology and Incidence

Often ECC follows prolonged bottle-feeding, especially at night, of juice, milk, formula, or other sweetened beverages. The extended contact time with the fermentable carbohydrate–containing beverages, coupled with the position of the tongue against the nipple, which causes pooling

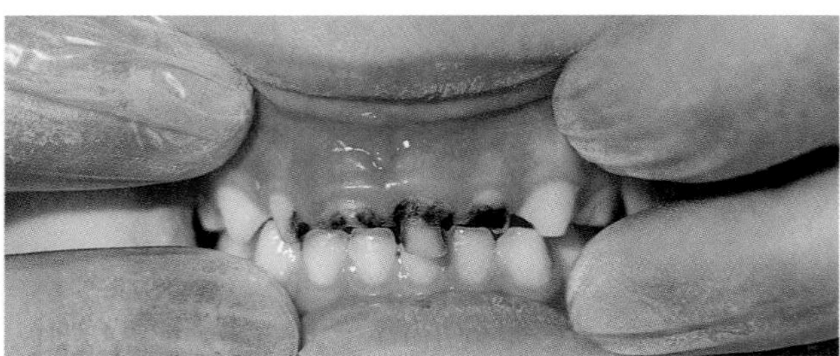

FIGURE 26-3 Early childhood caries. *(From Swartz MH:* Textbook of physical diagnosis, history, and examination, *ed 5, Philadelphia, 2006, Saunders.)*

of the liquid around the maxillary incisors, particularly during sleep, contributes to the decay process. The mandibular anterior teeth are usually spared (Figure 26-3) because of the protective position of the lip and tongue and the presence of a salivary duct in the floor of the mouth. In general, children from low-income families and minority populations experience the greatest amount of oral disease, the most extensive disease, and the most frequent use of dental services for pain relief; yet these children have the fewest overall dental visits (CDC, 2010).

Nutrition Care

Management of ECC includes diet and oral hygiene education for parents, guardians, and caregivers (Zero, 2010). Messages should be targeted to counter the health habits that contribute to this problem: poor oral hygiene, failure to brush a child's teeth at least daily, frequent use of bottles filled with sweetened beverages, and lack of fluoridated water. Dietary guidelines include removal of the bedtime bottle and modification of the frequency and content of the daytime bottles. Bottle contents should be limited to water, formula, or milk. Infants and young children should not be put to bed with a bottle. Teeth and gums should be cleaned with a gauze pad or washcloth after all bottle feedings. All efforts should be made to wean children from a bottle by 1 year of age. Educational efforts should be positive and simple, focusing on oral hygiene habits and promotion of a balanced, healthy diet. Between-meal snacks should include cariostatic foods. When foods are cariogenic, they should be followed by tooth brushing or rinsing the mouth. Parents and caregivers need to understand the causes and consequences of ECC and how they can be avoided.

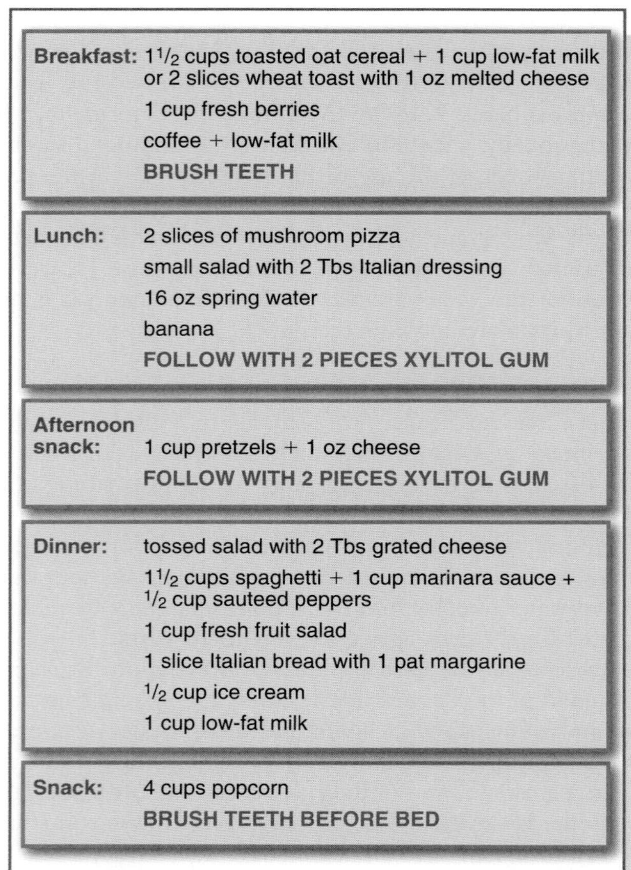

FIGURE 26-4 A balanced diet plan with low cariogenic risk.

CARIES PREVENTION

Caries prevention programs focus on a balanced diet, modification of the sources and quantities of fermentable carbohydrates, and the integration of oral hygiene practices into individual lifestyles (Zero, 2010). Meals and snacks should be followed with brushing, rinsing the mouth vigorously with water, or chewing sugarless gum for 15 to 20 minutes, preferably gum that contains xylitol (Splieth, 2009). Positive habits should be encouraged, including snacking on anticariogenic or cariostatic foods, chewing sugarless gum after eating or drinking cariogenic items, and having sweets with meals rather than as snacks. Despite the potential for a diet that is based on the dietary guidelines to be cariogenic, with proper planning and good oral hygiene a balanced diet low in cariogenic risk can be planned. See Figure 26-4 for a sample diet.

Practices to avoid include sipping carbonated beverages for extended periods; frequent snacking; and harboring candy, sugared breath mints, or hard candies in the mouth for extended periods. Over-the-counter chewable or liquid medications and vitamin preparations, such as chewable vitamin C or liquid cough syrup, may contain sugar and contribute to caries risk.

Fermentable carbohydrates such as candy, crackers, cookies, pastries, pretzels, snack crackers, chips, and even fruits should be eaten with meals. Notably, "fat-free" snack and dessert items and "baked" chips and snack crackers tend to have a higher simple sugar concentration than their higher fat-containing counterparts.

TOOTH LOSS AND DENTURES

Tooth loss (**edentulism**) and removable prostheses (dentures) can have a significant effect on dietary habits, masticatory function, olfaction, and nutritional adequacy. As dentition status declines, masticatory performance is compromised. Compromised masticatory function, from partial or complete edentulism or complete dentures, may have a negative effect on food choices, resulting in decreased intake of whole grains, fruits, and vegetables (Tsakos, 2010). This problem is more pronounced in older adults, whose appetite and intake may be compromised further by chronic disease, social isolation, and the use of multiple medications (see Chapter 9).

Dentures need to be checked periodically by a dental professional for appropriate fit. Changes in body weight or changes in alveolar bone over time possibly may alter the fit of the dentures. Counseling on appropriate food choices and textures is advocated.

Nutrition Care

Full dentures replace missing teeth but are not a perfect substitute for natural dentition. Both before and after denture placement, many individuals may experience difficulty biting and chewing, even after denture insertion. The foods found to cause the greatest difficulty for persons with complete dentures include fresh whole fruits and vegetables (e.g., apples and carrots), hard-crusted breads, and steak. Therefore dietary assessment and counseling related to oral health should be provided to the denture wearer. Simple guidelines should be provided for cutting and preparing fruits and vegetables to minimize the need for biting and reduce the amount of chewing. The importance of positive eating habits needs to be stressed as a component of total health. Overall, guidelines that reinforce the importance of a balanced diet should be part of the routine counseling given to all patients.

OTHER ORAL DISORDERS

Oral diseases extend beyond dental caries. Deficiencies of several vitamins (riboflavin, folate, B_{12}, and C) and minerals (iron and zinc) may be first detected in the oral cavity because of the rapid tissue turnover of the oral mucosa (see Appendix 30). Periodontal disease is a local and systemic disease. Select nutrients play a role, including vitamins A, C, E; folate; *β*-carotene; and the minerals calcium, phosphorus, and zinc. Oral cancer, often a result of tobacco and alcohol abuse, can have a significant effect on eating ability and nutritional status. This problem is compounded by the increased caloric and nutrient needs of persons with oral carcinomas. In addition, surgery, radiation therapy, and chemotherapy are modalities used to treat oral cancer that also can affect dietary intake, appetite, and the integrity of the oral cavity. Some but not all problems affecting the oral cavity are discussed here.

PERIODONTAL DISEASE

Pathophysiology

Periodontal disease is an inflammation of the gingiva with infection caused by oral bacteria and subsequent destruction of the tooth attachment apparatus. Untreated disease results in a gradual loss of tooth attachment to the bone. Progression is influenced by the overall health of the host and the integrity of the immune system. The primary causal factor in the development of periodontal disease is plaque. Plaque in the **gingival sulcus**, a shallow, V-shaped space around the tooth, produces toxins that destroy tissue and permit loosening of the teeth. Important factors in the defense of the gingiva to bacterial invasion are (1) oral hygiene, (2) integrity of the immune system, and (3) optimal nutrition. The defense mechanisms of the gingival tissue, epithelial barrier, and saliva are affected by nutritional intake and status. Healthy epithelial tissue prevents the penetration of bacterial endotoxins into subgingival tissue.

Nutritional Care

Deficiencies of vitamin C, folate, and zinc increase the permeability of the gingival barrier at the gingival sulcus, increasing susceptibility to periodontal disease. Severe deterioration of the gingiva is seen in individuals with scurvy or vitamin C deficiency. Although other nutrients, including vitamins A, E, β-carotene, and protein, have a role in maintaining gingival and immune system integrity, there are no scientific data to support supplemental uses of any of these nutrients to treat periodontal disease.

Although optimal nutrition may play a role in positive outcomes of periodontal treatment, nutrients alone are not a cure for the disease (Schifferle, 2005). In societies in which malnutrition and periodontal disease are prevalent, poor oral hygiene is also usually evident. In such instances it is difficult to determine whether malnutrition is the cause of the disease or one of many contributing factors, including poor oral hygiene, heavy plaque buildup, insufficient saliva, or coexisting illness.

The roles of calcium and vitamin D relate to the link between osteoporosis and periodontal disease, in which bone loss is the common denominator. The association between periodontal disease and systemic osteopenia and osteoporosis has been documented (Jeffcoat, 2005) (see Chapter 25). Because dairy foods are a rich source of calcium and vitamin D, researchers documented an inverse relationship between increased dairy food intake and decreased incidence of periodontal disease (Al-Zahrani, 2006). Although causal relationships have not been determined, the association of calcium and dairy foods with periodontal disease warrants advocating a sufficient intake of dairy foods in those who tolerate them. Management strategies for the patient or client with periodontal disease follow many of the same guidelines as for caries prevention listed in Box 26-2.

Severe periodontal disease may be treated surgically. Diet adequacy is particularly important both before and after periodontal surgery, when adequate nutrients are needed to regenerate tissue and support immunity to prevent infection. Adequacy of calories, protein, and micronutrients should be ensured. If the ability to consume one's regular diet is altered, a diet modified in consistency can be individually designed. Oral supplements can be used when necessary to attain adequate nutrient intake.

ORAL MANIFESTATIONS OF SYSTEMIC DISEASE

Acute systemic diseases such as cancer and infections, as well as chronic diseases such as diabetes mellitus, autoimmune diseases, and chronic kidney disease, are characterized by oral manifestations that may alter the diet and nutritional status. Cancer therapies, including irradiation of the head and neck region, chemotherapy, and surgeries to the oral cavity, have a significant effect on the integrity of the oral cavity and on an individual's eating ability, which may consequently affect nutrition status (see Chapter 37).

If the condition of the mouth adversely affects one's food choices, the person with chronic disease may not be able to follow the optimal diet for medical nutrition therapy. For example, poorly controlled diabetes may manifest in xerostomia or candidiasis, which may then affect the ability to consume a diet to appropriately control blood sugar, further deteriorating glucose control.

In addition, many medications alter the integrity of the oral mucosa, taste sensation, or salivary production (see Chapter 9). Phenytoin (Dilantin) may cause severe gingivitis. Many of the protease inhibitor drugs used to treat HIV and acquired immune deficiency syndrome (AIDS) are associated with altered taste and dry mouth. Care should be taken to assess the effects of medication on the oral cavity and minimize these effects using alterations in diet or drug therapy.

Diabetes Mellitus

Diabetes is associated with several oral manifestations, many of which occur only in periods of poor glucose control. These include burning mouth syndrome, periodontal disease, candidiasis, dental caries, and xerostomia (Lamster, 2008). The microangiopathic conditions seen in diabetes, along with altered responses to infection, contribute to risk of periodontal disease in affected persons. Tooth infection, more common in those with diabetes, leads to deterioration of diabetes control (Bender and Bender, 2003). Besides blood glucose control, dietary management for people with diabetes after any oral surgery procedures or placement of dentures should include modifications in the consistency, temperature, and texture of food to increase eating comfort, reduce oral pain, and prevent infections or decay while managing glucose control (see Chapter 31).

Fungal Infections

Oropharyngeal fungal infections may cause a burning, painful mouth and dysphagia. The ulcers that accompany viral infections such as herpes simplex and cytomegalovirus cause pain and can lead to reduced oral intake. Very hot and cold foods or beverages, spices, and sour or tart foods also may cause pain and should be avoided. Consumption of temperate, moist foods without added spices should be encouraged. Small, frequent meals followed by rinsing with lukewarm water or brushing to reduce the risk of dental caries are helpful. Once the type and extent of oral manifestations are identified, a nutrition care plan can be developed. Oral high calorie–high protein supplements in liquid or pudding form may be needed to meet nutrient needs and optimize healing.

Head and Neck Cancers

Head, neck, and oral cancers can alter eating ability and nutrition status because of the surgeries and therapies used to treat these cancers. Surgery, depending on the location and extent, may alter eating or swallowing ability, as well as the capacity to produce saliva. Radiation therapy of the head and neck area and chemotherapeutic agents can affect the quantity and quality of saliva and the integrity of the oral mucosa. Thick, ropey saliva is often the result of radiation therapy to the head and neck area, causing xerostomia. Dietary management focuses on the recommendations described earlier for xerostomia, along with modifications in food consistency following surgery (see Chapter 37).

HIV Infection and AIDS

Viral and fungal infections, stomatitis, xerostomia, periodontal disease, and Kaposi sarcoma are oral manifestations of HIV that can cause limitations in nutrient intake and result in weight loss and compromised nutrition status. These infections often are compounded by a compromised immune response, preexisting malnutrition, and gastrointestinal consequences of HIV infection (see Chapter 38). Viral diseases, including herpes simplex and cytomegalovirus, result in painful ulcerations of the mucosa.

Stomatitis, or inflammation of the oral mucosa, causes severe pain and ulceration of the gingiva, oral mucosa, and palate, which makes eating painful. **Candidiasis** on the tongue, palate, or esophagus can make chewing, sucking, and swallowing painful (odynophagia), thus compromising intake. Table 26-3 outlines the effects of associated oral infections.

Xerostomia

Xerostomia (dry mouth) is seen in poorly controlled diabetes mellitus, Sjögren's syndrome, other autoimmune diseases, and as a consequence of radiation therapy and certain medications (Box 26-3). Xerostomia from radiation therapy

BOX 26-3

Medications That May Cause Xerostomia

Antianxiety agents
Anticonvulsants
Antidepressants
Antihistamines
Antihypertensives
Diuretics
Narcotics
Sedatives
Serotonin reuptake inhibitors
Tranquilizers

TABLE 26-3

Effects of Oral Infections

Location	Problem	Effect	Diet Management
Oral cavity	Candidiasis, KS, herpes, stomatitis	Pain, infection, lesions, altered ability to eat, dysgeusia	Increase kilocalorie and protein intake; administer oral supplements; provide caries risk reduction education
	Xerostomia	Increased caries risk, pain, no moistening power, tendency of food to stick, dysgeusia	Moist, soft, nonspicy foods; "smooth" cool or warm foods and fluids; caries risk reduction education
Esophagus	Candidiasis, herpes, KS, cryptosporidiosis	Dysphagia, odynophagia	Try oral supplementation first; if that is unsuccessful, initiate NG feedings using silastic feeding tube or PEG
	CMV, with or without ulceration	Dysphagia, food accumulation	PEG

CMV, Cytomegalovirus; *KS*, Kaposi's sarcoma; *NG*, nasogastric; *PEG*, percutaneous endoscopic gastrostomy.

CLINICAL SCENARIO

Gina is a 74-year-old woman with a history of type 2 diabetes, hypertension, and arthritis. She complains of dry mouth and difficulty chewing; is partially edentulous; and states that she tends to choose soft, "mushy" foods. She states that her dentist told her she has periodontal disease and will need multiple tooth extractions and a full maxillary and partial mandibular denture. She takes glyburide, amlodipine (Norvasc), and celecoxib (Celebrex), and glucosamine and chondroitin. She is 5′1″ and weighs 176 lb. She lives alone, but receives assistance with food shopping and cooking from her family and friends. She claims to brush her teeth daily but rarely flosses because of her arthritic hands. She occasionally conducts self-monitoring fasting glucose fingersticks and states that her usual reading is 150 mg/dL.

Nutrition Diagnostic Statements

1. Chewing difficulty secondary to poor dentition and xerostomia as evidenced by patient report and choice of soft foods.
2. Altered nutrition-related laboratory value (glucose) secondary to diabetes and possibly food choices as evidenced by inadequate blood glucose control.

Nutrition Care Questions

1. What are the cultural, educational, and environmental influences affecting dental and nutritional health?
2. What are the diet counseling recommendations for the dental conditions?
3. What are the nutritional and dietary risk factors?
4. What are appropriate diet counseling recommendations for this patient?

may be more permanent than that from other causes (Kielbassa et al., 2006). Radiation therapy procedures to spare the parotid gland should be implemented when possible to reduce the damage to the salivary gland. Efforts to stimulate saliva production using pilocarpine and citrus-flavored, sugar-free candies may ease eating difficulty.

Individuals without any saliva at all have the most difficulty eating; artificial salivary agents may not offer sufficient relief. Lack of saliva impedes all aspects of eating, including chewing, forming a bolus, swallowing, and sensing taste; causes pain; and increases the risk of dental caries and infections. Dietary guidelines focus on the use of moist foods without added spices, increased fluid consumption with and between all meals and snacks, and judicious food choices.

Problems with chewy (steak), crumbly (cake, crackers, rice), dry (chips, crackers), and sticky (peanut butter) foods are common in persons with severe xerostomia. Alternatives should be suggested, or the foods should be avoided to avert dysphagia risk. Drinking water with a lemon or lime twist or citrus-flavored seltzers or sucking on frozen tart grapes, berries, or sugar-free candies may help. Good oral hygiene habits are important in reducing the risk of tooth decay and should be practiced after all meals and snacks. Flavored gums and mints containing xylitol may help to reduce the risk of associated decay.

USEFUL WEBSITES

American Academy of Pediatric Dentistry
http://www.aapd.org/
American Dental Association
http://www.ada.org/
American Dental Hygienists Association
http://www.adha.org/
American Academy of Periodontology
http://www.perio.org/
Diabetes and Oral health
http://www.nidcr.nih.gov/HealthInformation/DiseasesAndConditions/DiabetesAndOralHealth/default.htm
http://www.diabetes.org/living-with-diabetes/treatment-and-care/oral-health-and-hygiene/
HIV Dent
http://www.hivdent.org/
National Institute of Dental and Craniofacial Research
http://www.nidcr.nih.gov/
Oral Health America
http://oralhealthamerica.org/
Surgeon General Report on Oral Health
http://www.surgeongeneral.gov/library/oralhealth/
World Health Organization on Oral Health
http://www.who.int/oral_health/en/

REFERENCES

Alvarez JA, et al: Dental fluorosis: exposure, prevention and management, *Med Oral Patol Oral Cir Bucal* 14:E103, 2009.

Al-Zahrani MS: Increased intake of dairy products is related to lower periodontitis prevalence, *J Periodontol* 77:289, 2006.

American Dental Association: *Council on Access Prevention and Interprofessional Relations: fluoridation facts*, 2005. Accessed 22 April 2010 from http://www.ada.org/sections/newsAndEvents/pdfs/fluoridation_facts.pdf.

Bender IB, Bender AB: Diabetes mellitus and the dental pulp, *Journal of Endodontics* 29:383, 2003.

Centers for Disease Control and Prevention (CDC): *National Oral Health Surveillance System*, 2006. Accessed 22 April 2010 from http://apps.nccd.cdc.gov/nohss/IndicatorV.asp?Indicator=2.

Centers for Disease Control and Prevention (CDC): Improving oral health: preventing cavities, gum disease, tooth loss, and oral cancer, 2010. Accessed 22 April 2010 from http://www.cdc.gov/chronicdisease/resources/publications/AAG/doh.htm.

Chalmers JM, Ettinger RL: Public health issues in geriatric dentistry in the United States, *Dental Clinics of North America* 52:423, 2008.

Deshpande A, Jadad AR: The impact of polyol-containing chewing gums on dental caries: asystematic review of original randomized trials and observational studies, *J Am Dent Assoc* 139:1602, 2008.

Fontana M, Zero DT: Assessing patients' caries risk, *J Am Dent Assoc* 137:1231, 2006.

Holbrook WP, et al: Gastric reflux is a significant causative factor of tooth erosion, *J Dent Res* 88:422, 2009.

Jeffcoat M: The association between osteoporosis and oral bone loss, *J Periodontol* 76:2125S, 2005.

Kielbassa AM, et al: Radiation-related damage to dentition, *Lancet Oncol* 7:326, 2006.

Lamster IB, et al: The relationship between oral health and diabetes mellitus, *J Am Dent Assoc* 139:19S, 2008.

Marshall TA, et al: Comparison of the intakes of sugars by young children with and without dental caries experience, *J Am Dent Assoc* 138:39, 2007.

Morin K: Fluoride: action and use, *MCN Am J Matern Child Nurs* 31:127, 2006.

Moynihan P: The interrelationship between diet and oral health, *Proc Nutr Soc* 64:571, 2005.

Palmer C, Wolfe SH: Position of the American Dietetic Association: the impact of fluoride on health, *J Am Diet Assoc* 105:1620, 2005.

Quandt SA, et al: Food avoidance and food modification practices of older rural adults: association with oral health status and implications for service provision, *Gerontologist* 50:100, 2009.

Ramalingam L, et al: Adding casein phosphopeptide-amorphous calcium phosphate to sports drinks to eliminate in vitro erosion, *Pediatr Dent* 27:61, 2005.

Schifferle RE: Nutrition and periodontal disease, *Dent Clin North Am* 49:595, 2005.

Sohn WB, et al: Carbonated soft drinks and dental caries in the primary dentition, *J Dent Res* 85:262, 2006

Splieth CH, et al: Effect of xylitol and sorbitol on plaque acidogenesis, *Quintessence Int* 40:279, 2009.

Touger-Decker R, et al: Position of the American Dietetic Association: oral health and nutrition, *J Am Diet Assoc* 107:1418, 2007.

Tsakos GK, et al: Edentulism and fruit and vegetable intake in low-income adults, *J Dent Res* 89:462, 2010.

Walker GD, et al: Casein phosphopeptide-amorphous calcium phosphate incorporated into sugar confections inhibits the progression of enamel subsurface lesions in situ, *Caries Res* 44:33, 2010.

Weintraub JA, et al: Fluoride varnish efficacy in preventing early childhood caries, *J Dent Res* 85:172, 2006.

Wongkhantee SV, et al: Effect of acidic food and drinks on surface hardness of enamel, dentine, and tooth-coloured filling materials, *J Dent* 34:214, 2006.

Zero DT, et al: The biology, prevention, diagnosis and treatment of dental caries: scientific advances in the United States, *J Am Dental Assoc* 1:25S, 2010.

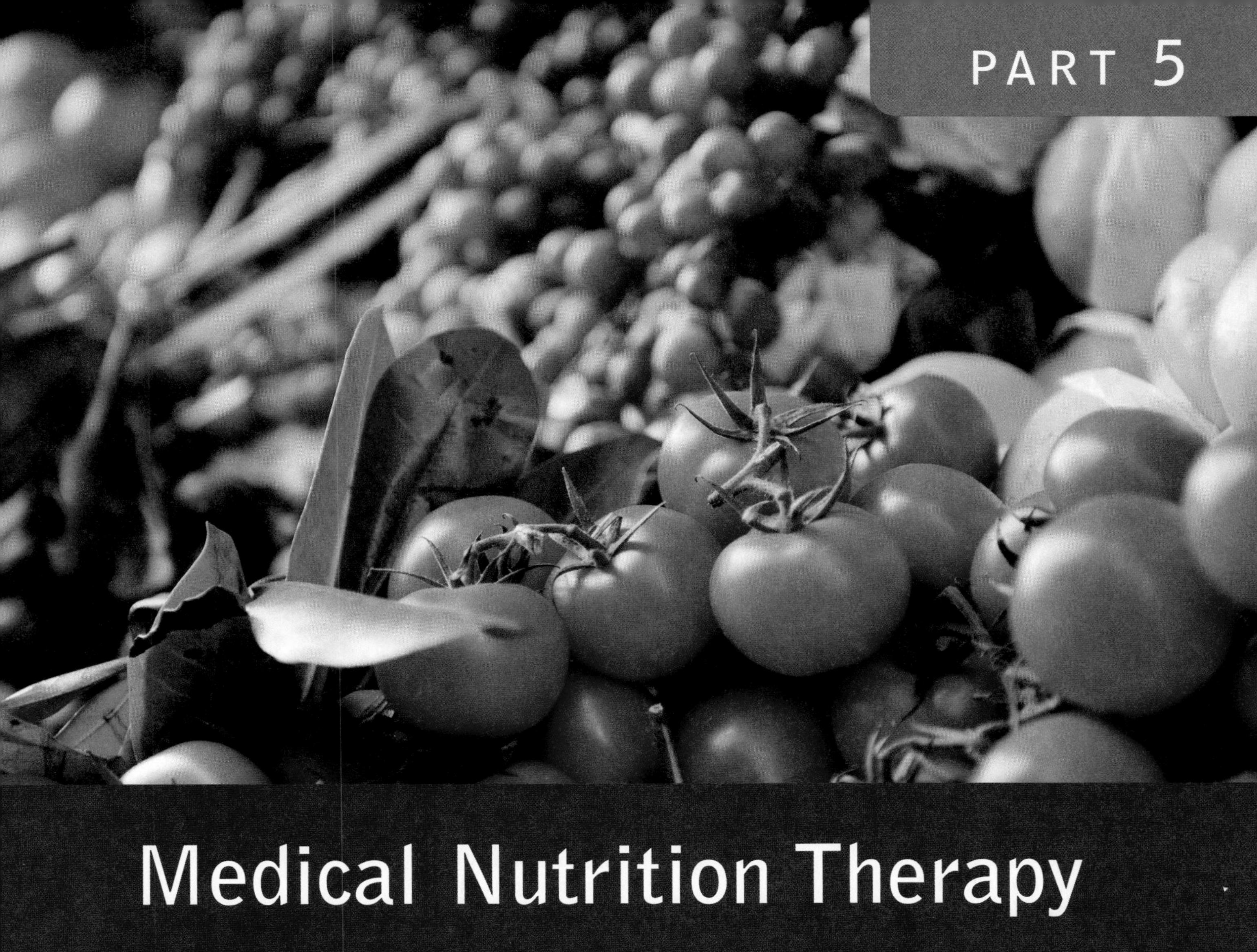

PART 5

Medical Nutrition Therapy

The chapters in this section reflect the evolution of nutritional science, from the identification of nutrient requirements and the practical application of this knowledge, to the concepts that relate nutrition to the prevention of chronic and degenerative diseases and optimization of health. The role of nutrition in reducing inflammation, now recognized as a contributor to chronic disease, supports the awareness of diet in disease prevention and management.

Medical nutrition therapy (MNT) includes the assessment, nutrition diagnosis, interventions, monitoring, and evaluation for established disease. In some cases, medical nutrition therapy is a powerful preventive measure. The list of diseases amenable to nutrition intervention continues to increase, especially because hundreds of conditions are now known to have a genetic component and a connection with the nutrient-gene expression pathway.

Sophisticated feeding and nourishment procedures place an increased responsibility on those who provide nutrition care. The nutrition-related disorders included here can be managed by changes in dietary practices based on current knowledge. The goal in all cases is to move the individual along the continuum of disease management toward better nutritional health and overall well-being.

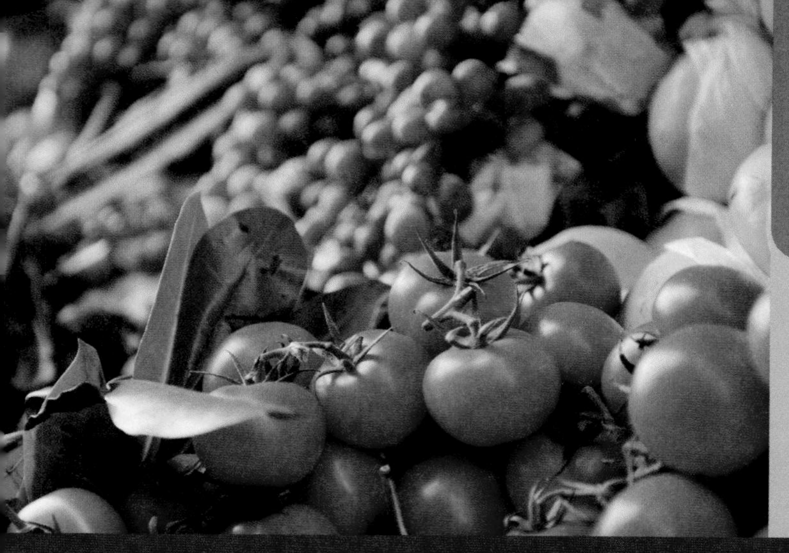

CHAPTER 27

L. Kathleen Mahan, MS, RD, CDE
Kathie Madonna Swift, MS, RD, LDN

Medical Nutrition Therapy for Adverse Reactions to Food: Food Allergies and Intolerances

KEY TERMS

adverse reaction to food (ARF)
allergen
anaphylaxis
antibodies
antigen
antigen presenting cell (APC)
atopic dermatitis (eczema)
atopy
basophils
B cells
CAP–fluorescein-enzyme immunoassay (FEIA)
cell-mediated immunity
conformational epitopes
cross reactivity
cytokine
double-blind, placebo-controlled food challenge (DBPCFC)
dysbiosis
elimination diet
eosinophilic esophagitis (EE)
eosinophilic gastroenteritis (EGE)
epitope
food allergen–specific serum IgE testing
food allergy
food and symptom diary
food challenge
food immunotherapy vaccine
food intolerance
food protein-induced enterocolitis syndromes (FPIES)
food sensitivity
granulocyte
gut-associated lymphoid tissue (GALT)
hapten
histamine
hypersensitivity
immunoglobulin (Ig)
IgE-mediated food allergy
immunoglobulin G (IgG)
leaky gut
lymphocyte
macrophage
mast cells
monocytes
nonallergic food sensitivities
oral allergy syndrome (OAS)
oral mucosal tolerance
pollen-food syndrome (PFS)
probiotics
profilins
radioallergosorbent test (RAST)
sensitivity related illness
sensitization
skin-prick test
specific oral tolerance induction (SOTI)
T cells
Th cells
Th1 cells
Th2 cells

Sections of this chapter were written by Sherry Hubbard, RD, for the previous edition of this text.

There is growing evidence that adverse reactions to food (ARFs) are more prevalent than in the past, with a defined increase in severity and scope. Changes in the modern diet and environmental influences interacting with genetic predisposition have been implicated in the escalation of ARFs and the parallel rise in other chronic disorders such as asthma and autoimmune diseases. Estimates suggest that 20% of the population alters their diet because of perceived ARFs (Sicherer and Sampson, 2010). ARFs are implicated in many conditions as a result of the involvement of major organ systems, including the digestive tract, the respiratory system, and the skin. The management of ARFs is complex because of the diverse response by which the body reacts to food constituents and the multifaceted nature of the mechanisms involved. The clinical relevance of ARFs should be carefully assessed and evaluated in the nutrition care process, because this can greatly affect a person's quality of life.

DEFINITIONS

It is important to comprehend the language of ARFs because it can be a source of confusion and misunderstanding. The following definitions are used in this chapter. **Adverse reactions to food (ARFs)** encompass both food allergies and food intolerances, both of which can result in distressing symptoms and adversely affect health.

Food allergy or **hypersensitivity** is an adverse immune mediated reaction to a food, usually a food protein or **hapten** (a small molecule that can elicit an immune response only when attached to a large carrier protein). The symptoms are caused by the individual's unique response to the food, not by the food itself. For example, a person who is allergic to a food such as peanuts can develop life-threatening **anaphylaxis** after consuming a very small amount of peanuts, whereas other individuals have no adverse response to eating peanuts. Furthermore, the symptoms of the allergy in one individual can differ greatly from those in another in response to the same food. It has been estimated that food allergy affects up to 4% of the population, with a greater prevalence in childhood that is estimated at almost 8% (Chafen et al., 2010; National Institute of Allergy and Infectious Diseases [NIAID], 2010). Symptoms of food allergy are noted in Box 27-1.

Food intolerance is an adverse reaction to a food that does not involve the immune system and occurs because of the way the body processes the food or components in the food. It may be caused by a toxic, pharmacologic, metabolic, digestive, psychologic, or idiopathic reaction to a food or chemical substances in that food. For example, an individual can be intolerant of milk not because of an allergy to milk protein, but because of an inability to digest lactose; see Chapter 29 for discussion of lactose intolerance).

Food sensitivity refers to an ARF or component of the food when it is not clear whether the reaction is due to food allergy or intolerance. The umbrella term food sensitivity has been used interchangeably with food allergy and food intolerance, but does not give any indication as to the cause of the person's symptoms (Joneja, 2003). An emerging hypothesis called **sensitivity-related illness** poses that an individual who is exposed to some type of toxicant or insult may then become sensitive to food, inhalants, or chemicals (Genuis, 2010).

ARFs illustrate the critical importance of appreciating "biochemical uniqueness" as a core clinical concept in an integrative nutrition assessment. Numerous factors, including genetics, intestinal barrier integrity, resident intestinal microflora, stress, psychological factors, and environmental and physiological influences, affect an individual's unique

BOX 27-1
Symptoms of Food Allergy

Gastrointestinal

Abdominal pain
Nausea
Vomiting
Diarrhea
Gastrointestinal bleeding
Protein-losing enteropathy
Oral and pharyngeal pruritus

Cutaneous

Urticaria (hives)
Angioedema
Eczema
Erythema (skin inflammation)
Itching
Flushing

Respiratory

Rhinitis
Asthma
Cough
Laryngeal edema
Milk-induced syndrome with respiratory disease (Heiner syndrome)
Airway tightening

Systemic

Anaphylaxis
Hypotension
Dysrhythmias

Conditions with Possible Allergy Component

Irritable bowel syndrome
Chronic-fatigue syndrome
Attention-deficit and hyperactivity disorders
Otitis media
Psychiatric disorders
Neurologic disorders
Fibromyalgia
Migraine headache

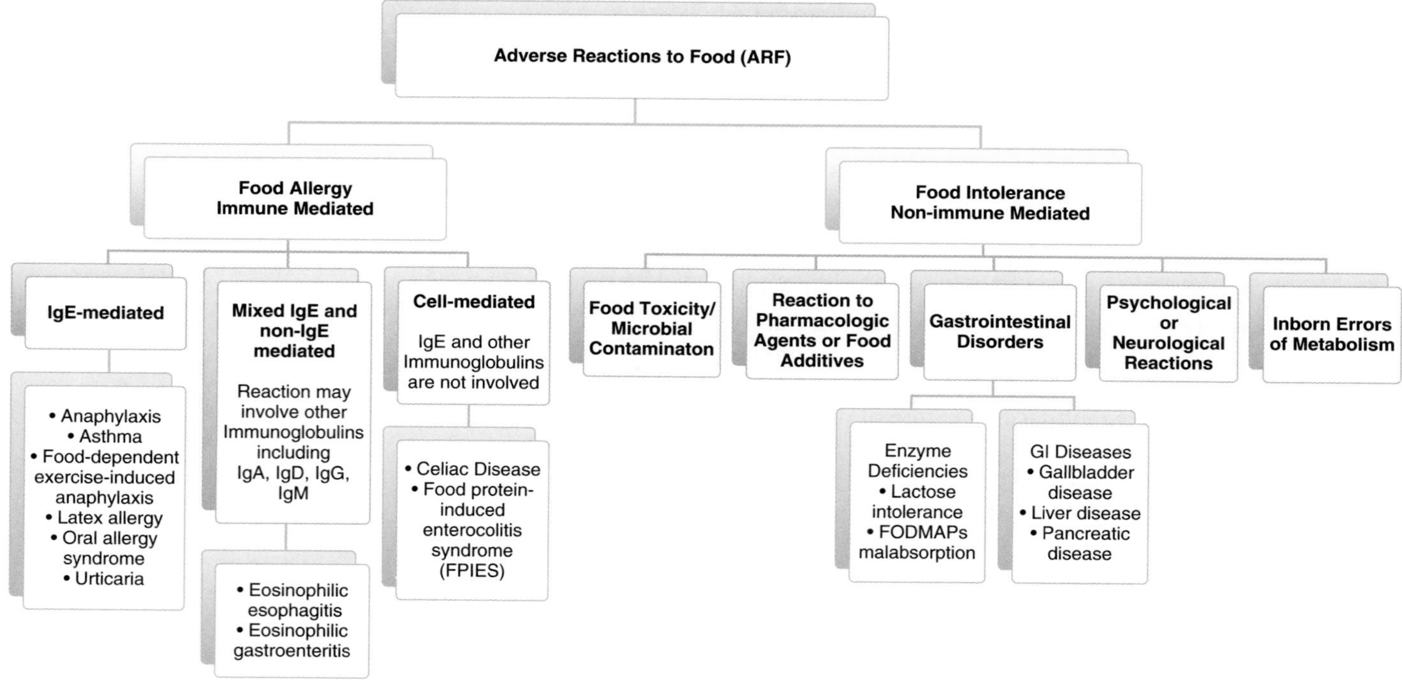

FIGURE 27-1 Adverse reactions to food.

response to food or a component of food and its ultimate interpretation by the body as either "friend" or "foe" (Figure 27-1).

The immune system functions to clear the body of foreign substances or **antigens** such as viruses, bacteria, cancer cells, and other pathogens and disease-causing agents. Normally, when food antigens interact with cells of the immune system, they are dispelled from the body without an adverse reaction, unlike when a pathogenic virus or bacterium is expelled and there is a noticeable inflammatory reaction from microbial infection. Food comes from foreign material, either plant or animal, that our immune systems typically perceive as "foreign but safe" as a result of a process of **oral mucosal tolerance** that occurs when we digest and absorb food. Tolerance indicates that an individual is clinically and immunologically tolerant of the food (NIAID and NIH, 2010).

ETIOLOGY

Heredity

Food allergy has a hereditary component that it is not yet clearly defined. **Atopy** is a condition of genetic predisposition to produce excessive immunoglobulin (Ig) E antibodies in response to an **allergen**. Atopic individuals, usually identified in infancy, and confirmed by positive skin-prick test, are characterized by severe IgE-mediated reactions to dander, pollens, food, or other environmental factors, which present as food allergy, **atopic dermatitis (eczema)**, atopic conjunctivitis, atopic rhinitis, or asthma. A study of Finnish children showed that up to the age of 4 years, children with two parents reporting any type of allergic reactions were three times as likely to have a food allergy as were children with allergy-free parents. Children with one allergic parent were twice as likely to have a food allergy (Pyrhönen et al., 2010). However, genetic susceptibility alone does not completely explain the prevalence of food allergy; other environmental influences (external, maternal, and gastrointestinal [GI] environment) and interactions between the host and the environment need to be considered.

Antigen Exposure

Exposure to food antigens in the digestive tract, followed by immune regulation or suppression, is a prerequisite for the development of tolerance to the food, or oral tolerance (Burks et al., 2008). Food allergy is believed to occur when oral tolerance fails. Ongoing research is focused on how oral tolerance develops and is maintained (Brandtzaeg, 2010). The amount of antigen and environmental factors also influence the development of food allergy. The effects of food antigens and other antigens may be additive. Clinical symptoms of food allergy may increase when inhalant allergies are exacerbated by seasonal or environmental changes. Similarly, the effects of environmental factors, such as early exposure to microbes, toxins, tobacco smoke, stress, exercise, and cold may exacerbate the clinical symptoms of food allergy.

Maternal Diet and Early Infant Feeding

The initial exposure to an antigen may occur during pregnancy or lactation or in early infancy. The food does not have to be ingested by the infant directly. Postnatal sensitization may occur with exposure to food allergens by inhalation, skin contact, or ingestion. In fact, there is increasing evidence that many allergic reactions to food are initiated by exposure to food antigens through routes other than the digestive tract. (Lack, 2008). Food allergen sensitization can be a result of exposure to a food antigen through breast milk. More likely, it occurs from environmental exposure (skin or air) causing initial sensitization that is followed by continued exposure to antigens from the mother's milk.

Gastrointestinal Microbiota

GI permeability and microbiota are critical influences in allergic disease. Both increased intestinal permeability; also referred to as "**leaky gut**" and the presence of excessive amounts of abnormal bacteria or "**dysbiosis**" influence gut immune function. This gut immune function is in the **gut-associated lymphoid tissue (GALT)**, the largest mass of lymphoid tissue in the body. GI permeability is thought to be greatest in early infancy and to decline with intestinal maturation. A leaky gut with altered permeability and possibly dysbiosis allows antigen penetration and presentation to the GALT lymphocytes and sensitization (Groschwitz and Hogan, 2009). Other conditions such as GI disease, malnutrition, prematurity, and immunodeficiency may also be associated with increased gut permeability and risk of development of food allergy. See Fig. 39-3 in Chapter 39.

PATHOPHYSIOLOGY

In allergy, the immune system unleashes defensive chemicals (inflammatory mediators) in response to something (in this case, food) that should not cause a response. The immune system mistakenly identifies food as a threat and mounts an attack against it. **Sensitization** occurs on the first exposure of the immune cells to the allergen and there are no symptoms of reaction. Thereafter, whenever that same foreign material enters the body, the immune system responds to this threat in the same manner. Because individuals can develop immunologic sensitization as evidenced by the production of allergen-specific IgE without having clinical symptoms upon exposure to those foods, a **IgE-mediated food allergy** requires both the presence of sensitization and the development of specific signs and symptoms on exposure to the food. Sensitization alone is not sufficient to define food allergy (NIAID and NIH, 2010; Boyce et al., 2011; Vickery et al., 2011) (Figure 27-2).

The combination of an allergen with allergen-specific IgE fixed to tissue mast cells or circulating **basophils** causes the release of chemical mediators, including **histamine**, enzymes, lipid-derived prostaglandins, interleukins, and others. When released, these inflammatory mediators can cause itching, pain, reddening, tissue swelling, contraction of smooth muscle, vasodilation, and fluid secretions. Manifestations, which are most often systemic, may involve multiple organs and systems (see *Pathophysiology and Care Management Algorithm:* Food Allergies).

Immune System Cells

Lymphocytes are the "command and control" cells of the immune system and include two important groups: **B cells**, arising from stem cells in the bone marrow, and **T cells**. T cells also originate from stem cells, but are later transported to the thymus gland where they mature. These two types of cells function as the basis for the humoral immune response and for cell-mediated immunity

Monocytes and **macrophages** are primarily phagocytes that engulf foreign material, break it apart, and display specific molecules of the material on their surfaces. making them **antigen-presenting cells (APC)**. The antigenic component displayed on the surface is an **epitope**, and is recognized by T cells. T cells respond by generating a cytokine message that stimulates their differentiation.

T cells, often called T "helper" cells (**Th cells**) differentiate into Th-1 cells or Th-2 cells which have different roles in the immune response under different circumstances, and secrete different sets of cytokines. **Th1 cells** regulate the activities of the B cells to produce antibodies and direct damage to target cells, resulting in the destruction of antigens. This function is useful in defending against bacteria, viruses, and other pathogenic cells. **Th2 cells** mediate the allergic response by regulating the production by B cells of IgE sensitized to food allergens.

These allergen-specific antibodies attach themselves to **mast cells** (in the lungs, skin, tongue and linings of the nose and intestinal tract) or basophils (in circulation). On second exposure to the allergen, the sensitized IgE antibodies and the allergen form antibody-antigen complexes that activate granulocytes

Granulocytes contain intracellular granules, or small vessels that are storage depots for defense chemicals or inflammatory mediators that protect the body from invading pathogens. When these granulocytes are activated, they degranulate and release these inflammatory mediators such as histamine, prostaglandins, leukotrienes, and cytokines. Each of the mediators has a specific effect on local tissues and at distant sites, resulting in the symptoms of allergy. Degranulation of other granulocytes such as neutrophils and eosinophils attracted to the reaction site by mediators such as chemokines causes release of additional inflammatory chemicals, which further enhance the allergic response, resulting in increased symptom severity.

The humoral immune response is mediated by **antibodies** and has a major role in food allergy. Antigen-specific antibodies are produced by the B lymphocytes (B cells) in response to the antigen presented. The union of an antigen and antibody results in the degranulation of mast cells or basophils and the release of chemical inflammatory mediators, or direct cellular damage, which in turn causes symptoms. Each antibody contains a globulin protein; because of their association with the immune system, they are referred to as **immunoglobulins (Ig)**. Five distinct classes of

PATHOPHYSIOLOGY AND CARE MANAGEMENT ALGORITHM

Food Allergies

ETIOLOGY

Common food allergens
Foods with high protein content, usually of plant or marine origin

Risk factors
- Heredity
- History of atopy
- Antigen exposure
- GI permeability
- Amount of antigen presented
- Environmental factors such as stress or toxins
- Microflora imbalance

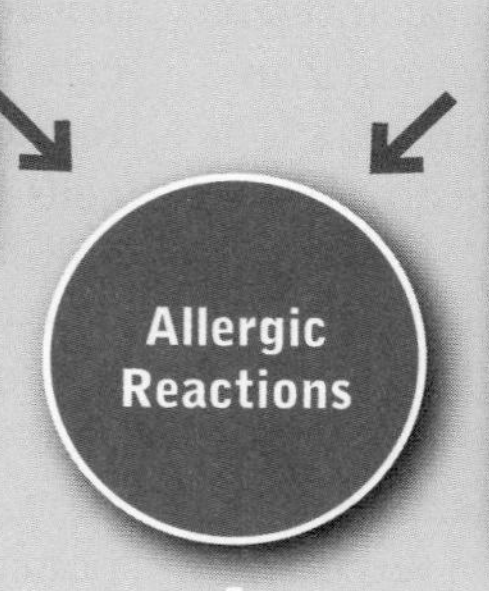

PATHOPHYSIOLOGY

IgE-mediated
Immediate hypersensitivity

Mixed IgE- and non-IgE mediated
Hypersensitivity

Cell-mediated
Delayed hypersensitivity

Release of inflammatory mediators

GI, Cutaneous, Respiratory, and Systemic Symptoms, Anaphylaxis

MANAGEMENT

Medical Management
- History
- Physical examination
- Biochemical and immunologic testing
- Treatment to optimize GI function

- Reintroduction of foods by food challenge (DBPCFC) to test for resolution of allergy (with treatment for anaphylaxis available)

- Epinephrine for management of acute reactions and anaphylaxis

Nutrition Management
- Assessment of nutrition status
- Food and symptom diaries
- Elimination diet for identification of potential allergens
- Education for avoidance of food allergens
- Personalized supplementation including vitamins, minerals, prebiotics, probiotics, and glutamine, etc. as necessary to optimize GI function

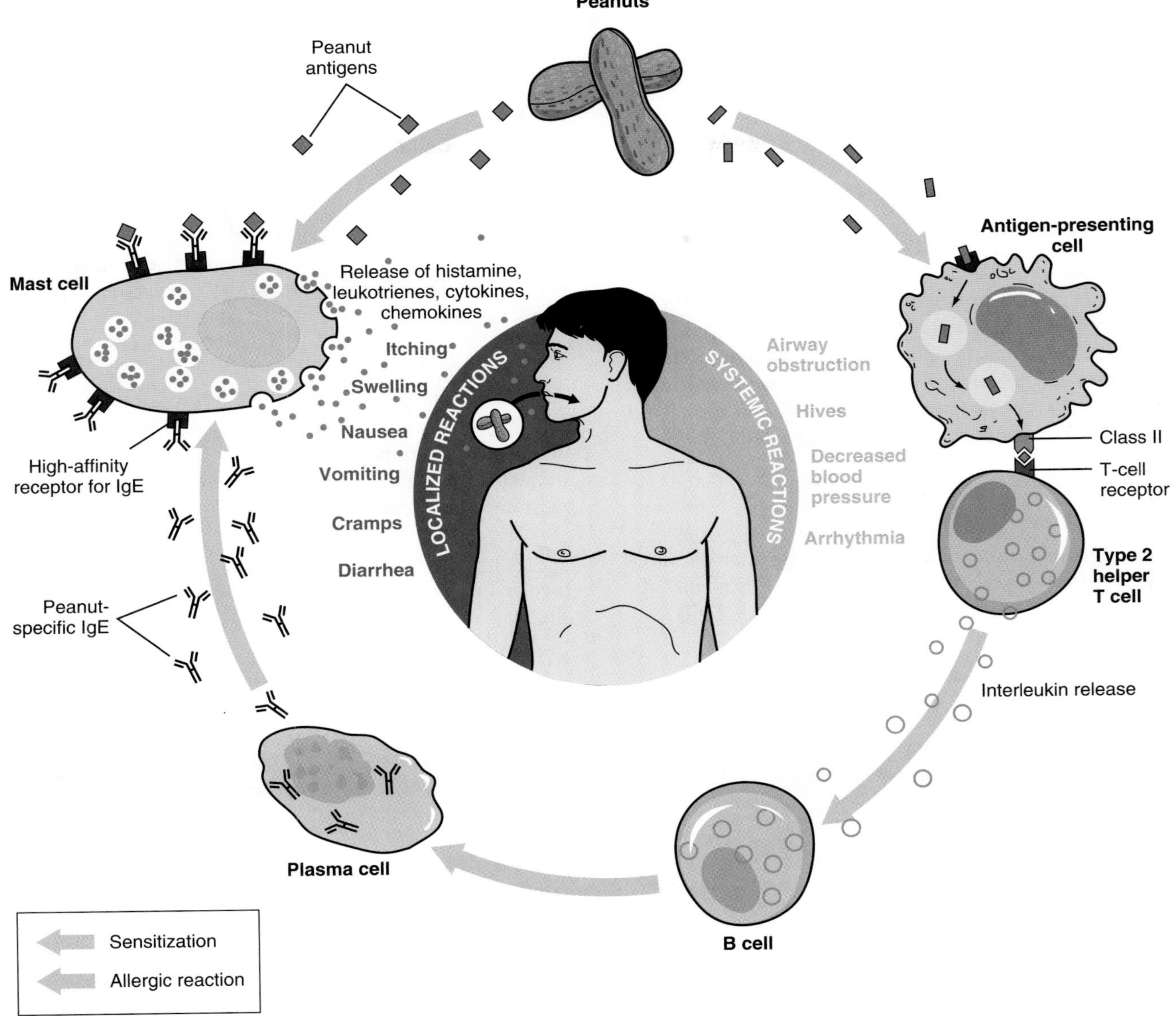

FIGURE 27-2 Sensitization process and IgE-mediated allergic reaction.

antibodies have been identified: IgA, IgD, IgE, IgG, and IgM. Each Ig has a specific function in immunity reactions (Box 27-2).

IgE-MEDIATED REACTIONS

IgE-mediated food allergic reactions usually are rapid in onset, occurring within minutes to a few hours of exposure. The methods of exposure include inhalation, skin contact and ingestion. A wide range of symptoms has been attributed to this type of food allergy; and frequently involve the GI, cutaneous, or respiratory systems, and can range from mild hives to life-threatening anaphylaxis Table 27-1).

A few foods account for the vast majority of IgE-mediated allergic reactions: milk, eggs, peanuts, tree nuts, soy, wheat, fish, and shellfish. However, any food is capable of eliciting an IgE-mediated reaction after a person has been sensitized to it. Food-induced anaphylaxis, oral allergy syndrome (OAS), immediate GI hypersensitivity, latex-food allergy syndrome, and exercise-induced anaphylaxis are IgE-mediated immune reactions.

Food-Induced Anaphylaxis

Food-induced anaphylaxis is an acute, often severe, and sometimes fatal immune response that usually occurs within a limited period following exposure to an antigen. Multiple organ systems are affected. Symptoms can include respiratory distress, abdominal pain, nausea, vomiting, cyanosis, arrhythmia, hypotension, angioedema, urticaria, diarrhea, shock, cardiac arrest, and death. The vast majority of fatal anaphylactic reactions to foods in adults in North America

BOX 27-2

The Immunoglobulins

IgM

The largest antibody; a first line defender that can mop up many antigens at one time.

IgA

Found in two forms—serum IgA and secretory IgA (sIgA). The latter is present in mucus secretions in the mouth, respiratory and gastrointestinal tracts, vagina, and colostrum in mammalian milk. It is the "first-line" defense immunoglobulin, which encounters any antigen entering from the external environment. Serum IgA is in the second highest amount in circulation, exceeded only by IgG.

IgG

Defends against pathogens and persists long after the threat is over; it may be responsible for some non-IgE mediated hypersensitivity reactions. Four subtypes include IgG1, IgG2, IgG3, and IgG4. IgG4 has been implicated in some types of adverse reactions to food. Food protein–specific IgG antibodies tend to rise in the first few months after the introduction of a food and then decrease even though the food may continue to be consumed. People with inflammatory bowel disorders such as celiac disease or ulcerative colitis often have high levels of IgG and IgM (Stapel et al., 2008).

IgE

The classic allergy antibody of hay fever, asthma, eczema, and food-induced anaphylaxis, oral allergy syndrome, and immediate gastrointestinal hypersensitivity reactions. Immediate allergic reactions usually involve IgE and are the most clearly understood mechanisms.

IgD

Involved in immunoglobulin class switching and its role in allergy is not well defined.

TABLE 27-1

Types of Allergic Reactions

Reaction/ Classification	IgE-Mediated	Mixed IgE- and Non-IgE–Mediated	Cell-Mediated
Mechanism	The allergen binds with sensitized IgE antibodies on mast cells or basophils. Upon binding, chemical inflammatory mediators are released from the cell.	Both antibodies and T-cells are associated with triggering inflammatory mediators and the development of symptoms.	T-cells interact directly with antigen and release inflammatory mediators.
Timing	Immediate hypersensitivity; minutes to 1 hour	Delayed onset >2 hr; chronic, relapsing	Delayed onset >2 hr; chronic, relapsing
Symptomology			
Systemic	Anaphylactic shock; food-dependent, exercised-induced anaphylaxis		
Cutaneous	Acute contact urticaria, angioedema, flushing, morbilliform rash, pruritus, urticaria	Atopic dermatitis	Contact dermatitis, dermatitis herpetiformis
Gastrointestinal	Immediate gastrointestinal food allergy, oral allergy syndrome	Eosinophilic esophagitis (EE), eosinophilic gastroenteritis (EGE)	Allergic proctitis, celiac disease, FPIES, infantile colic
Respiratory	Acute rhinoconjunctivitis, asthma	Asthma	Pulmonary hemosiderosis (Heiner syndrome)

FPIES, Food protein–induced enterocolitis syndrome; *Ig*, immunoglobulin.

involve peanuts or tree nuts; in children anaphylaxis to other foods such as egg and milk are reported more frequently. People with known anaphylactic reactions to food allergens should carry and be prepared to use injected epinephrine via an injectable adrenaline at all times. Epinephrine is the drug of choice to reverse an allergic reaction, even with asthma (Franchini et al, 2010). Delayed use of epinephrine has been associated with an increased risk of biphasic reactions in which a recurrence of symptoms 4 to 12 hours after the initial anaphylactic reaction may be fatal.

Oral Allergy Syndrome

The **oral allergy syndrome (OAS)**, or **pollen-food syndrome (PFS)**, results from direct contact with food allergens and is confined almost exclusively to the oropharynx and rarely involves other target organs (Hoffmann and Burks, 2008). Sensitization occurs through the respiratory system or skin (Fernandez-Rivas et al., 2006). The reaction to foods occurs as a result of the presence of an antigen within the food with a structure similar to that of the pollen. The primary sensitization is to the pollen, not the food. Symptoms are rapid and appear within minutes upon ingestion of the offending food. They include itching and irritation of oral tissues along with swelling and sometimes blisters, and most often subside within 30 minutes. OAS is most commonly seen in individuals with coexisting seasonal allergic rhinitis to birch, ragweed, or grass pollens following ingestion of specific fruits, vegetables, and some nuts. (Geroldinger-Simic et al, 2011.) The cooked fruit or vegetable is often tolerated because the reactions are caused by predominately heat-labile proteins cross-reacting with pollen proteins. However, this is not always the case and a careful history and questioning about the food is important (Kondo and Urisu, 2009). Box 27-3 lists the foods and pollens most commonly linked with OAS.

BOX 27-3

Foods and Pollens Involved in Oral Allergy Syndrome

Food	Pollen
Almonds	B
Apple	B
Apricot	B
Banana	R
Carrot	B
Celery	B
Chamomile	R
Cherry	B
Cucumber	R
Echinacea	R
Fennel	B
Fig	B, G
Green pepper	B
Hazelnut	B
Kiwi	B
Melon	R, G
Nectarine	B
Parsley	B
Parsnip	B
Peanut	G
Peach	B
Pear	B
Plum	B
Potato	B
Prune	B
Pumpkin seed	B
Tomato	G
Walnut	B
Zucchini	R

B = birch pollen; R = ragweed pollen; G = grass pollen.

Immediate Gastrointestinal Hypersensitivity

A range of GI symptoms can develop within minutes to 2 hours after ingestion of an offending food and may include nausea, vomiting, diarrhea, and abdominal pain. More than half of patients with food allergy have GI reactions that are mediated by IgE-dependent and independent mechanisms involving mast cells, eosinophils, and other immune cells (Bischoff and Crowe, 2005). The GI manifestations can involve eosinophilic esophagitis, or may occur in conjunction with allergic symptoms outside the digestive tract such as respiratory (wheezing) or skin symptoms (urticaria) (Sicherer and Sampson, 2010).

Profilins and Allergy to Latex

Allergy to latex or natural rubber is common. Up to 50% of latex-sensitive individuals can respond with allergic symptoms when exposed to cross-reactive food allergens (Blanco, 2003). In the pollen-food-latex syndrome, **cross reactivity** occurs between the food antigen and various latex antigens found in many items such as latex gloves, clothing, children's toys, and other articles in the immediate environment.

Profilins are proteins, present in all eukaryotic cells, that form allergens from pollen, latex, and plant foods (Santos and Van Ree, 2011). As a food allergen, profilin usually elicits mild oral allergy syndrome, is not modified by processing, but may be linked with allergy to melons, banana, tomato, and many of the OAS foods (see Box 27-3) (Santos and Van Ree, 2011; Condemi, 2002). Potential therapies such as curcumin may help control the allergic response (Kurup et al., 2007).

Food-Dependent, Exercise-Induced Anaphylaxis

Food-dependent, exercise-induced anaphylaxis (FDEIA) is a distinct form of physical allergy in which an offending food triggers an anaphylactic reaction only when the individual exercises within 2 to 4 hours after eating (DuToit, 2007). The food may not be problematic in the absence of exercise. It appears to be more common in adolescent girls and young women. Celery, seafood, a gliadin component in wheat, and other foods have been reported as offending agents (Morita et al., 2009). In FDEIA, the combination of a sensitizing food and exercise precipitates symptoms, possibly related to increased GI permeability, blood-flow redistribution, and increased osmolality (Robson-Ansley and Toit, 2010). The prevalence and causative agents and effective methods of diagnosis in FDEIA continue to be explored.

NON–IgE-MEDIATED OR MIXED ANTIBODY REACTIONS

The contribution of non–IgE-mediated immunologic reactions to food hypersensitivity continues to be investigated. It has been postulated that non-IgE antigen-antibody complexes may play a role in food-related inflammatory diseases. These include various forms of colitis, enteritis with bleeding, malabsorptive disorders, ulceration, and chronic pneumonitis (Heiner syndrome). Non–IgE-mediated antibody reactions may also be involved in celiac disease, protein-losing enteropathies, **eosinophilic esophagitis (EE)**, **eosinophilic gastroenteritis (EGE)**, and ulcerative colitis. Multiple components of the immune system are likely to be involved with different underlying mechanisms.

Eosinophilic Esophagitis and Eosinophilic Gastroenteritis

EE and EGE are characterized by eosinophilic infiltration of the esophagus, stomach, or intestines with peripheral eosinophilia. Both conditions can have serious consequences and distinction is important because it may influence therapy (Rothenberg, 2004). Many studies have indicated that food allergies are responsible, and almost half of the patients who present with EGE have atopic features (Eroglu et al., 2009; Roy-Ghanta et al., 2008). Identification of specific offending allergens is not always possible. A comprehensive elimination diet may improve symptoms of EE (Kagalwalla et al., 2006; Spergel et al., 2005). EGE can occur at any age and symptoms can easily be mistaken for functional GI disorders. Nutrition assessment is important with either condition because the implementation of an elimination diet aimed at identifying and excluding food antagonists can be most helpful.

CELL-MEDIATED REACTIONS

Cell-mediated immunity is non–IgE-mediated and acts in reponse to viruses, fungi, tumor cells, and other foreign cells through its production of the controller T lymphocytes (T helper or Th cells.) Th cells are involved in most aspects of the immune response, from directing other immune cells, to responding to the recognition of a foreign antigen. However they have no cytotoxic or phagocytotic activity themselves.

When an antigen stimulates a T-cell response, the T cells produce **cytokines** which cause them to differentiate into Th-1 cells or Th-2 cells. Specific cytokines secreted by allergen-driven Th2 cells may induce B cells to produce IgE antibodies. The IgE antibodies attach to specific receptors on the surface of mast cells or basophils. Coupling of the specific antigen with the IgE on the mast cell or basophil surface starts a series of reactions that result in the release of the inflammatory mediators stored within the mast cell and basophil granules.

Manipulating the Th1 and Th2 immune response for allergy prevention and possible protection against Th1 type autoimmune disease and Th2-mediated atopic disease is a current area of investigation. The model of Th1 and Th2 immunity will continue to evolve, moving beyond the simplistic interpretation of protective versus allergic response in view of more recent evidence on the complexities of T helper cells and cytokine production (Durrant and Metzger, 2010).

Food Protein–Induced Enterocolitis Syndromes (FPIES)

An example of a cell-mediated reaction is **food protein–induced enterocolitis syndrome (FPIES)** which is most commonly seen in formula-fed infants, and is typically provoked by cow's milk or soy protein-based formula (Mehr et al., 2009). A response to sheep or goat's milk is less common but can also occur (Järvinen and Chatchatee, 2009.)

Occasionally FPIES is seen in breast-fed infants, presumably caused by milk proteins from the mother's diet crossing into her milk. The infant reacts with emesis, diarrhea, poor growth, and lethargy. In protein-induced proctocolitis, bloody and mucus-laden stools are also seen. Food-specific IgE antibodies have no value in this diagnosis; confirmation of FPIES is challenging because it mimics other GI inflammatory disorders. Infants should be switched to an extensively hydrolyzed casein formula. If they do not tolerate that, they may require an elemental formula. Breast-fed infants should remain on the breast, and the mother should eliminate cow's milk from her diet. FPIES is usually transient and resolves after a few weeks to months.

FOOD INTOLERANCES

Food intolerances (**nonallergic food sensitivities**) are ARFs caused by nonimmunologic mechanisms including toxic, pharmacologic, metabolic, or idiosyncratic reactions. Food intolerances are much more common than food allergies. Clinically, it is important to distinguish food intolerance from immune-mediated food allergy. Symptoms caused by food intolerances are often similar to food allergy and include GI, cutaneous, and respiratory manifestations. See Table 27-2.

Lactose Intolerance

Intolerance to the disaccharide lactose is the most common ARF, and most cases result from a genetically influenced reduction of intestinal lactase. Half of the world's population has hypolactasia (Jarvela et al., 2009). Abdominal bloating and cramping, flatulence, and diarrhea occur usually several hours following lactose ingestion. Because the symptoms are similar, lactose intolerance is often confused with allergy to cow's milk; however, some individuals who are allergic to cow's milk can also have respiratory or

TABLE 27-2

Examples of Food Intolerances

Cause	Associated Food(s)	Symptoms
Gastrointestinal Disorders		
Enzyme Deficiencies		
Lactase	Foods containing lactose and mammalian milk	Bloating, flatulence, diarrhea, abdominal pain
Glucose-6 phosphate dehydrogenase	Fava or broad beans	Hemolytic anemia
Fructase	Foods containing sucrose or fructose	Bloating, flatulence, diarrhea, abdominal pain
Diseases		
Cystic fibrosis	Symptoms may be precipitated by many foods, especially high-fat foods or certain proteins	Bloating, loose stools, abdominal pain, malabsorption
Gallbladder disease	Symptoms may be precipitated by high-fat foods	Abdominal pain after eating
Pancreatic disease	Symptoms may be precipitated by eating	Anorexia, nausea, dysgeusia, and other gastrointestinal symptoms
Inborn Errors of Metabolism		
Phenylketonuria	Foods containing phenylalanine	Elevated serum phenylalanine levels, mental retardation
Galactosemia	Foods containing lactose or galactose	Vomiting, lethargy, failure to thrive
Psychological or Neurologic Reactions		
	Symptoms may be precipitated by any food	Wide variety of symptoms involving any system
Reactions to Pharmacologic Agents in Foods		
Vasoactive Amines		
Phenylethylamine	Chocolate, aged cheeses, red wine	Migraine headaches
Tyramine	Aged cheeses, brewer's yeast, Chianti wine, canned fish, bananas, eggplant, tomatoes, raspberries, plums	Migraine headaches, cutaneous erythema, urticaria and hypertensive crisis in patients taking monoamine oxidase inhibitors
Histamine	Aged cheeses, fermented foods (e.g., tofu, sauerkraut), many processed meats (e.g., sausage), canned fish, beer, red wine, champagne, ketchup	Erythema, headaches, decreased blood pressure
Histamine-releasing agents	Shellfish, egg whites, chocolate, strawberries, bananas, pineapple, tomatoes, spinach, nuts, peanuts	Urticaria, eczema, pruritus
Reactions to Food Additives		
Tartrazine or FD&C yellow no. 5	Artificially colored yellow or yellow-orange foods, soft drinks, some medicines	Hives, rash, asthma
Benzoic acid or sodium benzoate; BHA; BHT; nitrates	Soft drinks and some cheeses, some margarines, and many processed food products and foods with preservatives	Hives, rash, asthma
Monosodium glutamate (MSG)	Asian food and foods with MSG added as a flavor enhancer	Headaches, nausea, asthma, flushing, abdominal pain

Continued

TABLE 27-2

Examples of Food Intolerances—cont'd

Cause	Associated Food(s)	Symptoms
Sulfites		
Sodium sulfite, potassium sulfite, sodium metabisulfite, potassium metabisulfite, sodium bisulfite, potassium bisulfite, sulfur dioxide	Shrimp, avocado, instant potatoes, dried fruits and vegetables, and fresh fruits and vegetables treated with sulfites to prevent browning, acidic juices, wine, beer, and many processed foods	Acute asthma and anaphylaxis, loss of consciousness
Reactions to Microbial Contamination or Toxins in Foods		
Proteus, klebsiella or Escherichia coli bacteria cause histidine to break down to a histamine	Unrefrigerated scombroid fish (tuna, bonita, mackerel); heat-stable toxin produced	Scombroid fish poisoning (itching, rash, vomiting, diarrhea); anaphylactic type reaction

BHA, Butylated hydroxyanisole; *BHT*, butylated hydroxytoluene.

anaphylactic reactions. Deficiencies of lactase and other carbohydrate-digesting enzymes and their management are discussed further in Chapter 29.

Carbohydrate Intolerances

Carbohydrates, sugars, starches, and polysaccharides are complex in structure and must be broken down by enzymes for optimal digestion, absorption, and assimilation. Adverse reactions can occur if there is a deficiency of enzymes responsible for the breakdown of carbohydrates, especially disaccharides.

Maldigestion and malabsorption of the fructo-, oligo-, di-, and monosaccharides and polyols (FODMAPs) may also occur (Gibson and Shepherd, 2010). Included are the sugars and the polyols sorbitol, maltitol, and others. Intolerances lead to diarrhea, cramping, and flatulence. They appear to be more common in individuals who have an underlying functional GI disorder, such as irritable bowel syndrome. GI symptoms reported after the ingestion of fruit juice may be related to fructose intolerance, a problem from widespread use of high-fructose corn syrups in food manufacturing and processing (see Chapter 29 for discussion of the FODMAPs diet.) Tools are available for assessment of FODMAPs intake (Barrett and Gibson, 2010.)

Food Additives or Pharmacologic Reactions

An adverse reaction may be to a food additive or pharmacologically active component in that food. Research should clarify nutritional concerns, including underlying mechanisms, genetic susceptibilities, risks from medications, food processing techniques, and food labeling. A wide range of allergic-like symptoms can result from ingestion of biogenic amines such as histamine and tyramine; salicylates; carmine (cochineal extracts); artificial food dyes and colorings such as FD & C #5; and preservatives such as benzoic acid, sodium benzoate, butylated hydroxyanisole (BHA), butylated hydroxytoluene (BHT), nitrates, sulfites, and monosodium glutamate (MSG) (Joneja, 2003).

Ingestion of foods with a high histamine content, including fermented foods such as tofu and sauerkraut, aged cheeses, processed meats and fish, alcoholic beverages (champagne and red wine), and old food, may result in symptoms indistinguishable from food allergy, because histamine is an important mediator responsible for IgE-mediated hypersensitivity reactions. Foods such as strawberries, egg whites, shellfish, and some food additives (e.g., tartrazine) and preservatives (e.g., benzoates) stimulate histamine release from mast cells. Histamine intolerance or sensitivity may be suspected when an allergic cause has been ruled out (Maintz and Novak, 2007). A deficiency of the enzymes diamine oxidase or histamine-N-methyltransferase and a genetic defect in histamine metabolism have been implicated (Maintz and Novak, 2007).

Tyramine is formed from the amino acid tyrosine and can cause adverse reactions in individuals who are taking monoamine oxidase inhibitors (MAOIs), which inhibit the breakdown of tyramine. This is an example of a potentially serious ARF caused by a drug-food interaction. Fortunately, the MAOIs are used infrequently today. Tyramine is found in some fermented foods such as aged cheeses, wines, vinegars, and naturally in bananas, eggplant, raspberries, plums, and tomatoes. Ingestion may cause migraine headaches or chronic hives in tyramine-sensitive individuals, with the response being dose-dependent (Joneja, 2003). See Box 9-3 in Chapter 9 and Chapter 41.

Reactions to sulfites are most common in asthmatics and result in a range of symptoms in sulfite-sensitive individuals. These can include dermatitis, urticaria, hypotension, abdominal pain, diarrhea, and life-threatening asthmatic and anaphylactic reactions. Chronic respiratory and skin problems can also be due to sulfite sensitivity (Vally et al., 2009). The mechanisms remain unclear.

Adverse reactions to MSG were originally reported as the "Chinese restaurant syndrome" because of its use in Chinese cooking. Complaints of headache, nausea, flushing, abdominal pain, and asthma occurred after ingestion.

Glutamates are found naturally in tomatoes, Parmesan cheese, mushrooms, and other foods. Results from double-blind, placebo-controlled food challenges (DBPCFC) found symptoms from MSG to be neither persistent, clear, consistent, nor serious (Geha et al., 2000; Williams and Woessner, 2009). Considering the debate about this common flavoring agent, dietetic practitioners should be aware of MSG sensitivity.

Food Toxins and Microbial Contaminants

Other causes of food intolerance can be mistaken for food allergy. Food toxicity or food poisoning results from microbial contamination of food and can cause nausea, vomiting, diarrhea, abdominal pain, headache, and fever. Most episodes are self-limiting and should be distinguished from food allergy through a thorough history. Pseudoallergic or anaphylactoid reactions to food can result from ingredients that mimic the effects of mast cell degranulation, but do not involve the production of antibodies (Reese et al., 2009). Some adverse reactions are triggered by physiologic reactions to foods that result from a heightened sensory response to foods.

Unclear Adverse Reactions

The role of food allergy or intolerance in behavioral disorders (anxiety, depression, and mood disorders), neurologic disorders (migraine headache), musculoskeletal disorders (fibromyalgia, chronic fatigue syndrome), irritable bowel syndrome, and many other clinical conditions is emerging. Even if a food-symptom relationship is not proven but food avoidance is perceived as helpful because of personal experience, appropriate therapy can optimize nutritional status (Hepworth, 2010). Psychological ARFs exist and are often prevalent in individuals with underlying psychiatric disorders (Kelsay, 2003).

ASSESSMENT

Diagnosis of ARFs requires identification of the suspected food or food ingredient, proof that the food causes an adverse response, and verification of immune- or nonimmune-mediated response. The first diagnostic tool is the detailed clinical history, followed by appropriate testing. Biochemical tests can rule out nonallergenic causes of symptoms. Tests that may be useful include a complete blood count and differential; stool tests for reducing substances, ova, parasites, or occult blood; breath hydrogen tests; intestinal permeability tests; genetic tests for celiac disease and gluten sensitivity profiles ; tests for small intestinal bacterial overgrowth (SIBO); and a sweat chloride test for cystic fibrosis (see Chapters 8, 28, 29 and 35). Tests to diagnose adverse reactions to food and identify the immune response should not be used alone, but rather in conjunction with history, physical, and nutrition assessment. See Table 27-3 for a complete description of tests.

Immunologic Testing

Skin-Prick Test

In **skin-prick tests**, the skin is pricked and a food allergen is placed under the skin in contact with allergen-specific IgE (bound to the surface of cutaneous mast cells). These tests are the most economic immunologic tests, providing results within 15 to 30 minutes. Comparison with the positive control (histamine) and the negative control (usually the solute used for the antigen or saline) provide parameters necessary for accurate readings (see Figure 27-3). All skin-prick tests are compared with the control wheal. Test wheals that are 3 mm greater than the negative control usually indicate a positive result. Negative skin-prick tests have good negative predictive accuracy and suggest the absence of an IgE-mediated reaction. Positive skin-prick test results, however, indicate only the possibility of food allergy. In the patient with a suspected food allergy, the skin-prick test is useful in supporting the diagnosis. For children younger than 2 years of age, the skin test is reserved to confirm immunologic mechanisms after symptoms have been confirmed by a positive test result from a food challenge or when the history of the reaction is impressive.

In children with atopic dermatitis, skin-prick testing for food allergens is contraindicated because of the high reactivity of the skin, leading to false-positive reactions and the real danger of sensitization to the allergen through inflamed skin (Lack, 2008) (Figure 27-4).

All foods that test positive must correlate with a strong exposure history or be proven to cause allergic reactions through food challenges before they can be considered

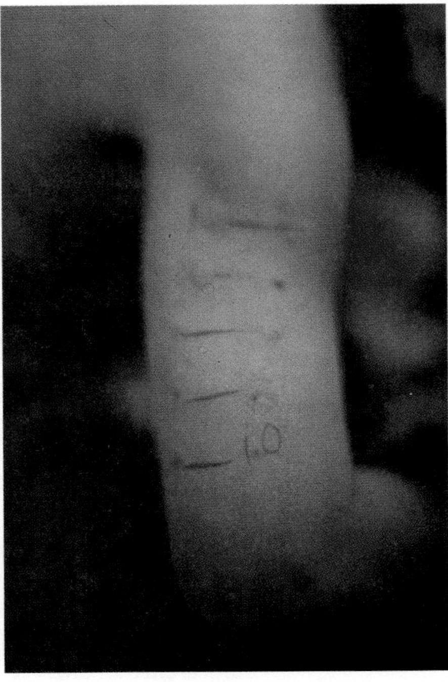

FIGURE 27-3 A skin-prick test showing the wheal and flare of the reaction to the allergen as compared with the reaction to the histamine control at the bottom.

TABLE 27-3

Tests Used in the Assessment of Adverse Reactions to Foods

	Skin Tests	
Skin testing (scratch, prick, or puncture)	A drop of antigen is placed on the skin, and the skin is then scratched or punctured to allow penetration; assesses IgE-mediated sensitization.	Screening test; cannot be relied on as sole diagnostic tool; a history of food-symptom relationship also important; more reliable for negative findings than positive; negative results confirm absence of IgE-mediated allergic response.
Atopy patch test	Small pads soaked with allergen are applied to unbroken skin for 48 hours and read at 72 hours.	Variable sensitivity and specificity; used to assess delayed or non-IgE reactions; no clinical value in diagnosis of food allergy.
Intradermal testing also called skin endpoint titration (SET)	In a clinical setting, a small amount of allergen is injected directly into subcutaneous layer of skin.	More sensitive than skin-prick testing, but with a greater risk of adverse reactions; not recommended as sole diagnostic tool.
Applied kinesiology also called muscle strength testing	Subject's arm is extended and foods to be tested are placed in the hand; test is considered to yield positive results if the arm moves more easily after the food has been placed in hand.	Nonstandardized; may result in false-positive or false-negative results; not validated for diagnostic use.
Sublingual testing	Drops of allergen extract are placed under the tongue and symptoms are recorded.	May result in false-positive results; not validated for diagnostic use.
Provocation testing and neutralization	Subcutaneous injection of allergen extract elicits symptoms; this is then followed by injection of a weaker or stronger preparation to neutralize symptom.	May result in false-positive results; not validated for diagnostic use.
	Blood Tests	
CAP-FEIA	Serum is mixed with food on a paper disk and then washed with radioactively labeled IgE. Compared with RAST, this test binds more allergen; best for assessing IgE-mediated reactions.	Reliable for only six foods: milk, eggs, wheat, cow's milk, peanuts, and soy.
RAST	Being replaced with CAP-FEIA test; assesses IgE-mediated sensitization.	More sensitive assays now replace RAST; cannot be relied on as sole diagnostic tool. High sIgE values may not guarantee allergic reactivity, whereas low sIgE values may not eliminate the potential for allergic reactivity.
ELISA	Much like RAST, except that no radioactive material is used; being replaced with CAP-FEIA; assesses IgE-mediated sensitization.	Same as for RAST. Cannot be relied on as sole diagnostic tool. High sIgE values may not guarantee allergic reactivity, whereas low sIgE values may not eliminate the potential for allergic reactivity.
ALCAT	Indirect measurement of the presence of prostaglandins, cytokines, and leukotrienes released from degranulation of leukocytes in presence of allergen; measures change of leukocyte via automated computer analysis.	No information on the immune mechanism leading to leukocyte degranulation. Negative results can indicate oral tolerance. Not validated for diagnostic use, but still used clinically; reliability still questionable.
MRT	Indirect measurement of the presence of prostaglandins, cytokines and leukotrienes released from degranulation of leukocytes in presence of allergen; measures volume change of leukocyte via automated computer analysis.	No information on the immune mechanism leading to leukocyte degranulation; negative results can indicate oral tolerance. Not validated for diagnostic use, but still used clinically; reliability still questionable.

TABLE 27-3

Tests Used in the Assessment of Adverse Reactions to Foods—cont'd

Specific IgG, IgM, IgA antibody assays	Techniques of precipitation hemagglutination complement fixation; requires special expertise.	Specific IgG not validated for diagnostic use; but still used clinically; reliability still questionable. Positive results may simply indicate previous exposure to the food.
Serum IgG4	Blood testing for food-specific IgG4.	Not validated for diagnostic use; tends to indicate previous exposure to the food, but still used clinically; reliability still questionable.
Cytotoxic testing	Allergen is mixed with whole blood or serum leukocyte suspension. Lysed leukocytes are then counted; a reduction of white blood cells or death of leukocytes indicates an immune response.	Nonstandardized; may result in false-positive or false-negative results; not widely validated for diagnostic use.
BAT	In vitro assessment using whole blood; measures the response of inflammatory markers following antigen exposure.	Still under investigation; no current defined clinical value in diagnosis of food allergy.
CRD	In vitro assessment; focused diagnosis of serum-specific IgE. Determines IgE binding patterns to specific peptides using microarray analysis.	Still under investigation; not commercially available for diagnosis of food allergy.
	Food Challenges	
DBPCFC	Allergen is disguised and given orally and patient monitored for reaction; patient and physician blinded; also tested with placebo.	"Gold standard" for food allergy testing.
Single-blind food challenge	Suspect food is disguised from patient and orally given by physician in a clinical setting.	Less time-consuming than DBPCFC; may be used in instances in which patient experiences symptoms secondary to fear or aversion to suspect food.
Open oral food challenge	Suspect food is orally given to patient in undisguised, natural form in gradual doses under medical supervision.	Less time-consuming than DBPCFC; should not be used in instances in which patient experiences symptoms secondary to fear or aversion to suspect food.
Food elimination diets	Suspect foods are eliminated from the diet for a set period to identify foods responsible for ARF. During gradual reintroduction symptoms are carefully observed.	May help identify foods responsible for ARF; strict, long-term elimination diets may require monitoring to ensure nutritional adequacy.

ALCAT, Antigen leukocyte cellular antibody test; *BAT,* basophil activation test; *CAP-FEIA,* CAP-fluorescein-enzyme immunoassay; *CRD,* component-resolved diagnostics; *DBPCFC,* double-blind, placebo-controlled food challenge; *ELISA,* enzyme-linked immunosorbent assay; *Ig,* immunoglobulin; *MD,* medical doctor; *MRT,* mediator release test; *RAST,* radioallergosorbent test; *sIg,* secretory immunoglobulin.

allergenic. The most common food allergens (milk, egg, peanut, soy, wheat, shellfish, fish, and tree nuts) account for most of the positive food skin-prick tests (Nowak-Wegrzyn and Sampson, 2006).

Serum Antibody Tests

Food allergen–specific serum IgE testing is used to identify foods that may be causing the allergic response. The **radioallergosorbent test (RAST)** and the enzyme-linked immunosorbent assay (ELISA), both IgE tests, are being replaced by the **CAP–fluorescein-enzyme immunoassay (FEIA)** The CAP-FEIA is a blood test that provides a quantitative assessment of allergen-specific IgE antibodies; higher levels of antibodies are predictors of clinical symptoms. The CAP-FEIA test has been approved for only six foods: egg, milk, peanut, fish, wheat, and soy (soy is still not as predictive) (Sampson, 2004). It is fairly effective as shown by testing known food-allergic children whose food allergies had been previously proven with DBPCFCs. Test results should be followed with either food elimination and challenge or DBPCFCs to complete the diagnostic process (Sampson, 2004). It should be noted that CAP-FEIA or skin testing

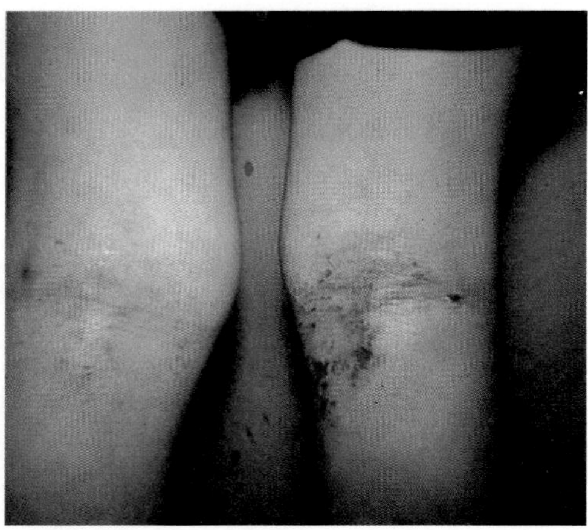

FIGURE 27-4 Atopic eczema: An immunoglobulin E–mediated skin reaction to a food allergen. Commonly seen on the back of knees and the inside of elbows.

results for IgE sensitization may remain positive even after the child has "outgrown" the allergy, and the food can be eaten without symptoms.

Other Tests

Many attempts have been made to suggest that **immunoglobulin G (IgG)** is an indicator of allergy, especially measured by the IgG4 fraction of the immunoglobulin. However, a positive IgG4 response to foods only indicates repeated exposure to components that are recognized as foreign proteins by the immune system; thus the clinical usefulness of IgG4 testing is questionable (Stapel et al., 2008).

Some tests indirectly measure the amount of cytokines released by lymphocytes and granulocytes upon degranulation in response to food antigen exposure. Examples of these tests are the antigen leukocyte cellular antibody test (ALCAT) and the mediator release test (MRT). These tests do not measure IgE-mediated responses. They may be useful in identifying problematic foods in cell-mediated or delayed reactions, but should be followed up with appropriate food elimination and clinical observation of the patient. (NIAID and NIH, 2010).

MEDICAL NUTRITION THERAPY

A nutrition-focused physical examination and a complete nutrition assessment (see Chapters 4, 6, 8 and Appendices 29 and 30) should be performed. Gathered information should include the time of food ingestion relative to the onset of symptoms, a description of the most recent symptoms, a list of suspected foods, and an estimate of the quantity of food required to cause a reaction. Prenatal history, early feeding practices, and exposure is also important in a thorough history.

Measurements for infants and children should be plotted on a growth chart and evaluated in relationship to earlier measurements. Because decreased weight-for-height measurements may be related to malabsorption or food allergy or intolerance, patterns of growth and their relationship to the onset of symptoms should be explored. Clinical signs of malnutrition should be assessed, including the evaluation of fat and muscle stores.

Food and Symptom Diary

A 7- to 14-day **food and symptom diary** is a very useful tool for uncovering ARFs (Figure 27-5). This diary can also be used to identify possible nutrient insufficiencies and deficiencies. The food and symptom diary should include the time the food is eaten, the quantity and type of food, all food ingredients if possible, the time symptoms appear relative to the time of food ingestion, and any supplements or medications taken before or after the onset of symptoms. Other influences such as stress, physical exercise, elimination and sleep patterns can provide valuable information in piecing together the factors that affect ARFs.

The location where the reaction occurred can even be informative, providing unexpected insights into possible food sources of allergen exposure. Or the information obtained can indicate something other than a food reaction. A reaction that appears to be caused by a food when the food allergen cannot be found may actually be caused by a pet or a chemical or other environmental factor. The more information obtained about the adverse reaction, the more useful the diary. The 1- to 2-week food and symptom diary also can serve as a baseline for future interventions.

Food-Elimination Diets

Food elimination is a useful tool in the diagnosis and management of ARFs when used in conjunction with a thorough history and nutrition assessment. With a standard **elimination diet**, suspect foods are eliminated from the diet for a specified period, usually 4 to 12 weeks, followed by a reintroduction and food-challenge phase. All forms (i.e., cooked, raw, and protein derivatives) of a suspected food are removed from the diet, and a food and symptom record is kept during the elimination phase. This record is used to ensure that all forms of suspected foods have been eliminated from the diet and to evaluate the nutritional adequacy of the diet. Elimination diets should be personalized, and may entail eliminating only one or two suspect foods at a time to see if there is improvement in symptoms. If multiple foods are suspected, a variation of the "strict" elimination diet shown in Table 27-4 could be used. Any food on the list that is suspect should be substituted with a food that is not likely to cause a reaction.

Elemental formulas, medical foods or hypoallergenic formulas can also be used for additional nutrition support with the elimination diet. An elemental formula provides high-quality calories in an easily digestible form and helps to optimize nutritional status. Because of low palatability and high cost, this should be reserved for the most restrictive cases.

After the designated elimination phase, foods are systematically reintroduced into the diet one at a time to determine any adverse reactions while the person is carefully monitored. If symptoms persist with careful avoidance of suspect

Name ____________

	DAY 1 DATE		DAY 2 DATE		DAY 3 DATE	
	FOOD	SYMPTOMS	FOOD	SYMPTOMS	FOOD	SYMPTOMS
Time: BREAKFAST						
Medications						
SUPPLEMENTS						
Snack Time:						
Time: LUNCH						
Medications						
SUPPLEMENTS						
Snack Time:						
Time: DINNER						
Medications						
SUPPLEMENTS						
Snack Time:						
MEDICATIONS						

FIGURE 27-5 Food and symptom diary.

foods, other causes for the symptoms should be considered. If a positive result has been obtained on a skin test or allergen-specific IgE blood test and symptoms improve unequivocally with the elimination of the food, that food should be eliminated from the diet until an oral food challenge is appropriate. The oral food challenge will prove or disprove a food symptom relationship. If symptoms improve with only the elimination of multiple foods, multiple food challenges are necessary.

Oral Food Challenge

An oral **food challenge** is conducted in a supervised medical setting once symptoms have resolved and when the person is not taking any antihistamines. Foods are challenged one at a time on different days while the person is carefully observed in a medical setting for the recurrence of symptoms, thus eliminating confusion. The three types of food challenges are an open food challenge, which allows the food to be given openly; a single-blind, placebo-controlled food challenge, in which the food is hidden from the patient with at least one placebo; and a **double-blind, placebo-controlled food challenge (DBPCFC)**, in which the food is hidden from the patient and the clinician and is presented with at least one to three placebos. Increasing amounts of the offending food should be given every 15 to 60 minutes until there is a convincing, but not life-threatening, response. The goal is to ingest 6 to 10 g of dry food or 80 mL of liquid food mixed in a masking food the patient tolerates (Nowak-Wegrzyn and Sampson, 2006). A person with a positive challenge response must be given appropriate medications to stop symptoms and be observed for an additional 1 to 2 hours. Those who are observed to have a negative challenge response should also be observed for an additional 1 to 2 hours because a reaction may occasionally occur later than expected. The amount of food tolerated under observation can then be offered at home.

The DBPCFC provides objective results by eliminating outside influences; it is the standard when attempting to establish a food and symptom relationship and to confirm a food allergy. Each DBPCFC must be personalized. Single foods (e.g., applesauce, grape juice) or tolerated food combinations can "hide" a suspect food. The product must mask any hint of the flavor, color, or texture of the suspect food or allergen. The patient should not be able to detect the differences between the "reactive" food and the placebo food. Because severe reactions can occur during a challenge, a physician must be in attendance with emergency supplies measured and ready to be administered.

After a negative DBPCFC, an open challenge should be given. In this challenge the patient is given a serving of the suspect food. Interestingly, reactions have occurred during the open challenge that did not occur in the blind challenge.

TABLE 27-4

Guidelines for Elimination Diets

- These guidelines emphasize foods that are naturally nutrient-rich.
- Guidelines should be personalized according to the patient's history and should eliminate other foods that are known allergens or foods that aggravate symptoms.
- Refer to label reading guidelines to avoid ingredients to be eliminated. See Boxes 27-4 through 27-10.
- Amounts should be individually tailored to energy needs.
- Suggest limiting number of spices to five to minimize dietary variables.

	Foods Allowed	Foods To Avoid
Elimination Diet Level I: Milk-, egg-, and wheat-free		
Animal proteins	Fish, shellfish, turkey, chicken, beef, pork	Eggs, egg substitutes containing egg whites and all products containing eggs (see Box 27-4)
Plant proteins	Beans, lentils, split peas, organic soybeans, and soy products	Nonorganic soy
Dairy alternatives	Nondairy beverage alternatives including soy beverages	Milk (cow, goat, sheep) and all products containing milk ingredients (see Box 27-5)
Grains	Amaranth, barley, buckwheat, corn, millet, oats, quinoa, rice, rye	Wheat, all forms of wheat (see Box 27-6)
Vegetables	All vegetables and starchy vegetables	Vegetable dishes containing milk, egg, or wheat (e.g., tempura, breaded, etc.)
Fruits	All fruits and 100% fruit juices	Fruit pies, pastries, cookies, etc., that contain milk, egg, or wheat
Fats and oils	Coconut oil, organic canola oil, grapeseed oil, olive oil, flaxseed oil, sesame oil, safflower oil, milk-free organic (nonhydrogenated) margarines	Butter, margarine, hydrogenated oils, shortening
Peanuts, nuts, and seeds	Peanuts, nuts, and natural nut butters, seeds and natural seed butters	Any peanut, nut, or seed product containing milk, egg, wheat (e.g., milk chocolate candy with nuts)
Beverages	Tea, herbal tea, coffee, decaffeinated tea, and coffee	Beverages containing milk (cow, goat, sheep)
Sweeteners	Cane or beet sugar, honey, maple syrup, blackstrap molasses	Artificial sweeteners
Other	Salt, pepper, herbs, and spices	Egg-, milk-, or wheat-containing condiments; all artificial ingredients, salad dressing, mayonnaise, spreads containing milk, egg, wheat
Elimination Diet Level 2: More Limited		
Eliminates top eight allergens (milk, egg, wheat, fish, shellfish, soybeans, peanuts, tree nuts) and corn, gluten, chocolate, sesame, coffee, tea, alcohol, and artificial ingredients		
Animal protein sources	Turkey, chicken, lean cuts beef, lamb, pork	Fish, shellfish, eggs, sausages, deli meats
Plant protein sources	Beans, lentils, split peas	Soybeans and soy products, peanuts, tree nuts
Dairy alternatives	Nondairy, soy-free, nut-free beverage alternatives (rice beverage, hempseed beverage)	Milk and all dairy alternative beverages containing soy, or tree nuts
Grains	Amaranth, buckwheat, millet, quinoa, rice, teff, tapioca, wild rice, gluten-free oat	Wheat, regular oats, barley, rye, corn, spelt, kamut, triticale
Vegetables	Most vegetables and starchy vegetables	Corn; vegetable dishes containing ingredients to avoid such as breaded, creamed, etc.
Fruits	Most fruits and 100% fruit juices	Fruit pies, pastries, cookies, etc., that contain ingredients to avoid

TABLE 27-4

Guidelines for Elimination Diets—cont'd

	Foods Allowed	Foods To Avoid
Fats and oils	Olive oil, coconut oil, flaxseed oil, grapeseed oil, organic canola oil, safflower oil, sunflower oil	Butter, margarine, vegetable oil, soy oil, corn oil, peanut oil, shortening, processed oils, sesame oil
Peanuts, nuts, and seeds	Seeds and seed butters	Peanuts and peanut-containing products, tree nuts and tree nut–containing products
Beverages	Herbal tea, 100% unsweetened fruit or vegetable juice, water, nondairy soy-free beverages	Coffee, caffeinated tea, other caffeinated beverages, alcoholic beverages, soft drinks
Sweeteners	Cane or beet sugar, honey, maple syrup, blackstrap molasses	Artificial sweeteners
Other	Salt, pepper, all spices	Chocolate, condiments containing any eliminated ingredient, all artificial ingredients, salad dressing, mayonnaise, spreads

Elimination Diet Level 3: Very few foods/Limited ingredients

Intended to be used in the short-term only.

- Animal proteins: Chicken, turkey, lamb
- Grains: Rice in any form including rice cakes and rice cereal
- Vegetables: Sautéed or steamed leafy green vegetables including spinach, kale, bok choy, collard greens, green beans, squash, sweet potatoes, potatoes
- Fruits: Pear
- Oils: Extra virgin olive oil
- Beverages: Water, herbal tea, vegetable broths (gluten-free)
- Sweeteners: Maple syrup

Occasionally symptoms may accompany the last presentation if the threshold is greater than indicated by the history. Most allergic reactions occur within 2 hours of the challenge. Non–IgE-mediated reactions may occur more than 24 hours after challenge. Monitoring of the patient should continue during this time.

If there is a clear history of a life-threatening anaphylactic reaction after eating a specific food, that food should not be challenged unless there is sufficient evidence that the person is no longer reacting to the allergen and skin test or allergen-specific IgE blood test results are negative, and then only in a controlled medical setting where epinephrine is available. Because of the risk of severe reactions and the lack of standardization of the testing procedure, many clinicians are questioning the use of the DBPCFC to document a food allergy reaction (Mullin et al., 2010).

Avoidance of Unsafe Food

Although many food intolerances may allow some ingestion of the offending food, food allergies usually do not. Total avoidance of the unsafe food (food allergen) is the only proven treatment for food allergy. **Food immunotherapy vaccine** is a possible future treatment meant to complement food allergen avoidance, but these vaccines are still experimental (Sicherer and Sampson, 2010).

Recent research has produced encouraging evidence that **specific oral tolerance induction (SOTI)** can be achieved by introducing the culprit food via the digestive tract in minute then increasing quantities for an extended period (Clark et al., 2009; Zapatero et al., 2008). Allergic individuals and their families need guidelines and suggestions for avoiding allergenic foods and ingredients, substituting permissible foods for restricted foods in meal planning and preparation, and selecting nutritionally adequate replacement foods (Joneja, 2007).

Additional food characteristics may be relevant. For example, recent studies suggest that 70% to 80% of young children allergic to milk or eggs can tolerate baked (heat-denatured) forms of the protein, but not the unbaked form. It is suggested that these children make IgE antibodies primarily to **conformational epitopes** (antigenic determinants on the surface of the food proteins that are recognized by the immune system) and represent those children who will naturally outgrow their food allergies (Sicherer and Sampson, 2010).

To help identify and avoid offending foods, allergy-specific lists that describe foods to avoid, state key words for ingredient identification, and present acceptable substitutes are useful and necessary in counseling (Boxes 27-4 through 27-8). Caretakers and school personnel working with the food-allergic child should be cautioned to read labels carefully before purchasing or serving food. The Food Allergy and Anaphylaxis Network, a nonprofit organization

Text continued on p. 582

BOX 27-4

Eliminating Eggs: Label Reading and Strategies

Foods and Ingredients to Avoid*

Albumin
Apovitellin
Avidin
Bernaise sauce
Dried eggs
Eggnog
Egg solids
Egg substitutes
Egg white[†]
Egg yolk
Flavoprotein
Frozen eggs
Globulin
Hollandaise sauce
Imitation egg product
Lecithin
Livetin
Lysozyme
Mayonnaise
Meringue
Ovalbumin
Ovoglobulin
Ovoglycoprotein
Ovomucin
Ovomucoid
Ovomuxoid
Ovovitellin
Powdered egg
Simplesse
Vitellin

Egg Substitutes (Equivalent to 1 Egg)

1½ tsp Ener G Egg Replacer (ENERG-G Foods, Inc.) + 1 Tbsp of water
1 packet plain gelatin + 1 c boiling water— use 3 Tbsp of this mixture
½ tsp baking powder + 1 Tbsp liquid + 1 Tbsp vinegar
2 Tbsp fruit puree (use in baking for binding, but not leavening); try apples or prunes
1 Tbsp ground flaxseed + 3 Tbsp of water
1 tsp yeast dissolved in ¼ c warm water
1 medium banana
1½ Tbsp water + 1½ Tbsp oil + 1 tsp baking powder
¼ c soft tofu, beaten
To achieve the emulsifying effect in baking: 2 Tbsp wholewheat flour + ½ tsp oil + ½ tsp baking powder + 2 Tbsp milk, water, or fruit juice.

*Eliminate the following foods, as well as any foods containing any of these ingredients.

[†]Egg whites and shells may be used as a clarifying agent in soup stocks, consommés, wine, alcoholic beverages, and coffee drinks.

BOX 27-5

Eliminating Cow's Milk: Label Reading and Strategies

Foods and Ingredients to Avoid*

Acidophilus milk
Ammonium caseinate
Artificial butter flavor
Butter
Butter fat
Butter oil
Calcium caseinate
Caramel candy
Carob candies
Casein
Casein hydrolysate
Cheese and cheese flavor (e.g., cheddar, Colby, cream, Edam, Gouda, Monterey Jack, mozzarella, Muenster, Neufchâtel, parmesan, provolone, ricotta, Romano, Swiss, cottage)
Chocolate milk
Condensed milk
Creamed candies
Cultured buttermilk
Curds
Custard
Delactosed whey
Dry milk (whole, low-fat, nonfat)
Eggnog
Evaporated milk
Ghee
Goat's milk[†]
Half & half cream
Hydrolysates (casein, milk protein, protein, whey, whey protein)
Ice cream
Lactalbumin, lactalbumin phosphate
Lactoferrin
Lactoglobin
Lactose

BOX 27-5

Eliminating Cow's Milk: Label Reading and Strategies—cont'd

Lactulose
Low-fat ice cream
Magnesium caseinate
Malted milk
Milk chocolate
Milk (whole, 2%, 1½%, 1%, ½%, skim, evaporated, condensed)
Milk protein
Nougat
Potassium caseinate
Pudding
Rennet casein
Semisweet chocolate
Sherbet, most types
Sodium caseinate
Sour cream
Sour cream dressings
Sour cream solids
Sour milk solids
Sweet whey
Sweetened condensed milk
Whey
Whey protein concentrate
Whipping cream
Yogurt, frozen
Yogurt, regular

Ingredients Potentially Made With Cow's Milk Products

Bavarian cream flavoring
Brown sugar flavoring
Butter flavoring
Caramel flavoring
Coconut cream flavoring
Natural flavoring
Recaldent, used in tooth-whitening chewing gums
Simplesse

Substitutes for 1 c of Cow's Milk in Recipes

1 c light-colored fruit juice (e.g., apple, orange, white grape)
1 c herbal tea
1 c milk-free infant formula
1 c soy milk
1 c hemp milk
1 c rice milk, oat milk or other grain milk
1 c almond milk or other nut milk
1 c water

Milk-Free Infant Formulas

Partially Hydrolyzed (Cow's Milk Protein) Infant Formula‡

Enfamil Gentlease Lipil (Mead Johnson Nutritionals) whey/casein protein blend
Gerber Good Start (Nestle) 100% whey protein

Extensively Hydrolyzed Infant Formula§

Enfamil Nutramigen with Enflora LGG (Mead Johnson)
Pregestimil Lipil (Mead Johnson)
Similac Expert Care Alimentum (Abbott Laboratories)

Free Amino-Acid Base Infant Formula¶

EleCare (Abbott Laboratories)
Enfamil Nutramigen AA (Mead Johnson)
Neocate products (Nutricia North America)

Soy Infant Formula¶

Enfamil ProSobee (Mead Johnson)
Gerber Good Start Soy PLUS (Nestle)
Similac Isomil Soy (Abbott Laboratories)

Organic Soy Infant Formula¶

Baby's Only Organic Soy (Nature's One)
Earth's Best Organic Soy (Hain Celestial Group)

Data from Bahna SL: Hypoallergenic formulas: optimal choices for treatment versus prevention, Ann Allergy Asthma Immunol 101:5, 2008; Greer FR et al: Effects of early nutritional interventions on the development of atopic disease in infants and children: the role of maternal dietary restriction, breastfeeding, timing of introduction of complementary foods, and hydrolyzed formulas, *Pediatrics* 121:183, 2008; Kneepkens CM, Meijer Y: Clinical practice: diagnosis and treatment of cow's milk allergy, Eur J Pediatr 168:891, 2009.

*Individuals who must avoid all cow's milk sources frequently need a calcium supplement.

†Goat's milk protein is similar to cow's milk protein. Those with cow's milk allergy may experience similar symptoms with goat's milk ingestion (Pessler and Nejat, 2004). Goat's milk is not recommended as a cow's milk substitute, especially in infants, because it has a high renal solute load and is very low in folic acid compared with cow's milk.

‡Partially hydrolyzed: Nonhypoallergenic; contains partially digested proteins that have a molecular weight greater than extensively hydrolyzed formula protein chains. May cause a reaction in one third to one half of individuals with a cow's milk protein allergy.

§Extensively hydrolyzed: Hypoallergenic; contains extensively digested casein or whey proteins that have a molecular weight less than partially hydrolyzed formula protein chains. Tolerated without an allergic reaction in 90% of individuals with a cow's milk protein allergy.

¶Free amino acid–based infant formula: Hypoallergenic; peptide-free formula that contains essential and nonessential amino acids. Usually tolerated by those allergic to extensively hydrolyzed formulas.

¶Soy formula: Should not be used in infants younger than 6 months old with food allergies.

BOX 27-6

Eliminating Wheat: Label Reading and Strategies

Foods and Ingredients to Avoid

All-purpose flour
Bran
Bread
Bread crumbs
Bread flour
Bulgar
Cake
Cake flour
Cereal extract
Cookies
Couscous
Cracked wheat
Durum flour
Durum wheat
Emmer
Enriched flour
Farina
Gluten
Graham flour
High-gluten flour
High-protein flour
Kamut
Kamut flour
Laubina
Leche alim
Malted cereals
Minchin
Multi-grain breads
Multi-grain flours
Pasta
Pastries
Pastry flour
Puffed wheat
Red wheat flakes
Rolled wheat
Semolina
Shredded wheat
Soft wheat flour
Spelt
Sprouted wheat
Tortillas
Triticale
Wheat (bran, germ, gluten, malt, meal, starch)
Wheat bread
Wheat bread crumbs
Wheat flakes
Wheat flour
Wheat pasta
Wheat protein beverage
Wheat protein powder
Wheat tempeh
White bread
White flour
Whole wheat berries
Whole wheat flour
Vital gluten
Winter wheat flour
Vitalia macaroni

Other Possible Sources of Wheat

Ale and beer
Baking mixes and baked products
Breaded or floured foods including batter-fried foods
Gelatinized starch
Hydrolyzed vegetable protein
Meats containing fillers including processed meats and meatloaf
Modified food starch
Modified starch
Starch
Soy sauce
Vegetable gum
Vegetable starch
Xanthan gum

Substitutions (Equivalent to 1 c Wheat Flour)

1 c rye meal
1-1¼ c rye flour
1 c potato flour
1⅓ c rolled oats or oat flour
½ c potato flour + 1/2 c rye flour
⅝ c potato starch
⅝ c rice flour + 1/3 c rye flour
Adding 1 tsp of xanthan gum to every cup of flour improves the texture of baked goods
Wheat-free and gluten-free flour products are available

Wheat-Free Alternatives

Amaranth
Barley (if not intolerant of gluten)
Buckwheat
Chickpea
Corn
Lentil
Millet
Oats (if not intolerant of gluten)
Quinoa
Rice
Rye (if not intolerant of gluten)
Tapioca

BOX 27-7

Eliminating Peanuts: Label Reading and Strategies

Foods and Ingredients to Avoid*

Arachis oil
Artificial tree nuts
Beer nuts
Cold-pressed peanut oil
Defattened peanuts
Egg rolls
Expelled or expressed peanut oil
Granulated peanuts
Ground nuts
High-protein food
Hydrolyzed plant protein
Hydrolyzed vegetable protein
Marzipan
Mixed nuts
Nougat
Nuts with artificial flavoring
Peanuts, all varieties
Peanut butter
Peanut flakes
Peanut flour
Peanut meal
Peanut oil

Additional Products That May Contain Peanuts†

Baked goods
Candy
Cashew butter
Cheesecake crusts
Chili
Chocolate candy
Dog food and treats
Egg rolls
Frozen desserts
Hamster feed
Ice cream
Livestock feed
Pie crusts
Salad dressing
Sauces
Soups
Stews
Sunflower seeds

*Eliminate all sources of peanuts from diet including cross contaminated food or utensils. There is a high risk of cross contamination when eating out, especially when dining at Asian, Chinese, Mexican, Thai, Mediterranean, and Indian restaurants.

†Peanut powder, peanut butter, and peanuts may be used as an ingredient or garnish for many dishes.

BOX 27-8

Eliminating Soy: Label Reading and Strategies

Foods and Ingredients to Avoid*

Chee-fan
Deep-fried mature soy seed
Edamame
Fermented soybean paste
Fermented soybeans
Hamanattoo
Immature green soy seed
Ketjap
Lecithin made from soy†
Miso
Natto
Shoyu sauce
Soy nuts
Soy protein (concentrate, hydrolyzed, isolate)
Soy protein shakes
Soy sauce
Soybean curd
Soybean flour
Soybean grits
Soybean milk
Soybean oil†
Soybean sprouts
Soy lecithin†
Sufu
Tamari
Tao-cho
Tao-si
Taotjo
Tempeh
Textured soy protein
Textured vegetable protein
Tofu
Whey-soy drink

Ingredients Potentially Made from Soybean Products

Hydrolyzed plant protein
Hydrolyzed vegetable protein

Continued

BOX 27-8

Eliminating Soy: Label Reading and Strategies—cont'd

Natural flavoring
Vegetable broth
Vegetable gum
Vegetable starch
Xanthan gum

Soy and Milk Substitutes

Fruit juices
Hemp, grain, or nut beverages

Soy-Free Infant Formulas

Partially hydrolyzed (cow's milk protein) infant formula[‡]

Enfamil Gentlease Lipil (Mead Johnson Nutritionals) whey-casein protein blend
Gerber Good Start (Nestle) 100% whey protein

Extensively Hydrolyzed Infant Formula[§]

Enfamil Nutramigen with Enflora LGG (Mead Johnson)
Pregestimil Lipil (Mead Johnson)
Similac Expert Care Alimentum (Abbott Laboratories)

Free Amino-Acid Base Infant Formula[¶]

EleCare (Abbott Laboratories)
Enfamil Nutramigen AA (Mead Johnson)
Neocate products (Nutricia North America)

Data from Kneepkens CM, Meijer Y: Clinical practice. Diagnosis and treatment of cow's milk allergy. Eur J Pediatr, 168:891, 2009.

*There is a high risk of cross-contamination when eating out, especially dining at Asian restaurants.

[†]Several studies indicate that soybean lecithin and soy oil are frequently tolerated by individuals who are soy allergic.

[‡]Partially hydrolyzed: Nonhypoallergenic; contains partially digested cow's milk proteins that have a molecular weight greater than extensively hydrolyzed formula protein chains.

[§]Extensively hydrolyzed: Hypoallergenic; contains extensively digested casein or whey proteins that have a molecular weight less than partially hydrolyzed formula protein chains.

[¶]Free amino-acid–based infant formula: Hypoallergenic; peptide-free formula that contains essential and nonessential amino acids. Usually tolerated by those allergic to extensively hydrolyzed formulas.

created to support the food-allergic child, has worked with board-certified allergists and dietitians to develop an excellent education program for day-care or school programs. Food substitutions can be challenging when working within school food program guidelines and special help may be necessary.

Food ingredients to be avoided may be hidden in the diet in unfamiliar forms. When a food-sensitive person ingests a hidden allergen, the most common reason is that the "safe" food was contaminated. This may happen as a result of using common serving utensils such as at an ice cream parlor, salad bar, or deli (where the meat slicer may be used to slice both meat and cheese). Manufacturing plants or restaurants may use the same equipment to produce two different products (e.g., peanut butter and almond butter); despite cleaning, traces of an allergen may remain on the equipment between uses. Alternatively, a restaurant may use the same oil to fry both potatoes and fish (Box 27-9).

In addition, the food may have been genetically modified, changing its allergenicity. Here again, label reading is essential. See *Focus On:* Genetically Modified (GM) Foods.

Another situation that may lead to the unknowing ingestion of an allergenic food occurs when one product is used to make a second product, and only the ingredients of the second product are listed on the food label. An example is the listing of mayonnaise as an ingredient in a salad dressing without specifically listing egg as an ingredient of the mayonnaise. Labels must be read often to ensure that ingredients have not changed in the processing of the food (Box 27-10).

BOX 27-9

Reasons Why Allergens May Contaminate a Food

- Common serving utensils used to serve different foods
- Manufacture of two different food products using the same equipment without proper cleaning in between
- Misleading or inaccurate labels (e.g., nondairy creamers that contain sodium caseinate)
- Ingredients added for a specific purpose are listed on the label only in general terms of their purpose rather than as a specific ingredient (e.g., egg white that is simply listed as an "emulsifier")
- Addition of an allergenic product to a second product that bears a label listing only the ingredients of the second product (e.g., mayonnaise, without noting eggs)
- Switching of ingredients by food manufacturers (e.g., a shortage of one vegetable oil prompting substitution with another)
- An ingredient that is present in a food but in such a low percentage that it does not have to be listed on a label

FOCUS ON

Genetically Modified (GM) Foods

Genetic engineering or modification (GM) is the process whereby a protein from one plant can be transferred to another. GM foods have been in the U.S. food supply for at least 15 years. Plants can be made to tolerate herbicides and thus be more insect resistant with changed taste, texture, and appearance. In addition GM can affect the allergenicity of the modified food in two ways: (1) by introducing allergens, or (2) by changing the level or nature of intrinsic allergens. Once a protein has been transferred, the allergenicity potential must be evaluated (Zolla, 2008). For example, GM soy and GM corn contain new transgenic proteins with allergenic properties; GM soy has up to seven times more of a known soy allergen than its non-GM counterpart (Pusztai and Bardocz, 2005). The safety evaluation of a GM food should include the gene source, how closely the new protein resembles known allergens, and how persons with known allergy to the protein transferred might react if exposed. The lack of evidence that GM food is unsafe cannot be interpreted as proof that it is safe.

There are also long-term concerns beyond those related to the presence of unknown protein allergens. A long-term study of both weaning and old mice consuming either GM corn or non-GM corn found that the mice consuming the GM corn had an increased presence of several cytokines that are specifically involved in inflammatory and allergic responses, and alterations in the numbers of B cells and T cells, indicating an abnormal response to the genetically altered corn (Finamore et al., 2008). Furthermore, it has been argued that GM foods should be subjected to the same testing and approval procedures as medicines (i.e., clinical trials) to ensure that any possibility of an adverse effect on human health from a GM food can be detected (Dona and Arvanitoyannis, 2009). Because using GM foods can complicate the elimination diet or, as already mentioned, aggravate an immune-mediated response, it may be prudent to advise those with documented food allergies to eat only organic forms of corn, soybeans, canola, and other foods for which there are GM versions in the food supply.

BOX 27-10

Allergen Labeling of Foods

Since January 1, 2006 the updated **Food Allergen Labeling and Consumer Protection Act (FALCPA)** requires the top allergens to be clearly listed by manufacturers as an ingredient or following the ingredient list on food labels. This includes ingredients in any amount and also mandates specific ingredients to be listed such as the type of nut or seafood.

The Food Allergen Labeling and Consumer Protection Act of 2004 (FALCPA) Effective January, 2006

Requirements of the Law

- **Top 8 allergens must be clearly listed** by manufacturers as an ingredient or following the ingredient list on food labels of any food product containing allergens
- Applies to all packaged foods sold in the United States
- Does not apply to USDA regulated products including meat, poultry products, and some egg products
- Does not list sources of possible contamination
- Does not apply to prescription medication or alcoholic beverages
- Does not apply to foods packaged or wrapped after being ordered by the consumer

Top Allergens

- Any ingredient containing or derived from the top 8 allergens—milk, eggs, fish, shellfish, tree nuts, peanuts, wheat, or soybeans
- For tree nuts, fish, and shellfish the specific type must be listed (example: walnut, pecan, shrimp, tuna)

Reading the Food Label

- Ingredients may be included within the food's ingredient list directly or in parentheses following the name, if an ingredient does not clearly identify the allergen
- Following the list of ingredients all food allergens may be listed in a **"Contains" statement**
- Manufacturers may voluntarily list potential unintended allergens that may be present due to cross contamination in a clear way that does not interfere with the required food ingredient list

When foods are removed from the diet, alternative nutrient sources must be provided. Table 27-5 defines the levels of nutritional risk based on the types of food removed from the diet. For example, when eggs are omitted, other foods must provide choline, vitamin D, protein, and energy.

Healing the Gut and Restoring Immune Balance

Because 70% of immune cells are located in the gut-associated lymphatic tissue (GALT), efforts to restore gut health should improve immune function and modulate allergic responses. Besides eliminating problematic foods, other measures include optimizing stomach acidity and enzyme function; identifying and treating intestinal pathogens such as bacteria, yeasts, and parasites; restoring intestinal barrier function; and repleting nutritional stores (see Chapters 28 and 29). Sometimes after the gut is healed it is possible to institute a rotation diet where foods identified as causing allergic reactions can be consumed on a planned "rotating" basis without symptoms developing. There is some preliminary research to suggest that rotation diets in combination with probiotics may be useful in the management of food intolerances in patients with diarrhea-dominant irritable bowel syndrome (Drisko, et al, 2006). See *Clinical Insight:* Rotation Diets—Where's the Science? Are they Clinically Useful?

CLINICAL INSIGHT

Rotation Diets—Where's the Science? Are they Clinically Useful?

By Janice V Joneja, PhD, CDR

With Ig-E Meditated Allergy

There is no published evidence-based research on the use of rotation diets in the management of Ig-E mediated food allergy. Available material on the subject relies on anecdotal reports, testimonials, and directives from practitioners based on theory and perception, but no science (Teuber and Porch-Curren, 2003).

There are numerous websites claiming relief from multiple allergies with a variety of diagnostic procedures and rotation diets. There is no evidence-based research to support their claims, but the description of the management strategy and testimonials from clients is very convincing. It is critical that dietitians be aware of these claims and the enormous incentive for the patient suffering sometimes debilitating symptoms, to believe them and follow their directives.

With Non-IgE mediated allergy and food sensitivities

Non- IgE immunologically-mediated food hypersensitivities may be dose-related. A rotation diet that restricts the number and quantity of foods known to contain the culprit component is often beneficial (Joneja, 2003). However, when the diet is used, there is no scientific basis for a 4, 5, 7 or even 30 day rotation of foods. All have been used clinically. Such diets need to be formulated on an individual basis to ensure that the dose of the reactive component is reduced to a minimum, while nutrients equivalent to those eliminated are supplied by alternative foods.

TABLE 27-5

Nutritional Risk in food Allergy Management

Level of Risk	Food Characteristics/Examples
Low risk	Any food that can easily be eliminated with minimum or no nutritional risk to the patient; protein, calorie, and nutrient consumption is adequate. *Example:* Avoidance of a specific fruit or vegetable
Moderate risk	Any food that may be encountered frequently throughout the food supply yet the elimination of which does not significantly limit food choices or vital nutrient sources; questionable adequacy of protein, calorie, and nutrient consumption. *Example:* Avoidance of fish, crustaceans, or tree nuts
Complex risk	Any food that permeates the food supply, providing a significant source of specific nutrients that are not readily available through other foods that are a part of the normal diet, the elimination of which results in a significant lifestyle and dietary change because of the difficulty of avoiding that food and products containing that food; adequate protein, calorie, and nutrient consumption unlikely. *Example:* Avoidance of wheat, soy, egg, milk, peanuts, or multiple foods

Nutritional Adequacy

The nutritional adequacy of the diet should be monitored on a regular basis by conducting an ongoing evaluation of the patient's growth, nutrition status, and food records. The omission of foods from the diet on the basis of proper or improper diagnosis can and has threatened the nutritional status of the allergic individual (Noimark and Cox, 2008). Malnutrition and poor growth may occur in children who consume inadequate elimination diets. Vitamin and mineral supplementation may be needed to prevent this, especially when multiple foods are omitted. Nutrition assessment needs to be done regularly. Because food is an important part of a person's culture, the social aspects of eating can make adherence to an elimination diet difficult. Continued support from health care providers is needed to minimize the effect of dietary changes on family and social life. The strategies listed in Box 27-11 can help families and individuals cope with food allergies.

It was previously thought that most children would "outgrow" their food allergies by 3 years of age; however, it is becoming apparent that this is not the case. Only 11% of egg-allergic and 19% of milk-allergic children resolved their allergies by 4 years of age. However, almost 80% resolved these allergies by age 16 (Savage et al., 2007; Skripak et al., 2007).

This is not true for peanut allergy, which is considered a persistent allergy lasting a lifetime for most children (Sicherer and Sampson, 2010). Sensitization procedures show some promise (Stahl and Rans, 2011.) While about 20% of children with peanut allergy will outgrow their early allergy to peanut, it appears that, once outgrown, frequent peanut ingestion is recommended to maintain the tolerance (NIAID, 2010.)

PREVENTING FOOD ALLERGY

Intensive research is being focused on the pathogenesis and prevention of allergic disease, including the role of genetics and environmental factors such as early dietary exposures and feeding practices. Allergy prevention guidelines have gradually shifted away from allergen avoidance to examination of the role of specific dietary factors in the development and prevention of allergic disease (Jennings and Prescott, 2010).

Pregnancy and Infancy

Allergen Exposure

The traditional approach for dietary allergy prevention has been avoidance of food allergens in the maternal diet and early postnatal period. However, there is a lack of evidence that maternal dietary restrictions during pregnancy help prevent atopic disease in infants. Food restriction to avoid antigen exposure while breast-feeding does not appear to prevent atopic disease, with the possible exception of atopic eczema (Greer et al., 2008). However, recent research indicates that exposure to food antigens in the "safe" environment of pregnancy and in breast milk is more likely to lead to tolerance rather than sensitization to those foods in the infant. Current trials on infant feeding are attempting to elucidate the concept of oral tolerance and define the effect that delayed introduction of solids and allergenic foods has on development of allergic disease.

BOX 27-11

Strategies for Coping with Food Allergy

Food Substitutions

Try to substitute item-for-item at meals. For example, if the family is eating pasta for dinner, substitution of a gluten free pasta may be better accepted for the gluten sensitive person than a dissimilar item.

Dining Out and Eating Away from Home

Eating meals away from home can be risky for individuals with food allergies. Whether at a fancy restaurant or a fast-food establishment, inadvertent exposure to an allergen can occur, even among the most knowledgeable individuals. Here are some precautions to take:

- Bring "safe" foods along to make eating out easier. For breakfast, bring along soy milk if others will be having cereal with milk.
- Alert the wait staff to the potential severity of the food allergy or allergies.
- Question the wait staff carefully about ingredients.
- Always carry medications.

Special Occasions

Call the host family in advance to determine what foods will be served. Offer to provide an acceptable dish that all can enjoy.

Grocery Shopping

Be informed about what foods are acceptable, and read labels carefully. Product ingredients change over time; continue to read the labels on foods, even if they were previously determined to be "safe" foods. Allow for the fact that shopping will take extra time.

Label Reading

Labeling legislation makes it easier for individuals with food allergies to identify certain potential allergens from the ingredient list on food labels. For example, when food manufacturers use protein hydrolysates or hydrolyzed vegetable protein, they must now specify the source of protein used (e.g., hydrolyzed soy or hydrolyzed corn). Although reactions to food colors or food dyes are rare, individuals who suspect an intolerance will find them listed separately on the food label, rather than categorized simply as "food color."

Breastfeeding

Breast milk contains a host of immunologically active compounds such as transforming growth factor–beta, lactoferrin, lysozymes, long-chain fatty acids, antioxidants, and secretory IgA (sIgA), all of which have an effect on immune development, including oral tolerance, and help to reinforce the gut-epithelial barrier (Brandtzaeg, 2009; Jennings and Prescott, 2010). Breastfeeding without any maternal dietary restrictions is strongly encouraged, although the exact role of breastfeeding in allergy prevention is unclear. There is evidence that exclusive breastfeeding for at least 3 months protects against wheezing in early life (Greer et al., 2008). For infants at high risk of developing atopic disease (infants with a first-degree relative with allergy) exclusive breastfeeding for at least 4 months is recommended (Host et al., 2008). Continuation of breastfeeding through the time when solid foods are introduced is believed to help prevent the development of food allergy (Greer et al., 2008).

Sensitivity to breast milk is rare but has been reported. Allergens in the mother's diet such as cow's milk, eggs, and peanuts can pass into the breast milk and cause sensitization and then an allergic reaction in the exclusively breast-fed infant. Food challenges to each food will determine food symptom relationships. The mother eats a suspect food before nursing, and the infant is observed for symptoms for up to 24 hours after nursing. If a food is judged to yield a positive test result through challenge, that food is eliminated from the mother's diet and she is encouraged to continue breastfeeding. The nutritional adequacy of the mother's diet should be monitored when food groups are omitted from her diet.

Choice of Infant Formula

In infants at high risk of developing atopic disease who are not exclusively breastfed for 4 to 6 months, a partially hydrolyzed or extensively hydrolyzed formula to replace a cow's milk formula is recommended. Extensively hydrolyzed formulas may be more protective than partially hydrolyzed formulas in prevention of atopic disease (Greer et al., 2008). Soy-based infant formulas offer no advantage for the purpose of allergy prevention and some infants may react adversely to these formulas. Amino acid–based formulas may be used in allergy, but have not been adequately studied for atopy prevention. See Boxes 27-5 and 27-8.

Solid Food Introduction

It is recommended that solid foods or complementary foods other than breastmilk or formula should not be introduced until 4 to 6 months of age. There is no convincing evidence that delaying introduction beyond this time prevents the development of atopic disease, and this also pertains to the introduction of foods that are considered to be highly allergenic such as peanuts, eggs, and fish (Greer et al., 2008, Jennings and Prescott, 2010). Although early exposure to some food antigens, such as wheat and gluten, is being promoted as a method of encouraging oral tolerance to them, this technique has not been proven to be effective (Poole et al., 2006).

Early Diet and Immunomodulatory Factors

Dietary factors in early life may influence asthma and allergic disease development. The immunoregulatory network in newborns is orchestrated not only by microbial products but also by dietary constituents such as vitamin A, vitamin D, ω-3 fatty acids, folate, and other micronutrients (Brandtzaeg, 2010).

Antioxidants

Diets high in antioxidants such as β-carotene, vitamin C, vitamin E, zinc, and selenium may prevent the development of food allergies. There have been positive associations found between maternal antioxidant status in pregnancy and cord blood immune responses (West et al, 2010). Higher maternal intake of green and yellow vegetables, citrus fruit, and β-carotene during pregnancy was significantly associated with a reduced risk of eczema, but not wheezing, in the infants. Maternal vitamin E consumption was inversely related to the risk of infantile wheeze, but not eczema (Miyake et al., 2010). Thus optimizing food sources of antioxidants from fruit and vegetable intake during pregnancy may be an effective effort for allergy risk reduction.

Folate

Folate deficiency has been associated with several disorders characterized by enhanced activation of the cellular, Th1-type immune response (Husemoen et al., 2006). An intriguing development has been the recognition of epigenetic effects of dietary folate in the development of asthma (Jennings and Prescott, 2010). Impaired folate metabolism may be related to the development of atopy, although the significance is not clear, because one study demonstrated that prenatal folate supplementation was associated with increased childhood wheezing (Miller, 2008), whereas another found the opposite (Matsui and Matsui, 2009).

Pre- and Probiotics

Prebiotics include the nondigestible, fermentable oligosaccharides that stimulate the growth and activity of bacteria in the colon, whereas **probiotics** are live microorganisms that impart health benefits to the host. Their role in allergy prevention has not been thoroughly studied and should elucidate the effect of the individual strain, timing, dose, and environmental factors that affect colonization and host genetic factors. By supplementing during pregnancy 1 month before delivery, or providing the infant with 6 months' treatment of probiotic therapy either from the nursing mother or with direct supplementation, the incidence of infant food allergy–related atopic eczema may be reduced (Rautava et al., 2005). However, administration of probiotics to infant feeds for prevention of allergic disease requires further investigation and studies have not yielded consistent results (Osborn and Sinn, 2007).

Polyunsaturated Fatty Acids (PUFA)

The role of polyunsaturated fatty acids (ω-3 and ω-6 PUFAs) in allergy development has been the subject of investigation

CLINICAL SCENARIO

Sally is 18 months old. At birth she was unable to tolerate cow's milk–based formulas. Each feeding resulted in diarrhea and vomiting. The pediatrician recommended that her mother switch to a partially hydrolyzed casein infant formula, which Sally tolerated well. Within 2 months she developed eczema that was treated with steroid creams. Cow's milk was introduced when Sally was 12 months of age. Skin symptoms increased remarkably. When eggs and later peanut butter were introduced, she experienced immediate wheezing; watery, swelling eyes; hives; increased itchiness; and diarrhea. Sally's parents are unaware of how to look for egg or peanut sources; thus Sally has experienced several trips to the emergency room. The last reaction was much more intense. Her family physician suspects egg and peanut allergies and has sent her to see a board-certified allergist and a registered dietitian.

Nutrition Diagnostic Statements

1. Food and nutrition-related knowledge deficit by parents related to food sources of eggs and peanuts as evidenced by serious reactions in their daughter following ingestion.
2. Intake of unsafe foods related to ingestion of egg- and peanut-containing foods as evidenced by serious reactions to foods.

Nutrition Care Questions

1. How many food allergen suspects are there, and what are they? Why?
2. What measures will her parents need to take if Sally is to lose sensitivity to any of the food allergens?
3. What other circumstances may arise that may warrant special instructions to caregivers?
4. How often should Sally be checked for sensitivity changes?
5. What would you tell Sally's parents to look for on food labels?
6. What nutrient substitutions must be considered?

because PUFAs have effects on immune function and inflammation. Some studies have suggested that maternal consumption of fish oil in pregnancy protects against the development of asthma, eczema, and allergic sensitization. However, a recent systematic review indicated that supplementation with ω-3 and ω-6 oils is unlikely to play an important role for the primary prevention of sensitization or allergic disease (Anandan et al., 2009). Further studies are needed to elucidate the role of fatty acids in allergy prevention and their role in the inflammatory cascade. In the meantime, inclusion of both plant (flaxseeds, hempseeds, chia seeds, purslane, organic soybeans, walnuts) and animal food sources (safe wild fish) of ω-3 PUFAs in the maternal diet can be encouraged.

Vitamin D

It has been proposed that the increase in the development of food allergy in children may be due to an increased prevalence of vitamin D deficiency. Deficiency of this vitamin in a developmentally critical period increases susceptibility to colonization of the gut with abnormal intestinal microbial flora and GI infections, contributing to an abnormally porous gut and inappropriate exposure of the immune system to dietary allergens. Vitamin D helps promote immunoregulation through T-cell differentiation and has been found to be associated with a reduced risk of infant wheezing (Jennings and Prescott, 2010). Preliminary studies suggest that early correction of vitamin D deficiency might promote mucosal immunity, healthy microbial ecology, and allergen tolerance, and may prevent food allergy development (Vassallo and Camargo, 2010).

USEFUL WEBSITES

Food Allergy and Anaphylaxis Network
www.foodallergy.org
The American Latex Allergy Association
http://www.latexallergyresources.org/
American Academy of Allergy, Asthma, and Immunology
www.aaaai.org
The Asthma and Allergy Foundation of America
www.aafa.org
Non-GMO Shopping Guide
www.nongmoshoppingguide.com

REFERENCES

Anandan C, et al: ω 3 and 6 oils for primary prevention of allergic disease: systematic review and meta-analysis, *Allergy* 64:840, 2009.

Barrett JS, Gibson PR: Development and validation of a comprehensive semi-quantitative food frequency questionnaire that includes FODMAP intake and glycemic index, *J Am Diet Assoc* 110:1469, 2010.

Bischoff S, Crowe SE: Gastrointestinal food allergy: new insights into pathophysiology and clinical perspectives, *Gastroenterology* 128:1089, 2005.

Blanco C: Latex-fruit syndrome, *Curr Allergy Asthma Rep* 3:47, 2003.

Boyce JA, et al: Guidelines for the diagnosis and management of food allergy in the United States: Summary of the NIAID-Sponsored Expert Panel Report, *J Am Diet Assoc* 111:17, 2011.

Brandtzaeg P: Food allergy: separating the science from the mythology, *Nat Rev Gastroenterol Hepatol* 7:380, 2010.

Brandtzaeg P: "ABC" of mucosal immunology, *Nestle Nutr Workshop Ser Pediatr Prog* 64:23, 2009.

Burks AW, et al: Oral tolerance, food allergy, and immunotherapy: implications for future treatment, *J Allergy Clin Immunol* 121:1344, 2008.

Chafen JJS, et al: Diagnosing and managing common food allergies: a systematic review, *JAMA* 303:1848, 2010.

Clark AT, et al: Successful oral tolerance induction in severe peanut allergy, *Allergy* 64:1218. 2009.

Condemi J: Allergic reactions to natural rubber latex at home, to rubber products, and to cross-reacting foods, *J Allergy Clin Immunol* 110:S107, 2002.

Dona A, Arvanitoyannis IS: Health risks of genetically modified foods, *Crit Rev Food Sci Nutr* 49:164, 2009.

Drisko J, et al: Treating irritable bowel syndrome with a food elimination diet followed by food challenge and probiotics, *J Am Coll Nutr* 25:514, 2006.

Durrant DM, Metzger DW: Emerging roles of T helper subsets in the pathogenesis of asthma, *Immunol Invest* 39:526, 2010.

DuToit G: Food-dependent exercise-induced anaphylaxis in childhood, *Pediatr Allergy Immunol* 18:455, 2007.

Eroglu Y, et al: Pediatric eosinophilic esophagitis: single-center experience in northwestern USA, *Pediatr Int* 51:531, 2009.

Fernandez-Rivas M, et al: Apple allergy across Europe: how allergen sensitization profiles determine the clinical expression of allergies to plant foods, *J Allergy Clin Immunol* 118:481, 2006.

Finamore A, et al: Intestinal and peripheral immune response to MON810 maize ingestion in weaning and old mice, *J Agriculture Food Chem* 56:11533, 2008.

Franchini S et al. Emergency treatment of asthma, *N Engl J Med.* 363:2567, 2010.

Geha R, et al: Multicenter, double-blind, placebo-controlled, multiple-challenge evaluation of reported reactions to monosodium glutamate, *J Allergy Clin Immunol* 106:973, 2000.

Genuis SJ: Sensitivity related illness: the escalating pandemic of allergy, intolerance and chemical sensitivity, *Sci Total Environ* 408:6047, 2010.

Gibson PR, Shepherd SJ: Evidence-based dietary management of functional gastrointestinal symptoms: the FODMAP approach, *J Gastroenterol Hepatol* 25:252, 2010.

Geroldinger-Simic M, et al: Birch pollen-related food allergy: clinical aspects and the role of allergen-specific IgE and IgG(4) antibodies, *J Allergy Clin Immunol* 127:616, 2011.

Greer FR, et al: Effects of early nutritional interventions on the development of atopic disease in infants and children: the role of maternal dietary restriction, breastfeeding, timing of introduction of complementary foods, and hydrolyzed formulas, *Pediatrics* 121:183, 2008.

Groschwitz KR, Hogan SP: Intestinal barrier function: molecular regulation and disease pathogenesis, *J Allergy Clin Immunol* 124:3, 2009.

Hepworth K: Eating disorders today—not just a girl thing, *J Christ Nurs* 27:236, 2010.

Hofmann A, Burks AW: Pollen food syndrome: update on the allergens, *Curr Allergy Asthma Rep* 8:413, 2008.

Host A, et al: Dietary prevention of allergic diseases in infants and small children. Amendment to previous published articles in Pediatric Allergy and Immunology 2004, by an expert group set up by the Section on Pediatrics, *Europ Acad Allergology Clin Immunology, Pediatr Allergy Immunol* 19:1, 2008.

Husemoen LL, et al: The association between atopy and factors influencing folate metabolism: is low folate status causally related to the development of atopy? *Int J Epidemiol* 35:954, 2006.

Järvinen KM, Chatchatee P. Mammalian milk allergy: clinical suspicion, cross-reactivities and diagnosis. *Curr Opin Allergy Clin Immunol* 9:251, 2009.

Jarvela I, et al: Molecular genetics of human lactase deficiencies, *Ann Med* 41:568, 2009.

Jennings S, Prescott SL: Early dietary exposures and feeding practices: role in pathogenesis and prevention of allergic disease? *Postgrad Med J* 86:94, 2010.

Joneja JMV: *Dealing with food allergies in babies and children*, Boulder, CO, 2007, Bull Publishing Company.

Joneja JMV: *Dealing with food allergies: a practical guide to detecting culprit foods and eating a healthy, enjoyable diet*, Boulder, CO, 2003, Bull Publishing Company.

Kagalwalla AF, et al: Effect of six-food elimination diet on clinical and histologic outcomes in eosinophilic esophagitis, *Clin Gastroenterol Hepatol* 4:1097, 2006.

Kelsay K: Psychological aspects of food allergy, *Curr Allergy Asthma Rep* 3:41, 2003.

Kondo Y, Urisu A: Oral allergy syndrome, *Allergol Int* 58:485, 2009.

Kurup VP, et al: Immune response modulation by curcumin in a latex allergy model, *Clin Mol Allergy* 5:1, 2007.

Lack G: Epidemiological risks for food allergy, *J Allergy Clin Immunol* 121:1331, 2008.

Maintz L, Novak N: Getting more and more complex: the pathophysiology of atopic eczema, *Eur J Dermatol* 17:267, 2007.

Matsui EC, Matsui W: Higher serum folate levels are associated with a lower risk of atopy and wheeze, *J Allergy Clin Immunol* 123:1253, 2009.

Mehr S, et al: Food protein-induced enterocolitis syndrome: 16-year experience, *Pediatrics* 123:e459, 2009.

Miller RL: Prenatal maternal diet affects asthma risk in offspring, *J Clin Invest* 118:3265, 2008.

Miyake Y, et al: Consumption of vegetables, fruit, and antioxidants during pregnancy and wheeze and eczema in infants, *Allergy* 65:758, 2010.

Morita E, et al: Food-dependent exercise-induced anaphylaxis-importance of omega-5 gliadin and HMW-glutenin as causative antigens for wheat-dependent exercise-induced anaphylaxis, *Allergol Int* 58:493, 2009.

Mullin GE, et al: Testing for food reactions: the good, the bad and the ugly, *Nutr Clin Prac* 25:192, 2010.

NIAID-Sponsored Expert Panel: Guidelines for the diagnosis and management of food allergy in the United States: Report of the NIAID-sponsored Expert Panel, *J Allerg Clin Immunol* 126(6 Suppl):S1, 2010. www.niaid.nih.gov/topics/foodallergy/clinical/pages/default.aspx. Accessed April, 2011.

Noimark L, Cox HE: Nutritional problems related to food allergy in childhood, *Pediatr Allergy Immunol* 19:188, 2008.

Nowak-Wegrzyn A, Sampson H: Adverse reactions to foods, *Med Clin North Am* 90:1, 2006.

Osborn DA, Sinn JK: Probiotics in infants for prevention of allergic disease and food hypersensitivity, *Cochrane Database Syst Rev* 17(4):CD006475, 2007.

Pessler F, Nejat M: Anaphylactic reaction to goat's milk in a cow's milk-allergic infant, *Pediatr Allergy Immunol* 15:183, 2004.

Poole JA, et al: Timing of initial exposure to cereal grains and the risk of wheat allergy, *Pediatrics* 117:2175, 2006.

Pusztai A, Bardocz S: GMO in animal nutrition: potential benefits and risks. In Mosenthin R, Zentek J, Zebrowska T, editors: *Biology of nutrition in growing animals*, St Louis, 2005, Elsevier.

Pyrhönen K, et al: Heredity of food allergies in an unselected child population: an epidemiological survey from Finland, *Pediatr Allergy Immunol* 22(1pt2):e124, 2011.

Rautava S, et al: New therapeutic strategy for combating the increasing burden of allergic disease: probiotics—a Nutrition, Allergy, Mucosal Immunology and Intestinal Microbiota (NAMI) Research Group report, *J Allergy Clin Immunol* 116:1, 2005.

Reese I, et al: Diagnostic approach for suspected pseudoallergic reaction to food ingredients, *J Dtsch Dermatol Ges* 7:70, 2009.

Robson-Ansley P, Toit GD: Pathophysiology, diagnosis and management of exercise-induced anaphylaxis, *Curr Opin Allergy Clin Immunol* 10:312, 2010.

Rothenberg ME: Eosinophilic gastrointestinal disorders (EGID), *J Allergy Clin Immunol* 113:11, 2004.

Roy-Ghanta S, et al: Atopic characteristics of adult patients with eosinophilic esophagitis, *Clin Gastroenterol Hepatol* 6:531, 2008.

Sampson H: Update on food allergy, *J Allergy Clin Immunol* 113:5, 2004.

Santos A, Van Ree R. Profilins: mimickers of allergy or relevant allergens? *Int Arch Allergy Immunol.* 155:191, 2011.

Savage JH, et al: The natural history of egg allergy, *J Allergy Clin Immunol* 120:1413, 2007.

Sicherer SH, Sampson HA: Food allergy, *J Allergy Clin Immunol* 125:S116, 2010.

Skripak JM, et al: The natural history of Ig-E mediated cow's milk allergy, *J Allergy Clin Immunol* 120:1172, 2007.

Spergel JM, et al: Treatment of eosinophilic esophagitis with specific food elimination diet directed by a combination of skin prick and patch tests, *Ann Allergy Asthma Immunol* 95:336, 2005.

Stahl MC, Rans TS: Potential therapies for peanut allergy, *Ann Allergy Asthma Immunol* 106:179, 2011.

Stapel SO, et al: Testing for IgG4 against foods is not recommended as a diagnostic tool: EAACI Task Force Report, *Allergy* 63:793, 2008.

Teuber SS, Porch-Curren C: Unproved diagnostic and therapeutic approaches to food allergy and intolerance. *Curr Opin Allergy Clin Immunol* 3:217, 2003.

Vally H, et al: Clinical effects of sulphite additives, *Clin Exp Allergy* 39:1643, 2009.

Vassallo MF, Camargo CA: Potential mechanisms for the hypothesized link between sunshine, vitamin D and food allergy in children, *J Allergy Clin Immunol* 126:217, 2010.

Vickery BP, et al: Pathophysiology of food allergy, *Pediatr Clin N Am*, 58:363, 2011.

West CE, et al: Role of diet in the development of immune tolerance in the context of allergic disease, *Curr Opinion Pediatr* 22:635, 2010.

Williams AN, Woessner KM: Monosodium glutamate 'allergy': menace or myth? *Clin Exp Allergy* 39:640, 2009.

Zapatero L, et al: Oral desensitization in children with cow's milk allergy, *J Invest Allergol Clin Immunol* 18:389, 2008.

Zolla L, et al: Proteomics as a complementary tool for identifying unintended side effects occurring in transgenic maize seeds as a result of genetic modifications, *J Proteome Res* 7:1850, 2008.

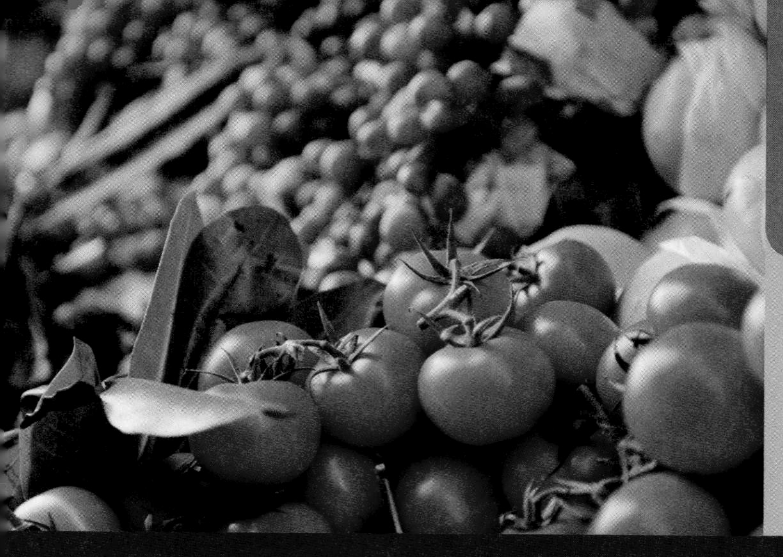

CHAPTER 28

Joseph S. Krenitsky, MS, RD
Nora Decher, MS, RD, CNSC

Medical Nutrition Therapy for Upper Gastrointestinal Tract Disorders

KEY TERMS

achalasia
achlorhydria
achylia gastrica
atrophic gastritis
Barrett's esophagus (BE)
bezoar
Billroth I
Billroth II
dumping syndrome
duodenal ulcer
dyspepsia
endoscopy
esophagogastroduodenoscopy (EGD)
epigastric
esophagitis
functional dyspepsia
fundoplication
gastrectomy
gastric ulcer
gastritis
gastroesophageal reflux disease (GERD)
gastroparesis
heartburn
Helicobacter pylori
hiatal hernia
lower esophageal sphincter (LES)
melena
odynophagia
parietal cells
parietal cell vagotomy
peptic ulcer
pyloroplasty
reactive hypoglycemia
Roux-en-Y
stress ulcer
truncal vagotomy
vagus nerve

Digestive disorders are among the most common problems in health care. More than 50 million visits are made annually to ambulatory care facilities for symptoms related to the digestive system. More than 10 million endoscopies and surgical procedures involving the gastrointestinal tract (GIT) are performed each year (Cherry et al., 2008). Dietary habits and specific food types can play an important role in the onset, treatment, and prevention of many GI disorders. Nutrition therapy is vital in prevention and treatment of malnutrition, deficiencies, and conditions that can develop from GIT disease, such as secondary osteoporosis or anemia. Additionally, diet and lifestyle modifications can improve nutritional well being and quality of life by decreasing symptoms, health care visits, and associated costs. Table 28-1 describes disorders of the upper GIT, their typical symptoms, and nutritional consequences.

ASSESSMENT PARAMETERS

Nutritional screening and careful evaluation of patients with upper GI disorders guide the patient's overall plan of care. Unintentional weight loss over time is the single most useful

TABLE 28-1

Upper Gastrointestinal Disorders and Nutritional Consequences

Gastrointestinal Condition	Common Symptoms	Possible Nutritional Consequences
Achalasia	Aperistalsis; delayed or incomplete relaxation of the lower esophageal sphincter in response to swallowing; dysphagia	Decreased nutritional intake leading to malnutrition, weight loss, nutrient deficiencies; considered a premalignant disorder
Cancer of the oral cavity, esophagus, or stomach	Asymptomatic, or difficulty chewing, swallowing, epigastric discomfort, delayed gastric emptying	Anorexia, decreased variety of foods, weight loss, change in food textures; may require surgery, radiation, chemotherapy, enteral feeding
Dumping syndrome after gastrectomy, pyloroplasty, fundoplication, Roux-en-Y gastric bypass surgery	Early satiety, bloating, nausea; weak, lightheaded, sweaty; later symptoms such as reactive hypoglycemia and possible cramping, diarrhea	Decreased intake, malabsorption of nutrients, weight loss, nutrient deficiencies
Duodenal ulcer	Pain several hours after meals; may be relieved by eating	Perceived food intolerances, increased or decreased food intake
Dyspepsia	Upper abdominal discomfort, bloating, especially after meals	Possible decreased intake of food variety or energy intake, gastric acid suppression may lead to nutrient malabsorption and deficiencies.
Esophageal stricture or tumor	Asymptomatic, or difficulty swallowing foods; solids may especially cause discomfort	Reduced energy and nutrient intake, weight loss.
Gastric ulcer	Vague epigastric discomfort associated with eating	Decreased intake in general, or of selected foods
GERD	Acid taste, increased belching, hoarseness, dry cough, burning sensation in upper middle of chest, sometimes spasm, difficulty swallowing, bloating	Reduced quality and quantity of dietary intake, gastric acid suppression may lead to nutrient malabsorption and deficiencies
Gastroparesis	Abdominal bloating, decreased appetite/ anorexia, nausea and vomiting, fullness, early satiety, halitosis, and postprandial hypoglycemia	Reduced energy and nutrient intake, decreased nutrient use resulting from hyperglycemia, dehydration Severe cases may benefit from feeding-tube placement.

GERD, Gastroesophageal reflux disease.

parameter, with severe malnutrition indicated by a loss of 2% or more of usual body weight in 1 week, 5% or more during 1 month, or 10% or more during 6 months. Other assessments of nutritional risk include percent of ideal body weight and body mass index. Patients who have severe weight loss benefit from beginning nutritional support early, sometimes prior to or during other medical treatments.

During the initial assessment, the clinician should also obtain an assessment of the patient's weight history, changes in appetite, nausea, vomiting, diarrhea, problems with chewing or swallowing, typical daily dietary intake, use of supplemental nutrition (oral, enteral, or parenteral), food allergies or intolerances, use of supplements (vitamins, minerals, herbs, probiotics, or protein powders), use of stool-bulking agents or laxatives, and medications. Intolerance to various foods, inadequate intake, and malabsorption can lead to nutrient deficiencies and increased morbidity. Common laboratory values, such as B_{12}, folate, ferritin, and 25-hydroxy vitamin D, may be useful in the initial assessment and monitoring. Other laboratory values may be useful, particularly when malabsorption or insufficient intake of certain nutrients is suspected. Patients with gastric surgeries or gastric acid suppression are at higher risk for nutrient deficiencies, such as iron or B_{12}. In patients with gastric surgeries, deficiencies may manifest early or develop over time.

THE ESOPHAGUS

The esophagus is a tubular organ, approximately 25 cm long, that is lined with both tubular and striated muscles. Swallowing triggers peristalsis—waves of coordinated muscles contractions. As a bolus of food is moved voluntarily from the mouth to the pharynx, the upper sphincter

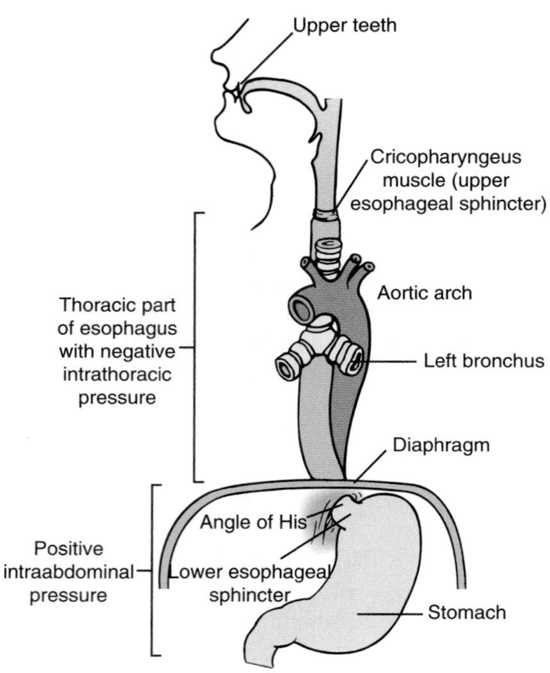

FIGURE 28-1 Normal esophagus. *(Modified from Price SA, Wilson LM: Pathophysiology: clinical concepts of disease processes, ed 6, St Louis, 2003, Mosby.)*

relaxes, the food moves into the esophagus, and peristaltic waves move the bolus down the esophagus; the **lower esophageal sphincter (LES)** relaxes to allow the food bolus to pass into the stomach (Figure 28-1). From start to finish, this process generally takes 5 seconds when in an upright position, and up to 30 seconds when in a supine position (Cordova-Fraga, 2008).

The normal esophagus has a multitiered defense system that prevents tissue damage from exposure to gastric contents, including LES contraction, normal gastric motility, esophageal mucus, tight cellular junctions, and cellular pH regulators. Dysphagia (difficulty in swallowing) may be by obstruction, inflammation, or abnormal upper esophageal sphincter function that causes derangement of the swallowing mechanism. Skeletomuscular disorders and motility disorders may result in dysphagia. For example, **achalasia** is characterized by a failure of esophageal neurons, resulting in loss of ability to relax the LES and normal peristalsis. **Odynophagia** (painful swallowing) may interfere with nutritional intake in some patients with oral or esophageal cancers.

Gastroesophageal Reflux and Esophagitis

Regurgitation occurs in approximately half of infants in the first few months of life; most cases resolve after the first year. Reflux of gastric contents into the esophagus is a normal physiologic event that occurs daily in healthy individuals (Orlando, 2008). In **gastroesophageal reflux disease (GERD)** episodes of reflux overwhelm esophageal protective mechanisms and result in symptoms such as **heartburn**, a burning sensation in the esophagus, or inflammation with erosion of the lining of the esophagus. Approximately 7% to 8% of the U.S. population experiences heartburn daily, and 20% to 40% of adults report symptoms of GERD at least once weekly. The prevalence of GERD in children may range from approximately 2% to 20% (Gold, 2006).

The types of GERD can be distinguished by **esophagogastroduodenoscopy (EGD)**, which uses a fiberoptic endoscope to directly visualize the esophagus, stomach, and duodenum. EGD can be useful in determining the success of treatment in erosive GERD (Yuan and Hunt, 2009). Erosive GERD is generally associated with more severe and prolonged symptoms, compared with the nonerosive esophageal reflux disease (Orlando, 2008). Some people experience GERD symptoms primarily in the evening (nocturnal GERD), which may occur as a result of decreased salivary secretions and swallowing, decreased GI motility, prolonged exposure to acid, and being in the supine position (Gerson and Fass, 2009).

Pathophysiology

The pathophysiology of GERD is complex. The most common underlying mechanisms are thought to be reduced LES pressure, inadequate esophageal tissue defense, direct mucosal irritants, decreased gastric motility, and increased intraabdominal pressure. LES pressure decreases during pregnancy (heartburn affects up to 80% of women in their third trimester), in women taking progesterone-containing oral contraceptives, and even in the late stage of a normal menstrual cycle (Dowswell and Neilson, 2008).

The pressure of the LES may be influenced by other conditions, including hiatal hernia, scleroderma (a disease that involves hardening and tightening of skin and connective tissues), and hypersecretory diseases such as Zollinger-Ellison syndrome. Transient LES relaxations, which are induced by distension of the proximal stomach (the same stimulus for belching) are common in GERD. Patients with chronic respiratory disorders, such as chronic obstructive pulmonary disease, are at risk for GERD because of frequent increases in intraabdominal pressure. Muscle relaxants and nonsteroidal antiinflammatory drugs (NSAIDs) are the primary offending medications implicated in GERD.

The presentation of GERD symptoms varies, but may include reflux of gastric secretions, heartburn, substernal pain, belching, and esophageal spasm. In children, vomiting, dysphagia, refusal to eat, or complaints of abdominal pain may be present (Hassall, 2005). Manifestations such as pharyngeal irritation, frequent throat clearing, hoarseness, and worsening of asthmatic symptoms may also occur. The frequency and severity of symptoms do not always predict the severity or complications of the disease, and may not correlate with endoscopic findings. Some patients have few overt symptoms and relatively significant disease; others may have considerable discomfort without erosive, longstanding consequences.

Prolonged acid exposure can result in **esophagitis** (inflammation of the esophagus), esophageal erosions, ulceration, scarring, stricture, and in some cases dysphagia (see

Pathophysiology and Care Management Algorithm: Esophagitis). Acute esophagitis may be caused by reflux, ingestion of a corrosive agent, viral or bacterial infection, intubation, radiation, or eosinophilic infiltration. Eosinophilic esophagitis is characterized by an isolated, severe eosinophilic infiltration of the esophagus manifested by GERD-like symptoms that may be caused by an immune response. See Chapter 27. Irritants such as smoking and large doses or chronic use of aspirin or NSAIDs can increase the risk of esophagitis (Pera et al., 2005).

The severity of the esophagitis resulting from gastroesophageal reflux is influenced by the composition, frequency, and volume of the gastric reflux; length of exposure of the esophagus to the gastric reflux; the health of the mucosal barrier; and the rate of gastric emptying. Symptoms of esophagitis and GERD may impair the ability to consume an adequate diet, and interfere with sleep, work, social events, and the overall quality of life.

A common contributor to gastroesophageal reflux and esophagitis is **hiatal hernia**. The presence of hiatal hernia is not synonymous with reflux, but it increases the likelihood of symptoms and complications. The esophagus passes through the diaphragm by way of the esophageal hiatus or ring. The attachment of the esophagus to the hiatal ring may become compromised, allowing a portion of the upper stomach to move above the diaphragm. The most common type of hiatal hernia is the sliding hernia, and the less common form is the paraesophageal hernia (Figure 28-2).

When acid reflux occurs with a hiatal hernia, the gastric contents remain above the hiatus longer than normal. The prolonged acid exposure increases the risk of developing more serious esophagitis (Orlando, 2008). Because increases in intragastric pressure force acidic stomach contents up into the esophagus, persons with hiatal hernia may experience difficulty when lying down or bending over. **Epigastric** pain occurs in the upper middle region of the abdomen after large, energy-dense meals. Weight reduction and decreasing meal size decreases the negative consequences of hiatal hernia.

Barrett's esophagus (BE) is a precancerous condition in which the normal squamous epithelium of the distal esophagus is replaced by an abnormal columnar epithelium known as *specialized intestinal metaplasia.* Certain risk factors may prompt physicians to consider testing for BE, including prolonged history of GERD symptoms (>5 years), white race, male sex, older age (>50 years), and family history of BE or adenocarcinoma of the esophagus. It is estimated that 5% to 15% of persons with GERD have BE (Lichtenstein et al., 2007; Pera et al., 2005). Both GERD and BE increase a patient's risk for adenocarcinoma of the esophagus. The incidence of adenocarcinoma of the esophagus is rising at a rate exceeding all other cancers in the US–4% to 10% annually (Okoro and Wang, 2010).

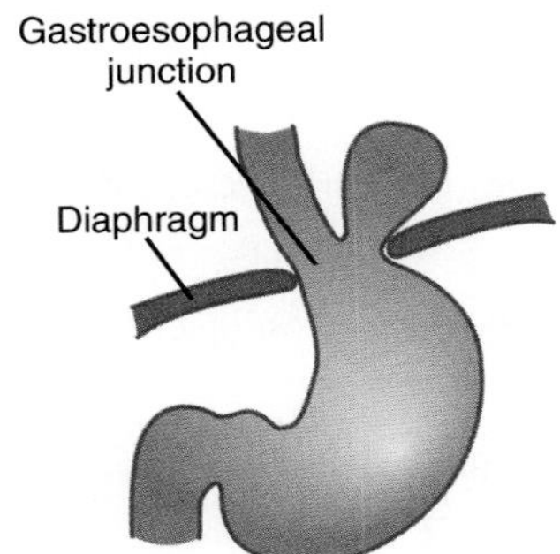

FIGURE 28-2 Hiatal hernia. *(Modified from Price SA, Wilson LM: Pathophysiology: clinical concepts of disease processes, ed 6, St Louis, 2003, Mosby.)*

Medical and Surgical Management

The primary medical treatment of esophageal reflux is suppression of acid secretion. Proton pump inhibitors (PPIs), which decrease acid production by the gastric parietal cell, are most effective (Rohof et al., 2009), but milder forms of reflux are sometimes managed by H_2 receptor (a type of histamine receptor on the parietal cell) antagonists and antacids. The aim in acid-suppression therapy is to raise the gastric pH above 4 during periods when reflux is most likely to occur. (See "Gastritis and Peptic Ulcers" later in this chapter for side effects.) Prokinetic agents, which increase propulsive contractions of the stomach, may be used in persons who have delayed gastric emptying. Refer to Table 28-2 for medications commonly used in upper GI disorders.

Raising the head of the bed by 6 to 8 inches can reduce likelihood of nocturnal reflux. Frequent bending over should be avoided. Obesity is a contributing factor to GERD and hiatal hernia because it increases intragastric pressure, and weight loss may reduce acid contact time in the esophagus, leading to decreased reflux symptoms. Box 28-1 lists modifications that are aimed at enhancing esophageal acid

BOX 28-1

Nutrition Care Guidelines for Reducing Gastroesophageal Reflux and Esophagitis

1. Avoid large, high-fat meals.
2. Avoid eating at least 3 to 4 hours before lying down.
3. Avoid smoking.
4. Avoid alcoholic beverages.
5. Avoid caffeine-containing foods and beverages.
6. Stay upright and avoid vigorous activity soon after eating.
7. Avoid tight-fitting clothing, especially after a meal.
8. Consume a healthy, nutritionally complete diet with adequate fiber.
9. Avoid acidic and highly spiced foods when inflammation exists.
10. Lose weight if overweight.

Data from National Digestive Diseases Information Clearinghouse. Accessed 17 February 2010 from http://digestive.niddk.nih.gov/.

PATHOPHYSIOLOGY AND CARE MANAGEMENT ALGORITHM

Esophagitis

ETIOLOGY

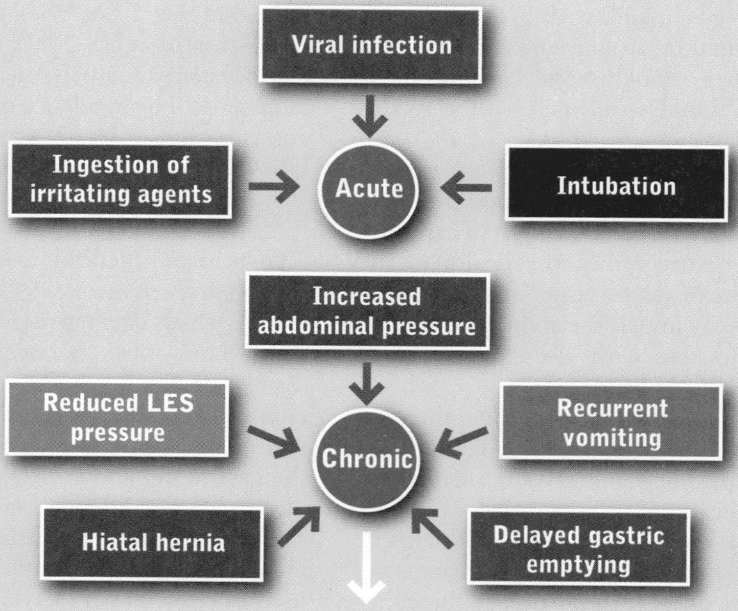

PATHOPHYSIOLOGY

Reflux of gastric acid and/or intestinal contents through the lower esophageal sphincter (LES) and into the esophagus

MANAGEMENT

Behavioral Modification

Avoid:

- Eating within 3-4 hours of retiring
- Lying down after meals
- Tight-fitting garments
- Cigarette smoking

Medical/Surgical Management

- Proton pump inhibitors
- Histamine-2 receptor antagonists
- Antacids
- Prokinetic agents
- Fundoplication

Nutrition Management

Goal:
Decrease exposure of esophagus to gastric contents
Avoid:

- Large meals
- Dietary fat
- Alcohol

Goal:
Decrease acidity of gastric secretions
Avoid:

- Coffee
- Fermented alcoholic beverages

Goal:
Prevent pain and irritation
Avoid:

- Any food that the patient feels exacerbates his/her symptoms clearance, minimizing the occurrence of reflux, or both. Lifestyle interventions alone are unlikely to suffice, except in mild cases of GERD.

Of patients with severe GERD, 5% to 10% do not respond to medical therapy. They may be treated surgically with **fundoplication**, a procedure in which the fundus of the stomach is wrapped around the lower esophagus to limit reflux. Use of tobacco products is contraindicated with reflux. Smoking tobacco products decreases LES pressure and prolongs acid clearance by decreasing salivation. Smoking also compromises GIT integrity and increases the risk of esophageal and other cancers (see *Clinical Insight:* Smoking and Gastrointestinal Function).

Medical Nutrition Therapy

Certain diet and lifestyle changes may relieve symptoms in some patients with GERD. The main factors are caffeine, alcohol, tobacco, and stress. Other dietary factors include

CLINICAL INSIGHT

Smoking and Gastrointestinal Function

The gastrointestinal effects of smoking include the reduction of lower esophageal and pyloric sphincter pressure, increased reflux, alteration of the nature of the gastric contents, inhibition of pancreatic bicarbonate secretion, accelerated gastric emptying of liquids, and lower duodenal pH. The acid secretory response to gastrin or acetylcholine is increased considerably. Smoking also impairs the ability of cimetidine and other drugs to lower the overnight acid secretion that is thought to play a key role in ulcerogenesis. Nicotine is responsible for many of the effects of tobacco use; but increased exposure to hydrocarbons, oxygen radicals, and a number of other substances is thought to also contribute to the overall effects. Finally, smoking impairs spontaneous healing and increases the risk and rapidity of ulcer recurrence, as well as the likelihood that the ulcer will perforate and require surgery.

Tobacco exposure may play a role in the development of inflammatory bowel disease (IBD). Smoking impairs the formation of granulomas in Crohn's disease (Leong et al., 2006). Passive and active smoking exposure in childhood (by age 10 to 15) seems to be associated with the development of IBD (Mahid et al., 2006).

TABLE 28-2

Some Common Medications Used in the Treatment of Upper Gastrointestinal Tract Disorders

Type of Medication	Common Names	Medication Function
Proton pump inhibitor	Omeprazole Lansoprazole Esomeprazole Pantoprazole Dexlansoprazole Rabeprazole	Inhibits acid secretion
H_2 blocker	Cimetidine Ranitidine Famotidine Nizatidine	Blocks the action of histamine on parietal cells, decreasing the production of acid
Prokinetic	Erythromycin Metoclopramide Domperidone	Increases contractility of the stomach and shortens gastric emptying time
Antisecretory	Octreotide (somatostatin analogue) Somatostatin	Inhibits release of insulin and other gut hormones. Slows rate of gastric emptying and small intestine transit time; increases intestinal water and sodium absorption
Antidumping	Acarbose	Delays carbohydrate digestion by inhibiting alpha-glycoside hydrolase, which interferes with conversion of starch to monosaccharides
Antigas agent	Simethicone	Lowers surface tension of gas bubbles
Antacids	Magnesium, calcium, or aluminum bound to carbonate or phosphate	Buffers gastric acid

dietary fat, chocolate, coffee, onions, peppermint, spices, citrus foods, wine, and carbonated beverages.

The role of spices in the pathologic conditions related to upper GI disorders is not clear. In patients with GI lesions, foods highly seasoned with chili powder and pepper may cause discomfort. The type of chili and amount of capsaicin consumed make the difference (Milke et al., 2006). Foods such as carminatives (peppermint and spearmint) may lower LES pressure. While fermented alcoholic beverages (such as beer and wine) stimulate the secretion of gastric acid and should be limited, coffee may be used in small amounts.

Limiting or avoiding aggravating foods may improve symptoms in some individuals. There is no need to eliminate foods if they do not affect symptoms (El-Serag et al., 2005). Chewing gum has been shown to increase salivary secretions, which help to raise esophageal pH, but no studies prove efficacy when compared with other lifestyle changes.

For patients with severe esophagitis, a low-fat, liquid diet initially minimizes esophageal distention, passes more easily through any strictured areas, and empties readily from the stomach. Foods with an acidic pH including citrus juices, tomatoes, and soft drinks cause pain when the esophagus is already inflamed and should be avoided.

Identification and treatment of the main mechanism underlying the GERD is the first line of therapy. Large, high-fat meals delay gastric emptying and prolong acid secretion; avoiding those conditions prior to going to bed is often useful. Lifestyle modifications, including change in dietary practices, weight loss, smoking cessation, and elevation of the head of the bed, can reduce symptoms (see Box 28-1).

Oral Cancer and Surgeries

Pathophysiology

The patient diagnosed with cancer of the oral cavity, pharynx, or esophagus may present with existing nutritional problems and dysphagia or odynophagia secondary to the tumor mass, obstruction, oral infection, or ulceration. Nutritional deficits may be compounded by the treatment, which commonly involves surgical resection, radiation, or chemotherapy. Chemotherapy may produce nausea, vomiting, and anorexia (see Chapter 37). Chewing, swallowing, salivation, and taste acuity are often altered. Extensive dental decay, osteoradionecrosis, and infections may also occur.

Surgery of the Mouth or Esophagus

Surgery of the mouth or esophagus may be necessary to remove tumors. Thus it may be necessary to provide nutrition using liquid supplements. Patients who are unable to take adequate nutrition orally for an extended time, such as those with extensive disease or those requiring major surgery, are likely to benefit from a gastrostomy tube placement. The enteral route of nutrition is preferred; however, if the GIT is not functional, parenteral nutrition can be provided (see Chapter 14).

Tonsillectomy. Tonsils are lymphatic tissue. Mild inflammation of the tonsils is considered a natural part of the efforts of the immune system to fight infection. Rarely, the physician may remove the tonsils if they are too large and obstruct the ability to breathe, or for the purpose of reducing the number and frequency of ear infections, tonsillitis, and sinusitis. Cold, mild-flavored, soft, moist foods bring the most comfort to the patient and offer the most protection against unexpected bleeding from the surgical area. The patient can typically consume a normal diet within 3 to 5 days.

Medical Nutrition Therapy

When the patient is unable to meet energy and protein needs orally for prolonged periods, tube feeding should be considered. Gastrostomy feedings can be total or supplemental; many nutritionally complete formulas are available (see Appendix 32). Enteral tube feedings are most commonly provided as ready-to-feed formulas, which are convenient and nutritionally complete. To add variety to the diet, ordinary foods such as fruits can be puréed and mixed with water until liquefied. Table foods may be prepared in a blender, but maintaining nutritional adequacy, sanitation, and a viscosity that will not clog feeding tubes is too labor-intensive to be practical for most patients or their families.

Fluid intake, artificial saliva solutions, and saline rinses may be used to prevent dry mouth. Topical anesthetics can be used to relieve pain. Because narcotic pain medications delay gastric emptying and constipation, extra fluids and a bowel regimen (stool softeners, laxatives) may be necessary.

THE STOMACH

The mucosa of the stomach and duodenum is protected from the proteolytic actions of gastric acid and pepsin by a coating of mucus secreted by glands in the epithelial walls from the lower esophagus to the upper duodenum. The mucosa is also protected from bacterial invasion by the digestive actions of pepsin and hydrochloric acid (HCl) and the mucus secretions. HCl is secreted by the parietal cells in response to stimuli by gastrin, acetylcholine, and histamine. The mucus contains acid-neutralizing bicarbonate, and additional bicarbonate is provided by the pancreatic juice secreted into the intestinal lumen. Production of mucus is stimulated by the action of prostaglandins.

Dyspepsia

Pathophysiology

Dyspepsia (indigestion) refers to nonspecific, persistent upper-abdominal discomfort or pain. The discomfort may be related to organic causes such as esophageal reflux, gastritis, peptic ulcer, gallbladder disease, or other identifiable pathologic conditions. Because of the variety of presentations and symptoms, dyspepsia may overlap with other problems such as GERD or irritable bowel syndrome, anxiety, and depression. Diet, stress, and other lifestyle factors may contribute to the symptoms.

Functional dyspepsia (nonulcer dyspepsia) describes persistent or recurrent upper GI discomfort, without underlying pathologic conditions. Symptoms of functional dyspepsia are reported in approximately 15% to 20% of adults per year and may include vague abdominal discomfort, bloating, early satiety, nausea, and belching. Underlying mechanisms are not entirely clear; visceral hypersensitivity to acid or distention, impaired gastric accommodation, altered brain-gut axis, and abnormal gastric motility and emptying have all been considered (Fajardo et al., 2005).

Medical Nutrition Therapy

Dietary and lifestyle management is the same as for GERD. Excessive volumes of food or high intake of fat, sugar, caffeine, spices, or alcohol are commonly implicated but have not been confirmed in all cases. Delayed emptying and increased sensation of fullness are common features. Reduction of dietary fat intake, use of smaller meals, diets of low caloric density, and achieving a healthy weight may be helpful (Pilichiewicz et al., 2009). Because alcoholic beverages may alter GI functions in a number of ways, limiting intake is recommended. Mild exercise enhances movement of foodstuffs through the GIT and increases one's sense of well being. Because periods of persistent stress may contribute to functional GI disorders, behavioral management and emotional support may also help. If symptoms persist, further evaluation should be pursued to identify the underlying cause.

Gastritis and Peptic Ulcers

Pathophysiology

Gastritis and peptic ulcers result when infectious, chemical, or neural abnormalities disrupt mucosal integrity of the stomach. The most common cause is ***Helicobacter pylori*** infection, a gram-negative bacteria that is somewhat resistant to the acidic medium of the stomach. *H. pylori* infection induces inflammation from both innate and systemic immune response. Olfactomedin 4 is a glycoprotein that has been found to be up-regulated in *H. pylori*–infected patients, leading to expression of proinflammatory cytokines or chemokines through Nod1- and Nod2-mediated nuclear factor (NF)-κB activation; this inhibits host immune response and contributes to persistence of *H. pylori* colonization (Liu et al., 2010).

The prevalence of *H. pylori* infection generally correlates with geography and the socioeconomic status of the population. It ranges from approximately 10% in developed countries to 80% to 90% in developing countries. Although gastritis is a characteristic observation, only 10% to 15% of those infected by the organism develop symptomatic ulceration, and approximately 1% develop gastric cancer (Ernst et al., 2006; Fennerty, 2005).

H. pylori infection is responsible for most cases of chronic inflammation of the gastric mucosa and peptic ulcer, gastric cancer, and **atrophic gastritis** (chronic inflammation with deterioration of the mucous membrane and glands) resulting in achlorhydria and loss of intrinsic factor (Israel and Peek, 2006; Selgrad et al., 2008). The infection does not resolve spontaneously, and risks of complications increase with duration of the infection. Other factors affect the risk of pathologic consequences, including the patient's age at onset of the initial infection, the specific strain and concentration of the organism, genetic factors related to the host, and the lifestyle and overall health of the patient. The infection is typically confined to the mucosa of the stomach. Treatment of *H. pylori* typically involves the use of two or three antibiotics and acid-suppressing medications. Doing so ameliorates the gastritis, reduces the conditions that favor carcinogenesis, and may improve digestive function (Bytzer and O'Morain, 2005; Guzzo et al., 2005) (see *Focus On:* The Changing Face of *Helicobacter pylori* and Gastric Cancer).

FOCUS ON

The Changing Face of *Helicobacter pylori* and Gastric Cancer

Traditionally, gastric cancer was considered a single disease. However, scientists now classify gastric cancer by its location in either the top inch of the stomach near the esophagus (gastric cardia) or the rest of the stomach (noncardia). This new classification of gastric cancers was adopted in part because of the role of *Helicobacter pylori*.

H. pylori appears to be a strong risk factor for noncardia gastric cancer; however, the role of *H. pylori* in the development of gastric cardia cancer remains controversial. A study of patients in Finland investigated *H. pylori* infection in patients from blood obtained at the time of enrollment, before the patients actually developed cancer (Kamangar et al., 2006). When patients who developed cancer were compared with age-matched controls who did not develop cancer, *H. pylori* infection resulted in an eightfold increase in the incidence of noncardia gastric cancer but a 60% decrease in the incidence of cardia gastric cancer.

The decrease in gastric cardia cancer with *H. pylori* infection was an unexpected finding because previous studies had not shown this. One reason that older studies may have had misleading results was that researchers did not check for the presence of *H. pylori* until after the diagnosis of gastric cancer, and *H. pylori* does not flourish on precancerous or malignant cells.

Population studies support the protective effect of *H. pylori* on gastric cardia cancer (Whiteman et al., 2010). Developed countries have seen a decrease in this infection in recent years because of increased information, testing, and effective treatment. Concomitantly, there has been a decreased incidence of noncardia gastric cancer, but an increase in the incidence of gastric cardia and esophageal cancers in these countries. The revelation that treating *H. pylori* infection decreases the risk for some cancers but may increase the risk of other cancers is prompting more research.

Other Forms of Gastritis

Chronic use of aspirin or other NSAIDs, steroids, alcohol, erosive substances, tobacco, or any combination of these factors may compromise mucosal integrity and increase the chance for acquiring acute or chronic gastritis. Eosinophilic gastritis may also contribute to some cases of gastritis (Whittingham and Mackay, 2005). See Chapter 27. Poor nutrition and general poor health may contribute to the onset and severity of the symptoms and can delay the healing process.

Acute gastritis refers to rapid onset of inflammation and symptoms. Chronic gastritis may occur over a period of months to decades, with waxing and waning of symptoms. Gastritis may manifest by a number of symptoms, including nausea, vomiting, malaise, anorexia, hemorrhage, and epigastric pain. Prolonged gastritis may result in atrophy and loss of stomach parietal cells, with a loss of secretion of HCl (**achlorhydria**) and intrinsic factor, resulting in pernicious anemia.

Recent studies emphasize the importance of considering side effects of chronic acid suppression either from disease or chronic use of acid-suppressing medication such as PPIs (Katz, 2010). These include reduction of gastric secretion of HCl, which has been shown to reduce absorption of nutrients such as B_{12}, calcium, and nonheme iron, which rely on intragastric proteolysis to make them bioavailable (McColl, 2009). Acid suppression may increase incidence of some bone fractures (Gray et al., 2010), as well as increase risk for intestinal infection, as gastric acidity is a front-line barrier to microbial invasion (Ali et al., 2009; Linsky et al., 2010).

Medical Treatment

Endoscopy is a common diagnostic tool (see *Focus On:* Endoscopy and Capsules). Treatment of gastritis includes the eradication of pathogenic organisms (e.g., *H. pylori*) and withdrawal of any provoking agents. Antibiotics and PPIs are the primary medical treatments.

Peptic Ulcers

Pathophysiology

Normal gastric and duodenal mucosa is protected from the digestive actions of acid and pepsin by the secretion of mucus, the production of bicarbonate, the removal of excess acid by normal blood flow, and the rapid renewal and repair of epithelial cell injury. **Peptic ulcer** refers to an ulcer that occurs as a result of the breakdown of these normal defense and repair mechanisms. Typically more than one of the mechanisms must be malfunctioning for symptomatic peptic ulcers to develop. Peptic ulcers typically show evidence of chronic inflammation and repair processes surrounding the lesion.

The primary causes of peptic ulcers are *H. pylori* infection, gastritis, the use of aspirin, other NSAIDs and corticosteroids, and severe illness (see "Stress Ulcers" later in this chapter) (see *Pathophysiology and Care Management*

FOCUS ON

Endoscopy and Capsules

The mucosa of the upper gastrointestinal (GI) tract can be viewed, photographed, and biopsied by means of endoscopy, a procedure that involves passing a flexible tube into the esophagus that has a light and camera on the distal end. It can be passed through the esophagus and into the stomach or upper small bowel. This procedure is called esophagogastroduodenoscopy (EGD). Inflammation, erosions, ulcerations, changes in the blood vessels, and destruction of surface cells can be identified. These changes can then be correlated with chemical, histologic, and clinical findings to formulate a diagnosis. This may be useful when physicians suspect certain conditions, such as complicated GERD (strictures, BE, esophageal varices, or gastroduodenal ulcers.) EGD can also be used for a number of therapeutic purposes such as cauterization at ulcer sites, dilation or deployment of stents in areas of stricture, and placement of percutaneous feeding tubes.

Endoscopy may be used in long-term monitoring of patients with chronic esophagitis and gastritis because of the possibility that they will develop premalignant lesions or carcinoma (Wong et al, 2010). Recently, capsules containing a miniaturized video camera, light, and radio transmitter that can be swallowed and the signal transmitted to a receiver worn on the waist of the patient, allow wireless capsule endoscopy. Capsule endoscopy can be used to view segments of the GIT that are not accessible by standard EGD, to screen for abnormalities or bleeding, check pH, and measure the time it takes to pass through different segments of the GIT.

The procedure is less invasive than normal endoscopy and provides the advantage of being able to observe, record, and measure GI function as the patient is ambulatory. However, the images from capsule endoscopy can be blurred by rapid intestinal transit or limited in number after battery failure in cases of slow transit. Additionally, reviewing the thousands of images obtained after each capsule endoscopy can be very time consuming.

Prototypes of the newest generation of capsule endoscopy allow the physician to magnetically guide the capsule to a specific location by having the patient lie on a special table. Future generations of capsule endoscopy are on the drawing boards to hopefully allow therapeutic measures to be accomplished in the small bowel via capsule endoscopy.

Algorithm: Peptic Ulcer) (Israel and Peek, 2006). Life stress may lead to behaviors that increase peptic ulcer risk. Excessive use of concentrated forms of ethanol can damage gastric mucosa, worsen symptoms of peptic ulcers, and interfere with ulcer healing. However, modest doses of alcoholic beverages in otherwise healthy persons do not appear to cause peptic ulcers. Consumption of beer and wine increases gastric secretions, whereas low concentrations of alcohol may not. Use of tobacco products decreases bicarbonate secretion, decreases mucosal blood flow, exacerbates inflammation, and is associated with additional complications of *H. pylori* infection. Other risk factors include gastrinoma and Zollinger-Ellison syndrome (see Chapter 30).

As a result of earlier screening for *H. pylori* and early recognition of the symptoms and risk factors associated with peptic ulcers, their incidence and prevalence and the number

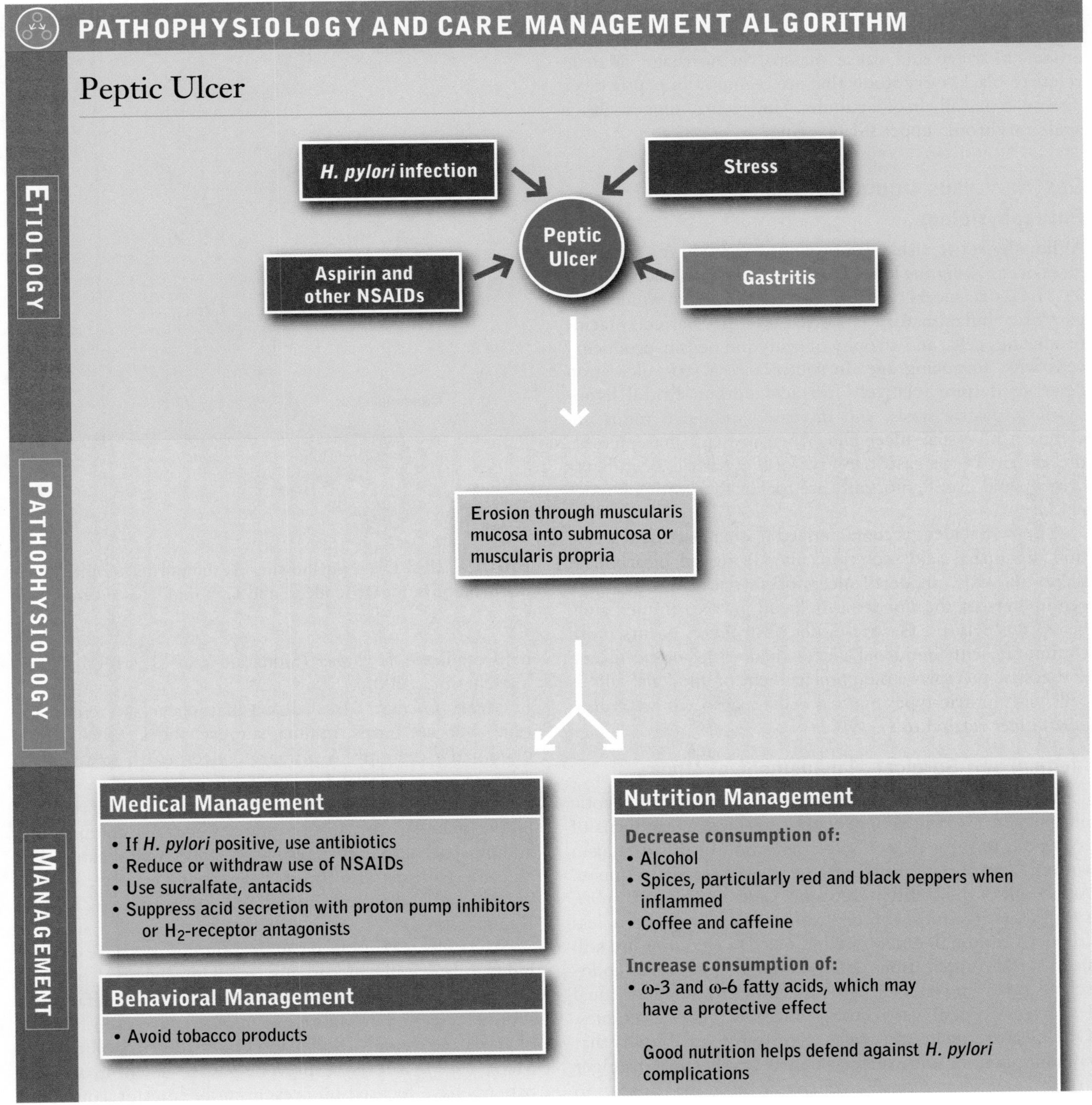

of surgical procedures related to them have decreased markedly in the last three decades.

Peptic ulcers normally involve two major regions: gastric and duodenal. Uncomplicated peptic ulcers in either region may present with signs similar to those associated with dyspepsia and gastritis. Abdominal pain or discomfort is characteristic of both gastric and duodenal ulcers, although anorexia, weight loss, nausea and vomiting, and heartburn may occur slightly more often in persons with gastric ulcers. In some patients peptic ulcers are asymptomatic.

Complications of hemorrhage and perforation contribute significantly to the morbidity and mortality of peptic ulcers. Ulcers can perforate into the peritoneal cavity or penetrate into an adjacent organ (usually the pancreas), or they may erode an artery and cause massive hemorrhage. **Melena** refers to black, tarry stools that are common in peptic ulcer disease, especially in older adults. Melena may suggest either acute or chronic upper GI bleeding.

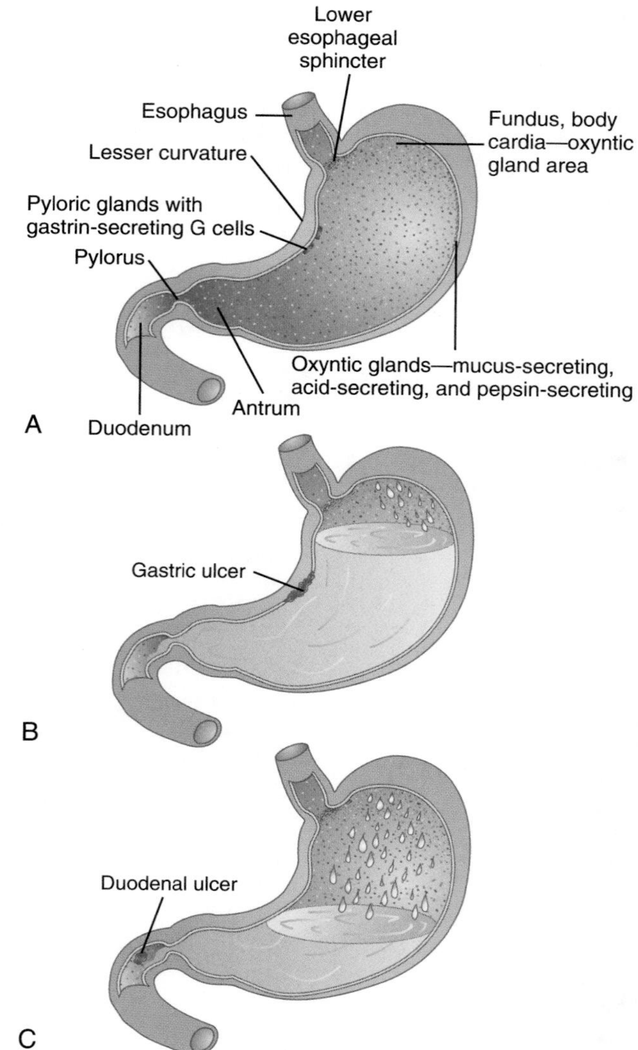

FIGURE 28-3 Diagram showing **A,** the normal stomach and duodenum; **B,** a gastric ulcer; and **C,** a duodenal ulcer.

Gastric versus Duodenal Ulcers

Pathophysiology

Although **gastric ulcers** can occur anywhere in the stomach, most occur along the lesser curvature of the stomach (Figure 28-3). Gastric ulcers typically are associated with widespread gastritis, inflammatory involvement of parietal (acid-producing) cells, and atrophy of acid- and pepsin-producing cells with advancing age. In some cases gastric ulceration develops despite relatively low acid output. Antral hypomotility, gastric stasis, and increased duodenal reflux are common in gastric ulcer and, when present, may increase the severity of the gastric injury. With a gastric ulcer, hemorrhage and overall mortality are higher than with a duodenal ulcer.

A **duodenal ulcer** is characterized by increased acid secretion, nocturnal acid secretion, and decreased bicarbonate secretion. Most duodenal ulcers occur within the first few centimeters of the duodenal bulb, in an area immediately below the pylorus. Gastric outlet obstruction occurs more commonly with duodenal ulcers than with gastric ulcers, and gastric metaplasia (i.e., replacement of duodenal villous cells with gastric-type mucosal cells) may occur with duodenal ulcer related to *H. pylori*.

Medical and Surgical Management of Ulcers

Peptic Ulcers. The primary cause of gastritis and peptic ulcers is *H. pylori* infection; therefore the primary focus of treatment in most cases is the eradication of this organism with the appropriate antibiotic and acid suppressive regimen. As a result of the ability to recognize and eradicate *H. pylori*, surgical intervention for peptic ulcer management is less frequent, although emergent and elective surgeries are still needed for complications. Interventions may include endoscopic, open, and laparoscopic procedures to treat individual lesions, to partial gastrectomy and selective vagotomies. One measure includes regular use of protective foods that contain phenolic antioxidants such as cranberries or ginger extracts (*Zingiber officinale*), which may have the capacity to help eradicate *H. pylori* (Siddaraju and Dharmesh, 2007; Vattem et al., 2005).

Stress Ulcers. **Stress ulcers** may occur as a complication of severe burns, trauma, surgery, shock, renal failure, or radiation therapy. A primary concern with stress ulceration is the potential for significant hemorrhage. Gastric ischemia with GI hypoperfusion, oxidative injury, reflux of bile salts and pancreatic enzymes, microbial colonization, and mucosal barrier changes have also been implicated. The true mechanisms are not completely understood, but the use of antioxidant compounds shows promise (Zhu and Kaunitz, 2008).

Stress ulcers that bleed can be a significant cause of morbidity in critically ill patients, but knowledge of effective prevention and treatment is still incomplete. Sucralfate, acid suppressives, and antibiotics as necessary are used for prophylaxis and therapy (Kallet and Quinn, 2005; Stollman and Metz, 2005). Efforts to prevent gastric ulcers in stressed patients have focused on preventing or limiting conditions leading to hypotension and ischemia and coagulopathies. Avoiding NSAIDs and large doses of corticosteroids is also beneficial. Providing oral or enteral feeding (when possible) increases GI vascular perfusion and stimulates secretion and motility.

Medical Nutrition Therapy

In persons with atrophic gastritis, vitamin B_{12} status should be evaluated because a lack of intrinsic factor and acid results in malabsorption of this vitamin (see Chapters 3 and 33). Low acid states result in reduced absorption of iron, calcium, and other nutrients because of the role of gastric acid in increasing their bioavailability. In the case of iron-deficiency anemia, other causes may be the presence of *H. pylori* and gastritis. Eradication of *H. pylori* has resulted in improved absorption of iron and increased ferritin levels (Hershko and Ronson, 2009).

For several decades dietary factors have gained or lost favor as a significant component in the cause and treatment of dyspepsia, gastritis, and peptic ulcer disease. There is little evidence that specific dietary factors cause or exacerbate gastritis or peptic ulcer disease. Protein foods temporarily buffer gastric secretions, but they also stimulate secretion of gastrin, acid, and pepsin. Milk or cream, which in the early days of peptic ulcer management was considered important in coating the stomach, is no longer considered medicinal.

The pH of a food has little therapeutic importance, except for patients with existing lesions of the mouth or the esophagus. Most foods are considerably less acidic than the normal gastric pH of 1 to 3. The pH of orange juice and grapefruit is 3.2 to 3.6, and the pH of commonly used soft drinks ranges from approximately 2.8 to 3.5. On the basis of their intrinsic acidity and amount consumed, fruit juices and soft drinks are not likely to cause peptic ulcers or appreciably interfere with healing. Some patients express discomfort with ingestion of acidic foods, but the response is not consistent among patients, and in some, symptoms may be related to heartburn.

Consumption of large amounts of alcohol may cause at least superficial mucosal damage and may worsen existing disease or interfere with treatment of the peptic ulcer. Modest consumption of alcohol does not appear to be pathogenic for peptic ulcers unless coexisting risk factors are also present. On the other hand, beers and wines significantly increase gastric secretions and should be avoided in symptomatic disease.

Both coffee and caffeine stimulate acid secretion and may also decrease LES pressure; however, neither has been strongly implicated as a cause of peptic ulcers outside of the increased acid secretion and discomfort associated with their consumption.

When very large doses of certain spices are fed orally or placed intragastrically without other foods, they increase acid secretion and cause small, transient superficial erosions, inflammation of the mucosal lining, and altered GI permeability or motility. Most often incriminated are chili, cayenne, and black peppers (Milke et al., 2006). Small amounts of chili pepper or its pungent ingredient, capsicum, may serve to increase mucosal protection by increasing production of mucus; but large amounts may cause superficial mucosal damage, especially when consumed with alcohol. Interestingly, another spice, curcumin, through its antiinflammatory activity that inhibits NF-κB pathway activation may be a chemopreventive candidate against *H. pylori*–related cancer (Zaidi et al., 2009).

The synergy of food combinations may inhibit the growth of *H. pylori.* Food provides an interesting alternative to therapies that include antibiotics, PPIs, and bismuth salts (Kennan et al., 2010). Studies suggest that green tea, broccoli sprouts, black currant oil, and kimchi (fermented cabbage) help with *H. pylori* eradication. Probiotics containing *lactobacillus* and *bifidobacterium* have also been studied for prevention, management, and eradication of *H. pylori* (Lionetti et al., 2010; Sachdeva and Nagpal, 2009). More controlled studies with different foods and combinations of probiotics would be beneficial.

Omega-3 and omega-6 fatty acids are involved in inflammatory, immune, and cytoprotective physiologic conditions of the GI mucosa, but they have not yet been found to be effective for treatment. Long-term clinical trials have not been performed. Overall, a high-quality diet without nutrient deficiencies may offer some protection and may promote healing. Persons being treated for gastritis and peptic ulcer disease should be advised to avoid foods that exacerbate their symptoms, and to consume a nutritionally complete diet with adequate dietary fiber from fruits and vegetables.

Carcinoma of the Stomach

Pathophysiology

Because symptoms are slow to manifest themselves and the growth of the tumor is rapid, carcinoma of the stomach is frequently overlooked until it is too late for a cure. Loss of appetite, strength, and weight frequently precede other symptoms. In some cases **achylia gastrica** (absence of HCl and pepsin) or achlorhydria (absence of HCl in gastric secretions) may exist for years before the onset of gastric carcinoma.

Consumption of fruits, vegetables, and selenium appears to have a modest role in the prevention of GI cancers, whereas alcohol consumption and overweight increase the risk (van den Brandt and Goldbohm, 2006). Other factors that may increase the risk of gastric cancer include chronic infection with *H. pylori*, smoking, intake of highly salted or pickled foods, or inadequate amounts of micronutrients (Lynch et al., 2005).

Malignant neoplasms of the stomach can lead to malnutrition as a result of excessive blood and protein losses or, more commonly, because of obstruction and mechanical interference with food intake. Most cancers of the stomach are treated by surgical resection; thus part of the nutritional considerations includes partial or total resection of the stomach, a **gastrectomy**.

Medical Nutrition Therapy

The dietary regimen for carcinoma of the stomach is determined by the location of the cancer, the nature of the functional disturbance, and the stage of the disease. Gastrectomy is one of the possible therapies, and some patients may experience difficulties with nutrition after surgery. The patient with advanced, inoperable cancer should receive a diet that is adjusted to his or her tolerances, preferences, and comfort. Anorexia is almost always present from the early stages. In the later stages of the disease, the patient may tolerate only a liquid diet. If a patient is unable to tolerate oral feeding, consideration should be given to using an alternate route, such as a gastric or intestinal feeding tube, or in the case of the inability to feed enterally, parenteral nutrition. The nutritional support for the patient should be in line with the patient's goals of care.

Gastric Surgeries

Gastric surgeries are performed less frequently today, because of increased recognition and improved treatment of *H. pylori* and acid secretion. However, partial or total gastrectomy may still be necessary for patients with ulcer disease that does not respond to therapy, or with malignancy (Figure 28-4). Gastric surgeries performed for weight loss, or bariatric surgeries, are becoming increasingly common. These surgeries, such as **Roux-en-Y**, gastric bypass, gastric banding, vertical banding gastroplasty, and jejunoileal bypass, are designed to induce malnutrition through volume restriction, malabsorption, or both (see Chapter 22).

Types of Surgeries

A partial gastrectomy involves removal of the gastrin-secreting antrum, as much as 75% of the distal stomach.

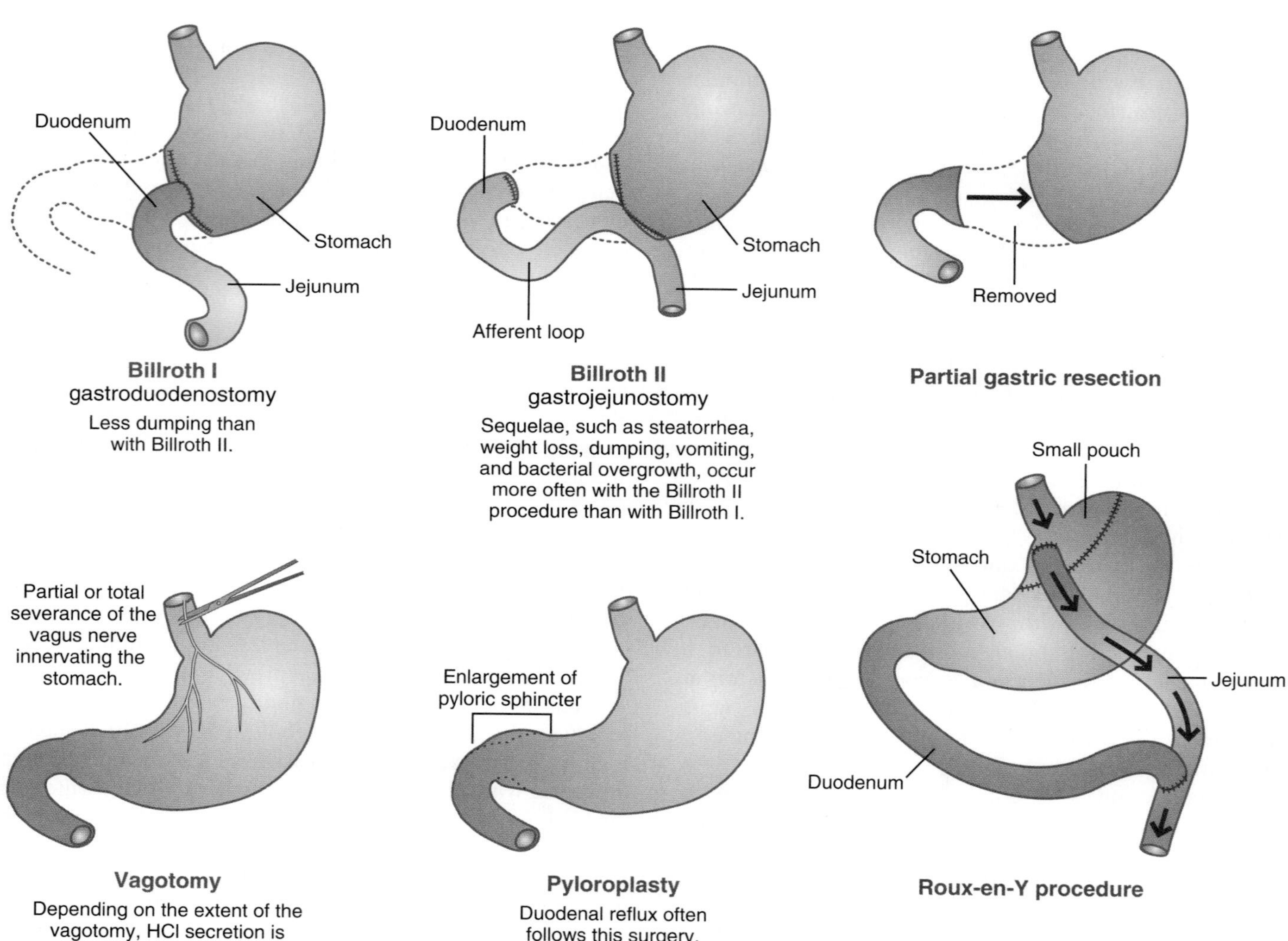

FIGURE 28-4 Gastric surgical procedures.

During surgery, the remnant stomach may be reattached to the duodenum, a **Billroth I**, or to the side of the jejunum, a **Billroth II**. In a Billroth II, the duodenal stump is preserved, allowing for the continued flow of bile and pancreatic enzymes into the intestines.

Vagotomy, with or without gastric resection, was developed after it was demonstrated that the **vagus nerve** was not only responsible for motility of the stomach but also stimulated the parietal cells in the proximal stomach to secrete acid. **Truncal vagotomy**, complete severing of the vagus nerve on the distal esophagus, decreases acid secretion by **parietal cells** in the stomach and decreases their response to gastrin, but it also creates poor gastric emptying. When truncal vagotomy is performed, a drainage procedure such as **pyloroplasty** is performed to allow better gastric emptying of solids. A **parietal cell vagotomy** (partial or selective) divides and severs only the vagus nerve branches that affect the proximal stomach where gastric acid secretion occurs, whereas the antrum and pylorus remain innervated, and gastric emptying can proceed more normally.

Total gastrectomy is performed for malignancies that affect the middle or upper stomach. The entire stomach is removed and usually reconstructed with the Roux-en-Y method. The total gastrectomy, by definition, involves a functional vagotomy, eliminating acid production.

Postoperative Medical Nutrition Therapy

After most types of gastric surgery, oral intake of foods and fluids is initiated as soon as it is determined that the patient's GIT is functioning. Small, frequent feedings of ice or water are initiated, followed by liquids and easily digested solid foods, after which the patient can progress to a regular diet. If the surgery requires an extended period for healing, or the patient is unable to tolerate an oral diet, the patient may be fed through a feeding tube, such as a jejunostomy (see Chapter 14).

Understanding the surgery performed and patient's resulting anatomy is paramount to providing proper nutritional care. Nutritional complications after gastric surgeries are varied. Complications such as obstruction, dumping, abdominal discomfort, diarrhea, and weight loss may occur, depending on the nature and extent of the disease and surgical interventions (see Figure 28-4). Patients may have difficulty regaining normal preoperative weight because of inadequate food intake related to (1) early satiety, (2) symptoms of dumping syndrome (see later in this chapter), or (3) malabsorption of nutrients.

Patients with certain gastric surgeries, such as Roux-en-Y, are set up for impaired digestion and absorption caused by a mismatch in timing of entry of food into the small intestine and the release of bile and pancreatic enzymes. Patients who were lactose tolerant before gastric surgery may experience relative lactase deficiency, either because food enters the small intestine further downstream or because the rate of transit through the proximal small intestine is increased. Because of the complications of reflux or dumping syndrome associated with traditional gastrectomies, other procedures are used, including truncal, selective, or parietal cell vagotomy, pyloromyotomy, antrectomy, Roux-en-Y esophagojejunostomy, loop esophagojejunostomy, and pouches or reservoirs made from jejunal or ileocecal segments (Tomita, 2005.)

Over the long term, anemia, osteoporosis, and select vitamin and mineral deficiencies may occur as a result of malabsorption or limited dietary intake. Iron deficiency may be attributable to loss of acid secretion. Gastric acid normally facilitates the reduction of iron compounds, allowing their absorption. Rapid transit and diminished contact of dietary iron with sites of iron absorption can also lead to iron-deficiency anemia.

Vitamin B_{12} deficiency may cause a megaloblastic anemia. If the amount of gastric mucosa is reduced, intrinsic factor may not be produced in quantities adequate to allow for complete vitamin B_{12} absorption, and pernicious anemia may result. Bacterial overgrowth in the proximal small bowel or in the afferent loop contributes to vitamin B_{12} depletion because bacteria compete with the host for use of the vitamin. Therefore after gastrectomy patients should receive prophylactic vitamin B_{12} supplementation (injections) or take synthetic oral supplementation.

Dumping Syndrome

Pathophysiology

The **dumping syndrome** is a complex GI and vasomotor response to the presence of larger-than-normal quantities of hypertonic foods and liquids in the proximal small intestine. Dumping syndrome usually occurs as a result of surgical procedures that allow excessive amounts of liquid or solid foods to enter the small intestine in a concentrated form. Milder forms of dumping may occur to varying degrees in persons without surgical procedures, and most of the symptoms can be reproduced in normal individuals by infusing a loading dose of glucose into the jejunum (Ukleja, 2005). Dumping may occur as a result of total or partial gastrectomy, manipulation of the pylorus, after fundoplication, vagotomy, and after some gastric bypass procedures for obesity (Ukleja, 2005). As a result of better medical management of peptic ulcers, use of selective vagotomies, and newer surgical procedures to avoid complications, classic dumping is less frequently encountered in clinical practice.

Symptoms can be divided into early, mid, and late stages of dumping of foods and beverages into the small intestine. Early dumping is characterized by both GI and vasomotor symptoms, whereas late dumping is predominantly characterized by vascular symptoms. Characteristics and severity of symptoms vary between patients. In early dumping, patients may experience abdominal fullness and nausea within 10-30 minutes of eating a meal. These symptoms are attributed to accelerated gastric emptying of hyperosmolar solution into the small bowel, and resultant fluid shifts from the circulation into the bowel. It is thought that patients with these early dumping symptoms are experiencing a decrease in peripheral vascular resistance and perhaps visceral pooling of blood.

In the intermediate stage, from 20 minutes to more than 1 hour after eating, patients may experience abdominal bloating, increased flatulence, crampy abdominal pain, and explosive diarrhea. These symptoms are likely related to the malabsorption of carbohydrates and other foodstuffs and the subsequent fermentation of the substrates entering the colon (see Chapter 29).

Late dumping, occurring from 1 to 3 hours after a meal, is characterized by vascular symptoms, related to **reactive hypoglycemia**. Rapid delivery, as well as hydrolysis and absorption of carbohydrates, produces an exaggerated rise in insulin level with a subsequent decline in blood glucose level (see Chapter 31). Patients may experience flushing, rapid heartbeat, faintness, and sweating, and feel the need to sit or lie down. They may feel anxious, weak, shaky, or hungry, and have difficulty concentrating. The rapid changes in blood glucose and the secretion of gut peptides, glucose insulinotropic polypeptide, and glucagon-like polypeptide-1 appear to be at least partly responsible for the late symptoms (Ukleja, 2005).

Medical Management

Medical intervention typically involves dietary changes as the initial treatment, and they are usually effective. In 3% to 5% of patients, severe dumping persists despite dietary change. In these patients, medications may be used to slow gastric emptying and delay transit of food through the GIT. Some, such as acarbose, inhibit alpha glycoside hydrolase and interfere with carbohydrate absorption, and octreotide, a somatostatin analogue, inhibits insulin release. See Table 28-2 for common medications. Rarely, surgical intervention is used to treat dumping syndrome.

Medical Nutrition Therapy

Patients with dumping syndrome may experience weight loss and malnutrition caused by inadequate intake, malabsoption or a combination of both. The prime objective of nutrition therapy is to restore nutrition status and quality of life. Proteins and fats are better tolerated than carbohydrates because they are hydrolyzed more slowly into osmotically active substances. Simple carbohydrates such as lactose, sucrose, and dextrose are hydrolyzed rapidly; thus quantities should be limited, but complex carbohydrates (starches) can be included in the diet. Liquids enter the jejunum rapidly; thus some patients may have problems tolerating liquids with meals. Patients with severe dumping may benefit from limiting the amount of liquids taken with meals, and taking liquids between meals, without solid food. Lying down immediately after meals may also decrease the severity of symptoms.

The use of fiber supplements, particularly pectin or gums (e.g., guar) can be beneficial in managing dumping syndrome because of their ability to form gels with carbohydrates and delay GI transit. Patients may need to be taught true portion sizes of foods, especially carbohydrate foods such as juices, soft drinks, desserts, and milk. The exchange lists given in Appendix 34 can be used to calculate carbohydrate intake and teach the patient about carbohydrate control.

BOX 28-2

Basic Guidelines for Dumping Syndrome

Small, more frequent meals
Less solid, more crushed foods
Limited fluids during meals
Fewer simple sugars
More complex carbohydrates
More soluble fiber
Increased amounts of fat in the diet
Lactose-free foods if needed

Postgastrectomy patients often do not tolerate lactose, but small amounts (e.g., 6 g or less per meal) may be tolerated at one time. Patients typically do better with cheeses or unsweetened yogurt than with fluid milk. Nondairy milks are also useful. Vitamin D and calcium supplements may be needed when intake is inadequate. Commercial lactase products are available for those with significant lactose malabsorption (see Chapter 29).

When steatorrhea (greater than 7% of dietary fat excreted in stool) exists, reduced fat formulas or pancreatic enzymes may be beneficial. Box 28-2 provides general nutrition guidelines for patients with dumping syndrome after gastric surgery; however, each diet must be adjusted based on a careful dietary and social history from the patient.

Gastroparesis

Pathophysiology

Gastroparesis, or delayed gastric emptying, is a complex and potentially debilitating condition. The nature of gastroparesis is complex in part because gastric motility is orchestrated by a variety of chemical and neurologic factors. Viral infection, diabetes, and surgeries are the most common causes for gastroparesis; however, more than 30% of cases are idiopathic. Numerous classes of clinical conditions are associated with gastroparesis, including mechanical obstructions, metabolic or endocrine disorders, acid-peptic diseases, gastritis, postgastric surgery, disorders of gastric smooth muscle, psychogenic disorders, and neuropathic disorders. Clinical symptoms may include abdominal bloating, decreased appetite and anorexia, nausea and vomiting, fullness, early satiety, halitosis, and postprandial hypoglycemia.

Diagnosis and Medical Management

The gold-standard measure of gastric emptying rate is scintigraphy, a nuclear test of gastric emptying. This consists of the patient ingesting a radionucleotide-labeled meal (such as an egg labeled with ^{99m}technetium), and scintigraphic images are taken over time (generally 4 hours) to assess the rate of gastric emptying.

Numerous symptoms of gastroparesis can affect oral intake, and the management of these symptoms generally improves nutritional status. Treatment of nausea and vomiting is perhaps the most vital, and prokinetics and antiemetics are the primary medical therapies (see Table 28-2). Metoclopramide and erythromycin are medications that may be used to promote gastric motility. Small bowel bacterial overgrowth, ileal brake (the slowing effect on intestinal transit and appetite of undigested nutrients, often fat, reaching the ileum), or formation of a bezoar (concentration of undigested material in the stomach) are other factors that may affect nutritional status.

Bezoar formation may be related to undigested food such as cellulose, hemicellulose, lignin and fruit tannins (phytobezoars), or medications (pharmacobezoars) such as cholestyramine, sucralfate, enteric coated aspirin, aluminum-containing antacids, and bulk-forming laxatives. Treatment of bezoars includes enzyme therapy (such as papain or cellulose), lavage, and sometimes endoscopic therapy to mechanically break up the bezoar. Most patients respond to some combination of medication and dietary intervention; however, unresponsive and more severe cases many benefit from placement of an enteral tube, such as a percutaneous endoscopic gastrostomy (PEG) with jejunal extension or a PEG and percutaneous endoscopic jejunostomy (Parrish and Yoshida, 2005). These tube combinations allow nutrition to bypass the stomach while providing an alternative route for venting of gastric secretions, which may relieve nausea and vomiting.

Medical Nutrition Therapy

The primary dietary factors that affect gastric emptying (in order of clinical importance) are volume, liquids versus solids, hyperglycemia, fiber, fat, and osmolality (Maljaars et al., 2007). Larger volumes of food that create stomach distension (approximately 600 mL) have been shown to delay gastric emptying and increase satiety (Oesch et al., 2006). Generally, patients benefit from smaller, more frequent meals. Patients with gastroparesis often have preserved emptying of liquids, as they empty, in part, by gravity and do not require antral contraction. Shifting the diet to more pureed and liquefied foods is often useful. A number of medications (such as narcotics and anticholinergics) slow gastric emptying. Moderate to severe hyperglycemia (serum blood glucose >200 mg/dL) may acutely slow gastric motility, with long-term detrimental effects on gastric nerves and motility. Laboratory data considered in initial assessment include glycosylated hemoglobin A1c (if diabetes is present), ferritin, vitamin B_{12}, and 25-OH vitamin D.

Fiber, particularly pectin, can slow gastric emptying and increase risk of bezoar formation in patients who are susceptible. It is prudent to advise patients to avoid high-fiber foods and fiber supplements. The size of the fibrous particles, not the amount of fiber, is more important in bezoar risk (e.g., potato skins versus bran). This and the resistance to chewing are factors in bezoar formation. Examination of the patient's dentition is very important because patients who have missing teeth, a poor bite, or are edentulous are at greater risk. People even with good dentition have swallowed and passed food particles up to 5-6 cm in diameter (potato skins, seeds, tomato skins, peanuts).

Fat is a powerful inhibitor of stomach emptying primarily mediated by cholecystokinin (Goetze et al., 2007); however, many patients tolerate fat well in liquid form. Fat should not be restricted in patients who are struggling to meet their daily caloric needs. Studies have demonstrated a slowing effect of highly osmotic foods on gastric emptying, but, compared with other interventions, dietary manipulation of osmolarity is not clinically effective (Parrish, 2007).

CLINICAL SCENARIO 1

Jim, a 45-year-old man, is an executive who travels extensively in his work. He recently visited his doctor complaining about upper gastrointestinal (GI) distress. He reports frequent bouts of heartburn in the middle of the night, and he has lost 15 lb during the last year without intentionally dieting. Jim also occasionally experiences heartburn soon after consumption of specific meals and foods. Jim's doctor diagnosed esophageal reflux, and x-ray studies revealed a hiatal hernia.

Jim has received a good deal of advice regarding specific foods and diets from a variety of sources, but he is confused about what he should eat. Jim is coming to you to discuss nutrition therapies.

Nutrition Diagnostic Statements

1. Involuntary weight loss related to heartburn and GI pain after some meals and foods as evidenced by 15-lb weight loss in the absence of dieting.
2. Food- and nutrition-related knowledge deficit related to appropriate foods for reflux as evidenced by confusion related to multiple sources of information.

Nutrition Care Questions

1. What is heartburn? Does hiatal hernia have anything to do with it?
2. Why might Jim experience heartburn in the middle of the night?
3. Why might Jim experience burning after consumption of certain foods or meals?
4. Why do you suppose Jim lost weight?
5. Do you recommend that he regain the weight?
6. What recommendations would you give for reducing Jim's symptoms?
7. Write a progress note using ADIME language.

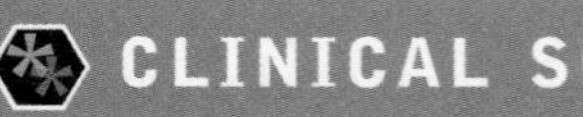

CLINICAL SCENARIO 2

Mr. Smith had his stomach removed 3 months ago as a result of gastric cancer. He is having difficulty with bloating, nausea, and light-headedness soon after meals. Later, after the meal, he often experiences lower abdominal cramping and diarrhea.

Nutrition Diagnostic Statement

Altered gastrointestinal function related to dumping symptoms following meals as evidenced by history of gastric carcinoma requiring resection of stomach.

Nutrition Care Questions

1. What do you think could be responsible for the different symptoms Mr. Smith is experiencing?
2. What additional information should you gather about Mr. Smith in your nutritional assessment?
3. Should you recommend laboratory work to check any vitamin or mineral levels?
4. Are there measures you can recommend to prevent his postprandial symptoms?

USEFUL WEBSITES

American Gastrointestinal Association
http://www.gastro.org/
American College of Gastroenterology
http://www.acg.gi.org/
International Foundation for Functional Gastrointestinal Disorders
http://www.aboutgimotility.org/
National Digestive Diseases Information Clearinghouse
http://digestive.niddk.nih.gov/
The Gastroparesis and Dysmotilities Association
http://www.digestivedistress.com/

REFERENCES

Ali T, et al: Long-term safety concerns with proton pump inhibitors, *Am J Med* 122:896, 2009.

Bytzer P, O'Morain C: Treatment of *Helicobacter pylori*, *Helicobacter* 10:40S, 2005.

Cherry DK, et al: National Ambulatory Medical Care Survey: 2006 summary, *Natl Health Stat Report* 3:1, 2008.

Cordova-Fraga T: Effects of anatomical position on esophageal transit time: a biomagnetic diagnostic technique, *World J Gastro* 14:5707, 2008.

Dowswell T, Neilson JP: Interventions for heartburn in pregnancy, *Cochrane Database Syst Rev* 4:CD007065, 2008.

El-Serag HB, et al: Dietary intake and the risk of gastro-oesophageal reflux disease: a cross sectional study in volunteers, *Gut* 54:11, 2005.

Ernst PB, et al: The translation of *Helicobacter pylori* basic research to patient care, *Gastroenterol* 130:188, 2006.

Fajardo NR, et al: Frontiers in functional dyspepsia, *Curr Gastroenterol Report* 7:289, 2005.

Fennerty MB: *Helicobacter pylori:* why it still matters in 2005, *Cleveland Clinic J Med* 72:S1, 2005.

Gerson LB, Fass R: A systematic review of the definitions, prevalence, and response to treatment of nocturnal gastroesophageal reflux disease, *Clin Gastro Hepatol* 7:372, 2009.

Goetze O, et al: The effect of macronutrients on gastric volume responses and gastric emptying in humans: a magnetic resonance imaging study, *Am J Physiol* 292:G11, 2007.

Gold BD: Is gastroesophageal reflux disease really a life-long disease: do babies who regurgitate grow up to be adults with GERD complications? *Am J Gastroenterol* 101:641, 2006.

Gray SL, et al: Proton pump inhibitor use, hip fracture, and change in bone mineral density in postmenopausal women: results from the Women's Health Initiative, *Arch Int Med* 170: 765, 2010.

Guzzo JL, et al: Severe and refractory peptic ulcer disease: the diagnostic dilemma: case report and comprehensive review, *Dig Dis Sci* 50:1999, 2005.

Hassall E: Decisions in diagnosing and managing chronic gastroesophageal reflux disease in children, *J Pediatr* 146:S3, 2005.

Hershko C, Ronson A: Iron deficiency, *Helicobacter* infection and gastritis, *Acta Haematol* 122:97, 2009.

Israel DA, Peek RM: The role of persistence in *Helicobacter pylori* pathogenesis, *Curr Opin Gastroenterol* 22:3, 2006.

Kallet RH, Quinn TE: The GIT and ventilator-associated pneumonia, *Resp Care* 50:910, 2005.

Kamangar F, et al: Opposing risks of gastric cardia and noncardia gastric adenocarcinomas associated with *Helicobacter pylori* seropositivity, *J Natl Cancer Inst* 98:1445, 2006.

Katz MH: Failing the acid test: benefits of proton pump inhibitors may not justify the risks for many users, *Arch Int Med* 170:747, 2010.

Kennan JI, et al: Individual and combined effects of foods on *Helicobacter pylori* growth, *Phytother Res* 24:1229, 2010.

Leong WL, et al: Association of intestinal granulomas with smoking, phenotype, and serology in Chinese patients with Crohn's's disease, *Am J Gastroenterol* 101:1024, 2006.

Lichtenstein DR, et al: Role of endoscopy in the management of GERD, *Gastro Endo* 66:219, 2007.

Linsky A, et al: Proton pump inhibitors and risk for recurrent Clostridium difficile infection, *Arch Int Med* 170:772, 2010.

Lionetti E, et al: Role of probiotics in pediatric patients with *Helicobacter pylori* infection: a comprehensive review of the literature, *Helicobacter* 15:79, 2010.

Liu W, et al: Olfactomedin 4 down-regulates innate immunity against *Helicobacter pylori* infection, *Proc Natl Acad Sci U S A* 107:11056, 2010.

Lynch HT, et al: Gastric cancer: new genetic developments, *J Surg Oncol* 90:114, 2005.

Mahid Suhal S, et al: Smoking and inflammatory bowel disease: a meta-analysis, *Mayo Clin Proc* 81:1462, 2006.

Maljaars J, et al: The GIT: neuroendocrine regulation of satiety and food intake, *Alimentary Pharmacol Ther* 26:241S, 2007.

McColl KE: Effect of proton pump inhibitors on vitamins and iron, *Am J Gastroenterol* 104:S5, 2009.

Milke P, et al: Gastroesophageal reflux in healthy subjects induced by two different species of chilli (Capsicum annum), *Dig Dis* 24:184, 2006.

Oesch S, et al: Effect of gastric distension prior to eating on food intake and feelings of satiety in humans, *Physiol Behav* 87:903, 2006.

Okoro NI, Wang KK: Changing faces of Barrett's esophagus: implications for adenocarcinoma, *Gastroenterol* 138:1620, 2010.

Orlando RC: Pathophysiology of gastroesophageal reflux disease, *J Clin Gastroenterol* 42:584, 2008.

Parrish CR, Yoshida CM: Nutrition intervention for the patient with gastroparesis: an update, *Pract Gastroenterol* 29:29, 2005.

Parrish CR: Nutrition concerns for the patient with gastroparesis, *Current Gastro Rep* 9:295, 2007.

Pera M, et al: Epidemiology of esophageal adenocarcinoma, *J Surg Oncol* 92:151, 2005.

Pilichiewicz AN, et al: Relationship between symptoms and dietary patterns in patients with functional dyspepsia, *Clin Gastro Hepatol* 7:317, 2009.

Rohof WO, et al: Pathophysiology and management of gastroesophageal reflux disease, *Minerva Gastroenterol Dietologica* 55:289, 2009.

Sachdeva A, Nagpal J: Effect of fermented milk-based probiotic preparations on *Helicobacter pylori* eradication: a systematic review and meta-analysis of randomized-controlled trials, *Eur J Gastroenterol & Hep* 1:45, 2009.

Selgrad M, et al: Dyspepsia and *Helicobacter pylori*, *Dig Dis* 26:210, 2008.

Siddaraju MN, Dharmesh SM: Inhibition of gastric H+, K+-ATPase and *Helicobacter pylori* growth by phenolic antioxidants of Zingiber officinale, *Mol Nutr Food Res* 51:324, 2007.

Stollman N, Metz DC: Pathophysiology and prophylaxis of stress ulcer in intensive care unit patients, *J Crit Care* 20:35, 2005.

Tomita R: A novel surgical procedure of vagal nerve, lower esophageal sphincter, and pyloric sphincter-preserving nearly total gastrectomy reconstructed by single jejunal interposition, and postoperative quality of life, *Hepato-Gastroenterol* 52:1895, 2005.

Ukleja A: Dumping syndrome: pathophysiology and treatment, *Nutr Clin Pract* 20:517, 2005.

Van den Brandt PA, Goldbohm RA: Nutrition in the prevention of gastrointestinal cancer, *Best Pract Res Clin Gastroenterol* 20:589, 2006.

Vattem DA, et al: Enhancing health benefits of berries through phenolic antioxidant enrichment: focus on cranberry, *Asia Pacific J Clin Nutr* 14:120, 2005.

Whiteman DC, et al: Association of *Helicobacter pylori* infection with reduced risk for esophageal cancer is independent of environmental and genetic modifiers, *Gastroenterol* 139:73, 2010.

Whittingham S, Mackay IR: Autoimmune gastritis: historical antecedents, outstanding discoveries, and unresolved problems, *Int Rev Immunol* 24:1, 2005.

Wong T, et al: Barrett's surveillance identifies patients with early esophageal adenocarcinoma. *Am J Med* 123:462, 2010.

Yuan Y, Hunt RH: Evolving issues in the management of reflux disease? *Curr Opin Gastroenterol* 25:342, 2009.

Zaidi SF, et al: Modulation of activation-induced cytidine deaminase by curcurmin in *Helicobacter pylori*-infected gastric epithelial cells, *Helicobacter* 14:588, 2009.

Zhu A, Kaunitz J: Gastroduodenal mucosal defense, *Curr Gastroenterol Rep* 10:548, 2008.

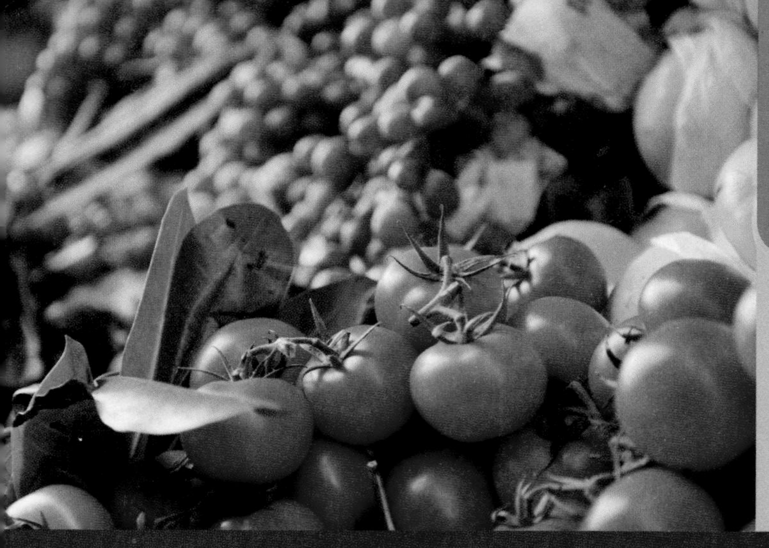

CHAPTER 29

Nora Decher, MS, RD, CNSC
Joseph S. Krenitsky, MS, RD

Medical Nutrition Therapy for Lower Gastrointestinal Tract Disorders

KEY TERMS

aerophagia
antibiotic-associated diarrhea (AAD)
celiac disease (CD)
colostomy
constipation
Crohn's disease
dermatitis herpetiformis
diarrhea
dietary fiber
diverticulitis
diverticulosis
encopresis
enterocutaneous (EC) fistula
fistula
flatulence
flatus
FODMAPs
functional GI disorder
glutamine
gluten
gluten intolerance
gluten-sensitive enteropathy
gluten sensitivity
high-fiber diet
hypolactasia
ileal pouch
ileostomy
inflammatory bowel disease (IBD)
irritable bowel syndrome (IBS)
J-pouch
lactose intolerance
medium-chain triglycerides (MCTs)
microscopic colitis
pouchitis
prebiotics
probiotics
refractory celiac disease
residue
short-bowel syndrome (SBS)
small intestine bacterial overgrowth (SIBO)
soluble fiber
S-pouch
steatorrhea
synbiotic
tropical sprue
ulcerative colitis (UC)
W-pouch

Dietary interventions for many diseases of the intestinal tract are primarily designed to alleviate symptoms and to correct nutrient deficiencies. However, nutrition interventions play a preventative and therapeutic role in several conditions, such as diverticular disease and treatment of some types of constipation. Celiac disease (CD) is the only gastrointestinal (GI) condition for which dietary modification is the primary treatment. Careful assessment of the nature and severity of the primary GI problem is necessary to identify the nutrition diagnosis and appropriate interventions. Assessment may include evaluating the frequency and amount of nutrients consumed, medical and surgical history, medications used, subjective experiences with foods, and depth of understanding of the relationship between diet and the GI problem. The GI assessment should include information on the duration and severity of the disorder; its effect on digestion, secretion, and absorption of nutrients; and its effect on symptoms and complications. Meal consistency, frequency, and size, as well as other characteristics of the diet, may then be altered to fit the patient's needs.

COMMON INTESTINAL PROBLEMS

It is important to understand some of the common GI processes and symptoms that occur in healthy people prior to discussing the nutrition issues relating to lower GI tract (GIT) disorders. The interaction of diet with intestinal gas, flatulence, constipation, and diarrhea provides insight when considering the more serious disorders.

Intestinal Gas and Flatulence

Pathophysiology

Air is commonly swallowed (**aerophagia**), and other gasses are produced within the GIT by digestive processes and bacteria. These gases are either expelled through belching (eructation) or passed rectally (**flatus**). Intestinal gases include nitrogen (N_2), oxygen (O_2), carbon dioxide (CO_2), hydrogen (H_2), and in some persons methane (CH_4). Some of these gasses are absorbed into the circulation and then exhaled from the lungs.

Approximately 200 mL of gas is present in the healthy GIT. Humans excrete an average of 700 mL of gas each day, but are capable of moving considerably more through the GIT. The amount of intestinal gas varies greatly among individuals and from one day to the next. When patients complain about "excessive gas," or **flatulence**, they may be referring to increased volume or frequency of belching or passage of rectal gas. They may also complain of abdominal distention or cramping associated with the accumulation of gases in the upper or lower GIT. However, the perception of gas and the degree of symptoms experienced by an individual do not necessarily correlate with the amount of gas that is actually in the GIT (Azpiroz, 2005; Morken et al., 2007). Inactivity, decreased GI motility, aerophagia, dietary components, and certain GI disorders can alter the amount of intestinal gas and individual symptoms. Aerophagia can be avoided to some degree by eating slowly, chewing with the mouth closed, limiting gum chewing, and refraining from drinking through straws. Movement of gas through the GIT may be enhanced with upright stance, mild exercise, or abdominal massage.

Gas production occurs in the stomach and small intestine from bacterial fermentation of carbohydrates, and can result in abdominal discomfort and distention. The colonies of bacteria in the small bowel are normally present in limited numbers, but various conditions can lead to overgrowth of bacteria, potentially causing diarrhea, bloating, distention, or other symptoms. Because the small intestine is less tolerant of gas than the colon, this distention may cause pain. The movement of gas into the small intestine and beyond is slowed by high-calorie, high-fat meals. Slowed excretion or retained gas may contribute to the perception of distention or bloating with large meals in normal circumstances and with the abdominal discomfort that is experienced in **functional GI disorders**, such as irritable bowel syndrome (IBS) (Azpiroz, 2005; Harder et al, 2006). Functional GI disorders present symptoms that are not explained by a known structural, infectious, or metabolic cause.

Increased amounts of H_2 and CO_2—and sometimes CH_4—in rectal gas can lower the fecal pH, causing excessive colonic bacterial fermentation and malabsorption of fermentable substrate. The amounts and types of gases produced may depend on the mix of microorganisms in the individual's colon. Consumption of large amounts of dietary fiber (especially soluble fiber), resistant starches, lactose in persons who are lactase deficient, or modest amounts of fructose or sugar alcohols (such as sorbitol) may result in increased gas production in the colon and increased flatulence (Beyer et al., 2005). In the United States consumption of fruit juices, fruit drinks, and high-fructose corn syrup (HFCS) in soft drinks and confections has increased significantly in recent years. Fructose is normally well absorbed when consumed in the form of sucrose or as small amounts of HFCS, but not so well when consumed as the only or predominant sugar in the diet (see Chapter 1). In children 10-20 g of fructose, or 25 g in adults, is sufficient to result in malabsorption.

Medical Nutrition Therapy

When assessing a patient it is important to differentiate between increased production of gas and gas that is not being passed. Likewise, it is important to consider why a patient may have new or increased symptoms. A thorough review of the patient's medical history considers predisposing factors and treatment of underlying conditions before implementing nutrition therapy.

One of the direct nutrition considerations is development of lactose intolerance. Recent viral or GI infection may provoke temporary or even permanent impairment in the ability to digest lactose, and appropriate diet modifications can improve symptoms. A dramatic change in diet, such as adoption of a high-fiber diet, can also alter gas production. Foods that contain raffinose (a complex sugar resistant to digestion), such as beans, cabbage, Brussels sprouts, broccoli, asparagus and some whole grains, can increase gas production.

Altered bowel flora occur over time after an increase in dietary fiber. Although there are no randomized studies regarding the best way to implement high-fiber diets, a gradual introduction of fiber with adequate fluid consumption appears to reduce complaints of gas. Inactivity, dysmotility, constipation, or partial obstruction may be contributing to the inability to move normal amounts of gas as produced. Increased physical activity or exercise may help, if an underlying obstruction or dysmotility is not present.

Constipation

Constipation, commonly defined as difficult or infrequent passage of stool (Cook et al., 2009), is one of the most common intestinal maladies in Western societies, and may occur in 5% to 25% of the population or more (Müller-Lissner, 2009). Prevalence of constipation has been reported in as high as 50% to 80% of patients taking opioids daily for chronic pain, and may occur despite laxative use (Bell et al., 2009; Tuteja et al., 2010).

Although several definitions for constipation are based on frequency, difficulty, or consistency of stool, the sensation of "feeling constipated" may be enough to warrant intervention. Often, patients are troubled more by the physical discomfort of straining, hard stools, or incomplete evacuation than by the infrequency of bowel movements. In adults, normal stool weight is approximately 100 to 200 g daily, and normal frequency may range from one stool every 3 days to three times per day. Normal transit time through the GIT ranges from approximately 18 to 48 hours.

Children normally have more frequent stools, ranging from an average of two to three stools daily for the first few months of life to approximately one and a half bowel movements daily by age 3. As many as one third of children from ages 6 to 12 years complain of constipation in any given year (Biggs and Dery, 2006). Children may exhibit vomiting, abdominal pain, anorexia, or **encopresis** (involuntary passage of stool or fecal soiling).

Pathophysiology

Constipation may be caused by lifestyle factors (inadequate hydration, lack of exercise) or other medical conditions. Treatments differ based on the cause of constipation. Box 29-1 outlines numerous factors that may contribute to constipation.

The most common causes of constipation in otherwise healthy persons include repeatedly ignoring the urge to defecate, lack of fiber in the diet, insufficient fluid intake, inactivity, or use of certain medications. Individuals who believe that it is necessary to have scheduled and frequent bowel movements, yet ignore dietary and other recommendations for maintaining laxation, may be at risk for overuse of medications. When the desired stool frequency or timing of defecation does not occur, they may try to compensate with the use of medications and enemas. Chronic use of stimulant laxatives may damage the structure and innervation of the colon. Opioid medications bind to motility receptors in the gut, and chronic use may lead to constipation, delayed gastric emptying, nausea, and abdominal pain (Holzer, 2009).

BOX 29-1

Causes of Constipation

Lifestyle

Lack of exercise or mobility
Ignoring the urge to defecate
Inadequate fiber
Laxative abuse

Dysmotility Disorders

Chronic intestinal pseudoobstruction
Hypothyroidism
Colonic inertia
Gastroparesis
Hirschprung's disease
Metabolic and endocrine abnormalities such as diabetes

Neuromuscular Disorders (Particularly in Immobile or Wheelchair-Bound Patients)

Amyotrophic lateral sclerosis
Multiple sclerosis
Muscular dystrophy
Friedreich ataxia
Scleroderma involving the gut
Cerebral palsy
Para- or quadriplegia

Chronic Use of Opiates

Oncology patients
Chronic pain patients
Narcotic bowel syndrome

Pelvic Floor Disorders

Pregnancy

Other Gastrointestinal Disorders

Diseases of the upper gastrointestinal tract
Diseases of the large bowel resulting in:
- Failure of propulsion along the colon (colonic inertia)
- Anorectal malformations or outlet obstruction

Irritable bowel syndrome (IBS)
Anal fissure or hemorrhoid

Data from DeLillo AR, Rose S: Functional bowel disorders in the geriatric patient: constipation, fecal impaction and fecal incontinence, Am J Coll Gastroenterol 95:901, 2000; Schiller, LR: Nutrients and constipation: cause or cure? Pract Gastroenterol 32:4,2008; Siddiqui MA, Castell DO: Gastrointestinal disorders in the elderly, Comp Ther 23:349, 1997.

Medical Treatment for Adults

It is important to first rule out serious neurologic, GI, or endocrine disorders, or constipation caused by medications. After this is done, the first approach to treat mild and functional constipation is to ensure adequate dietary fiber, exercise, and heeding the urge to defecate. Patients who depend on laxatives are usually encouraged to use milder products, reducing the dose until withdrawal is complete.

When constipation persists despite lifestyle interventions, medications that promote regular bowel movements may be prescribed (Emmanuel et al., 2009). Anionic surfactants such as docusate sodium or docusate potassium are used as stool softeners to make bowel movements easier to pass. Osmotic agents such as magnesium hydroxide, sorbitol, and lactulose draw fluid into the bowel. Polyethylene glycol is an isosmotic agent that treats constipation by keeping the water it is taken within the gut rather than it being absorbed. Bisacodyl and senna compounds have stimulant activity on bowel motility and also act to prevent water absorption. Lubiprostone is a prostaglandin E1 derivative that increases fluid secretion by the epithelial cells of the GIT (Ramkumar and Rao, 2005). Impactions of stool require evacuation and a more stringent preventive and maintenance program, including combinations of medications, fluids, activity, or enemas.

Medical Treatment for Infants and Children

Approximately 3% to 5% of all pediatric outpatient visits are related to chronic constipation. In the most severe cases of functional constipation with frequent stool retention, the rectum becomes insensitive to distention, and encopresis may result. After disease is ruled out, treatment includes laxatives, lubricants, adequate dietary fiber, and fluid. A careful history and physical examination followed by parent and child education, behavioral intervention, and appropriate use of laxatives often leads to dramatic improvement (Biggs and Dery, 2006) (see Chapter 18).

Medical Nutrition Therapy

Primary nutrition therapy for constipation in otherwise healthy people is consumption of adequate amounts of dietary fiber, both soluble and insoluble, as well as fluids. Fiber increases colonic fecal fluid, microbial mass (which accounts for 60% to 70% of stool weight), stool weight and frequency, and the rate of colonic transit. With adequate fluid, fiber may soften stools and make them easier to pass. Unfortunately, most adults and children in the United States chronically consume only about half the amount of fiber recommended by the Institute of Medicine (14 g/1000 kcal). Adult women should consume approximately 25 g of fiber daily, men approximately 38 g, and children from 19 to 25 g daily.

Dietary fiber refers to edible plant materials not digested by the enzymes in the GIT. It consists of cellulose, hemicelluloses, pectins, gums, lignin, starchy materials, and oligosaccharides that are partially resistant to digestive enzymes. Fiber can be provided in the form of whole grains, fruits, vegetables, legumes, seeds, and nuts. These foods are also high in **prebiotics**, substances that are not digested by humans and fuel colonic microflora. Appendix 41 lists the fiber content of foods.

Different from fiber, **residue** refers to the end result of digestive, secretory, absorptive, and fermentative processes. Increasing dietary fiber may result in increased fecal output, but increasing dietary lactose (a fiber-free food) in a person who is a lactose malabsorber also increases fecal weight (residue).

Every 10 g of carbohydrate reaching the colon may be fermented into as much as 1000 mL of gas. Thus transition to a diet pattern that meets guidelines for fiber often requires substantial change. A high-fiber therapeutic diet may need to exceed 25 to 38 g/day. The **high-fiber diet** in Box 29-2 provides more than the amount of fiber recommended. Amounts greater than 50 g/day are not necessary and may increase abdominal distention and excessive flatulence.

Bran and powdered fiber supplements may be helpful in persons who cannot or will not eat sufficient amounts of fibrous foods. Several of these concentrates are palatable and can be added to cereals, yogurts, fruit sauces, juices, or soups. Cooking does not destroy fiber, although the structure may change. Consumption of at least eight 8-oz glasses (~2 L) of fluids daily is recommended to facilitate the effectiveness of a high-fiber intake. Gastric obstruction and fecal impaction may occur when boluses of fibrous gels or bran are not consumed with sufficient fluid to disperse the fiber.

Recommendations for increased dietary fiber for laxation should not be implemented in patients with neuromuscular disorders, dysmotility syndromes, chronic opioid use, pelvic floor disorders or other serious GI disease (Schiller, 2008). In some conditions, such as neuromuscular disorders, a specific laxative medication regimen is a necessary part of care.

BOX 29-2

Guidelines for High-Fiber Diets

1. Increase consumption of whole-grain breads, cereals, and other products to 6-11 servings daily.
2. Increase consumption of vegetables, legumes, fruits, nuts, and edible seeds to 5-8 servings daily.
3. Consume high-fiber cereals, granolas, and legumes to bring fiber intake to 25 g in women or 38 g in men or more daily.
4. Increase consumption of fluids to at least 2 L (or approximately 2 qt) daily.

Note: Following these guidelines may cause an increase in stool weight, fecal water, and gas. The amount that causes clinical symptoms varies among individuals, depending on age and presence of gastrointestinal (GI) disease, malnutrition, or resection of the GI tract.

Diarrhea

Diarrhea is characterized by the frequent evacuation of liquid stools, usually exceeding 300 mL, accompanied by an excessive loss of fluid and electrolytes, especially sodium and potassium. Diarrhea occurs when there is accelerated transit of intestinal contents through the small intestine, decreased enzymatic digestion of foodstuffs, decreased absorption of fluids and nutrients, increased secretion of fluids into the GIT, or exudative losses.

Types of Diarrhea and Their Pathophysiology

Diarrhea may be related to inflammatory disease; infections with fungal, bacterial, or viral agents; medications; over consumption of sugars or other osmotic substances; or insufficient or damaged mucosal absorptive surface.

Exudative diarrheas are always associated with mucosal damage, which leads to an outpouring of mucus, fluid, blood, and plasma proteins, with a net accumulation of electrolytes and water in the gut. Prostaglandin and cytokine release may be involved. The diarrheas associated with

Crohn's disease, ulcerative colitis (UC), and radiation enteritis are often exudative

Osmotic diarrheas occur when osmotically active solutes are present in the intestinal tract and are poorly absorbed. Examples include the diarrhea that accompanies dumping syndrome or that which follows lactose ingestion in the person with a lactase deficiency.

Secretory diarrheas are the result of active intestinal secretion of electrolytes and water by the intestinal epithelium, resulting from bacterial exotoxins, viruses, and increased intestinal hormone secretion. Unlike osmotic diarrhea, fasting does not relieve secretory diarrhea.

Malabsorptive diarrhea results when a disease process impairs digestion or absorption to the point that fat and other nutrients appear in the stool in increased amounts. Excess fat in the stool is called **steatorrhea**. Diarrhea occurs because of the osmotic action of these nutrients and the action of the bacteria on the nutrients that pass into the colon. Malabsorptive diarrhea occurs when there is not enough healthy absorptive area, inadequate production or interrupted flow of bile and pancreatic enzymes, or there is rapid transit, such as in inflammatory bowel disease (IBD) or after extensive bowel resection. Box 29-3 lists diseases and conditions associated with malabsorption and diarrhea.

Medication-induced diarrheas are frequent in hospitalized and long-term care patients. Medications such as lactulose (used in the management of hepatic encephalopathy) and sodium polystyrene sulfonate with sorbitol (used to treat hyperkalemia) create increased bowel movements as part of their mechanism of action. Some antibiotics have direct effects on GI function (see Chapter 9). For example, as a motilin agonist, erythromycin increases lower GI motility; clarithromycin and clindamycin also increase GI secretions.

In the normal GIT, bacterial "salvage" from sloughed intestinal cells and undigested foodstuffs converts osmotically active molecules (carbohydrate and amino acids) to gases and short-chain fatty acids (SCFAs). Absorption of the SCFAs facilitates absorption of electrolytes and water from the colon. Broad-spectrum antibiotics decrease the number of bacteria in the bowel and may result in increased osmotically active molecules, reduced absorption of electrolytes and water, and diarrhea.

Some antibiotics allow opportunistic proliferation of pathogenic organisms normally suppressed by competitive organisms in the GIT. The organisms or the toxins produced by some opportunistic organisms can cause colitis and increased secretion of fluid and electrolytes. The treatment of *Escherichia coli* and several other organisms has been implicated in **antibiotic-associated diarrhea (AAD)** (Schroeder, 2005). Overall, infection with *Clostridium difficile* is the most common cause of AAD, especially among patients who receive antibiotics within health care facilities. *C. difficile* is the leading cause of nosocomial (hospital-acquired) diarrhea in the United States (O'Keefe, 2010). This infection may cause colitis, secretory diarrhea, severe dilation of the colon (toxic megacolon), perforation of the bowel wall, peritonitis, or even death (Sánchez-Pérez et al., 2010).

BOX 29-3

Diseases and Conditions Associated with Malabsorption

Inadequate Digestion

Pancreatic insufficiency
Gastric acid hypersecretion
Gastric resection

Altered Bile Salt Metabolism with Impaired Micelle Formation

Hepatobiliary disease
Interrupted enterohepatic circulation of bile salts
Bacterial overgrowth
Drugs that precipitate bile salts

Abnormalities of Mucosal Cell Transport

Biochemical or Genetic Abnormalities

Disaccharidase deficiency
Monosaccharide malabsorption
Specific disorders of amino acid malabsorption
Abetalipoproteinemia
Vitamin B12 malabsorption
Celiac disease

Inflammatory or Infiltrative Disorders

Crohn's disease
Amyloidosis
Scleroderma
Tropical sprue
Gastrointestinal allergy
Infectious enteritis
Whipple's disease
Intestinal lymphoma
Radiation enteritis
Drug-induced enteritis
Endocrine and metabolic disorders
Short-bowel syndrome (SBS)

Abnormalities of Intestinal Lymphatics and Vascular System

Intestinal lymphangiectasia
Mesenteric vascular insufficiency
Chronic congestive heart failure

Data from Beyer PL: Short bowel syndrome. In Coulston AM, Rock CL, Monson ER, editors: Nutrition in the prevention and treatment of disease, ed 1, San Diego, 2001, Academic Press; Branski D et al: Chronic diarrhea and malabsorption, Pediatr Clin North Am 43:307, 1996; Mitra AD et al: Management of diarrhea in HIV-infected patients, Int J STD AIDS 12:630, 2001; Fine KD: Diarrhea. In Feldman M, Sleisenger MH, Scharschmidt BF, editors: Gastrointestinal and liver disease, ed 6, Philadelphia, 1998, Saunders; Podolsky DK: Inflammatory bowel disease, N Engl J Med 347:417, 2002; Sundarum A et al: Nutritional management of short bowel syndrome in adults, J Clin Gastroenterol 34:207, 2002.

C. difficile occurs in 50% of hospitalized patients with a stay longer than 4 weeks (DeLegge and Berry, 2009). In the mid 1990s, the incidence of *C. difficile* was reported to be between 30-40 cases per 100,000 patients, but by 2005 the incidence doubled to 84 cases per 100,000 patients (DeLegge and Berry, 2009). Additionally, resistant strains of *C. difficile* are less susceptible to treatment with antimicrobials, and cause a more severe form of the disease with increased health care costs, and higher mortality (O'Keefe, 2010).

C. difficile is a spore-forming organism, and the spores are resistant to common disinfectant agents. The spore-forming ability of *C. difficile* allows the organism to be spread inadvertently to other patients by health care providers (iatrogenic infection) if strict infection control procedures are not followed. The presence of this infection is detected by analysis of a stool sample for the presence of the toxin produced by the organisms. Clindamycin, penicillins, and cephalosporins are associated most often with the development of *C. difficile* infection. Its occurrence depends on the number of antibiotics used, the duration of exposure to antibiotics, and the patient's overall health. Chronic suppression of stomach acid with proton-pump inhibitor medications during broad-spectrum antibiotic therapy may also increase susceptibility to *C. difficile* infection (Howell et al., 2010; Linsky et al., 2010).

With human immunodeficiency virus (HIV) and other immune deficiency states, several factors contribute to the diarrhea, including the toxic effects of medications, proliferation of opportunistic organisms, and the GI manifestations of the disease itself (Kulkarni et al., 2009) (see Chapter 38). Increased risk of opportunistic infection is also associated with use of antineoplastic agents (such as chemotherapy) or with malnutrition.

Medical Treatment

Because diarrhea is a symptom, not a disease, the first step in medical treatment is to identify and treat the underlying problem. The next goal is to manage fluid and electrolyte replacement. In cases of severe diarrhea, restoring fluid and electrolyte is first priority. Electrolyte losses, especially potassium and sodium, should be corrected early by using oral glucose electrolyte solutions with added potassium. Oral rehydration solutions (ORS) work because they contain concentrations of sodium and glucose that are optimal for interaction with the sodium-glucose transport (SGLT) proteins in the intestinal epithelial cells. With intractable diarrhea, especially in an infant or young child, parenteral feeding may be required. Parenteral nutrition (PN) may even be necessary if exploratory surgery is anticipated or if the patient is not expected to resume full oral intake within 5 to 7 days (see Chapter 14).

Supplementation with **probiotics** shows some promise to prevent recurrence of *C. difficile* but there is inadequate data to recommend probiotics as a primary treatment for *C. difficile* infections. (Gao et al., 2010; Lawrence et al., 2005 Pillai 2008); see *New Directions*: Probiotics for the Right Balance of Bugs.

NEW DIRECTIONS

Probiotics for the Right Balance of Bugs

Some gastrointestinal conditions such as *Clostridium difficile* infection, small intestine bacterial overgrowth, antibiotic-associated diarrhea, and perhaps even inflammatory bowel disease may result or have exacerbated symptoms when there are alterations to the colonies of microorganisms that exist in the small or large intestines. Exposure to broad-spectrum antibiotics causes dramatic alterations to native gastrointestinal (GI) flora, and placing the patient at risk for opportunistic GI infections. Concentrated cultures of live microorganisms such as lactobacillus, bifidobacteria, and *Saccharomyces boulardii* ingested as a supplement or in foods (yogurt or kefir) confer a health benefit on the host. It has been suggested that probiotics may restore the balance of intestinal microbes and improve symptoms and prevent or treat conditions such as antibiotic-associated diarrhea. Certain types of probiotics may be effective in reducing the duration of enterovirus-induced acute infectious diarrhea in pediatric and adult patients (Hickson et al., 2007) and in irritable bowel disease (Guyonnet et al., 2007).

One multicenter study investigated 64 patients with active or recurrent *C. difficile* infection. All patients were given a combination of oral antibiotics and 1 g/day of *S. boulardii* or a placebo for 4 weeks, then evaluated after another 4 weeks. The researchers found that patients treated with *S. boulardii* had a significantly lower risk for developing another *C. difficile* infection during the study period (Lawrence et al., 2005). Probiotics improved diarrhea by shortening duration by 1.4 days or reducing incidence by approximately 30%. There is insufficient evidence to recommend routine probiotic therapy as an adjunct to antibiotic therapy for *C. difficile* colitis (Pillai and Nelson, 2008). Improvement is not 100% in all people. Thus more controlled studies are needed (Aragon et al., 2010; Whorwell et al., 2006).

Products that combine probiotic microorganisms and a prebiotic fiber source have been described as **synbiotics** for their synergistic effects. However, there are no controlled studies that have systematically investigated the effectiveness of probiotics alone compared with synbiotics. There is a need for controlled studies to understand which strains of probiotics should be provided, as well as type and amount of prebiotic fibers.

Although there is a long history of safe use of many strains of probiotics in foods in healthy humans, there is a limited body of evidence on the use of large doses of concentrated probiotic supplements, especially of specific strains that exhibit greater resistance to gastric acid or have increased ability to proliferate in the GIT. There is very limited safety data to support the use of concentrated probiotic supplements in patients with immunocompromised states, critical illness, or when probiotics are administered directly into the small intestine, as with jejunal feeding tubes. There have been a number of case reports of hospitalized patients receiving concentrated strains of probiotics that have become septic because of infection in the bloodstream with the very same strain of probiotic being administered (Whelan and Myers, 2010). In a review of cases of adverse events related to probiotic administration in hospitalized patients, 25% of those adverse events resulted in the death of the patient (Whelan and Myers, 2010). In a large double-blind, randomized study of a high-dose multispecies probiotic administered via jejunal feeding tube in patients with severe acute pancreatitis, there were significantly more deaths in the patients who received probiotics compared with those receiving the inactive placebo (Besselink et al., 2008).

Probiotic preparations hold promise as an adjunctive or primary treatment in several gastrointestinal conditions, but there is a need for additional studies before routine use of these preparations is adopted, especially for hospitalized or immunocompromised patients. The studies to date have been relatively small, have used varying doses and strains of probiotic microorganisms, and there remains much to be learned about true effectiveness, differences between probiotic strains, possible benefits of coadministration of prebiotics, best doses, safety, and cost-benefit of using probiotics.

Medical Nutrition Therapy

All nutrition interventions related to diarrhea must be viewed within the context of the underling pathologic condition responsible for the diarrhea. Replacement of necessary fluids and electrolytes is the first step, using ORSs, soups and broths, vegetable juices, and isotonic liquids. Restrictive diets, such as the BRAT diet made up of bananas, rice, applesauce, and toast, are nutrient poor and there is no evidence that they are necessary during acute diarrheal illness. However, some clinicians recommend a progression of starchy carbohydrates such as cereals, breads, and low-fat meats, followed by small amounts of vegetables and fruits, followed by fats. The goal with this progression is to limit large amounts of hyperosmotic carbohydrates that may be maldigested or malabsorbed, foods that stimulate secretion of fluids, and foods that speed the rate of GI transit.

Sugar alcohols, lactose, fructose, and large amounts of sucrose may worsen osmotic diarrheas. Because the activity of the disaccharidases and transport mechanisms decrease during inflammatory and infectious intestinal disease, sugars may need to be limited, especially in children (Robayo-Torres et al., 2006). It is important to remember that malabsorption is only one potential cause of diarrhea, and diarrhea may occur without significant malabsorption of macronutrients (carbohydrate, fat, and protein). Absorption of most nutrients occurs in the small intestine; diarrhea related to colonic inflammation or disease preserves the absorption of most ingested nutrients.

Minimal fiber and low-residue diets are rarely indicated (Table 29-1). Patients are encouraged to resume a regular diet as tolerated that contains moderate amounts of soluble fiber. The metabolism of fiber and resistant starches by colonic bacteria leads to production of SCFAs, which in physiologic quantities serve as a substrate for colonocytes, facilitate the absorption of fluid and salts, and may help to regulate GI motility (Binder, 2010).

Fibrous material tends to slow gastric emptying, moderate overall GI transit, and pull water into the intestinal lumen. Providing fiber to patients with diarrhea does increase the volume of stool, and in some cases (such as small intestine bacterial overgrowth [SIBO]) can initially increase gas and bloating. Modest intake of prebiotic components and **soluble fibers** such as pectin or gum slows transit through the GIT.

Several probiotics have been tested for preventing AAD in children; risk reduction was higher from *Saccharomyces boulardii* than for *Lactobacillus GG* or *Lactobacillus bifidus* and *Streptococcus thermophilus* (Szajewska, 2006). Studies are needed to find the combination of probiotics, prebiotics, and antibiotics that works most effectively in each situation (Teitelbaum, 2005).

Severe and chronic diarrhea is accompanied by dehydration and electrolyte depletion. If also accompanied by prolonged infectious, immunodeficiency, or inflammatory disease, malabsorption of vitamins, minerals, and protein or fat may also occur, and nutrients may need to be replaced parenterally or enterally. In some forms of infectious diarrheas, loss of iron from GI bleeding may be severe enough to cause anemia. Nutrient deficiencies themselves cause mucosal changes such as decreased villi height and reduced enzyme secretion, further contributing to malabsorption. As the diarrhea begins to resolve, the addition of more normal amounts of fiber to the diet may help to restore normal mucosal function, increase electrolyte and water absorption, and increase the firmness of the stool.

Food in the lumen is needed to restore the compromised GIT after disease and periods of fasting. Early refeeding after rehydration reduces stool output and shortens the duration of illness. Micronutrient replacement or supplementation may also be useful for acute diarrhea, probably because it accelerates the normal regeneration of damaged mucosal epithelial cells.

Treating Diarrhea in Infants and Children

Acute diarrhea is most dangerous in infants and small children, who are easily dehydrated by large fluid losses. In these cases replacement of fluid and electrolytes must be aggressive and immediate. Standard ORS recommended by the World Health Organization and the American Academy of Pediatrics contain a 2% concentration of glucose (20 g/L),

TABLE 29-1

Food to Limit in a Low-Fiber (Minimal Residue) Diet

Food	Comments
Lactose (in lactose malabsorbers)	6-12 g is normally tolerated in healthy lactase-deficient individuals, but may not be in some individuals.
Fiber (quantities >20 g)	Modest amounts (10-15 g) may help maintain normal consistency of gastrointestinal (GI) contents and normal colonic mucosa in healthy states and GI disease.
Resistant starch (especially raffinose and stachyose found in legumes)	
Sorbitol, mannitol, and xylitol (excess, >10 g/day)	
Fructose (excess, 20-25 g/meal)	
Sucrose (excess, >25-50 g/meal)	Well tolerated in moderate amounts; large amounts may cause hyperosmolar diarrhea or decreased fecal pH with fermentation to short-chain fatty acids.
Caffeine	Increases GI secretions, colonic motility.
Alcoholic beverages (especially wine and beer)	Increase GI secretions.

GI, Gastrointestinal.

TABLE 29-2

Oral Rehydration Solution: Composition and Recipes

Element	Composition
Glucose (g/100 mL)	20
Sodium (mEq/L)	90
Potassium (mEq/L)	20
Chloride (mEq/L)	80
Bicarbonate (mEq/L)	30
Osmolarity (mOsm/L)	330
Recipes* (each makes 1 liter)	
2 cups Gatorade, 2 cups water, ¾ tsp salt	28 g glucose, 82 mEq Na, 1.5 eEq K
1 quart water, ¾ tsp salt, 6 teaspoons sugar	24 g glucose, 76 mEq Na, 0 mEq K

Data from Krenitsky J, McCray S: University of Virginia Health System Nutrition Support Traineeship Syllabus, Charlottesville, Va, 2010, University of Virginia Health System; World Health Organization: Guidelines for cholera control, WHO/COD/Ser/80.4, Rev 1, Geneva, 1986.

Recipes from Parrish CR: The Clinician's guide to short bowel syndrome, *Pract Gastroenterol* 29:67, 2005.

K, Potassium; *Na*, sodium.

*The solution should be made fresh every 24 hr.

45 to 90 mEq/L of sodium, 20 mEq/L of potassium, and a citrate base (Table 29-2).

Newer reduced-osmolarity solutions (200-250 mOsm/L) have advantages over the traditional WHO-recommended ORS in treating acute diarrhea in children (Atia and Buchman, 2009). The use of reduced-osmolarity ORS in children with acute diarrhea resulted in decreased need for intravenous therapy, significant reduction in stool output, and decreased vomiting when compared with standard WHO-recommended ORS (Atia and Buchman, 2009). Commercial solutions such as Pedialyte, Infalyte, Lytren, Equalyte, and Rehydralyte typically contain less glucose and slightly less salt and are available in pharmacies, often without prescription. Oral rehydration therapy is less invasive and less expensive than intravenous rehydration and, when used with children, allows parents to assist with their children's recovery.

A substantial proportion of children 9 to 20 months of age can maintain adequate intake when offered either a liquid or a semisolid diet continuously during bouts of acute diarrhea. Even during acute diarrhea, the intestine can absorb up to 60% of the food eaten. Some practitioners have been slow to adopt the practice of early refeeding after severe diarrhea in infants despite evidence that "resting the gut" is actually more damaging. Thus prescription of the typical hospital "full liquid" or "clear liquid" diet, which is commonly high in fructose, lactose, and other sugars, is inappropriate for recovery from diarrhea.

Gastrointestinal Strictures and Obstruction

Intestinal tumors or scarring from GI surgeries, IBD, peptic ulcer, or radiation enteritis may partially or completely obstruct the GIT or cause dysfunctional segments. Obstructions may be partial or complete, and may occur in the stomach (gastric outlet obstruction), small intestine or large intestine. Symptoms include bloating, abdominal distention and pain, and sometimes nausea and vomiting.

Pathophysiology

People with gastroparesis, Crohn's disease, scars, adhesions, dysmotility, or volvulus are all prone to obstruction. Partial or complete obstructions are not usually caused by foods in an otherwise healthy individual; however, when sections of the GIT are partially obstructed or not moving appropriately, foods may contribute to obstruction.

Although there are no controlled studies that have investigated different diets and the frequency of obstructive symptoms, it is believed that fibrous plant foods can contribute to obstructions because the fiber in the foods may not be completely chewed or reduced in size enough to pass through abnormal or narrowed segments of the GIT.

Medical Nutrition Therapy

Most clinicians would recommend patients prone to obstructions to chew food well and avoid excessive fiber intake. In addition, potato skins, citrus fruits, persimmons, and similar foods should be avoided by edentulous patients.

With a partial obstruction, the patient may be able to tolerate easily digestible foods and liquids, depending on the location of stricture or obstruction in the GIT. A more proximal (closer to the mouth) blockage may require a semisolid or liquid diet. However, the more distal (closer to the anus) the blockage, the less likely altering the consistency of the diet will help.

During complete obstruction, symptoms are more severe. Patients may be intolerant of oral intake and also of their own secretions. Intensive intervention, such as surgery, may be required for complete obstruction. In some cases, enteral feeding beyond the point of obstruction may be feasible, but if enteral feeding is not possible for a prolonged period, PN may be needed. Working with the patient and physician is necessary to determine the nature, site, and duration of the obstruction, so that nutrition therapy can be individualized.

DISEASES OF THE SMALL INTESTINE

Celiac Disease (Gluten-Sensitive Enteropathy)

Celiac disease (CD), or **gluten-sensitive enteropathy**, is characterized by a combination of four factors: (1) genetic susceptibility, (2) exposure to gluten, (3) an environmental "trigger," and (4) an autoimmune response. **Gluten** refers to specific peptide fractions of proteins (prolamines) found in wheat (glutenin and gliadin), rye (secalin), and barley (hordein). These peptides are generally more resistant to complete digestion by GI enzymes and may reach the small intestine intact. In a normal, healthy intestine, these peptides are harmless. However, in persons with CD these peptides travel from the intestinal lumen, across the intestinal epithelium, and into the lamina propria where they can trigger an inflammatory response that results in flattening of intestinal villi and elongation of the crypt cells (secretory cells), along with a more general systemic immune response (Kagnoff, 2007).

The term **gluten sensitivity** is commonly used to describe persons with nonspecific symptoms, without the immune response characteristic of CD or the consequential intestinal damage. **Gluten intolerance** describes individuals who have symptoms, and who may or may not have CD. These two terms are used to describe symptoms such as nausea, abdominal cramps, or diarrhea after ingesting gluten. Patients who experience these symptoms should generally be advised against following a gluten-free (GF) diet without having a workup to exclude or confirm a diagnosis of CD because (1) there may be an underlying medical condition for which a GF diet is not the treatment; (2) after following a GF diet for months or years, it is difficult to diagnose CD; and (3) although generally a healthy way to eat, a GF diet can be expensive and restrictive.

Pathophysiology

The "triggers" of CD are not well understood, but stressors (illness, inflammation, etc.) are thought to play a role. When CD remains untreated, the immune and inflammatory response eventually results in atrophy and flattening of villi. Over time, the process can cause enough damage to the intestinal mucosa to compromise normal secretory, digestive, and absorptive functions, leading to impaired micronutrient and macronutrient absorption (Chand and Mihas, 2006). Cells of the villi become deficient in the disaccharidases and peptidases needed for digestion and also in the carriers needed to transport nutrients into the bloodstream (see Figure 29-1). The disease primarily affects

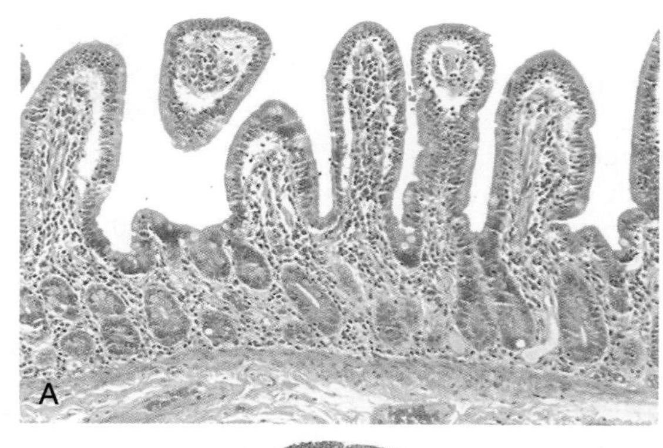

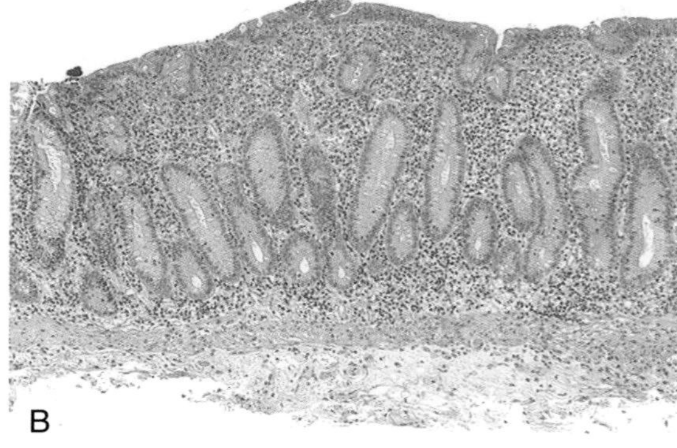

FIGURE 29-1 CD (gluten-sensitive enteropathy). **A,** Peroral jejunal biopsy specimen of diseased mucosa shows severe atrophy and blunting of villi, with a chronic inflammatory infiltrate of the lamina propria. **B,** Normal mucosal biopsy. *(From Kumar V and others: Robbins and Cotran pathologic basis of disease, ed 7, Philadelphia, 2005, Saunders.)*

the proximal and middle sections of the small bowel, although the more distal segments may also be involved (Bonamico et al., 2008).

The prevalence of CD has been underestimated in the past and now is considered to affect at least 1 in 133 persons in the United States. The onset and first occurrence of symptoms may appear any time from infancy to adulthood, but the peak in diagnosis occurs between the fourth and sixth decade. The disease may become apparent when an infant begins eating gluten-containing cereals. In some, it may not appear until adulthood, when it may be triggered or unmasked during GI surgery, stress, pregnancy, or viral infection. Or it may be discovered as a result of evaluation for another suspected problem. Approximately 20% of cases are diagnosed after the age of 60 years.

The presentation in young children is likely to include the more "classic" GI symptoms of diarrhea, steatorrhea, malodorous stools, abdominal bloating, apathy, fatigue, and poor weight gain. Although GI-related symptoms are often thought to be most common, an increasing number of patients present without GI symptoms. Fifty percent of celiac patients have few or no obvious symptoms, and some are overweight at presentation (Venkatasubramani et al., 2010). CD is frequently misdiagnosed as irritable bowel syndrome (IBS), lactase deficiency, gallbladder disease, or other disorders not necessarily involving the GIT, because the presentation and onset of symptoms vary so greatly.

Patients may present with one or more of a host of conditions associated with CD: anemias, generalized fatigue, weight loss or failure to thrive, osteoporosis, vitamin or mineral deficiencies, and (although rare) GI malignancy. **Dermatitis herpetiformis**, yet another manifestation of CD, presents as an itchy skin rash; its presence is diagnostic of CD. Box 29-4 lists conditions associated with CD. Persons who are diagnosed late in life, who cannot or will not comply with the diet, or who were diagnosed as children but told they would grow out of it are at a higher risk for experiencing long-term complications from CD (Nachman et al., 2010).

BOX 29-4

Symptoms and Conditions Associated with Celiac Disease

Nutritional

Anemia (iron or folate, rarely B12)
Osteomalacia, osteopenia, fractures (vitamin D deficiency, inadequate calcium absorption)
Coagulopathies (vitamin K deficiency)
Dental enamel hypoplasia
Delayed growth, delayed puberty, underweight
Lactase deficiency

Extraintestinal

Lassitude, malaise (sometimes despite lack of anemia)
Arthritis, arthralgia
Dermatitis herpetiformis
Infertility, increased risk of miscarriage
Hepatic steatosis, hepatitis
Neurologic symptoms (ataxia, polyneuropathy, seizures); may be partly nutrition related
Psychiatric syndromes

Associated Disorders

Autoimmune diseases: type 1 diabetes, thyroiditis, hepatitis, collagen vascular disease
Gastrointestinal malignancy
IgA deficiency

Data from Fasano A, Catassi C: Current approaches to diagnosis and treatment of celiac disease: an evolving spectrum, Gastroenterology 120:636, 2001; Hill ID et al: Celiac disease: working group report of the First World Congress of Pediatric Gastroenterology, Hepatology and Nutrition, J Pediatr Gastroenterol Nutr 35:785, 2002.

IgA, Immunoglobulin A.

Assessment

The diagnosis of CD is made by a combination of clinical, laboratory, and histologic evaluations. Persons suspected of having CD should be evaluated for the overall pattern of symptoms and family history. Biopsy of the small intestine is the gold standard for diagnosis (Chand and Mihas, 2006). An intestinal biopsy positive for CD generally shows villous atrophy, increased intraepithelial lymphocytes, and crypt cell hyperplasia. Biopsy is not used for initial screening because of its cost and invasiveness.

Several serologic tests are used for screening. These tests identify the presence of antibodies in the blood, such as anti-tissue transglutaminase (anti-TTG), and anti-endomysial antibodies, and deaminated gliadin peptide. The sensitivity and specificity of these tests are 90% to 99% (Rostom et al., 2005). There is a higher incidence of immunoglobulin (Ig) A deficiency in patients with CD; thus physicians often measure IgA levels if serologic findings are normal but the overall clinical picture suggests CD. Using capsule endoscopy to image the entire intestinal mucosa can show inflammation related to CD, but is not currently used in the initial diagnosis (El-Matary et al., 2009). Because dietary change alters diagnostic results, initial evaluation should be done *before* the person has eliminated gluten-containing foods from his or her diet. Serologic tests may also be used to monitor the response of a newly diagnosed patient treated with a GF diet.

Lifelong, strict adherence to a GF diet is the only known treatment for CD. See Box 29-5 for a list of safe, questionable and unsafe choices on the GF diet. The GF diet greatly diminishes the autoimmune process, and the intestinal mucosa usually reverts to normal or near normal. Within 2 to 8 weeks of starting the GF diet, most patients report that their clinical symptoms have abated. Histologic, immunologic, and functional improvements may take months to years, depending on the duration of the disease, age of the subject, and degree of dietary compliance. With strict

BOX 29-5

The Basic Gluten-Free Diet

Foods	Safe Choices	Questionable	Avoid
Grains and Flours	Amaranth, arrowroot, bean flours (such as garbanzo or fava bean flour), buckwheat, corn (maize) or cornstarch, flax, Job's tears, millet, potato, quinoa, ragi, rice, sorghum, soybean (soya), tapioca, teff	Carob-soy flour, buckwheat pancake mixes (often contain wheat flour), pure uncontaminated oats (note: a small percentage of people with celiac disease react to pure oats; discuss with your health care provider first)	Wheat (bulghur, couscous, durum, farina, graham, kamut, semolina, spelt, triticale, wheat germ), rye, barley, oats (except pure, uncontaminated oats), low gluten flour. Caution: "wheat free" does not necessarily mean "gluten free"
Cereals—Hot or Dry	Cream of rice, cream of buckwheat, hominy, gluten-free dry cereals, grits	Puffed rice or corn cereals (possible contamination); pure uncontaminated oats (small percentage of people with CD react to oats)	Those with wheat, rye, oats (except pure, uncontaminated), barley, barley malt, malt flavoring, wheat germ, bran
Potatoes, Rice, Starch	Any plain potatoes, sweet potatoes and yams, all types of plain rice, rice noodles, 100% buckwheat soba noodles, gluten-free pasta, polenta, hominy, corn tortillas, parsnips, yucca, turnips	Check labels for commercial potato or rice products with seasoning packets	Battered or deep-fried French fries (unless no other foods have been fried in the same oil), pasta, noodles, wheat starch, stuffing, flour tortillas, croutons
Crackers, Chips, Popcorn	Rice wafers or other gluten-free crackers, rice cakes; plain corn chips, tortilla chips, potato chips, and other root (taro, beet, etc.) chips, plain popcorn	Flavored chips	Crackers, graham crackers, rye crisps, matzo, croutons
Desserts	Sorbet, popsicles, Italian ice	Check labels on ice cream and pudding	Ice cream with bits of cookies, "crispies," pretzels, etc; pie crust, cookies, cakes, ice cream cones, and pastries made from gluten-containing flours
Milk and Yogurt	Any plain, unflavored milk or yogurt, buttermilk, cream, half and half	Flavored milks or yogurts (check labels)	Malted milk, yogurts with added "crunchies" or toppings
Cheese	Cheese (all styles including blue cheese and gorgonzola), processed cheese (i.e., American), cottage cheese	Cheese spreads or sauces (check labels)	
Eggs	All types of plain, cooked eggs	Eggs benedict (sauce usually made with wheat flour)	
Meat, Fish, Shellfish, Poultry	Any fresh, plain untreated meat, fish, shellfish, or poultry; fish canned in brine, vegetable broth, or water	Commercially treated, preserved, or marinated meats, luncheon meats, fish, shellfish; self-basting or cured poultry	Breaded or battered meats
Beans and Legumes	Any plain frozen, fresh, dried, or canned (no flavorings or sauces added) beans: garbanzo beans, kidney beans, lentils, pinto beans, edamame, lima, black beans, etc	Check labels for added ingredients—sauces may have gluten	

BOX 29-5

The Basic Gluten-Free Diet—cont'd

Foods	Safe Choices	Questionable	Avoid
Soy Products and Meat Analogs or Alternatives	Plain tempeh, tofu, edamame	Check labels on miso, soy sauce, seasoned tofu and tempeh, meat analogs (imitation meat substitutes), imitation seafood	Seitan; 3-Grain Tempeh
Nuts and Seeds	Any plain (salted or unsalted) nuts, seeds or nut butters, coconut	Dry-roasted nuts (check with manufacturer—may dust with flour during processing)	Nut butters with gluten containing ingredients
Fruits and Juices	Any plain fresh, canned, frozen fruits or juices, plain dried fruit	Pie fillings (often thickened with gluten containing flour)	Dried fruit dusted with flour
Vegetables	Any plain, fresh, canned or frozen vegetables including corn, peas, lima beans, etc.		Vegetables in gluten containing sauce or gravy
Soups	Homemade soups with known allowed ingredients	Check labels on all commercial soups	
Condiments, Jams, and Syrups	Ketchup, mustard, salsa, wheat-free soy sauce, mayonnaise, vinegar (except malt vinegar), jam, jelly, honey, pure maple syrup, molasses	Check labels on soy sauce, salad dressings, commercial sauces, soup base, marinades, coating mixes	Malt vinegar
Seasonings and Flavorings	Any *plain* herb or spice; salt; pepper; brown or white sugar; or artificial sweetener (i.e., Equal, Sweet-N-Low, Splenda)	Seasoning mixes, bouillon	
Fats	Butter, margarine, all pure vegetable oils (including canola), mayonnaise, cream	Check labels on salad dressings, sandwich spreads	
Baking Ingredients	Yeast, baking soda, baking powder, cream of tartar, regular chocolate baking chips		See grains and flours; Check label on grain sweetened, carob or vegan chocolate chips
Beverages	Coffee, tea, pure cocoa powder, sodas, Silk Soymilk, Rice Dream beverage	Check labels on flavored instant coffee mixes (such as swiss mocha, cappuccino); herbal teas, soy or rice drinks (may contain barley malt or rice syrup)	Malted beverages
Alcohol	Wine, all distilled liquor including vodka, tequila, gin, rum, whiskey and pure liqueurs, gluten-free beers (Redbridge, Bard's Tale Beer, ciders)	Drink mixes	Beer, ale, lager
Candies	Check labels—many are gluten-free		Candy from bulk food bins Licorice

Adapted from Parrish CR, Krenitsky J, McCray S: University of Virginia Health System Nutrition Support Traineeship Syllabus, Charlottesville, Va, 2010, University of Virginia Health System.

CD, Celiac disease.

dietary control, levels of the specific antibodies usually become undetectable within 3 to 6 months in most persons. In some individuals, recovery may be slow or incomplete.

A small percentage of patients are "nonresponders" to diet therapy. Inadvertent gluten intake is the most common offender, but another coexisting disorder may be present (such as pancreatic insufficiency, IBS, bacterial overgrowth, fructose intolerance, other GI maladies, or unknown causes). For nonresponders, intensive interviewing to identify a source of gluten contamination or treatment of another underlying disease may resolve the symptoms. Diagnosis of **refractory celiac disease** is made when patients do not respond or respond only temporarily to a GF diet, and all external causes have been ruled out, including inadvertent gluten ingestion. Patients with refractory disease may respond to steroids, azathioprine, cyclosporine, or other medications classically used to suppress inflammatory or immunologic reactions (see *Pathophysiology and Care Management Algorithm*: Celiac Disease).

Several novel treatments for CD are being studied for their potential as alternative therapies. Researchers seek to treat CD by reducing gluten exposure (by digestion from enzymes), decreasing uptake of gluten (by tightening junctions between intestinal epithelial cells), altering the immune response to gluten, or repairing intestinal injury.

Medical Nutrition Therapy

Elimination of gluten peptides from the diet is the only treatment of CD. The diet omits all dietary wheat, rye, and barley, which are the major sources of the prolamin fractions

In general, patients should be assessed for nutrient deficiencies before supplementation is initiated. In all newly diagnosed patients, the clinician should consider checking levels of ferritin, red blood cell folate, and 25-hydroxy vitamin D. If patients present with more severe symptoms, such as diarrhea, weight loss, malabsorption, or signs of nutrient deficiencies (night-blindness, neuropathy, prolonged prothrombin time, etc.), other vitamins such as fat-soluble vitamins (A, E, K) and minerals (zinc) should be checked.

The healing of the intestinal mucosa that occurs after initiation of a GF diet improves nutrient absorption, and many patients who eat well-balanced GF diets do not need nutritional supplementation. However, most specialty GF products are not fortified with iron and B vitamins like other grain products, so the diet may not be as complete without at least partial supplementation. Anemia should be treated with iron, folate, or vitamin B_{12}, depending on the nature of the anemia. Patients with malabsorption may benefit from a bone density scan to assess for osteopenia or osteoporosis. Calcium and vitamin D supplementation are likely to be beneficial in these patients. Electrolyte and fluid replacement is essential for those dehydrated from severe diarrhea.

Those who continue to have malabsorption should take a general vitamin-mineral supplement to at least meet DRI recommendations. Lactose and fructose intolerance sometimes occur secondary to CD, and sugar alcohols are not well absorbed, even in a healthy gut. A low-lactose or low-fructose diet may be useful in controlling symptoms, at least initially. Once the GIT returns to more normal function, lactase activity may also return, and the person can incorporate lactose and dairy products back into the diet.

In general, many fruits, vegetables, grains, meats, and dairy products that are plain and unseasoned are safe to eat. Oats were once thought to be questionable for persons with CD; however, extensive studies have shown that they are safe in the GF diet as long as they are pure, uncontaminated oats (Garsed and Scott, 2007). A very small population of patients with CD may not tolerate even pure oats. In general, patients do not need to be advised against including GF oats in their diet unless they have demonstrated intolerance to GF oats.

Flours made from corn, potatoes, rice, soybean, tapioca, arrowroot, amaranth, quinoa, millet, teff, and buckwheat can be substituted in recipes. Patients can expect differences in textures and flavors of common foods using the substitute flours, but new recipes can be quite palatable once the adjustment is made. In GF baked goods, gums such as xanthan, guar, and cellulose can be used to provide the elasticity needed to trap leavening gases in baked goods.

A truly GF diet requires careful scrutiny of the labels of all bakery products and packaged foods. Gluten-containing grains are not only used as a primary ingredient but may also be added during processing or preparation of foods. For example, hydrolyzed vegetable protein can be made from wheat, soy, corn, or mixtures of these grains.

The diet for the person with CD requires a major lifestyle change because of the change from traditional grains in the diet. A tremendous number of foods made with wheat (in particular breads, cereals, pastas, and baked goods) are a common part of a Western diet. However, there is increasing awareness among food companies and restaurants of the expanding demand for GF foods, and these businesses are responding. The individual and family members should all be taught about label reading, safe food additives, food preparation, sources of cross contamination (such as toasters, condiment jars, bulk bins, and buffets), and hidden sources of gluten (such as medications and communion wafers) to be compliant. Box 29-6 provides sources of hidden gluten and cross-contamination. Eating in cafeterias, restaurants, vending outlets, street markets, at friends' homes, and at social events can be challenging, especially initially.

To avoid misinterpretation of information, newly diagnosed patients should be started with an in-depth instruction from a registered dietitian on the GF diet, along with reliable resources for further guidance and support. Persons with CD generally need several education or counseling sessions with a registered dietitian knowledgeable in the disease management (American Gastroenterological Association, 2006; Case, 2005). Box 29-7 lists CD resources.

PATHOPHYSIOLOGY AND CARE MANAGEMENT ALGORITHM

Celiac Disease (Gluten-Sensitive Enteropathy or Nontropical Sprue)

ETIOLOGY

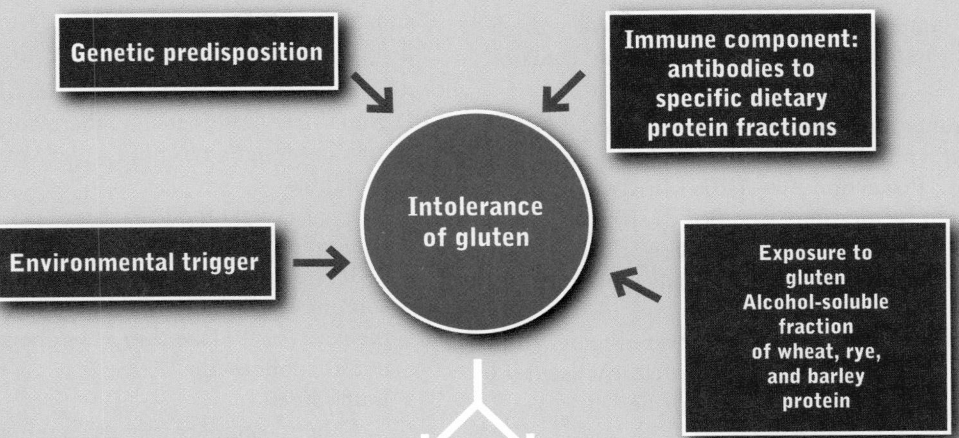

PATHOPHYSIOLOGY

Damage To Small Bowel

- Atrophy and flattening of villi
- Reduced area for absorption
- Cellular deficiency of disaccharidases and peptidases
- Reduced nutrient transport carriers

Extraintestinal Manifestations

- Anemia
- Bone loss
- Muscle weakness
- Polyneuropathy
- Endocrine disorders (e.g., infertility)
- Follicular hyperkeratosis
- Dermatitis herpetiformis

Intestinal Manifestations

- Chronic diarrhea
- Chronic constipation
- Malabsorption of vitamins and minerals

MANAGEMENT

Medical Management

- Electrolyte and fluid replacement
- Management of other co-morbid conditions

Nutrition Management

- Delete gluten sources (wheat, rye, barley) from diet
- Vitamin and mineral supplementation
- Substitute with corn, potato, rice, soybean, tapioca, arrowroot, and other non-gluten flours
- Calcium and vitamin D administration
- Read food labels carefully for hidden gluten-containing ingredients
- Supplementation with ω-3 fatty acids
- Guidance to support groups and reliable internet resources

BOX 29-6

Hidden Gluten Exposure and Cross-Contamination

Hidden Gluten Exposure

Unfortunately, gluten is not always obvious. Review the list below for some "unsuspected" products that may contain gluten.

- Over-the-counter and prescription medications
  The labeling requirements of the Food Allergen and Consumer Protection Act of 2004 (FALCPA) **do not** apply to medications. See Box 27-10 in Chapter 27. Check with your pharmacist or call the manufacturer to determine if there is any gluten in your medications.
  Note: **Dietary supplements** are covered under FALCPA regulations so wheat must be clearly listed if it is an ingredient in a vitamin, mineral or herbal supplement.
- Communion wafers
  Gluten-free recipes are available.
- Uncommon sources
  If laboratory values stay elevated and symptoms remain and, possible sources of gluten cannot be found in the diet, it may be worth checking into other sources such as toothpaste, mouthwash, or lipstick.

Cross-Contamination

Below are some of the most common sources of gluten contamination. A few crumbs that may not even be seen can cause damage to the intestine, so it is best to avoid these situations:

- Toasters used for gluten-containing foods
  Keep two toasters at home and designate one as gluten-free. Alternatively, there are now bags available that are designed to hold a piece of bread in the toaster.
- Bulk bins
  Prepackaged food is a safer bet.
- Condiment jars (peanut butter, jam, mayonnaise, etc.)
  It is best to keep a separate gluten-free jar for commonly used items and be sure to label it clearly. At the very least, make sure everyone in the house knows not to "double-dip."
- Buffet lines
  Other customers may use one serving utensil for multiple items. Food from one area may be spilled into another food container. It may be safer to order from the menu.
- Deep-fried foods
  Oil is typically used over and over to fry foods. It is highly likely that French fries (or other GF foods) are fried in the same oil as battered and breaded foods like fried chicken.

Adapted from Parrish CR, Krenitsky J, McCray S: University of Virginia Health System Nutrition Support Traineeship Syllabus, Charlottesville, Va, 2010, University of Virginia Health System.

GF, Gluten free.

Marked gut improvement and a return to normal histologic findings occurs in the majority of patients after an average of 2 years (Hutchinson et al., 2010). Patients who are able to follow the GF diet closely have a better overall response.

Tropical Sprue

Tropical sprue is an acquired diarrheal syndrome with malabsorption that occurs in many tropical areas (Nath, 2005). In addition to diarrhea and malabsorption, anorexia, abdominal distention, and nutritional deficiency as evidenced by night blindness, glossitis, stomatitis, cheilosis, pallor, and edema can occur. Anemia may result from iron, folic acid, and vitamin B_{12} deficiencies.

Pathophysiology

Diarrhea appears to be an infectious type, although the precise cause and the sequence of pathogenic events remains unknown. The syndrome may include bacterial overgrowth, changes in GI motility, and cellular changes in the GIT. Identified intestinal organisms may differ from one region of the tropics to the next. As in CD, the intestinal villi may be abnormal, but the surface cell alterations are much less severe. The gastric mucosa is atrophied and inflamed, with diminished secretion of hydrochloric acid and intrinsic factor.

Medical Treatment

Treatment of tropical sprue typically includes use of broad-spectrum antibiotics, folic acid, fluid, and electrolytes.

Medical Nutrition Therapy

Nutrition management includes restoration and maintenance of fluids, electrolytes, macronutrients, and micronutrients, and introduction of a diet that is appropriate for the extent of malabsorption (see "Diarrhea" earlier in this chapter). Along with other nutrients, B_{12} and folate supplementation may be needed if deficiency is identified. Nutritional deficiency increases susceptibility to infectious agents, further aggravating the condition.

INTESTINAL BRUSH-BORDER ENZYME DEFICIENCIES

Intestinal enzyme deficiency states involve deficiencies of the brush-border disaccharidases that hydrolyze disaccharides at the mucosal cell membrane. Disaccharidase deficiencies may occur as (1) rare congenital defects such as the

BOX 29-7

Celiac Disease Resources

Support Groups

Gluten Intolerance Group
Phone: 206-246-6652
E-mail: info@gluten.net
Website: www.gluten.net

Canadian Celiac Association
Phone: 800-363-7296
E-mail: customerservice@celiac.ca
Website: www.celiac.ca

Celiac Disease Foundation
Phone: 818-990-2354
E-mail: cdf@celiac.org
Website: www.celiac.org

Celiac Sprue Association
Phone: 877-272-4272
E-mail: celiacs@csaceliacs.org
Website: www.csaceliacs.org

Medical Centers

Beth Israel Deaconess Celiac Center
Boston, Massachusetts
www.bidmc.harvard.edu/celiaccenter

University of Maryland Center for Celiac Research
Baltimore, Maryland
www.celiaccenter.org

Celiac Disease Center at Columbia University
New York, New York
www.celiacdiseasecenter.columbia.edu

University of Chicago Celiac Disease Program
Chicago, Illinois
www.celiacdisease.net

Other Celiac Organizations/Resources

National Foundation for Celiac Awareness
www.celiacawareness.org

Celiac listserv
www.enabling.org/ia/celiac

Gluten-free Restaurant Awareness Program
www.glutenfreerestaurants.org

Celiac Disease for Dummies, book by Ian Blumer and Sheila Crowe

Celiac Disease and Gluten-free Support Center
www.celiac.com

Clan Thompson Celiac Site (free newsletter)
www.clanthompson.com

Gluten Free Diet—A Comprehensive Resource Guide, book by Shelley Case

Real Life with Celiac Disease: Troubleshooting and Thriving Gluten Free, book by Melinda Dennis and Daniel Leffler

Adapted from Parrish CR, Krenitsky J, McCray S: University of Virginia Health System Nutrition Support Traineeship Syllabus, Charlottesville, Va, 2010, University of Virginia Health System.

sucrase, isomaltase, or lactase deficiencies seen in the newborn; (2) generalized forms secondary to diseases that damage the intestinal epithelium (e.g., Crohn's disease or CD); or, most commonly, (3) a genetically acquired form (e.g., lactase deficiency) that usually appears after childhood but can appear as early as 2 years of age. For this chapter, only lactose malabsorption is described in detail (see Chapter 44 for a discussion of inborn metabolic disorders).

Lactose Intolerance

Lactose intolerance is the syndrome of diarrhea, abdominal pain, flatulence, or bloating occurring after lactose consumption. Secondary lactose intolerance can develop as a consequence of infection of the small intestine, inflammatory disorders, HIV, or malnutrition. In children it is typically secondary to viral or bacterial infections. Lactose malabsorption is commonly associated with other GI disorders, such as IBS, which is not surprising because lactose intolerance is so common.

Of the adult worldwide population, 70%, especially African, Hispanic, Asian, South American, and Native American populations, demonstrate lactose malabsorption. However, the prevalence of lactose intolerance in the United States has not yet been accurately estimated because of limitations in the current studies (Suchy et al., 2010). Typically, lactase activity declines exponentially at weaning to about 10% of the neonatal value. Lactose malabsorption and intolerance has been reported to be low in children below age six, but increases throughout childhood, peaking at age 10-16.

There is little evidence that lactose intolerance increases with increasing adult age (Suchy et al, 2010). Even in adults who retain a high level of lactase levels (75% to 85% of white adults of Western European heritage), the quantity of lactase is approximately half that of other saccharidases such as sucrase, α-dextrinase, or glucoamylase. The decline of lactase is commonly known as **hypolactasia**; the adult form involves down-regulation after weaning (Järvelä 2005) and may have a relationship with an increased risk of colon cancer in some populations (Rasinperä et al. 2005). See *Focus On:* Lactose Intolerance—NOT an Uncommon Anomaly.

FOCUS ON

Lactose Intolerance—NOT an Uncommon Anomaly

When lactose intolerance was first described in 1963, it appeared to be an infrequent occurrence, arising only occasionally in the white population. Because the capacity to digest lactose was measured in people from a wide variety of ethnic and racial backgrounds, it soon became apparent that disappearance of the lactase enzyme shortly after weaning, or at least during early childhood, was actually the predominant (normal) condition in most of the world's population. With a few exceptions, the intestinal tracts of adult mammals produce little, if any, lactase after weaning (the milks of pinnipeds—seals, walruses, and sea lions—do not contain lactose).

The exception of lactose tolerance has attracted the interest of geographers and others concerned with the evolution of the world's population. A genetic mutation favoring lactose tolerance appears to have arisen approximately 10,000 years ago, when dairying was first introduced. Presumably, it would have occurred in places where milk consumption was encouraged because of some degree of dietary deprivation and in groups in which milk was not fermented before consumption (fermentation breaks down much of the lactose into monosaccharides). The mutation would have selectively endured, because it would promote greater health, survival, and reproduction of those who carried the gene.

It is proposed that the mutation occurred in more than one location and then accompanied migrations of populations throughout the world. It continues primarily among whites from northern Europe and in ethnic groups in India, Africa, and Mongolia. The highest frequency (97%) of lactose tolerance occurs in Sweden and Denmark, suggesting an increased selective advantage in those able to tolerate lactose related to the limited exposure to ultraviolet light typical of northern latitudes. Lactose favors calcium absorption, which is limited in the absence of vitamin D produced by skin exposure to sunlight (see Chapter 3).

Dairying was unknown in North America until the arrival of Europeans. Thus Native Americans and all of the non-European immigrants are among the 90% of the world's population who tolerate milk poorly, if at all. This has practical implications with respect to group feeding programs such as school breakfasts and lunches. However, many lactose-intolerant people are able to digest milk in small to moderate amounts (Shaukat et al., 2010).

Pathophysiology

When large amounts of lactose are consumed, especially by persons who have little remaining lactase enzyme or with concurrent GI problems, loose stools or diarrhea can occur. As is the case with any malabsorbed sugar, lactose may act osmotically, and increase fecal water, as well as provide a substrate for rapid fermentation by intestinal bacteria, which may result in bloating, flatulence, and cramps. Malabsorption of lactose is due to a deficiency of lactase, the enzyme that digests the sugar in milk. Lactose that is not hydrolyzed into galactose and glucose in the upper small intestine passes into the colon, where bacteria ferment it to SCFAs, carbon dioxide, and hydrogen gas.

Medical Treatment

Lactose malabsorption is diagnosed by (1) an abnormal hydrogen breath test, or (2) an abnormal lactose tolerance test. During a hydrogen breath test, the patient is given a standard dose of lactose after fasting, and breath hydrogen is measured. If lactose is not digested in the small intestine, it passes into the colon where it is fermented by microbes to SCFAs, CO_2, and hydrogen. Hydrogen is absorbed into the bloodstream and is exhaled through the lungs. The breath hydrogen test shows increased levels 60 to 90 minutes after lactose ingestion.

During a lactose tolerance test, a dose of lactose is given and if the individual has sufficient lactase enzyme, blood sugar will rise, reflecting the digestion of lactose to galactose and glucose. If the individual is lactose intolerant (lactase deficient) blood sugar will not rise because the lactose is not absorbed; it passes into the colon and GI symptoms may appear. The lactose tolerance test was originally based on an oral dose of lactose equivalent to the amount in 1 quart of milk (50 g). Recently, doses lower than 50 g of lactose have been used to approximate more closely the usual consumption of lactose from milk products.

Demonstrated lactose malabsorption does not always indicate a person will be symptomatic. Many factors play a role, including the amount of lactose ingested, the residual lactase activity, the ingestion of food in addition to lactose, the ability of the colonic bacteria to ferment lactose, and the sensitivity of the individual to the lactose fermentation products (Suchy et al., 2010). Consumption of small amounts should be of little consequence because the SCFAs are readily absorbed and the gases can be absorbed or passed. Larger amounts, usually greater than 12 g/day, consumed in a single food (the amount typically found in 240 mL of milk) may result in more substrate entering the colon than can be disposed of by normal processes (Suchy et al., 2010). Because serving sizes of milk drinks are increasing and more than one source of lactose might be consumed in the same meal, the amounts of lactose consumed may be more important than in years past.

Medical Nutrition Therapy

Management of lactose intolerance requires dietary change. The symptoms are alleviated by reduced consumption of lactose-containing foods. Persons who avoid dairy products may need calcium and vitamin D supplementation or must be careful to get nondairy sources of these nutrients. A completely lactose-free diet is not necessary in lactase-deficient persons. Most lactose maldigesters can consume some lactose (up to 12 g/day) without major symptoms, especially when taken with meals or in the form of cheeses or cultured dairy products (Shaukat et al., 2010); see Chapter 3 and Table 29-3.

Many adults with intolerance to moderate amounts of milk can ultimately adapt to and tolerate 12 g or more of lactose in milk (equivalent to 240 mL of full-lactose milk) when introduced gradually, in increments, over several weeks. Incremental or continuous exposure to increasing quantities of fermentable sugar can lead to improved tolerance, not as a consequence of increased lactase enzyme production but perhaps by altered colonic flora. This has been shown with lactulose, a nonabsorbed carbohydrate that is biochemically similar to lactose (Bezkorovainy 2001).

TABLE 29-3

Lactose Content of Common Foods

Product	Serving Size	Approximate Lactose Content (grams)
Milk (nonfat, 1%, 2% whole), chocolate milk, acidophilis milk, buttermilk	1 cup	10-12
Butter, margarine	1 tsp	trace
Cheese	1 ounce	0-2
• Cheddar, sharp	1 ounce	0
• American, swiss, parmesan	1 ounce	1
• Bleu cheese	1 ounce	2
Cottage cheese	½ cup	2-3
Cream (light), whipped cream	½ cup	3-4
Cream cheese	1 ounce	1
Evaporated milk	1 cup	24
Half-and-half	½ cup	5
Ice cream	½ cup	6
Ice milk	½ cup	9
Nonfat dry milk powder (unreconstituted)	1 cup	62
Sherbet, orange	½ cup	2
Sour cream	½ cup	4
Sweetened condensed milk, undiluted	1 cup	40
Yogurt, cultured, low-fat*	1 cup	5-10

*Note: Although yogurt does contain lactose, cultured yogurt is generally well tolerated by those with lactose intolerance

Individual differences in tolerance may relate to the state of colonic adaptation. Regular consumption of milk by lactase-deficient persons may increase the threshold at which diarrhea occurs.

Lactase enzyme and milk products treated with lactase enzyme (e.g., Lactaid) are available for lactase maldigesters who have discomfort with milk ingestion. Commercial lactase preparations may differ in their effectiveness. Fermented milk products, such as aged cheeses and yogurts, are well tolerated because the lactose content is low. Tolerance of yogurt may be the result of a microbial galactosidase in the bacterial culture that facilitates lactose digestion in the intestine. The presence of galactosidase depends on the brand and processing method. Because this microbial enzyme is sensitive to freezing, frozen yogurt may not be as well tolerated. Although the addition of probiotics may change this, evidence is lacking (Levri et al., 2005).

Fructose Malabsorption

Consumption of fructose in the United States, especially from fruit juices, fruit drinks, and HFCS in soft drinks and confections, has increased significantly in recent years. The human small intestine has a limited ability to absorb fructose, compared with the ability to rapidly and completely absorb glucose. Breath hydrogen testing has revealed that up to 75% of healthy people will incompletely absorb a large quantity of fructose (50 g) taken alone (Barrett and Gibson, 2007). Absorption of fructose is improved when it is ingested with glucose (such as in sucrose) because glucose absorption stimulates pathways for fructose absorption.

Pathophysiology

Although fructose malabsorption is common in healthy people, its appearance appears to depend on the amount of fructose ingested. In one study, more than 50% of people had a positive breath hydrogen test after a 25-g load, whereas 73% had a positive breath hydrogen test after a 50-g load (Beyer et al., 2005). Although some degree of fructose malabsorption may be normal, those with coexisting GI disorders may be more likely to experience GI symptoms after fructose ingestion. Patients with IBS and visceral hypersensitivity may be more sensitive to gas, distension, or pain from fructose malabsorption, whereas those with SBBO may experience symptoms from normal amounts of fructose.

Medical Nutrition Therapy

People with fructose malabsorption and those patients with GI conditions that experience symptoms of fructose malabsorption may not have problems with foods containing balanced amounts of glucose and fructose, but may need to limit or avoid foods containing large amounts of free fructose (Beyer et al., 2005). Pear, apple, mango, and Asian pear are notable in that they have substantially more "free fructose" (more fructose than glucose) (Barrett and Gibson, 2007). Additionally, most dried fruits and fruit juices may pose a problem in larger amounts because of the amount of fructose provided per serving. Foods sweetened with HFCS (as opposed to sucrose) are also more likely to cause symptoms. Hepatic fructose metabolism is similar to ethanol, in that they both serve as substrates for de novo lipogenesis, thus promoting hepatic insulin resistance, dyslipidemia, and hepatic steatosis (Lustig, 2010). The degree of fructose intolerance and tolerance to the symptoms of fructose malabsorption are so variable that tolerable intake of these foods must generally be individualized with each patient.

INFLAMMATORY BOWEL DISEASES

The two major forms of **inflammatory bowel disease (IBD)** are Crohn's disease and ulcerative colitis (UC). Both Crohn's disease and UC are relatively rare disorders, but they result in frequent use of health care resources. The prevalence is approximately 130 cases per 100,000 persons for Crohn's disease and 100 per 100,000 for UC. The onset of IBD occurs most often in patients 15 to 30 years of age, but for some it occurs later in adulthood. Both sexes are equally affected. IBD occurs more commonly in developed areas of the world, in urban compared with rural environments, and in northern compared with southern climates.

Crohn's disease and **ulcerative colitis (UC)** share some clinical characteristics, including diarrhea, fever, weight loss, anemia, food intolerances, malnutrition, growth failure, and extraintestinal manifestations (arthritic, dermatologic, and hepatic). In both forms of IBD, the risk of malignancy increases with the duration of the disease. The reasons for the increased risk are not firmly established but are likely related to the increased inflammatory and proliferative state and nutritional factors. Although malnutrition can occur in both forms of IBD, it is more of a lifelong concern in patients with Crohn's disease. The features that distinguish the forms of the disease in terms of genetic characteristics, clinical presentation, and treatment are discussed in Table 29-4.

Crohn's Disease and Ulcerative Colitis

Crohn's disease may involve any part of the GIT, but approximately 50% to 60% of cases involve both the distal ileum and the colon. Only the small intestine or only the colon is involved in 15% to 25% of cases. Disease activity in UC is limited to the large intestine and rectum. In Crohn's disease, segments of inflamed bowel may be separated by healthy segments, whereas in UC the disease process is continuous (Figure 29-2). Mucosal involvement in Crohn's disease is transmural in that it affects all layers of the mucosa; in UC the disease normally is limited to the mucosa. Crohn's disease is characterized by abscesses, fistulas, fibrosis, submucosal thickening, localized strictures, narrowed segments of bowel, and partial or complete obstruction of the intestinal lumen. Bleeding is more common in UC.

Pathophysiology

The cause of IBD is not completely understood, but it involves the interaction of the GI immunologic system and genetic and environmental factors. The genetic susceptibility is now recognized to be diverse, with a number of possible gene mutations that affect risk and characteristics of

TABLE 29-4

Ulcerative Colitis versus Crohn's Disease

	Ulcerative Colitis	Crohn's Disease
Presentation	Bloody diarrhea	Perianal disease, abdominal pain (65%), mass in abdomen
Gross Pathology	Rectum always involved Moves continuously, proximally from rectum Thin wall Few strictures Diffuse ulceration	Rectum may not be involved Can occur anywhere along gastrointestinal tract Not continuous: "skip lesions" Thick wall Strictures common Cobblestone appearance
Histopathology	No granulomas Low inflammation Deeper ulcers (hence named ulcerative) Pseudopolyps Abscesses in crypts	Granulomas More inflammation Shallow ulcers Fibrosis
Extraintestinal Manifestations	Sclerosing cholangitis Pyoderma gangrenosum	Erythema nodosum Migratory polyarthritis Gallstones
Complications	Toxic megacolon Cancer Strictures and fistulas are very rare	Malabsorption Cancer Strictures or fistulas Perianal disease

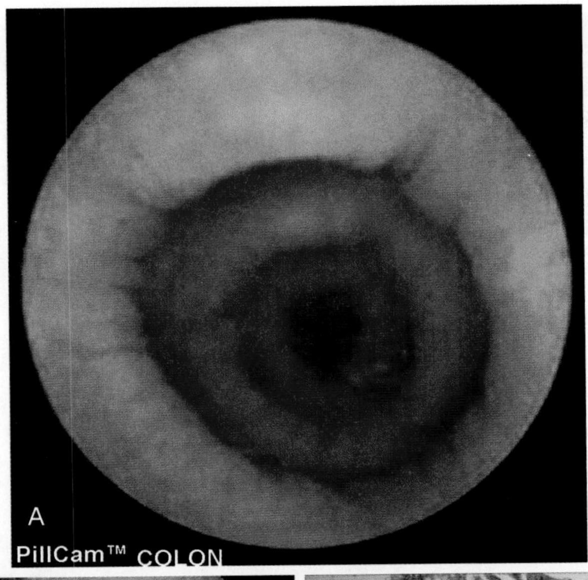

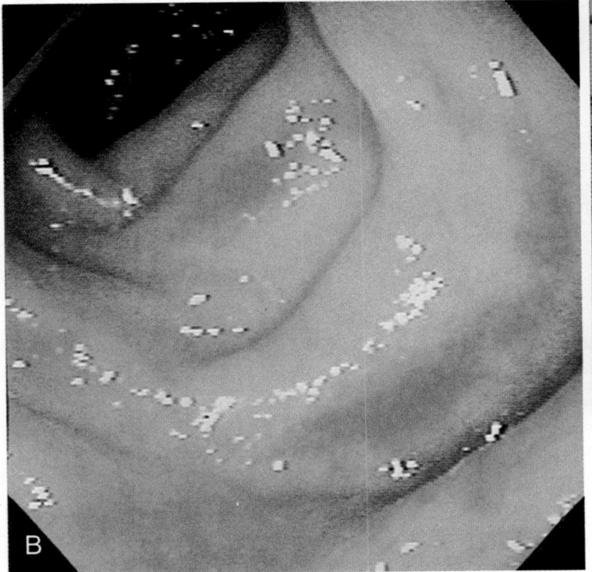

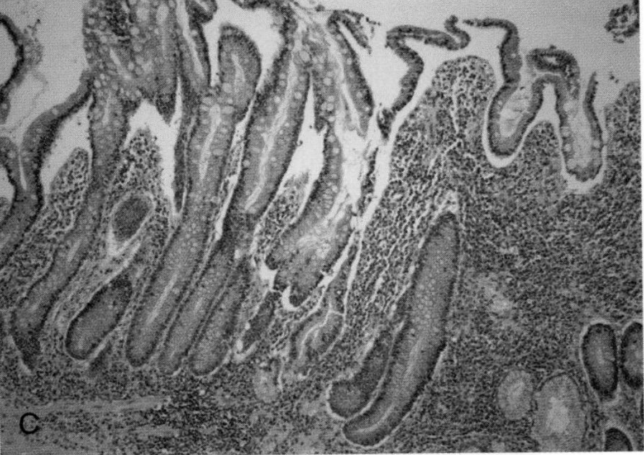

FIGURE 29-2 A, Normal colon, **B,** ulcerative colitis, **C,** Crohn's disease. *(A, From Fireman, Z., & Kopelman, Y. (2007). The colon—the latest terrain for capsule endoscopy. Digestive and Liver Disease, 39(10), 895-899. B, From Black JM, Hawks JH: Medical-surgical nursing: clinical management for positive outcomes, ed 8, St. Louis, 2009, Saunders. C, From McGowan, CE, Lagares-Garcia, JA, & and Bhattacharya, B. (2009). Retained capsule endoscope leading to the identification of small bowel adenocarcinoma in a patient with undiagnosed Crohn disease. Annals of Diagnostic Pathology, 13(6), 390-393.)*

the disease. The diversity in the genetic alterations among individuals may help explain differences in the onset, aggressiveness, complications, location, and responsiveness to different therapies as seen in the clinical setting (Shih and Targan, 2008). The major environmental factors include resident and transient microorganisms in the GIT and dietary components.

The genes affected (e.g., C677T mutation related to methylene-tetrahydrofolate reductase) normally play a role in the reactivity of the host GI immune system to luminal antigens such as those provided by intestinal flora and the diet. In animal models inflammatory disease does not occur without the intestinal flora. Normally, when an antigenic challenge or trauma occurs, the immune response rises to the occasion; it is then turned off and continues to be held in check after the challenge resolves. In IBD, increased exposure, decreased defense mechanisms, or decreased tolerance to some component of the GI microflora occur. Inappropriate inflammatory response and an inability to suppress it play primary roles in the disease. For example, one of the genes affected in Crohn's disease is the NOD_2/$CARD_{15}$ gene, which codes for a small peptide that interacts with a host of GI bacteria. Failure to produce that peptide may result in abnormal immune responses (Mueller and Macpherson, 2006).

The inflammatory response (e.g., increased cytokines and acute-phase proteins, increased GI permeability, increased proteases, and increased oxygen radicals and leukotrienes)

PATHOPHYSIOLOGY AND CARE MANAGEMENT ALGORITHM

Inflammatory Bowel Disease

ETIOLOGY

Genetic predisposition

Unknown "irritant" Viral? Bacterial? Autoimmune?

Abnormal activation of the mucosal immune response. Secondary systemic response

PATHOPHYSIOLOGY

Inflammatory Response

Damage to the cells of the small and/or large intestine with malabsorption, ulceration, or stricture

- Diarrhea
- Weight loss
- Poor growth
- Hyperhomocysteinemia
- Partial GI obstructions

MANAGEMENT

Medical Management

- Corticosteroids
- Antiinflammatory agents
- Immunosuppressants
- Antibiotics
- Anticytokine medications

Surgical Management

- Bowel resection that can result in short bowel syndrome (SBS)

Nutrition Management

- Oral enteral formula (tube-feed if necessary)
- Use of foods that are well tolerated
- Parenteral nutrition in patients with severe disease or obstruction
- Multivitamin supplement containing folic acid, B_{12}, and B_6
- ω-3 fatty acid supplementation
- Consider use of prebiotics and probiotics
- Modify fiber intake as necessary
- Tests for food intolerances

results in GI tissue damage (Sanders, 2005). In IBD either the regulatory mechanisms are defective or the factors perpetuating the immune and acute-phase responses are enhanced, leading to tissue fibrosis and destruction. The clinical course of the disease may be mild and episodic or severe and unremitting (see *Pathophysiology and Care Management Algorithm*: Inflammatory Bowel Disease).

Diet is an environmental factor that may trigger relapses of IBD. Foods, microbes, individual nutrients, and incidental contaminants provide a huge number of potential antigens, especially considering the complexity and diversity of the modern diet. Malnutrition can affect the function and effectiveness of the mucosal, cellular, and immune barriers; diet can also affect the type and relative composition of the resident microflora. Several nutrients (e.g., dietary lipids) can affect the intensity of the inflammatory response.

Food allergies and other immunologic reactions to specific foods have been considered in the pathogenesis of IBD and its symptoms; however, the incidence of documented food allergies, compared with food intolerances, is relatively small. The permeability of the intestinal wall to molecules of food and cell fragments is likely increased in inflammatory states, allowing the potential for increased interaction of antigens with host immune systems (Müller et al., 2005).

Food intolerances occur more often in persons with IBD than in the population at large, but the patterns are not consistent among individuals or even between exposures from one time to the next. Reasons for specific and nonspecific food intolerances are abundant and are related to the severity, location, and complications associated with the disease process. Partial GI obstructions, malabsorption, diarrhea, altered GI transit, increased secretions, food aversions, and associations are but a few of the problems experienced by persons with IBD. However, neither food allergies nor intolerances fully explain the onset or manifestations in all patients (see Chapter 27).

Medical Management

The goals of treatment in IBD are to induce and maintain remission and to improve nutrition status. Treatment of the primary GI manifestations appears to correct most of the extraintestinal features of the disease as well. The most effective medical agents include corticosteroids, antiinflammatory agents (aminosalicylates), immunosuppressive agents (cyclosporine, azathioprine, mercaptopurine), antibiotics (ciprofloxacin and metronidazole), and monoclonal tumor necrosis factor antagonists (anti-TNF) (infliximab, adalimumab, certolizumab, and natalizumab), agents that inactivate one of the primary inflammatory cytokines. Anti-TNF is normally used in severe cases of Crohn's disease and fistulas, but it has not been shown to be effective in UC.

Investigations of various treatment modalities for the acute and chronic stages of IBD are ongoing, and include new forms of existing drugs, as well as new agents targeted to regulate cytokines, eicosanoids, or other mediators of the inflammatory and acute-phase response (Caprilli et al., 2006; Travis et al., 2006). ω-3 fatty acid supplements (fish oil capsules) in Crohn's disease significantly reduce disease activity (Turner et al., 2009). Use of fish oil supplements in UC appears to result in a significant medication-sparing effect, with reductions in disease activity and increased time in remission reported (Seidner et al., 2005). Use of foods and supplements containing prebiotics and probiotic cultures are being investigated because each has the potential to alter both the GI microflora and the immunologic response at the gut level (Dotan and Rachmilewitz, 2005).

Surgical Management

In Crohn's disease, surgery may be necessary to repair strictures or remove portions of the bowel when medical management fails. Approximately 50% to 70% of persons with Crohn's disease will undergo surgery related to the disease. Surgery does not cure Crohn's disease, and recurrence often occurs within 1 to 3 years of surgery. The chance of needing subsequent surgery in the patient's life is approximately 30% to 70%, depending on the type of surgery and the age at first operation. Major resections of the intestine may result in varying degrees of malabsorption of fluid and nutrients. In extreme cases patients may have extensive or multiple resections, resulting in short-bowel syndrome (SBS) and dependence on PN to maintain adequate nutrient intake and hydration.

With UC, approximately 20% of patients have a colectomy and removal of the colon, and this resolves the disease. Inflammation does not occur in the remaining GIT. Whether a colectomy is necessary depends on the severity of the disease and indicators of increased cancer risk. After a colectomy for UC, surgeons may create an ileostomy with an external collection pouch and an internal abdominal reservoir fashioned with a segment of ileum or an ileoanal pouch, which spares the rectum, to serve as a reservoir for stool. The internal Koch pouch may also be used (see Chapter 14).

Medical Nutrition Therapy

Persons with IBD are at increased risk of nutrition problems for a host of reasons related to the disease and its treatment. Thus the primary goal is to restore and maintain the nutrition status of the individual patient. Foods, dietary and micronutrient supplements, enteral and PN may all be used to accomplish that mission. Oral diet and the other means of nutrition support may change during remissions and exacerbations of the disease.

Persons with IBD often have fears and misconceptions regarding GI symptoms and the role of food. Patients are also often confused by dietary advice from associates, various media, and health care providers. Education is a key form of nutrition intervention. There is no single dietary regimen for reducing symptoms or decreasing the flares in IBD. Diet and specific nutrients play a supportive role in maintaining nutrition status, limiting symptom exacerbations, and supporting growth in pediatric patients.

The ability of parenteral or enteral nutrition to induce remission of IBD has been debated for several years. Evaluation is confounded by the natural course of IBD with exacerbations and remissions, and by the genetic diversity of the patients. Studies have generally concluded that (1) nutrition support may bring about some clinical remission when used as a sole source of treatment; (2) "complete bowel rest" using PN is not necessarily required; (3) enteral nutrition has the potential to feed the intestinal epithelium and alter GI flora and is the preferred route of nutrition support; (4) enteral nutrition may temper some elements of the inflammatory process, serve as a valuable source of nutrients needed for restoration of GI defects, and be steroid sparing; (5) children benefit from the use of enteral nutrition to maintain growth and reduce the dependence on steroids that may affect growth and bone disease (Dray and Marteau, 2005; Lochs, 2006; Sanderson and Croft, 2005). Patients and caretakers must be very committed when using enteral nutrition formulas or tube feeding because it takes 4 to 8 weeks before one sees the clinical effects.

Timely nutritional support is a vital component of therapy to restore and maintain nutritional health. Malnutrition itself compromises digestive and absorptive function by increasing the permeability of the GIT to potential inflammatory agents. PN is not as nutritionally complete, has increased risk of infectious complications, and is more expensive than enteral nutrition. However, PN may be required in patients with persistent bowel obstruction, fistulas, and major GI resections that result in SBS where enteral nutrition is not possible.

Energy needs of patients with IBD are not greatly increased (unless weight gain is desired). Generally when disease activity increases basal metabolic rate, physical activity is greatly curtailed and overall energy needs are not substantially changed.

Protein requirements may be increased, depending on the severity and stage of the disease and the restoration requirements. Inflammation and treatment with corticosteroids induce a negative nitrogen balance and cause a loss of lean muscle mass. Protein losses also occur in areas of inflamed and ulcerated intestinal mucosa via defects in epithelial tight junctions. See Fig. 39-3 in Chapter 39. To maintain positive nitrogen balance, 1.3-1.5 g/kg/day of protein is recommended.

Supplemental vitamins, especially folate, B_6, and B_{12}, may be needed as well as minerals and trace elements to replace stores or for maintenance because of maldigestion, malabsorption, drug-nutrient interactions, or inadequate intake (Zezos et al., 2005). Diarrhea can aggravate losses of zinc, potassium, and selenium. Patients who receive intermittent corticosteroids may need supplemental calcium and vitamin D. Patients with IBD are at increased risk of osteopenia and osteoporosis; 25-OH vitamin D levels and bone density should be routinely monitored.

In daily life people with IBD may have intermittent "flares" of the disease characterized by partial obstructions, nausea, abdominal pain, bloating, or diarrhea. Many patients report specific, individualized food intolerances. Patients are sometimes advised to eliminate the foods they suspect are responsible for the intolerance. Often, the patient becomes increasingly frustrated as the diet becomes progressively limited and symptoms still do not resolve. Malnutrition is a significant risk in patients with IBD, and an overly restricted diet only increases the likelihood of malnutrition and weight loss.

During acute and severe exacerbations of the disease, the diet is tailored to the individual patient. In patients with rapid intestinal transit, extensive bowel resections, or extensive small bowel disease, absorption may be compromised. Here, excessive intake of lactose, fructose, or sorbitol may contribute to abdominal cramping, gas, and diarrhea; and high fat intake may result in steatorrhea. However, the incidence of lactose intolerance is no greater in patients with IBD than in the general population. Patients with IBD who tolerate lactose should not restrict lactose-containing foods because they can be a valuable source of high quality protein, calcium, and vitamin D.

Patients with strictures or partial bowel obstruction benefit from a reduction in dietary fiber or limited food particle size. Small, frequent feedings may be tolerated better than large meals. Small amounts of isotonic, liquid oral supplements may be valuable in restoring intake without provoking symptoms. In cases in which fat malabsorption is likely, supplementation with foods made with **medium-chain triglycerides (MCTs)** may be useful in adding calories and serving as a vehicle for fat-soluble nutrients. However, these products are expensive and may be less effective than more basic treatments.

Factors associated with of the development of IBD in epidemiologic studies include increased sucrose intake, lack of fruits and vegetables, a low intake of dietary fiber, use of red meat and alcohol, and altered ω-6/ω-3 fatty acid ratios. Yet dietary interventions to modify these factors during IBD flares have not resulted in significant improvements (Rajendran and Kumar, 2010).

The same foods that are responsible for GI symptoms (gas, bloating, and diarrhea) in a normal, healthy population are likely to be the triggers for the same symptoms in patients with mild stages of IBD or those in remission.

Patients receive nutritional information from a variety of sources, including support groups, Internet news groups, the audio and printed media, well-meaning friends, and food supplement salespersons. The information is sometimes inaccurate or exaggerated, or it may pertain only to one individual's situation. The health care provider can help patients sort out the role of foods in normal, everyday GI disturbances and in IBD and teach them how to evaluate valid nutrition information from unproven or exaggerated claims. Patients' participation in the management of their disease may help to reduce not only the symptoms of the disease but the associated anxiety level as well.

Probiotic foods and supplements have been investigated as potential therapeutic agents for IBD because of their ability to modify the microbial flora and modulate gut inflammatory response. High-dose probiotic supplements (e.g., VSL#3) improved disease activity in patients with UC who had **pouchitis**, inflammation in the ileal pouch surgically formed after colectomy (Holubar et al., 2010). However, a different probiotic supplement at a lower dose did not significantly reduce symptoms (Holubar et al., 2010). Probiotic supplements also appear to be useful for induction and extension of remissions in pediatric and adult UC (Guandalini, 2010; Mallon et al., 2007).

Although probiotics appear useful in UC, probiotic studies to date have not demonstrated significant improvement in Crohn's disease activity in adults or pediatric patients, nor do probiotic supplements appear to prolong remission in Crohn's disease (Butterworth et al., 2008; Guandalini, 2010).

Regular intake of prebiotic foods such as oligosaccharides, fermentable fibers, and resistant starches can alter the mixture of microorganisms in the colonic flora, feeding lactobacillus and bifidobacteria to provide competition to and theoretically suppress pathogenic or opportunistic microflora. Additionally, fermentation of prebiotics leads to increased production of SCFAs, theoretically creating a more acidic and less favorable environment for opportunistic bacteria.

Use of probiotics and prebiotics may serve to prevent small intestine bacterial overgrowth in predisposed individuals and to treat diarrhea. Additional study is needed to identify the dose, the most effective prebiotic and probiotic foods, the form in which they can be used for therapeutic and maintenance purposes, and their relative value compared with other therapies (Penner et al., 2005).

Microscopic Colitis

Injury of the colon caused by UC, Crohn's disease, infections, radiation injury, and ischemic insult to the colon all present with abnormalities such as edema, redness, bleeding, or ulcerations that are visible on colonoscopy examination. **Microscopic colitis** is characterized by inflammation that is not visible by inspection of the colon during colonoscopy, and is only apparent when the colon's lining is biopsied and then examined under a microscope.

There are two types of microscopic colitis. In lymphocytic colitis, there is an accumulation of lymphocytes within the lining of the colon. In collagenous colitis, there is also a layer of collagen (like scar tissue) just below the lining. Some experts believe that lymphocytic colitis and collagenous colitis represent different stages of the same disease. Symptoms include chronic, watery diarrhea, mild abdominal cramps, and pain.

More than 30% of patients report weight loss (Simondi et al., 2010). Patients with microscopic colitis can have diarrhea for months or years before the diagnosis is made. The cause of microscopic colitis is unknown. Microscopic colitis appears more frequently in patients aged 60-70 years, and collagenous colitis occurs more frequently in females (Jobse et al., 2009; Tysk et al., 2008).

Patients with CD are 70 times more likely than the normal population to develop microscopic colitis (Green et al., 2009). Patients with CD and microscopic colitis have more severe villous atrophy and frequently require steroids or immunosuppressant therapies in addition to a GF diet to control diarrhea. Research is underway to determine possible effective treatments for microscopic colitis, including corticosteroids and immunosuppressive agents. Medical nutrition therapy is supportive in nature with efforts to maintain weight and nutrition status, avoid symptom exacerbation, and maintain hydration.

Irritable Bowel Syndrome

Irritable bowel syndrome (IBS) is characterized by chronically recurring abdominal discomfort or pain and altered bowel habits. Other common symptoms include bloating, feelings of incomplete evacuation, presence of mucus in the stool, straining or increased urgency (depending on the type of presentation), and increased GI distress associated with psychosocial distress.

IBS is one of the most common reasons for primary care visits and consultations with gastroenterologists in the United States. IBS occurs in approximately 15% of women and 10% of men; however, it is estimated that only 25% to 50% of those with symptoms actually seek treatment. Typically, symptoms first occur between adolescence and the fourth decade of life, but many persons do not bring the problem to the attention of a physician. Persons with IBS often have increased absenteeism from school and work, decreased productivity, increased health care costs, and decreased quality of life as a result of their symptoms.

Diagnosis is based on international consensus criteria (Rome criteria) and diagnostic algorithms that help separate other medical or surgical disorders that manifest with similar symptoms (Malagelada, 2006). According to the criteria, symptoms of abdominal discomfort must be present for at least 3 days per month for the past 3 months, include at least two of three features: (1) discomfort relieved by defecation, (2) onset associated with a change in frequency of stool, and (3) onset associated with a change in form of the stool. Diagnosis further categorizes the syndrome into one of three subtypes: diarrhea predominant, constipation predominant, or mixed. Small intestinal bacterial overgrowth (SIBO) has been described in a significant number of patients with IBS, particularly diarrhea-predominant IBS (Ghoshal et al., 2010a). Positive hydrogen or lactulose breath tests have been reported in 22% to 54% of patients with IBS (Ford and Spiegel, 2009; Lombardo et al., 2010). Prevalence of CD has been reported as fourfold greater in individuals diagnosed with IBS than in individuals without IBS, likely because of misdiagnosis of IBS, and screening for CD has been determined to be cost-effective in this population (Ford and Spiegel, 2009).

Pathophysiology

The normal enteric nervous system is sensitive to the presence, chemical composition, and volume of foods in the GIT, and also responds to a variety of inputs from the central nervous system (see Chapter 1). Increased awareness and sensitivity of the GIT to internal and external stimuli and altered motility appear to be primary features of IBS (Malagelada, 2006). Persons with IBS have heightened enteric sensitivity and motility in response to usual GI and environmental stimuli. They react more significantly than normal persons to intestinal distention, dietary changes, and psychosocial factors. IBS is considered a functional disorder, because it is a diagnosis by exclusion and is based on symptoms, not structural or biochemical abnormality. It is commonly described as a "brain-gut disorder" because of the association with serotonin.

The mediators of GI responses may be abnormal secretion of peptide hormones or signaling agents (e.g., neurotransmitters secreted in response to the hormones); but altered handling of intestinal gas, microbial flora, SIBO, and other contributors affect some forms of IBS. Post-infectious IBS typically appears abruptly after gastroenteritis and is essentially managed with the same approach as other forms of IBS (Ghoshal et al., 2010b). In addition to stress and dietary patterns, factors that may worsen symptoms include (1) excess use of laxatives and other over-the-counter medications; (2) antibiotics; (3) caffeine; (4) previous GI illness; and (5) lack of regularity in sleep, rest, and fluid intake. In patients with a strong family history of allergy, hypersensitivity to certain foods may aggravate IBS; a trial of food elimination and challenge may be justified (see Chapter 27).

Medical Management

The first step in management of IBS and other functional GI disorders includes first validating the reality of the patient's complaints and establishing an effective clinician-patient relationship. Care should be tailored to help the patient deal with the symptoms and the factors that may trigger them. Education, medications, pain management, counseling, and diet each play a role in care. Depending on the predominant pattern and severity of the symptoms, medications may include those that affect GI motility, visceral hypersensitivity, or psychological symptoms. Relaxation and stress-reduction techniques may also be useful.

Osmotic laxatives are commonly used to treat constipation, although they have not been thoroughly studied. Agents that affect how the GIT responds to serotonin (5-hydroxytryptophane [5-HT], a major mediator in the sensory and motility functions of the enteric nervous system) are under investigation. Two major 5-HT receptors, 5-HT$_3$ antagonists, and 5-HT$_4$ agonists have been targeted for use in treating patients with different forms of IBS. 5-HT$_3$ antagonists have shown some success in women with diarrhea-predominant IBS, whereas 5-HT$_4$ agonists serve as prokinetic agents that stimulate peristalsis of the small and large intestine and are used in the management of constipation-predominant IBS. A number of other agents are being evaluated. Low-dose loperamide is commonly effective in patients who have diarrhea-predominant IBS.

Antispasmotic agents have been used to treat pain associated with IBS, but have not been thoroughly studied in randomized trials. Tricyclic antidepressants in low doses have been shown to reduce symptoms in some cases.

Medical Nutrition Therapy

The goals of nutrition therapy for IBS are to ensure adequate nutrient intake, tailor the diet for the specific GI pattern of IBS, and explain the potential roles of foods in the management of symptoms. There is little scientific evidence for restricting particular foods. Large meals and certain foods may be poorly tolerated, such as excess quantities of dietary fat, caffeine, lactose, fructose, sorbitol, and alcohol. This is especially true in persons with diarrhea-predominant IBS or mixed IBS.

Most fiber studies in the IBS population to date have numerous short-comings, such as a strong placebo effect (Heizer et al., 2009). Some patients with constipation-predominant IBS may benefit from fiber in the form of bulk laxatives (e.g., psyllium) (Bijkerk et al., 2009). Supplementation of insoluble fiber, such as wheat bran, may actually worsen symptoms. Consumption of adequate fluid is recommended, especially when powdered fiber supplements are used.

Food intolerances and allergies should be evaluated objectively because patients may unnecessarily limit large groups of foods, resulting in frustration and an incomplete diet (Kalliomäki, 2005; Seibold, 2005). In clinical practice, it can be very difficult to determine if a patient's symptoms are truly from an adverse reaction to food. Systematically eliminating and reintroducing foods can be useful in determining if a patient is truly reacting to a food. A double-blind, placebo-controlled food challenge may be helpful but it is time-consuming and labor intensive (Heizer et al., 2009). See Chapter 27.

Foods with fiber, resistant starches, and oligosaccharides may serve as prebiotic foods, which favor the maintenance of healthy microflora and resistance to pathogenic infections. Results of initial studies on the use of prebiotic and probiotic supplements have been mixed. More studies comparing types of organisms, doses, and subtypes of IBS are needed. Additionally, potential benefits of prebiotics may be outweighed by poor absorption.

Some probiotic supplements may offer benefits in IBS. However, the randomized controlled trials that have been conducted have been small and have produced variable results depending on the type and dose of the probiotic as well as the individual population studied (Aragon et al., 2010). One study evaluated different doses of *Bifidobacterium infantis* in women diagnosed with IBS (Whorwell et al., 2006). The group treated with the higher dose of probiotic reported a significant improvement in abdominal pain or discomfort, bloating and distension, sensation of incomplete evacuation, passage of gas, straining, and bowel habit satisfaction.

A diet low in fermentable oligo-, di-, and monosaccharides and polyols (**FODMAPs**) has been theorized to be useful (Shepherd et al., 2008). The low FODMAP diet limits foods that contain fructose, lactose, fructo- and galactooligosaccharides (fructans and galactans), and sugar alcohols (sorbitol, mannitol, xylitol and maltitol). FODMAPs are poorly absorbed in the small intestine, highly osmotic, and rapidly fermented by bacteria. Limiting the amount of FODMAPs per meal has been shown to reduce GI symptoms in patients with IBS (Gibson and Shepherd 2010). However, a cutoff value for acceptable amounts of FODMAPs has not been well defined, and is likely patient specific. See Table 29-5 for foods containing FODMAPs as well as dietary instructions.

Peppermint oil also shows promise. One randomized controlled trial showed significant improvement in abdominal symptoms for individuals supplementing with peppermint oil (Ford et al., 2008).

TABLE 29-5

Foods Containing FODMAPs, and Low FODMAP Diet Instructions

FODMAP	High FODMAP food
Fructose	Fruits: apples, pears, peaches, mango, sugar snap peas, watermelon, canned fruit in natural juice, dried fruit, fruit juice Sweeteners: honey, high fructose corn syrup,
Lactose	Milk (cow, goat and sheep), ice cream, soft cheeses (e.g., ricotta, cottage cheese)
Oligosaccharides (fructans or galactans)	Vegetables: artichokes, asparagus, beets, brussel sprouts, broccoli, cabbage, fennel, garlic, leeks, okra, onions, peas, shallots Cereals: wheat and rye (in large amounts) Legumes: chickpeas, lentils, kidney beans, baked beans Fruits: watermelon, apples, peaches, rambutan, persimmon
Polyols	Fruits: apples, apricots, cherries, longon, lychee, pears, nectarine, peaches, plums, prunes, watermelon Vegetables: avocado, cauliflower, mushrooms, snow peas Sweeteners: sorbitol, mannitol, maltitol, xylitol, and others ending in "-ol"

Low FODMAP Diet Instructions

- Avoid foods that contain fructose in excess of glucose (unless fructose malabsorption is not demonstrated).
- Try ingesting a source of glucose with fructose-containing foods (i.e., sucrose contains equal amounts of glucose and fructose).
- Limit amount of fructose at any one meal.
- Avoid foods that contain significant amounts of fructans and galactans.
- Restrict lactose-containing foods (unless lactose malabsorption is not demonstrated).
- Avoid polyol-containing foods.

Adapted from Gibson PR, Shepherd SJ: Evidence-based dietary management of functional gastrointestinal symptoms: the FODMAP approach, J Gastroenterol Hepatol 25:252, 2010.

FODMAP, Fermentable oligo-, di-, and monosaccharides and polyols.

The nutrition practitioner can work with the person with IBS to identify his or her concerns and perceptions, review the characteristics of the disease and the potential role of various foods, and teach the client how to reduce food-related symptoms. Sometimes clients become trapped in a vicious cycle in which anxiety about food, GI distress, and social embarrassment leaves them with an unnecessarily restrictive diet, declining nutrition status, and worsening symptoms. Reassurance and the gradual return to a good diet with limitations of only irritating foods can greatly improve quality of life.

Diverticular Disease

Diverticulosis is the condition of having saclike herniations (diverticula) in the colonic wall. The incidence of diverticulosis increases with age. Sigmoid involvement occurs in almost all cases; right-sided colonic involvement occurs in Asians, but it is rare in whites. Most persons are asymptomatic. However, 15% to 20 % of persons with diverticulosis experience colicky pain; approximately 5% experience inflammation and diverticulitis.

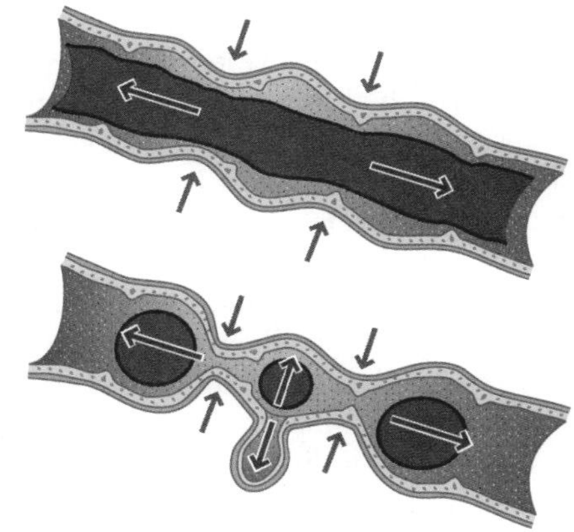

FIGURE 29-3 Mechanism by which low-fiber, low-bulk diets might generate diverticula. Where the colon contents are bulky *(top)*, muscular contractions exert pressure longitudinally. If the fecal contents are small in diameter *(bottom)*, contractions can produce occlusion and exert pressure against the colon wall, which may produce a diverticular hernia.

Pathophysiology

The cause of diverticulosis has not been clearly elucidated. A combination of colonic structure, motility, genetics, and a lifelong low-fiber intake results in increased intracolonic pressures (Parra-Blanco, 2006; Salzman and Lillie, 2005). The pressures result from attempts to propel small, dry, hard fecal material through the lumen of the bowel. Theoretically, circular muscles completely close around the fecal material when the stools are small and longitudinal muscles contract, attempting to push the contents distally. Increased pressure allows herniations of the mucosal wall to develop through weaker segments of the colon. See Fig. 29-3. This theory is supported by multiple human and animal studies. In general, diverticular disease is relatively rare in countries where a high-fiber diet is part of the lifelong pattern, and increasing where there is "Westernization" of the diet with high intake of refined foods (Salzman and Lillie, 2005). Lack of exercise may also contribute.

Medical and Surgical Treatment

Complications of diverticular disease range from painless, mild bleeding and altered bowel habits to diverticulitis. **Diverticulitis** includes a spectrum of inflammation, abscess formation, acute perforation, acute bleeding, obstruction, and sepsis. Treatment typically includes antibiotics and oral intake as tolerated. A modified diet or bowel rest may be indicated based on the patient's degree of illness, desire to eat, and likelihood of imminent surgery (Salzman and Lillie, 2005). Colon cleansers that cause hard stools, constipation, and straining are not recommended. Approximately 10% to 25% of patients with diverticulosis develop diverticulitis, and approximately one fourth to one third of those admitted to hospitals require surgery.

Medical Nutrition Therapy

At one time it was thought that "roughage" (dietary fiber) aggravated diverticular disease; thus the classic diet therapy was low in fiber. It is now recognized that a high-fiber diet, in combination with adequate hydration, promotes soft, bulky stools that pass more swiftly and require less straining with defecation. High-fiber intakes have been found to relieve symptoms for most patients, and exercise appears to aid in preventing constipation.

Patients may require extensive encouragement to adopt the high-fiber approach. Fiber intake should be increased gradually because it may cause bloating or gas. These side effects usually disappear within 2 to 3 weeks. Recommended intakes of dietary fiber, preferably from foods, are 25 g/day for adult women and 38 g/day for men. If an individual cannot or will not consume the necessary amount of fiber, methylcellulose and psyllium fiber supplements have been used with good results. Adequate fluid intake (e.g., 2 to 3 L daily) should accompany the high-fiber intake.

During an acute flare of diverticulitis, a low-residue diet or PN may be required initially, followed by a gradual return to a high-fiber diet. Historically, health care providers have advised patients with diverticular disease to avoid seeds, nuts, or skins of plant matter to prevent complications or after bouts of diverticulitis. A recent 18-year study found no association between nut, corn, or popcorn consumption and diverticular bleeding (Strate et al., 2008). In fact, the researchers reported an inverse association between nut and popcorn consumption and the risk of diverticulitis. There is no data to support restriction.

Intestinal Polyps and Colon Cancer

In the United States and worldwide, colorectal cancer is the third most common cancer in adults and is also the second most common cause of cancer death. However, the number of new cases of colon cancer decreased 3% for men and 2.2% for women during the past decade. There are approximately 142,500 new cases of colorectal cancer per year, and the incidence is higher in men than women (National Cancer Institute and U.S. National Institutes of Health, 2010). The highest rates are seen in whites of northern European origin. Rates in Africa and Asia are lower, but they tend to rise with migration and westernization.

Pathophysiology

Factors that increase the risk of colorectal cancer include family history, long-term presence of IBD, familial polyposis, adenomatous polyps, and several dietary components. Polyps are considered precursors of colon cancers (see Chapter 37 for more details). Patterns of dietary practices rather than specific nutrients may be more predictive of the risk of developing colorectal cancer. Dietary risk factors include increased meat, fat, and alcohol intake; obesity; and inadequate intake of several micronutrients, fruits, vegetables, and whole grains. Food preparation methods may also influence the carcinogenic potential of meats and fatty foods (McGarr et al., 2005; Raju and Cruz-Correa, 2006).

Use of aspirin and nonsteroidal antiinflammatory agents and exercise appear to be protective (Raju and Cruz-Correa, 2006).

Micronutrients considered protective in epidemiologic and cohort studies include vitamin D, folate, calcium, and selenium. There have been several types of supportive studies regarding the protective role of fruits and vegetables as a group, individual plant foods, high-fiber grains, ω-3 fatty acids, several antioxidants, and phytochemicals; but the data are not always consistent. The use of prebiotics and probiotics alters colonic microflora, induces glutathione transferase, increases butyrate content of the stool, reduces toxic and genotoxic compounds, and in animal models reduces the development of some precancerous lesions (McGarr et al., 2005).

Medical Management

Patients diagnosed with colorectal polyps or cancer may require moderate to significant interventions, including medications, radiation therapy, chemotherapy, colonic surgery, or enteral or PN support.

Medical Nutrition Therapy

Recommendations from cancer organizations that publish public health messages or consensus statements include notations that target colon cancer. These recommendations typically include sufficient exercise; weight maintenance or reduction; modest and balanced intake of lipids; adequate intake of micronutrients from fruits, vegetables, legumes, whole grains, and dairy products; and limited use of alcohol. Supplements are normally encouraged if the diet is not adequate. The diet for cancer survivors typically follows these prevention guidelines (see Chapter 37).

NUTRITIONAL CONSEQUENCES OF INTESTINAL SURGERY

Small Bowel Resections and Short-Bowel Syndrome

Short-bowel syndrome (SBS) can be defined as inadequate absorptive capacity resulting from reduced length or decreased functional bowel after resection. A loss of 70% to 75% of small bowel usually results in SBS, defined as 100-120 cm of small bowel without a colon, or 50 cm of small bowel with the colon remaining. A more practical definition of SBS is the inability to maintain nutrition and hydration needs with normal fluid and food intake, regardless of bowel length.

Patients with SBS often have complex fluid, electrolyte, and nutritional management issues (Parrish, 2005). Consequences of SBS include malabsorption of micronutrients and macronutrients, frequent diarrhea, steatorrhea, dehydration, electrolyte imbalances, weight loss, and growth failure in children. Other complications include gastric hypersecretion, oxalate renal stones, and cholesterol gallstones. Individuals who eventually need long-term PN have increased risk of catheter infection, sepsis, cholestasis, and liver disease, and reduced quality of life associated with chronic intravenous nutrition support (Diamanti et al., 2007).

Pathophysiology

The most common reasons for major resections of the intestine in adults include Crohn's disease, radiation enteritis, mesenteric infarct, malignant disease, and volvulus (Parrish, 2005). In the pediatric population most cases of SBS result from congenital anomalies of the GIT, atresia, volvulus, or necrotizing enterocolitis.

Duodenal Resection. Resections of the duodenum (≈10 in) are rare, which is fortunate as it is the preferred site for absorption of key nutrients such as iron, zinc, copper, and folate. The duodenum is a key player in the digestion and absorption of nutrients, as it is the portal of entry for pancreatic enzymes and bile salts. See Chapter 1.

Jejunal Resections. The jejunum (6-10 ft) is responsible for a large portion of nutrient absorption. Normally most digestion and absorption of food and nutrients occurs in the first 100 cm of small intestine. Jejunal enterohormones play key roles in digestion and absorption. Cholecystokinin (CCK) stimulates pancreatic secretion and gallbladder contraction, and secretin stimulates secretion of bicarbonate from the pancreas. Gastric inhibitory peptide slows gastric secretion and gastric motility, whereas vasoactive inhibitory peptide inhibits gastric and bicarbonate secretion. What remains to be digested or fermented and absorbed are small amounts of sugars, resistant starch, fiber, lipids, dietary fiber, and fluids. After jejunal resections, the ileum typically adapts to perform the functions of the jejunum. The motility of the ileum is comparatively slow, and hormones, secreted in the ileum and colon help to slow gastric emptying and secretions. Because jejunal resections result in reduced surface area and faster intestinal transit, the functional reserve for absorption of micronutrients, excess amounts of sugars (especially lactose), and lipids is reduced.

Ileal Resections. Significant resections of the ileum, especially the distal ileum, produce major nutritional and medical complications. The distal ileum is the only site for absorption of bile salts and the vitamin B_{12}-intrinsic factor complex. The ileum also absorbs a major portion of the 7-10 L of fluid ingested and secreted into the GIT daily (see Chapter 1). The ileocecal valve, at the junction of the ileum and cecum, maximizes nutrient absorption by controlling the rate of passage of ileal contents into the colon and preventing reflux of colonic bacteria, which may decrease risk for SIBO.

Although malabsorption of bile salts may appear to be benign, it creates a cascade of consequences. If the ileum cannot "recycle" bile salts secreted into the GIT, hepatic production cannot maintain a sufficient bile salt pool or the secretions to emulsify lipids. The gastric and pancreatic lipases are capable of digesting some triglycerides to fatty acids and monoglycerides, but, without adequate micelle formation facilitated by bile salts, lipids are poorly absorbed. This can lead to malabsorption of fats and fat-soluble vitamins A, D, E, and K. In addition, malabsorption of fatty acids results in their combination with calcium, zinc, and magnesium to form fatty acid–mineral soaps, thus leading to their malabsorption as well. To compound matters, colonic absorption of oxalate is increased, leading to hyperoxaluria and increased frequency of renal oxalate stones. Relative dehydration and concentrated urine, which are common with ileal resections, further increase the risk of stone formation (see Chapter 36).

The colon (≈5 ft long) is responsible for reabsorbing 1-1.5 L of electrolyte-rich (particularly sodium and chloride) fluid each day, but is capable of adapting to increase this capacity to 5-6 L daily. Preservation of colon is key to maintaining hydration status. If the patient has any colon left, malabsorption of bile salts can act as a mucosal irritant, increasing colonic motility with fluid and electrolyte losses. Consumption of high-fat diets with ileal resections and retained colon may also result in the formation of hydroxy fatty acids, which also increase fluid loss. Cholesterol gallstones occur because the ratio of bile acid, phospholipid, and cholesterol in biliary secretions is altered. Dependence on PN increases the risk of biliary "sludge," secondary to decreased stimulus for evacuation of the biliary tract (see Chapter 30).

Medical and Surgical Management of Resections

The first step in management is assessment of the remaining bowel length from patient records or interview. Assessment should quantify dietary intake as well as stool and urine output over 24 hours. Medications and hydration status should be assessed. Medications may be prescribed to slow GI motility, decrease secretions, or treat bacterial overgrowth. The primary "gut slowing" medications include loperamide, and, if needed, narcotic medications. Somatostatin and somatostatin analogs; glucagon-like polypeptide 2; growth hormone; and other hormones with antisecretory, antimotility, or trophic actions have been studied for use to slow both motility and secretions. Surgical procedures such as creation of reservoirs ("pouches") to serve as a form of colon, intestinal lengthening, and intestinal transplant have been performed to help patients with major GI resections (Shatnawei et al., 2010). Intestinal transplant is very complex and is reserved for gut failure, or when patients develop significant complications from PN.

Medical Nutrition Therapy

Most patients who have significant bowel resections require PN initially to restore and maintain nutrition status. The duration of PN and subsequent nutrition therapy will be based on the extent of the bowel resection, the health of the patient, and the condition of the remaining GIT. In general, older patients with major ileal resections, patients who have lost the ileocecal valve, and patients with residual disease in the remaining GIT do not fare as well. Enteral feeding provides a trophic stimulus to the GIT; PN is used to restore and maintain nutrient status. Some may require lifetime PN to maintain adequate fluid and nutrition status.

The more extreme and severe the problem, the slower the progression to a normal diet. Small, frequent, mini meals (6 to 10 per day) are likely to be better tolerated than larger feedings (Matarese et al., 2005; Parrish, 2005). Tube feeding may be useful to maximize intake when a patient would not typically eat, such as nighttime (see Chapter 14). Because of malnutrition and disuse of the GIT, the digestive and absorptive functions of the remaining GIT may be compromised, and malnutrition itself will delay postsurgical adaptation. The transition to more normal foods may take weeks to months, and some patients may never tolerate normal concentrations or volumes of foods.

Maximum adaptation of the GIT may take 1-2 years after surgery. Adaptation improves function, but it does not restore the intestine to normal length or capacity. Whole nutrients are the most important stimuli of the GIT. Other nutritional measures have also been studied as a means of hastening the adaptive process and decreasing malabsorption, but their evidence for use is limited. For example, **glutamine** is the preferred fuel for small intestinal enterocytes and thus may be valuable in enhancing adaptation. Nucleotides (in the form of purines, pyrimidine, ribonucleic acid) may also enhance mucosal adaptation, but unfortunately they are often lacking in parenteral and enteral nutritional products. SCFAs (e.g., butyrate, propionate, acetate) produced from microbial fermentation of carbohydrate and fibers are major fuels for the colonic epithelium.

Patients with jejunal resections and an intact ileum and colon will likely adapt quickly to normal diets. A normal balance of protein, fat, and carbohydrate sources is satisfactory. Six small feedings with avoidance of lactose, large amounts of concentrated sweets, and caffeine may help to reduce the risk of bloating, abdominal pain, and diarrhea. Because the typical American diet may be nutritionally lacking and use of some micronutrients may be marginal, patients should be advised that the quality of their diet is of utmost importance. A multivitamin and mineral supplement may be required to meet all their nutritional needs.

Patients with ileal resections require increased time and patience in the advancement from parenteral to enteral nutrition. Because of losses, fat-soluble vitamins, calcium, magnesium, and zinc may need to be supplemented. Dietary fat may need to be limited, especially in those with remaining colon. Small amounts at each feeding are more likely to be tolerated and absorbed.

MCT products add to the caloric intake and serve as a vehicle for lipid-soluble nutrients. Because boluses of MCT oil (e.g., taken as a medication in tablespoon amounts) may add to the patient's diarrhea, it is best to divide the doses equally in feedings throughout the day. Fluid and electrolytes, especially sodium, should be provided in small amounts and frequently.

In patients with SBS an oral diet or enteral nutrition plus the use of gut-slowing medications should be maximized to prevent dependence on PN. Frequent meals, removal of osmotic medications and foods, use of oral hydration therapies, and other interventions should be pursued. In some cases, overfeeding in an attempt to compensate for malabsorption results in further malabsorption, not only of ingested foods and liquids but also of the significant amounts of GI fluids secreted in response to food ingestion. Patients with an extremely short bowel may depend on parenteral solutions for at least part of their nutrient and fluid supply. Small, frequent snacks provide some oral gratification for these patients, but typically they can supply only a portion of their fluid and nutrient needs (see Chapter 14 for discussion of home PN).

Small Intestine Bacterial Overgrowth

Small intestine bacterial overgrowth (SIBO) is a syndrome characterized by over-proliferation of bacteria within the small bowel. There are a number of physiologic processes that normally limit the amount of small intestine bacterial colonies. Gastric acid, bile, and pancreatic enzymes have bacteriostatic and bactericidal action within the small bowel. Normal propulsive action of bowel motility "sweeps" bacteria into the distal bowel. The ileocecal valve prevents migration of the large numbers of colonic bacteria into the small intestine. SIBO has also been referred to as "blind loop syndrome" because one cause of bacterial overgrowth can result from stasis of the intestinal tract as a result of obstructive disease, strictures, radiation enteritis, or surgical procedures that leaves a portion of bowel without normal flow (a blind loop or Roux limb).

Pathophysiology

Frequently, more than one of the normal homeostatic defenses must be impaired before small intestine bacteria overproliferate to the point that symptoms develop. Chronic use of medications that suppress gastric acid allow more bacteria to survive passage into the small bowel. Liver diseases or chronic pancreatitis can decrease the production or flow of bile and pancreatic enzymes into the bowel. Gastroparesis, narcotic medications, or bowel dysmotility disorders decrease peristalsis and can impair the ability to propel bacterial to the distal bowel. Surgical resection of the distal ileum and ileocecal valve can result in retrograde proliferation of colonic bacteria.

One of the most common symptoms of SIBO is chronic diarrhea from fat maldigestion. Bacteria within the small bowel deconjugate bile salts resulting in impaired formation of micelles and thus impaired fat digestion and steatorrhea. Carbohydrate malabsorption occurs because of injury to the brush border secondary to the toxic effects of bacterial products and consequent enzyme loss. The expanding numbers of bacteria use the available vitamin B_{12} and other nutrients for their own growth, and the host becomes deficient. Bacteria within the small bowel produce folic acid as a byproduct of their metabolism, and vitamin B_{12} deficiency with normal or elevated serum folic acid is common. Bloating and distention are also frequently reported in SIBO, resulting from the action of bacteria on carbohydrates with production of hydrogen and methane within the small bowel.

Medical Treatment

Treatment is directed toward control of the bacterial growth with antibiotics, probiotics, prebiotics, and in some cases surgical modification of the blind loop.

Medical Nutrition Therapy

Part of the problem with bacterial overgrowth in the small intestine is that carbohydrates reaching the site where microbes are harbored serve as fuel for their proliferation, with subsequent increased production of gases and organic acids. At least theoretically a diet that limits refined carbohydrates that are readily fermented such as refined starches and sugars (e.g., lactose, fructose, alcohol sugars) and substitutes whole grains, and vegetables, can limit the proliferation and increase motility. See Table 29-5: Low FODMAP Diet.

Limited studies are available as to the effectiveness of diets and probiotic and prebiotic materials in the prevention and treatment of altered GI motility, strictures, abnormal anatomy of the GIT, and the presence of opportunistic organisms in the colon (*C. difficile* and other organisms). Because vitamin B_{12} may be lost in fermentation and some dietary nutrients may be lacking, an assessment of the medical problem and the patient's dietary intake is in order. If bile salts are being degraded, as in the case of blind loop syndrome, MCTs may be helpful if they provide a source of lipid and energy.

Fistulas

Pathophysiology

A **fistula** is an abnormal passage between two organs or between an organ and the skin. An **enterocutaneous (EC) fistula** is an abnormal passage beginning at the bowel and exiting at the skin. Fistulas may occur as a result of prenatal developmental error, trauma, surgery, or inflammatory or malignant disease processes. Most EC fistulas occur after surgery and usually manifest 7-10 days postoperatively. Fistulas of the intestinal tract can be serious threats to nutrition status because large amounts of fluid and electrolytes are lost and malabsorption and infection can occur.

Medical Treatment

Fluid and electrolyte balance must be restored, infection must be brought under control, and aggressive nutrition support may be necessary to permit spontaneous closure or to maintain optimal nutritional status prior to surgical closure.

Medical Nutrition Therapy

Nutrition management of patients with EC fistulas can be very challenging. Either PN, tube feeding, oral diet, or a combination, are used in patients with fistulas. The success rate of the chosen method depends on multiple variables, including the location of the fistula, the presence of abscesses or obstructions, the length of functional bowel, the ability to manage fistula output, and the patient's overall condition (Willcutts, 2010).

Ileostomy or Colostomy

Patients with severe UC, Crohn's disease, colon cancer, or intestinal trauma frequently require the surgical creation of an opening from the body surface to the intestinal tract to permit defecation from the intact portion of the intestine. When the entire colon, rectum, and anus must be removed, an **ileostomy**, or an opening of the ileum at the abdominal wall, is performed. If only the rectum and anus are removed, a **colostomy** can provide entrance to the colon. In some cases a temporary opening may be made to allow surgery and healing of more distal parts of the intestinal tract.

The opening, or stoma, eventually shrinks to the size of a nickel. The output from the stoma depends on its location. The consistency of the stool from an ileostomy is liquid (effluent), whereas that from a colostomy ranges from mushy to fairly well formed. Stool from a colostomy on the left side of the colon is firmer than that from a colostomy on the right side. Odor is a major concern of the patient with an ileostomy or colostomy; however, an ileostomy effluent usually has a weakly acidic odor that is not unpleasant.

Medical Treatment

Patients with a permanent colostomy or ileostomy require sympathetic understanding from the entire health care team. Acceptance of the condition and the problems involved in maintaining bowel regularity is usually difficult. Nursing personnel, especially enterostomal therapists (who specialize in the care of stomas), play a major role in supporting and teaching patients with ostomies. Having these patients meet other people who have undergone similar surgery may help with the adjustment. Eventually they may be encouraged by the realization that in the future they will not have the multiple hospitalizations or chronic disabilities that accompanied their intestinal disease.

Medical Nutrition Therapy

Malodorous stools may be caused by steatorrhea or partial digestion or bacterial fermentation of foodstuffs. SCFAs, sulfur-containing compounds, ammonia, methane, and other end products can produce odors. Because an individual patient may have different flora, types and amounts of gases and odors may differ among patients and with different dietary practices. Patients learn to observe their stools to determine which foods to eliminate; this differs from one patient to the next.

Foods that tend to cause odor from a colostomy are legumes, onions, garlic, cabbage, eggs, fish, some medications, as well as some vitamin and mineral supplements. Persistent odor may be attributable to poor stoma hygiene or to an ileostomy complication that allows bacterial overgrowth in the ileum. Deodorants are available, and modern pouch appliances are odor-proof. Gas production may cause the pouch to become tense and distended, and accidental dislodgment is likely. The nutritional recommendations for reducing flatulence, presented in this chapter, may be helpful for patients with colostomies.

The normal output from the ileum to the colon is in the range of 750 mL to 1.5 L in the intact GIT. After a colectomy and creation of an ileostomy, adaptation occurs within 1 to 2 weeks. Fecal output will lessen, and stools will become less liquid. Reduction in stool volume may not occur to the same extent in patients who have had an ileal resection in addition to a colectomy. Depending on the amount of ileum resected, the ileal output may be 1.5 to 5 times greater than that of the patient who has had only a colectomy. Patients with ileostomies have an above-average need for salt and water to compensate for excessive losses in stool. Inadequate water intake can result in small urine volumes and a predisposition for renal calculi. A normal diet provides adequate sodium, and patients should be instructed to drink at least 1 L more than their ostomy output daily.

The patient with a normal, functional ileostomy usually does not become nutritionally depleted. Surgical procedures such as ileostomy may require specific dietary changes but no greater energy intake; caloric expenditures in these patients are similar to those of normal subjects. Those who also undergo resection of the terminal ileum need vitamin B_{12} supplementation or intravenous injections. Patients with an ileostomy may have low vitamin C and folate intakes because of low fresh vegetable and fruit intakes, and they require supplementation.

Patients with ileostomies should be guided by physiologic reasons for intolerance of foods and not by anecdotal reports. Because gastric emptying may be more rapid and foodstuffs are not fermented to the same degree after colostomy, absorption of nutrients may be somewhat better from cooked, shredded, or pureed fruits and vegetables. Because it is possible for a food bolus to get caught at the point where the ileum narrows as it enters the abdominal wall, it is important to warn the patient to avoid very fibrous vegetables and to chew all food well. Other than this, patients with either an ileostomy or a colostomy should be encouraged to follow their normal diet, omitting only foods known to cause problems.

Ileal Pouch after Colectomy

Pathophysiology

As an alternative to creation of an ileostomy for persons who have had their colons removed, surgeons can create a reservoir using a portion of the distal ileum. Folds of the ileum are joined together to create a small pouch, which is then connected to the rectum and ileum. This is called an **ileal pouch**–anal anastomosis. The most common pouch is the **J-pouch**, but **S** and **W** pouches are sometimes created using additional folds of ileum. Like the colon, the pouch develops a microflora capable of at least partially fermenting fiber and carbohydrate. Because the reservoir is smaller than the colon, bowel movements are likely to occur more frequently than normal (i.e., between four and eight times daily). A Koch pouch is a type of applianceless ileostomy that uses an internal reservoir with a one-way valve, constructed from a loop of intestine, that is attached to the abdominal wall with a skin-level stoma. Patients must insert a tube or catheter into the stoma to open the valve and allow drainage of ileostomy contents. The technical difficulties of surgical construction and the potential for complications has led to decreased use of the Koch pouch in favor of the J-pouch with anal anastomosis.

Medical Treatment

Vitamin B_{12} injections are usually required because, as in SBBO, the microbes may compete for and bind intraluminal vitamin B_{12}. Other problems commonly reported include obstruction; inflammation of the pouch; and increased stool output, frequency, and gas. The incidence of obstruction may be lessened with attention to particle size of fibrous foods, chewing thoroughly, and consuming small meals frequently throughout the day. Stool frequency and volume do not return to normal, however. The normal, intact colon absorbs 80% to 90% of the liter or so of fluid entering from the ileum, leaving only 100 to 200 mL. After surgery the remaining ileum does adapt to a small degree by increasing efficiency of fluid absorption, but even after adaptation, fluid output is always in the range of 300 to 600 mL.

Pouchitis is an inflammation of the mucosal tissue forming the pouch. The associated pathologic changes have been described as being somewhat similar to that of IBD (e.g., UC). The cause of pouchitis is not entirely clear, but it may be related to selected bacterial overgrowth, bile salt malabsorption, or insufficient SCFA production. Antibiotics are the primary form of therapy, but experiments with different types of dietary fiber, prebiotics and probiotics, and other nutrient components have been used successfully to reduce the incidence (Guarner, 2005; Meier and Steuerwald, 2005).

CLINICAL SCENARIO

A 35-year-old woman, Sarah, was diagnosed with celiac disease 2 years ago and has presented to the Digestive Health Clinic with complaints of 3 weeks of diarrhea and abdominal pain. She reports losing weight, despite eating her typical diet. However, she reports recently starting a new job as a high school English teacher. She has been buying lunch at the school's cafeteria because they seem to have a good selection of hot foods that are gluten-free. Sarah reports she received education on a gluten-free diet from a registered dietitian when she was diagnosed. She seems to have a good understanding of the gluten-free diet and has connected with her local celiac support group.

Summary of "Typical Day" Diet History

Breakfast

1 cup gluten-free cereal with 4 oz 1% milk; 1 cup orange juice; 1 cup coffee with 2 T 1% milk and 1 tsp sugar

Lunch (from the Cafeteria)

Corn tortilla with 3 oz tuna and 1 oz melted cheddar cheese
4 oz trail mix (peanuts, cashews, raisins, and chocolate pieces)
1 banana
1 cup chocolate milk
20 oz water

Snack

12 baby carrots
2 T red pepper hummus
10 oz water

Dinner

5 oz grilled chicken breast, marinated in gluten-free marinade
1 cup chickpea, tomato, and spinach salad with 2 tsp olive oil or balsamic dressing
3 oz white wine
½ cup vanilla ice cream

Abnormal laboratory values: Tissue transglutaminase (TTG) immunoglobulin (Ig)A 60 (2 years ago), down to <4 (1 yr ago)
Diarrhea >5 days
Current Medications: loperamide (started 2 weeks ago), Fibercon (started 1 month ago)
Food intolerance to gluten

Nutrition Diagnostic Statement

Altered gastrointestinal function related to possible inadvertent gluten ingestion as evidenced by diarrhea.

Interventions

Recheck tTG- IgA
Review potential sources for cross-crosscontamination, including: food preparation, buffet lines, toasters, and bulk bins.
Review potential hidden gluten sources, including food binders, coatings, and flavorings (trail mix, chocolate milk); medications (Fibercon); and communion wafers.
Recommend patient check her medications with a pharmacist or the manufacturer, to ensure they are gluten-free.
Recommend patient speak with the cafeteria manager to determine what cooked foods are safe for her to eat.
Recommend patient consider bringing her own lunch to school until she has identified what foods are safe to eat at school.
Refer to a gastroenterologist, if symptoms do not resolve after above intervention.

Nutrition Care Questions

1. Categorize the interventions listed into those related to education, counseling, or care management.
2. Write a gluten-free menu plan that could work for one week.

Medical Nutrition Therapy

There are few controlled studies regarding diet and ileal pouch. Food intolerances are common but relatively mild (Steenhagen et al., 2006). The same dietary measures that are used by others to reduce excessive stool output (reduced caffeine, lactose avoidance in lactase-deficient persons, limitation of fructose and sorbitol) will likely reduce stool volume and frequency in persons with pouches. Adequate fluid and electrolyte intake are especially important because of the increase in intestinal losses.

Rectal Surgery

Nutrition care after rectal surgery such as hemorrhoidectomy should be directed toward maintaining an intake that will allow wound repair and prevent infection of the wound by feces. The frequency of stools is minimized by the use a minimum-residue diet (see Table 29-1). Chemically defined diets are low in residue, and their use can reduce stool volume and frequency to as little as 50 g every 6 days, making the surgical construction of a temporary colostomy unnecessary. A normal diet is resumed after healing is complete, and the patient is instructed about the benefits of eating a high-fiber diet to avoid constipation in the future.

USEFUL WEBSITES

Celiac Disease Resources
Celiac Disease Awareness
http://celiac.nih.gov/

Gluten Intolerance Group
http://www.gluten.net/
Celiac Disease Foundation
http://www.celiac.org/
Celiac Sprue Association
http://www.csaceliacs.org/
University of Virginia Division of Gastroenterology and Hepatology
www.uvahealth.com/celiacsupport
Crohn's and Colitis Foundation of America
http://www.ccfa.org/
Ileostomy, Colostomy, Pouches
National Digestive Diseases Information Clearinghouse
http://digestive.niddk.nih.gov/ddiseases/pubs/ileostomy/index.htm
Medline
http://www.nlm.nih.gov/medlineplus/tutorials/colostomy/htm/index.htm

REFERENCES

American Gastroenterological Association (AGA) Institute: Medical position statement on the diagnosis and management of celiac disease, *Gastroenterol* 131:1977, 2006.

Aragon G, Graham DB: Probiotic therapy for irritable bowel syndrome, *Gastroenterol Hepatol* 6:39, 2010.

Atia AN, Buchman AL: Oral rehydration solutions in non-cholera diarrhea: a review, *Am J Gastroenterol* 104:2596, 2009.

Azpiroz F: Intestinal gas dynamics: mechanisms and clinical relevance, *Gut* 54:893, 2005.

Barrett JS, Gibson PR: Clinical ramifications of malabsorption of fructose and other short-chain carbohydrates, *Practical Gastroenterol* 31:51, 2007.

Bell TJ, et al: The prevalence, severity, and impact of opioid-induced bowel dysfunction: results of US and European Patient Survey (PROBE 1), *Pain Med* 10:35, 2009.

Besselink MGH, et al: Probiotic prophylaxis in predicted severe acute pancreatitis: a randomised, double-blind, placebo-controlled trial, *Lancet* 371:651, 2008.

Beyer PL, et al: Fructose intake at current levels in the United States may cause gastrointestinal distress in normal adults, *J Am Diet Assoc* 105:1559, 2005.

Bezkorovainy A. Probiotics: determinants of survival and growth in the gut. *Am J Clin Nutr* 73:399S, 2001.

Biggs WS, Dery WH: Evaluation and treatment of constipation in infants and children, *Am Fam Physician* 73:469, 2006.

Bijkerk CJ et al: Soluble or insoluble fibre in irritable bowel syndrome in primary care? Randomised placebo controlled trial, *BMJ (Clinical Research Ed)* 339:b3154, 2009.

Binder HJ: Role of colonic short-chain fatty acid transport in diarrhea, *Ann Rev Physiol* 72:297, 2010.

Bonamico M, et al: Duodenal bulb biopsies in celiac disease: a multicenter study, *J Pediatr Gastroenterol Nutr* 47:618, 2008.

Butterworth AD, et al: Probiotics for induction of remission in Crohn's disease, Cochrane Database Syst Rev (Online) CD006634, 2008.

Caprilli R, et al: European evidence based consensus on the diagnosis and management of Crohn's disease: special situations, *Gut* 55(Suppl 1):i36, 2006.

Case S: The gluten-free diet: how to provide effective education and resources, *Gastroenterol* 128:S128, 2005.

Chand N, Mihas AA: Celiac disease: current concepts in diagnosis and treatment, *J Clin Gastroenterol* 40:3, 2006.

Cook IJ, et al: Chronic constipation: overview and challenges, *Neurogastroenterol Motil* 21(Suppl 2):1, 2009.

DeLegge MH, Berry A: Enteral feeding: should it be continued in the patient with clostridium difficile enterocolitis? *Practical Gastroenterol* 40, 2009.

Diamanti A, et al: Prevalence of life-threatening complications in pediatric patients affected by intestinal failure, *Transplant Proc* 39:1632, 2007.

Dotan I, Rachmilewitz D: Probiotics in inflammatory bowel disease: possible mechanisms of action, *Curr Opin Gastroenterol* 21:426, 2005.

Dray X, Marteau P: The use of enteral nutrition in the management of Crohn's disease in adults, *JPEN* 29:S166, 2005.

El-Matary W, et al: Diagnostic characteristics of given video capsule endoscopy in diagnosis of celiac disease: a meta-analysis, *J Laparoendosc Adv Surg Tech A* 19:815, 2009.

Emmanuel AV, et al: Pharmacological management of constipation. *Neurogastroenterol Motil* 21(Suppl 2):41, 2009.

Ford AC, et al: Yield of diagnostic tests for celiac disease in individuals with symptoms suggestive of irritable bowel syndrome: systematic review and meta-analysis, *Arch Intern Med* 169:651, 2009.

Ford AC, Spiegel BMR: Small intestinal bacterial overgrowth in irritable bowel syndrome: systematic review and meta-analysis, *Clin Gastroenterol Hepatol* 7:1279, 2009.

Ford AC, et al: Effect of fibre, antispasmodics, and peppermint oil in the treatment of irritable bowel syndrome: systematic review and meta-analysis, *BMJ* 337:a2313, 2008.

Gao XW, et al: Dose-response efficacy of a proprietary probiotic formula of *Lactobacillus acidophilus* CL1285 and *Lactobacillus casei* LBC80R for antibiotic-associated diarrhea and *Clostridium difficile*-associated diarrhea prophylaxis in adult patients, *Am J Gastroenterol*, 2010. Accessed 2010 from http://www.ncbi.nlm.nih.gov/pubmed/20145608.

Garsed K, Scott BB: Can oats be taken in a gluten-free diet? A systematic review, *Scand J Gastroenterol* 42:171, 2007.

Ghoshal UC, et al: Frequency of small intestinal bacterial overgrowth in patients with irritable bowel syndrome and chronic non-specific diarrhea, *J Neurogastroenterol Motil* 16:40, 2010a.

Ghoshal UC, et al: Bugs and irritable bowel syndrome: the good, the bad and the ugly, *J Gastroenterol Hepatol* 25:244, 2010b.

Gibson PR, Shepherd SJ: Evidence-based dietary management of functional gastrointestinal symptoms: The FODMAP approach, *J Gastroenterol Hepatol* 25:252, 2010.

Green PH: An association between microscopic colitis and celiac disease, *Clin Gastroenterol Hepatol* 7:1210, 2009.

Guandalini S: Update on the role of probiotics in the therapy of pediatric inflammatory bowel disease, *Expert Rev Clin Immunol* 6:47, 2010.

Guarner F: Inulin and oligofructose: impact on intestinal diseases and disorders, *Br J Nutr* 93(Suppl 1):S61, 2005.

Guyonnet D, et al: Effect of a fermented milk containing Bifidobacterium animalis DN-173 010 on the health-related quality of life and symptoms in irritable bowel syndrome in adults in primary care: a multicentre, randomized, double-blind, controlled trial, *Aliment Pharmacol Ther* 26:475, 2007.

Harder H, et al: Effect of high- and low-caloric mixed liquid meals on intestinal gas dynamics, *Dig Dis Sci* 51:140, 2006.

Heizer WD, et al: The role of diet in symptoms of irritable bowel syndrome in adults: a narrative review, *J Am Diet Assoc* 109:1204, 2009.

Hickson M, et al: Use of probiotic *Lactobacillus* preparation to prevent diarrhea associated with antibiotics: randomised double blind placebo controlled trial, *BMJ* 335:80, 2007.

Holubar SD, et al: Treatment and prevention of pouchitis after ileal pouch-anal anastomosis for chronic ulcerative colitis, Cochrane Database Syst Rev 6:CD001176, 2010.

Holzer P: Opioid receptors in the gastrointestinal tract, *Regul Pept* 155:11, 2009.

Howell MD, et al: Iatrogenic gastric acid suppression and the risk of nosocomial Clostridium difficile infection, *Arch Int Med* 170:784, 2010.

Hutchinson JM, et al: Long-term histological follow-up of people with coeliac disease in a UK teaching, *QJM* 103:511, 2010.

Järvelä IE: Molecular genetics of adult-type hypolactasia, *Ann Med* 37:179, 2005.

Jobse P, et al: Collagenous colitis: description of a single centre series of 83 patients, *Eur J Int Med* 20:499, 2009.

Kagnoff MF: Celiac disease: pathogenesis of a model immunogenetic disease, *J Clin Invest* 117:41, 2007.

Kalliomäki MA: Food allergy and irritable bowel syndrome, *Curr Opin Gastroenterol* 21:708, 2005.

Kulkarni SV, et al: Opportunistic parasitic infections in HIV/AIDS patients presenting with diarrhea by the level of immunosuppression, *Indian J Med Res* 130:63, 2009.

Lawrence SJ, et al: Probiotics for recurrent *Clostridium difficile* disease, *J Med Microbiol* 54:905, 2005.

Levri KM, et al: Do probiotics reduce adult lactose intolerance? A systematic review, *J Fam Pract* 54:613, 2005.

Linsky A, et al: Proton pump inhibitors and risk for recurrent *Clostridium difficile* infection, *Arch Int Med* 170:772, 2010.

Lochs H: To feed or not to feed? Are nutritional supplements worthwhile in active Crohn's disease? *Gut* 55:306, 2006.

Lombardo L, et al: Increased incidence of small intestinal bacterial overgrowth during proton pump inhibitor therapy, *Clin Gastroenterol Hepatol* 8:504, 2010.

Lustig RH: Fructose: metabolic, hedonic, and societal parallels with ethanol, *J Am Diet Assoc* 110:1307, 2010.

Malagelada JR: A symptom-based approach to making a positive diagnosis of irritable bowel syndrome with constipation, *Int J Clin Pract* 60:57, 2006.

Mallon P, et al: Probiotics for induction of remission in ulcerative colitis, Cochrane Database Syst Rev CD005573, 2007.

Matarese LE, et al: Short bowel syndrome: clinical guidelines for nutrition management, *Nutr Clin Pract* 20:493, 2005.

McGarr SE, et al: Diet, anaerobic bacterial metabolism, and colon cancer: a review of the literature, *J Clin Gastroenterol* 39:98, 2005.

Meier R, Steuerwald M: Place of probiotics, *Curr Opin Crit Care* 11:318, 2005.

Morken MH, et al: Intestinal gas in plain abdominal radiographs does not correlate with symptoms after lactulose challenge, *Eur J Gastroenterol Hepatol* 19:589, 2007.

Mueller C, Macpherson AJ Layers of mutualism with commensal bacteria protect us from intestinal inflammation, *Gut* 55:276-284, 2006.

Müller S, et al: Anti-saccharomyces cerevisiae antibody titers are stable over time in Crohn's patients and are not inducible in murine models of colitis, *World J Gastroenterol* 11:6988, 2005.

Müller-Lissner S: The pathophysiology, diagnosis, and treatment of constipation, *Deutsches Ärzteblatt International* 106:424, 2009.

Nachman F: Long-term deterioration of quality of life in adult patients with celiac disease is associated with treatment noncompliance, *Dig Liver Dis* 2010. Accessed 2010 from http://www.ncbi.nlm.nih.gov/pubmed/20399159.

Nath SK: Tropical sprue, *Curr Gastroenterol Reports* 7:343, 2005.

National Cancer Institute and U.S. National Institutes of Health: Colon and rectal cancer, 2010. Accessed 1 July 2010 from http://www.cancer.gov/cancertopics/types/colon-and-rectal.

O'Keefe SJD: Tube feeding, the microbiota, and Clostridium difficile infection, *World J Gastroenterol* 16:139, 2010.

Parra-Blanco A: Colonic diverticular disease: pathophysiology and clinical picture, *Digestion* 73(Suppl 1):47, 2006.

Parrish CR: The clinician's guide to short bowel syndrome, *Pract Gastroenterol* 29:67, 2005.

Penner R, Fedorak RN: Probiotics and nutraceuticals: nonmedicinal treatments of gastrointestinal diseases, *Curr Opin Pharmacol* 5:596, 2005.

Pillai A, Nelson R: Probiotics for treatment of Clostridium difficile-associated colitis in adults, Cochrane Database Syst Rev CD004611, 2008.

Rajendran N, Kumar D: Role of diet in the management of inflammatory bowel disease, *World J Gastroenterol* 16:1442, 2010.

Raju R, Cruz-Correa M: Chemoprevention of colorectal cancer, *Dis Colon Rectum* 49:113, 2006.

Ramkumar D, Rao SSC: Efficacy and safety of traditional medical therapies for chronic constipation: systematic review, *Am J Gastroenterol* 100:936, 2005.

Rasinperä H, et al: The C/C-13910 genotype of adult-type hypolactasia is associated with an increased risk of colorectal cancer in the Finnish population, *Gut* 54:643, 2005.

Robayo-Torres CC, et al: Disaccharide digestion: clinical and molecular aspects, *Clin Gastroenterol Hepatol* 4:276, 2006.

Rostom A, et al: The diagnostic accuracy of serologic tests for celiac disease: a systematic review, *Gastroenterol* 128:S38, 2005.

Salzman H, Lillie D: Diverticular disease: diagnosis and treatment, *Am Fam Phys* 72:1229, 2005.

Sánchez-Pérez M, et al: Toxic megacolon secondary to Clostridium difficile colitis. Case report, *Revista De Gastroenterologia De Mexico* 75:103, 2010.

Sanders DSA: Mucosal integrity and barrier function in the pathogenesis of early lesions in Crohn's disease, *J Clin Pathol* 58:568, 2005.

Sanderson IR, Croft NM: The anti-inflammatory effects of enteral nutrition, *J Parenter Enteral Nutr* 29:S134, 2005.

Schiller LR: Nutrients and constipation: cause or cure? *Pract Gastroenterol* 32:43, 2008.

Schroeder MS: *Clostridium difficile*-associated diarrhea, *Am Fam Physician* 71:921, 2005.

Seibold F: Food-induced immune responses as origin of bowel disease? *Digestion* 71:251, 2005.

Seidner DL, et al: An oral supplement enriched with fish oil, soluble fiber, and antioxidants for corticosteroid sparing in ulcerative colitis: a randomized, controlled trial, *Clin Gastroenterol Hepatol* 3:358, 2005.

Shatnawei A: Intestinal failure management at the Cleveland Clinic, *Arch Surg* 145:521, 2010.

Shaukat A: Systematic review: effective management strategies for lactose intolerance, *Ann Int Med* 2010. Accessed 2010 from http://www.ncbi.nlm.nih.gov/pubmed/20404262.

Shepherd SJ, et al: Dietary triggers of abdominal symptoms in patients with irritable bowel syndrome: randomized placebo-controlled evidence, *Clin Gastroenterol Hepatol* 6:765, 2008.

Shih DQ, Targan SR: Immunopathogenesis of inflammatory bowel disease, *World J Gastroenterol* 14:390, 2008.

Simondi D, et al: A retrospective study on a cohort of patients with lymphocytic colitis, *Revista Española De Enfermedades Digestivas* 102:381, 2010.

Steenhagen E, et al: Sources and severity of self-reported food intolerance after ileal pouch-anal anastomosis, *J Am Diet Assoc* 106:1459, 2006.

Strate LL, et al: Nut, corn, and popcorn consumption and the incidence of diverticular disease, *JAMA* 300:907, 2008.

Suchy FJ, et al: National Institutes of Health Consensus Development Conference: lactose intolerance and health, *Ann Int Med* 152:792, 2010.

Szajewska H, et al: Probiotics in the prevention of antibiotic-associated diarrhea in children: a meta-analysis of randomized controlled trials, *J Pediatr* 149:367, 2006.

Teitelbaum JE: Probiotics and the treatment of infectious diarrhea, *Pediatr Infect Dis J* 24:267, 2005.

Travis SPL, et al: European evidence based consensus on the diagnosis and management of Crohn's disease: current management, *Gut* 55 (Suppl 1):i16, 2006.

Turner D et al: ω 3 fatty acids (fish oil) for maintenance of remission in Crohn's disease, Cochrane Database Syst Rev CD006320, 2009.

Tuteja AK, Biskupiak J: Opioid-induced bowel disorders and narcotic bowel syndrome in patients with chronic non-cancer pain, *Neurogastroenterol Motil* 22:424, 2010.

Tysk C, et al: Diagnosis and management of microscopic colitis, *World J Gastroenterol* 14:7280, 2008.

Venkatasubramani N, et al: Obesity in pediatric celiac disease, *J Pediatr Gastroenterol Nutr* 2010. Accessed 2010 from http://www.ncbi.nlm.nih.gov/pubmed/20479683.

Whelan K, Myers CE: Safety of probiotics in patients receiving nutritional support: a systematic review of case reports, randomized controlled trials, and nonrandomized trials, *Am J Clin Nutr* 91:687, 2010.

Whorwell PJ, et al: Efficacy of an encapsulated probiotic Bifidobacterium infantis 35624 in women with irritable bowel syndrome, *Am J Gastroenterol* 101:1581, 2006.

Willcutts K: The art of fistuloclysis: nutritional management of enterocutaneous fistulas, *Pract Gastroenterol* 2010.

Zezos P, et al: Hyperhomocysteinemia in ulcerative colitis is related to folate levels, *World J Gastroenterol*, 11:6038, 2005.

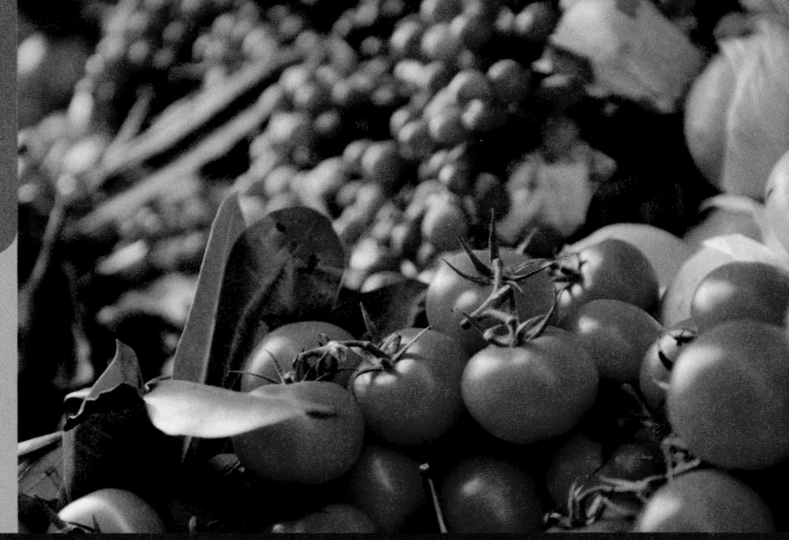

CHAPTER 30

Jeanette M. Hasse, PhD, RD, LD, CNSC, FADA
Laura E. Matarese, PhD, RD, LDN, CNSC, FADA

Medical Nutrition Therapy for Hepatobiliary and Pancreatic Disorders

KEY TERMS

alcoholic liver disease
aromatic amino acids (AAAs)
ascites
bile
branched-chain amino acids (BCAAs)
cholangitis
cholecystectomy
cholecystitis
choledocholithiasis
cholelithiasis
cholestasis
cirrhosis
fasting hypoglycemia
fatty liver
fulminant liver disease
hemochromatosis
hepatic encephalopathy
hepatic failure
hepatic osteodystrophy
hepatic steatosis
hepatitis
hepatorenal syndrome
jaundice
Kayser-Fleischer ring
Kupffer cells
nonalcoholic fatty liver disease (NAFLD)
nonalcoholic steatohepatitis (NASH)
pancreaticoduodenectomy (Whipple procedure)
pancreatitis
paracentesis
portal hypertension
portal systemic encephalopathy
primary biliary cirrhosis (PBC)
secondary biliary cirrhosis
steatorrhea
varices
Wernicke encephalopathy
Wilson's disease

The liver is of primary importance; one cannot survive without a liver. The pancreas and liver are essential to digestion and metabolism. Although it is important, the gallbladder can be removed, and the body will adapt comfortably to its absence. Knowledge of the structure and functions of these organs is vital. When they are diseased, the necessary medical nutrition therapy (MNT) is complex.

PHYSIOLOGY AND FUNCTIONS OF THE LIVER

Structure

The liver is the largest gland in the body, weighing approximately 1500 g. The liver has two main lobes: the right and left. The right lobe is further divided into the anterior and posterior segments; the right segmental fissure, which cannot be seen externally, separates the segments. The externally visible falciform ligament divides the left lobe into the medial and lateral segments. The liver is supplied with blood from two sources: the hepatic artery, which supplies approximately one third of the blood from the aorta; and the portal vein, which supplies the other two thirds and collects blood drained from the digestive tract.

Approximately 1500 mL of blood per minute circulates through the liver and exits via the right and left hepatic veins into the inferior vena cava. Just as there is a system of blood vessels throughout the liver, there also exists a series of bile ducts. **Bile**, which is formed in the liver cells, exits the liver through a series of bile ducts that increase in size as they approach the common bile duct. It is a thick, viscous fluid secreted from the liver, stored in the gallbladder, and released into the duodenum when fatty foods enter the duodenum. It emulsifies fats in the intestine and forms compounds with fatty acids to facilitate their absorption.

Functions

The liver has the ability to regenerate itself. Only 10% to 20% of functioning liver is required to sustain life, although removal of the liver results in death, usually within 24 hours. The liver is integral to most metabolic functions of the body and performs more than 500 tasks. The main functions of the liver include metabolism of carbohydrate, protein, and fat; storage and activation of vitamins and minerals; formation and excretion of bile; conversion of ammonia to urea; metabolism of steroids; and action as a filter and flood chamber.

The liver plays a major role in carbohydrate metabolism. Galactose and fructose, products of carbohydrate digestion, are converted into glucose in the hepatocyte or liver cell. The liver stores glucose as glycogen (glycogenesis) and then returns it to the blood when glucose levels become low (glycogenolysis). The liver also produces "new" glucose (gluconeogenesis) from precursors such as lactic acid, glycogenic amino acids, and intermediates of the tricarboxylic acid cycle (see Chapter 3).

Important protein metabolic pathways occur in the liver. Transamination and oxidative deamination are two such pathways that convert amino acids to substrates that are used in energy and glucose production as well as in the synthesis of nonessential amino acids. Blood-clotting factors such as fibrinogen; prothrombin; and serum proteins, including albumin, α-globulin, β-globulin, transferrin, ceruloplasmin, and lipoproteins are formed by the liver.

Fatty acids from the diet and adipose tissue are converted in the liver to acetyl-coenzyme A by the process of β-oxidation to produce energy. Ketones are also produced. The liver synthesizes and hydrolyzes triglycerides, phospholipids, cholesterol, and lipoproteins as well.

The liver is involved in the storage, activation, and transport of many vitamins and minerals. It stores all the fat-soluble vitamins in addition to vitamin B_{12} and the minerals zinc, iron, copper, and magnesium. Hepatically synthesized proteins transport vitamin A, iron, zinc, and copper in the bloodstream. Carotene is converted to vitamin A, folate to 5-methyl tetrahydrofolic acid, and vitamin D to an active form (25-hydroxycholecalciferol) by the liver.

In addition to functions of nutrient metabolism and storage, the liver forms and excretes bile. Bile salts are metabolized and used for the digestion and absorption of fats and fat-soluble vitamins. Bilirubin is a metabolic end product from red blood cell destruction; it is conjugated and excreted in the bile.

Hepatocytes detoxify ammonia by converting it to urea, 75% of which is excreted by the kidneys. The remaining urea finds its way back to the gastrointestinal tract (GIT). The liver also metabolizes steroids. It inactivates and excretes aldosterone, glucocorticoids, estrogen, progesterone, and testosterone. It is responsible for the detoxification of substances, including drugs and alcohol. Finally, the liver acts as a filter and flood chamber by removing bacteria and debris from blood through the phagocytic action of **Kupffer cells** located in the sinusoids and by storing blood backed up from the vena cava as in right heart failure.

Laboratory Assessment of Liver Function

Biochemical markers are used to evaluate and monitor patients having or suspected of having liver disease. Enzyme assays measure the release of liver enzymes, and other tests measure liver function. Screening tests for hepatobiliary disease include serum levels of bilirubin, alkaline phosphatase, aspartate amino transferase, and alanine aminotransferase. Table 30-1 elaborates common laboratory tests for liver disorders (see also Appendix 30).

DISEASES OF THE LIVER

Diseases of the liver can be acute or chronic, inherited or acquired. Liver disease is classified in various ways: acute viral hepatitis, fulminant hepatitis, chronic hepatitis, nonalcoholic steatohepatitis (NASH), alcoholic hepatitis and cirrhosis, cholestatic liver diseases, inherited disorders, and other liver diseases.

Acute Viral Hepatitis

Acute viral **hepatitis** is a widespread inflammation of the liver and is caused by hepatitis viruses A, B, C, D, and E (Figure 30-1, Table 30-2). Hepatitis A and E are the infectious forms, mainly spread by fecal-oral route. Hepatitis B, C, and D are the serum forms that are spread by blood and body fluids (Hoofnagle, 2007). Minor agents such as Epstein-Barr virus, cytomegalovirus, herpes simplex, yellow fever, and rubella can also cause an acute hepatitis.

The general symptoms of acute viral hepatitis are divided into four phases. The first phase, the early prodromal phase, affects approximately 25% of patients, causing fever, arthralgia, arthritis, rash, and angioedema. This is followed by the preicteric phase, in which malaise, fatigue, myalgia, anorexia, nausea, and vomiting occur. Some patients complain of epigastric or right upper quadrant pain. The third phase is the icteric phase, in which **jaundice** appears. Finally, during the

TABLE 30-1

Common Laboratory Tests Used to Test Liver Function

Laboratory Test	Comment
Hepatic Excretion	
Total serum bilirubin	When increased, may indicate bilirubin overproduction or defect in hepatic uptake or conjugation.
Indirect serum bilirubin	Unconjugated bilirubin; increased with excessive bilirubin production (hemolysis), immaturity of enzyme systems, inherited defects, drug effects.
Direct serum bilirubin	Conjugated bilirubin; increased with depressed bilirubin excretion, hepatobiliary disease, intrahepatic or benign postoperative jaundice and sepsis, and congenital conjugated hyperbilirubinemia.
Urine bilirubin	More sensitive than total serum bilirubin; confirms if liver disease is cause of jaundice.
Urine urobilinogen	Used when obstructive jaundice is expected; rarely used.
Serum bile acids	Reflects efficacy of ileal resorption and hepatic extraction of bile acids from portal circulation; levels increase with liver disease; little clinical use.
Cholestasis	
Serum alkaline phosphatase	Enzyme widely distributed in liver, bone, placenta, intestine, kidney, leukocytes; mainly bound to canalicular membranes in liver; increased levels suggest cholestasis but can be increased with bone disorders, pregnancy, normal growth, and some malignancies.
5′-Nucleotidase (5′-NT)	Enzyme present in canalicular and plasma membranes of hepatocytes; also in heart and pancreas; increases with liver disease.
Leucine aminopeptidase (LAP)	Cellular peptidase; usually increased in cholestasis and suggests hepatobiliary origin of elevation of alkaline phosphatase; may also increase with pregnancy.
γ-Glutamyl transpeptidase (GGT)	Enzyme associated with microsomes and plasma membranes in hepatocytes; also present in kidney, pancreas, heart, brain; increased with liver disease, but also after myocardial infarction, in neuromuscular disease, pancreatic disease, pulmonary disease, diabetes mellitus, and during alcohol ingestion.
Hepatic Enzymes	
Alanine aminotransferase (ALT, formerly SGPT)	Located in cytosol of hepatocyte; found in several other body tissues but highest in liver; increased with liver cell damage.
Aspartate aminotransferase (AST, formerly SGOT)	Located in cytosol and mitochondria of hepatocyte; also in cardiac and skeletal muscle, brain, pancreas, kidney, and leukocytes; increased with liver cell damage.
Serum lactic dehydrogenase	Located in liver, red blood cells, cardiac muscle, kidney; increased with liver disease but lacks sensitivity and specificity because it is found in most other body tissues.
Serum Proteins	
Prothrombin time (PT)	Most blood coagulation factors are synthesized in the liver; vitamin K deficiency and decreased synthesis of clotting factors increase prothrombin time and risk of bleeding.
Partial thromboplastin time (PTT)	Assesses the “intrinsic” clotting mechanism; reflects activity of all clotting factors except platelet factor E, factors VII and XII; complementary to PT.
Serum albumin	Main export protein synthesized in the liver and most important factor in maintaining plasma oncotic pressure; decreased synthesis occurs with liver dysfunction, thyroid and glucocorticoid hormone dysfunction, abnormal plasma colloid osmotic pressure, and toxins; increased losses occur with protein-losing enteropathy, nephrotic syndrome, burns, gastrointestinal bleeding, exfoliative dermatitis.

Continued

TABLE 30-1

Common Laboratory Tests Used to Test Liver Function—cont'd

Laboratory Test	Comment
Serum globulin	α_1 and α_2-globulins are synthesized in the liver; levels increase with chronic liver disease; limited diagnostic use in hepatobiliary disease.
Mitochondrial antibody	90% of patients with PBC have antibodies in their serum against a lipoprotein component of the inner mitochondrial membrane; also present in 25% of patients with chronic active hepatitis and postnecrotic cirrhosis.
Antinuclear and smooth-muscle antibodies	May be positive in patients with chronic active hepatitis (usually not associated with hepatitis B or C virus) and in a minority of patients with PBC; not organ- or species-specific.
Markers of Specific Liver Diseases	
Serum ferritin	Major iron storage protein; increased level sensitive indicator of genetic hemochromatosis.
Ceruloplasmin	Major copper-binding protein synthesized by liver; decreased in Wilson disease.
α-Fetoprotein	Major circulating plasma protein; increased with hepatocellular carcinoma.
α_1-Antitrypsin	Main function is to inhibit serum trypsin activity; decreased levels indicate α_1-antitrypsin deficiency, which can cause liver and lung damage.
Markers for Viral Hepatitis	
IgM anti-HAV	Marker for hepatitis A; indicates current or recent infection or convalescence.
IgG anti-HAV	Marker for hepatitis A; indicates current or previous infection and immunity.
HBsAg	Marker for hepatitis B; positive in most cases of acute or chronic infection.
HBeAg	Marker for hepatitis B; transiently positive during active virus replication; reflects concentration and infectivity of virus.
IgM or IgG anti-HBc	Marker for hepatitis B; positive in all acute and chronic cases; positive in carriers; not protective.
Anti-HBe	Marker for hepatitis B; transiently positive during convalescence and in some chronic cases and carriers; not protective; reflects low infectivity.
Anti-HBs	Marker for hepatitis B; positive late in convalescence; protective.
Anti-HCV	Marker for hepatitis C; positive 5-6 weeks after onset of hepatitis C virus; not protective; reflects infectious state.
HCV-RNA	Marker for hepatitis C.
IgM or IgG anti-HDV	Marker for hepatitis D; indicates infection; not protective.
IgM anti-HEV	Marker for hepatitis E; indicates current or recent infection; not protective.
IgG anti-HEV	Marker for hepatitis E; indicates current or previous infection and immunity.
Miscellaneous	
Ammonia	Liver converts ammonia to urea; may increase with hepatic failure and portal-systemic shunts.

Data from Baker AL: Liver chemistry tests. In Kaplowitz N, editor: Liver and biliary diseases, ed 2, Baltimore, 1996, Williams & Wilkins; Hoofnagle JH, Lindsay KL: Acute viral hepatitis. In Goldman L, Bennett JC, editors: Cecil textbook of medicine, ed 21, Philadelphia, 2000, Saunders; Kamath PS: Clinical approach to the patient with abnormal liver test results, Mayo Clin Proc 71:1089, 1996; Lindsay KL, Hoofnagle JH: Serologic tests for viral hepatitis. In Kaplowitz N, editor: Liver and biliary diseases, ed 2, Baltimore, 1996, Williams & Wilkins; Weisiger RA: Laboratory tests in liver disease. In Goldman L, Bennett JC, editors: Cecil textbook of medicine, ed 21, Philadelphia, 2000, Saunders.

Anti-HBe, Antibody to HBeAg; *HbeAg*, hepatitis B e-antigen; *Anti-HBs*, antibody to HBsAg; *HAV*, hepatic A virus; *HBc*, hepatitis B core; *HBsAg*, hepatitis B surface antigen; *HCV*, hepatitis C virus; *HDV*, hepatitis D virus; *HEV*, hepatitis E virus; *IgG*, immunoglobin G; *IgM*, immunoglobulin M; *PBC*, primary biliary cirrhosis; *RNA*, ribonucleic acid; *SGOT*, serum glutamic oxaloacetic transaminase; *SGPT*, serum glutamic pyruvic transaminase.

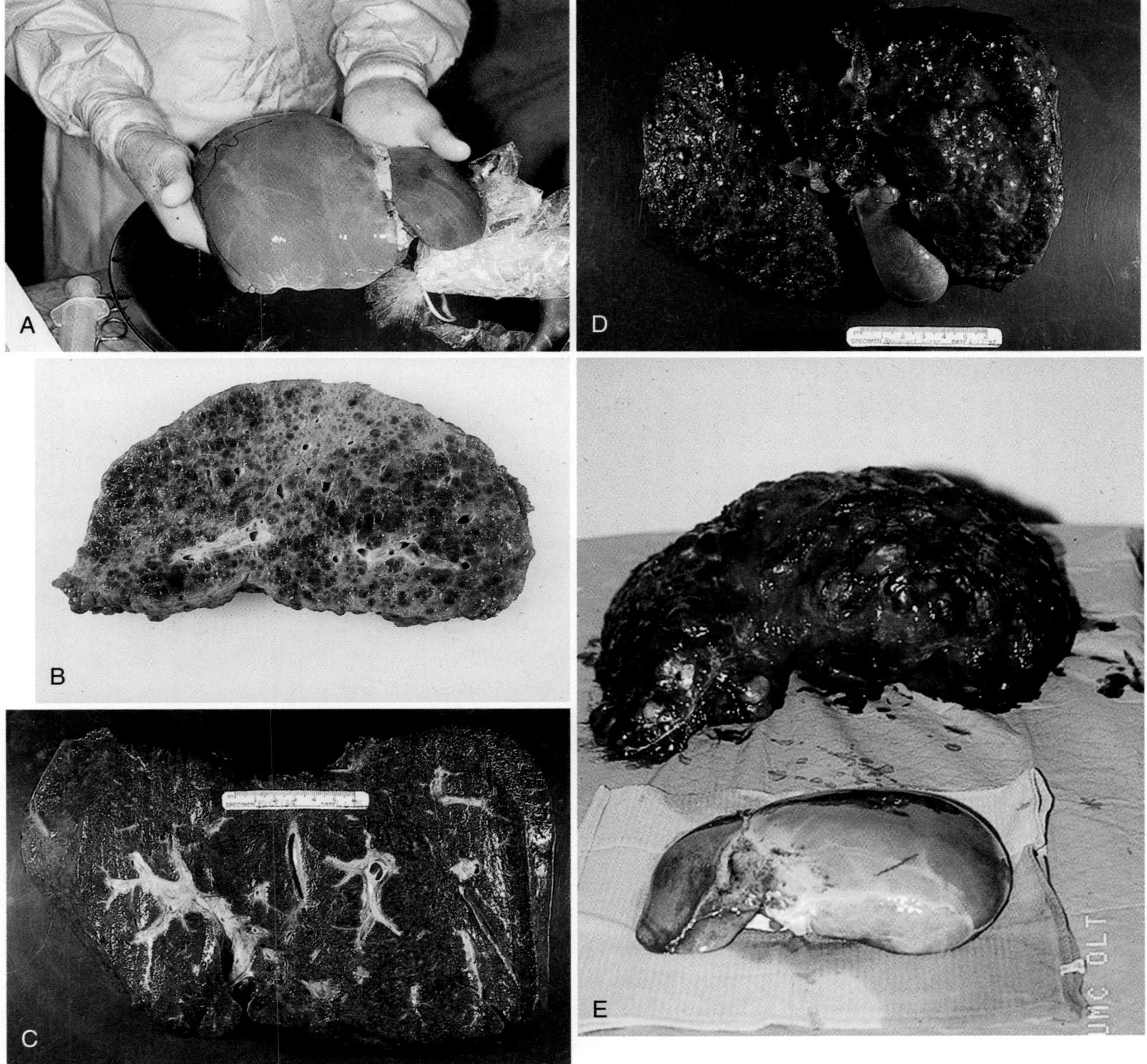

FIGURE 30-1 **A,** Normal liver. **B,** Liver with damage from chronic active hepatitis. **C,** Liver with damage from sclerosing cholangitis. **D,** Liver with damage from primary biliary cirrhosis. **E,** Liver with damage from polycystic liver disease *(background)* and normal liver *(foreground)*. *(Courtesy Baylor Transplant Institute, Baylor University Medical Center, Dallas, TX.)*

TABLE 30-2

Types of Viral Hepatitis

Virus	Transmission	Comments
Hepatitis A	Fecal-oral route; is contracted through contaminated drinking water, food, and sewage.	Anorexia is the most frequent symptom, and it can be severe. Other common symptoms include nausea, vomiting, right upper quadrant abdominal pain, dark urine, and jaundice (icterus). Recovery is usually complete, and long-term consequences are rare. Serious complications may occur in high-risk patients; subsequently, great attention must be given to adequate nutritional intake.
Hepatitis B & C	HBV and HCV are transmitted via blood, blood products, semen, and saliva. For example, they can be spread from contaminated needles, blood transfusions, open cuts or wounds, splashes of blood into the mouth or eyes, or sexual contact.	HBV and HCV can lead to chronic and carrier states. Chronic active hepatitis can also develop, leading to cirrhosis and liver failure.
Hepatitis D	HDV is rare in the United States and depends on the HBV for survival and propagation in humans.	HDV may be a coinfection (occurring at the same time as HBV) or a superinfection (superimposing itself on the HBV carrier state). This form of hepatitis usually becomes chronic.
Hepatitis E	HEV is transmitted via the oral-fecal route.	HEV is rare in the United States (typically only occurs when imported), but it is reported more frequently in many countries of southern, eastern, and central Asia; northern, eastern, and western Africa; and Mexico. Contaminated water appears to be the source of infection, which usually afflicts people living in crowded and unsanitary conditions. HEV is generally acute rather than chronic.
Hepatitis G/GB	HGV and a virus labeled GBV-C appear to be variants of the same virus.	Although HGV infection is present in a significant proportion of blood donors and is transmitted through blood transfusions, it does not appear to cause liver disease.

HBV, Hepatitis B virus; *HCV*, hepatitis C virus; *HDV*, hepatitis D virus; *HEV*, hepatitis E virus; *HGV*, hepatitis G virus.

convalescent phase, jaundice and other symptoms begin to subside.

Complete recovery is expected in more than 95% of hepatitis A cases, in 90% of acute hepatitis B cases, but in only 15% to 50% of acute hepatitis C cases. Chronic hepatitis does not usually develop with hepatitis E, and symptoms and liver function tests usually normalize within 6 weeks (Hoofnagle, 2007).

Fulminant Hepatitis

Fulminant hepatitis is a syndrome in which severe liver dysfunction is accompanied by hepatic encephalopathy, a clinical syndrome characterized by impaired mentation, neuromuscular disturbances, and altered consciousness. **Fulminant liver disease** is defined by the absence of preexisting liver disease and the development of hepatic encephalopathy within 2 to 8 weeks of the onset of illness. The causes of fulminant hepatitis include viral hepatitis in approximately 75% of cases, chemical toxicity (e.g., acetaminophen, drug reactions, poisonous mushrooms, industrial poisons), and other causes (e.g., Wilson's disease, fatty liver of pregnancy, Reye syndrome, hepatic ischemia, hepatic vein obstruction, and disseminated malignancies). Extrahepatic complications of fulminant hepatitis are cerebral edema, coagulopathy and bleeding, cardiovascular abnormalities, renal failure, pulmonary complications, acid-base disturbances, electrolyte imbalances, sepsis, and pancreatitis.

Chronic Hepatitis

To be diagnosed with chronic hepatitis, a patient must have at least a 6-month course of hepatitis or biochemical and clinical evidence of liver disease with confirmatory biopsy findings of unresolving hepatic inflammation (Hoofnagle, 2007). Chronic hepatitis can have autoimmune, viral, metabolic, or medicine or toxin causes. The most common causes of chronic hepatitis are hepatitis B, hepatitis C, and autoimmune hepatitis. Other causes are drug-induced liver disease, metabolic diseases, and NASH. Cryptogenic cirrhosis is cirrhosis of an unknown cause.

Clinical symptoms of chronic hepatitis are usually nonspecific, occur intermittently, and are mild. Common symptoms include fatigue, sleep disorders, difficulty concentrating, and mild right upper quadrant pain. Severe advanced disease can lead to jaundice, muscle wasting, tea-colored urine, ascites, edema, hepatic encephalopathy, gastrointestinal bleeding, splenomegaly, palmar erythema, and spider angiomata.

Nonalcoholic Fatty Liver Disease

Nonalcoholic fatty liver disease (NAFLD) is a spectrum of liver disease ranging from steatosis to steatohepatitis. It involves the accumulation of fat droplets in the hepatocytes and can lead to fibrosis, cirrhosis, and even hepatocellular carcinoma. Steatosis is the simple accumulation of fat within the liver. Causes of NAFLD include drugs, inborn errors of metabolism, and acquired metabolic disorders (type 2 diabetes mellitus, lipodystrophy, jejunal ileal bypass, obesity, and malnutrition) (Diehl, 2007). It is commonly associated with obesity, diabetes mellitus, dyslipidemia, and insulin resistance.

Nonalcoholic steatohepatitis (NASH) is associated with accumulation of fibrous tissue in the liver. A two-hit hypothesis has been proposed to explain why some patients who develop NAFLD do not progress to NASH, and others do. Insulin resistance may lead to steatosis, but some type of oxidative stress is theorized to cause the disease to progress to NASH.

Patients with NASH may be asymptomatic but can experience malaise, weakness, or hepatomegaly. The treatment is often gradual weight loss, insulin-sensitizing drugs such as thiazolidinediones or possibly metformin, and treatment of dyslipidemia. Extreme, rapid weight loss can accelerate NASH developing into cirrhosis and increase the chance of gallstone development.

Chronic liver disease and cirrhosis can develop in patients with NASH. The progression to cirrhosis is variable, depending on age and the presence of obesity and type 2 diabetes, which contribute to a worsening prognosis (Diehl, 2007). Some studies suggest that vitamin E, betaine, and *S*-adenosylmethionine may be beneficial in reducing NASH by reducing tumor necrosis factor–α activity.

Alcoholic Liver Disease

Alcoholic liver disease is the most common liver disease in the United States, with age-adjusted death rates of 4.2 per 100,000 people (National Institute on Alcohol Abuse and Alcoholism, 2005). Acetaldehyde is a toxic byproduct of alcohol metabolism that causes damage to mitochondrial membrane structure and function. Acetaldehyde is produced by multiple metabolic pathways, one of which involves alcohol dehydrogenase (see *Focus On:* Metabolic Consequences of Alcohol Consumption).

Several variables predispose some people to alcoholic liver disease. These include genetic polymorphisms of alcohol-metabolizing enzymes, gender (women more than men), simultaneous exposure to other drugs, infections with hepatotropic viruses, immunologic factors, and poor nutrition status. The pathogenesis of alcoholic liver disease progresses in three stages (Figure 30-2): hepatic steatosis (Figure 30-3), alcoholic hepatitis, and finally cirrhosis.

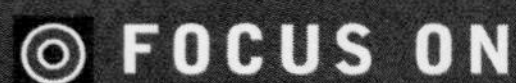

Metabolic Consequences of Alcohol Consumption

Ethanol is metabolized primarily in the liver by alcohol dehydrogenase. This results in acetaldehyde production with the transfer of hydrogen to nicotinamide adenine dinucleotide (NAD), reducing it to NADH. The acetaldehyde then loses hydrogen and is converted to acetate, most of which is released into the blood.

Many metabolic disturbances occur because of the excess of NADH, which overrides the ability of the cell to maintain a normal redox state. These include hyperlacticacidemia, acidosis, hyperuricemia, ketonemia, and hyperlipemia. The tricarboxylic acid (TCA) cycle is depressed because it requires NAD. The mitochondria, in turn, use hydrogen from ethanol rather than from the oxidation of fatty acids to produce energy via the TCA cycle, which leads to a decreased fatty acid oxidation and accumulation of triglycerides. In addition, NADH may actually promote fatty acid synthesis. Hypoglycemia can also occur in early alcoholic liver disease secondary to the suppression of the TCA cycle, coupled with decreased gluconeogenesis due to ethanol.

Hepatic Steatosis

Fatty infiltration, known as **hepatic steatosis** or **fatty liver**, is caused by a culmination of these metabolic disturbances: (1) an increase in the mobilization of fatty acids from adipose tissue; (2) an increase in hepatic synthesis of fatty acids; (3) a decrease in fatty acid oxidation; (4) an increase in triglyceride production; and (5) a trapping of triglycerides in the liver. Hepatic steatosis is reversible with abstinence from alcohol. Conversely, if alcohol abuse continues, cirrhosis can develop.

Alcoholic Hepatitis

Alcoholic hepatitis is generally characterized by hepatomegaly, modest elevation of transaminase levels, increased serum bilirubin concentrations, normal or depressed serum albumin concentrations, or anemia. Patients may also have abdominal pain, anorexia, nausea, vomiting, weakness, diarrhea, weight loss, or fever. If patients discontinue alcohol intake, hepatitis may resolve; however, the condition often progresses to the third stage. Nutrition support is the main treatment in addition to counseling or support to continue avoidance of alcohol. Molecular genetics may lead to new therapies in the future (Willner and Reuben, 2005).

Alcoholic Cirrhosis

Clinical features of alcoholic **cirrhosis**, the third stage, vary. Symptoms can mimic those of alcoholic hepatitis; or patients can develop gastrointestinal bleeding, hepatic encephalopathy, or **portal hypertension** (elevated blood pressure in the

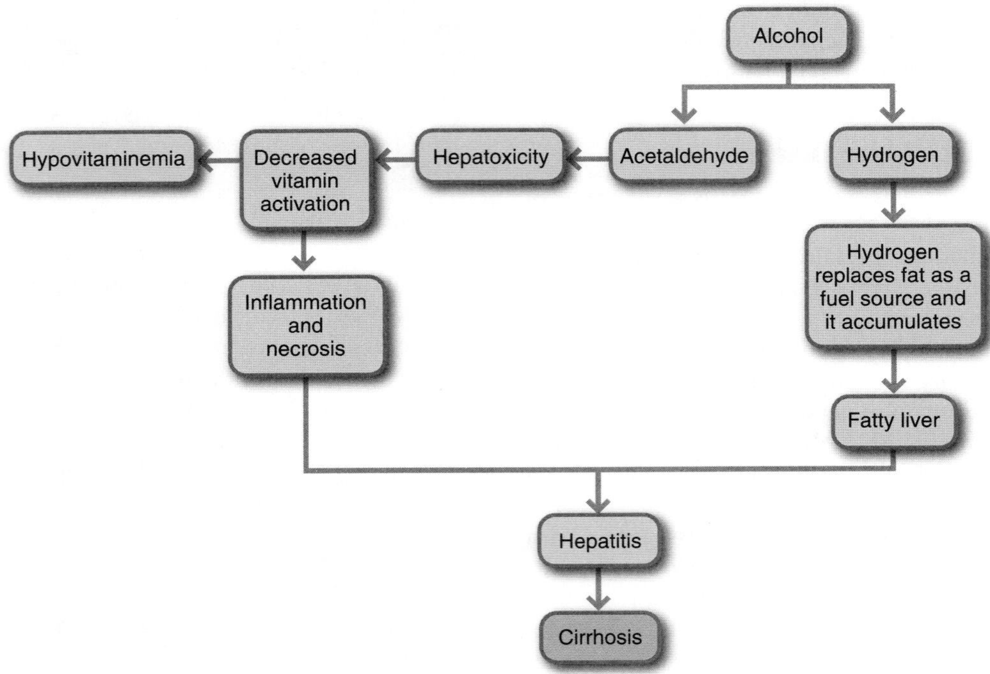

FIGURE 30-2 Complications of excessive alcohol consumption stem largely from excess hydrogen and from acetaldehyde. Hydrogen produces fatty liver and hyperlipemia, high blood lactic acid, and low blood sugar. The accumulation of fat, the effect of acetaldehyde on liver cells, and other factors as yet unknown lead to alcoholic hepatitis. The next step is cirrhosis. The consequent impairment of liver function disturbs blood chemistry, notably causing a high ammonia level that can lead to coma and death. Cirrhosis also distorts liver structure, inhibiting blood flow. High pressure in vessels supplying the liver may cause ruptured varices and accumulation of fluid in the abdominal cavity. Response to alcohol differs among individuals; in particular, not all heavy drinkers develop hepatitis and cirrhosis.

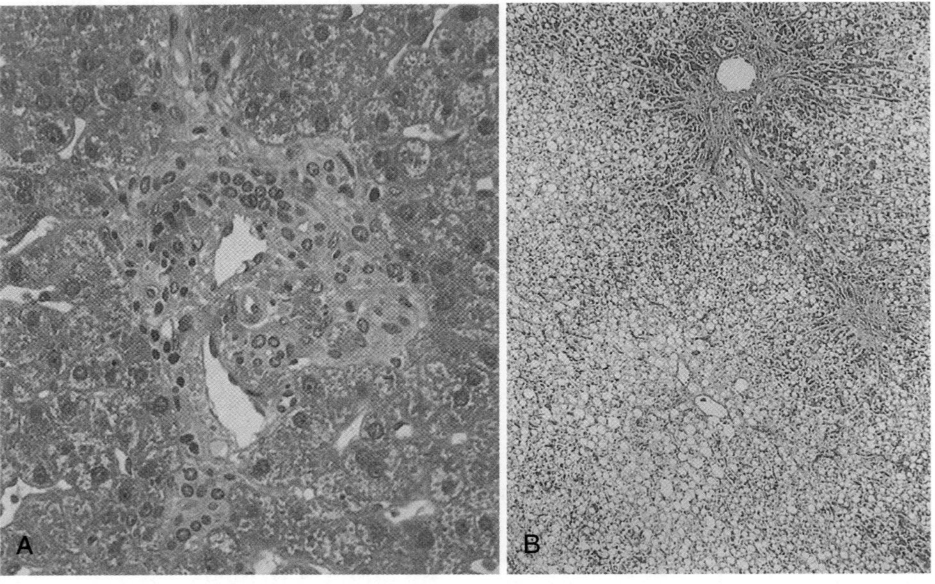

FIGURE 30-3 **A,** Microscopic appearance of a normal liver. A normal portal tract consists of the portal vein, hepatic arteriole, one to two interlobular bile ducts, and occasional peripherally located ductules. **B,** Acute fatty liver. This photomicrograph on low power exhibits fatty change involving virtually all the hepatocytes, with slight sparing of the liver cells immediately adjacent to the portal tract *(top)*. *(From Kanel G, Korula J: Atlas of liver pathology, Philadelphia, 1992, Saunders.)*

portal venous system caused by the obstruction of blood flow through the liver). They often develop **ascites**, the accumulation of fluid, serum protein, and electrolytes within the peritoneal cavity caused by increased pressure from portal hypertension and decreased production of albumin (which maintains serum colloidal osmotic pressure). A liver biopsy usually reveals micronodular cirrhosis, but it can be macronodular or mixed. Prognosis depends on abstinence from alcohol and the degree of complications already developed. Ethanol ingestion creates specific and severe nutritional abnormalities (see *Clinical Insight*: Malnutrition in the Alcoholic).

Cholestatic Liver Diseases

Primary Biliary Cirrhosis

Primary biliary cirrhosis (PBC) is a chronic cholestatic disease caused by progressive destruction of small and intermediate-size intrahepatic bile ducts. The extrahepatic biliary tree and larger intrahepatic ducts are normal. Ninety-five percent of patients with PBC are women. This disease progresses slowly, eventually resulting in cirrhosis, portal hypertension, liver transplantation, or death (Afdhal, 2007).

PBC is an immune-mediated disease in which serum autoantibodies, elevated immunoglobulin levels, circulating immune complexes, and depressed cell-mediated immune response are present. PBC typically presents with a mild elevation of liver enzymes with physical symptoms of pruritus and fatigue. Treatment with ursodeoxycholic acid can slow progression of the disease (Afdhal, 2007). Several nutritional complications from cholestasis can occur with PBC, including osteopenia, hypercholesterolemia, and fat-soluble vitamin deficiencies.

Sclerosing Cholangitis

Sclerosing cholangitis shows fibrosing inflammation of segments of extrahepatic bile ducts, with or without involvement of intrahepatic ducts. Progression of the disease leads to complications of portal hypertension, **hepatic failure** (liver function diminished to 25% or less), and cholangiocarcinoma. Primary sclerosing cholangitis (PSC) is the most common type. Like PBC, PSC may be an immune disorder because of its strong association with human leukocyte antigen haplotypes, autoantibodies, and multiple immunologic abnormalities. Of patients with PSC, 70% to 90% also have inflammatory bowel disease (especially ulcerative colitis), and men are more likely than women (2.3 : 1) to have PSC (Afdhal, 2007). Patients with PSC are also at increased risk of fat-soluble vitamin deficiencies resulting from steatorrhea associated with this disease. **Hepatic osteodystrophy** may occur from vitamin D and calcium malabsorption, resulting in secondary hyperparathyroidism, osteomalacia, or rickets. No treatment slows progression of the disease or improves survival. Ursodeoxycholic acid may improve laboratory values (serum bilirubin, alkaline phosphatase, and albumin), but has no effect on survival (Afdhal, 2007).

CLINICAL INSIGHT

Malnutrition in the Alcoholic

Several factors contribute to the malnutrition that is common in chronic alcoholics with liver disease:

1. Alcohol can replace food in the diet of moderate and heavy drinkers, displacing the intake of adequate calories and nutrients. In light drinkers, it is usually an additional energy source, or empty calories. Although alcohol yields 7.1 kcal/g, when it is consumed in large amounts it is not used efficiently as a fuel source. When individuals consume alcohol on a regular basis but do not fulfill criteria for alcohol abuse, they are often overweight because of the increased calories (alcohol addition). This is different from the heavy drinker who replaces energy-rich nutrients with alcohol (alcohol substitution).
2. In the alcoholic, impaired digestion and absorption are related to pancreatic insufficiency, as well as morphologic and functional alterations of the intestinal mucosa. Acute and chronic alcohol intake impairs hepatic amino acid uptake and synthesis into proteins, reduces protein synthesis and secretion from the liver, and increases catabolism in the gut.
3. Use of lipids and carbohydrates is compromised. An excess of reduction equivalents (e.g., nicotinamide adenine dinucleotide phosphate) and impaired oxidation of triglycerides result in fat deposition in the hepatocytes and an increase in circulating triglycerides. Insulin resistance is also common.
4. Vitamin and mineral deficiencies occur in alcoholic liver disease as a result of reduced intake and alterations in absorption, storage, and ability to convert the nutrients to their active forms (Leevy and Moroianu, 2005). Steatorrhea resulting from bile acid deficiency is also common in alcoholic liver disease affecting fat-soluble vitamin absorption. Vitamin A deficiency can lead to night blindness (Leevy and Moroianu, 2005). Thiamin deficiency is the most common vitamin deficiency in alcoholics and is responsible for Wernicke encephalopathy (Leevy and Moroianu, 2005). Folate deficiency can occur as a result of poor intake, impaired absorption, accelerated excretion, and altered storage and metabolism. Inadequate dietary intake and interactions between pyridoxal-5′-phosphate (active coenzyme of vitamin B6) and alcohol reduce vitamin B6 status. Deficiency of all B vitamins and vitamins C, D, E, and K is also common (Leevy and Moroianu, 2005). Hypocalcemia, hypomagnesemia, and hypophosphatemia are not uncommon among alcoholics; furthermore, zinc deficiency and alterations in other micronutrients can accompany chronic alcohol intake (Leevy and Moroianu, 2005).

Inherited Disorders

Inherited disorders of the liver include hemochromatosis, Wilson disease, α_1-antitrypsin deficiency, protoporphyria, cystic fibrosis, glycogen storage disease, amyloidosis, and sarcoidosis. The first three disorders most commonly result in liver failure.

Hemochromatosis

Hemochromatosis is an inherited disease of iron overload associated with the gene HFE. Patients with hereditary hemochromatosis absorb excessive iron from the gut and may store 20 to 40 g of iron compared with 0.3 to 0.8 g in normal persons (see Chapter 33). Increased transferrin saturation (≥45%) and ferritin (more than two times normal) suggest hemochromatosis. Hepatomegaly, esophageal bleeding, ascites, impaired hepatic synthetic function, abnormal skin pigmentation, glucose intolerance, cardiac involvement, hypogonadism, arthropathy, and hepatocellular carcinoma may develop. Early diagnosis includes clinical, laboratory, and pathologic testing, including elevated serum transferrin levels. Life expectancy is normal if phlebotomy is initiated before the development of cirrhosis or diabetes mellitus.

Wilson's Disease

Wilson's disease is an autosomal-recessive disorder associated with impaired biliary copper excretion. Copper accumulates in various tissues, including the liver, brain, cornea, and kidneys. **Kayser-Fleischer rings** are greenish-yellow pigmented rings encircling the cornea just within the corneoscleral margin, formed by copper deposits. Patients can present with acute, fulminant, or chronic active hepatitis and with neuropsychiatric symptoms. Low serum ceruloplasmin levels, elevated copper concentration in a liver biopsy, and high urinary copper excretion confirm the diagnosis (Kowdley, 2007).

Copper-chelating agents and zinc supplementation (to inhibit intestinal copper absorption and binding in the liver) are used to treat Wilson disease once it is diagnosed. Copper chelation improves survival but does not prevent cirrhosis; transplantation corrects the metabolic defect (Medici, 2006). A low-copper diet is no longer required, but could be implemented if other therapies are unsuccessful (see Table 30-3). If this disease is not diagnosed until onset of fulminant failure, survival is not possible without transplantation.

α_1-Antitrypsin Deficiency

α_1-Antitrypsin deficiency is an inherited disorder that can cause both liver and lung disease. α_1-Antitrypsin is a glycoprotein found in serum and body fluids; it inhibits neutrophil proteinases. Cholestasis or cirrhosis is caused by this deficiency and there is no treatment except liver transplantation.

Other Liver Diseases

Liver disease has several other causes. Liver tumors can be primary or metastatic, benign or malignant. Hepatocellular carcinoma usually develops in cirrhotic livers. The highest risk occurs in those with hepatitis B, hepatitis C, and

TABLE 30-3

Copper Content of Commonly Used Foods*

Food Groups	High (>0.2 mg/Portion Commonly Used†) (Avoid)	Moderate (0.1-0.2 mg/Portion) (No More Than 6 Servings/Day)	Low (<0.1 mg/Portion Commonly Used†) (May Be Eaten As Desired)
Meat and meat substitutes	Lamb; pork; pheasant; quail; duck; goose; squid; salmon; all organ meats including liver, heart, kidney, brain; all shellfish, including oysters, scallops, shrimp, lobster, clams, and crab; meat gelatin; soy protein meat substitutes; tofu; all nuts and seeds	All other fish (3 oz), dark meat turkey (3 oz), peanut butter (2 tbsp)	Beef, cheese, cottage cheese, eggs, light meat turkey; cold cuts and frankfurters that do not contain pork, dark turkey or organ meats, all others not listed on high or moderate list
Fats and oil	Avocado	Olives (2 medium); cream (½ c)	Butter, cream, margarine, mayonnaise, nondairy cream substitutes, oils, sour cream, salad dressings (made from allowed ingredients), all others not listed on high or moderate list
Milk	Chocolate, cocoa, soy milk		All other daily products, milk flavored with carob

TABLE 30-3

Copper Content of Commonly Used Foods*—cont'd

Food Groups	High (>0.2 mg/Portion Commonly Used†) (Avoid)	Moderate (0.1-0.2 mg/Portion) (No More Than 6 Servings/Day)	Low (<0.1 mg/Portion Commonly Used†) (May Be Eaten As Desired)
Starch	Dried beans, including soybeans, lima beans, baked beans, garbanzo beans, pinto beans; dried peas; lentils; millet; barley; wheat germ; bran breads and cereals; cereals with >0.2 mg of copper per serving (check label); soy flour; soy grits; sweet potatoes (fresh)	Whole-wheat bread (1 slice), potatoes in any form (½ c or 1 small), pumpkin (¾ c), melba toast (4), whole-wheat crackers (6), parsnips (⅔ c), winter squash (½ c), green peas (½ c), instant oatmeal (½ c), instant Ralston (½ c), cereals with 0.1-0.2 mg of copper per serving (check labels), dehydrated and canned soups (1 c)	Breads and pasta from refined flour, canned sweet potatoes, rice, regular oatmeal, cereals with <0.1 mg of copper per serving (check label), all others not listed on high or moderate list
Vegetables	Mushrooms, vegetable juice cocktail	Bean sprouts (1 c), beets (½ c), spinach (½ c cooked, 1 c raw), tomato juice and other tomato products (½ c), broccoli (½ c), asparagus (½ c)	All others, including fresh tomatoes
Fruits	Nectarines; dried fruits, including raisins, dates, and prunes (dried fruits are permitted if dried at home)	Mango (½ c), pears (1 medium), pineapple (½ c), papaya ¼ average)	All others
Desserts	Desserts that contain significant amounts of any foods high in copper		All others
Sugar and sweets	Chocolate, cocoa	Licorice (1 oz), syrups (1 oz)	All others including jams, jellies, and candies made with allowed fruits; carob; flavoring extracts
Miscellaneous	Brewer's yeast	Ketchup	
Beverages‡	Instant breakfast beverages, mineral water, alcohol§	Postum and other cereal beverages	All others, including fruit-flavored beverages; lemonade

From Pemberton CM et al: Mayo Clinic diet manual: a handbook of nutrition practices, ed 7, St Louis, 1994, Mosby.

*Copper content of the usual American diet varies, with estimates from 1 mg of copper a day to 5 mg/day. The concentration of copper in foods is affected by soil conditions, geographic location, species, diet, processing method, and contamination in processing. The exact copper content of foods is difficult to verify. It is estimated that avoiding high-copper foods and restricting moderate-copper foods result in a diet of approximately 1 mg/day. For practical purposes, diets are designed to limit foods with higher copper content rather than to achieve a specific level of copper in the diet.

†Portions commonly used are those generally accepted as typical portion sizes in various nutrient data source manuals.

‡A water sample from the patient's home water supply should be analyzed for copper content. Demineralized water should be used if the water contains more than 100 mcg/L.

§Although not necessarily high in copper, alcohol is discouraged because of its action as a hepatotoxin.

hereditary hemochromatosis. The liver can also be affected by systemic diseases such as rheumatoid arthritis, systemic lupus erythematosus, polymyalgia, temporal arteritis, polyarteritis nodosa, systemic sclerosis, and Sjögren's syndrome. When hepatic blood flow is altered, as in acute ischemic and chronic congestive hepatopathy, Budd-Chiari syndrome, and hepatic venoocclusive disease, dysfunction occurs. Individuals with hepatic or portal vein thromboses should be evaluated for a myeloproliferative disorder. Parasitic, bacterial, fungal, and granulomatous liver diseases also occur. Finally, cryptogenic cirrhosis is any cirrhosis for which the cause is unknown.

TREATMENT OF CIRRHOSIS AND ITS COMPLICATIONS

Cirrhosis has many clinical manifestations, as illustrated in Figure 30-4. Several major complications of cirrhosis

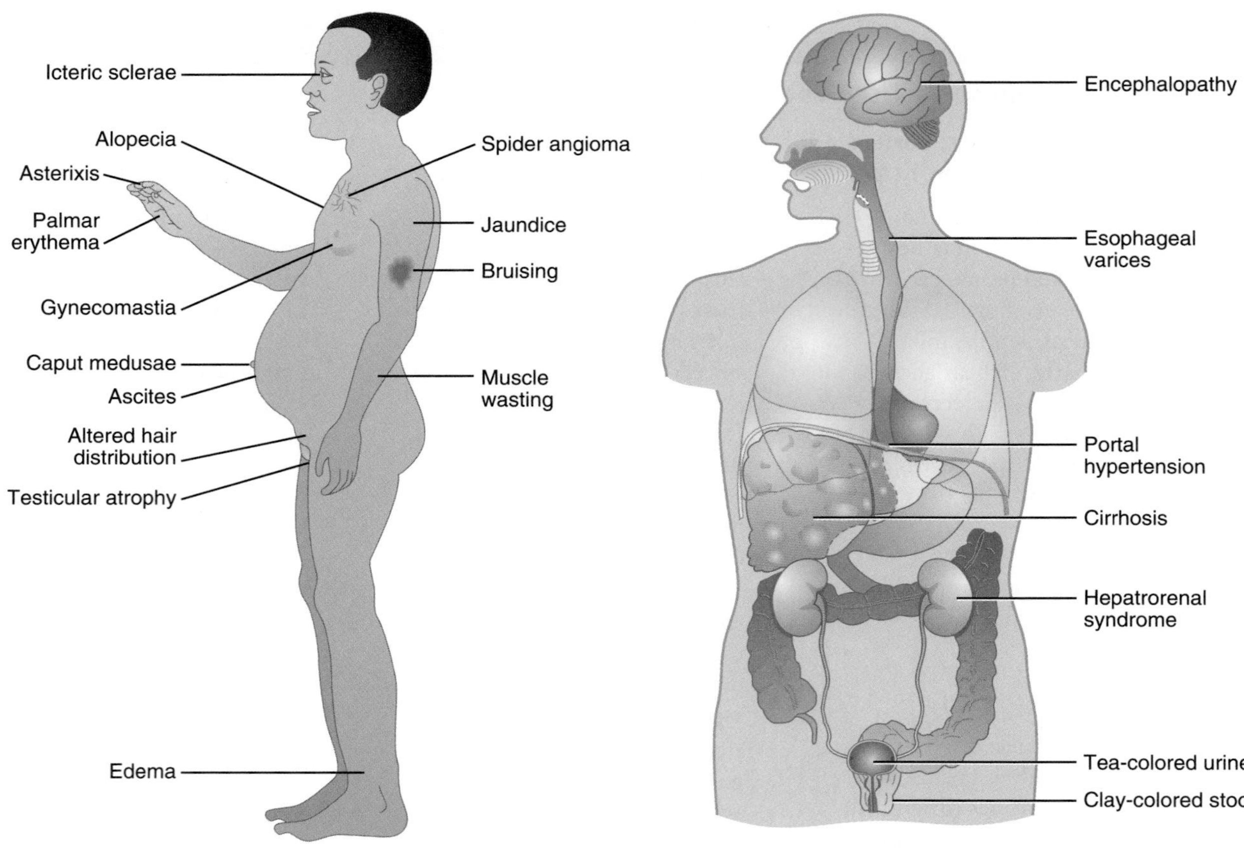

FIGURE 30-4 Clinical manifestations of cirrhosis.

and end-stage liver disease (ESLD), including malnutrition, ascites, hyponatremia, hepatic encephalopathy, glucose alterations, fat malabsorption, hepatorenal syndrome, and osteopenia, have nutritional implications. When appropriate nutrition therapy is provided to patients with liver disease, malnutrition can be reversed, and clinical outcomes improved. Studies to date have shown positive outcomes with oral and enteral nutrition (EN) in malnourished patients with cirrhosis, including improvement in nutrition status and clinical complications of cirrhosis such as ascites, encephalopathy, and infection (Campillo et al., 2005).

Nutrition Assessment

A specific nutrition assessment must be performed to determine the extent and cause of malnutrition. Many traditional markers of nutrition status are affected by liver disease and its consequences, making traditional assessment difficult. Table 30-4 summarizes the factors that affect interpretation of nutrition assessment parameters in patients with liver dysfunction.

Objective parameters that are helpful when monitored serially include anthropometric measurements and dietary intake evaluation (see Chapter 9). The best way to perform a nutrition assessment may be to combine these parameters with the subjective global assessment (SGA) approach, which has demonstrated an acceptable level of reliability and validity. This method uses a few readily available parameters obtained by an experienced clinician. The SGA gives a broad perspective, but it is not sensitive to changes in nutrition status. Other available parameters should also be reviewed. The SGA approach is summarized in Box 30-1.

Malnutrition

Moderate to severe malnutrition is a common finding in patients with advanced liver disease (Figure 30-5). This is extremely significant, considering that malnutrition plays a major role in the pathogenesis of liver injury and has a profound negative effect on prognosis. The prevalence of malnutrition depends on nutrition assessment parameters used, type and degree of liver disease, and socioeconomic status.

Numerous coexisting factors are involved in the development of malnutrition in liver disease (see *Pathophysiology and Care Management Algorithm:* Malnutrition in Liver Disease). Inadequate oral intake, a major contributor, is caused by anorexia, dysgeusia, early satiety, nausea, or vomiting associated with liver disease and the drugs used to treat it. Another cause of inadequate intake is dietary restriction.

TABLE 30-4

Factors That Affect Interpretation of Nutrition Assessment in Patients With End-Stage Liver Disease

Parameter	Factors Affecting Interpretation
Body weight	Affected by edema, ascites, and diuretic use.
Anthropometric measurements	Questionable sensitivity, specificity, and reliability. Multiple sources of error. Unknown if skinfold measurements reflect total body fat. References do not account for variation in hydration status and skin compressibility.
Creatinine-height index	Affected by malnutrition, aging, decreased body mass, and protein intake. Affected by renal function. Creatinine is a metabolic end product of creatine synthesized in the liver; therefore severe liver disease alters creatinine synthesis rates.
Nitrogen balance studies	Nitrogen is retained in the body in the form of ammonia. Hepatorenal syndrome can affect the excretion of nitrogen.
3-Methyl histidine excretion	Affected by dietary intake, trauma, infection, and renal function.
Visceral protein levels	Synthesis of visceral proteins is decreased.
Immune function tests	Affected by hydration status, malabsorption, and renal insufficiency. Affected by hepatic failure, electrolyte imbalances, infection, and renal insufficiency.
Bioelectrical impedance	Invalid with ascites and edema.

Modified from Hasse J: Nutritional aspects of adult liver transplantation. In Busuttil RW, Klintmalm GB, editors: Transplantation of the liver, ed 2, Philadelphia, 2005, Saunders.

BOX 30-1

Subjective Global Assessment Parameters for Nutrition Evaluation of Liver Disease Patients

History

Weight change (consider fluctuations resulting from ascites and edema)
Appetite
Taste changes and early satiety
Dietary intake (calories, protein, sodium)
Persistent gastrointestinal problems (nausea, vomiting, diarrhea, constipation, difficulty chewing or swallowing)

Physical Findings

Muscle wasting
Fat stores
Ascites or edema

Existing Conditions

Disease state and other problems that could influence nutrition status such as hepatic encephalopathy, gastrointestinal bleeding, renal insufficiency, infection

Nutritional Rating Based on Results

Well nourished
Moderately (or suspected of being) malnourished
Severely malnourished

From Hasse J: Nutritional aspects of adult liver transplantation. In Busuttil RW, Klintmalm GB, editors: Transplantation of the liver, ed 2, Philadelphia, 2005, Saunders.

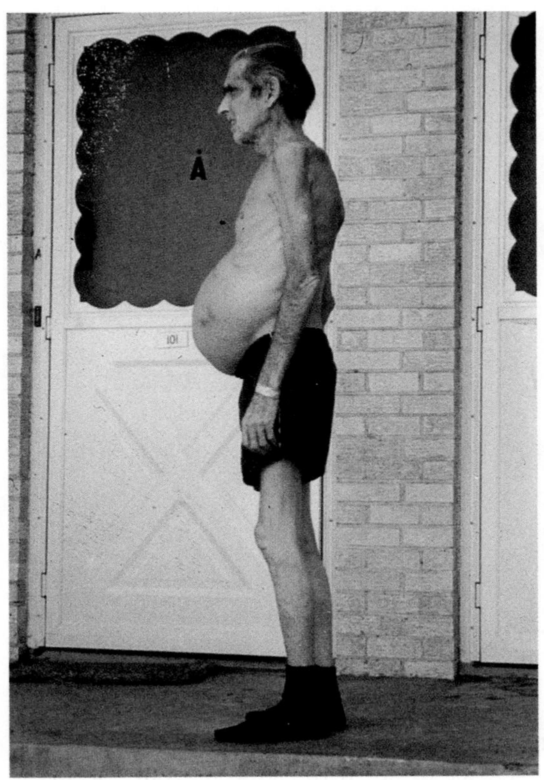

FIGURE 30-5 Severe malnutrition and ascites in a man with end-stage liver disease.

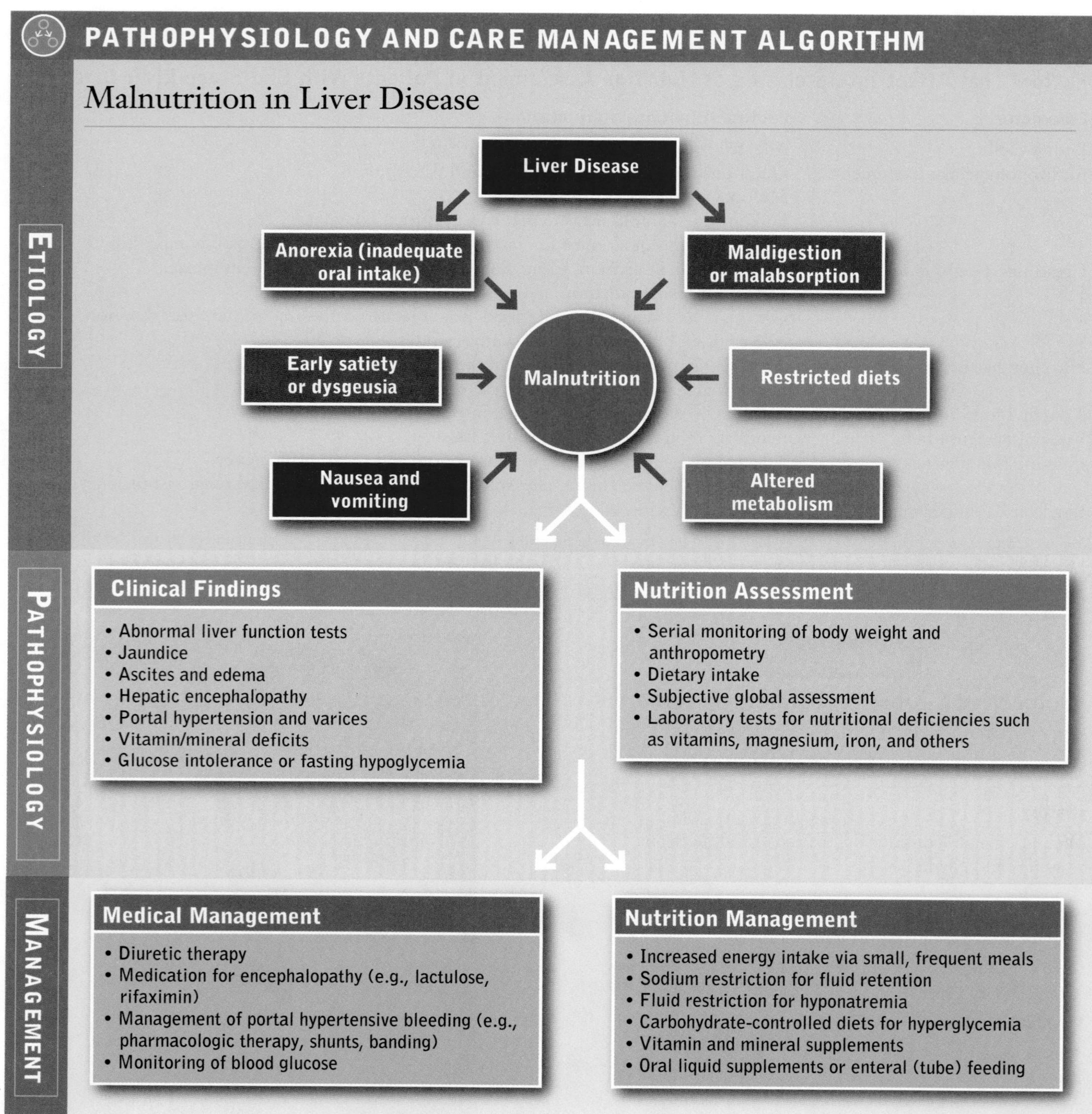

Maldigestion and malabsorption also play a role. **Steatorrhea**, presence of fat in the stool, is common in cirrhosis, especially if there is disease involving bile duct injury and obstruction. Medications may also cause specific malabsorptive losses. In addition, altered metabolism secondary to liver dysfunction causes malnutrition in various ways. Micronutrient function is affected by altered storage in the liver, decreased transport by liver-synthesized proteins, and renal losses associated with alcoholic and advanced liver disease. Abnormal macronutrient metabolism and increased energy expenditure can also contribute to malnutrition. Finally, protein losses can occur from large-volume **paracentesis** when fluid from the abdomen (ascites) is removed through a needle.

Nutrition Intake Problems

Because anorexia, nausea, dysgeusia, and other gastrointestinal symptoms are common, adequate nutrition intake is difficult to achieve. With ascites, early satiety is also a frequent complaint. Smaller, more frequent meals are better tolerated than three traditional meals. In addition, frequent feedings may also improve nitrogen balance and prevent hypoglycemia. Oral liquid supplements should be encouraged, and, when necessary, enteral tube feedings used. Adjunctive nutrition support should be given to malnourished patients with liver disease if their intake is less than dietary reference intake (DRI) levels of 0.8 g of protein and 30 calories/kg of body weight daily and if they are at risk for fatal complications from the disease. Esophageal varices are usually not a contraindication for tube feeding (Crippin, 2006).

Nutrient Requirements

Energy

Energy requirements vary among patients with cirrhosis. Several studies have measured resting energy expenditure (REE) in patients with liver disease to determine energy requirements. Some found that patients with ESLD had normal metabolism and that others had hypometabolism or hypermetabolism. Ascites or shunt placement may increase energy expenditure slightly.

In general, energy requirements for patients with ESLD and without ascites are approximately 120% to 140% of the REE. Requirements increase to 150% to 175% of REE if ascites, infection, and malabsorption are present or if nutritional repletion is necessary. This equates to approximately 25 to 35 calories per kilogram body weight. Estimated dry body weight should be used in calculations to prevent overfeeding. Oral nutritional supplements or tube feeding can increase or ensure optimal intake in malnourished patients, thus reducing complications and prolonging survival (Plauth et al., 2006).

Carbohydrates

Determining carbohydrate needs is challenging in liver failure because of the primary role of the liver in carbohydrate metabolism. Liver failure reduces glucose production and peripheral glucose use. The rate of gluconeogenesis is decreased, with preference for lipids and amino acids for energy. Alterations in the hormones insulin, glucagon, cortisol, and epinephrine are responsible in part for the preference for alternative fuels. In addition, insulin resistance can be present with liver dysfunction.

Lipid

In cirrhosis, plasma free fatty acids, glycerol, and ketone bodies are increased in the fasting state. The body prefers lipids as an energy substrate. Lipolysis is increased with active mobilization of lipid deposits, but the net capacity to store exogenous lipid is not impaired. A range of 25% to 40% of calories as fat is generally recommended.

Protein

Protein is by far the most controversial nutrient in liver failure, and its management is also the most complex. Cirrhosis has long been thought of as a catabolic disease with increased protein breakdown, inadequate resynthesis, depleted status, and muscle wasting. However, protein kinetic studies demonstrate increased nitrogen losses only in patients with fulminant hepatic failure or decompensated disease but not in stable cirrhosis.

Patients with cirrhosis also have increased protein use. Studies suggest that 0.8 g of protein/kg/day is the mean protein requirement to achieve nitrogen balance in stable cirrhosis. Therefore in uncomplicated hepatitis or cirrhosis without encephalopathy, protein requirements range from 0.8 to 1 g/kg of dry weight per day to achieve nitrogen balance.

To promote nitrogen accumulation or positive balance, at least 1.2 to 1.3 g/kg daily is needed. In situations of stress such as alcoholic hepatitis or decompensated disease (sepsis, infection, gastrointestinal bleeding, or severe ascites), at least 1.5 g of protein per kilogram per day should be provided.

Vitamins and Minerals

Vitamin and mineral supplementation is needed in all patients with ESLD because of the intimate role of the liver in nutrient transport, storage, and metabolism, in addition to the side effects of drugs (Table 30-5). Vitamin deficiencies can contribute to complications. For example, folate and vitamin B_{12} deficiencies can lead to macrocytic anemia. Deficiency of pyridoxine, thiamin, or vitamin B_{12} can result in neuropathy. Confusion, ataxia, and ocular disturbances can result from a thiamin deficiency.

Deficiencies of fat-soluble vitamins have been found in all types of liver failure, especially in cholestatic diseases in which malabsorption and steatorrhea occur. Impaired dark adaptation can occur from vitamin A deficiency. Hepatic osteodystrophy or osteopenia can develop from vitamin D deficiency. Therefore supplementation is necessary, and may require using water-soluble forms. Intravenous or intramuscular vitamin K is often given for 3 days to rule out vitamin K deficiency as the cause of a prolonged prothrombin times. Water-soluble vitamin deficiencies associated with liver disease include thiamin (which can lead to **Wernicke encephalopathy**), pyridoxine (B_6), cyanocobalamin (B_{12}), folate, and niacin (B_3). Large doses (100 mg) of thiamin are given daily for a limited time if deficiency is suspected.

Mineral nutriture is also altered in liver disease. Iron stores may be depleted in patients experiencing gastrointestinal bleeding; however, iron supplementation should be avoided by persons with hemochromatosis or hemosiderosis (see Chapter 33). Elevated serum copper levels are found in cholestatic liver diseases (i.e., PBC and PSC). Because copper and manganese are excreted primarily via bile, supplements should not contain these minerals. Manganese deposition has been noted to accumulate in brains of patients with cirrhosis leading to impaired motor function (Garcia-Tsao, 2007).

In Wilson's disease, excess copper in various organs causes severe damage. Oral chelating agents such as zinc acetate or *d*-penicillamine are the primary treatment. Dietary copper

TABLE 30-5

Vitamin and Mineral Deficits in Severe Hepatic Failure

Vitamin or Mineral	Predisposing Factors	Signs of Deficiency
Vitamin A	Steatorrhea, neomycin, cholestyramine, alcoholism	Night-blindness, increased infection risk
Vitamin B1 (thiamine)	Alcoholism, high CHO diet	Neuropathy, ascites, edema, CNS dysfunction
Vitamin B3 (niacin)	Alcoholism	Dermatitis, dementia, diarrhea, inflammation of mucous membranes
Vitamin B_6 (pyridoxine)	Alcoholism	Mucous membrane lesions, seborrheic dermatitis, glossitis, angular stomatitis, blepharitis, peripheral neuropathy, microcytic anemia, depression
Vitamin B_{12} (Cyanocobalamin)	Alcoholism, cholestyramine	Megaloblastic anemia, glossitis, CNS dysfunction
Folate	Alcoholism	Megaloblastic anemia, glossitis, irritability
Vitamin D	Steatorrhea, glucocorticoids, cholestyramine	Osteomalacia, rickets (in children), possible link to cancer or autoimmune disorders
Vitamin E	Steatorrhea, cholestyramine	Peripheral neuropathy, ataxia, skeletal myopathy, retinopathy, immune system impairment
Vitamin K	Steatorrhea, antibiotics, cholestyramine	Excessive bleeding; bruising
Iron	Chronic bleeding	Stomatitis, microcytic anemia, malaise
Magnesium	Alcoholism, diuretics	Neuromuscular irritability, hypokalemia, hypocalcemia
Phosphorus	Anabolism, alcoholism	Anorexia, weakness, cardiac failure, glucose intolerance
Zinc	Diarrhea, diuretics, alcoholism	Immunodeficiency, impaired taste acuity, wound healing, protein synthesis

CNS, central nervous system.

restriction (see Table 30-3) is not routinely prescribed unless other therapies are unsuccessful. A vegetarian diet may be useful as adjunctive therapy; copper is less available.

Zinc and magnesium levels are low in liver disease related to alcoholism, in part because of diuretic therapy. Calcium, as well as magnesium and zinc, may be malabsorbed with steatorrhea. Therefore the patient should take supplements of these minerals at least at the level of the DRI.

Herbal Supplements

There are multiple case reports of different herbal supplements resulting in liver failure. Terpenoid-containing dietary supplements have been implicated in causing severe and sometimes fatal hepatotoxicity, including teucrium polium (germander), Sho-saiko-to, *Centella asiatica*, and black cohosh (Chitturi and Farrell, 2008). Liver injury has also been caused by N-nitrosofenfluramine, ephedra alkaloids, Boh-Gol-Zhee, Kava, and pyrrolizidine alkaloids (Chitturi and Farrell, 2008).

Two herbal supplements have become popular in the treatment of liver disease. Milk thistle is popular among those suffering from viral hepatitis or alcoholic liver disease. The active component in milk thistle is silymarin. It is proposed to reduce free radical production and lipid peroxidation associated with hepatotoxicity. *S*-adenosyl-*L*-methionine (SAMe) is another popular complementary medicine product purported to act as a methyl donor for methylation reactions and participate in glutathione (an antioxidant) synthesis. A Cochrane review did not show any evidence to support or refute a beneficial effect of either milk thistle or SAMe in patients with alcoholic liver disease (Rambaldi et al., 2006, 2007).

Portal Hypertension

Pathophysiology and Medical Treatment

Portal hypertension increases collateral blood flow and can result in swollen veins (**varices**) in the GIT. These varices often bleed, causing a medical emergency. Treatment includes administration of α-adrenergic blockers to decrease heart rate, endoscopic banding or variceal ligation, and radiologic or surgical placement of shunts. During an acute bleeding episode, somatostatin analog may be administered to decrease bleeding, or a nasogastric tube equipped with an inflatable balloon is placed to tamponade bleeding vessels.

Medical Nutrition Therapy

During acute bleeding episodes, nutrition cannot be administered enterally. Parenteral nutrition (PN) is indicated if a patient will be taking nothing orally for at least 5 days. Repeated endoscopic therapies may cause esophageal strictures or impair a patient's swallowing. Finally, surgically or radiologically placed shunts may increase the incidence of encephalopathy and reduce nutrient metabolism because blood is shunted past the liver cells.

Ascites

Pathophysiology and Medical Treatment

Fluid retention is common, and ascites (accumulation of fluid in the abdominal cavity) is a serious consequence of liver disease. Portal hypertension, hypoalbuminemia, lymphatic obstruction, and renal retention of sodium and fluid contribute to fluid retention. Increased release of catecholamines, renin, angiotensin, aldosterone, and antidiuretic hormone secondary to peripheral arterial vasodilation causes renal retention of sodium and water.

Large-volume paracentesis may be used to relieve ascites. Diuretic therapy is often used and includes spironolactone and furosemide. These drugs are often used in combination for best effect. Major side effects of loop diuretics such as furosemide include hyponatremia, hypokalemia, hypomagnesemia, hypocalcemia, and hypochloremic acidosis. Conversely, spironolactone is potassium sparing. Therefore serum potassium levels must be monitored carefully and supplemented or restricted if necessary because deficiency or excess can contribute to metabolic abnormalities. Weight; abdominal girth; urinary sodium concentration; and serum levels of urea nitrogen, creatinine, albumin, uric acid, and electrolytes should be monitored during diuretic therapy.

Medical Nutrition Therapy

Dietary treatment for ascites includes sodium restriction in addition to diuretic therapy. Sodium is commonly restricted to 2 g/day (see Chapter 34 and Appendix 37 for discussion of low-sodium diets). More severe limitations may be imposed; however, caution is warranted because of limited palatability and the risk of overrestricting sodium. Adequate protein intake is also important when a patient undergoes frequent paracentesis.

Hyponatremia

Pathophysiology

Hyponatremia often occurs because of decreased ability to excrete water resulting from the persistent release of antidiuretic hormone, sodium losses via paracentesis, excessive diuretic use, or overly aggressive sodium restriction.

Medical Nutrition Therapy

Fluid intake is usually restricted to 1 to 1.5 L/day, depending on the severity of the edema and ascites. A moderate sodium intake should be continued because excessive sodium intake will worsen fluid retention and the dilution of serum sodium levels.

Hepatic Encephalopathy

Pathophysiology and Medical Treatment

Hepatic encephalopathy is a syndrome characterized by impaired mentation, neuromuscular disturbances, and altered consciousness. Gastrointestinal bleeding, fluid and electrolyte abnormalities, uremia, infection, use of sedatives, hyperglycemia or hypoglycemia, alcohol withdrawal, constipation, azotemia, dehydration, portosystemic shunts, and acidosis can precipitate hepatic encephalopathy. Subclinical or minimal hepatic encephalopathy also affects patients with chronic hepatic failure. Hepatic or **portal systemic encephalopathy** results in neuromuscular and behavioral alterations. Box 30-2 describes the four stages of hepatic encephalopathy.

BOX 30-2

Four Stages of Hepatic Encephalopathy

Stage	Symptoms
I	Mild confusion, agitation, irritability, sleep disturbance, decreased attention
II	Lethargy, disorientation, inappropriate behavior, drowsiness
III	Somnolent but arousable, incomprehensible speech, confused, aggressive behavior when awake
IV	Coma

There are three main theories regarding the mechanism by which hepatic encephalopathy occurs. Ammonia accumulation is considered an important causal factor in the development of encephalopathy. When the liver fails, it is unable to detoxify ammonia to urea, and ammonia is a direct cerebral toxin. Ammonia levels are elevated in the brain and bloodstream, leading to impaired neural function through cytotoxicity, cell swelling, and depletion of glutamate (Fitz, 2006). The main source of ammonia is its endogenous production by the GIT from the metabolism of protein and from the degradation of bacteria and blood from gastrointestinal bleeding. Exogenous protein is also a source of ammonia. Some clinicians suggest that dietary protein causes an increase in ammonia levels and subsequently hepatic encephalopathy, but this has not been proven in studies.

Drugs such as lactulose and rifaximin are given. Lactulose is a nonabsorbable disaccharide. It acidifies the colonic contents, retaining ammonia as the ammonium ion. It also acts as an osmotic laxative to remove the ammonia. Rifaximin is a nonabsorbable antibiotic that helps decrease colonic ammonia production.

Another suggested mechanism involves the γ-aminobutyric acid (GABA) receptor complex in contributing to neuronal inhibition in hepatic encephalopathy. Flumazenil or other benzodiazepine receptor antagonists may help reduce hepatic encephalopathy.

A final hypothesis is the "altered neurotransmitter theory." A plasma amino acid imbalance exists in ESLD in which the **branched-chain amino acids (BCAAs)** valine, leucine, and isoleucine are decreased. The BCAAs furnish as much as 30% of energy requirements for skeletal muscle, heart, and brain when gluconeogenesis and ketogenesis are depressed causing serum BCAA levels to fall. **Aromatic**

amino acids (AAAs) tryptophan, phenylalanine, and tyrosine, plus methionine, glutamine, asparagine, and histidine are increased, Plasma AAAs and methionine are released into circulation by muscle proteolysis, but the synthesis into protein and liver clearance of AAAs is depressed. This changes the plasma molar ratio of BCAAs to AAAs and may contribute to the development of hepatic encephalopathy. High levels of AAAs may limit the cerebral uptake of BCAAs because they compete for carrier-mediated transport at the blood-brain barrier.

Medical Nutrition Therapy

The practice of protein restriction in patients with low-grade hepatic encephalopathy is based on the premise that protein intolerance causes hepatic encephalopathy, but it has never been proven in a study. True dietary protein intolerance is rare except in fulminant hepatic failure, or in a rare patient with chronic endogenous hepatic encephalopathy. Unnecessary protein restriction may worsen body protein losses and must be avoided.

Patients with encephalopathy often do not receive adequate protein. More than 95% of patients with cirrhosis can tolerate mixed-protein diets up to 1.5 g/kg of body weight. Studies evaluating the benefit of supplements enriched with BCAAs and restricted in AAAs have varied in study design, sample size, composition of formulas, level of encephalopathy, type of liver disease, duration of therapy, and control groups. When high methodologic quality studies are evaluated, there are no significant improvements or survival benefits associated with giving extra BCAAs to patients.

Other theories postulate that vegetable proteins and casein may improve mental status compared with meat protein. Casein-based diets are lower in AAAs and higher in BCAAs than meat-based diets. Vegetable protein is low in methionine and ammoniagenic amino acids, but BCAA-rich. The high-fiber content of a vegetable-protein diet may also play a role in the excretion of nitrogenous compounds.

Finally, it has been proposed that probiotics and synbiotics (sources of gut-friendly bacteria and fermentable fibers) can be used to treat hepatic encephalopathy. Probiotics (see Chapter 29) may improve hepatic encephalopathy by reducing ammonia portal blood (Pereg et al., 2010) or by preventing production or uptake of lipopolysaccharides in the gut (Gratz et al., 2010). Thus they decrease inflammation and oxidative stress in the hepatocyte (thus increasing hepatic clearance of toxins including ammonia), and minimizing uptake of other toxins.

Glucose Alterations

Pathophysiology

Glucose intolerance occurs in almost two thirds of patients with cirrhosis, and 10% to 37% of patients develop overt diabetes. Glucose intolerance in patients with liver disease occurs because of insulin resistance in peripheral tissues. Hyperinsulinism also occurs in patients with cirrhosis, possibly because insulin production is increased, hepatic clearance is decreased, portal systemic shunting occurs, there is a defect in the insulin-binding action at the receptor site, or there is a postreceptor defect.

Fasting hypoglycemia, or low blood glucose, can occur because of the decreased availability of glucose from glycogen in addition to the failing gluconeogenic capacity of the liver when the patient has ESLD. Hypoglycemia occurs more often in acute or fulminant liver failure than in chronic liver disease. Hypoglycemia may also occur after alcohol consumption in patients whose glycogen stores are depleted by starvation because of the block of hepatic gluconeogenesis by ethanol.

Medical Nutrition Therapy

Patients with diabetes should receive standard medical and nutrition therapy to achieve normoglycemia (see Chapter 31). Patients with hypoglycemia should eat frequently to prevent this condition (see *Clinical Insight:* Fasting Hypoglycemia).

Fat Malabsorption

Pathophysiology

Fat absorption may be impaired in liver disease. Possible causes include decreased bile salt secretion (as in PBC, sclerosing cholangitis, and biliary strictures), administration of neomycin or cholestyramine, and pancreatic enzyme

CLINICAL INSIGHT

Fasting Hypoglycemia

Two-thirds of the glucose requirement in an adult is used by the central nervous system. During fasting, plasma glucose concentrations are maintained for use by the nervous system and the brain because liver glycogen is broken down, or new glucose is made from nonglucose precursors such as alanine. Fasting hypoglycemia occurs when there is reduced synthesis of new glucose or reduced liver glycogen breakdown.

Causes of fasting hypoglycemia include cirrhosis, consumption of alcohol, extensive intrahepatic cancer, deficiency of cortisol and growth hormone, or non–β cell tumors of the pancreas. The method for detecting it involves measuring plasma insulin when plasma glucose is low. The diagnostic hallmark of an insulinoma is altered insulin secretion in the presence of hypoglycemia. Fasting hypoglycemia may also be caused by spontaneously produced antibodies. All patients with liver or pancreatic disease should be monitored for fasting hypoglycemia. Nutrition therapy involves balanced meals with small, frequent snacks to avoid periods of fasting. Monitoring of blood glucose and insulin levels is required.

insufficiency. Stools may be greasy, floating, or light- or clay-colored, signifying malabsorption, which can be verified by a 72-hour fecal fat study (see Chapter 29 and Appendix 30).

Medical Nutrition Therapy

If significant steatorrhea is present, replacement of some of the long-chain triglycerides or dietary fat with medium-chain triglycerides (MCTs) may be useful. Because MCTs do not require bile salts and micelle formation for absorption, they are readily taken up via the portal route (see Chapter 29). Some nutrition supplements contain MCTs, which can be used in addition to liquid MCT oil (see Chapter 14).

Significant stool fat losses may warrant a trial of a low-fat (40 g/day) diet. If diarrhea does not resolve, fat restriction should be discontinued because it decreases the palatability of the diet and severely hampers adequate calorie intake.

Renal Insufficiency and Hepatorenal Syndrome

Pathophysiology, Medical and Nutrition Therapies

Hepatorenal syndrome is renal failure associated with severe liver disease without intrinsic kidney abnormalities. Hepatorenal syndrome is diagnosed when the urine sodium level is less than 10 mEq/L and oliguria persists in the absence of intravascular volume depletion. If conservative therapies, including discontinuation of nephrotoxic drugs, optimization of intravascular volume status, treatment of underlying infection, and monitoring of fluid intake and output fail, dialysis may be required. In any case, renal insufficiency and failure may necessitate alteration in fluid, sodium, potassium, and phosphorus intake (see Chapter 36).

Osteopenia

Pathophysiology

Osteopenia often exists in patients with PBC, sclerosing cholangitis, and alcoholic liver disease. Depressed osteoblastic function and osteoporosis also can occur in patients with hemochromatosis, and osteoporosis is prevalent in patients who have had long-term treatment with corticosteroids. Corticosteroids increase bone resorption; suppress osteoblastic function; and affect sex hormone secretion, intestinal absorption of dietary calcium, renal excretion of calcium and phosphorus, and the vitamin D system.

Medical Nutrition Therapy

Prevention or treatment options for osteopenia include weight maintenance, ingestion of a well-balanced diet, adequate protein to maintain muscle mass, 1500 mg of calcium per day, adequate vitamin D from the diet or supplements, avoidance of alcohol, and monitoring for steatorrhea, with diet adjustments as needed to minimize nutrient losses.

LIVER RESECTION AND TRANSPLANTATION

Liver resection and ablation are fairly common now that problem areas can be located by means of tomography and arteriography. As with any major surgery, protein and energy needs increase after liver resection. Needs are also increased for liver cell regeneration. EN is vital because of the role of portal hepatotropic factors necessary for liver cell proliferation. Optimal nutrition is most important for patients with poor nutrition status before hepatectomy (e.g., patients with hepatocellular carcinoma or cholangiocarcinoma).

Liver transplantation has become an established treatment for ESLD. Malnutrition is common in liver transplant candidates. Dietary intake can often be enhanced if patients eat small, frequent, nutrient-dense meals; oral nutritional supplements may also be well tolerated. Enteral tube feeding is indicated when oral intake is inadequate or contraindicated. Varices are not an absolute contraindication for placement of a feeding tube. Because PN can adversely affect liver function, EN is preferred. PN is reserved for patients without adequate gut function. (See Chapter 14.)

In the acute posttransplant phase, nutrient needs are increased to promote healing, deter infection, provide energy for recovery, and replenish depleted body stores. Nitrogen requirements are elevated in the acute posttransplant phase and can be met with early postoperative tube feeding. Probiotics and fiber added to tube feeding may reduce postoperative infection rate better than tube feeding or fiber alone (Rayes et al, 2005).

Multiple medications used after transplant have nutritional side effects such as anorexia, gastrointestinal upset, hypercatabolism, diarrhea, hyperglycemia, hyperlipidemia, sodium retention, hypertension, hyperkalemia, and hypercalciuria. Therefore dietary modification is based on the specific side effects of drug therapy (Table 30-6). During the posttransplant phase, nutrient requirements are adjusted to prevent or treat problems of obesity, hyperlipidemia, hypertension, diabetes mellitus, and osteopenia. Table 30-7 summarizes nutrient needs following liver transplantation.

PHYSIOLOGY AND FUNCTIONS OF THE GALLBLADDER

The gallbladder lies on the undersurface of the right lobe of the liver (Figure 30-6). The main function of the gallbladder is to concentrate, store, and excrete bile, which is produced by the liver. During the concentration process, water and electrolytes are resorbed by the gallbladder mucosa. The chief constituents of bile are cholesterol, bilirubin, and bile salts. Bilirubin, the main bile pigment, is derived from the release of hemoglobin from red blood cell destruction. It is transported to the liver, where it is conjugated and excreted via bile. Bile salts are made by liver cells from cholesterol and are essential for the digestion and absorption of fats, fat-soluble vitamins, and some minerals (see Chapter 1).

TABLE 30-6

Drugs Commonly Used After Liver Transplantation

Immunosuppressant Drug	Possible Nutritional Side Effects	Proposed Nutrition Therapy
Azathioprine	Macrocytic anemia	Give folate supplements.
	Mouth sores	Adjust food and meals as needed; monitor intake.
	Nausea, vomiting, diarrhea, anorexia, sore throat, stomach pain, decreased taste acuity	
Antithymocyte globulin (ATG), antilymphocyte globulin (ALG)	Nausea, vomiting	Adjust food and meals as needed; monitor intake.
Basiliximab	None reported	
Cyclosporine	Sodium retention	Decrease sodium intake.
	Hyperkalemia	Decrease potassium intake.
	Hyperlipidemia	Limit fat and simple carbohydrate intake.
	Hyperglycemia	Decrease simple carbohydrate intake.
	Decreased serum magnesium level	Increase magnesium intake; give supplements.
	Hypertension	Limit sodium intake.
	Nausea, vomiting	Adjust food and meals as needed; monitor intake.
Daclizumab	None reported	
Glucocorticoids	Sodium retention	Decrease sodium intake.
	Hyperglycemia	Decrease simple carbohydrate intake.
	Hyperlipidemia	Limit fat and simple carbohydrate intake.
	False hunger	Avoid overeating.
	Protein wasting with high doses	Increase protein intake.
	Decreased absorption of calcium and phosphorus	Increase calcium and phosphorus intake; give supplements as needed.
Muromonab-CD3	Nausea, vomiting, anorexia	Adjust food and meals as needed; monitor intake.
Mycophenolate mofetil, mycophenolic acid	Nausea, vomiting, diarrhea	Adjust food and meals as needed; monitor intake.
Sirolimus	Possible GI symptoms	Adjust food and meals as needed; monitor intake.
	Hyperlipidemia	Limit fat and simple carbohydrate intake.
Tacrolimus	Hyperglycemia	Decrease simple carbohydrate intake.
	Hyperkalemia	Decrease potassium intake.
	Nausea, vomiting	Adjust food and meals as needed; monitor intake.

GI, Gastrointestinal.

The primary transporter responsible for bile salt secretion is the bile salt export pump (BSEP). Overall, bile salts play a key role in a wide range of physiologic and pathophysiologic processes (Lam et al., 2010). Excreted into the small intestine via bile, bile salts are later resorbed into the portal system (enterohepatic circulation). This is the primary excretory pathway for the minerals copper and manganese.

Bile contains immunoglobulins that support the integrity of the intestinal mucosa. Fibroblast growth factor receptor (FGFR) 4 controls bile acid metabolism and protects the liver from fibrosis; FGFR1 and FGFR2 assist in regeneration of the liver (Böhm et al., 2010). Molecular crosstalk between bile acid–activated nuclear receptors and proinflammatory nuclear mediators provides new understanding of inflammation-induced cholestasis (Kosters and Karpen, 2010).

Bile is removed by the liver via bile canaliculi that drain into intrahepatic bile ducts. The ducts lead to the left and right hepatic ducts, which leave the liver and join to become the common hepatic duct. The bile is directed to the gallbladder via the cystic duct for concentration and storage.

TABLE 30-7

Nutrition Care Guidelines for Liver Transplant Patient

	Pretransplantation	Immediate Posttransplantation (First 2 Posttransplant Months)	Long-Term Posttransplantation
Calories & protein*	High calorie (basal + 20% or more) Moderate protein (1-1.5 g/kg)	Moderate calorie (basal + 15%-30%) High protein (1.2-1.75 g/kg)	Weight maintenance (basal + 10%-20%) Moderate protein (1 g/kg)
Fat	As needed	Approximately 30% of calories	Moderate fat (30% of calories)
Carbohydrate	Reduced simple carbohydrate if diabetes or obesity present	Reduced simple carbohydrate if diabetes present	Reduced simple carbohydrate, especially if diabetes or obesity present
Sodium	2 g/day	2-4 g/day (as indicated)	2-4 g/day (as indicated)
Fluid	Restrict to 1000-1500 mL/day (if hyponatremic)	As needed	As needed
Calcium	800-1200 mg/day	800-1200 mg/day	1200-1500 mg/day
Vitamins	Multivitamin/mineral supplementation to DRI levels; additional water- and fat-soluble vitamins as indicated	Multivitamin/mineral supplementation to DRI levels; additional water- and fat-soluble vitamins as indicated	Multivitamin/mineral supplementation to DRI levels

Modified from Porayko MK et al: Impact of malnutrition and its therapy on liver transplantation, Semin Liv Dis 11(4):305, 1991.
DRI, Dietary reference intake.
*Use estimated dry or ideal weight.

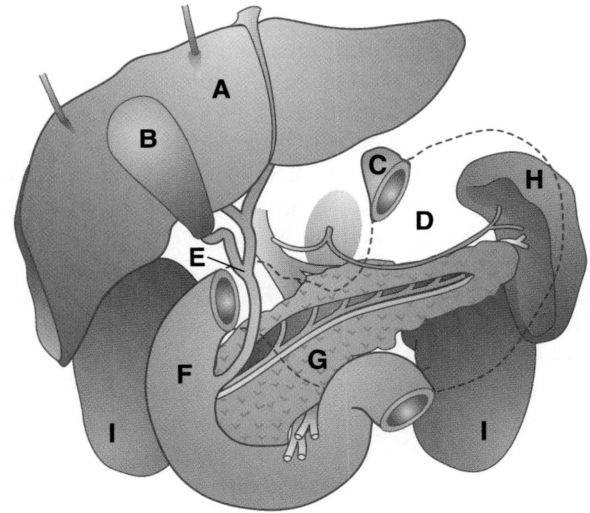

FIGURE 30-6 Schematic drawing showing relationship of organs of the upper abdomen. **A,** Liver (retracted upward); **B,** gallbladder; **C,** esophageal opening of stomach; **D,** stomach *(shown in dotted outline)*; **E,** common bile duct; **F,** duodenum; **G,** pancreas and pancreatic duct; **H,** spleen; **I,** kidneys. *(Courtesy Cleveland Clinic, Cleveland, Ohio, 2002.)*

The cystic duct joins the common hepatic duct to form the common bile duct. The bile duct then joins the pancreatic duct, which carries digestive enzymes.

During the course of digestion, food reaches the duodenum, causing the release of intestinal hormones such as cholecystokinin (CCK) and secretin. This stimulates the gallbladder and pancreas and causes the sphincter of Oddi to relax, allowing pancreatic juice and bile to flow into the duodenum at the ampulla of Vater to assist in fat digestion. For this reason diseases of the gallbladder, liver, and pancreas are often interrelated.

DISEASES OF THE GALLBLADDER

Disorders of the biliary tract affect millions of people each year, causing significant suffering and even death by precipitating pancreatitis and sepsis. A diverse spectrum of disease affects the biliary system, often presenting with similar clinical signs and symptoms. Treatment may involve diet, medication, or surgery.

Cholestasis

Pathophysiology and Medical Management

Cholestasis is a condition in which little or no bile is secreted or the flow of bile into the digestive tract is obstructed. This can occur in patients without oral or enteral feeding for a prolonged period, such as those requiring PN, and can predispose to acalculous cholecystitis. BSEP deficiency results in several different genetic forms of cholestasis and acquired forms of cholestasis such as drug-induced cholestasis and intrahepatic cholestasis of pregnancy (Lam et al., 2010). Prevention of cholestasis requires stimulation of biliary motility and secretions by at least minimum enteral feedings. If this is not possible, drug therapy is used.

Cholelithiasis

Pathophysiology

The formation of gallstones (calculi) is **cholelithiasis**. Virtually all gallstones form within the gallbladder. Gallstone disease affects millions of Americans each year and causes significant morbidity. In most cases gallstones are asymptomatic. Gallstones that pass from the gallbladder into the common bile duct may remain there indefinitely without causing symptoms, or they may pass into the duodenum with or without symptoms.

Choledocholithiasis develops when stones slip into the bile ducts, producing obstruction, pain, and cramps. If passage of bile into the duodenum is interrupted, cholecystitis can develop. In the absence of bile in the intestine, lipid absorption is impaired, and without bile pigments, stools become light in color (acholic). If uncorrected, bile backup can result in jaundice and liver damage (**secondary biliary cirrhosis**). Obstruction of the distal common bile duct can lead to pancreatitis if the pancreatic duct is blocked.

Most gallstones are unpigmented cholesterol stones composed primarily of cholesterol, bilirubin, and calcium salts. Bacteria also play a role in gallstone formation. Low-grade chronic infections produce changes in the gallbladder mucosa, which affect its absorptive capabilities. Excess water or bile acid may be absorbed as a result. Cholesterol may then precipitate out and cause gallstones (Volzke et al., 2005).

High dietary fat intake over a prolonged period may predispose a person to gallstone formation because of the constant stimulus to produce more cholesterol for bile synthesis required in fat digestion. Rapid weight loss (as with jejunoileal and gastric bypass and fasting or severe calorie restriction) is associated with a high incidence of biliary sludge and gallstone formation.

Indeed, cholelithiasis and fatty liver disease share risk factors including central obesity, insulin resistance, and diabetes (Weikert et al., 2010).

Risk factors for cholesterol stone formation include female gender, pregnancy, older age, family history, obesity and truncal body fat distribution, diabetes mellitus, inflammatory bowel disease, and drugs (lipid-lowering medications, oral contraceptives, and estrogens). Certain ethnic groups are at greater risk of stone formation, including Pima Indians, Scandinavians, and Mexican-Americans.

Pigmented stones typically consist of bilirubin polymers or calcium salts. They are associated with chronic hemolysis. Risk factors associated with these stones are age, sickle cell anemia and thalassemia, biliary tract infection, cirrhosis, alcoholism, and long-term PN (Abayli et al., 2005).

Medical & Surgical Management

Cholecystectomy is surgical removal of the gallbladder, especially if the stones are numerous, large, or calcified. The cholecystectomy may be done as a traditional open laparotomy or as a less invasive laparoscopic procedure. Recently, it has been noted that cholecystectomy is a predictor of the development of cirrhosis and is associated with elevated serum liver enzymes (Ioannou, 2010).

Chemical dissolution with the administration of bile salts, chenodeoxycholic acid, and ursodeoxycholic acid (litholytic therapy) or dissolution by extracorporeal shockwave lithotripsy may also be used less often than surgical techniques. Patients with gallstones that have migrated into the bile ducts may be candidates for endoscopic retrograde cholangiopancreatography techniques (Adler et al., 2005).

Medical Nutrition Therapy

No specific dietary treatment is available to prevent cholelithiasis in susceptible persons. Gallstones are more prevalent in low-fiber, high-fat, Westernized diets. Consumption of large amounts of animal protein and animal fat, especially saturated fat, and a lack of dietary fiber, promote gallstone development.

There may also be some benefit in replacing simple sugars and refined starches with high-fiber carbohydrates. Individuals consuming refined carbohydrates have a 60% greater risk for developing gallstones, compared with those who consumed the most fiber, in particular insoluble fiber (Tsai, 2005). Thus plant-based diets may reduce the risk of cholelithiasis. Vegetarian diets are high in fiber and low in fat, consisting primarily of unsaturated fat. Vitamin C, which is generally high in vegetarian diets, affects the rate-limiting step in the catabolism of cholesterol to bile acids and is inversely related to the risk of gallstones in women.

Weight cycling (repeatedly losing and regaining weight), fasting, and very-low-calorie diets increase the likelihood of cholelithiasis. Along with weight reduction, there is some evidence that physical activity will reduce the risk of cholecystitis. In cholecystitis, MNT includes a high-fiber, low-fat, plant-based diet to prevent gallbladder contractions. Data are conflicting as to whether intravenous lipids stimulate gallbladder contraction.

After surgical removal of the gallbladder, oral feedings can be advanced to a regular diet as tolerated. In the absence of the gallbladder, bile is secreted directly by the liver into the intestine. The biliary tract dilates, forming a "simulated pouch" over time, to allow bile to be held in a manner similar to the original gallbladder.

Cholecystitis

Pathophysiology

Inflammation of the gallbladder is known as **cholecystitis**, and it may be chronic or acute. It is usually caused by gallstones obstructing the bile ducts (calculous cholecystitis), leading to the backup of bile. Bilirubin, the main bile pigment, gives bile its greenish color. When biliary tract obstruction prevents bile from reaching the intestine, it backs up and returns to the circulation. Bilirubin has an affinity for elastic tissues; therefore when it overflows into the general circulation, it causes the yellow skin pigmentation and eye discoloration typical of jaundice.

Acute cholecystitis without stones (acalculous cholecystitis) may occur in critically ill patients or when the gallbladder and its bile are stagnant. Impaired gallbladder emptying in chronic acalculous cholecystitis appears to be due to diminished spontaneous contractile activity and decreased contractile responsiveness to CCK. The walls of the gallbladder become inflamed and distended, and infection can occur. During such episodes, the patient experiences upper-quadrant abdominal pain accompanied by nausea, vomiting, and flatulence.

Chronic cholecystitis is long-standing inflammation of the gallbladder. It is caused by repeated, mild attacks of acute cholecystitis. This leads to thickening of the walls of the gallbladder. The gallbladder begins to shrink and eventually loses the ability to perform its function: concentrating and storing bile. Eating foods that are high in fat may aggravate the symptoms of cholecystitis, because bile is needed to digest such foods. Chronic cholecystitis occurs more often in women than in men, and the incidence increases after the age of 40. Risk factors include the presence of gallstones and a history of acute cholecystitis.

Surgical Management

Acute cholecystitis requires surgical intervention unless medically contraindicated. Without surgery, the condition may either subside or progress to gangrene.

Medical Nutrition Therapy

Acute Cholecystitis. In an acute attack, oral feedings are discontinued. PN may be indicated if the patient is malnourished and it is anticipated that he or she will not be taking anything orally for a prolonged period. When feedings are resumed, a low-fat diet is recommended to decrease gallbladder stimulation. A hydrolyzed low-fat formula or an oral low-fat diet consisting of 30 to 45 g of fat per day can be given. Table 30-8 shows a fat-restricted diet.

Following cholecystectomy, patients may experience symptoms of gastritis secondary to duodenogastric reflux of bile acids. The reflux may also be responsible for symptoms in this postcholecystectomy syndrome. At present, there are no well-established pharmacologic approaches in the management of postcholecystectomy gastritis. The symptoms are not caused, but exacerbated, by the cholecystectomy. It has been proposed that the addition of soluble fiber to the diet will act as a sequestering agent and bind the bile in the stomach between meals to avoid gastritis.

Chronic Cholecystitis. Patients with chronic conditions may require a long-term, low-fat diet that contains 25% to 30% of total kilocalories as fat. Stricter limitation is undesirable because fat in the intestine is important for some stimulation and drainage of the biliary tract. The degree of food intolerance varies widely among persons with gallbladder disorders; many complain of foods that cause flatulence and bloating. For this reason it is best to determine with the patient which foods should be eliminated. See Chapter 29 for a discussion of potential gas-forming foods. Administration of water-soluble forms of fat-soluble vitamins may be of benefit in patients with chronic gallbladder conditions or in those in whom fat malabsorption is suspected.

Cholangitis

Pathophysiology and Medical Management

Inflammation of the bile ducts is known as **cholangitis**. Patients with acute cholangitis need resuscitation with fluids and broad-spectrum antibiotics. If the patient does not improve with conservative treatment, placement of a percutaneous biliary stent or cholecystectomy may be needed.

Sclerosing cholangitis can result in sepsis and liver failure. Most patients have multiple intrahepatic strictures, which makes surgical intervention difficult, if not impossible. Patients are generally on broad-spectrum antibiotics. Percutaneous ductal dilation may provide short-term bile duct patency in some patients. When sepsis is recurrent, patients may require chronic antibiotic therapy. See the section on sclerosing cholangitis in the liver disease section.

PHYSIOLOGY AND FUNCTIONS OF THE EXOCRINE PANCREAS

The pancreas is an elongated, flattened gland that lies in the upper abdomen behind the stomach. The head of the pancreas is in the right upper quadrant below the liver within the curvature of the duodenum, and the tapering tail slants upward to the hilum of the spleen. This glandular organ has both an endocrine and exocrine function. Pancreatic cells manufacture glucagon, insulin, and somatostatin for absorption into the bloodstream (endocrine function) for regulation of glucose homeostasis (see Chapter 31). Other cells secrete enzymes and other substances directly into the intestinal lumen, where they aid in digesting proteins, fats, and carbohydrates (exocrine function).

In most people the pancreatic duct, which carries the exocrine pancreatic secretions, merges with the common bile duct into a unified opening through which bile and pancreatic juices drain into the duodenum at the ampulla of Vater. Many factors regulate exocrine secretion from the pancreas. Neural and hormonal responses play a role, with the presence and composition of ingested foods being a large contributor. The two primary hormonal stimuli for pancreatic secretion are secretin and CCK (see Chapter 1).

Factors that influence pancreatic secretions during a meal can be divided into three phases: (1) the cephalic phase, mediated through the vagus nerve and initiated by the sight, smell, taste, and anticipation of food that leads to the secretion of bicarbonate and pancreatic enzymes; (2) gastric distention with food initiates the gastric phase of pancreatic secretion, which stimulates enzyme secretion;

TABLE 30-8

Fat-Restricted Diet*

Food Allowed	Food Excluded
Beverages	
Skim milk or buttermilk made with skim milk; coffee, tea, Postum, fruit juice, soft drinks, cocoa made with cocoa powder and skim milk	Whole milk, buttermilk made with whole milk, chocolate milk, cream in excess of amounts allowed under fats
Bread and Cereal Products	
Plain, nonfat cereals; spaghetti, noodles, rice, macaroni; plain whole grain or enriched breads, air-popped popcorn, bagels, English muffins	Biscuits, breads, egg or cheese bread, sweet rolls made with fat, pancakes, doughnuts, waffles, fritters, popcorn prepared with fat, muffins, natural cereals and breads to which extra fat is added
Cheese	
Cottage cheese, ¼ c to be used as substitute for 1 oz of cheese, or low-fat cheeses containing less than 5% butterfat	Whole-milk cheeses
Desserts	
Sherbet made with skim milk; nonfat frozen yogurt; nonfat frozen nondairy desserts; fruit ice; sorbet; gelatin; rice, bread, cornstarch, tapioca, or pudding made with skim milk; fruit whips with gelatin, sugar, and egg white; fruit; angel food cake; graham crackers; vanilla wafers; meringues	Cake, pie, pastry, ice cream, or any dessert containing shortening, chocolate, or fats of any kind, unless especially prepared using part of fat allowance
Eggs	
Three per week prepared only with fat from fat allowance; egg whites as desired; low-fat egg substitutes	More than one/day unless substituted for part of the meat allowed
Fats	
Choose up to the limit allowed among the following (1 serving in the amount listed equals 1 fat choice): 1 tsp butter or margarine 1 Tbsp reduced-fat margarine 1 tsp shortening or oil 1 tsp mayonnaise 2 tsp Italian or French dressing 1 Tbsp reduced-fat salad dressing 1 strip crisp bacon ⅛ avocado (4-inch diameter) 2 Tbsp light cream 1 Tbsp heavy cream 6 small nuts 5 small olives	Any in excess of amount prescribed on diet; all others
Fruits	
As desired	Avocado in excess of amount allowed on fat list
Lean Meat, Fish, Poultry, and Meat Substitutes	
Choose up to the limit allowed among the following: poultry without skin, fish, veal (all cuts), liver, lean beef, pork, and lamb, all with visible fat removed—1 oz cooked weight equals 1 equivalent; ¼ c water packed tuna or salmon equals 1 equivalent; tofu or tempeh—3 oz equals 1 equivalent	Fried or fatty meats, sausage, scrapple, frankfurters, poultry skins, stewing hens, spareribs, salt pork, beef unless lean, duck, goose, ham hocks, pig's feet, luncheon meats (unless reduced fat), gravies unless fat-free, tuna and salmon packed in oil, peanut butter

TABLE 30-8

Fat-Restricted Diet*—cont'd

Food Allowed	Food Excluded
Milk	
Skim, buttermilk, or yogurt made from skim milk	Whole, 2%, 1%, chocolate, buttermilk made with whole milk
Seasonings	
As desired	None
Soups	
Bouillon, clear broth, fat-free vegetable soup, cream soup made with skimmed milk, packaged dehydrated soups	All others
Sweets	
Jelly, jam, marmalade, honey, syrup, molasses, sugar, hard sugar candies, fondant, gumdrops, jelly beans, marshmallows, cocoa powder, fat-free chocolate sauce, red and black licorice	Any candy made with chocolate, nuts, butter, cream, or fat of any kind
Vegetables	
All plainly prepared vegetables	Potato chips; buttered, au gratin, creamed, or fried potatoes and other vegetables unless made with allowed fat; casseroles or frozen vegetables in butter sauce

Daily Food Allowances for 40-g–Fat Diet

Food	Amount	Approximate Fat Content (g)
Skim milk	2 c or more	0
Lean meat, fish, poultry	6 oz or 6 equivalents	18
Whole egg or egg yolks	3 per week	2
Vegetables	3 servings or more, at least 1 or more dark green or deep yellow	0
Fruits	3 or more servings, at least 1 citrus	0
Breads, cereals	As desired, fat-free	0
Fat exchanges*	4-5 exchanges daily	20-25
Desserts and sweets	As desired from permitted list	0
	Total Fat	38-43

*Fat content can be reduced further by reducing the fat exchanges. 1 Fat exchange = 5 g of fat.

and (3) the intestinal phase, mediated by the release of CCK, with the most potent effect.

DISEASES OF THE EXOCRINE PANCREAS

Pancreatitis

Pathophysiology and Medical Management

Pancreatitis is an inflammation of the pancreas and is characterized by edema, cellular exudate, and fat necrosis. The disease can range from mild and self-limiting to severe, with autodigestion, necrosis, and hemorrhage of pancreatic tissue. Ranson and colleagues (1974) identified 11 signs that could be measured during the first 48 hours of admission and that have prognostic significance (Box 30-3). By using these observations, one can determine the likely outcome of hospitalization. Surgical intervention may be necessary. Pancreatitis is classified as either acute or chronic, the latter with pancreatic destruction so extensive that exocrine and endocrine function are severely diminished, and maldigestion and diabetes may result.

The symptoms of pancreatitis can range from continuous or intermittent pain of varying intensity to severe upper abdominal pain, which may radiate to the back. Symptoms may worsen with the ingestion of food. Clinical presentation may also include nausea, vomiting, abdominal distention, and steatorrhea. Severe cases are complicated by hypotension, oliguria, and dyspnea. There is extensive destruction of pancreatic tissue with subsequent fibrosis, enzyme production is diminished, and serum amylase and lipase may

BOX 30-3

Ranson's Criteria to Classify the Severity of Pancreatitis

At Admission or Diagnosis

Age >55 yr
White blood cell count >16,000 m3
Blood glucose level >200 mg/100 mL
Lactic dehydrogenase >350 units/L
Aspartate transaminase >250 units/L

During the Initial 48 Hours

Hematocrit decrease of >10 mg/dL
Blood urea nitrogen increase of >5 mg/dL
Arterial PO2 <60 mm Hg
Base deficit >4 mEq/L
Fluid sequestration >6000 mL
Serum calcium level <8 mg/mL

Modified from Ranson JH et al: Prognostic signs and the role of operative management in acute pancreatitis, Surg Gynecol Obstet 139:69, 1974.

TABLE 30-9

Some Tests of Pancreatic Function

Test	Significance
Secretin stimulation test	Measures pancreatic secretion, particularly bicarbonate, in response to secretin stimulation
Glucose tolerance test	Assesses endocrine function of the pancreas by measuring insulin response to a glucose load
72-hr stool fat test	Assesses exocrine function of the pancreas by measuring fat absorption that reflects pancreatic lipase secretion

appear normal. However, absence of enzymes to aid in the digestion of food leads to steatorrhea and malabsorption. Table 30-9 describes several tests used to determine the extent of pancreatic destruction.

Medical Nutrition Therapy

Alcohol use, smoking, body weight, diet, genetic factors, and medications all affect the risk of developing pancreatitis. Thus diet modification has an important role after diagnosis. Dietary recommendations differ, depending on whether the condition is acute or chronic. Obesity appears to be a risk factor for the development of pancreatitis and an increased severity.

Depressed serum calcium levels are common. Hypoalbuminemia occurs, with subsequent third spacing of fluid. The calcium, which is bound to albumin, is thus affected and may appear artificially low. Another occurrence is "soap" formation in the gut by calcium and fatty acids, created by the fat necrosis that results in less calcium absorption. Checking an ionized calcium level is a method of determining available calcium.

Acute Pancreatitis. Pain associated with acute pancreatitis (AP) is partially related to the secretory mechanisms of pancreatic enzymes and bile. Therefore nutrition therapy is adjusted to provide minimum stimulation of these systems (see *Pathophysiology and Care Management Algorithm:* Pancreatitis). In the past the pancreas was put "at rest." During acute attacks all oral feeding is withheld, and hydration maintained intravenously. In less severe attacks, a clear liquid diet with negligible fat may be given in a few days. The patient should be monitored for any symptoms of pain, nausea, or vomiting. The diet should be progressed as tolerated to easily digested foods with a low fat content and then advanced as tolerated. Foods may be better tolerated if they are divided into six small meals (see Table 30-8).

Severe AP results in a hypermetabolic, catabolic state with immediate metabolic alterations in the pancreas and also in remote organs. Metabolic demands are similar to those of sepsis. Amino acids are released from muscle and used for gluconeogenesis. These patients often exhibit signs of malnutrition such as decreased serum levels of albumin, transferrin, and lymphocytes. Attention should be given to a nutrition regimen with adequate protein in an effort to achieve positive nitrogen balance.

Oral nutrition must be further delayed when the acute illness persists longer than a few days as evidenced by persistent or recurrent elevation of serum amylase, continued abdominal pain, and ileus; or when cessation of nasogastric suction is followed by return of symptoms, the presence of a complication such as pancreatic abscess or pseudocyst, or a suspected obstruction to the main pancreatic ducts.

The optimal route of nutrition in AP has been the subject of much controversy over the years. Failure to use the GIT in patients with AP may exacerbate the stress response and disease severity, leading to more complications and prolonged hospitalization; thus EN is preferred for nutrition therapy (McClave et al., 2006; Louie et al., 2005). There is a substantial cost savings with EN and fewer septic complications. Most patients with AP have a return of bowel function within 2 to 3 days following an attack and can advance quickly from intravenous fluids to diet.

Both PN and EN are equally effective in terms of days to normalization of serum amylase, days to resumption of oral feeding, serum albumin levels, nosocomial infections, and clinical outcome in patients with mild to moderate pancreatitis (Petrov, 2009). The favorable effect of either EN or PN on patient outcome may be enhanced by supplementation with modulators of inflammation and systemic immunity (McClave et al., 2006).

Aggressive nutrition support may include attempts to use the GIT. The location of the feeding and the composition of the formula determine the degree of pancreatic stimulation. Infusion into the jejunum eliminates the

PATHOPHYSIOLOGY AND CARE MANAGEMENT ALGORITHM

Pancreatitis

ETIOLOGY

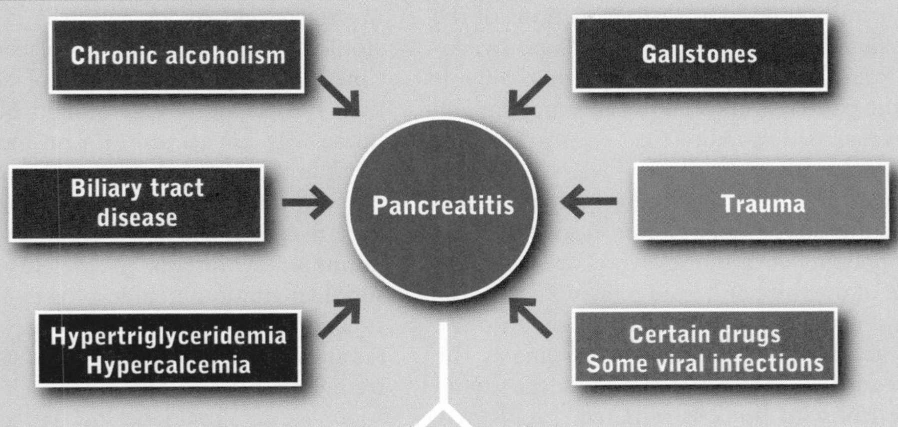

PATHOPHYSIOLOGY

Diagnosis

I: Apply Ranson's criteria
II: Tests of pancreatic function
- Secretin stimulation test
- Glucose tolerance test
- 72-hour stool fat test

Clinical Findings

Symptoms:
- Abdominal pain and distention
- Nausea
- Vomiting
- Steatorrhea

In severe form:
- Hypotension
- Oliguria
- Dyspnea

MANAGEMENT

Medical Management

Acute:
- Withhold oral feeding
- Give IV fluids
- Administer H_2-receptor antagonists, somatostatin

Chronic:
- Manage intestinal pH with:
  - Antacids
  - H_2-receptor antagonists
  - Proton pump inhibitors
- Administer insulin for glucose intolerance

Nutrition Management

Acute:
- Withhold oral and enteral feeding
- Support with IV fluids
- If oral nutrition cannot be initiated in 5 to 7 days, start tube feeding
- Once oral nutrition is started, provide
  - Easily digestible foods
  - Low-fat diet
  - 6 small meals
  - Adequate protein intake
  - Increased calories

Chronic:
- Provide oral diet as in acute phase
- TF can be used when oral diet is inadequate or as a treatment to reduce pain
- Supplement pancreatic enzymes
- Supplement fat-soluble vitamins and vitamin B_{12}

cephalic and gastric phases of exocrine pancreatic stimulation (McClave et al., 2006; Stanga et al., 2005). Although various formulations have been used in pancreatitis, no studies have determined the relative merits of standard, partially digested, elemental, or "immune-enhanced" formulations. Polymeric formulas infused at various sections of the gut stimulate the pancreas more than elemental and hydrolyzed formulas. Close observation for patient tolerance is important. When the patient is allowed to eat, supplemental pancreatic enzymes may be needed to treat steatorrhea. See Chapter 14) for jejunal feeding details.

In severe, prolonged cases, PN may be necessary. Patients with mild to moderate stress can tolerate dextrose-based solutions, whereas patients with more severe stress require a mixed fuel system of dextrose and lipid to avoid complications of glucose intolerance. Lipid emulsion should not be included in a PN regimen if hypertriglyceridemia is the cause of the pancreatitis. A serum triglyceride level should be obtained before PN with lipids is initiated. Lipids may be given to patients with triglyceride values less than 400 mg/dL. Because of the possibility of pancreatic endocrine abnormalities and a relative insulin resistance, close glucose monitoring is also warranted. H_2-receptor antagonists may be prescribed to decrease hydrochloric acid production, which will reduce stimulation of the pancreas. Somatostatin is considered the best inhibitor of pancreatic secretion and may be added to the PN solution.

Chronic Pancreatitis. In contrast to AP, chronic pancreatitis (CP) evolves insidiously over many years. CP is characterized by recurrent attacks of epigastric pain of long duration that may radiate into the back. The pain can be precipitated by meals. Associated nausea, vomiting, or diarrhea makes it difficult to maintain adequate nutrition status. Patients with CP are at increased risk of developing protein-calorie malnutrition because of pancreatic insufficiency and inadequate oral intake. Patients with CP admitted to a tertiary care center usually have malnutrition, increased energy requirements, weight loss, deficits of lean muscle and adipose tissue, visceral protein depletion, and impaired immune function.

The objective of therapy for patients is to prevent further damage to the pancreas, decrease the number of attacks of acute inflammation, alleviate pain, decrease steatorrhea, and correct malnutrition. Dietary intake should be as liberal as possible, but modifications may be necessary to minimize symptoms.

The first goal of MNT is to provide optimal nutrition support, and the second is to decrease pain by minimizing stimulation of the exocrine pancreas. Because CCK stimulates secretion from the exocrine pancreas, one approach is to decrease CCK levels. If postprandial pain is a limiting factor, alternative enteral therapies that minimally stimulate the pancreas are warranted. Nutrition counseling, antioxidants, and pancreatic enzymes may play a role in effective management of CP as well.

Idiopathic CP is often associated with a cystic fibrosis gene mutation, and therapies directed toward cystic fibrosis may benefit these patients. When pancreatic function is diminished by approximately 90%, enzyme production and secretion are insufficient; maldigestion and malabsorption of protein and fat thus become a problem. Large meals with high-fat foods and alcohol should be avoided.

The patient may present with weight loss despite adequate energy intake and will complain of bulky, greasy stools. Pancreatic enzyme replacement is mandatory at this time. Pancreatic enzyme replacements are given orally with meals; the dosage should be at least 30,000 units of lipase with each meal. To promote weight gain, the level of fat in the diet should be the maximum a patient can tolerate without increased steatorrhea or pain. Additional therapies that may be tried to maintain nutrition status and minimize symptoms in patients with maximum enzyme supplementation include a lower-fat diet (40 to 60 g/day) or substitution of some dietary fat with MCT oil to improve fat absorption and weight gain. Meals should be small and frequent.

The diet should be low fat, primarily from vegetable-based oils such as olive oil. Reduce significantly or eliminate trans-fatty acids, found in commercially baked goods. Substitution of dietary fat with MCT oil may relieve steatorrhea and lead to weight gain. Malabsorption of the fat-soluble vitamins may occur in patients with significant steatorrhea. Also, deficiency of pancreatic protease, necessary to cleave vitamin B_{12} from its carrier protein, could potentially lead to vitamin B_{12} deficiency. With appropriate supplemental enzyme therapy, vitamin absorption should be improved; however, the patient should still be monitored periodically for vitamin deficiencies. Water-soluble forms of the fat-soluble vitamins or parenteral administration of vitamin B_{12} may be necessary (see Chapter 33). There is some evidence that increasing intake of antioxidants (found in fruits and vegetables) may help protect against pancreatitis or alleviate symptoms of the condition.

Because pancreatic bicarbonate secretion is frequently defective, medical management may also include maintenance of an optimal intestinal pH to facilitate enzyme activation. Antacids, H_2-receptor antagonists, or proton pump inhibitors that reduce gastric acid secretion may be used to achieve this effect.

In chronic cases with extensive pancreatic destruction, the insulin-secreting capacity of the pancreas decreases, and glucose intolerance develops. Treatment with insulin and nutrition therapy is then required (see Chapter 31). Management is delicate and should focus on control of symptoms rather than normoglycemia.

Effort should be made to cater to the patient's tolerances and preferences for nutritional management; however, alcohol is prohibited because of the possibility of exacerbating the pancreatic disease. There is evidence that the progressive destruction of the pancreas will be slowed in the alcoholic patient who abstains from alcohol.

Pancreatic Surgery

A surgical procedure often used for pancreatic carcinoma is a **pancreaticoduodenectomy (Whipple procedure)**. A

CLINICAL SCENARIO

A 40-year-old man is admitted to the hospital with chief complaints of right upper quadrant pain, anorexia, nausea, dysgeusia, and frequent loose stools. On physical examination, he has mild peripheral edema with a slightly jaundiced appearance. No asterixis is noted. The patient's mental status is clear, but he appears lethargic. He reports no history of portal hypertension, ascites, or gastrointestinal bleeding. Muscle wasting is noted along with stomatitis. A liver biopsy shows steatosis and fibrosis. The patient has a significant alcohol abuse history spanning 15 years, suggesting alcoholic hepatitis. Abnormal laboratory values include elevated liver enzymes and total bilirubin; serum albumin, 2.5 g/dL; transferrin, 150 mg/dL; megaloblastic anemia profile; ammonia, 75 mmol/L. Nutritional data include height, 177.8 cm; weight, 67 kg; ideal body weight, 75 kg ± 10%; usual body weight, 82 kg (5 years ago), 73 kg (6 months ago).

Nutrition Diagnostic Statements

1. Involuntary weight loss related to postprandial pain as evidenced by 25-lb weight loss.
2. Excessive alcohol intake related to history of alcoholism as evidenced by 15-year heavy alcohol use.

Interventions

Initiate commercial beverage twice daily.
Initiate vitamin and mineral supplement.

Monitoring and Evaluation

Monitor food and beverage intake.
Assess food and nutrition knowledge.
Assess adherence to prescribed diet and alcohol abstinence.

cholecystectomy, vagotomy, or a partial gastrectomy may also be done during the surgery. The pancreatic duct is reanastomosed to the jejunum. Partial or complete pancreatic insufficiency can result, depending on the extent of the pancreatic resection. Most patients who have undergone pancreatic resection are at risk for vitamin and mineral deficiencies and will benefit from vitamin and mineral supplementation. Nutrition care is similar to that for CP.

USEFUL WEBSITES

National Institute on Alcohol Abuse and Alcoholism
http://www.niaaa.nih.gov
American Liver Foundation
http://www.liverfoundation.org
Transplant Living
http://www.transplantliving.org/

REFERENCES

Abayli B, et al: Helicobacter pylori in the etiology of cholesterol gallstones, *J Clin Gastroenterol* 39:134, 2005.

Adler DG, et al: Standards of Practice Committee of American Society for Gastrointestinal Endoscopy: ASGE guideline: the role of ERCP in diseases of the biliary tract and the pancreas, *Gastrointest Endosc* 62:1, 2005.

Afdhal NH: Diseases of the gallbladder and bile ducts. In Goldman L, et al, editors: *Cecil textbook of medicine*, ed 23, Philadelphia, 2007, Saunders.

Böhm F, et al: FGF receptors 1 and 2 control chemically-induced injury and compound detoxification in regenerating livers of mice, *Gastroenterology* 139:1385, 2010.

Campillo B, et al: Enteral nutrition in severely malnourished and anorectic cirrhotic patients in clinical practice, *Gastroenterol Clin Biol* 29:645, 2005.

Chitturi S, Farrell GC: Hepatotoxic slimming aids and other herbal hepatotoxins, *J Gastroenterol Hepatol* 23:366, 2008.

Crippin JS: Is tube feeding an option in patients with liver disease? *Nutr Clin Pract* 21:296, 2006.

Diehl AM: Alcoholic and nonalcoholic steatohepatitis. In Goldman L, et al., editors: *Cecil textbook of medicine*, ed 23, Philadelphia, 2007, Saunders.

Fitz JG: Hepatic encephalopathy, hepatopulmonary syndromes, hepatorenal syndrome, and other complications of liver disease. In Feldman M, editor: *Sleisenger and Fordtran's gastrointestinal and liver disease*, ed 8, Philadelphia, 2006, Saunders.

Garcia-Tsao G: Cirrhosis and its sequelae. In Goldman L, et al., editors: *Cecil textbook of medicine*, ed 23, Philadelphia, 2007, Saunders.

Gratz SW, et al: Probiotics and gut health: a special focus on liver diseases, *World J Gastroenterol* 16:403, 2010.

Hoofnagle JH: Hepatitis. In Goldman L, et al., editors: *Cecil textbook of medicine*, ed 23, Philadelphia, 2007, Saunders.

Ioannou GN: Cholelithiasis, cholecystectomy, and liver disease, *Am J Gastroenterol* 105:1364, 2010.

Kosters A, Karpen SJ: The role of inflammation in cholestasis: clinical and basic aspects, *Semin Liver Dis* 30:186, 2010.

Kowdley KV: Inherited and metabolic hepatic disorders. In Goldman L, et al., editors: *Cecil textbook of medicine*, ed 23, Philadelphia, 2007, Saunders.

Lam P, et al: The bile salt export pump: clinical and experimental aspects of genetic and acquired cholestatic liver disease, *Semin Liver Dis* 30:125, 2010.

Leevy CM, Moroianu SA: Nutritional aspects of alcoholic liver disease, *Clin Liver Dis* 9:67, 2005.

Louie BE, et al: 2004 MacLean-Mueller prize enteral or parenteral nutrition for severe pancreatitis: a randomized controlled trial and health technology assessment, *Can J Surg* 48:298, 2005.

McClave S, et al: Nutrition support in acute pancreatitis: a systematic review of the literature, *JPEN J Parenter Enteral Nutr* 30:143, 2006.

Medici V, et al: Diagnosis and management of Wilson's disease: results of a single center experience, *J Clin Gastroenterol* 40:936, 2006.

National Institute on Alcohol Abuse and Alcoholism. Age-specific and age-adjusted death rates for cirrhosis with and without mention of alcohol, United States, 1970-2005. October 2008. Available at: http://www.niaaa.nih.gov/Resources/DatabaseResources/QuickFacts/Liver/Pages/cirmrt3b.aspx. Accessed February 21, 2011.

Pereg D, et al: Probiotics for patients with compensated liver cirrhosis: a double-blind placebo-controlled study, *Nutrition* 6 May 2010. [Epub ahead of print.]

Petrov MS, et al: Systemic review: nutrition support in acute pancreatitis, *Alimen Pharmacol Ther* 28:704, 2009.

Plauth M, et al: ESPEN Guidelines on enteral nutrition: liver disease, *Clin Nutr* 25:285, 2006.

Rambaldi A, Gluud C: S-adenosyl-L-methionine for alcoholic liver diseases, Cochrane Database Syst Rev 2006, Issue 2. Art. No.: CD002235.

Rambaldi A, et al: Milk thistle for alcoholic and/or hepatitis B or C virus liver diseases, Cochrane Database Syst Rev 2007, Issue 4. Art. No.: CD003620.

Ranson JH, et al: Prognostic signs and the role of operative management in acute pancreatitis, *Surg Gynecol Obstet* 139:69, 1974.

Rayes N, et al: Supply of pre- and probiotics reduces bacterial infection rates after liver transplantation—a randomized, double-blind trial, *Am J Transplant* 5:125, 2005.

Stanga Z, et al: Effect of jejunal long-term feeding in chronic pancreatitis, *JPEN J Parenter Enteral Nutr* 29:12, 2005.

Tsai CJ, et al: Dietary carbohydrates and glycaemic load and the incidence of symptomatic gall stone disease in men, *Gut* 54:823, 2005.

Volzke H, et al: Independent risk factors for gallstone formation in a region with high cholelithiasis prevalence, *Digestion* 71:97, 2005.

Weikert C, et al: Presence of gallstones or kidney stones and risk of type 2 diabetes, *Am J Epidemiol* 171:447, 2010.

Willner IR, Reuben A: Alcohol and the liver, *Curr Opin Gastroenterol* 21:323, 2005.

CHAPTER 31

Marion J. Franz, MS, RD, LD, CDE

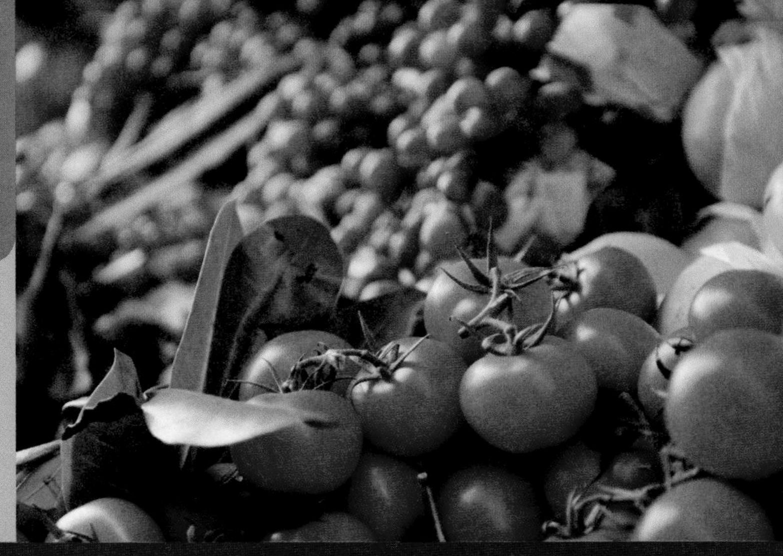

Medical Nutrition Therapy for Diabetes Mellitus and Hypoglycemia of Nondiabetic Origin

KEY TERMS

A1C
acanthosis nigricans
acceptable daily intake (ADI)
amylin
autonomic symptoms
carbohydrate counting
continuous glucose monitoring (CGM)
correction factor (CF)
counterregulatory (stress) hormones
dawn phenomenon
Diabetes Control and Complications Trial (DCCT)
diabetic ketoacidosis (DKA)
exchange lists
fasting hypoglycemia
gastroparesis
gestational diabetes mellitus (GDM)
glucagon
glucose-lowering medications
glucotoxicity
glycemic index (GI)
glycemic load (GL)
glycosylated hemoglobin (A1C)
honeymoon phase
hyperglycemia
hypoglycemia (or insulin reaction)
hypoglycemia of nondiabetic origin
hyperglycemic hyperosmolar state (HHS)
immune-mediated diabetes mellitus
incretins
insulin deficiency
insulin resistance
insulin secretagogues
latent autoimmune diabetes in adults (LADA)
lipotoxicity
macrosomia
macrovascular diseases
metabolic syndrome
microvascular diseases
neuroglycopenic symptoms
nutrition assessment
polydipsia
polyuria
postprandial (after a meal) blood glucose
postprandial (reactive) hypoglycemia
prediabetes
preprandial (fasting/premeal) blood glucose
self-monitoring of blood glucose (SMBG)
Somogyi effect
target blood glucose goals
type 1 diabetes mellitus (T1DM)
type 2 diabetes mellitus (T2DM)
United Kingdom Prospective Diabetes Study (UKPDS)
Whipple triad

Diabetes mellitus is a group of diseases characterized by high blood glucose concentrations resulting from defects in insulin secretion, insulin action, or both. Insulin is a hormone produced by the β-cells of the pancreas that is necessary for the use or storage of body fuels (carbohydrate, protein, and fat). Persons with diabetes do not produce adequate insulin; with **insulin deficiency**, **hyperglycemia** (elevated blood glucose) occurs.

Diabetes mellitus contributes to a considerable increase in morbidity and mortality rates, which can be reduced by early diagnosis and treatment. Direct medical expenditures such as inpatient care, outpatient services, and nursing home care total are astronomical and indirect costs such as disability, work loss, and premature mortality are equally high. Average medical expenditures among people with diabetes is double that of people who do not have diabetes. Thus providing medical nutrition therapy (MNT) for prevention and treatment of diabetes has tremendous potential to reduce these costs. Fortunately, people with diabetes can take steps to control the disease and lower the risk of complications and premature death.

INCIDENCE AND PREVALENCE

In 2007 total prevalence of diabetes in the United States for all ages was 23.6 million people, or 7.8% of the population. Of these, 17.9 million are diagnosed and 5.7 million undiagnosed. In 2007 1.6 million new cases of diabetes were diagnosed in people age 20 years or older (Centers for Disease Control and Prevention [CDC], 2007).

Much of the increase is because type 2 diabetes mellitus (T2DM) is no longer a disease that affects mainly older adults. Between 1990 and 1998, the prevalence of diabetes increased by 76% among people in their 30s. Among youth, the prevalence of T2DM also increased dramatically in recent decades.

The prevalence of T2DM is highest in ethnic groups in the United States. Diabetes has been diagnosed, in people aged 20 years or older, in 14.2% of American Indians and Alaska Natives, 11.8% of non-Hispanic blacks, 10.4% of Hispanics, and 7.5% of Asian Americans. Among Hispanics, rates were 12.6% for Puerto Ricans, 11.9% for Mexican Americans, and 8.2% for Cubans (CDC, 2007). In addition, another 57 million people (25% of adults 20 years or older and 35% of adults 60 years or older) have **prediabetes**, which includes impaired glucose tolerance (IGT) (2-hour postchallenge glucose of 140-199 mg/dL) and impaired fasting glucose (IFG) (fasting plasma glucose [FPG] 100-25 mg/dL) (CDC, 2007). Persons with prediabetes are at high risk for conversion to T2DM and cardiovascular disease (CVD) if lifestyle prevention strategies are not implemented.

CATEGORIES OF GLUCOSE INTOLERANCE

Assigning a type of diabetes to an individual often depends on the circumstances present at the time of diagnosis, and many individuals do not easily fit into a single category. Thus it is less important to label the particular type of diabetes than it is to understand the pathogenesis of the hyperglycemia and to treat it effectively (American Diabetes Association [ADbA], 2011a). What is clear is the need to intervene early with lifestyle interventions, beginning with prediabetes and continuing through the disease process. Categories of glucose intolerance are listed in Table 31-1.

Prediabetes

Individuals with a stage of impaired glucose homeostasis that includes IFG and IGT are often referred to as having prediabetes, indicating their relatively high risk for the development of diabetes and CVD. People at risk have IFG, IGT, both, or a hemoglobin A1C (A1C) of 5.7% to 6.4% and should be counseled about strategies, such as weight loss and physical activity, to lower their risks.

Type 1 Diabetes

At diagnosis, people with **type 1 diabetes mellitus (T1DM)** are often lean and experience excessive thirst, frequent urination, and significant weight loss. The primary defect is pancreatic β-cell destruction, usually leading to absolute insulin deficiency and resulting in hyperglycemia, **polyuria** (excessive urination), **polydipsia** (excessive thirst), weight loss, dehydration, electrolyte disturbance, and ketoacidosis. The rate of β-cell destruction is quite variable, proceeding rapidly in infants and children and slowly in others (mainly adults). The capacity of a healthy pancreas to secrete insulin is far in excess of what is needed normally. Therefore the clinical onset of diabetes may be preceded by an extensive asymptomatic period of months to years, during which β-cells are undergoing gradual destruction (see *Pathophysiology and Care Management Algorithm:* Type 1 Diabetes Mellitus).

T1DM accounts for 5% to 10% of all diagnosed cases of diabetes. Persons with T1DM depend on exogenous insulin to prevent ketoacidosis and death. Although it may occur at any age, even in the eighth and ninth decades of life, most cases are diagnosed in people younger than 30 years of age, with a peak incidence at around ages 10 to 12 years in girls and ages 12 to 14 years in boys (ADbA, 2011a). T1DM has been increasing 3% to 4% per year in children and youth, and even more in young children younger than age 5.

T1DM has two forms: immune-mediated and idiopathic. **Immune-mediated diabetes mellitus** results from an autoimmune destruction of the β-cells of the pancreas, the only cells in the body that make the hormone insulin. *Idiopathic T1DM* refers to forms of the disease that have no known cause, found mostly in persons of African or Asian origin (ADbA, 2011a).

Risk factors for T1DM may be genetic, autoimmune, or environmental. The genetic predisposition to T1DM is the result of the combination of human leukocyte antigen (HLA)–DQ coded genes for disease susceptibility offset by genes that are related to disease resistance (ADbA, 2011a). However, the genetic factors that confer susceptibility or

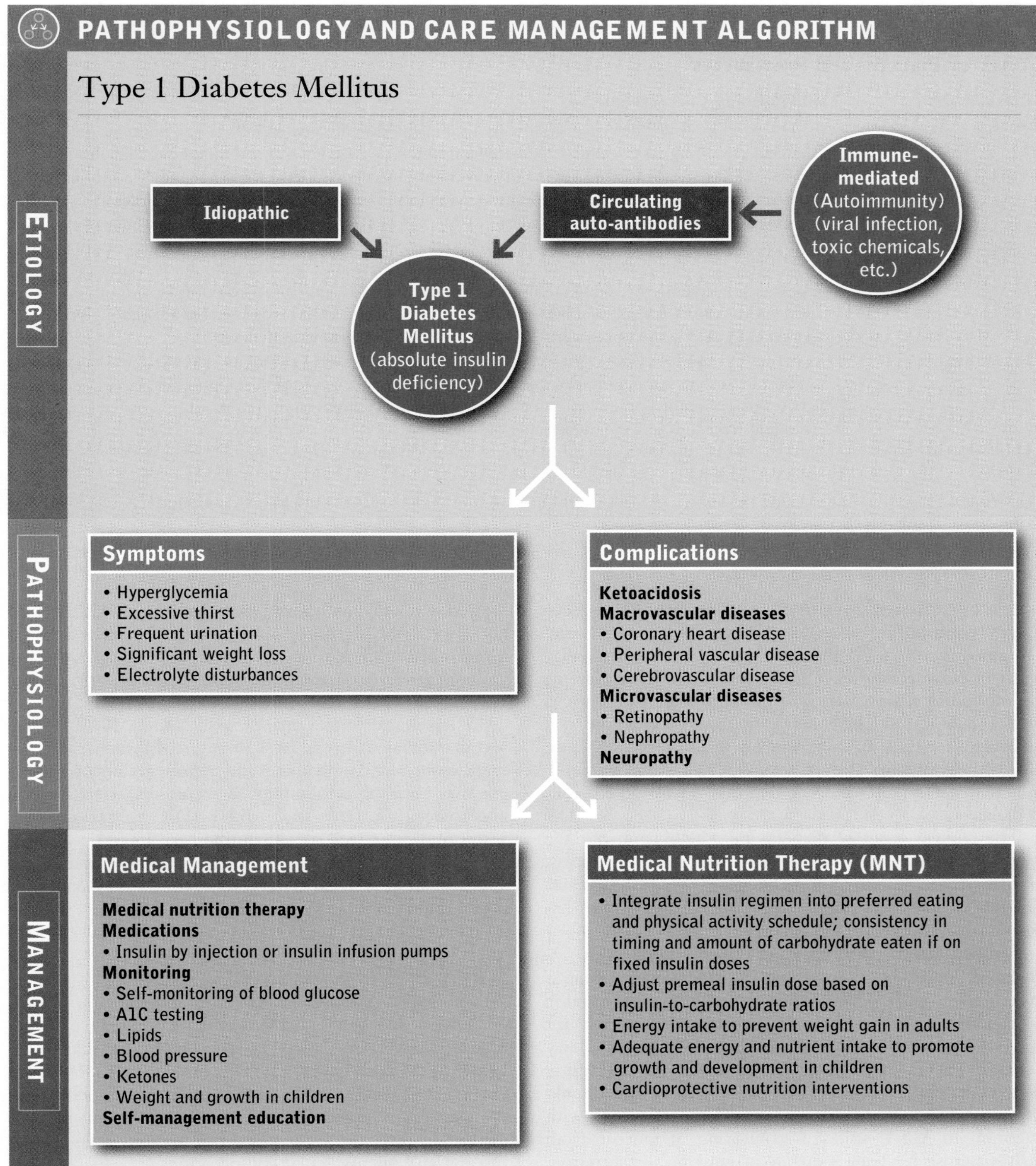

protection remain unclear. A 50% discordance rate of T1DM exists between identical twins, suggesting that specific genes are necessary but not sufficient for its development. A trigger, likely environmental, is necessary for the expression of the genetic propensity. At this time there are no known means to prevent T1DM.

Pathophysiology

Regardless of the trigger, early T1DM is first identified by the appearance of active autoimmunity directed against pancreatic β-cells and their products. At diagnosis, 85% to 90% of patients with T1DM have one or more circulating autoantibodies to islet cells, endogenous insulin, or other

TABLE 31-1

Types of Diabetes and Prediabetes

Classification	Distinguishing Characteristics
Type 1 diabetes	Characterized by β-cell destruction, usually leading to absolute insulin deficiency; immune-mediated diabetes (resulting from cellular-mediated autoimmune destruction) and idiopathic diabetes (no known causes) are two forms. Affected persons are usually children and young adults, although it can occur at any age, and depend on exogenous insulin to prevent ketoacidosis and death. Immune-mediated type 1 diabetes accounts for 5% to 10% of all diagnosed cases of diabetes.
Type 2 diabetes	Results from a progressive insulin secretory defect (insulin deficiency) on the background of insulin resistance. Affected persons are often older than 30 years at diagnosis, although it is now occurring frequently in young adults and children. Initially, individuals do not depend on exogenous insulin for survival but often require it as the disease progresses for adequate glycemic control. Type 2 diabetes accounts for ~90% to 95% of those with diabetes.
Prediabetes	Fasting or glucose tolerance test results above normal, but not diagnostic of diabetes. These persons should be monitored closely because they have an increased risk of developing diabetes.
GDM	Diabetes diagnosed in some women during pregnancy. Approximately 7% of all pregnancies (ranging from 1% to 14%, depending on the population) are complicated by GDM.
Other specific types	Diabetes that results from specific genetic syndromes, surgery, drugs, malnutrition, infections, or other illnesses.

Data from American Diabetes Association: Diagnosis and classification of diabetes mellitus (Position Statement), Diabetes Care 34:S63, 2011.

GDM, Gestational diabetes mellitus.

antigens that are constituents of islet cells. Antibodies identified as contributing to the destruction of β-cells are (1) islet cell autoantibodies; (2) insulin autoantibodies, which may occur in persons who have never received insulin therapy; (3) antibodies against islet tyrosine phosphatase (known as IA-2 and IA-2β); and (4) autoantibodies to glutamic acid decarboxylase (GAD), a protein on the surface of β-cells. GAD autoantibodies appear to provoke an attack by the T cells (killer T lymphocytes), which may destroy the β-cells in diabetes.

The clinical onset of diabetes may be abrupt, but the pathophysiologic insult is a slow, progressive process. Hyperglycemia and symptoms develop only after greater than 90% of the secretory capacity of the β-cell mass has been destroyed.

Frequently, after diagnosis and the correction of hyperglycemia, metabolic acidosis, and ketoacidosis, endogenous insulin secretion recovers. During this **honeymoon phase** exogenous insulin requirements decrease dramatically for up to 1 year or longer, and good metabolic control may be easily achieved. However, the need for increasing exogenous insulin replacement is inevitable and should always be anticipated. Intensive insulin therapy along with attention to MNT and self-monitoring of glucose from early diagnosis has been shown to prolong insulin secretion. Within 5 to 10 years after clinical onset, β-cell loss is complete, and circulating islet cell antibodies can no longer be detected.

Amylin, a glucoregulatory hormone is also produced in the pancreatic β-cell and co-secreted with insulin. Amylin complements the effects of insulin by regulating postprandial glucose levels and suppressing glucagon secretion. T1DM is an amylin-deficient state. Individuals with T1DM are also prone to other autoimmune disorders such as Grave's disease, Hashimoto's thyroiditis, Addison's disease, vitiligo, celiac disease, autoimmune hepatitis, myasthenia gravis, and pernicious anemia.

Latent autoimmune diabetes in adults (LADA) may account for as many as 10% of cases of insulin-requiring diabetes in older individuals and represents a slowly progressive form of autoimmune diabetes that is frequently confused with T2DM. Adults with LADA have HLA genetic susceptibility as well as autoantibodies. They may retain sufficient β-cell function so as to not require insulin for approximately six years, but eventually require intensive insulin interventions (Rosario, 2005).

Type 2 Diabetes

Type 2 diabetes mellitus (T2DM) accounts for 90% to 95% of all diagnosed cases of diabetes and is a progressive disease that, in many cases, is present long before it is diagnosed. Hyperglycemia develops gradually and is often not severe enough in the early stages for the person to notice any of the classic symptoms of diabetes. Although undiagnosed, these individuals are at increased risk of developing macrovascular and microvascular complications.

Risk factors for T2DM include genetic and environmental factors, including a family history of diabetes; older age; obesity, particularly intraabdominal obesity; physical inactivity; a prior history of gestational diabetes; prediabetes; and race or ethnicity. Adiposity and a longer duration of obesity are powerful risks factors for T2DM, and even small weight losses are associated with a change in glucose levels toward normal in persons with prediabetes. Nevertheless, T2DM is found in persons who are not obese, and many obese persons never develop T2DM. Therefore obesity combined with a genetic predisposition may be necessary for T2DM to occur (see *Pathophysiology and Care Management Algorithm:* Type 2 Diabetes Mellitus).

Pathophysiology

T2DM is characterized by a combination of insulin resistance and β-cell failure. Endogenous insulin levels may be normal, depressed, or elevated; but they are inadequate to overcome concomitant **insulin resistance** (decreased tissue sensitivity or responsiveness to insulin). As a result, hyperglycemia ensues.

Insulin resistance is first demonstrated in target tissues, mainly muscle, liver, and adipose cells. Initially there is a compensatory increase in insulin secretion (hyperinsulinemia), which maintains glucose concentrations in the normal or prediabetic range. In many persons the pancreas is unable to continue to produce adequate insulin, hyperglycemia occurs, and the diagnosis of diabetes is made. Therefore insulin levels are always deficient relative to elevated glucose levels before hyperglycemia develops.

Hyperglycemia is first exhibited as an elevation of **postprandial (after a meal) blood glucose** caused by insulin resistance at the cellular level and is followed by an elevation in fasting glucose concentrations. As insulin secretion decreases, hepatic glucose production increases, causing the increase in **preprandial (fasting) blood glucose** levels. The insulin response is also inadequate in suppressing alpha-cell glucagon secretion, resulting in glucagon hypersecretion and increased hepatic glucose production. Compounding the problem is **glucotoxicity**, the deleterious effect of hyperglycemia on both insulin sensitivity and insulin secretion; hence the importance of achieving near-euglycemia in persons with T2DM.

Insulin resistance is also demonstrated at the adipocyte level, leading to lipolysis and an elevation in circulating free fatty acids. In particular, excess intraabdominal obesity, characterized by an excess accumulation of visceral fat around and inside abdominal organs, results in an increased flux of free fatty acids to the liver, leading to an increase in insulin resistance. Increased fatty acids also cause a further decrease in insulin sensitivity at the cellular level, impair pancreatic insulin secretion, and augment hepatic glucose production (**lipotoxicity**). These defects contribute to the development and progression of T2DM and are also primary targets for pharmacologic therapy.

Persons with T2DM may or may not experience the classic symptoms of uncontrolled diabetes, and they are not prone to develop ketoacidosis. The progressive loss of β-cell secretory function means that persons with T2DM will require more medications over time to maintain the same level of glycemic control; eventually exogenous insulin will be required. Insulin is also required sooner for control during periods of stress-induced hyperglycemia, such as during illness or surgery.

Gestational Diabetes Mellitus

Gestational diabetes mellitus (GDM) occurs in approximately 7% of all pregnancies (ranging from 1% to 14% depending on the population studied), resulting in more than 200,000 cases annually (ADbA, 2011a). After delivery, approximately 90% of all women with GDM become normoglycemic but are at increased risk of developing GDM earlier in subsequent pregnancies. Immediately after pregnancy, 5% to 10% of women with GDM are diagnosed with T2DM. Women who have had GDM have a 40% to 60% chance of developing diabetes in the next 5 to 10 years (CDC, 2007). Lifestyle modifications aimed at reducing or preventing weight gain and increasing physical activity after pregnancy may reduce the risk of subsequent diabetes.

Previously GDM was defined as any degree of glucose intolerance with onset or first recognition during pregnancy. However, the number of pregnant women with undiagnosed diabetes has increased and therefore it has now been recommended that high-risk women found to have diabetes at their initial prenatal visit receive a diagnosis of overt, not gestational, diabetes (ADbA, 2011b). The majority of cases of GDM will be diagnosed during the second or third trimester of pregnancy because of the increase in insulin-antagonist hormone levels and normal insulin resistance that occurs at this time.

An oral glucose challenge was previously used as an indication of the need for diagnostic testing for GDM. However, new guidelines have been proposed. Women at high risk should be tested during the first trimester. Women with an A1C of greater than 6.5%, a fasting glucose of more than 126 mg/dL (7 mmol/L), or a 1-hour glucose or more than 200 mg/dL (11.1 mmol/L) likely had diabetes before becoming pregnant and should be treated for GDM. Screening should be done during the 24th to 28th week of pregnancy using a 75-g oral glucose tolerance test (OGTT). A fasting glucose of more than 92 mg/dL (5.1 mmol/L), a 1-hour glucose of more than 180 mg/dL (10 mmol/L), or a 2-hour glucose of 153 mg/dL (8.4 mmol/L) or more is diagnostic of GDM.

During pregnancy, treatment to normalize maternal blood glucose levels reduces the risk of adverse maternal, fetal, and neonatal outcomes. Extra glucose from the mother crosses the fetal placenta and the fetus's pancreas responds by releasing extra insulin to cope with the excess glucose. The excess glucose is converted to fat, which results in **macrosomia**. The fetus may become too large for a normal birth, resulting in the need for cesarean delivery. Neonatal hypoglycemia at birth is another common problem. The above-normal levels of maternal glucose have caused the fetus to produce extra insulin. However, after birth the extra glucose is no longer available to the fetus; until his or her pancreas can adjust, the neonate may require extra glucose through intravenous feedings for a day or two to keep blood glucose levels normal.

GDM does not cause congenital anomalies. Such malformations occur in women with diabetes prior to pregnancy who have uncontrolled blood glucose levels during the first

PATHOPHYSIOLOGY AND CARE MANAGEMENT ALGORITHM

Type 2 Diabetes Mellitus

ETIOLOGY

Genetic factors

Risk factors (obesity, older age, race or ethnicity, prediabetes, history of gestational diabetes)

Environmental factors

Intake of excessive calories and physical inactivity

Type 2 Diabetes Mellitus (insulin resistance; insulin deficiency)

PATHOPHYSIOLOGY

Symptoms (variable)

- Hyperglycemia
- Fatigue
- Excessive thirst
- Frequent urination

Clinical Findings

- Abnormal patterns of insulin secretion and action
- Decreased cellular uptake of glucose and increased postprandial glucose
- Increased release of glucose by liver (gluconeogenesis) resulting in fasting hyperglycemia
- Central obesity
- Hypertension
- Dyslipidemia

MANAGEMENT

Medical Management

Medical nutrition therapy
Physical activity
Medications
- Glucose-lowering medications
- Insulin

Monitoring
- Self-monitoring of blood glucose
- A1C testing
- Lipids
- Blood pressure
- Weight

Self-management education

Medical Nutrition Therapy (MNT)

- Lifestyle strategies (food/eating and physical activity) that improve glycemia, dyslipidemia, and blood pressure
- Nutrition education (carbohydrate counting and fat modification) and counseling
- Energy restriction
- Blood glucose monitoring to determine adjustments in food or medications
- Cardioprotective nutrition interventions

six to eight weeks of pregnancy when fetal organs are being formed. Because GDM doesn't appear until later in pregnancy, the fetal organs were formed before hyperglycemia became a problem.

When optimal blood glucose levels are not being maintained with MNT or the rate of fetal growth is excessive, pharmacologic therapy is needed (American Dietetic Association [ADA], 2009a). Research supports the use of insulin, insulin analogs, metformin, and glyburide during pregnancy. Women with GDM should be screened for diabetes 6 to 12 weeks postpartum and should be followed with subsequent screening for the development of diabetes or prediabetes (ADbA, 2011b).

Other Types of Diabetes

This category includes diabetes associated with specific genetic syndromes (such as maturity-onset diabetes of youth), diseases of the exocrine pancreas (such as cystic fibrosis), drug- or chemical-induced (such as in the treatment of acquired immune deficiency syndrome or after organ transplantation), surgery, infections, and other illnesses. Such types of diabetes may account for 1% to 5% of all diagnosed cases of diabetes (ADbA, 2011a).

SCREENING AND DIAGNOSTIC CRITERIA

Testing or screening for diabetes should be considered in all adults who are overweight (body mass index [BMI] of 25 kg/m^2 or more) and who have one or more additional risk factors for T2DM in the following list. In those without these risk factors, testing should begin at age 45 years. If tests are normal, testing should be done at 3-year intervals; A1C, FPG, or 2-hour OGTT can be used to test for either prediabetes or diabetes (ADbA, 2011b). Additional risk factors for diabetes are:

- Physical inactivity
- First-degree relative with diabetes
- Members of a high-risk population (African American, Latino, Native American, Asian-American, and Pacific Islander)
- Women who have delivered a baby weighing more than 9 lb or have been diagnosed with GDM
- Hypertensive (blood pressure 140/90 mm Hg or more or taking medication for hypertension)
- High-density lipoprotein (HDL) cholesterol level of less than 35 mg/dL (0.9 mmol/L) or a triglyceride level of more than 250 mg/dL (2.82 mmol/L)
- Women with polycystic ovary syndrome (PCOS)
- A1C of 5.7% or more, IGT, or IFG on previous testing
- Severe obesity
- **Acanthosis nigricans** (gray-brown skin pigmentations)
- History of CVD

Consistent with screening recommendations for adults, children and youth at increased risk for T2DM should be tested. The age of initiation of screening is age 10 years or at onset of puberty, and the frequency is every 3 years (ADbA, 2011b). Youth who are overweight (BMI greater than the 85th percentile for age and sex, weight for height greater than the 85th percentile, or weight of more than 120% of ideal for height) and have any two of the following risk factors should be screened: family history of T2DM, members of high-risk ethnic populations, signs of insulin resistance (acanthosis nigricans, hypertension, dyslipidemia, PCOS, small for gestational age birthweight, or maternal history of diabetes or GDM during the child's gestation.)

Diagnostic criteria for diabetes and prediabetes are summarized in Table 31-2. Four diagnostic methods may be used to diagnose diabetes and each, in the absence of unequivocal hyperglycemia, must be confirmed on a subsequent day by repeat testing. It is preferable that the same test be repeated for confirmation (ADbA, 2011b).

The use of A1C for diagnosing diabetes was not previously recommended. However, the A1C assay is now highly standardized and is a reliable measure of chronic glucose levels. The A1C test reflects longer-term glucose concentrations and is assessed from the results of **glycosylated hemoglobin** (simplified as **A1C**) tests. When hemoglobin and other proteins are exposed to glucose, the glucose becomes attached to the protein in a slow, nonenzymatic, and concentration-dependent fashion. Measurements of A1C therefore reflect a weighted average of plasma glucose concentration over the preceding weeks. In nondiabetic persons A1C values are 4% to 6%; these values correspond to mean blood glucose levels of approximately 70 to 126 mg/dL (3.9 to 7 mmol/L). A1C values vary less than FPG and testing is more convenient as patients are not required to be fasting or to undergo an OGTT. For conditions with abnormal red cell turnover, such as pregnancy or anemias from hemolysis and iron deficiency, the diagnosis of diabetes must use glucose criteria exclusively (ADbA, 2011b).

MANAGEMENT OF PREDIABETES

In no other disease does lifestyle—healthy and appropriate food choices and physical activity—play a more important role in both prevention and treatment than in diabetes. Studies comparing lifestyle modifications to medication have provided support for the benefit of weight loss (reduced energy intake) and physical activity as the first choice to prevent or delay diabetes. Clinical trials comparing lifestyle interventions to a control group have reported risk reduction for T2DM from lifestyle interventions ranging from 29% to 67% (ADbA, 2011b). Two frequently cited studies are the Finnish Diabetes Prevention Study and the Diabetes Prevention Program in which lifestyle interventions focused on a weight loss of 5% to 10%, physical activity of at least 150 min/week of moderate activity, and ongoing counseling and support. Both reported a 58% reduction in the incidence of T2DM in the intervention group compared with the control group and persistent reduction in the rate of conversion to T2DM within 3 to

TABLE 31-2

Diagnosis of Diabetes Mellitus and Impaired Glucose Homeostasis (Prediabetes)

Diagnosis	Criteria
Diabetes	A1C ≥ 6.5%* OR FPG ≥ 126 mg/dL (≥7 mmol/L)* OR 2-hour PG ≥ 200 mg/dL (≥11.1 mmol/L) during an OGTT* OR In patients with classic symptoms of hyperglycemia or hyperglycemic crisis, a random PG ≥ 200 mg/dL (≥11.1 mmol/L)
Prediabetes	FPG 100-125 mg/dL (5.6-7 mmol/L) [Impaired fasting glucose] OR 2-hour PG 140-199 mg/dL (7.8-11 mmol/L) [Impaired glucose tolerance] OR A1C 5.7%-6.4%
Normal	FPG < 100 mg/dL (<5.6 mmol/L) 2-hour PG < 140 mg/dL (<7.8 mmol/L)

Data from American Diabetes Association: Diagnosis and classification of diabetes mellitus (Position Statement), Diabetes Care 34:S63, 2011.

A1C, Hemoglobin A1C; *FPG*, fasting plasma glucose; *OGTT*, oral glucose tolerance test; *PG*, plasma glucose (measured 2 hours after an OGTT with administration of 75 g of glucose).

*In the absence of unequivocal hyperglycemia, criteria should be confirmed by repeat testing.

14 years postintervention follow-up (Diabetes Prevention Program, 2009; Li, 2008; Lindström, 2006).

Medical Management

Use of the pharmacologic agents metformin, α-glucosidase inhibitors, orlistat, and thiazolidinediones (TZDs) has been shown to decrease incidence of diabetes by various degrees (ADbA, 2011b). At this time, metformin is the only drug that should be considered for use in diabetes prevention. It is the most effective in those with a BMI of at least 35 kg/m^2 and who are younger than age 30. For other drugs, issues of cost, side effects, and lack of persistence of effect are of concern.

Medical management must include lifestyle changes. Physical activity is important to prevent weight gain and maintain weight loss. For cardiovascular fitness and to reduce risk of T2DM, recommendations include moderate-intensity aerobic physical activity for a minimum of 30 minutes 5 days per week (150 min/week) (i.e., walking 3 to 4 miles/hour) or vigorous-intensity aerobic physical activity for a minimum of 20 minutes 3 days per week (90 min/week). Muscle-strengthening activities involving all major muscle groups 2 or more days per week are also recommended (U.S. Department of Health and Human Services, 2008). Physical activity independent of weight loss improves insulin sensitivity.

Bariatric Surgery and Prediabetes

For morbidly obese individuals, bariatric surgery can reduce the incidence of diabetes. Because improvement in glucose occurs rapidly and before significant weight loss, decreased risk may be related to diversion of nutrients away from the gastrointestinal tract (Guidone et al., 2006) or by changes from bariatric surgery on the signaling mechanism of the gut to pancreatic islet cells, muscles, fat, liver, and other organs (Wilson and Pories, 2010).

Medical Nutrition Therapy for Prediabetes

Goals of MNT for prediabetes emphasize the importance of food choices that facilitate moderate weight loss (Box 31-1). Because of the effects of obesity on insulin resistance, weight loss is an important goal (see Chapter 22). In addition, studies have reported a relationship between higher levels of total dietary fat and greater insulin resistance.

Whole grains and dietary fiber are associated with reduced risk of diabetes. Increased intake of whole grain–containing foods improves insulin sensitivity independent of body weight, and increased intake of dietary fiber has been associated with improved insulin sensitivity and improved ability to secrete insulin adequately to overcome insulin resistance (Mayer-Davis et al., 2006). Moderate consumption of alcohol (1 to 3 drinks per day [15 to 45 g alcohol]) is linked with decreased risk of T2DM, coronary heart disease (CHD), and stroke. But the data do not support recommending alcohol consumption to persons at risk for diabetes who do not already drink alcoholic beverages (ADbA, 2008).

MANAGEMENT OF DIABETES

Two classic clinical trials have demonstrated beyond a doubt the clear link between glycemic control and the

BOX 31-1

Goals of Medical Nutrition Therapy for Diabetes Mellitus

Goals of Medical Nutrition Therapy That Apply to Persons at Risk for Diabetes or with Prediabetes:

1. To decrease risk of diabetes and cardiovascular disease by promoting healthy food choices and physical activity leading to moderate weight loss that is maintained

Goals of Medical Nutrition Therapy for Persons with Diabetes

1. To the extent possible, achieve and maintain:
   - Blood glucose levels in the normal range or as close to normal as is safely possible
   - A lipid and lipoprotein profile that reduces the risk for vascular disease
   - Blood pressure levels that reduce the risk for vascular disease
2. To prevent, or at least slow the rate of, development of the chronic complications of diabetes by modifying nutrient intake and lifestyle as appropriate
3. To address individual nutrition needs, taking into account personal and cultural preferences and willingness to change
4. To limit food choices only based on evidence and to maintain the pleasure of eating

Goals of Nutrition Therapy That Apply to Specific Situations:

1. For youth with type 1 diabetes, youth with type 2 diabetes, pregnant and lactating women, and older adults with diabetes, to meet the nutritional needs of these unique times in the life cycle
2. For individuals treated with insulin or insulin secretagogues, to provide self-management training for safe conduct of exercise, prevention and treatment of hypoglycemia, and treatment of acute illness

Adapted from American Diabetes Association: Nutrition recommendations and interventions for diabetes (position statement), Diabetes Care 31:S61, 2008.

development of complications in persons with T1DM and T2DM, as well as the importance of nutrition therapy in achieving control. The **Diabetes Control and Complications Trial (DCCT)** studied approximately 1400 persons with T1DM treated with either intensive (multiple injections of insulin or use of insulin infusion pumps guided by blood glucose monitoring results) or conventional (one or two insulin injections per day) regimens. Patients who achieve control similar to the intensively treated patients can expect a 50% to 75% reduction in the risk of progression to retinopathy, nephropathy, neuropathy, and fewer long-term cardiovascular complications (Diabetes Control and Complications Trial, 2005). Another study, the **United Kingdom Prospective Diabetes Study (UKPDS)** demonstrated conclusively that glucose and blood pressure control decreased the risk of long-term complications in T2DM. A reduction in energy intake was at least as important, if not more important, than the actual weight lost.

Medical Management

There is a progressive nature in T2DM. The "diet" doesn't fail; the pancreas fails to secrete enough insulin to maintain adequate glucose control. As the disease progresses, MNT alone is not enough to keep A1C level at 7% or less. Therapy needs to be intensified over time. Medication, and often insulin, need to be combined with nutrition therapy.

The management of all types of diabetes includes MNT, physical activity, monitoring, medications, and self-management education. An important goal of treatment is to provide the patient with the necessary tools to achieve the best possible control of glycemia, lipidemia, and blood pressure to prevent, delay, or arrest the microvascular and macrovascular complications while minimizing hypoglycemia and excess weight gain (ADbA, 2011b). Optimal control of diabetes also requires the restoration of normal carbohydrate, protein, and fat metabolism.

Insulin is both anticatabolic and anabolic and facilitates cellular transport (Table 31-3). In general, the **counterregulatory (stress) hormones** (glucagon, growth hormone, cortisol, epinephrine, and norepinephrine) have the opposite effect of insulin.

The American Diabetes Association's (ADbA) glycemic treatment goals for persons with diabetes are listed in Table 31-4. Achieving goals requires open communication and appropriate self-management education. Patients can assess day-to-day glycemic control by **self-monitoring of blood glucose (SMBG)** and measurement of urine or blood ketones. Longer-term glycemic control is assessed by A1C testing. Lipid levels and blood pressure must also be monitored (Table 31-5). Lipids should be measured annually, and blood pressure should be monitored at every diabetes management visit (ADbA, 2011b).

Medical Nutrition Therapy for Diabetes

MNT is integral to total diabetes care and management. Effective integration of MNT into the overall management of diabetes requires a coordinated team effort, including a registered dietitian (RD) who is knowledgeable and skilled in implementing current nutrition therapy recommendations for diabetes. MNT requires an individualized approach and effective nutrition self-management education and counseling. Monitoring glucose, A1C and lipid levels, blood pressure, weight, and quality-of-life issues is essential in evaluating the success of nutrition-related recommendations. If desired outcomes from MNT are not met, changes in overall diabetes care and management should be recommended (ADbA, 2008).

The American Dietetic Association (ADA) published evidence-based nutrition practice guidelines (EBNPG) for T1DM and T2DM in adults in their Evidence Analysis Library (ADA, 2008) and in print (Franz et al., 2010a). The

TABLE 31-3

Action of Insulin on Carbohydrate, Protein, and Fat Metabolism

Effect	Carbohydrates	Protein	Fat
Anticatabolic (prevents breakdown)	Decreases breakdown and release of glucose from glycogen in the liver	Inhibits protein degradation, diminishes gluconeogenesis	Inhibits lipolysis, prevents excessive production of ketones and ketoacidosis
Anabolic (promotes storage)	Facilitates conversion of glucose to glycogen for storage in liver and muscle	Stimulates protein synthesis	Facilitates conversion of pyruvate to free fatty acids, stimulating lipogenesis
Transport	Activates the transport system of glucose into muscle and adipose cells	Lowers blood amino acids in parallel with blood glucose levels	Activates lipoprotein lipase, facilitating transport of triglycerides into adipose tissue

TABLE 31-4

Recommendations for Glycemic Control for Adults with Diabetes

Glycemic Control	Criteria
A1C	<7.0%*
Preprandial capillary plasma glucose	70-130 mg/dL (3.9-7.2 mmol/L)
Peak postprandial capillary plasma glucose†	<180 mg/dL (<10 mmol/L)

Modified from American Diabetes Association: Standards of medical care in diabetes—2011 (Position Statement), Diabetes Care 34:S31, 2011.

A1C, Hemoglobin A1C.

*Referenced to a nondiabetic range of 4%-6% using a DCCT-based assay.

†Postprandial glucose measurements should be made 1-2 hours after the beginning of the meal, generally peak levels in patients with diabetes.

TABLE 31-5

Recommendations for Lipid and Blood Pressure for Adults with Diabetes

Lipids/Blood Pressure	Criteria
LDL cholesterol	<100 mg/dL (<2.6 mmol/L)*
HDL cholesterol	
Men	>40 mg/dL (>1.1 mmol/L)
Women	>50 mg/dL (>1.4 mmol/L)
Triglycerides	<150 mg/dL (<1.7 mmol/L)
Blood Pressure	<130/80 mm Hg

Modified from American Diabetes Association: Standards of medical care in diabetes—2011 (Position Statement), Diabetes Care 34:S31, 2011.

CVD, Cardiovascular disease; *HDL*, high-density lipoprotein; *LDL*, low-density lipoprotein.

*In individuals with overt CVD, a lower LDL cholesterol goal of <70 mg/dL (1.8 mmol/L), using a high dose of a statin, is an option.

ADbA nutrition recommendations are summarized in their annual standards of care (ADb, 2010b) and in a position statement (ADbA, 2008). Although numerous studies have attempted to identify the optimal percentages of macronutrients for the meal plan of persons with diabetes, it is unlikely that one such combination of macronutrients exists. The best mix appears to vary, depending on individual circumstances (ADbA, 2008). If guidance is needed, the RD should encourage consumption of macronutrients based on the dietary reference intakes (DRIs) for healthy eating (ADA, 2008), which recommend that adults should consume 45% to 65% of total energy from carbohydrate, 20% to 35% from fat, and 10% to 35% from protein.

Goals and Desired Outcomes

The goals for MNT for diabetes emphasize the role of lifestyle in improving glucose control, lipid and lipoprotein profiles, and blood pressure. To date, Medicare reimburses qualified dietitian providers for providing evidence-based MNT for diabetes management to eligible participants. Improving health through food choices and physical activity is the basis of all nutrition recommendations for the treatment of diabetes (see Box 31-1). Interventions include reduced energy and fat intake, carbohydrate counting, simplified meal plans, healthy food choices, individualized meal-planning strategies, exchange lists, low-fat vegan diet, insulin-to-carbohydrate ratios, physical activity, and behavioral strategies.

Besides being skilled and knowledgeable in assessing and implementing MNT, RDs must also be aware of expected outcomes from MNT, when to assess outcomes, and what feedback, including recommendations, should be given to referral sources. Furthermore, the effect of MNT on A1C will be known by 6 weeks to 3 months, at which time the RD must assess whether the goals of therapy have been met by changes in lifestyle or whether changes or additional medications are needed (ADA, 2008).

Research supports MNT as an effective therapy in reaching diabetes treatment goals. Clinical trials and outcomes studies have reported decreases in A1C levels at 3 to 6 months ranging from 0.25% to 2.9% (average 1% to 2%) with higher reductions seen in T2DM of shorter duration (Franz et al., 2008). These outcomes are similar to those from oral **glucose-lowering medications**. MNT is reported to reduce low-density lipoprotein (LDL) cholesterol by 9% to 12% compared with baseline values or to a Western-type diet (Van Horn et al., 2008). After initiation of MNT, improvements are apparent in 3 to 6 months. MNT provided by RDs for hypertension report an average reduction in blood pressure of approximately 5 mm Hg for both systolic and diastolic blood pressure (ADA, 2009b).

Carbohydrate Intake

Sugars, *starch*, and *fiber* are the preferred carbohydrate terms. Blood glucose levels after eating are primarily determined by the rate of appearance of glucose from carbohydrate digestion and absorption into the bloodstream and the ability of insulin to clear glucose from the circulation. Low-carbohydrate diets might seem to be a logical approach to lowering postprandial glucose. However, foods that contain carbohydrates (whole grains, fruits, vegetables, and low-fat milk) are excellent sources of vitamins, minerals, dietary fiber, and energy. Therefore these foods are important components of a healthy diet for all Americans, including those with diabetes (ADbA, 2008).

The long-held belief that sucrose must be restricted based on the assumption that sugars are more rapidly digested and absorbed than starches is not justified. The total amount of carbohydrate eaten at a meal, regardless if the source is starch or sucrose, is the primary determinant of postprandial glucose levels. The glycemic effect of carbohydrate foods cannot be predicted based on their structure (i.e., starch versus sugar) owing to the efficiency of the human digestive tract in reducing starch polymers to glucose. Starches are rapidly metabolized into 100% glucose during digestion, in contrast to sucrose, which is metabolized into only approximately 50% glucose and approximately 50% fructose. Fructose has a very low glycemic response, which has been attributed to its slow rate of absorption and its storage in the liver as glycogen (see Chapters 3 and 9, and Appendix 43).

Although numerous factors influence glycemic response to foods, monitoring total grams of carbohydrates, whether by use of carbohydrate counting, exchanges, or experienced-based estimation remains a key strategy in achieving glycemic control (ADA, 2008; ADbA, 2011b). Numerous studies have reported that when individuals are allowed to choose from a variety of starches and sugars, the glycemic response is nearly identical if the total amount of carbohydrate is similar.

Day-to-day consistency in the amount of carbohydrate eaten at meals and snacks is reported to improve glycemic control, especially in persons on either MNT alone, glucose-lowering medications, or fixed insulin regimens. In persons with T1DM or T2DM who adjust their mealtime insulin doses or who are on insulin pump therapy, insulin doses should be adjusted to match carbohydrate intake, known as the *insulin-to-carbohydrate ratios* (ADA, 2008). Several methods are used to estimate the nutrient content of foods.

In **carbohydrate counting** food portions contributing 15 g of carbohydrates (regardless of the source) are considered as one carbohydrate serving. Testing premeal and postmeal glucose levels is important for making adjustments in either food intake or medication to achieve glucose goals.

Exchange lists group foods into lists—carbohydrates, which includes starches, fruits, milk, sweets, desserts, and other carbohydrates, and nonstarchy vegetables; meat and meat substitutes; fats; and free foods. Each food list is a group of measured foods of approximately the same nutritional value. Combination foods such as casseroles, pizza, and soups, which fit into more than one food group, and fast foods are also listed. In addition, symbols are used to identify foods that are high in fiber, contain extra fat, or are high in sodium.

Glycemic Index and Glycemic Load

The **glycemic index (GI)** of food was developed to compare the physiologic effects of carbohydrates on glucose. The GI index measures the relative area under the postprandial glucose curve of 50 g of digestible carbohydrates compared with 50 g of a standard food, either glucose or white bread. When bread is the reference food, the GI index for the food is multiplied by 0.7 to obtain the value that is comparable to glucose being used as the reference food (glycemic index of glucose = 100, white bread = 70). The index does not measure how rapidly blood glucose levels increase. The peak glucose response for individual foods (Brand-Miller et al., 2009) and meals, either high or low glycemic index, occurs at approximately the same time.

The estimated **glycemic load (GL)** of foods, meals, and dietary patterns is calculated by multiplying the GI by the amount of carbohydrates in each food and then totaling the values for all foods in a meal or dietary pattern. In studies comparing low- and high-GI diets, total carbohydrate is first kept consistent. However, for some individuals use of the GI and GL may provide an additional modest benefit (ADbA, 2010b).

A major problem with the GI is the variability of response to a specific carbohydrate food. For example, Australian potatoes are reported to have a high GI, whereas potatoes in the United States and Canada have moderate GIs (Fernandes et al., 2005). The mean glycemic response and standard deviation of 50 g of carbohydrate from white bread tested in 23 subjects was 78 ± 73 with an individual coefficient of variation (CV) of 94%. Although the average GI of bread from three tests was 71%, the range of GI values was broad, ranging from 44 to 132 and the CV 34% (Vega-López et al., 2007).

Studies, primarily of short duration, report mixed effects on A1C levels (ADA, 2008). These studies are complicated by differing definitions of "high GI" or "low GI" diets or quartiles; GIs in the low GI diets range from 38% to 77% and in the high GI diets from 63% to 98%. More recently, two trials, each one year in duration, reported no significant differences in A1C levels from low GI versus high GI diets

(Wolever et al., 2008) or ADbA diets (Ma et al., 2008). Furthermore, most people likely already consume a moderate GI diet. It is unknown whether further lowering of the dietary GI can be achieved in the long term.

Fiber

Evidence is lacking to recommend a higher fiber intake for people with diabetes than for the population as a whole. Thus recommendations for fiber intake for people with diabetes are similar to the recommendations for the general public. Although diets containing 44 to 50 g of fiber daily improve glycemia, more usual fiber intakes (less than 24 g daily) have not shown beneficial effects. It is unknown if individuals living at home can daily consume the amount of fiber needed to improve glycemia. However, consuming foods containing 25 to 30 g of fiber per day, with special emphasis on soluble fiber sources (7-13 g) is recommended as part of cardioprotective nutrition therapy (ADA, 2008).

Grams of fiber (and sugar alcohols) are included on food labels and are calculated as having approximately half the energy (2 kcal/g) of most other carbohydrates (4 kcal/g). Adjustments in carbohydrate intake values is practical only if the amount per serving is more than 5 g. In that case, counting half of the carbohydrate grams from fiber (and sugar alcohols) would be useful in calculating exchanges and food choices for food labels or recipes and for individuals who are using insulin-to-carbohydrate ratios for managing their diabetes (Wheeler, 2008).

Sweeteners

Even though sucrose restriction cannot be justified on the basis of its glycemic effect, it is still good advice to suggest that persons with diabetes be careful in their consumption of foods containing large amounts of sucrose. Sucrose intakes of 10% to 35% of total energy intake do not have a negative effect on glycemic or lipid responses when substituted for isocaloric amounts of starch (ADA, 2008). If sucrose is included in the food and meal plan, it should be substituted for other carbohydrate sources or, if added, be adequately covered with insulin or other glucose-lowering medications. Care should be taken to avoid excess energy intake (ADbA, 2008).

There appears to be no significant advantage of alternative nutritive sweeteners such as fructose versus sucrose. Fructose provides 4 kcal/g, as do other carbohydrates, and even though it does have a lower glycemic response than sucrose and other starches, large amounts (15% to 20% of daily energy intake) of fructose have an adverse effect on plasma lipids. However, there is no reason to recommend that persons with diabetes avoid fructose, which occurs naturally in fruits and vegetables as well as in foods sweetened with fructose (ADbA, 2008).

Reduced-calorie sweeteners approved by the Food and Drug Administration (FDA) include sugar alcohols (erythritol, sorbitol, mannitol, xylitol, isomalt, lactitol, and hydrogenated starch hydrolysates) and tagatose. They produce a lower glycemic response and contain, on average, 2 calories/g. As for fiber, persons using insulin-to-carbohydrate ratios can subtract one half of sugar alcohol grams from total carbohydrate when the grams are more than 5 (Wheeler et al., 2008). There is no evidence that the amounts of sugar alcohols likely to be consumed will reduce glycemia or energy intake (ADbA, 2008.) Although their use appears to be safe, some people report gastric discomfort after eating foods sweetened with these products, and consuming large quantities may cause diarrhea, especially in children.

Saccharin, aspartame, neotame, acesulfame potassium, and sucralose are nonnutritive sweeteners currently approved by the FDA. All such products must undergo rigorous testing by the manufacturer and scrutiny from the FDA before they are approved and marketed to the public. For all food additives, including nonnutritive sweeteners, the FDA determines an **acceptable daily intake (ADI)**, defined as the amount of a food additive that can be safely consumed on a daily basis during a person's lifetime without risk. The ADI generally includes a 100-fold safety factor and greatly exceeds average consumption levels. For example, aspartame actual daily intake in persons with diabetes is 2 to 4 mg/kg of body weight daily, well below the ADI of 50 mg/kg daily.

In December 2008 the FDA stated that the stevia-derived sweetener, Rebaudioside A, is generally recognized as safe and it is currently being marketed. All FDA-approved nonnutritive sweeteners, when consumed within the established daily intake levels, can be used by persons with diabetes, including pregnant women (ADbA, 2008). As new so-called "natural" and other sweeteners appear in the market, people with diabetes should be aware that many do contain energy and carbohydrate, as do foods sweetened with them, that need to be accounted for.

Protein Intake

The amount of protein usually consumed by persons with diabetes (15% to 20% of energy intake) has minimal acute effects on glycemic response, lipids, and hormones, and no long-term effect on insulin requirements, and therefore does not need to be changed. Exceptions are in persons who consume excessive protein choices high in saturated fatty acids, have a protein intake less than the recommended daily allowance, or in the presence of diabetic nephropathy (ADA, 2008). Although nonessential amino acids undergo gluconeogenesis, in well-controlled diabetes the glucose produced does not appear in the general circulation. Although protein has no long-term effect on insulin needs, it is just as potent a stimulant of acute insulin release as carbohydrate. Furthermore, protein does not slow the absorption of carbohydrates and adding protein to the treatment of hypoglycemia does not prevent subsequent hypoglycemia.

Short-term studies with small numbers of subjects with diabetes suggest that diets with protein contents greater than 20% of total energy may improve glucose and insulin concentrations, reduce appetite, and improve satiety. However, such diets appear to be difficult to follow and the long-term effects of increased protein intake on regulation of energy intake, satiety, and weight loss have not been adequately studied.

Dietary Fat

Studies in persons with diabetes demonstrating the effects of specific percentages of dietary saturated and *trans*-fatty acids and specific amounts of cholesterol on CVD risk are limited. However, persons with diabetes are considered to have a risk of CVD similar to those with a past history of CVD. Therefore after focusing on achieving glycemic control, cardioprotective nutrition interventions should be implemented in the initial series of encounters (ADA, 2008). See Chapter 34 for recommendations for the prevention and treatment of CVD.

In metabolic studies in which energy intake is maintained so that subjects do not lose weight, diets high in either carbohydrates or monounsaturated fat lower LDL cholesterol equivalently. The concern has been the potential of a high-carbohydrate diet (more than 55% of energy intake) to increase triglycerides and postprandial glucose compared with a high–monounsaturated fat diet. However, in other studies when energy intake is reduced, the adverse effects of high-carbohydrate diets are not observed. Therefore energy intake appears to be a factor in determining the effects of a high-carbohydrate versus a high–monounsaturated fat diet.

There is evidence from the general population that foods containing ω-3 polyunsaturated fatty acids are beneficial and two to three servings of fish per week are recommended. Although most studies in persons with diabetes who have used ω-3 supplements show beneficial lowering of triglycerides, an accompanying rise in LDL cholesterol also has been noted. If supplements are used, the effects on LDL cholesterol should be monitored.

Alcohol

The same precautions that apply to alcohol consumption for the general population apply to persons with diabetes. Abstention from alcohol should be advised for people with a history of alcohol abuse or dependence; for women during pregnancy; and for people with medical problems such as liver disease, pancreatitis, or advanced neuropathy. If individuals choose to drink alcohol, daily intake should be limited to one drink or less for adult women and two drinks or less for adult men (1 drink = 12 oz beer, 5 oz of wine, or 1½ oz of distilled spirits). Each drink contains approximately 15 g of alcohol. The type of alcoholic beverage consumed does not make a difference (ADbA, 2008).

Moderate amounts of alcohol ingested with food have minimum, if any, acute effect on glucose and insulin levels. Alcoholic beverages should be considered an addition to the regular food and meal plan for all persons with diabetes. No food should be omitted, given the possibility of alcohol-induced hypoglycemia and because alcohol does not require insulin to be metabolized. Excessive amounts of alcohol (three or more drinks per day) on a consistent basis contribute to hyperglycemia, which improves as soon as alcohol use is discontinued.

In persons with diabetes, light to moderate amounts of alcohol (1 to 2 drinks per day; 15 to 30 g of alcohol) are associated with a decreased risk of CHD, perhaps because of the concomitant increase in HDL cholesterol and improved insulin sensitivity associated with alcohol consumption. Ingestion of light to moderate amounts of alcohol does not raise blood pressure, whereas excessive, chronic ingestion of alcohol does raise blood pressure and may be a risk factor for stroke.

Micronutrients

No clear evidence has been established for benefits from vitamin or mineral supplements in persons with diabetes (compared with the general population) who do not have underlying deficiencies (ADbA, 2008). In select groups such as the elderly, pregnant or lactating women, strict vegetarians, or those on calorie-restricted diets, a multivitamin supplement may be needed.

Because diabetes may be a state of increased oxidative stress, there has been interest in prescribing antioxidant vitamins in people with diabetes. Clinical trial data not only indicate the lack of benefit from antioxidants on glycemic control and progression of complications but also provide evidence of the potential harm of vitamin E, carotene, and other antioxidant supplements. Routine supplementation with antioxidants such as vitamins E and C and carotene is not advised because of lack of evidence of effectiveness and concern related to long-term safety (ADbA, 2008).

Dietary Supplements

Alpha-lipoic acid (ALA), which functions as an antioxidant, may have potential benefits for persons with diabetes and peripheral neuropathy. Short-term trials of intravenous and oral ALA reported improvements in symptoms of neuropathy. A long-term, multicenter trial is currently assessing the role of ALA given orally to determine whether ALA slows the progression of neuropathy versus only improving the neuropathy symptoms.

Several small studies have suggested a role for chromium supplementation in the management of glucose intolerance, gestational diabetes, body weight, and corticosteroid-induced diabetes. A systematic review of 41 studies regarding the effect of chromium supplementation on glucose metabolism and lipid levels reported no significant effect of chromium on lipid or glucose metabolism in people without diabetes and inconsistent effects in subjects with diabetes. However, the evidence is limited by the overall poor quality and heterogeneity of available studies (Balk et al., 2007). In addition, there is no benefit of chromium picolinate supplementation in reducing body weight. Benefit from chromium supplementation has not been clearly demonstrated and therefore is not recommended (ADbA, 2008).

Physical Activity and Exercise

Physical activity involves bodily movement produced by the contraction of skeletal muscles that requires energy expenditure in excess of resting energy expenditure. Exercise is a subset of physical activity: planned, structured, and repetitive bodily movement performed to improve or maintain one or more components of physical fitness. Aerobic exercise consists of rhythmic, repeated, and continuous movements of the same large muscle groups for at least 10 minutes at a time. Examples include walking, bicycling, jogging, swimming, and many sports. Resistance exercise consists of activities that use muscular strength to move a weight or work against a resistive load. Examples include weight lifting and exercises using resistance-providing machines.

Physical activity should be an integral part of the treatment plan for persons with diabetes. Exercise helps all persons with diabetes improve insulin sensitivity, reduce cardiovascular risk factors, control weight, and improve well being. Given appropriate guidelines, the majority of people with diabetes can exercise safely. The activity plan varies depending on interest, age, general health, and level of physical fitness.

Despite the increase in glucose uptake by muscles during exercise, glucose levels change little in individuals without diabetes. Muscular work causes insulin levels to decline while counterregulatory hormones (primarily glucagon) rise. As a result, the increased glucose use by the exercising muscles is matched with increased glucose production by the liver. This balance between insulin and counterregulatory hormones is the major determinant of hepatic glucose production, underscoring the need for insulin adjustments in addition to adequate carbohydrate intake during exercise for people with diabetes.

In persons with T1DM, the glycemic response to exercise varies, depending on overall diabetes control, plasma glucose and insulin levels at the start of exercise; timing, intensity, and duration of the exercise; previous food intake; and previous conditioning. An important variable is the level of plasma insulin during and after exercise. Hypoglycemia can occur because of insulin-enhanced muscle glucose uptake by the exercising muscle.

In persons with T2DM, blood glucose control can improve with physical activity, largely because of decreased insulin resistance and increased insulin sensitivity, which results in increased peripheral use of glucose not only during but also after the activity. This exercise-induced enhanced insulin sensitivity occur independent of any effect on body weight. Structured exercise interventions of at least 8 weeks' duration are reported to lower A1C. Exercise also decreases the effects of counterregulatory hormones; this in turn reduces the hepatic glucose output, contributing to improved glucose control.

Potential Problems with Exercise

Hypoglycemia is a potential problem associated with exercise in persons taking insulin or **insulin secretagogues**. Hypoglycemia can occur during, immediately after, or many hours after exercise. Hypoglycemia has been reported to be more common after exercise, especially exercise of long duration, strenuous activity or play, or sporadic exercise, than during exercise. This is because of increased insulin sensitivity after exercise and the need to replete liver and muscle glycogen, which can take up to 24 to 30 hours (see Chapter 23). However, hypoglycemia can also occur during or immediately after exercise. Blood glucose levels before exercise reflect only the value at that time, and it is unknown if this is a stable blood glucose level or a blood glucose level that is dropping. If blood glucose levels are dropping before exercise, adding exercise can contribute to hypoglycemia during exercise. Furthermore, hypoglycemia on the day before exercise may increase the risk of hypoglycemia on the day of exercise as well.

Hyperglycemia can also result from exercise of high intensity, likely as a result of the effects of counterregulatory hormones. When a person exercises at what for him or her is a high level of exercise intensity, there is a greater-than-normal increase in counterregulatory hormones. As a result, hepatic glucose release exceeds the rise in glucose use. The elevated glucose levels may also extend into the postexercise state. Hyperglycemia and worsening ketosis can also result in persons with T1DM who are deprived of insulin for 12 to 48 hours and are ketotic. Vigorous activity should probably be avoided in the presence of ketosis (ADbA, 2011b). However, high-intensity exercise is more likely to be the cause of hyperglycemia than insulin deficiency.

Exercise Guidelines

The variability of glucose responses to exercise contributes to the difficulty in giving precise guidelines for exercising safely. Frequent blood glucose monitoring before, during, and after exercise helps individuals identify their response to physical activities. To meet their individual needs, patients must modify general guidelines to reduce insulin doses before (or after) or ingest carbohydrates after (or before) exercise.

Carbohydrate for Insulin or Insulin Secretagogue Users. During moderate-intensity exercise, glucose uptake is increased by 8 to 13 g/hour; this is the basis for the recommendation to add 15 g carbohydrate for every 30 to 60 minutes of activity (depending on the intensity) over and above normal routines. Moderate exercise for less than 30 minutes usually does not require any additional carbohydrate or insulin adjustment. Added carbohydrates should be ingested if preexercise glucose levels are less than 100 mg/dL (5.6 mmol/L). Supplementary carbohydrate is generally not needed in individuals who are not treated with insulin or insulin secretagogues (ADbA, 2011b).

In all persons, blood glucose levels decline gradually during exercise, and ingesting a carbohydrate feeding during prolonged exercise can improve performance by maintaining the availability and oxidation of blood glucose. For the exerciser with diabetes whose blood glucose levels may drop sooner and lower than the exerciser without diabetes, ingesting carbohydrate after 40 to 60 minutes of exercise is important and may also assist in preventing hypoglycemia. Drinks containing 6% or less of carbohydrates empty from the stomach as quickly as water and have the advantage of providing both needed fluids and carbohydrates (see Chapter 23). Consuming carbohydrates immediately after exercise optimizes repletion of muscle and liver glycogen stores. For the exerciser with diabetes, this takes on added importance because of increased risk for late-onset hypoglycemia.

Insulin Guidelines. It is often necessary to adjust the insulin dosage to prevent hypoglycemia. This occurs most often with moderate to strenuous activity lasting more than 45 to 60 minutes. For most persons a modest decrease (of approximately 1 to 2 units) in the rapid- or short-acting insulin during the period of exercise is a good starting point. For prolonged vigorous exercise, a larger decrease in the total daily insulin dosage may be necessary. After exercise, insulin dosing may also need to be decreased.

Precautions for Persons with Type 2 Diabetes. Persons with T2DM may have a lower Vo_{2max} and therefore need a more gradual training program. Rest periods may be needed, but this does not impair the training effect from physical activity. Autonomic neuropathy or medications, such as for blood pressure, may not allow for increased heart rate, and individuals must learn to use perceived exertion as a means of determining exercise intensity. Blood pressure may also increase more in persons with diabetes than in those who do not have diabetes, and exercise should not be undertaken if systolic blood pressure is greater than 180 to 200 mm Hg (ADbA, 2010b).

Heat Intolerance. When persons with diabetes live and exercise in hot climates, they may experience "heat unawareness" because of their impaired ability to sweat and sense thirst. It is important to suggest adequate hydration techniques to counteract this effect.

Exercise Recommendations

People with diabetes should be advised to perform at least 150 min/week of moderate-intensity aerobic physical activity (50% to 70% of maximum heart rate) or at least 90 min/week of vigorous aerobic exercise (more than 70% of maximum heart rate.) The physical activity should be distributed over at least 3 days/week and with no more than 2 consecutive days without physical activity. In the absence of contraindications, people with T2DM should be encouraged to perform resistance exercise three times a week, targeting all major muscle groups, progressing to three sets of 8 to 10 repetitions at a weight that cannot be lifted more than eight to ten times. There is an additive benefit of combined aerobic and resistance training in adults with T2DM (ADbA, 2011b).

It is recommended that providers assess patients for conditions that might contraindicate certain types of exercise or predispose to injury. High-risk patients should be encouraged to start with short periods of low-intensity exercise and increase the intensity and duration slowly (ADbA, 2011b).

Medications

A consensus statement on the approach to management of hyperglycemia in T2DM has been published by the ADbA and the European Association for the Study of Diabetes (Nathan et al., 2009). Interventions at the time of diagnosis include lifestyle (MNT and physical activity) and metformin. If A1C is 7% or more, the next well-validated therapies are to add either a sulfonylurea or basal insulin. The alternative path is to add the less well-validated therapies of pioglitazone or an incretin glucagon-like peptide 1 (GLP-1) agonist. The overall objective is to achieve and maintain glycemic control and to change interventions, including the use of insulin, when therapeutic goals are not being met (ADbA, 2011b).

All persons with T1DM and many persons with T2DM who no longer produce adequate endogenous insulin need replacement of insulin. In persons with T2DM, insulin may be needed to restore glycemia to near normal. Circumstances that require the use of insulin in T2DM include the failure to achieve adequate control with administration of oral medications; periods of acute injury, infection, extreme heat exposure, surgery, or pregnancy.

Glucose-Lowering Medications for Type 2 Diabetes

Understanding that T2DM is a progressive disease is important for the understanding of treatment choices. Assisting individuals with diabetes to understand the disease process also helps them to understand and accept changes in medications that occur over time. Diabetes is first diagnosed when there is insufficient insulin available to maintain euglycemia and as insulin deficiency progresses medications and eventually insulin will be required to achieve glycemic goals. This is not a "diet failure" or a "medication failure" but rather a failure of the insulin secreting capacity of the β-cells.

Glucose-lowering medications target different aspects of the pathogenesis of T2DM—insulin resistance at the cellular level, incretin system defects, endogenous insulin deficiency, elevated levels of glucagon, and excessive hepatic glucose release. Because the mechanisms of action differ, the medications can be used alone or in combination. Table 31-6 lists the generic and brand names of glucose-lowering medications for persons with T2DM, their principal sites of action, and expected decreases in A1C when used as monotherapy.

Biguanides. Metformin suppresses hepatic glucose production, is not associated with hypoglycemia, may cause small weight losses when therapy begins, and is relatively inexpensive. The most common side effects are gastrointestinal, which often disappear with time. To minimize these effects, the medication should be taken with food consumption and the smallest dose (500 mg) given twice a day for a week and gradually increased to maximum doses. A rare side effect is severe lactic acidosis, which can be fatal. Acidosis usually occurs in patients who use alcohol excessively, have renal dysfunction, or have liver impairments (Nathan et al., 2009).

Sulfonylureas. The sulfonylureas promote insulin secretion by the beta cells of the pancreas. First- and second-generation sulfonylurea drugs differ from one another in their potency, pharmacokinetics, and metabolism. Disadvantages of their use include weight gain and the potential

TABLE 31-6

Glucose-Lowering Medications for Type 2 Diabetes

Class and Generic Names	Recommended Dose	Principal Action	Mean Decrease in A1C
Class: Biguanide			
Metformin (Glucophage) Metformin Extended Release (Glucophage XR)	500-850 mg tid or 1000 mg bid 500-2000 mg once daily	Decrease hepatic glucose production	1.5% to 2%
Class: Sulfonylureas (Second-generation)			
Glipizide (Glucotrol) Glipizide (Glucotrol XL) Glyburide (Glynase Prestabs) Glimepiride (Amaryl)	2.5-20 mg single or divided dose; single dose for XL 12 mg daily 4-8 mg daily	Stimulate insulin secretion from the β-cells	1% to 2%
Class: Thiazolidinediones			
Pioglitazone (Actos)	15-45 mg daily	Improve peripheral insulin sensitivity	1% to 2%
Class: GLP-1 Agonists			
Exenatide (Byetta) Liraglutide (Victoza)	Initially dosed at 5 mcg twice a day—at breakfast and lunch; increased to 10 mcg twice a day Once daily at any time, independent of meals; initially 0.6 mg/day for 1 week, then increased to 1.2 mg/day; maximum dose 1.8 mg/day	Enhances glucose-dependent insulin secretion and suppresses postprandial glucagon secretion	0.5% to 0.9%
Class: Alpha Glucosidase Inhibitors			
Acarbose (Precose) Miglitol (Glyset)	25-100 mg three times daily with meals 25-100 mg three times daily with meals	Delay carbohydrate absorption	0.5% to 1%
Class: Glinides			
Repaglinide (Prandin) Nateglinide (Starlix)	0.5-4 mg before meals 120 mg before meals	Stimulate insulin secretion from β-cells	1% to 2%
Class: Amylin Agonists			
Pramlintide (Symlin)	Initially dosed at 60 mcg before meals; dose increased directly to 120 mcg if no clinically significant nausea occurs after 3-7 days	Decreases glucagon production, which decreases mealtime hepatic glucose release and prevents postprandial hyperglycemia	0.4% to 0.7%
Class: DPP-4 Inhibitors			
Sitaglipton (Januvia) Saxagliptin (Onglyza)	100 mg once daily 5 mg once daily	Enhance the effects of GLP-1 and GIP by preventing degradation	0.5% to 0.8%
Insulin			
Insulin	No dose limit	Supplements endogenous insulin	Unlimited

Adapted from Nathan DM et al: Medical management of hyperglycemia in type 2 diabetes: a consensus algorithm for initiation and adjustment of therapy, Diabetes Care 32:193-203, 2009.

A1C, Hemoglobin A1C; *bid*, twice daily; *DPP*, dipeptidyl peptidase; *GIP*, glucose-dependent insulinotropic peptide; *GLP*, glucagon-like peptide; *tid*, three times daily.

to cause hypoglycemia. They have the advantage of being inexpensive.

Thiazolidinediones. TZDs or glitazones decrease insulin resistance in peripheral tissues and thus enhance the ability of muscle and fat cells to take up glucose. TZDs also have a favorable effect on lipids and do not independently cause hypoglycemia. Adverse effects include weight gain and edema.

Glucagon-like Peptide-1 Agonist. Exenatide (Byetta) and liraglutide (Victoza) are incretin mimetic or incretin-like agents that have many of the same glucose-lowering effects as the body's naturally occurring incretin, GLP-1. **Incretins** are hormones made by the gastrointestinal tract and released during nutrient absorption, which increase glucose-dependent insulin secretion, slow gastric emptying, decrease glucagon production, and decrease appetite. GLP-1 agonists are associated with reduction in A1C and modest weight loss. Typically exenatide is injected twice a day, at breakfast and at the evening meal and liraglutide is injected once a day, at any time, independent of meals. They often cause gastrointestinal disturbances, which tend to abate over time (Nathan et al., 2009.) A once-weekly injection of a GLP-1 agonist is currently being tested.

Alpha Glucosidase Inhibitors. Acarbose (Precose) and miglitol (Glyset) are alpha-glucosidase inhibitors that work in the small intestine to inhibit enzymes that digest carbohydrates, thereby delaying carbohydrate absorption and lowering postprandial glycemia. They do not cause hypoglycemia or weight gain when used alone, but they can frequently cause flatulence, diarrhea, cramping, or abdominal pain. Symptoms may be alleviated by initiating therapy at a low dose and gradually increasing the dose to therapeutic levels.

Glinides. The meglitinides differ from the sulfonylureas in that they have short metabolic half-lives, which result in brief episodic stimulation of insulin secretion. They are given before meals, decreasing postprandial glucose excursions and less risk of hypoglycemia. Nateglinide only works in the presence of glucose and is a somewhat less potent secretagogue. Risk of weight gain is similar to sulfonylureas (Nathan et al., 2009).

Dipeptidyl Peptidase 4 Inhibitors. GLP-1 and glucose-dependent insulinotropic peptide, the main intestinal stimulants of insulin are rapidly degraded by dipeptidyl peptidase 4 (DPP-4) inhibitors. DPP-4 inhibitors prolong their half-lives. They are relatively well tolerated, are weight-neutral, and do not cause hypoglycemia when used as monotherapy (Nathan et al., 2009).

Amylin Agonists (Pramlintide). Pramlintide is a synthetic analog of the β-cell hormone amylin. It is injected before meals slowing gastric emptying and inhibiting glucagon production resulting in a decrease in postprandial glucose excursions. It is approved for use as adjunctive therapy with regular insulin or rapid-acting insulin (Nathan et al., 2009).

Insulin. For persons with T2DM the transition to insulin often begins with a long-acting or premixed insulin given at bedtime or before the evening meal to control fasting glucose levels. However, eventually many patients with T2DM require a more physiologic insulin regimen at bedtime or an evening meal to achieve control (see following section). If large doses of insulin are required, oral medications such as insulin sensitizers are often combined with the insulin regimen.

Insulin

Insulin has three characteristics: onset, peak, and duration (Table 31-7). U-100 is the concentration of insulin available in the United States. This means it has 100 units of insulin per milliliter of fluid (100 units/mL). U-100 syringes deliver U-100 insulin; however, insulin pens are now being used more frequently as an alternative to the traditional syringe-needle units.

Rapid-acting Insulins. Rapid-acting insulins include insulin lispro (Humalog), insulin aspart (Novolog), and insulin glulisine (Apidra) and are used as bolus (mealtime) insulins. They are insulin analogs that differ from human insulin in amino acid sequence but bind to insulin receptors and thus function in a manner similar to human insulin. All have an onset of action within 15 minutes, a peak in activity at 60 to 90 minutes, and a duration of 3 to 5 hours. They result in fewer hypoglycemic episodes compared with regular insulin.

Regular Insulin. Regular insulin is a short-acting insulin with an onset of action 15 to 60 minutes after injection and a duration of action ranging from 5 to 8 hours. For best results the slow onset of regular insulin requires it to be taken 30 to 60 minutes before meals.

Intermediate-acting Insulin. Neutral protamine Hagedorn (NPH) is the only available intermediate-acting insulin; Lente insulin has been discontinued. Its appearance is cloudy, and its onset of action is about 2 hours after injection, with a peak effect from 6 to 10 hours.

Long-acting Insulins. Insulin glargine (Lantus) and insulin determir (Levemir) are long-acting insulins; Ultralente has been discontinued. Insulin glargine is an insulin analog that, because of its slow dissolution at the injection site, results in a relatively constant and peakless delivery over 24 hours. Because of its acidic pH, it cannot be mixed with any other insulin in the same syringe before injection and is usually given at bedtime. However, glargine can be given before any meal, but, whichever time is chosen, it must be given consistently at that time. Insulin determir is absorbed from the subcutaneous tissue relatively quickly but then binds to albumin in the bloodstream, resulting in a prolonged action time of approximately 17 hours. Therefore it may need to be given twice a day. Basal insulin analogs decrease the chances of hypoglycemia, especially nocturnal hypoglycemia (Rosenstock et al., 2005).

Premixed Insulins. Premixed insulins include 70% NPH/30% regular, 75% lispro protamine (NPL [addition of neutral protamine to lispro to create an intermediate-acting insulin])/25% lispro, 50% lispro protamine and 50% lispro, and 70% protamine (addition of neutral protamine to aspart to create an immediate-acting insulin)/30% aspart. Persons using premixed insulins must eat at specific

TABLE 31-7

Action Times of Human Insulin Preparations

Type of Insulin	Onset of Action	Peak Action	Usual Effective Duration	Monitor Effect In
Rapid-Acting	<15 min	1-2 hr	3-5 hr	1-2 hr
Insulin lispro (Humalog) Insulin aspart (NovoLog) Insulin glulisine (Apidra)				
Short-Acting				
Regular	0.5-1 hr	2-3 hr	3-6 hr	≈4 hr
Intermediate-Acting				
NPH	2-4 hr	4-10 hr	10-16 hr	8-12 hr
Long-Acting				
Insulin glargine (Lantus)	2-4 hr	Peakless	20-24 hr	10-12 hr
Insulin determir (Levemir)	2-4 hr	Peakless	18-24 hr	10-12 hr
Mixtures				
70/30 (70% NPH, 30% regular)	0.5 to 1 hr	Dual	10-16 hr	
Humalog Mix 75/25 (75% NPL, 25% lispro)	<15 min	Dual	10-16 hr	
Humalog Mix 50/50 (50% protamine lispro, 50% lispro)	<15 min	Dual	10-16 hr	
Novolog Mix 70/30 (70% NPA, 30% aspart)	<15 min	Dual	10-16 hr	

Adapted from Reactive and Fasting Hypoglycemia 4th Edition © 2007 International Diabetes Center at Park Nicollet, Minneapolis, MN. All rights reserved. Used with permission. 1-888-637-2675.

NPA, Neutral protamine aspart; *NPH*, neutral protamine Hagedorn; *NPL*, neutral protamine lispro.

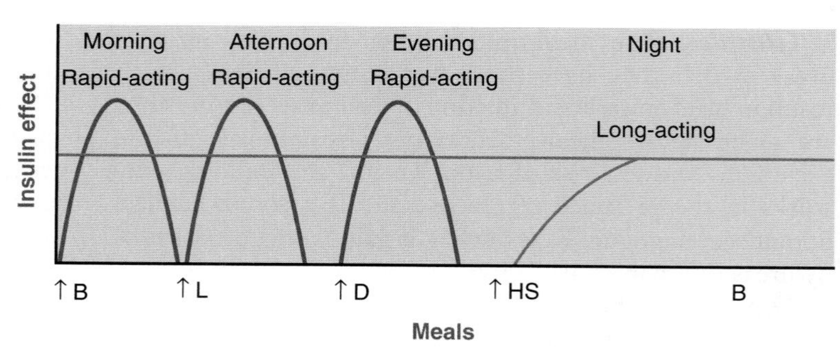

FIGURE 31-1 Time actions of flexible insulin regimens. *(Modified from Kaufman FR: Medical management of type 1 diabetes, ed 5, Alexandria, Va, 2008, American Diabetes Association.)*

times and be consistent in carbohydrate intake to prevent hypoglycemia.

Insulin Regimens. All persons with T1DM and those with T2DM who no longer produce adequate endogenous insulin need replacement of insulin that mimics normal insulin action. After individuals without diabetes eat, their plasma glucose and insulin concentrations increase rapidly, peak in 30 to 60 minutes, and return to basal concentrations within 2 to 3 hours. To mimic this, rapid-acting (or short-acting) insulin is given before meals, and this is referred to as *bolus* or *mealtime insulin* (Figure 31-1).

Mealtime insulin doses are adjusted based on the amount of carbohydrate in the meal. An insulin-to-carbohydrate ratio can be established for an individual that will guide decisions on the amount of mealtime insulin to inject. Basal or background insulin dose is that amount of insulin required in the postabsorptive state to restrain endogenous glucose output primarily from the liver. Basal insulin also limits lipolysis and excess flux of free fatty acids to the liver. Long-acting insulins are used for basal insulin. The type and timing of insulin regimens should be individualized, based on eating and exercise habits and blood glucose concentrations.

These physiologic insulin regimens allow increased flexibility in the type and timing of meals. For normal-weight persons with T1DM, the required insulin dosage is approximately 0.5 to 1 unit/kg of body weight per day. Approximately 50% of the total daily insulin dose is used to provide for basal or background insulin needs. The remainder (rapid-acting insulin) is divided among the meals either proportionately to the carbohydrate content or by giving approximately 1 to 1.5 units of insulin per 10 to 15 g of carbohydrates consumed. The larger amount is usually needed to cover breakfast carbohydrates as a result of the presence in the morning of higher levels of counterregulatory hormones. Persons with T2DM may require insulin doses in the range of 0.5 to 1.2 units/kg of body weight daily. Large doses, even more than 1.5 units/kg of body weight daily, may be required at least initially to overcome prevailing insulin resistance.

Insulin pump therapy provides basal rapid-acting or short-acting insulin pumped continuously by a mechanical device in micro amounts through a subcutaneous catheter that is monitored 24 hours a day. Both lispro and aspart work well in insulin pumps, resulting in improved glycemia and less hypoglycemia than with regular insulin. Boluses of the insulin are given before meals. Pump therapy requires a committed and motivated person who is willing to do a minimum of four blood glucose tests per day, keep blood glucose and food records, and learn the technical features of pump use.

Self-Management Education

Diabetes management is a team effort. Persons with diabetes must be at the center of the team because they have the responsibility for day-to-day management. RDs, nurses, physicians, and other health care providers contribute their expertise to developing therapeutic regimens that help the person with diabetes achieve the best metabolic control possible. The goal is to provide patients with the knowledge, skills, and motivation to incorporate self-management into their daily lifestyles. Dietitians can demonstrate their specialized diabetes knowledge by obtaining certification beyond the RD credential. Two diabetes care certifications available to RDs are the certified diabetes educator, a specialty certification, and board certified-advanced diabetes management, an advanced practice certification.

Monitoring

The health care team, including the individual with diabetes, should work together to implement blood glucose monitoring and establish individual **target blood glucose goals** (see Table 31-4).

Self-monitoring of Blood Glucose

SMBG is used on a day-to-day basis to manage diabetes effectively and safely; however, measurement of A1C levels provides the best available index of overall diabetes control. Patients can perform SMBG up to eight times per day—before breakfast, lunch, and dinner; at bedtime; 1 to 2 hours after meals; and during the night or whenever needed to determine causes of hypoglycemia or hyperglycemia. For patients using multiple insulin injections or insulin pump therapy, SMBG is recommended three or more times daily, generally prior to each meal. For persons using less frequent insulin injections, noninsulin therapies, or MNT alone, SMBG may be useful as a guide to the success of the therapy (ADbA, 2011b). For these persons, SMBG is often performed one to four times a day, often before breakfast and before and 2 hours after the largest meal but only 3 or 4 days per week.

The ADA EBNPG for diabetes reviewed the evidence on glucose monitoring and recommended that for persons with T1DM or T2DM on insulin therapy, at least three to four glucose tests per day are needed to determine the accuracy of the insulin doses and to guide adjustments in insulin doses, food intake, and physical activity. Once established, some insulin regimens require less frequent SMBG. For persons on MNT alone or MNT in combination with glucose-lowering medications, frequency and timing depend on diabetes management goals and therapies.

Self management education and training is necessary to use SMBG devices and data correctly (ADA, 2008). Individuals need to be taught how to adjust their management program based on the results of SMBG. The first step in using such records is to learn how to identify patterns in blood glucose levels taken at the same time each day that are outside the target range—generally high readings for three or more days in a row or low readings two days in a row. The next step is to determine if a lifestyle factor (meal times, carbohydrate intake, quantity and time of physical activity) or medication dose adjustment is needed.

If changes in medication doses such as insulin are needed, adjustments are made in the insulin (or mediations) acting at the time of the problem glucose readings. After pattern management is mastered, algorithms for insulin dose changes to compensate for an elevated or low glucose value can be used. A commonly used formula determines the insulin sensitivity, or **correction factor (CF)**, which defines how many milligrams per deciliter a unit of rapid-acting (or short-acting) insulin will lower blood glucose levels over a 2- to 4-hour period (Kaufman, 2008). The CF is determined by using the "1700 rule," in which 1700 is divided by the total daily dose (TDD) of insulin the individual typically takes. For example, if the TDD is 50 units of insulin, the CF = 1700/50 = 35. In this case, 1 unit of insulin should lower the individual's blood glucose level by 35 mg/dL (2 mmol/L).

In using blood glucose monitoring records, it should be remembered that factors other than food affect blood glucose concentrations. An increase in blood glucose can be the result of insufficient insulin or insulin secretagogue; too much food; or increases in glucagon and other counterregulatory hormones as a result of stress, illness, or infection. Factors that contribute to hypoglycemia include too much insulin or insulin secretagogue, not enough food, unusual amounts of exercise, and skipped or delayed meals. Urine glucose testing, used in the past, has so many limitations that it should not be used.

It is now possible to do **continuous glucose monitoring (CGM)**, which measures glucose in interstitial fluid and provides readings every 5 to 10 minutes. Other features include alarms for glucose highs and lows and the ability to download data and track trends over time. The ADbA recommends that CGM in conjunction with intensive insulin regimens can be a useful tool to lower A1C in selected adults (age 25 years and older) with T1DM. Evidence is less strong for A1C lowering in children, teens, and younger adults (ADbA, 2011b). After reviewing the evidence, the ADA EBNPG for diabetes concluded that persons experiencing unexplained elevations in A1C or unexplained hypoglycemia may benefit from use of CGM or more frequent SMBG (ADA, 2008).

A1C Monitoring

A1C tests should be done at least twice a year in persons who are meeting treatment goals and have stable glycemic control. They should be done quarterly in persons whose therapy has changed or who are not meeting glycemic goals. In persons without diabetes A1C values are 4% to 6%. These values correspond to mean plasma glucose levels of approximately 70-126 mg/dL (3.9-7 mmol/L). Correlation between A1C levels and average glucose levels have recently been verified (ADbA, 2011b). An A1C of 6% reflects an average glucose level of 126 mg/dL. In general, each 1% change in A1C reflects a change of approximately 28-29 mg/dL.

Ketone, Lipid, and Blood Pressure Monitoring

Urine or blood testing can be used to detect ketones. Testing for ketonuria or ketonemia should be performed regularly during periods of illness and when blood glucose levels consistently exceed 240 mg/dL (13.3 mmol/L). The presence of persistent, moderate, or large amounts of ketones, along with elevated blood glucose levels, requires insulin adjustments. Persons with T2DM rarely have ketosis; however, ketone testing should be done when the person is seriously ill.

For most adults, lipids should be measured at least annually; however, in adults with low-risk lipid values, assessments may be repeated every 2 years. Blood pressure should be measured at every routine diabetes visit (ADbA, 2011b).

IMPLEMENTING THE NUTRITION CARE PROCESS

The nutrition care process articulates the consistent and specific steps used to deliver MNT (ADA, 2011). For some individuals with diabetes MNT will be implemented in individual sessions and for others in group sessions. Providing nutrition interventions in groups is becoming increasingly more important; however, group interventions must also allow for individualization of MNT and evaluation of outcomes. The following sections review implementation of individual MNT.

The ADA EBNPG recommend that MNT be provided by a RD in an initial series of three to four encounters each lasting 45 to 90 minutes. This series, beginning at diagnosis of diabetes or at first referral to an RD for MNT for diabetes, should be completed within 3 to 6 months and the RD should determine if additional encounters are needed after the initial series based on the nutrition assessment of learning needs and progress toward desired outcomes. At least one follow-up encounter is recommended annually to reinforce lifestyle changes and to evaluate and monitor outcomes that affect the need for changes in MNT or medication. The RD should again determine if additional MNT encounters are needed. Although glycemic control is the primary focus for diabetes management, cardioprotective nutrition interventions for the prevention and treatment of CVD should also be implemented in the initial series of encounters (ADA, 2008).

Nutrition Assessment

The **nutrition assessment** involves obtaining information before and during the encounter needed to identify nutrition-related problems. Assessment data can be obtained from the referral source or the patient's medical records and from the patient. Patient data can be collected from forms the patient completes before the first encounter or directly from the patient. By collecting as much date as possible before the first session, completion of the assessment and implementation of interventions can begin more efficiently. Nutrition assessment is an ongoing process that involves not only initial data collection, but also reassessment and analysis of patient data and needs. Box 31-2 provides a summary of assessment categories.

The ADA EBNPG for diabetes highlights three specific assessment recommendations. First, the RD should assess food intake (focusing on carbohydrate), medication, metabolic control (glycemia, lipids, and blood pressure), anthropometric measurements, and physical activity as the basis for the implementation of the nutrition prescription, goals, and interventions. Second, the RD should assess glycemic control and focus MNT to achieve and maintain blood glucose levels in the target range. However, the need for cardioprotective nutrition interventions should also be assessed. Third, the RD should assess the relative importance of weight management for persons with diabetes who are overweight of obese. They note that although modest

BOX 31-2

Nutrition Assessment

Nutrition Assessment Categories

Biochemical data, medical tests, and procedures, which include laboratory data such as for A1C, glucose, lipids, kidney function, and blood pressure measurements

Anthropometric measurements, which include height, weight, body mass index, waist circumference, growth rate, and rate of weight change

Client History, Which Includes

General patient information, such as age, gender, race and ethnicity, language, literacy, and education

Medical and health history and medical treatment, including goals of medical therapy and prescribed medications related to medical condition for which medical nutrition therapy is being implemented

Readiness to change nutrition-related behaviors

Weight management goals

Physical activity history and goals

Social history, such as social and medical support, cultural and religious beliefs, and socioeconomic status

Other medical or surgical treatments, therapy, and alternative medicine

Food and nutrition history

Food intake, nutrition and health knowledge and beliefs

Food availability

Supplement use

Modified from Franz MJ, et al: American Dietetic Association pocket guide to lipid disorders, hypertension, diabetes, and weight management, Chicago, Il, 2010, American Dietetic Association.

weight loss has been shown to improve insulin resistance in overweight and obese insulin-resistant individuals, research on sustained weight loss interventions lasting 1 year or longer reports inconsistent effects on A1C (ADA, 2008).

Nutrition Diagnosis

The nutrition diagnosis identifies and describes a specific nutrition problem that can be resolved or improved through treatment or intervention by an RD (see Chapter 11). Patients may have more than one nutrition diagnoses, in which case the RD must to prioritize them in the nutrition intervention step. The nutrition diagnostic language includes three domains: (1) intake problems related to the quantity of intake versus requirements; (2) clinical findings and problems related to medical (or physical) condition; and (3) behavioral-environmental findings and problems related to knowledge, attitudes and beliefs, physical environment, and access to food. A nutrition diagnosis is formatted according to problem, etiology, and signs and symptoms (PES). Examples of diabetes-related nutrition diagnoses are listed in Box 31-3.

BOX 31-3

Examples of PES Statements Related to Diabetes Mellitus

Nutrition Diagnosis: Inconsistent Carbohydrate Intake

Inconsistent carbohydrate intake (P) related to incorrect application of carbohydrate counting (E) as evidenced by food records revealing two additional carbohydrate servings for many meals and wide fluctuations in blood glucose levels, most days of the week (S)

Nutrition Diagnosis: Inconsistent Carbohydrate Intake

Inconsistent carbohydrate intake (P) related to inconsistent timing of meals (E) as evidenced by wide fluctuations in blood glucose levels (S)

Nutrition Diagnosis: Excessive Carbohydrate Intake

Excessive carbohydrate intake (P) compared with insulin dosing related to inaccurate carbohydrate counting (E) as evidenced by the number of carbohydrate servings per meal noted in food record and postmeal glucose levels consistently >200 mg/dL (S)

Nutrition Diagnosis: Inappropriate Intake of Food Fats

Excessive saturated fat intake (P) related to lack of knowledge of saturated fat content of foods (E) as evidenced by self-report of high saturated fat intake (S)

Nutrition Diagnosis: Altered Laboratory Values

Altered blood glucose values (P) related to insufficient insulin (E) as evidenced by hyperglycemia despite very good eating habits (S)

Nutrition Diagnosis: Overweight or Obesity

Overweight (P) related to excessive energy intake with limited physical activity (E) as evidenced by a body mass index of 30 and food history indicating consumption of 2800 kcal per day vs 2200 calories (estimated needs) and sedentary lifestyle (S)

Nutrition Diagnosis: Food- and Nutrition-Related Knowledge Deficit

Food- and nutrition-related knowledge deficit (P) related to lack of exposure to information (E) as evidenced by new diagnosis of diabetes (or prediabetes, lipid disorder, hypertension) (S)

Nutrition Diagnosis: Not Ready for Lifestyle Change

Not ready for lifestyle change (P) related to denial of need to change in precontemplation (E) as evidenced by reluctance to begin participation in physical activity program (S)

Modified from Franz MJ, Boucher JL, Pereira RF: American Dietetic Association pocket guide to lipid disorders, hypertension, diabetes, and weight management, Chicago, Il, 2010, American Dietetic Association.

Nutrition Intervention

Nutrition interventions include two distinct steps: planning the nutrition goals and implementing the actual interventions. Planning involves prioritizing the nutrition diagnoses, conferring with the persons with diabetes and others, reviewing current nutrition practice guidelines for diabetes, setting goals, determining the nutrition prescription, and choosing specific intervention strategies.

Implementation is the action phase. In the food and nutrient delivery phase, an individualized food and meal plan is developed. and specific nutrient recommendations as needed are included. Nutrition education involves the transfer of knowledge to the specific deficits identified in the nutrition diagnosis statements. Nutrition counseling involves behavior and attitude change through the use of strategies that promote behavior changes and motivation and intention to change. However, nutrition care must also be coordinated with other health care providers who can assist in the implementation of the nutrition prescription and nutrition therapy. If home care is needed, follow-up should take place.

Nutrition Therapy Interventions for Specific Populations

Type 1 Diabetes and Patients Requiring Insulin Therapy. The first priority is to integrate an insulin regimen into the usual eating habits and physical activity schedule. With the many insulin options now available (rapid- and long-acting insulins), an insulin regimen can be planned that will conform to an individual's preferred meal routines and food choices (ADbA, 2008). It is no longer necessary to create unnatural or artificial divisions of meals and snacks.

Physiologic insulin regimens that mimic natural insulin secretion involve multiple injections (three or more insulin injections per day) or use of an insulin infusion pump. These types of insulin regimens allow increased flexibility in choosing when and what to eat. Mealtime insulin doses are adjusted to match carbohydrate intake (insulin-to-carbohydrate ratios.) This can be accomplished by comprehensive nutrition education and counseling on interpretation of blood glucose patterns, nutrition-related medication management, and collaboration with the health care team (ADA, 2008). For persons who receive fixed insulin regimens such as with the use of premixed insulins or those who do not adjust their mealtime insulin doses, day-to-day consistency in the timing and amount of carbohydrates eaten is recommended.

Attention must also be paid to total energy intake as well as carbohydrate intake. Weight gain may adversely affect glycemia, lipids, blood pressure, and general health; thus prevention of weight gain in adults is desirable.

Type 2 Diabetes with MNT Alone or with Glucose-Lowering Medications. The first priority is to adopt lifestyle interventions that improve the metabolic abnormalities of glycemia, dyslipidemia, and hypertension. Lifestyle interventions independent of weight loss that can improve glycemia include reduced energy intake and increased energy expenditure through physical activity. Because many persons also have dyslipidemia and hypertension, limitation of saturated and *trans*-fatty acids, cholesterol, and sodium is recommended. These interventions should be implemented as soon as the diagnosis of diabetes is made.

MNT interventions for established T2DM differ from interventions for prevention. Because of the progressive nature of T2DM, MNT interventions progress from prevention of obesity, to the prevention or delay of T2DM, to strategies for improved metabolic control. Modest weight loss is beneficial in persons with insulin resistance, but, as the disease progresses to insulin deficiency, medications usually need to be combined with MNT. Emphasis should be on blood glucose control, improved food choices, increased physical activity, and moderate energy restriction rather than weight loss alone because it is unclear whether weight loss alone will improve glycemic control (ADA, 2008).

The first step in food and meal planning is teaching which foods are carbohydrates (fruits, grains, starchy vegetables, milk, sweets), average portion sizes, and how many servings to select at meals (and snacks, if desired). Limiting fats, especially saturated and *trans*-fats, encouraging physical activity, and using blood glucose monitoring to adjust food and eating patterns and medications are also important components of successful MNT for T2DM. Frequent follow-up with an RD can provide the problem-solving techniques, encouragement, and support that lifestyle changes require.

Physical activity improves insulin sensitivity, acutely lowers blood glucose in persons with diabetes, and may also improve cardiovascular status. By itself it has only a modest effect on weight; however, it is essential for long-term weight maintenance. Cardiorespiratory fitness in persons with diabetes appears to be more important than thinness in relation to all-cause and cardiovascular mortality. Therefore it is important to counsel patients to increase physical activity and fitness levels.

Weight-loss drugs may be beneficial in the treatment of overweight persons with T2DM and can help achieve a 5% to 10% weight loss when combined with lifestyle modifications. It is generally recommended that they be used only in people with a BMI greater than 27.

Bariatric surgery can be an effective weight-loss treatment for severely obese patients with T2DM and can result in marked improvements in glycemia. Bariatric surgery should be considered for adults with BMI of more than 35 kg/m^2 and T2DM, especially if the diabetes and associated comorbidities are difficult to control with lifestyle and pharmacologic therapy (ADbA, 2011b; see Chapter 22).

Type 1 Diabetes in Youth. Involvement of a multidisciplinary team, including a physician, RD, nurse, and behavioral specialist, all trained in pediatric diabetes, is the best means of achieving optimal diabetes management in youth. However, the most important team members are the child or adolescent and his or her family.

A major nutrition goal for children and adolescents with T1DM is maintenance of normal growth and development. Possible causes of poor weight gain and linear growth include poor glycemic control, inadequate insulin, and overrestriction of calories. The last may be a consequence of the common erroneous belief that restricting food, rather than adjusting insulin, is the way to control blood glucose. Other reasons unrelated to diabetes management include thyroid abnormalities and malabsorption syndromes. Excessive weight gain can be caused by excessive caloric intake, overtreatment of hypoglycemia, or overinsulinization. Other causes include low physical activity levels and hypothyroidism, accompanied by poor linear growth (Silverstein et al., 2005).

The nutrition prescription is based on the nutrition assessment. Newly diagnosed children often present with weight loss and hunger; as a result, the initial meal plan must be based on adequate calories to restore and maintain appropriate body weight. In about 4 to 6 weeks the initial caloric level may need to be modified to meet more usual caloric requirements. Nutrient requirements for children and adolescents with diabetes appear to be similar to those of children and adolescents without diabetes. The DRIs can be used to determine energy requirements (Institute of Medicine, 2002). However, it may be preferable to use a food and nutrition history of typical daily intake, providing that growth and development are normal, to determine an individual child's or adolescent's energy needs.

Consultation with an RD to develop and discuss the medical nutrition plan is encouraged (Silverstein et al., 2005). Because energy requirements change with age, physical activity, and growth rate, an evaluation of height, weight, BMI, and the nutrition plan must be updated at least every year. Good metabolic control is essential for normal growth and development (for growth charts see Appendixes 9 through 16). However, withholding food or having the child eat consistently without an appetite for food in an effort to control blood glucose should be discouraged. Calories should be adequate for growth and restricted if the child becomes overweight.

Individualized food and meal plans, insulin regimens using basal (background) and bolus (mealtime) insulins, and insulin algorithms or insulin pumps can provide flexibility for children with T1DM and their families. This approach accommodates irregular meal times and schedules and varying appetites and activity levels (ADbA, 2008). Blood glucose records are essential to assist in making appropriate changes in insulin regimens. Daily eating patterns in young children generally include three meals and two or three snacks, depending on the length of time between meals and the child's physical activity level. Children often prefer smaller meals and snacks. Snacks can prevent hypoglycemia between meals and provide adequate calories. Older children and teens may prefer only three meals. Blood glucose monitoring data are then used to integrate an insulin regimen into the meal, snack, and exercise schedules.

After the appropriate nutrition prescription has been determined, the meal planning approach can be selected. A number of meal planning approaches can be used. Carbohydrate counting for food planning provides youth and their families with guidelines that facilitate glycemic control while still allowing the choice of many common foods that children and adolescents enjoy. However, whatever approach to food planning is used, the youth and family must find it understandable and applicable to their lifestyle.

Type 2 Diabetes in Youth. Childhood obesity has been accompanied by an increase in the prevalence of T2DM among children and adolescents. IGT has been shown to be highly prevalent in obese youth, irrespective of ethnic group, and is associated with insulin resistance. Once T2DM develops, β-cell failure is also a factor. Thus T2DM in youth appears to follow a progressive pattern similar to T2DM in adults.

Successful lifestyle treatment of T2DM in children and adolescents involves cessation of excessive weight gain, promotion of normal growth and development, and the achievement of blood glucose and A1C goals. Nutrition guidelines should also address comorbidities such as hypertension and dyslipidemia. Offer behavior modification strategies to decrease intake of high-caloric, high-fat, and high-carbohydrate foods (extra-large desserts) and drinks (regular soda and other high-sugar beverages) while encouraging healthy eating habits and regular physical activity for the entire family (ADbA, 2008). In addition, metformin is used when lifestyle strategies alone have not achieved target glucose goals. Youth with T2DM may also require insulin therapy to achieve adequate glycemic control.

Preexisting Diabetes and Pregnancy. Normalization of blood glucose levels during pregnancy is very important for women who have preexisting diabetes or who develop GDM. Table 31-8 lists glucose goals for pregnancy. The MNT goals are to assist in achieving and maintaining optimal blood glucose control and to provide adequate maternal and fetal nutrition throughout pregnancy, energy intake for appropriate maternal weight gain, and necessary

TABLE 31-8

Plasma Glucose Goals during Pregnancy

Preexisting Diabetes (Type 1 or Type 2)	Gestational Diabetes
Premeal, bedtime, and overnight glucose 60-99 mg/dL (3.3-5.4 mmol/L)	Preprandial ≤ 95 mg/dL (5.3 mmol/L)
Peak postprandial glucose 100-129 mg/dL (5.4-7.1 mmol/L)	1 h postmeal ≤ 140 mg/dL (7.8 mmol/L)
A1C < 6.0%	2 h postmeal ≤ 120 mg/dL (6.7 mmol/L)

Modified from American Diabetes Association: Standards of medical care—2011 (Position Statement), Diabetes Care 34:S21, 2011b.

A1C, Hemoglobin A1C.

vitamins and minerals (ADbA, 2008). Nutrition recommendations during pregnancy and lactation appear to be similar for women with and without diabetes; therefore the DRIs can be used to determine energy and nutrient requirements during pregnancy and for lactation (Institute of Medicine, 2002).

Preconception counseling and the ability to achieve near-normal blood glucose levels before pregnancy have been shown to be effective in reducing the incidence of anomalies in infants born to women with preexisting diabetes to nearly that of the general population. As a result of hormonal changes during the first trimester, blood glucose levels are often erratic. Although caloric needs do not differ from those preceding pregnancy, the meal plan may need to be adjusted to accommodate the metabolic changes. Women should be educated about the increased risk of hypoglycemia during pregnancy and cautioned against overtreatment.

The need for insulin increases during the second and third trimesters of pregnancy. At 38 to 40 weeks' postconception, insulin needs and levels peak at two to three times prepregnancy levels. Pregnancy-associated hormones that are antagonistic to the action of insulin lead to elevated blood glucose levels. For women with preexisting diabetes, this increased insulin need must be met with increased exogenous insulin.

Meal plan adjustments are necessary to provide the additional calories required to support fetal growth, and weight should be monitored. During pregnancy the distribution of energy and carbohydrate intake should be based on the woman's food and eating habits and blood glucose responses. Insulin regimens can be matched to food intake, but maintaining consistency of times and amounts of food eaten are essential to avoid hypoglycemia caused by the continuous fetal draw of glucose from the mother. Smaller meals and more frequent snacks are often needed. A late-evening snack is often necessary to decrease the likelihood of overnight hypoglycemia and fasting ketosis. Records of food intake and blood glucose values are essential for determining whether glycemic goals are being met and for preventing and correcting ketosis.

Regular follow-up visits during pregnancy are needed to monitor caloric and nutrient intake, blood glucose control, and whether there is starvation ketosis. Urine or blood ketones during pregnancy may signal starvation ketosis that can be caused by inadequate energy or carbohydrate intake, omission of meals or snacks, or prolonged intervals between meals (e.g., more than 10 hours between the bedtime snack and breakfast). Ketonemia during pregnancy has been associated with reduced IQ scores in children, and women should be instructed to test for ketones periodically before breakfast.

Gestational Diabetes Mellitus. MNT for GDM primarily involves a carbohydrate-controlled meal plan that promotes optimal nutrition for maternal and fetal health with adequate energy for appropriate gestational weight gain, achievement and maintenance of normoglycemia, and absence of ketosis. Specific nutrition and food recommendations are determined and modified based on individual assessment and blood glucose records. Monitoring blood glucose, fasting ketones, appetite, and weight gain can aid in developing an appropriate, individualized meal plan and in adjusting the meal plan throughout pregnancy.

Nutrition practice guidelines for gestational diabetes have been developed and field-tested (ADA, 2009a). All women with GDM should receive MNT at diagnosis of GDM. Monitoring records guide nutrition therapy and are used to determine if additional therapy is needed. Insulin, metformin, or glyburide therapy is added if glucose goals exceed target range (see Table 31-8) on two or more occasions in a 1- to 2-week period without some obvious explanation. Lack of weight gain and ketone testing can be useful in determining whether women are undereating to keep glucose levels within target range in an effort to avoid insulin therapy.

Carbohydrates should be distributed throughout the day into three small to moderate size meals and two to four snacks. All women require a minimum of 175 g of carbohydrates daily (Institute of Medicine, 2002). An evening snack is usually needed to prevent accelerated ketosis overnight. Carbohydrates are not as well tolerated at breakfast as they are at other meals because of increased levels of cortisol and growth hormones. To compensate, the initial food plan may have approximately 30 g of carbohydrate at breakfast. To satisfy hunger, protein foods can be added because they do not affect blood glucose levels.

Although caloric restriction must be viewed with caution, a modest energy restriction to slow weight gain is recommended for overweight or obese women with GDM. A slight calorie restriction results in a slowing of maternal weight gain in obese women with GDM without causing maternal or fetal compromise or ketonuria (ADA, 2009a). Energy intake of less than approximately 1700 to 1800 kcal/day is not advised. Weight gain during pregnancy for women with GDM should be similar to that of women without diabetes.

Exercise assists in overcoming peripheral resistance to insulin and in controlling fasting and postprandial hyperglycemia and may be used as an adjunct to nutrition therapy to improve maternal glycemia. The ideal form of exercise is unknown, but a brisk walk after meals is often recommended.

Women with GDM (and women with preexisting diabetes) should be encouraged to breastfeed because breastfeeding is associated with a reduced incidence of future T2DM (Stuebe, 2005). For women with GDM who are overweight or obese or with above-recommended weight gain during pregnancy, weight loss is advised after delivery. Weight loss reduces the risks of recurrent GDM or future development of T2DM (ADA, 2009a).

Older Adults. The prevalence of diabetes and prediabetes increases dramatically as people age. Many factors predispose older adults to diabetes: age-related decreases in insulin production and increases in insulin resistance, adiposity, decreased physical activity, multiple prescription medications, genetics, and coexisting illnesses. A major factor appears to be insulin resistance. Controversy persists as to whether the insulin resistance is itself a primary change or whether it is attributable to reduced physical activity, decreased lean body mass (sarcopenia), and increased adipose tissue, which are common in older adults. Furthermore, medications used to treat coexisting diseases may complicate diabetes therapy in older persons.

Despite the increase in glucose intolerance with age, aging per se should not be a reason for suboptimal control of blood glucose. Even if it is incorrectly assumed that preventing long-term diabetic complications is not relevant to the care of older adults, persistent hyperglycemia has deleterious effects on the body's defense mechanisms against infection. It also increases the pain threshold by exacerbating neuropathic pain, and it has a detrimental effect on the outcome of cerebrovascular accidents.

Nutrition recommendations for older adults with diabetes must be extrapolated from what is known from the general population and should address nutrition-related cardiovascular risk factors common in older adults and encourage consumption of a variety of foods. Because of the loss of lean body mass and exercise patterns, the energy requirements of older adults are 20% to 30% lower than those of younger adults (ADbA, 2008). Physical activity can significantly reduce the decline in aerobic capacity that occurs with age, improve risk factors for atherosclerosis, slow the decline in age-related lean body mass, decrease central adiposity, and improve insulin sensitivity; thus it should be encouraged.

Malnutrition, not obesity, is the more prevalent nutrition-related problem in older adults. It often remains subclinical or unrecognized because the result of malnutrition—excessive loss of lean body mass—resembles the signs and symptoms of the aging process. Both malnutrition and diabetes adversely affect wound healing and defense against infection, and malnutrition is associated with depression and cognitive deficits. The most reliable indicator of poor nutrition status in older adults is a change in body weight; involuntary weight gain or loss of more than 10 pounds or 10% of body weight in less than 6 months indicates a need to evaluate the reason for the change in weight.

It is essential that older adults, especially those in long-term care settings, receive a diet that meets their nutritional needs, enables them to attain or maintain a reasonable body weight, helps control blood glucose, and is palatable. Dietary restriction is not warranted for older residents in long-term health facilities. Residents should be served the regular, unrestricted menu with consistency in the amount and timing of carbohydrates (ADbA, 2008). A multivitamin and mineral supplement to meet the DRIs may be necessary.

Hyperglycemia and dehydration can lead to a serious complication of diabetes in older adults: **hyperglycemic hyperosmolar state (HHS)**. Patients with HHS have a very high blood glucose level (ranging from 400 to 2800 mg/dL, [22.2-155.6 mmol/L] with an average of 1000 mg/dL [55.6 mmol/L]) without ketones. Patients are markedly dehydrated, and mental alterations range from mild confusion to hallucinations or coma. Patients who have HHS have sufficient insulin to prevent lipolysis and ketosis. Treatment consists of hydration and small doses of insulin to control hyperglycemia.

The Nutrition Prescription

To develop, educate, and counsel patients regarding the nutrition prescription, it is essential to learn about the patient's lifestyle and eating habits. Food and eating histories can be done several ways, with the objective being to determine a schedule and pattern of eating that will be the least disruptive to the lifestyle of the individual with diabetes and, at the same time, will facilitate improved metabolic control. With this objective in mind, asking the individual either to record or report what, how much, and when he or she typically eats during a 24-hour period may be the most useful. Another approach is to ask the patient to keep and bring a 3-day or 1-week food intake record. The request to complete a food record can be made when an appointment with the RD is scheduled. It is also important to learn about the patient's daily routine and schedule. The following information is needed: (1) time of waking; (2) usual meal and eating times; (3) work schedule or school hours; (4) type, amount, and timing of exercise; and (5) usual sleep habits.

Using the assessment data and food and nutrition history information, a preliminary food and meal plan can then be designed, and, if the patient desires, sample menus provided. Developing a food and meal plan does not begin with a set calorie or macronutrient prescription; instead, it is determined by modifying the patient's usual food intake as necessary. The worksheet in Figure 31-2 can be used to record the usual foods eaten and to modify the usual diet as necessary. The macronutrient and caloric values for the food lists are listed on the form and in Table 31-9; see Appendix 34 for portion sizes of the foods on the food lists. These tools are useful in evaluating nutrition assessments.

Using the form in Figure 31-2, the RD begins by totaling the number of servings from each food list and multiplying this number by the grams of carbohydrate, protein, and fat contributed by each. Next the grams of carbohydrate, protein, and fat are totaled from each column; the grams of carbohydrates and protein are then multiplied by 4 (4 kcal/g of carbohydrates and protein), and the grams of fat are multiplied by 9 (9 kcal/g of fat). Total calories and percentage of calories from each macronutrient can then be determined. Numbers derived from these calculations are then rounded off. Figure 31-3 provides an example of a preliminary food and meal plan. In this example the nutrition prescription is the following: 1900 to 2000 calories, 230 g of carbohydrates (50%), 90 g of protein (20%), 65 g of fat (30%). The number of carbohydrate choices for each meal and snack is the total of the starch, fruit, and milk servings. Vegetables, unless starchy or eaten in very large amounts (three or more servings per meal), are generally considered "free foods." The carbohydrate choices are circled under each meal and snack column.

The next step is to evaluate the preliminary meal plan. First and foremost, does the patient think it is feasible to

Food Group	Meal/Snack/Time Breakfast	Snack	Lunch	Snack	Dinner	Snack	Total servings/ day	CHO (g)	Protein (g)	Fat (g)	Calories
Starches								15	3	1	80
Fruit								15			60
Milk								12	8	1	100
Vegetables								5	2		25
Meats/ Substitutes									7	5(3)	75(55)
Fats										5	45
CHO Choices							Total grams				
							Calories/ gram	X4=	X4=	X9=	Total calories
							Percent calories				

Calculations are based on medium-fat meats and skim/very low-fat milk. If diet consists predominantly of low-fat meats, use the factor 3 g instead of 5 g fat; if predominantly high-fat meats, use 8 g fat. If low-fat (2%) milk is used, use 5 g fat; if whole milk is used, use 8 g fat.

FIGURE 31-2 Worksheet for assessment and design of a meal or food plan. *CHO*, Carbohydrate.

TABLE 31-9

Macronutrient and Caloric Values for Food Lists*

The following chart shows the macronutrients and calories from each list.

Food List	Carbohydrate (grams)	Protein (grams)	Fat (grams)	Calories
Carbohydrates				
Starch: breads, cereals and grains, starchy vegetables, crackers, snacks, and beans, peas, and lentils	15	0-3	0-1	80
Fruits	15	—	—	60
Milk				
Fat-free, low-fat, 1%	12	8	0-3	100
Reduced-fat, 2%	12	8	5	120
Whole	12	8	8	160
Sweets, Desserts, and Other carbohydrates	15	Varies	Varies	Varies
Nonstarchy Vegetables	5	2	—	25
Meat and Meat Substitutes				
Lean	—	7	0-3	55
Medium-fat	—	7	4-7	75
High-fat	—	7	8+	100
Plant-based protein	—	7	Varies	Varies
Fats	—	—	5	45
Alcohol	Varies	—	—	100

From American Diabetes Association and American Dietetic Association: Choose Your Foods: Exchange Lists for Diabetes, Alexandria, Va, Chicago, Il, 2008, American Diabetes Association, American Dietetic Association.

*See Appendix 34.

	Meal/Snack/Time										
	Breakfast	Snack	Lunch	Snack	Dinner	Snack	Total servings/ day	CHO (g)	Protein (g)	Fat (g)	Calories
Food Group	7:30 AM	10:00	12:00	3:00	6:30	10:00					
Starches	2	1	2–3	1	2–3	1–2	10	15 150	3 30	1 10	80
Fruit	1		1		1	0–1	3	15 45			60
Milk	1				1		2	12 24	8 16	1 2	100
Vegetables			✓		✓			5 10	2 4		25
Meats/ Substitutes			2–3		3–4		6		7 42	5(3) 30	75(55)
Fats	1	0–1	1–2	0–1	1–2	0–1	5			5 25	45
CHO Choices	3–4 CHO	1 CHO	3–4 CHO	1 CHO	4–5 CHO	1–2 CHO	Total grams	229	92	67	
							Calories/ gram	X4= 916	X4= 368	X9= 603	Total calories
							Percent calories	50	19	30	1900–2000

1900–2000 calories
230 g CHO-50%
90 g protein-20%
65 g fat-30%

Calculations are based on medium-fat meats and skim/very low-fat milk. If diet consists predominantly of low-fat meats, use the factor 3 g, instead of 5 g fat; if predominantly high-fat meats, use 8 g fat. If low-fat (2%) milk is used, use 5 g fat; if whole milk is used, use 8 g fat.

FIGURE 31-3 An example of a completed worksheet from the assessment, the nutrition prescription, and a sample 1900- to 2000-calorie meal plan. *CHO*, Carbohydrate.

implement the meal plan into his or her lifestyle? Second, is it appropriate for diabetes management? Third, does it encourage healthful eating?

To discuss feasibility, the food and meal plan is reviewed with the patient in terms of general food intake. Timing of meals and snacks and approximate portion sizes and types of foods are discussed. Calorie levels are only approximate and adjustments in calories can be made during follow-up visits. A meal-planning approach can be selected later that will assist the patient in making his or her own food choices. At this point it needs to be determined whether this meal plan is reasonable.

To determine the appropriateness of the meal plan for diabetes management, distribution of the meals or snacks must be assessed along with the types of medications prescribed and treatment goals. For patients with T2DM receiving MNT alone or MNT with glucose-lowering medications, often the meal plan begins with three or four carbohydrate servings per meal for adult women and four or five for adult men and, if desired, one or two for a snack. Results of blood glucose monitoring before the meal and 2 hours after the meal, plus feedback from the patient, are used to assess if these recommendations are feasible and realistic and to determine if target glucose goals are being achieved.

For patients who require insulin, the timing of eating is important because insulin must be synchronized with food consumption (see "Medications" earlier in the chapter). If the eating pattern is determined first, an insulin regimen can be selected that will fit with it. To prevent overnight hypoglycemia, some patients may require a bedtime snack. The best way to ensure that the meal plan encourages healthful eating is to encourage patients to eat a variety of foods from all the food groups. The Dietary Guidelines for Americans, with its suggested number of servings from each food group, can be used to compare the patient's meal plan with the nutrition recommendations for all Americans (see Chapter 12).

Nutrition Education and Counseling

Implementation of MNT begins with the RD selecting from a variety of interventions (reduced energy and fat intake, carbohydrate counting, simplified meal plans, healthy food choices, individualized meal planning strategies, exchange lists, insulin-to-carbohydrate ratios, and physical activity and behavioral strategies) (ADA, 2008). All of these interventions have been shown to lead to improved metabolic outcomes. Furthermore, nutrition education and counseling must be sensitive to the personal needs, willingness to change, and ability to make changes of the individual with diabetes. No single meal-planning approach has been shown to be more effective than any other, and the meal-planning approach selected should allow individuals with diabetes to select appropriate foods for meals and snacks.

A popular approach to meal planning is carbohydrate counting. It can be used as a basic meal-planning approach or for more intensive management. Carbohydrate-counting educational tools are based on the concept that after eating it is the carbohydrate in foods that is the major predictor of postprandial blood glucose levels. One carbohydrate serving contributes 15 g of carbohydrates. Basic carbohydrate counting emphasizes the following topics: basic facts about carbohydrates, primary food sources of carbohydrate, average portion sizes and the importance of consistency and accurate portions, amount of carbohydrates that should be eaten, and label reading. Advanced carbohydrate counting emphasizes the importance of record keeping, calculating insulin-to-carbohydrate ratios, and pattern management.

An important goal of nutrition counseling is to facilitate changes in existing food and nutrition-related behaviors and the adoption of new ones. The combined use of behavior change theories may potentially have a greater effect than any individual theory or technique used alone (Franz et al., 2010b). The following "five As" can guide the education and counseling sessions: ask, assess, advise, agree, and arrange. The "ask" step emphasizes the importance of questions as the RD aims to develop a relationship with the client. Motivational interviewing techniques are used initially and throughout all of the encounters.. In the "assess" step, the RD evaluates the client's readiness to change. Different intervention strategies may be needed for individuals at different stages of the change process (see Chapter 15). The "advise" step uses a client-centered framework that adapts nutrition interventions to meet the client's needs, wants, priorities, preferences, and expectations. In the "agree" step the RD facilitates the client's process of setting his or her own short-term goals related to nutrition, physical activity, or glucose monitoring (if appropriate) and helps outline the client's potential methods for accomplishing lifestyle changes. In the "arrange" step, plans for follow-up are identified to evaluate responses to nutrition interventions. The patient is also given information on how to call or e-mail with questions and concerns. In making plans for the next encounter, the patient is asked to keep a 3-day or weekly food record with blood glucose–monitoring data.

Nutrition Monitoring and Evaluation

Food intake, medication, metabolic control (glycemia, lipids, and blood pressure), anthropometric measurements, and physical activity should be monitored and evaluated (ADA, 2008). Medical and clinical outcomes should be monitored after the second or third visit to determine whether the patient is making progress toward established goals. If no progress is evident, the individual and RD need to reassess and perhaps revise nutrition interventions. Blood glucose monitoring results can be used to determine whether adjustments in foods and meals will be sufficient to achieve blood glucose goals or if medication additions or adjustments need to be combined with MNT. Nutrition care must be coordinated with an interdisciplinary team.

Documentation in the patient's medical record serves as a communication tool for members of the health care team. The medical record also serves as a legal document of what was done and not done and supports reimbursement of nutrition services billed to insurance carriers. There are many different formats available for medical record documentation. The appropriate format depends on where the RD practices and whether electronic health records are used. Regardless of the specific format, the RD can document using the ADIME content (Writing Group of the Nutrition Care Process, 2008).

Follow-Up Encounters

Successful nutrition therapy involves a process of assessment, problem solving, adjustment, and readjustment. Food records can be compared with the meal plan, which will help to determine whether the initial meal plan needs changing, and can be integrated with the blood glucose–monitoring records to determine changes that can lead to improved glycemic control.

Nutrition follow-up visits should provide encouragement and ensure realistic expectations for the patient. A change in eating habits is not easy for most people, and they become discouraged without appropriate recognition of their efforts. Patients should be encouraged to speak freely about problems they are having with food and eating patterns. Furthermore, there may be major life changes that require changes in the meal plan. Job and schedule changes, travel, illness, and other factors all have affect the meal plan.

ACUTE COMPLICATIONS

Hypoglycemia and diabetic ketoacidosis (DKA) are the two most common acute complications related to diabetes.

Hypoglycemia

A low blood glucose, or **hypoglycemia** (or **insulin reaction**), is a common side effect of insulin therapy, although patients taking insulin secretagogues can also be affected. **Autonomic symptoms** arise from the action of the autonomic nervous system and are often the first signs of mild hypoglycemia. Adrenergic symptoms include shakiness, sweating, palpitations, anxiety, and hunger. **Neuroglycopenic symptoms**, related to an insufficient supply of glucose to the brain, can also occur at similar glucose levels as autonomic symptoms but with different manifestations. The earliest signs of neuroglycopenia include a slowing down in performance and difficulty concentrating and reading. As blood glucose levels drop further, the following symptoms occur: frank mental confusion and disorientation, slurred or rambling speech, irrational or unusual behaviors, extreme fatigue and lethargy, seizures, and unconsciousness. Symptoms differ for different people but tend to be consistent from episode to episode for any one person. Several common causes of hypoglycemia are listed in Box 31-4.

BOX 31-4

Common Causes of Hypoglycemia

Inadvertent or deliberate errors in medication (generally insulin) dosages
Excessive insulin or oral secretagogue dosages
Improper timing of insulin in relation to food intake
Intensive insulin therapy
Inadequate food intake
Omitted or inadequate meals or snacks
Delayed meals or snacks
Unplanned or increased physical activities or exercise
Prolonged duration or increased intensity of exercise
Alcohol intake without food

Adapted from Kaufman F: Medical management of type 1 diabetes, ed 5, Alexandria, Va, 2008, American Diabetes Association.

BOX 31-5

Treatment of Hypoglycemia

- Immediate treatment with carbohydrates is essential.
- If the blood glucose level falls below 70 mg/dL (3.9 mmol/L), treat with 15 g of carbohydrates, which is equivalent to:
  - 15 g carbohydrate from glucose tablets (3) or glucose gel
  - 4 to 6 ounces of fruit juice or regular soft drinks
  - 6 saltine crackers
  - 1 tablespoon of syrup or honey
- Retest in approximately 10 to 15 minutes. If the blood glucose level remains <70 mg/dL (<3.9 mmol/L), treat with an additional 15 g of carbohydrates.
- Repeat testing and treatment until the blood glucose level returns to within normal range.
- If it is more than 1 hour to the next meal, test again 60 minutes after treatment as additional carbohydrate may be needed.

Adapted from Kaufman F: Medical management of type 1 diabetes, ed 5, Alexandria, Va, 2008, American Diabetes Association.

In general, a blood glucose of 70 mg/dL (3.9 mmol/L) or lower should be treated immediately. Treatment of hypoglycemia requires ingestion of glucose or carbohydrate-containing food. Although any carbohydrate will raise glucose levels, glucose is the preferred treatment. Commercially available glucose tablets have the advantage of being premeasured to help prevent overtreatment. Ingestion of 15 to 20 g of glucose is an effective but temporary treatment. Initial response to treatment should be seen in approximately 10 to 20 minutes; however, blood glucose should be evaluated again in approximately 60 minutes because additional carbohydrate may be necessary (Box 31-5).

The form of carbohydrates (i.e., liquid or solid) used to treat does not make a difference. If patients are unable to swallow, administration of subcutaneous or intramuscular glucagon may be needed. Parents, roommates, and spouses should be taught how to mix, draw up, and administer glucagon so that they are properly prepared for emergency situations. Kits that include a syringe prefilled with diluting fluid are available.

SMBG is essential for prevention and treatment of hypoglycemia. Changes in insulin injections, eating, exercise schedules, and travel routines warrant increased frequency of monitoring. Some patients experience hypoglycemia unawareness, which means that they do not experience the usual symptoms of hypoglycemia. Patients need to be reminded of the need to treat hypoglycemia, even in the absence of symptoms. Short-term relaxation of glycemic targets generally assists in the correction of hypoglycemia unawareness (ADbA, 2011b).

Hyperglycemia and Diabetic Ketoacidosis

Hyperglycemia can lead to **diabetic ketoacidosis (DKA)**, a life-threatening but reversible complication characterized by severe disturbances in carbohydrate, protein, and fat metabolism. DKA is always the result of inadequate insulin for glucose use. As a result, the body depends on fat for energy, and ketones are formed. Acidosis results from increased production and decreased use of acetoacetic acid and 3-β-hydroxybutyric acid from fatty acids. These ketones spill into the urine; hence the reliance on testing for ketones.

DKA is characterized by elevated blood glucose levels (greater than 250 mg/dL but generally less than 600 mg/dL) and the presence of ketones in the blood and urine. Symptoms include polyuria, polydipsia, hyperventilation, dehydration, the fruity odor of ketones, and fatigue. SMBG, testing for ketones, and medical intervention can all help prevent DKA. If left untreated, DKA can lead to coma and death. Treatment includes supplemental insulin, fluid and electrolyte replacement, and medical monitoring. Acute illnesses such as flu, colds, vomiting, and diarrhea, if not managed appropriately, can lead to the development of DKA. Patients need to know the steps to take during acute illness to prevent DKA (Box 31-6). During acute illness, oral ingestion of approximately 150 to 200 g of carbohydrates per day (45 to 50 g every 3 to 4 hours) should be sufficient, along with medication adjustments, to keep glucose in the goal range and to prevent starvation ketosis (ADbA, 2008).

Fasting hyperglycemia is a common finding in persons with diabetes. The amount of insulin required to normalize blood glucose levels during the night is less in the predawn period (from 1:00 to 3:00 AM) than at dawn (4:00 to 8:00 AM). The increased need for insulin at dawn causes a rise in fasting blood glucose levels referred to as the **dawn phenomenon**. It results if insulin levels decline between predawn and dawn or if overnight hepatic glucose output becomes excessive as is common in T2DM. To identify the dawn phenomenon, blood glucose levels are monitored at bedtime and at 2:00 to 3:00 AM. With the dawn phenomenon, predawn blood glucose levels will be in the low range of normal but

BOX 31-6

Sick-Day Guidelines for Persons with Diabetes

1. During acute illnesses, usual doses of insulin and other glucose-lowering medications are required. The need for insulin continues, or may even increase, during periods of illness. Fever, dehydration, infection, or the stress of illness can trigger the release of counterregulatory or "stress" hormones, causing blood glucose levels to become elevated.
2. Blood glucose levels and urine or blood testing for ketones should be monitored at least four times daily (before each meal and at bedtime). Blood glucose readings exceeding 250 mg/dL and the presence of ketones are danger signals indicating that additional insulin is needed.
3. Ample amounts of liquid need to be consumed every hour. If vomiting, diarrhea, or fever is present, small sips—1 or 2 tablespoons every 15 to 30 min—can usually be consumed. If vomiting continues and the individual is unable to take fluids for longer than 4 hours, the health care team should be notified.
4. If regular foods are not tolerated, liquid or soft carbohydrate-containing foods (such as regular soft drinks, soup, juices, and ice cream) should be eaten. Eating approximately 10 to 15 g of carbohydrate every 1-2 hours (or 50 g of carbohydrate every 3 to 4 hours) is usually sufficient.
5. The health care team should be called if illness continues for more than 1 day.

Adapted from Kaufman F: Medical management of type 1 diabetes, ed 5, Alexandria, Va, 2008, American Diabetes Association.

not in the hypoglycemic range. For patients with T2DM, metformin is often used because it decreases hepatic glucose output. For persons with T1DM, administering insulin that does not peak at 1:00 to 3:00 AM such as a long-acting insulin should be considered.

Hypoglycemia followed by "rebound" hyperglycemia is called the **Somogyi effect**. This phenomenon originates during hypoglycemia with the secretion of counterregulatory hormones (glucagon, epinephrine, growth hormone, and cortisol) and is usually caused by excessive exogenous insulin doses. Hepatic glucose production is stimulated, thus raising blood glucose levels. If rebound hyperglycemia goes unrecognized and insulin doses are increased, a cycle of overinsulinization may result. Decreasing evening insulin doses or, as for the dawn phenomenon, taking a long-acting insulin should be considered.

LONG-TERM COMPLICATIONS

Long-term complications of diabetes include macrovascular diseases, microvascular diseases, and neuropathy. **Macrovascular diseases** involve diseases of large blood vessels; **microvascular diseases** associated with diabetes involve the small blood vessels and include nephropathy and retinopathy. In contrast, diabetic neuropathy is a condition characterized by damage to the nerves. MNT is important in managing several long-term complications of diabetes. Nutrition therapy is also a major component in reducing risk factors for chronic complications, especially those related to macrovascular disease.

Macrovascular Diseases

Insulin resistance, which may precede the development of T2DM and macrovascular disease by many years, induces numerous metabolic changes known as the **metabolic syndrome** (see Chapters 9 and 32). It is characterized by intraabdominal obesity or the android distribution of adipose tissue (waist circumference greater than 102 cm [40 in] in men and greater than 88 cm [35 in] in women) and is associated with dyslipidemia, hypertension, glucose intolerance, and increased prevalence of macrovascular complications. Other risk factors include genetics, smoking, sedentary lifestyle, high-fat diet, renal failure, and microalbuminuria.

Macrovascular diseases, including CHD, peripheral vascular disease, and cerebrovascular disease are more common, tend to occur at an earlier age, and are more extensive and severe in people with diabetes. Persons with diabetes have the same CVD risk equivalent as persons with preexisting CVD and no diabetes (Buse et al., 2007). Furthermore, in women with diabetes the increased risk of mortality from heart disease is greater than in men, in contrast to the nondiabetic population, in which heart disease mortality is greater in men than in women.

Dyslipidemia

Patients with diabetes have an increased prevalence of lipid abnormalities that contribute to higher rates of CVD. In T2DM the prevalence of an elevated cholesterol level is approximately 28% to 34%. Approximately 5% to 14% of patients with T2DM have high triglyceride levels; also, lower HDL cholesterol levels are common. Persons with T2DM typically have smaller, denser LDL particles, which increase atherogenicity even if the total LDL cholesterol level is not significantly elevated. Lifestyle intervention, including MNT, increased physical activity, weight loss, and smoking cessation should always be implemented. MNT should focus on the reduction of saturated and *trans*-fatty acids and cholesterol (see Chapter 33).

Hypertension

Hypertension is a common comorbidity of diabetes, with approximately 73% of adults with diabetes having blood pressure of 130/80 mm Hg or higher or using prescription medications for hypertension (CDC, 2007). Treatment of hypertension in persons with diabetes should be vigorous to reduce the risk of macrovascular and microvascular disease. Blood pressure should be measured at every routine visit with a goal for blood pressure control of less than 130/80 mm Hg. Patients with systolic blood pressure of 130 to 139 mm Hg or a diastolic blood pressure of 80 to 89 mm Hg should be given MNT for hypertension (see Chapter 33).

Microvascular Diseases

Nephropathy

In the United States and Europe diabetic nephropathy has become the most common single cause of end-stage renal disease (ESRD), accounting for approximately 40% of new cases. Approximately 20% to 40% of patients with diabetes develop evidence of nephropathy, but in T2DM a considerably smaller number progress to ESRD. However, because of the much greater prevalence of T2DM, such patients constitute more than half of the patients with diabetes currently starting on dialysis.

The earliest clinical evidence of nephropathy is the appearance of low but abnormal urine albumin levels (30 to 299 mg/24 hr), referred to as *microalbuminuria* or *incipient nephropathy*. Microalbuminuria is also a marker of increased CVD risk. Without specific interventions, progression to overt nephropathy or clinical albuminuria (300 mg/24 hr or more) occurs over a period of years. An annual screening for microalbuminuria should be performed in patients who have had T1DM for more than 5 years, and in all patients with T2DM at diagnosis and during pregnancy (ADbA, 2010b). The preferred screening method is by measurement of albumin-to-creatinine ratio in a random spot collection. Two of three tests within a 3 to 6 month period should be abnormal before a patient is designated as having microalbuminuria. Serum creatinine should be measured at least annually in all adults with diabetes regardless of the degree of urine albumin excretion. The serum creatinine is used to estimate glomerular filtration rate (GFR) and stage the level of chronic kidney disease, if present. Studies have found decreased GFR in the absence of increased urine albumin excretion in a substantial percentage of adults with diabetes.

Although diabetic nephropathy cannot be cured, the clinical course of the disease can be modified. To reduce the risk or slow the progression of nephropathy, glucose and blood pressure control should be optimized. In the treatment of both microalbuminuria and macroalbuminuria, either angiotensin-converting enzyme inhibitors or angiotensin receptor blockers should be used, except during pregnancy. If one class is not tolerated, the other should be substituted, and their combination will decrease albuminuria more than use of either agent alone (ADbA, 2011b).

Research on low-protein diets delaying the progression of renal disease has been controversial. In eight trials with duration greater than 6 months, the low-protein diets (prescribed 0.6 g/kg/day; actual intake 0.9 g/kg/day) compared with usual protein diets (1.3 g/kg/day) were not significantly associated with a change in GFR or creatinine clearance rate, but did result in a decline in urinary protein excretion (Pan et al., 2008).

The ADA EBNPG recommends a protein intake of less than 1 g/kg/day for persons with diabetic nephropathy. Studies implementing lower-protein diets in the management of diabetic nephropathy are inconclusive. For persons with late-stage diabetic nephropathy, hypoalbuminemia (an indicator of malnutrition) and energy intake must be monitored and changes in protein and energy intake made to correct deficits. A protein intake of approximately 0.7 g/kg/day has been associated with hypoalbuminemia, whereas a protein intake of approximately 0.9 g/kg/day has not (ADA, 2008). With microalbuminuria there may be additional benefits in lowering phosphorus to 500 to 1000 mg/day along with the low-protein diet. Although several studies have explored the potential of plant versus animal protein, the data are inconclusive (see Chapter 36).

Retinopathy

Diabetic retinopathy is estimated to be the most frequent cause of new cases of blindness among adults 20 to 74 years of age. Glaucoma, cataracts, and other disorders of the eye also occur earlier and more frequently with diabetes (ADbA, 2011b). Laser photocoagulation surgery can reduce the risk of further vision loss but usually does not restore lost vision—thus a screening program to detect diabetic retinopathy is important. Adults and adolescents with T1DM should have an initial dilated and comprehensive eye examination by an ophthalmologist or optometrist within 5 years after the onset of diabetes and patients with T2DM should be examined shortly after the diagnosis of diabetes. Subsequent examinations for both groups should be done annually. Less frequent examinations may be considered (every 2 to 3 years) if the eye examination is normal (ADbA, 2011b).

There are three stages of diabetic retinopathy. The early stage of *nonproliferative diabetic retinopathy (NPDR)* is characterized by microaneurysms, a pouchlike dilation of a terminal capillary, lesions that include cotton-wool spots (also referred to as *soft exudates*), and the formation of new blood vessels as a result of the great metabolic need of the retina for oxygen and other nutrients supplied by the bloodstream. As the disease progresses to the middle stages of moderate, severe, and very severe NPDR, gradual loss of the retinal microvasculature occurs, resulting in retinal ischemia. Extensive intraretinal hemorrhages and microaneurysms are common reflections of increasing retinal nonperfusion.

The most advanced stage, termed *proliferative diabetic retinopathy*, is the final and most vision-threatening stage of diabetic retinopathy. It is characterized by the onset of ischemia-induced new vessel proliferation at the optic disk or elsewhere in the retina. The new vessels are fragile and prone to bleeding, resulting in vitreous hemorrhage. With time the neovascularization tends to undergo fibrosis and contraction, resulting in retinal traction, retinal tears, vitreous hemorrhage, and retinal detachment. Diabetic macular edema, which involves thickening of the central (macular) portion of the retina, and glaucoma, in which fibrous scar tissue increases intraocular pressure, are other clinical findings in retinopathy.

Neuropathy

Chronic high levels of blood glucose are also associated with nerve damage and 60% to 70% of people with diabetes have mild to severe forms of nervous system damage (CDC, 2007). Intensive treatment of hyperglycemia reduces the risk and slows progression of diabetic neuropathy, but does not reverse neuronal loss. Peripheral neuropathy usually affects the nerves that control sensation in the feet and hands. Autonomic neuropathy affects nerve function controlling various organ systems. Cardiovascular effects include postural hypotension and decreased responsiveness to cardiac nerve impulses, leading to painless or silent ischemic heart disease. Sexual function may be affected, with impotence the most common manifestation.

Damage to nerves innervating the gastrointestinal tract can cause a variety of problems. Neuropathy can be manifested in the esophagus as nausea and esophagitis, in the stomach as unpredictable emptying, in the small bowel as loss of nutrients, and in the large bowel as diarrhea or constipation.

Gastroparesis is characterized by delayed gastric emptying in the absence of mechanical obstruction of the stomach (Camilleri, 2007). Symptoms are reported by 5% to 12% of persons with diabetes. It results in delayed or irregular contractions of the stomach, leading to various gastrointestinal symptoms such as feelings of fullness, bloating, nausea, vomiting, diarrhea, or constipation. Gastroparesis should be suspected in individuals with erratic glucose control.

The first step in management of patients with neuropathy should be to aim for stable and optimal glycemic control. MNT involves minimizing abdominal stress. Small, frequent meals may be better tolerated than three full meals a day; and these meals should be low in fiber and fat. If solid foods are not well tolerated, liquid meals may need to be recommended. For patients using insulin, as much as possible, the timing of insulin administration should be adjusted to match the usually delayed nutrient absorption. Insulin injections may even be required after eating. Frequent blood glucose monitoring is important to determine appropriate insulin therapy.

Prokinetic agents most commonly used to treat gastroparesis include metoclopramide and erythromycin. Antiemetic agents may be helpful for the relief of symptoms. In very severe cases, generally with unintentional weight loss, a feeding tube is placed in the small intestine to avoid the stomach. Gastric electric stimulation with electrodes surgically implanted in the stomach may be used when medications fail to control nausea and vomiting.

HYPOGLYCEMIA OF NONDIABETIC ORIGIN

Hypoglycemia of nondiabetic origin has been defined as a clinical syndrome with diverse causes in which low levels of plasma glucose eventually lead to neuroglycopenia. *Hypoglycemia* means low (hypo) blood glucose (glycemia). Normally the body is remarkably adept at maintaining fairly steady blood glucose levels—usually between 60 and 100 mg/dL (3.3 to 5.6 mmol/L), despite the intermittent ingestion of food. Maintaining normal levels of glucose is important because body cells, especially the brain and central nervous system, must have a steady and consistent supply of glucose to function properly. Under physiologic conditions the brain depends almost exclusively on glucose for its energy needs. Even with hunger, either because it has been many hours since food was eaten or because the last meal was small, blood glucose levels remain fairly consistent.

Pathophysiology

In a small number of people, blood glucose levels drop too low. Symptoms are often felt when blood glucose is below 65 mg/dL (3.6 mmol/L). If the brain and nervous system are deprived of the glucose they need to function, symptoms such as sweating, shaking, weakness, hunger, headaches, and irritability can develop. Symptoms of hypoglycemia have been recognized at plasma glucose levels of approximately 60 mg/dL, and impaired brain function has occurred at levels of approximately 50 mg/dL.

Hypoglycemia can be difficult to diagnose because these typical symptoms can be caused by many different health problems. For example, adrenaline (epinephrine) released as a result of anxiety and stress can trigger the symptoms similar to those of hypoglycemia. The only way to determine whether hypoglycemia is causing these symptoms is to measure blood glucose levels while an individual is experiencing the symptoms. Hypoglycemia can best be defined by the presence of three features known as the **Whipple triad**: (1) a low plasma or blood glucose level, (2) symptoms of hypoglycemia at the same time, and (3) amelioration of the symptoms by correction of the hypoglycemia.

A fairly steady blood glucose level is maintained by the interaction of several mechanisms. After eating, food is broken down into glucose and enters the bloodstream. As blood glucose levels rise, the pancreas responds by releasing the hormone insulin, which allows glucose to leave the bloodstream and enter various body cells, where it fuels the body's activities. Glucose is also taken up by the liver and stored as glycogen for later use.

When glucose concentrations from the last meal decline, the body goes from a "fed" to a "fasting" state. Insulin levels decrease, which keeps the blood glucose levels from falling too low. Stored glucose is released from the liver back into the bloodstream with the help of **glucagon** from the pancreas. Normally the body's ability to balance glucose, insulin, and glucagon (and other counterregulatory hormones) keeps glucose levels within the normal range. Glucagon provides the primary defense against hypoglycemia; without it, full recovery does not occur. Epinephrine is not necessary for counterregulation when glucagon is present. However, in the absence of glucagon, epinephrine has an important role.

Types of Hypoglycemia

Two types of hypoglycemia can occur in people who do not have diabetes. If blood glucose levels fall below normal limits within 2 to 5 hours after eating, this is **postprandial (reactive) hypoglycemia**. It can be caused by an exaggerated or late insulin response caused by either insulin resistance or elevated GLP-1; alimentary hyperinsulinism; renal glycosuria; defects in glucagon response; high insulin sensitivity; rare syndromes such as hereditary fructose intolerance, galactosemia, leucine sensitivity; or a rare β-cell pancreatic tumor (insulinoma), causing blood glucose levels to drop too low. Alimentary hyperinsulinism is common after gastric surgery, associated with rapid delivery of food to the small intestine, rapid absorption of glucose, and exaggerated insulin response. These patients respond best to multiple, frequent feedings.

The ingestion of alcohol after a prolonged fast or the ingestion of large amounts of alcohol and carbohydrates on an empty stomach ("gin-and-tonic" syndrome) may also cause hypoglycemia within 3 to 4 hours in some healthy persons.

Idiopathic reactive hypoglycemia is characterized by normal insulin secretion but increased insulin sensitivity and, to some extent, reduced response of glucagon to acute hypoglycemia symptoms. The increase in insulin sensitivity associated with a deficiency of glucagon secretion leads to hypoglycemia late postprandially. Idiopathic reactive hypoglycemia has been inappropriately overdiagnosed by both physicians and patients, to the point that some physicians doubt its existence. Although rare, it does exist but can be documented only in persons with hypoglycemia that occurs spontaneously and who meet the criteria of Whipple triad.

Fasting hypoglycemia, or postabsorptive hypoglycemia, is often related to an underlying disease. This food-deprived hypoglycemia may occur in response to having gone without food for 8 hours or longer and can be caused by conditions that upset the body's ability to balance blood glucose. These include eating disorders and other serious underlying medical conditions, including hormone deficiency states (e.g., hypopituitarism, adrenal insufficiency, catecholamine or glucagon deficiency), acquired liver disease, renal disease, certain drugs (e.g., alcohol, propranolol, salicylate), insulinoma (of which most are benign, but 6% to 10% can be malignant), and other nonpancreatic tumors. Taking high doses of aspirin may also lead to fasting hypoglycemia. Factitious hypoglycemia, or self-administration of insulin or sulfonylurea in persons who do not have diabetes, is a cause as well. Symptoms related to fasting hypoglycemia tend to be particularly severe and can include a loss of mental acuity, seizures, and unconsciousness. If the underlying problem can be resolved, hypoglycemia is no longer a problem.

Diagnostic Criteria

One of the criteria used to confirm the presence of hypoglycemia is a blood glucose level of less than 50 mg/dL (2.8 mmol/L.) Previously the OGTT test was the standard test for this condition; however, this test is no longer used. Recording fingerstick blood glucose measurements during spontaneous, symptomatic episodes at home is used to establish the diagnosis. An alternative method is to perform a glucose test in a medical office setting, in which case the patient is given a typical meal that has been documented in the past to lead to symptomatic episodes; the Whipple triad can be confirmed if symptoms occur. If blood glucose levels are low during the symptomatic period and if the symptoms disappear on eating, hypoglycemia is probably a responsible diagnosis. It is essential to make a correct diagnosis in patients with fasting hypoglycemia because the implications are serious.

Management of Hypoglycemia

The management of hypoglycemic disorders involves two distinct components: (1) relief of neuroglycopenic symptoms by restoring blood glucose concentrations to the normal range, and (2) correction of the underlying cause. The immediate treatment is to eat foods or beverages containing carbohydrates. As the glucose from the breakdown of carbohydrates is absorbed into the bloodstream, it increases the level of glucose in the blood and relieves the symptoms. If an underlying problem is causing hypoglycemia, appropriate treatment of this disease or disorder is essential.

Almost no research has been done to determine what type of food-related treatment is best for the prevention of hypoglycemia. Traditional advice has been to avoid foods containing sugars and to eat protein- and fat-containing foods. Recent research on the GI and sugars has raised questions about the appropriateness of restricting only sugars because these foods have been reported to have a lower GI than many of the starches that were encouraged in the past. Restriction of sugars may contribute to a decreased intake in total carbohydrates, which may be more important than the source of the carbohydrates.

The goal of treatment is to adopt eating habits that will keep blood glucose levels as stable as possible (International Diabetes Center, 2007). To stay symptom free, it is important for individuals to eat five to six small meals or snacks per day. Doing this provides manageable amounts of glucose to the body. Recommended guidelines are listed in Box 31-7.

Patients with hypoglycemia may also benefit from learning carbohydrate counting and, to prevent hypoglycemia, eating three to four carbohydrate servings (15 g of carbohydrate per serving) at meals and one to two for snacks (see Appendix 34). Foods containing protein that are also low in saturated fat can be eaten at meals or with snacks. These foods are expected to have minimum effect on blood glucose levels and can add extra food for satiety and calories. However, because both protein and carbohydrate stimulate insulin release, a moderate intake may be advisable.

BOX 31-7

Guidelines for Preventing Hypoglycemic Symptoms in People Who Do Not Have Diabetes

1. Eat small meals, with snacks interspersed between meals and at bedtime. This means eating five to six small meals rather than two to three large meals to steady the release of glucose into the bloodstream.
2. Spread the intake of carbohydrate foods throughout the day. Most individuals can eat two to four servings of carbohydrate foods at each meal and one to two servings at each snack. If carbohydrates are removed from the diet completely, the body loses its ability to handle carbohydrates properly, so this is not recommended. Carbohydrate foods include starches, fruits and fruit juices, milk and yogurt, and foods containing sugar.
3. Avoid or limit foods high in sugar and carbohydrate, especially on an empty stomach. Examples of these foods are regular soft drinks, syrups, candy, fruit juices, regular fruited yogurts, pies, and cakes.
4. Avoid beverages and foods containing caffeine. Caffeine can cause the same symptoms as hypoglycemia and make the individual feel worse.
5. Limit or avoid alcoholic beverages. Drinking alcohol on an empty stomach and without food can lower blood glucose levels by interfering with the liver's ability to release stored glucose (gluconeogenesis). If an individual chooses to drink alcohol, it should be done in moderation (one or two drinks no more than twice a week), and food should always be eaten along with the alcoholic beverage.

Modified from International Diabetes Center: Reactive and fasting hypoglycemia, Minneapolis, 2007, International Diabetes Center.

CLINICAL SCENARIO

Nutrition Assessment

Client History

Debra Smith, a 45-year-old women with known diagnosis of T2DM for 3 years, has been referred for nutrition counseling. She has not had a medical check-up for 2 years, although she reports continuing to take metformin. She is on no lipid or blood pressure medications. She returns at this time with a primary complaint of chronic fatigue. She states she hasn't returned for any follow-up visits because the only advice she gets is to lose weight, which she has tried to do numerous times without success. Food and nutrition history includes a usual intake of about 2,300 calories and frequent skipping of meals, especially breakfast. She eats few fruits and vegetables and because she has been told to avoid carbohydrate foods, she eats 5-6 oz of meat per meal, contributing to a high saturated fat intake. She drinks a glass of wine only on special occasions. She is willing to try to make some changes in her eating habits. She also reports being physically inactive but is willing to start a walking program.

Biochemical Data

Hemoglobin A1C: 8.3%
Low-density lipoprotein cholesterol: 119 mg/dL
Triglycerides: 275 mg/dL
High-density lipoprotein cholesterol: 34 mg/dL
Blood pressure: 148/88 mm Hg

Anthropometric Data

Height 64 in; weight 175 lb; body mass index 30

Medications

Metformin (Glucophage) 1000 mg twice daily

Nutrition Diagnostic Statements

Food- and nutrition-related knowledge deficit related to no education or counseling for appropriate medical nutrition therapy as evidenced by food history of inappropriate food choices despite belief that she is making appropriate choices.

Inconsistent carbohydrate intake related to lack of knowledge of appropriate food choices as evidenced by food history with either limited or excessive carbohydrate food choices at meals.

Nutrition Interventions

Nutrition prescription: Carbohydrate counting beginning with 3 to 4 carbohydrate servings per meal
Nutrition education: Update patient's knowledge of appropriate nutrition therapy for diabetes beginning with glycemic outcomes; at follow-up visits address cardioprotective nutrition interventions; encourage physical activity starting with short walks
Nutrition counseling: Collaborate with patient to identify behavior change goals

Nutrition Monitoring and Evaluation

Food and blood glucose monitoring records
Weight change
Physical activity
Schedule follow-up session in 4 weeks

USEFUL WEBSITES

American Association of Diabetes Educators
http://www.diabeteseducator.org/
American Diabetes Association
http://www.diabetes.org/
American Dietetic Association
ADA Evidence Analysis Library:
http://www.adaevidencelibrary.com
ADA Diabetes Type 1 and Type 2 for Adults Evidence-Based Nutrition Practice Guidelines:
http://www.adaevidencelibrary.com/topic.cfm?cat=3251
ADA Gestational Diabetes Mellitus Evidence-Based Nutrition Practice Guidelines:
http://www.adaevidencelibrary.com/topic.cfm?format_tables=0&cat=3731
Diabetes Care and Education Practice Group
http://www.dce.org/
DCE Patient Education Handouts:
http://www.dce.org/pub_publications/education.asp
International Diabetes Center, Minneapolis, Minnesota
http://idcdiabetes.org
IDC Publishing:
http://www.idcpublishing.com
Joslin Diabetes Center
Resources for Healthcare Professionals:
http://www.joslin.org/
National Diabetes Education Program
http://www.ndep.nih.gov
National Institute of Diabetes and Digestive Kidney Diseases
http://www.niddk.nih.gov

REFERENCES

American Diabetes Association (ADbA): Diagnosis and classification of diabetes mellitus (Position Statement), *Diabetes Care* 34(Suppl 1):S63, 2011a.

American Diabetes Association (ADbA): Standards of medical care in diabetes—2011 (Position Statement), *Diabetes Care* 34(Suppl 1):S11, 2011b.

American Diabetes Association (ADbA): Nutrition recommendations and interventions for diabetes (Position Statement), *Diabetes Care* 31(Suppl 1):S61, 2008.

American Dietetic Association (ADA): Diabetes type 1 and type 2 for adults evidence-based nutrition practice guidelines, 2008. Accessed 2 June 2010 from http://www.adaevidencelibrary.com/topic.cfm?=3251&auth=1.

American Dietetic Association (ADA): Gestational diabetes mellitus (GDM) evidence-based nutrition practice guidelines, 2009a. Accessed 2 June 2010 from http://www.adaevidencelibrary.com/topic.cfm?format_tables=0&cat=3731.

American Dietetic Association (ADA): Effectiveness of MNT for hypertension, 2009b. Accessed 2 June 2010 from http://www.adaevidencelibrary.com/conclusion.cfm?conclusion_statement_id=251204.

American Dietetic Association (ADA): *International dietetics & nutrition terminology (IDNT) reference manual. standardized language for the nutrition care process*, ed 3, Chicago, 2011, American Dietetic Association.

Balk EM, et al: Effect of chromium supplementation on glucose metabolism and lipids: a systematic review of randomized controlled trials, *Diabetes Care* 30:2154, 2007.

Brand-Miller JC, et al: Glycemic index, postprandial glycemia, and the shape of the curve in healthy subjects: analysis of a database of more than 1000 food, *Am J Clin Nutr* 89:97, 2009.

Buse JB, et al: Primary prevention of cardiovascular diseases in people with diabetes mellitus: a scientific statement from the American Heart Association and the American Diabetes Association, *Diabetes Care* 30:162, 2007.

Camilleri M: Diabetic gastroparesis, *N Engl J Med* 356:820, 2007.

Centers for Disease Control and Prevention (CDC): *National diabetes fact sheet: general information and national estimates on diabetes in the United States, 2007*, Atlanta, Ga, 2007, U.S. Department of Health and Human Services, Centers for Disease Control and Prevention.

Diabetes Control and Complications Trial/Epidemiology of Diabetes Interventions and Complications (DCCT/EDIC) Study Research Group: Intensive diabetes treatment and cardiovascular disease in patients with type 1 diabetes, *N Engl J Med* 353:2643, 2005.

Diabetes Prevention Program Research Group: 10-year follow-up of diabetes incidence and weight loss in the Diabetes Prevention Program Outcome Study, *Lancet* 374:1677, 2009.

Fernandes G, et al: Glycemic index of potatoes commonly consumed in North America, *J Am Diet Assoc* 105:557, 2005.

Franz MJ, et al: Evidence-based nutrition practice guidelines for diabetes and scope and standards of practice, *J Am Diet Assoc* 108:S52, 2008.

Franz MJ, et al: The American Dietetic Association evidence-based nutrition practice guidelines for type 1 and type 2 diabetes in adults: evidence and recommendations, *J Am Diet Assoc* 110, December, 2010a.

Franz MJ, et al: *American Dietetic Association pocket guide to lipid disorders, hypertension, diabetes, and weight management*, Chicago, Il, 2010b, American Dietetic Association.

Guidone C, et al: Mechanisms of recovery from type 2 diabetes after malabsorptive bariatric surgery. *Diabetes* 55:2025, 2006.

Institute of Medicine: *Dietary reference intakes: energy, carbohydrate, fiber, fat, fatty acids, cholesterol, protein, and amino acids*, Washington, DC, 2002, National Academies Press.

International Diabetes Center: *Reactive and fasting hypoglycemia*, Minneapolis, 2007, International Diabetes Center.

Kaufman FR: *Medical management of type 1 diabetes*, ed 5, Alexandria, VA, 2008, American Diabetes Association.

Li GP, et al: The long-term effect of lifestyle interventions to prevent diabetes in the China Da Qing Diabetes Prevention Study: a 20-year follow-up study, *Lancet* 371:1783, 2008.

Lindström J, et al: Sustained reduction in the incidence of type 2 by lifestyle intervention: follow-up of the Finnish Diabetes Prevention Study, *Lancet* 368:1673, 2006.

Ma Y, et al: A randomized clinical trial comparing low-glycemic index versus ADA dietary education among individuals with type 2 diabetes, *Nutrition* 24:45, 2008.

Mayer-Davis EJ, et al: Towards understanding of glycemic index and glycemic load in habitual diet: associations with glycemia in the Insulin Resistance Study, *Br J Nutr* 95:397, 2006.

Nathan DM, et al: Medical management of hyperglycemia in type 2 diabetes: a consensus algorithm for the initiation and adjustment of therapy, *Diabetes Care* 32:193, 2009.

Pan Y, et al: Low-protein diet for diabetic nephropathy: a meta-analysis of randomized controlled trials, *Am J Clin Nutr* 88:660, 2008.

Rosario PWS, et al: Comparison of clinical and laboratory characteristics between adult-onset type 1 diabetes and latent autoimmune diabetes in adults, *Diabetes Care* 28:1803, 2005.

Rosenstock J, et al: Reduced hypoglycemia risk with insulin glargine: a meta-analysis comparing insulin glargine with human NPH insulin in type 2 diabetes, *Diabetes Care* 28:950, 2005.

Silverstein J, et al: Care of children and adolescents with type 1 diabetes: a statement of the American Diabetes Association, *Diabetes Care* 28:186, 2005.

Stuebe AM, et al: Duration of lactation and incidence of type 2 diabetes, *JAMA* 294:2601, 2005.

U.S. Department of Health and Human Services: 2008 physical activity guidelines for Americans, 2008. Accessed from http://www.health.gov/paguidelines/.

Van Horn L, et al: The evidence for dietary prevention and treatment of cardiovascular disease, *J Am Diet Assoc* 108:287, 2008.

Vega-López S, et al: Interindividual variability and intra-individual reproducibility of glycemic index values for commercial white bread, *J Am Diet Assoc* 30:1412, 2007.

Wheeler ML, et al: *Choose your foods: exchange lists for diabetes*, sixth edition, 2008: description and guidelines for use, *J Am Diet Assoc* 108:883, 2008.

Wilson JB, Pories WS: Durable remission of diabetes after bariatric surgery: what is the underlying pathway, *Insulin* 5:46, 2010.

Wolever TMS, et al: The Canadian Trial of Carbohydrates in Diabetes, a 1-y controlled trial of low-glycemic index dietary carbohydrate in type 2 diabetes: no effect on glycated hemoglobin but reduction in C-reactive protein, *Am J Clin Nutr* 87:114, 2008.

Writing Group of the Nutrition Care Process/Standardized Language Committee: nutrition care process part ii: using the international dietetics and nutrition terminology to document the nutrition care process, *J Am Diet Assoc* 108:1287, 2008.

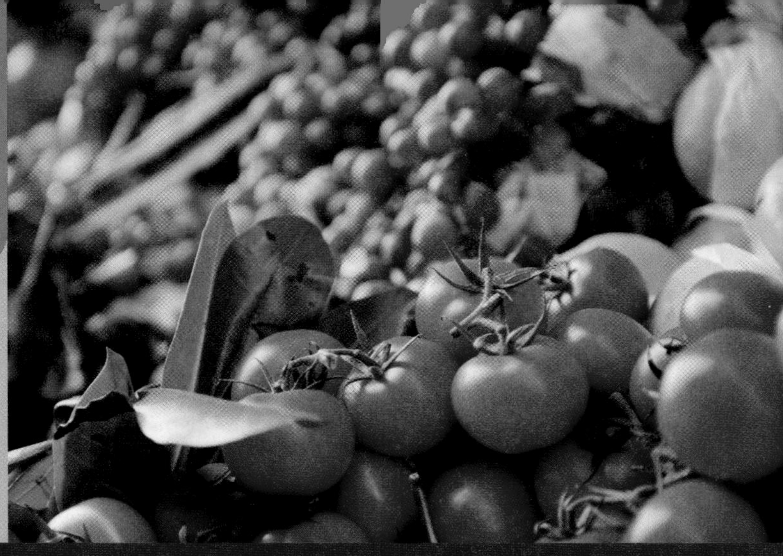

CHAPTER 32

Sheila Dean, DSc, RD, LD, CCN, CDE

Medical Nutrition Therapy for Thyroid and Related Disorders

KEY TERMS

5′-deiodinase
adrenal fatigue
autoimmune thyroid disorders (AITDs)
calcitonin
cortisol
cretinism
euthyroid sick syndrome
goitrin
Graves' disease
Hashimoto's thyroiditis
hyperthyroidism
hypothalamus
hypothalamic-pituitary-thyroid (HPT) axis
hypothyroidism
pituitary gland
polycystic ovary syndrome (PCOS)
reverse T3 (rT3)
Schmidt's syndrome
thyroid-binding globulin (TBG)
thyroglobulin antibodies (TGB Ab)
thyroid peroxidase (TPO)
thyroid peroxidase antibodies (TPO Ab)
thyroid-stimulating hormone (TSH)
thyrotropin-releasing hormone (TRH)
thyroxine (T4)
triiodothyronine (T3)
tyrosine

Diabetes mellitus appears to be the most common endocrine-related chronic disease (American Diabetes Association [ADbA], 2007). However, according to the American Association of Clinical Endocrinologists (2005), 27 million Americans have thyroid-related disorders and more than half remain undiagnosed. Furthermore, individuals with diabetes tend to have a higher prevalence of thyroid disorders.

Thyroid-related diseases are often poorly diagnosed, and there is much about their treatment that requires greater clarification and study. For example, radiation exposure of the thyroid at a young age is a risk factor for the development of thyroid cancer, lasting for a lifetime after exposure (Sinnott et al., 2010). Efforts to reduce exposure from medical x-ray examinations can protect the thyroid gland.

Genetic factors promote the endocrine autoimmune diseases. Recent genome-wide association studies (GWAS) have enabled identification of relevant immune response pathways; the same allele that predisposes to a certain autoimmune disease can be protective in another (Wiebolt et al., 2010). Thus endocrine GWAS are needed, especially for Graves' disease, Hashimoto's thyroiditis, and Addison's disease. Each of these disorders has stages beginning with genetic susceptibility, environmental triggers, and active autoimmunity, followed by metabolic derangements with overt symptoms of disease (Michels and Eisenbarth, 2010). Research is needed to clarify how nutrients interact with genetics, especially in the **autoimmune thyroid disorders (AITDs)**.

THYROID PHYSIOLOGY

The thyroid gland is a small, butterfly-shaped gland found just below the Adam's apple. Although it weighs less than an ounce, it produces hormones that influence essentially every organ, tissue, and cell in the body, thus having an enormous effect on health. The thyroid gland responds to stimulation by **thyroid-stimulating hormone (TSH)**, a hormone secreted by the pituitary gland. When stimulated, the thyroid gland produces two main hormones: **thyroxine (T4)**, a thyroid hormone named for its four molecules of iodine, and **triiodothyronine (T3)**, a thyroid hormone named for its three molecules of iodine. T3 is the most predominant and active form of thyroid hormone that the body can use. The thyroid gland regulates many processes in the body, including fat and carbohydrate metabolism, body temperature, and heart rate. The thyroid also produces **calcitonin**, a hormone that helps regulate the amount of blood calcium. Last, **reverse T3 (rT3)** an isomer of T3, is derived from T4 through the action of deiodinase. The body cannot use rT3.

The synthesis of these hormones requires **tyrosine**, a key amino acid involved in the production of thyroid hormone, and the trace mineral iodine. Within the cells of the thyroid gland, iodide is oxidized to iodine by hydrogen peroxide, a reaction termed the *organification* of iodide. Two additional molecules of iodine bind to the tyrosyl ring in a reaction that involves **thyroid peroxidase (TPO)**, an enzyme in the thyroid responsible for thyroid hormone production. Completed thyroid hormones are released into the circulation; however, metabolic effects of thyroid hormones result when the hormones ultimately occupy specific thyroid receptors. It is estimated a cell needs five to seven times more T4 to bind to the nuclear receptors to have a physiologic effect compared with T3.

The biosynthetic processes resulting in generation of thyroid hormones within the thyroid gland are controlled by feedback mechanisms within the **hypothalamic-pituitary-thyroid axis (HPT axis)**. The HPT axis is part of the endocrine system responsible for the regulation of metabolism. As its name suggests, it depends on the **hypothalamus** (a tiny, cone-shaped structure located in the lower center of the brain that communicates between the nervous and endocrine systems), the **pituitary gland** (the master gland of the endocrine system located at the base of the brain), and the thyroid gland (Figure 32-1).

The hypothalamus produces and secretes **thyrotropin-releasing hormone (TRH)**, which travels to the pituitary gland, stimulating it to release TSH, which signals the thyroid gland to upregulate its synthetic machinery. Although T4, T3, and rT3 are generated within the thyroid gland, T4 is quantitatively the major secretory product. All T4 found in circulation is generated in the thyroid unless exogenously administered. Production of T3 and rT3 within the thyroid is relegated to very small quantities and is not considered significant compared with their peripheral production (Figure 32-2).

When T4 is released from the thyroid, it is primarily in a bound form with **thyroid-binding globulin (TBG)**, a protein that transports thyroid hormones through the bloodstream, with lesser amounts bound to T4-binding prealbumin. It is estimated that only 0.03% to 0.05% of T4 within the circulatory system is in a free or unbound form; this unbound T4 is called *free T4*. In peripheral tissues, approximately 70% of T4 produced is either deiodinated and converted to T3 or rT3, or eliminated. As mentioned, T3 is considered to be the most metabolically active thyroid hormone. Although some T3 is produced in the thyroid, approximately 80% to 85% is generated outside the thyroid, primarily by conversion of T4 in the liver and kidneys. The pituitary and nervous system are capable of converting T4 to T3, so are not reliant on T3 produced in the liver or kidney. Within the liver and kidney, the enzyme responsible for production of T3 is a selenium-dependent enzyme called **5′-deiodinase**, an enzyme that removes one molecule of iodine from T4 to form either T3 or rT3 (Figure 32-3).

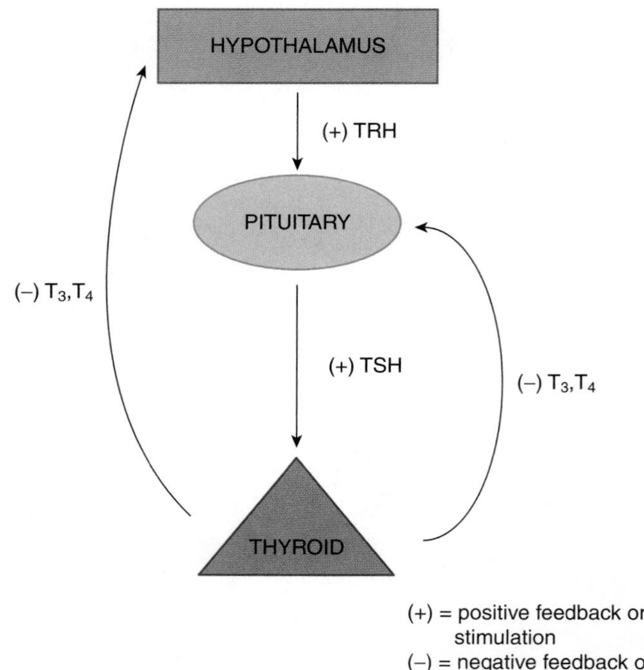

FIGURE 32-1 The hypothalamus-pituitary-thyroid axis.

ASSESSMENT IN THYROID DISORDERS

Assessment begins with an evaluation of thyroid status based on laboratory data such as a full thyroid panel. It may also include a diet history to evaluate micronutrients pertaining to thyroid health along with an evaluation of calorie and carbohydrate intake. Additionally, an assessment of dietary intake of goitrogenic foods may be warranted.

Laboratory Norms: Functional versus Pathological Ranges

A typical (statistical) reference range for TSH in many laboratories is approximately 0.2-5.5 mIU/L. Individuals with TSH values greater than 2 mIU/L have an increased risk of developing overt hypothyroidism during the next 20 years. Subclinical autoimmune thyroid disease is so

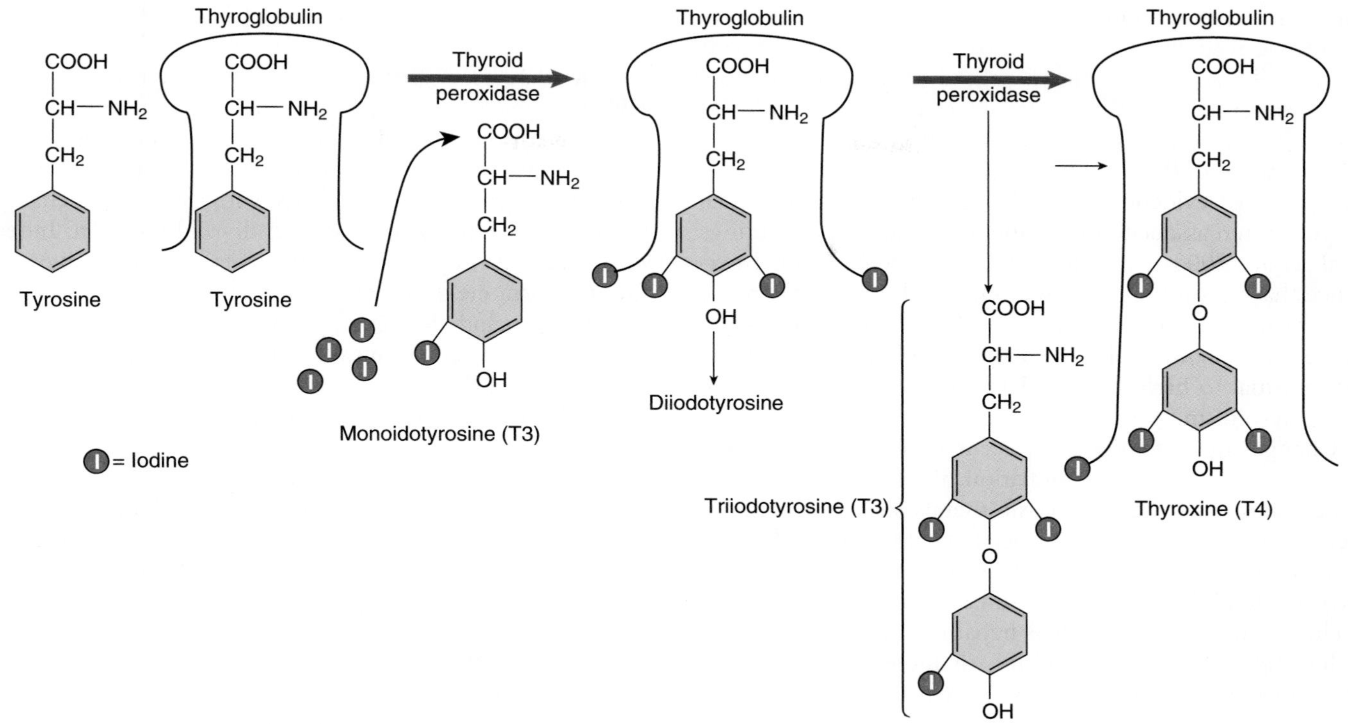

FIGURE 32-2 Constructing thyroid hormones. (1) Accumulation of the raw materials tyrosine and iodide (I-), (2) fabrication or synthesis of the hormone, and (3) secretion of free hormone into the blood.

Hypothalamus sends Thyroid Releasing Hormone (TRH) to the pituitary gland.

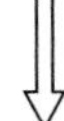

Pituitary gland releases Thyroid Stimulating Hormone (TSH) to the thyroid gland.

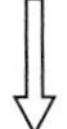

TSH stimulates Thyroid Peroxidase (TPO) activity to use iodine and tyrosine to create T4 and T3 hormones.

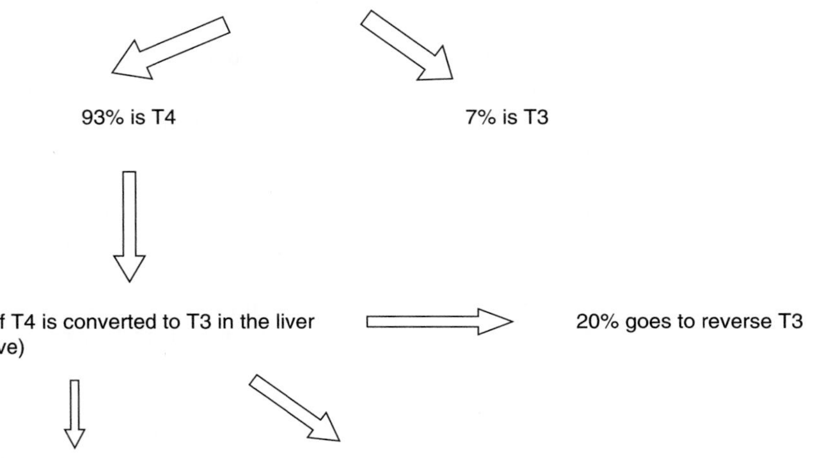

FIGURE 32-3 Thyroid metabolism.

common in the population that laboratory reference ranges derived from testing apparently healthy subjects could easily be misconstrued for those with disease. Importantly, several studies have detected an increase in TPO antibody positivity with TSH concentrations outside the narrow range of 0.2-1.9 mIU/L (Downs et al., 2008). This fact provides evidence that TSH in the upper reference range is often associated with abnormal pathologic findings (Hak et al., 2000; Saravanan et al., 2002). Additional evidence that thyroid function within the laboratory reference ranges can be associated with adverse outcomes is shown in Table 32-1. Conversely, decreased TSH levels combined with normal to high T4 or T3 levels may be suggestive of hyperthyroidism.

Changes in 5′-deiodination occur in a number of situations, such as stress, poor nutrition, illness, selenium deficiency, and drug therapy. Toxic metals such as cadmium, mercury and lead have been associated with impaired hepatic 5′-deiodination in animal models. Free radicals are also involved in inhibition of 5′-deiodinase activity. In the course of chronic liver disease such as hepatic cirrhosis, alterations in hepatic deiodination resulting in increased rT3 and a simultaneous decrease in T3 levels have also been observed (Box 32-1).

TABLE 32-1

Variation In Thyroid Function within Reference Range and Adverse Outcomes

TSH > 2 mIU/L*	Increased 20-year risk of hypothyroidism
TSH > 2 mIU/L*	Increased frequency of thyroid autoantibodies
TSH > 4 mIU/L*	Increased risk of heart disease
TSH 2-4 mIU/L*	Cholesterol values respond to thyroxine replacement
Free T4 < 10.4 pmol/L†	Impaired psychomotor development of infant if occurs in first trimester of pregnancy

T3, Triiodothyronine; *T4*, thyroxine; *TSH*, thyroid-stimulating hormone.

*Typical reference ranges: TSH 0.2-5.5 mIU/L

†Typical reference ranges: free T4 9.8-25 pml/L

BOX 32-1

5′-Deiodinase Inhibitors

Selenium deficiency
Inadequate protein, excess carbohydrates
High insulin
Chronic illness
Stress (cortisol)
Cd, Hg, Pb and other heavy metal toxins
Compromised liver or kidney function

HYPOTHYROIDISM

Of the detected cases of underactive thyroid (**hypothyroidism**), more than half are due to an autoimmune disorder called **Hashimoto's thyroiditis**, in which the immune system attacks and destroys thyroid gland tissue. A common clinical presentation of patients with functional changes of the endocrine system is altered thyroid function. Indeed *subclinical* hypothyroidism represents the first signs of thyroid hormone dysfunction for many individuals. Typical symptoms include low energy, cold hands and feet, fatigue, hypercholesterolemia, muscle pain, depression, and cognitive deficits (Box 32-2). Evaluating thyroid hormone metabolism is needed before thyroid hormone replacement therapy.

Women are five to eight times more likely than men to suffer from hypothyroidism. In addition, individuals who have celiac disease may be at risk (see *Clinical Insight:* Was It Gluten That Caused Her Hypothyroidism?)

Pathophysiology

Hashimoto's thyroiditis is an autoimmune disorder in which the immune system attacks and destroys the thyroid gland. It is the most common form of hypothyroidism. The enlarged, chronically inflamed thyroid gland becomes nonfunctional, with reactive parts of the gland deteriorating after several years. Thyroid autoantibodies indicate the body's immune system is attacking itself and whether an autoimmune thyroid condition is present, be it hypothyroidism or hyperthyroidism.

Specific antibody tests identify Hashimoto's thyroiditis. **Thyroid peroxidase antibodies (TPO Ab)** are immune cells

BOX 32-2

Common Symptoms of Hypothyroidism and Hyperthyroidism

Hypothyroidism	Hyperthyroidism
Fatigue	Heat intolerance, sweating
Forgetfulness	Weight loss
Depression	Alterations in appetite
Heavy menses	Frequent bowel movements
Dry, course hair	Changes in vision
Mood swings	Fatigue and muscle weakness
Weight gain	Menstrual disturbance
Hoarse voice	Impaired fertility
Dry, course skin	Mental disturbances
Constipation	Sleep disturbances
	Tremors
	Thyroid enlargement

From Shomon M: Thyroid disease symptoms—hypothyroidism and hyperthyroidism, 2008. Accessed July 15, 2010 from http://thyroid.about.com/cs/basics_starthere/a/symptoms.htm.

CLINICAL INSIGHT

Was It Gluten That Caused Her Hypothyroidism?

A case report described a 23-year-old woman with a diagnosis of hypothyroidism caused by Hashimoto's thyroiditis and autoimmune Addison's disease who was found in evaluation to have elevated antiendomysium antibody levels. During a 3-month period on a gluten-free diet, the patient demonstrated remarkable clinical improvement in both her GI related symptoms and, more importantly, in her thyroid function. She required progressively less thyroid and adrenal replacement therapy. After 6 months her endomysium antibody level became negative, her antithyroidal antibody titer decreased significantly, and thyroid medication was discontinued. This case report points out the important effect of a hypoallergenic diet on thyroid function in relation to the potential reduction of antithyroidal antibodies.

A number of studies show the importance of gluten in the induction of endocrine autoantibodies and organ system dysfunction in adolescent celiac patients (Cassio et al., 2010; Meloni et al., 2009). Furthermore, the genetic risk for celiac disease is largely related to human leukocyte antigen genotypes, which in turn is largely accountable for its link to autoimmune thyroid disease (Barker and Liu, 2008). It has been reported that gluten-dependent diabetes and thyroidal-related antibodies were found in patients with celiac disease, but were abolished after a gluten-free diet was followed (Duntas, 2009). Similarly, there is a high prevalence of thyroid disorders in untreated adult patients with celiac disease; gluten withdrawal through dietary avoidance may single-handedly reverse this abnormality. This is another important dietary variable that can modify thyroid hormone activity. Because rice has low antigenicity and is gluten-free, a rice-based diet may be desirable in these patients.

that indicate the immune system is attacking TPO in the thyroid gland. The TPO Ab test is the most important, because TPO is the enzyme responsible for the production of thyroid hormones, and the most frequent target of attack in Hashimoto's. **Thyroglobulin antibodies (TGB Ab)** are immune cells that indicate the immune system in attacking thyroglobulin in the thyroid gland. Sometimes this test is necessary as well because it is the second most common target for Hashimoto's disease.

Schmidt's syndrome refers to hypothyroidism with other endocrine disorders, including Addison's disease (adrenal insufficiency), hypoparathyroidism, and diabetes mellitus, all of which may be autoimmune in nature. **Euthyroid sick syndrome** is hypothyroidism, associated with a severe systemic illness that causes decreased peripheral conversion of T4 to T3, an increased conversion of T3 to the inactive rT3, and decreased binding of thyroid hormones. Conditions commonly associated with this syndrome include protein-calorie malnutrition, surgical trauma, myocardial infarction, chronic renal failure, diabetic ketoacidosis, anorexia nervosa, cirrhosis, thermal injury, and sepsis. Once the underlying cause is treated, the condition is usually resolved (see *Pathophysiology and Care Management Algorithm:* Thyroid Dysfunction).

Triggers

Adrenal Stress and Oxidative Stress. Low thyroid function is almost always secondary to some other condition, often **adrenal fatigue** (Abdullatif and Ashraf, 2006). Adrenal fatigue (adrenal stress) denotes a syndrome caused by the decreased ability of the adrenal glands to respond adequately to stress (Wilson, 2008). The adrenal glands are the two glands that sit over the kidneys and are primarily responsible for governing the body's adaptations to stress of any kind. Chronic adrenal stress causes the following:

- Affects communication between the brain and hormone-secreting glands. The hypothalamus and pituitary gland direct hormone production, including that of the thyroid. When the hypothalamus and pituitary weaken because of chronic adrenal stress, they are not able to communicate well with the thyroid gland.
- Increases thyroid-binding protein activity, so that thyroid hormones cannot get into cells to do their job.
- Hampers the conversion of T4 to active forms of T3 that the body can use.
- Interferes with the detoxification pathways through which unnecessary thyroid hormones exit the body, leading to thyroid hormone resistance.
- Causes cells to lose sensitivity to thyroid hormones.
- Weakens the immune barriers of the digestive tract, lungs, and brain; promotes poor immune regulation.

These factors increase the risk for triggering Hashimoto's or exacerbating it. These are some of the ways adrenal stress directly affect thyroid function.

Chronic adrenal stress affects other systems of the body, which in turn, decrease thyroid function. For example, the adrenal hormone **cortisol** plays a big role in thyroid health. Cortisol raises blood sugar when it drops too low. When

PATHOPHYSIOLOGY AND CARE MANAGEMENT ALGORITHM

Thyroid Dysfunction

Etiology

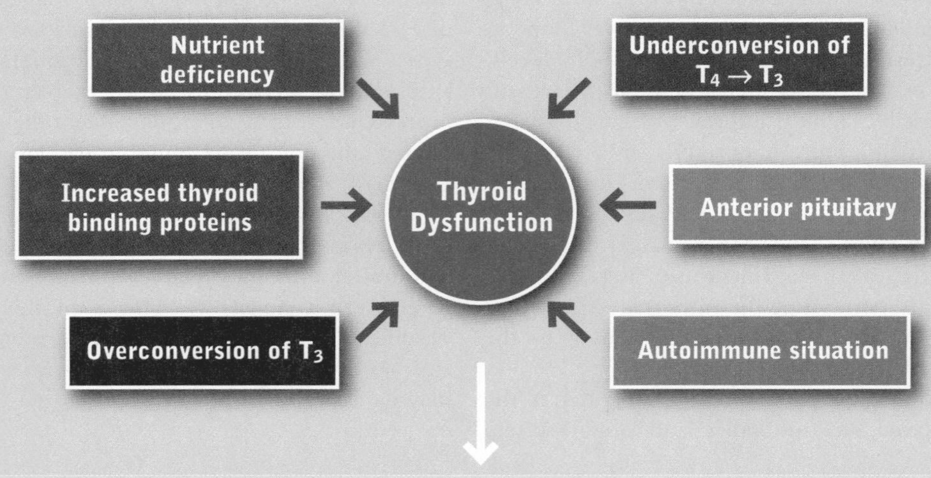

- Nutrient deficiency
- Underconversion of $T_4 \rightarrow T_3$
- Increased thyroid binding proteins
- Anterior pituitary
- Overconversion of T_3
- Autoimmune situation

→ Thyroid Dysfunction

Pathophysiology

Hypothyroidism

- Tissue resistance to T_3
- Need to lost other characterizations
- Weight gain
- Dry skin
- Hair loss
- Tiredness/fatigue
- Constipation

Hyperthyroidism

- Need to list
- Characterizations here
- Weight loss
- Popping eyes

Management

Medical Management

1. Drug therapy

Nutrition

Assessment

- Full thyroid panel
- Diet history to evaluate micronutrient intake csp vit D, Iodine, zinc, selenium
- History of presence of stressors, toxins, autoantibodies, infection

Management

- Supplementation with appropriate nutrients
- Anti-inflammating diet
- Elimination diet to possible food sensitivity

Medical Management

1. Drug therapy
2. Radioactive Iodine
3. Surgical removal

this happens repeatedly, it exhausts the adrenal and thyroid glands, as well as the hypothalamus and the pituitary gland. Over time, this exhaustion leads to functional hypothyroidism. Additionally, constant cortisol production weakens the gastrointestinal (GI) tract, making it more susceptible to inflammation, dysbiosis, and infection. Thus a vicious cycle weakens the thyroid.

Aging. Maintaining thyroid hormone function throughout the aging process appears to be an important hallmark of healthy aging. The incidence of hypothyroidism (underactive thyroid) increases with age. By age 60, 9% to 17% of men and women have an underactive thyroid. The absence of circulating thyroid autoantibodies in healthy centenarians is noted. Because unhealthy aging is associated with a progressively increasing prevalence of organ-specific and non–organ-specific autoantibodies, the absence of these antibodies may represent a significantly reduced risk for cardiovascular disease and other chronic age-related disorders.

Pregnancy. Thyroid dysfunction has been related to obstetrical complications such as premature delivery, gestational hypertension, preeclampsia, and placental abruption. Nearly 1 out of 50 women in the United States is diagnosed with hypothyroidism during pregnancy. Out of every 100 miscarriages, 6 are associated with thyroid hormone deficiency during pregnancy; up to 18% of women are diagnosed with postpartum thyroiditis; and approximately 25% of women develop permanent hypothyroidism (De Vivo et al., 2010; Yassa et al., 2010).

The World Health Organization (WHO) recently increased the recommended iodine intake during pregnancy from 200 to 250 mcg/d and suggested that a median urinary iodine (UI) concentration of 150-249 mcg/L indicates adequate iodine intake in pregnant women. In areas of severe iodine deficiency, maternal and fetal hypothyroxinemia can cause cretinism and adversely affect cognitive development in children. To prevent fetal damage, iodine should be given before or early in pregnancy. In countries or regions where less than 90% of households are using iodized salt and the median UI concentration in school-age children is less than 100 mcg/L, the WHO recommends iodine supplementation in pregnancy and infancy (Zimmermann, 2009).

Medical Management

When the thyroid is underactive (hypothyroidism) because of autoimmune disease (Hashimoto's disease), radioactive iodine treatment, congenital defects, or surgical removal (thyroidectomy), the conventional pharmacologic approach for treatment is prescription thyroid hormone replacement medication. Table 32-2 provides an overview of key forms of thyroid hormone replacement. With the further elucidation of the effects of genetics, new agents are likely to become available as adjunct therapy (Anderson, 2008).

Medical Nutrition Therapy

It is well established that several nutrients are involved in thyroid health, particularly iodine and selenium. Because of the critical role of iodine in the synthesis of thyroid hormone, this trace mineral has received the most attention historically with respect to thyroid disorders. Other deficiencies of micronutrients such as iron, selenium, vitamin A, and

TABLE 32-2

Pharmacologic Treatments for Hypothyroidism

Medication Brand Name	Medication Generic Name	Use and Comments
Synthroid, Levoxyl	levothyroxine—(synthetic T4)	Most commonly prescribed synthetic form of thyroid hormone replacement drug (thyroxine).
Cytomel	liothyronine—(synthetic T3)	Synthetic form of T3, which can also be compounded. Sometimes prescribed in addition to T4.
Armour Thyroid	desiccated natural thyroid	Prepared from dried or powdered porcine (pig) or mixed beef and pork thyroid gland for therapeutic use. Available by prescription and frequently used as an alternative to synthetic thyroid drugs. All brands contain a mixture of approximately 80% T4 and 20% T3. Difficult to standardize
Thyrolar	liotrix—(synthetic T4-T3 combination)	Synthetic combination of T4 and T3 Sometimes used in lieu of Armour Thyroid because of problem with standardization.

From Shomon M: *All about thyroid drugs*, 2007. Accessed May 16, 2011 from http://thyroid.about.com/cs/thyroiddrugs/a/overview.htm.
T3, Triiodothyronine; *T4*, thyroxine.

possibly zinc may interact with iodine nutriture and thyroid function (Hess, 2010).

Fasting or Restrictive Diets. Calorie and carbohydrate restriction may substantially reduce thyroid hormone activity. There is a wide range of variation between individuals; genetics, obesity, gender, and the macronutrient content of the hypocaloric diet influence the response. Nutritional status and energy expenditure both influence thyroid function centrally at the level of TSH secretion, deiodination, and possibly elsewhere. Because an increase of rT3 is found at the expense of T3 during caloric restriction, it is possible that the hepatic pathways play a substantial role in metabolic control during energy balance. However, when caloric restriction is longer than three weeks, T4 and rT3 levels return to normal values.

Fasting also exerts a powerful influence on the metabolism of thyroid hormones. Mild elevations in endogenous cortisol levels might be partly responsible. Ketones generated from calorie deprivation do not appear to suppress T3 generation and hepatic 5′-deiodinase activity. However, it is not clear whether ketones have a similar effect in a calorie-sufficient diet. On a low-calorie diet, elimination of rT3 by 5′-deiodination is decreased. Calories and energy balance might also influence thyroid hormone metabolism during increased caloric consumption, during which the clearance of rT3 by 5′-deiodination is actually increased. On a low-calorie diet, elimination of rT3 by 5′-deiodination is decreased; however, the clearance of rT3 by 5′-deiodination is actually increased with a high calorie diet.

Goitrogens. Cyanogenic plant foods (cauliflower, broccoli, cabbage, Brussel sprouts, mustard seed, turnip, radish, bamboo shoot, and cassava) exert antithyroid activity through inhibition of TPO. The hydrolysis of some glucosinolates found in cruciferous vegetables (e.g., progoitrin) may yield **goitrin**, a compound known to interfere with thyroid hormone synthesis. The hydrolysis of indole glucosinolates results in the release of thiocyanate ions, which can compete with iodine for uptake by the thyroid gland. Increased exposure to thiocyanate ions from cruciferous vegetable consumption, however, does not increase the risk of hypothyroidism unless accompanied by iodine deficiency.

Soybean, an important source of protein in many developing countries, also has goitrogenic properties when iodine intake is limited. The isoflavones, genistein and daidzein, inhibit the activity of TPO and can lower thyroid hormone synthesis. Furthermore, soybean interrupts the enterohepatic cycle of thyroid hormone metabolism. However, high intakes of soy isoflavones do not appear to increase the risk of hypothyroidism when iodine consumption is adequate.

Since the addition of iodine to soy-based formulas in the 1960s, there have been no further reports of hypothyroidism developing in soy formula-fed infants. Soybeans are by far the most concentrated source of isoflavones in the human diet. Small amounts are found in a number of legumes, grains, and vegetables. Average dietary isoflavone intakes in Asian countries, in particular in Japan and China, range from 11-47 mg/day because of intake of the traditional foods made from soybeans, including tofu, tempeh, miso, and matte, whereas intakes are considerably lower in Western countries (2 mg/day). Soy products (meat substitutes, soy milk, soy cheese, and soy yogurt), however, are gaining popularity in Western countries. Although research has not determined the exact effect of soy on the metabolic fate of thyroid hormones, excessive soy consumption is best approached cautiously in those with suspected impairment of thyroid metabolic pathways.

Iodine. As a trace element, iodine is present in the human body in amounts of 10-15 mg and 70% to 80% of it is located in the thyroid gland (Melse-Boonstra and Jaiswal, 2010) (see Chapter 3). Ninety percent of it is organically bound to thyroglobulin (Tg). Iodide is actively absorbed in the thyroid gland to help produce the biochemically active thyroid hormones, T4 and T3 (see Figure 32-2).It is estimated the thyroid gland must capture a minimum of 60 mcg of iodide (the ionic form of iodine) daily to ensure an adequate supply for the production of thyroid hormone (Gropper et al., 2009). Inadequate intake of iodine impairs thyroid function and results in a spectrum of disorders. Randomized controlled intervention trials in iodine deficient populations have shown that providing iron along with iodine results in greater improvements in thyroid function and volume than providing iodine alone (Hess, 2010). It is also vital to thyroid function, as it is a major cofactor and stimulator for the enzyme TPO.

In autoimmune Hashimoto's, supplementing with iodine may exacerbate the condition. Because iodine stimulates production of TPO, this in turn increases the levels of TPO antibodies (TPO Abs) dramatically, indicating an autoimmune flare-up. Some people develop symptoms of an overactive thyroid, whereas others have no symptoms despite tests showing an elevated level of TPO Abs. Therefore one must be cautious regarding the use of iodine. Furthermore, although iodine deficiency is the most common cause of hypothyroidism for most of the world's population (Melse-Boonstra and Jaiswal, 2010), in the United States and other westernized countries, Hashimoto's accounts for the majority of cases (Ebert, 2010; Sloka et al., 2005).

Although the risk of iodine deficiency for populations living in iodine-deficient areas without adequate iodine fortification programs is well recognized, concerns have been raised that certain subpopulations may not consume adequate iodine in countries considered iodine-sufficient. Vegetarian and nonvegetarian diets that exclude iodized salt, fish, and seaweed have been found to contain very little iodine. Furthermore, UI excretion studies suggest that iodine intakes are declining in Switzerland, New Zealand, and the United States, possibly because of increased adherence to dietary recommendations to restrict salt intake for reducing the incidence of hypertension.

Severe iodine deficiency during pregnancy has been shown to increase the risk of stillbirths, spontaneous abortions, and congenital abnormalities. The most severe is **cretinism**, which is a state of mental retardation mostly in combination with dwarfism, deaf-mutism, and spasticity (Chen and Hetzel, 2010). These conditions are largely irreversible. The consequences of severe iodine deficiency during pregnancy on pregnancy outcome and early infant development have been described extensively (Zimmermann, 2009); other details can be found in Chapter 16.

Iron. Historically, it has been thought that low thyroid function may cause anemia. Recent studies suggest that low thyroid function may be secondary to low iron status or anemia. The reason for this is because TPO is a glycosylated heme enzyme that is iron-dependent. The insertion of heme iron into TPO is necessary for the enzyme to translocate to the apical cell surface of thyrocytes (or thyroid epithelial cells), thus assisting TPO to catalyze the two initial steps of thyroid hormone synthesis (Zimmermann, 2006). A full assessment of iron status could likely help to identify the cause of many cases of thyroid malfunction (Titchenal et al., 2009).

Selenium. Selenium, as selenocysteine, is a cofactor for 5′-deiodinase. If selenium is deficient, the deiodinase activity is impaired, resulting in a decreased ability to deiodinate T4 to T3. In animals, deficiencies of selenium are associated with impaired 5′-deiodinase activity in the liver and kidney, as well as reduced T3 levels. Evidence suggests a strong linear association between lower T3/T4 ratios and reduced selenium status, even among individuals considered to be euthyroid based on standard laboratory parameters. This association is particularly strong in older adults, possibly as the result of impaired peripheral conversion. An inverse relationship between T3 and breast cancer is associated with decreased selenium status, even when plasma T4 and TSH concentrations may be similar. This combination of factors strongly suggests that low T3 may be due to faulty conversion of T4 to T3 expected in selenium deficiency.

Selenium participates in the antioxidant network. It assists in detoxification as part of glutathione peroxidase, an enzyme whose main biologic role is to protect the organism from oxidative damage. Several studies reported on the benefit of selenium treatment both in Hashimoto's thyroiditis and Graves' disease.

Evidence also suggests that high intakes of selenium might exert a detrimental influence on thyroid hormone metabolism. Although individuals exposed to high dietary levels of selenium typically have normal levels of T4, T3, and TSH, a significant inverse correlation has been found between T3 and selenium. Some researchers have hypothesized the activity of 5′-deiodinase might become depressed after a high dietary intake of selenium, suggesting a safe level of dietary selenium at or below 500 mcg daily (Kohrle and Gartner, 2009).

POLYCYSTIC OVARY SYNDROME

Polycystic ovary syndrome (PCOS) is a common endocrine disorder of unknown cause that affects an estimated 3% to 12% of women of reproductive age in Western societies (Moran et al., 2010). The condition is characterized by reproductive issues such as amenorrhea or other menstrual irregularities, anovulation, enlarged ovaries with multiple cysts, and infertility. More generalized symptoms include acne, hirsutism (excessive or abnormal distribution of hair growth), male-pattern baldness, obesity, and sleep apnea (Table 32-3).

Pathophysiology

Biochemical and endocrine abnormalities in women with PCOS include elevated levels of androgens (dehydroepiandrosterone, testosterone, and androstenedione), hyperinsulinemia (which results from insulin resistance), impaired glucose tolerance, and hyperlipidemia. Hyperandrogenism is responsible for many of the symptoms of PCOS, such as reproductive and menstrual abnormalities, hirsutism, and acne. Elevated androgen levels, in turn, appear to be due in part to hyperinsulinemia, which triggers the increase in androgen production. Thus interventions that improve insulin resistance and hyperinsulinemia may reverse some of the manifestations of PCOS.

TABLE 32-3

Nutrition Treatment For Polycystic Ovary Syndrome

Obesity	• Institute weight management program of diet and exercise.
Insulin resistance	• Restrict refined carbohydrates (low glycemic index diet) and total calories. • Increase high fiber foods. • Recommend small, frequent meals. • Monitor carefully to ascertain benefit from high- versus low-carbohydrate diet. • Consider supplementation with chromium picolinate.
Low serum 25 hydroxy vitamin D	• Administer vitamin D_3 (cholecalciferol).
Clomiphene-citrate resistant infertility	• Use short-term NAC as adjunct.
Laboratory or clinical evidence of hypothyroidism	• Institute thyroid hormone replacement. • Use foods or supplements with selenium and iodine.

NAC, N-acetylcysteine.

The insulin resistance seen in women with PCOS is unique in that it occurs independent of body weight to some extent and is not always corrected by weight loss. It appears to result from a postreceptor defect in an insulin-mediated signaling pathway (Diamanti-Kandarkis and Papavassiliou, 2006). Conventional treatment of PCOS includes diet and exercise to promote weight loss. In women who are obese, weight loss may improve insulin resistance, decrease androgen levels and hirsutism, and restore ovulation in some cases. Low–glycemic index diets have historically been recommended without evidence of their clinical effectiveness. However, the capacity of dietary carbohydrates to increase postprandial blood sugar response may be an important consideration for optimizing metabolic and clinical outcomes in PCOS. Furthermore, independent of weight loss, a low–glycemic index diet appears to result in greater improvements in health, including improved insulin sensitivity, improved menstrual regularity, better emotion scores (on a questionnaire designed to detect changes in quality of life), and decreased markers of inflammation as compared with a conventional low-fat diet when matched closely for macronutrient and fiber content (Marsh et al., 2010).

Medical Management

Hypothyroidism occurs in some cases of PCOS. Laboratory tests for thyroid function are frequently normal in patients with clinical evidence of hypothyroidism, and treatment with thyroid hormone results in clinical improvement in many patients. Therefore an empirical trial of thyroid hormone should be considered for patients with PCOS who have clinical evidence of hypothyroidism.

Thyroid antibody status should be taken into account when considering empirical treatment with thyroid hormone in women with PCOS. Metformin is frequently prescribed to improve insulin resistance, and treatment with this drug may lead to resumption of ovulation. Other therapies include the drugs clomiphene citrate (to induce ovulation) and spironolactone (an antiandrogen), as well as oral contraceptives (to treat menstrual irregularities and hirsutism).

Medical Nutrition Therapy

Nutritional interventions that may be beneficial for women with PCOS include dietary modifications designed to enhance insulin sensitivity. This includes restricting refined carbohydrates and total calories; consuming high-fiber foods; and eating small, frequent meals. Some patients with insulin resistance fare better on a diet high in complex carbohydrates (approximately 60% of total calories), whereas others respond better to a low-carbohydrate diet (≤40% of total calories). Additionally, supplementation with vitamin D_3 (800-1200 IU/day), and chromium picolinate (200-1000 mcg/day) has been reported to improve glucose tolerance, insulin secretion, and insulin sensitivity (Lydic et al., 2006). Short-term treatment with N-acetylcysteine (600 mg twice a day) may be useful as an adjunct to clomiphene citrate in women with clomiphene citrate-resistant infertility (Rizk et al., 2005). In addition, treatment with thyroid hormone may be beneficial for women who have laboratory or clinical evidence of hypothyroidism (Table 32-3).

HYPERTHYROIDISM

Graves' disease is an autoimmune disease in which the thyroid is diffusely enlarged (goiter) and overactive, producing an excessive amount of thyroid hormones. It is the most common cause of **hyperthyroidism** (overactive thyroid) in the United States. Physical symptoms frequently include red, dry, swollen, puffy, and bulging eyes (exophthalmos), heat intolerance, difficulty sleeping, and anxiety (see Box 32-2). However the most common sign of Graves' disease is goiter or thyroid enlargement (Figure 32-4).The excessive thyroid hormones may cause a serious metabolic imbalance, thyrotoxicosis. The prevalence of maternal thyrotoxicosis is approximately 1 case per 500 persons, with maternal Graves' disease being the most common cause (American Thyroid Association, 2008).

Pathophysiology

Commonly, patients have a family history involving a wide spectrum of autoimmune thyroid diseases, such as Graves' disease, Hashimoto's thyroiditis, or postpartum thyroiditis. In Graves's disease, the TRH receptor itself is the primary autoantigen and is responsible for the manifestation of hyperthyroidism. The thyroid gland is under continuous stimulation by circulating autoantibodies against the TRH receptor, and pituitary TSH secretion is suppressed because of the increased production of thyroid hormones. These thyroid-stimulating antibodies cause release of thyroid hormone and Tg and they also stimulate iodine uptake, protein synthesis, and thyroid gland growth.

The Tg and TPO Abs appear to have little role in Graves' disease. However, as mentioned earlier, they are markers of Hashimoto's autoimmune disease against the thyroid. A TSH antibody—typically referred to as *thyroid-stimulating immunoglobulin*—test is used to identify hyperthyroidism, or Graves' disease.

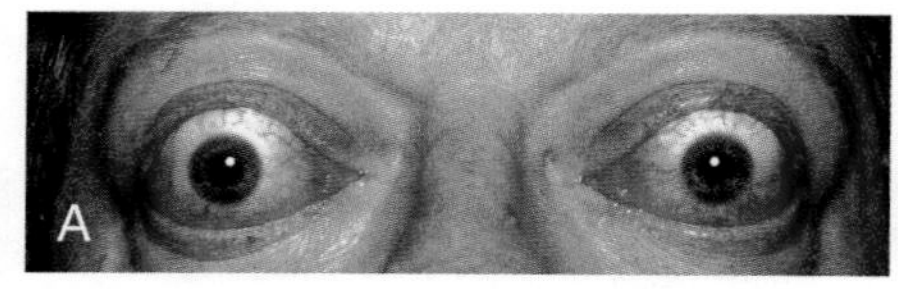

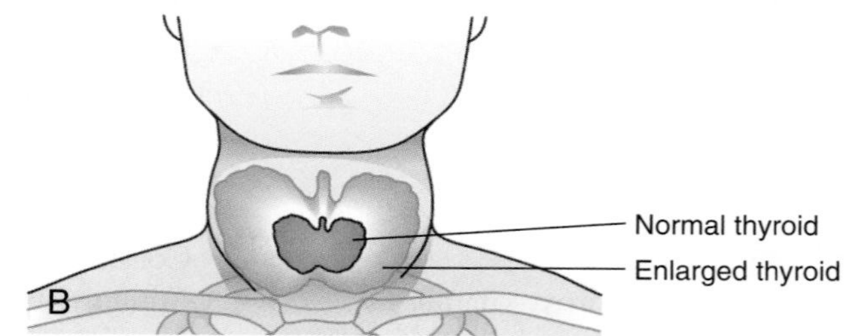

FIGURE 32-4 A, Exophthalmos. *(From SPL/Photo Researchers, Inc.)* **B,** Thyroid enlargement. *(From Buck C: 2011 ICD-9-CM, for Hospitals, Volumes 1, 2 and 3, Professional Edition, St. Louis, 2011, Saunders.)*

Triggers

Graves' disease is an autoimmune disorder, influenced by a combination of environmental and genetic factors. Genetic factors contribute to approximately 20% to 30% of overall susceptibility. Other factors include infection, excessive iodide intake, stress, female gender, steroids, and toxins. Smoking has been implicated in the worsening of Graves' ophthalmopathy. Graves' disease has also been associated with infectious agents such as *Yersinia enterocolitica* and *Borrelia burgdorferi.*

Genetics. Several autoimmune thyroid disease susceptibility genes have been identified and appear to be specific to either Graves' disease or Hashimoto's thyroiditis, whereas others confer susceptibility to both conditions. The genetic predisposition to thyroid autoimmunity may interact with environmental factors or events to precipitate the onset of Graves' disease. *HLA-DRB1* and *HLA-DQB1* appear to be associated with Graves' disease susceptibility.

Stress. Stress can be a factor for thyroid autoimmunity. Acute stress-induced immunosuppression may be followed by immune system hyperactivity, which could precipitate autoimmune thyroid disease. This may occur during the postpartum period, in which Graves' disease may occur 3-9 months after delivery. Estrogen may influence the immune system, particularly the β-cells. Trauma to the thyroid has also been reported to be associated with Graves' disease. This may include surgery of the thyroid gland, percutaneous injection of ethanol, and infarction of a thyroid adenoma.

Medical Management

For patients with sustained forms of hyperthyroidism, such as Graves's disease or toxic nodular goiter, antithyroid medications can be used. The goal with this form of drug therapy is to prevent the thyroid from producing hormones (Table 32-4).

The effects of immunotherapy are also being evaluated (Michels and Eisenbarth, 2010). See *Pathophysiology and Care Management Algorithm:* Thyroid Dysfunction.

MANAGING IMBALANCES OF THE HYPOTHALAMUS-PITUITARY-THYROID AXIS

The thyroid has a relationship to hypothalamic, pituitary, immune, adrenal, and cardiovascular functions that affect clinical, cellular, and molecular outcomes. A checklist of considerations is found in Box 32-3, and is discussed here.

1. *Provide adequate precursors for the formation of T4.* Iodide is a limiting nutrient in many individuals for the production of T4. Adequate levels of organic iodide, which can come from sea vegetables, iodized salt, and seafood, are important in T4 production. Adequate dietary protein intake is important in establishing proper protein calorie nutrition. Supplementation with tyrosine does not appear to have a beneficial effect on elevating thyroid hormones.
2. *Reduce antithyroidal antibodies.* A variety of food antigens could induce antibodies that crossreact with the thyroid gland. A food elimination diet using gluten-free grains and possible elimination of casein, the predominant milk protein, might be considered for hypothyroidism of unexplained origin. It has also been suggested that environmental toxins may play a role in inducing autoimmune thyroiditis and thyroid dysfunction. Implementing nutritional support and providing adequate levels of vitamin D to support the immune system may be beneficial.

TABLE 32-4

Treatments for Hyperthyroidism

Medication Brand Name	Medication Generic Name	Use and Comments
Tapazole	methimazole (MMI)	• Both drugs interfere with the thyroid gland's production of hormones. • Both have side effects which include rash, itching, joint pain, and fever.
Northyx	propylthiuracil (PTU)	• Liver inflammation or reduction in white blood cells may occur. • Underlying hyperthyroidism can return when patient is no longer taking the medication.
Radioactive iodine		• Most widely recommended permanent treatment of hyperthyroidism. • Thyroid cells absorb radioactive iodine, which damages or kills them. • If too many of the thyroid cells are damaged, remaining thyroid does not produce enough hormone, resulting in hypothyroidism and supplemental thyroid hormone may be necessary.
Surgical Treatment		
• Thyroid is either partially or completely removed. • Not as common as pharmacologic modes of treatment.		

BOX 32-3

Factors Promoting Thyroid Health In Adults

Consider

Protein: 0.8 g/kg/day
Iodine (once autoimmune disease has been ruled out): 150 mcg/day
Selenium (as L-selenomethionine): 75-200 mcg/day
Zinc (as zinc citrate): 10 mg/day
Vitamin D (as D3 or cholecalciferol): 400 IU/day
Vitamin E (as d-alpha tocopherol succinate): 100 IU/day
Vitamin C (as ascorbic acid): 100-500 mg/day
Guggulsterones (from guggul extract):100 mg/day
Ashwaganda: 100 mg/day

Reduce or Eliminate

Gluten (found in wheat, rye, oats, and barley)
Processed soy
Excessive uncooked goitrogenic foods

3. *Improve the conversion of T4 to T3.* Nutritional agents that help support proper deiodination by the type 1 5′-deiodinase enzyme include selenomethionine (as L-selenomethionine) and zinc (as zinc glycinate or zinc citrate). Human studies have repeatedly demonstrated consequent reduced concentrations of thyroid hormones when a zinc deficiency is present (Blazewicz et al., 2010). In children with Down syndrome, zinc sulfate may reduce thyroidal antibodies, improve thyroid function, and reduce the incidence of subclinical hypothyroidism.
4. *Enhance T3 influence on mitochondrial bioenergetics.* A number of important nutritional relationships improve thyroid hormones' effect on the mitochondria. Selenium supplementation in animals can improve the production of T3 and lower autoantibodies to thyroid hormones, while improving energy production. Supplementation with selenomethionine results in improved deiodination of T4, which may improve adenosine triphosphate formation by supporting improved mitochondrial activity. Food sources of selenium include the Brazil nut, snapper, cod, halibut, yellow fin tuna, salmon, sardines, shrimp, mushrooms, and barley.
5. *Monitor use of botanical products.* Based on animal studies, it appears that certain botanical preparations influence thyroid activity. The most significant products include *Commiphora mukul* (guggulsterones, from guggul extract) and *Withania somnifera* (ashwagandha). *Commiphora mukul* demonstrates strong thyroid stimulatory action. Its administration (1 mg/100 g body weight) increases iodine uptake by the thyroid, increases TPO activity, and decreases lipid peroxidation, suggesting that increased peripheral generation of T3 might be mediated by this plant's antioxidant effects. *Withania somnifera* (ashwagandha) root extract (1.4 g/kg) may increase T3 and T4 concentrations without changing 5′-deiodinase activity.
6. *Avoid disruption of thyroid hormone metabolism from flavonoids.* Flavonoids, both natural and synthetic, have the potential to disrupt thyroid hormone metabolism. Synthetic flavonoid derivatives can decrease serum T4 concentrations and inhibit both the conversion of T4 toT3 and the metabolic clearance of rT3 by the selenium-dependent 5′-deiodinase. Naturally occurring flavonoids appear to have a similar inhibitory effect. Of the naturally occurring flavonoids, luteolin (most often found in leaves, but also seen in celery, thyme, dandelion, green pepper, thyme, perilla, camomile tea, carrots, olive oil, peppermint, rosemary, and oregano) is the most active inhibitor of 5′-deiodinase activity. Because isolated or concentrated flavonoids are increasingly used as therapeutic interventions, more research on the potential influence of these substances on thyroid hormone metabolism is desirable.
7. *Use caution with supplements.* Lipoic acid reduces the conversion of T4 to T3. Because it is usually not a therapeutic advantage to decrease peripheral activation of T3 subsequent to T4 therapy, use of lipoic acid supplements in hypothyroid patients receiving exogenous hormone therapy should be approached with caution.
8. *Maintain vitamin sufficiency.* One nutrient that is critically important for establishing immune balance and preventing the production of autoantibodies is vitamin D. Vitamin D is considered a prohormone with antiproliferative, differentiating, and immunosuppressive activities. Vitamin D is an effective immune modulator (Baeke et al., 2010) and may suppress the development of autoimmune diseases, such as arthritis and multiple sclerosis. Conversely, a vitamin D deficiency is associated with numerous autoimmune conditions, including Hashimoto's. More than 90% of people with autoimmune thyroid disease have a genetic defect affecting their ability to metabolize vitamin D (Lin et al.,2006; Stefanic et al., 2008). Vitamin D also appears to work with other nutritional factors to help regulate immune sensitivity and may protect against development of autoantibodies. After exposure to heavy metals, decreases in a variety of hepatic antioxidant lipid peroxidation (the oxidative degradation of lipids) systems have been observed. Ascorbic acid has been shown to be effective in preventing cadmium-induced decreases in T3 and hepatic 5′-deiodination.

OTHER ENDOCRINE SYSTEM DISORDERS

Cushing's Syndrome

In Cushing's syndrome, too much cortisol remains in the bloodstream over a long period. The exogenous form occurs when individuals take steroids or other similar medications and ceases when the medication is stopped. Endogenous Cushing's syndrome is rare and occurs as the result of a tumor on the adrenal or pituitary gland. Weight gain, easy bruising, depression, muscle loss, and weakness are common symptoms. A weight management protocol may be needed.

Addison's Disease

Primary adrenal insufficiency, also known as Addison's disease, is rare. In this condition, insufficient steroid hormones are produced in spite of adequate levels of the hormone ACTH. Regulation of blood glucose levels and stress management are affected. Loss of appetite, fatigue, low blood pressure, nausea and vomiting, and darkening of skin on the face and neck may occur. Patients with Addison's disease should not restrict their salt intake unless they have concurrent hypertension. Those patients who live in warm climates and therefore have increased losses through perspiration, may need to increase salt intake.

CLINICAL SCENARIO

Frank is a 72-year-old man from Jamaica who moved to the United States 2 years ago. He has been diagnosed with hypothyroidism this past year. He comes to your clinic with his medicine and traditional folk remedies, including Synthroid, garlic, and chamomile. His diet history indicates daily use of chicken, rice, celery, dandelion, green pepper, mango, and papaya. He states that he has been very tired lately, has little energy, and has constipation. His hormone levels on his last medical report were thyroxine (T4): 1.7, triiodothyronine (T3): 75, and thyroid-stimulating hormone (TSH) : 15, indicative that his hypothyroidism is still not well controlled.

Nutrition Diagnostic Statement

Food-drug interaction related to mixing Synthroid with foods and herbs that aggravate thyroid function as evidenced by fatigue, constipation, high TSH, and low serum T3 and T4.

Nutrition Care Questions

1. What other information do you need for a more thorough assessment?
2. What advice would you offer Frank about his diet?
3. What foods and herbs conflict with Synthroid?
4. Because traditional folk remedies are commonly used, how do you plan to discuss these issues with Frank?

USEFUL WEBSITES

American Association of Clinical Endocrinologists
http://www.aace.com/

American Thyroid Association
http://www.thyroid.org/

Endocrine Web
http://www.endocrineweb.com/

Thyroid Disease Information
http://thyroid.about.com/

REFERENCES

Abdullatif H, Ashraf A: Reversible subclinical hypothyroidism in the presence of adrenal insufficiency, *Endocr Pract* 12:572, 2006.

American Association of Clinical Endocrinologists: *Facts about thyroid disease*, 2005. Accessed 16 August 2010 from http://www.aace.com/public/awareness/tam/2005/pdfs/thyroid_disease_fact_sheet.pdf.

American Diabetes Association (ADbA): *Diabetes Statistics*, 2007. Accessed July 15, 2010 from http://www.diabetes.org/diabetes-basics/diabetes-statistics/.

American Thyroid Association: *Iodine deficiency*, 2008 Accessed July 15, 2010 from http://www.thyroid.org/patients/patient_brochures/iodine?deficiency.html.

Anderson MS: Update in endocrine autoimmunity, *J Clin Endocrinol Metab* 93:3663, 2008.

Baeke F, et al: Vitamin D: modulator of the immune system, *Curr Opin Pharmacol* 10:482, 2010.

Barker J, Liu E: Celiac disease: pathophysiology, clinical manifestations, and associated autoimmune conditions, *Adv Pediatr* 55:349, 2008.

Blazewicz A, et al: Determination of cadmium, cobalt, copper, iron, manganese, and zinc in thyroid glands of patients with diagnosed nodular goitre using ion chromatography, *J Chromatogr B Analyt Technol Biomed Life Sci* 878:34, 2010.

Cassio A, et al: Long-term clinical significance of thyroid autoimmunity in children with celiac disease, *J Pediatr* 156:292, 2010.

Chen Z, Hetzel B: Cretinism revisited, *Best Pract Res Clin Endocrinol Metab* 24:39, 2010.

De Vivo A, et al: Thyroid function in women found to have early pregnancy loss, *Thyroid* 20:633, 2010.

Diamanti-Kandarakis E, Papavassiliou A: Molecular mechanisms of insulin resistance in polycystic ovary syndrome, *Trends Mol Med* 12:324, 2006.

Downs H, et al: Clinical inquiries: How useful are autoantibodies in diagnosing thyroid disorders? *J Fam Pract* 57:615, 2008.

Duntas L: Does celiac disease trigger autoimmune thyroiditis? *Nat Rev Endocrinol* 5:190, 2009.

Ebert E: The thyroid and the gut, *J Clin Gastroenterol* 44:402, 2010.

Gropper S, et al: *Advanced nutrition and human metabolism*, Belmont, CA, 2009, Wadsworth Cengage Learning.

Hak AE, et al: Subclinical hypothyroidism is an independent risk factor for atherosclerosis and myocardial infarction in elderly women: the Rotterdam study, *Ann Intern Med* 132:270, 2000.

Hess S: The impact of common micronutrient deficiencies on iodine and thyroid metabolism: the evidence from human studies, *Best Pract Res Clin Endocrinol Metab* 24:117, 2010.

Kohrle J, Gartner R: Selenium and Thyroid, *Best Pract Res Clin Endocrinol Metab* 23:815, 2009.

Lin W, et al: Vitamin D receptor gene polymorphisms are associated with risk of Hashimoto's thyroiditis in Chinese patients in Taiwan, *J Clin Lab Anal* 20:109, 2006.

Lydic M, et al: Chromium picolinate improves insulin sensitivity in obese subjects with polycystic ovary syndrome, *Fertil Steril* 86:243, 2006.

Marsh K, et al: Effect of a low glycemic index compared with a conventional healthy diet on polycystic ovary syndrome, *Am J Clin Nutr* 92:83, 2010.

Meloni A, et al: Prevalence of autoimmune thyroiditis in children with celiac disease and effect of gluten withdrawal, *J Pediatr* 155:51, 2009.

Melse-Boonstra A, Jaiswal N: Iodine deficiency in pregnancy, infancy and childhood and its consequences for brain development, *Best Pract Res Clin Endocrinol Metab* 24:29, 2010.

Michels AW, Eisenbarth GS: Immunologic endocrine disorders, *J Allergy Clin Immunol* 125:S226, 2010.

Moran L, et al: Polycystic ovary syndrome and weight management, *Womens Health* 6:271, 2010.

Rizk A, et al: N-acetyl-cysteine is a novel adjuvant to clomiphene citrate in clomiphene citrate-resistant patients with polycystic ovary syndrome, *Fertil Steril* 83:367, 2005.

Saravanan P, et al: Psychological well-being in patients on "adequate" doses of L-thyroxine: results of a large controlled community based questionnaire study, *Clin Endocrinol* 57:577, 2002.

Shomon M: *All about thyroid drugs*, 2007. Accessed July 15, 2010 fromhttp://thyroid.about.com/cs/thyroiddrugs/a/overview.htm.

Shomon M: *Thyroid disease symptoms—hypothyroidism and hyperthyroidism*, 2008. Accessed from http://thyroid.about.com/cs/basics_starthere/a/symptoms.htm.

Sinnott B, et al: Exposing the thyroid to radiation: a review of its current extent, risks, and implications, *Endocr Rev* 31:756, 2010.

Sloka J, et al: Co-occurrence of autoimmune thyroid disease in a multiple sclerosis cohort, *J Autoimmune Dis* 2:9, 2005.

Stefanic M, et al: Association of vitamin D receptor gene 3′-variants with Hashimoto's thyroiditis in the Croatian population, *Int J Immunogenet* 35:125, 2008.

Titchenal A, et al: Iron plays an important role for the thyroid, 2009. Accessed July 10, 2010 from http://www.nutritionatc.hawaii.edu/HO/2009/415.htm.

Wiebolt J, et al: Endocrine autoimmune disease: genetics become complex, *Eur J Clin Invest* 40:1144, 2010.

Wilson J: *Adrenal fatigue: the 21st century stress syndrome*, Petaluma, CA, 2008, Smart Publications.

Yassa L, et al: Thyroid Hormone Early Adjustment in Pregnancy (the THERAPY) Trial, *J Clin Endocrinol Metab* 95:3234, 2010.

Zimmermann M: Iodine deficiency in pregnancy and the effects of maternal iodine supplementation on the offspring: a review, *Am J Clin Nutr* 89:668S, 2009.

Zimmermann M: The influence of iron status on iodine utilization and thyroid function, *Ann Rev Nutr* 26:367, 2006.

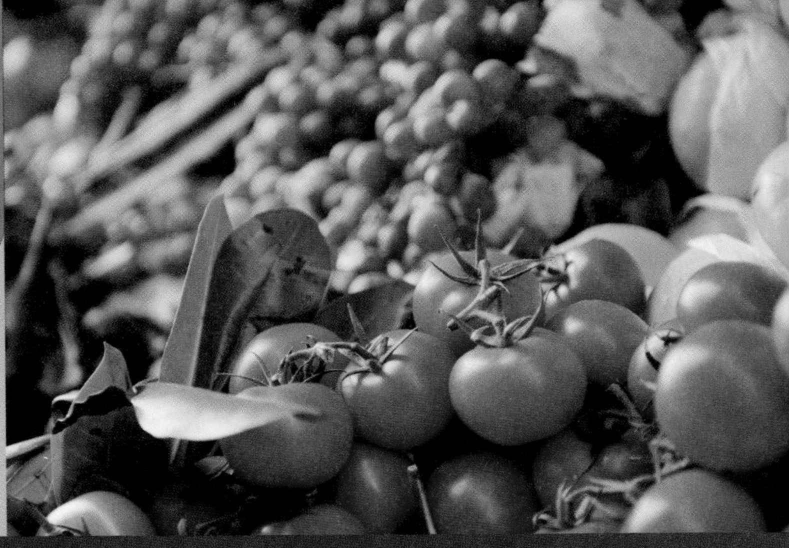

CHAPTER 33

Tracy Stopler, MS, RD
Susan Weiner, MS, RD, CDE

Medical Nutrition Therapy for Anemia

KEY TERMS

anemia
aplastic anemia
ferritin
ferroprotein
hematocrit
heme iron
hemochromatosis
hemoglobin
hemolytic anemia
hepcidin
holotranscobalamin II (holo TCII)
hypochromic
intrinsic factor (IF)
iron-deficiency anemia
koilonychia
macrocytic anemia
meat-fish-poultry (MFP) factor
megaloblastic anemia
microcytic anemia
nonheme iron
pagophagia
pernicious anemia
plasma
protoporphyrin
reticulocytosis
restless legs syndrome (RLS)
serum
sickle cell anemia (SCA)
sideroblastic (pyridoxine-responsive) anemia
soluble serum transferrin receptors (STFRs)
thalassemia
total iron-binding capacity (TIBC)
transferrin
transferrin receptor
transferrin saturation

It is important for nutrition professionals to understand the myriad terms related to blood disorders. **Hemoglobin** is a conjugated protein containing four heme groups and globin; it is the oxygen-carrying pigment of the erythrocytes. The **hematocrit** is the volume percentage of erythrocytes in the blood. **Plasma** is the liquid portion of whole blood containing coagulation factors; **serum** is the liquid portion of whole blood without coagulation factors.

Anemia is a deficiency in the size or number of red blood cells (RBCs) or the amount of hemoglobin they contain. This deficiency limits the exchange of oxygen and carbon dioxide between the blood and the tissue cells. Anemia classification is based on cell size—*macrocytic* (larger than normal), *normocytic* (normal), and *microcytic* (small)—and on hemoglobin content—*hypochromic* (pale color from deficiency of hemoglobin) and *normochromic* (normal color; (Table 33-1). **Macrocytic anemia** presents with larger-than-normal RBCs, plus increased mean corpuscular volume (MCV) and mean corpuscular hemoglobin concentration (MCHC). **Microcytic anemia** is

TABLE 33-1

Morphologic Classification of Anemia

Morphologic Type of Anemia	Underlying Abnormality	Clinical Syndromes and Causes	Treatment
Macrocytic (MCV > 94; MCHC > 31)			
Megaloblastic	Vitamin B_{12} deficiency	Pernicious anemia	Vitamin B_{12}
	Folic acid deficiency	Nutritional megaloblastic anemias, sprue, and other malabsorption syndromes	Folic acid
	Inherited disorders of DNA synthesis	Orotic aciduria	Treatment based on the nature of the disorder
	Drug-induced disorders of DNA synthesis	Chemotherapeutic agents, anticonvulsants, oral contraceptives	Discontinue offending drug and administer folic acid
Nonmegaloblastic	Accelerated erythropoiesis	Hemolytic anemia	Treatment of underlying disease
	Increased membrane surface area		Treatment of underlying disease
Hypochromic Microcytic (MCV < 80; MCHC < 31)			
	Iron deficiency	Chronic loss of blood, inadequate diet, impaired absorption, increased demands	Ferrous sulfate and correction of underlying cause
	Disorders of globin synthesis	Thalassemia	Nonspecific
	Disorders of porphyrin and heme synthesis	Pyridoxine-responsive anemia	Pyridoxine
	Other disorders of iron metabolism		Treatment based on nature of disorder
Normochromic Normocytic (MCV 82-92; MCHC > 30)			
	Recent blood loss	Various	Transfusion, iron, correction of underlying condition
	Overexpansion of plasma volume	Pregnancy	Restore homeostasis
	Hemolytic diseases	Overhydration	Treatment based on the nature of the disorder
	Hypoplastic bone marrow	Aplastic anemia	Transfusion
		Pure red blood cell aplasia	Androgens
	Infiltrated bone marrow	Leukemia, multiple myeloma, myelofibrosis	Chemotherapy
	Endocrine abnormality	Hypothyroidism, adrenal insufficiency	Treatment of underlying disease
	Chronic disorders		Treatment of underlying disease
	Renal disease	Renal disease	Treatment of underlying disease
	Liver disease	Cirrhosis	Treatment of underlying disease

Modified from Wintrobe MM et al: Clinical hematology, ed 8, Philadelphia, 1981, Lea & Febiger.

DNA, Deoxyribonucleic acid; *MCHC*, Mean corpuscular hemoglobin concentration: concentration of hemoglobin expressed in grams per deciliter (g/dL); *MCV*, mean corpuscular volume: volume of one red blood cell expressed in femtoliters (fL).

characterized by smaller-than-normal erythrocytes and less circulating hemoglobin, as in iron deficiency anemia and thalassemia.

Most anemias are caused by a lack of nutrients required for normal erythrocyte synthesis, principally iron, vitamin B_{12}, and folic acid. These anemias that result from an inadequate intake of iron, protein, certain vitamins (B_{12}, folic acid, pyridoxine, and ascorbic acid), copper, and other heavy metals are called *nutritional anemias*. Other anemias result from conditions such as hemorrhage, genetic abnormalities, chronic disease states, or drug toxicity, and have varying degrees of nutritional consequence.

IRON-RELATED BLOOD DISORDERS

Iron status can range from overload to deficiency and anemia. Routine measurement of iron status is necessary because approximately 6% of Americans have a negative iron balance, approximately 10% have a gene for positive balance, and approximately 1% have iron overload. Deviations from normal iron status are summarized in Box 33-1. Iron overload disease develops in persons with stage II positive balance after years of iron overload have caused progressive damage to tissues and organs (Figure 33-1).

Iron status has a variety of indicators. Serum ferritin is an iron apoferritin complex, one of the chief storage forms of iron. Serum ferritin levels are in equilibrium with body iron stores. Very early (stage I) positive iron balance may best be recognized by measuring **total iron-binding capacity (TIBC)**, the capacity of transferrin to take on or become saturated with iron. Conversely, measurement of serum or plasma ferritin levels may best reveal early (stage I or II) negative iron balance, although serum TIBC may be as good an indicator (see Chapter 8). **Transferrin saturation** is the measure of the amount of iron bound to transferrin and is a gauge of iron supply to the tissues; the percent saturation = serum iron/TIBC × 100.

Iron-Deficiency Anemia

Iron-deficiency anemia is characterized by the production of small (microcytic) erythrocytes and a diminished level of circulating hemoglobin. This microcytic anemia is actually the last stage of iron deficiency, and it represents the end point of a long period of iron deprivation.

Pathophysiology

There are many possible causes of iron-deficiency anemia (see *Pathophysiology and Care Management Algorithm:* Iron Deficiency Anemia). The condition can arise from:

1. Inadequate dietary intake secondary to a poor diet without supplementation
2. Inadequate absorption resulting from diarrhea, achlorhydria, intestinal disease such as celiac disease, atrophic gastritis, partial or total gastrectomy, or drug interference
3. Inadequate utilization secondary to chronic gastrointestinal disturbances
4. Increased iron requirement for growth of blood volume, which occurs during infancy, adolescence, pregnancy, and lactation
5. Increased excretion because of excessive menstrual blood (in females); hemorrhage from injury; or chronic blood loss from a bleeding ulcer, bleeding hemorrhoids, esophageal varices, regional enteritis, ulcerative colitis, parasitic or malignant disease
6. Defective release of iron from iron stores into the plasma and defective iron use caused by a chronic inflammation or other chronic disorder

With few exceptions, iron-deficiency anemia in adult men is the result of blood loss. Large losses of menstrual blood can cause iron deficiency in women, many of whom are unaware that their menses are unusually heavy.

Because anemia is the last manifestation of chronic, long-term iron deficiency, the symptoms reflect a malfunction of a variety of body systems. Inadequate muscle function is reflected in decreased work performance and exercise tolerance. Neurologic involvement is manifested by behavioral changes such as fatigue, anorexia, and pica, especially **pagophagia** (ice eating). Abnormal cognitive development in children suggests iron deficiency before it has developed into overt anemia.

Growth abnormalities, epithelial disorders, and a reduction in gastric acidity are also common. A possible sign of early iron deficiency is reduced immunocompetence, particularly defects in cell-mediated immunity and the phagocytic activity of neutrophils, which may lead to frequent infections. **Restless legs syndrome (RLS)** with leg pain or discomfort may result from a lack of iron in the brain; this alters dopamine production and movement. Besides iron deficiency, kidney failure, Parkinson disease, diabetes, rheumatoid arthritis, or pregnancy can aggravate RLS (National Heart, Blood and Lung Institute, 2010).

As iron-deficiency anemia becomes more severe, defects arise in the structure and function of the epithelial tissues,

BOX 33-1

Altered Iron Status

Stages I and II negative iron balance (i.e., iron depletion): In these stages iron stores are low and there is no dysfunction. In stage I negative iron balance, reduced iron absorption produces moderately depleted iron stores. Stage II negative iron balance is characterized by severely depleted iron stores. More than 50% of all cases of negative iron balance fall into these two stages. When persons in these two stages are treated with iron, they never develop dysfunction or disease.

Stages III and IV negative iron balance (i.e., iron deficiency): Iron deficiency is characterized by inadequate body iron, dysfunction, and disease. In stage III, dysfunction is not accompanied by anemia, but anemia does occur with stage IV.

Stages I and II positive iron balance: Stage I positive iron balance usually lasts for several years with no accompanying dysfunction. Supplements of iron or vitamin C promote progression to dysfunction or disease, whereas iron removal prevents progression to disease.

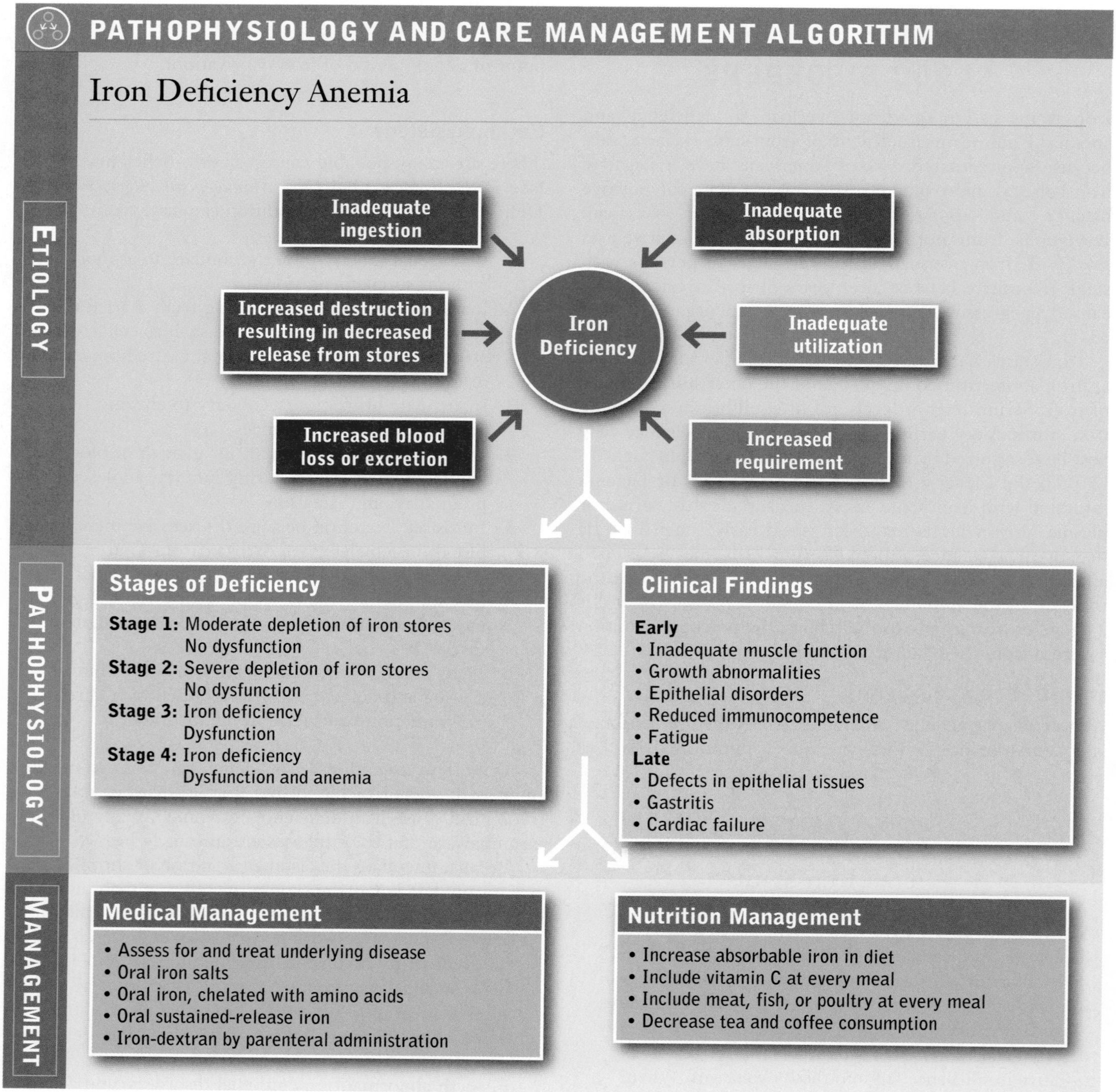

PATHOPHYSIOLOGY AND CARE MANAGEMENT ALGORITHM

Iron Deficiency Anemia

ETIOLOGY

Iron Deficiency ← causes:
- Inadequate ingestion
- Inadequate absorption
- Increased destruction resulting in decreased release from stores
- Inadequate utilization
- Increased blood loss or excretion
- Increased requirement

PATHOPHYSIOLOGY

Stages of Deficiency

Stage 1: Moderate depletion of iron stores
No dysfunction
Stage 2: Severe depletion of iron stores
No dysfunction
Stage 3: Iron deficiency
Dysfunction
Stage 4: Iron deficiency
Dysfunction and anemia

Clinical Findings

Early
- Inadequate muscle function
- Growth abnormalities
- Epithelial disorders
- Reduced immunocompetence
- Fatigue

Late
- Defects in epithelial tissues
- Gastritis
- Cardiac failure

MANAGEMENT

Medical Management
- Assess for and treat underlying disease
- Oral iron salts
- Oral iron, chelated with amino acids
- Oral sustained-release iron
- Iron-dextran by parenteral administration

Nutrition Management
- Increase absorbable iron in diet
- Include vitamin C at every meal
- Include meat, fish, or poultry at every meal
- Decrease tea and coffee consumption

especially of the tongue, nails, mouth, and stomach. The skin may appear pale, and the inside of the lower eyelid may be light pink instead of red. Mouth changes include atrophy of the lingual papillae, burning, redness, and in severe cases a completely smooth, waxy, and glistening appearance of the tongue (glossitis). Angular stomatitis may also occur, as may a form of dysphagia. Gastritis occurs frequently and may result in achlorhydria. Fingernails can become thin and flat, and eventually **koilonychia** (spoon-shaped nails) may be noted (Figure 33-2).

Progressive, untreated anemia results in cardiovascular and respiratory changes that can eventually lead to cardiac failure. Some behavioral symptoms respond to iron therapy before the anemia is cured, suggesting they may be the result of tissue depletion of iron-containing enzymes rather than from a decreased level of hemoglobin.

	(IRON EXCESS)*			(IRON INSUFFICIENCY)			
				NEGATIVE BALANCE			
	POSITIVE BALANCE		NORMAL	DEPLETION		DEFICIENCY	
	STAGE II Iron overload EXCESS	STAGE I Positive iron balance	Normal	STAGE I Early negative iron balance	STAGE II Iron depletion	STAGE III Damaged metabolism: iron-deficient erythropoiesis	STAGE IV Clinical damage: iron deficiency anemia
Iron stores / Circulating iron / Erythron iron							
RE marrow Fe	4+	3+	2-3+	1+	0-1+	0	0
Transferrin IBC (mcg/100ml)†	<300	<300	330 ± 30	300-360	360	390	410
Plasma ferritin (mcg/L)‡	>300	>150	100 ± 60	<25	20	10	<10
Iron absorption (%)	>15	10-15	5-10	10-15	10-15	10-20	10-20
Plasma iron (mcg/100ml)†	>175	>150	115 ± 50	<120	115	<60	<40
Transferrin saturation (%)†	>60	>45	35 ± 15	30	30	<15	<15
Sideroblasts (%)	40-60	40-60	40-60	40-60	40-60	<10	<10
RBC protoporphyrin	30	30	30	30	30	100	200
Erythrocytes	Normal	Normal	Normal	Normal	Normal	Normal	Microcytic/ hypochromic
Serum transferrin receptors	Normal	Normal	Normal	Normal-High	High	Very high	Very high
Ferritin-iron (haloferritin) (ng/ml)§	Very high	High	Normal	Normal-Low	Low	Very low	Very low

*Randall Lauffer of Harvard and Joe McCord of University of Colorado–Denver hold that *any* storage iron is excessive because of its potential to promote excessive free radical generation. (Herbert V et al: Most free radical injury is iron related, *Stem Cells* 12:289, 1994.)
†Inflammation reduces transferrin (and the plasma iron on it), because transferrin is a reverse acute-phase reactant.
‡Inflammation produces elevated ferritin, because ferritin protein is an acute-phase reactant.
§Ferritin-iron is unaffected by inflammation, so it is reliable when ferritin, transferrin, and plasma iron are not.
Dallman (pediatrician) definition of negative balance: less absorbed than *excreted.*
Herbert (internist) definition of negative balance: less absorbed than *needed.*

FIGURE 33-1 Sequential stages of iron status. *IBC,* Iron-binding capacity; *RBC,* red blood cell; *RE,* reticuloendothelial cells. *(Copyright Victor Herbert, 1995.)*

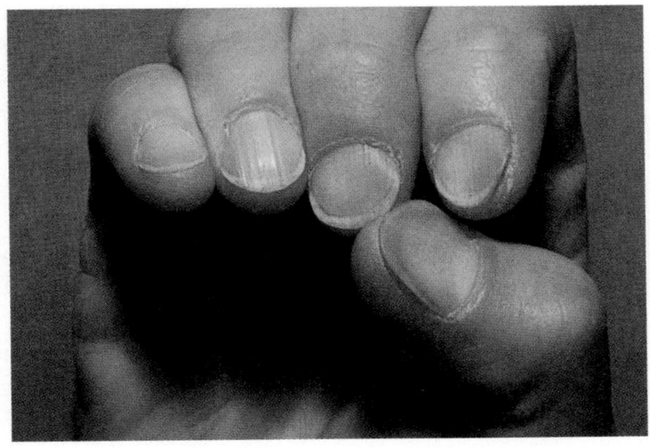

FIGURE 33-2 Fingernails with cuplike depressions (koilonychia) are a sign of iron deficiency in adults. *(From Callen JP et al: Color atlas of dermatology, Philadelphia, 1993, Saunders.)*

Diagnosis

A definitive diagnosis of iron-deficiency anemia requires more than one method of iron evaluation; **ferritin**, iron and transferrin are the most useful. The evaluation should also include an assessment of cell morphology. By itself, hemoglobin concentration is unsuitable as a diagnostic tool in cases of suspected iron-deficiency anemia for three reasons: (1) it is affected only late in the disease, (2) it cannot distinguish iron deficiency from other anemias, and (3) hemoglobin values in normal individuals vary widely.

After absorption, iron is transported by plasma **transferrin**—a β1-globulin (protein) that binds iron derived from the gastrointestinal tract, iron storage sites, or hemoglobin breakdown—to the bone marrow (hemoglobin synthesis), endothelial cells (storage), or placenta (fetal needs). Transferrin molecules are generated on the surface of RBCs in response to the need for iron. With iron deficiency, so many **transferrin receptors** are on the cell surface looking for iron that some of them break off and float in the serum. Their presence is an early measurement of developing iron deficiency; a higher quantity of **soluble serum transferrin receptors (STFRs)** means greater deficiency of iron. Progressive stages of iron deficiency can be evaluated by measurements, as shown in Table 33-2.

Protoporphyrin is the iron-containing portion of the respiratory pigments that combines with protein to form hemoglobin or myoglobin. The zinc protoporphyrin (ZnPP)/heme ratio is measured to assess iron deficiency. However, this ZnPP/heme ratio and hemoglobin levels are affected by chronic infection and other factors that can produce a condition that mimics iron-deficiency anemia when, in fact, iron is adequate.

TABLE 33-2

Biochemical Evaluation of Iron Deficiency

Measure	Comment
Quantity of serum or plasma ferritin	The most sensitive indicator of negative iron balance
Quantity of serum or plasma iron	
Quantity of total circulating transferrin	
Percent saturation of circulating transferrin	This measures the iron supply to the tissues. It is calculated by dividing serum iron by the TIBC; levels less than 16% are considered inadequate for erythropoiesis.
Percent saturation of ferritin with iron	
Quantity of STFR	STFR measures early iron deficiency.

STFR, Soluble serum transferrin receptor; *TIBC*, total iron-binding capacity.

Medical Management

Treatment of iron-deficiency anemia should focus primarily on the underlying cause, although this is often difficult to determine. The goal is repletion of iron stores.

Oral Supplementation. The chief treatment for iron-deficiency anemia involves oral administration of inorganic iron in the ferrous form. Although the body uses both ferric and ferrous iron, the reduced ferrous is easier on the gut and better absorbed. At a dose of 30 mg, absorption of ferrous iron is three times greater than if the same amount were given in the ferric form. Chelated forms of iron (combined with amino acids) are more bioavailable than nonchelated iron. Chelated iron is less affected by phytate, oxalate, phosphate, and calcium (all iron absorption inhibitors). Chelated iron causes less gastrointestinal disturbances than elemental iron because it is needed in lower doses when it is absorbed into mucosal cells (Ashmead, 2001).

Iron is best absorbed when the stomach is empty; however, under these conditions it tends to cause gastric irritation. Gastrointestinal side effects can include nausea, epigastric discomfort and distention, heartburn, diarrhea, or constipation. If these side effects occur, the patient is told to take the iron with meals instead of on an empty stomach; however, this sharply reduces the absorbability of the iron. Gastric irritation is a direct result of the high quantity of free ferrous iron in the stomach.

Health professionals usually prescribe oral iron for 3 months (three times daily) to treat iron deficiency. Depending on the severity of the anemia and the patient's tolerance, the daily dose of elemental iron should be 50 to 200 mg for adults and 6 mg/kg of body weight for children. Ascorbic acid greatly increases both iron absorption and gastric irritation through its capacity to maintain iron in the reduced state.

Absorption of 10 to 20 mg of iron per day permits RBC production to increase to approximately three times the normal rate and, in the absence of blood loss, hemoglobin concentration to rise at a rate of 0.2 g/dL daily. Increased **reticulocytosis** (an increase in the number of young RBCs) is seen within 2 to 3 days after iron administration, but affected persons may report subjective improvements in mood and appetite sooner. The hemoglobin level will begin to increase by day 4. Iron therapy should be continued for 4 to 5 months, even after restoration of normal hemoglobin levels, to allow for repletion of body iron reserves.

Parenteral Iron-Dextran. If iron supplementation fails to correct the anemia, (1) the patient may not be taking the medication as prescribed; (2) bleeding may be continuing at a rate faster than the erythroid marrow can replace blood cells; or (3) the supplemental iron is not being absorbed, possibly as a result of malabsorption secondary to steatorrhea, celiac disease, or hemodialysis. In these circumstances parenteral administration of iron in the form of iron-dextran may be necessary. Although replenishment of iron stores by this route is faster, it is more expensive than, and not as safe as oral administration.

Medical Nutrition Therapy

In addition to iron supplementation, attention should be given to the amount of absorbable dietary iron consumed. A good source of iron contains a substantial amount of iron in relation to its calorie content and contributes at least 10% of the recommended dietary allowance (RDA) for iron. Liver; kidney; beef; dried fruits; dried peas and beans; nuts; green leafy vegetables; and fortified whole-grain breads, muffins, cereals, and nutrition bars are among the foods that rank highest in iron content (see Appendix 54). It is estimated that 1.8 mg of iron must be absorbed daily to meet the needs of 80% to 90% of adult women and adolescent boys and girls.

Bioavailability of Dietary Iron. Because typical Western diets generally contain 6 mg/1000 kcal of iron, the bioavailability of iron in the diet is more important in correcting or preventing iron deficiency than the total amount of dietary iron consumed. The rate of absorption depends on the iron status of the individual, as reflected in the level of iron stores. The lower the iron stores, the greater the rate of iron absorption. Individuals with iron-deficiency anemia absorb approximately 20% to 30% of dietary iron compared with the 5% to 10% absorbed by those without iron deficiency.

Form of Iron. **Heme iron** (approximately 15% of which is absorbable) is the organic form in meat, fish, and poultry, and is known as the **meat-fish-poultry (MFP) factor**. It is much better absorbed than nonheme iron. **Nonheme iron** can be found in MFP, as well as in eggs, grains, vegetables, and fruits, but it is not part of the heme molecule. The absorption rate of nonheme iron varies between 3% and 8%, depending on the presence of dietary enhancing factors, specifically ascorbic acid and meat, fish, and poultry. Ascorbic acid is not only a powerful reducing agent, but it also binds iron to form a readily absorbed complex. The mechanism by which the MFP factor potentiates the absorption of nonheme iron in other foodstuffs is unknown.

Inhibitors. Iron absorption can be inhibited to varying degrees by factors that chelate iron, including carbonates, oxalates, phosphates, and phytates (unleavened bread, unrefined cereals, and soybeans). Factors in vegetable fiber may inhibit nonheme iron absorption. If taken with meals, tea and coffee can reduce iron absorption by 50% through the formation of insoluble iron compounds with tannin. Iron in egg yolk is poorly absorbed because of the presence of phosvitin.

IRON OVERLOAD

Excess iron is stored as ferritin and hemosiderin in the macrophages of the liver, spleen, and bone marrow. The body has a limited capacity to excrete iron. Approximately 1 mg of iron is excreted daily through the gastrointestinal tract, urinary tract, and skin. To maintain a normal iron balance, the daily obligatory loss must be replaced by the absorption of heme and nonheme food iron. Persons with iron overload excrete increased amounts of iron, especially in the feces, to compensate partially for the increased absorption and higher stores.

Excessive iron intake usually stems from accidental incorporation of iron into the diet from environmental sources. In developing countries the iron overload can result from eating foods cooked in cast-iron cooking vessels or contaminated by iron-containing soils. In developed countries it likely results from excessive intake of iron-supplemented foods or multivitamin and mineral supplementation.

Uncommon disorders associated with iron overload or toxicity include thalassemias, sideroblastic anemia, chronic hemolytic anemia, ineffective erythropoiesis, transfusional iron overload (secondary to multiple blood transfusions), porphyria cutanea tarda, aplastic anemia, and alcoholic cirrhosis. **Aplastic anemia** is a normochromic-normocytic anemia accompanied by a deficiency of all the formed elements in the blood; it can be caused by exposure to toxic chemicals, ionizing radiation, and medications, although the cause is often unknown.

Brain iron increases with age, is higher in men, and is abnormally elevated in neurodegenerative diseases, including Alzheimer disease and Parkinson disease (Bartzokis et al., 2010). Several gene variants affect iron metabolism and may contribute to early onset of these conditions.

Hemochromatosis

Hemochromatosis is the most common form of iron overload that causes progressive hepatic, pancreatic, cardiac, and other organ damage. People with this condition absorb three times more iron from their food than those without hemochromatosis. This disease, associated with the HFE gene, is often underdiagnosed. Persons who have two affected genes (homozygotes) will die of iron overload unless they donate blood frequently. Otherwise, the excessive iron absorption continues unabated.

Asians and Pacific Islanders have the highest levels of iron in their blood of all racial and ethnic groups, but they have the lowest prevalence of the gene mutation found with the typical form of hemochromatosis (Adams et al., 2005). The Hemochromatosis and Iron Overload Screening Study notes that non-Hispanic whites have the highest prevalence of the C282Y mutation of the hereditary iron (HFE) gene, followed by Native Americans, Hispanics, blacks, Pacific Islanders, and Asians.

In women, monthly menses slow the associated organ damage until after menopause (Adams et al., 2005). Men are particularly susceptible to hemochromatosis because they have no physiologic mechanisms for losing iron such as menstruation, pregnancy, or lactation.

Pathophysiology

Hepcidin is a peptide synthesized in the liver that functions as the principal regulator of systemic iron homeostasis. It regulates iron transport from iron-exporting tissues into plasma. Hepcidin deficiency underlies most known forms of hereditary hemochromatosis (Nemeth and Ganz, 2006). Hepcidin inhibits the cellular efflux of iron by binding to and inducing the degradation of **ferroprotein**, the sole iron exporter in iron-transporting cells. Hepcidin controls plasma iron concentration and tissue distribution of iron by inhibiting intestinal iron absorption, iron recycling by macrophages, and iron mobilization from hepatic stores.

Hepcidin synthesis is increased by iron loading and decreased by anemia and hypoxia. Its synthesis is also greatly increased during inflammation, trapping iron in macrophages, decreasing plasma iron concentrations, and causing iron-restricted erythropoiesis that is characteristic of anemia of chronic disease. There is evidence that the mutation of the HFE gene leading to hemochromatosis is also associated with increased levels of gastrin in the stomach, leading to increased levels of gastric acid and thus increased absorption of iron (Smith et al., 2006).

In hemochromatosis iron absorption is enhanced, resulting in a gradual, progressive accumulation of iron. Most affected persons do not know they have it. In its early stages iron overload may result in symptoms similar to iron deficiency such as fatigue and weakness; later it can cause chronic abdominal pain, aching joints, impotence, and menstrual irregularities.

A progressive, positive iron balance may result in a variety of serious problems, including hepatomegaly, skin pigmentation, arthritis, heart disease, hypogonadism, diabetes mellitus, and cancer. Individuals with abnormally high iron levels are more likely to develop cancer of the colon. Iron is a prooxidant that can be used for tumor cell growth and proliferation. There also seems to be increased risk for age-related macular degeneration and Alzheimer disease because of the oxidant effect of iron overload (Connor and Lee, 2006; Dunaief, 2006).

Assessment

If an iron overload is suspected, the following screening tests should be performed: serum ferritin level (storage iron), serum iron concentration, TIBC, and percent of transferrin saturation ([serum iron/TIBC] × 100). Iron overload may be present if the percent of transferrin saturation is greater than 50 in women and 60 in men, and if the serum iron level is greater than 180 mg/dL. Deoxyribonucleic acid (DNA) testing, using blood or cheek cell samples, is also available for early detection of hemochromatosis. Liver biopsy is the gold standard for the diagnosis of iron overload.

Medical Management

The patient with iron overload may simultaneously be anemic as a result of damage to the bone marrow, an inflammatory disorder, cancer, internal bleeding, or chronic infection. Iron supplements should not be taken until the cause is known.

For patients with significant iron overload, weekly phlebotomy for 2 to 3 years may be required to eliminate all excess iron. Treatment for iron overload may also involve iron depletion with intravenous desferrioxamine-B, a chelating agent that is excreted by the kidneys, or with calcium disodium ethylenediaminetetraacetic acid (EDTA). Mortality is preventable if excess body iron is removed by phlebotomy therapy before hepatic cirrhosis develops. Patients diagnosed as having hemochromatosis should inform all blood relatives so they can be evaluated.

Medical Nutrition Therapy

Individuals with iron overload should ingest less heme iron from meat, fish, and poultry compared with nonheme iron from plant foods. Persons with iron overload should also avoid alcohol and vitamin C supplements because both enhance iron absorption. In addition, vitamin C supplements may cause release of harmful free radical–generating excess iron from body stores.

Affected persons should avoid foods that are highly fortified with iron (i.e., many breakfast cereals, fortified "energy" or sports bars, and many meal-replacement drinks or shakes that are fortified with vitamins and minerals). They should also avoid iron supplements or multiple vitamin and mineral supplements that contain iron. The dietary requirement for iron should not be exceeded, and perhaps the intake of iron should be less in some persons. The dietary reference intakes (DRIs) for iron are summarized on the inside front cover. The RDA for women in their child-bearing years is 18 mg; for pregnant women, 27 mg; and the RDA for adult men and women 51 years of age and older is 8 mg.

MEGALOBLASTIC ANEMIAS

Megaloblastic anemia reflects a disturbed synthesis of DNA, which results in morphologic and functional changes in erythrocytes, leukocytes, platelets, and their precursors in the blood and bone marrow. This anemia is characterized by the presence of large, immature, abnormal, RBC progenitors in the bone marrow; 95% of cases are attributable to folic acid or vitamin B_{12} deficiency. Two disorders of cobalamin metabolism arise from mutations of the methionine synthase and methionine synthase reductase genes; these disorders feature both megaloblastic anemia and neurologic manifestations.

Both vitamins are essential to the synthesis of nucleoproteins. Hematologic changes are the same for both; however, the folic acid deficiency is the first to appear. Normal body folate stores are depleted within 2 to 4 months in individuals consuming folate-deficient diets. By contrast, vitamin B_{12} stores are depleted only after several years of a vitamin B_{12}–deficient diet. In persons with vitamin B_{12} deficiency, folic acid supplementation can mask B_{12} deficiency (Figure 33-3). In correcting the anemia, the vitamin B_{12} deficiency may remain undetected, leading to the irreversible neuropsychiatric damage that is only corrected with B_{12} supplementation (see Chapters 3 and 8).

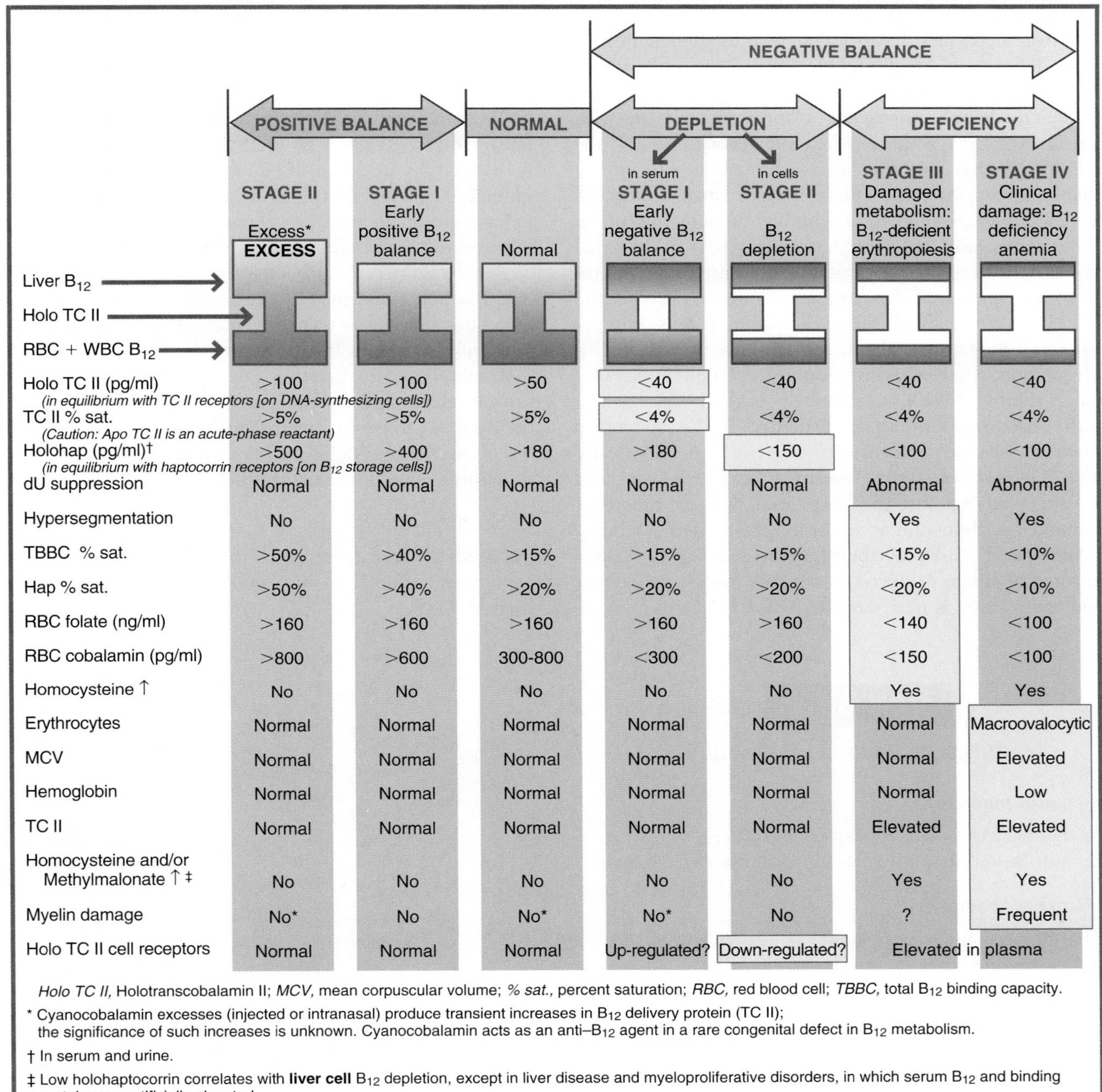

	POSITIVE BALANCE		NORMAL	DEPLETION		DEFICIENCY	
	STAGE II Excess*	STAGE I Early positive B_{12} balance	Normal	in serum STAGE I Early negative B_{12} balance	in cells STAGE II B_{12} depletion	STAGE III Damaged metabolism: B_{12}-deficient erythropoiesis	STAGE IV Clinical damage: B_{12} deficiency anemia
Holo TC II (pg/ml) (in equilibrium with TC II receptors [on DNA-synthesizing cells])	>100	>100	>50	<40	<40	<40	<40
TC II % sat. (Caution: Apo TC II is an acute-phase reactant)	>5%	>5%	>5%	<4%	<4%	<4%	<4%
Holohap (pg/ml)† (in equilibrium with haptocorrin receptors [on B_{12} storage cells])	>500	>400	>180	>180	<150	<100	<100
dU suppression	Normal	Normal	Normal	Normal	Normal	Abnormal	Abnormal
Hypersegmentation	No	No	No	No	No	Yes	Yes
TBBC % sat.	>50%	>40%	>15%	>15%	>15%	<15%	<10%
Hap % sat.	>50%	>40%	>20%	>20%	>20%	<20%	<10%
RBC folate (ng/ml)	>160	>160	>160	>160	>160	<140	<100
RBC cobalamin (pg/ml)	>800	>600	300-800	<300	<200	<150	<100
Homocysteine ↑	No	No	No	No	No	Yes	Yes
Erythrocytes	Normal	Normal	Normal	Normal	Normal	Normal	Macroovalocytic
MCV	Normal	Normal	Normal	Normal	Normal	Normal	Elevated
Hemoglobin	Normal	Normal	Normal	Normal	Normal	Normal	Low
TC II	Normal	Normal	Normal	Normal	Normal	Elevated	Elevated
Homocysteine and/or Methylmalonate ↑ ‡	No	No	No	No	No	Yes	Yes
Myelin damage	No*	No	No*	No*	No	?	Frequent
Holo TC II cell receptors	Normal	Normal	Normal	Up-regulated?	Down-regulated?	Elevated in plasma	

Holo TC II, Holotranscobalamin II; *MCV,* mean corpuscular volume; *% sat.,* percent saturation; *RBC,* red blood cell; *TBBC,* total B_{12} binding capacity.

* Cyanocobalamin excesses (injected or intranasal) produce transient increases in B_{12} delivery protein (TC II); the significance of such increases is unknown. Cyanocobalamin acts as an anti–B_{12} agent in a rare congenital defect in B_{12} metabolism.

† In serum and urine.

‡ Low holohaptocorrin correlates with **liver cell** B_{12} depletion, except in liver disease and myeloproliferative disorders, in which serum B_{12} and binding proteins are artificially elevated.

There may be hematopoietic cell and glial cell B_{12} depletion **prior to** liver cell depletion, and those cells may be in stage III or IV negative B_{12} balance, whereas liver cells are still in stage II.

FIGURE 33-3 Sequential stages of vitamin B_{12} status. *(From Herbert V: Staging vitamin B_{12}. In Ziegler EE, Filer LJ, editors: Present knowledge in nutrition, ed 7, Washington, DC, 1996, International Life Sciences Institute Press.)*

Folic Acid Deficiency Anemia

Etiology

Folic acid deficiency anemia is associated with tropical sprue, can affect pregnant women, and occurs in infants born to mothers with folic acid deficiency. Folic acid deficiency in early pregnancy can also result in an infant with a neural tube defect (see Chapter 16). Prolonged inadequate diets, faulty absorption and use of folic acid, and increased requirements resulting from growth are believed to be the most frequent causes. Other causes include gluten-induced enteropathy (childhood and adult celiac disease), idiopathic steatorrhea, nontropical sprue and drugs (anticonvulsants, barbiturates, cycloserine, ethanol, sulfasalazine, cholestyramine and metformin), and amino acid excess (glycine and methionine).

Because alcohol interferes with the folate enterohepatic cycle, most alcoholics have a negative folate balance or a folate deficiency. Alcoholics constitute the only group that generally has all six causes of folic acid deficiency simultaneously: inadequate ingestion, absorption, and use with increased excretion, requirement, and destruction of folic acid. Box 33-2 describes the causes of folate deficiency.

Folate absorption takes place in the small intestine. Enzyme conjugases (e.g., pteroylpolyglutamate hydrolase, the folate conjugase), found in the brush border of the small intestine, hydrolyze the polyglutamates to monoglutamates and reduce them to dihydrofolate and tetrahydrofolic acid (THFA) in the small intestinal epithelial cells (enterocytes). From the enterocytes these forms are transported to the circulation, where they are bound to protein and transported as methyl THFA into the cells of the body.

In the absence of vitamin B_{12}, 5-methyl THFA, the major circulating and storage form of folic acid, is metabolically inactive. To be activated the 5-methyl group is removed, and THFA is cycled back into the folate pool, where it functions as the main 1-carbon-unit acceptor in mammalian biochemical reactions. THFA may then be converted to the coenzyme form of folate required to convert deoxyuridylate to thymidylate, which is necessary for DNA synthesis.

MTHFR Allele. A genetic defect found in 10% of whites is the methylenetetrahydrofolate reductase (MTHFR) deficiency. (See Chapters 5 and 8.) The allele is problematic in pregnancy, and may contribute to miscarriages, anencephaly, or neural defects. Because MTHFR irreversibly reduces 5,10-methylenetetrahydrofolate to 5-methyltetrahydrofolate, its deficiency may result in developmental delay, motor and gait dysfunction, seizures, neurologic impairment, extremely high levels of homocysteine, clotting disorders, and other conditions.

Methylfolate Trap. Vitamin B_{12} deficiency can result in a folic acid deficiency by causing folate entrapment in the metabolically useless form of 5-methyl THFA (Figure 33-4). The lack of vitamin B_{12} to remove the 5-methyl unit means that metabolically inactive methyl THFA is trapped. It cannot release its 1-carbon methyl group to become THFA, the basic 1-carbon carrier that picks up 1-carbon units from one molecule and delivers them to another. Hence a functional folic acid deficiency results.

Pathophysiology

Folate deficiency develops in four stages: two that involve depletion, followed by two marked by deficiency (Figure 33-5):

BOX 33-2

Causes of Folate Deficiency

Inadequate Ingestion

Poor diet (lack of or overcooked fruits and vegetables), vitamin B_{12} or vitamin C deficiency, chronic alcoholism

Inadequate Absorption

Gluten-induced enteropathy or celiac disease, tropical sprue, drug interactions, congenital defects

Inadequate Utilization

Antagonists, anticonvulsants, enzyme deficiency, both vitamin B_{12} and vitamin C deficiency, chronic alcoholism, excess glycine and methionine

Increased Requirement

Extra tissue demand, infancy, increased hematopoiesis, increased metabolic activity, Lesch-Nyhan syndrome, drugs

Increased Excretion

Vitamin B_{12} deficiency, liver disease, kidney dialysis, chronic exfoliative dermatitis

Increased Destruction

Dietary oxidants

Modified from Herbert V, Das KC: Folic acid and vitamin B_{12}. In Shils ME et al., editors: Modern nutrition in health and disease, ed 8, vol 1, Philadelphia, 1994, Lea & Febiger.

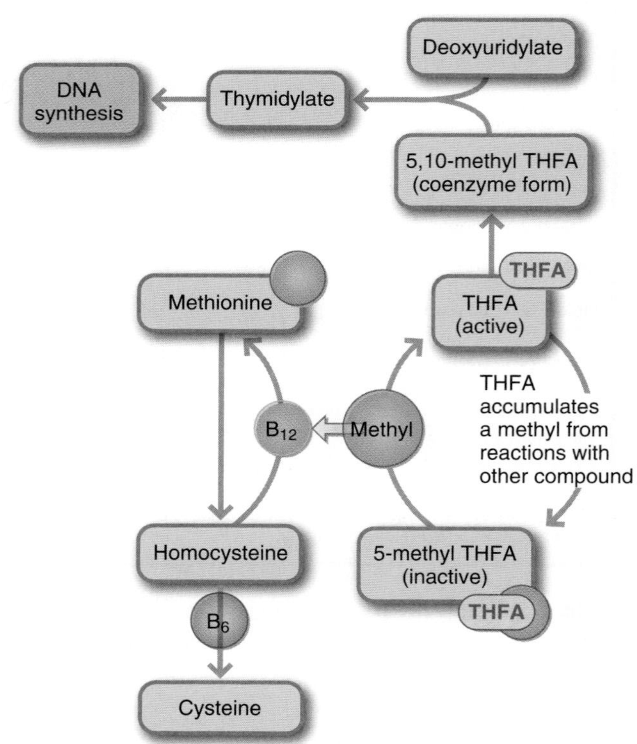

FIGURE 33-4 Methylfolate trap. A deficiency of vitamin B_{12} can result in a deficiency of folic acid because folate is trapped in the form of 5-methyltetrahydrofolate (5-methyl THFA), which cannot be converted to THFA and methyl groups donated by the vitamin B_{12}–dependent pathway. *DNA*, Deoxyribonucleic acid.

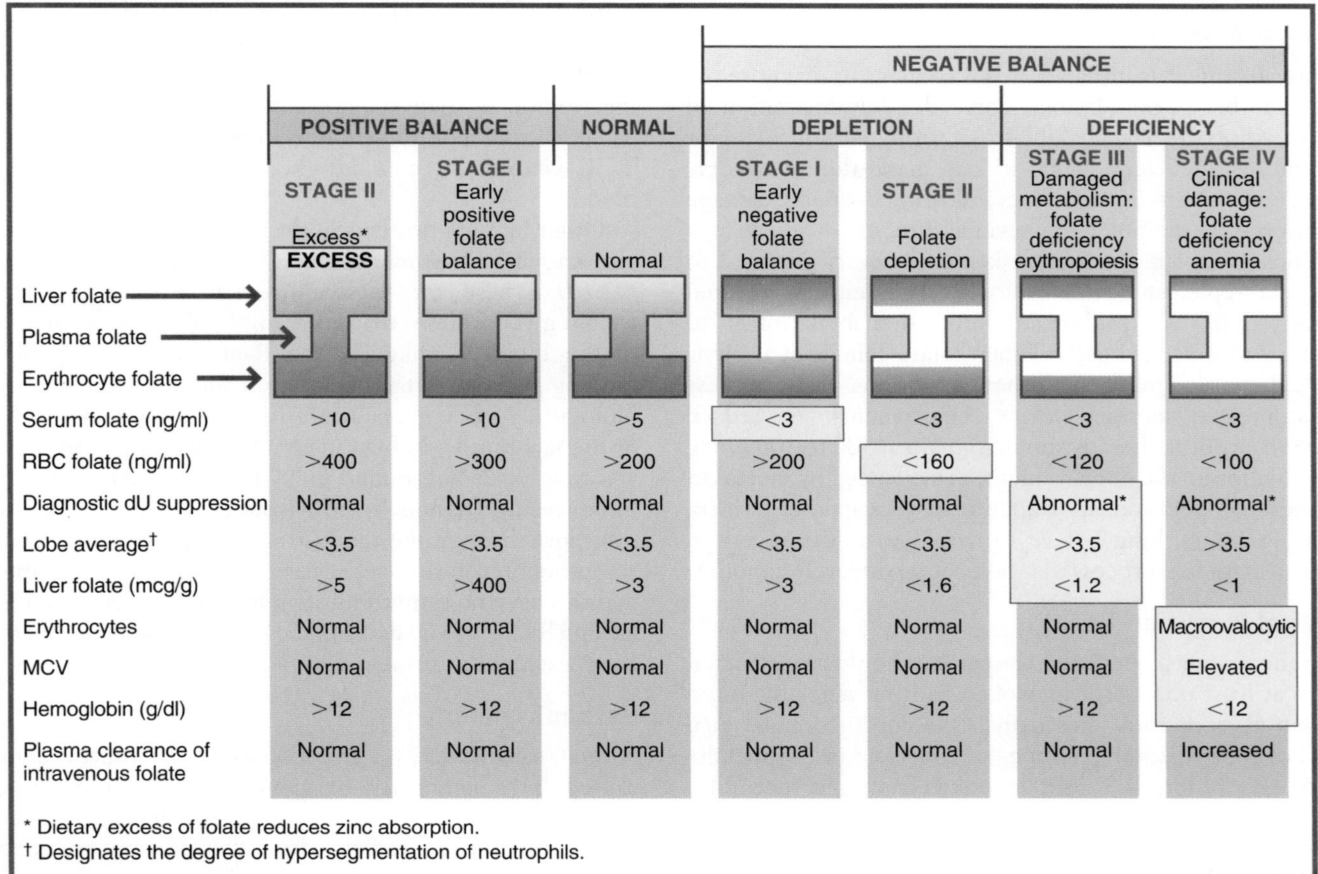

	POSITIVE BALANCE		NORMAL	NEGATIVE BALANCE: DEPLETION		NEGATIVE BALANCE: DEFICIENCY	
	STAGE II Excess* EXCESS	STAGE I Early positive folate balance	Normal	STAGE I Early negative folate balance	STAGE II Folate depletion	STAGE III Damaged metabolism: folate deficiency erythropoiesis	STAGE IV Clinical damage: folate deficiency anemia
Serum folate (ng/ml)	>10	>10	>5	<3	<3	<3	<3
RBC folate (ng/ml)	>400	>300	>200	>200	<160	<120	<100
Diagnostic dU suppression	Normal	Normal	Normal	Normal	Normal	Abnormal*	Abnormal*
Lobe average†	<3.5	<3.5	<3.5	<3.5	<3.5	>3.5	>3.5
Liver folate (mcg/g)	>5	>400	>3	>3	<1.6	<1.2	<1
Erythrocytes	Normal	Normal	Normal	Normal	Normal	Normal	Macroovalocytic
MCV	Normal	Normal	Normal	Normal	Normal	Normal	Elevated
Hemoglobin (g/dl)	>12	>12	>12	>12	>12	>12	<12
Plasma clearance of intravenous folate	Normal	Normal	Normal	Normal	Normal	Normal	Increased

* Dietary excess of folate reduces zinc absorption.
† Designates the degree of hypersegmentation of neutrophils.

FIGURE 33-5 Sequential stages of folate status. *dU*, Deoxyuridine; *MCV*, mean corpuscular volume; *RBC*, red blood cell. *(From Herbert V: Folic acid. In Shils ME, Olson JA, Shike M, editors: Modern nutrition in health and disease, ed 9, Philadelphia 1998, Lea & Febiger.)*

Stage 1: Characterized by early negative folate balance (serum depletion to less than 3 ng/mL).

Stage 2: Characterized by negative folate balance (cell depletion), with a decrease in erythrocyte folate levels to less than 160 ng/mL.

Stage 3: Characterized by damaged folate metabolism, with folate-deficient erythropoiesis. This stage is characterized by slowed DNA synthesis, manifested by an abnormal diagnostic deoxyuridine (dU) suppression test correctable in vitro by folates, granulocyte nuclear hypersegmentation, and macroovalocytic red cells.

Stage 4: Characterized by clinical folate-deficiency anemia, with an elevated MCV and anemia.

Because of their interrelated roles in the synthesis of thymidylate in DNA formation, a deficiency of either vitamin B_{12} or folic acid results in a megaloblastic anemia. The immature nuclei do not mature properly in the deficient state; and large (macrocytic), immature (megaloblastic) RBCs are the result. The common clinical signs of folic acid deficiency include fatigue, dyspnea, sore tongue, diarrhea, irritability, forgetfulness, anorexia, glossitis, and weight loss.

Assessment

Normal body folate stores are depleted within 2 to 4 months on a folate-deficient diet, resulting in a macrocytic, megaloblastic anemia with a decreased number of erythrocytes, leukocytes, and platelets. Folate-deficiency anemia is manifested by very low serum folate (<3 ng/mL) and RBC folate levels of less than 140-160 ng/mL. Whereas a low serum folate level merely diagnoses a negative balance at the time the blood is drawn, an red cell folate (RCF) level measures actual body folate stores and thus is the superior measurement for determining folate nutriture. To differentiate folate deficiency from vitamin B_{12} deficiency, levels of serum folate, RCF, serum vitamin B_{12}, and vitamin B_{12} bound to transcobalamin II (TCII) can be measured simultaneously using a radioassay kit. Also diagnostic for folate deficiency is an elevated level of formiminoglutamic acid in the urine, as well as the dU suppression test in bone marrow cells or peripheral blood lymphocytes. See Chapter 8.

Medical Management

Before treatment is initiated, it is important to diagnose the cause of the megaloblastosis correctly. Administration of folate will correct megaloblastosis from either folate or vitamin B_{12} deficiency, but it can mask the neurologic damage of vitamin B_{12} deficiency, allowing the nerve damage to progress to the point of irreversibility.

A dosage of 1 mg of folate taken orally every day for 2 to 3 weeks replenishes folate stores. Maintaining repleted stores requires an absolute minimum oral intake of 50 to 100 mcg of folic acid daily. When folate deficiency is complicated by alcoholism or other conditions that suppress hematopoiesis, increase folate requirements, or reduce folate absorption, therapy should remain at 500 to 1000 mcg daily. Symptomatic improvement, as evidenced by increased alertness, cooperation, and appetite, may be apparent within 24 to 48 hours, long before hematologic values revert to normal, a gradual process that takes approximately a month.

Medical Nutrition Therapy

After the anemia is corrected, the patient should be instructed to eat at least one fresh, uncooked fruit or vegetable or to drink a glass of fruit juice daily. One cup of orange juice supplies approximately 135 mcg of folic acid (see Appendix 46 for a list of foods). Fresh, uncooked fruits and vegetables are good sources of folate because folate can easily be destroyed by heat. In 1998 the Food and Drug Administration required that grains be fortified with folic acid. The DRIs for folate are RDAs and are summarized on the inside front cover of this text. The RDA for adults is 400 mcg daily. The Dietary Guidelines for Americans recommend that women of childbearing age who may become pregnant and those in their first trimester of pregnancy consume adequate synthetic folic acid (600 mcg/day) from fortified foods and supplements in addition to consuming a variety of foods containing folate.

Vitamin B_{12} Deficiency and Pernicious Anemias

Intrinsic factor (IF) is a glycoprotein in the gastric juice that is necessary for the absorption of dietary vitamin B_{12}. Secreted by parietal cells of the gastric mucosa, IF is necessary for the absorption of exogenous vitamin B_{12}. Ingested vitamin B_{12} is freed from protein by gastric acid and gastric and intestinal enzymes. The free vitamin B_{12} attaches to salivary R-binder, which has a higher affinity for the vitamin than does IF. An acid pH (2.3) is needed, such as that found in the healthy stomach.

The release of pancreatic trypsin into the proximal small intestine destroys R-binder and releases vitamin B_{12} from its complex with R-protein. With an alkaline pH (6.8) in the intestine, IF binds the vitamin B_{12}. The vitamin B_{12}–IF complex is then carried to the ileum. In the ileum, with the presence of ionic calcium (Ca^{2+}) and a pH (>6), the complex attaches to the surface vitamin B_{12}–IF receptors on the ileal cell brush border. Here, the vitamin B_{12} is released and attaches to **holotranscobalamin II (holo TCII)**. Holo TCII is vitamin B_{12} attached to the β-globulin, the major circulating vitamin B_{12} delivery protein. Like IF, holo TCII plays an active role in binding and transporting vitamin B_{12}. The TCII–vitamin B_{12} complex then enters the portal venous blood.

Other binding proteins in the blood include haptocorrin, also known as *transcobalamin I (TCI)* and *transcobalamin III (TCIII)*. These are α-globulins, larger macromolecular-weight glycoproteins that make up the R-binder component of the blood. Unlike IF, the R-proteins are capable of binding not only vitamin B_{12} itself but also to many of its biologically inactive analogs. Although approximately 75% of the vitamin B_{12} in human serum is bound to haptocorrin and roughly 25% is bound to TCII, only TCII is important in delivering vitamin B_{12} to all the cells that need it. After transport through the bloodstream, TCII is recognized by receptors on cell surfaces. Patients with haptocorrin abnormalities have no symptoms of vitamin B_{12} deficiency. Those lacking TCII rapidly develop megaloblastic anemia. Vitamin B_{12} is excreted in urine.

Pathophysiology

Pernicious anemia is a megaloblastic, macrocytic anemia caused by a deficiency of vitamin B_{12}, most commonly from a lack of IF. Rarely, vitamin B_{12} deficiency anemia occurs in strict vegetarians whose diet contains no vitamin B_{12} except for traces found in plants contaminated by microorganisms capable of synthesizing vitamin B_{12}. Other causes include antibody to IF in saliva or gastric juice; small intestinal disorders affecting the ileum such as celiac disease, idiopathic steatorrhea, tropical sprue, cancers involving the small intestine; drugs (paraaminosalicylic acid, colchicine, neomycin, metformin, antiretrovirals); and long-term ingestion of alcohol or calcium-chelating agents (Table 33-3).

Stages of Deficiency

As a result of normal enterohepatic circulation (i.e., excretion of vitamin B_{12} and analogs in bile and resorption of vitamin B_{12} in the ileum), it generally takes decades for strict vegetarians who are not receiving vitamin B_{12} supplementation to develop a vitamin B_{12} deficiency. Serum B_{12}, homocysteine, and methylmalonic acid levels are not as effective as predictors of B_{12}-responsive neurologic disorders; patients with unexplained leukoencephalopathy should be treated proactively because even long-standing deficits may be reversible (Graber et al., 2010).

Stage 1: Early **negative vitamin B_{12} balance** begins when vitamin B_{12} intake is low or absorption is poor, depleting the primary delivery protein, TCII. A low TCII (<40 pg/mL) may be the earliest detectable sign of a vitamin B_{12} deficiency (Serefhanoglu et al., 2008). This is a vitamin B_{12} predeficiency stage.

TABLE 33-3

Causes of Vitamin B_{12} Deficiency

Inadequate ingestion	Poor diet resulting from a vegan diet and lack of supplementation, chronic alcoholism, poverty
Inadequate absorption	Gastric disorders, small intestinal disorders, competition for absorption sites, pancreatic disease, HIV or AIDS
Inadequate utilization	Vitamin B_{12} antagonists, congenital or acquired enzyme deficiency, abnormal binding proteins
Increased requirement	Hyperthyroidism, increased hematopoiesis
Increased excretion	Inadequate vitamin B_{12} binding protein, liver disease, renal disease
Increased destruction	Pharmacologic doses of ascorbic acid by antioxidants

AIDS, Acquired immune deficiency syndrome; *HIV*, human immunodeficiency virus.

Stage 2: Vitamin B_{12} depletion shows a low B_{12} on TCII and a gradual lowering of B_{12} in haptocorrin (holohap <150 pg/mL), the storage protein.

Stage 3: Damaged metabolism and vitamin B_{12}–deficient erythropoiesis includes an abnormal dU suppression, hypersegmentation, a decreased TIBC and holohap percent saturation, a low RCF level (<140 ng/mL), and subtle neuropsychiatric damage (impaired short-term and recent memory).

Stage 4: Clinical damage occurs, including vitamin B_{12} deficiency anemia; includes all preceding parameters, including macroovalocytic erythrocytes, elevated MCV, elevated TCII levels, increased homocysteine (see Chapter 34) and methylmalonic acid levels, and myelin damage. Leukoencephalopathy and autonomic dysfunction occur with very low serum B_{12} levels (<200 pg/mL); psychiatric changes, neuropathy, and dementia may also occur (Graber et al., 2010).

Clinical Findings

Pernicious anemia affects not only the blood but also the gastrointestinal tract and the peripheral and central nervous systems. This distinguishes it from folic acid deficiency anemia. The overt symptoms, which are caused by inadequate myelinization of the nerves, include paresthesia (especially numbness and tingling in the hands and feet), diminution of the senses of vibration and position, poor muscular coordination, poor memory, and hallucinations. If the deficiency is prolonged, the nervous system damage may be irreversible, even with initiation of vitamin B_{12} treatment.

Helicobacter pylori causes peptic ulcer disease and chronic gastritis. Both conditions are associated with hypochlorhydria, reduced production of IF by epithelial cells in the stomach, vitamin B_{12} malabsorption, and pernicious anemia. There is also a correlation between autoimmune gastritis and pernicious anemia. More than 90% of patients with pernicious anemia have parietal cell antibodies (PCAs) and 50% to 70% have elevated IF antibodies. Serum vitamin B_{12} levels of the *H. pylori*–infected patients are significantly lower than that of uninfected patients (Sarari et al., 2008).

A study on *H. pylori* infection and autoimmune type atrophic gastritis examined serum markers for gastric atrophy (pepsinogen I, pepsinogen I/II, and gastrin) and autoimmunity. Positive serum autoimmune markers (IF antibodies and PCA) suggest that *H. pylori* contributes to autoimmune gastritis and pernicious anemia (Veijola et al., 2010).

Vitamin B_{12} deficiency is an important modifiable risk factor for osteoporosis in both men and women. Adults with vitamin B_{12} levels below 148 pg/mL have a lower average bone mineral density and greater risk for osteoporosis (Tucker and Mayer, 2005).

Reduced vitamin B_{12} status and elevated homocysteine concentrations are common. These alterations are problematic among vegans (Elmadfa and Singer, 2009). B_{12}-folate-homocysteine interactions aggravate heart disease and may lead to adverse pregnancy outcomes (Moreiras et al., 2009).

Diagnosis

Vitamin B_{12} stores are depleted after several years without vitamin B_{12} intake. A low holo-TCII value (<40 pg/mL) is a sign of early B_{12} deficiency. Radioassays measure more than one component within the same biologic medium. The Becton-Dickinson SimulTRAC Radioassay Kit measures the levels of serum vitamin B_{12} and serum folate simultaneously in a single test tube.

Other laboratory tests that may be helpful in diagnosing a vitamin B_{12} deficiency and determining its cause include measurements of unsaturated B_{12} binding capacity, IF antibody (IFAB), the Schilling test, the dU suppression test, and tests to determine serum homocysteine and serum methionine levels (see Chapter 8). The IFAB and Schilling urinary excretion tests can determine whether the deficiency is caused by a lack of IF. The IFAB assay is performed on a patient's serum, whereas the Schilling test requires that the patient first swallow radioactive B_{12} alone and then a second time with IF.

The vitamin B_{12} assay is performed on the patient's urine after both steps of the Schilling test are completed. Patients with pernicious anemia excrete very little vitamin B_{12} during the first step because little or no vitamin B_{12} is absorbed. However, during the second step the urinary excretion becomes almost normal because more vitamin B_{12} is absorbed with the addition of the IF. Vitamin B_{12} deficiency secondary to malabsorption syndrome is manifested by a decrease in urinary excretion of B_{12} that remains unchanged with IF administration.

Medical Management

Treatment usually consists of an intramuscular or subcutaneous injection of 100 mcg or more of vitamin B_{12} once per week. After an initial response is elicited, the frequency of administration is reduced until remission can be maintained indefinitely with monthly injections of 100 mcg. Very large oral doses of vitamin B_{12} (1000 mcg daily) are also effective, even in the absence of IF, because approximately 1% of vitamin B_{12} will be absorbed by diffusion. Initial doses should be increased when vitamin B_{12} deficiency is complicated by debilitating illness such as infection, hepatic disease, uremia, coma, severe disorientation, or marked neurologic damage. A response to treatment is evidenced by improved appetite, alertness, and cooperation, followed by improved hematologic results, as manifested by marked reticulocytosis within hours of an injection.

Medical Nutrition Therapy

A high-protein diet (1.5 g/kg of body weight) is desirable both for liver function and for blood regeneration. Because green leafy vegetables contain both iron and folic acid, the diet should contain increased amounts of these foods. Meats (especially beef and pork), eggs, milk, and milk products are particularly rich in vitamin B_{12} (see Appendix 46).

For those individuals prescribed metformin for treatment of diabetes, 10% to 30% have reduced vitamin B_{12} absorption. Metformin negatively affects the calcium-dependent membrane and the B_{12}-IF complex by decreasing the absorbability by the ileal cell surface receptors. Increased intake of calcium reverses the vitamin B_{12} malabsorption (see Chapter 9).

The Dietary Guidelines for Americans recommend that people older than age 50 consume vitamin B_{12} in its crystalline form (i.e., fortified cereals or supplements) to overcome the effects of atrophic gastritis. The DRIs for B_{12} are RDAs and are summarized on the inside front cover. The RDA for adult men and women is 2.4 mcg daily.

OTHER NUTRITIONAL ANEMIAS

Anemia of Protein-Energy Malnutrition

Protein is essential for the proper production of hemoglobin and RBCs. Because of the reduction in cell mass and thus oxygen requirements in protein-energy malnutrition (PEM), fewer RBCs are required to oxygenate the tissue. Because blood volume remains the same, this reduced number of RBCs with a low hemoglobin level (**hypochromic**, normocytic anemia), which can mimic an iron-deficiency anemia, is actually a physiologic (nonharmful) rather than harmful anemia. In acute PEM, the loss of active tissue mass may be greater than the reduction in the number of RBCs, leading to polycythemia. The body responds to this RBC production, which is not a reflection of protein and amino acid deficiency but of an oversupply of RBCs. Iron released from normal RBC destruction is not reused in RBC production but is stored, so that iron stores are often adequate. Iron-deficiency anemia can reappear with rehabilitation when RBC mass expands rapidly.

The anemia of PEM may be complicated by deficiencies of iron and other nutrients and by associated infections, parasitic infestation, and malabsorption. A diet lacking in protein is usually deficient in iron, folic acid, and, less frequently, vitamin B_{12}. The nutrition counselor plays an important role in assessing recent and typical dietary intake of these nutrients.

Copper-Deficiency Anemia

Copper and other heavy metals are essential for the proper formation of hemoglobin. Ceruloplasmin, a copper-containing protein, is required for normal mobilization of iron from its storage sites to the plasma. In a copper-deficient state, iron cannot be released; this leads to low serum iron and hemoglobin levels, even in the presence of normal iron stores. Other consequences of copper deficiency suggest that copper proteins are needed for use of iron by the developing erythrocyte and for optimal functions of the erythrocyte membrane (see Chapter 3). The amounts of copper needed for normal hemoglobin synthesis are so minute that they are usually amply supplied by an adequate diet; however, copper deficiency may occur in infants who are fed cow's milk or a copper-deficient infant formula. It may also be seen in children or adults who have a malabsorption syndrome or who are receiving long-term total parenteral nutrition that does not supply copper.

Sideroblastic (Pyridoxine-Responsive) Anemia

Sideroblastic anemia is characterized by a derangement in the final pathway of heme synthesis, leading to a buildup of iron-containing immature RBCs. It has four primary characteristics: (1) microcytic and hypochromic RBCs; (2) high serum and tissue iron levels (causing increased transferrin saturation); (3) the presence of an inherited defect in the formation of δ-aminolevulinic acid synthetase, an enzyme involved in heme synthesis (pyridoxal-5-phosphate is necessary in this reaction); and (4) a buildup of iron-containing immature RBCs (sideroblasts, for which the anemia is named). The iron that cannot be used for heme synthesis is stored in the mitochondria of immature RBCs. These iron-laden mitochondria do not function normally, and the development and production of RBCs become ineffective. The symptoms are those of both anemia and iron overload. The neurologic and cutaneous manifestations of vitamin B_6 deficiency are not observed. The anemia responds to the administration of pharmacologic doses of pyridoxine and thus is referred to as ***vitamin B_6 (pyridoxine)–responsive anemia***, to distinguish it from anemia caused by a dietary vitamin B_6 deficiency.

Treatment consists of a therapeutic trial dose of 50 to 200 mg daily of pyridoxine or pyridoxal phosphate, which is 25 to 100 times the RDA. If the anemia responds to one or the other, pyridoxine therapy is continued for life. However, the anemia is only partially corrected; a normal hematocrit value is never regained. Patients respond to this treatment to varying degrees, and some may achieve near-normal hemoglobin levels.

Acquired sideroblastic anemias such as those attributable to drug therapy (isoniazid, chloramphenicol), copper deficiency, hypothermia, and alcoholism are not responsive to vitamin B_6 (pyridoxine) administration.

Vitamin E–Responsive Hemolytic Anemia

Hemolytic anemia occurs when defects in RBC membranes lead to oxidative damage and eventually to cell lysis.

This anemia is caused by shortened survival of mature RBCs. Vitamin E, an antioxidant, is involved in protecting the membrane against oxidative damage, and one of the few signs noted in vitamin E deficiency is early hemolysis of RBCs (see Chapter 3). Vitamin E–responsive hemolytic anemia in neonates is discussed in Chapter 43.

NONNUTRITIONAL ANEMIAS

Anemia of Pregnancy

A physiologic anemia is the anemia of pregnancy, which is related to increased blood volume and usually resolves with the end of the pregnancy; however, demands for iron during pregnancy are also increased so that inadequate iron intake may also play a role (see Chapter 16 for further discussion).

Anemia of Chronic Disease

Anemia of chronic disease occurs from inflammation, infection, or malignancy because there is decreased RBC production, possibly as a result of disordered iron metabolism. Ferritin levels are normal or increased, but serum iron levels and TIBC are low. It is important that this form of anemia, which is mild and normocytic, not be mistaken for iron-deficiency anemia; iron supplements should not be given. Recombinant erythropoietin therapy usually corrects this anemia. See Chapters 6 and 39.

Sickle Cell Anemia

Pathophysiology

Sickle cell anemia (SCA), a chronic hemolytic anemia also known as *hemoglobin S disease*, affects 1 of 600 African Americans in the United States as a result of homozygous inheritance of hemoglobin S. This results in defective hemoglobin synthesis, which produces sickle-shaped RBCs that get caught in capillaries and do not carry oxygen well. The disease is usually diagnosed toward the end of the first year of life.

In addition to the usual symptoms of anemia, SCA is characterized by episodes of pain resulting from the occlusion of small blood vessels by the abnormally shaped erythrocytes. The occlusions frequently occur in the abdomen, causing acute, severe abdominal pain. The hemolytic anemia and vasoocclusive disease result in impaired liver function, jaundice, gallstones, and deteriorating renal function. The constant hemolysis of erythrocytes increases iron stores in the liver; however, iron-deficiency anemia and SCA can coexist. Iron overload is less common and is usually a problem only in those who have received multiple blood transfusions.

Typically serum homocysteine levels are elevated, which may be due to low concentrations of vitamin B_6. Children with SCA were found to have these lower vitamin B_6 levels despite B_6 intakes comparable to those of unaffected children.

Medical Management

No specific treatment exists for SCA other than relieving pain during a crisis, keeping the body oxygenated, and possibly administering an exchange transfusion. It is important that SCA not be mistaken for iron-deficiency anemia, which can be treated with iron supplements, because iron stores in the patient with SCA secondary to transfusions are frequently excessive.

Zinc can increase the oxygen affinity of both normal and sickle-shaped erythrocytes. Thus zinc supplements may be beneficial in managing sickle cell disease, especially because decreased plasma zinc is common in children with the SS genotype sickle cell disease and is associated with decreased linear and skeletal growth, muscle mass, and sexual maturation. Zinc supplementation (as little as 10 mg daily) may also prevent the deficit in growth that appears in these children (Zemel et al., 2007). Because zinc competes with copper for binding sites on proteins, the use of high doses of zinc may precipitate copper deficiency.

Medical Nutrition Therapy

Children with SCA and their families should receive instruction about how they can develop a well-balanced food plan providing enough calories and protein for growth and development. Their dietary intake may be low because of the abdominal pain characteristic of the disease. They also have increased metabolic rates, leading to a need for a higher caloric intake. This hypermetabolism is probably due to a constant inflammation and oxidative stress (Akohoue et al., 2007; Hibbert et al., 2005). Therefore their diets must be high enough in calories to meet these needs and must provide foods high in folate and the trace minerals zinc and copper (see Appendix 58 for sources of these minerals). In addition, they may be low in vitamins A, C, D, and E, folate, calcium and fiber. The diet should be high in folate (400 to 600 mcg daily) because the increased production of erythrocytes needed to replace the cells being continuously destroyed also increases folic acid requirements.

When assessing the nutrition status of patients with SCA, the questions related to the use of vitamin and mineral supplements, the consumption of alcohol (which increases iron absorption), and sources of protein (animal sources being high in both zinc and iron) in the diet must be given special attention. A multivitamin and mineral supplement containing 50% to 150% of the RDA for folate, zinc, and copper (not iron) is recommended.

Dietary fluid and sodium intake influence the risk for vasoocclusive events in SCA; increasing fluid intake and limiting high-sodium foods should be discussed (Fowler et al., 2010). Intake of 2 to 3 quarts of water daily is recommended. Finally, it is important to remember that patients with sickle cell disease may require higher than RDA amounts of protein.

If it is necessary for the diet to be low in absorbable iron, the diet should emphasize vegetable proteins. Iron-rich foods, such as liver, iron-fortified formula, iron-fortified cereals, and iron-fortified energy bars are excluded. Substances such as alcohol and ascorbic acid supplements, both of which enhance iron absorption should be avoided. However, it is important to remember that iron deficiency may be present in some patients with SCA owing to repeated phlebotomies, excessive transfusions, or hematuria secondary to renal papillary necrosis. This should be assessed, and the diet adjusted appropriately.

Hypochromic Microcytic Transient Anemia (Sports Anemia)

Increased RBC destruction, along with decreased hemoglobin, serum iron, and ferritin concentrations, may occur at the initiation and early stages of a vigorous training program. Once called *march hemoglobinuria*, this anemia was believed to arise in soldiers as a result of mechanical trauma incurred by erythrocytes (RBCs) during long marches. The RBCs in the capillaries are compressed every time the foot lands until they burst, releasing hemoglobin. It was thought that a similar situation existed in runners, especially long-distance runners; however, it is now thought that it is a physiologic anemia (i.e., a transient problem of blood volume and dilution) (see Chapter 24 for further discussion).

Athletes who have hemoglobin concentrations below those needed for optimal oxygen delivery may benefit from consuming nutrient and iron-rich foods; ensuring that their diets contain adequate protein; and avoiding tea, coffee, antacids, H_2-blockers, and tetracycline, all of which inhibit iron absorption. No athlete should take iron supplements unless true iron deficiency is diagnosed based on a complete blood cell count with differential, serum ferritin level, serum iron level, TIBC, and percent saturation of iron-binding capacity. Athletes who are female, vegetarian, involved in endurance sports, or entering a growth spurt are at risk for iron-deficiency anemia and therefore should undergo periodic monitoring.

Thalassemias

Thalassemias (α and β) are severe inherited anemias characterized by microcytic, hypochromic, and short-lived RBCs resulting from defective hemoglobin synthesis, which affects mostly persons in the Mediterranean region. The ineffective erythropoiesis leads to an increase in plasma volume, progressive splenomegaly, and bone marrow expansion with the result of facial deformities, osteomalacia, and bone changes. Ultimately there is increased iron absorption and progressive iron deposition in tissues, resulting in oxidative damage. The accumulation of iron causes dysfunction of the heart, liver, and endocrine glands. Because these patients require transfusions to stay alive, they must also have regular chelation therapy to prevent the damaging buildup of iron that can occur. Impaired growth in children accompanying thalassemia major can be partially corrected by increasing caloric intake.

CLINICAL SCENARIO

Dana is a 30-year-old mother of a 2-year-old and is now planning to become pregnant with her second child. Struggling to lose the last 10 pounds from her first pregnancy, her diet of choice over this past year has been a version of the low-carbohydrate diet. Dana's food intake lacks variety and balance. She is low on fruits, vegetables, and grains. She complains of diarrhea, loss of appetite, weakness, and irritability. Her blood work reveals a normal hemoglobin level but a low serum folate level. She has scheduled an appointment to see you.

Nutrition Diagnostic Statement

Inadequate B vitamin intake related to consumption of very low-carbohydrate diet as evidenced by low serum folate level.

Nutrition Care Questions

1. What are the risks of following a low-carbohydrate diet, especially before pregnancy?
2. What folate-containing, nutrient-dense foods could be included in her diet that would be beneficial to her pending pregnancy?
3. What supplements, if any, and in what amounts, would you recommend to Dana?
4. Which websites can you refer Dana to for her to learn more about the role of folate and neural tube defects?
5. What information do you need to gather before developing a plan for Dana? Of what would this plan consist?

USEFUL WEBSITES

Anemia Institute for Research and Education
http://www.anemiainstitute.org
Anemia Lifeline
http://www.anemia.com/
Iron Disorders Institute
http://www.irondisorders.org/
Iron Overload Disease Association
http://www.ironoverload.org/

REFERENCES

Adams PC, et al: Hemochromatosis and iron-overload screening in a racially diverse population, *N Engl J Med* 352:1769, 2005.

Akohoue SA, et al: Energy expenditure, inflammation and oxidative stress in steady-state adolescents with sickle cell anemia, *Pediatr Res* 61:233, 2007.

Ashmead D: The absorption and metabolism of iron amino acid chelate, *Archivos Latino Americano De Nutricion* 51:1, 2001.

Bartzokis G, et al: Prevalent iron metabolism gene variants associated with increased brain ferritin iron in healthy older men, *J Alzheimers Dis* 20:333, 2010.

Connor JR, Lee SY: HFE mutations and Alzheimer's disease, *J Alzheimers Dis* 10:267, 2006.

Dunaief JL: Iron induced oxidative damage as a potential factor in age-related macular degeneration: the Cogan Lecture, *Invest Opthamol Vis Sci* 47:4660, 2006.

Elmadfa I, Singer I: Vitamin B_{12} and homocysteine status among vegetarians: a global perspective, *AM J Clin Nutr* 89:1693S, 2009.

Fowler JT, et al: Dietary water and sodium intake of children and adolescents with sickle cell anemia, *J Pediatr Hematol Oncol* 32:350, 2010.

Graber JJ, et al: Vitamin B_{12}-responsive severe leukoencephalopathy and autonomic dysfunction in a patient with "normal" serum B12 levels, *J Neurol Neurosurg Psychiatry* 81:1369, 2010.

Hibbert JM, et al: Proinflammatory cytokines and the hypermetabolism of children with sickle cell disease, *Exp Biol Med (Maywood)* 230:68, 2005.

Moreiras GV, et al: Cobalamin, folic acid, and homocysteine, *Nutr Rev* 67:69S, 2009.

Nemeth E, Ganz T: Regulation of iron metabolism by hepcidin, *Ann Rev Nutr* 26:323, 2006.

National Heart, Blood and Lung Institute (NHBLI): What is restless legs syndrome. Accessed 9 August 2010 from http://www.nhlbi.nih.gov/health/dci/Diseases/rls/rls_WhatIs.html.

Serefhanoglu S, et al: Measuring holotranscobalamin II, an early indicator of negative B_{12} balance, by radioimmunoassay in patients with ischemic cerebrovascular disease, *Ann Hematol* 87:391, 2008.

Sarari A, et al: Helicobacter pylori, a causative agent of vitamin B_{12} deficiency, *J Infect Dev Ctries* 2:346, 2008.

Smith KA, et al: Circulating gastrin is increased in hemochromatosis, *FEBS Lett* 580:6195, 2006.

Tucker K, Mayer M: Low plasma vitamin B_{12} is associated with lower bone mineral density: the Framingham Osteoporosis Study, *J Bone Miner Res* 20:152, 2005.

Veijola L: Association of autoimmune type atrophic corpus gastritis with *Helicobacter pylori* infection, *World J Gastroenterol* 16.1:83, 2010.

Zemel BS, et al: Effects of delayed pubertal development, nutritional status, and disease severity on longitudinal patterns of growth failure in children with sickle cell disease, *Pediatr Res* 61:607, 2007.

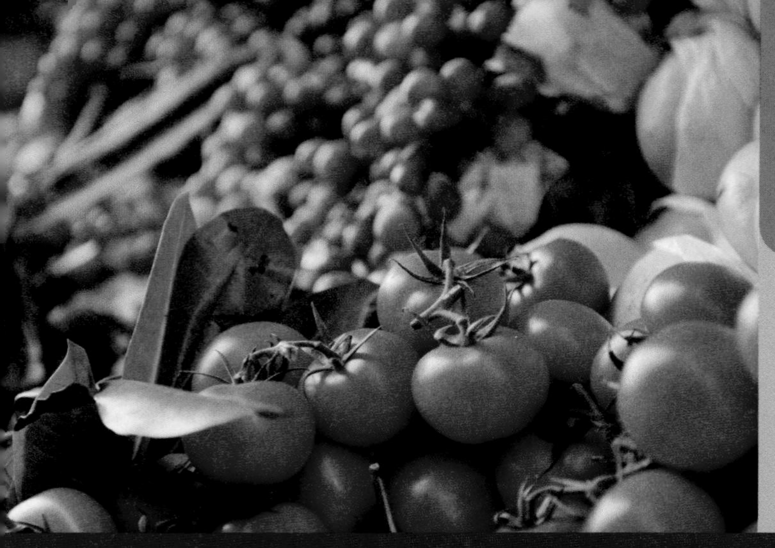

CHAPTER 34

Janice L. Raymond, MS, RD, CD
Sarah C. Couch, PhD, RD, LD

Medical Nutrition Therapy for Cardiovascular Disease

KEY TERMS

3-hydroxy-3-methylglutaryl–coenzyme A (HMG-CoA)
angina
angiography
apolipoproteins
atheroma
atherogenesis
atherosclerotic heart disease (ASHD)
atherothrombosis
bile acid sequestrant
blood pressure
cardiac cachexia
cardiac catheterization
cardiovascular disease (CVD)
C-reactive protein (CRP)
chylomicron
coronary heart disease (CHD)
diastolic blood pressure (DBP)
Dietary Approaches to Stop Hypertension (DASH)
dyslipidemia
dyspnea
edema
essential hypertension
familial combined hyperlipidemia (FCHL)
familial dysbetalipoproteinemia
familial hypercholesterolemia (FH)
fatty streak
foam cells
heart failure (HF)
high-density lipoprotein (HDL)
homocysteine
hypercholesterolemia
hypertension
hypertriglyceridemia
intermediate-density lipoprotein (ILD)
ischemia
left ventricular hypertrophy (LVH)
lipoprotein
low-density lipoprotein (LDL)
metabolic syndrome
myocardial infarction (MI)
nitric oxide
orthopnea
plaque
prehypertension
renin-angiotensin system (RAS)
secondary hypertension
statins
stroke
syncope
systolic blood pressure (SBP)
Therapeutic Lifestyle Changes (TLC) Diet
thrombus
***Trans*-fatty acids**
very-low-density lipoprotein (VLDL)
xanthoma

Sections of this chapter were written by Debra Krummel, PhD, RD for the previous edition of this text.

Cardiovascular disease (CVD) is a group of interrelated diseases that include coronary heart disease (CHD), atherosclerosis, hypertension, ischemic heart disease, peripheral vascular disease, and heart failure (HF). These diseases are interrelated and often coexist. An estimated 81,100,000 adult Americans (one in three) have one or more types of CVD (Box 34-1).

CVD remains the number one killer of both men and women in the United States; one of every 2.9 deaths is attributed to CVD. In 2010 it is estimated that 1.26 million Americans had a new or recurrent coronary attack. Every 25 seconds an American suffers a coronary event and about every minute someone will die from one (American Heart Association [AHA], 2010). The lifetime risk for CVD in American men is two in three and for women is one in two (AHA, 2010).

Of all causes of death, CHD, cancer, and stroke are the leaders (AHA, 2010). **Coronary heart disease (CHD)** involves the narrowing of small vessels that oxygenate the heart muscle. **Myocardial infarction (MI)**, or **ischemia**, in one or more of the coronary arteries with tissue damage, is the main form of heart disease responsible for CVD deaths. Heart disease and stroke cause the most deaths in both sexes of all ethnic groups, increasing with age. Until the age of 65 years, black men have the highest rates of CHD deaths; thereafter white men have the highest rates. Black women have higher rates than white women at all ages. Among whites older than age 18, 12.1% have CVD. In the same age group 10.2% of African Americans have heart disease and in Hispanics the incidence is 8.1%. The incidence in adult Native Americans is 12.1%, in Native Hawaiians or other Pacific Islanders it is 19.7 %, and in Asians it is 5.2%. This chapter discusses the incidence, pathophysiologic findings, prevention, and treatment of each of the CVDs.

ATHEROSCLEROSIS AND CORONARY HEART DISEASE

Atherogenesis is the process leading to development of atherosclerosis. It is a chronic, local, inflammatory response to risk factors, such as high levels of low-density lipoprotein (LDL) cholesterol, that are injurious to the arterial wall (Badimon et al., 2006; Heinecke, 2006 et al.). Hence lesion formation, progression, and eventual **plaque** rupture result from the release of inflammatory cytokines. Proinflammatory (e.g., tumor necrosis factor-alpha [TNF-α], interleukin [IL]-6, and C-reactive protein [CRP]) and antiinflammatory cytokines (e.g., IL-9, IL-10) are the key proteins that must be balanced to prevent plaque rupture and subsequent clinical events (Tedgui and Mallat, 2006).

BOX 34-1

Types and Incidence of Cardiovascular Disease in the United States

Hypertension: 74,500,000
Coronary heart disease: 17,600,000
Myocardial infarction: 8,500,000
Angina pectoris: 10,200,000
Heart failure: 5,800,000
Stroke: 6,400,000

Because of comorbidities, it is not possible to add these numbers together to reach a total (AHA, 2010).

Pathophysiology

Atherosclerotic heart disease (ASHD) involves narrowing and loss of elasticity in the blood vessel wall caused by accumulation of plaque. Plaque forms when inflammation stimulates a response by phagocytic white blood cells (monocytes). Once in the tissue, monocytes evolve into macrophages that ingest oxidized cholesterol, and become **foam cells** and then **fatty streaks** in these vessels. Intracellular microcalcification occurs, forming deposits within the vascular smooth muscle cells of the surrounding muscular layer (Figure 34-1).

A protective fibrin layer (**atheroma**) forms between the fatty deposits and the artery lining. Atheromas produce enzymes that cause the artery to enlarge over time, thus compensating for the narrowing caused by the plaque. This "remodeling" of the shape and size of the blood vessel may result in an aneurysm. Atheromas can rupture or break off, forming a **thrombus**, where they attract blood platelets and activate the clotting system in the body. This response can result in a blockage and restricted blood flow.

Only high-risk or vulnerable plaque forms thrombi. Vulnerable plaque are lesions with a thin fibrous cap, few smooth muscle cells, many macrophages (inflammatory cells), and a large lipid core (Figure 34-2). Arterial changes begin in infancy and progress asymptomatically throughout adulthood if the person has risk factors, is susceptible to arterial thrombosis, or has a genetic susceptibility (Naghavi et al., 2006) (Figure 34-3). Consequently, atherosclerosis is a "silent" disease because many individuals are asymptomatic until the first, often fatal, MI.

The clinical outcome of impaired arterial function arising from atherosclerosis depends on the location of the impairment. In the coronary arteries atherosclerosis causes **angina** or chest pain, MI, and sudden death; in the cerebral arteries it causes **strokes** and transient ischemic attacks; and in the peripheral circulation it causes intermittent claudication, limb ischemia, and gangrene (Figure 34-4). Thus atherosclerosis is the underlying cause of many forms of CVD.

Cholesterol is delivered into cell walls by **low-density lipoprotein (LDL)**, especially smaller particles. To attract and stimulate the macrophages, the cholesterol must be released from the LDL particles and oxidized, a key step in the ongoing inflammatory process. Additionally, macrophages must move excess cholesterol quickly into **high-density lipoprotein (HDL)** particles to avoid becoming foam cells and dying. **Dyslipidemia** refers to a blood lipid profile that increases the risk of developing atherosclerosis.

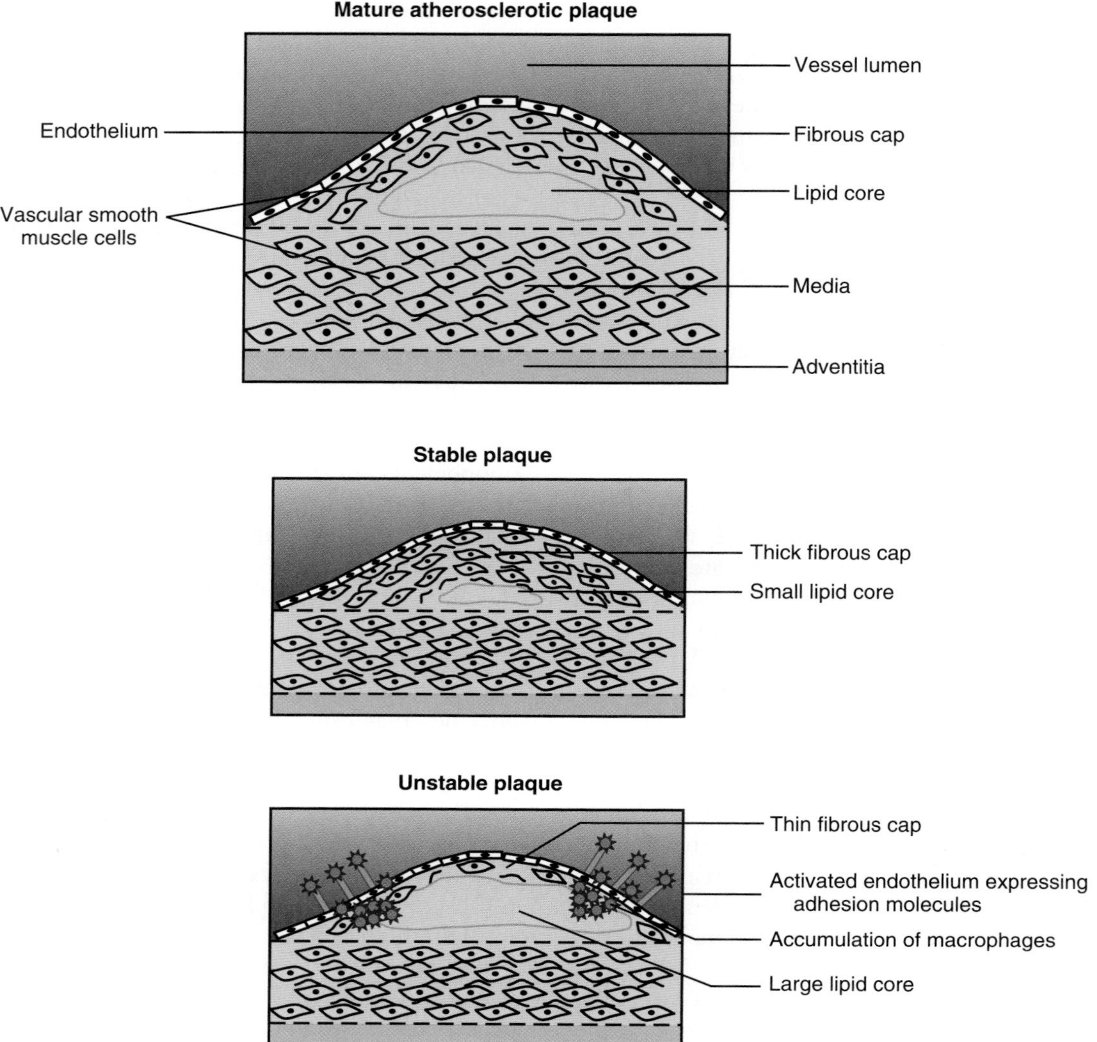

FIGURE 34-1 The structure of mature, stable, and unstable plaque. *(From Rudd JHF et al: Imaging of atherosclerosis—can we predict plaque rupture? Trends Cardiovasc Med 15:17, 2005.)*

Typically it is a condition in which LDL levels are elevated and HDL levels are low. Three important biochemical measurements in CVD include lipoproteins, total cholesterol, and triglycerides.

Lipoproteins

Because lipid is not water soluble, it is carried in the blood bound to protein. These complex particles, called **lipoproteins**, vary in composition, size, and density. Lipoproteins measured in clinical practice—chylomicrons, very-low-density lipoprotein (VLDL), low-density lipoproteins (LDL), and high-density lipoproteins (HDL)—consist of varying amounts of triglyceride, cholesterol, phospholipid, and protein. Each class of lipoprotein actually represents a continuum of particles. The ratio of protein to fat determines the density; thus particles with higher levels of protein are the most dense (e.g., HDLs have more protein than LDLs). The physiologic role of lipoprotein includes transporting lipid to cells for energy, storage, or use as substrate for synthesis of other compounds such as prostaglandins, thromboxanes, and leukotrienes.

The largest particles, **chylomicrons**, transport dietary fat and cholesterol from the small intestine to the liver and periphery. Once in the bloodstream, the triglycerides within the chylomicrons are hydrolyzed by lipoprotein lipase (LPL), located on the endothelial cell surface in muscle and adipose tissue. **Apolipoproteins** carry lipids in the blood and also control the metabolism of the lipoprotein molecule. Apo C-II, one of the apolipoproteins, is a cofactor for LPL. When approximately 90% of the triglyceride is hydrolyzed, the particle is released back into the blood as a remnant. The liver metabolizes these chylomicron remnants, but some deliver cholesterol to the arterial wall and thus are considered atherogenic. Consumption of high-fat meals produces more chylomicrons and remnants. When fasting plasma studies are done, chylomicrons are normally absent.

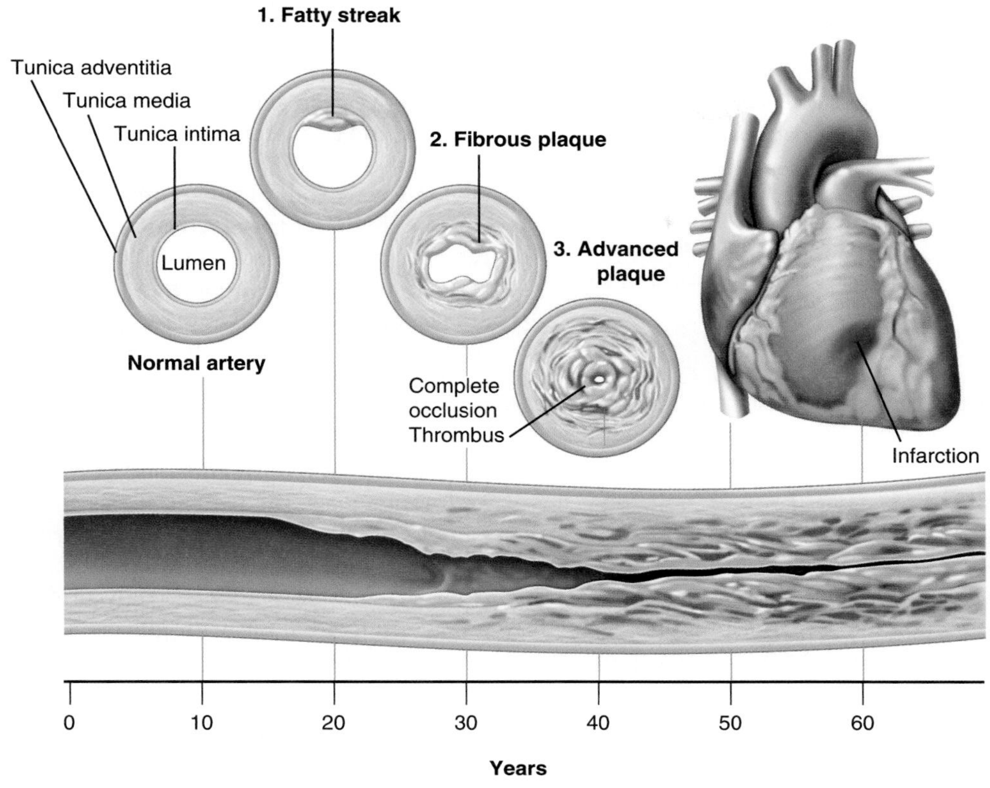

FIGURE 34-2 Natural progression of atherosclerosis. *(From Harkreader H: Fundamentals of nursing: caring and clinical judgment, Philadelphia, 2007, Saunders.)*

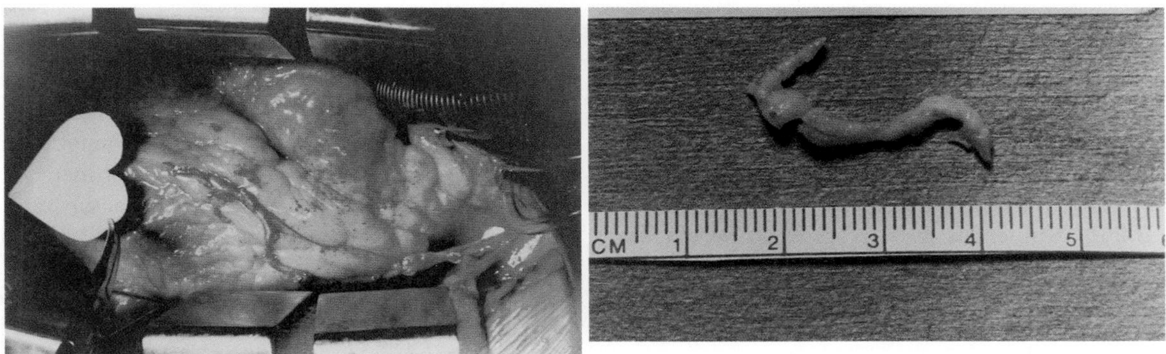

FIGURE 34-3 Plaque that can be surgically removed from the coronary artery. *(Photographs courtesy Ronald D. Gregory and John Riley, MD.)*

Very-low-density lipoprotein (VLDL) particles are synthesized in the liver to transport endogenous triglyceride and cholesterol. Triglyceride accounts for 60% of the VLDL particle. The large, buoyant VLDL particle is believed to be nonatherogenic. Vegetarian and low-fat diets increase the formation of large VLDL particles. Smaller VLDL particles (i.e., remnants) are formed from triglyceride hydrolysis by LPL. Normally these remnants, called **intermediate-density lipoproteins (IDLs)**, are atherogenic and are taken up by receptors on the liver or converted to LDLs. In **metabolic syndrome**, the remnants are atherogenic (Olufadi and Byrne, 2006). Some of the smaller LDL particles stay in the blood, are oxidized, and are then taken into the arterial wall. Clinically, a total triglyceride level is a measurement of the triglycerides carried on both the VLDL and the IDL remnants.

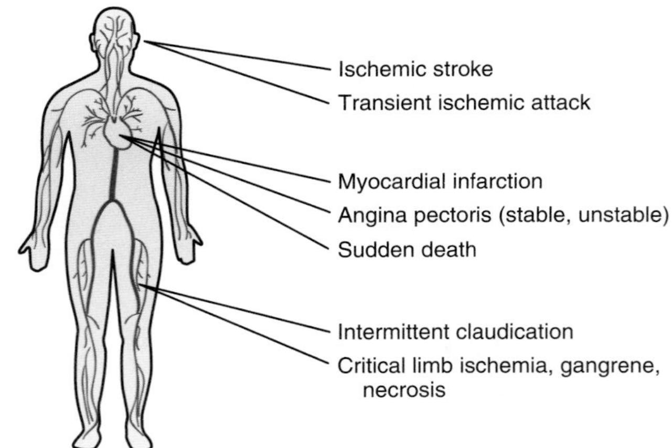

FIGURE 34-4 Major clinical manifestations of atherothrombotic disease. *(From Viles-Gonzalez JF et al: Atherothrombosis: a widespread disease with unpredictable and life-threatening consequences, Eur Heart J 25:1197, 2004.)*

LDL is the primary cholesterol carrier in blood, formed by the breakdown of VLDL. After LDL formation, 60% is taken up by LDL receptors on the liver, adrenals, and other tissues. The remainder is metabolized via nonreceptor pathways. Both the number and activity of these LDL receptors are major determinants of LDL cholesterol levels in the blood. Apo B-100 (apo B) constitutes 95% of the apolipoproteins in LDL. Persons with a high triglyceride level usually have high apo B levels, giving these particles a longer time to deposit lipid in the arterial wall (Marcovina and Packard, 2006). High LDL cholesterol is specifically associated with atherosclerosis.

HDL particles contain more protein than any of the other lipoproteins, which accounts for their metabolic role as a reservoir of the apolipoproteins that direct lipid metabolism. Apo A-I, the main apolipoprotein in HDL, is an antiinflammatory, antioxidant protein that also helps to remove cholesterol from the arterial wall to the liver (Barter and Rye, 2006). Numerous groups promote evaluation of apo A-I or the ratio of apo B to apo A-I to determine risk and treatment (Marcovina and Packard, 2006; Walldius and Jungner, 2006). The lower the ratio, the lower the CHD risk. Both apo C and apo E on HDL are transferred to chylomicrons. Apo E helps receptors metabolize chylomicron remnants and also inhibits appetite (Gotoh et al., 2006). Therefore high HDL levels are associated with low levels of chylomicrons; VLDL remnants; and small, dense LDLs. Subsequently, high HDL implies lower atherosclerotic risk, except in patients with **familial hypercholesterolemia (FH)** who can have a triglyceride-enriched HDL_3 fraction that is proatherogenic (Ottestad et al., 2006).

Total Cholesterol

A total cholesterol measurement captures cholesterol contained in all lipoprotein fractions: 60% to 70% is carried on LDL, 20% to 30% on HDL, and 10% to 15% on VLDL. Studies have consistently shown that a high serum cholesterol level (specifically high LDL cholesterol) is one of the key causes of CHD, stroke, and mortality.

Triglycerides

The triglyceride-rich lipoproteins include chylomicrons, VLDLs, and any remnants or intermediary products formed in metabolism. Of these triglyceride-rich lipoproteins, chylomicrons and VLDL remnants are known to be atherogenic because they activate platelets, the coagulation cascade, and clot formation (Olufadi and Byrne, 2006). All contain the apo B lipoprotein. Fasting triglyceride levels are classified as normal (<150 mg/dL), borderline high (150 to 199 mg/dL), high (200 to 499 mg/dL), and very high (<500 mg/dL) (National Cholesterol Education Program [NCEP], 2002).

Patients with familial dyslipidemias have high triglyceride levels (**hypertriglyceridemia**). Triglycerides in the very high range place the patient at risk for pancreatitis. These patients usually have hyperchylomicronemia and require diets very low in fat (i.e., 10% to 15% of calories derived from fat) and medications. Triglyceride measurements are now considered along with glucose intolerance, hypertension, low HDL cholesterol, and high LDL cholesterol as part of the metabolic syndrome.

GENETIC HYPERLIPIDEMIAS

The study and identification of the genes responsible for the familial forms of hyperlipidemia have provided insight into the roles of enzymes, apolipoproteins, and receptors on cells involved in lipid metabolism. Several forms of hyperlipidemia have strong genetic components and are described here.

Familial Hypercholesterolemia

FH (type IIa hyperlipidemia) is a monogenetic disorder that is seen around the world, with an estimated 10,000,000 people being affected. It is major risk factor for CHD; 85% of men and 50% of women with FH will have a coronary event before the age of 65 years unless the **hypercholesterolemia** is successfully treated (Civeira, 2004). Defects in the LDL receptor gene cause FH; 800 mutations have been identified and screening is possible (Lombardi et al., 2006). Early detection is critical. Treatment with statin drugs improves arterial function and structure (Masoura, 2011). Ultrasound of the Achilles tendon for **xanthomas** (cholesterol deposits from LDL) correctly identifies the majority of FH patients.

Polygenic Familial Hypercholesterolemia

Polygenic FH is the result of multiple gene defects. The apo E-4 allele is common in this form. The diagnosis is based on two or more family members having LDL cholesterol levels above the 90th percentile without any tendon xanthomas. Usually these patients have lower LDL cholesterol levels than patients with the nonpolygenic form, but they remain at high risk for premature disease. The treatment is lifestyle change in conjunction with cholesterol-lowering drugs.

Familial Combined Hyperlipidemia

Familial combined hyperlipidemia (FCHL) is a disorder in which two or more family members have serum LDL cholesterol or triglyceride levels above the 90th percentile. Several lipoprotein patterns may be seen in patients with FCHL. These patients can have (1) elevated LDL levels with normal triglyceride levels (type IIa), (2) elevated LDL levels with elevated triglyceride levels (type IIb), or (3) elevated VLDL levels (type IV). Often these patients have the small, dense LDL associated with CHD. Consequently all forms of FCHL cause premature disease; approximately 15% of patients who have an MI before the age of 60 have FCHL. The defect in FCHL is hepatic overproduction of apo B-100 (VLDL) or a defect in the gene that produces hepatic lipase, the liver enzyme involved in triglyceride removal from the bloodstream. Patients with FCHL usually have other risk factors such as obesity, hypertension, diabetes, or metabolic syndrome. If lifestyle measures are ineffective, treatment includes medication. Patients with elevated triglyceride levels also need to avoid alcohol.

Familial Dysbetalipoproteinemia

Familial dysbetalipoproteinemia (type III hyperlipoproteinemia) is relatively uncommon. Catabolism of VLDL and chylomicron remnants is delayed because apo E-2 replaces apo E-3 and apo E-4. For dysbetalipoproteinemia to be seen, other risk factors such as older age, hypothyroidism, obesity, diabetes, or other dyslipidemias such as FCHL must be present. Total cholesterol levels range from 300 to 600 mg/dL, and triglyceride levels range from 400 to 800 mg/dL. This condition creates increased risk of premature CHD and peripheral vascular disease. Diagnosis is based on determining the isoforms of apo E. Treatment involves weight reduction, control of hyperglycemia and diabetes, and dietary restriction of saturated fat and cholesterol. If the dietary regimen is not effective, drug therapy is recommended.

Medical Diagnosis

Noninvasive tests such as electrocardiograms, treadmill stress tests, thallium scans, and echocardiography are used initially to establish a cardiovascular diagnosis. A more definitive, invasive test is **angiography (cardiac catheterization)**, in which a dye is injected into the arteries and radiographic images of the heart are obtained. Most narrowing and blockages from atherosclerosis are readily apparent on angiograms; however, neither smaller lesions nor lesions that have undergone remodeling are visible.

Magnetic resonance imaging scans show the smaller lesions and can be used to follow atherosclerosis progression or regression following treatments. To predict MI or stroke, measuring the intimal thickness of the carotid artery may be used. Intracoronary thermography helps to determine the presence of vulnerable plaque.

Finally, the calcium in atherosclerotic lesions can be assessed. Electron beam computed tomography can measure calcium in the coronary arteries; persons with a positive scan are far more likely to have a future coronary event than those with a negative scan. Despite these findings, atherosclerosis imaging in asymptomatic individuals is a controversial public health topic because of the costs associated with screening (O'Malley, 2006; Raggi, 2006).

Approximately two thirds of cases of acute coronary syndromes (unstable angina and acute MI) happen in arteries that are minimally or mildly obstructed. This illustrates the role of thrombosis in clinical events. In the ischemia of an infarction, the myocardium or other tissue is deprived of oxygen and nourishment. Whether the heart is able to continue beating depends on the extent of the musculature involved, the presence of collateral circulation, and the oxygen requirement.

Prevention and Management of Risk Factors

The identification of risk factors for atherosclerosis, CHD, and stroke has been a landmark achievement. The primary prevention of these disorders involves the assessment and management of the risk factors in the asymptomatic person. Persons with multiple risk factors are the target population, especially those with modifiable factors (Box 34-2).

Risk factor reduction has been shown to reduce CHD in persons of all ages. Approximately one quarter of the decline in CHD is attributable to improved treatment; more than half is from the reduction in risk factors. Many coronary events could be prevented with adoption of a healthy lifestyle (eating a heart-healthy diet, exercising regularly, managing weight, and not using tobacco) and adherence to lipid and hypertension drug therapy (Chiuve et al., 2006). The Framingham Study, conducted over several decades, has given much useful information to researchers (see *Focus On:* Framingham Heart Study). An algorithm also used to screen for risk factors is shown in Figure 34-5.

In the medical model, primary prevention of CHD and stroke involves altering similar risk factors toward a healthy patient profile. For ischemic stroke, atherosclerosis is the underlying disease. Therefore optimal lipid levels, as determined by the National Cholesterol Education Program (NCEP) for hypercholesterolemia, are also the target levels to prevent stroke. Guidelines for cholesterol management were released as the *Third Report of the Expert Panel on Detection, Evaluation, and Treatment of High Blood Cholesterol in Adults* (*Adult Treatment Panel* or *ATP III*). In the past the recommended dietary approach was a Step I and Step II diet, but this has been replaced by the **Therapeutic Lifestyle Changes (TLC) Diet**. Updates of the NCEP guidelines are due by the fall of 2011.

Although the National Heart, Lung and Blood Institute created the NCEP, the American Heart Association (AHA) has endorsed it. AHA suggests that primary prevention of CHD should begin in children older than age 2 (Gidding et al., 2009). Dietary recommendations for children are a bit more liberal than those for adults. Activity is emphasized in maintaining ideal body weight. Early

FOCUS ON

Framingham Heart Study

Since 1948 various leading investigators (Dr. Joseph Mountain, Dr. Thomas Dawber, Dr. William Kannel, and Dr. William Castelli) have been studying the population (28,000) of Framingham, Massachusetts, to determine the prevalence and incidence of cardiovascular disease and factors related to its development. This is the largest epidemiologic study of cardiovascular disease in the world. Initial study participants (n = 5209) were healthy adults between 30 and 62 years of age. The study continues today, looking at the children and grandchildren of the original cohort. Through this cohort study, the concept of risk factors and thus prevention was born. Modifiable risk factors not only predict disease in healthy adults but also contribute to the disease process in those who have atherosclerotic disease. The seven major risk factors identified by the Framingham study are age, sex, blood pressure, total and high-density lipoprotein cholesterol, smoking, glucose intolerance, and left-ventricular hypertrophy (Opie et al., 2006).

Milestones of the Framingham Study

1960 Cigarette smoking found to increase the risk of heart disease.
1961 Cholesterol level, blood pressure, and electrocardiogram abnormalities found to increase the risk of heart disease.
1967 Physical activity found to reduce the risk of heart disease, and obesity found to increase the risk of heart disease.
1970 High blood pressure found to increase the risk of stroke.
1976 Menopause found to increase the risk of heart disease.
1978 Psychosocial factors found to affect heart disease.
1988 High levels of high-density lipoprotein cholesterol found to reduce risk of death.
1994 Enlarged left ventricle (one of two lower chambers of the heart) found to increase the risk of stroke.
1996 Progression from hypertension to heart failure described.
2006 Genetic Research Study begins to identify genes underlying cardiovascular diseases in 9000 participants from three generations.
2008 Discovery and publication of four risk factors that raise probability of developing precursor of heart failure; new 30-year risk estimates developed for serious cardiac events.
2009 Researchers find parental dementia may be linked to poor memory in middle-aged adults.

In 1971 the offspring study was begun to measure the influence of heredity and environment on the offspring of the original cohort. The younger group appears to be more health conscious because they have lower rates of smoking, lower blood pressures, and lower cholesterol levels than their parents at the same age. The Generation III Cohort Study of the grandchildren is presently underway.

Data from http://www.framingham.com/heart/timeline.htm. Accessed March 19, 2011.

BOX 34-2

Cardiovascular Disease Risk Factors

Major Risk Factors

Hypertension
Age (older than 45 years for men, 55 years for women)
Diabetes mellitus
Estimated glomerular filtration rate <60 mL/min
Microalbuminuria
Family history of premature cardiovascular disease (men <55 years of age, or women <65 years of age)

Modifiable Cardiovascular Risk Factors

Lipoprotein profile
- Low-density lipoprotein cholesterol, elevated
- Total triglycerides, elevated
- High-density lipoprotein (HDL) cholesterol, low

Inflammatory markers
Fibrinogen
C-reactive protein

Lifestyle Risk Factors

Tobacco use, particularly cigarettes
Physical inactivity
Poor diet
Stress
Insufficient sleep
Excessive alcohol consumption

Related Conditions

Hypertension
Obesity (body mass index >30 kg/m2)
Metabolic syndrome (including reduced HDL, elevated triglycerides, abdominal obesity)

Modified from National Institutes of Health, National Heart, Lung, and Blood Institute National High Blood Pressure Education Program: The Seventh Report of the Joint National Committee on Prevention, Detection, Evaluation, and Treatment of High Blood Pressure, NIH Publication No. 04-5230, August 2004.

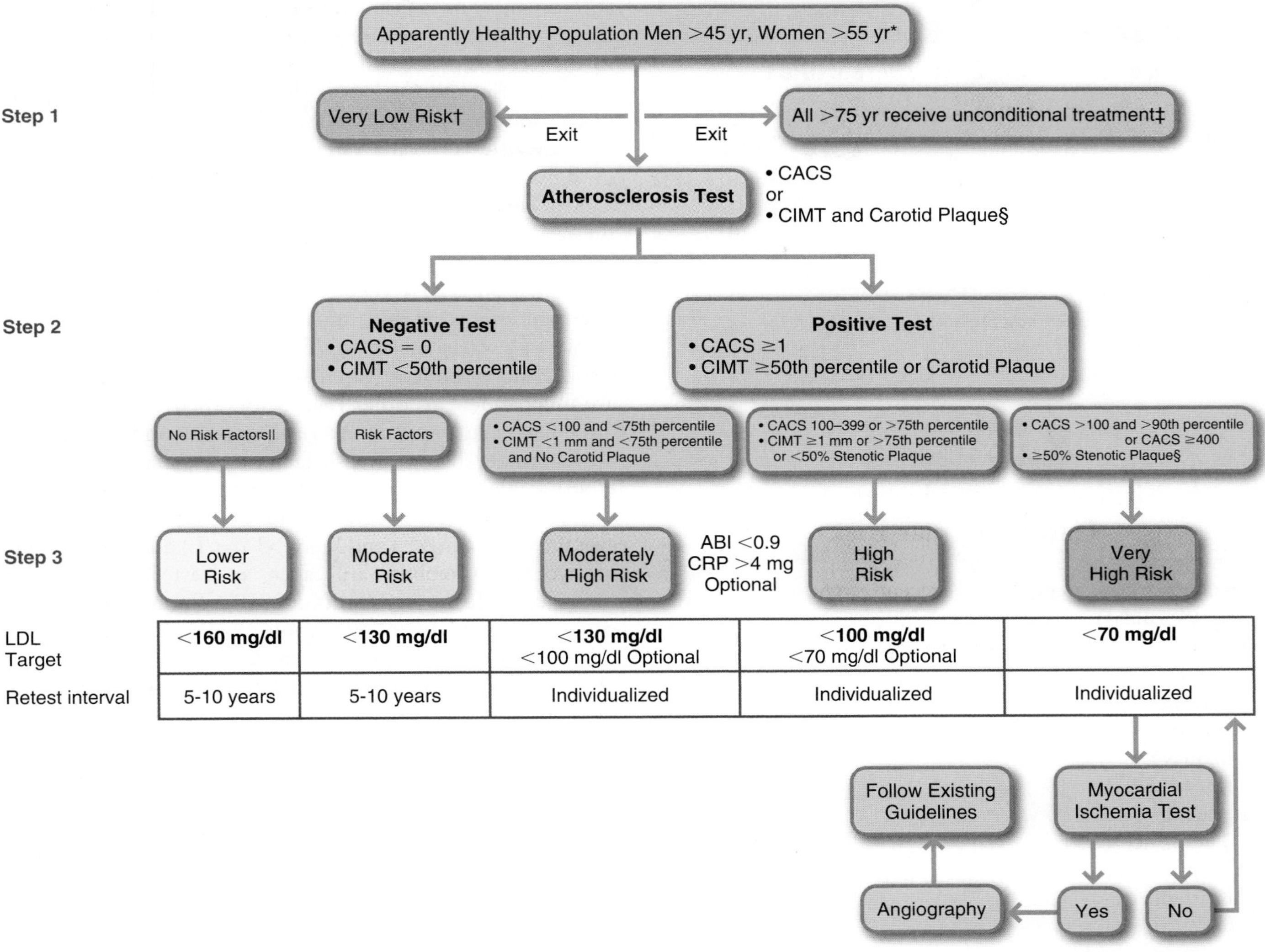

FIGURE 34-5 Flow chart of the first Screening for Heart Attack Prevention and Education (SHAPE) Guideline. *ABI*, Ankle-brachial index; *CACS*, coronary artery calcium score; *CIMT*, carotid intima-media thickness; *CRP*, C-reactive protein; *LDL*, low-density lipoprotein.
*No history of angina, heart attack, stroke, or peripheral arterial disease.
†Population age older than 75 years is considered high risk and must receive therapy without testing for atherosclerosis.
‡Must not have any of the following: total cholesterol level 200 mg/dL (5.18 mmol/L), blood pressure higher than 120/80 mm Hg, diabetes mellitus, smoking, family history of coronary heart disease, or the metabolic syndrome.
§Pending the development of standard practice guidelines.
¶High cholesterol, high blood pressure, diabetes, smoking, family history of coronary heart disease, or the metabolic syndrome.
¶For stroke prevention, follow existing guidelines. *(From Vulnerable plaque to vulnerable patient. Part III: Executive summary of the screening for heart attack prevention and education [SHAPE] task force report, Am J Cardiol 98[2A]:2H, 2006.)*

screening for dyslipidemia is recommended for children with a family history of hypercholesterolemia or CHD. Goals for total cholesterol levels for 2- to 19-year-olds are shown in Table 34-1.

For adults, a desirable lipoprotein profile is a total cholesterol level of less than 200 mg/dL, LDL cholesterol less than 130 mg/dL, HDL cholesterol greater than 40 mg/dL, and triglyceride level less than 150 mg/dL (NCEP, 2002). An LDL cholesterol level less than 100 mg/dL is recommended for persons with two or more risk factors (high-risk patients). See Fig. 34-5 for AHA recommendations.

Inflammatory Markers

Increasing knowledge about the role of inflammation in CVD gives credence to the use of inflammatory markers to indicate the presence of atherosclerosis in asymptomatic individuals or the extent of atherosclerosis in patients with symptoms. Several markers have been suggested (Box 34-3),

TABLE 34-1

Cholesterol Levels for 2- to 19-Year-Olds

Levels	Total Cholesterol (mg/dL)	LDL-C (mg/dL)
Acceptable	<170	<110
Borderline	170-199	110-129
High	≥200	≥130

Modified from Fletcher B et al: Managing abnormal blood lipids: a collaborative approach, Circulation 112:3184, 2005.

LDL-C, Low-density lipoprotein cholesterol.

BOX 34-3

Inflammatory Markers for Cardiovascular Risk

Genetic markers: angiotensin II receptor type-1 polymorphism
Oxidized low-density lipoprotein cholesterol
  Adhesion molecules
  Selectins
Free fatty acids
Cytokines
  Interleukin-1
Interleukin-6
  Tumor necrosis factor-α
Acute-phase reactants
  Fibrinogen
  C-reactive protein
  Serum amyloid A
White blood cell count
Erythrocyte sedimentation rate

Derived from Fung MM et al: Early inflammatory and metabolic changes in association with AGTR1 polymorphisms in prehypertensive subjects, Am J Hypertens 23 September 2010. [Epub ahead of print]; Pearson TA et al: Markers of inflammation and cardiovascular disease: application to clinical and public health practice: a statement for healthcare professionals from the Centers for Disease Control and Prevention and the American Heart Association, Circulation 107:499, 2003.

and research continues to look at the effects of diet on these biomarkers (Esposito and Giugliano, 2006). A recent study showed that the plasma levels of ω-3 fatty acids were inversely associated with the inflammatory markers CRP, IL-6, fibrinogen, and homocysteine (Kalogeropoulos, 2010). In addition, genetic factors also play a role.

Fibrinogen. Most MIs are the result of an intracoronary thrombosis. Prospective studies have shown that plasma fibrinogen is an independent predictor of CHD risk. Factors associated with an elevated fibrinogen are smoking, diabetes, hypertension, obesity, sedentary lifestyle, elevated triglycerides, and genetic factors. More clinical trials are needed to determine if fibrinogen is involved in atherogenesis or is just a marker of vascular damage. Blood thrombogenicity increases with high LDL cholesterol and in diabetes. To date the most widely studied preventive factor for thrombogenesis is the use of aspirin; 75 mg/day of aspirin reduces total CHD, nonfatal MI, and CVD events but does not have any effect on stroke or cardiovascular mortality (Bartolucci and Howard, 2006).

C-Reactive Protein. **C-reactive protein (CRP)** is synthesized in the liver as the acute-phase response to inflammation. Thus in a normal individual without infection or inflammation, CRP levels are very low <0.6 mg/dL. Because atherogenesis is an inflammatory process, CRP has been shown to be elevated (>3 mg/dL) in people with angina, MI, stroke, and peripheral vascular disease; the elevated levels are independent of other risk factors (Scirica et al., 2006). CRP has been found in arterial atheroma and therefore is now considered both a risk factor and a causal agent for **atherothrombosis** (Scirica et al., 2006).

CRP levels are categorized for risk as low (<1 mg/L); average (2 to 3 mg/L) and high (>3 mg/L) after the average of two measurements are taken at least 2 weeks apart (American Heart Association, 2010). Because CRP is a general measure of inflammation, it is not specific to the heart or vascular system and therefore an increased level requires further investigation to determine the source of the inflammation.

Few studies have investigated the effects of dietary variables on CRP, but higher intakes of fruits and vegetables tend to lower CRP levels. For instance, the "Daniel Fast" has shown improvement in multiple cardiovascular indicators, including CRP. This is a 21-day diet without animal products and preservatives that highlights fruits, vegetables, whole grains, legumes, nuts, and seeds (Bloomer et al., 2010). Dietary intervention trials are needed.

Homocysteine. **Homocysteine**, an amino acid metabolite of methionine, is a risk factor. It was first observed that children who were deficient in cystathionine B synthase, the essential enzyme for breakdown of homocysteine, had premature atherosclerosis in some veins. Although the original homocysteine hypothesis for atherothrombotic disease has fallen out of favor, prior studies did not comprehensively adjust for confounding factors. Indeed, elevated total homocysteine (tHcy) independently increases the odds of stroke, especially in younger individuals (Towfighi et al., 2010). Tests for folate alleles in susceptible individuals are useful, giving vitamins B_6, B_{12}, and methylated folate when needed.

Modifiable Lifestyle Factors

The AHA supports diet and lifestyle recommendations to reduce risk of CVD, shown in Box 34-4.

Poor Diet Quality

It is known that diet is the predominant environmental cause of coronary atherosclerosis and that diet modification unequivocally can reduce risk of CHD. Not surprisingly, caloric intake increased by approximately 300 kcal between 1985 and 2000 (Thom et al., 2006). A major environmental,

BOX 34-4

American Heart Association Lifestyle Goals for Risk Reduction

- Consume an overall healthy diet.
- Aim for a healthy body weight.
- Aim for recommended levels of low-density lipoprotein cholesterol, high-density lipoprotein cholesterol, and triglycerides.
- Aim for a normal blood pressure.
- Aim for a normal blood glucose level.
- Be physically active.
- Avoid use of and exposure to tobacco products.

From Lichtenstein AH et al: Diet and lifestyle recommendations revision 2006: a scientific statement from the American Heart Association Committee, Circulation 114:83, 2006. Reprinted with permission. Circulation. 2006; 114:82-96. © American Heart Association, Inc.

dietary contributor to obesity is the increase in portion sizes that has occurred during the last 20 years. Most Americans consume less than the recommended amount of fiber (Anderson, 2009); only 22% of adults consume five servings of fruits and vegetables daily. Nutrition diagnoses common in this population include the following (Brindle, 2006):

- Excessive energy intake
- Excessive fat intake (saturated)
- Inadequate vitamin intake (e.g., B-complex)
- Inadequate mineral intake (e.g., potassium, calcium)
- Inadequate intake of bioactive substances (e.g., stanols or sterols)
- Excessive alcohol intake
- Food- and nutrition-related knowledge deficit
- Undesirable food choices
- Limited adherence to nutrition-related recommendations
- Inadequate physical activity
- Obesity or overweight

Physical Inactivity

Physical inactivity and a low level of fitness are independent risk factors for CHD. Physical activity is associated with CVD, independent of the common cardiometabolic risk factors of obesity, serum lipids, serum glucose and hypertension, in both men and women (McGuire, 2009). Despite public health recommendations to increase activity levels, 40% of Hispanic women, 34% of black women, 32% of American Indian and Alaskan Native women, and 22% of white women reported no leisure-time physical activity in the Behavioral Risk Factor Surveillance System survey (2007). Approximately 20% of all men were inactive. With the high prevalence of obesity, physical activity is a high priority. Physical activity lessens CHD risk by retarding atherogenesis, increasing vascularity of the myocardium, increasing fibrinolysis, increasing HDL cholesterol, improving glucose tolerance and insulin sensitivity, aiding in weight management, and reducing blood pressure.

Stress

Stress activates a neurohormonal response in the body that results in increased heart rate, blood pressure, and cardiac excitability. The stress hormone angiotensin II is released following stimulation of the sympathetic nervous system (SNS); exogenous infusion of angiotensin II accelerates the formation of plaque (Mehta and Griendling, 2007). The INTERHEART study found that the effect of stress is comparable to that of hypertension.

Tobacco Use

The increased risk of CVD and stroke from cigarette smoking has been recognized for more than 40 years, with definitive evidence presented in several Surgeon General reports. Smoking is the number one cause of preventable death in the United States; 35% of deaths from tobacco use are from CVD (Thom et al., 2006). Smoking is synergistic with other risk factors (i.e., the risk of CHD is much higher with multiple risk factors) and directly influences acute coronary events, including thrombus formation, plaque instability, and arrhythmias (abnormal heart rhythm). Thus tobacco causes subclinical atherosclerosis. Women who smoke and use oral contraceptives have 10 times the risk of developing CHD than women who do not smoke and who do not use contraceptives. Risk also increases with the number of cigarettes smoked each day; low-tar brands do not reduce the risk. Furthermore, any exposure, including second-hand smoke, increases the risk (Thom et al., 2006).

Controllable Risk Factors

Diabetes

Diabetes is both a disease and a risk factor. The prevalence of diabetes mirrors that of obesity in the United States. Since 1990, a 61% increase in the prevalence of diabetes has been observed, and it is becoming more prevalent in obese children (Thom et al., 2006). Any form of diabetes increases the risk for CHD, with occurrence at younger ages. Most people with diabetes die from CVD. Similarly, 75% of people with diabetes have more than two risk factors for CHD (McCollum et al., 2006). Some of the increased risk for CHD seen in diabetic patients is attributable to the concurrent presence of other risk factors, such as dyslipidemia, hypertension, and obesity. Thus diabetes is now considered a CHD risk factor (see Chapter 31).

Hypertension

Hypertension is a significant risk factor for CHD, stroke, and HF.

Metabolic Syndrome

Since the early findings of the Framingham study, it has been known that a clustering of risk factors markedly increases the risk of CVD. See Chapter 22 for an in-depth discussion of metabolic syndrome.

Obesity

Obesity has now reached epidemic levels in children and adults in many developed countries. Body mass index (BMI) and CHD are positively related; as BMI goes up, the risk of CHD also increases. The prevalence of overweight and obesity is the highest that it has ever been in the United States; 65% of adults are overweight, and 31% are obese (Blumenthal et al., 2010). Obesity rates vary by race and ethnicity in women. Non-Hispanic black women have the highest prevalence, followed by Mexican-American women, American Indians and Alaskan natives, and non-Hispanic whites. In men the rates of obesity vary from 25% to 28% of the population. The epidemic of obesity and diabetes could reverse the downward trend in CHD mortality if it is not soon controlled, especially given the increasing rates seen in children and adolescents (Thompson et al., 2007) (see Chapter 22).

Carrying excess adipose tissue greatly affects the heart through the many risk factors that are often present: hypertension, glucose intolerance, inflammatory markers (IL-6, TNF-α, CRP), obstructive sleep apnea, prothrombotic state, endothelial dysfunction, and dyslipidemia (small LDL, increased apo B, low HDL, high triglyceride levels) (Poirier et al., 2006). Many inflammatory proteins are now known to come from the adipocyte (Berg, Scherer, 2006). These concurrent risk factors may help to explain the high morbidity and mortality rates observed in people who are obese.

Weight distribution (abdominal versus gynoid) is also predictive of CHD risk, glucose tolerance, and serum lipid levels. Central adiposity has also been strongly related to markers of inflammation, especially CRP. Therefore a waist circumference of less than 35 inches for women and 40 inches for men is recommended.

Small weight losses (10 to 20 lb) can improve LDL cholesterol, HDL cholesterol, triglycerides, high blood pressure, glucose tolerance, and CRP levels, even if an ideal BMI is not achieved. Weight loss has also been correlated with lower CRP levels. However, to restore vascular function, the amount of weight that must be lost, the time of weight maintenance, or the amount of improvement in endothelial function that lessens cardiovascular events is still unknown.

Nonmodifiable Risk Factors

Age and Sex

With increasing age, higher mortality rates from CHD are seen in both genders. However, gender is a factor for the assessment of risk. The incidence of premature disease in men 35 to 44 years of age is three times as high as the incidence in women of the same age. Therefore being older than 45 years of age is considered a risk factor for men (NCEP, 2002). For women the increased risk comes after the age of 55 years, which is after menopause for most women. Overall the increased risk for CHD parallels increase in age.

Family History and Genetics

A family history of premature disease is a strong risk factor, even when other risk factors are considered. A family history is considered to be positive when MI or sudden death occurs before the age of 55 years in a male first-degree relative or the age of 65 in a female first-degree relative (parents, siblings, or children). The presence of a positive family history, although not modifiable, influences the intensity of risk factor management.

Menopausal Status

Endogenous estrogen confers protection against CVD in premenopausal women, probably by preventing vascular injury. Loss of estrogen following natural or surgical menopause is associated with increased CVD risk. Rates of CHD in premenopausal women are low except in women with multiple risk factors. During the menopausal period total cholesterol, LDL cholesterol, and triglyceride levels increase; HDL cholesterol level decreases, especially in women who gain weight.

Medical Nutrition Therapy

Medical nutrition therapy (MNT), which includes discussion of physical activity, is the primary intervention for patients with elevated LDL cholesterol (Box 34-5). Physicians are encouraged to refer patients to registered dietitians (RDs) to help patients meet goals for therapy based on LDL cholesterol levels.

With diet, exercise, and weight reduction, patients can often reach serum lipid goals and reduce body inflammation. The complexity of changes, number of changes, and motivation of the patient will dictate how many patient visits it will take for the adherent client to be successful.

BOX 34-5

Nutritional Factors That Affect Low-density Lipoprotein Cholesterol

Increase

Saturated and *trans*-fatty acids
Dietary cholesterol
Excess body weight

Decrease

Polyunsaturated fatty acids
Viscous fiber
Plant stanols/sterols
Weight loss
Isoflavone-containing soy protein (limited evidence)
Soy protein

From Fletcher B et al: Managing abnormal blood lipids: a collaborative approach, Circulation 112:3188, 2005.

An initial visit of 45 to 90 minutes followed by two to six visits of 30 to 60 minutes each with the RD is recommended (American Dietetic Association [ADA] Evidence Library, 2006). Consequently these interventions are tried before drug therapy and also continue during pharmacologic treatment to enhance effectiveness of the medication (see *Pathophysiology and Care Management Algorithm:* Atherosclerosis).

Therapeutic Lifestyle Changes

The TLC dietary pattern is used for primary and secondary prevention of CHD; its updated version can be found in Table 34-2. The AHA recommends diet and lifestyle changes to reduce CVD risk in all people older than the age of 2 (Lichtenstein et al., 2006). Recommendations include saturated fat less than 7% of calories and total fat content 25% to 35% of calories.

Consuming 30% to 35% of calories from fat while maintaining a low saturated fatty acid (SFA) and *trans*-fatty acid intake is the dietary pattern recommended for individuals with insulin resistance or metabolic syndrome. This higher fat intake, emphasizing polyunsaturated fatty acids (PUFAs) and monounsaturated fatty acids (MUFA), can lower triglycerides, and raise HDL cholesterol and lower LDL cholesterol without exacerbating blood glucose levels.

Planned MNT requires a 3- to 6-month time frame. Lowering SFAs and trans-fats is the first level of behavior change. The TLC diet is followed for 6 weeks. At visit two the LDL response is evaluated and therapy is intensified if warranted. Adjuncts such as plant sterols and stanols, and fiber are incorporated into education at the second visit (dietary compliance must be monitored during this period). At visit three, metabolic syndrome treatment begins if target LDL is not reached. Once the maximum LDL reduction has occurred, management of metabolic syndrome or the cluster of risk factors becomes the target for MNT interventions.

Increasing physical activity, decreasing energy intake, and weight loss are critical for normalizing multiple risk factors. Behavioral strategies for weight management and cardiovascular risk reduction have been provided in Box 34-6. Learning outcomes for the client include planning meals that fit the TLC plan, reading food labels, modifying recipes, preparing or purchasing appropriate foods, and choosing healthier choices when dining out.

Along with the TLC dietary pattern, the Dietary Approaches to Stop Hypertension (DASH) pattern, discussed later in this chapter, is also very appropriate for CVD prevention and treatment. These dietary patterns emphasize grains, cereals, legumes, vegetables, fruits, lean meats, poultry, fish, and nonfat dairy products.

Because animal fats provide approximately two thirds of the SFAs in the American diet, these foods are limited. High-fat choices are omitted, but low-fat choices can be included. Similarly with dairy products, nonfat choices are recommended. Meat is limited to 5 oz/day. Lean meats are high in protein, zinc, and iron; thus if patients wish to consume meat, a 5-oz portion or less can be fit into the dietary plan if other low SFA choices are made. Eggs are restricted to four per week; however, eggs do not contribute to high cholesterol levels in the same way as other animal protein. Most people should add the recommended two servings of fatty fish per week.

For highly motivated patients who want to avoid drug therapy, sometimes very-low-fat diets are effective for reaching blood lipid goals. These diets can also be used as an adjunct to drug therapy for secondary prevention and possible regression of lesions. Such diets contain minimum

TABLE 34-2

Therapeutic Lifestyle Change Dietary Pattern

Nutrient	Recommended Intake
Total fat	25%-35% of total calories
Saturated fat	Less than 7% of total calories
Trans-fatty acids	Zero or as low as possible
Polyunsaturated fat	Up to 10% of total calories
Monounsaturated fat	Up to 20% of total calories
Carbohydrate†	50% to 60% of total calories, especially from whole grains, fruits and vegetables
Fiber	25-30 g/day (soluble forms such as psyllium at 10-25 g)
Plant sterols	2 g/day
Protein	Approximately 15% of total calories
Cholesterol	Less than 200 mg/day
Total calories (energy)	Balance energy intake and expenditure to maintain desirable body weight/prevent weight gain. Daily energy expenditure should include at least moderate physical activity of approximately200 kcal/day).

Updated by authors in 2010 from National Heart, Lung, and Blood Institute: Detection, evaluation, and treatment of high blood cholesterol in adults (adult treatment panel III), Final report, U.S. Department Of Health and Human Services, NIH Publication No. 02-5215, Bethesda, Md, September 2002.

†Refined carbohydrates should be limited.

PATHOPHYSIOLOGY AND CARE MANAGEMENT ALGORITHM

Atherosclerosis

ETIOLOGY

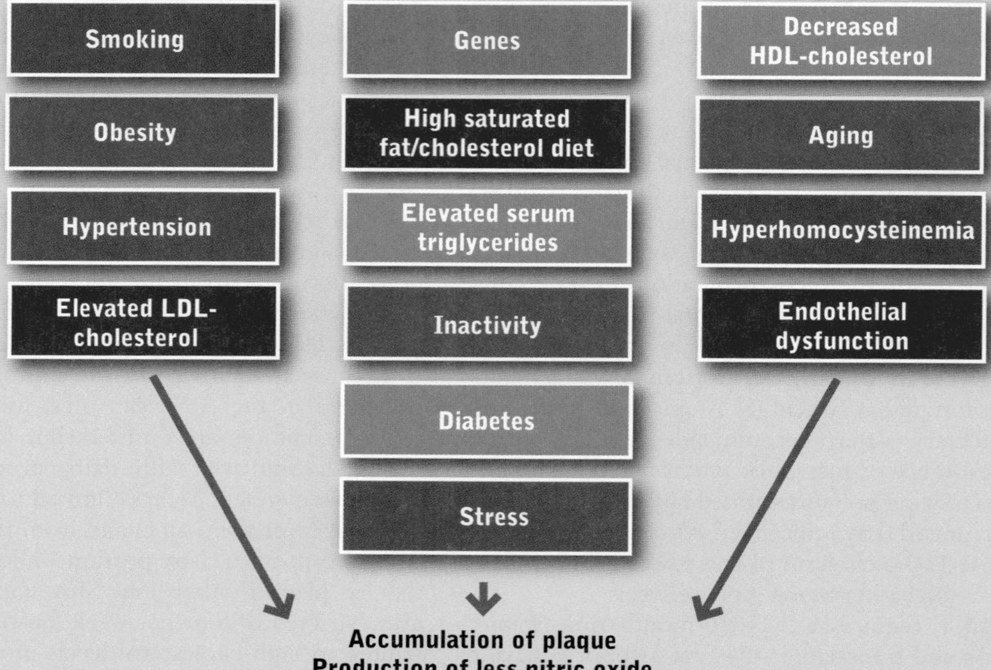

Accumulation of plaque
Production of less nitric oxide
Oxidized LDL cholesterol taken up by macrophages
Formation of foam cells and fatty streaks

PATHOPHYSIOLOGY

Clinical Findings

- Elevated serum total cholesterol
- Elevated LDL cholesterol
- Elevated serum triglycerides
- Elevated C-reactive protein
- Low HDL-cholesterol

Nutrition Assessment

- BMI evaluation
- Waist circumference; waist to hip ratio (WHR)
- Dietary assessment for: SFA, *trans*-fatty acids, ω-3 fatty acids, fiber, sodium, alcohol, and refined carbohydrates

MANAGEMENT

Medical Management

- Bile acid sequestrants
- HMG CoA reductase inhibitors (statins)
- Triglyceride-lowering medication
- Blood pressure—lowering medication
- Medication for glucose management
- Percutaneous coronary intervention (PCI)
  - Balloon
  - Stent
- Coronary artery bypass graft (CABG)
- Antiplatelet Therapy

Nutrition Management

- TLC dietary pattern—7% kcal from SFA
- AHA dietary pattern—7% kcal from SFA
- DASH dietary pattern
- Weight reduction if needed
- Increase dietary fiber to 25–30 g/day or more
- Add stanols and sterols (2–3 g/day) in multiple doses
- Add ω-3 fats
- Add fruits and vegetables for antioxidants
- Reduce dietary cholesterol—<200 mg/day
- CoQ_{10} for those on statin drugs

BOX 34-6

American Heart Association Diet Recommendations for Cardiovascular Disease Risk Reduction

- Balance calorie intake and physical activity to achieve or maintain a healthy body weight.
- Consume a diet rich in vegetables and fruits.
- Choose whole-grain, high-fiber foods.
- Consume fish, especially oily fish, at least twice a week.
- Limit intake of saturated fat to <7% of energy, *trans*-fat to <1% of energy, and cholesterol to <300 mg/day by:
  - Choosing lean meats and vegetable alternatives.
  - Selecting fat-free (skim), 1%-fat, and low-fat dairy products.
  - Minimizing intake of partially hydrogenated fats.
- Minimize intake of beverages and foods with added sugars.
- Choose and prepare foods with little or no salt.
- Consume alcohol in moderation.
- When eating food that is prepared outside of the home, follow the American Heart Association Diet and Lifestyle Recommendations.

Modified from Lichtenstein AH et al: Diet and lifestyle recommendations revision 2006: a scientific statement from the American Heart Association Committee, Circulation 114:83, 2006. Reprinted with permission. Circulation. 2006;114:82-96. © American Heart Association, Inc.

amounts of animal products; thus SFA (<3%), cholesterol (<5 mg/day), and total fat (<10%) intakes are very low. The emphasis is on low-fat grains, legumes, fruits, vegetables, and nonfat dairy foods. Because egg whites are allowed, the plan is a lacto-ovo-vegetarian regimen.

For more than 40 years epidemiologic studies, experimental studies, and clinical trials have shown that numerous dietary risk factors affect serum lipids, atherogenesis, and CHD. To ensure nutritional adequacy, consulting with an RD is recommended. Key discussion points follow.

Saturated Fatty Acids. The predominant sources of SFAs in the American diet are animal foods (meat and dairy). SFAs are restricted because they have the most potent effect on LDL cholesterol, which rises in a dose-response fashion when increasing levels of SFAs are consumed. In the National Health and Nutrition Examination Survey (NHANES) IV, the mean consumption of SFAs was 11% of kilocalories, versus the goal of less than 7% of energy. SFAs raise serum LDL cholesterol by decreasing LDL receptor synthesis and activity. Regardless of form, all fatty acids lower fasting triglycerides if they replace carbohydrate in the diet.

Trans-fatty Acids. **Trans-fatty acids** (stereoisomers of the naturally occurring *cis*-linoleic acid) are produced in the hydrogenation process used in the food industry to increase shelf life of foods and to make margarines, made from oil, firmer. Most *trans*-fatty acids intake comes from partially hydrogenated vegetable oils. These fatty acids are limited because they raise LDL cholesterol (Basu et al., 2006). No more than 1% of calories (approximately 1-3 g/day) should come from *trans*-fatty acids (Lichtenstein et al., 2006).

Monounsaturated Fatty Acids. Oleic acid (C18:1) is the most prevalent MUFA in the American diet. Substituting oleic acid for carbohydrate has almost no appreciable effect on blood lipids. However, replacing SFAs with MUFAs (as would happen when substituting olive oil for butter) lowers serum cholesterol levels, LDL cholesterol levels, and triglyceride levels to about the same extent as PUFAs. The effects of MUFAs on HDL cholesterol depend on the total fat content of the diet. When intakes of both MUFA (>15% of total kilocalories) and total fat (>35% of kilocalories) are high, HDL cholesterol does not change or increases slightly compared with levels with a lower-fat diet. Oleic acid as part of the Mediterranean diet (Figure 34-6) has been shown to have antiinflammatory effects.

In epidemiologic studies, high-fat diets of people in Mediterranean countries have been associated with low blood cholesterol levels and CHD incidence. Among other factors, the main fat source is olive oil, which is high in MUFA. This observation led to many studies on the benefits of high-fat and high-MUFA diets. A Mediterranean-type step I diet may reduce recurrent CVD by 50% to 70% and has been shown to positively affect lipoprotein levels in high-risk populations (Carter et al., 2010). This diet emphasizes fruits, root vegetables (carrots, turnips, potatoes, onions, radishes), leafy green vegetables, breads and cereals, fish, foods high in α-linolenic acid (flax, canola oil), vegetable oil products (salad dressing and other products made with nonhydrogenated oils), and nuts and seeds (walnuts and flaxseed).

Red wine is considered a key part of the Mediterranean diet. Resveratrol, a polyphenolic compound, is found in the skin of red grapes. Resveratrol in large quantities appears to lower blood pressure by increasing nitric oxide levels. Its role in smaller quantities found in the 1-2 glasses of red wine recommended in the Mediterranean diet is not yet clear (Carter, 2010). Grape juice is another good source of resveratrol.

Polyunsaturated Fatty Acids. The essential fatty acid linoleic acid (LA) is the predominant PUFA consumed in the American diet; its effect depends on the total fatty acid profile of the diet. When added to study diets, large amounts of LA diminish HDL serum cholesterol levels. High intakes of ω-6 PUFAs may exert adverse effects on the function of vascular endothelium or stimulate production of proinflammatory cytokines. Thus a low ratio of ω-6:ω-3 PUFAs is recommended (Basu et al., 2006; Gebauer et al., 2006). Replacing PUFAs for carbohydrate in the diet results in a decline in serum LDL cholesterol. When SFAs are replaced with PUFAs in a low-fat diet, LDL and HDL cholesterol levels are lowered. Overall, eliminating SFAs is twice as effective in lowering serum cholesterol levels as increasing PUFAs.

FIGURE 34-6 The Traditional Healthy Mediterranean Diet Pyramid. *(Courtesy Oldways Preservation and Exchange Trust, www.oldwayspt.org.)*

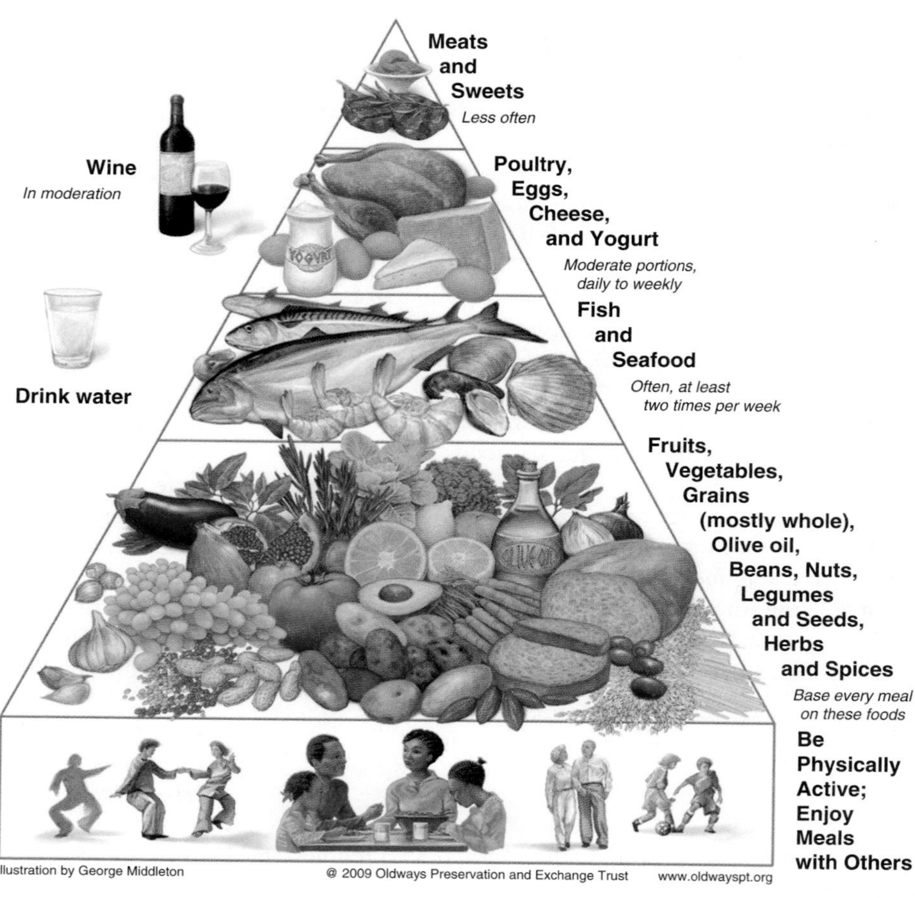

Omega-3 Fatty Acids. The main ω-3 fatty acids (eicosapentaenoic acid [EPA] and docosahexaenoic acid [DHA]) are high in fish oils, fish oil capsules, and ocean fish. Many studies have shown that eating fish is associated with a decreased CVD risk. The recommendation for the general population for fish consumption is to eat fish high in ω-3 fatty acids (salmon, tuna, mackerel, sardines) at least twice a week (Psota et al., 2006). For patients who have CVD, 1 g of EPA and DHA combined is recommended from fish if possible but, if not, then from supplements (Lichtenstein et al., 2006). Patients who have hypertriglyceridemia need 2 to 4 g of EPA and DHA per day for effective lowering. Omega-3 fatty acids lower triglyceride levels by inhibiting VLDL and apo B-100 synthesis, thereby decreasing postprandial lipemia.

An ω-3 fatty acid from vegetables, α-linolenic acid (ALA), has antiinflammatory effects. CRP levels are reduced when patients consume 8 g of ALA daily (Basu et al., 2006). Omega-3 fatty acids are cardioprotective because they interfere with blood clotting and alter prostaglandin synthesis. Omega-3 fat stimulates production of **nitric oxide**, a substance that stimulates relaxation of the blood vessel wall (vasodilation). Unfortunately, high intakes prolong bleeding time, a common condition among Eskimo populations with high ω-3 fat dietary intakes and low incidence of CHD.

Total Fat. Total fat intakes are related to obesity, which affects many of the major risk factors for atherosclerosis. Also, high-fat diets increase postprandial lipemia and chylomicron remnants, both of which are associated with increased risk of CHD. When fat is reduced in the diet and carbohydrate is the replacement source of calories, triglycerides and HDL levels are affected. Low-fat diets (<25% of total kilocalories from fat) raise triglyceride levels and lower HDL cholesterol levels. However, research on the role of fat in prevention and treatment of CVD is now aimed at moderate-fat diets with a low ω-6:ω-3 fat ratio that includes MUFA, such as from nuts. Nuts are part of a heart-healthy diet; a 37% lower risk of CHD in those consuming nuts at least four times a week has been noted (Kelly and Sabate, 2006).

Dietary Cholesterol. Dietary cholesterol raises total cholesterol and LDL cholesterol but to a lesser extent than SFAs. The AHA and TLC dietary patterns contain no more than 200 mg of cholesterol each day. There is a threshold beyond which addition of cholesterol to the diet has minimal effects. When cholesterol intakes reach 500 mg/day, only small increments in blood cholesterol occur. Cholesterol responsiveness also varies widely among individuals. Some people are hypo-responders (i.e., their plasma cholesterol level does not increase after dietary cholesterol challenge), whereas others are hyper-responders (i.e., their plasma cholesterol level responds more strongly than expected to a cholesterol challenge). Hyper-responders may have the apo E-4 allele and poor rates of conversion of cholesterol to bile acids, which causes elevated LDL cholesterol. Feeding cholesterol to animals enriches lipoproteins, which are atherogenic beyond just the rise in serum cholesterol. The effect of dietary cholesterol on inflammatory factors has been inconsistent (Basu et al., 2006).

Fiber. High intake levels of dietary fiber are associated with significantly lower prevalence of CHD and stroke (Anderson, 2009). The AHA, TLC, and DASH dietary patterns emphasize fruits, vegetables, legumes, and whole grains, so they contain adequate fiber to lower LDL cholesterol. In particular, the soluble fibers in pectins, gums, mucilages, algal polysaccharides, and some hemicelluloses lower LDL cholesterol. The quantity of fiber needed to produce the lipid-lowering effect varies by food source; higher quantities of legumes are needed than of pectin or gums. Proposed mechanisms for the hypocholesterolemic effect of soluble fiber include the following: (1) the fiber binds bile acids, which lowers serum cholesterol as it repletes the bile acid pool; and (2) bacteria in the colon ferment the fiber to produce acetate, propionate, and butyrate, which inhibit cholesterol synthesis. The role of fiber, if any, on inflammatory pathways is not well established (Erkkila and Lichtenstein, 2006). Minerals, vitamins, and antioxidants that are components of a high-fiber diet further enrich the diet.

Insoluble fibers such as cellulose and lignin have no effect on serum cholesterol levels. Of the total recommended fiber intake (25 to 30 g daily for adults), approximately 6 to 10 g should be from soluble fiber. This level is easy to achieve with the recommended five or more servings of fruits or vegetables per day and six or more servings of grains (if whole grains and high-fiber cereals are chosen).

Antioxidants. Two dietary components that affect the oxidation potential of LDL cholesterol are the level of LA in the particle and the availability of antioxidants. Vitamins C, E, and β-carotene at physiologic levels have antioxidant roles in the body. Vitamin E is the most concentrated antioxidant carried on LDLs, the amount being 20 to 300 times greater than any other antioxidant. A major function of vitamin E is to prevent oxidation of PUFAs in the cell membrane. The AHA does not recommend vitamin E supplementation for CVD prevention. However, RRR-α-tocopherol, the natural form of vitamin E, shows promise as an antiinflammatory agent (Basu et al., 2006). Foods with concentrated amounts of catechins have been found to improve vascular reactivity. Red grapes, red wine, tea (especially green tea), chocolate, and olive oil should be in any preventive eating plan (Kay et al., 2006).

Stanols and Sterols. Since the early 1950s plant stanols and sterols isolated from soybean oils or pine tree oil have been known to lower blood cholesterol by inhibiting absorption of dietary cholesterol. When esterified and made into margarines, 2 to 3 g/day may lower cholesterol up to 20%. ATP)–III includes stanols as part of dietary recommendations for lowering LDL cholesterol in adults. Because these esters can also affect the absorption of and cause lower β-carotene, α-tocopherol, and lycopene levels, further safety studies are needed for use in normocholesterolemic individuals, children, and pregnant women.

Weight Loss. Weight loss improves endothelial function measured using different methods (Brook, 2006). In a group of patients with extreme obesity (BMI = 52), flow-mediated dilation, which is an estimate of endothelial function, improved after the patients lost a mean of 23 kg (Williams et al., 2005). Overall, it is not known how much weight has to be lost, how long the effect lasts, and whether the improvement in endothelial function reduces coronary events (Brook, 2006).

Medical Management

Pharmacologic Management

Determination of drug therapy depends on risk category and attainment of the LDL cholesterol goal. Many drugs are available for LDL lowering (see Chapter 9). Regardless of the drug used or category of risk, the TLCs underpin all treatment. The classes of drugs include the following: (1) **bile acid sequestrants** such as cholestyramine (adsorbs bile acids); (2) nicotinic acid; (3) **statins**, or **3-hydroxy-3-methylglutaryl–coenzyme A (HMG-CoA)** reductase inhibitors, which inhibit the rate-limiting enzyme in cholesterol synthesis; (4) fibric acid derivatives; and (5) probucol. Classes 1, 2, and 3 have been the first choices for treatment.

Medical Intervention

Medical interventions such as percutaneous coronary intervention (PCI) are now performed in patients with asymptomatic ischemia or angina. PCI, previously known as *percutaneous transluminal coronary angioplasty*, is a procedure that uses a catheter with a balloon that, once inflated, breaks up plaque deposits in an occluded artery. Coronary stenting involves a wire mesh tube inserted to hold an artery open; it can release medication that prevents clotting (Thom et al., 2006).

PCI is often possible because of earlier detection of blockages. The most common problem with PCI is restenosis of the artery. A recent study examined more than 2200 patients, half of whom received intervention of medication and lifestyle changes such as quitting smoking, exercise, and nutrition, and half of whom received lifestyle changes as well as angioplasty. After 5 years it was observed that the number who had heart attacks, was hospitalized, or died because of their heart problems was virtually identical in both groups. Angioplasty did not appear to provide an additional benefit verus lifestyle changes combined with medication (Boden et al., 2007).

Because PCI is performed with the patient under local anesthesia in a cardiac catheterization laboratory, recovery is quicker than with coronary artery bypass graft (CABG) surgery. In CABG surgery, an artery from the chest is used to redirect blood flow around a diseased vessel. Candidates for CABG usually have more than two occluded arteries. CABG surgeries have decreased since 1995 because more PCI procedures are being done. These surgeries improve survival time, relieve symptoms, and markedly improve the quality of life for patients with CHD. However, CABG does not cure atherosclerosis; the new grafts are also susceptible to atherogenesis. Consequently restenosis is common within 10 years of surgery. Risk factor modification, including at a minimum TLCs and probably more aggressive dietary changes, is needed to stop progression.

In the postoperative period CABG patients, like others undergoing major surgery, are in a catabolic state; therefore adequate nutritional intake via oral routes is essential. Patients with complications may be at risk for developing cardiac cachexia, which is often associated with HF. Patients are usually discharged with the TLC, AHA, or DASH dietary pattern.

HYPERTENSION

Hypertension is persistently high arterial **blood pressure**, the force exerted per unit area on the walls of arteries. To be defined as hypertension, the **systolic blood pressure (SBP)**, the blood pressure during the contraction phase of the cardiac cycle, has to be 120 mm Hg or higher; or the **diastolic blood pressure (DBP)**, the pressure during the relaxation phase of the cardiac cycle, has to be 80 mm Hg or higher; this is reported as more than 120/80 mm Hg. If an individual has a blood pressure of 120 mm Hg and a DBP of 80 mm Hg, this is read as a blood pressure of 120/80.

In the Seventh Report of the Joint National Committee on Prevention, Detection, Evaluation, and Treatment of High Blood Pressure, hypertension is classified in stages, based on the risk of developing CVD (Table 34-3). Individuals diagnosed with **prehypertension** have a SBP between 120 and 139 mm Hg or a DBP between 80 and 89 mm Hg, and they are at high risk for developing hypertension and CVD. Stage 1 hypertension (140 to 159/90 to 99 mm Hg) is the most prevalent level seen in adults; this is the group most likely to have a MI or stroke. The defining point for hypertension is arbitrary because any level of elevated blood pressure is associated with increased incidence of CVD and renal disease. Therefore normalization of blood pressure is important for all stages of hypertension.

Hypertension is a common public health problem in developed countries. In the United States one in three adults has high blood pressure (AHA, 2010). Untreated hypertension leads to many degenerative diseases, including HF, end-stage renal disease, and peripheral vascular disease. It is often called a "silent killer" because people with hypertension can be asymptomatic for years and then have a fatal stroke or heart attack. Although no cure is available, hypertension is easily detected and usually controllable. Some of the decline in CVD mortality during the last two decades has been attributed to the increased detection and control of hypertension. The emphasis on lifestyle modifications has given diet a prominent role in both the primary prevention and management of hypertension.

Of those persons with high blood pressure, 90% to 95% have **essential hypertension** (hypertension of unknown cause) or primary hypertension. The cause involves a complex interaction between poor lifestyle choices and gene expression. Lifestyle factors that have been implicated include poor diet (i.e., high sodium, low fruit and vegetable intake), smoking, physical inactivity, stress, and obesity. Vascular inflammation has also been implicated (Savoia and Schiffrin, 2007). Many genes play a role in hypertension; most relate to the renal or neuroendocrine control of blood pressure. Evaluations of 2.5 million genotyped polymorphisms have identified CYP17A1, CYP1A2, FGF5, SH2B3, MTHFR, ZNF652, and PLCD3 genes in hypertensive individuals, primarily of European or Asian ancestry (Newton-Cheh et al., 2009). Hypertension that arises as the result of another disease, usually endocrine, is referred to as **secondary hypertension**. Depending on the extent of the underlying disease, secondary hypertension can be cured.

Prevalence and Incidence

Approximately 74 million American adults age 20 and older have hypertension or are taking antihypertensive medication (AHA, 2010). Prevalence rates for hypertension have remained somewhat stable during the last 8 years, but are still almost double the *Healthy People 2010* goal; more than 30% of the adult U.S. population has high blood pressure (Egan et al., 2010). Non-Hispanic black adults have a higher age-adjusted prevalence of hypertension (43% of men; 44.8% of women) than non-Hispanic whites (34.3% of men; 31.1% of women), Mexican-Americans (25.9% of men; 31.6% of women), or Native Americans (25.3% men and women) (AHA, 2010, AHA, 2007). The prevalence of high blood pressure in blacks is one of the highest rates seen anywhere in the world. Because blacks develop hypertension earlier in life and maintain higher blood pressure levels, their risk of fatal stroke, heart disease, or end-stage kidney disease is higher than in whites (AHA, 2010).

A person of any age can have hypertension. Approximately 16% of boys and 9% of girls have elevated blood pressure (Ostchega et al., 2009). With aging, the prevalence of high blood pressure increases (Figure 34-7). Before the age of 45 more men than women have high blood pressure, and after age 65 the rates of high blood pressure among women in each racial group surpass those of the men in their group (AHA, 2010). Because the prevalence of hypertension rises with increasing age, more than half the older adult population (>65 years of age) in any racial group has hypertension. Although lifestyle interventions targeted to older persons may reduce the prevalence of hypertension, early intervention programs provide the greatest long-term

TABLE 34-3

Classification and Management of Blood Pressure for Adults Ages 18 Years or Older

Classification*				Management*		
					Initial Drug Therapy	
	Systolic BP (mm Hg)*		Diastolic BP (mm Hg)*	Lifestyle Modification	Without Compelling Indication	With Compelling Indications
Normal	<120	and	<80	Encourage		
Prehypertension	120-139	or	80-89	Yes	No antihypertensive drug indicated	Drugs for compelling indications†
Stage 1 hypertension	140-159	or	90-99	Yes	Thiazide-type diuretics for most; may consider ACE inhibitor, ARB, β-blocker, CCB, or combination	Drugs for compelling indications Other antihypertensive drugs (diuretics, ACE inhibitor, ARB, β-blocker, CCB) as needed
Stage 2 hypertension	≥160	or	≥100	Yes	Two-drug combination for most (usually thiazide-type diuretic and ACE inhibitor or ARB or β-blocker or CCB)‡	Drugs for compelling indications Other antihypertensive drugs (diuretics, ACE inhibitor, ARB, β-blocker, CCB) as needed

From Chobanian AV et al and the National High Blood Pressure Education Program Coordinating Committee: The Seventh Report of the Joint National Committee on Prevention, Detection, Evaluation, and Treatment of High Blood Pressure, JAMA 89:2560, 2003.

ACE, Angiotensin-converting enzyme; *ARB*, angiotensin-receptor blocker; *BP*, blood pressure; *CCB*, calcium channel blocker.

*Treatment determined by highest BP category.

†Treat patients with chronic kidney disease or diabetes to blood pressure goal of less than 130/80 mm Hg.

‡Initial combined therapy should be used cautiously in those at risk for orthostatic hypotension.

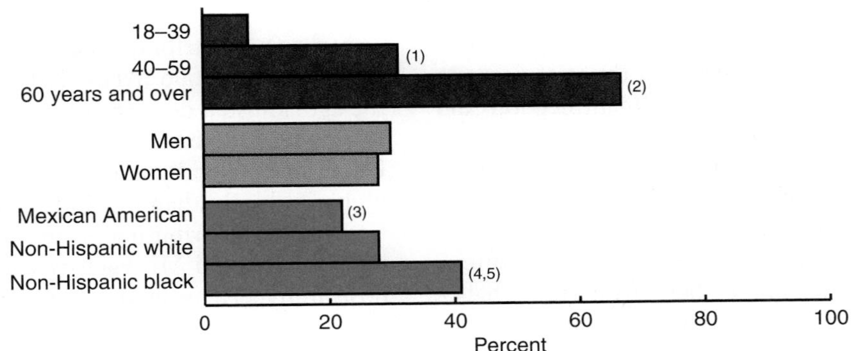

[1]Statistically significant difference between ages 18–39 and 40–59 years.
[2]Statistically significant difference between ages 40–59 and 60 years and over.
[3]Statistically significant difference between the non-Hispanic white and Mexican-American populations.
[4]Statistically significant difference between the non-Hispanic white and non-Hispanic black populations.
[5]Statistically significant difference between the non-Hispanic black and Mexican-American populations.
SOURCE: CDC/NCHS, National Health and Nutrition Examination Survey.

FIGURE 34-7 Age specific and age-adjusted prevalence of hypertension in adults: United States, 2005-2006. *(Ostchega Y, Yoon SS, Hughes J, Louis T. Hypertension awareness, treatment, and control—continued disparities in adults: United States, 2005-2006. NCHS data brief no. 3, Hyattsville, MD: National Center for Health Statistics. 2008.)*

TABLE 34-4

Manifestations of Target Organ Disease from Hypertension

Organ System	Manifestations
Cardiac	Clinical, electrocardiographic, or radiologic evidence of coronary artery disease; left ventricular hypertrophy; left ventricular malfunction or cardiac failure
Cerebrovascular	Transient ischemic attack or stroke
Peripheral	Absence of one or more pulses in extremities (except for dorsalis pedis) with or without intermittent claudication; aneurysm
Renal	Serum creatinine >130 μmol/L (1.5 mg/dL), proteinuria (1+ or greater); microalbuminuria
Retinopathy	Hemorrhages or exudates, with or without papilledema

From the Joint National Committee on Prevention, Detection, Evaluation, and Treatment of High Blood Pressure: Fifth report (JNC V), Arch Intern Med 153:149, 1993.

BOX 34-7

Risk Factors and Adverse Prognosis in Hypertension

Risk Factors

Black race
Youth
Male gender
Persistent diastolic pressure >115 mm Hg
Smoking
Diabetes mellitus
Hypercholesterolemia
Obesity
Excessive alcohol intake
Evidence of end organ damage

Cardiac

Cardiac enlargement
Electrocardiographic signs of ischemia or left ventricular strain
Myocardial infarction
Heart failure

Eyes

Retinal exudates and hemorrhages
Papilledema

Renal

Impaired renal function

Nervous system

Cerebrovascular accident

From Fisher ND, Williams GH: Hypertensive vascular disease. In Kasper DL et al., editors: Harrison's principles of internal medicine, ed 16, New York, 2005, McGraw-Hill.

potential for reducing overall blood pressure-related complications (Gidding et al., 2009).

The relationship between blood pressure and risk of CVD events is continuous, independent of other risk factors. The higher the blood pressure, the greater the chance of target organ damage, including left ventricular hypertrophy (LVH), HF, stroke, chronic kidney disease, and retinopathy (ADA, 2009). As many as 30% of adults with hypertension have treatment-resistant hypertension, which means that their blood pressure remains high despite the use of three or more antihypertensive drugs from different classes (Calhoun et al., 2008). Treatment-resistant hypertension puts an individual at greater risk of target organ damage. Older age and obesity are two of the strongest risk factors associated with the condition. Identification and reversal of lifestyle factors contributing to treatment resistance, along with diagnosis and appropriate treatment of secondary causes and use of effective multidrug regimens are essential treatment strategies.

Adults with diabetes have CVD death rates two to four times higher than adults without diabetes (American Diabetes Association, 2007). Consequently, national guidelines have set the target blood pressure goal for antihypertensive therapy for individuals with diabetes at 130/80 mm Hg, lower than that recommended for the general population. With the increased prevalence of diabetes, this is an important public health problem to address.

Although hypertensive patients are often asymptomatic, hypertension is not a benign disease. Cardiac, cerebrovascular, and renal systems are affected by chronically elevated blood pressure (Table 34-4). High blood pressure was the primary or a contributory cause in 326,000 of the 2.4 million U.S. deaths in 2006 (AHA, 2010). Between 1996 and 2006 the age-adjusted death rate from hypertension increased by 19.5%; overall deaths from hypertension increased by 48%. Death rates from hypertension are approximately 3.2 times higher in blacks than in whites (AHA, 2010). Hypertension is a major contributing factor to atherosclerosis, stroke, renal failure, and MI. Factors associated with a poor prognosis in hypertension are shown in Box 34-7.

Pathophysiology

Blood pressure is a function of cardiac output multiplied by peripheral resistance (the resistance in the blood vessels to the flow of blood). Thus the diameter of the blood vessel markedly affects blood flow. When the diameter is decreased (as in atherosclerosis) resistance and blood pressure increase. Conversely, when the diameter is increased (as with vasodilator drug therapy), resistance decreases and blood pressure is lowered.

Many systems maintain homeostatic control of blood pressure. The major regulators are the SNS for short-term control and the kidney for long-term control. In response to a fall in blood pressure, the SNS secretes norepinephrine, a vasoconstrictor, which acts on small arteries and arterioles to increase peripheral resistance and raise blood pressure. Conditions that result in overstimulation of the SNS (i.e., certain adrenal disorders or sleep apnea) result in increased blood pressure (Khayat et al., 2009). The kidney regulates blood pressure by controlling the extracellular fluid volume and secreting renin, which activates the **renin-angiotensin system (RAS)** (Figure 34-8). Abnormal blood pressure is usually multifactorial. In most cases of hypertension, peripheral resistance increases. This resistance forces the left ventricle of the heart to increase its effort in pumping blood through the system. With time, LVH and eventually HF can develop.

Common genetic variants of the RAS gene, including angiotensin-converting enzyme (ACE) and angiotensinogen, have shown relationships with hypertension (Norton et al., 2010). An increased production of these proteins may increase production of angiotensin II, the primary mediator of the RAS, thus increasing blood pressure. Angiotensin II may also trigger low-grade inflammation within the blood vessel wall, a condition that predisposes to hypertension (Savoia and Schiffrin, 2007).

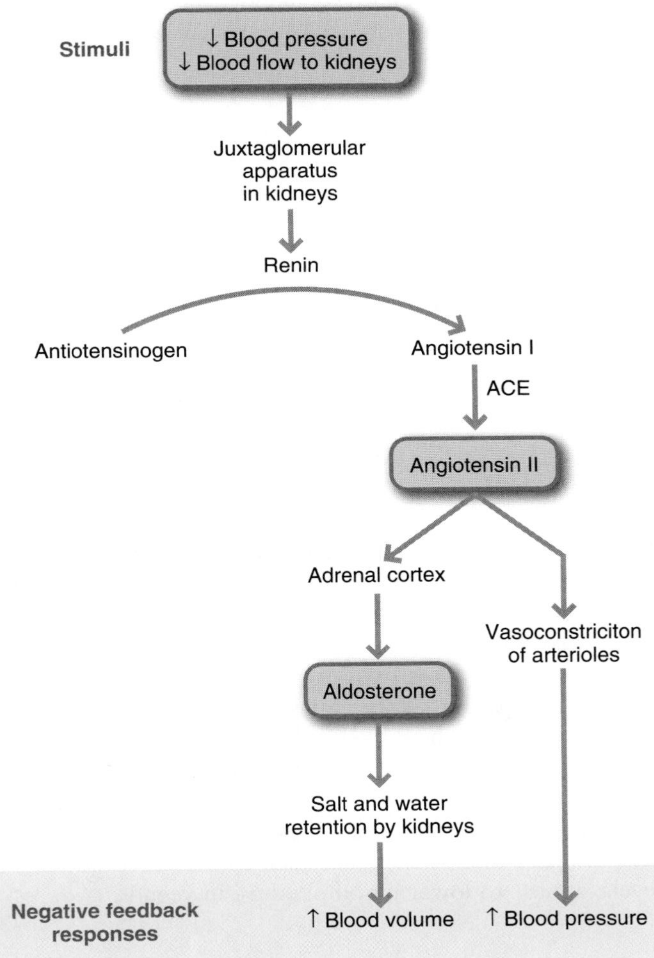

FIGURE 34-8 Renin-angiotensin cascade. *ACE*, Angiotensin-converting enzyme. *(Reprinted with permission from Fox SI: Human physiology, ed 6, New York, 1999, McGraw-Hill.)*

Hypertension often occurs with other risk factors for CVD including visceral (intraabdominal) obesity, insulin resistance, high triglycerides, and low HDL cholesterol levels. The coexistence of three or more of these risk factors leads to metabolic syndrome. It is unclear whether one or more of these risk factors precedes the others or whether they occur simultaneously. Accumulation of visceral fat synthesizes increased amounts of angiotensinogen, which activates the RAS and increases blood pressure (Mathieu et al., 2009). Also, angiotensin II, the primary mediator of the RAS, promotes the development of large dysfunctional adipocytes, which produce increased amounts of leptin and reduced quantities of adiponectin. Higher levels of leptin and lower amounts of circulating adiponectin activate the SNS, a key component of the hypertensive response (Depres, 2006).

Primary Prevention

Positive changes in hypertension awareness, treatment, and control have occurred during the last several years. Based on analysis of NHANES data from 2007-2008, 81% of people with hypertension are aware that they have it (Egan et al., 2010), up from 72% in 1999-2004. Current hypertension treatment and control rates have also increased; this 50% control rate meets the *Healthy People 2010* objective, and reflects increased awareness, treatment and control of hypertension. In 2008 women, younger adults (aged 18-39 years), and Hispanic individuals had lower rates of blood pressure control compared with men, younger individuals, and non-Hispanic whites. Improving hypertension treatment through targeted intervention programs should have a positive effect on CVD outcomes. Blood pressure treatment guidelines highlight the importance of evaluating patients for the presence of multiple CVD risk factors and individualizing lifestyle modification and drug therapies accordingly.

Primary prevention can improve quality of life and the associated costs. One strategy is to reduce blood pressure in those with prehypertension (above 120/80) but below the cutoff points for stage 1 hypertension. A downward shift of 3 mm Hg in SBP would decrease the mortality from stroke by 8% and from CHD by 5% (Appel, 2006). Persons at highest risk should be strongly encouraged to adopt healthier lifestyles.

Changing lifestyle factors have documented efficacy in the primary prevention and control of hypertension. These factors were systematically reviewed and categorized by the American Dietetic Association (ADA) in 2009 (Table 34-5). A strong recommendation (i.e., high benefit/risk ratio with supporting evidence) is made for reducing intake of dietary sodium and increasing intake of fruits and vegetables. The ADA Practice Guidelines also recommend weight reduction

TABLE 34-5

Evidence Analysis Library Recommendations on Blood Pressure and Hypertensive Adults

Food or Nutrient	Recommendation	Rating
Fruits and vegetables	Fruits and vegetables should be recommended at a level of five to ten servings per day for significant BP reduction.	Strong
Sodium	Sodium intake should be limited to no more than 2300 mg/day; if adherent to this recommendation and BP target not achieved, a further reduction in dietary sodium to 1600 mg/day should be encouraged in combination with a DASH dietary pattern. Approximate SBP reduction range 2-8 mm Hg.	Strong
DASH diet	Individuals should adopt the DASH dietary pattern, which is rich in fruits, vegetables, low-fat dairy, and nuts; low in sodium, total fat, and saturated fat; and adequate in calories for weight management. Approximate SBP reduction range 8-14 mm Hg.	Consensus
Physical activity	Individuals should be encouraged to engage in aerobic physical activity for at least 30 minutes per day on most days of the week, as it reduces SBP. Approximate SBP reduction range 4-9 mm Hg.	Consensus
Weight management	Optimal body weight should be achieved and maintained (BMI 18.5-24.9) to reduce BP. Approximate SBP reduction range 5-20 mm Hg/10 kg.	Consensus
Alcohol	For individuals who can safely consume alcohol, consumption should be limited to no more than two drinks (24 oz beer, 10 oz wine, or 3 oz of 80-proof liquor) per day in most men and to no more than one drink per day in women. Approximate SBP reduction range 2-4 mm Hg.	Consensus
Calcium	The effect of increasing calcium intake with lowered blood pressure is unclear; although some research indicates minimal benefit.	Fair
Magnesium	The effect of increasing magnesium intake with lowered blood pressure is unknown; although some research indicates minimal benefit.	Fair
Omega-3 fatty acids	Studies investigating increased consumption of ω-3 fatty acids have not demonstrated a beneficial effect on BP.	Fair
Potassium	Studies support a modest relationship between increasing intake of potassium and a lower sodium-potassium ratio with lowered blood pressure.	Fair

BMI, Body mass index; *BP*, blood pressure; *DASH*, Dietary Approaches to Stop Hypertension; *SBP*, systolic blood pressure.
Recommendations listed are for those rated by the American Dietetic Association as strong, fair, and consensus; for those with weak ratings consult the American Dietetic Association Evidence Analysis Library for Hypertension (2009) http://www.adaevidencelibrary.com/topic.cfm?cat=3259.

if overweight; limiting alcohol intake; adopting a dietary pattern that emphasizes fruits, vegetables, and low-fat dairy products; and increasing physical activity. These recommendations are consensus recommendations based on expert opinion. A fair recommendation is made for increasing dietary potassium, magnesium, and calcium to recommended levels based on the dietary reference intakes (DRI). Evidence is not clear for modifications in dietary fats to lower blood pressure.

Fats

Although dietary lipids do not seem to affect blood pressure, they strongly affect CVD risk; thus the TLC diet is recommended. Although fatty acids may not directly affect blood pressure, an olive oil–enriched diet may reduce the need for antihypertensive medication. Both the amount and type of fat have been studied with respect to blood pressure. In several large prospective observational studies and clinical trials, intake of total fat and specific fatty acids had little effect on blood pressure (Cicero et al., 2009). Supplementation with large doses of fish oil (average 3.7 g/day) can give a modest reduction in SBP and DBP, especially in older hypertensive persons.

Fewer vegans have hypertension than omnivores, even though their salt intake is not significantly different. The vegan diet tends to be higher in PUFAs, among other nutrients, and lower in total fat, SFAs, and cholesterol. PUFAs are precursors of prostaglandins, whose actions affect renal sodium excretion and relax vascular musculature. Thus factors other than dietary fat, such as increased potassium levels, appear to lower blood pressure in vegans.

Protein

Although soy protein may contribute to the lowering of blood pressure, the effect of increased soy food intake on blood pressure remains controversial (ADA, 2009).

Dietary Patterns Emphasizing Fruits and Vegetables

Several dietary patterns have been shown to lower blood pressure. Vegetarian dietary patterns have been associated with lower SBP in observational studies and clinical trials. Average SBP reductions of 5 to 6 mm Hg have been reported. Specifically, the **Dietary Approaches to Stop Hypertension (DASH)** Diet Study shows that this low-fat dietary pattern (including lean meats and nuts and emphasizing fruits, vegetables, and nonfat dairy products) decreased SBP. The DASH diet is found to be more effective than just adding fruits and vegetables to a low-fat dietary pattern (Appel et al., 2006). Although the DASH diet is safe and currently advocated for preventing and treating prehypertension and hypertension, the diet is high in potassium, phosphorus, and protein, depending on how it is planned. For this reason the DASH diet is not advisable for individuals with end-stage renal disease (Appel et al., 2006).

The OmniHeart Trial examined the effects of three versions of the DASH diet on blood pressure and serum lipids. The diets studied included the original DASH diet, a high-protein version of the DASH diet (25% of energy from protein, approximately half from plant sources), and a DASH diet high in unsaturated fat (31% of calories from unsaturated fat, mostly monounsaturated). Although each diet lowered SBP, substituting some of the carbohydrate (approximately 10% of total calories) in the DASH diet with either protein or monounsaturated fat achieved the best reduction in blood pressure and blood cholesterol (Appel et al., 2006; Miller et al., 2006). This could be achieved by substituting nuts for some of the fruit, bread, or cereal servings.

Because many hypertensive patients are overweight, hypocaloric versions of the DASH diet have also been tested for efficacy in promoting weight loss and blood pressure reduction. A hypocaloric DASH diet versus a low-calorie, low-fat diet produces a greater reduction in SBP and DBP. More recently, the ENCORE study showed that the addition of exercise and weight loss to the DASH diet resulted in greater blood pressure reductions, greater improvements in vascular function, and reduced left ventricular mass compared with the DASH diet alone (Blumenthal et al., 2010).

Weight Reduction

There is a strong association between BMI and hypertension among men and women in all race or ethnic groups and in most age groups. The risk of developing elevated blood pressure is two to six times higher in overweight than in normal-weight persons (National Institutes of Health [NIH], 2004). Risk estimates from population studies suggest that 30% or more of cases of hypertension can be directly attributed to obesity (AHA, 2010). Weight gain during adult life is responsible for much of the rise in blood pressure seen with aging.

Some of the physiologic changes proposed to explain the relationship between excess body fat and blood pressure are overactivation of the SNS and RAS and vascular inflammation (Mathieu et al., 2009). Visceral fat in particular promotes vascular inflammation by inducing cytokine release, proinflammatory transcription factors, and adhesion molecules (Savoia and Schiffrin, 2007). Low-grade inflammation occurs in the vasculature of individuals with elevated blood pressure; whether it precedes the onset of hypertension is unclear. Weight loss, exercise, and a Mediterranean-style diet are quite beneficial.

Virtually all clinical trials on weight reduction and blood pressure support the efficacy of weight loss on lowering blood pressure. Reductions in blood pressure can occur without attainment of desirable body weight in most participants. Larger blood pressure reductions are achieved in participants who lost more weight and were also taking antihypertensive medications. This latter finding suggests a possible synergistic effect between weight loss and drug therapy. Although weight reduction and maintenance of a healthy body weight is a major effort, interventions to prevent weight gain are needed prior to midlife. In addition, BMI is recommended as a screening tool in adolescence for future health risk.

Sodium

Evidence from a variety of studies supports lowering blood pressure and CVD risk by reducing dietary sodium. For example, in the Trials of Hypertension Prevention more than 2400 individuals with moderately elevated blood pressure were randomly assigned to either cut their sodium by 750 to 1000 milligrams per day or to follow general guidelines for healthy eating for 18 months to 4 years. In 10 to 15 years after the studies ended, individuals who cut their sodium experienced a 25% to 30% lower risk of heart attacks, strokes, or other cardiovascular events compared with the group that did not (Cook et al., 2007). Several randomized trials have confirmed these positive effects of sodium reduction on blood pressure and cardiovascular outcomes for normotensive and hypertensive individuals.

The DASH sodium trials tested the effects of three different levels of sodium intake (1500 mg, 2300 mg, and 3300 mg/day) combined with either a typical U.S. diet or the DASH diet in persons with prehypertension or stage 1 hypertension (Appel, 2006). The lowest blood pressures were achieved by those eating the 1500-mg sodium level in the DASH diet. In both the DASH diet and the typical American diet groups, the lower the sodium, the lower the blood pressure. Such data provide the basis for current dietary guidelines to limit sodium intake to 1500 mg/day for those with higher than optimal blood pressure (U.S. Department of Health and Human Services, 2005) (see Chapter 12). For those with normal blood pressure, the Dietary Guidelines for Americans recommend an intake of less than 2300 mg of sodium, the equivalent of 6 grams of salt, each day. This goal is supported by the ADA Practice Guidelines (ADA, 2009) and other organizations.

There is heterogeneity in individual responsiveness to sodium. Some persons with hypertension show a greater decrease in their blood pressures in response to reduced sodium intake than others. The term *salt-sensitive hypertension* has been used to identify these individuals. *Salt-resistant hypertension* refers to individuals with hypertension whose blood pressures do not change significantly with lowered salt intakes. Salt sensitivity varies, with individuals having greater or lesser degrees of blood pressure reduction. In general, individuals who are more sensitive to the effects of salt and sodium tend to be individuals who are black, obese, and middle-aged or older, especially if they have diabetes, chronic kidney disease, or hypertension. Currently, there are no practical methods for identifying the salt-sensitive individual from the salt-resistant individual.

Calcium

Higher dairy versus supplemental calcium is associated with lower risk of hypertension (Wang et al., 2008). Analyses of the effects of calcium on blood pressure report modest reductions in SBP and DBP in hypertensive patients (Dickinson, 2006b). Mechanistically, a low calcium intake increases intracellular calcium concentration. This in turn increases 1,25-vitamin D_3 and parathyroid hormone levels, causing calcium influx into vascular smooth muscle cells and greater vascular resistance (Kris-Etherton et al., 2009). Alternatively, peptides derived from milk proteins, especially fermented milk products, may function as ACEs, thereby lowering blood pressure. The DASH trial found that 8-week consumption of a diet high in fruits, vegetables, and fiber; three servings of low-fat dairy products/day; and lower total and saturated fat could lower SBP and DBP by 5.5 and 3 mm Hg greater, respectively, than the control diet. The fruit and vegetable diet without dairy foods results in blood pressure reductions approximately half that of the DASH diet. The ADA Practice Guidelines recommend a diet rich in fruits, vegetables, and low-fat dairy products (versus calcium supplements) for the prevention and management of elevated blood pressure (ADA, 2009). An intake of dietary calcium to meet the DRI is recommended.

Magnesium

Magnesium is a potent inhibitor of vascular smooth-muscle contraction and may play a role in blood pressure regulation as a vasodilator. High dietary magnesium is often correlated with lower blood pressure (Sontia and Touyz, 2007). Less consistent findings have been reported from trials of magnesium supplementation (Dickinson et al., 2006b). The DASH dietary pattern emphasizes foods rich in magnesium, including green leafy vegetables, nuts, and whole-grain breads and cereals. Overall food sources of magnesium rather than supplemental doses of the nutrient are encouraged to prevent or control hypertension (ADA, 2009).

Potassium

Higher potassium intakes are usually associated with lower blood pressures, often dose-responsive. Specifically, supplemental doses of potassium in the range of 1900 to 4700 mg/day will lower blood pressure approximately 2 to 6 mm Hg DBP and 2 to 4 mm Hg SBP (Dickinson et al., 2006a). The effects of potassium are greater in those with higher initial blood pressure, in blacks compared with whites, and in those with higher intakes of sodium. Higher potassium intake is also associated with a lower risk of stroke. More significant effects are found for improved diet, aerobic exercise, alcohol and sodium restriction, and fish oil supplements than for potassium supplements (Dickinson et al., 2006a).

The large number of fruits and vegetables recommended in the DASH diet makes it easy to meet the dietary potassium recommendations—approximately 4.7 g/day (ADA, 2009). In individuals with medical conditions that could impair potassium excretion (e.g., chronic renal failure, diabetes, and congestive HF), a lower potassium intake (< 4.7 g/day) is appropriate to prevent hyperkalemia.

Physical Activity

Less active persons are 30% to 50% more likely to develop hypertension than their active counterparts. Despite the benefits of activity and exercise in reducing disease, many Americans remain inactive. Hispanics (33% men, 40% women), blacks (27% men, 34% women), and whites (18% men, 22% women) all have a high prevalence of sedentary lifestyles (AHA, 2010). Exercise is beneficial to blood pressure. Increasing the amount of low- to moderate-intensity physical activity to 30 to 45 minutes most days of the week is an important adjunct to other strategies.

Alcohol Consumption

Excessive alcohol consumption is responsible for 5% to 7% of the hypertension in the population (Appel et al., 2006). A three drink/day amount (a total of 3 oz of alcohol) is the threshold for raising blood pressure and is associated with a 3-mm Hg rise in SBP. For preventing high blood pressure, alcohol intake should be no more than two drinks per day (24 oz of beer, 10 oz of wine, or 3 oz of 80-proof whiskey) in men, and no more than one drink a day is recommended for lighter-weight men and for women.

Medical Management

The goal of hypertension management is to reduce morbidity and mortality from stroke, hypertension-associated heart disease, and renal disease. The three objectives for evaluating patients with hypertension are to (1) identify the possible causes, (2) assess the presence or absence of target organ disease and clinical CVD, and (3) identify other CVD risk factors that will help guide treatment. The presence of risk factors and target organ damage determines treatment priority.

Lifestyle modifications are definitive therapy for some and adjunctive therapy for all persons with hypertension. Several months of compliant lifestyle modifications should be tried before drug therapy is initiated. An algorithm for treatment of hypertension is shown in Figure 34-9. Even if lifestyle modifications cannot completely correct the blood

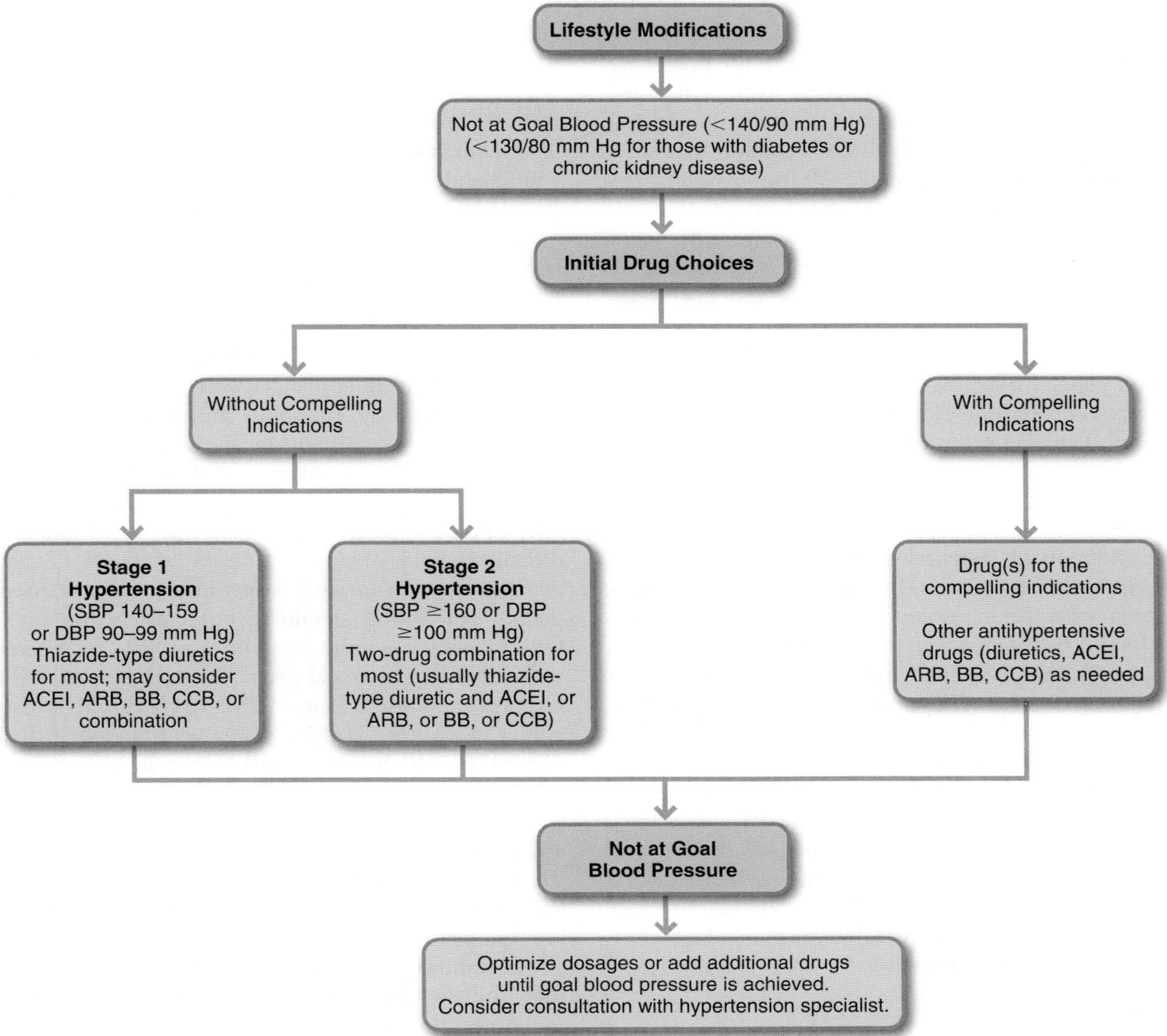

FIGURE 34-9 Algorithm for treatment of hypertension. *ACEI,* angiotensin-converting enzyme inhibitor; *ARB,* angiotensin-receptor blocker; *BB,* β-blocker; *CCB,* calcium channel blocker; *DBP,* diastolic blood pressure; *SBP,* systolic blood pressure. *(From National Institutes of Health, National Heart, Lung and Blood Institute National High Blood Pressure Education Program: The Seventh Report of the Joint National Committee on Prevention, Detection, Evaluation, and Treatment of High Blood Pressure, NIH Publication No. 04-5230, August 2004).*

pressure, they help increase the efficacy of pharmacologic agents and improve other CVD risk factors. Management of hypertension requires a lifelong commitment.

Pharmacologic therapy is necessary for many individuals, especially if blood pressure remains elevated after 6 to 12 months of lifestyle changes. Most patients with hypertension more severe than stage 1 hypertension require drug treatment; however, lifestyle modifications remain a part of therapy in conjunction with medications. The standard treatment for hypertension includes diuretics and β-blockers, although other drugs (β-ACE inhibitors, α-receptor blockers, and calcium antagonists) are equally effective. All these drugs can affect nutrition status (see Chapter 9).

Diuretics lower blood pressure in some patients by promoting volume depletion and sodium loss. Thiazide diuretics increase urinary potassium excretion, especially in the presence of a high salt intake, thus leading to potassium loss and possible hypokalemia. Except in the case of a potassium-sparing diuretic such as spironolactone or triamterene, additional potassium is usually required.

A number of medications either raise blood pressure or interfere with the effectiveness of antihypertensive drugs. These include oral contraceptives, steroids, nonsteroidal antiinflammatory drugs, nasal decongestants and other cold remedies, appetite suppressants, cyclosporine, tricyclic antidepressants, and monoamine-oxidase inhibitors (see Chapter 9 and Appendix 31).

Medical Nutrition Therapy

The appropriate course of nutrition therapy for managing hypertension should be guided by data from a detailed nutrition assessment. Weight history; leisure-time physical activity; and assessment of dietary sodium, alcohol, saturated fat, and other patterns (e.g., intake of fruits, vegetables, and low-fat dairy products) are essential components of the medical and diet history. Nutrition assessment should include evaluation of the individual in the following specific domains to determine nutrition problems and diagnoses: food and nutrient intake; knowledge, beliefs, and attitudes; behavior; physical activity and function; and appropriate biochemical data. Following are the components of the current recommendations for managing elevated blood pressure. See Table 34-6 for a list of approaches sometimes used.

Energy Intake

For each kilogram of weight lost, reductions in SBP and DBP of approximately 1 mm Hg are expected. Hypertensive patients who weigh more than 115% of ideal body weight should be placed on an individualized weight-reduction program that focuses on both hypocaloric dietary intake and exercise (see Chapter 22). A modest caloric reduction is associated with a significant lowering of SBP and DBP, and LDL cholesterol levels. Hypocaloric diets that include a low-sodium DASH dietary pattern have produced more significant blood pressure reductions than low-calorie diets emphasizing only low-fat foods. Another benefit of weight loss on blood pressure is the synergistic effect with drug therapy. Weight loss should be an adjunct to drug therapy because it may decrease the dose or number of drugs necessary to control blood pressure.

DASH Diet

The DASH diet is used for both preventing and controlling high blood pressure (see Appendix 33). Successful adoption of this diet requires many behavioral changes: eating twice the average number of daily servings of fruits, vegetables, and dairy products; limiting by one-third the usual intake of beef, pork, and ham; eating half the typical amounts of fats, oils, and salad dressings; and eating one-quarter the number of snacks and sweets. Lactose-intolerant persons may need to incorporate lactase enzyme or use other strategies to replace milk. Assessing patients' readiness to change and engaging patients in problem solving, decision making, and goal setting are behavioral strategies that may improve adherence (Appel et al., 2006).

The high number of fruits and vegetables consumed on the DASH diet is a marked change from typical patterns of Americans. To achieve the 8 to 10 servings, two to three fruits and vegetables should be consumed at each meal. Importantly, because the DASH diet is high in fiber, gradual increases in fruit, vegetables, and whole-grain foods should be made over time. Slow changes can reduce potential short-term gastrointestinal disturbances associated with a high-fiber diet such as bloating and diarrhea. The DASH pattern is in the current AHA nutrition guidelines (Appel et al., 2006). Servings for different calorie levels are shown in Appendix 33.

Salt Restriction

The Dietary Guidelines for Americans recommend that young adults consume less than 2400 mg of sodium per day. People with hypertension, blacks, and middle-age and elderly people—almost half the population—are advised to consume no more than 1500 mg/day (U.S. Department of Agriculture [USDA], 2005). The DASH-Sodium trial showed that people consuming diets of 1.5 g/day of sodium had greater blood pressure benefits than those with higher intakes. Lower-sodium diets were also shown to maintain low blood pressure over time and enhance the efficacy of certain blood pressure–lowering medications. Although it may be advisable for individuals with elevated blood pressure to restrict sodium to adequate intake (AI) levels, adherence to diets containing less than 2 g/day of sodium is very difficult to achieve.

In addition to advice to select minimally processed foods, dietary counseling should include instruction on reading food labels for sodium content, avoidance of discretionary salt in cooking or meal preparation (1 tsp salt = 2400 mg sodium), and use of alternative flavorings to satisfy individual taste. The DASH eating plan is rich in fruits and vegetables, which are naturally lower in sodium that many other foods.

Because most dietary salt comes from processed foods and eating out, changes in food preparation and processing can help patients reach the sodium goal. Sensory studies show that commercial processing could develop and revise recipes using lower sodium concentrations and reduce added sodium without affecting consumer acceptance. The food industry has begun this effort to reduce sodium in the American diet. See *Focus On:* Sodium and the Food Industry.

Potassium-Calcium-Magnesium

Consuming a diet rich in potassium has been shown to lower blood pressure and blunt the effects of salt on blood pressure in some individuals (Appel et al., 2006). The recommended intake of potassium for adults is 4.7 g/day (National Academies of Science, Institute of Medicine, 2004). Potassium-rich fruits and vegetables include leafy green vegetables, fruits, and root vegetables. Examples of such foods include oranges, beet greens, white beans, spinach, bananas, and sweet potatoes. Although meat, milk, and cereal products contain potassium, the potassium from these sources is not as well-absorbed as that from fruits and vegetables (USDA, 2005).

Increased intakes of calcium and magnesium may have blood pressure benefits, although there is not enough data at present to support a specific recommendation for increasing levels of intake (ADA, 2009). Rather, recommendations suggest meeting the AI intake for calcium and the recommended dietary allowance for magnesium from food sources rather than supplements. The DASH diet plan encourages

FOCUS ON

Sodium and the Food Industry

Most foods sold in supermarkets and restaurants are high in salt. The dramatic differences in sodium from brand to brand suggest that many companies could easily achieve significant reductions without sacrificing taste. According to the Center for Science in the Public Interest (Liebman, 2010), processed foods and restaurant foods contribute approximately 80% of the sodium in Americans' diets; 10% comes from salt added during cooking at home or at the table; the remaining 10% is naturally occurring. Americans now consume approximately 4000 mg of sodium per day—about twice the recommended amount. To help address this problem, the National Academy of Science and Institute of Medicine (2010) issued a report calling for urgent government action to reduce salt in packaged and restaurant foods. The report recommends five strategies to reduce sodium levels in America's food supply. The primary strategy is to set a mandatory national sodium level standard for foods. The interim strategy is voluntary reduction of sodium content in foods by food manufacturers. Supporting strategies are for government agencies, public health and consumer organizations, and the food industry to administer activities to support both the reduction of sodium in the food supply and consumers' intake of sodium. Federal agencies are recommended to improve the data collection, monitoring, and surveillance of sodium intake measurement, salt taste preference, and sodium content of foods.

foods that would be good sources of both nutrients, including low-fat dairy products, dark green leafy vegetables, beans, and nuts.

Lipids

Current recommendations for lipid composition of the diet are recommended to help control weight and decrease the risk of CVD. Omega-3 fatty acids are not highlighted, because their consumption does not appear to lower blood pressure (ADA, 2009). However, the research continues.

Alcohol

The diet history should contain information about alcohol consumption. Alcohol intake should be limited to no more than two drinks daily in men, which is equivalent to 2 oz of 100-proof whiskey, 10 oz of wine, or 24 oz of beer. Women or lighter-weight men should consume half this amount.

Exercise

Moderate physical activity, defined as 30 to 45 minutes of brisk walking on most days of the week, is recommended as an adjunct therapy in hypertension. Overweight or obese hypertensive patients should strive for 300 to 500 kcal expended in exercise per day or 1000 to 2000 kcal/week to promote weight loss or weight control. Because exercise is strongly associated with success in weight-reduction and weight-maintenance programs, any increase in activity level should be encouraged. Daily moderate-intensity physical activity lasting 60 to 90 minutes is recommended for individuals trying to maintain a new lower weight after having lost weight (USDA, 2005).

Treatment of Hypertension in Children and Adolescents

The prevalence of primary hypertension among children in the United States is increasing in concert with rising obesity rates and increased intakes of high-calorie, high-salt foods (Mitsnefes, 2006). Hypertension tracks into adulthood and has been linked with carotid intimal-medial thickness, LVH, and fibrotic plaque formation. Secondary hypertension is more common in preadolescent children, mostly from renal disease; primary hypertension caused by obesity or a family history of hypertension is more common in adolescents (Luma and Spiotta, 2006). In addition, it has been noted that intrauterine growth retardation leads to hypertension in childhood (Shankaran, 2006).

High blood pressure in youth is based on a normative distribution of blood pressure in healthy children. Hypertension is defined as an SBP or DBP of greater than the 95th percentile for age, sex, and height. The designation for prehypertension in children is SBP or DBP of greater than the 90th percentile. Therapeutic lifestyle changes are recommended as an initial treatment strategy for children and adolescents with prehypertension or hypertension. These lifestyle modifications include regular physical activity, avoiding excess weight gain, limiting sodium, and consuming a DASH-type diet.

Weight reduction is considered the primary therapy for obesity-related hypertension in children and adolescents. Unfortunately, sustained weight loss is difficult to achieve in this age group. The Framingham Children's Study showed that children with higher intakes of fruits, vegetables (a combination of four or more servings per day), and dairy products (two or more servings per day) had lower SBP compared with those with lower intakes of these foods. Couch and colleagues (2008) showed that adolescents with prehypertension and hypertension could achieve a significant reduction in SBP in response to a behaviorally oriented nutrition intervention emphasizing the DASH diet. Because adherence to dietary interventions may be particularly challenging among children and teenagers, innovative nutrition intervention approaches that address the unique needs and

TABLE 34-6

Complementary and Alternative Approaches to Lowering Blood Pressure

Common Name	Scientific Name	Effect on BP and Mechanism of Action	Side Effects and Risks
Coenzyme Q_{10}	Ubiquinone	Decreases SBP and DBP via a direct effect on the vascular endothelium and smooth muscle.	May cause gastrointestinal discomfort, nausea, flatulence, and headaches.
Vitamin C and Vitamin E taken in combination as supplement	Ascorbic Acid α-tocopherol	Decreases SBP and DBP, decreases arterial stiffness, and improves endothelial function by improving antioxidant status.	Vitamin E supplementation alone may increase BP.
Vitamin D	1,25-Dihydroxy vitamin D_3	Decreases SBP via suppression of renin expression and vascular smooth muscle cell proliferation.	Hypercalcemia may occur depending on level of supplementation.
Fish oil	Omega-3 polyunsaturated fatty acid	At very high doses in hypertensive individuals, SBP and DBP reductions may occur by increasing the endothelium-dependent vasodilatory response; it may also increase the bioavailability of NO in the vascular wall.	May cause gastrointestinal discomfort, belching, bad breath and altered taste.
Garlic	Allium sativum	Reduces SBP and DBP in individuals with hypertension via vasodilation resulting from activation of potassium channels; may also be due to activation of NOS.	May cause bad breath and body odor.
Resveratrol	Trans-3,4′,5-trihydroxystilbene	Reduces systolic BP in animals via enhanced NOS expression in the aorta.	Unknown
Mistletoe	*Viscum album*	Reduces systolic BP in animals via a sympathetic mechanism.	Unknown
Hawthorn berry	*Crataegus oxycantha, Crataegus monogyna*	Exerts a mild, gradual BP lowering effect. The mechanism is unclear.	Unknown
Mulberry	*Morus alba*	Reduces SBP and DBP animals. The mechanism is unclear.	Unknown
Roselle	*Hibiscus sabdariffa*	Lowers SBP in pre- and mildly hypertensive adults via calcium channel activation.	None
Dogbane plant	*Rauwolfia serpentine*	Reduces SBP by depleting catecholamines and serotonin from central and peripheral synapses.	None
Quercetin	3,3′,4′,5,7-pentahydr oxyflavone	Reduced SBP via a direct vasodilator effect; also may cause an increase in the bioavailability and biological activity of NO.	May cause joint discomfort with long-term use and gastrointestinal upset unless taken with meals. May increase estradiol and reduce the effectiveness of other forms of estrogen.

Data from Fragakis AS, Thomson C: The health professional's guide to popular dietary supplements, ed 3, 2007, American Dietetic Association, Chicago, IL.

BP, Blood pressure; *DBP*, diastolic blood pressure; *NO*, nitric oxide; *NOS*, nitric oxide synthase; *SBP*, systolic blood pressure.

circumstances of this age-group are important considerations in intervention design (see Chapters 18 and 19).

Treatment of Blood Pressure in Older Adults

More than half of the older population has hypertension; this is not a normal consequence of aging. The lifestyle modifications discussed previously are the first step in treatment of older adults, as with younger populations. The Trial of Nonpharmacologic Interventions in the Elderly study found that losing weight (8 to 10 lb) and reducing sodium intake (to 1.8 g/day) can lessen or eliminate the need for drugs in obese, hypertensive older adults. Although losing weight and decreasing sodium in older adults are very effective in lowering blood pressure, knowing how to facilitate these changes and promote adherence remains an obstacle for health professionals.

Blood pressure should be controlled regardless of age, initial blood pressure level, or duration of hypertension (NIH, 2004). Severe sodium restrictions are not adopted because these could lead to volume depletion in older patients with renal damage. Drug treatment in the older adult is supported by very strong data.

HEART FAILURE

Normally the heart pumps adequate blood to perfuse tissues and meet metabolic needs (Figure 34-10). In **heart failure (HF)**, formerly called *congestive heart failure*, the heart cannot provide adequate blood flow to the rest of the body, causing symptoms of fatigue, shortness of breath (**dyspnea**), and fluid retention. Diseases of the heart (valves, muscle, blood vessels) and vasculature can lead to HF (see *Pathophysiology*

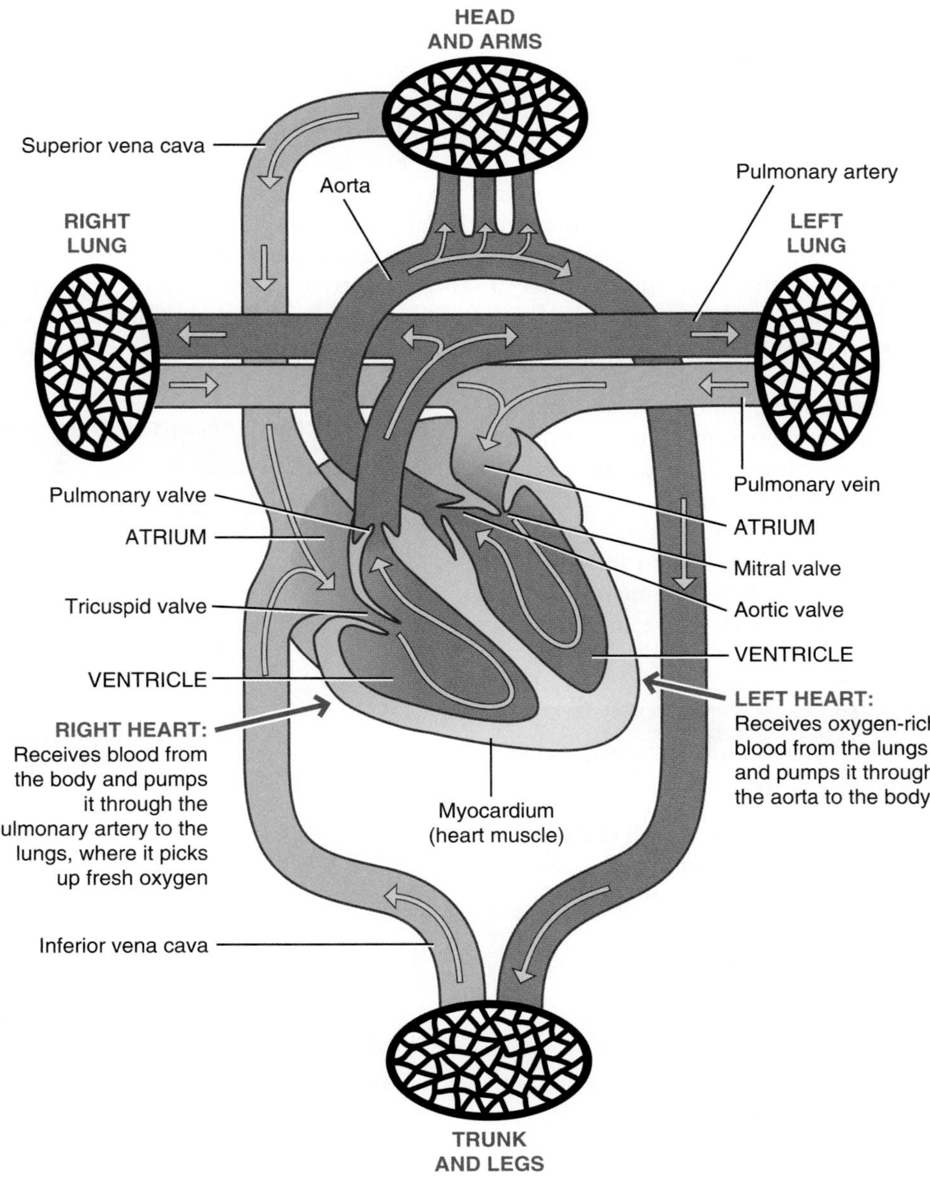

FIGURE 34-10 Structure of the heart pump.

and Care Management Algorithm: Heart Failure). HF can be right-sided, left-sided, or can affect both sides of the heart. It is further categorized as *systolic failure* when the heart cannot pump, or eject, blood efficiently out of the heart or *diastolic failure,* meaning the heart cannot fill with blood as it should.

HF is a major public health problem that affects more than 5 million Americans. The prevalence of HF increases with age. HF affects almost 10 per 1,000 population after age 65 (AHA, 2010). Black women have the highest rates of HF, followed by black men, Mexican-American men, white men, white women, and Mexican-American women (Thom et al., 2006). The incidence of new cases of HF has risen during the last 20 years because of an aging population, the increased number of people being saved from a MI, and the increase in obesity. In 2006 the overall death rate for HF was 89.2 per 100,000 population (AHA, 2010). The death rate per 100,000 for white men was 103.7, black men 105.9, white women 80.3, and black women 84.4. Unlike other CVDs, the number of people being discharged with an HF diagnosis rose from 877,000 in 1996 to 1,106,000 in 2006 (AHA, 2010).

Pathophysiology

The progression of HF is similar to that of atherosclerosis because there is an asymptomatic phase when damage is silently occurring (stages A and B) (Figure 34-11). HF is initiated by damage or stress to the heart muscle either of acute MI or insidious (hemodynamic pressure or volume overloading) onset. See Table 34-7 for classifications of HF.

The progressive insult alters the function and shape of the left ventricle such that it hypertrophies in an effort to sustain blood flow, a process known as *cardiac remodeling.* Symptoms do not usually arise until months or years after cardiac remodeling begins. Many compensatory mechanisms from the SNS, RAS, and cytokine system are activated to restore homeostatic function. Proinflammatory cytokines, such as TNF-αα, IL-1, and IL-6 are increased in blood and the myocardium and have been found to regulate cardiac remodeling.

Another substance, B-natriuretic peptide (BNP), is secreted by the ventricles in response to pressure and is predictive of the severity of HF and mortality at any level of BMI (Horwich et al., 2006). Patients are asymptomatic during these first two stages. BNP is often highly elevated in patients with HF (greater than 100 pg/mL is abnormal, and some patients have levels over 3000 pg/mL). Nesiritide (recombinant human BNP) provides symptomatic and hemodynamic improvement in acute decompensated HF and is now standard procedure (Arora et al., 2006).

Eventually overuse of compensatory systems leads to further ventricle damage, remodeling, and worsening of symptoms (stage C). HF patients have elevated levels of norepinephrine, angiotensin II, aldosterone, endothelin, and vasopressin; all of these are neurohormonal factors that increase the hemodynamic stress on the ventricle by causing sodium retention and peripheral vasoconstriction. These neurohormones and the proinflammatory cytokines contribute to disease progression; hence current studies focus on inhibition of these undesirable pathways and promotion of desirable ones.

For the final stages of HF, there is a subjective scale used to classify symptoms based on the degree of limitation in daily activities (Table 34-8). The severity of symptoms in this classification system is weakly related to the severity of left ventricular dysfunction; therefore treatment encompasses both improving functional capacity and lessening progression of the underlying disease.

TABLE 34-7

Classifications of Heart Failure

Class I	No undue symptoms associated with ordinary activity and no limitation of physical activity
Class II	Slight limitation of physical activity; patient comfortable at rest
Class III	Marked limitation of physical activity; patient comfortable at rest
Class IV	Inability to carry out physical activity without discomfort; symptoms of cardiac insufficiency or chest pain at rest

Modified from Hunt SA et al: ACC, AHA, 2005, Guideline update for the diagnosis and management of chronic heart failure in the adult: a report of the American College of Cardiology/American Heart Association Task Force, J Am Coll Cardiol 46:e1, 2005.

TABLE 34-8

Skeletal Muscle Changes in Heart Failure

Functio laesa	Weakness Fatigability
Structural	Loss of muscle mass Atrophy, fibrosis, no ≠ apoptosis Fiber type switch type I–type llb Loss of mitochondria Endothelial damage
Blood flow	Capillary density ↓? Vasodilation Peak leg blood flow ↓
Metabolism	Proteolysis Oxidative metabolism ↓ Acidosis glycolysis ≠
Inflammation	Cytokine and oxidative markers
Neuroendocrine	GH, IGF-1, epinephrine, norepinephrine, cortisol
Inactivity	TNF-α ≠≠
Genetic factors	Myostatin, IGF

From Strassburg S et al: Muscle wasting in cardiac cachexia, Int J Biochem Cell Biol 37:1938, 2005.

GH, Growth hormone; *IGF,* insulin-like growth factor; *TNF-α,* tumor necrosis factor-α.

PATHOPHYSIOLOGY AND CARE MANAGEMENT ALGORITHM

Heart Failure

ETIOLOGY

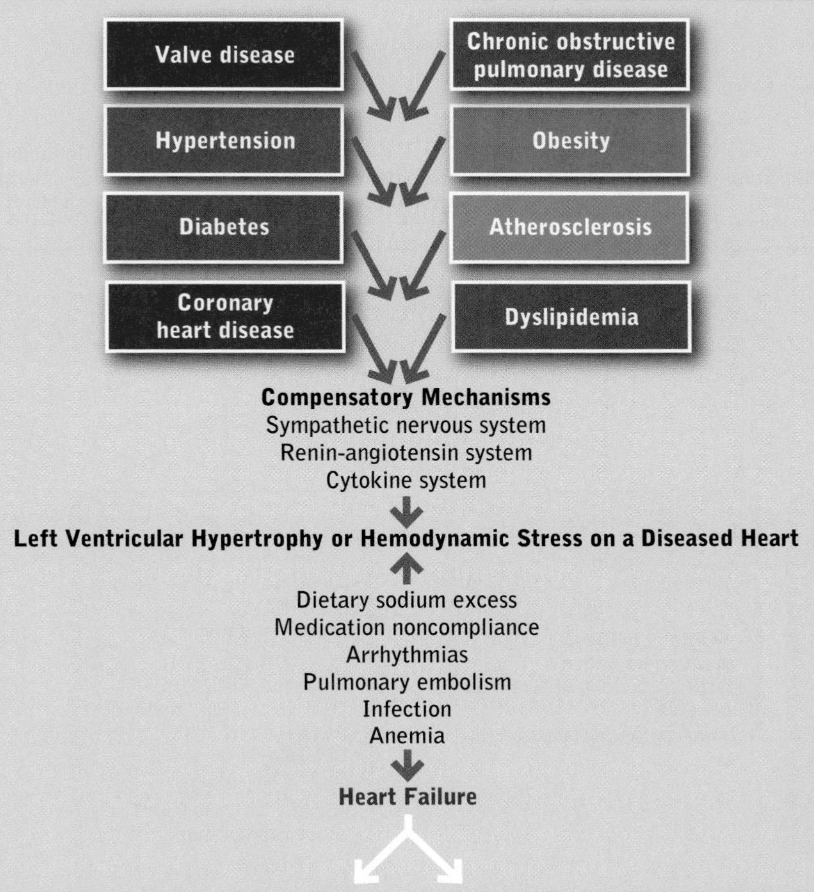

Valve disease
Chronic obstructive pulmonary disease
Hypertension
Obesity
Diabetes
Atherosclerosis
Coronary heart disease
Dyslipidemia

Compensatory Mechanisms
Sympathetic nervous system
Renin-angiotensin system
Cytokine system

↓

Left Ventricular Hypertrophy or Hemodynamic Stress on a Diseased Heart

↑

Dietary sodium excess
Medication noncompliance
Arrhythmias
Pulmonary embolism
Infection
Anemia

↓

Heart Failure

PATHOPHYSIOLOGY

Clinical Findings

- Shortness of breath
- Fatigue
- Fluid retention
- Peripheral vasoconstriciton
- Elevated B-natriuretic peptide
- Mental confusion
- Memory loss
- Anxiety
- Insomnia
- Syncope and headache
- Dry cough

Nutrition Assessment

- Anorexia
- Nausea, abdominal pain and feeling of fullness
- Constipation
- Malabsorption
- Malnutrition
- Cardiac cachexia
- Hypomagnesemia
- Hyponatremia

MANAGEMENT

Medical Management

- ACE inhibitors
- Angiotensin receptor blockers
- Aldosterone blockers
- β-blockers
- Digoxin
- Vasodilators
- Implantable defibrillator
- Heart transplant

Nutrition Management

- Diet low in saturated fat, *trans* fat, cholesterol
- Restricted sodium diet—<2 gm/day
- Increased use of whole grains, fruits, vegetables
- Limit fluid to 2 L per day
- Lose to or maintain appropriate weight
- Magnesium supplementation
- Thiamin supplementation
- Increase physical activity as tolerated
- Avoid tobacco
- Avoid alcohol

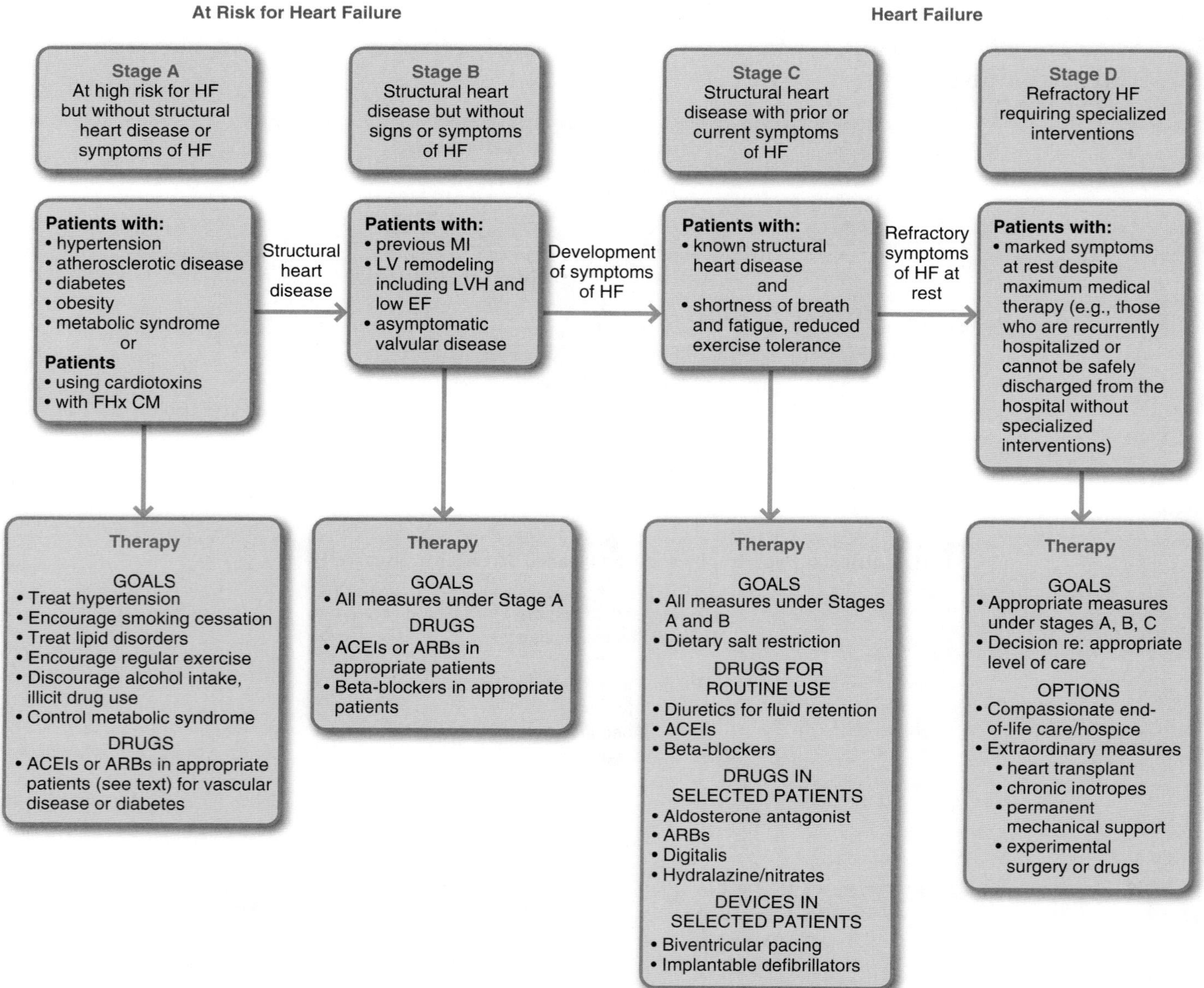

FIGURE 34-11 Stages of heart failure and recommended therapy by stage. *ACEI*, Angiotensin-converting enzyme inhibitor; *ARB*, angiotensin receptor blocker; *CM*, cardiomyopathy; *EF*, ejection fraction; *FHx*, family history; *HF*, heart failure; *IV*, intravenous; *MI*, myocardial infarction; *LV*, left ventricular; *LVH*, left ventricular hypertrophy. *(Source: Hunt SA et al: ACC/AHA 2005 guideline update for the diagnosis and management of chronic heart failure in the adult: a report of the American College of Cardiology/American Heart Association Task Force, J Am Coll Cardiol 46: el, 2005.)*

In HF the heart can compensate for poor cardiac output by (1) increasing the force of contraction, (2) increasing in size, (3) pumping more often, and (4) stimulating the kidneys to conserve sodium and water. For a time this compensation maintains near-normal circulation, but eventually the heart can no longer maintain a normal output (decompensation). Advanced symptoms can develop in weeks or months, and sudden death can occur at any time.

Three symptoms—fatigue, shortness of breath, and fluid retention—are the hallmarks of HF. Shortness of breath on exertion, or effort intolerance, is the earliest symptom. This shortness of breath gets worse and occurs at rest (**orthopnea**) or at night (paroxysmal nocturnal dyspnea). Fluid retention can manifest as pulmonary congestion or peripheral edema. Evidence of hypoperfusion includes cool forearms and legs, sleepiness, declining serum sodium level caused by fluid overload and worsening renal function.

Decreased cranial blood supply can lead to mental confusion, memory loss, anxiety, insomnia, **syncope** (loss of oxygen to the brain causing brief loss of consciousness), and headache. The latter symptoms are more common in older patients and often are the only symptoms; this can lead to a delay in diagnosis. Often the first symptom in older adults is a dry cough with generalized weakness and anorexia.

Cardiac cachexia is the end result of HF in 10% to 15% of patients. It is defined as involuntary weight loss of at least 6% of nonedematous body weight during a 6-month period (Springer et al., 2006). Unlike normal starvation, which is characterized by adipose tissue loss, this cachexia is characterized by a significant loss of lean body mass. This decrease in lean body mass further exacerbates HF because of the loss of cardiac muscle and the development of a heart that is soft and flabby. In addition, there are structural, circulatory, metabolic, inflammatory, and neuroendocrine changes in the skeletal muscle of patients with HF (Delano and Moldawer, 2006). Differences between younger and older patients are listed in Table 34-9.

Cardiac cachexia is a serious complication of HF with a poor prognosis and high mortality rate. Symptoms that reflect inadequate blood supply to the abdominal organs include anorexia, nausea, a feeling of fullness, constipation, abdominal pain, malabsorption, hepatomegaly, and liver tenderness. All of these contribute to the high prevalence of malnutrition observed in hospitalized patients with HF. Lack of blood flow to the gut leads to loss of bowel integrity; bacteria and other endotoxins may enter the bloodstream and cause cytokine activation. Proinflammatory cytokines such as TNF-α and adiponectin are highest in patients with cardiac cachexia. An increased level of TNF-α is associated with a lower BMI, smaller skinfold measurements, and decreased plasma total protein levels, indicative of a catabolic state.

Adiponectin levels are high in HF and are a marker for wasting and a predictor of mortality. As with TNF-α, adiponectin levels are also inversely correlated with BMI. Treatments for muscle wasting are being explored (Springer et al., 2006).

TABLE 34-9

Heart Failure in Middle Age versus Older Adulthood

	Middle Age	Older Adulthood
Prevalence	<1%	≈10%
Sex	Men > Women	Women > Men
Cause	CAD	Hypertension
Clinical features	Typical	Atypical
LVEF	Reduced	Normal
Comorbidities	Few	Multiple
RCTs	Many	Few
Therapy	Evidence-based	Empiric
Physician treating HF	Cardiologist	Primary care

From Rich MW: Office management of heart failure in the elderly, AM J Med 118:342, 2005.

CAD, Coronary artery disease; *HF*, heart failure; *LVEF*, left ventricular ejection fraction; *RCT*, randomized clinical trial.

Risk Factors

The Framingham Study (see *Focus On:* Framingham Heart Study) showed the risk factors for HF were hypertension, diabetes, CHD, and **left ventricular hypertrophy (LVH)** (enlargement of the left ventricle of the heart). Antecedent hypertension is present in 75% of HF cases (AHA, 2010). Individuals who have diabetes mellitus and ischemic heart disease more frequently develop HF compared with patients without diabetes (Rosano et al., 2006). Diabetes is an especially strong risk factor for HF in women. The prevalence of both hypertension and diabetes increases with age, making the elderly particularly vulnerable to HF. Another large cohort study of older adults (70 to 79 years) showed that waist circumference and percentage of body fat were the strongest predictors of who would develop HF (Nicklas et al., 2006). Numerous changes in cardiovascular structure and function also place the elderly at high risk for developing HF (Box 34-8).

Prevention

Because long-term survival rates for persons with HF are low, prevention is critical. HF is categorized into four stages ranging from persons with risk factors (stage A—primary prevention) to persons with advanced HF (stage D—severe disease). For stages A and B the aggressive treatment of underlying risk factors and diseases such as dyslipidemia, hypertension, and diabetes is critical to prevent structural damage to the myocardium and the appearance of HF symptoms. Such prevention has been very effective. Even patients who experience an MI can reduce the risk of HF with antihypertensive therapy.

For stages C and D, secondary prevention strategies to prevent further cardiac dysfunction are warranted. These strategies include the use of ACE inhibitors (first line of therapy), angiotensin receptor blockers, aldosterone blockers, β-blockers, and digoxin. Early detection, correction of

BOX 34-8

Principal Effects of Aging on Cardiovascular Structure and Function

Increased vascular stiffness
Increased myocardial stiffness
Decreased β-adrenergic responsiveness
Impaired mitochondrial ATP production
Decreased baroreceptor responsiveness
Impaired sinus node function
Impaired endothelial function
Net Effect: Marked reduction in cardiovascular reserve

From Rich MW: Office management of heart failure in the elderly, Am Med 118:342, 2005.

ATP, Adenosine triphosphate.

asymptomatic left ventricular dysfunction, and aggressive management of risk factors are needed to lower the incidence and mortality of HF.

New research is studying the effects of cardiotonic steroids, including marinobufagenin, a group of hormones found in plasma and urine of patients with HF, MI, and chronic renal failure (Tian et al., 2010). If there are preventive measures, studies will identify them.

Medical Management

Therapy recommendations correspond to the stage of HF. For patients at high risk of developing HF (stage A), treatment of the underlying conditions (hypertension, dyslipidemia, thyroid disorders, arrhythmias), avoidance of high-risk behaviors (tobacco, excessive alcohol, illicit drug use), and lifestyle changes (weight reduction, exercise, reduction of sodium intake, heart-healthy diet) are recommended. All these recommendations are carried through the other stages. In addition, an implantable defibrillator, which shocks the heart when it stops, can be placed in patients at risk of sudden death. Pharmacologic treatment of HF is the hallmark of therapy with progressive stages. The last stage also includes surgically implanted ventricular-assist devices, heart transplantation, and continual intravenous therapy.

The short-term goals for the treatment of HF are to relieve symptoms, improve the quality of life, and reduce depression if it is present. The long-term goal of treatment is to prolong life by lessening, stopping, or reversing left ventricular dysfunction. Medical management is tailored to clinical and hemodynamic profiles with evidence of hypoperfusion and congestion. In some cases surgical procedures are needed to alleviate the HF caused by valvular disease; medical management is limited in these instances.

Initial management of HF includes a restricted sodium diet (less than 2000 mg daily) and regular activity, as symptoms permit. Bed rest is no longer recommended except for those with acute failure. The heart becomes deconditioned with less exercise, whereas with regular exercise capacity can be increased. Standard fluid restrictions are to limit total fluid intake to 2 L (2000 mL) daily. When patients are severely decompensated, a more restrictive fluid intake (1000 to 1500 mL daily) may be warranted for adequate diuresis. A sodium-restricted diet should be maintained despite low-sodium blood levels because in this case the sodium has shifted from the blood to the tissues. Serum sodium appears low in a patient who is fluid overloaded because of dilution; diuresis improves the levels by decreasing the amount of water in the vascular space.

An ACE inhibitor is the first line of pharmacologic treatment for HF. As the stages progress, a β-blocker or angiotensin receptor blocker may be added. In Stages C and D selected patients may also take a diuretic, aldosterone antagonists, digitalis, and vasodilators (e.g., hydralazine). Basically these medications reduce excess fluid, dilate blood vessels, and increase the strength of the heart's contraction. Several of these medications have neurohormonal benefits along with their primary mechanism of action. For example, ACE inhibitors (e.g., captopril, enalapril) not only inhibit the RAS (see Chapter 36) but also improve symptoms, quality of life, exercise tolerance, and survival. Similarly, spironolactone has both diuretic and aldosterone-blocking functions that result in reduced morbidity and mortality in patients. Most of these medications can affect nutrition status (see Chapter 9 and Appendix 31).

Medical Nutrition Therapy

The RD provides MNT, which includes assessment, establishing a nutrition diagnosis, and interventions (education, counseling). As part of a multidisciplinary team (physician, pharmacist, psychologist, nurse, and social worker), the RD positively affects patient outcomes. Reduced readmission to the hospital, fewer days in the hospital, improved compliance with restricted sodium and fluid intakes, and improved quality of life scores are the goals in HF patients.

Nutrition screening for HF in older adults can help prevent disease progression and improve disease management, overall health, and quality-of-life outcomes. The first step in screening is determination of body weight. Altered fluid balance complicates assessment of body weight in the patient with HF. Weights should be taken before eating and after voiding at the same time each day. A dry weight (weight without edema) should be determined on the scale at home. Patients should record daily weights and advise their care providers if weight gain exceeds more than 1 lb a day for patients with severe HF, more than 2 lb a day for patients with moderate HF, and more than 3 to 5 pounds with mild HF. Restricting sodium and fluids along with diuretic therapy may restore fluid balance and prevent full-blown HF.

Dietary assessments in HF patients reveal that more than half have malnutrition, usually related to the cardiac cachexia mentioned earlier. Negative energy balance and negative nitrogen balances can be noted. In overweight patients caloric reduction must be carefully monitored to avoid excessive and rapid body protein catabolism. Nutrition education to promote behavior change is a critical component of MNT. The benefits of MNT should be communicated to patients.

The total diet must be addressed in patients with HF because underlying risk factors are often present; dietary changes to modify these risk factors are an important component of MNT. For dyslipidemia or atherosclerosis, a heart-healthy diet low in SFAs, *trans*-fatty acids, and cholesterol and high in fiber, whole grains, fruits, and vegetables is recommended. For persons with hypertension, the DASH diet is recommended. Both of these dietary patterns emphasize lower-sodium foods and higher intake of potassium. Total energy expenditure is higher in HF patients because of the catabolic state, adequate protein and energy should be provided.

Salt Restriction

Edema in patients with decompensated HF results from impaired cardiac function. Inadequate blood flow to the kidneys leads to aldosterone and vasopressin (antidiuretic hormone) secretion. Both these hormones act to conserve fluid, thus trying to restore blood flow. Aldosterone promotes sodium resorption, and vasopressin promotes water conservation in the distal tubules of the nephron. Sodium and fluid thus accumulate in the tissues. Even asymptomatic patients with mild HF and no edema can retain sodium and water if consuming a high-salt diet.

The degree of restriction depends on the individual. For the healthy elderly population (older than 71 years), the AI is 1200 mg (50 mmol)/day. Recommendations for HF patients vary between 1200 and 2400 mg/day. For patients taking large doses of lasix (80 mg/day), a sodium intake of less than 2 g/day is recommended to optimize the effects of the diuretic. Severe restrictions (500 mg/day) are unpalatable and nutritionally inadequate. See *Focus On:* Sodium and Salt Measurement Equivalents.

Adherence to sodium restrictions can be problematic for many individuals, and individualized instruction is recommended. Ethnic differences in sodium consumption must be considered. Some cultures have traditional diets that are very high in sodium such as Kosher and Asian diets. In some cases regional cooking, like in some areas in the southern United States, depends heavily on salt.

Positive outcomes (i.e., decreased urinary sodium excretion, less fatigue, less frequent edema) have been observed in HF patients receiving MNT. The type of sodium restriction prescribed should be the least restrictive diet that will still achieve the desired results. The first step is to minimize or eliminate the use of table salt and high-sodium foods (Box 34-9) (see Appendix 37 for further explanation of the sodium-restricted diet).

Poor adherence to low-sodium diets occurs in part as a result of lack of knowledge about sodium and lower-sodium food choices by the patient, and perception that the diet interferes with the social aspects of eating. Lack of cooking skills or adequate cooking facilities is another obstacle because it leads patients to eat premade foods that tend to be high in salt. Memory loss, severe fatigue, and economic issues are all challenges to following a low-sodium diet. In addition, food labels, although informative, may be hard for many patients or their caregivers to comprehend (Box 34-10).

Alcohol

In excess, alcohol contributes to fluid intake and raises blood pressure. Many cardiologists recommend avoiding alcohol. Chronic alcohol ingestion may lead to cardiomyopathy and HF (Li and Ren, 2006). Although heavy drinking should be discouraged, moderate drinking may lower the risk of HF through beneficial effects of alcohol on coronary artery disease. Quantity, drinking patterns, and genetic factors influence the relationship between alcohol consumption and HF (Djousse and Gaziano, 2008). If alcohol is consumed, intake should not exceed one drink per day for women and two drinks per day for men. A drink is equivalent to 1 oz of alcohol (1 oz of distilled liquor), 5 oz of wine, or 12 oz of beer.

FOCUS ON

Sodium and Salt Measurement Equivalents

Sodium chloride is approximately 40% (39.3%) sodium and 60% chloride. To convert a specified weight of sodium chloride to its sodium equivalent, multiply the weight by 0.393. Sodium is also measured in milliequivalents (mEq). To convert milligrams of sodium to mEq, divide by the atomic weight of 23. To convert sodium to sodium chloride (salt), multiply by 2.54. Millimoles (mmol) and milliequivalents (mEq) of sodium are the same. For example:

1 tsp of salt = approximately 6 g NaCl = 6096 mg NaCl
6096 mg NaCl × 0.393 = 2396 mg Na (approximately 2400 mg)
2396 mg Na/23 = 104 mEq Na
1 g Na = 1000 mg/23 = 43 mEq or mmol
1 tsp of salt = 2400 mg or 104 mEq Na

BOX 34-9

Top Ten Categories of High-Sodium Foods

1. Smoked, processed, or cured meats and fish (e.g., ham, bacon, corned beef, cold cuts, hot dogs, sausage, salt pork, chipped beef, pickled herring, anchovies, tuna, and sardines)
2. Tomato juices and tomato sauce, unless labeled otherwise
3. Meat extracts, bouillon cubes, meat sauces, *MSG, and taco seasoning
4. Salted snacks (potato chips, tortilla chips, corn chips, pretzels, salted nuts, popcorn, and crackers)
5. Prepared salad dressings, condiments, relishes, ketchup, Worcestershire sauce, barbecue sauce, cocktail sauce, teriyaki sauce, soy sauce, commercial salad dressings, salsa, pickles, olives, and sauerkraut
6. Packaged mixes for sauces, gravies, casseroles, and noodle, rice, or potato dishes; macaroni and cheese; stuffing mix
7. Cheeses (processed and cheese spreads)
8. Frozen entrees and pot pies
9. Canned soup
10. Foods eaten away from home

**MSG*, Monosodium glutamate.

Note: Reading labels is most important; some brands are lower in sodium than others.

BOX 34-10

Food Labeling Guide for Sodium

Sodium-free	Less than 5 mg per standard serving; cannot contain any sodium chloride
Very low sodium	35 mg or less per standard serving
Low sodium	140 mg or less per standard serving
Reduced sodium	At least 25% less sodium per standard serving than in the regular food
Light in sodium	50% less sodium per standard serving than in the regular food
Unsalted, without added salt, or no salt added	No salt added during processing; the product it resembles is normally processed with salt
Lightly salted	50% less added sodium than is normally added; product must state "not a low-sodium food" if that criterion is not met

Data from U.S. Food and Drug Administration: Scouting for sodium and other nutrients important to blood pressure, FDA Consumer Publication No. 95-2284, 1995.

Caffeine

Until now caffeine has been considered detrimental to patients with HF because it contributes to irregular heartbeats. However, a study in the Netherlands suggests that moderate intake of either tea or coffee reduces CHD risk; tea actually reduces CHD deaths (deKonig Gans, 2010). Researchers in the United States followed 130,054 men and women and found that those who reported drinking four or more cups of coffee each day had an 18% lower risk of hospitalization for heart rhythm disturbances. Those who reported drinking one to three cups each day had a 7% reduction in risk (Klatsky, 2010). The antioxidant effects of coffee and tea may be beneficial.

Calcium

Patients with HF are at increased risk of developing osteoporosis because of low activity levels, impaired renal function, and prescription drugs that alter calcium metabolism (Zittermann et al., 2006). Cachectic HF patients have lower bone mineral density and lower calcium levels than HF patients without cachexia (Anker, 2006). Caution must be used with calcium supplements because they may aggravate cardiac arrhythmias. Before transplant, most HF patients only have subtle changes in bone.

Coenzyme Q_{10}

Levels of coenzyme Q_{10} (CoQ_{10}) are often lower in HF patients; it is postulated that repletion can prevent oxidative stress and further myocardial damage (Sanders, 2006). However, in two randomized control trials in patients with class III and IV symptoms, CoQ_{10} had limited benefit (Levy and Kohlhaas, 2006). Routine supplementation is not recommended by the AHA at this time. However, HF is known to be associated with key deficiencies of micronutrients that are required for cardiac function and further studies are needed (Soukoulis, 2009). It should be noted that patients on statins (HMG-CoA reductase inhibitors) may have a different reason to consider supplementation. HMG-CoA reductase inhibitors are a class of cholesterol lowering drugs that are known to interfere with synthesis of CoQ_{10} (see Chapter 9).

D-Ribose

D-ribose is a component of ATP for cellular metabolism and energy production. Myocardial ischemia lowers cellular energy levels, integrity, and function. The failing heart is energy-starved. D-ribose is being tested to correct this deficient cellular energy as a naturally occurring carbohydrate (Shecterle et al., 2010).

Energy

The energy needs of patients with HF depend on their current dry weight, activity restrictions, and the severity of the HF. Overweight patients with limited activity must achieve and maintain an appropriate weight that will not stress the myocardium. For the obese patient, hypocaloric diets (1000 to 1200 kcal daily) reduce the stress on the heart and facilitate weight reduction. However, the nutrition status of the obese patient must be assessed to ensure that the patient is not malnourished. In patients with severe HF, energy needs are increased by 30% to 50% more than basal level as a result of the increased energy expenditure of the heart and lungs; 31 to 35 kcal/kg of body weight is often used as the starting point for determining caloric requirements. Patients with cardiac cachexia may require further increases in energy to 1.6 to 1.8 times the resting energy expenditure for nutritional repletion.

Fats

Fish consumption and fish oils rich in ω-3 fatty acids can lower elevated triglyceride levels, prevent atrial fibrillation, and perhaps even reduce mortality rates in HF patients (Roth and Harris, 2010). Intake of at least 1 g daily of ω-3 fatty acids from either oily fish or fish-oil supplements can be safely recommended. Interestingly, recent evidence suggests that high saturated fat feeding in mild to moderate HF preserves contractile function and prevents the switch from fatty acid to glucose metabolism, thus serving a cardioprotective role (Chess et al., 2009; Christopher et al., 2010).

Feeding Strategies

Patients with HF often tolerate small, frequent feedings better than larger, infrequent meals because the latter are more tiring to consume, can contribute to abdominal distention, and markedly increase oxygen consumption. All these factors tax the already stressed heart. Caloric supplements can help to increase energy intake; however, this intervention may not reverse this form of malnutrition (Anker et al., 2006).

Folate, Vitamin B_6, and Vitamin B_{12}

High dietary intakes of folate and vitamin B_6 have been associated with reduced risk of mortality from HF and stroke in some populations (Cui et al., 2010). Elevated tHcy levels should be lowered when possible.

Magnesium

Magnesium deficiency is common in patients with HF as a result of poor dietary intake and the use of diuretics, including furosemide. As with potassium, the diuretics used to treat HF increase magnesium excretion. Magnesium deficiency aggravates changes in electrolyte concentration by causing a positive sodium and negative potassium balance. Because deficient magnesium status is associated with poorer prognosis, blood magnesium levels should be measured in HF patients and treated accordingly. Magnesium supplementation (800 mg/day) produces small improvements in arterial compliance (Fuentes et al., 2006). Poor dietary intake of magnesium has been associated with elevated CRP, a product of inflammation. Hypermagnesemia may be found in some cases of renal failure, HF, and high doses of furosemide.

Thiamin

Patients with HF are at risk for thiamin deficiency because of poor food intake; use of loop diuretics, which increases excretion; and advanced age. Thiamin deficiency is diagnosed using erythrocyte thiamin pyrophosphate levels in 33% of HF patients (Hanninen et al., 2006). Loop diuretics can deplete body thiamin and cause metabolic acidosis. Thiamin status should be assessed in HF patients on loop diuretics, and appropriate supplementation recommended if necessary. Thiamin supplementation (e.g., 200 mg/day) can improve left ventricular ejection fraction (fraction of blood pumped out of the ventricles with each heart beat) and symptoms.

Vitamin D

Patients with a polymorphism of the vitamin D receptor gene have higher rates of bone loss than HF patients without this genotype. Vitamin D may improve inflammation in HF patients (Vieth and Kimball, 2006). In a double-blind, randomized, placebo-controlled trial, supplementation with vitamin D (50 mcg or 2000 international units of vitamin D_3 per day) for 9 months increased the antiinflammatory cytokine IL-10 and decreased the proinflammatory factors in HF patients (Schleithoff et al., 2006). As a steroid hormone, vitamin D regulates gene expression and inversely regulates renin secretion (Meems et al., 2010). However, it remains unclear if vitamin D supplementation is truly needed in HF patients.

CARDIAC TRANSPLANTATION

Cardiomyopathies represent a heterogeneous group of diseases that often lead to progressive HF; types include dilated cardiomyopathy, hypertrophic cardiomyopathy, restrictive cardiomyopathy, and arrhythmogenic right ventricular cardiomyopathy (Wexler et al., 2009). Cardiac transplantation is the only cure for refractory, end-stage HF. Because the number of donor hearts is limited, careful selection of recipients with consideration of the likelihood for adherence to lifelong therapeutic regimen and their quality of life is imperative (D'Amico, 2005). Nutrition support before and after transplantation is crucial to decrease morbidity and mortality. Thus the nutrition care of the heart transplant patient can be divided into three phases: pretransplant, immediate posttransplant, and long-term posttransplant.

Pretransplant Medical Nutrition Therapy

A comprehensive nutrition assessment of the pretransplant patient should include a history, physical and anthropometric assessment, and biochemical testing. Recommended lifestyle changes prior to transplantation include restricting alcohol consumption, losing weight, exercising, quitting smoking, and eating a low-sodium diet (Wexler et al., 2010). Extremes in body weight (<80% or >140% of ideal body weight) increase the patient's risk for infection, diabetes, morbidity, and higher mortality. Pretransplant comorbidities such as hyperlipidemia and hypertension also reduce survival rates. If oral intake is inadequate, an enteral feeding should be tailored to the nutritional and comorbid conditions of the patient.

Immediate Posttransplant Nutrition Support

The nutritional goals in the acute posttransplant patient are to (1) provide adequate protein and calories to treat catabolism and promote healing, (2) monitor and correct electrolyte abnormalities, and (3) achieve optimal blood glucose control (Hasse, 2001). In the immediate posttransplant period nutrient needs are increased, as is the case after any major surgery. Protein needs are increased because of steroid-induced catabolism, surgical stress, anabolism, and wound healing.

Patients progress from clear liquids to a soft diet given in small, frequent feedings. Enteral feeding may be appropriate in the short term, especially if complications arise. Nutrient intake is often maintained by using liquid supplements and foods of high caloric density, especially in patients with poor appetite. Weight gain to an ideal weight is the nutritional goal for patients who were cachectic before transplant. The increase in cardiac function helps to halt the presurgical cachectic state. Hyperglycemia can be exacerbated by the stress of the surgery and the immunosuppressive drug regimen. Dietary adjustments can be made to aid in glucose control (see Table 34-10).

Long-Term Posttransplant Nutrition Support

Comorbid conditions that often occur after transplantation include hypertension, excessive weight gain, hyperlipidemia,

TABLE 34-10

Short-Term Posttransplant Nutrient Recommendations

Nutrient	Recommendations	Comment
Protein	1.5-2.0 g/kg	Protein catabolism is increased due to because of surgery and corticosteroids. Protein is required for wound healing; infection prevention; and losses from drains, wounds, etc.
Calories	130%-150% of REE	Upper range for underweight patients; lower range for overweight patients.
Carbohydrate	50%-70% of nonprotein calories	Medications may cause hypoglycemia; treat with sliding-scale insulin.
Lipid	30%-50% of nonprotein calories	Higher range is recommended only when hyperglycemia is severe and not under control with insulin alone.
Fluid	1 mL/calorie	Monitor output from urine, drains, etc.
Sodium	2-4 g/day	Restrict if edema is present.
Phosphorus, magnesium, bicarbonate	Individualize	Monitor biochemical parameters.

From Hasse JM: Nutrition assessment and support of organ transplant recipients, JPEN 25(3):120, 2001.
REE, Resting energy expenditure.

CLINICAL SCENARIO

Tom is a 55-year-old single man with hypertension (blood pressure 145/92), high low-density lipoprotein cholesterol (241) and low high-density lipoprotein cholesterol (38). He reports that he often eats in his car so he frequents fast-food restaurants. He works long hours and, other than gardening on the weekends, he does not exercise. He is 5′10″ and 220 lbs. His breakfast is usually a cheese-egg biscuit, white toast with butter, bacon, and coffee without milk or cream. Lunch is a fried luncheon meat sandwich with mayonnaise, potato chips, and a piece of fruit pie with ice cream. Dinner is often fried chicken, mashed potatoes with gravy, creamed vegetables, and some type of whipped cream dessert.

Using the following list, what are Tom's nutritional diagnoses? Which should be the top priority?

Nutrition Diagnostic Term

Excessive energy intake
Excessive intake of fats
Excessive alcohol intake
Inadequate fiber intake
Inadequate calcium intake
Inadequate magnesium intake
Inadequate potassium intake
Excessive sodium intake
Overweight or obesity
Food- and nutrition-related knowledge deficit
Undesirable food choices
Physical inactivity

Nutrition Care Questions

Which interventions would be most beneficial for Tom?
What signs and symptoms would you want to monitor and evaluate?

osteoporosis, and infection. Hypertension is managed by diet, exercise, and medications. Minimizing excessive weight gain is important because patients who become obese after transplantation are at higher risk for rejection and lower rates of survival.

Increases in total LDL cholesterol and triglycerides are a consequence of immunosuppressive drug therapy and increase the risk of HF after transplantation Along with a heart-healthy diet, patients also need a lipid-lowering drug regimen to normalize blood lipids. Statins are recommended in the early and long-term postoperative periods. Because of their LDL-lowering effect, stanols or sterols may be helpful to reduce statin dosages (Goldberg et al., 2006).

Before transplantation, patients are likely to have osteopenia because of their lack of activity and cardiac cachexia. After transplantation, patients are susceptible to steroid-induced osteoporosis. Patients require optimal calcium and vitamin D intake to slow bone loss; weight-bearing exercise and antiresorptive drug therapy are often necessary. Infection must be avoided because of the necessity of lifelong use of immunosuppressive drugs. Food safety should be discussed.

USEFUL WEBSITES

American Association of Cardiovascular and Pulmonary Rehabilitation
http://www.aacvpr.org/
American Dietetic Association, Evidence Analysis Library
http://www.eatright.org/
American Heart Association
http://www.heart.org/
NCEP Adult Treatment Panel Guidelines
http://www.nhlbi.nih.gov/guidelines/cholesterol/atp_iii.htm

REFERENCES

American Diabetes Association: *National Diabetes Factsheet*, Alexandria, VA, 2007, American Diabetes Association.

American Dietetic Association: *Hypertension, ADA Evidence Analysis Library*, Chicago, IL, 2009, ADA.

American Heart Association: *Heart Disease and Stroke Statistics: 2010 Update At-A-Glance*, Dallas, Texas, 2010, American Heart Association.

American Heart Association Statistics Committee and Stroke Statistics Committee. AHA Statistics Update: Heart Disease and Stroke Statistics—2007 Update, *Circulation* 115:e69-171, 2007.

Anderson JW, et al: Health benefits of fiber, *Nutrition Reviews* 67:188, 2009.

Anker SD, et al: ESPEN guidelines on enteral nutrition: cardiology and pulmonology evidence-based recommendations, *Clin Nutr* 25:311, 2006.

Appel LJ, et al: Dietary approaches to prevent and treat hypertension: a scientific statement from The American Heart Association, *Hypertension* 47:296, 2006.

Arora RR, et al: Short- and long-term mortality with nesiritide, *Am Heart J* 152:1084, 2006.

Badimon L, et al: Cell biology and lipoproteins in atherosclerosis, *Curr Mol Med* 6:439, 2006.

Bartolucci AA, Howard G: Meta-analysis of data from the six primary prevention trials of cardiovascular events using aspirin, *Am J Cardiol* 98:746, 2006.

Barter P, Rye K: Homocysteine and cardiovascular disease, *Circulation Res* 99:565, 2006.

Basu A, et al: Dietary factors that promote or retard inflammation, *Arterioscler Thromb Vasc Biol* 26:995, 2006.

Behavioral Risk Factor Surveillance System: Prevalence of heart disease—United States, 2005, CDC, *MMWR* 56(6):113, 2007.

Berg AH, Scherer PE: Adipose tissue, inflammation and cardiovascular disease, *Circ Res* 96:939, 2006.

Bloomer RJ, et al: Effect of a 21 day Daniel Fast on metabolic and cardiovascular disease risk factors in men and women, *Lipids Health Dis* 9:94, 2010.

Blumenthal JA, et al: Effects of the DASH diet alone and in combination with exercise and weight loss on blood pressure and cardiovascular biomarkers in men and women with high blood pressure: the ENCORE study, *Arch Int Med* 126, 2010.

Boden WE, et al: Optimal medical therapy with or without PCI for stable coronary disease, *N Engl J Med* 356:1503, 2007.

Brindle P, et al: Accuracy and impact of risk assessment in the primary prevention of cardiovascular disease: a systematic review, *Heart* 92:1752, 2006.

Brook RD: Obesity, weight loss, and vascular function, *Endocrine* 29:21, 2006.

Calhoun DA, et al: Resistant hypertension: diagnosis, evaluation, and treatment: a scientific statement from the American Heart Association Professional Education Committee of the Council for High Blood Pressure Research, *Circulation* 117: e510, 2008.

Carter SJ, et al: Relationship between Mediterranean diet score and atherothrombotic risk: findings from the Third National Health and Nutrition Examination Survey (NHANES-III), 1988-1994, *Atherosclerosis* 4:630, 2010.

Chess DJ, et al: A high-fat diet increases adiposity but maintains mitochondrial oxidative enzymes without affecting development of heart failure with pressure overload, *Am J Physiol Heart Circ Physiol* 297:1585, 2009.

Chiuve SE, et al: Healthy lifestyle factors in the primary prevention of coronary heart disease among men: benefits among users and nonusers of lipid-lowering and antihypertensive medications, *Circulation* 114:160, 2006.

Christopher BA, et al: Myocardial insulin resistance induced by high fat feeding in heart failure is associated with preserved contractile function, *Am J Physiol Heart Circ Physiol* 299:H1917, 2010.

Chobanian AV, et al: The Seventh Report of the Joint National Committee on the Prevention, Evaluation and Treatment of High Blood Pressure: the JNC 7 report, *JAMA* 289:2560, 2003.

Cicero AF, et al: ω-3 polyunsaturated fatty acids: their potential role in blood pressure prevention and management, *Curr Vasc Pharmacol* 3:330, 2009.

Civeira F, et al: Guidelines for the diagnosis and management of heterozygous familial hypercholesterolemia, *Atherosclerosis* 173:55, 2004.

Cook NR, et al: Long term effects of dietary sodium reduction on cardiovascular disease outcomes: observational follow-up of the trials of hypertension prevention (TOHP), *BMJ* 334:885, 2007.

Couch SC, et al: The efficacy of a clinic-based behavioral nutrition intervention emphasizing a DASH-type diet for adolescents with elevated blood pressure, *J Pediatr* 152:494, 2008.

Cui R, et al: Dietary folate and vitamin B_6 and B_{12} intake in relation to mortality from cardiovascular diseases: Japan collaborative cohort study, *Stroke* 41:1285, 2010.

D'Amico CL: Cardiac transplantation: patient selection in the current era, *J Cardiovasc Nurs* 20:S4, 2005.

DeKonig Gans JM, et al: Tea and coffee consumption and cardiovascular morbidity and mortality, *Arterioscler Thromb Vasc Biol* 10:1161, 2010.

Delano MJ, Moldawer L: The origins of cachexia in acute and chronic inflammatory diseases, *Nutr Clin Pract* 21:68, 2006.

Despres JP, Lemieux I: Abdominal obesity and metabolic syndrome, *Nature* 444:881, 2006.

Djousse L, Gaziano JM: Alcohol consumption and heart failure: a systematic review, *Curr Atheroscler Rep* 10:117, 2008.

Dickinson HO, et al: Lifestyle interventions to reduce raised blood pressure: a systematic review of randomized, controlled trials, *J Hypertens* 24:215, 2006a.

Dickinson HO, et al: Magnesium supplementation for the management of essential hypertension in adults, *Cochrane Database Syst Rev* 3:CD004640, 2006b.

Egan BM, et al: US trends in prevalence, awareness, treatment, and control of hypertension, 1988-2008, *JAMA* 303:2043, 2010.

Erkkila AT, Lichtenstein AH: Fiber and cardiovascular disease risk: how strong is the evidence? *J Cardiovasc Nurs* 21:3, 2006.

Esposito K, Giugliano D: Diet and inflammation: a link to metabolic and cardiovascular diseases, *Eur Heart J* 27:15, 2006.

Fuentes J, et al: Acute and chronic oral magnesium supplementation: effects on endothelial function, exercise function, exercise capacity, and quality of life in patients with symptomatic heart failure, *Congest Heart Fail* 12:9, 2006.

Gebauer SK, et al: ω-3 fatty acid dietary recommendations and food sources to achieve essentiality and cardiovascular benefits, *Am J Clin Nutr* 83:1526s, 2006.

Gidding SS, et al: Implementing the American Heart Association pediatric and adult nutrition guidelines: a scientific statement from the American Heart Association Nutrition Committee of the Council on Nutrition, Physical Activity and Metabolism, Council on Cardiovascular Disease in the Young, Council on Arteriosclerosis, Thrombosis and Vascular Biology, Council on Cardiovascular Nursing, Council on Epidemiology and Prevention, and Council for High Blood Pressure Research, *Circulation* 119:1161, 2009.

Goldberg AC, et al: Effect of plant stanol tablets on low-density lipoprotein lowering in patients on statin drugs, *Am J Cardiol* 97:376, 2006.

Gotoh K, et al: Apolipoprotein A-IV interacts synergistically with melanocortins to reduce food intake, *Am J Physiol Regul Integr Comp Physiol* 290:R202, 2006.

Hanninen SA, et al: The prevalence of thiamin deficiency in hospitalized patients with congestive heart failure, *J Am Coll Cardiol* 47:354, 2006.

Hasse J: Nutrition assessment and support of organ transplant recipients, *JPEN J Parenter Enteral Nutr* 25:120, 2001.

Heinecke JW: Lipoprotein oxidation in cardiovascular disease: chief culprit or innocent bystanders? *J Exp Med* 203:813, 2006.

Horwich TB, et al: B-type natriuretic peptide levels in obese patients with advanced heart failure, *J Am Coll Cardiol* 47:85, 2006.

Kay CD, et al: Effects of antioxidant rich foods on vascular reactivity: review of the clinical evidence, *Curr Atheroscler Rep* 8:510, 2006.

Kalogeropoulos N, et al: Unsaturated fatty acids are inversely associated and ω-6/ω-3 ratios are positively related to inflammation and coagulation markers in plasma of apparently healthy adults, *Clin Chim Acta* 411:584, 2010.

Kelly JH, Sabate J: Nuts and coronary heart disease: an epidemiological perspective, *Br J Nutr* 96:S61, 2006.

Khayat R, et al: Obstructive sleep apnea: the new cardiovascular disease. Part 1: obstructive sleep apnea and the pathogenesis of vascular disease, *Heart Failure Reviews* 14:143, 2009.

Klatsky AL: Coffee drinking and caffeine associated with reduced risk of hospitalization for heart rhythm disturbances. Presented at *AHA 50th Annual Conference on Cardiovascular Disease, Epidemiology and Prevention*, 5 March 2010, San Francisco, Calif.

Kris-Etherton PM, et al: Milk products, dietary patterns and blood pressure management, *J Am Coll Nutr* 28:103S, 2009.

Levy HB, Kohlhaas HK: Considerations for supplementing with coenzyme Q during statin therapy, *Ann Pharmacother* 40:290, 2006.

Li Q, Ren J: Cardiac overexpression of metallothionein attenuates chronic alcohol intake-induced cardiomyocyte contractile dysfunction, *Cardiovasc Toxicol* 6:173, 2006.

Lichtenstein AH, et al: Diet and lifestyle recommendations revision 2006: a scientific statement from the American Heart Association Nutrition Committee, *Circulation* 114:82, 2006.

Liebman B: Salt: shaving salt, saving lives. *Nutrition Action Newsletter* April 2010. Accessed 2 July 2010 from http://www.cspinet.org/nah/articles/salt.html.

Lombardi MP, et al: Molecular genetic testing for familial hypercholesterolemia in the Netherlands: a stepwise screening strategy enhances the mutation detection rate, *Genet Test* 10:77, 2006.

Luma GB, Spiotta RT: Hypertension in children and adolescents, *Am Fam Physician* 73:1558, 2006.

Marcovina S, Packard CJ: Measurement and meaning of apolipoprotein A-I and apolipoprotein B plasma levels, *J Intern Med* 259:437, 2006.

Masoura C, et al: Arterial endothelial function and wall thickness in familial hypercholesterolemia and familial combined hyperlipidemia and the effect of statins. A systemic review and meta-analysis, *Atherosclerosis* 214:129, 2011.

Mathieu P, et al: The link among inflammation, hypertension and cardiovascular disease. *Hypertension* 53:577, 2009.

McCollum M, et al: Prevalence of multiple cardiac risk factors in U.S. adults with diabetes, *Curr Med Res Opin* 22:1031, 2006.

McGuire K, et al: Ability of physical activity to predict cardiovascular disease beyond commonly evaluated cardiometabolic risk factors, *Am J Cardiol* 104:1522, 2009.

Meems LM, et al: Vitamin D biology in heart failure: molecular mechanisms and systematic review, *Curr Drug Targets* 12:29, 2011.

Mehta P, Griendling K: Angiotensin II signaling: physiological and pathological effects in the cardiovascular system, *Am J Physiol Cell Physiol* 292:C82, 2007.

Miller ER III, et al: The effects of macronutrients on blood pressure and lipids: an overview of the DASH and Omni Heart Trials, *Curr Atheroscler Rep* 8:460, 2006.

Mitsnefes MM: Hypertension in children and adolescents, *Pediatr Clin North Am* 53:493, 2006.

Naghavi M, et al: From vulnerable plaque to vulnerable patient. Part III: Executive summary of the Screening for Heart Attack Prevention and Education (SHAPE) Task Force Report, *Am J Cardiol* 98:2, 2006.

National Cholesterol Education Program (NCEP): Expert Panel on Detection, Evaluation, and Treatment of High Blood Cholesterol in Adults (Adult Treatment Panel III) final report, *Circulation* 106:3143, 2002.

National Academy of Science, Institute of Medicine: Strategies to reduce sodium intake in the United States. Accessed 2 July 2010 from http://www.iom.edu/sodiumstrategies/.

National Academy of Science, Institute of Medicine: *Dietary reference intakes: water, potassium, sodium chloride and sulfate*, ed 1, Washington, DC, 2004, National Academies Press.

National Institutes of Health; National Heart, Lung and Blood Institute; National High Blood Pressure Education Program: *The 7th Report of the Joint National Committee on Prevention, Detection, and Treatment of High Blood Pressure*, NIH Publication 04-5230, August 2004.

Newton-Cheh C, et al: Genome-wide association study identifies eight loci associated with blood pressure, *Nat Genet* 41:666, 2009.

Nicklas B, et al: Abdominal obesity is an independent risk factor for chronic heart failure in older people, *J Am Geriatr Soc* 54:413, 2006.

Norton GR, et al: Gene variants of the renin-angiotensin system and hypertension: from a trough of disillusionment to a welcome phase of enlightenment? *Clin Sci (Lond)* 118:487, 2010.

Olufadi R, Byrne CD: Effects of VLDL and remnant particles on platelets, *Pathophysiol Haemost Thromb* 35:281, 2006.

O'Malley PG: Atherosclerosis imaging of asymptomatic individuals, *Arch Intern Med* 166:1065, 2006.

Opie LH, et al: Controversies in stable coronary artery disease, *Lancet* 367:69, 2006.

Ostchega Y, et al: Trends in elevated blood pressure among children and adolescents: data from the National Health and Nutrition Examination Survey, 1988-2006, *Am J Hyperten* 22:59, 2009.

Ottestad IO, et al: Triglyceride-rich HDL3 from patients with familial hypercholesterolemia are less able to inhibit cytokine release or to promote cholesterol efflux, *J Nutr* 136:877, 2006.

Pearson T, et al: Markers of inflammation and cardiovascular disease: application to clinical and public health practice: a statement for healthcare professionals from the Centers for Disease Control and Prevention and the American Heart Association, *Circulation* 107:499, 2003.

Poirier P, et al: Obesity and cardiovascular disease: pathophysiology, evaluation, and effect of weight loss, *Circulation* 113:898, 2006.

Psota TL, et al: Dietary ω-3 fatty acid intake and cardiovascular risk, *Am J Cardiol* 98:3, 2006.

Raggi P: Noninvasive imaging of atherosclerosis among asymptomatic individuals, *Arch Intern Med* 166:1068, 2006.

Roth EM, Harris WS: Fish oil for primary and secondary prevention of coronary heart disease, *Curr Atheroscler Rep* 12:66, 2010.

Rosano GM, et al: Metabolic therapy for patients with diabetes mellitus and coronary artery disease, *Am J Cardiol* 98:14, 2006.

Savoia C, Schiffrin E: Vascular inflammation in hypertension and diabetes: molecular mechanisms and therapeutic interventions, *Clin Sci (London)* 112:375, 2007.

Sanders S, et al: The impact of coenzyme Q_{10} on systolic function in patients with chronic heart failure, *J Card Fail* 12:464, 2006.

Shecterle LM, et al: The patented uses of D-ribose in cardiovascular diseases, *Recent Pat Cardiovasc Drug Discov* 5:138, 2010.

Schleithoff SS, et al: Vitamin D supplementation improves cytokine profiles in patients with congestive heart failure: a double-blind, randomized, placebo-controlled trial, *Am J Clin Nutr* 83:754, 2006.

Scirica BM, et al: Is C-reactive protein an innocent bystander or proatherogenic culprit, *Circulation* 113:2128, 2006.

Shankaran S, et al: Fetal origin of childhood disease: intrauterine growth restriction in term infants and risk for hypertension at 6 years of age, *Arch Pediatr Adolesc Med* 160:977, 2006.

Sontia B, Touyz RM: A role of magnesium in hypertension, *Arch Bioch Biophys* 458:33, 2007.

Soukoulis V, et al: Micronutrient deficiencies an unmet need in heart failure, *J Am Coll Cardiol* 54:1660, 2009.

Springer J, et al: Prognosis and therapy approaches of cardiac cachexia, *Curr Opin Cardiol* 3:229, 2006.

Tedgui A, Mallat Z: Cytokines in atherosclerosis: pathogenic and regulatory pathways, *Physiol Rev* 86:515, 2006.

Thom T, et al: Heart disease and stroke statistics—2006 update from the American Heart Association Statistics Committee, *Circulation* 113:e85, 2006.

Thompson DR, et al: Childhood overweight and cardiovascular disease risk factors: the National Heart, Lung and Blood Institute Growth and Health Study, *J Pediatr* 150:18, 2007.

Tian J, et al: Renal ischemia regulates marinobufagenin release in humans, *Hypertension* 56:914, 2010.

Towfighi A, et al: Pronounced association of elevated serum homocysteine with stroke in subgroups of individuals: a nationwide study, *J Neurol Sci* 298:153, 2010.

US Department of Agriculture, United States Department of Health and Human Services: Dietary Guidelines for Americans 2005. Accessed 3 March 2010 from www.healthierus.gov/dietaryguidelines.

Vieth R, Kimball S: Vitamin D in congestive heart failure, *Am J Clin Nutr* 83:731, 2006.

Walldius G, Jungner I: The apoB/apoA-I ratio: a strong, new risk factor for cardiovascular diseases and a target for lipid-lowering therapy—a review of the evidence, *J Intern Med* 259:493, 2006.

Wang L, et al: Blood pressure response to calcium supplementation: a meta-analysis of randomized controlled trials, *J Hum Hypertension* 20:571, 2008.

Wexler RK, et al: Cardiomyopathy: an overview, *Am Fam Physician* 79:778, 2009.

Williams IL, et al: Endothelial function and weight loss in obese humans, *Obes Surg* 15:1055, 2005.

Zittermann A, et al: Markers of bone metabolism in congestive heart failure, *Clin Chim Acta* 366:27, 2006.

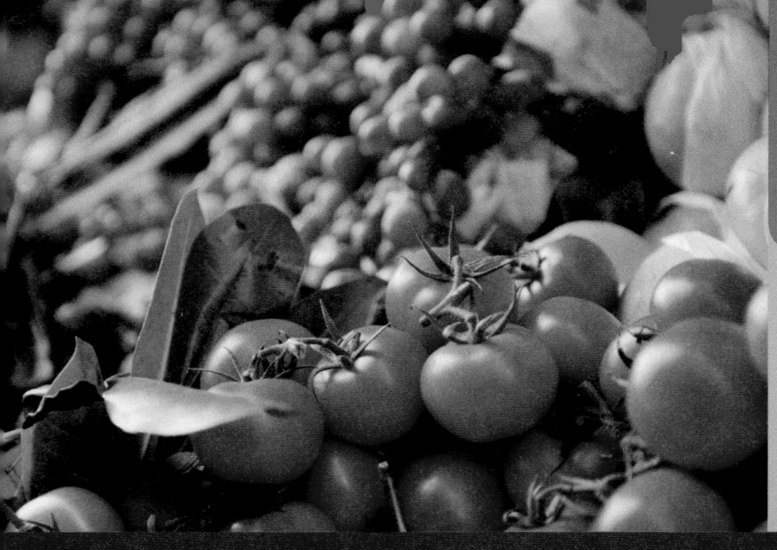

CHAPTER 35

Donna H. Mueller, PhD, RD, FADA, LDN

Medical Nutrition Therapy for Pulmonary Disease

KEY TERMS

acute respiratory distress syndrome
asthma
bronchopulmonary dysplasia (BPD)
chronic bronchitis
chronic lung disease of prematurity (CLD)
chronic obstructive pulmonary disease (COPD)
cor pulmonale
cystic fibrosis (CF)
distal intestinal obstruction syndrome (DIOS)
dyspnea
elastase
emphysema
hypercapnia
osteopenia
pancreatic enzyme replacement therapy (PERT)
pancreatic insufficiency (PI)
pulmonary aspiration
pulmonary function tests
pulse oximetry
respiratory quotient (RQ)
spirometry
surfactant
sweat test
tachypnea
tuberculosis (TB)

During fetal life, from birth to maturity and throughout adulthood, the pulmonary system is intertwined with nutrition. An optimal pulmonary system enables the body to obtain the oxygen needed to meet its cellular demands for energy from macronutrients, and to remove metabolic byproducts. Optimal nutrition permits the proper growth and development of the respiratory organs, supporting structures of the skeleton and muscles, and related nervous, circulatory, and immunologic systems. Overall, a person's nutritional well being and proper metabolism of nutrients are essential for the formation, development, growth, maturity, and protection of healthy lungs and associated processes throughout life.

THE PULMONARY SYSTEM

The respiratory structures include the nose, pharynx, larynx, trachea, bronchi, bronchioles, alveolar ducts, and alveoli (Figure 35-1). Supporting structures include the skeleton and the muscles (e.g., the intercostal, abdominal, and diaphragm muscles). Within a month after conception, pulmonary structures are recognizable. The pulmonary system grows and matures during gestation and childhood. No new alveoli are produced after approximately age 20. As aging occurs there is a loss of lung capillaries and the lungs lose elasticity.

Gas exchange is the major function of the pulmonary system (Figure 35-2). The lungs enable the body to obtain the oxygen needed to meet its cellular metabolic demands and to remove the carbon dioxide (CO_2) produced by these processes. Healthy nerves, blood, and lymph are needed to supply oxygen and nutrients to all tissues. The lungs also filter, warm, and humidify inspired air.

The lungs have several metabolic functions. For example, they help regulate the body's acid-base balance. The body's pH partially is maintained by the proper balance of CO_2 and O_2. The lungs synthesize arachidonic acid, that ultimately may be converted to prostaglandins or leukotrienes,

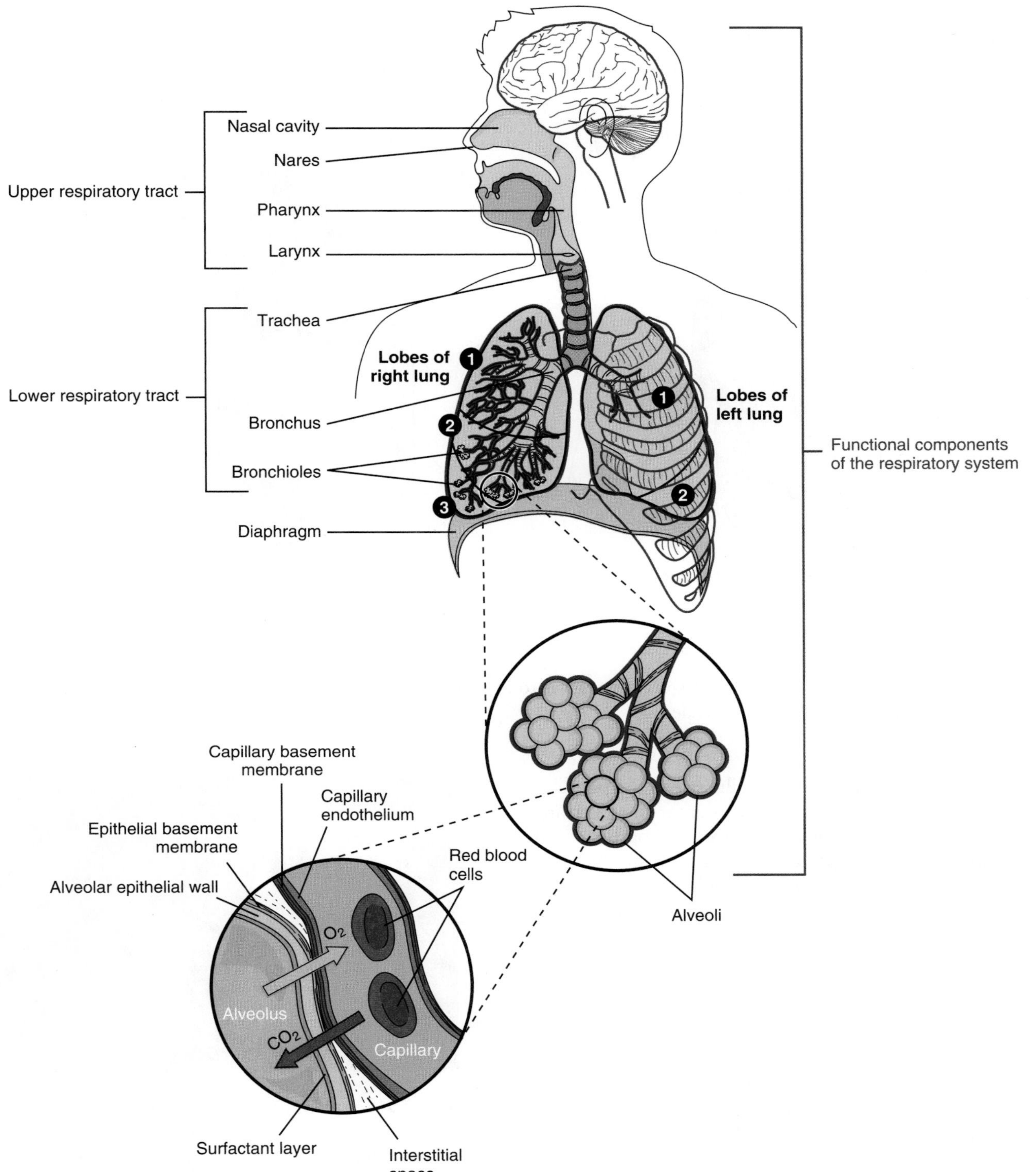

FIGURE 35-1 The anatomy of the pulmonary system is highly complex and interdependent.

a possible cause of bronchoconstriction in asthma. The lungs convert angiotension I to angiotensin II by the angiotension-converting enzyme (ACE) found mainly in the numerous capillary beds of the lungs. Angiotensin II increases blood pressure.

The alveolar cells secrete **surfactant**, a compound synthesized from proteins and phospholipids that serves to maintain the stability of pulmonary tissue by reducing the surface tension of fluids that coat the lung.

The lungs are an important part of the body's immune defense system because inspired air is laden with particles and microorganisms. Mucus keeps the airways moist and traps the particles and microorganisms from inspired air. Most cells that line the trachea, bronchi, and bronchioles

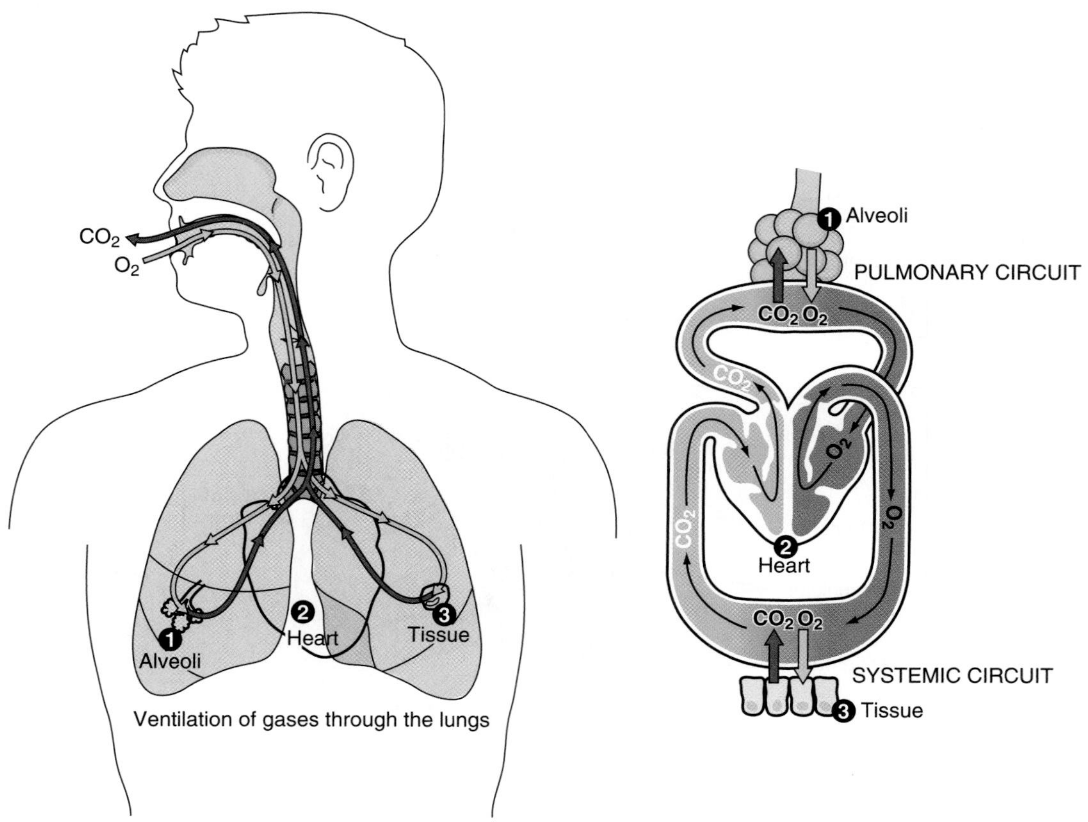

FIGURE 35-2 The major function of the respiratory tract is to provide the oxygen for cellular metabolism and to remove the carbon dioxide that is produced but not needed.

have cilia. These constantly beating cilia sweep the particles upward toward the pharynx so they can enter the gastrointestinal tract. Each time a person swallows, the particle- and microorganism-containing mucus passes into the digestive tract. The epithelial surface of the alveoli contains macrophages. By the process of phagocytosis, these alveolar macrophages engulf inhaled inert materials and microorganisms and digest them.

Medical Treatment

Pulmonary system disorders may be categorized as *primary*, such as tuberculosis (TB), bronchial asthma, and cancer of the lung; or *secondary* when associated with cardiovascular disease, obesity, human immunodeficiency virus (HIV) infection, sickle cell disease, and scoliosis. Conditions may also be acute or chronic. Examples of acute conditions include aspiration pneumonia, airway obstruction from foods like peanuts, and allergic anaphylaxis from consumption of shellfish. Examples of chronic conditions include cystic fibrosis (CF) and lung cancer.

The assessment of pulmonary status generally starts with physical examination using percussion and auscultation. These bedside techniques provide important information to the clinician on breathing. Numerous diagnostic and monitoring tests such as imaging procedures, arterial blood gas determinations, sputum cultures, and biopsies can also be employed. Signs and symptoms of pulmonary disease include

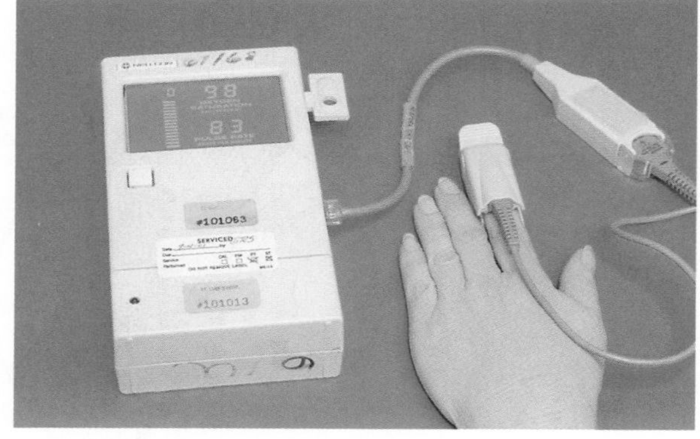

FIGURE 35-3 A pulse oximeter is an inexpensive and non-invasive instrument used to monitor a person's blood oxygen level. *(From Potter PA, Perry AG: Fundamentals of nursing, ed 7, St. Louis, 2009, Mosby.)*

cough, early satiety, anorexia, weight loss, **dyspnea** (shortness of breath), and fatigue.

Pulmonary function tests are used to diagnose or monitor the status of lung disease; they are designed to measure the ability of the respiratory system to exchange oxygen and CO_2. **Pulse oximetry** is one such test. A small device called a *pulse oximeter*, which uses light waves to measure the oxygen saturation of arterial blood, is placed on the end of the finger (Figure 35-3). Normal for a young, healthy person is 95%

to 99%. **Spirometry** is another common pulmonary function test. This involves breathing into a spirometer that gives information on lung volume and the rate at which air can be inhaled and exhaled.

Medical Nutrition Therapy in Pulmonary Disease

Individualized nutrition assessment, diagnosis, and intervention, followed by routine monitoring and evaluation, are integral components of care for each patient with pulmonary disease. Concomitant assessment of the cardiovascular, renal, neurologic, and hematologic systems is important because diseases often produce complications affecting pulmonary anatomy, physiologic findings, and biochemistry. Nutrition assessment precedes any nutrition intervention or medical treatment, unless the treatment is emergent.

Effect of Malnutrition on the Pulmonary System

The relationship between malnutrition and respiratory disease has long been recognized. Malnutrition adversely affects lung structure, elasticity, and function; respiratory muscle mass, strength, and endurance; lung immune defense mechanisms; and control of breathing. For example, protein and iron deficiencies result in low hemoglobin levels which diminish the oxygen-carrying capacity of the blood. Low levels of calcium, magnesium, phosphorus, and potassium compromise respiratory muscle function at the cellular level. Hypoproteinemia contributes to the development of pulmonary edema by decreasing colloid osmotic pressure, allowing body fluids to move into the interstitial space. Decreased levels of surfactant contribute to the collapse of alveoli, thereby increasing the work of breathing. The supporting connective tissue of the lungs is composed of collagen, which requires ascorbic acid for its synthesis. Normal airway mucus is a substance consisting of water, glycoproteins, and electrolytes, and thus requires adequate nutritional intake.

Pulmonary disease substantially increases energy requirements. This factor explains the rationale for including body composition and weight parameters in medical, surgical, pharmacologic, and nutrition research studies. Weight loss from inadequate energy intake is significantly correlated with a poor prognosis in persons with pulmonary diseases. Malnutrition leading to impaired immunity places any patient at high risk for developing respiratory infections. Malnourished patients with pulmonary disease who are hospitalized are likely to have lengthy stays and are susceptible to increased morbidity and mortality.

The complications of pulmonary diseases or their treatments can make adequate intake and digestion difficult. Absorption and metabolism of most nutrients are affected. As pulmonary disease progresses, several conditions may interfere with food intake and overall nutrition status. For example, abnormal production of sputum, vomiting, **tachypnea** (rapid breathing), hemoptysis, thoracic pain, nasal polyps, anemia, depression, and altered taste secondary to medications are often present. Weight loss, low body mass index (BMI), and other adverse effects are listed in Box 35-1.

BOX 35-1

Adverse Effects of Lung Disease on Nutrition Status

Increased Energy Expenditure

Increased work of breathing
Chronic infection
Medical treatments (e.g., bronchodilators, chest physical therapy)

Reduced Intake

Fluid restriction
Shortness of breath
Decreased oxygen saturation while eating
Anorexia resulting from chronic disease
Gastrointestinal distress and vomiting

Additional Limitations

Difficulty preparing food due to fatigue
Lack of financial resources
Impaired feeding skills (for infants and children)
Altered metabolism
Food-drug interaction

ASPIRATION

Pulmonary aspiration involves the movement of food or fluid into the lungs, which can result in pneumonia or even death. Besides liquids, foods that are most easily aspirated include those that have a round shape such as nuts, popcorn, hard candy, and hot dog pieces; or chunks of inadequately chewed foods such as meat or raw vegetables. Infants and toddlers are at increased risk for aspiration, as are older adults and persons with oral, upper gastrointestinal, neurologic, or muscular abnormalities. In addition, close attention must be given to people receiving enteral tube feedings (see Chapter 14). Because the primary reason for aspiration pneumonia is excessive lung secretions, pulmonary treatments and suctioning are critical to preventing aspiration.

ASTHMA

Asthma, a disease of bronchial hyperresponsiveness and airway inflammation, has increased in prevalence during the last three decades. The syndrome appears to result from complex interactions among genetic, immunologic, and environmental factors. It is characterized by (1) increased mucus secretion that can obstruct the airways, (2) inflammation and swelling, and (3) smooth muscle tightening that results in smaller airways. Asthma is characterized by airflow obstruction and is a leading cause of hospitalization and death worldwide (DHHS, 2010; Stevenson and Birrell, 2010).

Pathophysiology

Genetic attributes, environmental exposures, and gene-environmental interactions all play a role in asthma. Respiratory infections caused by viruses, *Chlamydophila* or *Mycoplasma*, have been hypothesized to have significant roles in the pathogenesis (Guilbert and Denlinger, 2010). Host immunity is also critical. A healthy diet during pregnancy and during the early years, and prolonged breastfeeding may decrease the risk of asthma in childhood. In children genetically at high risk of asthma, being overweight at age 1 year is often associated with a decreased risk of asthma and better lung function at ages 6 and 8 years; however, being overweight beyond infancy may confer a higher risk for asthma (Zhang et al., 2010). Thus obesity should be avoided after the toddler stage.

Medical Treatment

Asthma is categorized as *allergic (extrinsic)* and *nonallergic (intrinsic)*. Allergic asthma is more common and is generally triggered by inhalation of pollen, pet dander, air pollution, cigarette smoke, or other inhalants. Nonallergic asthma may be triggered by factors such as ear infections, stress, viruses, and exercise. Asthmatic symptoms may be aggravated by exposure to allergens such as shrimp or sulfites (see Chapter 27); rhinoviruses; and botanicals such as citronella in insect repellents, rusty-leafed rhododendron in natural honeys, and strawberry leaf in herbal teas.

Eosinophilic airway inflammation is commonly observed; therefore removal of potential triggers and known sensitizers is an important measure. A life-threatening situation with flat airways, known as *status asthmaticus*, can result without proper intervention. Corticosteroid therapy is often prescribed, but chronic use may place the individual at risk for osteopenia, bone fractures, or steroid-induced hyperglycemia. New research proposes use of sublingual immunotherapy and other novel treatments (Peden and Bush, 2011.)

Medical Nutrition Therapy

Food and individual nutrients have possible roles in the treatment of asthma. Examples include soy, ω-3 fatty acids and ω-6 fatty acids (decreasing the production of bronchoconstrictive leukotrienes), antioxidant nutrients (protecting the airway tissues from oxidative stress), vitamin D (a molecular antiinfective nutrient), magnesium (a smooth-muscle relaxant and antiinflammatory agent), and methylxanthine bronchodilators such as caffeine (Baines et al., 2009; Barros, et al., 2008; Bede, et al., 2008; Kalhan, et al., 2008; Kazaks, et al., 2010; Lindemann, 2009; Schubert, et al., 2009). The dilemma for the nutrition care provider is the paucity of evidence-based research to support practice procedures (Allan and Devereux, 2011; Kealoha, 2009; Raviv and Smith, 2010; Sorkness, 2009). Scientific nutrition studies aimed at producing evidence-based results are desperately needed.

One illustration is the often-asked question: "Does milk cause an increase in mucus production in asthma?" A literature review found no cause-and-effect relationship, and avoiding dairy foods could lead to inadequate intake of nutrients (Wüthrich et al., 2005). However, until scientists clearly demonstrate the biologic foundations of people's perceptions, clinicians will be asked the question and be expected to determine the proper course of treatment.

Nutrition assessment and therapy must take into account routinely prescribed medications. These include bronchodilators that relax the airway smooth muscle and antiinflammatory agents that suppress airway inflammation. Pulmonary patients experience side effects such as dry mouth and throat, nausea, early satiety, vomiting, diarrhea, increased serum glucose levels, sodium retention, hypokalemia, hand tremors, headache, and dizziness. Another possible side effect of medications or chronic coughing is gastroesophageal reflux. Chronic steroid use causes bone demineralization. Bone density tests should be part of the nutritional assessment when these drugs are chronically used (see Chapter 9).

Nutrition therapy should include individual evaluation for environmental or food triggers and strategies for their avoidance if necessary. In addition, there is need for a diet of wholesome foods to provide optimal energy and balance of nutrients; proper ratio of ω-3 and ω-6 fatty acids and phytonutrients; correction of diagnosed energy and nutrient deficiencies or excesses; careful attention to medication-food-nutrient interactions; frequent monitoring to maintain healthy pulmonary status; and education of the patient, family, and community (American Academy of Allergy, Asthma, and Immunology, 2005).

CHRONIC LUNG DISEASE OF PREMATURITY AND BRONCHOPULMONARY DYSPLASIA

Chronic lung disease of prematurity (CLD) and **bronchopulmonary dysplasia (BPD)** are closely related. Newborn lungs appear unable to respond to adverse situations. Immature lungs often cannot synthesize surfactant that permits inflation for gas exchange.

Pathophysiology

CLD and BPD are the result of incomplete recovery from lung injury during the neonatal period. CLD and BPD occur most frequently in infants who are extremely premature or of low birth weight (see Chapter 43). Other risk factors include perinatal infection, meconium aspiration, tracheoesophageal fistula, and generalized infections. Signs and symptoms of CLD and BPD include hypercapnia, tachypnea, wheezing, dyspnea, recurrent respiratory infections, **cor pulmonale** (right ventricular enlargement and heart failure), and a characteristic radiographic appearance of the lungs.

Medical Treatment

Because the pathophysiologic conditions of CLD and BPD are incompletely understood, medical treatment and

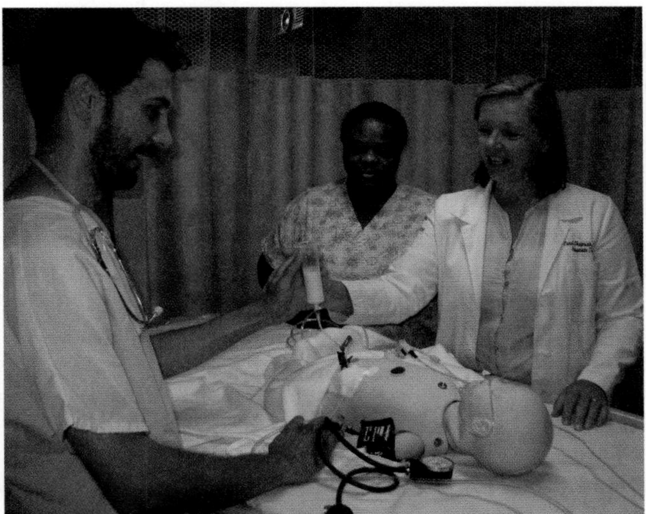

FIGURE 35-4 Demonstration of how to gastrostomy feed a baby with bronchopulmonary dysplasia.

nutrition intervention are empirically based and often have limited scientific rationale (Van Marter, 2009). Infants with severe disease often require prolonged intensive medical care, provided by an interdisciplinary team. Figure 35-4 shows student members of the interdisciplinary team practicing tube feeding a simulated infant with BPD. Therapies such as parenteral nutrition or enteral tube feedings, mechanical ventilation, supplemental oxygen, and medications may be required long after discharge from the hospital.

Medical Nutrition Therapy

Because of the fragile nature of affected infants, careful and consistent nutrition assessment is imperative. Infant growth is followed closely because it is a major outcome indicator of medical and nutrition therapy. Because lung size is stature-dependent, linear growth is important for the growth of healthy lung tissue and for the resolution of the condition. Observations of growth patterns of infants with CLD and BPD suggest that these infants have delayed growth, thereby requiring careful assessment of both respiratory and nutrition status (Box 35-2).

Possible reasons for growth failure among infants include increased energy needs combined with inadequate dietary intake, gastroesophageal reflux, emotional deprivation, and chronic hypoxia. Growth should be evaluated and compared with that of other infants of the same postconceptional age (see Chapter 43). Infants with CLD and BPD have special short- and long-term nutritional requirements related to both their prematurity and their pulmonary status. The general goals of nutrition care are to supply adequate nutrient intakes, promote linear growth, maintain fluid balance, and develop age-appropriate feeding skills. Meeting energy and nutrient needs is a major challenge in the care of infants and toddlers with BPD.

BOX 35-2

Components of Nutrition Assessment for Infants with Bronchopulmonary Dysplasia

History

Birth weight
Gestational age
Medical history
Nutrition history
Previous growth pattern

Medical Status

Respiratory status
Oxygen saturation
Use of medications
Emesis
Stool pattern
Urine output
Urine specific gravity
Ventilator dependency

Nutrition-Biochemical Measures

Anthropometrics
- Weight
- Length
- Growth percentiles
- Head circumference

Biochemical
- Hemoglobin
- Hematocrit
- Serum electrolytes
- C-reactive protein
- Transthyretin

Feeding History

Volume of intake
Frequency of feedings
Behavior during feedings
Formula composition
Use of solid foods
Developmental feeding milestones
Swallowing difficulty
Gastroesophageal reflux

Environmental Concerns

Parent-child interaction
Home facilities
Access to safe food supply
Community resources
Economic resources
Access to food and nutrients

Energy

Increased energy needs are well recognized in infants with CLD and BPD. Resting energy expenditure for infants with CLD and BPD has been documented to be 25% to 50% greater than that in age-matched controls. Energy needs also vary during the course of the disease. In the acute phase, when infants are kept in controlled temperature environments, are fed parenterally, remain relatively inactive, and are not growing or are growing slowly, energy requirements may be 50 to 85 kcal/kg daily. In contrast, during the convalescent phase, when infants are growing rapidly, being fed orally, and using additional energy for temperature regulation, activity, and the work of breathing, they may require 120 to 130 kcal/kg or more daily.

Macronutrients

Protein intake should be within the advised range for infants of comparable postconceptional age. As the caloric density of the diet is increased by the addition of fat and carbohydrate, protein should provide 7% or more of total calories because lesser amounts may be inadequate for growth.

Additions of fat or carbohydrate are made to formula only after it has been concentrated to 24 kcal/oz to keep protein at an acceptable level. See Box 43-2 in Chapter 43. Fat provides essential fatty acids (EFAs) and helps meet energy demands when tolerance for fluid and CO_2 load is limited. Excessive amounts of carbohydrate increase the **respiratory quotient (RQ)** (the ratio of CO_2 expired to the volume of oxygen inspired) and the output of CO_2. This would seem to make the work of breathing more difficult; however, the clinical application of manipulating nutrient mix to change RQ is controversial. Ongoing calculation of the proportions of the macronutrients related to respiratory status are major considerations in any nutritional evaluation.

Fluid

To maintain fluid balance, infants with CLD and BPD may require fluid restriction, sodium restriction, and diuretics, all of which have nutritional implications. When fluid intake is restricted, the use of parenteral lipids or calorically dense enteral feedings may help the infant meet energy needs. When calorically dense formulas are used (>24 kcal/oz), the adequacy of fluid intake and urinary output must be monitored closely.

Vitamins and Minerals

Adequate supplies of all vitamins and minerals are essential. Special attention is focused on those related to prematurity, infections, oxygen therapy, and drug-nutrient interactions. Adequate vitamin K is essential for bone development and should be monitored, especially when colon microflora are insufficient for the synthesis of this vitamin. Vitamin A is essential because of its role in the proper development and maintenance of the epithelial cells of the respiratory tract. In fact, some reports support the conclusion that vitamin A (either as an oral or intramuscular supplement) prevents or fully treats CLD and BPD, whereas others reject that conclusion (Darlow, 2007; Van Marter, 2009).

Mineral intake and retention should be monitored and supplemented as needed to maintain normal levels. Determination of mineral requirements is complicated by lack of adequate stores as a result of prematurity (e.g., iron, zinc, and calcium), growth delay, and the multiple medications prescribed for infants and toddlers with CLD and BPD. Medications may include diuretics, bronchodilators, antibiotics, cardiac antiarrhythmics, and corticosteroids. Collectively, these medications are associated with increased urinary loss of minerals, especially chloride, potassium, and calcium. Additional chloride losses may occur in infants with chronic CO_2 retention and respiratory acidosis because of metabolic correction for the acidosis. Deficiencies of chloride or potassium are associated with muscle weakness and impaired growth (see Chapter 7). For infants sensitive to sodium loads, lower-sodium formulas can be used, and the sodium content of medications, water, and foods must be considered (see Chapter 34).

Infants with CLD and BPD are at risk for **osteopenia** (inadequate bone mineralization). Besides limited nutrient intake, other risk factors include inadequate stores of calcium and phosphorus related to prematurity, intermittent respiratory acidosis, chronic use of certain medications, and insufficient physical activity. See Chapter 25.

Feeding Strategies

Feeding difficulties frequently occur among infants with CLD and BPD. Risk factors include a history of unpleasant oral experiences (e.g., intubation, frequent suctioning, or recurrent vomiting), a history of parenteral and enteral nutrition, delayed introduction of solids, and discomfort or choking associated with eating solids. Infants may tire easily while breast-feeding or bottle-feeding. Useful approaches that facilitate feeding acceptance include providing a pleasant and calm mealtime environment, providing oral stimulation during tube feedings, using consistent and appropriate feeding techniques, and gradually introducing progressive texture and flavor changes.

Barriers to adequate intake include anorexia, fatigue, poor coordination of breathing and swallowing, and inability to suck. To meet energy needs, calorically dense formulas, small and frequent feedings, use of a soft nipple, and nasogastric or gastrostomy tube feedings may be needed. Gastroesophageal reflux is also common and may result in vomiting with expulsion of feedings, which leads to inadequate nutritional intake. Treatment includes upright positioning, medications such as antacids or histamine H_2-receptor antagonists, and thickening of formula. In severe cases surgical fundoplication may be necessary.

CHRONIC OBSTRUCTIVE PULMONARY DISEASE

Chronic obstructive pulmonary disease (COPD) is characterized by slow, progressive obstruction of the airways. COPD may be subdivided into two categories: **emphysema** (type I), which is characterized by abnormal, permanent enlargement and destruction of the alveoli; and **chronic bronchitis** (type II), in which there is a productive cough with inflammation of the bronchi and other lung changes. Tobacco smoking or continual contact with second-hand smoke are the primary causative factors. Environmental air pollution (including cooking in a confined, unventilated space) and genetic susceptibility are other possible causal factors.

Pathophysiology

Patients with emphysema are thin and often cachectic. They are generally older and have mild hypoxemia but normal hematocrit values. Cor pulmonale (right ventricular enlargement and failure of the heart) develops late in the course of the disease. Conversely, patients with chronic bronchitis are of normal weight and, indeed, are often overweight. Hypoxemia is prominent in these patients, hematocrit values are increased, and cor pulmonale develops early.

Medical Treatment

Medical and surgical treatment approaches for persons with COPD are codified and periodically updated based on the latest research (Global Initiative for Chronic Obstructive Lung Disease, 2009). The four goals for effective management are to (1) assess and monitor disease, (2) reduce risk factors, (3) maintain stable COPD, and (4) manage any exacerbations. Early, accurate diagnosis is key to treatment. Once the disease progresses, in addition to pulmonary rehabilitation programs and oxygen therapy, numerous medications are prescribed, mainly bronchodilators, glucocorticosteroids, and mucolytic agents, along with antibiotics to treat infections. Surgical treatments for advanced COPD, including lung transplantation, may be options for some patients.

Medical Nutrition Therapy

Medical nutrition therapy (MNT) for people with COPD has been evaluated and recommendations have been made. (American Dietetic Association, 2010). The primary goals of nutrition care for patients with COPD are to facilitate nutritional well being, maintain an appropriate ratio of lean body mass to adipose tissue, correct fluid imbalance, manage drug-nutrient interactions, and prevent osteoporosis.

After fluid status, energy is a primary consideration. Because maintaining energy balance is crucial for combating this progressive disorder, accurate evaluation of both energy intake and energy expenditure is essential. On the energy intake side, decreased food intake is common. Morning headache and confusion from **hypercapnia** (excessive CO_2 in the blood) may interfere with food preparation or intake. Other pertinent assessments focus on blood oxygen saturation, fatigue, anorexia, difficulty chewing and swallowing from dyspnea, constipation from low-fiber food selections, or diarrhea. Diarrhea occurs from impaired peristalsis, secondary to lack of oxygen to the gastrointestinal tract.

On the other hand, energy expenditure is generally elevated because of airflow obstruction, thus increasing the energy needs from the increased work of breathing. Gas diffusing capacity, CO_2 retention, respiratory inflammation, and biochemical mediators such as hormones and cytokines also affect energy expenditure. Common outcomes are reduced respiratory and skeletal muscle strength and endurance along with increased muscle fatigability, altered pulmonary accessory muscle function, and increased susceptibility to infections. Malnourished patients with COPD, including those diagnosed with pulmonary cachexia, have a worse prognosis than those who are well nourished (King, 2008).

Nutritional depletion may be evidenced clinically by low body weight for height and reduced triceps fatfold measurements. Decreases in lean body mass may occur, even when actual weight appears stable. Calculation of BMI may be insufficient to detect alterations. Instead, determination of body composition helps to differentiate lean muscle mass from adipose tissue and overhydration from dehydration. In patients with cor pulmonale and the resultant fluid retention, weight maintenance or gain from fluid may camouflage actual wasting of lean body mass. Thus for patients retaining fluids, careful interpretation of both anthropometric measurements and biochemical indicators of nutrition status is necessary, especially because the latter are depressed by hemodilution (see Chapters 6 and 8).

The medication profile should be assessed for food and nutrient interactions. Examples of drugs with potential nutritional implications are bronchodilators, expectorants, and corticosteroids (see Chapter 9).

Energy

Meeting energy needs can be difficult. For patients participating in pulmonary inpatient or outpatient rehabilitation programs, adjusted energy requirements depend on the intensity and frequency of exercise therapy. Actual energy needs may be increased or decreased (Weekes, 2009). It is crucial to remember that energy balance and nitrogen balance are intertwined. Consequently, maintaining optimal energy balance is essential to preserving visceral and somatic proteins. Preferably, indirect calorimetry should be used to determine energy needs and to prescribe and monitor the provision of sufficient, but not excessive calories (American Dietetic Association, 2010). When energy equations are used for prediction of needs, increases for physiologic stress must be included. Caloric needs may vary significantly from one person to the next, and even in the same individual (see Chapter 2).

Macronutrients

In stable COPD, requirements for water, protein, fat, and carbohydrate are determined by the underlying lung disease, oxygen therapy, medications, weight status, and any acute fluid fluctuations. Attention to the metabolic side effects of malnutrition and the role of individual amino acids is necessary (Baldi, 2010). Determination of a specific patient's macronutrient needs is made on an individual basis, with close monitoring of outcomes.

Sufficient protein of 1.2 to 1.7 g/kg of dry body weight is necessary to maintain or restore lung and muscle strength, as well as to promote immune function. A balanced ratio of protein (15% to 20% of calories) with fat (30% to 45% of calories) and carbohydrate (40% to 55% of calories) is important to preserve a satisfactory RQ from substrate metabolism use (see Chapter 2). Repletion but not overfeeding is particularly critical in patients with compromised ability to exchange gases as excess feeding of calories results in CO_2 that must be expelled. Other concurrent disease processes such as cardiovascular or renal disease, cancer, or diabetes mellitus affect the total amounts, ratios, and kinds of protein, fat, and carbohydrate prescribed.

Vitamins and Minerals

As with macronutrients, vitamin and mineral requirements for individuals with stable COPD depend on the underlying pathologic conditions of the lung, other concurrent diseases, medical treatments, weight status, and bone mineral density. For people continuing to smoke tobacco, additional vitamin C is necessary. Research indicates that people who smoke approximately one pack of cigarettes per day appear to require approximately 16 mg more ascorbate per day, whereas those who smoke two packs need approximately 32 mg more than the recommended dietary allowance.

The role of minerals such as magnesium and calcium in muscle contraction and relaxation may be important for people with COPD. Intakes at least equivalent to the dietary reference intake (DRI) should be provided. Depending on bone mineral density test results, coupled with food intake history and glucocorticoid medications use, additional vitamins D and K also may be necessary (see Chapter 25).

Patients with cor pulmonale and subsequent fluid retention require sodium and fluid restriction. Depending on the diuretics prescribed, increased dietary intake of potassium may be required (see Chapter 9).

Feeding Strategies

Interdisciplinary team involvement is paramount. A modified oral diet is usually preferred. Adequate exercise, fluids, and easily-chewed dietary fiber enhance gastrointestinal motility. When abdominal bloating is a problem, limitation of foods associated with gas formation may help (see Chapter 29).

Patients and their families benefit from specific suggestions for enhancing appetite, promoting oral intake, and lessening fatigue when cooking or eating. Some suggestions are resting before meals, eating small portions of nutrient-dense foods, and planning medications and breathing treatments around mealtimes. For many patients using oxygen at mealtimes, eating slowly, chewing foods well, and engaging in social interaction all can enhance food intake, nutrient metabolism, and enjoyment of the experience. To prevent aspiration, special caution must be given to proper sequencing of breathing with swallowing as well as to proper sitting posture during eating. Patients with disease-related physical limitations may require assistance with food shopping, meal preparation, and linkage with community resources such as congregate meal programs or home-delivered meals (Fig. 35-5).

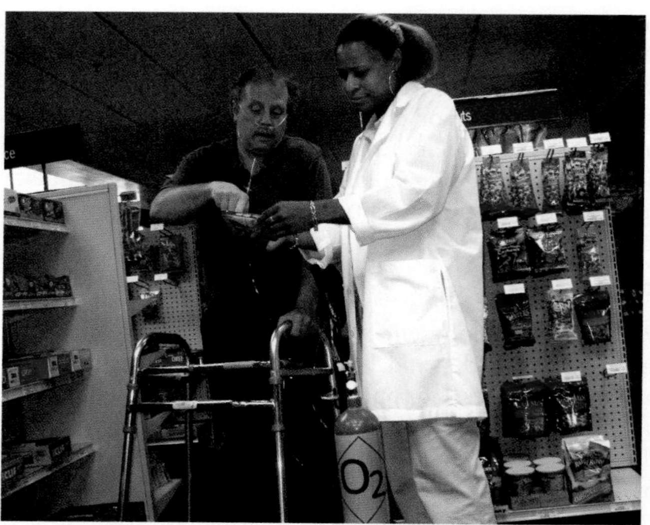

FIGURE 35-5 An individual with chronic obstructive pulmonary disease and oxygen being shown how to read a label.

Enteral tube feeding can be used to increase total caloric and nutrient intake for some patients with COPD. Decisions to implement this method of nutrition support should take into consideration the goal of the nutrition therapy, the ability of the caregivers, the attitude of the patient, and the cost (see Chapter 14).

CYSTIC FIBROSIS

Cystic fibrosis (CF) is a complex multisystem disorder that is inherited in an autosomal-recessive fashion. The underlying genetic basis of the disease has been identified, with more than 1400 mutations noted. CF remains one of the most common lethal genetic disorders in the white population, and it is expressed in other population groups as well. Approximately 2% to 5% of white populations are heterozygotes, with a CF incidence of 1:3500 live births.

CF was once thought to be only a pediatric disease, but the number of people surviving to or being diagnosed at 18 years or older is approximately 42%. Survival has dramatically improved because of scientific advancements and improvements in diagnostic and treatment procedures, including nutrition. The median age of patients is approximately 37 years. Many women with CF have delivered healthy infants, and some have chosen to breastfeed their unaffected infants.

Pathophysiology

Expression of the CF gene is largely restricted to epithelial cells. In CF, almost all exocrine glands are affected and secrete abnormally thick, tenacious mucus that obstructs glands and ducts in various organs. The clinical features are dominated by involvement of the respiratory tract, sweat and salivary glands, intestine, pancreas, liver, and reproductive tract. Pulmonary complications include acute and chronic bronchitis, bronchiectasis, pneumonia, atelectasis, and peribronchial and parenchymal scarring. Infection with *Staphylococcus aureus* and *Pseudomonas aeruginosa* is typical. Pneumothorax and hemoptysis are common. In advanced stages, cor pulmonale or infection with *Burkholderia cepacia* may be present, signifying a poor prognosis.

Medical Treatment

Several methods are available for diagnosing CF. For families with previously identified CF, prenatal analysis may be possible. Several countries and most states in the United States conduct routine neonatal screening for the disease. Genotyping is available and is a routine procedure. The most reliable clinical diagnostic test, known as the **sweat test**, is performed by pilocarpine iontophoresis.

CF can have a profound effect on the digestive system. Infants born with meconium ileus have the diagnosis of probable CF until differentiated from other causes. Approximately 85% to 90% of persons with CF have **pancreatic insufficiency (PI)**, in which plugs of thick mucus reduce the quantity of digestive enzymes released from the pancreas into the small intestine. The resultant enzyme insufficiency causes maldigestion of food and malabsorption of nutrients. Decreased bicarbonate secretion can further reduce digestive enzyme activity. Decreased bile acid resorption contributes to fat malabsorption.

Distal intestinal obstruction syndrome (DIOS), recurrent intestinal impaction, sometimes occurs in children and adults. Prevention of DIOS involves intake of adequate enzymes, fluids, and dietary fiber and regular exercise; treatment includes adding stool softeners, laxatives, hyperosmolar enemas, or intestinal lavage.

The presence of excessive mucus lining the small intestinal tract may interfere with nutrient absorption by the microvilli. Gastrointestinal complications include bulky, foul-smelling stools; cramping and intestinal obstruction; rectal prolapse; and liver involvement. As the disease progresses, damage to the endocrine portion of the pancreas causes impaired glucose tolerance and development of CF-related diabetes mellitus (Moran, 2010). Pancreatic enzyme replacement therapy is essential (see *Focus On:* PERT Therapy).

Medical Nutrition Therapy

Because of the numerous intricate manifestations and complications, nutritional requirements and care must be individually determined for each patient. MNT must be coordinated with other treatments, including a variety of different kinds of medicines and chest physical therapy. The goals of nutrition care in CF are to control maldigestion and malabsorption, provide adequate nutrients, promote optimal growth or maintain weight for height, support pulmonary function, and prevent nutritional deficiencies. Individuals at especially high risk include infants, children, adolescents, and pregnant or lactating women, even when they are medically stable. They should have a nutrition assessment. Comprehensive MNT for people with CF has been evaluated scientifically, with recommendations published (Michel, 2009; Stallings, 2008). Periodic updated practice guidelines are available online from the various international CF organizations and should be consulted for the latest information.

Maldigestion and malabsorption, as well as the progressive complications of the disease, make it difficult to meet increased nutrient needs. Factors interfering with adequate intake and retention of nutrients include dyspnea, coughing and cough-induced vomiting, gastrointestinal discomfort, anorexia during episodes of infection, possible impaired sense of smell and taste, and glucosuria. Growth retardation and difficulty maintaining desired weight for height are common problems. Before diagnosis, infants with CF often demonstrate growth failure. With treatment, growth generally improves. When energy and nutrient intakes are adequate, growth nearly appropriate for age usually can be achieved (Leonard, 2010) (see *Pathophysiology and Care Management Algorithm:* Cystic Fibrosis).

As lung disease progresses, growth velocity in children and weight for height in adults may decline. The long-term relationship between nutrition support, growth, and survival is not known; however, improved nutrition status on a long-term basis continues to be suggested as a contributing factor to increased survival. Adults have similar medical, surgical, psychosocial, and nutrition assessment concerns, but they also have regular adult life issues. Thus they require nutrition information delivered by different educational approaches than those used with children (Morton, 2009; Watson, 2008).

FOCUS ON

PERT Therapy

Pancreatic enzyme replacement therapy (PERT) is the first step taken to correct maldigestion and malabsorption. The microspheres, designed to withstand the acidic environment of the stomach, release enzymes in the duodenum, where they digest protein, fat, and carbohydrate. The quantity of enzymes to be taken with food depends on the degree of pancreatic insufficiency; the quantity of food eaten; the fat, protein, and carbohydrate content of food consumed; and the type of enzymes used. Enzyme dosage per meal or snack is adjusted empirically to control gastrointestinal symptoms, including steatorrhea, and to promote growth appropriate for age. Following the manufacturer's directions about storage and administration of a particular brand of enzyme is important to emphasize. If gastrointestinal symptoms cannot be controlled, enzyme dosage, patient adherence, and enzyme type should be reevaluated. Fecal **elastase** (protein-digesting enzyme secreted by the pancreas and involved in hydrolysis of peptide bonds), fecal fat, or nitrogen balance studies may help to evaluate the adequacy of enzyme supplementation.

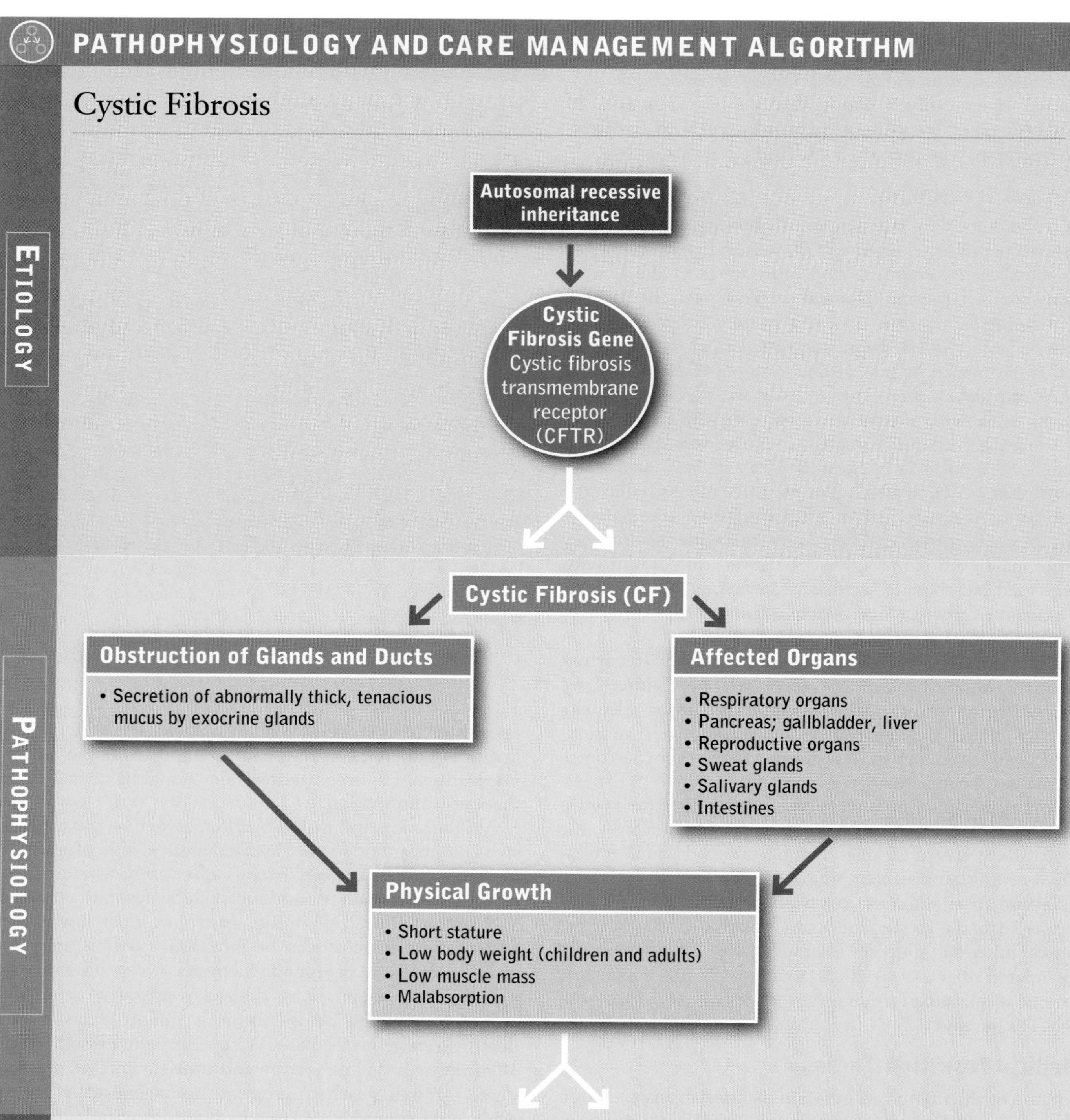
PATHOPHYSIOLOGY AND CARE MANAGEMENT ALGORITHM
Cystic Fibrosis
ETIOLOGY
Autosomal recessive inheritance
Cystic Fibrosis Gene
Cystic fibrosis transmembrane receptor (CFTR)
PATHOPHYSIOLOGY
Cystic Fibrosis (CF)
Obstruction of Glands and Ducts
• Secretion of abnormally thick, tenacious mucus by exocrine glands
Affected Organs
• Respiratory organs
• Pancreas; gallbladder, liver
• Reproductive organs
• Sweat glands
• Salivary glands
• Intestines
Physical Growth
• Short stature
• Low body weight (children and adults)
• Low muscle mass
• Malabsorption
MANAGEMENT
Medical Management
• Genotyping
• Oral or IV antibiotics
• Aerosol antibiotics
• Inhaled medications
• Chest and physical therapy
Nutrition Management
• Monitor ongoing nutrition status
• Supply pancreatic enzyme replacement therapy (PERT)
• Meet increased energy requirements
• Provide vitamin and mineral supplementation

Macronutrients

Energy needs vary widely from individual to individual, even in the same individual throughout the course of life based on gender, age, basal metabolic rate, physical activity, respiratory infection, severity of lung disease, and severity of malabsorption. When laboratory methods to determine energy requirements are unavailable, equations for calculating caloric recommendations are convenient to use (Magoffin, 2008). Patients with CF should not be encouraged to decrease their activity levels, but rather to increase their energy intake instead. Relatively healthy children with CF usually are able to maintain normal growth and energy stores when they eat a high-energy, moderate-fat diet complemented with sufficient pancreatic enzyme replacement therapy (PERT).

Dietary protein levels are increased in CF as a result of malabsorption; however, when energy needs are adequately met, individuals with CF generally can meet their protein needs. At least 15% to 20% of the total calories consumed as proteins or the appropriate DRI for protein for the individual's gender, age, and height is suggested.

Fat intake should provide 35% to 40% or more of total kilocalories as tolerated. Dietary fat helps to provide the required energy, EFAs (i.e., linoleic acid and linolenic acid), and fat-soluble vitamins. Moreover, fat limits the volume of food required to meet energy demands and improves the palatability of the diet. Indications of fat intolerance include an increase in the number of stools, greasy stools, or abdominal cramping.

EFA deficiencies may be present, even among patients who are treated adequately with pancreatic enzymes to control malabsorption (Strandvik, 2010). Although clinical signs of EFA deficiency are rare, blood and tissue lipid levels may be abnormal (Aldamiz-Echievarria, 2009). Even if the visible signs of EFA deficiency (e.g., the typical skin lesions) are not noticeable, the clinician should consider routinely testing for abnormal blood lipid profiles. In addition, at-risk patients need to be encouraged to include sources of EFAs (e.g., canola, flaxseed, soybean, or corn oil, or fish) as part of their daily fat intake.

As the disease progresses, changes in carbohydrate intake may be necessary. Lactose intolerance may become evident (see Chapter 29), and pancreatic endocrine involvement may require carbohydrate adjustments.

Vitamins and Minerals

With pancreatic enzyme replacement, the water-soluble vitamins appear to be adequately absorbed in patients with CF. Requirements under normal conditions can usually be met by diet plus a standard age-appropriate multivitamin and mineral supplement; however, monitoring individual variations is important.

Even with pancreatic enzyme supplementation, fat-oluble vitamins usually remain inadequately absorbed. Low serum concentrations of vitamin A despite increased hepatic stores have been documented in CF, suggesting impaired mobilization and transport of the vitamin from the liver. Decreased levels of vitamin D metabolites have also been observed. This is one of several factors that may be related to the decreased bone mineral content seen in populations with CF. Low vitamin E levels have been associated with hemolytic anemia and abnormal neurologic findings. Individuals with CF may be at risk for vitamin K deficiency secondary to long-term use of antibiotics or liver disease, as well as malabsorption. Thus vitamin regimens should be adjusted based on routine serum monitoring of the individual.

Mineral intake should meet the gender and age recommendations according to the DRI. Special attention must be given to some of the minerals. Sodium requirements for infants, children, and adults are increased in CF because of increased losses in sweat. When sodium intake is inadequate, lethargy, vomiting, and dehydration may occur. Adequate salt is consumed by most children and adults who eat a typical North American diet with processed foods; however, supplemental salt is required under some conditions. Infants require extra salt because of the low-sodium content of breast milk, formula, and infant foods (Coates et al., 2009). Children and adults need additional salt during periods of fever, hot weather, or physical exertion. Table salt or proprietary electrolyte replacement solutions are used.

Other minerals are not routinely supplemented, although mineral status should be evaluated on an individual basis. Decreased bone mineralization starts during childhood and must be assessed and addressed (Haworth, 2010). Low iron stores and low magnesium levels have been described in CF. Plasma zinc levels may be low in cases of moderate to severe malnutrition.

Feeding Strategies

Diet modification focuses on meeting the increased nutritional requirements of CF. Along with adequate dietary modification, positive eating behaviors must be established (Stark et al., 2010). Parent educational materials are available online from the Cystic Fibrosis Foundation. For infants with CF and their families, the immunologic and psychosocial benefits of breast-feeding are well established, and breast-feeding should be encouraged. For the infant with pancreatic insufficiency, enzyme microspheres can be added to a small amount of baby food or placed directly in the infant's mouth. Supplementation with high-calorie formula may be necessary to meet growth goals. For formula-fed infants, standard formulas (20-27 kcal/oz) given with supplemental enzymes are usually adequate.

For children and adults, intake can be enhanced by regular and enjoyable mealtimes, larger food portions at meals, extra snacks, and foods selected for high-nutrient density. Homemade or proprietary nutritional supplements such as fortified beverages and puddings also can help the individual with CF attain nutritional goals.

Supplementation by feeding tube is an alternative for those unable to meet nutritional needs by the oral route. Formulas are provided by continuous infusion through a nasogastric, gastrostomy, or jejunostomy tube, often while the person sleeps. Elemental (predigested) and nonelemental formulas with enzymes may be effective. See Chapter 14.

Intensive supplementation has been associated with improved weight gain, slowed decline in pulmonary function, decreased incidence of respiratory infection, and improved sense of well being. Although the short-term benefits of supplementation have been well documented, nutrition status is likely to regress when supplementation is discontinued. The long-term effect of intensive supplementation on the course of the disease has not been determined. Parenteral nutrition is best used for short-term support in patients with clearly evident needs such as those recuperating from gastrointestinal surgery.

LUNG CANCER

The primary sites of lung cancer are usually the bronchi, with subsequent metastasis to other organs such as the bone, brain, liver, or skin. As new screening technologies become commonplace, early detection and diagnosis should improve.

Pathophysiology

Lung cancer is often associated with persistent tobacco smoking for many years, but other inhaled pollutants may initiate the malignant condition.

Medical Treatment

Currently the medical treatment of lung cancer involves radiation therapy, chemotherapy, and surgery, which are accompanied by various nutritional side effects. Patients with lung cancer experience the added stress of respiratory fatigue and diminished lung residual capacity. Smoking cessation sessions are part of most wellness programs and offer ideal settings for nutrition education.

Medical Nutrition Therapy

In cigarette smokers, food components and specific nutrients have been investigated as either preventive or therapeutic modalities for lung cancer. High-dose β-carotene supplements may have a negative effect, whereas increased consumption of fruits and vegetables may be beneficial (Hercberg, 2005). The possible role of whole foods or their various components, or botanicals, in lung cancer initiation, promotion, or treatment receives worldwide attention (Lambert et al., 2005).

Because of the pulmonary constraints in people with lung cancer, purchasing and preparing foods may be overwhelming tasks. Eating may become an unpleasant activity because of severe pain, dyspnea, and dyspepsia. Weight loss, along with associated declines in other anthropometric and laboratory indicators of cancer-related malnutrition, portends a worsening prognosis. Thus, providing foods, beverages, and nutritional supplements in the forms and at the times best tolerated by the patient is essential. Administering oral medications with calorically dense nutritional supplements is another means of supplying needed nutrients (Cranganu and Camporeale, 2009).

PNEUMONIA

Pneumonia usually occurs as an infection from bacteria, viruses, or fungi, or as a consequence of aspiration of food, fluid, or secretions such as saliva. Aspiration is common in infants, children, and adults who are frail, have frequent coughing spasms, are unable to effectively chew or swallow their foods and beverages, or have inadequate head and neck control during eating.

Pathophysiology

The infection or foreign material cause the alveoli to become inflamed. These air sacs fill with fluid or pus, which results in symptoms including cough (with phlegm), fever, chills, and labored breathing.

Medical Nutrition Therapy

The role of vitamin A in treating pneumonia in children yielded conflicting results based on study designs (Mathew, 2010). Because of their role in inflammation and immunity, EFAs in adults were investigated, and showed a possible protective effect against pneumonia by the ingestion of α-linolenic and linoleic acids (Merchant et al., 2005).

Optimal nutrition status and proper feeding techniques aid in preventing this pulmonary infection. Suggestions for preventing aspiration of secretions or food and fluids are in Chapter 41 and Appendix 35. Once pneumonia occurs, the goals of nutrition care are to provide adequate fluids and energy. Small, frequent meals of nourishing foods usually are better tolerated, coupled with proper positioning during eating.

RESPIRATORY FAILURE

Respiratory failure (RF) occurs when the pulmonary system is unable to perform its functions. The causes may be traumatic, surgical, or medical. Multiple organ dysfunction syndrome (see Chapter 39) is the term used to denote abnormal interaction among the organ systems, culminating in relentless dysfunction of all organ systems.

Pathophysiology

Acute respiratory distress syndrome is a common complication of critical illness. Ultimately, in RF from any cause, the patient requires oxygen provided through a nasal cannula or by mechanical ventilator support for varying lengths of time and at various levels of oxygen.

Medical Treatment

Central factors in failure to wean from oxygen support or mechanical ventilation are respiratory muscle weakness and retention of CO_2. The prognosis is precarious for patients with underlying chronic pulmonary disease such as CF or emphysema, or for those who are otherwise medically compromised, malnourished, or older. Lung transplantation (or cardiopulmonary transplantation) may be a viable option for some patients.

Medical Nutrition Therapy

Nutritional needs vary widely within this group of patients, depending on the underlying disease process, prior nutrition status, and the patient's age. Hypercatabolism or hypermetabolism may be present.

As with most pulmonary diseases, body composition fluctuation is the hallmark nutrition assessment indicator for persons with RF. Most patients become severely underweight. Thus a series of accurate anthropometric measurements is crucial during the entire course of treatment, sometimes spanning the patient's lifetime (see Chapter 6). When at all possible, more accurate estimations of energy requirements are recommended with the use of indirect calorimetry measurements (see Chapter 2). Accurate interpretation of laboratory results may be confounded by fluid imbalances, medications, and ventilator support. Other nutritionally relevant factors to assess include immunocompetence, chronic mouth breathing, aerophagia, dyspnea, exercise tolerance, and depression.

The goals of nutrition care in patients with RF are to meet basic nutritional requirements, preserve lean body mass, restore respiratory muscle mass and strength, maintain fluid balance, improve resistance to infection, and facilitate weaning from oxygen support and mechanical ventilation by providing energy substrates without exceeding the capacity of the respiratory system to clear CO_2. Methods to provide nutrition support depend on the underlying disease, whether the patient is acutely or chronically ill, and whether ventilator support is necessary (see Chapter 14).

Energy

Because of hypercatabolism and hypermetabolism, energy needs are elevated in RF, and sufficient energy must be supplied to prevent the use of the body's own reserves of protein and fat. Energy requirements fluctuate and thus are best determined by continuous individual assessment. To estimate initial caloric requirements using prediction equations, see Chapter 2. Indirect calorimetry is considered the "gold standard" because it is the most accurate estimation of energy needs. Overfeeding in this population is particularly deleterious. By general agreement the most important factor is to provide adequate but not excessive energy.

Macronutrients

Because the patient with RF may be in negative nitrogen balance, protein should be supplied to restore balance; however, enterally supplied protein does affect the RQ. The basic requirements for carbohydrate and fat as actual nutrients for nourishment are influenced by the underlying organ system decompensation, the patient's respiratory status, and the ventilation methods used. Controversy persists concerning the optimal ratio of protein, fat, and carbohydrate supplied to patients with RF. Protein is calculated as 1.5 to 2 g/kg of dry body weight. Nonprotein calories are evenly divided between fat and carbohydrate. Daily monitoring of each patient's intake is crucial.

Water requirements must be individualized based on the method of oxygen delivery and environmental factors, coupled with knowledge of underlying disease processes and prescribed medications.

Vitamins and Minerals

Exact requirements for specific vitamins and minerals in RF are unknown. It is assumed that vitamins and minerals need to be supplied at least at the levels of the DRI plus repletion, based on the gender and age of the patient. The intake of vitamins and minerals necessary for anabolism, wound healing, and immunity, and those with antioxidant functions may need to be increased. For example, during anabolism mineral balance must be monitored in an anticipatory manner to prevent the refeeding syndrome (see Chapter 14). Minerals that function as electrolytes need to be monitored closely, especially because of fluid imbalances and the occurrence of respiratory acidosis or alkalosis. As a side effect of medications, potassium, calcium, and magnesium may be lost in the urine.

Feeding Strategies

Diet composition and food selections should be planned to accommodate the nutritional requirements, individual preferences, and living arrangements of the patient. Some people participate in pulmonary rehabilitation programs. Most patients who are not intubated or who have tracheostomies will be able to meet all or most of their nutritional needs by mouth. Small portions and favorite foods enhance oral food intake. Consumption must be monitored to maintain appropriate calorie levels and a suitable ratio of protein, fat, and carbohydrate.

Provision of adequate oxygen is crucial for proper digestion and absorption of food. Patients receiving inadequate oxygen may complain of anorexia, early satiety, malaise, bloating, and constipation or diarrhea. Intubated patients usually require enteral tube feedings or parenteral feedings. In a hospital setting establishing a nutrition protocol increases the likelihood of appropriate enteral feeding, thus yielding better outcomes such as decreased duration of mechanical ventilation. The use of specially formulated pulmonary proprietary products should be reserved for patients fitting the specified criteria (see Chapter 14). Otherwise effort and expense may not provide the expected results.

TUBERCULOSIS

Tuberculosis (TB) traditionally was diagnosed among economically disadvantaged population groups (e.g., immigrants, homeless persons, and children) or those living in close quarters (e.g., prisoners, refugees, and armed forces). At high risk are health care workers; residents in assisted living facilities, skilled nursing homes, or hospitals; and people who are immunocompromised such as those with cancer, chronic renal disease, or HIV (see Chapters 36 through 38).

Pathophysiology

Tuberculosis (TB) is a bacterial disease caused by mycobacteria, specifically *Mycobacterium tuberculosis*, *M. bovis*, or *M. africanum*. The disease is spread from inhalation of organisms dispersed as droplets from the sputum of infected persons (the bacteria-laden droplets can float in the air for several hours). TB yields prolonged cytokine production. Increased levels of interferon gamma, interleukin (IL)-10, and IL-6 are accompanied by a modest increase in the levels of cortisol, prolactin, and thyroid hormones and decreased testosterone and dehydroepiandrosterone levels (Bottasso et al., 2009).

TB produces profound abnormalities on the immune system. Although most people infected by the tubercle bacillus (90%) do not develop the disease during their lifetime, when there are coinfections with HIV, malnutrition, or diabetes, the risk of developing active disease increases considerably.

Medical Treatment

Pharmacologically, this pulmonary infection is treated with multiple medications, especially antibiotics. First-line drugs are isoniazid, rifampicin, ethambutol, and pyrazinamide. Each has drug-food-nutrient interactions (see Chapter 9). Because tubercle bacilli increasingly are becoming resistant to drug therapy; strains with increased virulence have emerged. New therapies are constantly under review.

Medical Nutrition Therapy

Signs and symptoms of TB with nutritional relevance include undernutrition, weight loss, night sweats, fatigue, dyspnea, and hemoptysis (Campbell and Bah-Sow, 2006; Villamor et al., 2006). People with chronic infections may need higher caloric intakes. Unless otherwise contraindicated, people with TB routinely require increased energy intake and fluids. Research has not found a role for vitamin A or zinc supplementation specifically, but vitamin C may have merit. Providing access to food and also to high-calorie, high-protein oral supplements is a less expensive, feasible medical option (Abba K, et al., 2008). Many patients require assistance with activities of daily living, such as shopping for food and meal preparation.

Because isoniazid absorption is reduced by food, it should be administered 1 hour before or 2 hours after meals. It depletes pyridoxine (vitamin B_6) and interferes with vitamin D metabolism, which in turn can decrease absorption of calcium and phosphorus. Patients thus require increased vitamins B_6 and D (Yamshchikov, et al., 2010), and minerals from meals or supplements.

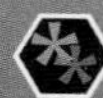

CLINICAL SCENARIO

Rick is a 63-year-old widower who is a retired commercial carpet installer. He started smoking when he was 15, and he smoked two packs per day until 7 years ago. You have an appointment with Rick during his next session at the Outpatient Pulmonary Rehabilitation Program. Significant findings are weight 124 lb, height 5′4″, blood pressure 127/65, heart rate 82, respiratory rate 18, temperature 98.6° F, oxygen saturation 95, carbon dioxide 54, forced vital capacity (FVC) 1.04 (28% predicted), forced expiratory volume in 1 second (FEV1) 0.37 (12% predicted), FEV1/FVC ratio 36, and forced expiratory flow 25%-76% 0.19 (67% predicted). History and physical examination reveal severe dyspnea on exertion, including showering, carrying packages, making the bed, and pushing a vacuum cleaner; orthopnea (two or three pillows); and decreased breath sounds. Prescribed medications include theophylline (300 mg twice daily), prednisone (20 mg once daily in the morning), fluticasone (Flovent; 220 mg, four puffs twice daily), albuterol and ipratropium (Atrovent; two puffs as needed), trimethoprim and sulfamethoxazole (Bactrim DS; 1 tablet every 12 hours), and furosemide (Lasix; as needed). Over-the-counter medications include vitamin C (250 mg twice daily), vitamin E (400 units daily), and calcium (500 mg daily). He had a blood test and his potassium was low; his diet history reveals almost no potassium intake.

Nutrition Diagnostic Statement

Food-medication interaction related to low potassium intake while on diuretic as evidenced by latest serum potassium.

Nutrition Care Questions

1. What other nutrition assessment information do you need before you see Rick?
2. What are the interrelationships between chronic obstructive pulmonary disease, food intake, and nutrient metabolism?
3. Are there any food-drug interactions that are a concern for Rick?
4. What are the principles of medical nutrition therapy for Rick? Explain the scientific rationale for each.
5. Write out a day's schedule to include mealtimes, medication administration times, and activities of daily living. Include the foods you might suggest for fulfilling the nutrition prescription. Verify by performing a computerized nutrient analysis.
6. What do you think of Rick's nutrient supplementation program? Would you have Rick change it?
7. You are planning a session on nutrition for the clients and their families who participate in the Outpatient Pulmonary Rehabilitation Program. What topics would you cover? What educational techniques would you use?

USEFUL WEBSITES

American Association for Respiratory Care
http://www.aarc.org
American Lung Association
http://www.lungusa.org
American Thoracic Society
http://www.thoracic.org
Cystic Fibrosis Foundation
http://www.cff.org
Cystic Fibrosis Genetic Analysis Consortium (Cystic Fibrosis Mutation Database)
http://www.genet.sickkids.on.ca/cftr
National Asthma Education and Prevention Program
http://www.nhlbi.nih.gov/guidelines/asthma
National Cancer Institute (Lung Cancer)
http://www.cancer.gov/cancertopics/types/lung
National Institute of Diabetes and Digestive and Kidney Diseases—Cystic Fibrosis Research
http://www.niddk.nih.gov

REFERENCES

Abba K, et al: Nutritional supplements for people being treated for active tuberculosis, *Cochrane Database Syst Rev* (4), 2008. Art. No.: CD006086. DOI: 10.1002/14651858.CD006086.pub2.

Aldamiz-Echievarria L, et al: Persistence of essential fatty acid deficiency in cystic fibrosis despite nutritional therapy, *Pediatric Res* 66:585, 2009.

Allan K, Devereux, G: Diet and asthma; nutrition implications from prevention to treatment, *J Am Diet Assoc* 111:258, 2011.

American Academy of Allergy, Asthma, and Immunology (AAAAI): Attaining optimal asthma control: A practice parameter, 2005. Accessed 22 October 2010 from www.aaaai.org.

American Dietetic Association, Evidence Analysis Library: COPD, 2010. Accessed 22 October 2010 from www.eatright.org.

Baines KL, et al: The nutrigenomics of asthma: molecular mechanisms of airway neutrophilia following dietary antioxidant withdrawal, *OMICS: Journal of Integrative Biology* 13:355, 2009.

Baldi S, et al: Fat-free mass change after nutritional rehabilitation in weight losing COPD: role of insulin, C-reactive protein and tissue hypoxia, *Int J COPD* 5:29, 2010.

Barros R, et al: Adherence to the Mediterranean diet and fresh fruit intake are associated with improved asthma control, *Allergy* 63:917, 2008.

Bede O, et al: Effects of magnesium supplementation on the glutathione redox system in atopic asthmatic children, *Inflammation Res* 57:279, 2008.

Bottasso O, et al: Immunoendocrine alterations during human tuberculosis as an integrated view of disease pathology, *Neuroimmunomodulation* 16:68, 2009.

Campbell IA, Bah-Sow O: Pulmonary tuberculosis: diagnosis and treatment, *Br Med J* 332:1194, 2006.

Coates AJ, et al: Evaluation of salt supplementation in CF infants, *J Cys Fibr* 8:382, 2009.

Cranganu A, Camporeale J: Nutrition aspects of lung cancer, *Nutr Clin Pract* 24:688, 2009.

Darlow BA, et al: Vitamin A supplementation to prevent mortality and short and long-term morbidity in very low birthweight infants, *Cochrane Database Syst Rev* 2007. CD000501.

DHHS (Department of Health and Human Services:) Action against asthma: a strategic plan for the Department of Health and Human Services. Accessed 22 October 2010 from http://www.aspe.hhs.gov/sp/asthma/.

Global Initiative for Chronic Obstructive Lung Disease (GOLD): Global strategy for the diagnosis, management, and prevention of chronic obstructive pulmonary disease, Executive summary, updated 2009. Accessed 22 October 2010 from http://www.goldcopd.org/.

Guilbert TW, Denlinger LC: Role of infection in the development and exacerbation of asthma, *Expert Rev Respir Med* 4:71, 2010.

Hercberg S: The history of β-carotene and cancers: from observational to intervention studies. What lessons can be drawn for future research on polyphenols? *Am J Clin Nutr* 81:218S, 2005.

Haworth, CS: Impact of cystic fibrosis on bone health, *Curr Opin Pulm Med* 16:616, 2010.

Kalhan R, et al: A mechanism of benefit of soy genistein in asthma: inhibition of eosinophil p38-dependent leukotriene synthesis, *Clin Exper Allergy* 38:103, 2008.

Kazaks AG, et al: Effect of oral magnesium supplementation on measures of airway resistance and subjective assessment of asthma control and quality of life in men and women with mild to moderate asthma: a randomized placebo controlled trial, *J Asthma* 47:83, 2010.

Kealoha, MK: What's new in alternative therapies for asthmatic children? *J Comm Health Nurs* 26:198, 2009.

King DA, et al: Nutritional aspects of chronic obstructive pulmonary disease, *Proc Am Thoracic Soc* 5:519, 2008.

Lambert JD, et al: Inhibition of carcinogenesis by polyphenols: evidence from laboratory investigations, *Am J Clin Nutr* 81:284S, 2005.

Leonard A, et al: Description of a standardized nutrition classification plan and its relation to nutritional outcomes in children with cystic fibrosis, *J Ped Psycol* 35:6, 2010.

Lindemann J, et al: Clinical study of the effects on asthma-related QOL and asthma management of a medical food in adult asthma patients, *Curr Med Res Opin* 25:2865, 2009.

Magoffin A, et al: Longitudinal analysis of resting energy expenditure in patients with cystic fibrosis, *J Pediatr* 152:703, 2008.

Mathew JL: Vitamin A supplementation for prophylaxis or therapy in childhood pneumonia: a systematic review of randomized controlled trials, *Indian Pediatr* 47:255, 2010.

Merchant AT, et al: Intake of ω-6 and ω-3 fatty acids and fish and risk of community-acquired pneumonia in U.S. men, *Am J Clin Nutr* 82:668, 2005.

Michel SH, et al: Nutrition management of pediatric patients who have cystic fibrosis, *Pediatr Clin N Am* 56:1123, 2009.

Moran A, et al: Clinical care guidelines for cystic fibrosis-related diabetes, *Diabetes Care* 33:2697, 2010.

Morton AM, et al: Symposium 6: Young people, artificial nutrition and transitional care. The nutritional challenges of the young adult with cystic fibrosis: transition, *Proc Nutr Soc* 68:430, 2009.

Peden DB, Bush RK. Advances in environmental and occupational respiratory disease in 2010, *J Allergy Clin Immunol* 127:696, 2011.

Raviv S, Smith LJ: Diet and asthma, *Curr Opin Pulm Med* 16:71, 2010.

Schubert R, et al: Effect of ω-3 polyunsaturated fatty acids in asthma after low-dose allergen challenge, *Int Arch Allergy Immunol* 148:321, 2009.

Sorkness RL: CAM and respiratory disease, *Nutr Clin Pract* 24:609, 2009.

Stallings VA, et al: Evidence-based practice recommendations for nutrition-related management of children and adults with cystic fibrosis and pancreatic insufficiency: results of a systematic review, *J Am Diet Assoc* 108:832, 2008.

Stark LJ, et al: The effects of an intensive behavior and nutrition intervention compared to standard of care on weight outcomes in CF, *Pediatr Pulmonol* 00:1, 2010.

Stevenson CS, Birrell MA: Moving towards a new generation of animal models for asthma and COPD with improved clinical relevance, *Pharmacol Ther* 130:93, 2011.

Strandvik B: Fatty acid metabolism in cystic fibrosis: prostaglandins, *Leukot Essent Fatty Acids* 83:121, 2010.

Van Marter LJ: Epidemiology of bronchopulmonary dysplasia, *Semin Fetal Neonatal Med* 14:358, 2009.

Villamor E, et al: Wasting and body composition of adults with pulmonary tuberculosis in relation to HIV-1 coinfection, socioeconomic status, and severity of tuberculosis, *Eur J Clin Nutr* 60:163, 2006.

Weekes CE, et al: Dietary counseling and food fortification in stable COPD: a randomized trial, *Thorax* 64:326, 2009.

Watson H, et al: A randomized controlled trial of a new behavioral home-based nutrition education program, “Eat Well with CF,” in adults with cystic fibrosis, *J Am Diet Assoc* 108:847, 2008.

Wüthrich B, et al: Milk consumption does not lead to mucus production or occurrence of asthma, *J Am Coll Nutr* 24:6:547S, 2005.

Yamshchikov AV, et al: Vitamin D status and antimicrobial peptide cathelicidin (LL-37) concentrations in patients with active pulmonary tuberculosis, *Am J Clin Nutr* 92:603, 2010.

Zhang Z, et al: Early childhood weight status in relation to asthma development in high-risk children, *J Allergy Clin Immunol* 126:1157, 2010.

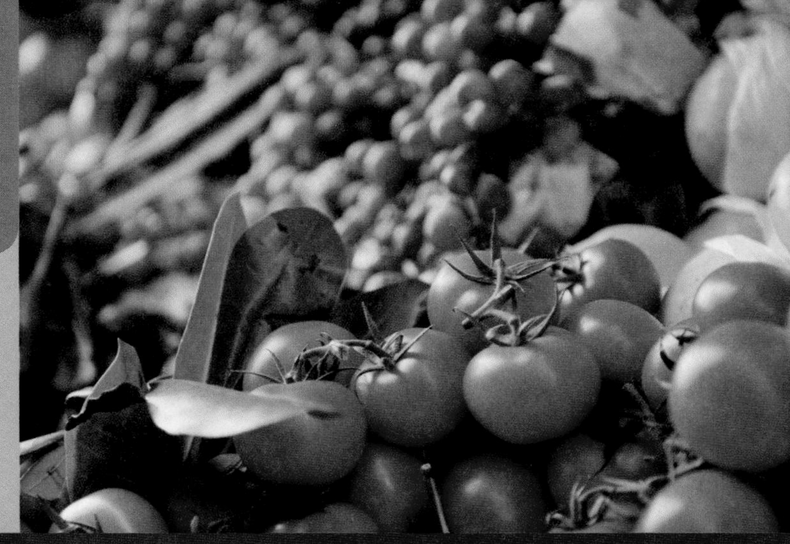

CHAPTER 36

Katy G. Wilkens, MS, RD
Veena Juneja, MSc, RD
Elizabeth Shanaman, RD, BS

Medical Nutrition Therapy for Renal Disorders

KEY TERMS

acute glomerulonephritides
acute kidney injury (AKI)
acute renal failure (ARF)
adynamic (low turnover) bone disease
antidiuretic hormone (ADH)
azotemia
calciphylaxis
chronic interstitial nephritis
chronic kidney disease (CKD)
continuous renal replacement therapy (CRRT)
continuous venovenous hemodialysis (CVVHD)
continuous venovenous hemofiltration (CVVH)
dialysate
end-stage renal disease (ESRD)
erythropoietin (EPO)
faconi syndrome
fistula
glomerular filtration rate (GFR)
hemodialysis (HD)
hypercalciuria
hyperoxaluria
intradialytic parenteral nutrition (IDPN)
intraperitoneal nutrition (IPN)
Kidney Dialysis Outcome Quality Initiative (KDOQI)
kinetic modeling
Kt/V
metastatic calcification
nephritic syndrome
nephrolithiasis
nephrotic syndrome
oliguria
osteitis fibrosa cystica
osteomalacia
peritoneal dialysis (PD)
phosphate binders
protein digestibility corrected amino acid score (PDCAAS)
protein-nitrogen appearance (PNA) rate
pyelonephritis
renal failure
renal osteodystrophy
renal replacement therapy (RRT)
renal tubular acidosis (RTA)
renin-angiotensin mechanism
syndrome of inappropriate anti-diuretic hormone (SIAH)
ultrafiltrate
urea reduction ratio (URR)
uremia
vasopressin

PHYSIOLOGY AND FUNCTION OF THE KIDNEYS

The main function of the kidney is to maintain the balance of fluids, electrolytes, and organic solutes. The normal kidney performs this function over a wide range of fluctuations in sodium, water, and solutes. This task is accomplished by the continuous filtration of blood with alterations in secretion and reabsorption of this filtered fluid. The kidney receives 20% of cardiac output, filtering approximately 1600 L/day of blood and producing 180 liters of fluid called **ultrafiltrate**. Through active processes of reabsorbing certain components and secreting others, composition of this ultrafiltrate is changed into the 1.5 L of urine excreted in an average day.

Each kidney consists of approximately 1 million functioning nephrons (Figure 36-1), consisting of a glomerulus connected to a series of tubules. Tubules consist of different segments: the proximal convoluted tubule, loop of Henle, distal tubule, and collecting duct. Each nephron functions independently and contributes to the final urine, although all are under similar control and coordination. If one segment of a nephron is destroyed, that complete nephron is no longer functional.

The glomerulus is a spherical mass of capillaries surrounded by a membrane, Bowman's capsule. The glomerulus produces the ultrafiltrate, which is then modified by the next segments of the nephron. Production of ultrafiltrate is mainly passive and relies on the perfusion pressure generated by the heart and supplied by the renal artery.

The tubules reabsorb the vast majority of components that compose the ultrafiltrate. Much of this process is active and requires a large expenditure of energy in the form of adenosine triphosphate (ATP). The tubule is a unique structure; differences in permeability between the various segments and hormonal responses allow the tubule to produce the final urine, which can vary widely in concentration of electrolytes, osmolality, pH, and volume. Ultimately, this urine is funneled into common collecting tubules and into the renal pelvis. The renal pelvis narrows into a single ureter per kidney, and each ureter carries urine into the bladder, where it accumulates before elimination.

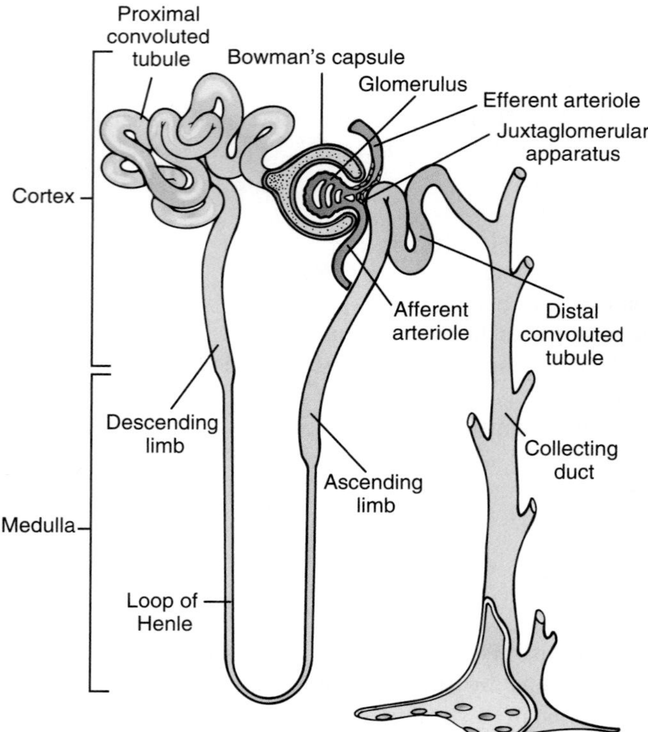

FIGURE 36-1 The nephron. *(Modified from Thibodeau GA, Patton KT: The human body in health and disease, ed 4, St Louis, 2005, Mosby.)*

The kidney has almost unlimited ability to regulate water homeostasis. Its ability to form a large concentration gradient between its inner medulla and outer cortex allows the kidney to excrete urine as dilute as 50 mOsm or as concentrated as 1200 mOsm. Given a daily fixed solute load of approximately 600 mOsm, the kidney can get rid of as little as 500 mL of concentrated urine or as much as 12 L of dilute urine. Control of water excretion is regulated by **vasopressin** (**antidiuretic hormone [ADH]**), a small peptide hormone secreted by the posterior pituitary. An excess of relative body water, indicated by a low osmolality, leads to prompt shut-off of all vasopressin secretion. Likewise, a small rise in osmolality brings about marked vasopressin secretion and water retention. However, the need to conserve sodium sometimes leads to a sacrifice of the homeostatic control of water for the sake of volume. See *Focus On:* Syndrome of Inappropriate Antidiuretic Hormone.

The minimum urinary volume capable of eliminating a relatively fixed 600 mOsm of solute is 500 mL, assuming that the kidney is capable of maximum concentration. Urinary volume of less than 500 mL/ day is called **oliguria**; it is impossible for such a small urine volume to eliminate all of the daily waste.

The majority of the solute load consists of nitrogenous wastes, primarily the end products of protein metabolism. Urea predominates in amount, depending on the protein content of the diet. Uric acid, creatinine (Cr), and ammonia are present in small amounts. If normal waste products are not eliminated appropriately, they collect in abnormal quantities in the blood, known as **azotemia**. The ability of the kidney to adequately eliminate nitrogenous waste products is defined as *renal function*. Thus **renal failure** is the inability to excrete the daily load of wastes.

The kidney also performs functions unrelated to excretion. One of these involves the **renin-angiotensin mechanism**, a major control of blood pressure. Decreased blood volume causes cells of the glomerulus (the juxtaglomerular apparatus) to react by secreting renin, a proteolytic enzyme.

FOCUS ON

Syndrome of Inappropriate Antidiuretic Hormone

Syndrome of inappropriate antidiuretic hormone (SIAH) is seen when there is an excessive amount of antidiuretic hormone released from the pituitary gland. Common causes include head injury, meningitis, cancer, infection, and hypothyroidism. The result is hyponatremia caused by hemodilution. It is characterized by a serum sodium less than 135 mEq/L and a urine sodium concentration greater than 20 mEq/L. If left untreated it can result in seizures and coma. It is treated with fluid restriction, generally less than 1800 mL/ day, and may require intravenous sodium administration. Oral sodium supplementation is contraindicated.

Renin acts on angiotensinogen in the plasma to form angiotensin I, which is converted to angiotensin II, a powerful vasoconstrictor and a potent stimulus of aldosterone secretion by the adrenal gland. As a consequence, sodium and fluid are reabsorbed, and blood pressure is returned to normal.

The kidney also produces the hormone **erythropoietin (EPO)**, a critical determinant of erythroid activity in the bone marrow. Deficiency of EPO is the primary cause of the severe anemia present in chronic renal disease.

Maintenance of calcium-phosphorus homeostasis involves the complex interactions of parathyroid hormone (PTH); calcitonin; active vitamin D; and three effector organs: the gut, kidney, and bone. The role of the kidney includes production of the active form of vitamin D—1,25-dihydroxycholecalciferol (1,25-$[OH]_2D_3$)—as well as elimination of both calcium and phosphorus. Active vitamin D promotes efficient absorption of calcium by the gut and is one of the substances necessary for bone remodeling and maintenance. Active vitamin D also suppresses PTH production, which is responsible for mobilization of calcium from bone (see Chapter 25).

RENAL DISEASES

The manifestations of renal disease are significant. They can be ordered by degree of severity: (1) kidney stones, (2) acute kidney injury (AKI), (3) chronic kidney disease (CKD), and (4) end-stage renal disease (ESRD) (National Kidney Foundation, 2002). Objectives of nutritional care depend on the abnormality being treated.

Kidney Stones (Nephrolithiasis)

Nephrolithiasis, the presence of kidney stones, is a significant health problem in the United States. It is characterized by frequent occurrences between the ages of 30 and 50, predominance in males, and a high recurrence rate. The risk doubles in those with a family history of kidney stones; stone formers often have first-degree relatives with kidney stones. Increased frequency of obesity, diabetes, and metabolic syndrome have resulted in increasing rates of nephrolithiasis among women, decreasing the male/female ratio from 1.7 : 1 to 1.3 : 1 (Zilberman, 2010). One Canadian study found significant differences in occurrence rates among ethnic groups, with highest rates in those of Arabic and West Indian descent and the lowest rates among those of East Asian or African descent (Mente, 2007). However, low urine volume is the single most important risk factor for nephrolithiasis.

Pathophysiology

Kidney stone formation is a complex process that consists of saturation; supersaturation; nucleation; crystal growth or aggregation; crystal retention; and stone formation in the presence of promoters, inhibitors, and complexors in urine. A typical metabolic evaluation is described in Table 36-1.

Calcium stones are the most common: 60% of stones are calcium oxalate, 10% calcium oxalate and calcium phosphate, and 10% calcium phosphate. Other stones are 5% to 10% uric acid, 5% to 10% struvite, and 1% cystine.

Obese stone formers excrete increased amount of sodium, calcium, uric acid, and citrate, and have lower urine pH. Obesity is the strongest predictor of stone recurrence in first-time stone formers. As body weight increases, the excretion of calcium, oxalate, and uric acid also increases. Patients with higher body mass index (BMI) have a decrease in ammonia excretion and impaired hydrogen ion buffering (Li et al., 2009). With increasing BMI, uric acid stones become more dominant than calcium oxalate stones, especially in men (Eisner, 2010b).

Uric acid stones are common in the presence of type 2 diabetes. Hyperinsulinemia may also contribute to the development of calcium stones by increasing urinary calcium excretion (Maalouf et al., 2010b). Weight control may be considered one of the preventive modalities and in stone formers, a BMI of 18 to 25 kg/m^2 is recommended.

With malabsorptive bariatric procedures such as Roux-en-Y gastric bypass (RYGB), urolithiasis is higher than in obese controls, probably because of the increased prevalence of hyperoxaluria and hypocitraturia in RYGB patients (Maalouf et al., 2010a). However, restrictive gastric surgery (i.e., gastric banding or sleeve gastrectomy) is not associated with increased risk of kidney stones (Semins et al., 2010).

Agents added intentionally or unintentionally to food or drug products have led to the appearance of new types of stones containing melamine and indinavir (Zilberman, 2010). See Table 36-2.

Calcium Stones. One third to one half of patients with calcium stones are hypercalciuric. **Hypercalciuria** describes a value of calcium in excess of 300 mg (7.5 mmol) per day in men, 250 mg (6.25 mmol) per day in women, or 4 mg (0.1 mmol)/kg/day for either in random urine collections of outpatients on unrestricted diets. Causes of hypercalciuria may include primary hyperparathyroidism, sarcoidosis, excess vitamin D intake, hyperthyroidism, glucocorticoid use, or renal tubular acidosis (RTA).

Idiopathic hypercalciuria (IH) seems to have a genetic basis. IH can be triggered by an excessive dietary calcium intake, increased intestinal absorption of calcium that may or may not be vitamin D–mediated, decreased renal tubular reabsorption of calcium, or prolonged bed rest. Increased gut absorption of calcium is noted in essentially all patients with IH. However, urinary calcium is higher than normal at any level of net calcium absorption, suggesting that some of the urine calcium is derived from the bone. When challenged with a very-low-calcium diet, the loss of more calcium in the urine than is in the diet results in abnormal bone mineral wasting. Patients with IH tend toward negative phosphorus balance even on normal intakes. The defective phosphate metabolism may lead to increased 1,25$(OH)_2D_3$ levels, and increased intestinal calcium absorption.

Bone loss can be high in patients with IH in whom low calcium intake exaggerates bone loss from increased net acid excretion (NAE). For decades low-calcium diets were recommended to reduce the hypercalciuria in these stone-formers. However, chronic prolonged calcium restriction,

TABLE 36-1

Baseline Information and Metabolic Evaluation of Urolithiasis

Information	Description and Data
History of urolithiasis	History of onset, frequency Family history Spontaneous passage or removal Retrieval, analysis of stone Current status with radiologic examination
Medical history, investigation	Hyperparathyroidism Renal tubular acidosis Urinary tract infection Sarcoidosis Hypertension Osteoporosis Inflammatory bowel disease, malabsorption syndrome, intestinal bypass surgery for obesity Metabolic syndrome or insulin resistance Diabetes mellitus Obesity
Blood tests	Serum—calcium, phosphorus, creatinine, uric acid, CO_2, albumin, parathyroid hormone, Hgb A1c
Urinalysis	Urine analysis with pH Urine culture
24-hr urine collection	Volume, calcium, oxalate, uric acid, sodium Citrate, magnesium, phosphorus Urea Creatinine Qualitative cystine
Medications and vitamins	Thiazide, allopurinol, vitamin C, vitamin B_6, vitamin D, cod liver oil, calcium carbonate, glucocorticoid therapy, potassium citrate
Occupation history and strenuous exercise	Dermal water losses Dehydration Low urine volume Type of job and activity level
Environment	Hard water area
Dietary evaluation	Intake of calcium, oxalate, animal protein, salt, purines, fructose, potassium Fruits and vegetables (related to urine pH) Herbal products Volume of fluid intake Type of fluids containing citrate, caffeine, phosphoric acid; mineral water; sports drinks

CO_2, Carbon Dioxide; *Hgb A1c*, hemoglobin A1c.

TABLE 36-2

Causes and Composition of Renal Stones

Pathogenetic Causes	Composition of Stone
Hypercalciuria, hyperoxaluria, hyperuricosuria, or hypocitraturia	Calcium oxalate
Primary hyperparathyroidism	Calcium oxalate
Cystinuria	Cystine
Infection	Struvite
Acid urine pH	Uric acid
Hyperuricosuria	Uric acid
Renal tubular acidosis	Calcium phosphate
Alkaline urine pH	Calcium phosphate

Modified from: Asplin JR: Evaluation of a kidney stone patient, Seminars in Nephrol 28(2):99, 2008.

deficient calcium intake, and increased losses from hypercalciuria decrease bone mineral density at the spine and cortical sites. Thus vertebral fracture risk increases fourfold among urolithiasis patients in comparison with the general population.

Undesirable bone resorption may be enhanced by a high protein intake of nondairy origin. An inadequate calcium with high protein intake induces metabolic acidosis, increases calcium excretion, and lowers urinary pH. This acid load inhibits the renal reabsorption of calcium. A reduction in nondairy animal protein may be recommended; see *Clinical Insight:* Urinary pH—How Does Diet Affect It?

Calcium supplements do not have the same protective effect as dietary calcium. A trial of combined calcium–vitamin D supplementation to prevent bone loss and fractures led to higher rates of stone formation in women (Jackson et al., 2006). If taken as a supplement, timing is important. Calcium supplements taken with meals increase urinary calcium and citrate but decrease urinary oxalate; thus the increase in citrate and decrease in oxalate counterbalance the effects of elevated urinary calcium. Therefore, if used by patients who cannot tolerate dairy products because of lactose intolerance, allergies, or preference, calcium supplements should be taken with meals. Urine calcium should be measured prior to starting the supplement and afterward to see the effect; if urine calcium increases, patients should increase fluid intake to dilute the urine concentration of calcium.

Patients may select 700-800 mg of calcium from dairy choices and consume the rest from nondairy foods to make up the total needed per day, according to age group and dietary reference intake (DRI) recommendations. Calcium

CLINICAL INSIGHT

Urinary pH—How Does Diet Affect It?

By Sheila Dean, DSc, RD, LD, CCN, CDE

Dietary intake can influence the acidity or alkalinity of the urine (Berardi, 2008). It has been shown that excessive dietary protein (particularly high in sulfur containing amino acids such as methionine and cysteine), and chloride, phosphorous, and organic acids are the main sources of dietary acid load. When these animal proteins such as meat and cheese, are eaten concomitantly with other acid producing foods, and not balanced out with alkaline producing foods such as fruit and vegetables, there is an increased risk of chronic acidosis. Acidosis (which is not to be confused with acidemia) has been linked to inflammatory related chronic diseases such as urolithiasis, hypertension, insulin resistance, low immune function and osteoporosis (Minich, 2007).

Consequently, when working with higher protein intakes it is important to provide a diet balanced in high alkaline foods. The most abundant alkaline foods are plant based foods; particularly vegetables and fruit abundant in alkalinizing micronutrients such as magnesium, calcium, sodium, and potassium. A more alkaline diet consisting of a higher fruit and vegetable intake is associated with a low potential renal acid load (PRAL) (Remer, 1995) Lower consumption of meat which is also associated with a lower PRAL may thus ameliorate not only the elevated blood pressure of hypertension but also the concurrent excess of morbidity and mortality of the concurrent cardiac, vascular and metabolic aspects of the hypertensive state.

Remer and Manz developed a physiologically based model to calculate the PRAL of selected, frequently consumed foods. By means of these PRAL data, the daily net acid excretion can be calculated, allowing for an accurate prediction of the effects of diet on acid load. This has been a reason to recommend animal protein limited diets, in order to control the dietary source of acids (Kiwull-Schone, 2008). The following food lists serve as a guide to influencing potential renal acid load (PRAL).

Potentially Acidic Foods

Protein: meat, fish, fowl, shellfish, eggs, all types of cheese, peanut butter, peanuts
Fat: bacon, butternuts, walnuts, pumpkin seeds, sesame seeds, sunflower seeds, creamy salad dressings
Carbohydrate: all types of bread including cornbran, oats, macaroni, ricebran, rye, wheat and especially wheat gluten
Sweets: gelatin desserts (dry mix with and without aspartame), pudding (instant, dry mix)

Potentially Basic or Alkaline Foods

Fat: dried beechnuts, dried chestnuts, acorn
Vegetables: all types including lentils but especially beets, beet greens, Swiss chard, dandelion greens, kale, leeks, mustard greens, spinach, turnip greens
Fruit: all types, especially currants, dates, figs, bananas, dried apricots, apples, prunes, raisins
Spices/Herbs: all types, especially fresh dill weed and dried spices/herbs such as spearmint, basil, coriander, curry powder, oregano, parsley
Sweets: sorghum syrup, sugar (brown), molasses, cocoa (dry powder)
Beverages: coffee

Neutral Foods

Fats: butter, margarine, oils
Dairy: milk
Vegetables: corn
Sweets: sugar (white), most syrups, honey
Beverages: water, tea

should be taken in divided doses, choosing a source with each meal to maximize oxalate binding. Any low-fat dairy choices are good options.

Oxalate Stones. **Hyperoxaluria** (>40 mg of oxalate in urine per day) plays an important role in calcium stone formation and is observed in 10% to 50% of recurrent stone formers. Primary hyperoxaluria is a feature of an autosomal-recessive genetic defect of a hepatic enzyme that results in overproduction of oxalate and a urinary oxalate concentration three to eight times normal. Multiple stones occur in these children, causing renal failure and early death.

Patients with inflammatory bowel diseases or gastric bypass often develop hyperoxaluria because of fat malabsorption. The bile acids produced during the digestive process normally are reabsorbed in the proximal gastrointestinal (GI) tract, but when this fails to occur, bile salts and fatty acids increase colonic permeability to oxalate. The unabsorbed fatty acids also bind calcium to form soaps, decreasing availability of calcium in a soluble form. With less calcium available to bind oxalate in the gut and prevent its absorption, serum oxalate and thus urinary oxilate levels increase.

Urinary oxalate also comes from endogenous synthesis, proportional to lean body mass. Ascorbic acid accounts for 35% to 55%, and glyoxylic acid accounts for 50% to 70% of urinary oxalate. In patients with CKD, excessive vitamin C intake may lead to stone formation. Oxalate synthesis is not increased with a high protein diet (Knight et al., 2009). Because pyridoxine acts as a cofactor in the conversion of glyoxylate to glycine, its deficiency could increase endogenous oxalate production.

The bioavailability of food oxalate and urine oxalate are affected by salt forms of oxalate, food processing and cooking methods, meal composition, and the presence of *Oxalabacter formigenes* in the GI tract (Massey, 2007). Stone-forming patients who lack this bacteria have significantly higher urinary oxalate excretion and stone episodes compared with patients colonized with the bacteria (Hatch and Freel, 2008).

Administration of *Oxalobacter formigenes* as enteric-coated capsules significantly reduces urine oxalate in patients with primary hyperoxaluria. Dietary advice for reducing urinary oxalate should include both use of this probiotic and reduction of dietary oxalate and simultaneous consumption of calcium-rich food or supplement to reduce oxalate absorption (Massey, 2007) (Box 36-1).

Uric Acid Stones. Uric acid is an end product of purine metabolism from food, de novo synthesis, and tissue catabolism. Approximately half of the purine load is from endogenous sources and is constant. Exogenous dietary sources provide the other half, accounting for the variation in urinary uric acid. The solubility of uric acid depends on urine volume, the amount excreted, and urine pH (Table 36-3). Uric acid stones form when urine is supersaturated with undissociated uric acid, which occurs at urinary pH less than 5.5.

The most important feature in uric acid stone formers is low urine pH resulting from increased NAE and impaired buffering caused by reduced urinary ammonium excretion.

BOX 36-1

Foods to Avoid for a Low Oxalate Diet

Rhubarb
Spinach
Strawberries
Chocolate
Wheat bran and whole-grain wheat products
Nuts (almonds, peanuts, or pecans)
Beets
Tea (green, black, iced, or instant)
High doses of turmeric

Data from Siener R et al: Oxalate content of cereals and cereal products, J Agric Food Chem 54:3008, 2006.

TABLE 36-3

Effect of Urine pH on Stone Formation

pH	State of Urate	Likely Stone Development
<5.5	Undissociated urate	Uric acid stones
5.5-7.5	Dissociated urate	Calcium oxalate stones
>7.5	Dissociated urate	Calcium phosphate stones

The former can be a result of low intake of alkali-producing foods or increased consumption of acid-producing foods. See *Clinical Insight:* Urine pH—How Does Diet Affect It?

Inflammatory bowel disease results in chronically acidic urine, usually from dehydration. GI bicarbonate loss from diarrhea may predispose these patients to uric acid stones. Uric acid stones are also associated with lymphoproliferative and myeloproliferative disorders, with increased cellular breakdown that releases purines and thus increases uric acid load. Diabetes, obesity, and hypertension appear to be associated with nephrolithiasis; diabetes is a common factor in uric acid stone development (Lieske et al., 2006). Besides diabetes management for patients with uric acid lithiasis and hyperuricosuric calcium oxalate stones, dietary purines should also be restricted.

Meat, fish, and poultry are rich in purines and acid ash, and thus should be used in moderation. Foods specifically high in purines should be avoided, including organ meats, anchovies, herrings, sardines, meat-based broth, and gravy (see Box 40-3 in Chapter 40). Dietary noncompliance or persistence of hyperuricosuria warrants use of medication such as allopurinol. Uric acid stones are the only stones amenable to dissolution therapy by urine alkalinization to a pH of 6 to 6.5. Potassium citrate has been used as the therapy of choice. Sodium bicarbonate increases urinary monosodium urate and calcium and should not be used.

Cystine Stones. Cystine stones represent 1% to 2% of urinary calculi and are caused by homozygous cystinuria. Cystine stones affect approximately 1 in 15,000 persons in the United States. Whereas normal individuals daily excrete

20 mg or less of cystine in their urine, stone-forming cystinuric patients excrete more than 250 mg/day. Cystine solubility increases when urine pH exceeds 7; therefore an alkaline urine pH must be maintained 24 hours per day, even while the patient sleeps. This is almost always achieved with the use of medication. Fluid intake of more than 4 L daily is recommended to prevent cystine crystallization. Lower sodium intake may be useful in reducing cystine in the urine.

Melamine and Indinavir Stones. Kidney stones, ARF, and death have been reported in young children who received melamine-contaminated infant formula. Melamine is an organic base synthesized from urea. When added to liquid milk or milk powder, it deceptively increases the protein content. Melamine precipitates in the distal renal tubules, forming crystals and sandlike stones. Hydration and urine alkalinization help with stone passage.

The treatment of human immunodeficiency virus infection with protease inhibitors has led to the appearance of another previously unknown urinary calculus: indinavir. Hypocitraturia is universal in all patients with indinavir stones as well as decreased solubility in a low urine volume with a low pH. These stones are soft, gelatinous, radiolucent, and are not amenable to basket removal or ureteroscopy. Intravenous (IV) hydration and temporary cessation of indinavir should be the first choice of treatment (Zilberman, 2010).

Struvite Stones. Struvite stones are composed of magnesium ammonium phosphate and carbonate apatite. They are also known as triple-phosphate or infection stones. Unlike most urinary stones, they occur more commonly in women than in men, at a ratio of 2 : 1. They form only in the presence of bacteria such as *Pseudomonas*, *Klebsiella*, *Proteus mirabilis*, and *Urealyticum* that carry urease, a urea-splitting enzyme. Urea breakdown results in ammonia and carbon dioxide (CO_2) production, thus raising urine pH and the level of carbonate. Struvite stones grow rapidly to large staghorn calculi in the renal pelvic area. The mainstay of treatment is extracorporeal shockwave lithotripsy (ECSWL) with adjunctive culture-specific antimicrobial therapy that uses urease inhibitors. The goal is to eliminate or prevent urinary tract infections by regularly screening and monitoring urine cultures.

Medical Management

Uric acid and struvite stones are the only type amenable to dissolution therapy in the form of ECSWL. Shockwave lithotripsy and endourologic techniques have almost replaced the open surgical procedures of stone removal of 20 years ago. Struvite stones are also treated with adjunctive culture-specific antimicrobial therapy that uses urease inhibitors. Management strategies are now aimed at kidney stone prevention (Asplin, 2008).

Medical Nutrition Therapy

After corrective treatment, nutrition assessment is needed to determine risk factors for stone recurrence. The risk in both men and women rises with increasing urine calcium and oxalate and decreases with increasing citrate and urine volume. There is a continuum of risk related to increasing urinary calcium and urinary oxalate. (Curhan and Taylor, 2008). Because urine chemistries change from day to day based on changes in the environment and diet, two 24-hour urine specimens are needed based on a usual diet, one during a week day and one on the weekend. Specific medical nutrition therapy (MNT) is then based on comprehensive metabolic evaluations. Nutrition counseling and metabolic monitoring can be quite effective (Table 36-4).

When a patient passes a stone, it should be determined if it is a new stone or a preexisting one and advisement given accordingly (Asplin, 2008). The effectiveness of any MNT should be monitored with evaluation of subsequent 24-hour urine collections. This gives the nutritionist and patient a measure of the effect of dietary changes. Once diet therapy is initiated, the goal is to prevent new stones from forming and preexisting stones from growing. See *Pathophysiology and Care Management Algorithm:* Kidney Stones.

Fluid and Urine Volume. A low urine volume is by far the most common abnormality noted on metabolic evaluation of stone formers, and its correction with a high fluid intake should be the focus in all types of kidney stones. The objective is to maintain urinary solutes in the undersaturated zone to inhibit nucleation; this increases urine volume and reduces solute load. The goal is the amount of urine flow rather than a specified fluid intake. High urine flow rate tends to wash out any formed crystals, and a urine volume of 2 to 2.5 L/day should prevent stone recurrence. Fluid intake should change based on different rates of extrarenal fluid loss that affect rate of urine flow.

Achieving a urine volume of 2 to 2.5 L/day usually requires an intake of 250 mL of fluid at each meal, between meals, at bedtime, and when arising to void at night. Hydration during sleep hours is important to break the cycle of the "most-concentrated" morning urine. Half of this daily 2.5 L should be taken as water. Even higher fluid intake, perhaps as much as 3 L/day, may be necessary to compensate for any GI fluid loss, excessive sweating from strenuous exercise, or an excessively hot or an excessively dry environment, such as a commercial airplane cabin.

Cranberry juice acidifies urine and is useful in the treatment of struvite stones. Black currant juice increases urinary citrate and oxalate and, because of its urine alkalinizing effect, may prevent the occurrence of uric acid stones.

Tea, coffee, beer, and wine have been associated with reduced risk of stone formation. The oxalate content of tea brewed from regular black or green tea is 300-1500 μmol/L. Because of the high oxalate content of tea, it should be taken with generous amounts of added milk; milk appears to reduce oxalate absorption by binding it in the gut lumen as calcium oxalate, making it less absorbable. Herbal teas have much lower oxalate content of 31-75 μmol/L and are an acceptable alternative (Massey, 2007). Soft drinks and colas that contain phosphoric acid should be avoided because of their urine acidifying effect.

Animal Protein. Epidemiologic studies find a correlation between improved standard of living, high animal protein intake, and the rising incidence of kidney stones.

TABLE 36-4

Recommendations for Diet and 24-Hour Urine Monitoring in Kidney Stone Disease

Diet Component	Intake Recommendation	24-Hour Urine
Protein	Normal intake: avoid excess	Monitor urinary urea
Calcium	Normal intake:1000 mg if age < 50 years; 1200 mg if age > 50 years Divide intake between three or more eating sessions	Calcium < 150 mg/L (<3.75 mmol/L)
Oxalate	Avoid moderate- to high-oxalate foods initially; further restrict if necessary	Oxalate < 20 mg/L (<220 μmol/L)
Fluid	2.5 L or more; assess type of fluids consumed; provide guidelines	Volume > 2 L/day
Purines	Avoid excessive protein intake; avoid specific high-purine foods	Uric acid < 2 mmol/L (<336 mg/L)
Vitamin C	< 500 mg/day	Monitor urinary oxalate
Vitamin D; cod liver oil	Supplements not recommended	
Vitamin B_6	40 mg or more per day reduces risk. No recommendation made	
Sodium	<100 mmol/day	Monitor urinary sodium

From: Curhan GC, Taylor EN: 24-h uric acid excretion and the risk of kidney stones, Kidney Internat 73:489, 2008.

Meat, fish, poultry eggs, cheese, and grains are the primary contributors of acid; see *Clinical Insight:* Urine pH—How Does Diet Affect It? An adequate-calcium, low animal–protein, low-salt diet (less than 4 g) reduces oxalate excretion more than a traditional low oxalate diet (Nouvenne et al., 2009).

Oxalate. Because much less oxalate than calcium exists in urine (ratio 1 : 5), changes in oxalate concentration have a greater effect than changes in urinary calcium. However, oxalate absorption, which is 3% to 8% of the amount in food, is affected by the amount of dietary calcium. On very low calcium intakes of less than 200 mg/day, oxalate absorption rises; it falls when a higher calcium (1200 mg) is ingested.

Dietary counseling to reduce oxalate absorption is beneficial for stone-forming individuals who have large intakes of high-oxalate foods and who excrete more than 30 mg (350 μmol) of oxalate per day. The American Dietetic Association recommends restriction of oxalate to approximately 60 mg/day. To keep the diet plan simple, the patient is told to avoid those foods that are high in oxalate as the first step.

When these foods are avoided, other foods eaten will often only add up to the 50-60 mg, the daily dietary target. In addition, the patient is advised to add calcium to each meal to bind oxalate. The total calcium intake for the day can be divided between at least three meals or as many eating occasions as possible. It takes 150 mg of calcium to bind 100 mg of oxalate. Patients should include approximately 150 mg calcium in each meal, such as that found in ½ cup milk, ice cream, pudding, yogurt, or ¾ oz cheese (Marcason, 2006; Massey, 2007).

Potassium. Stone formers often have a low to normal potassium intake and high sodium intake. Potassium intake is inversely related to the risk of kidney stones. Estimation of fruit and vegetable intake should be included in the metabolic evaluation. Stone formers should be encouraged to increase the potassium in their diets by choosing low-oxalate fruit and vegetables many times throughout the day (Domrongkitchaiporn et al., 2006; see Appendix 56). See Box 36-1.

Magnesium. Magnesium is a low-molecular-weight inhibitor that forms soluble complexes with oxalate. Like calcium, it inhibits oxalate absorption and may have a role to play in hyperoxaluric patients.

Phosphate. Excess urine phosphate contributes to calcium phosphate stone risk, but it is not as important a risk factor as urinary pH, which determines how much phosphate will be in the form of hydrogen phosphate (HPO_4) (Asplin, 2008). Calcium phosphate stones tend to occur in pregnant women in the second and third trimester of pregnancy.

Sodium. The daily amount of sodium chloride in modern diets reaches excessive levels of up to 10 g/day. The amount of sodium in the urine and hypercalciuria are directly correlated because sodium and calcium are reabsorbed at common sites in the renal tubule. Because the risk for nephrolithiasis is significantly higher in hypertensive individuals compared with normotensive individuals, sodium intake should be lowered to less than 2300 mg/day in patients with hypercalciuria (Asplin, 2008; Nouvenne et al, 2009; Straub and Hautmann, 2005). Consumption of a diet modeled on the Dietary Approaches to Stop Hypertension diet reduces the risk for kidney stones (Taylor et al., 2009). See Appendix 33.

Citrate. Citrate inhibits urinary stones by forming a complex with calcium in urine. Thus less calcium is available to bind urinary oxalate, which helps prevent the formation of calcium oxalate or calcium phosphate stones. Distal RTA

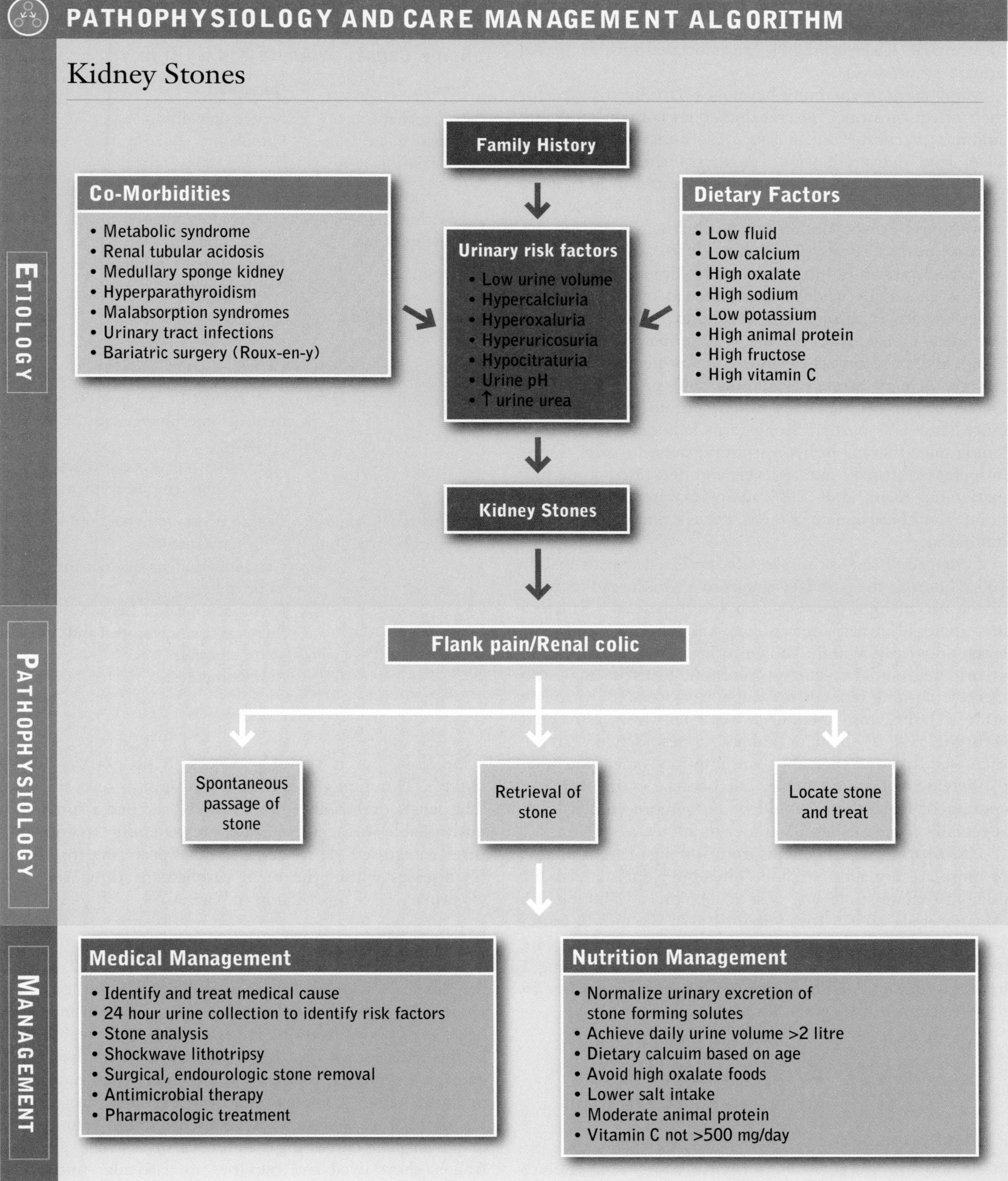
PATHOPHYSIOLOGY AND CARE MANAGEMENT ALGORITHM
Kidney Stones
ETIOLOGY
Family History
Co-Morbidities
• Metabolic syndrome
• Renal tubular acidosis
• Medullary sponge kidney
• Hyperparathyroidism
• Malabsorption syndromes
• Urinary tract infections
• Bariatric surgery (Roux-en-y)
Urinary risk factors
• Low urine volume
• Hypercalciuria
• Hyperoxaluria
• Hyperuricosuria
• Hypocitraturia
• Urine pH
• ↑ urine urea
Dietary Factors
• Low fluid
• Low calcium
• High oxalate
• High sodium
• Low potassium
• High animal protein
• High fructose
• High vitamin C
Kidney Stones
PATHOPHYSIOLOGY
Flank pain/Renal colic
Spontaneous passage of stone
Retrieval of stone
Locate stone and treat
MANAGEMENT
Medical Management
• Identify and treat medical cause
• 24 hour urine collection to identify risk factors
• Stone analysis
• Shockwave lithotripsy
• Surgical, endourologic stone removal
• Antimicrobial therapy
• Pharmacologic treatment
Nutrition Management
• Normalize urinary excretion of stone forming solutes
• Achieve daily urine volume >2 litre
• Dietary calcuim based on age
• Avoid high oxalate foods
• Lower salt intake
• Moderate animal protein
• Vitamin C not >500 mg/day

is an acidosis accompanied by hypokalemia. RTA, malabsorption syndrome with enteric hyperoxaluria, and excessive meat intake (lower urine pH) are associated with decreased urinary citrate levels.

Many citrate-containing beverages have been tested for their effect on urine. Several diet sodas contain moderate amounts of citrate and malate; malate increases the total alkali load delivered, which augments citraturia (Eisner, 2010a). One commercial sports drink tested in non–stone formers increased urine citrate as much as 170 mg/day, but many sports drinks contain too much fructose and do not increase urinary citrate (Goodman, 2009).

Hypocitraturia is most commonly idiopathic, but may also be caused by acidosis accompanied by hypokalemia, malabsorption syndrome with enteric hyperoxaluria, excessive meat intake, and acid ash (Zuckerman and Assimos, 2009). Half of recurrent calcium stone formers have hypocitraturia (urinary citrate of <300 mg/day), predominantly of dietary origin. Normal daily urinary citrate level should be more than 640 mg/day. Long-term lemonade or lime or lemon juice therapy in hypocitraturic stone formers results in increased urinary citrate levels and decreased stone formation rate (Kang et al., 2007). Mineral water, with its magnesium and bicarbonate content, raises urine pH and stone inhibition.

Fructose. Fructose intake has increased approximately 2000% during the past 30 years from a widespread increase in the use of high-fructose corn syrup in foods. Fructose may increase urinary excretion of calcium and oxalate. It is the only carbohydrate known to increase the production of uric acid and its urinary excretion. Fructose may also increase insulin resistance, which is associated with low urine pH. Fructose intake has been positively associated with the risk of incident kidney stones (Taylor, 2008). Increased fruit and vegetable consumption is recommended to increase potassium intake, but because of the fructose content of fruit, there should be even more emphasis on vegetables (Asselman and Verkoelen, 2008).

Vitamins. Health benefits from 500 mg of ascorbic acid or more are not substantiated. Thus individuals at risk for calcium oxalate stones are wise to not exceed 500 mg/day (Massey et al., 2005; Moyad et al., 2009). Vitamin B_6 in the form of pyridoxal phosphate is a required cofactor in oxalate metabolism; marginal B_6 status should be avoided. Using 2 to 10 mg/day of vitamin B_6 may reduce urinary oxalate in some calcium oxalate stone formers.

TABLE 36-5

Some Causes of Acute Kidney Injury

Causes	Condition
1. Prerenal inadequate renal perfusion	Severe dehydration Circulatory collapse
2. Intrinsic diseases within the renal parenchyma	Acute tubular necrosis • trauma, surgery • septicemia Ischemic acute tubular necrosis Nephrotoxicity • antibiotics, contrast agents, and other drugs Local reaction to drugs Vascular disorders • bilateral renal infarction Acute glomerulonephritis of any cause • poststreptococcal infection • systemic lupus erythematosus
3. Postrenal urinary tract obstruction	Benign prostatic hypertrophy with urinary retention Carcinoma of the bladder or prostate Retroperitoneal or pelvic cancer Bilateral ureteral stones and obstruction Rhabdomyolysis

ACUTE KIDNEY INJURY (ACUTE RENAL FAILURE)

Pathophysiology

Acute kidney injury (AKI), formerly **acute renal failure (ARF)**, is characterized by a sudden reduction in **glomerular filtration rate (GFR)**, the amount of filtrate per unit in the nephrons, and altered ability of the kidney to excrete the daily production of metabolic waste. AKI can occur in association with oliguria (decreased output of urine) or normal urine flow, but it typically occurs in previously healthy kidneys. Duration varies from a few days to several weeks. The causes of AKI are numerous, and can occur simultaneously (Table 36-5). These causes are generally classified into three categories: (1) Inadequate renal perfusion (prerenal), (2) diseases within the renal parenchyma (intrinsic), and (3) urinary tract obstruction (postrenal).

Medical Management

The ratio of blood urea nitrogen (BUN) to Cr can be used diagnostically to assess the location of damage to the kidney. Depending on where the insult occurs, BUN is increased because of poor filtration, and is more actively reabsorbed. In this situation, with a BUN/Cr ratio greater than 20:1, damage is prerenal (before the kidney). When damage is intrinsic (within the kidney), the BUN/Cr ratio decreases to less than 10:1. Generally, if careful attention is directed at diagnosing and correcting the prerenal or obstructive causes, AKI is short lived and requires no particular nutritional intervention.

Intrinsic AKI can result from causes listed in Table 36-5; of these, a prolonged episode of ischemia leading to ischemic acute tubular necrosis is the most devastating. Typically patients develop this illness as a complication of an overwhelming infection, severe trauma, surgical accident, or cardiogenic shock. The clinical course and outcome depends mainly on the underlying cause. Patients with AKI caused by drug toxicity generally recover fully after they stop taking the drug. On the other hand, the mortality rate associated with ischemic acute tubular necrosis caused by shock is approximately 70%. Typically these patients are highly catabolic, and extensive tissue destruction occurs in the early stages. Hemodialysis (HD) is used to reduce the acidosis, correct the uremia, and control hyperkalemia.

If recovery is to occur, it generally takes place within 2 to 3 weeks after the insult is corrected. The recovery (diuretic) phase is characterized first by an increase in urine output and later by a return of waste elimination. During this period dialysis may still be required, and careful attention must be paid to fluid and electrolyte balance and appropriate replacement.

Medical Nutrition Therapy

Nutritional care in AKI is particularly important because the patient not only has uremia, metabolic acidosis, and fluid and electrolyte imbalance, but also usually suffers from physiologic stress (e.g., infection or tissue destruction) that increases protein needs. The problem of balancing protein and energy needs with treatment of acidosis and excessive nitrogenous waste is complicated and delicate. In the early stages of AKI the patient is often unable to eat. Mortality in AKI is high, especially among those who are malnourished (Strejc, 2005). Early attention to nutritional support and early dialysis improves patient survival.

At the onset of AKI, depending on severity, some patients can be treated with medical management, other patients require **renal replacement therapy (RRT)** with standard HD or peritoneal dialysis (PD) to remove wastes and fluids until kidney function returns. In significant AKI, a patient in the intensive care unit (ICU) may require continuous treatments, rather than periodic dialysis. **Continuous renal replacement therapy (CRRT)** is the broad category term that includes a whole host of modalities. Most often used are **continuous venovenous hemofiltration (CVVH)** and **continuous venovenous hemodialysis (CVVHD)**, which use a small ultrafiltration membrane to produce an ultrafiltrate that can be replaced by parenteral nutrition (PN) fluids. This treatment allows parenteral feeding without fluid overload. Less often used are continuous arteriovenous hemofiltration, continuous arteriovenous hemodialysis, and continuous venovenous hemodiafiltration. These modalities differ in the type of blood access used, as well as type of filtration (diffuse versus convective, or both).

Protein. The amount of protein recommended is influenced by the underlying cause of AKI and the presence of other conditions. A range of recommended levels can be found in the literature, from 0.5-0.8 g/kg for nondialysis patients to 1-2 g/kg for dialyzed patients. With CRRT protein losses are high, and estimated protein needs increase to 1.5-2.5 g/kg. As the patient's overall medical status stabilizes and improves, metabolic requirements decrease. During this stable period before renal function returns, a minimum protein intake of 0.8-1 g/kg of body weight should be given. This remains dependent on the patient's overall status and comorbidities and should be evaluated individually.

Energy. Energy requirements are determined by the underlying cause of AKI and comorbidity. Energy needs can be measured at the bedside by indirect calorimetry in most ICUs (see Chapter 2). If this equipment is not available, calorie needs should be estimated at 30 to 40 kcal/kg of dry body weight per day. Excessive calorie intake can lead to excess CO_2 production, depressing respiration (see Chapter 35). If PD or CRRT with a glucose containing solution is used, the amount of glucose absorbed can add significantly to the daily energy intake and should be calculated. Large intakes of carbohydrate and fat are needed to prevent the use of protein for energy production. For patients who receive PN, high concentrations of both carbohydrate and lipid can be administered to fulfill these needs as long as respiratory status is monitored.

A high-calorie, low-protein diet may be used in cases in which dialysis or hemofiltration is unavailable. In addition to the usual dietary sources of refined sweets and fats, special high-calorie, low-protein, and low-electrolyte formulas have been developed to augment the diet. However, care must be taken with these products because hyperglycemia is not uncommon as a result of glucose intolerance, and additional insulin is often needed

Fluid and Sodium. During the early (often oliguric) phase of AKI, meticulous attention to fluid status is essential. Ideally fluid and electrolyte intake should balance the net output. With negligible urine output, significant contributions to total body water output include emesis and diarrhea, body cavity drains, and skin and respiratory losses. If fever is present, skin losses can be excessive; whereas if the patient is on humidified air, almost no losses occur. Because of the numerous IV drugs, blood, and blood products necessitated by the underlying disease, the challenge in managing patients at this point becomes how to cut fluid intake as much as possible while providing adequate protein and energy.

Sodium is restricted, based on decreased urinary production. In the oliguric phase when the sodium output is very low, intake should be low as well, perhaps as low as 20 to 40 mg/day. However, limiting sodium is often impossible because of the requirement for many IV solutions (including IV antibiotics, medications for blood pressure, and PN). The administration of these solutions in electrolyte-free water in the face of oliguria quickly leads to water intoxication (hyponatremia). For this reason, all fluid above the daily calculated water loss should be given in a balanced salt solution.

Potassium. Most of the excretion of potassium and the control of potassium balance are normal functions of the kidney. When renal function is impaired, potassium balance should be scrutinized carefully. In addition to dietary sources, all body tissues contain large amounts of potassium; thus tissue destruction can lead to tremendous potassium overload. Potassium levels can shift abruptly and need to be monitored frequently. Potassium intake needs to be

TABLE 36-6

Summary of Medical Nutrition Therapy for Acute Kidney Injury

Nutrient	Amount
Protein	0.8-1 g/kg IBW increasing as GFR returns to normal; 60% should be HBV protein
Energy	30-40 kcal/kg of body weight
Potassium	30-50 mEq/day in oliguric phase (depending on urinary output, dialysis, and serum K^+ level); replace losses in diuretic phase
Sodium	20-40 mEq/day in oliguric phase (depending on urinary output, edema, dialysis, and serum Na^+ level); replace losses in diuretic phase
Fluid	Replace output from the previous day (vomitus, diarrhea, urine) plus 500 mL
Phosphorus	Limit as necessary

GFR, Glomerular filtration rate; *HBV*, high biologic value; *IBW*, ideal body weight; *K^+*, potassium; *Na^+*, sodium.

individualized according to serum levels (see Appendices 36 and 56). The primary mechanism of potassium removal during AKI is dialysis. Control of serum potassium levels between dialysis administrations rely mainly on IV infusions of glucose, insulin, and bicarbonate, all of which serve to drive potassium into cells. Exchange resins such as sodium polystyrene sulfonate (Kayexalate), which exchange potassium for sodium in the GI tract, can be used to treat high potassium concentrations, but for many reasons these resins are less than ideal. Table 36-6 summarizes MNT for AKI.

CHRONIC KIDNEY DISEASE

A wide range of kidney lesions are characterized by a slow, steady decline in renal function. A number of the diseases discussed earlier lead to renal failure in some patients, whereas other patients have a benign course without loss of renal function. It is unclear why some patients remain stable with **chronic kidney disease (CKD)** for many months to years while others progress rapidly to renal failure and dialysis. The nature of this progressive loss of function has been the subject of an enormous amount of basic and clinical research during the past several decades and the subject of several excellent reviews (Remuzzi et al., 2006; Wenjun et al., 2009).

Pathophysiology

Once approximately one half to two thirds of kidney function has been lost, regardless of the underlying disease, progressive further loss of kidney function ensues. This is true even in diseases in which the underlying cause has been eliminated completely, such as in vesicoureteral reflux, cortical necrosis of pregnancy, or analgesic abuse. It is thought that, in response to a decreasing GFR, the kidney undergoes a series of adaptations to prevent this decline. Although in the short term this leads to improvement in filtration rate, in the long term it leads to an accelerated loss of nephrons and progressive renal insufficiency (Remuzzi et al., 2006). The nature of these adaptations involves a change in the hemodynamic characteristics of the remaining glomeruli, specifically leading to increased glomerular pressure. Factors that increase glomerular pressure tend to accelerate this process, whereas factors that decrease glomerular pressure tend to alleviate it.

Diabetes is the leading risk factor for CKD followed by hypertension. The National Kidney Foundation (NKF) divides CKD into five stages related to the estimated GFR (eGFR) (Table 36-7). Stages 1 and 2 are early stages with markers like proteinuria, hematuria, or anatomic issues. Stages 3 and 4 are considered advanced stages. Stage 5 results in death unless dialysis or transplantation is initiated.

Medical Management

The prevalence of CKD is now estimated at approximately one in nine adults in the United States, or 20 million Americans. This estimated prevalence of CKD is 11% of the population. Many states now urge clinical laboratories reporting serum Cr to also report the patient's eGFR, the rate at which the kidneys are filtering wastes. The formula, which takes into account the patient's sex, age, race, and Cr, is more accurate than the older Cockcroff-Gault formula sometimes used to calculate Cr clearance (Rigalleau et al., 2006). Patients having their eGFR calculated who have a low number do not necessarily have CKD. They must have repeated values over 3 months apart that are consistently low.

An online eGFR calculator can be found at the NKF site at http://www.kidney.org/professionals/kdoqi/gfr_calculator.cfm. With screening tools like the calculated eGFR and a greater awareness of the progressive nature of CKD, more attention has focused on its social, medical, and financial effects. For example, CKD is strongly linked with cardiovascular disease; see *Clinical Insight:* Chronic Kidney Disease and Heart Disease—A Deadly Union.

Medical Nutrition Therapy

With each level of CKD, a different nutritional therapy may be proposed. The primary objectives of MNT are to manage the symptoms associated with the syndrome (edema, hypoalbuminemia, and hyperlipidemia), decrease the risk of progression to renal failure, and maintain nutritional stores. Patients are primarily treated with statins to correct hyperlipidemia, low-sodium diets, and diuretics (Appel, 2006).

TABLE 36-7

Stages of Chronic Kidney Disease

Stage	eGFR	Description
1	90-130 mL/min	Kidney damage, but normal to increased kidney function
2	60-89 mL/min	Mild decrease in kidney function
3	30-59 mL/min	Moderate decrease in kidney function
4	15-29 mL/min	Severe decrease in kidney function
5	Less than 15 mL/min	Kidney failure with treatment necessary, defined as end-stage renal disease

eGFR, Estimated glomerular filtration rate.

CLINICAL INSIGHT

Chronic Kidney Disease and Heart Disease—A Deadly Union

The presence of chronic kidney disease (CKD) increases the risk category for those with coronary vascular disease (CVD), and exacerbates existing CVD. An alarming fact is that most patients with CKD die from heart disease before they develop end-stage renal disease. Recommendations are that CKD patients should decrease their cardiovascular risks: quit smoking, increase exercise, limit intake of fat, and reach and maintain a normal body weight.

Fortunately, intervention makes a difference. The United States Renal Data System Dialysis *M/M* Study included 2,264 patients with CKD. More than half had not seen a nephrologist in the year prior to needing dialysis, and a third had their first nephrologist encounter less than 4 months prior to starting dialysis. This late referral to nephrologists resulted in low serum albumin and hematocrit levels. Patients who had seen a nephrologist at least 2 years before dialysis had a decrease in mortality. Thus patients who have CKD and receive early nutrition counseling may postpone the need for dialysis, or come to dialysis better nourished. The expertise of the renal dietitian has been recognized by the Center for Medicare Services, allowing for physician-ordered medical nutrition therapy by registered dietitian providers for Americans with CKD who are not on dialysis.

Patients with an established severe protein deficiency who continue to lose protein may require an extended time of carefully supervised nutritional care. The diet should attempt to provide sufficient protein and energy to maintain a positive nitrogen balance and to produce an increase in plasma albumin concentration and disappearance of edema. In most cases, sufficient intake from carbohydrate and fats are needed to spare protein for anabolism.

Some of the more common nutrition diagnoses in the CKD population include:

- Inadequate mineral intake
- Excessive mineral intake
- Imbalance of nutrients
- Excessive fluid intake
- Impaired nutrient utilization
- Altered nutrition-related laboratory values
- Food-medication interaction
- Food- and nutrition-related knowledge deficit

Depending on the nutrition diagnosis, MNT interventions are adjusted for various intakes of minerals, protein, and fluids.

Protein. The recommended dietary protein level for CKD patients has changed over time. Historically, these patients received diets high in protein (up to 1.5 g/kg/day) in an attempt to increase serum albumin and prevent protein malnutrition. However, studies have shown that a reduction of protein intake to as low as 0.8 mg/kg/day may decrease proteinuria without adversely affecting serum albumin. Dietary protein has been championed as a factor that increases glomerular pressure and thus leads to accelerated loss of renal function. Numerous studies in experimental models of moderate renal insufficiency demonstrate a significant decline in this process with protein restriction. Clinical studies demonstrate a role for protein restriction in the management of patients with mild to moderate renal insufficiency to preserve renal function. To allow for optimal protein use, 50% to 60% of the protein should be from sources of high biologic value (HBV). The description for HBV protein has been expanded to include proteins with a high **protein digestibility corrected amino acid score (PDCAAS)** (see Chapter 3).

A large multicenter trial, Modification of Diet in Renal Disease, attempted to determine the role of protein, phosphorus restriction, and blood pressure control in the progression of renal disease. Thus the National Institute of Diabetes and Digestive and Kidney Diseases (NIDDKD) developed recommendations for the management of patients with progressive renal disease or pre-ESRD. Those recommendations for dietary protein intake in progressive renal failure are 0.8 g/kg/day with 60% HBV for patients whose GFR is greater than 55 mL/min, and 0.6 g/kg/day with 60% HBV for patients whose GFR is 25 to 55 mL/min.

The NKF's **Kidney Dialysis Outcome Quality Initiative (KDOQI)** panel suggests that patients whose GFR is less than 25 mL/min and who have not yet begun dialysis should be maintained on 0.6 g/kg/day of protein and 35 kcal/kg/day. If patients cannot maintain an adequate caloric intake on this protein recommendation, their protein intake should be increased to 0.75 g/kg/day. In both cases approximately 50% of the protein should be of HBV.

The potential benefits of protein restriction in the patient with moderate renal insufficiency must be weighed against the potential hazards of such treatment (i.e., protein malnutrition). If protein is restricted, careful monitoring and anthropometric studies should be carried out periodically as directed by the KDOQI guidelines.

Systemic hypertension, which aggravates the progressive loss of renal function, must be well controlled to produce benefits from protein restriction. Also important in the control of the progression of renal failure in people with diabetes is good blood glucose control. In a national multicenter trial, the Diabetes Control and Complications Trial showed that blood glucose control was more important than protein restriction in delaying the onset of renal failure in individuals who have diabetes (see Chapter 31).

Energy. Energy intake should be approximately 35 kcal/kg/day for adults to spare protein for tissue repair and maintenance.

Sodium. Edema, the most clinically apparent manifestation, indicates total body sodium overload. Additionally, because of low oncotic pressure from hypoalbuminemia, the volume of circulating blood may be reduced. Attempts to severely limit sodium intake or to use diuretics constantly may cause marked hypotension, exacerbation of coagulopathy, and deterioration of renal function. Therefore control of edema in this group of diseases should be with dietary intake of 2-3 g of sodium daily. The use of elastic full-length support hose may also be beneficial.

Potassium. Variability in disease states, individual intakes, and use of medications that may decrease potassium, such as diuretics, make potassium management possible. Many patients in early stage CKD take potassium-wasting diuretics and require supplementation. When urine output drops below 1 L/day, these same patients may require a potassium restriction as the kidney is no longer able to excrete all potassium ingested. This typically occurs rather late in stage 4 CKD.

Phosphorus. The importance of controlling phosphate in patients with early stage disease is often overlooked. Serum phosphorous levels elevate at the same rate as eGFR decreases. Early initiation of phosphate reduction therapies is advantageous for delaying hyperparathyroidism and bone disease. Unfortunately, patients are often asymptomatic during the early phase of hyperparathyroidism and hyperphosphatemia; they may not attend to their modified diets or understand the need to take phosphate binders with meals.

Those with an eGFR of less than 60 should be evaluated for renal bone disease, and benefit from phosphorus restriction. Ongoing monitoring of patient's phosphorus and use of **phosphate binders** is recommended. The diet is typically modified to allow no more than 1000 mg of phosphates daily, a limit that allows approximately 1-2 dairy foods per day. Because of the decrease in protein intake, the control of phosphorus is somewhat easier to manage. Patients who are in later stages of CKD, and intolerant of red meats because of uremic taste alterations, are often able to substitute milk foods for meat and still maintain a limited phosphate intake.

Lipids. The important consequence of dyslipidemia is cardiovascular disease. Pediatric patients with frequently relapsing or resistant nephrotic syndrome are at particular risk for premature atherosclerosis. Certain lipid-lowering agents in combination with a cholesterol-lowering diet can reduce total cholesterol, low-density lipoprotein cholesterol, and triglycerides in these patients (see Chapter 34). Lowering protein intake in adult patients may also lower fat and cholesterol intake from animal sources.

Vitamins. CKD patients are routinely recommended a water-soluble renal customized vitamin supplement, because restrictions may cause the diet to be inadequate.

DISEASES OF THE TUBULES AND INTERSTITIUM

To a great extent, the functions of the kidney tubules make them susceptible to injury. The enormous energy requirements and expenditures of the tubules for active secretion and reabsorption often leave this part of the kidney particularly vulnerable to ischemic injuries. Many toxic drugs can destroy or damage various segments of the tubules. The high-solute concentration generated in the medullary interstitium exposes it to damage from oxidants and precipitation of calcium-phosphate product (extraosseous calcification) and favors the sickling of red blood cells in sickle cell anemia. Indeed, a wide variety of diseases or disorders of the tubules and interstitium exist. They share common manifestations and can be considered together with respect to nutritional management.

Chronic interstitial nephritis can occur as a result of analgesic abuse, sickle cell disease, diabetes mellitus, or vesicoureteral reflux, and manifests primarily as inability to concentrate the urine and as mild renal insufficiency. A hereditary disorder of the interstitium, *medullary cystic disease*, also presents with this picture. Dietary management consists of adequate fluid intake, which can require several liters of extra fluid. This is generally quite well tolerated by the patient, except when intercurrent illness occurs.

Fanconi syndrome is characterized by an inability to reabsorb the proper amount of glucose, amino acids, phosphate, and bicarbonate in the proximal tubule, thus causing urinary excretion of these substances. Adults with this syndrome present with acidosis, hypokalemia, polyuria, or osteomalacia, whereas children present with polyuria, growth retardation, rickets, and vomiting. No specific medical treatment is available to treat Fanconi syndrome; therefore dietary treatment is the main form of management. Replacement therapy usually consists of large volumes of water and dietary supplements of bicarbonate, potassium, phosphate, calcium, and vitamin D.

Renal tubular acidosis (RTA), a defect in tubular handling of bicarbonate, can be caused by either a defect in the distal tubule (type 1) or a proximal tubular defect (type 2). Distal RTA leads to severe osteomalacia, kidney stones, or even nephrocalcinosis (calcification of the kidney). Distal RTA is treated with small amounts of bicarbonate, 70 to 100 mEq/day, with complete resolution of disease manifestations. Isolated proximal RTA in the adult is a benign disease, which is often made worse with bicarbonate and therefore should not be treated.

Pyelonephritis, a bacterial infection of the kidney, does not require extensive dietary management. However, in chronic cases the use of cranberry juice to reduce bacteriuria is useful (Kontiokari et al., 2005; Jepson, 2008). Concentrated tannins or proanthocyanidins in cranberry juice and blueberry juice may inhibit the adherence of *Escherichia coli* bacteria to the epithelial cells of the urinary tract.

GLOMERULAR DISEASES

The functions of the glomerulus that are important with respect to disease are production of an adequate ultrafiltrate and prevention of certain substances from entering this ultrafiltrate.

Nephritic Syndrome

Pathophysiology

Nephritic syndrome incorporates a group of diseases characterized by inflammation of the capillary loops of the glomerulus. These **acute glomerulonephritides** are sudden in onset, brief, and may proceed to complete recovery, development of chronic nephrotic syndrome, or ESRD. The primary manifestation of these diseases is hematuria (blood in the urine), a consequence of the capillary inflammation that damages the glomerular barrier to blood cells. The syndrome is also characterized by hypertension and mild loss of renal function. The most common presentation follows a streptococcal infection and is usually, although not always, self-limiting. Other causes include primary kidney diseases such as immunoglobulin A nephropathy (IgA); hereditary nephritis; and secondary diseases such as systemic lupus erythematosus (SLE), vasculitis, and glomerulonephritis (GN) associated with endocarditis, abscesses, or infected ventriculoperitoneal shunts.

Nephrotic Syndrome

Pathophysiology

Nephrotic syndrome comprises a group of diseases that derive from a loss of the glomerular barrier for protein. Large urinary protein losses lead to hypoalbuminemia with consequent edema, hypercholesterolemia, hypercoagulability, and abnormal bone metabolism. More than 95% of the cases of nephrotic syndrome stem from three systemic diseases: (1) diabetes mellitus, (2) SLE, and (3) amyloidosis; and from four diseases that are primarily of the kidney: (1) minimum change disease (seen only with electron microscopy), (2) membranous nephropathy, (3) focal glomerulosclerosis, and (4) membranoproliferative glomerulonephritis. Although renal function can deteriorate during the course of these diseases, it is not a consistent feature.

END-STAGE RENAL DISEASE

End-stage renal disease (ESRD) reflects the kidney's inability to excrete waste products, maintain fluid and electrolyte balance, and produce hormones. As renal failure slowly progresses, the level of circulating waste products eventually leads to symptoms of uremia (see *Pathophysiology and Care Management Algorithm:* Chronic Kidney Disease and End-Stage Renal Disease). **Uremia** is a clinical syndrome of malaise, weakness, nausea and vomiting, muscle cramps, itching, metallic taste in the mouth, and neurologic impairment that is brought about by an unacceptable level of nitrogenous wastes in the body.

Pathophysiology

ESRD can result from a wide variety of different kidney diseases. Currently 90% of patients reaching ESRD have chronic (1) diabetes mellitus, (2) hypertension, or (3) glomerulonephritis. The manifestations are somewhat nonspecific and vary by patient. No reliable laboratory parameter corresponds directly with the beginning of symptoms. However, as a rule of thumb, BUN of more than 100 mg/dL and Cr of 10 to 12 mg/dL are usually quite close to this threshold.

Medical Treatment

Once the patient progresses from stage 4 to stage 5 CKD, options for treatment for ESRD include dialysis, transplantation, or medical management progressing to death. Patients do best if they have some control and choice over their options.

Dialysis

Patients may choose to dialyze in an outpatient dialysis facility or they may prefer HD at home using either conventional daily or nocturnal dialysis. They may choose PD and have a choice of continuous ambulatory peritoneal dialysis (CAPD) or continuous cyclic peritoneal dialysis (CCPD),

PATHOPHYSIOLOGY AND CARE MANAGEMENT ALGORITHM

Chronic Kidney Disease and End-Stage Renal Disease

ETIOLOGY

Hypertension

Glomerulonephritis

Diabetes mellitus

Other Disorders (i.e., polycystic kidney disease, congenital anomalies, etc.)

CKD Chronic Kidney Disease

CKD Medical Management

- Blood pressure control
- Blood sugar control
- Immunosuppressant therapy
- Erythropoietin
- Active vitamin D

CKD Nutrition Management

- Sodium restriction
- Possible protein restriction
- Monitor etectrolytes and acid base balance
- Phosphate binders
- Decrease cardiac risk factors

PATHOPHYSIOLOGY

End-Stage Renal Disease (renal failure)

Inability to

- Excrete waste products
- Maintain fluid and electroyte balance
- Produce hormones

Uremia

Unacceptable level of nitrogenous wastes

Symptoms

- Malaise
- Weakness
- Nausea and vomiting
- Muscle cramps and itching
- Metallic taste in mouth
- Neurologic impairment

MANAGEMENT

ESRD Medical Management

- Dialysis
- Kidney transplantation
- Immunosuppressant therapy
- Psychologic support
- Conservative treatment and preparation for death
- Erythropoietin
- Active vitamin D

ESRD Nutrition Management

Goals

- Prevent nutrient deficiencies
- Control edema and serum electrolytes
  - Sodium and potassium restriction
- Prevent renal osteodystrophy
  - Use of phosphate binders, low phosphorus diet, and calcium supplementation
- Provide a palatable and attractive diet

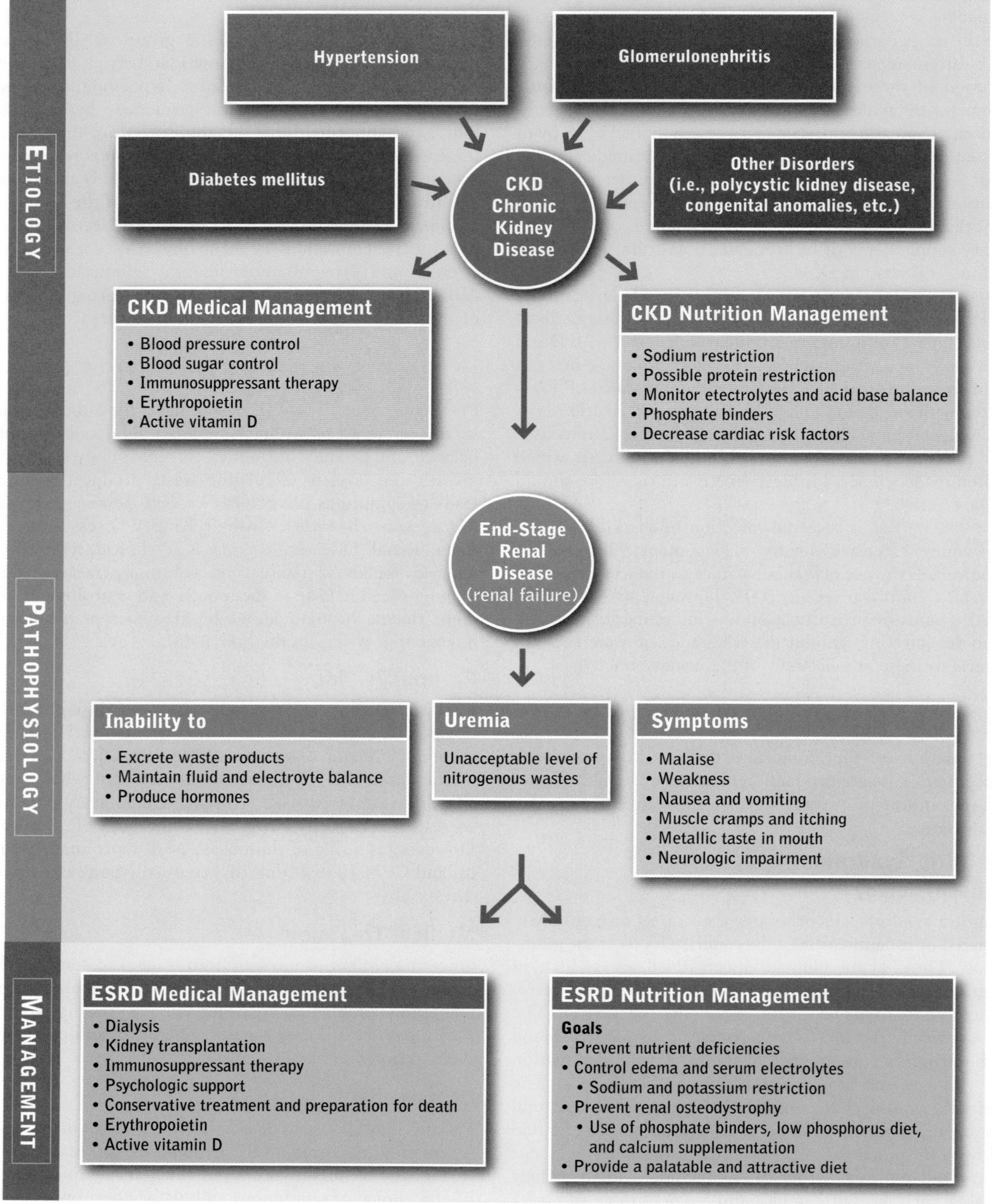

or combinations of the two. Patients, families, and their physicians together evaluate the therapy that best meets the patient's needs. Factors that come into account in this decision are availability of family or friends to assist with therapy, type of water supply to the home, capability of the patient or involved family (including eyesight and ability to perform sterile technique), previous abdominal surgeries, membrane characteristics of the individual's peritoneal membrane, body size, cardiac status, presence of poor vascular access, desire to travel, and a host of other considerations.

HD requires permanent access to the bloodstream through a **fistula** created by surgery to connect an artery and a vein (Figure 36-2). If the patient's blood vessels are fragile, an artificial vessel called a *graft* may be surgically implanted. Large needles are inserted into the fistula or graft before

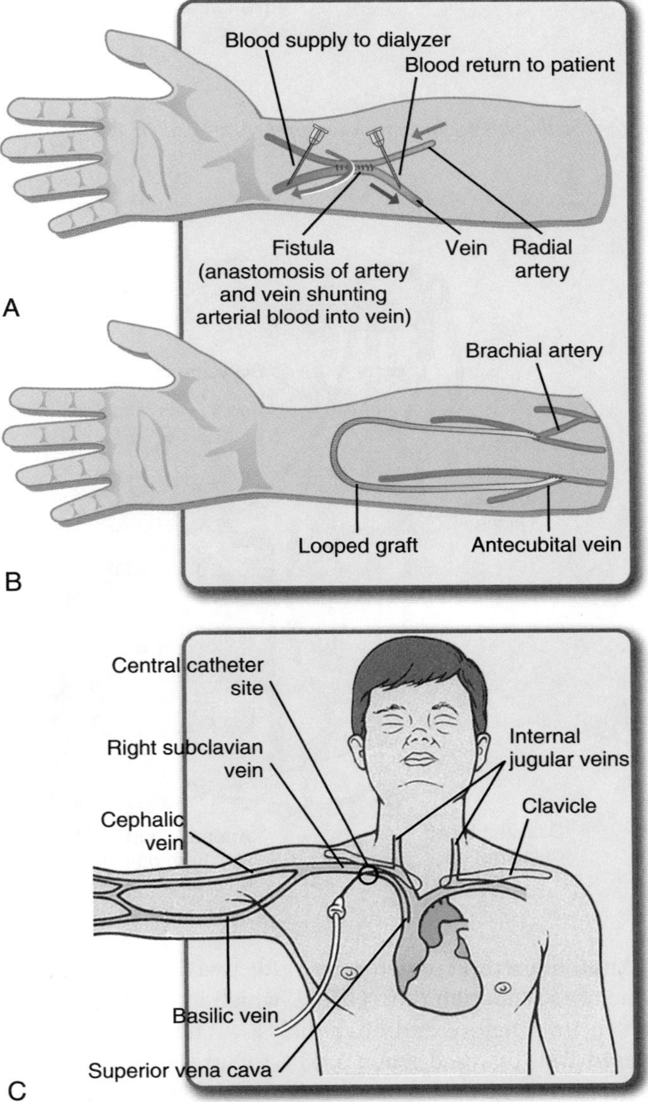

FIGURE 36-2 Types of access for hemodialysis. **A,** Arteriovenous fistula. **B,** Artificial loop graft. **C,** Subclavian catheter (usually temporary). *(From Lewis SL et al: Medical-surgical nursing: assessment and management of clinical problems, ed 7, St Louis, 2007, Mosby.)*

each dialysis and removed when dialysis is complete. Temporary access through subclavian catheters is common until the patient's permanent access can be created or can mature; however, problems with infection make these catheters undesirable.

The **hemodialysis (HD)** fluid and electrolyte content is similar to that of normal plasma. Waste products and electrolytes move by diffusion, ultrafiltration, and osmosis from the blood into the dialysate and are removed (Figure 36-3) (Himmelfarb and Ikizler, 2010). Outpatient HD usually requires treatment of 3 to 5 hours three times per week in a dialysis unit (Figure 36-4). Newer therapies can shorten the duration of treatment by increasing its frequency. Patients on these more frequent dialysis therapies have lower mortality rates, approaching that of transplantation. Patients on daily dialysis at home typically have treatments lasting from 2 to 3.5 hours 5 to 6 days a week, whereas some home dialysis patients receive nocturnal dialysis 3 to 6 times a week for 8 hours, while they sleep.

Peritoneal dialysis (PD) makes use of the body's own semipermeable membrane, the peritoneum. A catheter is surgically implanted in the abdomen and into the peritoneal cavity. **Dialysate** containing a high-dextrose concentration is instilled into the peritoneum, where diffusion carries waste products from the blood through the peritoneal membrane and into the dialysate; water moves by osmosis. This fluid is then withdrawn and discarded, and new solution is added.

Several types of PD exist. In CAPD, the dialysate is left in the peritoneum and exchanged manually, by gravity. Exchanges of dialysis fluid are done four to five times daily, making it a 24-hour treatment (Figure 36-5). In CCPD, patient treatments are done at night by a machine that does the exchanges. During the day these patients may keep a single dialysate exchange in the peritoneal cavity for extended periods (called a *long dwell*), perhaps the entire day. Several combinations of CAPD and CCPD are possible and are referred to here as *PD*.

Advantages of PD are avoidance of large fluctuations in blood chemistry, longer residual renal function, and the ability of the patient to achieve a more normal lifestyle. Complications include peritonitis, hypotension that requires fluid and sodium replacement, and weight gain. Tissue weight gain is experienced by most patients as a result of absorbing 400 to 800 calories per day from the glucose in the dialysate. This may be desirable in patients who are underweight, but eventually dietary intake or activity have to be modified to account for the energy absorbed from dialysate. Icodextrin (Extraneal, Baxter) is a long-chain, nonabsorbable sugar available for long dwell times. It offers superior fluid removal (ultrafiltration) without excess dextrose absorption. This can be useful for patients with diabetes and those with excessive tissue weight gain, but can cause other complications and is costly.

Evaluation of Dialysis Efficacy

Kinetic modeling is a method for evaluating the efficacy of dialysis that measures the removal of urea from the patient's

Diffusion is the passage of particles through a semipermeable membrane. Tea, for example, diffuses from a tea bag into the surrounding water.

Osmosis is the movement of fluid across a semipermeable membrane from a lower concentration of solutes to a higher concentration of solutes. (The water moves into the teabag.)

Diffusion and Osmosis can occur at the same time. (Particles move out and fluid moves in at the same time.)

Filtration is the passage of fluids through a membrane.

Ultrafiltration provides additional pressure to squeeze extra fluid through the membrane.

FIGURE 36-3 Dialysis: how it works. *(Modified from Core curriculum for the dialysis technician: a comprehensive review of hemodialysis, AMGEN, Inc.)*

FIGURE 36-4 Hemodialysis. Treatment is usually for 3 to 5 hours, three times per week.

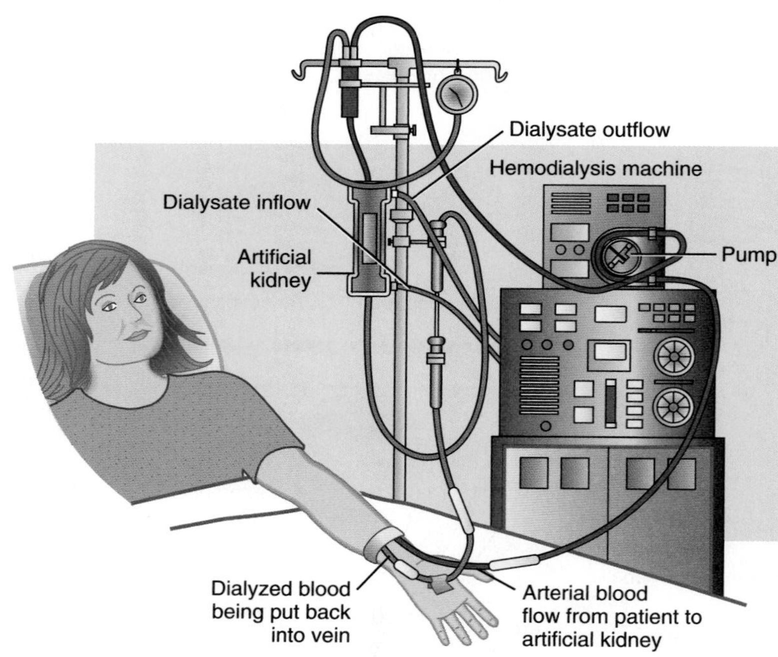

blood over a given period. This formula, often called **Kt/V** (where *K* is the urea clearance of the dialyzer, *t* is the length of time of dialysis, and *V* is the patient's total body water volume), should ideally produce a result higher than 1.4 per HD, or 3.2 per week. These calculations are somewhat complex and are typically calculated using a computer program. A more accurate method for determining adequacy of HD is the eKt/V where *e* stands for *equilibrated* and takes into account the amount of time it takes for urea to equilibrate across cell membranes after dialysis has stopped. An acceptable eKt/V is 1.2 or greater.

Another method to determine effective dialysis treatment is the **urea reduction ratio (URR)**, which looks at the reduction in urea before and after dialysis. The patient is considered well dialyzed when a 65% or greater reduction in the serum urea occurs during dialysis. Unlike Kt/V, this calculation can be done quickly at the patient's bedside by the practitioner. The method for calculating the efficacy of PD is somewhat different, but a weekly Kt/V of 2 is the goal. The Kt/V can be altered by several patient- and dialysis-associated variables. The calculations for Kt/V can also be used to determine the patient's **protein-nitrogen**

appearance (PNA) rate, which is a simplified nitrogen balance test in the dialysis patient. The PNA values should be between 0.8 and 1.4. Patients on short daily HD and nocturnal HD require different calculations to estimate their Kt/V.

Medical Nutrition Therapy

Goals of medical nutrition therapy in the management of ESRD are intended to:

1. Prevent deficiency and maintain good nutrition status (and, in the case of children, growth) through adequate protein, energy, vitamin, and mineral intake (Table 36-8).
2. Control edema and electrolyte imbalance by controlling sodium, potassium, and fluid intake.
3. Prevent or retard the development of renal osteodystrophy by controlling calcium, phosphorus, vitamin D, and PTH.
4. Enable the patient to eat a palatable, attractive diet that fits his or her lifestyle as much as possible.
5. Coordinate patient care with families, dietitians, nurses, and physicians in acute care, outpatient, or skilled nursing facilities.
6. Provide initial nutrition education, periodic counseling and long-term monitoring of patients.

Table 36-9 presents a guide for teaching patients about their blood values and control of their disease. Because dialysis is done at home or in an outpatient unit, all most all patients with ESRD assume responsibility for their own diets. Most long-term patients know their diets very well (Figure 36-6), having been instructed many times by renal dietitians at their dialysis units.

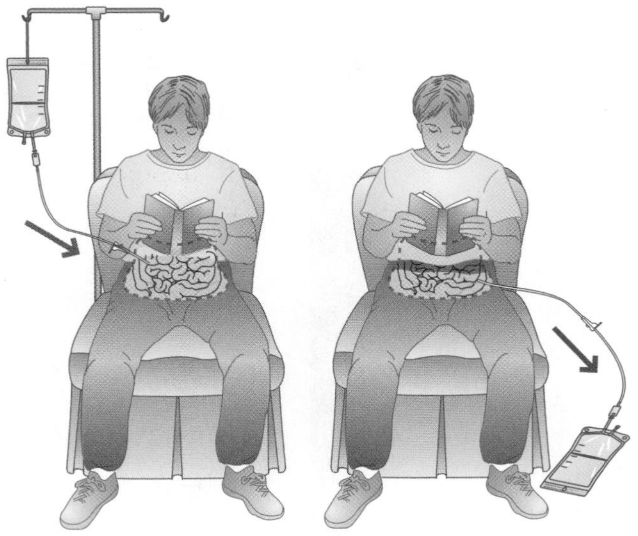

FIGURE 36-5 Continuous ambulatory peritoneal dialysis; 20-minute exchanges are given four to five times daily every day.

Protein

Dialysis is a drain on body protein, so protein intake must be increased accordingly. Protein losses of 20 to

Text continued on p. 822

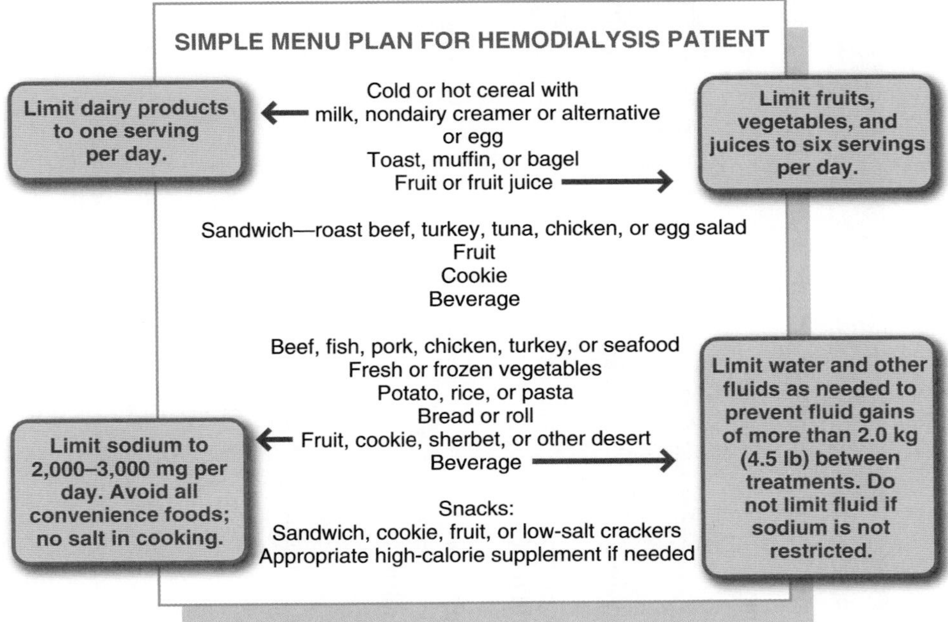

FIGURE 36-6 A simple menu plan for a patient on hemodialysis. The diet should allow for less than 4% fluid weight gain between dialyses.

TABLE 36-8

Nutrient Requirements of Adults with Renal Disease Based on Type of Therapy

Therapy	Energy	Protein	Fluid	Sodium	Potassium	Phosphorus
Impaired renal function	30-35 kcal/kg IBW	0.6-1.0 g/kg IBW	*Ad libitum*	Variable, 2-3 g/day	Variable, usually *ad libitum* or increased to cover losses with diuretics	0.8-1.2 g/day or 8-12 mg/kg IBW
Hemodialysis	35 kcal/kg IBW	1.2 g/kg IBW	750-1000 mL/day urine output	2-3 g/day	2-3 g/day or 40 mg/kg IBW	0.8-1.2 g/day or <17 mg/kg IBW
Peritoneal dialysis (CAPD)(CCPD)	30-35 kcal/kg IBW	1.2-1.5 g/kg BW	*Ad libitum* (minimum of 2000 mL/day urine output)	2-4 g/day	3-4 g/day	0.8-1.2 g/day
Transplant, 4-6 weeks after transplant	30-35 kcal/kg IBW	1.3-2 g/kg IBW	*Ad libitum*	2-3 g/day	Variable; may require restriction with cyclosporine-induced hyperkalemia	Calcium 1.2 g/day No need to limit phosphorus
6 weeks or longer after transplant	To achieve/maintain IBW: • Limit simple CHO • Fat < 35%/cals • Cholesterol < 400 mg/day • PUFA/SFA ratio > 1	1 g/kg BW	*Ad libitum*	2-3 g/day	Variable	Calcium 1.2 g/day No need to limit phosphorus

Modified from National Kidney Foundation: DOQI clinical practice guidelines for nutrition in chronic renal failure, Am J Kidney Dis 35(suppl 2), 2000; Wiggins K: Guidelines for nutrition care of renal patients, ed 3, Chicago, 2002, American Dietetic Association.

CAPD, Continuous ambulatory peritoneal dialysis; *CCPD*, continuous cyclical peritoneal dialysis; *IBW*, ideal body weight; *PUFA*, polyunsaturated fat; *SFA*, saturated fat.

TABLE 36-9

Guide to Blood Values in End-Stage Renal Disease Patients

This guide is to help in understanding laboratory reports. In the following table, the normal values are for people with good kidney function. Acceptable values for dialysis patients are also given. Many things affect blood values. Diet is only one of these. Underlying disease, adequacy of treatment, medications, and complications all may affect laboratory values.

Substance	Normal Values	Normal for People on Dialysis	Function	Diet Changes
Sodium	135-145 mEq/L	135-145 mEq/L	Found in salt and many preserved foods. A diet high in sodium causes thirst. When patients drink too much fluid, it may actually dilute their sodium, and serum levels will appear low. If patients eat too much sodium and do not drink water, sodium may be high. Too much sodium and water raise blood pressure and can cause fluid overload, pulmonary edema, and congestive heart failure.	High: Check fluid status. If high fluid gains, tell patient to eat fewer salty foods. If low fluid gains, make sure patient is gaining about 1.5 kg between dialyses (or < 4% body weight) and is not dehydrated (this is rare). Low: If high fluid gains, tell patient to eat less salt and fluid. Check fluid status—patient is probably drinking too much fluid. Limit weight gains to less than 4% of body weight between runs, and ask patient to eat fewer salty foods and limit fluid to 3 C plus urine output.
Potassium	3.5-5.5 mEq/L	3.5-5.5 mEq/L	Found in most high-protein foods, milk, fruits, and vegetables. Affects muscle action, especially the heart. High levels can cause the heart to stop. Low levels can cause symptoms such as muscle weakness and atrial fibrillation.	High: Ascertain that no other causes, such as gastrointestinal bleeding, trauma, or medications are creating high potassium values. Tell patient to avoid foods with more than 250 mg/serving and limit daily intake to 2000 mg. Consider lowering potassium in dialysate bath. Recheck blood level next treatment. Low: Add one high-potassium food/day, and recheck blood level. Consider raising potassium in dialysate bath if diet changes not working.
Urea nitrogen (BUN)	7-23 mg/dL	50-100 mg/dL	Waste product of protein breakdown. Unlike creatinine, this is affected by the amount of protein in the diet. Dialysis removes urea nitrogen.	High: Patient is probably underdialyzed. Check eKt/V. Check nPNA. Low: Underdialysis is also a cause. BUN may decrease if patient not eating because of uremic symptoms. Also decreases with loss of muscle.
Creatinine	0.6-1.5 mg/dL	Less than 15 mg/dL	A normal waste product of muscle breakdown. This value is controlled by dialysis. Patients have a higher amount because they are not dialyzing 24 hours a day, 7 days a week, as they would with normal kidney function.	Dialysis normally controls creatinine. Low creatinine may indicate good dialysis or low body muscle. Check the clearance of urea during dialysis (Kt/V) to assess dialysis adequacy. If patient losing weight, will break down more muscle, so creatinine may be higher. Patient may need to eat more protein and calories to stop weight loss.

Continued

TABLE 36-9

Guide to Blood Values in End-Stage Renal Disease Patients—cont'd

Substance	Normal Values	Normal for People on Dialysis	Function	Diet Changes
URR	N/A	Above 65% (or 0.65)	A measure of reduction of urea that occurs during a dialysis treatment. Postdialysis BUN is subtracted and divided by predialysis BUN to give a percentage.	No diet changes, but catabolism or anabolism will affect values, as with Kt/V and equilibrated clearance of urea during dialysis (eKt/V).
eKt/V	N/A	Above 1.2	A mathematic formula that attempts to quantify how well a patient is dialyzed. Represents the clearance of urea by the dialyzer, multiplied by the minutes of treatment, and divided by the volume of water the patient's body holds.	No diet changes. Low: Values below 1.2 are associated with increased morbidity and mortality. High: Higher values are associated with better outcomes.
Kt/V		Above 1.4 for hemodialysis Above 2 for peritoneal dialysis	Not adjusted for urea equilibration. See above.	No diet changes. See above.
nPNA	N/A	0.8-1.4	A calculation used to look at the rate of protein turnover in the body. Assumes patient is not catabolic because of infection, fever, surgery, or trauma. A good indicator of stable patient's protein intake, when combined with dietary history and albumin. The term *normalized* means that values have been adjusted to the patient's "normal" or ideal weight.	High: Patient may need to decrease protein intake. Have patient consult with nutritionist. Patient may be catabolic. Patient may be eating large amounts of protein. Low: Patient may need to increase protein intake. If patient is putting out urine, a small urine volume can make a big difference in results. Have patient keep a 48-hour urine collection.
Albumin	3.5-5 g/dL (bromcresol green) 3-4.5 g/dL (bromcresol purple)	3.5-5 g/dL Above 3.4 g/dL	Good measure of health in dialysis patients. Protein is lost with all dialysis. If albumin is below 2.9, fluid will "leak" from blood vessels into the tissue, thus causing edema. When fluid is in the tissue, it is more difficult to remove with dialysis. Low albumin is closely associated with increased risk of death in dialysis patients.	Low: Increase intake of protein-rich foods: meat, fish, chicken, eggs. A protein supplement may be needed. Intravenous albumin corrects short-term problems with oncotic pressure but does not change serum albumin levels.
Calcium	8.5-10.5 mg/dL	8.5-10.5 mg/dL	Found in dairy products. Dialysis patients' intakes are usually low. Active vitamin D is needed for absorption. The calcium value multiplied by the phosphorus value should not exceed 59, or patient will get calcium deposits in soft tissue. Because it is bound to albumin, calcium can be falsely lower if albumin is low. Ionized calcium is a more accurate test in this case.	High: Check with doctor if patient is taking calcium supplement or a form of active vitamin D These should be temporarily stopped. Low: If albumin is low, suggest an ionized calcium be drawn. Patient may need a calcium supplement between meals and active vitamin D. Check with physician.

Phosphorus	2.5-4.8 mg/dL	3-6 mg/dL	Found in milk products, dried beans, nuts, and meats. Used to build bones and helps the body produce energy. Acceptable levels depend on variety of factors, including calcium, PTH levels, and the level of phosphorus in diet. If calcium and PTH levels are normal, a slightly higher-than-normal level of phosphorus is acceptable.	High: Limit milk and milk products to 1 serving/day. Remind patient to take phosphate binders as ordered with meals and snacks. Noncompliance with binders is the most common cause of high phosphorus. Low: Add 1 serving milk product or other high-phosphorus food per day or decrease phosphate binders.
PTH intact (I-PTH)	10-65 pg/mL	200-300 pg/mL	A high level of PTH indicates that calcium is being pulled out of bone to maintain serum calcium levels. This syndrome is called secondary hyperparathyroidism. Leads to osteodystrophy. Pulsed doses of oral or IV vitamin D usually lower PTH.	High: Check whether patient taking oral or IV active vitamin D. Contact patient's physician regarding therapy. If patient has no symptoms (high phosphorus, bone pain, fractures), treat less aggressively. Low: No treatment available.
Aluminum	0-10 mcg/L	Less than 40 mcg/L	Patients taking aluminum hydroxide phosphate binders may develop aluminum toxicity, which can cause bone disease and dementia. Value should be checked every 6 months.	High: Discontinue aluminum hydroxide treatment.
Magnesium	1.5-2.4 mg/dL	1.5-2.4 mg/dL	Magnesium is normally excreted in the urine and can become toxic to dialysis patient. High levels may be caused by antacids or laxatives that contain magnesium such as Milk of Magnesia or Maalox.	No dietary changes, except to use nontoxic methods such as fiber to aid in relief of constipation. If magnesium is used as a phosphate binder, levels will need to be checked more often.
Ferritin	Male: 20-350 mcg/L Female: 6-350 mcg/L	300-800 mcg/L with EPO; 50 mcg/L without EPO	This is the way iron is stored in the liver. If iron stores are low, red blood cell production is decreased.	Low: Iron in food is not well absorbed. Most patients need an IV iron supplement. Patients should not take oral iron at same time as phosphate binders.
CO_2	22-25 mEq/L	22-25 mEq/L	Dialysis patients are often acidotic because they do not excrete metabolic acids in their urine. Acidosis may increase the rate of muscle and bone catabolism.	Low: Review eKt/V, BUN, nPNA. Oral sodium bicarbonate may be given to raise CO_2, but it presents a significant sodium load to patient.
Glucose	65-114 mg/dL	Same for nondiabetic patients Less than 300 mg/dL (patients with diabetes)	Because the kidney metabolizes insulin, low blood sugar levels caused by a longer half-life of insulin are possible. For patients with diabetes: a high blood sugar may increase thirst.	Most people need 6 to 11 servings of breads and starches or cereals per day and 2 to 4 servings of fruit per day to provide energy. Patients with diabetes should avoid concentrated sweets, unless blood sugar level is low.

Developed by Katy G. Wilkens, MS, RD, Northwest Kidney Centers, Seattle, Washington.

BUN, Blood urea nitrogen; *CO_2*, carbon dioxide; *DHT*, dihydrotachysterol; *EPO*, erythropoietin; *IV*, intravenous; *N/A*, not applicable; *nPNA*, normalized protein nitrogen appearance; *PTH*, parathyroid hormone; *URR*, urea reduction ratio.

30 g can occur during a 24-hour PD, with an average of 1 g/hour. Those receiving PD need 1.2 to 1.5 g/kg of body weight. At least 50% should be HBV protein. Patients who receive HD three times per week require a daily protein intake of 1.2 g/kg of body weight. Patients on dialysis who have low albumin levels have much higher mortality rates; thus emphasis is placed on adequate protein intake. Serum BUN and serum Cr levels, uremic symptoms, and weight should be monitored; and the diet should be adjusted accordingly.

In renal failure, prealbumin, which is metabolized by the kidney, is not a good nutritional marker, as values are routinely elevated. Albumin is a limited indicator of protein nutriture, but is routinely used in evaluating ESRD patients' nutritional status. Federal mandates require intervention at levels below 4 g/dL. However, because of the complexity of either acute or chronic inflammation, albumin remains predictive of poor survival in ESRD. Hypoalbuminemia is multifactorial and may be related to poor nutrition, inflammation, or comorbid disease. When interpreting albumin values, it is important to know the laboratory's methodology for measuring serum albumin, because different laboratory techniques give different results in renal failure (see Table 36-9).

Most patients find it challenging to consume adequate protein because uremia itself causes taste aberrations, notably to red meats. Some patients cannot even tolerate the smell of meat cooking. Often this protein aversion makes it difficult to achieve recommended high biological value protein intake. Patients may tolerate eggs, tofu, and "white" meats better. They can also use spices to hide the taste of meats, or serve animal proteins cold, to minimize the urea taste. Nutritional supplements may be helpful in some patients, and, occasionally, the phosphate restriction may need to be lifted to allow the consumption of dairy products to meet protein needs. As with all the nutritional parameters, meeting patient needs must be individualized.

Energy

Energy intake should be adequate to spare protein for tissue protein synthesis and to prevent its metabolism for energy (Byham-Gray, 2006). Depending on the patient's nutrition status and degree of stress, between 25 and 40 kcal/kg of body weight should be provided, with the lower amount for transplantation and PD patients and the higher level for the nutritionally depleted patient. Tools have been developed to allow the renal dietitian to assess the quality of the patient's nutrition status. The Subjective Global Assessment (Box 6-5) technique has been modified in this population to recognize the basic physiologic and immunologic changes in ESRD.

Fluid and Sodium Balance

The kidney's ability to handle sodium and water in ESRD must be assessed frequently through measurement of blood pressure, edema, fluid weight gain, serum sodium level, and dietary intake. The vast majority of dialysis patients need to restrict sodium and fluid intakes. Excessive sodium intake is responsible for increased thirst, increased fluid gain, and resultant hypertension. Even those patients who do not experience these symptoms but produce minimal amounts of urine will benefit from a reduced sodium intake to limit their thirst and prevent large intradialytic fluid gains.

In the patient who is maintained on HD, sodium and fluid intake are regulated to allow for a weight gain of 4 to 5 lb (2 to 3 kg) from increased fluid in the vasculature between dialyses. The goal is a fluid gain of less than 4% of body weight. A sodium intake of 87 to 130 mEq (2 to 3 g) daily and a limit on fluid intake (usually about 750 mL/day plus the amount equal to the urine output) is usually sufficient to meet these guidelines. Only fluids that are liquid at room temperature are included in this calculation. The fluid contained in solid foods is not included in the 750 mL limit. Solid foods in the average diet contribute approximately 500 to 800 mL/day of fluid. This fluid in solid food is calculated to approximately replace the 500 mL/day net insensible water loss.

An 86- to 130-mEq (2- to 3-g) sodium diet requires no salt in cooking; no salt at the table; no salted, smoked, or cured meat or fish; and no salted snack foods, canned soups, or high-sodium convenience foods. In today's increasing convenience food–oriented marketplace, it is estimated that 75% to 90% of sodium intake is consumed in convenience foods, with only 10% to 25% added to foods in cooking or at the table. It is important to remember that the most effective way to reduce the renal patient's thirst and fluid intake is to decrease sodium intake. It is salt intake that drives fluid consumption. Appendix 37 gives the details of a low-sodium meal plan. Many physicians and dietitians believe it is unethical to restrict fluid in patients who are not on a restricted sodium diet, because feelings of thirst become overwhelming to the patient with a high sodium intake.

When educating about fluid balance, the health care provider must teach the patient how to deal with thirst without drinking. Sucking on a few ice chips, cold sliced fruit, or sour candies or using artificial saliva are all good suggestions. In approximately 15% to 20% of patients, hypertension is not alleviated even after meticulous attention to fluid and water balance. In these patients hypertension is usually perpetuated by a high level of renin secretion and requires medication for control.

Although most patients with ESRD retain sodium, a small number may lose it. Examples of conditions with a salt-losing tendency are polycystic disease of the kidney, medullary kidney disease, chronic obstructive uropathy, chronic pyelonephritis, and analgesic nephropathy. To prevent hypotension, hypovolemia, cramps, and further deterioration of renal function, extra sodium may be required. A diet for these types of patients may contain 130 mEq (3 g) or more of sodium per day, which is the amount in a normal diet without added salt. Adding salt or salty foods can satisfy the need for extra sodium. The number of patients who require this higher sodium intake is small, but these patients exemplify the need for individual consideration of the diet prescription and a thorough understanding of the patient's underlying disease and present diet.

Patients receiving frequent dialysis treatments, either daily PD, short daily, or daily nocturnal dialysis may have higher allowance for sodium and fluid, based on an individual evaluation of their dry weight and laboratory values.

Potassium

Potassium usually requires restriction, depending on the serum potassium level, urine output, medications, and the frequency of HD. The daily intake of potassium for most Americans is 75 to 100 mEq (3 to 4 g). This is usually reduced in ESRD to 60 to 80 mEq (2.3 to 3.1 g) per day and is reduced for the anuric patient on dialysis to 51 mEq (2 g) per day. Some patients (i.e., those on high-flux dialysis or with increased dialysis times or frequencies such as PD, short daily or nocturnal) will be able to tolerate higher intakes. Again, a close monitoring of the patient's laboratory values, K^+ content of the dialysate, and dietary intake is essential.

The potassium content of foods is listed in Box 7-1 in Chapter 7, and in Appendixes 36 and 56. When counseling HD patients on a low-potassium diet, one should take care to point out that some low-sodium foods contain potassium chloride as a salt substitute rather than sodium chloride. Nutrition labels for products such as salt substitutes, Lite-Salt, and low-sodium herb mixtures must all be checked carefully to be sure they do not contain dangerous levels of potassium. Low-sodium soy sauces, low-sodium soups, and other special dietary products may need particular review by a trained professional. Reviewing such practices not only with the patient but with other people who may be cooking for the patient, such as a church group or neighbors who may use salt substitutes is advisable.

When a thorough diet history does not reveal the reason for elevated serum potassium, other nondietetic sources of potassium should be researched. Examples include poor dialysis adequacy or missed dialysis treatments, too high a concentration of potassium in the dialysate bath, very elevated blood sugar in patients with diabetes, acidosis, constipation, significant GI bleeding, some medications, blood transfusions, major trauma, chemotherapy, or radiation therapy. Occasionally, blood samples are handled improperly, resulting in hemolysis and falsely elevated potassium levels.

Phosphorus

More than 99% of excess phosphate is excreted in the urine. However, as GFR decreases, phosphorus is retained in the plasma. Because of the large molecular weight of the phosphate molecule, it is not easily removed by dialysis and patients experience net "gain" of about one half of the phosphate they consume daily. Phosphate intake is lowered by restricting dietary sources to 1200 mg/day or less. The difficulty in implementing the phosphorus restriction comes from the necessity for a high-protein diet. High protein foods, such as meats, contain high levels of phosphorus in the form of ATP. Additionally, other sources of protein—dairy products, nuts, and legumes—are also high in phosphorus. Thus high phosphorus foods cannot be eliminated without restricting protein, creating a challenge to balance intake with dietary intervention alone.

The American diet, which contains highly processed foods, has resulted in increases in both the types and amounts of phosphorus available for absorption, making compliance with a phosphorus restriction more difficult. Naturally occurring phosphate in food is only approximately 60% absorbed. Commonly used phosphate additives such as trisodium phosphate, disodium phosphate, and dicalcium phosphate are nearly 100% absorbed, making the processed diet a likely contributor to elevated phosphorus levels. Dietary intervention should focus on a balance of limiting dairy, nuts, beans, and processed foods while still encouraging enough HBV proteins to meet dietary needs.

Because dietary restrictions alone are not adequate to control serum phosphorus, nearly all patients who undergo dialysis require phosphate-binding medications. Phosphate binders such as calcium carbonate, calcium acetate, sevelamer carbonate and lanthanum carbonate are routinely used with each meal or snack to bind to phosphorus in the gut. These medications bind excess dietary phosphate and transport it through the GI tract for elimination, thus preventing its absorption into the blood. Side effects of taking these medications over long periods are common. Some may cause GI distress, diarrhea, or gas. Severe constipation, leading to intestinal impaction is a potential risk of excessive use of some types of phosphate binders; occasionally this may lead to perforation of the intestine resulting in peritonitis or death. Common medications are listed in Table 36-10.

Calcium and Parathyroid Hormone

In ESRD, the body's ability to maintain phosphorus-calcium balance is complicated by calcium and PTH controls. As GFR decreases, the serum calcium level declines for several reasons. First, decreased ability of the kidney to convert to inactive vitamin D to its active form, 1,25-$(OH)_2D3$ leads to poor GI absorption of calcium. Second, the need for serum calcium increases as serum phosphate levels increase. Both of these causes lead to hypertrophy of the parathyroid gland, which is responsible for calcium homeostasis. The resultant oversecretion of PTH increases resorption of bone to provide a calcium source.

The resulting metabolic bone disease, **renal osteodystrophy**, is essentially one of four types: (1) **osteomalacia**, (2) **osteitis fibrosa cystica**, (3) **metastatic calcification**, or (4) adynamic bone disease. With a deficit of calcium available from dietary absorption, the low calcium level triggers the release of PTH from the parathyroid glands. This acts to increase release of calcium from the bones by stimulating osteoclast activity. This can lead to osteomalacia or bone demineralization, as a result of lack of osteoblast stimulation to replace lost calcium in the bones.

Ongoing low calcium causes the parathyroid glands to continue producing PTH in an attempt to elevate serum calcium levels. In time this leads to secondary hyperparathyroidism, where even the baseline production of PTH by these enlarged glands is enough to cause severe bone

TABLE 36-10

Common Medications and Nutritional Supplements for Patients with End-Stage Renal Disease

Phosphate Binders

• Taken with meals and snacks to prevent dietary phosphorus absorption

Calcium carbonate	TUMS, Os-Cal, Calci-Chew, Calci-Mix
Calcium acetate	PhosLo
Mg/Ca^{++} carbonate	MagneBind
Sevelamer carbonate	Renvela
Lanthanum carbonate	Fosrenol
Aluminum hydroxide	AlternaGEL

Vitamins

• Increased need for water-soluble vitamins because of losses during dialysis
• Fat-soluble vitamins A, and K are not supplemented
• Vitamin E may be supplemented

Dialysis Recommendations

Vitamin C	60 mg (not to exceed 200 mg daily)
Folic acid	1 mg
Thiamin	1.5 mg
Riboflavin	1.7 mg
Niacin	20 mg
Vitamin B_6	10 mg
Vitamin B_{12}	6 mcg
Pantothenic acid	10 mg
Biotin	0.3 mg

Brand names include Nephrocap, Neph-ron FA, Nephplex, Nephrovites, and Dia-tx

Iron

• Iron needs are increased because of EPO therapy

IV iron	Iron dextran (Infed), Iron gluconate (Ferrlecit), Iron sucrose (Venofer)

EPO

• Stimulates bone marrow to produce red blood cells

IV or IM	Epogen

Activated Vitamin D

• Used for the management of hyperparathyroidism

Oral	Calcitriol (Rocaltrol), doxercalciferol (Hectorol)
IV	Calcitriol (Calcijex), paricalcitol (Zemplar)

Biphosphonates

• Inhibit bone resorption by blocking osteoclast activity

Oral	Alendronate (Fosamax)
IV	pamidronate (Aredia)

Calcium Supplements

TUMS, Os-Cal, Calci-Chew

Phosphorus Supplements

Kphos neutral, NutraPhos, NutraPhos K

Calcimimetics

• Mimic calcium and bind to parathyroid gland

Cinacalcet (Sensipar)

Cation Exchange Resin

• For the treatment of hyperkalemia

Oral or rectal	SPS (Kayexalate)

Developed by Fiona Wolf, RD, and Thomas Montemayor, RPh, Northwest Kidney Centers, Seattle, Washington, 2010.

Ca^{++}, Calcium; *CHO*, cholesterol; *EPO*, epoetin; *ESRD*, end-stage renal disease; *IV*, intravenous; *IM*, intramuscular; *MVI*; Multiple Vitamin Injection; *SPS*, sodium polystyrene sulfonate.

demineralization (osteitis fibrosis cystica), which is characterized by dull, aching bone pain.

Even though the serum calcium level is elevated in response to PTH, serum phosphate concentration remains high as the GFR falls lower. If the product of serum calcium multiplied by the serum phosphate level is greater than 70, metastatic calcification is imminent. Metastatic calcification occurs when calcium phosphate, removed from bones, is deposited in nonbone cells. This extraskeletal calcification may develop in joints, soft tissue, and vessels.

Calciphylaxis occurs when calcium phosphate is deposited in wound tissues with resultant vascular calcification, thrombosis, nonhealing wounds, and gangrene. It is frequently fatal. Clinical management aims to keep the calcium × phosphorus product below 55 by preventing transient elevations in serum phosphate concentration (National Kidney Foundation, 2003). Phosphorus intake must be controlled to as great a degree as possible to avoid aggravation of the delicate situation posed by hyperparathyroidism, phosphate retention, vitamin D deficiency, and hypocalcemia in renal failure.

Many patients on dialysis suffer from hypocalcemia, despite calcium supplementation. Because of this, the routine drug of choice is active vitamin D, 1,25-$(OH)_2D_3$, available as calcitriol (Rocaltrol and Calcijex). Analogs such as doxercalciferol (Hectorol) and paricalcitol (Zemplar) are also effective in lowering PTH and raising calcium levels, but with less enhancement of gut absorption of calcium than the 1,25 forms. Other mechanisms for controlling PTH include the medication cinacalcet (Sensipar), a calcimimetic or calcium-imitating drug, which binds to sites on the parathyroid gland and gives the gland a false impression that calcium levels are elevated. The drug is effective in suppressing PTH production and may also lower calcium levels dramatically, with significant consequences. Overall, close monitoring is essential.

In more extreme cases of hyperparathyroidism, use of surgical excision of portions of the parathyroid glands can be used in an attempt to restore balance. This creates the risk of low PTH, and can lead to **adynamic (low turnover) bone disease**, characterized by decreased levels of bone turnover and suppression of both osteoclasts and osteoblasts. This condition is unique to ESRD, in which oversuppression of the parathyroid gland and too much active vitamin D lead to decreased bone formation and fragile bones with very little matrix. Usually diagnosed by a low PTH level, this disease results in a high risk of nonhealing fractures. Oversuppression of the parathyroid gland by use of vitamin D or its analogs can mimic this as well.

Overall the dietary balance of phosphorus, the use of phosphate binders and vitamin D analogs, the removal of phosphate by dialysis, and intense monitoring of laboratory values all contribute to bone management in ESRD.

Lipid

Atherosclerotic cardiovascular disease is the most common cause of death among patients maintained on long-term dialysis (Bennett et al., 2006). This appears to be a function of both underlying disease (e.g., diabetes mellitus, hypertension, nephrotic syndrome) and a lipid abnormality common among patients with ESRD. The patient with ESRD typically has an elevated triglyceride level with or without an increase in cholesterol. The lipid abnormality likely represents both increased synthesis of very-low-density lipoprotein and decreased clearance as well as increased reliance on animal-based proteins.

Treatment of hyperlipidemia with diet or pharmacologic agents remains controversial. Epidemiologic evidence demonstrating increased incidence of atherosclerotic coronary disease is balanced by studies that demonstrate that patients with clearly defined clinical evidence of atherosclerosis at the initiation of dialysis are at no increased risk for a cardiovascular event. Although routine treatment appears unwarranted, a good case can be made for dietary and pharmacologic treatment of patients with ESRD with underlying lipid disorders and evidence of atherosclerosis. Lipid-lowering drugs, including most statins, may have a significant effect on better management (see Chapter 34).

On the other hand, low cholesterol levels can be a significant predictor of mortality in ESRD. They can indicate poor oral intake, and may be a useful tool in diagnosing malnutrition. Use of lipid-lowering drugs should be monitored and cut back if needed in these patients, particularly if they are underweight or suffering from malnutrition.

Iron and Erythropoietin

The anemia of chronic renal disease is caused by an inability of the kidney to produce EPO, the hormone that stimulates the bone marrow to produce red blood cells, an increased destruction of red blood cells secondary to circulating uremic waste products; and blood loss with dialysis or blood sampling. A synthetic form of EPO, recombinant human EPO (rHuEPO), is used to treat this form of anemia. Clinical trials have demonstrated a dramatic improvement in correcting anemia and restoring a general sense of well being (Locatelli F, 2006).

Use of EPO increases red blood cell production 2.5-fold. Almost always accompanying the rise in hematocrit is an increased need for iron that requires IV supplementation. Oral iron alone is not effective in maintaining adequate iron stores in patients who take EPO. Unless a documented allergic reaction exists, almost all patients taking EPO require periodic IV or intramuscular iron. For patients who are allergic to IV iron, several better-tolerated forms are now available as iron dextran (Infed), iron gluconate (Ferrlecit), and iron sucrose (Venofer).

Serum ferritin is an accurate indicator of iron status in renal failure. Patients who have received several transfusions and who are storing extra iron may have high serum ferritin levels of 800 to 5000 ng/mL (a normal level is 68 ng/mL for women and 150 ng/mL for men; see Appendix 30). In patients who are receiving EPO, ferritin should be kept above 300 ng/mL but below 800 ng/mL. When ferritin values fall below 100 ng/mL, IV iron is usually given. The percent of transferrin saturation is another useful indicator of iron status in these patients and should be between 25% to 30%.

Vitamins

Water-soluble vitamins are rapidly lost during dialysis. In general, ascorbic acid and most B vitamins are lost through dialysate at approximately the same rate they would have been lost in the urine (depending on the type and duration of treatment), with the exception of folate, which is highly dialyzable. Patients who still produce urine may be at increased risk of loss of water-soluble vitamins. Folate is recommended to be supplemented at 1 mg/day based on extra losses. Because vitamin B_{12} is protein-bound, losses of this B vitamin during dialysis are minimal. Altered metabolism and excretory function, as well as drug administration, also may alter vitamin levels. Little is known about GI absorption of vitamins in uremia, but it may be significantly decreased. Uremic toxins may interfere with the activity of some vitamins, such as inhibition of phosphorylation of pyridoxine and its analogs.

Another cause of decreased vitamin intake in uremia is the restriction of dietary phosphorus and potassium. Water-soluble vitamins are usually abundant in high-potassium foods such as citrus fruits and vegetables and high-phosphorus foods such as milk. Diets for patients on dialysis tend to be low in folate, niacin, riboflavin, and vitamin B_6. With frequent episodes of anorexia or illness, vitamin intake is decreased further. Whereas levels of water-soluble vitamins decrease as a result of dialysis, replacement of fat-soluble vitamins is not usually required in renal disease.

Several vitamin supplements that fit the needs of the uremic patient or the dialysis patient are now available by prescription: Nephrocaps, Nephplex, Dialyvite, and Renal Caps. An over-the-counter supplement containing the vitamin B complex and vitamin C is often used and can be less expensive than a prescription, but additional supplements of folic acid and pyridoxine may be needed.

Niacin has been found to be helpful in lowering phosphate levels in ESRD patients. It interferes with the sodium-phosphate pump in the GI lumen, causing decreased transport of phosphate, and thus works with a different mechanism than phosphate binders, (Cheng, S, 2006, 2008). It is usually dosed once daily, increasing compliance.

Nutrition Support in End-Stage Renal Disease

Enteral Tube Feeding

Patients with ESRD who require enteral tube feeding often do quite well on standard formulas used for most tube-fed patients (see Chapter 14). Patients should receive standard formulas before they try a "specialty" formula because the former are usually less expensive and typically have lower osmolality than the specific renal products. If electrolyte or fluid concerns arise, patients can be changed to one of the formulas now available that are specifically designed for renal patients: Nepro or Novasource Renal. If patients are receiving renal products only, they may develop problems with a low phosphorus or potassium levels as these products are often used in conjunction with oral intake.

Parenteral Nutrition

PN in ESRD is similar to PN used for other malnourished patients with respect to protein, carbohydrates, and fat, but differs in use of vitamins and minerals. Most researchers agree that vitamin needs for ESRD during PN differ from normal requirements; however, they do not agree on recommendations for individual nutrients. Folate, pyridoxine, and biotin should be supplemented. Vitamin A should not be provided parenterally unless retinol-binding protein is monitored because it is elevated in patients with ESRD. Because there is currently no parenteral vitamin that is specifically designed for patients with renal failure, a standard vitamin preparation is usually administered. Little information related to parenteral trace mineral supplementation is available. Because most trace minerals, including zinc, chromium, and magnesium, are excreted in the urine, a close monitoring of these minerals in the serum seems to be appropriate.

Intradialytic Parenteral Nutrition

Malnourished patients with chronic renal failure who are on HD have easy access to PN because of the direct blood access required by the dialysis therapy itself. **Intradialytic PN (IDPN)** can be administered if necessary without additional invasive procedures or need for a separate port. It is typically administered through a connection to the venous side of the extracorporeal circuit during dialysis. Because of the high blood flow rate achieved through use of the surgically created fistula and the high blood pump speeds that are attained, hypertonic glucose and protein can be administered without danger of phlebitis. Lipids may also be administered. Reimbursement issues are complex because IDPN is a supplemental feeding that requires the patient to have at least a functioning GI tract and only supplies an average of 1000 calories every HD treatment (Table 36-11).

Complications are similar to those encountered in usual PN, with the exception of postdialysis hypoglycemia caused by the abrupt ending of the glucose supply. To avoid this problem, glucose administration typically is tapered up and down during the first and last half hour of the 3- to 5-hour treatment. Insulin is given often, and can be given in the bag of the dextrose–amino acid solution, so that the patient does not become hypoglycemic if the infusion must be stopped. Blood sugar levels are typically monitored during the therapy. Some patients may benefit from a complex carbohydrate snack toward the end of the treatment to avoid posttreatment rebound hypoglycemia. Amino acid losses through the dialysate average approximately 10%.

Another method of nutrition support in PD patients is called **intraperitoneal nutrition (IPN)** using a peritoneal dialysate solution that contains amino acids instead of

TABLE 36-11

Regimen for Intradialytic Parenteral Nutrition Administered During Hemodialysis Therapy

Infusion	Quantity	Calories (kcal)	Volume (mL)
70% dextrose	350 g dextrose[†]	1190	500
15% amino acids	37.5 g protein	Protein should not be counted as calories	250
20% lipid emulsion	50 g fat	450	250
TOTAL		1640	1000*

Monitor serum glucose, sodium, potassium, bicarbonate, phosphate, triglycerides

Developed by Katy G. Wilkens, MS, RD, Northwest Kidney Centers, Seattle, Wash.

*Additional volume may include insulin and vitamins.

[†]3.4 kcal/gm because of hydration in IDPN solution.

dextrose. Typically one bag of this solution is used per day. Some patients experience side effects from this treatment. Reimbursement issues are significant.

End-Stage Renal Disease in Patients with Diabetes

Because renal failure is a complication of diabetes, approximately 40% to 50% of all new patients starting dialysis have diabetes (Zhang et al., 2005). The need to control blood sugar in these patients requires specialized diet therapy. The diet for diabetes management (see Chapter 31) can be modified for the patient on dialysis. In addition, the diabetic patient on dialysis often has other complications such as retinopathy, neuropathy, gastroparesis, and amputation, all of which can place this patient at high nutritional risk. The NKF has established guidelines for managing diabetes in the presence of CKD (National Kidney Foundation, 2007; Nelson and Tuttle, 2007), which can be accessed at www.kidney.org.

Increased osmolality caused by high serum levels of glucose may cause water and potassium to be pulled out of cells, with resultant hyperkalemia. Interpretation of commonly used laboratory values will change when a diabetic patient develops renal failure, because the hemoglobin A1c is affected by the shortened half life of red blood cells in uremia (Rigalleau et al., 2006).

Chronic Kidney Disease and End-Stage Renal Disease in Children

Although CKD may occur in children at any age, from the newborn infant to the adolescent, it is a relatively uncommon diagnosis. Causal factors in children include congenital defects, anatomic defects (urologic malformations or dysplastic kidneys), inherited disease (autosomal-recessive polycystic kidney disease), metabolic disorders that eventually result in renal failure (cystinosis or methylmalonic aciduria), or acquired conditions or illnesses (untreated kidney infections, physical trauma to kidneys, exposure to nephrotoxic chemicals or medications, hemolytic anemia due to *Escherichia coli* 0157 ingestion, or glomerular nephritis).

As with all children, the major concern is to promote normal growth and development. Without aggressive monitoring and encouragement, the child with renal failure rarely meets his or her nutritional requirements. If the renal disease is present from birth, nutrition support needs to begin immediately to avoid losing the growth potential of the first few months of life. Growth in children with CKD is usually delayed. Although no specific therapy ensures normal growth, factors capable of responding to therapy include metabolic acidosis, electrolyte depletion, osteodystrophy, chronic infection, and protein-calorie malnutrition. Energy and protein needs for children with chronic renal disease are at least equivalent to the DRIs for normal children of the same height and age. If nutrition status is poor, energy needs may be even higher to promote weight gain and linear growth.

Feeding by tube is required in the presence of poor intake, particularly in the critical growth period of the first 2 years of life. Gastrostomy tubes are almost always placed in these children to enhance nutritional intake and facilitate growth. PN is rarely initiated unless the GI tract is nonfunctional. For the nutritional requirements of children with renal failure see the Kidney Disease Outcome Quality Initiative at www.kdoqi.org.

Control of calcium and phosphorus balance is especially important for maintaining good growth. The goal is to restrict phosphorus intake while promoting calcium absorption with the aid of 1,25-$(OH)_2D_3$. This helps prevent renal osteodystrophy, which can cause severe growth retardation. Use of calcium carbonate formulations to supplement the dietary intake enhances calcium intake while binding excess phosphorus. Persistent metabolic acidosis is often associated with growth failure in infancy. In chronic acidosis the titration of acid by the bone causes calcium loss and contributes to bone demineralization. Bicarbonate may be added to the infant formula to counteract this effect.

Restriction of protein in pediatric diets is controversial. The so-called "protective" effect on kidney function must be weighed against the clearly negative effect of possible protein malnutrition on growth (National Kidney Foundation, 2009). The recommended dietary allowance for protein for age is usually the minimum amount given.

Each child's diet should be adjusted to his or her food preferences, family eating patterns, and biochemical needs. This is often not an easy task. In addition, care must be taken not to place too much emphasis on the diet to avoid its becoming a manipulative tool and an attention-getting device. Special encouragement, creativity, and attention are required to help the child with CKD consume the necessary energy. When possible, CCPD is given intermittently during the day and continuously at night as it allows liberalization of the diet. The child is more likely to meet nutritional requirements with fewer dietary restrictions and therefore experience better growth. See www.kidney.org for further tips on pediatric renal nutrition support.

Other treatments that help renal disease in children include the use of rHuEPO and recombinant deoxyribonucleic acid–produced human growth hormone. EPO is usually started when the child's serum hemoglobin falls below 10 g/dL, with a goal of maintaining hemoglobin between 11 and 12 g/dL. Correction of anemia with the use of rHuEPO may increase appetite, intake, and feeling of well being, but it has not been found to affect growth, even with seemingly adequate nutrition support.

Medical Nutrition Therapy for Transplantation

The nutritional care of the adult patient who has received a transplanted kidney is based mainly on the metabolic effects of the required immunosuppressive therapy. Medications typically used for the long term include azathioprine (Imuran), corticosteroids (e.g., prednisone), calcineurin inhibitors (cyclosporine A, Gengraf, SangCya, Sandimmune], tacrolimus [Prograf, F506]), sirolimus (Rapamune), mycophenolate mofetil (CellCept), and mycophenolic acid (Myfortic). Corticosteroids are associated with accelerated protein catabolism, hyperlipidemia, sodium retention, weight gain, hyperglycemia, osteoporosis and electrolyte disturbances. Calcineurin inhibitors are associated with hyperkalemia, hypertension, hyperglycemia, and hyperlipidemia. The doses of these medications used after transplantation are decreased over time until a "maintenance level" is reached.

During the first 6 weeks after surgery, a high-protein diet is often recommended (1.2-1.5 g/kg ideal body weight [IBW]) with an energy intake of 30-35 kcal/kg IBW, to prevent negative nitrogen balance. A moderate sodium restriction of 2-3 g/day during this period minimizes fluid retention and helps to control blood pressure (Keven, K. 2006). After recovery, protein intake should be decreased to 1 g/kg IBW, with calorie intake providing sufficient energy to maintain or achieve an appropriate weight for height. A balanced low-fat diet aids in lowering cardiac complications (National Kidney Foundation, 2009). Sodium intakes are individualized based on fluid retention and blood pressure (see Appendix 37).

Hyperkalemia warrants a temporary dietary potassium restriction. Following transplantation, many patients exhibit hypophosphatemia and mild hypercalcemia caused by bone resorption; this is associated with persistent hyperparathyroidism and the effects of steroids on calcium, phosphorus, and vitamin D metabolism. The diet should contain adequate amounts of calcium and phosphorus (1200 mg of each daily) and cholecalciferol (vitamin D_3, 2000 IU daily). Supplemental phosphorus may also be necessary to correct hypophosphatemia.

Hydration must also be monitored closely after transplantation. Because most kidney recipients required a fluid restriction while on dialysis, they need to be reminded of the importance of maintaining fluid intake after transplant. Typically, patients are encouraged to drink 2 L/day, but their overall needs depend on their urine output.

The majority of transplant recipients have elevated serum triglycerides or cholesterol for a variety of reasons. Intervention consists of medications, calorie restriction for those who are overweight, cholesterol intake limited to less than 300 mg/day, and limited total fat (see Chapter 34). In patients with glucose intolerance, limiting carbohydrates and a regular exercise regimen are appropriate. Tissue weight gain with resultant obesity is common after transplantation. Medication side effects, fewer dietary restrictions, and the lack of physical exercise can all contribute to post-transplant weight gain.

Education of Patients with End-Stage Renal Disease

For effective intervention, it is important to look at the long-range goals for educating the patient with ESRD about his or her nutritional needs. The average patient survives on dialysis 7 to 10 years. Patients with a relatively benign diagnosis may look forward to life spans of 20 to 40 years, particularly if they receive kidney transplants as a part of their treatment. The challenge for the dietitian is educating the patient with a chronic disease who will be primarily responsible for implementing the nutritional recommendations for the rest of his or her life. Thus intervention for ESRD and that for diabetes share many similarities.

Exchange lists are not always used in educating the patient about a renal diet. Rather a booklet, *The National Renal Diet* available from the American Dietetic Association (see "Useful Websites" later in this chapter), provides information about food sources of nutrients, adapting patients' usual intakes to meet requirements based on their laboratory values, and reducing the intake of certain foods when blood values rise. A sample diet for the patient receiving dialysis can be found in Appendix 36.

Counseling for Patients with End-Stage Renal Disease

It is incumbent on the registered dietitian (RD) to develop a long-standing rapport with the patient and family and to serve as an ally to help them make the best nutritional choices over an extended period. Understanding the burdens of a complex, challenging, ever-changing diet suggests the transfer of information to the renal patient and family in a workable, flexible, and easily understood manner. Skills for this task are just as challenging, if not more so, than maintaining a patient's iron status or keeping the patient at a good body weight. Empathy and use of techniques such as motivational interviewing or cognitive behavioral therapy are essential tools.

Coordination of Care in End-Stage Renal Disease

The position of the RD in the care of dialysis patients is unique because it is a federally mandated position. So, too, is the RD's place on the mandated interdisciplinary health care team that exists within each dialysis unit. The team approach is an important aspect of all health care; however, its importance is magnified in the dialysis team, which consists of the patient, renal nurse, renal social worker, nephrologist, and renal dietitian. Care of these complex, long-term ESRD patients requires the skill and compassion of each member of the health care team working together (Unruh et al., 2005). Advanced levels of practice are available for dietitians who wish to be certified as renal RDs; they can be certified through examination by the American Dietetic Association, and become a Board Certified Specialist in Renal Nutrition.

Emergency Diets for Dialysis Patients

When power outages, flooding, storms, hurricanes, or earthquakes threaten a community, they threaten the most vulnerable people in that community. Patients on HD require power and water sources to do their own treatments at home. If they travel to a dialysis unit, they need access to transportation. Because of poor outcomes in recent natural disasters, the federal government's ESRD program has specified that patients and care givers must be familiar with alternative nutritional therapies when dialysis is not available because of a natural or manmade emergency. Box 36-2 demonstrates the type of nutrient and practical information that must be considered when patients may be without

BOX 36-2

Emergency Dialysis Diet Plan

This plan will work for short periods (5 days or less) when patients cannot dialyze.

The Emergency Diet Plan does not replace dialysis; it should be used only in case of an emergency.

Guidelines

1. Limit meat to 3-4 oz/day.
2. Avoid all high-potassium fruits and vegetables.
3. Consume one to two 8-oz cups of fluid per day.
4. Choose low-salt foods.
5. Do not use salt or salt substitute.
6. Use fats and sugars for extra calories.
7. If the power is off for a day, foods in refrigerator should be eaten first.
8. Patients should eat food from the freezer while they still have ice crystals in the center.
9. Patients should have a portable Emergency Kit they can take with them to a disaster relief center. Sample foods are listed in the following diet plan.

Emergency Diet Plan

If a food is not on this list, patients should not eat it.

Meat and Protein Foods (three to four 1-oz choices/day)

1 egg
1 ounce meat, fish, tofu or poultry
¼ cup unsalted or rinsed canned fish or poultry
2 tablespoons unsalted peanut butter
¼ cup cottage cheese
½ can Ensure Plus, Boost Plus or Nepro

Starch (six to ten choices/day)

1 slice white bread
½ English muffin or bagel
5 unsalted crackers
2 graham crackers
6 shortbread cookies, vanilla wafers
1 cup unsalted rice, noodles, pasta
1 cup puffed wheat, rice, shredded wheat
1 cup of rice or pasta

Vegetables (one choice/day)

½-cup serving of green beans, summer squash, corn, beets, carrots, or peas
Should be fresh or frozen, not canned

Fruits (three to four choices/day)

1 small apple
15 grapes
½ cup serving of berries, cherries, applesauce, canned pears or canned pineapple

Fats and Oil (six or more choices/day)

1 tsp butter, margarine, oil or mayonnaise

Fluids (one to two choices/day)

1 cup water, coffee, tea, soda pop
½ cup Ensure Plus, Boost Plus or Nepro
½ cup serving of milk, half and half, soy, or rice milk
Cranberry, apple, or grape juice; or Kool-Aid

Emergency Kit

Have the following things stored in a box or bag easily accessible:

Foods listed in the Emergency Diet Plan
Can opener
Two gallon jugs of distilled water
Bleach, 1 Tbsp/gallon of water to sterilize
Flashlight and extra batteries
Sharp knife
Aluminum foil
Plastic mixing containers and lids
Measuring cup
Fork, knife, spoon
Battery-operated transistor radio
One-week supply of personal medicines kept in a handy place, including blood pressure medications and phosphate binders (insulin and some other medications must be kept refrigerated or cold)

Storage Tips

1. Store things in a clean, dry place such as a new garbage can or rubber tub.
2. Label and date when food is put in storage.
3. Change all food and water once a year. Eat unused food or donate to a food bank.

Dialysis Emergency Diet information from Katy Wilkens, MS, RD. Copyright Northwest Kidney Centers, 2011. For more emergency diet info see www.nwkidney.org or your local Network Coordinating Council website.

dialysis for days, or because they must be evacuated to a site that cannot meet their urgent nutritional needs.

Medical Management (Conservative Treatment) or Palliative Care

The decision to forego or discontinue dialysis and opt for end-of-life care is a difficult and emotional one. Factors such as religious practices, age, quality of life, and comorbid disease all play a role. Patients who are poor candidates for dialysis or transplantation may benefit from a low-protein, low-sodium diet to minimize physical symptoms, such as shortness of breath and uremia. Palliative care can be offered with the goal of balancing patient wishes for food choice with these complex side effects.

CLINICAL SCENARIO

A 67-year-old white man is seen by his primary care physician. The patient lives with a significant other; has an active lifestyle (golfing, biking, swimming); and a history of hemicolectomy, diverticulitis, and hypertension. His weight is 240 lb. His laboratory values show serum creatinine of 3.3 mg/dL, blood urea nitrogen of 72, albumin of 4.1, potassium of 5.5, phosphate of 6.7, calcium of 8.3, and his parathyroid hormone is 365. Blood pressure is 160/92.

Nutrition Diagnostic Statement

Altered laboratory values related to hypertension as evidenced by estimated glomerular filtration rate (eGFR) calculation.

Nutrition Care Questions

1. What is the patient's calculated eGFR?
2. What is the patient's stage of chronic kidney disease (CKD)?
3. What is the first goal for teaching?
4. What referral would you make to the patient's primary care provider?
5. What dietary factors would you address based on laboratory values?
6. What is the goal for protein intake for this patient?
7. How would you assess for improvement or stability of his CKD?
8. What would you expect for this patient during the next few years if no diet intervention is followed?

USEFUL WEBSITES

American Dietetic Association and the National Renal Diet
www.eatright.org
www.Ikidney.com
Life Options
www.lifeoptions.org
National Institute of Diabetes and Digestive and Kidney Diseases
www.niddk.nih.gov/health/kidney/kidney.htm
National Kidney Foundation
www.kidney.org
Kidney Disease Outcome Quality Initiative
www.kdoqi.org
Nationwide End-Stage Renal Network
www.esrdnetwork.org
Northwest Kidney Centers
www.nwkidney.org
Renal Network
www.renalnet.org
United States Renal Data Systems
http://www.usrds.org/

REFERENCES

Appel GB: Improved outcomes in nephrotic syndrome, *Cleve Clin J Med* 73:161, 2006.

Asplin JR: Evaluation of a kidney stone patient, *Semin Nephrol* 28:99, 2008.

Asselman M, Verkoelen CF: Fructose intake as a risk factor for kidney stone disease, *Kidney Int* 73:139, 2008.

Bennett SJ, et al: Nutrition in chronic heart failure with coexisting chronic kidney disease, *J Cardiovasc Nurs* 21:56, 2006.

Berardi JM, et al: Plant based dietary supplement increases urinary pH, *J Int Soc Sports Nutr* 5:20, 2008.

Byham-Gray LD: Weighing the evidence: energy determinations across the spectrum of kidney disease, *J Ren Nutr* 16(1):17, 2006.

Cheng S, et al: A randomized, double-blind, placebo-controlled trial of niacinamide for reduction of phosphorus in hemodialysis patients, *Clin J Am Soc Nephrol* 3:1131, 2008.

Cheng S, Coyne DW: Niacin and niacinamide for hyperphosphatemia in patients undergoing dialysis, *Int Urol Nephrol* 38:171, 2006.

Curhan GC, Taylor EN: 24-h uric acid excretion and the risk of kidney stones, *Kidney Int* 73:489, 2008.

Domrongkitchaiporn S, et al: Hypocitraturia in recurrent calcium stone formers: focusing on urinary potassium excretion, *Am J Kidney Dis* 48:546, 2006.

Eisner BH, et al: Citrate, malate and alkali content in commonly consumed diet sodas: implications for nephrolithiasis treatment, *J Urol* 183:2419, 2010a.

Eisner BH, et al: Relationship between body mass index and quantitative 24-hour urine chemistries in patients with nephrolithiasis, *Urology* 75:1289, 2010b.

Goodman JW, et al: Effect of two sports drinks on urinary lithogenicity, *Urol Res* 37:41, 2009.

Hatch M, Freel RW: The roles and mechanisms of intestinal oxalate transport in oxalate homeostasis, *Semin Nephrol* 28:143, 2008.

Himmelfarb J, Ikizler TA: Hemodialysis, *N Engl J Med* 363:1833, 2010.

Jackson RD, et al: Calcium plus vitamin D supplementation and the risk of fractures, *N Engl J Med* 354:669, 2006.

Jepson R: Review: cranberry products may prevent urinary tract infection in women with recurrent infections, *Evid Based Nurs* 11:74, 2008.

Kang DE, et al: Long-term lemonade based dietary manipulation in patients with hypocitraturic nephrolithiasis, *J Urol* 177:1358, 2007.

Keven K, et al: The impact of daily sodium intake on posttransplant hypertension in kidney allograft recipients, *Transplant Proc* 38:1323, 2006.

Kiwull-Schone H, et al: Food composition and acid-base balance: alimentary alkali depletion and acid load in herbivores, *J Nutr* 138:431S, 2008.

Knight J, et al: Increased protein intake on controlled oxalate diets does not increase urinary oxalate excretion, *Urol Res* 37:63, 2009.

Kontiokari T, et al: Cranberry juice and bacterial colonization in children—a placebo-controlled randomized trial, *Clin Nutr* 24:1065, 2005.

Li WM, et al: Association of body mass index and urine pH in patients with urolithiasis, *Urol Res* 37:193, 2009.

Lieske JC, et al: Diabetes mellitus and the risk of urinary tract stones: a population-based case controlled study, *Am J Kidney Dis* 48:897, 2006.

Locatelli F, et al: Nutritional-inflammation status and resistance to erythropoietin therapy in haemodialysis patients, *Nephrol Dial Transplant* 21:991, 2006.

Maalouf NM, et al: Hypocitraturia and hyperoxaluria after Roux-en-Y gastric bypass surgery, *J Urol* 183:1026, 2010a.

Maalouf NM, et al: Metabolic basis for low urine pH in type 2 diabetes, *Clin J Am Soc Nephrol* 5:1277, 2010b.

Marcason W: Where can I find information on the oxalate content of foods? *J Am Diet Assoc* 106:627, 2006.

Massey LK, et al: Ascorbate increases human oxaluria and kidney stone risk, *J Nutr* 135:1673, 2005.

Massey LK: Food oxalate: Factors affecting measurement, biological variation, and bioavailability, *J Am Diet Assoc* 107:1191, 2007.

Mente A, et al: Ethnic differences in relative risk of idiopathic nephrolithiasis in north America, *J Urol* 178:1992, 2007.

Minich D, et al: Acid-alkaline balance: role in chronic disease and detoxification, *Alter Ther* 13:62, 2007.

Moyad MA, et al: Vitamin C with metabolites reduce oxalate levels compared to ascorbic acid: a preliminary and novel clinical urologic finding, *Urol Nurs* 29:95, 2009.

National Kidney Foundation: KDOQI Clinical Practice Guideline for Nutrition in Children with CKD: 2008 Update, *Am J Kidney Dis* 53(Suppl 2):S1-S124, 2009.

National Kidney Foundation: Kidney Dialysis Outcome Quality Initiative (KDOQI) clinical practice guidelines for bone metabolism and disease in chronic kidney disease, *Am J Kidney Dis* 42(Suppl 3):S1-S202, 2003. These guidelines, as well as other KDOQI guidelines, can be accessed online at www.kdoqi.org.

National Kidney Foundation: K/DOQI Clinical Practice Guidelines for Chronic Kidney Disease: Evaluation, Classification and Stratification, *Am J Kidney Dis* 39(Suppl 1):S1-S266, 2002. These guidelines, as well as all other KDOQI guidelines, can be accessed online at www.kdoqi.org.

National Kidney Foundation: KDOQI. Clinical practice guidelines and clinical practice recommendations for diabetes and chronic kidney disease, *Am J Kidney Dis* 49(Suppl 2):S1-S180, 2007.

Nelson RG, Tuttle KR: The new KDOQI clinical practice guidelines and clinical practice recommendations for diabetes and CKD, *Blood Purif* 25:112, 2007.

Nouvenne A, et al: Effects of a low-salt diet on idiopathic hypercalcuria in calcium-oxalalate stone formers: a 3-mo randomized controlled trial, *Am J Clin Nutr* 91:365, 2009.

Remer T, et al: Potential renal acid load of foods and its influence on urine pH, *J Am Diet Assoc* 95:791, 1995.

Remuzzi G, et al: Mechanisms of progression and regression of renal lesions of chronic nephropathies and diabetes, *J Clin Invest* 116:288, 2006.

Rigalleau V, et al: Cockcroft-Gault formula is biased by body weight in diabetic patients with renal impairment, *Metabolism* 55:108, 2006.

Semins MJ, et al: The effect of restrictive bariatric surgery on urinary stone risk factors, *Urology* 76:826, 2010.

Straub M, Hautmann RE: Developments in stone prevention, *Curr Opin Urol* 15:119, 2005.

Strejc JM: Considerations in the nutritional management of patients with acute renal failure, *Hemodial Int* 9:135, 2005.

Taylor EN, Curhan GC: Fructose consumption and the risk of kidney stones, *Kidney Int* 73:207, 2008.

Taylor EN, et al: DASH-style diet associates with reduced risk of kidney stones, *J Am Soc Nephrol* 20:2253, 2009.

Unruh ML, et al: Choices for healthy outcomes in caring for end-stage renal disease (CHOICE) study, *Am J Kidney Dis* 46:1107, 2005.

Wenjun Ju, et al: Renal gene and protein expression signatures for prediction of kidney disease progression, *Am J Pathol* 174:2073, 2009.

Zhang R, et al: Kidney disease and the metabolic syndrome, *Am J Med Sci* 330:319, 2005.

Zilberman DE, et al: The impact of societal changes on patters of urolithiasis, *Curr Opin Urol* 20:148, 2010.

Zuckerman JM, Assimos DG: Hypocitraturia: pathophysiology and medical management, *Rev Urol* 11:134, 2009.

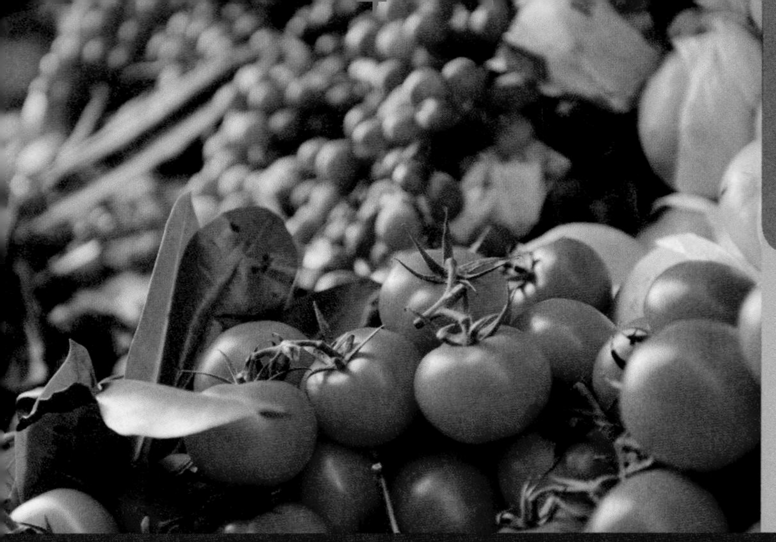

CHAPTER 37

Barbara L. Grant, MS, RD, CSO, LD
Kathryn K. Hamilton, MA, RD, CSO, CDN

Medical Nutrition Therapy for Cancer Prevention, Treatment, and Recovery

KEY TERMS

alternative medicine
angiogenesis
antiangiogenic therapy
antioxidants
apoptosis
biotherapy
cancer cachexia
cancer vaccines
carcinogen
carcinogenesis
chemoprevention
chemotherapy
classification
complementary therapy
control
cure
cytokines
drug resistance
dumping syndrome
emetogenic
epidemiologic studies
graft-versus-host disease (GVHD)
hematopoietic cell transplantation (HCT)
hematopoietic growth factors
hospice
initiation
integrative medicine
macrobiotic diet
malignant neoplasm
metabolic therapy
metastasis
monoclonal antibodies
mucositis
myelosuppression
N-nitroso compounds (NOCs)
neoplasm
neutropenia
nutrition impact symptoms
oncogenes
oncology
osteoradionecrosis
palliate (palliative care)
pancytopenia
phytochemicals
progression
promotion
radiation enteritis
radiation therapy
rate of tumor growth
sinusoidal obstructive syndrome (SOS)
staging
TNM staging system
trismus
tumor
tumor burden
tumor markers
tumor necrosis factor-α (cachectin)
tumor suppressor genes

Cancer involves the abnormal division and reproduction of cells that can spread throughout the body. Usually thought of as a single disease, cancer actually consists of more than 100 distinct types. The American Cancer Society (ACS) predicts the lifetime risk for developing cancer in the United States is slightly less than half of men and a little more than one third of women (American Cancer Society [ACS], 2009a). Annually in the United States, cancer is responsible for almost one out of every four deaths (ACS, 2009a). Evidence suggests that one third of the more than 560,000 cancer deaths may be attributed to nutrition and lifestyle behaviors such as poor diet, physical inactivity, alcohol use, and overweight and obesity. Almost an additional 171,000 cancer deaths are caused by tobacco use (ACS, 2010). It is estimated that 50% to 70% of cancer deaths are potentially preventable by decreasing high-risk behaviors; with approximately 30% of cancer deaths attributed to tobacco use and at least an additional 30% to poor nutrition (Brawer et al, 2009).

The cost of cancer care in the United States has doubled in the past 20 years to more than $48 billion annually (NCI, 2010a). Private insurance pays for 50% of the cost, Medicare coverage accounts for 34%, and Medicaid payment and other public programs cover the difference. Most medical care spending for cancer has shifted away from an inpatient care setting to outpatient care and treatment.

For dietetic professionals with interest in practicing in the area of oncology, the Standards of Practice and Standards of Professional Performance for Oncology Nutrition Practice provide guidance (Robien et al., 2010).

ETIOLOGY

The most prevalent types of cancer diagnosed in the United States are prostate, lung and bronchus, colorectal, and urinary bladder cancers for men; and breast, lung and bronchus, colorectal, and uterine cancers for women. The ACS established *2015 Challenge Goals* to improve cancer prevention and early detection efforts for lowering cancer incidence and mortality rates. These national recommendations outline specific measures to expand the use of established screening guidelines for the early detection of cancer, and ways to influence individual health behaviors such as protection from the sun, reducing tobacco use, maintaining a healthy body weight, improving diet, and increasing regular physical activity (ACS, 2010).

Overall, fewer Americans are dying from cancer, a trend that began more than 15 years ago. For many, cancer is now a chronic disease, like heart disease and diabetes. According to the National Cancer Institute (NCI), there are 11.7 million Americans living with a history of cancer; this means they are cancer free, are living with evidence of disease, or are undergoing cancer treatment (National Cancer Institute [NCI], 2010g). As a result of improvements in early detection of cancer and the development of new anticancer therapies, the relative survival rate for all cancers is now 66%, up from 50% in the 1970s (ACS, 2009a; NCI, 2010g). *The Annual Report to the Nation on the Status of Cancer, 1975-2006*, released in December 2009, found that rates of new diagnoses and rates of death from common cancers have declined significantly for men and women overall, as well as for most racial and ethnic populations. Although cancer rates continue to be higher for men than for women, men have experienced greater declines in cancer mortality. For colorectal cancer, the third most frequently diagnosed cancer in both men and women, overall rates have declined. Unfortunately, the incidence in men and women younger than 50 years old remains a concern.

PATHOPHYSIOLOGY

Carcinogenesis is the origin or development of cancer. **Oncology** is the study of all forms of cancer, and an oncologist is the medical doctor who specializes in cancer. Researchers believe changes in gene function cause normal cells to transform into cancerous cells. Thus the study of genetic material and its function (*genomics*) is of great scientific interest in cancer and its treatment. See *Pathophysiology and Care Management Algorithm:* Cancer.

Oncogenes are altered genes that promote tumor growth and change programmed cell death (**apoptosis**). **Tumor suppressor genes** are the opposite of oncogenes; these genes become deactivated in cancer cells. This loss in function can lead to unregulated cell growth and, ultimately, cancer. Examples of tumor suppressor genes include adenomatosis polyposis coli (APC), breast cancer types BRCA1 and BCRA2; and tumor suppressor p53, a protein that is involved in preventing cancer. Only approximately 5% of all cancers have been shown to occur as result of inherited genetic alterations. Factors observed in families with hereditary cancers include:

- A cancer diagnosis at an earlier age than normal for certain kinds of cancer
- Individuals with one type of cancer being diagnosed with a second type of cancer
- Certain types of cancers observed in specific ethnic populations (e.g., individuals of Ashkenazi Jewish ancestry with breast and ovarian cancer)
- Recognized cancer syndromes such as hereditary nonpolyposis colorectal cancer or Lynch syndrome, which cause individuals to be at greater risk for developing gastrointestinal (GI), ovarian, uterine, brain, or skin cancer (NCI, 2010b)

Genetic counselors assist individuals and their families to evaluate their risk of hereditary predisposition, that is, testing positive for gene mutations.

Phases of Carcinogenesis

A **carcinogen** is a physical, chemical, or viral agent that induces cancer. **Carcinogenesis** is a biologic, multistage process that proceeds on a continuum in three distinct phases: initiation, promotion, and progression. **Initiation** involves transformation of cells produced by the interaction

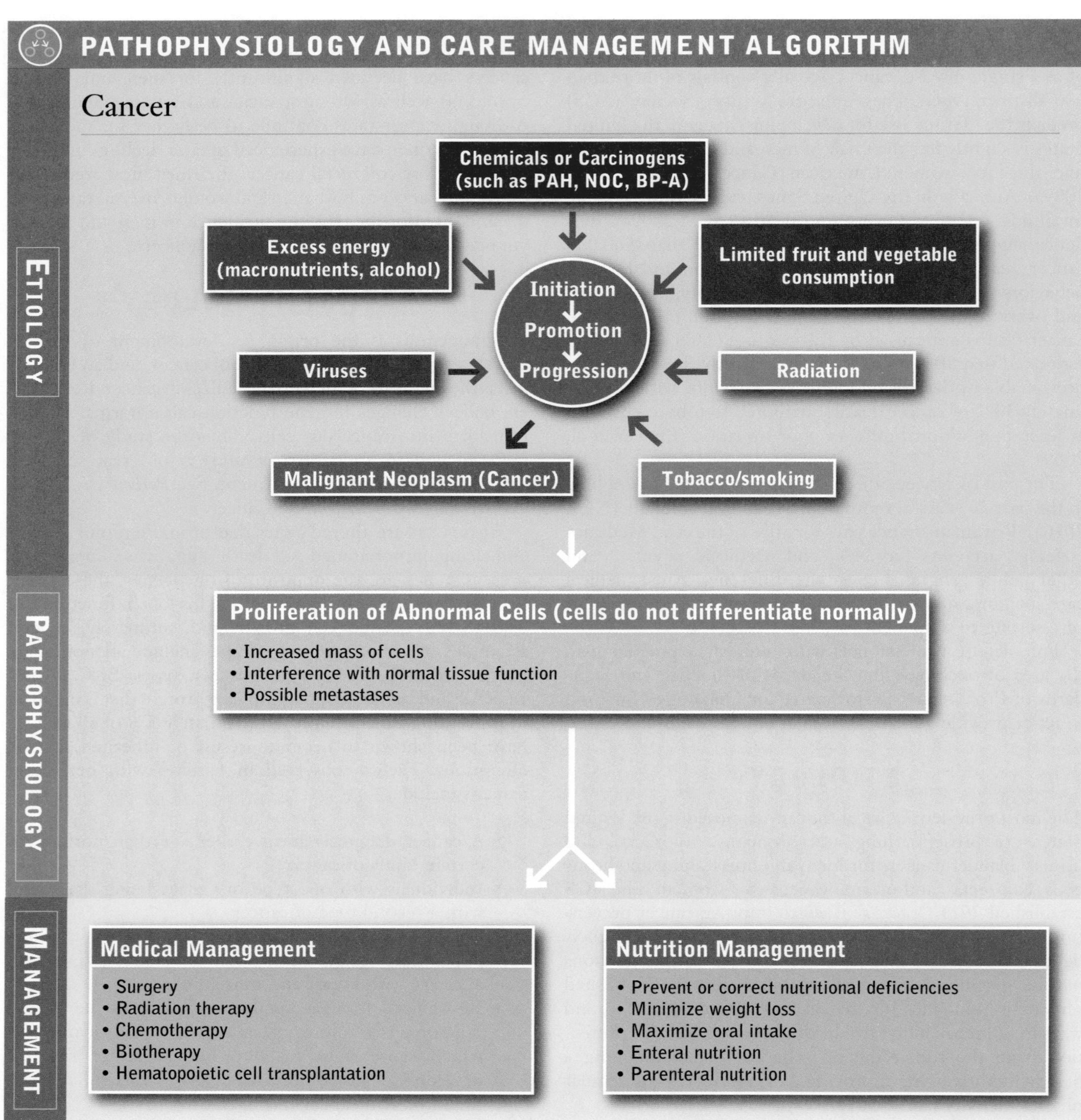

of chemicals, radiation, or viruses with cellular deoxyribonucleic acid (DNA). Transformation occurs rapidly, but cells can remain dormant for a variable period until they are activated by a promoting agent. After the initial cellular damage has occurred, transformation from normal cells to a detectable cancer can take many years or even decades. During **promotion**, initiated cells multiply and escape the mechanisms set in place to protect the body from the growth and spread of such cells. A **neoplasm**, new and abnormal tissue with no useful function, is established. In the third phase (**progression**), tumor cells aggregate and grow into a fully **malignant neoplasm** or a **tumor**.

In the process known as **metastasis**, the neoplasm has the capacity for tissue invasion that can spread to distant tissues and organs. For a cancer to metastasize, it must develop its own blood supply to sustain its growth of rapidly dividing abnormal cells. In normal cells, **angiogenesis** promotes the formation of new blood vessels that are essential to supply the body's tissues with oxygen and nutrients. In cancer cells, tumor angiogenesis occurs when tumors release substances that aid in the development of new blood vessels needed for their growth and metastasis.

NUTRITION AND CARCINOGENESIS

Nutrition may modify the carcinogenic process at any stage, including carcinogen metabolism, cellular and host defense, cell differentiation, and tumor growth. Gene expression can be promoted or altered by nutrients during pregnancy, childhood, and throughout a lifetime. Thus nutrition and diet contribute approximately 35% to causal factors for cancer (Greenwald et al., 2006). The strong influence of diet and nutrients is readily seen in studies of migration between cultures. Patterns of cancer occurrence often change over time to resemble that of the new country. For example, in Japan mortality from breast and colon cancer is low, and mortality from stomach cancer is high; the reverse is true among Japanese individuals living in the United States. After two or three generations, the cancer patterns become similar.

Studies looking at the role of nutrition and diet as causal factors of cancer seek to identify relationships between the diets of population groups and categories of individuals and the incidence of specific cancers. Sets of individuals are compared in case control, cohort, or cross-sectional studies. The strongest evidence comes from consistent findings of these different types of **epidemiologic studies** in diverse populations. In cancer research, epidemiologists look at human populations and evaluate how many people are diagnosed with cancer, what types of cancer occur in different populations and cultures, and what factors such as diet and lifestyle play a role in the development of the cancers.

The sheer complexity of diet presents a difficult challenge. There are literally thousands of chemicals in a normal diet; some are well known, and others are little known and unmeasured. Some naturally occurring dietary carcinogens are natural pesticides produced by plants for protection against fungi, insects, or animal predators, or mycotoxins that are secondary metabolites produced by molds in foods (e.g., aflatoxins, fumonisins, or ochratoxin). Food preparation and preservation methods may also provide dietary carcinogens. Thus diets contain both inhibitors and enhancers of carcinogenesis. Dietary carcinogen inhibitors include **antioxidants** (e.g., vitamin C, vitamin A and the carotenoids, vitamin E, selenium, zinc) and **phytochemicals**. See Table 37-1 and Table 12-5. Dietary enhancers of carcinogenesis may be the fat in red meat or the polycyclic aromatic hydrocarbons (PAHs) that form with the grilling of meat at high heat. Complicating the study of nutrition, diet, and cancer is the fact that when one major component of the diet is altered, other changes take place simultaneously. For example, decreasing animal protein also decreases animal fat. This makes the interpretation of research findings difficult because the effects cannot be clearly associated with a single factor.

Cancer cells can have a long latency or dormant period. This makes the diet at the time of cancer cell initiation or promotion—not at the time of diagnosis—most important. Some prospective epidemiologic studies attempt to deal with this challenge by measuring diet at one point in time and following the same subjects for several years. Studies done with laboratory animals test this effect, and since the early part of the last century, laboratory scientists have shown that various nutritional manipulations influence the occurrence of cancerous tumors in animals. Epidemiologic research, together with animal studies, provide a viable method for discovering the links between nutrition and cancer in humans.

Alcohol

Alcohol consumption is associated with increased cancer risk for cancers of the mouth, pharynx, larynx, esophagus, lung, colon, rectum, liver, and breast (both pre- and postmenopausal women) (World Cancer Research Fund [WCRF] and American Institute for Cancer Research [AICR], 2007). For cancers of the mouth, pharynx, larynx, and esophagus, daily consumption of two to three drinks

TABLE 37-1

Cancer-Protective Phytochemicals in Vegetables and Fruits

Color	Phytochemical	Vegetables and Fruits
Red	Lycopene	Tomatoes and tomato products, pink grapefruit, watermelon
Red and purple	Anthocyanins, polyphenols	Berries, grapes, red wine, plums
Orange	α- and β-carotene	Carrots, mangos, pumpkin
Orange and yellow	β-cryptoxanthin, flavonoids	Cantaloupe, peaches, oranges, papaya, nectarines
Yellow and green	Lutein, zeaxanthin	Spinach, avocado, honeydew, collard and turnip greens
Green	Sulforaphanes, indoles	Cabbage, broccoli, Brussels sprouts, cauliflower
White and green	Allyl sulphides	Leeks, onion, garlic, chives

increases risk two to three times compared with nondrinkers. When combined with tobacco use, the sum total risk is higher than the risk for just alcohol or tobacco alone, again compared with nondrinkers (Baan et al., 2007; WCRF and AICR, 2007). In addition, malnutrition associated with alcoholism is also likely to be important in the increased risk for certain cancers. In the United States, if people choose to drink, men are recommended to limit alcohol intake to two drinks per day and women to one drink per day. Serving sizes of popular alcoholic drinks include beer (12 oz), wine (5 oz), spirits/liquors (1.5 oz of 80-proof spirits). Three to four alcoholic drinks or more per week after breast cancer diagnosis may increase recurrence risk, especially among postmenopausal and overweight or obese women (Kwan, 2010).

Energy Intake and Body Weight

In animal studies chronic restriction of food inhibited the growth of most experimentally induced cancers and the occurrence of many spontaneous cancers. This effect was observed even when underfed animals ingested more dietary fat than control animals ingested. Caloric restriction, without malnutrition, appears to have a positive effect on cancer prevention in animals; it is unclear whether that effect translates to humans (Longo et al., 2010).

Obesity is a risk factor for cancer and may account for 6% of all cancers (Polednak, 2008). Currently 68% of all American adults are overweight or obese (Flegal et al., 2010). See Chapter 22. Obesity increases the risk for developing and dying from cancer (Schelbert, 2009). The relationship between body weight, body mass index (BMI), or relative body weight and site-specific cancer has been widely investigated; a positive association has been seen with cancers of the esophagus, pancreas, gallbladder, liver, breast (postmenopausal), endometrium, kidney, colon, and rectum (Toles et al., 2008; WCRF and AICR, 2007). For men, increased BMI correlates with esophageal, thyroid, colon, and kidney cancers; a weaker association exists between BMI and malignant melanoma, multiple myeloma, rectal cancer, leukemia, and non-Hodgkin's lymphoma (NHL) (Brawer et al., 2009). In women, stronger correlations are found between increased BMI and endometrium, gallbladder, kidney, and esophageal cancers; and a weaker association between increased BMI and leukemia, thyroid, postmenopausal breast, pancreas, and colon cancers and NHL. Bariatric surgery using gastric bypass may reduce cancer mortality by as much as 60% (Brawer et al., 2009).

The median adult BMI should be between 21 and 23 depending on the normal range with different populations (WCRF and AICR, 2007). Body weight throughout childhood should be at the lower end of normal BMI, because excessive weight in adolescence has been correlated with twofold increased risk of death for colon cancer in adulthood (Anderson et al., 2009). Being overweight or obese also appears to increase risk of cancer recurrence and decrease cancer survival (Anderson et al., 2009).

Obesity, age, hyperglycemia, and the incidence of metabolic syndrome play a role in the circulating levels of insulin-like growth factor-1 (IGF-1), a potentially cancer-causing compound. IGF-1 is a polypeptide secreted primarily by the liver and plays a key role in normal growth and development. It can promote the development and progression of prostate, breast, lung, and colon cancer. It has been hypothesized to stimulate the growth of cancer cells and inhibit their death (Blackburn, 2007; Pollack, 2008). IGF-1 secretion is increased when insulin levels are elevated. Obesity and high simple carbohydrate intakes potentially increase insulin resistance and raise circulating insulin levels. This area of research connects several known risk factors between nutrition, diet, and cancer (Parekh et al., 2010).

Overweight and obese cancer survivors are at risk for recurrence and for developing additional problems after surgery, including impaired wound healing, lymphedema following lymph node dissections, second cancers, heart disease, and diabetes mellitus (Anderson et al., 2009). Regular physical activity reduces mortality, especially in women and older individuals (Teucher, 2010). All types of physical activity help to protect against colon cancer, postmenopausal breast cancer, and endometrial cancer (Teucher, 2010). Therefore the ACS encourages all Americans to strive for 45-60 minutes of moderate to vigorous physical activity most days of the week (Doyle et al., 2006). Achieving and maintaining a reasonable weight should be a primary health goal for all cancer survivors (Doyle et al., 2006).

Fat

Research shows a link between some types of cancers and the amount of fat in the diet. Diets high in fat often contain significant amounts of meat. The link between meat and colorectal cancer risk results from a number of possible mechanisms: production of carcinogens from a high-fat diet, from heterocyclic amines (HCAs) and or polycyclic aromatic hydrocarbons (PAHs) from cooking; formation of carcinogenic **N-nitroso compounds (NOCs)** from processing and the influence of heme-iron are also suspected (WCRF and AICR, 2007).

Diets high in fat also tend to be high in calories, and contribute to overweight and obesity conditions. Because dietary fat intake is correlated with intake of other nutrients and dietary components, it is difficult to distinguish between the effects of dietary fats and protein, total calories, and fiber. Saturated fat in red meats may be associated with an increased risk of colorectal, endometrial, and possibly lymphoid and hematologic cancers (Ferguson, 2010; WCRF and AICR, 2007). Two large prospective randomized studies in the area of diet and breast cancer survival showed mixed results. The Women's Intervention Nutrition Study (WINS) found that an intervention that reduced dietary fat to 20% of total calories and caused a modest reduction in body weight may favorably influence breast cancer prognosis. However, the Women's Healthy Eating and Living (WHEL) study, which was very high in vegetables, fruit, and fiber and low in fat, demonstrated no significant survival benefit (Pierce et al., 2007).

Eating more ω-3 fatty acids (foods such as fatty fish, flaxseed oil, walnuts, certain algae) in relation to ω-6 fatty acids (polyunsaturated fats like corn oil, safflower oil, and sunflower oil) may potentially reduce risk of colon and prostate cancers (Berquin et al., 2008). Fish is a healthier protein selection than red meat, is lower in fat, and is a potentially rich source of ω-3 fatty acids. If choosing red meat, it is recommended to select leaner cuts and smaller portions. Poultry or legumes are also desirable alternatives to beef, veal, pork, and lamb.

Fiber, Carbohydrates, and Glycemic Index

Higher-fiber foods such as complex carbohydrates and whole grains are an important part of a healthy diet. The intake of dietary fiber can influence the intake of meat, dietary fat, and simple carbohydrates. Unfortunately, the studies on dietary fiber and cancer have been inconsistent, so dietary fiber was not included in the oncology section of the Evidence Analysis Library of the American Dietetic Association (American Dietetic Association [ADA], 2010a). Epidemiologic studies looking at the possible relationship between dietary fiber and large-bowel cancer showed no effect of a low-fat, high-fiber, high-fruits, and high-vegetables diet on adenoma recurrence years after randomization (ADA, 2008.) Dietary fiber may play a role in preventing breast cancer through nonestrogen pathways among postmenopausal women, but more research needs to be done (Park et al., 2009). However, fiber-rich fruits and vegetables are excellent sources of vitamins, minerals, and phytochemicals. Legumes and lentils have both fiber and additional nutrients worth consuming.

Nonnutritive and Nutritive Sweeteners

The Food and Drug Administration (FDA) has approved five nonnutritive sweeteners (acesulfame-K, aspartame, neotame, saccharin, and sucralose) for use in the food supply, and regulates them as food additives. They appear to be safe when used in moderation. Described as "high-intensity" sweeteners, nonnutritive sweeteners provide little or no energy because they sweeten in minute amounts. Nonnutritive sweeteners have been investigated primarily in relation to potential adverse health concerns, including long-term safety and carcinogenicity, but multiple studies during the past 20 years have indicated that when consumed in reasonable amounts, they are safe. Newer sugar substitutes on the market include Stevia, sugar alcohols (e.g., mannitol, sorbitol, xylitol), and blue agave. Stevia, a nonnutritive sweetener, is considered a dietary supplement but has approval from the FDA. Sugar alcohols are not considered nonnutritive sweeteners even though they are used in a similar way. Blue agave is the juice from the *Agave tequiliana* plant; the jury is still out on this sweetening option.

Protein

Most diets that contain significant amounts of protein also contain significant amounts of meat and fat, and insignificant amounts of fiber. The effect of protein on carcinogenesis depends on the tissue of origin and the type of tumor, as well as on the type of protein and the calorie content of the diet. In general, tumor development is suppressed by diets that contain levels of protein below that required for optimal growth and development; whereas it is enhanced by protein levels two to three times the amount that is required. The effects may be attributable to specific amino acids, a general effect of protein, or, in the case of low-protein diets, depressed food intake. Epidemiologic studies have found limited and conflicting results. Recommendations for lowering cancer risk and improving overall health encourage intake of plant foods and limiting foods from animal sources, including red meat and processed meats and poultry (WCRF and AICR, 2007).

Smoked, Grilled, and Preserved Foods

Nitrates are added as preservatives to processed meats. Nitrates can be readily reduced to form nitrites, which in turn can interact with dietary substrates such as amines and amides to produce N-nitroso compounds (NOCs): nitrosamines and nitrosamides, which are known mutagens and carcinogens. Nitrates or nitrites are used in smoked, salted, and pickled foods. Sodium and potassium nitrates are present in a variety of foods, and give hot dogs and processed deli meats their pink color, but the main dietary sources are vegetables and drinking water.

NOCs are also produced endogenously in the stomach and colon of people who eat large amounts of red meat. Studies looking at the detrimental effects of smoked foods have not demonstrated a clear, consistent connection between these foods and stomach cancer (WCRF and AICR, 2007). Diets with high amounts of fruits and vegetables that contain vitamin C and phytochemicals that can retard the conversion of nitrites to NOCs should be encouraged (Kushi et al., 2006).

Charring or cooking meat at high temperatures over an open flame (400° F or more) can cause the formation of polycyclic aromatic hydrocarbons (PAHs) and heterocyclic amines. PAHs have shown clear indications of mutagenicity and carcinogenicity. Normal roasting or frying food does not produce large amounts of PAHs compared with the amount produced when cooking over open flames. Animal proteins that produce the greatest dripping of fat on to the flames register the highest PAH formation. For example, grilled beef produces larger amounts of PAHs than grilled chicken, which produces higher amounts than oven-grilled chicken. The source of the flame can also influence PAH production; charcoal grilling promotes the most, followed by flame gas, and finally oven grilling (Farhadian et al., 2010).

Toxic Environments

The Environmental Protection Agency (EPA) was established in 1970, for the purpose of overseeing the acute and long-term health threats caused by substances in the environment. As part of this protection, the Toxic Substances Control Act passed in 1976 required manufacturers to submit health and safety information on all new chemicals. However, many were grandfathered in with the passage of this law and are still untested.

Everyday activities expose people to a myriad of chemicals through the air, and water, food, and beverages. In fact, 740 cancers per million people are estimated to be caused by these very common exposures (Chey, 2008). Health care practitioners grapple with assessing exposure to so many different agents. A good environmental history can be performed at clinical visits and then quickly reviewed for outdoor air pollutants such as nitrogen dioxide, ozone, and carbon monoxide which pose health risks. Exposure to heavy metals, pesticides, herbicides, and occupational exposures may also be noted. In addition to determining the patient's environmental exposure, practitioners must also determine exposure of family members or others living in the same household. Oxidative stress caused by these environmental exposures can be alleviated by changes in lifestyle, including smoking and diet. High intakes of antioxidant-rich foods and a nutrient-rich diet (not supplementation) is suggested (Kushi et al., 2006).

Toxicity from Bisphenol A

Bisphenol A (BPA) is an industrial chemical used since the 1960s in the manufacturing of many hard plastic bottles and the epoxy linings of metal-based food and beverage cans. It is also an ingredient in the production of epoxy resin used in paints and adhesives. Studies done when the product was developed indicated it was safe to use in food and beverage containers. However, recent studies employing novel approaches to test for subtle effects raised health concerns especially in developing fetuses, infants, and children (Layton, 2010). The National Toxicology Program at the National Institutes of Health (NIH) and the FDA are responding to growing evidence that BPA might increase the risk for cancer (FDA, 2010).

The shift in opinion likely resulted from a change in organizations evaluating the safety and the evaluative tools used (Beronius, 2010). The current goal is to reduce the use and exposure to BPA through several actions: encouraging the production of BPA-free baby bottles, using alternatives to the glue used in food containers, and increasing the oversight on the use of BPA in manufacturing and testing. The U.S. Department of Health and Human Services (USDHHS) supports eliminating it from infant and all food-related product production. Originally it was thought to leach from the plastic only when exposed to heat; now it is believed to leach even with cold temperatures. Exposure to BPA is so widespread in the food and beverage supply that it is estimated that 90% of Americans have traces of it in their urine (Layton, 2010).

NUTRIENTS FOR CANCER PREVENTION

Eating behaviors play a very important role in health promotion and disease prevention. **Chemoprevention** involves specific compounds or drugs used to prevent, delay, or retard the development of cancer (Kashfi, 2009). Nonsteroidal antiinflammatory drugs may protect against colon cancer. Other natural products currently being investigated include the hundreds of polyphenols in fruits and vegetables, green tea, curcumin from curry, and resveratrol from grapes and berries. Phenolic acid, flavonoids, stilbenes, and lignans are the most abundant polyphenols; the chemopreventive potential of these compounds comes from their ability to modulate epigenetic alterations in cancer cells. The epigenetic modification step occurs early in the development of a cancer cell, at a time when it is potentially reversible. Scientists are not completely clear how this process works. Yet it is reasonable to recommend a health-promoting diet rich in fruits, vegetables, soy, therapeutic culinary herbs such as turmeric and cinnamon, green tea, and coffee (Link et al., 2010). For this reason, health organizations have diet and lifestyle recommendations to reduce cancer risk. See Box 37-1.

BOX 37-1

Cancer Prevention Recommendations

American Cancer Society

1. Adopt a physically active lifestyle. Adults should engage in at least 30 minutes of moderate to vigorous physical activity, above usual activities, on 5 or more days of the week and 45 to 60 minutes of intentional activity at least 5 days per week.
2. Achieve and maintain a healthy body weight throughout life.
3. Eat a variety of healthful, colorful foods, with an emphasis on plant sources.
4. Limit consumption of alcohol.

American Institute for Cancer Research

Body Fatness: Be as lean as possible within the normal range of body weight.

Physical Activity: Be physically active as part of everyday life.

Foods and Drinks that Promote Weight Gain: Limit consumption of energy-dense foods. Avoid sugary drinks.

Plant Foods: Eat mostly foods of plant origin.

Animal Foods: Limit intake of red meat and avoid processed meat.

Alcoholic Beverages: Limit alcoholic beverages.

Preservation, Processing, Preparation: Limit consumption of salt. Avoid moldy cereals (grains) or pulses (legumes).

Dietary Supplements: Aim to meet nutritional needs through diet alone.

Breastfeeding: Mothers to breastfeed; children to be breastfed.

Cancer Survivors: Follow the same recommendations.

Data from Kushi LH et al: American Cancer Society guidelines on nutrition and physical activity for cancer prevention: reducing the risk of cancer with healthy food choices and physical activity, CA Cancer J Clin 56:310, 2006; World Cancer Research Fund (WCRF), American Institute for Cancer Research (AIRC): Food, nutrition, physical activity, and the prevention of cancer: a global perspective, Washington, DC, 2007, WCRF and AIRC.

Calcium and Vitamin D

Calcium supplementation and dairy, especially milk, may be associated with lower colorectal cancer risk. However, other studies suggest an increased risk for aggressive forms of prostate cancer with significant dairy intake or calcium supplementation (Chung et al., 2009; Huncharek et al., 2009). The relationships need to be explored further before clear recommendations can be made.

Vitamin D deficiencies are being detected in all age groups prompting exploration of the role of vitamin D in cancer prevention. For years, public health messages have encouraged use of sun screens and less direct exposure to the sun. Because of this there is reduced conversion of vitamin D on the skin surface and this may be responsible for the increase in deficiencies. Studies have reported that higher serum 25-hydroxyvitamin D (25 (OH) D) levels are associated with lower incidence rates of colon, breast, ovarian, renal, pancreatic, aggressive prostate, and others cancers. Until more is learned about the interaction between vitamin D_3 and cancer prevention, taking 2000 IU of vitamin D per day to achieve serum 25(OH)D levels of 40-60 ng/mL is considered safe (Garland, 2009; Garland et al, 2011).

Coffee and Tea

Coffee contains various antioxidant and phenolic compounds, some of which have been shown to have anticancer properties. Coffee also contains caffeine, a compound in the alkaloid phytochemical family. Coffee as a major source of antioxidants in the American diet may have a protective effect against cancer.

Tea is also a good source of phenols and antioxidants. Green tea is made from leaves that have been cooked, pressed, dried and not roasted, and because of this green tea, more so than black tea contains catechins that possess biologic activity with antioxidant, antiangiogenesis, and antiproliferative properties that are relevant to cancer prevention (Kuzuhara, 2008).

Folate and Folic Acid

Folate, from foods, affects DNA methylation, synthesis, and repair. Folate-associated one-carbon metabolism may play an important role in colorectal carcinogenesis because of gene variations. (Levine et al., 2010). Several epidemiologic studies suggest that higher folate intake is also associated with decreased pancreatic cancer risk (Oaks et al., 2010). However, excessive folate may also contribute to deleterious effects in certain cancers (Bailey et al., 2010). More research is needed to evaluate variables such as genetic polymorphisms, and folate from food versus folic acid from supplements.

Fruits and Vegetables

Fruit intake is protective against cancers of the mouth, pharynx, larynx, esophagus, cervix, lung and stomach (WCRF and AICR, 2007). Health benefits from vegetables are more difficult to quantify. Nonstarchy vegetables such as spinach, tomatoes, and peppers probably provide protection against mouth, pharynx, larynx, and esophageal cancers; all vegetables, but particularly green and yellow ones, probably protect against stomach cancer (WCRF and AICR, 2007). Most countries have recommendations for the consumption of vegetables and fruits that vary, but generally are for three or more servings of vegetables and two or more servings of fruit daily with a serving being approximately 80 g or ½ cup (WCRF and AICR, 2007).

Anticarcinogenic agents found in fruits and vegetables include antioxidants such as vitamins C and E, selenium, and phytochemicals. Phytochemicals include carotenoids, flavonoids, isoflavones, lignans, organosulfides, phenolic compounds, and monoterpenes. It is still unclear which specific substances of fruits and vegetables are the most protective against cancer (Russo, 2007). These substances have both complementary and overlapping mechanisms, including the induction of detoxification enzymes, inhibition of nitrosamine formation, provision of substrate for formation of chemotherapy agents, dilution and binding of carcinogens in the digestive tract, alteration of hormone metabolism, and antioxidant effects. It appears extremely unlikely that any one substance is responsible for all of the observed associations. See Table 12-5 and Table 37-1 for discussion of chemoprotective agents in fruits and vegetables.

Soy and Phytoestrogens

Soy is a plant-based protein, and it contains phytoestrogens (very weak plant-based estrogens) and isoflavones such as genistein and daidzein. Diets containing modest amounts of soy protect against breast cancer (Lee et al., 2010,) especially if the soy foods have been consumed before reaching adulthood apparently due to exposure to the weak estrogenic effects of isoflavones early in life (Lee et al., 2010). However, the use of soy remains controversial for women already diagnosed with hormone-sensitive cancers (e.g., breast, endometrium) and for postmenopausal women.

Commercially prepared soy supplement powders and foods made from soy products can, but may not always contain isoflavones at much higher concentrations than traditional whole soy foods such as edamame beans, tofu, or soy milk (Gardner et al., 2008; U.S. Department of Agriculture (USDA), 2010). The ACS advises breast cancer survivors to limit the consumption of soy foods to no more than three servings daily, and to avoid using prepared soy supplement powders and products (Doyle et al., 2006). Unlike the advice for women, men with hormone-sensitive cancer such as prostate cancer may benefit from regular consumption of soy foods. Prostate cancer is a testosterone driven cancer and estrogens (or phytoestrogens) are agonists.

MEDICAL DIAGNOSIS AND STAGING OF CANCER

Assessing symptoms of cancer at the earliest stage is critical for treatment effectiveness and survival. Table 37-2 summarizes constitutional or systemic symptoms of cancer and metastatic disease. Many symptoms of early or metastatic cancer affect an individual's ability to eat, digest, or absorb. According to the ACS, the following early warning signs and symptoms of cancer are described using the acronym "CAUTION"

Change in bowel or bladder habits
A sore that does not heal
Unusual bleeding or discharge
Thickening or lump in breast or elsewhere
Indigestion or difficulty in swallowing or chewing
Obvious change in a wart or mole
Nagging cough or hoarseness

TABLE 37-2

Signs and Symptoms of Cancer

Constitutional Symptoms of Cancer	Signs and Symptoms of Metastatic Cancer
Anorexia	Pain
Fatigue	Enlarged lymph nodes or body organs
Weight loss	Cough with or without hemoptysis
Fever	Bone pain with or without fracture
Sweating	Neurological symptoms
Anemia	

Data from National Cancer Institute (NCI): Dictionary of terms, 2010d. Accessed 23 October 2010 from http://www.cancer.gov/dictionary/.

When symptoms or screening tests suggest cancer, physicians use the following to establish a definitive diagnosis: evaluation of an individual's medical, social and family histories, physical examination, laboratory tests, imaging procedures, and tissue biopsy. Laboratory evaluation is composed of analysis of blood, urine, and other body fluids. In particular, oncologists evaluate **tumor markers** (e.g., α-fetoprotein [AFP], cancer antigen [CA] 125, CA 19-9, carcinoembryonic antigen [CEA], prostate-specific antigen [PSA]) and other substances in blood or body fluids that can be elevated in cancer. Imaging procedures and studies help determine a diagnosis (Table 37-3). Pathologists perform cytologic examinations by analyzing body fluids, sputum, urine, or tissue under a microscope. To detect malignant cells, they use a histopathologic examination to review specially stained tissue, flow cytometry to count and examine cells and chromosomes, immunohistochemistry to review antibodies for specific cell proteins, and cytogenetics to visualize genetic defects.

Oxidative damage to lipids in cellular membranes, proteins, and DNA is often permanent. Thus biomarkers may be used to estimate the DNA damage after exposure to cancer-causing agents such as tobacco smoke, asbestos fibers, heavy metals, and PAHs. 8-hydroxy-2′-deoxyguanosine (8-OHdG) is a new biomarker for the measurement of endogenous oxidative DNA damage and risk for cancer (Valavanidis et al., 2009). See Table 8-5 in Chapter 8.

Staging is used to identify how much a cancer has spread throughout the body. The stage of the cancer at the time of diagnosis is a strong predictor of survival and it directs

TABLE 37-3

Imaging Studies for Cancer Diagnosis and Disease Monitoring

Type of Imaging	Description and Use in Cancer Diagnosis and Treatment
CT Scan	**Description:** A CT scan is a radiographic procedure in which a series of detailed pictures of areas inside the body are taken from different angles. Images are created by a computer and are linked to an x-ray machine. **Use:** A CT scan is used to evaluate for abnormalities of possible cancer in a general anatomic area such as the head, chest, abdomen, or pelvis. Radiologists use CT scans to visualize suspicious lesions, internal organs, and lymph nodes.
MRI Scan	**Description:** An MRI scan is an imaging procedure that uses radio waves and a powerful magnet linked to a computer to create detailed pictures of areas inside the body. This type of scanning often creates better images of body organs and soft tissue than other type of scanning methods. **Use:** Images produced show differences between normal and cancerous tissue. In particular, an MRI scan is used to evaluate suspicious areas of the brain, spinal cord, and liver.
PET Scan	**Description:** A PET scan is a procedure in which a small amount of radioactive glucose is injected into a vein and a scanner is used to make detailed, computerized pictures of areas where glucose is used in the body. **Use:** Cancerous cells have an enhanced rate of glycolysis (they use more glucose than normal cells). Areas of glucose metabolism with high activity or "hot spots" appearing on the PET scan generally correlate to findings of cancer.

Data from American Cancer Society: Cancer glossary, 2010a. Accessed 10 June 2010 from http://www.cancer.org/CancerGlossary/index; National Cancer Institute (NCI): *Dictionary of terms,* 2010d. Accessed 23 October 2010 from http://www.cancer.gov/dictionary/.

CT, Computed tomography; *MRI,* magnetic resonance imaging; *PET,* positron emission tomography.

oncologists to the most effective treatment plan. Cancer staging is most frequently described as stage I, II, III, or IV—stage I being the least amount of disease and stage IV being the most advanced. The **tumor-node-metastasis (TNM) staging system** is also commonly used by oncologists. *T* stands for the size of the tumor, *N* stands for nodes or whether it has spread into lymph nodes, and *M* stands for metastasis, or whether the cancer has spread to distant organs.

For **classification**, tumors are often referred to as *solid* cancers, and hematologic-related cancers of the blood are frequently called *liquid* cancers. The classification of tumors is based on their tissue of origin, their growth properties, and their invasion of other tissues. Tumors that are not malignant are typically described as *benign*.

Because cancer occurs in cells that are replicating, the patterns of cancer are quite different in children and adults. In early life the brain, nervous system, bones, muscles, and connective tissues are still growing; therefore cancers involving these tissues are more prevalent in children than in adults. Common childhood cancers include neuroblastoma; medulloblastoma; osteosarcoma; and soft tissue sarcomas such as rhabdomyosarcoma, schwannoma, and germ cell tumors. Conversely, adult cancers frequently involve epithelial tissues that cover and line the body's internal and external surfaces. Cancers of the epithelial tissues include cancers of the skin, and circulatory, digestive, endocrine, reproductive, respiratory, and urinary systems. Cancers arising from these tissues are referred to as *carcinomas* and common types are classified as *adenocarcinomas*, *basal cell carcinomas*, *papillomas*, and *squamous cell carcinomas*.

Leukemias, lymphomas, and myelomas are cancers of the immune system and can occur in either children or adults. Leukemias arise most frequently from white blood cells of the bone marrow. Lymphomas are cancers that develop in the lymphatic system—its nodes, glands, and organs. Myeloma is cancer that originates in the plasma cells of the bone marrow and most frequently occurs in older adults.

Other types of cancer are related to infectious causes and cancer experts recommend antibiotics, vaccines, and changes in behavior for their prevention (ACS, 2009a). Examples include hepatocellular carcinoma linked to hepatitis B virus (HBV) exposure and alcoholic-related cirrhosis, oropharyngeal and cervical cancer incidence linked to human papillomavirus infection (HPV), and stomach cancer caused by chronic inflammation by *Helicobacter pylori*. See Chapter 28.

MEDICAL TREATMENT

Cancer treatment in the United States and in more than 115 countries is guided by evidence-based standards known as the *National Comprehensive Cancer Network (NCCN) Clinical Practice Guidelines in Oncology* (2010). The NCCN Guidelines encompass evidenced-based care for 97% of all cancers treated in oncology practice. Also listed with these guidelines are evidence-based recommendations for providing supportive care (e.g., management for cancer and cancer treatment–related pain, fatigue, and nausea).

Conventional modalities include antineoplastic therapy (e.g., chemotherapy, biotherapy, antiangiogenic agents, or hormonal agents), radiation therapy, and surgery used alone or in combination with other cancer therapies. Solid tumors and hematologic malignant diseases such as leukemias, lymphomas, and multiple myelomas may be treated with **hematopoietic cell transplantation (HCT)**.

Chemotherapy is the use of chemical agents or medications to systematically treat cancer. Biotherapy is the use of biologic agents to produce anticancer effects indirectly by inducing, enhancing, or suppressing an individual's own immune response. Antiangiogenic agents are used to inhibit the development of new blood vessels needed by cancers (tumor vasculature) and thus prevent their growth, invasion, and spread. Hormonal therapy is systemic therapy used for the treatment of hormone-sensitive cancers (e.g., breast, ovarian, prostate) by blocking or reducing the source of a hormone or its receptor site.

Radiation oncologists work in the area of therapeutic **radiation therapy**, which uses high-energy (ionizing radiation) in multiple fractionated doses, or radioactive chemicals to treat cancer. Surgery involves the surgical removal of cancerous tissue.

Response to cancer treatment is defined as *complete* or *partial response* (improvement), *stable disease* (same), or *disease progression* (worsening). Factors that affect an individual's response to treatment include **tumor burden** (the larger the tumor, the greater risk of metastatic disease), **rate of tumor growth** (rapidly growing tumors are usually more responsive to therapy), and **drug resistance** (tumors mutate as they grow, and with successive mutations new cancer cells become more likely to be resistant to therapy). Other factors contributing to an individual's response to cancer treatment include comorbid diseases (e.g., diabetes, renal disease, cardiopulmonary disease), age, performance status, support system, bone marrow reserve, and overall general health (NCI, 2010d; Polovich et al., 2009).

Goals of Treatment

The goal of cancer treatment may be to cure, control, or palliate. **Cure** is a complete response to treatment. Even if a treatment cannot cure a cancer, often there can be cancer **control** that extends life when a cure is not possible. Control measures may obscure microscopic metastases after tumors are surgically removed, reduce the size of tumors before surgery or radiation therapy, or alleviate symptoms and side effects of cancer. If a cancer cannot be cured or controlled, **palliative care** is offered. Palliative care helps individuals be as comfortable as possible. Palliation is designed to relieve pain and manage symptoms of illness; lessen isolation, anxiety and fear; and help maintain independence as long as possible (National Hospice and Palliative Care Organization [NHPCO], 2010). **Hospice** is care for individuals with a life expectancy of months and focuses on relieving symptoms, controlling pain, and providing support to patients and their families. Patients are made as comfortable as possible through the end of their lives.

MEDICAL NUTRITION THERAPY

Dietetic professionals should use the nutrition care process steps when providing medical nutrition therapy (MNT) (ADA, 2011). To further assist clinicians working in the cancer care setting the American Dietetic Association has developed the *Oncology Toolkit* with MNT protocols for breast, colorectal, esophageal, gastric, head and neck, hematologic, lung, and pancreatic cancers (ADA, 2010b). It also includes instructional and documentation forms using the nutrition care process (NCP) and standardized language to help individualize nutrition care with recommendations based on the current state of science.

Nutrition Screening and Assessment

With the recent shift of cancer care from the hospital setting to outpatient settings, nutrition screening and assessment should continue throughout the continuum of care. Ideally, nutrition screening and assessment for risk of nutrition problems should be interdisciplinary, instituted at the time of diagnosis, and reevaluated and monitored throughout treatment and recovery. The patient-generated Subjective Global Assessment has been adapted for use with cancer patients and incorporates sections completed by the patient or caregiver on weight history, food intake, symptoms, and functioning. Sections completed by a health care member (e.g., physician, nurse, registered dietitian, social worker) evaluate weight loss, disease, metabolic stress, and include a nutrition-focused physical examination. Nutritional risk and intervention are then determined by a scoring system (Charney and Cranganu, 2010).

Other tools are the Activities of Daily Living (ADL) tool, the Common Toxicity Criteria (CTC), and the Karnofsky Performance Scale (KPS) Index. The ADL tool assesses routine activities that people do each day without assistance such as bathing, dressing, and walking. CTC is an outcome measure used in cancer centers that compares acute toxicities of cancer treatment, and KPS is a scoring index that associates an individual's functional status with disease status and survival (McCallum, 2006).

In-depth assessment is undertaken to obtain more information and to identify nutrition problems. Careful review of the individual's appetite and oral intake is required, with an assessment of symptoms (e.g., nausea, vomiting, and diarrhea), weight status, comorbidities, and laboratory studies. A nutrition-focused physical examination is recommended to fully evaluate nutrition status and degree of risk (Fuhrman, 2009). Components of this type of assessment include a general survey of the body, review of vital signs and anthropometrics, and an evaluation of subcutaneous fat stores, muscle mass, and fluid status.

Energy

Determining individualized energy needs is vital to helping people maintain their weight and prevent weight loss associated with cancer. Methods used to estimate energy requirements for adults include using standardized equations or measuring resting metabolic rate using indirect calorimetry (Russell and Malone, 2009). See Chapter 2 for methods for determining energy requirements such as the Mifflin-St. Jeor and Ireton-Jones equations. To ensure that adequate energy is being provided. the individual's diagnosis, presence of other diseases, intent of treatment (e.g., curative, control, or palliation), anticancer therapies (e.g., surgery, chemotherapy, biotherapy, or radiation therapy), presence of fever or infection, and other metabolic complications need consideration. Established guidelines for quickly estimating energy needs of people with cancer based on body weight are shown in Table 37-4.

TABLE 37-4

Estimating Energy Needs of People with Cancer

Condition	Energy Needs
Cancer, nutritional repletion, weight gain	30-40 kcal/kg/day
Cancer, normometabolic	25-30 kcal/kg/day
Cancer, hypermetabolic, stressed	35 kcal/kg/day
Hematopoietic cell transplant	30-35 kcal/kg/day
Sepsis	25-30 kcal/kg/day
Obese	21-25 kcal/kg/day

Data from Gottschlich MM, editor: The A.S.P.E.N. nutrition support core curriculum: a case-based approach—the adult patient. Silver Spring, MD, 2007, American Society for Parenteral and Enteral Nutrition; Hurst JD, Gallagher AL: Energy, protein, micronutrient, and fluid requirement. In Elliott L et al., editors: The clinical guide to oncology nutrition, ed 2, Chicago, 2006, American Dietetic Association.

Protein

An individual's need for protein is increased during times of illness and stress. Additional protein is required by the body to repair and rebuild tissues affected by cancer therapy, and to maintain a healthy immune system (Hurst and Gallagher, 2006). Adequate energy should be provided, or the body will use its lean body mass as a fuel source. When determining protein requirements, dietetic professionals need to consider the degree of malnutrition, extent of disease, degree of stress, and ability to metabolize and use protein (Russell and Malone, 2009). For example, a cancer patient with a hematopoietic cell transplant may require 1.5-2 g/kg/day. A patient with severe stress may need 1.5-2.5 g/kg/day. Daily protein requirements are generally calculated using actual body weight.

Fluid

Fluid management in cancer care must ensure adequate hydration and electrolyte balance, and prevent dehydration and hypovolemia. Altered fluid balance may occur with fever, ascites, edema, fistulas, profuse vomiting or diarrhea, multiple concurrent intravenous (IV) therapies, impaired renal function, or medications such as diuretics. Individuals need close monitoring for dehydration (e.g., intracellular fluid losses caused by inadequate intake of fluid because of mucositis or anorexia) and hypovolemia (e.g., extracellular fluid losses from fever or GI fluids such as vomiting, diarrhea or malabsorption). Signs and symptoms of dehydration include fatigue, acute weight loss, hypernatremia, poor skin turgor, dry oral mucosa, dark or strong smelling urine, and decreased urine output. To carefully assess for hypovolemia, levels of serum electrolytes, blood urea nitrogen and creatinine should also be evaluated. A general guideline for estimating fluid needs for all adults without renal concerns is 30-35 mL/kg/day (Hurst and Gallagher, 2006). Another guideline is 1 mL fluid per 1 kcal of estimated calorie needs (Russell and Malone, 2009). In some instances, individuals undergoing cancer therapy may require IV fluid hydration to meet their treatment-related fluid needs.

Vitamins and Minerals

Individuals diagnosed with cancer often take large amounts of vitamin and mineral supplements because they believe that these products can enhance their immune system or even reverse the course of their disease. Others may see dietary supplementation as a way to make up for existing nutritional deficiencies at the time of diagnosis caused by poor diet and lifestyle choices. If individuals are experiencing difficulty with eating and treatment-related side effects, a multivitamin and mineral supplement that provides no more than 100% of the dietary reference intakes (DRIs) is considered safe (Doyle et al., 2006). In contrast, the American Institute for Cancer Research (AICR) encourages all people (including cancer survivors) not to use dietary supplements for cancer prevention, citing evidence that high-dose dietary supplementation can have cancer-promoting effects (WCRF and AICR, 2007). Whether for primary or secondary prevention, all individuals should consume vitamin and minerals from the foods they eat rather than use dietary supplements. In some instances during and after a cancer diagnosis, supplementation or restriction of specific micronutrients may be required above or below DRI levels, depending on medical diagnosis and laboratory analysis (e.g., iron supplementation for iron-deficiency anemia).

Supplement Use

The majority of cancer survivors use dietary supplements during all phases of anticancer treatment (Hardy, 2008). Despite increased use, oncology practitioners ask that patients avoid use of dietary supplements during treatment. Specifically, controversy continues over whether the use of antioxidant dietary supplements such as vitamins A, C, E, β-carotene, zinc, and selenium actually inhibits or enhances the antitumor effects of radiation therapy and chemotherapy (ACS, 2009b). Several randomized trials showed some potential for reducing treatment dose-limiting toxicities (Block et al., 2008). However, well-designed studies evaluating larger numbers of individuals are needed.

Cancer survivors should carefully evaluate the need and wisdom of taking dietary supplements both during and after treatment (Miller, 2008) and should avoid using antioxidant supplements while undergoing treatment until further research supports their use (ACS, 2009b; Hardy, 2008; WCRF and AICR, 2007). Individuals diagnosed with cancer should be encouraged to consume antioxidants from a variety of colorful food sources such as fruits, vegetables, and whole grains as a way to safely consume these naturally occurring, health-promoting phytonutrients, vitamins, and minerals (Grant et al., 2010).

Nutrition Diagnosis

Nutrition diagnosis identifies the specific nutrition problems that can be resolved or improved through nutrition intervention. (ADA, 2011). See Chapter 11. The following are examples of nutrition diagnoses using the "problem, etiology, and signs and symptoms" system developed for the cancer care setting:

Intake Domain

- Inadequate oral intake *related to* pelvic radiation therapy *as evidenced by* diarrhea and 2.5-pound weight loss in the preceding week
- Inadequate enteral nutrition (EN) infusion *related to* intolerance of EN *as evidenced by* nausea, abdominal distention, and weight loss of 3 pounds in the preceding 5 days
- Malnutrition *related to* cancer cachexia *as evidenced by* wasting of temporalis and interosseous muscles, and weight loss of more than 7.5% in 3 months

Clinical Domain

- Altered GI function *related to* recent ileostomy surgery *as evidenced by* 2 L/day ostomy diarrhea output, and the need for daily IV hydration during the preceding week
- Altered GI function *related to* biweekly chemotherapy *as evidenced by* nausea, vomiting, and anorexia in the preceding 4 days
- Swallowing difficulty *related to* an obstructing esophageal tumor *as evidenced by* dysphagia, odynophagia, and 10-pound weight loss in the preceding month

Behavioral-Environmental Domain

- Limited access to nutrition-related supplies *related to* lack of insurance and financial resources *as evidenced by* not using the prescribed amount of tube feeding formula and continued weight loss to 80% of usual weight during the preceding month
- Intake of unsafe food *related to* exposure to contaminated food while neutropenic *as evidenced by* hospitalization, diarrhea, and positive stool culture for salmonella
- Undesirable food choices *related to* an unwillingness to apply nutrition information *as evidenced by* ongoing diarrhea and diet history of continued high fiber food intake while undergoing pelvic radiation therapy

Nutrition Intervention

Nutrition intervention outlines specific actions to manage a nutrition diagnosis. It includes two distinct, interrelated components—planning and implementing nutrition interventions (ADA, 2011). The *Oncology Toolkit* recommends careful appraisal if the planned nutrition intervention will negatively affect patient safety or possibly interfere with the cancer treatment (ADA, 2010b). The *Toolkit* also advises evaluation of the nutrition intervention's likely effectiveness for improving nutrition status, possible financial burden, and patient acceptance

Intervention goals should be specific, achievable, and individualized to encourage cooperation. Goals need to be directed toward an objective measure such as body weight or some other meaningful index. Another goal is to minimize the effects of "nutrition impact symptoms" and to maximize the individual's nutritional parameters. **Nutrition impact symptoms** can be defined as symptoms and side effects of cancer and cancer treatment that directly affect the nutrition status. Consultation with the individual, caregivers, or family members regarding expected problems and their possible solutions should be initiated early in the course of cancer therapy and should continue in conjunction with follow-up nutrition assessment and care.

The adverse nutritional effects of cancer can be severe and may be compounded by the effects of the treatment regimens and the psychological effects of cancer. The result is often a profound depletion of nutrient stores and deterioration in nutrition status. Malnutrition, anorexia (loss of appetite), and weight loss are all significant issues in cancer care and are often present in many individuals at the time of diagnosis, even in children (Goldman et al., 2006). More than 50% of people with cancer lose body weight and more than one third lose more than 5% of their usual body weight (Skipworth, 2007). Studies consistently show that even small amounts of weight loss (less than 5% of body weight) before treatment is associated with a poorer prognosis and decreased quality of life, thus reinforcing the importance of early MNT (Fearon, 2008).

Oral Nutrition Management Strategies

Ideally the route of feeding is oral, although individuals may experience symptoms that affect this. Strategies for modifying dietary intake may be necessary, and depend on the specific eating problem and the individual's nutritional status. Food and its presentation may need modification. Liquid medical food supplements may be recommended for those unable to consume enough energy and protein to maintain weight and nutrition status (see Chapter 14). Education materials with suggestions for improving oral intake and managing treatment-related side effects include *Eating Hints* (NCI, 2010e), *Chemotherapy and You* (NCI, 2010c), and *Radiation Therapy and You* (NCI, 2010f). Table 37-5 outlines examples of nutrition intervention strategies.

Managing Anorexia and Alterations in Taste and Smell

Sometimes even before diagnosis, and then throughout cancer treatment, individuals may report anorexia, early satiety, and decreased food intake. Alterations in taste and smell are commonly experienced as well. Taste alterations can be associated with the disease itself, certain chemotherapy agents, radiation therapy, or surgery to the head and neck. Chemotherapy-induced, learned taste aversions have been reported in both adults and children. Individuals may also develop a heightened sense of smell that results in sensitivity to food preparation odors and aversions to nonfood items such as soaps or perfumes. These sensation abnormalities do not consistently correlate with the tumor site, extent of tumor involvement, tumor response to therapy, or food preferences and intake. Nutrition interventions that decrease the aroma of foods, such as serving foods cold instead of hot, may be helpful (NCI, 2010e).

Managing Alterations in Energy Metabolism

Energy metabolism is intimately related to carbohydrate, protein, and lipid metabolism, all of which are altered by tumor growth. Tumors exert a consistent demand for glucose, exhibit a characteristically high rate of anaerobic metabolism, and yield lactate as the end product. This expanded lactic acid pool requires an increased rate of host gluconeogenesis via Cori cycle activity, which is increased in some people with cancer but not in others. Both protein breakdown and lipolysis take place at increasing rates to maintain high rates of glucose synthesis. There is glucose intolerance and insulin resistance, characterized by excess fatty acid oxidation and decreased uptake and use of glucose by muscle.

Alterations in protein metabolism appear to be directed toward providing adequate amino acids for tumor growth. Most notable is the loss of skeletal muscle protein caused by increased protein breakdown, as well as decreased protein synthesis.

Managing Cancer Cachexia

A common secondary diagnosis in people with advanced cancer is a variant of protein-energy malnutrition. This syndrome is termed **cancer cachexia** and is characterized by progressive weight loss, anorexia, generalized wasting and weakness, immunosuppression, altered basal metabolic rate, and abnormalities in fluid and energy metabolism. There is also increased loss of adipose tissue, which is related to an increased rate of lipolysis, rather than a decrease in lipogenesis. Increased levels of lipid-mobilizing factor and proteolysis-inducing factor secreted by tumor cells will lead to increased loss of both fat and muscle mass. Individuals at the time of diagnosis with breast or hematologic cancers rarely present with significant weight loss, whereas individuals with lung, esophageal, or head and neck cancers often exhibit substantial weight loss. Cancer cachexia is caused in part by **cytokines** (immune-modulating agents), produced by the cancer itself or by the immune system in response to the cancer. Cytokines can cause metabolic changes and wasting that is similar to changes seen in inflammation. Proinflammatory cytokines include **tumor necrosis factor (TNF)-α (cachectin)** and TNF-β, interleukin (IL)-1, IL-6, and interferon-$\tilde{\alpha}$. These cytokines have overlapping physiologic activities, which makes it likely that no single substance is the sole cause. Resting energy expenditure (REE) is elevated, which is in contrast to the REE in chronic starvation wherein the body adapts to conserve energy and preserve body tissue. Cancer cachexia often increases closer to the time of death.

TABLE 37-5

Nutrition Intervention Strategies for Patients with Cancer

Side Effect or Symptom	Strategies
Weight loss	• Eat small, more frequent, nutrient dense meals and snacks. • Add protein and calories to favorite foods. • Use protein and calorie-containing supplements (e.g., whey or soy powder, nutritional supplements). • Keep nutrient dense foods close at hand and snack frequently.
Poor appetite or anorexia	• Capitalize on times when feeling best. • Eat meals and snacks in a pleasant atmosphere. • Keep nutrient dense foods close at hand and snack frequently. • Be as physically active as able.
Nausea and vomiting	• Sip on cool or room temperature clear liquids in small amounts. • Avoid high fat, greasy, spicy, or overly sweet foods. • Avoid foods with strong odors. • Eat bland, soft, easy-to-digest foods on scheduled treatment days.
Diarrhea	• Consume plenty of clear liquids such as water, clear juices, broth, gelatin, popsicles, sports drinks. • Decrease intake of high fiber foods such as nuts, raw fruits and vegetables, and whole-grain breads and cereals. • Avoid sugar alcohol–containing foods such as sugar-free candies and gums (e.g., mannitol, xylitol, sorbitol). • Eat applesauce, bananas, canned peaches, white rice or pasta, which are easy to digest and can firm up the stool.
Constipation	• Increase intake of high fiber foods such as whole grains, fresh or cooked fruits and vegetables, especially those with skins and seeds, dried fruits, beans, and nuts. • Drink plenty of healthy fluids to keep the digestive system moving. • Try to eat and snack at the same time each day. • Try to increase physical activity as able.
Sore throat	• Eat soft, moist foods with extra sauces, dressings, or gravies. • Avoid dry, coarse, or rough foods. • Avoid alcohol, citrus, caffeine, tomatoes, vinegar, and hot peppers. • Experiment with food temperatures (e.g. warm, cool, or icy) to find which temperature is the most soothing.
Sore mouth, mucositis, or thrush	• Maintain good oral hygiene (e.g., rinse mouth frequently, keep mouth clean). • Eat soft, moist foods with extra sauces, dressings, and gravies. • Avoid alcohol, citrus, caffeine, tomatoes, vinegar and hot peppers; and dry, coarse, or rough foods. • Try foods at room temperature or chilled.
Fatigue	• Consume easy-to-prepare, easy-to-eat foods. • Keep nutrient dense snacks close at hand and snack frequently. • Drink plenty of healthy fluids to keep the digestive system moving. • Be as physically active as possible.
Neutropenia	• Wash hands frequently and keep kitchen surfaces and utensils clean. • Do not eat raw or undercooked animal products, including meat, pork, game, poultry, eggs, and fish. • Wash all fresh fruits and vegetables. • "When in doubt, throw out" and "No oldy or moldy."
Altered taste or smell	• Maintain good oral hygiene (e.g., rinse mouth frequently, keep mouth clean). • Try marinades and spices to mask strange tastes. • Use plastic utensils if metallic tastes are a problem. • Try cooler foods, rather than warmer foods.
Thickened saliva	• Sip on liquids throughout the day to keep the oral cavity moist. • Thin oral secretions with club soda, seltzer water, or papaya nectar. • Try guaifenesin to help thin oral secretions. • Try using a cool mist humidifier while sleeping.
Xerostomia	• Sip on liquids throughout the day to keep the oral cavity moist. • Try tart foods to stimulate saliva, if open sores are not present. • Eat soft, moist foods with extra sauces, dressings, or gravies. • Maintain good oral hygiene (e.g., rinse mouth frequently, keep mouth clean).

Data from Elliott L et al., editors: The clinical guide to oncology nutrition, ed 2, Chicago, 2006, American Dietetic Association; Grant BL et al., editors: American Cancer Society's complete guide to nutrition for cancer survivors, ed 2, Atlanta, 2010, American Cancer Society; Grant BL, Hamilton KK, editors: Management of nutrition impact symptoms in cancer and educational handouts, Chicago, 2005, American Dietetic Association; National Cancer Institute (NCI): Eating hints, 2010e. Accessed 20 October 2010 from http://www.cancer.gov/publications/.

Pharmacotherapy

The pharmacologic management of cachexia and anorexia requires careful evaluation based on the patient's treatment goals and prognosis, and on close monitoring of symptoms. Prescribed medications sometimes prevent adequate intake. Ideally these agents are prescribed in combination with nutrition counseling and physical activity. A number of pharmacologic agents are under investigation, including appetite stimulants, metabolic agents, cytokine blockers, prokinetic agents, and anabolic agents. Several trials have shown improved appetite and increased energy intake and body weight in cancer patients treated with megestrol acetate, a progestational agent. Prolonged use of corticosteroids is associated with negative side effects such as osteoporosis, fluid retention, adrenal suppression, glucose intolerance, electrolyte imbalance, or even arm- and leg-muscle wasting. Oxandrolone, a synthetic anabolic steroid, combined with a resistance exercise program, may increase total body weight and lean tissue weight. Growth hormones have been studied in patients with wasting associated with human immunodeficiency virus, but few data are available regarding their use with cancer.

Managing Other Cancer-Related Metabolic Abnormalities

Metabolic alterations vary by tumor type. An individual's immunologic function can be impaired, apparently as the result of the disease, cancer treatment, or progressive malnutrition. In addition to the cancer-induced metabolic effects, the mass of the tumor may anatomically alter the physiology of specific organ systems. The activities of several enzyme systems involved with digestion and absorption can be affected, as can certain endocrine functions.

Critical imbalances in fluid and electrolyte status can occur in people who have cancers or are undergoing cancer treatments that promote excessive diarrhea, vomiting, or malabsorption. Profuse and often severe diarrhea can result from partial bowel obstructions and endocrine-secreting tumors such as those secreting serotonin (carcinoid tumors), calcitonin, or gastrin (Zollinger-Ellison syndrome). The use of antimetabolites, alkylating agents, and antibiotics may also lead to the development of severe diarrhea. In some instances, people who are immunocompromised or have undergone GI surgery may experience profuse diarrhea that is caused by intestinal pathogens such as *Clostridium difficile*.

Persistent vomiting is associated with intestinal obstruction, radiation therapy to the stomach and abdomen or brain, highly **emetogenic** (nausea-causing) chemotherapy agents, intracranial tumors, and advanced cancer (Grant, 2006). Careful assessment and evaluation of the cause of the diarrhea or vomiting is critical for effective management. Malabsorption may be caused by treatment-related pancreatic dysfunction, postsurgical short gut syndrome, acute or chronic **radiation enteritis** (inflammation of the GI tract tissues secondary to radiation), excess serotonin, steatorrhea, or chronic diarrhea.

Hypercalcemia may occur in individuals with bone metastases, caused by the osteolytic activity of tumor cells releasing calcium into the extracellular fluid. Hypercalcemia is potentially fatal, and is associated most commonly with multiple myeloma, lung cancer, and advanced breast and prostate cancer. Nausea, weakness, fatigue, lethargy, and confusion occur. Medical management of hypercalcemia includes rehydration and use of antihypercalcemic agents. Calcium supplementation from dietary supplements and antacids should be avoided. Restricting the intake of foods containing calcium is not indicated because the consumption of these foods has little effect in the overall management of hypercalcemia.

NUTRITIONAL IMPACT OF CANCER TREATMENTS

Chemotherapy

Chemotherapy uses chemical agents or medications to treat cancer. Classifications of chemotherapy cytotoxic agents include alkylating agents, antimetabolites, antitumor antibiotics, miscellaneous agents, nitrosoureas, and plant alkaloids (Wilkes and Barton-Burke, 2010). Once in the bloodstream, these agents are carried through the body to reach as many cancer cells as possible. Routes of administration for chemotherapy include:

- Oral: capsule, pill, or liquid
- Intravenous (IV): delivery of medication via an injection or an indwelling catheter into a vein
- Intraperitoneal: delivery of medication via a catheter directly into the abdominal cavity
- Intravesicular: delivery of medication via a Foley catheter directly into the bladder
- Intrathecal: delivery of medication via an injection into the central nervous system using an Ommaya reservoir or a lumbar puncture (Polovich et al., 2009)

Whereas surgery and radiation therapy are used to treat localized tumors, chemotherapy is a systemic therapy that affects the malignant tissue and normal cells as well. Cells of the body with a rapid turnover such as bone marrow, hair follicles, and the mucosa of the alimentary tract are the most affected. As a result, nutrition intake and nutrition status can be adversely affected. Nutrition-related symptoms include **myelosuppression** (suppression of bone marrow production of neutrophils, platelets, and red blood cells), anemia, fatigue, nausea and vomiting, loss of appetite, mucositis, changes in taste and smell, xerostomia (mouth dryness), dysphagia, and altered bowel function such as diarrhea or constipation (Table 37-6).

The severity of the side effects depends on the specific agents used, dosage, duration of treatment, number of treatment cycles, accompanying drugs, individual response, and current health status. The timely and appropriate use of supportive therapies such as antiemetics, antidiarrheals, hematopoietic agents, and antibiotics, as well as dietary changes, is important. Many people experience significant side effects, especially in "dose-intensive" multiple-agent

TABLE 37-6

Nutrition-Related Effects of Antineoplastic Agents: Chemotherapy, Biotherapy, Hormone Therapy, and Anti-angiogenic Agents

Agent Classification	Common Nutrition Impact Symptom
Chemotherapy	
Alkylating Agents	
• Cisplatin (Platinol), cyclophosphamide (Cytoxan), oxaliplatin (Eloxatin), temozolomide (Temodar)	• Myelosuppression, anorexia, nausea, vomiting, fatigue, renal toxicity
Antitumor Antibiotics	
• Bleomycin (Blenoxane), mitomycin (Mutamycin)	• Myelosuppression, anorexia, nausea, vomiting, fatigue, diarrhea, mucositis
Antimetabolites	
• Capecitabine (Xeloda), 5-fluorouracil (5-FU), gemcitabine (Gemzar), methotrexate	• Myelosuppression, anorexia, nausea, vomiting, fatigue, diarrhea, mucositis
Plant Alkaloids	
• Camptosar (Irinotecan), etoposide (VP-16), docetaxel (Taxotere), paclitaxel (Taxol), vinorelbine (Navelbine)	• Myelosuppression, anorexia, nausea, vomiting, fatigue, peripheral neuropathy
Miscellaneous	
• Procarbazine (Mutalane)	• Myelosuppression, nausea, vomiting, diarrhea, MAO inhibitor/avoid foods high in tyramine
Biotherapy	
Cytokines	
• Interferon-alfa (Intron A), interleukin (IL-2)	• Myelosuppression, anorexia, fatigue, nausea, flu-like symptoms, chills
Monoclonal Antibodies	
• Cetuximab (Erbitux), rituximab (Rituxan), trastuzumab (Herceptin)	• Infusion reaction of chills, fever, headache, hypotension; myelosuppression; nausea; vomiting; rash
Small Molecule Inhibitors	
• Erlotinib (Tarceva), Imatinib mesylate (Gleevec)	• Fever, chills, rash, diarrhea, fatigue, anorexia
Hematopoietic Growth Factors	
• Epoetin alfa (Procrit), pegfilgrastim (Neulasta)	• Fever, bone pain, flu-like symptoms, nausea
Hormone Therapy	
Antiandrogens	
• Bicalutamide (Casodex)	• Hot flashes, nausea, alterations in elimination (diarrhea or constipation)
Antihormones	
• Leuprolide (Lupron)	• Hot flashes, edema, nausea, anorexia
Antiestrogens	
• Anastrozole (Arimidex), tamoxifen (Novadex)	• Thrombophlebitis/embolism, fluid retention, hot flashes, nausea, joint discomfort, diarrhea
Progestins	
• Megestrol acetate (Megace)	• Increased appetite, weight gain, fluid retention
Antiangiogenic Agents	
• Bevacizumab (Avastin)	• Hemorrhage, hypertension, diarrhea, abdominal pain, myelosuppression, wound healing complications

Data from Polovich M et al: Chemotherapy and biotherapy guidelines and recommendations for practice, Pittsburgh, 2009, Oncology Nursing Society; Wilkes GM, Barton-Burke M: 2010 oncology nursing drug handbook, Boston, 2010, Jones and Bartlett.

chemotherapy regimens; **neutropenia** (reduced white blood cells or neutrophils) and myelosuppression are the primary factors limiting chemotherapy administration. Commonly experienced chemotherapy induced toxicities affecting the GI system include mucositis, nausea, vomiting, diarrhea, and constipation. Chemotherapy related taste abnormalities can lead to anorexia and decreased oral intake. Symptoms of GI toxicity are usually temporary; however, some multiagent chemotherapy regimens may lead to lasting GI side effects.

Diarrhea

Diarrhea is a common side effect of certain chemotherapy agents. Left unmanaged, it can lead to depletion of fluids, electrolytes, malnutrition, and even hospitalization (Muehlbauer et al., 2009). The intestinal mucosa and digestive processes can be affected, thus altering digestion and absorption to some degree. Protein, energy, and vitamin metabolism may be impaired. Total lymphocyte count is often depressed and does not accurately reflect nutrition status after chemotherapy administration.

Nausea and Vomiting

Chemotherapy induced nausea and vomiting are commonly classified as anticipatory (occurs before receiving treatment), acute (occurs within the first 24 hours after receiving treatment), or delayed (occurs 1 to 4 days after treatment), each of which is characterized by distinct pathophysiologic events and requires different therapeutic interventions (NCCN, 2010). Effective agents for treatment-related nausea and vomiting are the serotonin antagonists (e.g., ondansetron, granisetron, and dolasetron), neurokinin-1 (NK-1) receptor antagonists (e.g., aprepitant), dopamine antagonists (e.g., metoclopramide, prochlorperazine), and corticosteroids such as dexamethasone (Polovich et al., 2009; Tipton et al., 2007). Other antiemetic agents include cannabinoids (e.g., dronabinol, nabilone) and anxiolytics (e.g., lorazepam).

Food-Drug Interactions

Dietetic professionals can gain valuable insights regarding possible drug-nutrient interactions and contraindications by reviewing product medication inserts, pharmacy resource books, and medication databases or by consulting with pharmacy personnel (see Chapter 9 and Appendix 31). Some chemotherapy agents can cause potentially severe adverse events (Grant and Byron, 2006); for example:

- Individuals with certain types of lung cancer who are being treated with pemetrexed (Alimta) require vitamin B_{12} and folic acid supplementation throughout the duration of their therapy to avoid significant anemia associated with this chemotherapy agent.
- A severe hypertensive event is possible when tyramine-rich foods and beverages are consumed while taking procarbazine (Mutalane), a chemotherapy agent commonly used to treat brain cancer (see Chapter 9).
- Individuals with colon cancer receiving oxaliplatin (Eloxatin) should not drink, eat, or handle cold drinks or foods for up to 5 days because of treatment-related dysesthesias or transient paresthesias of the hands, feet, and throat.
- In order to prevent unnecessary gastric upset, individuals taking the medication, capecitabine (Xeloda), must take the medication within 30 minutes of eating food or a meal. Conversely, medications such as erlotinib (Tarceva) should not be taken with food and it can cause a rash and profound diarrhea unless taken on an empty stomach.

Oral Changes

People with altered taste acuity (dysgeusia, hypogeusia, ageusia) may benefit from increased use of flavorings and seasonings during food preparation. Meat aversions may require the elimination of red meats, which tend to be strong in flavor, or the substitution of alternative protein sources. Herpes simplex virus and *Candida albicans* (thrush) account for most oral infections. In addition to causing oral infections, some agents, especially corticosteroids, can cause hyperglycemia and can lead to excessive losses of urinary protein, potassium, and calcium.

Mucositis

Oral **mucositis**, an inflammation of the mucous membranes lining the oropharynx and esophagus, is a common side effect of some types of chemotherapy (Figure 37-1). Although many interventions exist, most strategies lack scientific evidence (Harris et al., 2008). General care guidelines include recommending daily oral care (e.g., keeping the mouth clean, avoidance of tobacco, alcohol, and irritating foods) and the use of bland rinses (e.g., baking soda or saline rinses). Bland liquids and soft solids are usually better tolerated in individuals with oral or esophageal mucositis and strong-flavored, acidic, or spicy foods should also be avoided. Commercially prepared liquid medical food supplements can be useful.

Biotherapy

Biotherapy is immunotherapy, a group of cancer treatment drugs prescribed to stimulate the body's own immune system and natural defenses to treat cancer. Biotherapy is sometimes used by itself, but it is most often given in combination with chemotherapy drugs. Different kinds of biotherapy drugs used to help the immune system recognize cancer cells and strengthen its ability to destroy them include:

- **Cytokines** such as interferon and IL-2 for treatment of malignant melanoma and metastatic melanoma
- **Monoclonal antibodies** such as trastuzumab (Herceptin) for treatment of specific types of breast cancer, and rituximab (Rituxan) for treatment of NHL
- **Cancer vaccines** made from an individual's own cancer or substances from tumor cells are currently under

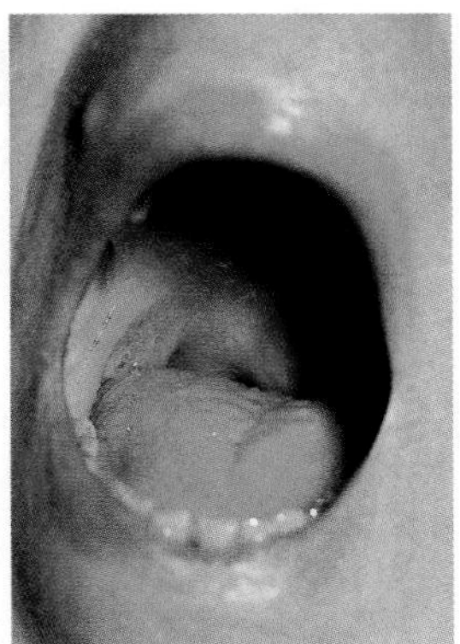

FIGURE 37-1 Oral mucositis. *(From Kanski JL: Clinical diagnosis in ophthalmology, ed 1, 2006, Elsevier.)*

investigation in clinical cancer trials (Wilkes and Barton-Burke, 2010).

Other types of biotherapy drugs are groups of proteins that cause blood cells to grow and mature (NCI, 2010d). These drugs are called **hematopoietic growth factors** and they include supportive care medications such as darbepoetin (Aranesp) or epoetin alfa (Procrit) to stimulate red blood cell production, and filgrastim (Neupogen) or pegfilgrastim (Neulasta) to stimulate the production of neutrophils in the bone marrow (Polovich et al., 2009). Individuals receiving these agents may experience fatigue, chills, fever, and flulike symptoms.

Hormone Therapy

Hormone therapy adds, blocks, or removes hormones to slow or stop the growth of hormone-sensitive breast or prostate cancer (NCI, 2010d). Examples of these agents include tamoxifen (Nolvadex) and anastrozole (Arimidex) for breast cancer and leuprolide (Lupron) or bicalutamide (Casodex) for prostate cancer (Wilkes and Barton-Burke, 2010). Side effects commonly include hot flashes, decreased libido, and bone pain.

Antiangiogenic Therapy

Antiangiongenic therapy prevents or reduces the growth of new blood vessels, and prevents tumor invasion. These agents are most frequently used in combination with other chemotherapy agents to maximize their effectiveness. An example of an antiangoiogenic agent used to treat colon or breast cancer is bevacizumab (Avastin).

Radiation Therapy

Radiation therapy, ionizing radiation used in multiple fractionated doses, is used to cure, control, or palliate cancer. Radiation therapy can be delivered externally into the body from a megavoltage machine or with brachytherapy by placing a radioactive source (implant) in or near the tumor to deliver a highly localized dose. Advances in technology to deliver radiation therapy with precise accuracy include radiation surgery (e.g., stereotactic radiosurgery) and intensity-modulated radiation therapy (IMRT). Whereas chemotherapy is a systemic therapy, radiation therapy affects only the tumor and the surrounding area. The side effects of radiation therapy are usually limited to the specific site being irradiated. Chemotherapy agents may also be given in combination with radiation therapy to produce a radiation-enhancing effect. People receiving multimodality therapy often experience side effects sooner and with greater intensity.

The acute side effects of radiation therapy when used alone generally occur around the second or third week of treatment, and usually resolve within 2 to 4 weeks after the radiation therapy has been completed. Late effects of radiation therapy may happen several weeks, months, or even years after treatment. Commonly experienced nutrition-related symptoms include fatigue, loss of appetite, skin changes, and hair loss in the area being treated (Table 37-7).

Radiation to the Head and Neck

Treatment for head and neck cancer usually includes a multimodality approach with aggressive chemotherapy, radiation therapy, and often surgery. Radiation therapy to the head and neck can cause acute nutrition-related symptoms: sore mouth, altered taste and smell, dysphagia and odynophagia, mucositis, xerostomia, anorexia, fatigue, and weight loss (Havrila et al., 2010). Prophylactic placement of percutaneous endoscopic gastrostomy (PEG) feeding tubes can help to reduce treatment-associated weight loss and malnutrition (Cady, 2007).

Salivary stimulants and substitutes or oral lubricants are beneficial for temporary relief of xerostomia (diminished salivation or loss of salivation) caused by head and neck radiation therapy or certain types of medications (e.g., pain medications). In addition, liquids and foods with sauces and gravies are usually well tolerated. Late effects of radiation therapy may include dental caries, permanent xerostomia, **trismus** (an inability to fully open the mouth), and **osteoradionecrosis** of the jaw (necrosis of the bone caused by exposure to radiation therapy).

Before beginning therapy, individuals should undergo a dental evaluation and thorough teeth cleaning and receive instruction in good oral hygiene and care, including daily brushing and rinsing (National Institute of Dental and Craniofacial Research, 2010). After therapy has been completed, individuals should continue to have close dental monitoring and follow-up. Individuals may also benefit from a referral to a speech therapist for assessment and evaluation of swallowing function.

Radiation to the Thorax

Nutrition-related symptoms of radiation therapy to the thorax (chest) can include heartburn and acute esophagitis,

TABLE 37-7

Nutrition-Related Effects of Radiation Therapy

Site of Radiation Therapy	Common Nutrition-Related Symptom
Central nervous system (brain and spinal cord)	**Acute Effects**
	Nausea, vomiting Fatigue Loss of appetite Hyperglycemia associated with corticosteroids
	Late Effects (>90 days after treatment)
	Headache, lethargy
Head and neck (tongue, larynx, pharynx, oropharynx, nasopharynx, tonsils, salivary glands)	**Acute Effects**
	Xerostomia Mucositis Sore mouth and throat Dysphagia, odynophagia Alterations in taste and smell Fatigue Loss of appetite
	Late Effects (>90 days after treatment)
	Mucosal atrophy and dryness Salivary glands—xerostomia, fibrosis Trismus Osteoradionecrosis Alterations in taste and smell
Thorax (esophagus, lung, breast)	**Acute Effects**
	Esophagitis Dysphagia, odynophagia Heartburn Fatigue Loss of appetite
	Late Effects (>90 days after treatment)
	Esophageal—fibrosis, stenosis, stricture, ulceration Cardiac—angina on effort, pericarditis, cardiac enlargement Pulmonary—dry cough, fibrosis, pneumonitis
Abdomen and pelvis (stomach, ovaries, uterus, colon, rectum)	**Acute Effects**
	Nausea, vomiting Changes in bowel function—diarrhea, cramping, bloating, gas Changes in urinary function—increased frequency, burning sensation with urination Acute colitis or enteritis Lactose intolerance Fatigue Loss of appetite
	Late Effects (>90 days after treatment)
	Diarrhea, malabsorption, maldigestion Chronic colitis or enteritis Intestinal—stricture, ulceration, obstruction, perforation, fistula Urinary—hematuria, cystitis

Data from: Bruner DW et al: Manual for radiation oncology and nursing practice and education, ed 3, Pittsburgh, 2005, Oncology Nursing Society; Havrila C et al: Medical and radiation oncology. In Marian M, Roberts S, editors: Clinical nutrition for oncology patients, Sudbury, MA, 2010, Jones and Bartlett.

accompanied by dysphagia and odynophagia. Late effects include possible esophageal fibrosis and stenosis. When this occurs, individuals are generally only able to swallow liquids, and the use of medical food supplements and nutrition support enteral nutrition (EN) may be necessary to meet nutritional needs. Often, individuals undergo esophageal dilations or swallowing therapy and rehabilitation to improve swallowing function.

Radiation to the Abdomen or Pelvis

Radiation therapy to the abdomen or pelvis may cause gastritis or enteritis that can be accompanied by nausea, vomiting, diarrhea, and anorexia (Muehlbauer et al., 2009. Late effects can include lasting GI damage such as malabsorption of disaccharides (e.g., lactose), fats, vitamins, minerals, and electrolytes. Proactive management includes encouraging affected individuals to consume soluble fiber, to increase intake of hydrating liquids, and to avoid eating high non-soluble fiber or lactose containing foods. To alleviate symptoms, medications such as antidiarrheals like loperamide and antimotility agents (e.g., metoclopramide) may be given to reduce intestinal motility.

Chronic radiation enteritis can develop with diarrhea, ulceration, or obstruction, intensifying the risk of malnutrition. Chronic radiation enteritis combined with or without significant bowel resection can result in bowel dysfunction (see Chapter 29 regarding short bowel syndrome [SBS]). The severity of this condition depends on the length and location of the nonfunctional or resected bowel, and generally is diagnosed when the individual has less than 150 cm of small intestine remaining. The sequelae of SBS include malabsorption, malnutrition, dehydration, weight loss, fatigue, and lactose intolerance (Havrila et al., 2010).

Initially parenteral nutrition (PN) may be required, and frequent monitoring of fluids and electrolytes may be necessary for weeks or months. Individuals with SBS may require an oral diet restricted to defined formula tube feedings or to frequent small meals high in protein, low in fat and fiber, and lactose-free. Dietary supplements that contain vitamin B_{12}; folic acid; thiamin; calcium; and vitamins A, E, and K are often indicated to prevent deficiencies. Serum concentrations of various minerals should also be monitored and adjusted as needed.

Total-Body Irradiation

Total-body irradiation (TBI) is a technique of radiation therapy that is used in hematopoietic cell transplantation (HCT) to eliminate malignant cells, to ablate the bone marrow and make room for the engraftment of the infused hematopoietic cells, and to suppress the immune system to decrease the risk of rejection. Commonly encountered side effects are fever, nausea, vomiting, headache, mucositis, parotitis (inflammation of the parotid glands), xerostomia, diarrhea, anorexia, fatigue, and associated weight loss.

Surgery

The surgical resection or removal of any part of the alimentary tract (mouth to anus), as well as the malignant disease process, can potentially impair normal digestion and absorption (Huhmann and August, 2010). Surgery may be used as a single mode of cancer treatment, or it may be combined with preoperative or postoperative adjuvant chemotherapy or radiation therapy. After surgery, individuals commonly experience fatigue, temporary changes in appetite and bowel function caused by anesthesia, and pain. They often require additional energy and protein for wound healing and recovery. Most side effects are temporary and dissipate after a few days following surgery. However, some surgical interventions have long-lasting nutritional implications (Table 37-8). When performing a nutrition assessment, it is very important to understand which part of the alimentary tract has been affected or surgically removed so the appropriate nutrition intervention can be recommended. Refer to Chapter 1 for a review gastrointestinal physiology.

Head and Neck Cancer

Individuals with head and neck cancer often have difficulty with chewing and swallowing caused by the cancer itself or the specific surgical intervention required to remove cancerous tissues. There can be additional problems because of history of smoking and alcohol abuse, illicit drug use, and subsequent poor nutrition intake, which place them at high risk for malnutrition and postoperative complications. Surgery often necessitates temporary or long-term reliance on EN support (e.g., PEG tube feedings). See Chapter 14. Individuals who resume oral intake often have prolonged dysphagia and require modifications of food consistency and extensive training in chewing and swallowing. Referrals to a speech therapist can yield dramatic positive results through evaluation and individualized instruction in swallowing and positioning techniques, as well as evaluation for aspiration risk.

Esophageal Cancer

Surgical intervention for treatment of esophageal cancer often requires partial or total removal of the esophagus. The stomach is commonly used for esophageal reconstruction. A feeding jejunostomy tube, which allows for early postoperative tube feedings, can be placed before an individual undergoes surgery or at the time of surgery. Usually the individual is able to progress to oral intake with specific dietary recommendations to minimize nutrition-related symptoms, which include reflux, dumping syndrome (discussed later in this chapter), dysmotility, gastroparesis, early satiety, vomiting, and fluid and electrolyte imbalances (Huhmann and August, 2010). Postsurgical recommendations include a low-fat diet with small, frequent feedings of energy-dense foods and avoidance of large amounts of fluids at any one time (see Chapter 28).

TABLE 37-8

Nutrition-Related Effects of Surgery in Cancer Treatment

Anatomic Site	Nutrition Impact Symptoms
Oral cavity	Difficulty with chewing and swallowing
	Aspiration potential
	Sore mouth and throat
	Xerostomia
	Alteration in taste and smell
Larynx	Alterations in normal swallowing, dysphagia
	Aspiration potential
Esophagus	Gastroparesis
	Indigestion, acid reflux
	Alterations in normal swallowing, dysphagia
	Decreased motility
	Anastomotic leak
Lung	Shortness of breath
	Early satiety
Stomach	Dumping syndrome
	Dehydration
	Early satiety
	Gastroparesis
	Fat malabsorption
	Vitamin and mineral malabsorption (vitamin B_{12} and D; calcium, iron)
Gallbladder and bile duct	Gastroparesis
	Hyperglycemia
	Fluid and electrolyte imbalance
	Fat malabsorption
	Vitamin and mineral malabsorption (vitamin A, D, E, and K; magnesium, calcium, zinc, iron)
Liver	Hyperglycemia
	Hypertriglyceridemia
	Fluid and electrolyte malabsorption
	Vitamin and mineral malabsorption (vitamin A, D, E, K, B_{12} and folic acid, magnesium, zinc)
Pancreas	Gastroparesis
	Fluid and electrolyte imbalance
	Hyperglycemia
	Fat malabsorption (vitamin A, D, E, K and B_{12}; calcium, zinc, iron)
Small bowel	Chyle leak
	Lactose intolerance
	Bile acid depletion
	Diarrhea
	Fluid and electrolyte imbalance
	Vitamin and mineral malabsorption (vitamin A, D, E, K, and B_{12}; calcium, zinc, iron)
Colon and rectum	Increased transit time
	Diarrhea
	Dehydration
	Bloating, cramping, gas
	Fluid and electrolyte imbalance
	Vitamin and mineral malabsorption (vitamin B_{12}, sodium, potassium, magnesium, calcium)
Ovaries and uterus	Early satiety
	Bloating, cramping, and gas
Brain	Nausea, vomiting
	Hyperglycemia associated with corticosteroids

Data from Elliott L et al., editors: The clinical guide to oncology nutrition, ed 2, Chicago, 2006, American Dietetic Association; Huhmann MB, August D: Surgical oncology. In Marian M, Roberts S, editors: Clinical nutrition for oncology patients, Sudbury, MA, 2010, Jones and Bartlett.

Gastric Cancer

Surgery is the most common treatment for cancer of the stomach, although chemotherapy and radiation therapy can be used before or after surgery to improve survival. Surgical interventions include partial, subtotal, or total gastrectomy. Placement of a jejunostomy feeding tube at surgery is advisable, and enteral nutrition (EN) support using a jejunal feeding tube is generally feasible within a few days after surgery.

Postgastrectomy syndrome encompasses a myriad of symptoms, including dumping syndrome, fat malabsorption, gastric stasis, lactose intolerance, anemias, and metabolic bone disease (osteoporosis, osteopenia, osteomalacia). **Dumping syndrome** is a common complication of gastric surgery, manifested by the rapid transit of foods or liquids, and the dilutional response of the small remaining stomach to highly osmotic bolus feedings. Individuals may experience GI and vasomotor symptoms such as abdominal cramps, diarrhea, nausea, vomiting, flushing, faintness, diaphoresis, and tachycardia (Huhmann and August, 2010). Individuals experiencing dumping syndrome should limit simple carbohydrates and liquids at meal times. See Chapter 28 for further recommendations for managing dumping syndrome.

Malabsorption is another complication of gastric surgery; deficiency of iron, folic acid, and less commonly vitamin B_{12} can lead to anemia. Micronutrient deficiencies of calcium and fat-soluble vitamins are also common (Huhmann and August, 2010). Individuals benefit from consumption of six to eight small meals per day, with fluids taken between meals. There may be fat intolerance, especially if the vagal nerve is severed. Administration of pancreatic enzymes with meals may help when the duodenal mixing of food and pancreatic juices is inadequate.

Pancreatic Cancer

Cancer of the pancreas, with or without surgical resection, can have significant nutritional consequences. The Whipple procedure and the pylorus-sparing pancreatic duodenectomy are the most common pancreatic cancer surgeries. Postsurgical complications include delayed gastric emptying, early satiety, glucose intolerance, bile acid insufficiency, diarrhea, and fat malabsorption. Pancreatic enzyme replacement, the use of small, more frequent low-fat meals and snacks, and avoidance of simple carbohydrates aid digestion and absorption.

Cancers of the Intestinal Tract

Partial or total resections of the intestinal tract because of colorectal cancer or carcinoid syndrome may induce profound losses of fluid and electrolytes secondary to decreased transit time and diarrhea, the severity of which is related to the length and site of the resection. Resections of as little as 15 cm of the terminal ileum can result in bile salt losses that exceed the liver's capacity for resynthesis, and vitamin B_{12} absorption is affected. With depletion of the bile salt pool, steatorrhea develops. Nutrition intervention strategies consist of a diet low in fat, osmolality, lactose, and oxalates (see Chapters 29).

Hematopoietic Cell Transplantation (HCT)

HCT is performed for the treatment of certain hematologic cancers such as leukemia, lymphoma, and multiple myeloma. The stem cells used for HCT arise from bone marrow, peripheral blood, or umbilical cord blood. The preparative regimen includes cytotoxic chemotherapy, with or without total-body irradiation (TBI). This treatment regimen is followed by intravenous (IV) infusion of hematopoietic cells from the individual (autologous) or from a histocompatible related or unrelated donor (allogeneic) or from an identical twin (syngeneic) (National Marrow Donor Program, 2010).

HCT procedures can significantly affect nutrition status. Dietetic professionals should conduct a thorough nutrition assessment of the individual before the initiation of therapy and reassessments and monitoring throughout the entire transplant course. The acute toxicities of immunosuppression that can last for 2 to 4 weeks after the transplant include nausea, vomiting, anorexia, dysgeusia, stomatitis, oral and esophageal mucositis, fatigue, and diarrhea. In addition, immunosuppressive medications can also adversely affect nutrition status.

Individuals typically have little or no oral intake and the GI tract is compromised during the first few weeks following transplant. Parenteral nutrition (PN) has become a standard component of care (Robien, 2010). Gastrostomy tubes are useful for long-term nutrition support; the PN should be reserved for individuals who are unable to tolerate oral or enteral feeding (ADA, 2010a). In addition, administration of optimal levels of PN is often complicated by the frequent need to interrupt it for the infusion of antibiotics, blood products, and IV medications. Careful monitoring and the use of more concentrated nutrient solutions, increased flow rates and volumes, and double- or triple-lumen catheters are needed.

Autologous HCT involves the use of the individual's own stem cells to reestablish hematopoietic stem cell function after the administration of high-dose chemotherapy. In some cases the use of mobilized stem cell progenitors has replaced autologous bone marrow as the source of hematopoietic progenitors for transplantation. Their use has shortened the period of **pancytopenia** (reduction in the cellular components of the blood), when individuals are at risk for bleeding, serious infections, or sepsis. These advances, along with improved prophylactic antibiotic regimens that are relatively easy to administer, have allowed individuals to receive autologous marrow transplantation in the outpatient setting. The reduced cost of transplantation has made it available to an increased number of people.

Because a majority of people receive much of their care outside the hospital, regular nutrition assessment and monitoring are important (Robien, 2010). The HCT procedure is associated with severe nutritional consequences that require prompt, proactive intervention. Nausea, vomiting, and diarrhea are caused by the cytotoxic conditioning regimen and may later accompany antibiotic administration. Complications of delayed-onset nutrition-related symptoms include varying degrees of mucositis, xerostomia, and dysgeusia. Mucositis, which is often severe and extremely painful, develops in more than 75% of transplant patients (see Figure 37-1).

Nutritional Precautions with Neutropenia

Individuals receiving HCT become immunocompromised and require supportive therapy, including medications and dietary changes to prevent infection. Of note, some cancer centers continue to prescribe a low-microbial or low-bacteria diet for people with low white blood cell counts (neutropenia). However, there is no clear evidence to support a strict "neutropenic" diet (only cooked foods) to reduce overall rates of infection or death (Gardner et al., 2008). Thus individuals should be instructed on food safety practices (Grant et al., 2010; Seattle Cancer Care Alliance [SCCA], 2010) that include:

- Avoidance of foods that contain unsafe levels of bacteria (raw meats, spoiled or moldy foods, and unpasteurized beverages)
- Thorough hand washing
- Special handling of raw meats, game, poultry, and eggs, utensils, cutting boards, and countertops
- Avoidance of untested well water
- Storage of foods at appropriate temperatures (below 40° F and above 140° F).

Graft-versus-Host Disease (GVHD)

Graft-versus-host disease (GVHD) is a major complication seen primarily after allogeneic transplants, in which the donated "donor" stem cells react against the tissues of the transplant recipient "host." The functions of several target organs (skin, liver, gut, lymphoid cells) are disrupted and are susceptible to infection. Acute GVHD can occur within the first 100 days after the transplant and may be seen as early as 7 to 10 days posttransplant. It may resolve, or it may develop into a chronic form that requires long-term treatment and dietary management. Skin GVHD is characterized by a maculopapular rash. GVHD of the liver, evidenced by jaundice and abnormal liver function tests, often accompanies GI GVHD and further complicates nutrition management.

The symptoms of acute GI GVHD can be severe; individuals may experience gastroenteritis, abdominal pain, nausea, vomiting, and large volumes of secretory diarrhea. Immunosuppressive medications and a phased dietary regimen should be instituted (Charuhas, 2006; SCCA, 2010). The first phase consists of total bowel rest and the use of PN until diarrhea subsides. Nitrogen losses associated with diarrhea can be severe and are compounded by the high-dose corticosteroids used to treat GVHD. The second phase reintroduces oral feedings of beverages that are isosmotic, low-residue, and lactose-free so as to compensate for the loss of intestinal enzymes secondary to alterations in the intestinal villi and mucosa. If these beverages are tolerated, phase three includes the reintroduction of solids that contain low levels of lactose, fiber, fat, and total acidity and no gastric irritants. In phase four dietary restrictions are progressively reduced as foods are gradually introduced and tolerance is established. Phase five includes the resumption of the individual's regular diet.

Chronic GVHD can develop up to 3 months after transplant and is observed with increased frequency in nonidentical related donors and unrelated donors. Chronic GVHD can affect the skin, oral mucosa (ulcerations, stomatitis, xerostomia), and the GI tract (anorexia, reflux symptoms, diarrhea) and can cause changes in body weight.

Another transplant-related complication is **sinusoidal obstructive syndrome (SOS)** (also known as venoocclusive disease), characterized by chemotherapy- or radiation therapy–induced damage to the hepatic venules. It can develop 1 to 3 weeks after transplant. Symptoms of right upper quadrant discomfort, hepatomegaly, fluid retention, and jaundice can occur; in severe cases individuals may experience progressive hepatic failure leading to encephalopathy and multiple-organ system failure. Nutrition support requires concentrated parenteral nutrients, careful fluid and electrolyte management, close monitoring, and adjustment of macronutrients and micronutrients based on the tolerance and response of each individual. The use of branched-chain amino acid formula is controversial. Serum ammonia level may not be a reliable indicator of protein tolerance, or of the development of encephalopathy (see Chapter 30.

Other acute or chronic complications of HCT include osteoporosis, pulmonary disease, impaired renal function, rejection of the graft, growth abnormalities in children, sepsis, and infection. Nutrition-related symptoms associated with HCT may persist; individuals receiving outpatient marrow transplantation require frequent monitoring and intervention.

NUTRITION MONITORING AND EVALUATION

Dietetic professionals must determine and quantify their patients' nutrition care goals by monitoring progress, measuring and evaluating outcomes and changes, and documenting this information throughout the process. See Chapter 11.

Physical Activity

Physical activity is an important part of cancer care. The effect of cancer and cancer treatment on the individual's quality of life should be addressed throughout cancer treatment and continue until the individual is able to successfully resume activities of daily living. Recovery from cancer treatment also requires physical activity to rebuild muscle; regain strength, energy and flexibility; and help relieve symptoms of stress, anxiety, and even depression. Physical activity and exercise may be helpful in strengthening the immune system. However, before participating in any type of physical activity and exercise program, individuals should be advised to undergo evaluation by qualified professionals, who can then design an individualized physical assessment and activity plan. The American College of Sports Medicine (ACSM) now offers a certification program for trainers working with people diagnosed with cancer (a Certified Cancer Exercise Trainer) (ACSM, 2010). In addition, community-based programs such as the YMCA's LiveStrong are available across the United States and offer physical activity and exercise opportunities to support cancer survivors; see www.livestrong.org/ymca.

PEDIATRIC CANCER

Like adults, children with cancer can experience malnutrition and nutrition-related symptoms as a result of their cancer and its treatment. The incidence of malnutrition ranges from 6% to 50% in the pediatric population, depending on the type, stage, and location of the cancer. It usually has greater severity in the presence of more aggressive cancers in later stages of the disease.

Psychogenic food refusal in children requires interventions that address underlying psychological issues. Families and caregivers often express their fears of dying through an extreme preoccupation with eating and maintaining weight. Creative efforts are required to minimize the psychological effects of fear, unpleasant hospital routines, unfamiliar foods, learned food aversions, and pain. Nutrition intervention strategies that use oral intake should stress the maximum use of favorite, nutrient-dense foods during times when intake is likely to be best and food aversions are least likely to occur. Oral medical foods can be useful, but their acceptance is often a problem; thus children should be offered a selection from which to choose.

EN support by nasogastric tube is indicated for selected children who are able to cooperate and who have functional GI tracts. Some children have even been taught to pass their own nasogastric tube for intermittent or nighttime feedings. It should be remembered, however, that aspiration is always a potential risk. PN is indicated for children who are receiving intense treatment associated with severe GI toxicity, and for children with favorable prognoses who are malnourished or have a high risk of developing malnutrition. PN is seldom indicated for children with advanced cancer associated with significant deterioration or with diseases that are unresponsive to therapy.

Universally accepted, evidenced-based guidelines for children diagnosed with cancer do not exist. However, the American Society for Parenteral and Enteral Nutrition (ASPEN) has established standards for the nutrition screening and specialized nutrition support for all hospitalized pediatric patients (Wessel et al., 2005). The nutritional requirements of pediatric patients with cancer are similar, with an adjustment for activity, to those of normal growing children. Often pediatric patients with cancer are not bedridden, but are as active as their healthy peers. Factors that may alter nutrient requirements in cancer include the effect of the disease on host metabolism; the catabolic effects of cancer therapy; and physiologic stress from surgery, fever, malabsorption, and infection. Fluid requirements are increased during anticancer therapy or in the presence of fever, diarrhea, or renal failure. Micronutrients may require supplementation during periods of poor intake, stress, or malabsorption.

The best long-term indicator of adequate nutrient intake is growth. Children have increased nutritional requirements for growth and development that must be met despite extended periods of cancer treatment (see Chapters 17 through 19). A special vulnerability exists during the adolescent growth spurt. Ewing sarcoma is frequently associated with malnutrition.

Another reason why children with advanced cancer are at greater risk of severe nutritional depletion than adults is the frequent use of more aggressive, multimodality treatment. The long-term nutritional effects of cancer and its treatment in children are not well documented. Deficiencies in energy and protein can be expected to affect growth adversely, although the effects may be temporary, and catch-up growth depends on how much energy children are able to consistently consume (Corrales and Utter, 2005; Ringwald-Smith et al., 2006). However, some cancer treatment regimens may have an effect on growth and development that is independent of nutritional deprivation. HCT is now an accepted and increasingly successful intensive therapy for a wide range of disorders in children. Many supportive therapies may be safely managed in the outpatient arena, thus reducing the period of hospitalization.

NUTRITION RECOMMENDATIONS FOR CANCER SURVIVORS

From the time of diagnosis through the balance of life, the ACS defines anyone living with a cancer diagnosis as a *cancer survivor* (Doyle et al., 2006). The ACS guidelines as well as the WCRF and AICR recommendations provide sound diet, nutrition, and physical activity advice for primary cancer prevention and health for all individuals, including cancer survivors. In addition, the ACS has published a Guide for Informed Choices for Nutrition and Physical Activity for cancer survivors. The ACS specifically declined to call these a set of "guidelines" or "recommendations" because the evidence in this area of study is not as plentiful as in the primary prevention realm.

Cancer survivors represent one of the largest groups of people living with a chronic disease. It is estimated that there were 11 million survivors in the United States in 2009, and a projected number of 20 million in 2020 (Cancer Facts and Figures, 2009). The majority of individuals with cancer are able to return to full function and regain quality of life. This trend is expected to continue because of recent awareness in cancer prevention, advances in cancer detection, development of more effective cancer treatments, and advancements in determining the genetic causes of cancer. Nutrition can be a very important component in the long-term survival plan.

COMPLEMENTARY AND INTEGRATIVE ONCOLOGY

Integrative, *complementary*, and *alternative medicine* describe therapies used by persons interested in the promotion of health or symptom management. **Complementary therapies** are typically noninvasive, inexpensive, and useful in controlling symptoms and improving quality of life during and after cancer treatment; they are used in addition to conventional medicine. Conversely, **alternative medicine** is used instead of conventional anticancer treatment; it can be expensive, possibly harmful, and may interfere with treatments or medications. **Integrative medicine** or integrative oncology is emerging as the preferred term to differentiate between alternative therapies that are unproven and potentially unsafe, and therapies that are more evidenced-based (Belk, 2006; Wesa et al., 2008). Integrative medicine works to integrate evidence-based complementary therapies into conventional cancer treatment. Integrative medicine uses strategies to promote self-empowerment, individual responsibility, and lifestyle changes that can potentially reduce risk for both cancer recurrence and second primary tumors (Sagar, 2009). Most experts agree that a large proportion of cancer survivors participate in these modalities; several studies report more than 90% participate in some form of CAM during and after treatment (Hardy, 2008).

The health care team working in oncology needs to be informed on the different therapies and knowledgeable regarding resources used to evaluate and educate the individuals in their care. Some cancer centers are fortunate; increasing consumer demand has encouraged health care institutions to create "Integrative Medicine" departments with onsite complementary services. Cancer survivors look for open, honest discussions or recommendations from their health care team. Medical, nursing, and nutrition assessments should include open-ended questions on dietary supplement use, such as, "What vitamins, minerals, herbs, or other dietary supplements are you currently taking?" and questions regarding the additional integrative or complementary therapies they are following at this time. The core components to discuss CAM therapies involve understanding and respecting the need people have to do something for themselves; having a willingness to listen to, explore, and respond frankly to questions; taking the time to discuss the options and offer advice; summarizing the discussion; documenting the dialog; and monitoring the progress of the therapy.

The NIH established a National Center for Complementary and Alternative Medicine (NCCAM) in 1999 and works to create a framework in which to evaluate and research CAM. See Box 37-2.

Dietary Supplements

The most common form of CAM practiced in the United States is the use of dietary supplements. Consumers spend in excess of $23 billion every year on natural products marketed to maintain or enhance health (Ashar, 2008). The largest percentage (18%) use nonvitamin, nonmineral natural products such as fish oil supplements and ginseng (Barnes, 2008). That number jumps significantly when surveying cancer survivors, in whom significant use occurs (Hardy, 2008). A primary motivation is symptom management but most also hope for tumor suppression (Wesa et al., 2008).

Nondisclosure of use is a common occurrence, with a reported 53% of individuals receiving chemotherapy not

BOX 37-2

The National Center for Complementary and Alternative Medicine (NCCAM) Categories of Medical Systems

Whole Medical Systems: Western and non-Western practices of medicine built on complete systems of theory and practice. Examples include homeopathic medicine, naturopathic medicine, traditional Chinese medicine, and ayurvedic medicine.

Mind-Body Therapies: Mind-body therapies "utilize a variety of methods to enhance the mind's capacity to affect bodily function and symptoms." Examples include meditation, guided imagery, prayer, yoga, and music therapy.

Biologically Based Practices: These practices use substances found in nature and includes therapeutic diets, herbs and botanicals, and other dietary supplements.

Manipulative and Body-based Practices: Treatments of this type involve manipulation of one of more parts of the body. Examples are chiropractic medicine, massage therapy, and reflexology.

Energy Medicine: The two types of therapy in this domain: biofield and bioelectric magnetic-based, work to affect the purported energy field that surrounds and penetrates the body. The existence of such fields has not been scientifically proven. Biofield therapies include qi gong, Reiki, and therapeutic touch. Bioelectric magnetism includes the unconventional use of pulsed fields and magnetic fields.

Data from National Center for Complementary and Alternative Medicine (NCCAM): Main page, 2010. Accessed 23 October 2010 from http://nccam.nih.gov/.

discussing use of dietary supplements with their health care team (Hardy, 2008). Unfortunately, many people view dietary supplements as natural, inexpensive alternatives for prescription medications or a quick, easy remedy to an underlying medical problem. Distrust of the medical system, fear of being "fired" or dismissed by their doctor, or anticipated ignorance from the health care team may prevent cancer survivors from discussing use of dietary supplements. Ashar and Lee outline five steps: 1) inquire about use, 2) evaluate the supplement, 3) discuss any relevant regulatory issues, 4) discuss available safety and efficacy data, and 5) compare risks and benefits of use to available conventional therapies (Ashar et al., 2008). Although time consuming, conversations that include most or all of these steps will not only help open lines of communication between health care provider and survivor, but also help prevent an adverse event or poor treatment decisions. Table 37-9 lists some of the commonly used supplements.

Diet Therapies

Metabolic therapy is a term used for a variety of cancer management methods, including unproven and disproved diagnostic methods and treatments (ACS, 2009b). Metabolic practitioners generally claim that diseases, including cancer, are caused by an accumulation of toxic substances in the body. They allege that, if these toxins are removed, the body can heal itself naturally. Three basic steps are common to metabolic therapy: detoxification, strengthening of the immune system, and the use of special modalities to attack cancer. These therapy regimens generally include colonic cleansing with coffee, wheat grass, or other substances;

TABLE 37-9

Potential Adverse Events with Integrative Therapies Commonly Used by Cancer Survivors

Dietary Supplement	Claim and Common Uses	Potential Adverse Event
Echinacea	Boosts the immune system.	May cause inflammation of the liver if used in conjunction with other medications such as anabolic steroids, methotrexate (chemotherapy), or others.
Garlic	Helps lower cholesterol.	May increase risk for excessive bleeding, especially when used with certain anticlotting agents.
Ginger	Helps with nausea.	May increase risk for excessive bleeding, especially when used with certain anticlotting agents.
Ginkgo	Helps increase blood circulation and oxygenation. Enhances memory and mental concentration.	May increase risk for excessive, bleeding especially when used with certain anticlotting agents.
Ginseng	Increases physical stamina and mental concentration.	May increase risk for excessive bleeding, especially when used with certain anticlotting agents; may increase heart rate and high blood pressure; may increase bleeding in women after menopause.
Goldenseal	Helps reduce inflammation and promote good bowel function.	May worsen swelling or high blood pressure.
Licorice	Helps soothe the stomach.	Certain licorice mixtures may cause high blood pressure, increase swelling, and cause electrolyte imbalances.
Saw palmetto	Helps with enlarged prostate and urinary inflammation.	May interact with other hormone therapies.
St. John's wort	Helps with mild to moderate depression, anxiety, or sleep disorders.	May decrease effectiveness of all currently marketed medication using cytochrome P450 pathway in the liver: HIV and AIDS medications (NNRTIs and PIs), carbamazepine, cyclosporine, irinotecan (Camptosar) for chemotherapy, midazolam (Versed), nifedipine (Procardia), simvastatin (Zocor), theophylline, warfarin (Coumadin).
Valerian	Helps as mild sedative or sleep aid, or muscle relaxant.	May increase effects of certain antiseizure medications or prolong effects of anesthetic agents.

Data from Natural Standards, 2010.

AIDS, Acquired immune deficiency syndrome; *HIV*, human immunodeficiency virus; *NNRTI*, nonnucleoside reverse transcriptase inhibitor; *PI*, protease inhibitor.

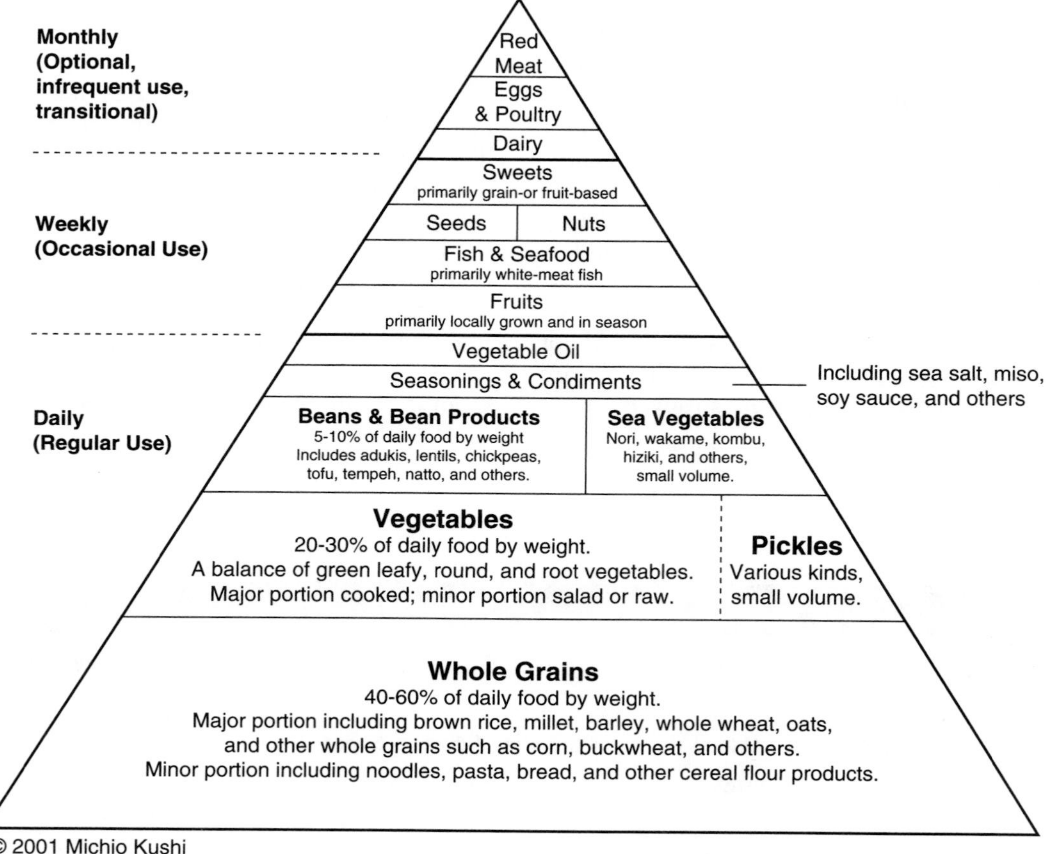

FIGURE 37-2 The Great Life Pyramid proposed for a macrobiotic diet. http://www.holistic-cooking.co.uk/WhatIsMacrobiotics.htm *(© Michio Kushi and permission given by Kushi Institute.)*

special diets; and vitamin and mineral supplementation. Complications of colonic irrigation include electrolyte imbalance, toxic colitis, bowel perforation, and sepsis. Most regimens promote "natural" and "organic" foods and recommend restriction of animal products, refined flours and sugars, and foods that are processed or contain artificial ingredients. Examples of metabolic therapies include the Gerson therapy, the Gonzalez regimen, the Livingston-Wheeler therapy and the Issels treatment. The special diets associated with cancer care promote the idea that food is medicine. Diet plans are individualized and food specifically chosen and prepared.

The **macrobiotic diet** and lifestyle is a program promoting natural healing, popularized in the United States by Michio Kushi in the late 1970s. This macrobiotic diet derives 40% to 60% of its calories from whole grains; 20% to 30% from vegetables; and the remainder from beans, bean products, sea vegetables, fruit, seeds, nuts, white-meat fish, and very occasionally seafood, poultry, red meat, eggs, and dairy (Kushi et al., 2006) (Figure 37-2). Research has determined that the diet is naturally deficient in calcium and vitamin B_{12}. The macrobiotic diet has not been scientifically proven to treat or cure cancer.

Orthomolecular Medicine

Orthomolecular medicine (OM) is the practice of restoring an optimal environment in the body by correcting imbalances and deficiencies, another alternative medicine practice in cancer care. The treatment is based on the theory that by correcting imbalances and deficiencies, the body will regain health. This has not been proven in clinical trials, and instead is extrapolated from basic science. Infusions or supplementation may involve large doses of vitamins, minerals, essential fatty acids, fiber, amino acids, or enzymes. Orthomolecular practitioners (often medical doctors) consider a number of CAM practices to be consistent with OM philosophy and may incorporate parts of naturopathic medicine, nutrition, acupuncture, mind-body therapies, and manipulative and body-based practices such as massage into their treatments.

Advanced Cancer and Palliative Care

Palliative care is the active total care of an individual when curative measures are no longer considered an option by either the medical team or the individual. Hospice care focuses on relieving symptoms and supporting individuals with a life expectancy of months, not years (NHPCO, 2010). The objectives are to provide for optimal quality of life; relieve physical symptoms; alleviate isolation, anxiety, and fear associated with advanced disease; and to help patients maintain independence as long as possible (McCallum and Fornari, 2006). The goals of nutrition intervention should focus on managing nutrition-related symptoms such as pain, weakness, loss of appetite, early satiety, constipation, weakness, dry mouth, and dyspnea (McCallum and Fornari, 2006). Another important goal is maintaining strength and energy to enhance quality of life, independence, and ability to perform activities of daily living. Nutrition should be provided "as tolerated or as desired" along with emotional support and awareness of and respect for individual needs and wishes. Thus the pleasurable aspects of eating should be emphasized, without concern for quantity or nutrient and energy content.

The use of nutrition support and hydration in individuals with advanced, incurable cancer is a difficult and often controversial issue and should be determined on a case-by-case basis. Advance directives are legal documents that guide health care providers regarding the specific wishes of individuals, outlining the extent of their desired medical care, including the provision of artificial nutrition and hydration. Whenever providing nutrition care, consideration should be given to advanced directives that may be in place.

CLINICAL SCENARIO 1

Janice is a 55-year-old mother of four children. Recently she was diagnosed with breast cancer (estrogen-receptor positive). Surgery, radiation therapy to her breast and five years of tamoxifen are planned for treatment of her disease. In the next 3 weeks she will undergo a lumpectomy, followed by 5 to 6 weeks of external-beam radiation therapy. She is 5′8″ tall, weighs 185 lb, and has a history of mild hypertension that has been controlled with dietary measures. She currently does not engage in regular physical activity but is motivated to make changes in her lifestyle to improve her fitness and overall health. She also is attracted to the use of multiple vitamins/minerals and dietary supplements, and complementary and alternative therapies for reducing her cancer recurrence risk and managing treatment-related side effects and postmenopausal symptoms.

Nutrition Diagnostic Statement 1

Physical inactivity related to lack of regular exercise plan as evidenced by patient reports of no exercise

Nutrition Diagnostic Statement 2

Food- and nutrition-related knowledge deficit related to medical nutrition therapy related to cancer treatment and secondary prevention as evidenced by patient requesting more information

Nutrition Care Questions

1. What recommendations would you give Janice to prepare her for surgery?
2. After radiation therapy and surgery, what side effects might Janice experience? List some dietary strategies Janice may follow if she experiences the following: fatigue, intermittent queasiness, a slight difficulty in swallowing (esophagus is in the radiation field), and an increased caloric intake (mostly caused by her need to "take care of" herself, which results in weight gain).
3. Is Janice at her ideal body weight? If not, what suggestions would you recommend? Consider her hypertension, planned surgery, and radiation therapy.
4. What dietary recommendations, if any, are appropriate for patients receiving tamoxifen?
5. What guidance should be provided with regard to the appropriate use of vitamin and mineral supplements and ways to evaluate alternative therapies? How does soy affect estrogen-receptor–positive forms of breast cancer? How should she manage hot flashes now that she is advised not to take estrogen replacement therapy?

CLINICAL SCENARIO 2

Michael is a 58-year-old man with a recent diagnosis of esophageal cancer. He has experienced gastroesophageal reflux (GERD) for the past 5 years and had been advised to undergo an endoscopic examination to rule out Barrett's esophagus, but he never followed up on his doctor's referral. He lost 40 pounds in the four months prior to his diagnosis because of lack of appetite and progressive difficulty swallowing solid foods. Prediagnosis, his diet consisted of drinking "muscle drinks" his son purchased at the local gym. He has been very pleased with his weight loss, but knew something was wrong.

Michael underwent an esophagogastrectomy 1 month ago and received some nutrition information from the inpatient registered dietitian right before he was discharged, but he

Continued

CLINICAL SCENARIO 2—cont'd

reports that he never read it. He has lost an additional 20 pounds in the past month, and has been admitted once for dehydration caused by lack of fluid intake and because of continued symptoms related to postsurgical dumping syndrome.

His current food and nutrition history includes small meals with a usual intake of approximately 1500 calories daily. He eats three times a day. He reports he does not have the energy to prepare food so while his wife is at work, he relies on frozen meals warmed in the microwave and canned soup. He has a sweet tooth and, because eating is difficult, he rewards himself with ice cream or a cookie after each meal. His beverages include whole milk, apple juice, and a "finger" of scotch each night. He finally has agreed to see the outpatient registered dietitian because he feels dehydrated again, has no energy, and needs to get back to work.

Biochemical Data

Albumin: 3.0 mg/dL
Blood urea nitrogen: 18 mg/dL
Creatinine: 0.6 mg/dL
Blood pressure: 110/60
Pulse rate of 90

Anthropometric Data

Height: 72″
Weight history: Usual body weight: 200 lb, preoperative weight: 160 lb, 1 month postoperative weight: 140lb
Body mass index: 19

Medications

Metoclopramide (Reglan) 30 minutes before each meal
Atorvastatin (Lipitor)
Metoprolol (Toprol)
Hydrochlorothiazide

Dietary Supplements

One-A-Day for Men

Nutrition Diagnostic Statements

1. Food- and nutrition-related knowledge deficit related to lack of education and counseling for appropriate medical nutrition therapy as evidenced by food history with inappropriate food choices.
2. Altered gastrointestinal function related to esophagogastrectomy as evidenced by weight loss, dehydration, and dumping syndrome.
3. Inadequate protein and energy intake related to postsurgery recovery as evidenced by decreased food and beverage intake, weight loss, and muscle wasting causing decreased creatinine.

Nutrition Interventions

Nutrition prescription: Small frequent meals consisting of energy-dense, lower-fat foods and limited simple carbohydrates; majority of fluid consumption between meals (sips during meals okay to aid in chewing and swallowing).

Nutrition education: Update Michael's knowledge of appropriate nutrition therapy following an esophagogastrectomy. Discuss tolerance of different food groups; sources of protein; energy-dense, easy-to-prepare menu options; and healthy beverage selections, including advising him to discontinue consumption of daily alcoholic beverage; and goal caloric intake needed for slow, steady weight gain. Suggest he consider eating every 2 hours, on the even hour, to create an external reminder to eat. Recommend he review his hypertension medication types and doses with his physicians because his need for medication may have changed with his significant weight loss.

At follow-up visits address weight-gain progress, bowel function, food and beverage intake and tolerance; encourage physical activity (physician approved) starting with short walks to regain muscle strength. JE needs to be accompanied by a friend or family member on these walks.

Nutrition counseling: Coordinate with patient and wife to ensure appropriate foods and beverages are available for consumption. Discuss expected acute and long-term side effects from surgery. Establish slow, steady weight gain and physical activity goals for next 3 months.

Nutrition Monitoring and Evaluation

1. Body weight trends
2. Hydration status
2. Serum albumin levels and creatinine levels (over 3 months)
3. Physical activity
4. Schedule follow-up session in 2 weeks, with optional phone call between visits

USEFUL WEBSITES

American Cancer Society
www.cancer.org

American Institute for Cancer Research
www.aicr.org

National Cancer Institute
www.cancer.gov

National Center for Complementary and Alternative Medicine (NCCAM)
http://nccam.nih.gov

Oncology Nutrition Practice Group
www.oncologynutrition.org

Survivorship Resources
http://www.iom/edu/en/Reports/2005/From-Cancer-Patient-to-Cancer-Survivor-Lost-in-Transition.aspx

REFERENCES

American Cancer Society: *Cancer facts & figures, 2009*, Atlanta, 2009a, American Cancer Society.

American Cancer Society: *Cancer glossary*, 2010a. Accessed 10 June 2010 from http://www.cancer.org/CancerGlossary/index.

American Cancer Society: *Cancer prevention & early detection facts & figures, 2010*, Atlanta, 2010, American Cancer Society.

American Cancer Society: *Complete guide to complementary and alternative cancer therapies*, ed 2, Atlanta, 2009b, American Cancer Society.

American College of Sports Medicine (ACSM): Certified cancer exercise trainer, 2010. Accessed 26 October 2010 from www.acsm.org.

American Dietetic Association(ADA): *Evidence analysis library: oncology evidence-based nutrition practice guidelines*, Chicago, 2010a, American Dietetic Association.

American Dietetic Association (ADA): *International dietetics & terminology: reference manual, standardized language for the nutrition care process*, Chicago, 2011, American Dietetic Association.

American Dietetic Association (ADA): *Oncology toolkit*, Chicago, 2010b, American Dietetic Association.

American Dietetic Association (ADA): Position of the American Dietetic Association: Health Implications of Dietary Fiber, *J American Dietetic Association* 108, 2008.

Anderson AS, et al: Obesity Management-An Opportunity for Cancer Prevention, *Surgeon* 7:5, 2009.

Ashar BH, et al: Advising patients who use dietary supplements, *Am J Med* 121, 2008.

Bailey RL, et al: Total folate and folic acid intake from foods and dietary supplements in the United States: 2003-2006, *Am J Clin Nutr* 91:231, 2010.

Baan R, et al: Carcinogenicity of alcoholic beverages, *Lancet Oncology* 8, 2007.

Barnes PM, et al: *Complementary and alternative medicine use among adults and children: United States, 2007*, National Health Statistics Reports, US Department of Health and Human Services, Centers for Disease Control, 10, 2008

Belk LB: Primer on integrative oncology, *Hematol Oncol Clin N Am* 20, 2006.

Beronius A, et al: Risk to all or none? A comparative analysis of controversies in the health risk assessment of bisphenol A, *Reprod Toxicol* 29:1, 2010

Berquin IM, et al: Multi-targeted therapy of cancer by omega-3 fatty acids, *Science Direct* 269, 2008.

Blackburn GL, et al: Metabolic Syndrome and the Onset of Cancer, *American Journal of Clinical Nutrition* 86:3, 2007.

Block KI, et al: Impact of antioxidant supplementation on chemotherapeutic efficacy: a systematic review of the evidence from randomized controlled trials, *Cancer Treat Rev* 123:1227, 2008.

Brawer R, et al: Obesity and Cancer, *Primary Care Clinical Office Practice* 36, 2009.

Bruner DW, et al: *Manual for radiation oncology and nursing practice and education*, ed 3, Pittsburgh, 2005, Oncology Nursing Society.

Cady J: Nutritional support during radiotherapy for head and neck: the role of prophylactic feeding tube placement, *J Clin Onc Nurs* 11:875, 2007.

Cancer facts and figures, 2009. Accessed 12 December 2009 from www.cancer.org.

Charney P, Cranganu A: Nutrition screening and assessment in oncology. In Marian M, Roberts S, editors: *Clinical nutrition for oncology patients*, Sudbury, MA, 2010, Jones and Bartlett.

Charuhas PM: Medical nutrition therapy in bone marrow transplantation. In Elliott L, et al., editors: *The clinical guide to oncology nutrition*, ed 2, Chicago, 2006, American Dietetic Association.

Chey H, et al: Toxins in everyday life, *Prim Care Clin Office Pract* 35, 2008.

Chung M, et al: Vitamin D and Calcium: systematic review of health outcomes, *Evid Rep Tech Assess* 183, 2009.

Corrales KM, Utter SL: Growth failure. In Samour PQ, King K, editors, *Handbook of pediatric nutrition*, ed 3, Sudbury, MA, 2005, Jones and Bartlett.

Doyle C, et al: The 2006 Nutrition, Physical Activity and Cancer Survivorship Advisory Committee. Nutrition and physical activity during and after cancer treatment: an American Cancer Society guide for informed choices. *CA Cancer J Clin* 56:323-353, 2006.

Elliott L, et al., editors: *The clinical guide to oncology nutrition*, ed 2, Chicago, 2006, American Dietetic Association.

Farhadian A, et al: Determination of polycyclic aromatic hydrocarbons in grilled meat, *Food Control* 21, 2010.

Fearon KC: Cancer cachexia: developing multimodal therapy for a multidimensional problem, *Eur J Cancer* 44:1124, 2008.

Ferguson LR: Meat and Cancer, *Meat Science* 84:308, 2010.

Flegel KM, et al: Prevalence and trends in obesity among US adults, 1999-2008, *JAMA* 303:3, 2010.

Food and Drug Administration (FDA): News and events: bisphenol A (BPA): update on bisphenol A (BPA) for use in food, January 2010. Accessed 3 November 2010 from www.fda.gov.

Fuhrman MP: Nutrition-focused physical assessment. In Charney P, Malone A, editors: *Nutrition assessment*, Chicago, 2009, American Dietetic Association.

Gardner A, et al: Randomized comparison of cooked and non-cooked diet in patient undergoing remission induction therapy for acute myeloid leukemia, *J Clin Oncol* 26:5684, 2008.

Garland CF, et al: Vitamin D for cancer prevention: global perspective, *Annual of Epidemiology* 19:468, 2009.

Garland CF, et al: Vitamin d supplement doses and serum 25 hydroxy d in the range associated with cancer prevention, *Anticancer Res* 31:607, 2011.

Goldman A, et al: Symptoms in children/young people with progressive malignant disease: United Kingdom Children's Cancer Study Group/Paediatric Oncology Nurses Forum survey, *Pediatrics* 117:1179, 2006.

Gottschlich MM, editor: *The A.S.P.E.N. nutrition support core curriculum: a case-based approach—the adult patient*, Silver Spring, MD, 2007, American Society for Parenteral and Enteral Nutrition.

Grant B, Byron J: Nutritional implications of chemotherapy. In Elliott L, et al., editors: *The clinical guide to oncology nutrition*, ed 2, Chicago, 2006, American Dietetic Association.

Grant BL, et al., editors: *American Cancer Society's complete guide to nutrition for cancer survivors*, ed 2, Atlanta, 2010, American Cancer Society.

Grant BL, Hamilton KK, editors: *Management of nutrition impact symptoms in cancer and educational handouts*, Chicago, 2005, American Dietetic Association.

Greenwald P, et al: The challenge of nutrition in cancer. In Blackburn V, et al, editors: *Nutritional oncology*, St Louis, 2006, Elsevier.

Hardy ML: Dietary supplement use in cancer care: help or harm, *Hematol Oncol Clin N Am* 22, 2008.

Harris DJ, et al: Putting evidence into practice: evidence-based interventions for the management of oral mucositis, *J Clin Onc Nurs* 12:141, 2008.

Havrila C, et al: Medical and radiation oncology. In Marian M, Roberts S, editor: *Clinical nutrition for oncology patients*, Sudbury, MA, 2010, Jones and Bartlett.

Huhmann MB, August D: Surgical oncology. In Marian M, Roberts S, editor: *Clinical nutrition for oncology patients*, Sudbury, MA, 2010, Jones and Bartlett.

Huncharek M, et al: Colorectal cancer risk and dietary intake of calcium, vitamin D and dairy products: a meta-analysis of 26,355 cases from 60 observational studies, *Nutr Cancer* 61:1, 2009.

Hurst JD, Gallagher AL: Energy, protein, micronutrient, and fluid requirement. In Elliott L, et al., editors: *The clinical guide to oncology nutrition*, ed 2, Chicago, 2006, American Dietetic Association.

Kashfi K: Anti-inflammatory agents as cancer therapeutics, *Adv Pharmacol* 57, 2009.

Kushi LH, et al: American Cancer Society guidelines on nutrition and physical activity for cancer prevention: reducing the risk of cancer with healthy food choices and physical activity, *CA Cancer J Clin* 56:310, 2006.

Kuzuhara T, et al: Green tea catechin as a chemical chaperone in cancer prevention, *Cancer Letter* 261, 2008.

Kwan M, et al: Alcohol Consumption and Breast Cancer Recurrence and Survival Among Women with Early–State Breast Cancer: The Life After Cancer Epidemiology Study, *J Clin Oncol* 10:1200, 2010.

Layton L: Reversing itself, FDA expresses concerns over health risks from BPA, *Washington Post Saturday*, 16 January 2010.

Lee SA, et al: Adolescent and adult soy food intake and breast cancer risk: results from the Shanghai women's health study, *Breast Dis* 21:2, 2010

Levine AJ, et al: A candidate gene study of folate-associated one carbon metabolism genes and colorectal cancer risk, *Cancer Epidemiol Biomarkers Prev* 19:1812, 2010.

Link A, et al: Cancer chemoprevention by dietary polyphenols: promising role for epigenetics, *Biochem Pharmacol* 80:1, 2010.

Longo V, et al: Calorie restriction and cancer prevention: metabolic and molecular mechanisms, *Trends in Pharmacological Sciences* 31:2, 2010.

McCallum PD: Nutrition screening and assessment in oncology. In Elliott L et al., editors: *The clinical guide to oncology nutrition*, ed 2, Chicago, 2006, American Dietetic Association.

McCallum PD, Fornari A: Nutrition therapy in palliative care. In Elliott L, et al., editors: *The clinical guide to oncology nutrition*, ed 2, Chicago, 2006, American Dietetic Association.

Miller M, et al: Dietary supplement use in individuals living with cancer and other chronic conditions: a population-based study, *J Am Diet Assoc* 108:3, 2008.

Muehlbauer PM, et al: Putting evidence into practice: evidence-based interventions to prevent, manage and treat chemotherapy and radiotherapy-induced diarrhea, *J Clin Onc Nurs* 13:336, 2009.

National Cancer Institute (NCI): *Cancer bulletin—cost of cancer care has doubled in the past 20 years*, 2010a. Accessed 23 October 2010 from http://www.cancer.gov/ncicancerbulletin/051810/page10.

National Cancer Institute (NCI): *Cancer genetics overview PDQ (Health Professional Version)*, 2010b. Accessed 23 October 2010 from http://www.cancer.gov/cancertopics/pdq/genetics/overview/healthprofessional.

National Cancer Institute (NCI): *Chemotherapy and you*, 2010c. Accessed 18 October 2010 from http://www.cancer.gov/publications/.

National Cancer Institute (NCI): *Dictionary of terms*, 2010d. Accessed 23 October 2010 from http://www.cancer.gov/dictionary/.

National Cancer Institute (NCI): *Eating hints*, 2010e. Accessed 20 October 2010 from http://www.cancer.gov/publications/.

National Cancer Institute (NCI): *Radiation therapy and you*, 2010f. Accessed 23 October 2010 from http://cancer.gov/publications/.

National Cancer Institute (NCI): *SEER stat fact sheets—cancer of all sites*, 2010g. Accessed 23 October 2010 from http://seer.cancer.gov/statfacts/html/all.print.html#incidence-mortality.

National Center for Complementary and Alternative Medicine (NCCAM): *Main page*, 2010. Accessed 23 October 2010 from http://nccam.nih.gov/.

National Comprehensive Cancer Network (NCCN): *NCCN clinical practice guidelines in oncology (NCCN guidelines)*, 2010. Accessed 24 October 2010 from http://www.nccn.org/clinical.asp.

Natural Standards Database (subscription) www.naturalstandard.com; accessed 11.10.

National Hospice and Palliative Care Organization (NHPCO): *How can palliative care help?* 2010. Accessed 23 October 2010 from http://www.nhpco.org.

National Institute of Dental and Craniofacial Research (NIDCR): *Cancer treatment and oral health*, 2010. Accessed 23 October 2010 from http://www.nidcr.nih.gov/OralHealth/Topics/CancerTreatment/.

National Marrow Donor Program (NMDP): *Types of transplants*, 2010. Accessed 23 October 2010 from http://www.marrow.org.

Oaks BM, et al: Folate intake, post-folic acid grain fortification, and pancreatic cancer risk in the Prostate, Lung, Colorectal, and Ovarian Cancer Screening Trial, *Am J Clin Nutr* 91:449, 2010.

Park Y, et al: Dietary Fiber intake and risk of breast cancer in postmenopausal women: the National Institutes of Health-AARP Diet and Health Study, *American Journal of Clinical Nutrition* 90, 2009.

Parekh N, et al: Lifestyle, Anthropometric, and Obesity-Related Physiologic Determinants of Insulin-like Growth Factor-1 in the Third National Health and Nutrition Examination Survey (1988-1994), *Annuals of Epidemiology* 20:3, 2010.

Polednak AP: Estimating the number of US incident cancers attributable to obesity and the impact on temporal trends in incidence rates for obesity-related cancers, *Cancer Detection and Prevention* 32:190, 2008.

Pierce JP, et al: Influence of a diet very high in vegetables, fruit and fiber and low in fat following treatment for breast cancer: the Women's Healthy Eating and Living (WHEL) randomized trial, *JAMA* 298:3, 2007.

Pollack M: Insulin, insulin-like growth factors and neoplasia, *Best Pract Res Clin Endocrinol Metab* 22:4, 2008.

Polovich M, et al: *Chemotherapy and biotherapy guidelines and recommendations for practice*, Pittsburgh, 2009, Oncology Nursing Society.

Ringwald-Smith K, et al: Medical nutrition therapy in pediatric oncology. In Elliott L, et al., editors: *The clinical guide to oncology nutrition*, ed 2, Chicago, 2006, American Dietetic Association.

Robien K: Hematological malignancies. In Marian M, Roberts S, editors: *Clinical nutrition for oncology patients*, Sudbury, MA, 2010, Jones and Bartlett.

Robien K, et al: American Dietetic Association: revised standards of practice and standards of professional performance for registered dietitians (generalist, specialty, and advanced) in oncology nutrition care, *J Am Diet Assoc* 110:310, 2010.

Russo GL: Ins and Outs of Dietary Phytochemical in Cancer Prevention, *Biochemical Pharmacology* 74, 2007.

Russell M, Malone A: Nutrient requirements. In Charney P, Malone A, editors: *Nutrition assessment*, Chicago, 2009, American Dietetic Association.

Sagar SM: The role of integrative medicine in a tertiary prevention survivorship program, *Prev Med* 40, 2009.

Schelbert KB: Comorbities of obesity, *Prim Care* 36:271, 2009.

Seattle Cancer Care Alliance (SCCA): Diet guidelines for immunosuppressed patients, 2010. Accessed 30 September 2010 from http://www.seattlecca.org/general-oncology-diet-guidelines.cfm.

Skipworth RJ, et al: Pathophysiology of cancer cachexia: much more than host-tumour interaction? *Clin Nutr* 266:667, 2007.

Teucher B, et al: Obesity: Focus on all-cause mortality and cancer, *Maturitas* 65, 2010.

Toles M, et al: Nutrition and the cancer survivor: evidence to guide oncology nursing practice, *Semin Oncol Nurs* 24:3, 2008.

Tipton JM, et al: Putting evidence into practice: evidence-based interventions to prevent, manage and treat chemotherapy-induced nausea and vomiting, *J Clin Onc Nurs* 11:70, 2007.

U.S. Department of Agriculture (USDA): *USDA-Iowa State University database on the isoflavone content of foods*, 2010. Accessed 23 October 2010 from http://www.nal.usda.gov/fnic/foodcomp/Data/isoflav/isfl_doc.pdf.

Valavanidis A, et al: 8-hydroxy-2′-deoxyguanosine (8-OHdG): a critical biomarker of oxidative stress and carcinogenesis, *J Environ Sci Health C Environ Carcinog Ecotoxicol Rev* 27:120, 2009.

Wesa K, et al: Integrative oncology: complementary therapies for cancer survivors, *Hematol Oncol Clin N Am* 22, 2008.

Wessel J, et al: American Society for Parenteral and Enteral Nutrition: task force on standards for specialized nutrition support for hospitalized pediatric patients, *Nutr Clin Pract* 20:103, 2005.

Wilkes GM, Barton-Burke M: *2010 oncology nursing drug handbook*, Boston, 2010, Jones and Bartlett.

World Cancer Research Fund (WCRF), American Institute for Cancer Research (AICR): *Food, nutrition, physical activity, and the prevention of cancer: a global perspective*, Washington, DC, 2007, WCRF and AICR.

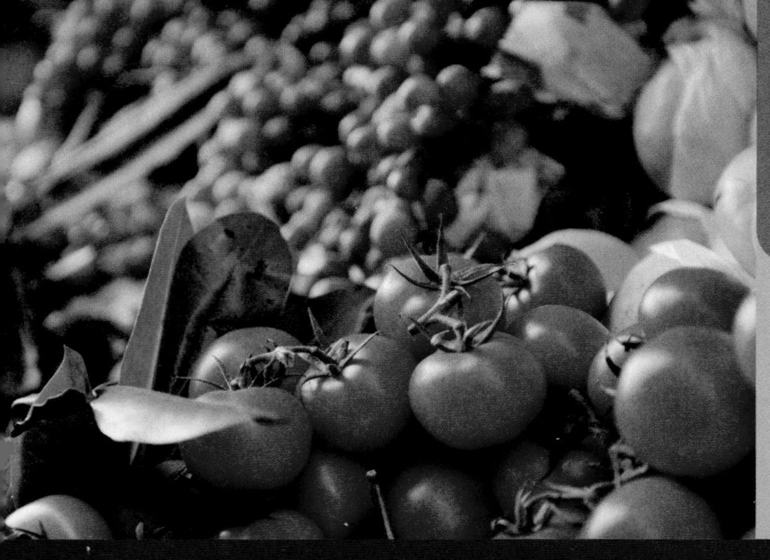

CHAPTER 38

Kimberly R. Dong, MS, RD
Cindy Mari Imai, MS, RD

Medical Nutrition Therapy for HIV and AIDS

KEY TERMS

acquired immune deficiency syndrome (AIDS)
acute HIV infection
antiretroviral therapy (ART)
asymptomatic HIV infection
CD4+ cells
CD4 count
clinical latency
drug resistance
HIV-associated lipodystrophy syndrome (HALS)
human immunodeficiency virus (HIV)
long-term nonprogression
opportunistic infections (OIs)
seroconversion
symptomatic HIV infection
T-helper lymphocyte cells
viral load

Acquired immune deficiency syndrome (AIDS) is caused by the human immunodeficiency virus (HIV). HIV affects the body's ability to fight off infection and disease, which can ultimately lead to death. Medications used to treat HIV have enhanced the quality of life and increased life expectancy of HIV-infected individuals. These antiretroviral therapy (ART) medications slow the replication of the virus but do not eliminate HIV infection. With increased access to ART, people are living longer with HIV. Unfortunately, health issues such as cardiovascular disease and insulin resistance are increasingly prevalent in this population.

Nutritional status plays an important role in maintaining a healthy immune system and delaying the progression of HIV to AIDS. To develop appropriate nutrition recommendations, the nutrition professional should be familiar with the pathophysiology of HIV infection, the medication and nutrient interactions, and the barriers to adequate nutrition. Mental health status and illicit drug use should be considered since it may affect nutrition intake.

EPIDEMIOLOGY AND TRENDS

Global Status of HIV and AIDS

The first cases of AIDS were described in 1981. Soon after, HIV was isolated and identified as the core agent leading to AIDS. Since then, the number of people with HIV has gradually increased, leading to a global pandemic affecting socioeconomic development worldwide. The continuing rise in the population of people living with HIV is reflective of new HIV infections and the widespread use of ART, which has delayed the progression of HIV infection to death. At the end of 2008 an estimated 33.4 million people were living with HIV or AIDS. There were 2.7 million new infections reported, an average of 7400 infections daily, and 2 million HIV-related deaths (Joint United Nations Programme on HIV/AIDS [UNAIDS] and the World Health Organization [WHO], 2009).

Despite increased prevention efforts and availability of ART, geographic variations in HIV infection is evident. The

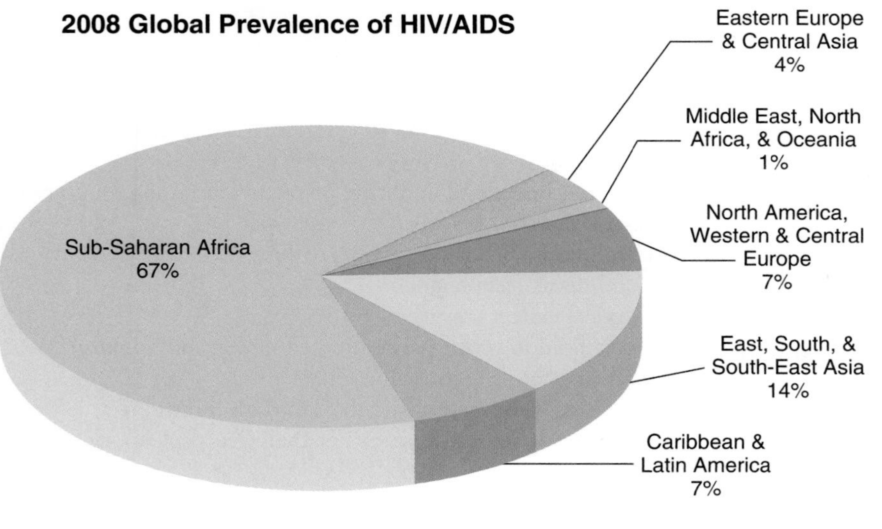

FIGURE 38-1 Global prevalence of HIV and AIDS. *(UNAIDS and WHO:* 2009 AIDS epidemic update. *Accessed 12 July 2010 from http://data.unaids.org/pub/Report/2009/JC1700_Epi_Update_2009_en.pdf. From UNAIDS/ONUSIDA 2009.)*

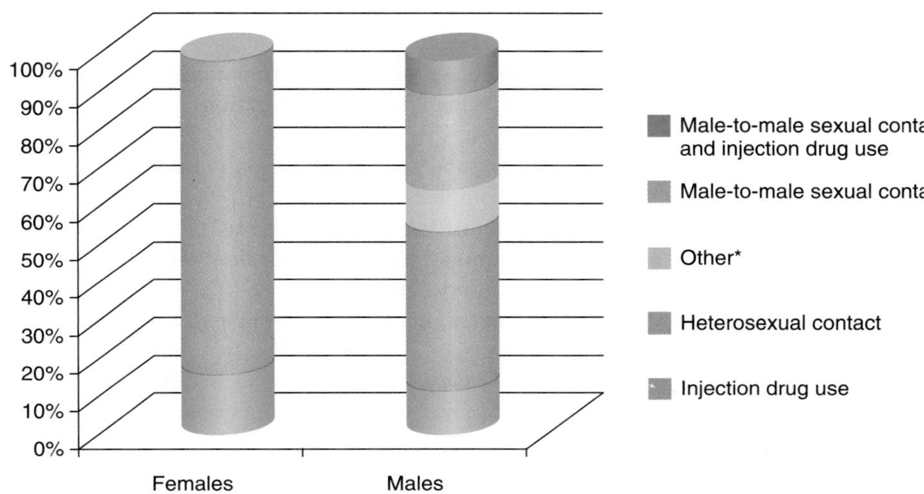

FIGURE 38-2 Estimated Percentage of HIV diagnoses by route of transmission in the United States, 2008. *(Centers for Disease Control and Prevention (CDC): HIV surveillance report, 2008a. Accessed from 12 July 2010 from http://www.cdc.gov/hiv/surveillance/resources/reports/2008report/pdf/2008SurveillanceReport.pdf.)*

majority of infections continue to occur in the developing world (Figure 38-1) where more than 97% occur in low- and middle-income countries (UNAIDS and WHO, 2009). Sub-Saharan Africa remains the region most heavily affected by HIV, accounting for two thirds of current HIV infections and 72% of HIV-related deaths (UNAIDS and WHO, 2009). However, increases in new infections are being seen in higher-income countries in eastern Europe such as Ukraine and the Russian Federation. Within sub-Saharan Africa, heterosexual transmission is the most prevalent mode of HIV transmission (UNAIDS and WHO, 2009). In other regions, populations affected by HIV include injection drug users, men who have sex with men, sex workers, and clients of sex workers.

The United States

Within the United States, more than 1.2 million people are living with HIV or AIDS and 21% may be unaware of their HIV status (Centers for Disease Control and Prevention [CDC], 2006, UNAIDS, 2008). Although more people are living with a diagnosis of HIV or AIDS, incidence has remained relatively stable since the 1990s. In 2008 men accounted for 75% of all diagnoses of HIV infection. The rate of new infections in men has been trending up since 2005, whereas the rate among women has remained stable (CDC, 2010). The largest percentage of persons living with HIV infection is among those aged 40-44; this same group accounts for the highest rate of new HIV infections. Ethnic populations disproportionately affected by HIV include blacks and Latinos, who accounted for 52% and 25% of HIV diagnoses, respectively, in 2008 (CDC, 2010). The most common route of transmission among men is male-to-male sexual contact and among women is heterosexual contact (Figure 38-2).

PATHOPHYSIOLOGY AND CLASSIFICATION

Primary infection with **human immunodeficiency virus (HIV)** is the underlying cause of AIDS. HIV invades the genetic core of the **CD4+ cells**, **T-helper lymphocyte cells**, which are the principal agents involved in protection against infection.

HIV infection causes a progressive depletion of CD4+ cells, which eventually leads to immunodeficiency.

HIV infection progresses through four clinical stages: acute HIV infection, clinical latency, symptomatic HIV infection, and progression of HIV to AIDS. The two main biomarkers used to assess disease progression are HIV ribonucleic acid (RNA) (**viral load**) and CD4+ T-cell count (CD4 count).

Acute HIV infection is the time from transmission of HIV to the host until the production of detectable antibodies against the virus (**seroconversion**) occurs. Half of individuals experience physical symptoms such as fever, malaise, myalgia, pharyngitis, or swollen lymph glands at 2-4 weeks following infection, but these generally subside after 1-2 weeks. Because of the nonspecific clinical features and short diagnostic window, acute HIV infection is rarely diagnosed. HIV seroconversion occurs within 3 weeks to 3 months after exposure. If HIV testing is done before seroconversion occurs, a "false negative" may result despite HIV being present. During the acute stage, the virus replicates rapidly and causes a significant decline in CD4+ cell counts. Eventually, the immune response reaches a viral setpoint where viral load stabilizes and CD4+cell counts return closer to normal.

A period of **clinical latency** or **asymptomatic HIV infection**, then follows. Further evidence of illness may not be exhibited for as long as 10 years postinfection. The virus is still active and replicating, although at a decreased rate compared with the acute stage, and CD4+ cell counts continue to steadily decline. In 3% to 5% of HIV-infected individuals, **long-term nonprogression** occurs, in which CD4+ cell counts remain normal and viral loads can be undetectable for years without medical intervention (Department of Health and Human Services [DHHS], 2010). It has been suggested that this unique population has different and fewer receptor sites for the virus to penetrate cell membranes (Wanke et al., 2009).

In the majority of cases, HIV slowly breaks down the immune system, making it incapable of fighting the virus. When CD4+ cell counts fall below 500 cells/ mm^3 individuals are more susceptible to developing signs and symptoms such as persistent fevers, chronic diarrhea, unexplained weight loss, and recurrent fungal or bacterial infections, all of which are indicative of **symptomatic HIV infection**.

As immunodeficiency worsens and CD4 counts fall to even lower levels, the infection becomes symptomatic and progresses to AIDS. The progression of HIV to AIDS increases risk of **opportunistic infections (OIs)**, which generally do not occur in individuals with healthy immune systems. The CDC classifies AIDS cases as positive laboratory confirmation of HIV infection in persons with a CD4+ cell count less than 200 cells/mm^3 (or less than 14%) or documentation of an AIDS-defining condition (Box 38-1).

HIV is transmitted via direct contact with infected body fluids like blood, semen, preseminal fluid, vaginal fluid, and breast milk. Cerebrospinal fluid surrounding the brain and spinal cord, synovial fluid surrounding joints, and amniotic fluid surrounding a fetus are other fluids that can transmit HIV. Saliva, tears, and urine do not contain enough HIV for transmission. Sexual transmission is the most common way HIV is transmitted and injection drug use is the second most prevalent method of transmission (see Figure 38-2).

BOX 38-1

2008 CDC Case Definition AIDS-Defining Clinical Conditions

Bacterial infections, multiple or recurrent (among children <13 years)
Candidiasis (bronchi, trachea, or lungs)
Candidiasis (esophagus)
Cervical cancer (invasive)
Coccidioidomycosis (disseminated or extrapulmonary)
Cryptococcosis (extrapulmonary)
Cryptosporidiosis (intestinal, >1 month duration)
Cytomegalovirus disease (other than liver, spleen, or nodes)
Cytomegalovirus retinitis (with loss of vision)
Encephalopathy (HIV related)
Herpes simplex: chronic ulcers (>1 month duration)
Herpes simplex: bronchitis, pneumonitis, or esophagitis
Histoplasmosis (disseminated or extrapulmonary)
Isosporiasis (intestinal, >1 month duration)
Kaposi's sarcoma
Lymphoid interstitial pneumonia or pulmonary lymphoid hyperplasia complex
Lymphoma, Burkitt (or equivalent term)
Lymphoma, immunoblastic (or equivalent term)
Lymphoma, primary (brain)
Mycobacterium avium complex (disseminated or extrapulmonary)
Mycobacterium kansasii (disseminated or extrapulmonary)
Mycobacterium tuberculosis (any site, pulmonary, disseminated, or extrapulmonary)
Pneumocystis jiroveci pneumonia
Pneumonia (recurrent)
Progressive multifocal leukoencephalopathy
Salmonella septicemia (recurrent)
Toxoplasmosis (brain)
Wasting syndrome attributed to HIV: >10% involuntary weight loss of baseline body weight plus (1) diarrhea (two loose stools per day for ≥30 days) or (2) chronic weakness and documented fever (≥30 days, intermittent or constant) in the absence of concurrent illness or condition other than HIV infection that could explain the findings (e.g., cancer, tuberculosis).

Source: Schneider E et al: Revised surveillance case definitions for HIV infection among adults, adolescents, and children aged <18 months and for HIV infection and AIDS among children aged 18 months to <13 years—United States, 2008. MMWR Recomm Rep 57(RR-10):1, 2008.

AIDS, Acquired immune deficiency syndrome; *CDC*, Centers for Disease Control and Prevention; *HIV*, human immunodeficiency virus.

Most people have HIV-1 infection, which, unless specified, is the type discussed in this chapter. HIV-1 mutates readily and has become distributed unevenly throughout the world in different strains, subtypes, and groups. HIV-2, first isolated in western Africa, is less easily transmitted and the time between infection and illness takes longer.

MEDICAL MANAGEMENT

HIV-related morbidity and mortality stem from the HIV virus weakening the immune system as well as the virus's effects on organs (such as the brain and kidney). If untreated, the HIV virion (virus particle) can replicate at millions of particles per day and rapidly progress through the stages of HIV disease. The introduction of three-drug combination ART in 1996 transformed the treatment of patients infected with HIV and has significantly decreased AIDS-defining conditions and mortality. Most drugs are formulated as individual medications, but increasingly many are available as fixed-dose combinations to simplify treatment regimens, decrease pill burden, and potentially improve patient medication adherence.

CD4 count is used as the major indicator of immune function in people with HIV infection. It is used to determine when to initiate ART and is the strongest predictor of disease progression. CD4 counts are generally monitored every 3 to 4 months. In addition, HIV RNA (viral load) is monitored on a regular basis because it is the primary indicator to gauge the efficacy of ART. Table 38-1 provides the current guidelines on when to initiate ART.

The fundamental goals of ART are to achieve and maintain viral suppression, reduce HIV-related morbidity and mortality, improve the quality of life, and restore and preserve immune function. This can generally be achieved within 12-24 weeks if there are no complications with adherence, or resistance to medications (DHHS, 2010). Because the guidelines for HIV management evolve rapidly, it is beneficial to frequently check for updated recommendations.

Classes of Antiretroviral Therapy Drugs

Currently **antiretroviral therapy (ART)** includes more than 20 antiretroviral agents from six mechanistic classes of drugs:

- Nucleoside and nucleotide reverse transcriptase inhibitors (NRTIs)
- Nonnucleoside reverse transcriptase inhibitors (NNRTIs)
- Protease inhibitors (PIs)
- Fusion inhibitors
- CCR5 (chemokine receptor 5) antagonists
- Integrase strand transfer inhibitors (INSTIs)

The most widely studied combination regimen for treatment of naïve patients consists of two NRTIs plus either one NNRTI or a PI (with or without ritonavir boosting). Recently, a regimen consisting of raltegravir was approved for treatment-naïve patients, making the combination of an INSTI with two NRTIs another option (DHHS, 2010).

Although a reasonable number of different antiretroviral medications are currently available for the treatment of HIV infections, there is a growing need for new drugs that have fewer long-term toxicities and greater potency. However, because eradication of HIV is not yet possible, and the need for treatment is lifelong, adverse effects of medications, including metabolic complications and other toxicities, become increasingly important because they may lead to nonadherence to the prescribed regimen. Nonadherence to ART can lead to **drug resistance**.

Predictors of Adherence

When initiating ART, patients must be willing and able to commit to lifelong treatment and should understand the benefits and risks of therapy and the importance of adherence. The patient's understanding about HIV disease and the specific regimen prescribed is critical. A number of factors have been associated with poor adherence, including low levels of literacy, certain age-related challenges (e.g., vision loss, cognitive impairment), psychosocial issues (e.g.,

TABLE 38-1

Indications for the Initiation of ART in HIV-infected Individuals

Clinical Category	CD4 Count	Recommendation
Asymptomatic, AIDS	<350 cells/mm^3	Treat
Asymptomatic	350-500 cells/mm^3	Treatment recommended
Asymptomatic	>500 cells/mm^3	Some clinicians recommend initiating therapy and some view treatment as optional
Symptomatic (AIDS, severe symptoms)	Any value	Treat
Pregnancy, HIV-associated nephropathy, HBV coinfection when treatment of HBV is indicated	Any value	Treat

From National Institutes of Health: Guidelines for the use of antiretroviral agents in HIV-1-infected adults and adolescents, 2009. Accessed 23 October 2010 from http://www.aidsinfo.nih.gov/contentfiles/AdultandAdolescentGL.pdf.

AIDS, Acquired immune deficiency syndrome; *ART*, antiretroviral therapy; *HBV*, hepatitis B virus; *HIV*, human immunodeficiency virus.

depression, homelessness, low social support, stressful life events, dementia, or psychosis), active substance use, stigma, difficulty with taking medication (e.g., trouble swallowing pills, daily schedule issues), complex regimens (e.g., pill burden, dosing frequency, food requirements), adverse drug effects, and treatment fatigue (DHHS, 2010).

When using boosted PIs and efavirenz, their longer half-lives may permit more lapses in adherence since drug levels stay high in the body for many days (Bangsberg, 2006; Raffa, 2008). However, these drugs are more likely to contribute to drug resistance if discontinued due to rapid viral mutation. Continued encouragement is needed to help patients adhere as closely as possible to the prescribed doses for all ART regimens.

Illicit Drug Use

In the United States, injection drug use is the second most common mode of HIV transmission. The most commonly used illicit drugs associated with HIV infection are heroin, cocaine, methamphetamine, and amyl nitrate (poppers). The chaotic lifestyle associated with drug use is associated with poor or inadequate nutrition, food insecurity, and depression. This complicates treatment of HIV if the individual is using drugs, and can potentially lead to poor adherence with ART medications. Special considerations should be taken into account if the liver is damaged from drug use or coinfection with hepatitis, and increased nutrient excretion from diuresis and diarrhea (Hendricks, 2009; Tang, 2010).

Injection drug use is strongly linked with transmission of bloodborne infections such as HIV, hepatitis B virus, and hepatitis C virus (HCV), especially if needles are reused or shared (see *Focus On:* HIV and Hepatitis C Virus Coinfection). Coinfection of HIV and HCV increases the risk of cirrhosis. Chronic HCV infection also complicates HIV treatment because of ART-associated hepatotoxicity.

Food-Drug Interactions

Some ART medications require attention to dietary intake. It is important to ask individuals with HIV to report all medications, including vitamins, supplements, and recreational substances that they consume to fully assess their needs and prevent drug interactions and nutrient deficiencies. Some nutrients can affect how drugs are absorbed or metabolized. Interactions between food and drugs can influence the efficacy of the drug or may cause additional or worsening adverse effects. For example, grapefruit juice and PIs both compete for the cytochrome P450 enzymes; thus individuals taking PIs who also drink grapefruit juice may have either increased or decreased blood levels of the drug. Tables 38-2, 38-3, 38-4, and 38-5 provide potential nutrient interactions with ART medications.

Some ART medications can cause diarrhea, fatigue, gastroesophageal reflux, nausea, vomiting, dyslipidemia, and insulin resistance. Timing is also important for ART efficacy, so patients with HIV must take medications on a schedule. Some medications indicate that they must be taken with food or on an empty stomach. Sometimes food needs to be taken within a specific time frame of administering a medication.

FOCUS ON

HIV and Hepatitis C Virus Coinfection

An estimated 200,000 to 300,000 people in the United States have human immunodeficiency virus (HIV) and hepatitis C virus (HCV). According to the CDC, 50% to 90% of HIV-infected injection drug users are also infected with HCV (CDC, 2007). Although it is unknown if HCV accelerates HIV disease progression, it has been shown to damage the liver more quickly in HIV-infected persons. In the presence of hepatic impairment, the metabolism and excretion of antiretroviral medications may be impaired, affecting the efficacy of HIV treatment. In addition, three classes of anti-HIV medications (nucleoside and nucleotide reverse transcriptase inhibitors, nonnucleoside reverse transcriptase inhibitors, and protease inhibitors) are associated with hepatotoxicity. Therefore it is important for HIV-infected patients to be tested for HCV to appropriately manage treatment and prolong healthy liver function.

HCV is viewed as an opportunistic infection (not an acquired immune deficiency syndrome–defining illness) in HIV-infected persons because it is associated with higher titers of HCV, more rapid progression to liver disease, and increased risk of cirrhosis (CDC, 2007). Nutrition recommendations (see Chapter 30) and dosing and choice of HIV medications must be adjusted for those with liver failure.

MEDICAL NUTRITION THERAPY

For people living with HIV, adequate and balanced nutrition intake is essential to maintain a healthy immune system and prolong lifespan. It has been documented that both children and adults who are living with HIV have lower fat-free and total fat mass (American Dietetic Association, 2010). Proper nutrition may help maintain lean body mass, reduce the severity of HIV-related symptoms, improve quality of life, and enhance adherence and effectiveness of ART. Therefore medical nutrition therapy (MNT) is integral to successfully manage HIV. See *Pathophysiology and Care Management Algorithm:* Human Immunodeficiency Virus Disease.

A registered dietitian (RD) can help the patient manage many of the necessary requirements for medications, minimize adverse effects, and address nutritional concerns. Some common nutrition diagnoses in this population include:

- Inadequate oral food and beverage intake
- Increased nutrient needs
- Swallowing difficulty

Text continued on p. 873

TABLE 38-2

Medication Interactions and Common Adverse Effects with NRTI Medications

Medication Name	Timing Considerations	Common Adverse Effects with Nutrition Implications
emtricitabine (Emtriva, FTC)*	Timing of food intake is not a consideration. Snacks may limit GI upset.	NRTIs in general can potentially lead to anemia, loss of appetite, low vitamin B_{12}, low copper, low zinc, and low carnitine.
lamivudine (Epivir, 3TC)†	Timing of food intake is not a consideration. Snacks may limit GI upset.	NRTIs in general can potentially lead to anemia, loss of appetite, low vitamin B_{12}, low copper, low zinc, and low carnitine.
zidovudine (Retrovir, ZDV, AZT)†	Timing of food intake is not a consideration.	Constipation Taste alterations Macrocytic anemia or neutropenia NRTIs in general can potentially lead to anemia, loss of appetite, low vitamin B_{12}, low copper, low zinc, and low carnitine.
abacavir, lamivudine, and zidovudine (Trizivir)†	Timing of food intake is not a consideration.	Nausea Vomiting Diarrhea Abdominal pain Fat maldistribution NRTIs in general can potentially lead to anemia, loss of appetite, low vitamin B-12, low copper, low zinc, and low carnitine.
didanosine (Videx, Videx EC, DDL)‡	Take 30 minutes before or 2 hours after a meal. Do not mix with acids such as grapefruit juice, oranges, or other citrus; tomatoes or tomato juice. Do not take antacids with magnesium or aluminum within 2 hours.	Pancreatitis Nausea NRTIs in general can potentially lead to anemia, loss of appetite, low vitamin B_{12}, low copper, low zinc, and low carnitine.
tenofovir (Viread, TDF)*	Timing of food intake is not a consideration.	Diarrhea Nausea Vomiting Flatus Renal issues NRTIs in general can potentially lead to anemia, loss of appetite, low vitamin B_{12}, low copper, low zinc, and low carnitine.
stavudine (Zerit, Zerit XR, d4T)‡	Timing of food intake is not a consideration. Snacks may limit GI upset.	Hyperlipidemia Lipodystrophy: significantly associated with lipoatrophy Pancreatitis Mouth and esophageal ulcers NRTIs in general can potentially lead to anemia, loss of appetite, low vitamin B_{12}, low copper, low zinc, and low carnitine.
abacavir (Ziagen, ABC)†	Timing of food intake is not a consideration. Snacks may limit GI upset.	Alcohol can increase drug levels Nausea Vomiting Diarrhea Loss of appetite NRTIs in general can potentially lead to anemia, loss of appetite, low vitamin B_{12}, low copper, low zinc, and low carnitine.

Hammer SH et al: 2006 recommendations of the International AIDS Society-USA Panel, *JAMA* 296:827, 2006.

National Institutes of Health: Guidelines for the use of antiretroviral agents in HIV-1-infected adults and adolescents, 2009. Accessed 23 October 2010 at http://www.aidsinfo.nih.gov/contentfiles/AdultandAdolescentGL.pdf.

GI, Gastrointestinal; *NRTI,* nucleoside and nucleotide reverse transcriptase inhibitor.

*Made by Gilead (www.gilead.com).

†Made by Glaxosmithkline (www.gsk.com)

‡Made by Bristol-Myers Squibb Company (www.bms.com)

TABLE 38-3

Medication Interactions and Common Adverse Effects with NNRTI Medications

Medication Name	Timing Considerations	Common Adverse Effects with Nutrition Implications
etravirine (Intelence, ETV)* delavirdine (Rescriptor, DLV)†	Take after a meal. Timing of food intake is not a consideration. Avoid St. John's wort.	Nausea Fat maldistribution Constipation Decreased appetite Diarrhea Dry mouth Flatus Hypertriglyceridemia Hyperglycemia
efavirenz (Sustiva)‡	Take on empty stomach.§ Take at bedtime to decrease adverse effects.	Taste alterations Potential loss of appetite Flatus Hypertriglyceridemia
nevirapine (Viramune, NVP)¶	Timing of food intake is not a consideration. Snacks may limit GI upset.	Nausea Loss of appetite Liver toxicity

Hammer SH et al: 2006 recommendations of the International AIDS Society-USA Panel, *JAMA* 296:827, 2006.

National Institutes of Health: Guidelines for the use of antiretroviral agents in HIV-1-infected adults and adolescents, 2009. Accessed 23 October 2010 from http://www.aidsinfo.nih.gov/contentfiles/AdultandAdolescentGL.pdf.

*Made by Tibotec Therapeutics (www.tibotectherapeutics.com).

†Made by Pfizer (www.pfizer.com).

‡Made by Bristol-Myers Squibb Company (www.bms.com).

§*Empty stomach* refers to 1 hour before meals or 2 hours after meals.

¶Made by Boehringer Ingelheim Pharmaceuticals, Inc (www.Boehringer-ingelheim.com).

TABLE 38-4

Medication Interactions and Common Adverse Effects with Protease Inhibitor Medications

Medication Name	Timing Considerations	Common Adverse Effects with Nutrition Implications
amprenavir (Agenerase)*	Take on an empty stomach.† Low-fat food limits GI upset. Avoid high-fat meals. Avoid grapefruit juice. Increase fluid intake. Avoid taking antacids within 2 hours.	Anemia Gas Nausea Vomiting Diarrhea Hyperlipidemia Fat maldistribution
tipranavir (Aptivus, TPV)‡	Take with fatty meal.	Hyperlipidemia (especially hypertriglyceridemia) Hyperglycemia Fat maldistribution Hepatotoxicity
indinavir (Crixivan)§	Avoid grapefruit juice. Avoid St. John's wort. Unboosted: Take on empty stomach but if not tolerated, may take with nonfat milk, low-fat meal, or light snack. RTV-boosted: Timing of food intake is not a consideration.	Loss of appetite Nausea Hyperlipidemia Metallic taste Hyperglycemia Fat maldistribution

TABLE 38-4

Medication Interactions and Common Adverse Effects with Protease Inhibitor Medications—cont'd

Medication Name	Timing Considerations	Common Adverse Effects with Nutrition Implications
lopinavir, ritonavir (Kaletra)¶	Take without regard to food.	Nausea Vomiting Diarrhea Hyperlipidemia (especially hypertriglyceridemia) Hyperglycemia Fat maldistribution
fosamprenavir (Lexiva, fAPV)*	Timing of food intake is not a consideration.	Diarrhea Nausea Vomiting Hyperlipidemia Hyperglycemia Fat maldistribution
ritonavir Norvir, RTV)¶	Take with a full meal to limit GI upset.	Nausea Vomiting Diarrhea Hyperlipidemia (primarily hypertriglyceridemia) Hyperglycemia Fat maldistribution
darunavir (Prezista)¶	Take with a meal or light snack.	Nausea Diarrhea Hyperlipidemia Hyperglycemia Fat maldistribution
atazanavir (Reyataz, ATV)**	Take with a light meal. Avoid taking with any mediation that interferes with acid secretion (antacids, H2 blockers, and proton pump inhibitors).	Hyperglycemia Fat maldistribution Hyperbilirubinemia
fortovase (FTV) soft gel, invirase (INV) (Saquinavir)††	Avoid garlic supplements. FTV: Take with full meals to lessen adverse effects. INV: Take within 2 hours after a full meal. Grapefruit juice increases absorption.	Gas Mouth/esophageal ulcers Nausea Diarrhea Hyperlipidemia Hyperglycemia Fat maldistribution
nelfinavir (Viracept)‡‡	Take with meals or snack. Increase fluid intake.	Diarrhea Hyperlipidemia Hyperglycemia Fat maldistribution

Hammer SH et al: 2006 recommendations of the International AIDS Society—USA Panel, *JAMA* 296:827, 2006.

National Institutes of Health: Guidelines for the use of antiretroviral agents in HIV-1-infected adults and adolescents, 2009. Accessed 23 October 2010 from http://www.aidsinfo.nih.gov/contentfiles/AdultandAdolescentGL.pdf.

GI, Gastrointestinal.

*Made by Galaxosmithkline (www.gsk.com).

†"Empty stomach" refers to 1 hour before meals or 2 hours after meals. Examples of low-fat food are fruit, cereal, nonfat milk, nonfat or low-fat yogurt. Light snack: <300 calories. Light meal: approximately 350 calories. Full meal or fatty meal: 900-1200 calories, 40%-50% of calories from fat for fatty meal.

‡Made by Boehringer Ingelheim Pharmaceuticals, Inc (www.Boehringer-ingelheim.com).

§Made by Merck (www.merck.com).

¶Made by Abbott Laboratories (www.abbott.com).

¶Made by Tibotec Therapeutics (www.tibotectherapeutics.com).

**Made by Bristol-Myers Squibb Company (www.bms.com).

††Made by Roche Laboratories, Inc (www.roche.com).

‡‡Made by Pfizer (www.pfizer.com).

PATHOPHYSIOLOGY AND CARE MANAGEMENT ALGORITHM

Human Immunodeficiency Virus Disease

ETIOLOGY

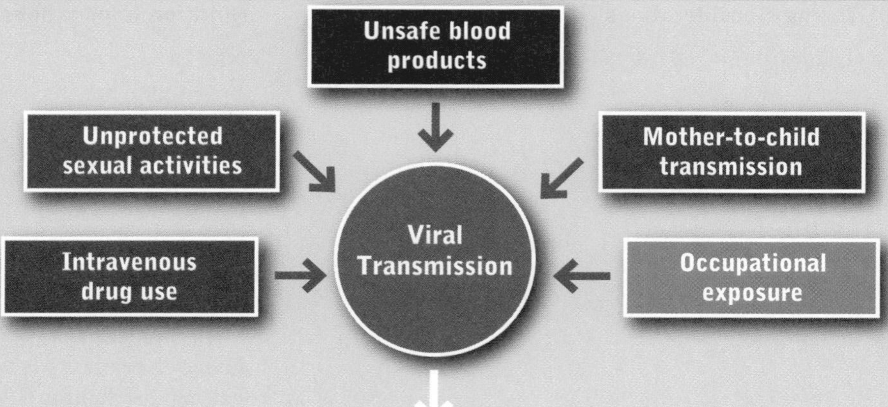

PATHOPHYSIOLOGY

Clinical Findings

Acute HIV infection (Acute retroviral syndrome) Fever, fatigue, rash, headache, generalized lymphadenopathy, pharyngitis, myalgia, nausea/vomiting, diarrhea, night sweats, adenopathy, oral ulcers, genital ulcers, neurological symptoms, malaise, anorexia, weight loss, wasting syndrome

Seroconversion

HIV Positive Test HIV rapid tests; ELISA test, Western blot; PCR test

Asymptomatic HIV infection Abnormal metabolism, change of body composition (body cell mass loss with/without weight loss, lipoatrophy, lipohypertrophy), vitamin B_{12} deficiency, susceptibility to pathogens

Symptomatic HIV infection Weight loss, thrush, fever, loss of LBM with/without weight loss, diarrhea, oral hairy leukoplakia, herpes zoster, peripheral neuropathy, idiopathic thrombocytopenic purpura, pelvic inflammatory disease

Asymptomatic AIDS

Symptomatic AIDS (AIDS defined conditions) CD4 cell count $<200/mm^3$, opportunistic infectious diseases (pneumocystitis jirovecii, pneumonia, others), Kaposi's sarcoma, lymphoma, HIV associated dementia, HIV associated wasting, vitamins/minerals deficiencies

MANAGEMENT

Medical Management

Treat possible co-morbidities
Hyperglycemia, hyperlipidemia, hypertension, body composition changes, pancreatitis, kidney and liver diseases, hypothyroidism, hypogonadism, osteopenia, hepatitis-C

Monitoring
Fasting blood lipid, fasting glucose/insulin level, protein status, blood pressure, TSH/testosterone level, CD4 cell count, and viral load

Medication
Antiretroviral therapy, lipid lowering agents, antidiabetic agents, antihypertensive agents, appetite stimulants, hormone replacement therapy, treatment for coinfectious diseases (i.e. hepatitis), prophylaxis and treatment for opportunistic infectious diseases

Nutrition Management

- Complete nutrition assessment 2-6 times/year. See Fig. 38-3
- Emphasize importance of early/ongoing nutritional intervention
- Promote adequate intake of nutrients and fluids
- Emphasize importance of food and water safety and sanitation
- Emphasize regular exercise and physical activity
- If psycho-social economic barriers to food, give resources
- Dietary multiple vitamin and mineral supplements
- Inform patient of possible side effects, symptoms and/or complications
- Monitor/manage metabolic abnormalities
- Small, frequent, nutrient-dense meals
- If mouth ulcers present, foods made need to be mashed or ground
- Appetite stimulants if necessary
- Parenteral nutrition if necessary
- Anabolic therapies

TABLE 38-5

Medication Interactions and Common Adverse Effects with Entry Inhibitor, INSTIs, and Combination Medications

Class of Medication	Medication Name	Timing Considerations	Common Adverse Effects with Nutrition Implications
Fusion inhibitors	enfuvirtide (Fuzeon, T20)*	Take without regard to food.	Nausea Vomiting
CCR5 antagonists	selzentry (Maraviroc, MVC)†	Take without regard to food.	Abdominal pain Hepatotoxicity
Integrase inhibitors	isentress (Raltegravir, RAL)‡	Take without regard to food.	Nausea Diarrhea
Combinations	efavirenz, tenofovir, and emtricitabine (Atripla)§	Take on empty stomach. Take at bedtime to decrease adverse effects.	Nausea Vomiting Gas

Hammer SH et al: 2006 recommendations of the International AIDS Society—USA Panel, *JAMA* 296:827, 2006.

National Institutes of Health: Guidelines for the use of antiretroviral agents in HIV-1-infected adults and adolescents, 2009. Accessed 23 October 2010 from http://www.aidsinfo.nih.gov/contentfiles/AdultandAdolescentGL.pdf.

INSTI, Integrase strand transfer inhibitor.

*Made by Roche Laboratories, Inc (www.roche.com).

†Made by Pfizer (www.pfizer.com).

‡Made by Merck (www.merck.com).

§Made by Gilead (www.gilead.com).

- Altered gastrointestinal (GI) function
- Food-medication interaction
- Involuntary weight loss
- Overweight and obesity
- Food- and nutrition-related knowledge deficit
- Oversupplementation
- Impaired ability to prepare foods or meals
- Inadequate access to food
- Intake of unsafe foods

All individuals with HIV infection should have access to a RD or other qualified nutrition professional. Patients should undergo a baseline nutrition assessment once they are diagnosed with HIV. Follow-up should be ongoing and take into consideration the multifactorial complications that may affect patient care. The American Dietetic Association recommends that a RD should provide at least one to two MNT encounters per year for individuals with asymptomatic HIV infection and at least two to six MNT encounters per year for symptomatic but stable HIV infection. Individuals diagnosed with AIDS usually need to be seen more often as they may require nutrition support (see Chapter 14).

Ultimately, MNT should be individualized and frequency of nutrition counseling should be determined by the patient's needs. The major goals of MNT for persons living with HIV infection are to optimize nutritional status, immunity, and well-being; to maintain a healthy weight and lean body mass; to prevent nutrient deficiencies and reduce the risk of comorbidities; and to maximize the effectiveness of medical and pharmacologic treatments. Thus screening should be performed on all patients medically diagnosed with HIV to identify those at risk for nutritional deficiencies or in need of MNT.

Patients who exhibit the various HIV-related symptoms or conditions listed in Figure 38-3 should be referred to a dietitian with expertise in managing this disease. A comprehensive nutrition assessment should be performed at the initial visit. In addition, regular monitoring and evaluation are essential to detect and manage any undesirable nutritional consequences of medical treatments or the disease process. Adverse nutrition implications are summarized in Table 38-6. Key factors for assessment are listed in Table 38-7.

Medical Factors

HIV infection should be confirmed by laboratory testing and not based on patient report (CDC, 2008b). The presence of comorbidities such as heart disease, diabetes, hepatitis, and OIs may complicate the patient's treatment profile. The assessment should include the patient's past medical history and pertinent immediate family history for heart disease, diabetes, cancers, or other disorders. Metabolic issues such as dyslipidemia and insulin resistance are common in people with HIV, and should be monitored. Biochemical measurements should be documented to determine course of HIV treatment, need for ART, efficacy of ART, and underlying malnutrition and nutrient deficiencies. Some common biochemical measurements include CD4 count, viral load, albumin, hemoglobin, iron status, lipid profile, liver function, renal function, glucose, insulin, and vitamin levels. See Table 38-8 for a list of common conditions associated with HIV and their nutritional implications.

I. Nutrition Screen and Referral Criteria for Adults with HIV/AIDS

Today's Date ________

Name ________ **Phone** ________ **Messages:** ☐ **Yes** ☐ **No** ☐ **Discreet**

Gender ________ **Language** ________ **DOB** ___/___/___ **Age** ______ **File #** ________

Medicaid Waiver Client? ☐ **Yes** ☐ **No** **Insurance** ________ **Case Managed By** ________

Referred By ________ **Date** ________ **Phone** ________

Screen every six months and/or per status change. Automatically refer to a registered dietitian for any of the following:
(Check and circle all that apply)

A. Medical Diagnosis and Nutrition Assessment

1. ☐ Newly diagnosed HIV infection
2. ☐ Newly diagnosed with AIDS
3. ☐ Any change in disease, diet or nutritional status
4. ☐ No nutrition assessment by a registered dietitian or not seen by a registered dietitian in six months

B. Physical Changes and Weight Concerns

1. ☐ ≥3% unintentional weight loss from usual body weight in the last 6 months or since last visit
(% wt. loss formula: usual body weight − current body wt/usual body wt × 100)
2. ☐ Visible wasting, <90% ideal body weight, BMI <20 kg/m^2, or decrease in body cell mass (BCM)
3. ☐ Uses anabolic steroids or growth hormone for weight, muscle gain or metabolic complications
4. ☐ Lipodystrophy: lipoatrophy, central fat adiposity and/or fat accumulation on the neck, upper back, breasts or other areas
5. ☐ Abdominal obesity: Waist circumference >102 cm or 40 inches (men) and >88 cm or 35 inches (women)
6. ☐ Client or MD initiated weight management, or obesity: BMI >30 kg/m^2

C. Oral/GI Symptoms

1. ☐ Uses an appetite stimulant or suppressant
2. ☐ Loss of appetite, desire to eat or poor oral intake of food or fluid for >3 days
3. ☐ Missing teeth, severe dental caries, difficulty chewing and/or swallowing
4. ☐ Mouth sores, thrush, or mouth, tooth or gum pain
5. ☐ Persistant diarrhea, constipation or change in stools (color, consistency, frequency, smell)
6. ☐ Persistant nausea or vomiting
7. ☐ Persistant gas, bloating or heartburn
8. ☐ Changes in perception of taste or smell
9. ☐ Food allergies or food intolerances (fat, lactose, wheat, etc.)
10. ☐ Medication involving food or meal modification
11. ☐ Receives or needs evaluation for oral supplement or enteral or parental nutrition

D. Metabolic Complications and Other Medical Conditions

1. ☐ Diabetes mellitus, impaired glucose tolerance, impaired fasting glucose, insulin resistance, or history of hypoglycemia or hyperglycemia
2. ☐ Hyperlipidemia: cholesterol >200 mg/dL, triglycerides ≥150 mg/dL, LDL >100 g/dL, and/or HDL <40 mg/dL (men), <50 mg/dL (women)
3. ☐ Hypertension: two BP readings 120-139/80-90 mm Hg or diagnosed with HTN
4. ☐ Hepatic disease: Hepatitis C, Hepatitis B, cirrhosis, steatotosis, or other: ________
5. ☐ Osteopenia/osteoporosis risk, e.g., elevated alkaline phosphatase, DEXA of the hip and spine low T-scores
6. ☐ Other conditions: renal disease, anemia, heart disease, pregnancy, cancer or other: ________
7. ☐ Albumin <3.5 mg/dL, prealbumin <19 mg/dL, or cholesterol <120 mg/dL
8. ☐ Scheduled chemotherapy or radiation therapy

E. Barriers to Nutrition, Living Environment, Functional Status

Usually or always needs assistance with:	Patient is:	
1. ☐ Eating	4. ☐ Homebound	7. ☐ Has limited or no cooking skills
2. ☐ Preparing food	5. ☐ Homeless	8. ☐ Income at or below Federal Poverty Guidelines
3. ☐ Shopping for food and necessities	6. ☐ Unable to secure food	9. ☐ Has no stove or refrigerator

F. Behavioral Concerns or Unusual Eating Behaviors

1. ☐ Disordered eating, e.g., binges, purges, purposely skips meals, avoids eating when hungry, pica
2. ☐ Alcoholic consumption: >2/day (men), >1/day (women), or with contraindicated condition
3. ☐ Substance abuse, e.g., alcohol, tobacco, drugs
4. ☐ Vegetarianism
5. ☐ Client initiated vitamin and/or mineral supplementation, or complimentary or alternative diet or related therapies

FIGURE 38-3 Nutrition screen and referral criteria for adults with HIV and AIDS. *(From ADA MNT Evidence Based Guides for Practice © 2005, American Dietetic Association, March 2005. For interim revisions see www.hivaidsdpg.org.)*

TABLE 38-6

Nutrition Recommendations for General Adverse Effects

Adverse Effect	Nutrition Recommendations
Nausea, vomiting	Eat small, frequent meals. Avoid drinking liquids with meals. Drink cool, clear liquids. Try dry crackers or toast. Try bland foods such as potatoes, rice, or canned fruits. Limit high-fat, greasy foods or foods that have strong odors such as ripe cheese or fish. Eat foods at room temperature or cooler. Wear loose-fitting clothes. Rest sitting up after meals. Keep a log of when nausea and vomiting occur and which foods seem to trigger it.
Diarrhea	Try plain carbohydrates such as white rice, rice congee, noodles, crackers, or white toast. Try low-fiber fruits like bananas and applesauce. Drink fluids that will replace electrolytes such as broths and oral hydration drinks. Try small, frequent meals. Avoid fatty, greasy foods. Avoid highly spiced foods. Avoid sugary items such as soda and fruit juice. Avoid milk and milk products. Limit caffeine.
Loss of appetite	Eat small, frequent meals. Focus on nutrient-dense foods such as milkshakes, lean protein, eggs, nut butters, vegetables, fruits, and whole grains. Try to eat in a pleasant environment
Taste alterations	Add spices and herbs to foods. Avoid canned foods or canned oral supplements.
Hyperlipidemia	NCEP diet (refer to Chapter 34).
Hyperglycemia	Diet for patients with diabetes (refer to Chapter 31)
Mouth and esophageal ulcers and sore throat	Try soft foods such as oatmeal, rice, applesauce, scrambled eggs, milkshakes, or yogurt. Avoid acidic foods such as citrus, vinegar, spicy, salty, or hot foods. Moisten foods with gravy or sauces. Drink liquids with meals. Avoid acidic beverages. Try foods and beverages at room temperature.
Pancreatitis	Focus on low-fat foods and limit fat at each meal. See Chapter 30. May need pancreatic enzymes to aid in digestion.
Weight loss	Eat small, frequent meals. See Chapter 22. Focus on nutrient-dense foods such as milkshakes, lean protein, eggs, nut butters, vegetables, fruits, whole grains, trail mixes, and tofu. Add rice, barley, and legumes to soups. Add dry milk powder or protein powder to casseroles, hot cereals, and milkshakes Try oral supplements

NCEP, National Cholesterol Education Program.

TABLE 38-7

Factors to Consider in Nutrition Assessment

Medical	Stage of HIV disease Comorbidities Opportunistic infections Metabolic complications Biochemical measurements

Continued

TABLE 38-7

Factors to Consider in Nutrition Assessment—cont'd

Physical	Changes in body shape Weight or growth concerns Oral or gastrointestinal symptoms Functional status (i.e., cognitive function, mobility) Anthropometrics
Social	Living environment (support from family and friends) Behavioral concerns or unusual eating behaviors Mental health (i.e., depression)
Economical	Barriers to nutrition (i.e., access to food, financial resources)
Nutritional	Typical intake Food shopping and preparation Food allergies and intolerances Vitamin, mineral, and other supplements Alcohol and drug use

HIV, Human immunodeficiency virus.

TABLE 38-8

HIV-related Conditions with Specific Nutrition Implications

Condition	Brief Description	Nutrition Implications
PCP	Potentially fatal fungal infection	Difficulty chewing and swallowing caused by shortness of breath
TB	Bacterial infection that attacks the lungs	Prolonged fatigue, anorexia, nutrient malabsorption, altered metabolism, weight loss
Cryptosporidiosis	Infection of small intestine caused by parasite	Watery diarrhea, abdominal cramping, malnutrition and weight loss, electrolyte imbalance
Kaposi's Sarcoma	Type of cancer causing abnormal tissue growth under the skin	Difficulty chewing and swallowing caused by lesions in oral cavity or esophagus Diarrhea or intestinal obstruction caused by lesions in intestine
Lymphomas	Abnormal, malignant growth of lymph tissue	
Brain	Changes in motor and cognitive abilities	Inability to prepare food and coordinate movement
Small bowel	Malabsorption	Weight loss, diarrhea, loss of appetite
Cytomegalovirus (disseminated)	Infection caused by herpes virus	Loss of appetite, weight loss, fatigue, enteritis, colitis
Candidiasis	Infection caused by fungi or yeast	Oral sores in mouth, difficulty chewing and swallowing, change in taste
HIV-induced enteropathy	Idiopathic, direct or indirect effect of HIV on enteric mucosa	Chronic diarrhea, weight loss, malabsorption, changes in cognition and behavior
HIV encephalopathy (AIDS dementia)	Degenerative disease of brain cause by HIV infection	Loss of coordination and cognitive function, inability to prepare food
Pneumocystis jirovecii pneumonia	Infection caused by fungi	Fever, chills, shortness of breath, weight loss, fatigue
Mycobacterium avium complex (disseminated)	Bacterial infection in lungs or intestine, spreads quickly through bloodstream	Fever, cachexia, abdominal pain, diarrhea, malabsorption

Coyne-Meyers K, Trombley LE: A review of nutrition in human immunodeficiency virus infection in the era of highly active antiretroviral therapy, Nutr Clin Prac 19:340, 2004.

Falcone EL et al: Micronutrient concentrations and subclncal atherosclerosis in adults with HIV, Am J Clin Nutr 91:1213, 2010.

McDermid JM et al: Mortality in HIV infection is independently predicted by host iron status and SLC11A1 and HP genotypes, with new evidence of a gene-nutrient interaction, Am J Clin Nutr 90:225, 2009.

Pitney CL et al: Selenium supplementation in HIV-infected patients: is there any potential clinical benefit? J Assoc Nurses AIDS Care 20:326, 2009.

Rodriguez M et al: High frequency of vitamin D deficiency in ambulatory HIV-positive patients, AIDS Res Hum Retroviruses 25:9, 2009.

AIDS, Acquired immune deficiency syndrome; *HIV*, human immunodeficiency virus; *PCP*, Pneumocystis pneumonia; *TB*, tuberculosis.

Physical Changes

The physical presentation of the patient should be considered during initial and follow-up assessments. Patients with HIV are aware of changes in their body shape and are instrumental in identifying these changes. Health care professionals should remember to ask patients about body shape changes every 3 to 6 months. Changes in body shape and fat redistribution can be monitored by anthropometric measurements. Commonly these are taken as circumferences around the waist, hip, mid-upper arm, and thigh, and as skinfold measurements of the tricep, subscapular, suprailiac, thigh, and abdomen. See Chapter 6. If a dorsocervical fat pad (fat behind the neck) is present, measurement of the neck diameter can help track changes in this area. These physical changes are referred to as **HIV-associated lipodystrophy syndrome (HALS)**. Unintentional weight changes should be monitored closely because they can indicate progression of HIV disease. Peripheral neuropathy is a potential side effect, most frequently associated with NRTIs. The resulting nerve damage causes stiffness, numbness, or tingling generally in the lower extremities. Patients experiencing neuropathy may be unable to work or be physically active.

Social and Economic Factors

Depending on a patient's mental status, psychosocial issues may take precedence over nutrition counseling. Depression is common, so the need to treat and provide services for mental health issues should be monitored. When individuals are unable to care for themselves, discussion with caretakers may be necessary to understand the patient's nutrition history. Particular habits, food aversions, timing of meals with medications, and related concerns should be documented.

Access to safe, affordable, and nutritious food should be evaluated. Common barriers include cost, location of supermarkets, lack of transportation, and lack of knowledge of healthier choices. In addition, because medications are costly, they often compete with food for available resources.

Nutrient Recommendations

When collecting the diet history, a review of current intake, changes in intake, limitations with food access or preparation, food intolerances or allergies, supplement use, current medications, and alcohol and recreational drug use will help determine the potential for any nutrient deficiencies and assist in making individualized recommendations.

Adequate nutrition intake can help patients with HIV with symptom management and improve the efficacy of medications, disease complications, and overall quality of life. Refer to Figure 38-3 for a sample nutrition screening form. Note that a one-size-fits-all approach does not address the complexity of HIV. RDs must provide recommendations to improve nutritional status, immunity, and quality of life, address drug-nutrient interactions or side effects, and identify barriers to desirable food intake (Box 38-2).

BOX 38-2

Education Needed by HIV Patients

Pregnancy, Lactation, Infancy, and Childhood

- Nutrition and food choices for healthy pregnancy and lactation
- Transmission risk in breastfeeding and replacement feeding alternatives
- Growth failure and developmental delay in children
- Support for normal growth trends in children

General Lifestyle Tips for Adults

- Basic nutrition concepts and healthy habits
- Physical activity recommendations
- Body image and altered body weight and shape
- Nutrition and food-related knowledge related to cultural or ethnic practices

Nutrition Interactions

- Prevention, restoration, and maintenance of optimal body composition with an emphasis on lean tissues
- Medication-nutrition interactions
- Management of barriers to nutritional wellness, nutrition-related side effects of treatments, and symptoms requiring attention
- Review of oral beverage or nutrient supplements
- Review of potential interactions with nonprescription medications and herbal supplements
- Evaluation of interactions with alcohol and recreational drugs

Life Skills and Socioeconomic Issues

- Safe food handling and water sources
- Access to adequate food choices
- Food preparation skills and abilities.

Adapted from American Dietetic Association: Position paper on nutrition intervention and Human Immunodeficiency Virus infection, J Am Diet Assoc 110:1105, 2010.

HIV, Human immunodeficiency virus.

In the early stages of nutrition therapy for HIV, the focus was on treatment and prevention of unintentional weight loss and wasting. Now with access to ART, new nutrition issues have arisen caused by HALS. HIV-related death from OIs has shifted to other chronic disease conditions such as heart disease and diabetes in healthier individuals who are living with HIV (Leyes, 2008).

Energy and Fluid

When determining energy needs, it is important to establish if the individual needs to gain, lose, or maintain weight. Other factors such as altered metabolism, nutrient deficiencies, severity of disease, comorbidities, and OIs should be taken into account when evaluating energy needs. Calculating energy and protein needs for this population is difficult because of other issues with wasting, obesity, HALS, and lack of accurate prediction equations. Some research suggests that resting energy expenditure is increased by approximately 10% in adults with asymptomatic HIV (Polo, 2007). After an OI, nutritional requirements increase by 20% to 50% in both adults and children (WHO, 2005a). Continuous medical and nutrition assessment is necessary to make adjustments as needed. Individuals with well-controlled HIV are encouraged to follow the same principles of healthy eating and fluid intake recommended for everyone.

Protein

The current recommended dietary reference intake (DRI) is 0.8 g of protein per kilogram of body weight per day for healthy individuals. Deficiency of protein stores and abnormal protein metabolism occur in HIV and AIDS, but no evidence exists for increased protein intake over and above that necessary to accompany the required increase in energy (WHO, 2005b). For people with HIV who have adequate weight and are not malnourished, protein supplementation may not be sufficient to improve lean body mass (Sattler, 2008). However, with an OI, an additional 10% increase in protein intake is recommended because of increased protein turnover (WHO, 2005b). If other comorbidities such as renal insufficiency, cirrhosis, or pancreatitis are present, protein recommendations should be adjusted accordingly.

Fat

There is evidence that dietary fat requirements are different with HIV infection (WHO, 2005b). General heart-healthy guidelines should be the focus for dietary fat intake. Recent research has focused on immune function and ω-3 fatty acids. There is some research to suggest increasing the intake of ω-3 fatty acids in individuals with HIV who have elevated serum triglycerides. See below.

Micronutrients

Vitamins and minerals are important for optimal immune function. Nutrient deficiencies can affect immune function and lead to disease progression. Micronutrient deficiencies are common in people with HIV infection as a result of malabsorption, drug-nutrient interactions, altered metabolism, gut infection, and altered gut barrier function. Vitamin A, zinc, and selenium serum levels are often low during times of response to infection, so it is important to assess dietary intake to determine whether correction of serum micronutrients is warranted (Coyne-Meyers and Trombley, 2004).

There are benefits to correcting some depleted serum levels of micronutrients. Low levels of vitamins A, B_{12}, and zinc are associated with faster disease progression (Coyne-Meyers and Trombley, 2004). Higher intakes of vitamins C and B have been associated with increased CD4 counts and slower disease progression to AIDS (Coyne-Meyers and Trombley, 2004). The Nutrition for Healthy Living study found that minorities and women tend to have lower micronutrient intakes and may benefit from nutrition counseling and dietary assessment (Jones, 2006).

Studies on micronutrients are difficult to interpret because there are a variety of study designs and outcomes. Serum micronutrient levels reflect conditions such as acute infection, liver disease, technical parameters, and recent intake. Adequate micronutrient intake through consumption of a balanced, healthy diet should be encouraged. However, diet alone may not be sufficient in people with HIV. A multivitamin and mineral supplement that provides 100% of the DRI may also be recommended. Megadosing on some micronutrients such as vitamins A, B_6, D, E, and copper, iron, niacin, selenium, and zinc may be detrimental to health outcomes and may not warrant protection against prevention of chronic diseases. At this time, there is no evidence to support micronutrient supplementation in adults with HIV-infection above the recommended levels of the DRI (Kawai, 2010, WHO, 2005c). See Table 38-9 for a summary.

SPECIAL CONSIDERATIONS

Wasting

Wasting implies unintentional weight loss and loss of lean body mass, which have been strongly associated with an increased risk of disease progression and mortality. Despite the efficacy of ART, wasting continues to be a common problem in the HIV population. Wasting may be caused by a combination of factors including inadequate dietary intake, malabsorption, and increased metabolic rates from viral replication or complications from the disease (WHO, 2005b). Until the underlying cause of weight loss is discovered, it will remain difficult to target effective nutrition therapy.

Obesity

Obesity in people with HIV has also been noted (Hendricks, 2006). Unintentional weight loss in HIV infection has been associated with mortality, but there needs to be more careful review in overweight or obese HIV-infected individuals. In the era of ART, it is no longer believed that continuously gaining body weight is a protective cushion against HIV-related wasting and progression to AIDS.

Some of the ART medications increase the risk of hyperlipidemia, insulin resistance, and diabetes. It is important to monitor these risk factors and provide nutrition recommendations to maintain a healthy weight. Physical activity, aerobic exercise, and resistance training are recommended to work synergistically with optimal nutrition intake to achieve a healthy weight and maintain lean body mass.

HIV-Associated Lipodystrophy Syndrome (HALS)

HALS refers to the metabolic abnormalities and body shape changes seen in patients with HIV, similar to the metabolic syndrome found in the general population. The typical body shape changes include fat deposition (generally visceral adipose tissue in the abdominal region or as a dorsocervical fat pad and breast hypertrophy) or fat atrophy seen as loss of subcutaneous fat in the extremities, face, and buttocks. The metabolic abnormalities include hyperlipidemia

TABLE 38-9

Common Micronutrient Deficiencies and Indications for Supplementation

Vitamin or Mineral	Potential Cause for Deficiency	Results of Vitamin Deficiency	Supplementation Indications
B_{12}	Malabsorption Inadequate intake	Increased risk of progression to AIDS Dementia Peripheral neuropathy Myelopathy Diminished performance (information processing and problem-solving skills)	Little evidence of benefits to supplementation beyond correcting low serum levels
A	Inadequate intake	Increased risk of progression to AIDS	Necessary to correct low levels Should not exceed DRI when serum levels are normal High intakes beyond correcting low levels can be detrimental to health and potentially increase risk of mortality from AIDS (Coyne-Meyers and Trombley, 2004) Needs more research
β-carotene	Inadequate intake Fat malabsorption	Potential relationship with oxidative stress Potentially weakens Immune function	Recommend only amounts found in multivitamin supplement Needs more research
E	Inadequate intake	Potential increased progression to AIDS Oxidative stress Impaired immune response High intake: may be associated with increased surrogate markers of atherosclerosis	Needs more research
D	Inadequate intake Inadequate exposure to sunshine	Immune suppression	Correct low levels Needs more research
Selenium	Inadequate intake	Potential increased progression to AIDS Weakened immune function Oxidative stress	Multivitamin providing DRI recommended Higher doses not recommended at this time until further research
Zinc	Inadequate intake	Increased risk for HIV-related mortality Weakened immune system Impaired healing processes Lower CD4 counts	Recommend supplementing to intakes of DRI High levels above DRI may lead to faster disease progression Needs more research
Iron	Low levels during initial asymptomatic HIV infection caused by inadequate absorption Inadequate intake	Anemia Progression and mortality in HIV infection High levels of iron potentially increase viral load Increase susceptibility to and severity from other infections such as TB	Correct low levels as needed Recommend intakes at DRI Needs more research

Coyne-Meyers K, Trombley LE: A review of nutrition in human immunodeficiency virus infection in the era of highly active antiretroviral therapy, Nutr Clin Prac 19:340, 2004.

Falcone EL et al: Micronutrient concentrations and subclinical atherosclerosis in adults with HIV, Am J Clin Nutr 91:1213, 2010.

McDermid JM et al: Mortality in HIV infection is independently predicted by host iron status and SLC11A1 and HP genotypes, with new evidence of a gene-nutrient interaction, Am J Clin Nutr 90:225, 2009.

Pitney CL et al: Selenium supplementation in HIV-infected patients: is there any potential clinical benefit? J Assoc Nurses AIDS Care 20:326, 2009.

Rodriguez M et al: High frequency of vitamin D deficiency in ambulatory HIV-positive patients, AIDS Res Hum Retroviruses 25:9, 2009.

AIDS, Acquired immune deficiency syndrome; *DRI*, dietary reference intake; *TB*, tuberculosis.

(particularly high triglycerides and low-density lipoprotein [LDL] cholesterol and low high-density lipoprotein [HDL] cholesterol) and insulin resistance. There is no consensus on the clinical definition of HALS and the manifestations vary greatly from patient to patient. Each part of the syndrome may occur independently or simultaneously.

The cause of HALS is multifactorial and includes duration of HIV infection, duration of ART medications, age, gender, race and ethnicity, increased viral load, and increased body mass index. Physical changes should be discussed with the health care team. It is important to monitor these changes by taking anthropometric measurements. Monitoring trends with body weight is important; however, doing so will not likely identify body shape changes. Generally, there is a shift in body composition even though weight remains stable. Taking waist, hip, arm, mid-upper arm, and thigh circumference measurements and tricep, subscapular, suprailiac, abdominal, and thigh skinfold measurements are useful in monitoring exact locations of either fat hypertrophy or atrophy.

Nutrition interventions associated with HALS are limited. For nutrition recommendations, the guidelines set by the National Cholesterol Education Program and American Diabetes Association are followed (see Chapters 31 and 34). Recommendations for physical activity, including aerobic exercise and resistance training, should complement dietary intake. In addition, special focus should be on achieving adequate dietary fiber intake. This can potentially decrease the risk of fat deposition (Dong et al., 2006; Hendricks, 2003) and improve glycemic control.

For patients who have high triglycerides, ω-3 fatty acids may be useful. Omega-3 fatty acids decrease serum triglycerides and may reduce inflammation and improve depression. In some studies, 2-4 g of fish oil supplements per day have been shown to lower serum triglyceride levels in patients with HIV (Wohl, 2005; Woods, 2009). Potential side effects from supplementation include GI distress, hyperglycemia, and increased LDL cholesterol levels. Use of supplements should be monitored and discussed with the health care team.

HIV IN WOMEN

Around the world, 15.7 million women are living with HIV or AIDS. In the United States, women accounted for more than 10,000 (25%) of the estimated number of new HIV infections in 2008 (CDC, 2010). The highest rate of new HIV infection is seen in African American women, which is 15 times as high as that of white women and nearly 4 times that of Hispanic women (CDC, 2010).

Although HIV-infected women are a minority in the United States, there are several factors that put them at higher risk of contracting HIV. Biologically, women are more likely to get HIV during unprotected vaginal sex because the lining of the vagina provides a larger area that can be exposed to HIV-infected semen. Barriers to receiving appropriate medical care also exist. Social and cultural stigma, lack of financial resources, responsibility to care for others, and fear of disclosure may prevent women from seeking proper care.

Preconception and Prenatal Considerations

HIV-infected women of child-bearing age should receive counseling prior to conception to learn how to decrease the risk of mother-to-child transmission. Current recommendations include prenatal screening for HIV, initiation of ART during pregnancy, and ART for the child once it is born. In the United States, these interventions have reduced the risk of mother-to-child transmission to less than 2% (DHHS, 2010a). Similar to HIV-negative women, adequate nutritional status and nutrient deficiencies should be monitored during pregnancy. Supplementation of vitamins B, C, and E have been shown to reduce the incidence of adverse pregnancy outcomes (e.g., low birth weight, fetal death) and decrease rates of mother-to-child transmission in women with compromised immune and nutrition status (Kawai, 2010). It is important to note if women have deficient serum vitamin A levels prior to supplementation, since different serum levels may affect risk of HIV transmission. Benefits may only be noted in those needing repletion of low levels.

Postpartum and Other Considerations

In the United States breastfeeding is not recommended for HIV-infected women, including those on ART, where safe, affordable, and feasible alternatives are available and culturally appropriate (DHHS, 2009). In developing countries, recommendations may differ depending on safety and availability of formula and access to clean drinking water.

HIV IN CHILDREN

An estimated 430,000 new HIV infections occurred globally among children younger than the age of 15 in 2008 (UNAIDS and WHO, 2009). In the United States an estimated 200 HIV-infected children are born each year. The majority of these infections stem from mother-to-child transmission in utero, during delivery, or through consumption of HIV-infected breastmilk. Recently, premastication (chewing foods or medicine before administering to a child) was reported as a route of transmission through blood in saliva (CDC, 2011).

Growth is the most valuable indicator of nutritional status in childhood. Poor growth may be an early indicator for progression of HIV disease. Growth failure can result from HIV infection itself and HIV-associated OIs (Guillen, 2007). Weight and height of HIV-infected children generally lags behind uninfected children of the same age. Loss of lean body mass with no changes in total body weight can also occur. To appropriately measure body changes, serial anthropometric measurements should be recorded, along with tracking of height and weight on growth charts (Sabery et al., 2009).

HIV treatment has improved the clinical outcomes for children, with ART initiation resulting in significant catch-up in weight and height but not to the level of uninfected children. The presence of HALS seen in adults is also common in children. With the increasing number of years on ART, more morphologic and metabolic abnormalities, as described in the section on HALS, are being documented in children (Sabery and Duggan, 2009). Multivitamin and micronutrient supplementation may be beneficial at the DRI levels for children who are malnourished. Research does not currently support any supplementation at higher doses.

COMPLEMENTARY AND ALTERNATIVE THERAPIES

In general, any treatment method that is not practiced in conventional medicine is considered complementary and alternative medicine (CAM). Dietary supplements, herbal treatments, megavitamins, acupuncture, yoga, and meditation are just a few of the therapies that are categorized as CAM. See Chapter 13.

The use of CAM is prevalent in patients with HIV infection. On average 60% of people living with HIV use CAM to treat HIV-related health concerns (Littlewood, 2008). People experiencing greater HIV symptom severity and longer disease duration are more likely to use CAM in an attempt to delay disease progression and alleviate side effects of HIV infection and treatment (Bormann, 2009). In addition, CAM use is more common in men who have sex with men, nonminorities, the better educated, and less impoverished individuals (Littlewood, 2008).

Despite the high percentage of CAM use, only one third of patients disclose CAM use to their health care providers (Liu, 2009). Some patients with HIV have noted benefits with taking dietary supplements; however, potential interactions with ART medications should be addressed (Hendricks, 2007). Therefore it is important that each patient be questioned carefully about use of alternative therapies, particularly those taken orally or subcutaneously. Information should be collected on the brands, dosage, frequency, timing, duration, and cost of the supplements. This should be compared with additional clinical information such as current medications, biochemical parameters, and nutrition intake. Each item should be researched for potential drug-drug and drug-nutrient interactions because they may interfere with ART use. For example, garlic and St. John's wort (*Hypericum perforatum*) decrease blood levels of ART medications, decreasing the efficacy of ART and potentially leading to drug resistance.

A key point in counseling patients who are using alternative therapies is to understand why they choose to use them. Most studies have found that there may not be any additional benefit to supplementing beyond correcting deficiencies. Food should be recommended first and patients should keep in mind that more is not always better. Caution should be used because dietary supplement labels can make a statement of nutrition support and health benefit, but it must be accompanied by the disclaimer, "This statement has not been evaluated by the Food and Drug Administration (FDA). This product is not intended to diagnose, treat, cure, or prevent any disease." Adverse event reporting for dietary supplements is voluntary, leading to a underreporting or underestimation of events.

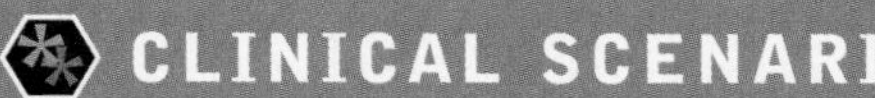

CLINICAL SCENARIO

EW is a 42-year-old male who has been HIV positive for 20 years. His viral load is undetectable and his CD4+ count is 643. His current HIV antiretroviral regimen is raltegravir (Isentress), atazanavir (Reyataz), ritonavir (Norvir), and emtricitabine (Emtriva); he also takes atorvastatin (Lipitor) and ranitidine (Zantac). His height is 5′9″ and his weight is 188 lb. His fasting lipid profile is total cholesterol 184 mg/dL, triglycerides 304 mg/dL, high-density lipoprotein 25 mg/dL, and low-density lipoprotein 96 mg/dL. Since his last visit 6 months ago, he has noticed changes in his body composition including loss of buccal fat and increasing abdominal girth. He lives by himself and doesn't like to cook; he also receives one meal per day from a community program. He walks 30 minutes daily. Upon taking a 24-hour recall, you find his caloric intake to be 2700 kcal/day.

Nutrition Diagnostic Statement

Excessive dietary intake caused by frequent intake of prepackaged meals as evidenced by diet history.

Nutrition Care Questions

1. What factors might be contributing to the body shape changes that the patient is experiencing?
2. What nutrition and lifestyle interventions would you recommend to address his nutrition diagnosis?
3. What are some biochemical and nutritional parameters you would monitor to determine if the nutrition intervention was successful?
4. How would you evaluate your desired nutrition outcomes to determine if the goals have been met?
5. The patient has also been complaining of nausea and diarrhea. What recommendations do you suggest for these symptoms? Are there any drug-nutrient interactions to be aware of?

USEFUL WEBSITES

American Dietetic Association Infectious Disease Dietetic Practice Group
http://www.hivaidsdpg.org/

Clinical Guidelines on HIV/AIDS Treatment, Prevention, and Research
http://www.aidsinfo.nih.gov

Centers for Disease Control and Prevention HIV Research, Prevention, and Surveillance
http://www.cdc.gov/hiv

Joint United Nations Programme on HIV/AIDS
http://www.unaids.org/

The National Center for Complementary and Alternative Medicine
http://www.nccam.nih.gov

REFERENCES

American Dietetic Association: Position paper on nutrition intervention and human immunodeficiency virus infection, *J Am Diet Assoc* 110:1105, 2010.

Bangsberg DR: Less than 95% adherence to nonnucleoside reverse-transcriptase inhibitor therapy can lead to viral suppression, *Clin Infect Dis* 43:939, 2006.

Bormann J, et al: Predictors of complementary/alternative medicine use and intensity of use among men with HIV infection from two geographic areas in the United States, *J Assoc Nurses AIDS Care* 20:468, 2009.

Centers for Disease Control and Prevention (CDC): *Coinfection with HIV and hepatitis C virus*, 2007. Accessed 12 July 2010 from http://www.cdc.gov/hiv/resources/factsheets/coinfection.htm.

Centers for Disease Control and Prevention (CDC): *HIV in the United States: an overview*, 2010. Accessed 12 July 2010 from http://www.cdc.gov/hiv/topics/surveillance/resources/factsheets/pdf/us_overview.pdf.

Centers for Disease Control and Prevention (CDC): *HIV prevalence estimates—United States*, 2006. Accessed 12 July 2010 from http://www.cdc.gov/mmwr/preview/mmwrhtml/mm5739a2.htm

Centers for Disease Control and Prevention (CDC): *HIV surveillance report*, 2008a. Accessed 12 July 2010 from http://www.cdc.gov/hiv/surveillance/resources/reports/2008report/pdf/2008SurveillanceReport.pdf.

Centers for Disease Control and Prevention (CDC): Revised surveillance case definitions for HIV infection among adults, adolescents, and children aged <18 months and for HIV infection and AIDS among children aged 18 months to <13 years—United States, *MMWR* 57(No.RR-10):1, 2008b.

Centers for Disease Control and Prevention (CDC): Premastication of food by caregivers of HIV-exposed children—nine U.S. sites, 2009–2010, *MMWR Morb Mortal Wkly Rep* 2011; 60(9):273-275.

Coyne-Meyers K, Trombley LE: A review of nutrition in human immunodeficiency virus infection in the era of highly active antiretroviral therapy, *Nutr Clin Prac* 19:340, 2004.

Department of Health and Human Services (DHHS): *Panel on antiretroviral guidelines for adults and adolescents: working guidelines for the use of antiretroviral agents in HIV-1-infected adults and adolescents*. Accessed 12 July2010 from http://aidsinfo.nih.gov/contentfiles/AdultandAdolescentGL.pdf.

Department of Health and Human Services (DHHS): *Panel on Treatment of HIV-Infected Pregnant Women and Prevention of Perinatal Transmission. Recommendations for Use of Antiretroviral Drugs in Pregnant HIV-1-Infected Women for Maternal Health and Interventions to Reduce Perinatal HIV Transmission in U.S.*, 2010a. Accessed12 July 2010 from http://aidsinfo.nih.gov/ContentFiles/PerinatalGL.pdf

Dong KR, et al: Dietary glycemic index of human immunodeficiency virus-positive men with and without fat deposition, *J Am Diet Assoc* 106:728, 2006.

Falcone EL, et al: Micronutrient concentrations and subclincal atherosclerosis in adults with HIV, *Am J Clin Nutr* 91;1213, 2010.

Guillen S, et al: Impact on weight and height with the use of HAART in HIV-infected children, *Pediatr Infectious Dis J* 26:334, 2007.

Hammer SH, et al: 2006 recommendations of the International AIDS Society—USA Panel, *JAMA* 296:827, 2007.

Hendricks K, Gorbach S: Nutrition issues in chronic drug users living with HIV infection, *Addiction Sci Clin Prac* 5(1):16, 2009.

Hendricks KM, et al: Dietary supplement use and nutrient intake in HIV-infected persons, *AIDS Reader* 1:1, 2007.

Hendricks KM, et al: Obesity in HIV-infection: dietary correlates, *J Am Coll Nutr* 25:321, 2006.

Hendricks KM, et al: High-fiber diet in HIV-positive men is associated with lower risk of developing fat deposition, *Am J Clin Nutr* 78:790, 2003.

Jones CY, et al: Micronutrient levels and HIV disease status in HIV-infected patients on highly active antiretroviral therapy in the Nutrition for Healthy Living cohort, *J Acquir Immune Defic Syndr* 43:475, 2006.

Kawai K, et al: A randomized trial to determine the optimal dosage of multivitamin supplements to reduce adverse pregnancy outcomes among HIV-infected women in Tanzania, *Am J Clin Nutri* 91:391, 2010.

Leyes P, et al: Use of diet, nutritional supplements and exercise in HIV-infected patients receiving combination antiretroviral therapies: a systematic review, *Antiretroviral Ther* 13:149, 2008.

Littlewood R, Vanable P: Complementary and alternative medicine use among HIV+ people: research synthesis and implications for HIV care, *AIDS Care* 20:1002, 2008.

Liu C, et al: Disclosure of complementary and alternative medicine use to health care providers among HIV-infected women, *Care STDS* 23:965, 2009.

McDermid JM, et al: Mortality in HIV infection is independently predicted by host iron status and SLC11A1 and HP genotypes, with new evidence of a gene-nutrient interaction, *Am J Clin Nutr* 90:225, 2009.

Pitney CL, et al: Selenium supplementation in HIV-infected patients: is there any potential clinical benefit? *J Assoc Nurses AIDS Care* 20:326, 2009.

Polo R, et al: Recommendations from SPNS/GEAM/SENBA/SENPE/AEDN/SEDCA/GESIDA on nutrition in the HIV-infected patient, *Nutr Hosp* 22:229, 2007.

Raffa JD, et al: Intermediate highly active antiretroviral therapy adherence thresholds and empirical models for the development of drug resistance mutations, *J Acquir Immune Defic Syndr* 47:397, 2008.

Rodriguez M, et al: High frequency of vitamin D deficiency in ambulatory HIV-positive patients, *AIDS Res Hum Retroviruses* 25:9, 2009.

Sabery N, Duggan C: A.S.P.E.N. clinical guidelines: nutrition support of children with human immunodeficiency virus infection, *JPEN J Parenteral Enteral Nutrition* 33:588, 2009.

Sabery N, et al: Pediatric HIV. In Hendricks K, et al, editors: *Nutrition management of HIV and AIDS*, Chicago, 2009, American Dietetic Association.

Sattler FR, et al: Evaluation of high-protein supplementation in weight-stable HIV-positive subjects with a history of weight loss: a randomized, double-blind, multicenter trial, *Am J Clin Nutr* 88:1313, 2008.

Tang AM, et al: Heavy injection drug use is associated with lower percent body fat in a multi-ethnic cohort of HIV-positive and HIV-negative drug users from three US cities, *Am J Drug Alcohol Abuse* 36:78, 2010.

Joint United Nations Programme on HIV/AIDS (UNAIDS): 2008 Report on the global AIDS epidemic. Accessed 12 July 2010 from http://www.unaids.org/en/KnowledgeCentre/HIVData/GlobalReport/2008/2008_Global_report.pdf.

Joint United Nations Programme on HIV/AIDS (UNAIDS) and World Health Organization (WHO): 2009 AIDS epidemic update. Accessed 12 July 2010 from http://data.unaids.org/pub/Report/2009/JC1700_Epi_Update_2009_en.pdf.

Wanke C, et al: Overview of HIV/AIDS today. In Hendricks K, et al, editors: *Nutrition management of HIV and AIDS*, Chicago, 2009, American Dietetic Association.

Wohl DA: Fish oils curb hypertriglyceridemia in HIV patients, *Clin Infect Dis* 41:1498, 2005.

Woods MN, et al: Effect of a dietary intervention and n-3 fatty acid supplementation on measures of serum lipid and insulin sensitivity in persons with HIV, *Am J Clin Nutr* 90:1566, 2009.

World Health Organization (WHO): Executive Summary of a scientific review: Consultation on Nutrition and HIV/AIDS in Africa: Evidence, lessons and recommendations for action. Durban, South Africa, 2005a. Accessed on 26 July 2010 from http://www.who.int/nutrition/topics/Executive_Summary_Durban.pdf

World Health Organization (WHO): Macronutrients and HIV/AIDS: a review of current evidence: Consultation on Nutrition and HIV/AIDS in Africa: evidence, lessons, and recommendations for action. Durban, South Africa, 2005b. Accessed on 26 July 2010 from http://www.who.int/nutrition/topics/PN1_Macronutrients_Durban.pdf

World Health Organization (WHO): Micronutrients and HIV/AIDS: a review of current evidence: Consultation on Nutrition and HIV/AIDS in Africa: evidence, lessons, and recommendations for action. Durban, South Africa, 2005c. Accessed on 26 July 2010 from http://www.who.int/nutrition/topics/PN2_Micronutrients_Durban.pdf

World Health Organization (WHO): Rapid advice: revised WHO principles and recommendations on infant feeding in the context of HIV, 2009. Accessed 12 July 2010 from http://whqlibdoc.who.int/publications/2009/9789241598873_eng.pdf

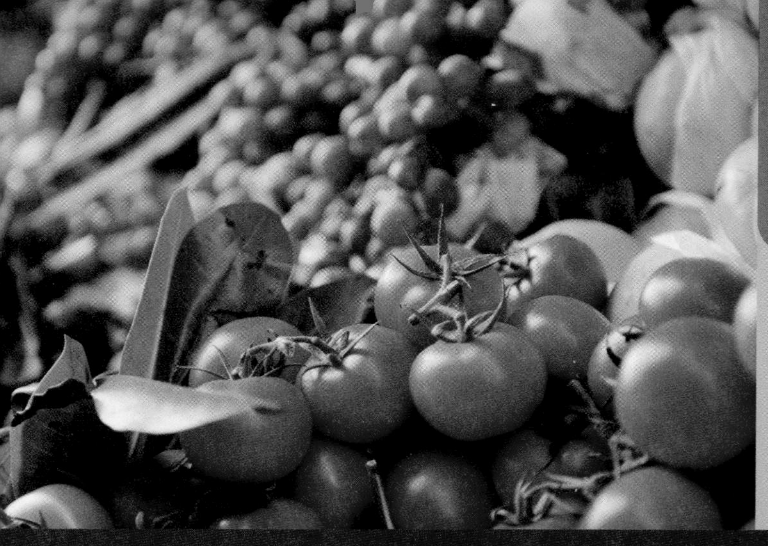

CHAPTER 39

Marion F. Winkler, PhD, RD, LDN, CNSC
Ainsley M. Malone, MS, RD, CNSC

Medical Nutrition Therapy for Metabolic Stress: Sepsis, Trauma, Burns, and Surgery

KEY TERMS

abdominal compartment syndrome
acute-phase proteins
adrenocorticotropic hormone
catecholamines
cortisol
counter-regulatory hormones
cytokines
ebb phase
epithelial barrier function (EBF)
flow phase
hemodynamic
ileus
interleukin-1 (IL-1)
interleukin-6 (IL-6)
multiple organ dysfunction syndrome (MODS)
nutrition support therapy
sepsis
shock
systemic inflammatory response syndrome (SIRS)
tight junctions
tumor necrosis factor (TNF)

Trauma from motor vehicle accidents, gunshots, stab wounds, falls, and burns are major causes of disability and death. Unintentional injuries and motor vehicle accidents are ranked as the fifth leading cause of death after heart disease, cancer, stroke, and chronic lower respiratory diseases. Injury results in profound metabolic alterations, beginning at the time of injury and persisting until wound healing and recovery are complete. Whether the event involves **sepsis** (infection), trauma, burns, or surgery, the systemic response is activated. The physiologic and metabolic changes that follow may lead to shock and other negative outcomes (Figure 39-1). Variable responses relate in part to the patient's age, previous state of health, preexisting disease, type of infection, and presence of multiple organ dysfunction syndrome (MODS).

METABOLIC RESPONSE TO STRESS

The metabolic response to critical illness, traumatic injury, sepsis, burns, or major surgery is complex and involves most metabolic pathways. Accelerated catabolism of lean body or skeletal mass occurs, which clinically results in net negative nitrogen balance and muscle wasting. The response to critical illness, injury, and sepsis characteristically involves both ebb and flow phases. The **ebb phase**, occurring immediately following injury, is associated with hypovolemia, shock, and tissue hypoxia. Typically decreased cardiac output, oxygen consumption, and body temperature occur in this phase. Insulin levels fall in direct response to the increase in glucagon, most likely as a signal to increase hepatic glucose production (Table 39-1).

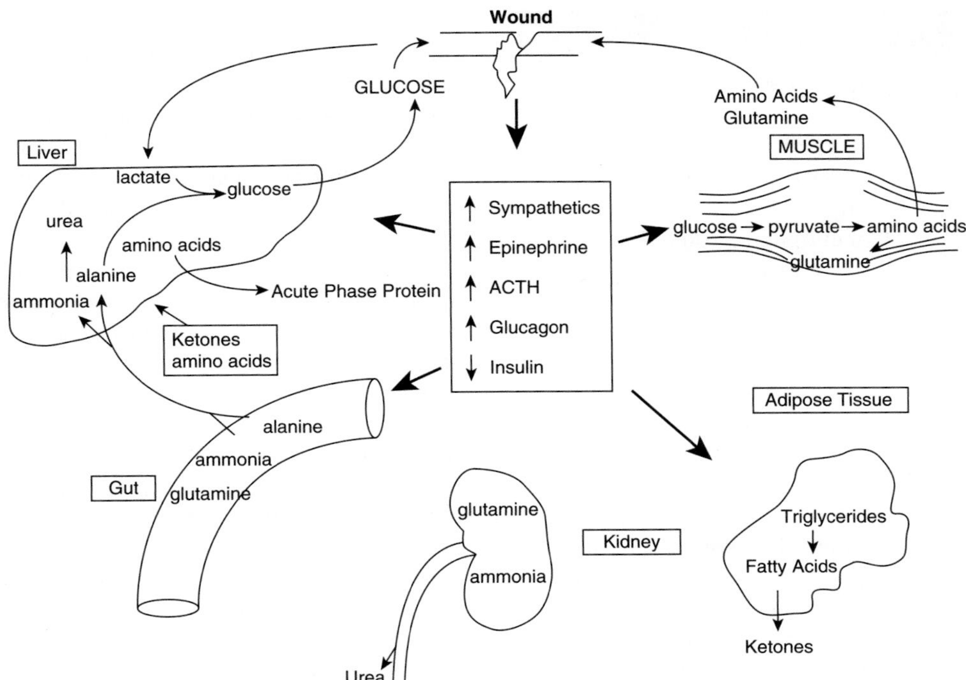

FIGURE 39-1 Neuroendocrine and metabolic consequences of injury, ACTH, adrenocorticotropic hormone. *(Reprinted from Lowry SF and Perez JM in Modern Nutrition in Health and Disease, Lippincott Williams & Wilkins, Philadelphia, PA, 2006, 1381-1400.)*

TABLE 39-1

Characteristics of Metabolic Phases Occurring After Severe Injury

	Flow Phase	
EBB-Phase Response	**Acute Response**	**Adaptive Response**
Hypovolemic Shock	**Catabolism Predominates**	**Anabolism Predominates**
↓ Tissue perfusion ↓ Metabolic rate ↓ Oxygen consumption ↓ Blood pressure ↓ Body temperature	↑ Glucocorticoids ↑ Glucagon ↑ Catecholamines Release of cytokines, lipid mediators Production of acute-phase proteins ↑ Excretion of nitrogen ↑ Metabolic rate ↑ Oxygen consumption Impaired use of fuels	Hormonal response gradually diminishes ↓ Hypermetabolic rate Associated with recovery Potential for restoration of body protein Wound healing depends in part on nutrient intake

From Enteral nutrition support in critical care, Columbus, OH, 1994, Ross Products Division, Abbott Labs.

Increased cardiac output, oxygen consumption, body temperature, energy expenditure, and total body protein catabolism characterize the **flow phase** that follows fluid resuscitation and restoration of oxygen transport. Physiologically, a marked increase occurs in glucose production, free fatty acid release, circulating levels of insulin, **catecholamines** (epinephrine and norepinephrine released by the adrenal medulla), glucagon, and cortisol. The magnitude of hormonal response appears to be associated with the severity of injury.

Hormonal and Cell-Mediated Response

Metabolic stress is associated with an altered hormonal state that results in an increased flow of substrate but poor use of carbohydrate, protein, fat, and oxygen. **Counter-regulatory hormones**, which are elevated after injury and sepsis, play a role in accelerated proteolysis. Glucagon promotes gluconeogenesis, amino acid uptake, ureagenesis, and protein catabolism. **Cortisol**, which is released from the adrenal cortex in response to stimulation by **adrenocorticotropic**

TABLE 39-2

Metabolic Responses During Stress

Organ	Response
Liver	↑ Glucose production ↑ Amino acid uptake ↑ Acute-phase protein synthesis ↑ Trace metal sequestration
Central nervous system	Anorexia Fever
Circulation	↑ Glucose ↑ Triglycerides ↑ Amino acids ↑ Urea ↓ Iron ↓ Zinc
Skeletal muscle	↑ Amino acid efflux (especially glutamine), leading to loss of muscle mass
Intestine	↓ Amino acid uptake from both luminal and circulating sources, leading to gut mucosal atrophy
Endocrine	↑ Adrenocorticotropic hormone ↑ Cortisol ↑ Growth hormone ↑ Epinephrine ↑ Norepinephrine ↑ Glucagon ↑ Insulin (usually)

From Michie HR: Metabolism of sepsis and multiple organ failure, World J Surg 20:461, 1996.

hormone secreted by the anterior pituitary gland, enhances skeletal muscle catabolism and promotes hepatic use of amino acids for gluconeogenesis, glycogenolysis, and acute-phase protein synthesis (Table 39-2).

After injury or sepsis, energy production increasingly depends on protein. Branched-chain amino acids (BCAAs leucine, isoleucine, and valine) are oxidized from skeletal muscle as a source of energy for the muscle; carbon skeletons are made available for the glucose-alanine cycle and muscle glutamine synthesis. The mobilization of **acute-phase proteins**, those secretory proteins in the liver that are altered in response to injury or infection, results in rapid loss of lean body mass and an increased net negative nitrogen balance, which continues until the inflammatory response resolves. Breakdown of protein tissue also causes increased urinary losses of potassium, phosphorus, and magnesium. Lipid metabolism is also altered in stress and sepsis. Increased circulation of free fatty acids is thought to result from increased lipolysis caused by elevated catecholamines and cortisol, as well as a marked elevation in the ratio of glucagon to insulin.

Most notable is the hyperglycemia observed during stress. This initially results from a marked increase in glucose production and uptake secondary to gluconeogenesis and elevated levels of hormones, including epinephrine, that diminish insulin release. Stress also initiates the release of aldosterone, a corticosteroid that causes renal sodium retention, and vasopressin (antidiuretic hormone), which stimulates renal tubular water resorption. The action of these hormones results in conservation of water and salt to support the circulating blood volume, noted in Table 39-2.

The response to injury is also regulated by metabolically active **cytokines** (proinflammatory proteins) such as **interleukin (IL)-1**, **IL-6**, and **tumor necrosis factor (TNF)**, which are released by phagocytic cells in response to tissue damage, infection, inflammation, and some medications. IL-6 is secreted by T cells and macrophages to stimulate the immune response to trauma or other tissue damage leading to inflammation; it has both proinflammatory and anti-inflammatory actions. Cytokines are thought to stimulate hepatic amino acid uptake and protein synthesis, accelerate muscle breakdown, and induce gluconeogenesis. IL-1 appears to have a major role in stimulating the acute-phase response. The vagus nerve helps to regulate cytokine production through a "cholinergic anti-inflammatory pathway," releasing nicotinic acetylcholine receptor alpha 7 to reduce excessive cytokine activity (Galloswitsch-Puerta and Tracey, 2005).

As part of the acute-phase response, serum iron and zinc levels decrease, and levels of ceruloplasmin increase, primarily because of sequestration and, in the case of zinc, increased urinary zinc excretion. The net effect of the hormonally and cell-mediated response is an increase in oxygen supply and a greater availability of substrates for metabolically active tissues.

STARVATION VERSUS STRESS

The metabolic response to critical illness is very different from simple or uncomplicated starvation, in which loss of muscle is much slower in an adaptive response to preserve lean body mass. Stored glycogen, the primary fuel source in early starvation, is depleted in approximately 24 hours. After the depletion of glycogen, glucose is available from the breakdown of protein to amino acids, depicted in Figure 39-2. The depressed glucose levels lead to decreased insulin secretion and increased glucagon. During the adaptive state of starvation, protein catabolism is reduced, and hepatic gluconeogenesis decreases.

Lipolytic activity is also different in starvation and in stress. After 1 week of fasting or food deprivation, a state of ketosis—in which ketone bodies supply the bulk of energy needs, thus reducing the need for gluconeogenesis and conserving body protein to the greatest possible extent—develops. In late starvation, as in stress, ketone body production is increased, and fatty acids serve as a major energy source for all tissues except the glucose-obligated brain, nervous system, and red blood cells.

Starvation is characterized by decreased energy expenditure, diminished gluconeogenesis, increased ketone body production, and decreased ureagenesis. Conversely, energy

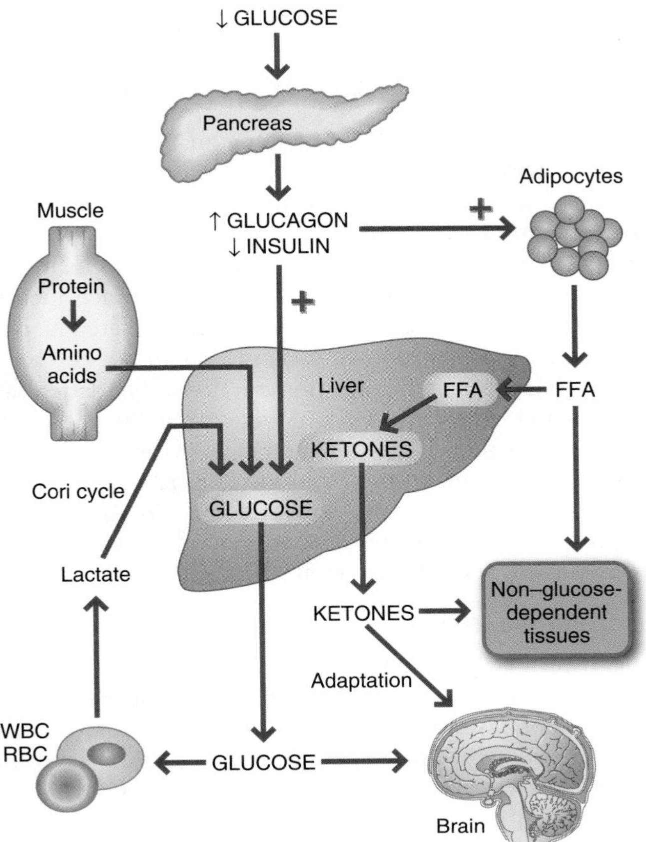

FIGURE 39-2 Metabolic changes in starvation. *FFAs*, Free fatty acids; *RBCs*, red blood cells; *WBCs*, white blood cells. *(From Simmons RL, Steed DL: Basic science review for surgeons, Philadelphia, 1992, Saunders.)*

expenditure in stress is markedly increased, as are gluconeogenesis, proteolysis, and ureagenesis. As discussed, the stress response is activated by hormonal and cell mediators—counter-regulatory hormones such as catecholamines, cortisol, and growth hormone. This mediator activation does not occur in starvation.

SYSTEMIC INFLAMMATORY RESPONSE SYNDROME AND MULTIPLE ORGAN DYSFUNCTION SYNDROME

Pathophysiology

Sepsis and the systemic inflammatory response syndrome (SIRS) often complicate the course of a critically ill patient. The term *sepsis* is used when a patient has a documented infection and an identifiable organism. Bacteria and their toxins lead to a stronger inflammatory response. Other microorganisms that lead to an inflammatory response include viruses, fungi, and parasites.

Systemic inflammatory response syndrome (SIRS) describes the widespread inflammation that can occur in infection, pancreatitis, ischemia, burns, multiple trauma, hemorrhagic shock, or immunologically mediated organ injury. The inflammation is usually present in areas remote from the primary site of injury, affecting otherwise healthy tissue. Each condition leads to release of cytokines, proteolytic enzymes, or toxic oxygen species (free radicals) and activation of the complement cascade. The American College of Chest Physicians (ACCP)–Society of Critical Care Medicine (SCCM) consensus conference definitions of sepsis are shown in Box 39-1.

BOX 39-1

Diagnosis for Systemic Inflammatory Response Syndrome (SIRS)

Site of infection established and at least two of the following are present:

- Body temperature above 38° C or less than 36° C
- Heart rate more than 90 beats/min
- Respiratory rate greater than 20 breaths/min (tachypnea)
- $Paco_2$ of less than 32 mm Hg (hyperventilation)
- White blood cell count above 12,000/mm^3 or less than 4000/mm^3
- Bandemia—the presence of more than 10% bands (immature neutrophils) in the absence of chemotherapy-induced neutropenia and leukopenia

Data from Bone et al: ACCP/SCCM Consensus Conference: Definitions for sepsis and organ failure and guidelines for the use of innovative therapies in sepsis, Chest 101:1664, 1992.

A common complication of SIRS is the development of **multiple organ dysfunction syndrome (MODS)**. The syndrome generally begins with lung failure and is followed by failure of the liver, intestines, and kidney in no particular order. Hematologic and myocardial failures usually manifest later; however, central nervous system changes can occur at any time. MODS can be primary as the direct result of injury to an organ from trauma. Examples of primary MODS include pulmonary contusion, renal failure caused by rhabdomyolysis, or coagulopathy from multiple blood transfusions. Secondary MODS occurs in the presence of inflammation or infection in organs remote from the initial injury.

Patients with SIRS and MODS are clinically hypermetabolic and exhibit high cardiac output, low oxygen consumption, high venous oxygen saturation, and lactic acidemia. Patients generally have a strong positive fluid balance associated with massive edema and a decrease in plasma protein concentrations.

Multiple hypotheses have been proposed to explain the development of SIRS or MODS. In some studies, SIRS leading to MODS appears to be mediated by excessive production of proinflammatory cytokines and other mediators of inflammation. The gut hypothesis suggests that the trigger is injury or disruption of the gut barrier function, with corresponding translocation of enteric bacteria into the mesentery lymph nodes, liver, and other organs. Unique gut-derived factors carried in the intestinal lymph but not the portal vein usually lead to acute injury- and shock-induced SIRS and MODS (Deitch et al., 2006).

Shock results in gut hypoperfusion; the hypoperfused gut is a source of proinflammatory mediators. Early gut hypoperfusion causes an **ileus** or lack of peristalsis in both the stomach and small bowel, and late infections cause further worsening of this gut dysfunction. Early enteral feeding is thought to restore gut function and influence the clinical course. The mechanism for this effect is due to the enhanced functional and structural integrity of the gut (Society of Critical Care Medicine [SCCM] and American Society for Parenteral and Enteral Nutrition [A.S.P.E.N., 2009).

Enteral nutrition (EN) may have a role in maintaining **tight junctions** between the intraepithelial cells, stimulating blood flow and inducing the release of trophic factors (Figure 39-3). Maintenance of villous height supports the secretory immunocytes that make up the gut-associated lymphoid tissue (Kang & Kudsk, 2007). With central parenteral nutrition (PN), mucosal atrophy and a loss of **epithelial barrier function (EBF)** may occur. A rise in interferon gamma and decline in IL-10 contribute to the loss of EBF in animal models along with a dramatic decline in the expression of tight junction and adherens junction proteins (Yang et al., 2009). Studies in animals suggest that glutamine added to the parenteral solution may protect the EBF (Nose et al., 2010).

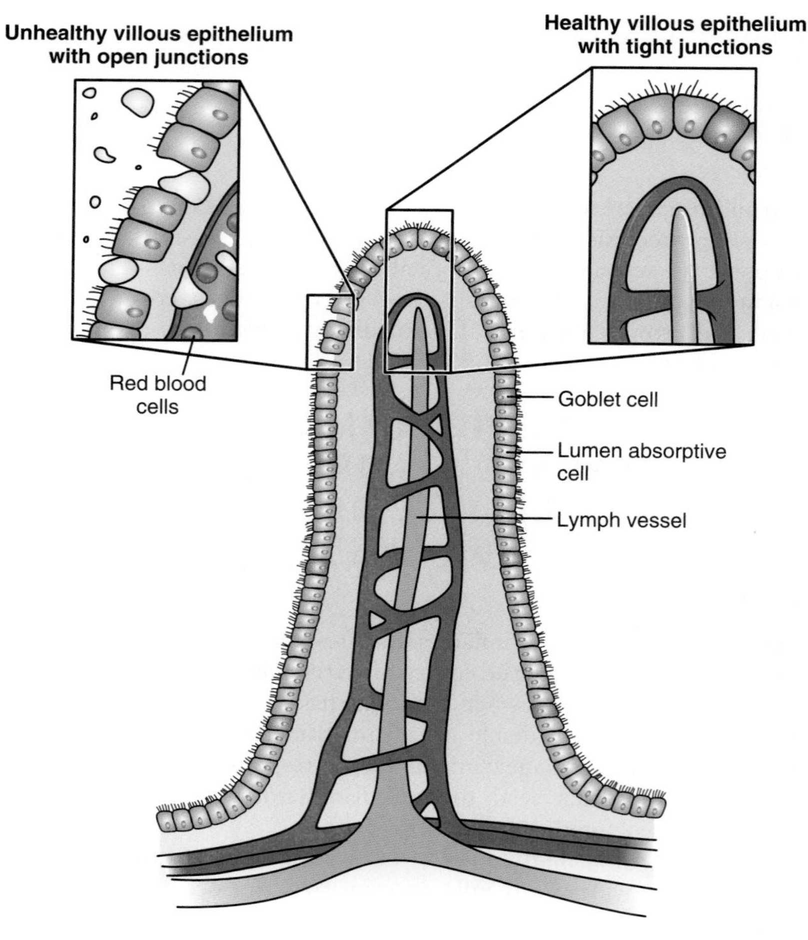

FIGURE 39-3 Tight junction in the intestinal villus, supporting gut membrane integrity.

MALNUTRITION: THE ETIOLOGY-BASED DEFINITION

The historical approach to defining malnutrition in the patient undergoing the stress response has recently been reevaluated. In an effort to provide consistency in its definition, an international group of nutrition support leaders developed an etiology basis for the definition of malnutrition for hospitalized adult patients. This approach focuses on the following three etiologies: starvation-related malnutrition, chronic disease–related malnutrition, or acute disease–related malnutrition (Figure 39-4). The latter category includes those patients experiencing SIRS and MODS and is characterized by a heightened cytokine response which in turn leads to profound losses in fat-free mass. Of note, in this setting, despite adequate provision of nutrition support therapy, repletion of lean body mass cannot occur (Jensen et al., 2009; Jensen et al., 2010).

Medical Nutrition Therapy

The critically ill patient typically enters an intensive care unit (ICU) because of a cardiopulmonary diagnosis, intraoperative or postoperative complication, multiple trauma, burn injury, or sepsis. Traditional methods of assessing nutritional status are often of limited value in the ICU setting. The severely injured patient is usually unable to

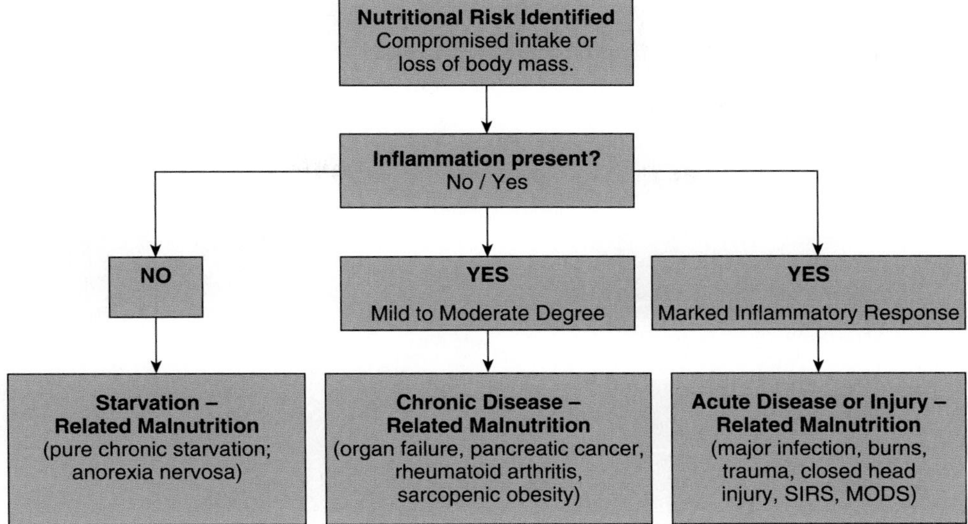

FIGURE 39-4 Diagram of Malnutrition Definitions. *(Adapted from Jensen GL et al: Malnutrition syndromes: a conundrum versus continuum, JPEN J Parenter Enteral Nutr 33:710, 2009; and Jensen G et al: Adult starvation and disease-related malnutrition: a proposal for etiology-based diagnosis in the clinical practice setting from the International Consensus Guideline Committee, JPEN J Parenter Enteral Nutr 34:156, 2010.)*

provide a dietary history. Values for weight may be erroneous after fluid resuscitation, and anthropometric measurements are not easily attainable, nor are they sensitive to acute changes. Hypoalbuminemia reflects severe illness, injury, and inflammation; thus serum albumin should not be used as a marker of nutritional status. Other plasma proteins such as prealbumin and transferrin often drop precipitously, related not to nutrition status but to an inflammation-induced decrease in hepatic synthesis and changes caused by compartmental shifts in body fluid. This is part of the acute-phase response in which secretory and circulating proteins are altered in response to inflammation or injury.

The critical role of physical assessment cannot be overlooked. Loss of lean body mass and accumulation of fluid are common to the ICU patient, and the ability to recognize these, as well as other important physical parameters is essential. In general, assessment focuses on the preadmission, preoperative, or preinjury nutrition status; presence of any organ system dysfunction; the need for early nutrition support therapy; and options that exist for enteral or parenteral access. Care planning should consider these factors. When monitoring critically ill patients, one must focus on laboratory data, not to define or determine nutrition status but to design the nutrition prescription (see Chapter 14).

Because the patient is so ill, oral intake of food or fluid may be severely limited. Therefore some common nutrition diagnoses include:

- Inadequate oral food and beverage intake (requiring other mode of nutrient or fluid administration)
- Inadequate or excessive intake from EN or PN infusion (for body requirements in nonambulatory patient)
- Inappropriate infusion of EN or PN (for example, using PN when EN is possible)
- Inadequate or excessive fluid intake (from intravenous [IV] infusions, nutrient solutions, tube flushes)
- Increased nutrient needs (such as protein for wound healing)
- Excessive carbohydrate intake (as when giving a parenteral solution to a chronically malnourished patient, with potential for refeeding syndrome)
- Abnormal nutrition-related laboratory values
- Altered gastrointestinal (GI) function (such as vomiting, diarrhea, constipation).

Nutrition Support Therapy

Nutrition support therapy incorporates early EN when feasible, appropriate macro- and micronutrient delivery, and glycemic control. Favorable expected outcomes from these practices include reduced disease severity, decreased length of time in the ICU, and decreased infectious morbidity and overall mortality.

The traditional goals of nutrition support therapy during sepsis and after injury include minimization of starvation, prevention or correction of specific nutrient deficiencies, provision of adequate calories to meet energy needs while minimizing associated metabolic complications, and fluid and electrolyte management to maintain adequate urine output and normal homeostasis (see *Pathophysiology and Care Management Algorithm:* Hypermetabolic Response).

Today, goals focus more on attempting to attenuate the metabolic response to stress, preventing oxidative cellular injury, and modulating the immune response (SCCM and A.S.P.E.N., 2009). The first emphasis of care in the ICU is establishing **hemodynamic** stability (maintenance of airway and breathing, adequate circulating fluid volume and tissue oxygenation, and acid-base neutrality). It is important to follow the patient's heart rate, blood pressure, cardiac

PATHOPHYSIOLOGY AND CARE MANAGEMENT ALGORITHM

Hypermetabolic Response

ETIOLOGY

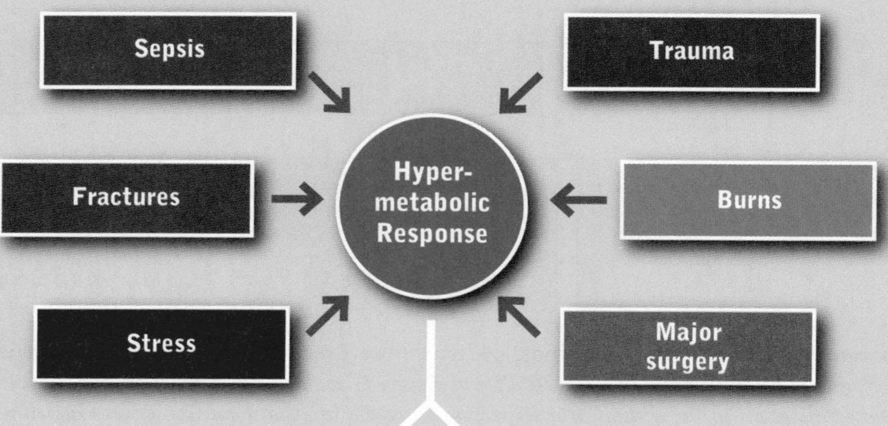

PATHOPHYSIOLOGY

EBB Phase

Hypovolemia
Shock
Tissue hypoxia
Decreased:
- Cardiac output
- O_2 consumption
- Body temperature

Flow Phase

Acute-phase proteins
Hormonal responses
Immune responses (cell-mediated and antibody)
Increased:
- Cardiac output
- O_2 consumption
- Body temperature
- Energy expenditure
- Protein catabolism

MANAGEMENT

Medical Management

- Treat cause of hypermetabolism
- Hemodynamic stability

Nutrition Management

- Minimize catabolism
- Meet energy requirements, but do not overfeed
  - Use indirect calorimetry if possible
  - Non-obese: 25-30 kcal/kg/day
  - Obese: 14-18 kcal/kg/day of actual body weight
- Meet protein, vitamin, and mineral needs
- Establish and maintain fluid and electrolyte balance
- Plan nutrition therapy (oral, enteral, and/or parenteral nutrition)
- Need for pharmaconutrients
- Physical therapy
- Exercise

output, mean arterial pressure, and oxygen saturation to assess hemodynamic stability and whether nutrition support therapy can commence.

Glycemic control and its relationship to improved outcomes has been the focus of extensive study. It is now recognized that more moderate (150-180 mg/dL), rather than tight (80-110 mg/dL), control is associated with positive outcomes in critically ill patients (American Dietetic Association, 2010). Dietitians must recognize the significant contribution of dextrose in PN formulas and its influence on glycemic control.

Nutritional Requirements

Energy. Ideally, indirect calorimetry (IC) should be used to determine energy requirements for critically ill patients. Oxygen consumption is an essential component in the determination of energy expenditure. Septic and trauma patients have substantial increases in energy expenditure associated with the magnitude of injury. IC can be performed serially as a patient's clinical status changes (Compher et al., 2006); this allows a more accurate assessment of energy requirements during a patient's stay in the ICU (see Chapter 2). IC is not appropriate for all patients, however, and should be performed and interpreted by experienced clinicians (Compher et al., 2006). High oxygen requirements, the presence of a chest tube, acidosis, and the use of supplemental oxygen are factors that may produce invalid results. In these situations measurement of energy expenditure by IC is not recommended (Malone, 2002).

In the absence of a metabolic cart for IC, energy requirements may be calculated as 25-30 kcal/kg/day (SCCM and A.S.P.E.N., 2009) or by using one of the many published predictive equations (see Chapter 2). Avoidance of overfeeding in the critically ill patient is important. Although adequate energy is essential for metabolically stressed patients, excess calories can result in complications such as hyperglycemia, hepatic steatosis, and excess carbon dioxide production, which can exacerbate respiratory insufficiency or prolong weaning from mechanical ventilation.

The amount of energy to provide critically ill obese patients is of current interest. Improved glycemic control and positive clinical outcomes occur in obese patients provided with 22 kcal/kg/day of ideal weight in conjunction with increased protein (Choban and Dickerson, 2005). There is some debate in practice as to what value should be used for weight in predictive equations. Actual body weight is a better predictor of energy expenditure than ideal body weight in obese individuals (Breen and Ireton-Jones, 2004). A recent evidence analysis review found the Penn State Equation, using actual body weight, to be 70% accurate in predicting energy expenditure if IC is unavailable (Frankenfield et al., 2007).

Research suggests that hypocaloric, high-protein nutrition support therapy or "permissive underfeeding" in critically ill obese patients results in achievement of net protein anabolism and minimizes complications resulting from overfeeding. Dickerson (2005) summarized a review of studies using hypocaloric specialized nutrition support in obese patients in the ICU. Although there is no agreement as to what constitutes hypocaloric feeding, studies suggest that this approximates 14-18 kcal/kg/day of actual body weight or 22 kcal/kg/day of ideal body weight (SCCM and A.S.P.E.N., 2009). More research is needed to validate hypocaloric feeding as the standard approach to nutrition support in obese patients, especially because of the wide variability in body composition (Port and Apovian, 2010).

Protein. Determination of protein requirements is difficult for critically ill patients. Patients typically require 1.2-2 g/kg/day depending on their baseline nutritional status, degree of injury and metabolic demand, and abnormal losses (e.g., through open abdominal wounds or burned skin) (SCCM and A.S.P.E.N., 2009). Administration of excessive amounts of protein will not decrease the characteristic net negative nitrogen balance seen among hypermetabolic patients.

Vitamins, Minerals, and Trace Elements. No specific guidelines exist for the provision of vitamins, minerals, and trace elements in metabolically stressed individuals. Micronutrient needs are elevated during acute illness because of increased urinary and cutaneous losses and diminished GI absorption, altered distribution, and altered carrier protein concentrations. With increased caloric intake there may be an increased need for B vitamins, particularly thiamin and niacin. Catabolism and loss of lean body tissue increase the loss of potassium, magnesium, phosphorus, and zinc. GI and urinary losses, organ dysfunction, and acid-base imbalance necessitate that mineral and electrolyte requirements be determined and adjusted individually. Fluid and electrolytes should be provided to maintain adequate urine output and normal serum electrolytes.

Feeding Strategies. The preferred route for nutrient delivery is an oral diet. However, critically ill patients are often unable to eat because of endotracheal intubation and ventilator dependence. Furthermore, oral feeding may be delayed by impairment of chewing, swallowing, by anorexia induced by pain-relieving medications, or by posttraumatic shock and depression. Patients who are able to eat may not be able to meet the increased energy and nutrient requirements associated with metabolic stress and recovery. They often require combinations of oral nutritional supplements, enteral tube nutrition, and PN. When EN fails to meet nutritional requirements or when GI feeding is contraindicated, PN support should be initiated (Figure 39-5).

Timing and Route of Feeding. EN is the preferred route of feeding for the critically ill patient who cannot eat food and who has good intestinal function. Feedings should be initiated early within the first 24-48 hours of ICU admission and advanced toward goal during the next 48-72 hours (SCCM and A.S.P.E.N., 2009). Intake of 50% to 65% of goal calories during the first week of hospitalization is thought to be sufficient to achieve the clinical benefit of EN. This practice is intended for patients who are hemodynamically stable. In the setting of hemodynamic instability (large volume requirements or use of high-dose catecholamine agents), tube feeding should be withheld until the patient is

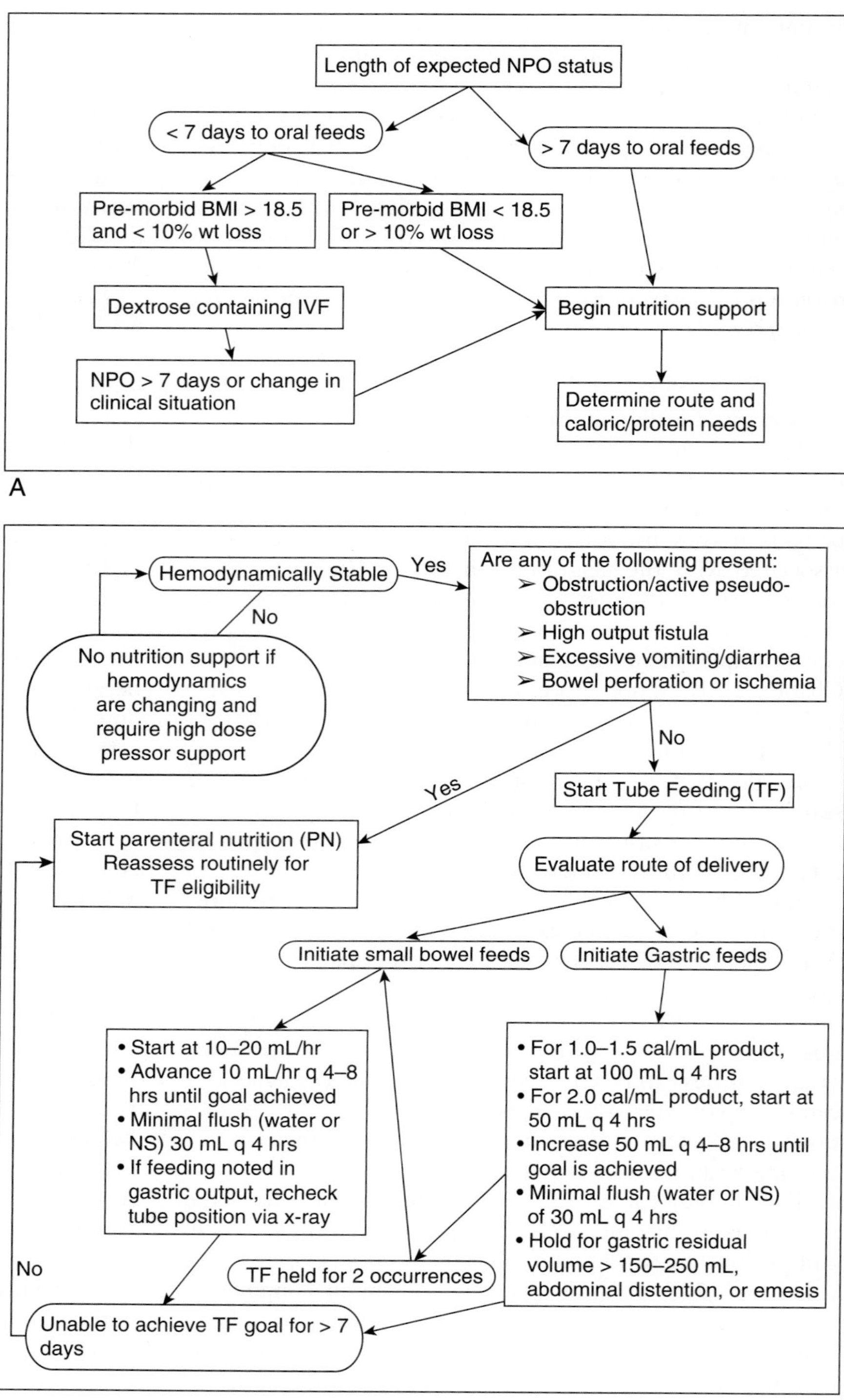

FIGURE 39-5 Timing and determining the route of nutrition support in the critically ill patient. **A,** Timing of nutrition support initiation. **B,** Determining optimal route of nutrition support. *(Reprinted with permission from Beth Taylor.)*

fully resuscitated or stable to minimize risk of ischemic or reperfusion injury (see Figure 39-5).

Either gastric or small-bowel feedings can be used. Small-bowel feedings are indicated when gastric residuals exceed 250 mL. Nasoenteric or surgically placed feedings tubes can be placed intraoperatively for patients with severe head, major thoracic, or spinal injury; facial injury requiring jaw wiring; proximal gastric or esophageal injuries, and major pancreatic or duodenal injury; and severe trauma with plans for repeated surgeries.

Enteral tolerance should be monitored by assessing level of pain, presence of abdominal distention, passage of flatus and stool, physical examination and, if appropriate, abdominal x-ray examination. Steps to reduce aspiration risk should be implemented, including elevating the head of the bed and use of promotility agents. The cause of diarrhea, when present, should be determined. Patients should be evaluated for intake of hyperosmolar medications and broad-spectrum antibiotics, and should be assessed for infectious diarrhea.

PN is indicated for patients in whom EN is unsuccessful or contraindicated. Supplemental PN is appropriate after 7-10 days of enteral feeding in situations in which goal requirements cannot be met (SCCM and A.S.P.E.N., 2009). For patients with preexisting malnutrition, PN should be used within 5-7 days of surgery and continue into the postoperative period.

Formula Selection. Choosing an enteral product should be based on fluid, energy, and nutrient requirements, as well as GI function. Most standard polymeric enteral formulas can be used to feed the critically ill patient. Some critically ill patients demonstrate intolerance to standard diets because of the fat content of the formula and temporarily require a lower-fat diet or a product containing a higher ratio of medium-chain triglycerides. Several commercially available products are marketed specifically for patients with trauma and metabolic stress. These products typically have higher protein content and a higher ratio of BCAAs or additional glutamine or arginine.

Immune modulating enteral formulations that contain arginine, glutamine, nucleic acids, antioxidants, and ω-3 fatty acids have potential beneficial effects and favorable outcomes for critically ill patients who have undergone GI surgery, as well as for trauma and burn patients. These formulations should not be routinely used for ICU patients with sepsis because they may worsen the inflammatory response (SCCM and A.S.P.E.N., 2009). Insoluble fiber should be avoided in critically ill patients; however, soluble fiber may be beneficial for the hemodynamically stable, critically ill patient who develops diarrhea (SCCM and A.S.P.E.N., 2009). Patients at high risk for bowel ischemia should not receive fiber-containing formulas or diets.

TRAUMA AND THE OPEN ABDOMEN

Following major abdominal trauma, bowel distention, and states of shock, some patients experience increased intraabdominal pressure leading to hypoperfusion and ischemia of the intestines and other peritoneal and retroperitoneal structures. **Abdominal compartment syndrome** occurs when there is increased intraabdominal pressure, often following major abdominal trauma or sepsis. This condition has profound consequences, including hemodynamic instability and respiratory, renal, and neurologic abnormalities. Because the abdominal cavity has become too small, management consists of emergent decompressive laparotomy to relieve the intraabdominal pressure (Walker and Criddle, 2003). Closure of the abdomen is not performed and instead a temporary sterile dressing may be applied.

Patients with an open abdomen have severe metabolic alterations, increased loss of fluids, and elevated nutritional requirements. The open abdomen may also be a significant source of protein loss depending on the amount of drainage (Cheatham et al., 2007). There has been some controversy as to whether patients with an open abdomen can be enterally fed. As long as the patient is hemodynamically stable and does not require large-volume fluid resuscitation or increasing doses of pressor agents, enteral feeding should be possible (Byrnes et al., 2010; Collier et al., 2007; Dissanaike et al., 2008). Ideally, a nasojejunal feeding tube should be positioned at the time of surgery to facilitate early EN support therapy.

Management of intestinal fistulas and large draining wounds are also challenging both surgically and nutritionally. These patients have metabolic abnormalities associated with losses of fluid, electrolytes, and nutrients. The priorities for management of intestinal fistulas are to restore blood volume, replace fluid and electrolyte losses, treat sepsis, control fistula drainage, protect the surrounding skin, and provide optimal nutrition support therapy. The use of PN has decreased mortality associated with fistulas and is associated with spontaneous fistula closure; however, these same outcomes are possible with EN if a feeding tube can be placed through or distal to the fistula site. See Chapter 14.

MAJOR BURNS

Pathophysiology

Major burns result in severe trauma. Energy requirements can increase as much as 100% above resting energy expenditure (REE), depending on the extent and depth of the injury (Figure 39-6). Exaggerated protein catabolism and increased urinary nitrogen excretion accompany this hypermetabolism. Protein is also lost through the burn wound exudate. Burn patients are particularly susceptible to infection, and this markedly increases requirements for both energy and protein. Because patients with major burns may develop an ileus and are anorexic, nutrition support therapy can be a real challenge. In children, healing after burn and trauma requires not only restoration of oxygen delivery and adequate calories to support metabolism and repair, but awareness of how children differ from adults in metabolic rate, growth requirements, and physiological response (Cook and Blinman, 2010).

Medical Management

Fluid and Electrolyte Repletion

The first 24 to 48 hours of treatment for thermally injured patients are devoted to fluid resuscitation. Several formulas have been developed to calculate the volume of resuscitation fluid needed. These formulas are based on the physiologic response of the body to thermal injury and are a good starting point for resuscitation. Generally half of the calculated volume for the first 24 hours is given during the first 8 hours following burn injury and the remaining half in the next 16 hours. Urine output is used to titrate the rate of IV fluid replacement.

The volume of fluid needed is based on the age and weight of the patient and the extent of the injury designated by percentage of total body surface area (TBSA) burned.

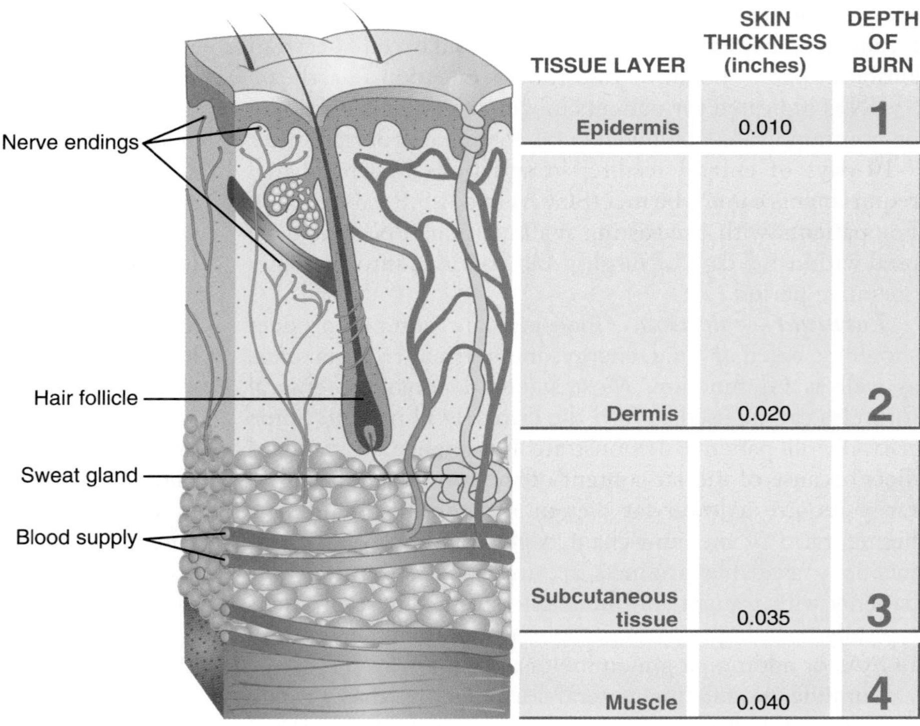

FIGURE 39-6 Interpretation of burn classification based on damage to the integument.

Once resuscitation is complete, ample fluids must be given to cover both maintenance requirements and evaporative losses that continue through open wounds. Evaporative water loss can be estimated at 2 to 3.1 mL/kg of body weight per 24 hours per percent of TBSA burn. Serum sodium, osmolar concentrations, and body weight are used to monitor fluid status. Providing adequate fluids and electrolytes as soon as possible after injury is paramount for maintaining circulatory volume and preventing ischemia.

Wound Management

Wound management depends on the depth and extent of the burn. Current surgical management promotes use of topical antimicrobial agents and biologic and synthetic dressings, early debridement, excision, and grafting. Energy expenditure may be reduced slightly by the practice of covering wounds as early as possible to reduce evaporative heat and nitrogen losses and prevent infection.

Ancillary Measures

Passive and active range of motion exercises should be started early in the hospital to prevent contracture formation. Physical and occupational therapy helps maintain function and prevents muscle wasting and atrophy. A warm environment minimizes heat loss and the expenditure of energy to maintain body temperature. Thermal blankets, heat lamps, and individual heat shields are often used to maintain environmental temperature near 30° C (86° F). Minimizing fear and pain with reassurance from the staff and adequate pain medication can also reduce catecholamine stimulation and help avoid increases in energy expenditure. Treatments such as biofeedback, guided imagery, and good sleep hygiene are helpful. Finally, antacids are given to patients with major burns to prevent formation of stress-related Curling ulcers in the gastric or duodenal mucosa.

Medical Nutrition Therapy

A burn patient has greatly accelerated metabolism and needs increased energy, carbohydrates, proteins, fats, vitamins, minerals, and antioxidants to heal and prevent detrimental sequelae (Chan and Chan, 2009). A healthy liver is also essential. Hepatic acute phase proteins are strong predictors for postburn survival through their roles in gluconeogenesis, glycogenolysis, lipolysis, and proteolysis (Jeschke, 2009).

The goals of nutrition support therapy following major burn injury include provision of adequate calories to meet energy needs while minimizing associated metabolic complications, prevention or correction of specific nutrient deficiencies, and fluid and electrolyte management for adequate urine output and normal homeostasis. Adequate surgical care, infection control, and nutrition should be available as soon as possible after the burn (Dylewski et al., 2010). Delays in admission to an organized burn unit can be detrimental, especially for children, because malnutrition is a common concern.

Achievement of enteral access and provision of a sufficient volume of enteral nutrients early in the hospital course of a critically ill burned patient affords an opportunity to improve the outcome of that patient. Enteral feeding provides a conduit for the delivery of immune stimulants and serves as effective prophylaxis against stress-induced gastropathy and GI hemorrhage. Tube placement beyond the stomach into the small bowel in hypermetabolic, severely ill patients prone to ileus and disordered gut motility may aid delivery of enteral nutrients while reducing risk of aspiration. Placement of enteral tubes during surgery has been practiced at some burn centers in an effort to minimize the length of time a burn patient is without nutrition support therapy. See Box 39-2 for the nutritional care goals for the burned person.

Energy

Increased energy needs of the burned patient vary according to the size of the burn with severe injuries often approaching two times predicted energy expenditure. Once a burn exceeds 50% to 60% TBSA, minimum increases in energy expenditure do not usually occur. Measuring energy expenditure via indirect calorimetry is the most reliable method for assessing energy expenditure in burned patients. Increasing energy requirements by 20% to 30% is necessary to account for energy expenditure associated with wound care and physical therapy. The Ireton-Jones equation is frequently used for assessing energy expenditure in the burned patient because it accounts for burn injury and ventilatory status (Ireton-Jones and Jones, 2002) (Box 39-3).

Additional calories may be required to meet the needs because of fever, sepsis, multiple traumas, or the stress of surgery. Although weight gain may be desirable for the severely underweight patient, this is generally not feasible until acute illness has resolved. Generally, caloric goals should not exceed more than 2 times the REE.

Weight maintenance should be the goal for overweight patients until the healing process is complete. Obese individuals may be at higher risk of wound infection and graft disruption. The energy requirement for the obese burned person is probably more than that calculated when ideal body weight is used but less than that calculated when actual body weight is used. IC is the most accurate method of determining the energy needs of the obese person who is burned.

Protein

The protein needs of burned patients are elevated because of losses through urine and wounds, increased use in gluconeogenesis, and wound healing. Recent evidence promotes the feeding of high amounts of protein. Providing 20% to 25% of total calories as protein of high biologic value is also recommended.

The adequacy of energy and protein intake is best evaluated by monitoring wound healing, graft take, and basic nutrition assessment parameters. Wound healing or graft take may be delayed if weight loss exceeds 10% of the usual weight. An exact evaluation of weight loss may be difficult to obtain because of fluid shifts or edema or because of differences in the weights of dressings or splints. The coordination of weight measurement with dressing changes or hydrotherapy may allow recording of a weight without dressings and splints (Mayes and Gottschlich, 2003). Generally the fluid gained during the resuscitation period is lost within 2 weeks. Trends in weight change can then be identified.

Nitrogen balance often is used to evaluate the efficacy of a nutritional regimen, but it cannot be considered accurate without accounting for wound losses, which is difficult to accomplish in a clinical setting. Nitrogen excretion should begin to decrease as wounds heal or are grafted or covered. However, serum albumin levels usually remain depressed until major burns are healed. Proteins with shorter half-lives such as prealbumin, retinol-binding protein, and transferrin help to assess the resolution of the inflammatory response and the adequacy of nutrition support therapy of burn patients (see Chapter 8).

BOX 39-2

Medical Nutrition Therapy Goals for Burned Patients

1. Minimize metabolic stress response by:
   - Controlling environmental temperature
   - Maintaining fluid and electrolyte balance
   - Controlling pain and anxiety
   - Covering wounds early
2. Meet nutritional needs by:
   - Providing adequate calories to prevent weight loss of greater than 10% of usual body weight
   - Providing adequate protein for positive nitrogen balance and maintenance or repletion of circulating proteins
   - Providing vitamin and mineral supplementation as indicated
3. Prevent Curling stress ulcer by:
   - Providing antacids or continuous enteral feedings

BOX 39-3

Ireton-Jones Equations

Ireton-Jones equation for obese patients:

$$EE = 606\ S + 9\ W - 12\ A + 400\ V + 1444$$

Ireton-Jones equation for ventilator patients:

$$EE = 1925 - 10\ A + 5\ W + 281\ S + 292\ T + 851\ B$$

Key

EE: energy expenditure in kcal/day (no stress correction required).
A: age in years
S: sex (1 = male, 0 = female)
T: trauma (0 = absent, 1 = present)
B: burn (0 = absent, 1 = present)
W: weight in kg (actual)
V: ventilator (0 = absent, 1 = present)

Micronutrients and Antioxidants

Vitamin needs generally increase for burn patients, but exact requirements have not been established. Supplements may be needed for patients who are eating food; however, most patients who receive tube feeding or PN receive amounts of vitamins in excess of the dietary reference intakes because of the high calorie intake. Vitamin C is involved in collagen synthesis and immune function and may be required in increased amounts for wound healing. Doses of 500 mg twice daily are the routine protocol at some burn centers (Mayes and Gottschlich, 2003). Vitamin A is also an important nutrient for immune function and epithelialization. Provision of 5000 units of vitamin A per 1000 calories of EN is often recommended (Mayes and Gottschlich, 2003).

Electrolyte imbalances that involve serum sodium or potassium are usually corrected by adjusting fluid therapy. Hyponatremia may be seen in patients whose evaporative losses are reduced drastically by the application of dressings or grafts; who have had changes in maintenance fluids; or who have been treated with silver nitrate soaks, which tend to draw sodium from the wound. Restricting the oral consumption of free water and sodium-free fluids may help correct hyponatremia. Hypokalemia often occurs after the initial fluid resuscitation and during protein synthesis. Slightly elevated serum potassium may indicate inadequate hydration.

Depression of serum calcium levels may be seen in patients with burns that involve more than 30% TBSA. Hypocalcemia often accompanies hypoalbuminemia. Calcium losses may be exaggerated if the patient is immobile or being treated with silver nitrate soaks. Early ambulation and exercise should help minimize these losses. Administration of calcium supplements may be necessary to treat symptomatic hypocalcemia.

Hypophosphatemia has also been identified in patients with major burns. This occurs most commonly in patients who receive large volumes of resuscitation fluid along with parenteral infusion of glucose solutions and large amounts of antacids for stress ulcer prophylaxis. Serum levels need to be monitored, and appropriate phosphate supplementation provided. Magnesium levels may also require attention because a significant amount of magnesium can be lost from the burn wound. Supplemental phosphorus and magnesium are often given parenterally to prevent GI irritation.

A depressed serum zinc level has been reported in burn patients, but whether this represents total body zinc nutriture or is an artifact of hypoalbuminemia is unclear, because zinc is bound to serum albumin. Zinc is a cofactor in energy metabolism and protein synthesis. Supplementation with 220 mg of zinc sulfate is appropriate (Mayes and Gottschlich, 2003). The anemia initially seen following a burn is usually unrelated to iron deficiency and is treated with packed red blood cells.

Methods of Nutrition Support Therapy

Methods of nutrition support therapy need to be implemented on an individual basis. Most patients with burns of less than 20% TBSA are able to meet their needs with a regular high-calorie, high-protein oral diet. Often the use of concealed nutrients such as protein added to puddings, milks, and gelatins is helpful because consuming large volumes of foods can be overwhelming to the patient. Patients should have immediate access to food and fluids at the bedside. They should be encouraged to consume calorically dense, high-protein drinks. Involving family and caregivers during mealtimes helps to promote good oral intake. Research is needed to identify ideal timing and forms of nutrition for critically ill infants and children, as this is currently not available (Joffe et al., 2009).

Patients with major burns, elevated energy expenditure, or poor appetites may require tube feeding or PN. Enteral feeding is the preferred method of nutrition support therapy for burn patients, but PN may be necessary with early excision and grafting to avoid the frequent interruptions of tube feeding required for anesthesia. Because ileus is often present only in the stomach, severely burned patients can be successfully fed by tube into the small bowel. PN may be needed for patients with persistent ileus who do not tolerate tube feedings or who have a high risk of aspiration. With careful monitoring, central lines for PN can be maintained through burn wounds. See Chapter 14.

SURGERY

The delivery of correctly formulated and safely administered nutritional and metabolic support is a matter of life or death in surgical and critical care units; obese patients have a higher surgical risk (Blackburn et al., 2010). Although surgical morbidity correlates best with the extent of the primary disease and the nature of the operation performed, malnutrition may also compound the severity of complications. A well-nourished patient usually tolerates major surgery better than a severely malnourished patient. Malnutrition is associated with a high incidence of operative complications, morbidity, and death. If a malnourished patient is expected to undergo major upper GI surgery and EN is not feasible, PN should be initiated 5-7 days preoperatively and continued into the postoperative period if the duration of therapy is anticipated to be longer than 7 days (SCCM and A.S.P.E.N., 2009). See Chapter 14.

Medical Nutrition Therapy

Preoperative Nutrition Care

The routine practice of ordering that a patient take nothing by mouth (NPO) at midnight prior to surgery has been discontinued in many settings. The American Society of Anesthesiologists historically recommended withholding solids for 6 hours preoperatively and clear liquids for 2 hours prior to induction of anesthesia. This practice was intended to minimize aspiration and regurgitation, but two Cochrane reviews suggest that patients may be allowed to take fluids up until a few hours before surgery without causing increased morbidity (Brady et al., 2003; Brady et al., 2009). The use of a carbohydrate-rich beverage in the preoperative period has been shown to enhance glycemic control; and decrease losses of nitrogen, lean body mass, and muscle strength following abdominal and colorectal surgery (Svanfeldt et al., 2007).

In emergency patients, preoperative fasting is not possible and surgery should be timed according to urgency; patients are treated as if the stomach is full (Søreide and Ljundqvist, 2006).

Postoperative Nutrition Care

Postoperative patients who are critically ill and in the ICU should receive early EN unless there is an absolute contraindication (SCCM and A.S.P.E.N., 2009). This practice following major GI surgery is associated with reduced infection and decreased hospitalization (Lewis et al., 2009). The use of immune-enhanced formulas is associated with a decrease in wound complications in patients who have undergone GI surgery (Mizock, 2010). If oral feeding is not possible or an extended NPO period is anticipated, an access device for enteral feeding should be inserted at the time of surgery. Combined gastrostomy-jejunostomy tubes offer significant advantages over standard gastrostomies because they allow for simultaneous gastric drainage from the gastrostomy tube and enteral feeding via the jejunal tube. Studies are underway to evaluate the effect of the use of fish oil with nutrition therapy to improve surgical outcomes in older adults after major surgery; early results show promise for reducing systemic inflammation, loss of lean muscle, and weight loss (Miller et al., 2010).

The timing of introduction of solid food after surgery depends on the patient's degree of alertness and condition of the GI tract. A general practice has been to progress over a period of several meals from clear liquids to full liquids and finally to solid foods. However, no physiologic reason exists for solid foods not to be introduced as soon as the GI tract is functioning and a few liquids are tolerated (Lewis et al., 2009). Surgical patients can be fed a regular solid-food diet rather than a clear liquid diet.

CLINICAL SCENARIO

Chronological Clinical Scenario with Suggested Answers

First Assessment

A 57-year-old man with pancreatitis of unknown cause was admitted to a hospital where he was managed conservatively, ingesting nothing by mouth (NPO) for 9 days without enteral or parenteral nutrition therapy. On hospital day 9 he was found to have pseudocysts and was transferred to a tertiary care center for further management.

Screening and Assessment Data:

Height = 71″ (180 cm)
Weight = 150 lb (68 kg)
Body mass index = 21 kg/m^2
Weight change in the 6 months prior to admission: yes
Amount of weight lost: 25 lb
Decreased intake in the previous 2 weeks: yes
Gastrointestinal symptoms persisting for more than 2 weeks: yes
Physical examination: temporal wasting
Radiologic examination: moderately dilated small bowel loops consistent with adynamic ileus
Maximum body temperature previous 24 hr (T_{max}) 37° C
Currently receiving 0.45% normal saline + 30 mEq KCl/L @ 125 mL/hr
Intake/Output = 4000/3800 mL

Laboratory Values

Sodium: 130 mmol/dL
Potassium: 3.4 mmol/dL
Chloride: 100 mmol/dL
Carbon dioxide: 20 mmol/dL
Blood urea nitrogen: 23 mg/dL
Creatinine: 0.8 mg/dL
Calcium: 8 mg/dL
Magnesium: 1.9 mg/dL
Phosphorus: 2.2 mg/dL
Albumin: 3 gm/dL

1. Write pertinent nutrition diagnosis statements (problem, etiology, and signs and symptoms [PES] format) in order of priority for this patient.
   Malnutrition related to inadequate oral food and beverage intake during a prolonged period as evidenced by 14% weight loss during 6 months and intake remains nil.
   Altered nutrition-related laboratory values related to the metabolic response to stress and a lack of electrolyte intake in diet and intravenous fluids as evidenced by low serum sodium, potassium, and phosphorus.
2. Should he be started on parenteral nutrition (PN)? Explain.
   By the information presented in the case, he should be started on PN because he is malnourished, has been NPO for 9 days, and does not appear to be ready to begin enteral feeding (secondary to ileus). It will be important to discuss enteral feeding via jejunal access with the physicians once ileus has resolved.

Continued

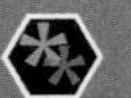

CLINICAL SCENARIO—cont'd

Chronological Clinical Scenario with Suggested Answers

3. Calculate his nutritional needs.
   His caloric requirement should be estimated using the Mifflin-St. Jeor equation, although the equation will not account for whatever level of hypermetabolism exists, and there are no studies to guide the choice of the "stress factor." The Mifflin-St. Jeor equation should be used because it is the most accurate of all the equations used for obese or nonobese, healthy people. The patient is not in a state that would justify the use of the available critical care equations. Actual body weight should be used.
   Mifflin-St. Jeor equation result for this patient is 1525 kcals/day.
   Protein requirement may be set at 1.5 g/kg body weight or 102 g/day.

First Change of Status with Reassessment

On hospital day 4 (day 13 of total hospitalization), the patient's body temperature spikes to 39° C and he is found to have infected pseudocysts. He goes to the operating room for drainage of pseudocysts and irrigation and debridement of the pancreas. Afterwards he is admitted to the intensive care unit sedated and mechanically ventilated. Current status is noted:

T_{max} 39.3 degrees centigrade
VE = 15.6 L/min (minute ventilation)
PN continues
Intravenous fluids: 0.45% normal saline solution 50 mL/hr
Intake/output = 6200/3000 mL

Laboratory Values

Sodium: 135 mmol/dL
Potassium: 3.8 mmol/dL
Chloride: 100 mmol/dL
Carbon dioxide: 29 mmol/dL
Blood urea nitrogen: 33 mg/dL
Creatinine: 1.0 mg/dL
Glucose: 210 mg/dL
Calcium: 8.4 mg/dL
Magnesium: 1.5 mg/dL
Phosphorus: 2.3 mg/dL
Albumin: 2.3 gm/dL
Arterial blood gas: 7.31/50/115/30

4. Upon monitoring, what is his metabolic state?
   He has become hypermetabolic and probably hypercatabolic.
   Hyperglycemia has worsened.
   Electrolyte depletion (phosphorus, magnesium).
5. What is his acid-base status?
   He has a respiratory acidosis (elevated arterial carbon dioxide pressure and decreased pH) with rising bicarbonate (attempted compensation for the respiratory acidosis, which has not been sufficient to return the pH to the normal range).
6. Write updated PES statements:
   Increased nutrient needs (energy and protein) related to a systemic inflammatory response as evidenced by fever and elevated minute ventilation.
   Altered nutrition-related laboratory values (hyperglycemia) related to stress metabolism and glucose intake as evidenced by blood glucose of 210 mg/dL.
   Altered nutrition-related laboratory values related to the metabolic response to stress and sepsis as evidenced by low serum sodium, phosphorus, and magnesium. Note: his hyponatremia could be a result of fluid overload rather than inadequate sodium intake.
7. Is the patient's blood glucose control adequate? If not, why and what should be done?
   His blood glucose is not adequately controlled. There is evidence that when glucose levels are controlled between 180-215 mg/dL, survival is better.
   The dextrose load in his PN should be reduced or a standardized insulin protocol should be instituted, or both. In addition, energy intake should be assessed to confirm absence of overfeeding because this could result in hyperglycemia. Medication administration should also be monitored because some can significantly contribute to elevated glucose levels (i.e., intravenous steroids).
8. Why is his serum albumin level falling?
   Decreased acute-phase proteins are a response to the inflammatory process his body has mounted to try to reestablish homeostasis.
9. Recalculate his nutritional needs.
   Protein requirement has probably increased (2 g/kg body weight or 136 g/day). Metabolic rate calculated by the Penn State equation is 2330 kcal:
   Penn State Equation:

$$HBE(1.1) + Ve(32) + T_{max}(140) - 5340$$

$$1500(1.1) + 15.6(32) + 39.3(140) - 5340$$

$$1667 + 499 + 5502 - 5340 = 2330$$

CLINICAL SCENARIO—cont'd

Chronological Clinical Scenario with Suggested Answers

HBE is Harris Benedict using actual weight, *Ve* is minute ventilation in L/min, T_{max} is maximum body temperature in the past 24 hours in degrees centigrade.

Second Change of Status with Reassessment

On hospital day 6, the patient returned to the operating room for further debridement. During the surgery, a nasojejunal tube was placed. Postoperatively he remains febrile with elevated minute ventilation, and requires fluid administration to maintain adequate blood pressure. On rounds, the dietitian asks whether the patient is stable enough to start tube feeding through the nasojejunal tube. The critical care team believes that despite his early postoperative state, the patient is sufficiently stable hemodynamically to initiate a trophic tube feeding.

10. What feeding formula should be used? Is an immune-enhancing tube feeding formula indicated?

Commercial immune-enhancing formulas that combine several nutrients thought to enhance immune function are not indicated for routine use, and may be contraindicated in the severely critically ill, such as this patient.

Most of the studies of enteral feeding in pancreatitis use peptide-based feeding formulas; it is reasonable to do the same in this case. However, it is possible that a polymeric formula would work as well. If a 1.0 kcal/mL formula is chosen, the infusion volume will be approximately 3 L/day; if a 1.5 kcal/mL formula is chosen, the volume will be approximately 2 L/day.

An enteral feeding with a peptide formula was initiated via nasojejunal access and gradually advanced to goal rate during the next 3-4 days. Tolerance was demonstrated via no change in abdominal distention, pain, or nausea and vomiting. As the feeding advanced, the PN was gradually weaned, then discontinued when goal enteral feeding was achieved.

USEFUL WEBSITES

American Society for Parenteral and Enteral Nutrition A.S.P.E.N.
http://www.nutritioncare.org

American Burn Association
http://www.ameriburn.org

Burn Nutrition
http://www.burnsurgery.com/Modules/burnmetabolism/pt2/index_nutrition.htm

Surgical Nutrition: Tutorial
http://www.surgical-tutor.org.uk/default-home.htm?core/ITU/nutrition.htm~right

REFERENCES

American Dietetic Association: *Critical illness: glucose control. Evidence-analysis library*. Accessed 25 October 2010 from http://www.adaevidencelibrary.com/topic.cfm?cat=4083&auth=1.

A.S.P.E.N. Society of Critical Care Medicine (SCCM) and American Society for Parenteral and Enteral Nutrition (A.S.P.E.N.): Guidelines for the provision and assessment of nutrition support therapy in the adult critically ill patients, *JPEN J Parenter Enteral Nutr* 33:277, 2009.

Blackburn GL: Nutrition support in the intensive care unit: an evolving science, *Arch Surg* 145:533, 2010.

Brady M, et al: Preoperative fasting for adults to prevent perioperative complications, *Cochrane Database Syst Rev* 4:CD004423, 2003.

Brady M, et al: Preoperative fasting for preventing perioperative complications in children, *Cochrane Database Syst Rev* Oct 7(4):CD005285, 2009.

Breen H, Ireton-Jones C: Predicting energy needs in obese patients, *Nutr Clin Pract* 19:284, 2004.

Byrnes MC, et al: Early enteral nutrition can be successfully implemented in trauma patients with an "open abdomen," *Am J Surg* 199:359, 2010.

Chan MM, Chan GM: Nutritional therapy for burns in children and adults, *Nutrition* 25:261, 2009.

Cheatham ML, et al: Nitrogen balance, protein loss, and the open abdomen, *Crit Care Med* 35:127, 2007.

Choban PS, Dickerson RN: Morbid obesity and nutrition support: is bigger different? *Nutr Clin Pract* 20:480, 2005.

Collier B, et al: Feeding the open abdomen, *JPEN J Parenter Enteral Nutr* 31:410, 2007.

Compher C, et al: Best practice methods to apply to measurement of resting metabolic rate in adults: a systematic review, *J Am Diet Assoc* 106:881, 2006.

Cook RC, Blinman TA: Nutritional support of the pediatric trauma patient, *Semin Pediatr Surg* 19:242, 2010.

Deitch EA, et al: Role of the gut in the development of injury- and shock-induced SIRS and MODS: the gut-lymph hypothesis, a review, *Front Biosci* 11:520, 2006.

Dickerson RN: Hypocaloric feeding of obese patients in the intensive care unit, *Curr Opin Clin Nutr Metabol Care* 8:189, 2005.

Dissanaike S, et al: Effect of immediate enteral feeding on trauma patients with an open abdomen: protection from nosocomial infections, *J Am Coll Surg* 207:690, 2008.

Dylewski ML, et al: Malnutrition among pediatric burn patients: a consequence of delayed admissions, *Burns* 36:1185, 2010.

Frankenfield D, et al: Prediction of resting metabolic rate in critically ill adult patients: results of a systematic review of the evidence, *J Am Diet Assoc* 107:1552, 2007.

Galloswitsch-Puerta M, Tracey KJ: Immunologic role of the cholinergic anti-inflammatory pathway and the nicotinic acetylcholine alpha 7 receptor, *Ann NY Acad Sci* 1062:209, 2005.

Ireton-Jones C, Jones JD: Improved equations for predicting energy expenditure in patients: the Ireton-Jones equations, *Nutr Clin Pract* 17:29, 2002.

Jensen GL, et al: Malnutrition syndromes: a conundrum versus continuum, *JPEN J Parenter Enteral Nutr* 33:710, 2009.

Jensen G, et al: Adult starvation and disease-related malnutrition: a proposal for etiology-based diagnosis in the clinical practice setting from the International Consensus Guideline Committee, *JPEN J Parenter Enteral Nutr* 34:156, 2010.

Jeschke MG: The hepatic response to thermal injury: is the liver important for postburn outcomes? *Mol Med* 15:337, 2009.

Joffe A, et al: Nutritional support for critically ill children, *Cochrane Database Syst Rev* Apr 15(2):CD005144, 2009.

Kang W, Kudsk KA: Is there evidence that the gut contributes to mucosal immunity in humans? *JPEN J Parenter Enteral Nutr* 31:246, 2007.

Lewis SJ, et al: Early enteral nutrition within 24 h of intestinal surgery versus later commencement of feeding: a systematic review and meta-analysis, *J Gastrointest Surg* 13:569, 2009.

Malone AM: Methods of assessing energy expenditure in the intensive care unit, *Nutr Clin Pract* 17:21, 2002.

Mayes T, Gottschlich MM: Burns and wound healing. In Matarase LE, Gottschlich MM, editors: *Contemporary nutrition support practice: a clinical guide*, ed 2, Philadelphia, 2003, Saunders.

Miller MD, et al: A Trial Assessing N-3 as Treatment for Injury-induced Cachexia (ATLANTIC trial): does a moderate dose fish oil intervention improve outcomes in older adults recovering from hip fracture? *BMC Geriatr* 10:76, 2010.

Mizock BA: Immunonutrition and critical illness: an update, *Nutrition* 26:701, 2010.

Nose K, et al: Glutamine prevents total parenteral nutrition-associated changes to intraepithelial lymphocyte phenotype and function: a potential mechanism for the preservation of epithelial barrier function, *J Interferon Cytokine Res* 30:67, 2010.

Port AM, Apovian C: Metabolic support of the obese intensive care unit patient: a current perspective, *Curr Opin Clin Nutr Metab Care* 13:184, 2010.

Søreide E, Ljungqvist O: Modern preoperative fasting guidelines: a summary of the present recommendations and remaining questions, *Best Pract Res Clin Anaesthesiol* 20:483, 2006.

Svanfeldt M, et al: Randomized clinical trial of the effect of preoperative oral carbohydrate treatment on postoperative whole-body protein and glucose kinetics, *Br J Surg* 94:1342, 2007.

Walker J, Criddle LM: Pathophysiology and management of abdominal compartment syndrome, *Am J Crit Care* 12:367, 2003.

Yang H, et al: Enteral versus parenteral nutrition: effect on intestinal barrier function, *Ann NY Acad Sci* 1165:338, 2009.

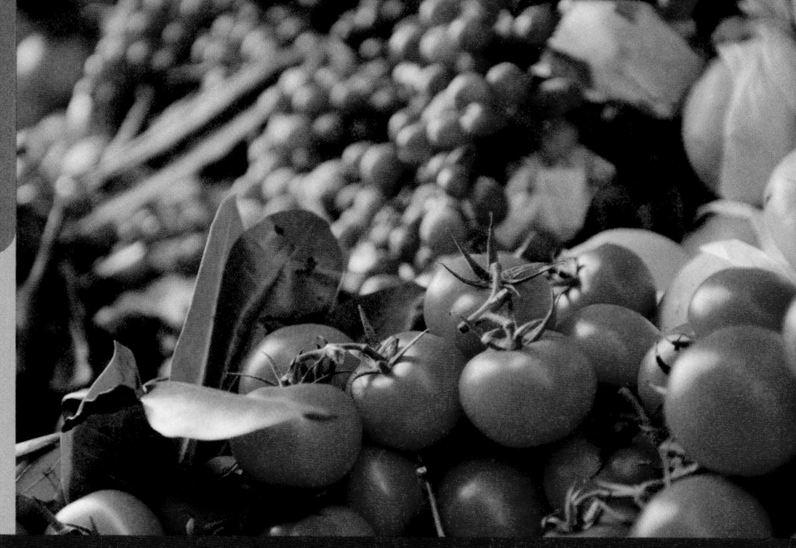

CHAPTER 40

F. Enrique Gómez, PhD
Martha Kaufer-Horwitz, DSc, NC

Medical Nutrition Therapy for Rheumatic Disease

KEY TERMS

activities of daily living (ADLs)
anti-inflammatory diet
anti-nuclear antibodies (ANA)
arachidonic acid (ARA)
biologic response modifiers
capsaicinoids
chronic fatigue syndrome (CFS)
c-reactive protein (CRP)
cytokines
disease-modifying anti-rheumatic drugs (DMARDs)
eicocanoids
fibromyalgia
gout
juvenile rheumatoid arthritis
osteoarthritis (OA)
prostaglandins (PGs)
prostanoids
purines
Raynaud's syndrome
rheumatic disease
rheumatoid arthritis (RA)
rheumatoid cachexia
rheumatoid factor (RF)
scleroderma
Sjögren's syndrome (SS)
synovial fluid
systemic lupus erythematosus (SLE)
temporomandibular disorders (TMDs)

Rheumatic disease and related conditions include more than 100 different manifestations of inflammation and loss of function of connective tissue and supporting body structures, including joints, tendons, ligaments, bones, muscles, and sometimes internal organs. Rheumatic disease is thought to have an autoimmune component. Because no identifiable cause or cure is known, pharmacotherapy, physical and occupational treatment, and medical nutrition therapy (MNT) play important roles in managing the symptoms. Table 40-1 provides an overview of the disorders and their management.

Rheumatic disease affects all population groups. According to the National Arthritis Data Workgroup, osteoarthritis (OA) affects 27 million Americans; gout, 3 million; fibromyalgia, 5 million; rheumatoid arthritis (RA), 1.5 million; Sjögren's syndrome (SS), 1 to 4 million; and systemic lupus erythematosus (SLE), 161,000 to 322,000 (Helmick et al., 2008; Lawrence et al., 2008). Estimates for the number of people in the United States with systemic sclerosis is 49,000. Arthritis and the related disorders are among the most prevalent chronic disease conditions in the United States and are associated with total direct and indirect costs to the U.S. economy of $128 billion per year in medical care and lost wages (Centers for Disease Control and Prevention [CDC], 2007).

Arthritis is a generic term that comes from the Greek word *Arthro*, which means "joint," and the suffix *-itis*, which means "inflammation." There are two distinct categories of disease: systemic, autoimmune rheumatic disease and nonsystemic OA. The more debilitating and autoimmune arthritis group includes RA, **juvenile rheumatoid arthritis**,

Sections of this chapter were written by Kristine Duncan, RD for the previous edition of this text.

TABLE 40-1

Summary of Medical Nutrition Therapy for Rheumatic Diseases

Disease	Medical Nutrition Therapy	Alternative Therapy	Supplements or Herbs That Can Be Safely Considered	Therapies without Adequate Evidence
Rheumatoid arthritis	Vegetarian, vegan, Mediterranean diet; anti-inflammatory diet; appropriate calories for maintenance of normal body weight; RDA for protein unless malnutrition present; moderate-fat diet with emphasis on ω-3 PUFAs and fish 1-2 times per week; modifications as needed for jaw pain, anorexia	Exercise, meditation, tai chi, spiritual practice, relaxation techniques	Supplement diet as needed to meet DRI for antioxidant nutrients and, calcium, folate, vitamins B_6, B_{12}, D; GLA; fish oils; rosemary, tumeric, curcumin, curry, ginger and other culinary herbs	China root, willow bark, valerian, feverfew, boswellia, copper or copper salts, devil's claw, thunder god vine, fasting, DHEA
Osteoarthritis	Weight management; diet adequate in calcium, folate, vitamins B_6, D, K; magnesium; anti-inflammatory diet (Box 40-2)	Exercise, acupuncture; SAM-e	Supplement diet as needed to meet DRI for antioxidant nutrients and, calcium, folate, vitamins B_6, B_{12}, and D; glucosamine, chondroitin; oils; diacercin; avocado soybean unsaponifiables, hyaluronic acid	Shark cartilage
Gout	Weight management; purine-controlled diet; adequate fluid consumption; alcohol, particularly beer, restricted or eliminated; fructose from sweetened beverages and juices restricted.	Exercise; alkaline-ash foods; see Clinical Insight box on Urinary pH in Chapter 36		
Lupus	Tailor diet to individual needs; calories to maintain IBW; restriction of protein, fluid, and sodium if renal involvement; check for gluten intolerance		Supplement diet as needed to meet DRI for antioxidant nutrients	
Scleroderma	Adequate fluid; high-energy, high-protein supplements as needed to prevent/correct weight loss; moist foods; modifications for GERD if needed			
Fibromyalgia and chronic fatigue syndrome	Vegetarian diets, vegan diet, weight control, ω-3 fatty acids	Moderate intensity graded exercise, cognitive behavioral therapy, stress management, massage	Riboflavin (B_2), CoQ_{10}, carnitine	Biofeedback, relaxation, chlorella, homeopathy, acupuncture, guaifenesin, magnesium, SAM-e
Sjögren's syndrome	Balanced diet with adequate B_6 or vitamin supplementation; restrict sugary foods and beverages; modify food consistency and size to improve chewing and swallowing processes			
TMD	Balanced diet with soft foods in small pieces, to improve chewing and reduce pain			

DHEA, Dehydroepiandrosterone; *DRI*, Dietary reference intake; *GERD*, gastroesophageal reflux disease; *GLA*, Gamma-linolenic acid; *IBW*, ideal body weight; *PUFA*, polyunsaturated fatty acid; *RDA*, recommended dietary allowance; *SAM-e*, *S*-adenosyl-L-methionine; *TMD*, temporomandibular disorder.

gout, SS, fibromyalgia, SLE, and scleroderma. The OA group includes OA, bursitis, and tendonitis. Other rheumatic diseases include spondyloarthropathies, polymyalgia rheumatica, and polymyositis.

Body changes associated with aging—including decreased somatic protein, body fluids, and bone density, and an increase in total body fat—may contribute to the onset and progression of arthritis. The aging body mass causes changes in neuroendocrine regulators, immune regulators, and metabolism, which affect the inflammatory process. Therefore recent increases in the frequency of these conditions may be the result of aging of the U.S. population. By 2030 approximately 20% of Americans (approximately 72 million people) will be older than 65 years and subsequently will be at high risk for rheumatic disease (National Institute of Arthritis and Musculoskeletal and Skin Diseases [NIAMS], 2006).

Unfortunately, the cause of most rheumatic conditions remains unknown. In addition, some forms of rheumatic conditions can affect other organs such as the skin or blood vessels. Rheumatic conditions have no known cure and are usually chronic, but may present as acute episodes with short or intermittent duration. Chronic arthritic conditions are associated with alternating periods of remission without symptoms, and flares with worsening symptoms that occur without any identifiable cause. Risk factors include repetitive joint injury, inherited cartilage weakness, genetic susceptibility, family history, gender, and environmental factors.

BOX 40-1

Production of Eicosanoids from Omega-3 and Omega-6 PUFAs

Eicosapentaenoic Acid (20:5, ω-3)

Thromboxane A_3: Weak vasoconstrictor and weak platelet aggregator
Prostacyclin PGI_3: Vasodilator and platelet antiaggregator
Leukotriene B_5: Weak inflammation inducer and weak chemotactic agent

Arachidonic Acid (20:4, ω-6)

Thromboxane A_2: Vasoconstrictor and potent platelet aggregator
Prostaglandin E_2: Vasodilator and platelet antiaggregator
Leukotriene B_4: Inflammation inducer and potent leukocyte chemotaxis and adherence inducer

Dihomo-γ-linolenic acid DGLA (20:3, ω-6)

Thromboxane A_1: Anti-inflammatory, pain reducer
Prostaglandin E_1: Vasodilator, inhibits monocyte and neutrophil function, prevents platelet aggregation
Leukotriene B_3: Very weak pro-inflammatory effects

From Galli C: Effects of fat and fatty acid intake on inflammatory and immune responses: A critical review, Ann Nutr Metab 55:123, 2009.

PUFA, Polyunsaturated fatty acid.

PATHOPHYSIOLOGY AND INFLAMMATION

Inflammation plays an important role in health and disease. The inflammatory process normally occurs to protect and repair tissue damaged by infections, injuries, toxicity, or wounds via accumulation of fluid and cells. Once the cause is resolved, the inflammation usually subsides. Whether inflammation is due to stress on the joints (OA) or to an autoimmune response (RA), an uncontrolled inflammatory reaction causes more damage than repair.

Polyunsaturated fatty acids (PUFAs) play an important role in inflammation as precursors of a potent group of modulators of inflammation termed **eicosanoids** (*eicos* means "20" in Greek). Eicosanoids include the **prostaglandins (PGs)**, thromboxanes (Txs) and leukotrienes (LTs) among others. PG and Tx are the product of the enzyme cyclooxygenase (COX) and are termed **prostanoids**, whereas LTs are the product of the enzyme lipoxygenase. For the synthesis of prostanoids, the COX reaction consumes two double bonds from the original PUFA, whereas lipoxygenase reaction consumes none (Box 40-1; see Chapter 6).

Depending on the PUFA used as substrate, different eicosanoids are produced: **arachidonic acid (ARA)** (20:4, ω-6) is the precursor of the series 2 of PG and Tx, and the series 4 of LT. If eicosapentaenoic acid (20:5, ω-3) is the substrate, series 3 of PG and Tx and series 5 of LT are produced. Finally, dihomo-γ-linoleic acid (DGLA) (20:3, ω-6) is the precursor of series 1 of PG and Tx, and of series 3 of LT.

The series 2 compounds (PG_2 and Tx_2) are the most abundant because ARA is abundant in plasma membranes of cells involved in inflammation (macrophages, neutrophils, fibroblasts), and are the most potent inflammatory eicosanoids. On the other hand, PG_1 and Tx_1, derived from DGLA, have antiinflammatory activities. Thus diets enriched with PUFAs that enhance the synthesis of antiinflammatory prostanoids are, at least theoretically, desirable for the long-term management of rheumatic disease, but usually do not replace the use of medications.

MEDICAL DIAGNOSIS AND TREATMENT

A thorough history of symptoms and a detailed physical examination are the cornerstones for an accurate diagnosis. However, laboratory testing can help to further refine the diagnosis and identify appropriate treatment.

Biochemical Assessment

Acute-phase proteins are plasma proteins whose concentration increases of more than 25% during inflammatory states.

Two acute-phase proteins traditionally used to screen for and monitor rheumatic disease are **rheumatoid factor (RF)** and **C-reactive protein (CRP)**, although they are nonspecific and may also indicate an infection or even a recent cardiac event. The term RF is used to refer to a group of self-reacting antibodies (an abnormal IgM against normal IgG), found in the sera of rheumatic patients. The American College of Rheumatology (ACR) recommends periodic measurements of RF and CRP in addition to a detailed assessment of symptoms and functional status, and radiographic examination to determine the current level of disease activity in these patients.

Antinuclear antibodies (ANA) appear to be present in many autoimmune diseases and can assist with proper diagnosis when used correctly; antineutrophil cytoplasmic antibodies and myositis-specific antibodies can provide information about the presence of rheumatic disease as well. Measurements of RF and anticyclic citrullinated peptide antibodies may provide unique data in the management of RA (Colgazier and Sutej, 2005). Routine blood testing can include complement, a complete blood count, creatinine, hematocrit, and a white blood cell count, in addition to analysis of urine or **synovial fluid** secreted by the synovial membrane in the joints.

Pharmacotherapy

Many of the drugs used in treating rheumatic diseases provide relief from pain and inflammation, with hopes of controlling symptoms rather than providing a cure. Analgesics such as acetaminophen (Tylenol) are effective pain relievers. Drugs commonly used to reduce inflammation affect the synthesis of PGs by inhibiting COX activity, thus diminishing PG production. Glucocorticoid therapy decreases the release of ARA from cell membrane phospholipids by binding to the receptor in the cell cytoplasm. This forms a complex that moves into the nucleus as a transcription factor and interferes with expression for the enzyme phospholipase.

Nonsteroidal antiinflammatory drugs (NSAIDs), which include ibuprofen (Advil or Motrin) and naproxen (Aleve), slow down the body's production of PGs by inhibiting COX-1 enzyme activity. They are considered useful tools in the management of most rheumatic disorders; however, long-term use of NSAIDs may cause gastrointestinal problems such as gastritis, ulcers, abdominal burning, pain, cramping, nausea, gastrointestinal bleeding, or even renal failure (Table 40-2; see Chapter 9 and Appendix 31). COX-2 inhibitors (COX-2 selective NSAIDs) such as celecoxib (Celebrex) have been shown to provide relief comparable to other NSAIDs with potentially less gastrointestinal and cardiovascular toxicity. Naproxen and celecoxib appear to be safer than other NSAIDs (Food and Drug Administration, 2005).

Biologic response modifiers are a class of drugs that selectively target different elements of the disease, and include those directed against interleukin (IL)-1 such as anakinra (Kineret), or against tumor necrosis factor (TNF)–α, like adalimumab (Humira), etanercept (Enbrel), and infliximab (Remicade). These molecules are administered by injection (vein or subcutaneous) because they are proteins and oral administration would destroy their biologic activities. The main drawback is their high cost, as high as $30,000 dollars per patient per year (American College of Rheumatology [ACR], 2006). Patients taking these drugs should be monitored for chronic infections.

Corticosteroids (cortisone [Cortone], prednisone [Deltasone], methylprednisolone [Medrol], and hydrocortisone [Cortef]) suppress the immune system and decrease inflammation, making them desirable treatments for many of the rheumatic diseases. Possible side effects of corticosteroids include hypertension, hyperglycemia, weight gain, and osteoporosis. Low-dose steroids control most of the inflammatory features of early polyarticular RA. Dehydroepiandrosterone (DHEA), a hormone made by the adrenal glands, has failed to show efficacy.

As the most potent of the antiinflammatory drugs used to treat RA, steroids have extensive catabolic effects that can result in negative nitrogen balance. Hypercalciuria and reduced calcium absorption can increase the risk of osteoporosis (see Chapters 9 and 25). Concomitant calcium (1 g/day) and vitamin D (at least 1000 IU/day) and monitoring of bone status may be suggested to minimize osteopenia. Care must be taken to avoid serum calcium levels greater than 11 mg/dL and 25-OH vitamin D levels less than 35 ng/mL. Edema often occurs and may require diet modification, including a sodium- and fluid-restricted diet. Other side effects of steroid use include cushingoid syndrome and gastrointestinal bleeding.

UNCONFIRMED THERAPIES

Because modern medicine cannot promise a cure or even permanent relief of symptoms, many persons turn to alternative approaches for help. With growing access to the Internet, patients have a greater exposure to remedies and controversial treatments. In a recent survey, rheumatologists in the United States showed a widespread favorable opinion toward many alternative therapies for patients with rheumatic diseases (Manek et al., 2010).

Favorable effects of self-help treatments are often reported anecdotally, but as a rule no cause-and-effect relationships are documented. Any amelioration can usually be attributed to the placebo effect or to characteristic cycles of worsening followed by periods of improvement. Therapies that are scientifically proven safe and effective can be promoted, whereas caution is needed in regard to therapies for which the science is limited.

Some remedies have their roots in medicine. Salicylates in aspirin are derived from willow bark; they have been around as a medicinal remedy for pain and inflammation for centuries. Willow bark and ginger may relieve pain because their chemical composition is similar to NSAIDs, but excessive blood thinning is a concern (Marcus, 2005). Additional research is needed on valerian, feverfew, boswellia, and curcumin before recommendations can be made for

TABLE 40-2

Nutritional Side Effects of Arthritis Medications

	NSAIDs						
Side Effects	**Traditional NSAIDs**	**COX-2s**	**Salicylates**	**Biologic Response Modifiers**	**Analgesics**	**Corticosteroids**	**DMARDs**
GI ulceration/bleeding	X*	X†	X			X	
Dyspepsia	X	X	X				X
Nausea and vomiting	X	X	X		X		X
Oral ulcers							X
Diarrhea	X	X	X				X
Polyuria						X	
Polydipsia						X	
Constipation					X		
Dry mouth					X		
Loss of appetite					X		X
Abdominal and stomach cramps	X	X	X	X			X
Metallic taste in mouth							X
Irritation and soreness of tongue							X
Irritated or bleeding gums							X
Folate antagonism							X
Increased excretion or decreased absorption of vitamin C	X		X				
Iron loss	X						
Potassium loss						X	
Vitamin B_6 loss						X	X
Increased potassium level	X						
Magnesium loss						X	
Edema	X	X	X			X	
Liver disease							X
Gallbladder disease							X
Renal disease							X
Proteinuria							X
Change in blood pressure				X		X	X
Hyperglycemia						X	
Osteoporosis						X	
Weight gain						X	
Urinary retention					X		
Thrombotic cardiovascular events		X					

Data from ACR: Guidelines for the management of rheumatoid arthritis, Arthritis Rheum 46:2, 2002; Arthritis Foundation: Arthritis today, 2005 drug guide; Boullata JI, Armenti VT, editors: Handbook of drug-nutrient interactions, Totowa, NJ, 2004, Humana Press.

*Less with diclofenac sodium with misoprostol, but increased risk of abdominal pain and diarrhea.

†Less than traditional NSAIDs.

COX, Cyclooxygenase; *DMARD*, disease-modifying antirheumatic drug; *GI*, gastrointestinal; *NSAID*, nonsteroidal antiinflammatory drug.

their usefulness in treating RA (National Center for Complementary and Alternative Medicine [NCCAM], 2009).

Although much of the dietary experimentation is harmless except for the costs, some self-treatment modalities can be harmful. It is best to avoid copper or copper salts, shark cartilage, devil's claw, echinacea, guaifenesin, alfalfa, wild yam, and methylsulfonylmethane (MSM). Both comfrey and alfalfa are herbs that have been promoted as potential cures for arthritis, yet both have been deemed toxic by the scientific community. Meditation, tai chi, relaxation techniques, thermotherapy and spiritual practice may offer pain reduction. Biofeedback, relaxation, chlorella supplements, magnet

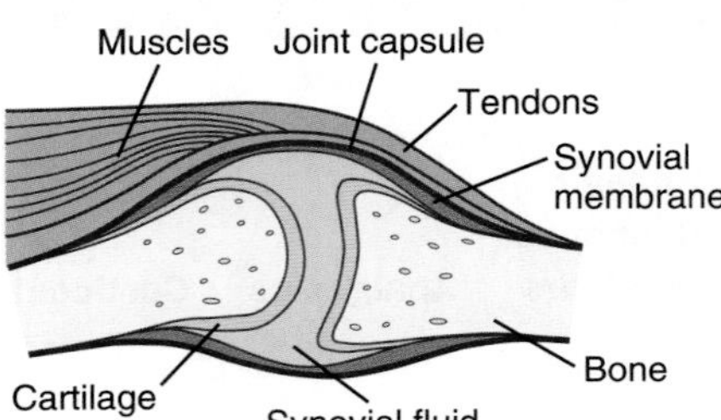

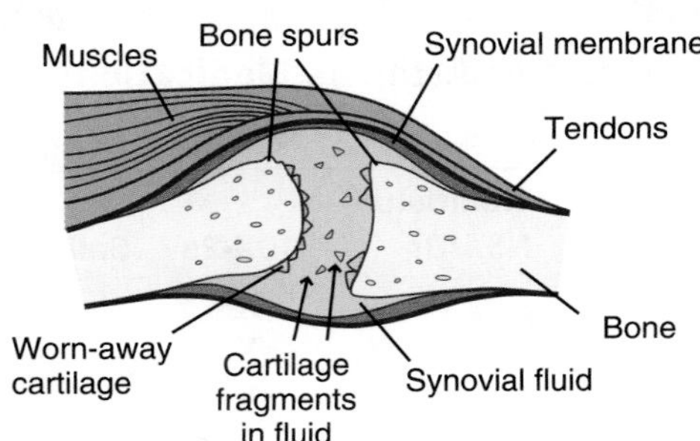

FIGURE 40-1 A healthy joint and a joint with severe osteoarthritis. *(From National Institute of Arthritis and Musculoskeletal and Skin Diseases:* Handout on health: osteoarthritis, *National Institutes of Health, Department of Health and Human Services, NIH Publication Number 06-4617, July 2002, revised May 2006.)*

therapies, homeopathy, botanical oils, and dietary modifications need further study before general recommendations can be made.

OSTEOARTHRITIS

Osteoarthritis (OA), formally known as *degenerative arthritis* or *degenerative joint disease*, is the most prevalent form of arthritis. Obesity, aging, female gender, white ethnicity, greater bone density, and repetitive-use injury associated with athletics have been identified as risk factors. OA is not systemic or autoimmune in origin, but involves cartilage destruction with asymmetric inflammation. It is caused by joint overuse, whereas RA is a systemic autoimmune disorder that results in symmetric joint inflammation.

Pathophysiology

OA is a chronic joint disease that involves the loss of habitually weight-bearing articular (joint) cartilage. This cartilage normally allows bones to glide smoothly over one another. The loss can result in stiffness, pain, swelling, loss of motion, and changes in joint shape, in addition to abnormal bone growth, which can result in osteophytes (bone spurs) (Huskisson, 2008) (see Figure 40-1 and the *Pathophysiology and Care Management Algorithm:* Osteoarthritis).

The joints most often affected in OA are the distal interphalangeal joints, the thumb joint, and, in particular, the joints of the knees, hips, ankles, and spine, which bear the bulk of the body's weight (Figure 40-2). The elbows, wrists, and ankles are less often affected. OA generally presents as pain that worsens with weight bearing and activity and improves with rest, and patients often report morning stiffness or "gelling" of the affected joint after periods of inactivity. Diseases of the joints influenced by congenital and mechanical derangements may contribute to OA as well. Inflammation occurs at times but is generally mild and localized.

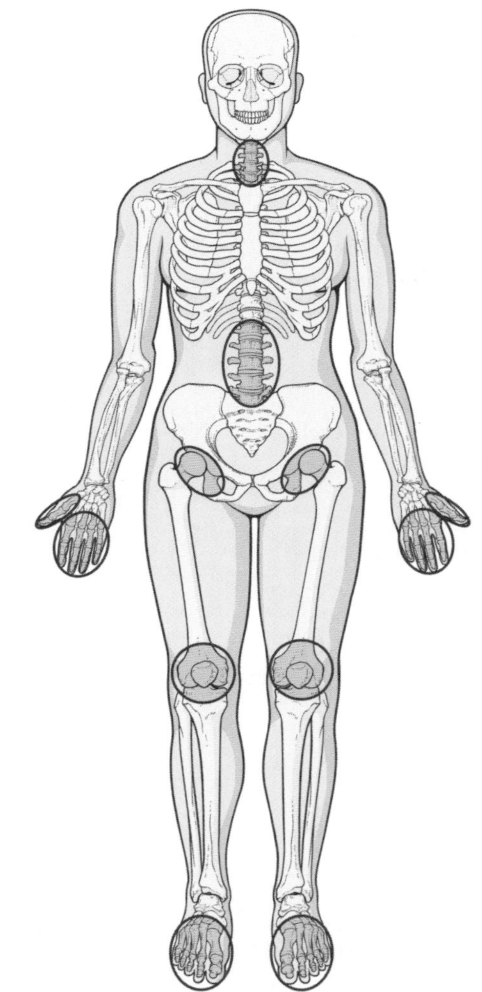

FIGURE 40-2 Joints commonly affected by osteoarthritis.

Medical and Surgical Management

The patient's medical history and level of pain should determine the most appropriate treatment. This should include nonpharmacologic modalities (patient education, physical and occupational therapy), pharmacologic agents, and surgical procedures with the goals of pain control, improved function and health-related quality of life, and avoidance of toxic effects from treatment (Huskisson, 2010). Weight loss and/or achievement of ideal body weight (body mass index

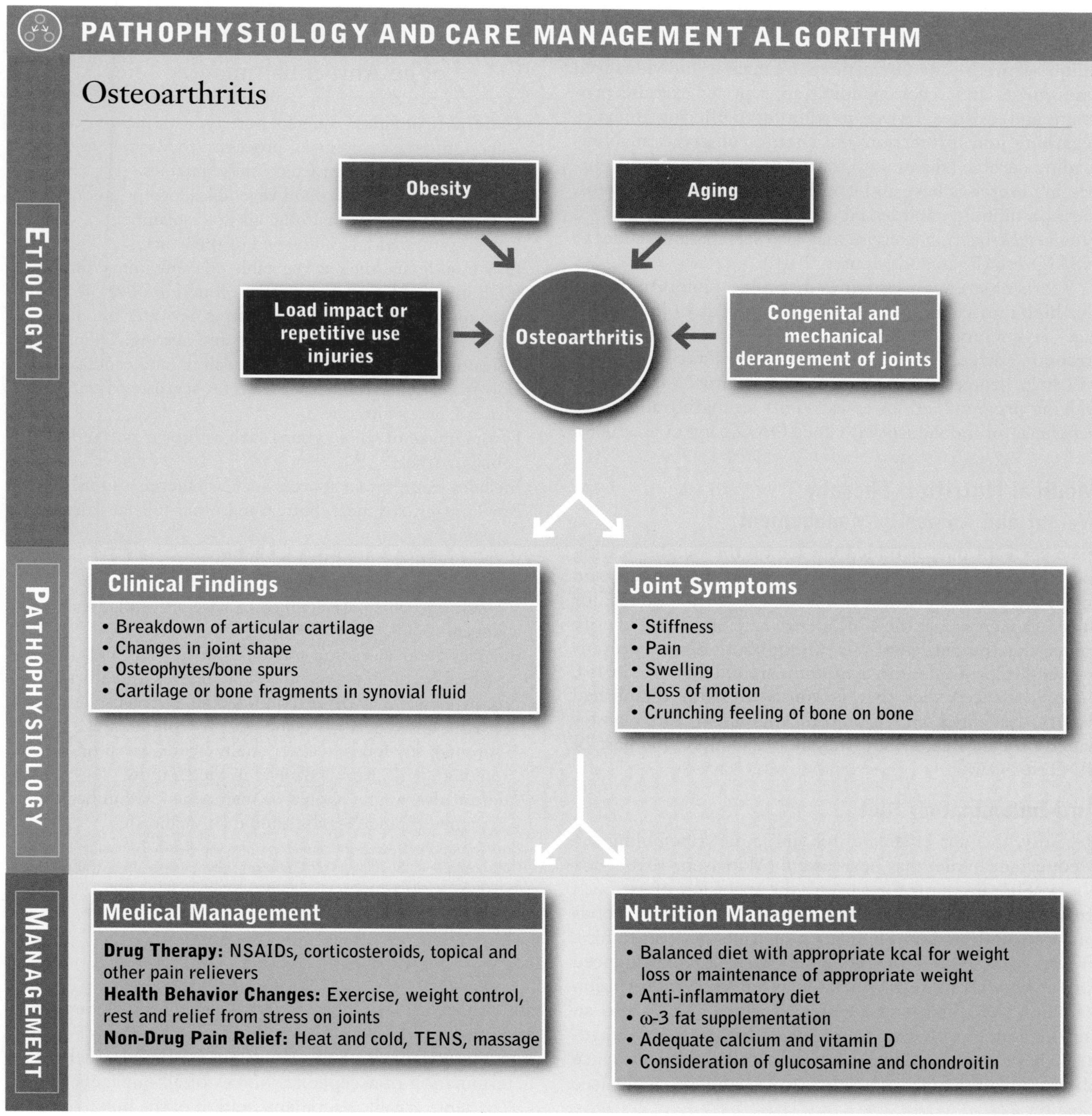

[BMI] of 18.5-24.9) should be part of the medical treatment as it improves OA dramatically. See Chapter 22.

Patients with severe symptomatic OA pain who have not responded adequately to medical treatment and who have been progressively limited in their **activities of daily living (ADLs)**, such as walking, bathing, dressing, and toileting, should be evaluated by an orthopedic surgeon. Surgical options include arthroscopic debridement (with or without arthroplasty), total joint arthroplasty, and osteotomy. Surgical reconstruction has been quite successful but should not be viewed as a replacement for overall good nutrition, maintenance of healthy body weight, and exercise.

Exercise

OA limits the ability to increase energy expenditure through exercise. It is critical that the exercise be done with correct form so as not to cause damage or exacerbate an existing problem. Physical and occupational therapists can provide unique expertise for OA patients by making individualized assessments and recommending appropriate exercise programs and assistive devices, in addition to offering guidance regarding joint protection and energy conservation. Non-loading aerobic (swimming), range-of-motion, and weight-bearing exercises have all been shown to reduce symptoms, increase mobility, and lessen continuing damage from OA. Nonweight-bearing exercise may also serve as an adjunct to NSAID use (Egan and Mentes, 2010).

Sports or strenuous activities that subject joints to repetitive high impact and loading increase the risk of joint cartilage degeneration. Therefore increased muscle tone and strength, correct form, general flexibility, and conditioning will help protect these joints in the habitual exerciser. A walking program and lower-extremity strength training are beneficial for individuals with knee OA (Zhang et al., 2008).

Medical Nutrition Therapy

Weight and Adiposity Management

Excess weight puts an added burden on the weight-bearing joints. Epidemiologic studies have shown that obesity and injury are the two greatest risk factors for OA. The risk for knee OA increases as the BMI increases. Controlling obesity can reduce the burden of OA through both disease prevention and improvement in symptoms (Holliday et al., 2010). A well-balanced diet that is consistent with established dietary guidelines and promotes attainment and maintenance of a desirable body weight is an important part of MNT for OA.

Anti-Inflammatory Diet

Recently, the **anti-inflammatory diet**, a diet resembling the Mediterranean diet, has been useful (Marcason, 2010) (Box 40-2). The diet aims for variety, the inclusion of as much fresh food as possible, the least amount of processed foods and fast food, and an abundance of fruits and vegetables. When combined with moderate exercise, diet-induced weight loss has been shown to be an effective intervention for knee OA (Egan and Mentes, 2010). There is also an anti-inflammatory effect from weight loss in OA management because the reduced fat mass results in the presence of less inflammatory mediators from adipose tissue (see Chapter 22).

Vitamins and Minerals

Cumulative damage to tissues mediated by reactive oxygen species has been implicated as a pathway that leads to many of the degenerative changes seen with aging. However, large doses of dietary antioxidants, including vitamin C, the tocopherols (vitamin E), β-carotene, and selenium have shown no benefit for the management of symptomatic OA (Canter et al., 2007; Rosenbaum et al., 2010).

Many patients with OA consume deficient levels of calcium, and vitamin D. Low serum levels of vitamin D are being studied for their role in OA progression (McAlindon and Biggee, 2005). Improving intake to at least dietary reference intake (DRI) levels is important. Comprehensive nutrition interviewing and counseling should include a determination of acceptable sources of all nutrients for the OA patient, as well as supplementation of the diet to achieve the recommended levels with special attention given to vitamin B_6, vitamin D, vitamin K, folate, and magnesium.

BOX 40-2

The Anti-inflammatory Diet

General principles: Aims for variety, with plenty of fresh food, the least amount of processed foods and "fast foods," and abundant fruits and vegetables.

Includes plenty of fruits and vegetables, except onions and potatoes, which contain the alkaloid solanine.

Low in saturated fat and devoid of trans fats.

Low in ω-6 fats, such as vegetable oils and animal fat.

High in ω-3 PUFAs such as those found in olive oil, flax, walnuts, pumpkin seeds and fatty cold-water oily fish like salmon, sardines, mackerel, and herring. Other healthy oils include grapeseed, walnut, and canola.

Low in refined carbohydrates such as sucrose, pasta, white bread, and white rice.

Favors intake of whole grains such as brown rice and bulgur wheat.

Includes lean protein sources such as chicken and fish.

Low in eggs, red meat, butter, and other full-fat dairy products

Low in refined and processed foods.

Includes spices such as ginger, curry, turmeric, and rosemary, which are claimed to have anti-inflammatory effects.

Includes good sources of phytonutrients: fruits and vegetables of all colors, especially berries, tomatoes, orange and yellow fruits, and dark leafy greens; cruciferous vegetables (cabbage, broccoli, brussels sprouts); soy foods, tea (especially white, green or oolong), dark plain chocolate in moderation.

Additionally, weight should be maintained within healthy parameters, and exercise should be included.

Data from Sears B: Anti-inflammatory diets for obesity and diabetes, J Am Coll Nutr 28:482S, 2009; Web MD: Anti-inflammatory diet: road to good health? Accessed from www.webmd.com/diet/guide/anti-inflammatory-diet-road-to-good-health.

PUFA, Polyunsaturated fatty acid.

Alternative Therapies

A variety of alternative therapies have been proposed to manage pain in OA, including topical aids, manipulative therapies, and acupuncture. **Capsaicinoids**, derived from chili peppers, have a fatty acid receptor that stimulates, then blocks, small-diameter pain fibers by depleting them of the neurotransmitter substance P, thought to be the principal chemomediator of pain impulses from the periphery. Capsaicin, applied with glyceryl trinitrate to reduce onsite burning, can reduce pain in OA patients (Kosuwon, 2010). Certain pulsed electromagnetic fields can also affect the growth of bone and cartilage with potential use in OA, and use of static magnets may provide temporary pain relief under certain circumstances (Pittler et al., 2007).

According to the Arthritis Foundation (AF), *S*-adenosyl-L-methionine (SAM-e) has also shown promise for reducing pain and improving mobility in people with OA at doses of 600 to 1200 mg/day, but should not be taken without a doctor's supervision (Arthritis Foundation [AF], 2007). A systematic review and meta-analysis also found benefit for OA patients treated with acupuncture (Kwon et al., 2006).

Other alternative therapies used to help lessen the need for medication are glucosamine sulfate, chondroitin sulfate, oils, and herbs. Other modalities include diacerein, avocado soybean unsaponifiables, and hyaluronic acid that have a symptomatic effect and low toxicity, but overall effects are small (Zhang et al., 2007). Advocates of these alternative modalities cite reports of progressive and gradual decline of joint pain and tenderness, improved mobility, sustained improvement after drug withdrawal, and a lack of toxicity associated with short-term use of these agents (AF, 2005a).

Glucosamine and Chondroitin

Sodium chondroitin sulfate (chondroitin sulfate) and glucosamine hydrochloride (glucosamine) are both involved in cartilage production, but their mechanism for eliminating pain has not been identified. Limited data suggest that glucosamine sulfate administered orally, intravenously, intramuscularly, or intraarticularly may produce a gradual and progressive reduction in joint pain and tenderness, as well as improved range of motion and walking speed (Huskisson, 2008). Glucosamine has produced consistent benefits, including greater than 50% improvement in symptom scores in patients with OA. In some cases glucosamine may be equal or superior to ibuprofen (McAlindon and Biggee, 2005). Together glucosamine and chondroitin rank third among all top-selling nutritional products in the United States.

The National Institutes of Health (NIH) undertook the Glucosamine/Chondroitin Arthritis Intervention Trial (GAIT), the first, large-scale, multicenter clinical trial in the United States to test the effects of these supplements on knee OA. A dose of 1500 mg of glucosamine (500 mg, three times daily) with 1200 mg of chondroitin (400 mg, three times daily) resulted in statistically significant pain relief for a small subset of participants who had moderate to severe pain, but not for those in the mild pain subset. Compared with 54% of those taking placebo, 79% of those taking glucosamine and chondroitin reported a 20% or greater reduction in pain. Because of the small sample size, these findings are considered preliminary (National Institutes of Health [NIH], 2008). Although it is not effective for all afflicted individuals, a safe dose of glucosamine and chondroitin sulfate is 1500 mg/day and 1200 mg/day in divided doses, respectively (AF, 2005a). GAIT and other studies have found no change in glucose tolerance (NIH, 2006). A metaanalysis report that looked at more than 3000 human subjects found no adverse effects of oral glucosamine administration on blood, urine, or fecal parameters and no serious or fatal side effects (Anderson et al., 2005). In contrast, chondroitin is chemically similar to commonly used blood thinners and could cause excessive bleeding if used in combination with blood thinners. Chondroitin may also elicit a reaction in those with shellfish allergies.

RHEUMATOID ARTHRITIS

Rheumatoid arthritis (RA) is a debilitating and frequently crippling autoimmune disease with overwhelming personal, social, and economic effects. Although less common than OA, RA is usually more severe. RA affects the interstitial tissues, blood vessels, cartilage, bone, tendons, and ligaments, as well as the synovial membranes that line joint surfaces. RA occurs more frequently in women than in men. The peak onset commonly occurs between 20 and 45 years of age.

Numerous remissions and exacerbations generally follow its onset, although for some people it lasts just a few months or years and then goes away completely. Although any joint may be affected by RA, involvement of the small joints of the extremities—typically the proximal interphalangeal joints of the hands and feet—is most common (Figure 40-3).

Pathophysiology

RA is a chronic, autoimmune, systemic disorder in which **cytokines** and the inflammatory process play a role. RA has articular manifestations that involve chronic inflammation that begins in the synovial membrane and progresses to subsequent damage in the joint cartilage (*Pathophysiology and Care Management Algorithm:* Rheumatoid Arthritis). Although the exact cause of RA is still unknown, certain genes have been discovered that play a role. The likely trigger is a viral or bacterial infection. It has been suggested

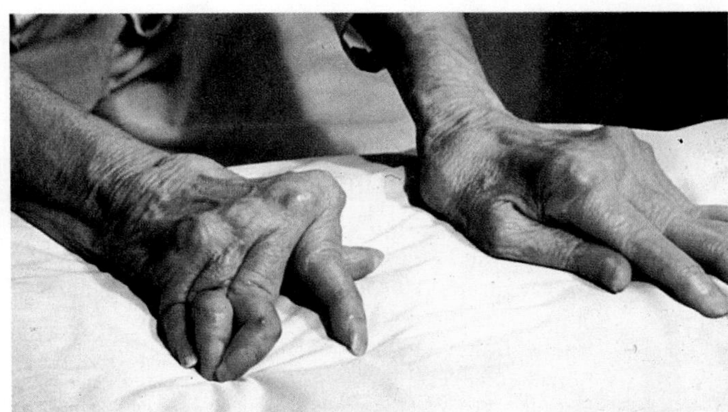

FIGURE 40-3 A patient with advanced rheumatoid arthritis. The twisted hands and the puffiness of the metacarpal joints are typical of the disease. *(From Damjanov I: Pathology for the health-related professions, ed 3, Philadelphia, 2006, Saunders.)*

that drinking large amounts of tea may increase the risk of developing RA (Walitt et al, 2010); however, other studies have suggested that teas are protective. More research is clearly needed.

Medical Management

The appearance of rheumatoid factor (RF), may precede symptoms of RA. Pain, stiffness, swelling, loss of function, and anemia are common. The swelling or puffiness is caused by the accumulation of synovial fluid in the membrane lining the joints and inflammation of the surrounding tissues (Figure 40-4).

RA patients are at increased risk for cardiovascular disease, explained by the systemic inflammatory response (Snow and Mikuls, 2005). This is especially significant considering findings regarding COX-2 selective NSAIDs. In

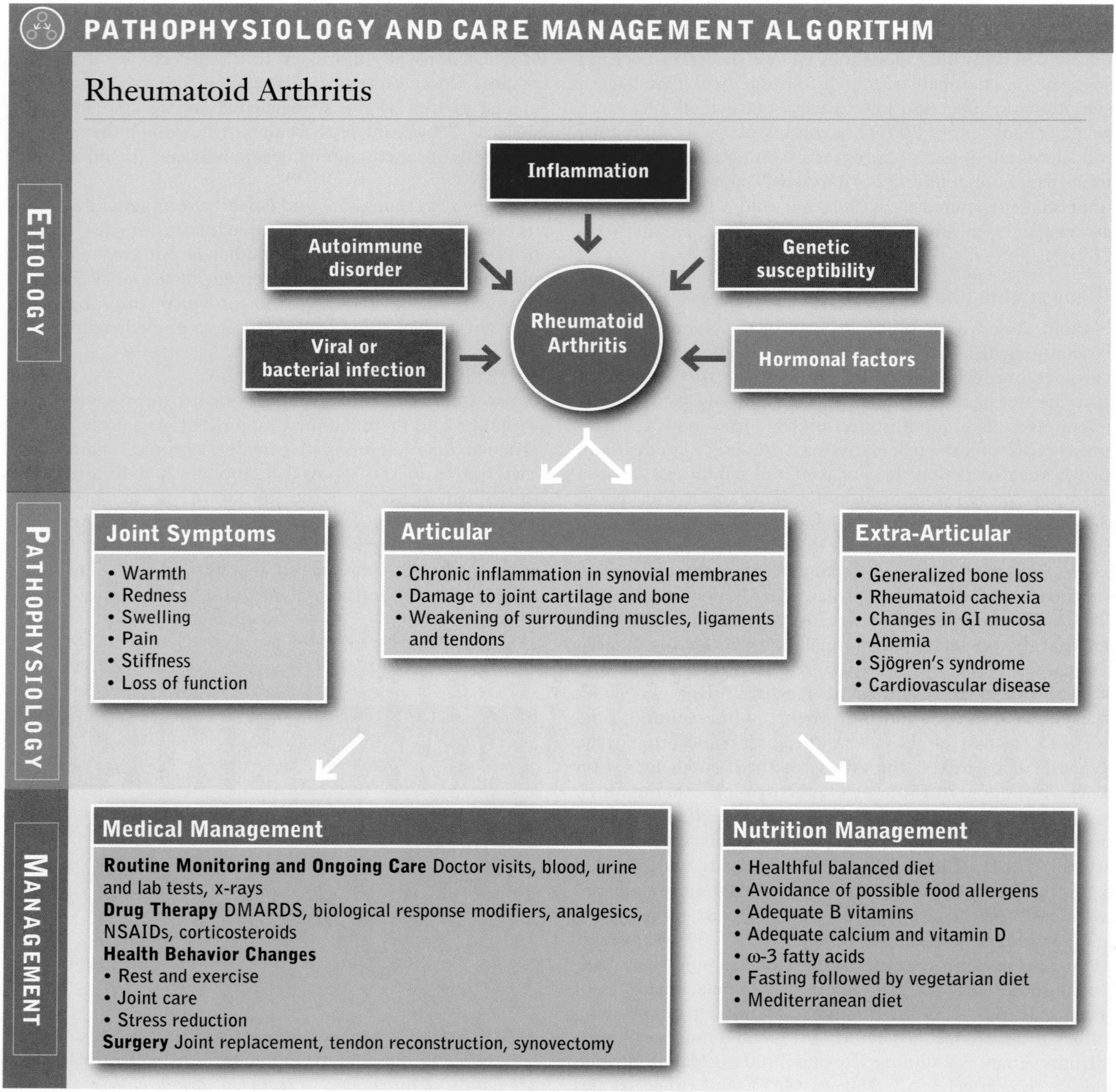

PATHOPHYSIOLOGY AND CARE MANAGEMENT ALGORITHM

Rheumatoid Arthritis

ETIOLOGY

Inflammation → Rheumatoid Arthritis

Autoimmune disorder → Rheumatoid Arthritis

Genetic susceptibility → Rheumatoid Arthritis

Viral or bacterial infection → Rheumatoid Arthritis

Hormonal factors → Rheumatoid Arthritis

PATHOPHYSIOLOGY

Joint Symptoms
- Warmth
- Redness
- Swelling
- Pain
- Stiffness
- Loss of function

Articular
- Chronic inflammation in synovial membranes
- Damage to joint cartilage and bone
- Weakening of surrounding muscles, ligaments and tendons

Extra-Articular
- Generalized bone loss
- Rheumatoid cachexia
- Changes in GI mucosa
- Anemia
- Sjögren's syndrome
- Cardiovascular disease

MANAGEMENT

Medical Management

Routine Monitoring and Ongoing Care Doctor visits, blood, urine and lab tests, x-rays

Drug Therapy DMARDS, biological response modifiers, analgesics, NSAIDs, corticosteroids

Health Behavior Changes
- Rest and exercise
- Joint care
- Stress reduction

Surgery Joint replacement, tendon reconstruction, synovectomy

Nutrition Management
- Healthful balanced diet
- Avoidance of possible food allergens
- Adequate B vitamins
- Adequate calcium and vitamin D
- ω-3 fatty acids
- Fasting followed by vegetarian diet
- Mediterranean diet

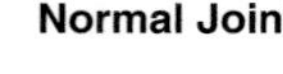

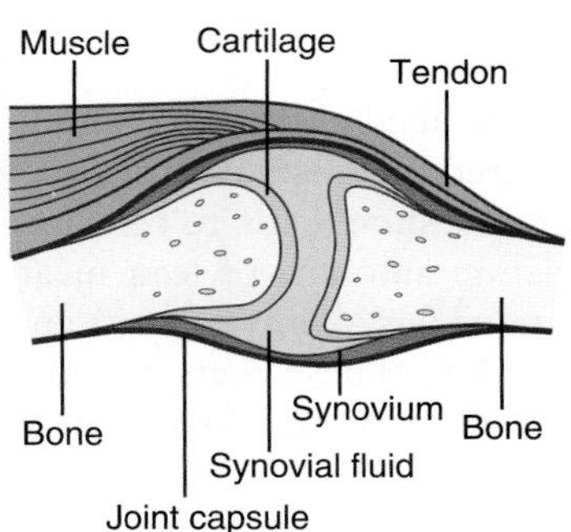

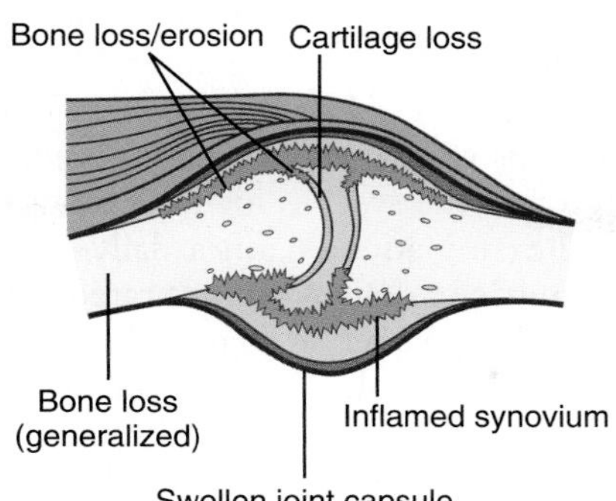

FIGURE 40-4 Comparison of a normal joint and one affected by rheumatoid arthritis, which has swelling of the synovium. *(From National Institute of Arthritis and Musculoskeletal and Skin Diseases: Handout on health: rheumatoid arthritis, NIH Publication Number 04-4179, January 1998, Revised May 2004. National Institutes of Health, Department of Health and Human Services.)*

fact, many of the drugs used to treat RA can result in hyperhomocysteinemia, hypertension, and hyperglycemia, all risk factors for cardiovascular disease. Conveniently, treatment aimed at reducing inflammation may benefit both diseases (Snow and Mikuls, 2005).

Pharmacologic Therapy

Medications to control pain and inflammation are the mainstay of treatment for RA. Salicylates and NSAIDs are often the first line of treatment, and methotrexate (MTX) is commonly prescribed as well, but these drugs may cause significant side effects. The choice of drug class and type is based on patient response to the medication, incidence and severity of adverse reactions, and patient compliance. Drug-nutrient side effects can occur with any of the drugs. Side effects of drug use may influence ingestion, digestion, and absorption, and hence nutrition status. See Chapter 9 and Appendix 31.

Salicylates are commonly used. However, chronic aspirin ingestion is associated with gastric mucosal injury and bleeding, increased bleeding time, and increased urinary excretion of vitamin C. Taking aspirin with milk, food, or an antacid often alleviates the gastrointestinal symptoms. Vitamin C supplementation is prescribed when serum levels of ascorbic acid are abnormally low. See Appendix 30.

Disease-modifying antirheumatic drugs (DMARDs) may be prescribed because of their unique ability to slow or prevent further joint damage caused by arthritis. These include MTX, sulfasalazine (Azulfidine), hydroxychloroquine (Plaquenil), azathioprine (Imuran), and leflunomide (Arava). In fact, the ACR recommends that the majority of patients with newly diagnosed RA be prescribed a DMARD within 3 months of diagnosis. Depending on which drug is selected, side effects can include myelosuppression or macular or liver damage. A main adverse effect of the DMARD MTX treatment is folate antagonism. Treatment with MTX induces a significant rise in serum homocysteine, which is corrected by folic acid supplementation and a properly balanced diet. Supplementation is advised to offset the toxicity of this drug, for protection against gastrointestinal disturbances, and for maintenance of red blood cell production without reducing the efficacy of MTX therapy. Long-term supplementation in patients on MTX is important to prevent neutropenia, mouth ulcers, nausea, and vomiting (see Appendix 31 and Chapters 9 and 31).

D-penicillamine is another DMARD, which acts as immunosuppressor by reducing the number of T cells, inhibiting macrophage function and decreasing IL-1 and RF production. Additional DMARDs include gold salt therapy and antimalarials and may lead to a remission in RA symptoms. Proteinuria may occur with administration of gold and D-penicillamine; therefore toxicity must be monitored continually. Minocycline (Minocin) is an antibiotic often used to treat mild RA (Cannon, 2009).

Surgery

Surgical treatment for RA may be considered if pharmacologic and nonpharmacologic treatment cannot adequately control the pain or maintain acceptable levels of functioning. Common surgical options include synovectomy, joint replacement, and tendon reconstruction.

Exercise

Physical and occupational therapy are often part of the initial therapy for newly diagnosed RA, but may also be integrated into the treatment plan as the disease progresses and ADLs are affected. To maintain joint function, recommendations may be given for energy conservation, along with range-of-motion and strengthening exercises. Although the patient may be reluctant at first, individuals with RA can participate in conditioning exercise programs without increasing fatigue or joint symptoms while improving joint mobility, muscle strength, aerobic fitness, and psychological well-being.

A loss of body cell mass that accompanies RA, called **rheumatoid cachexia**, involves the skeletal muscle, viscera, and immune system. This can lead to muscle weakness and loss of function, which may hasten morbidity and mortality in RA. Physical activity, including both aerobic exercise and strength training, seems to help. Any exercise program for an RA patient must take into account the individual's disease status.

Medical Nutrition Therapy

The nutrition care process and model serves as a guide for implementing MNT with RA patients. See Chapter 11. A comprehensive nutrition assessment of individuals with RA is essential, with a review of systems to determine the systemic effects of the disease process. A physical examination provides diagnostic signs and symptoms of nutrient deficiencies. Current weight and history of weight change over time are the least expensive, least invasive, and most reliable assessment tools to use. Weight change is an important measure of RA severity. The characteristic progression of malnutrition in RA is attributed to excessive protein catabolism evoked by inflammatory cytokines and by disuse atrophy resulting from functional impairment (Fukuda et al., 2005).

The diet history should review the usual diet; the effect of the handicap; types of food consumed; and changes in food tolerance secondary to oral, esophageal, and intestinal disorders. The effect of the disease on food shopping and preparation, self-feeding ability, appetite, and intake also needs to be assessed. The use of elimination or other diets purported to treat or cure arthritis should be identified (Smedslund, 2010). See Chapters 4, 6, and 8.

Articular and extraarticular manifestations of RA affect the nutrition status of individuals in several ways. Articular involvement of the small and large joints may limit the ability to perform nutrition-related ADLs, including shopping for, preparing, and eating food. Involvement of the temporomandibular joint can affect the ability to chew and swallow and may necessitate changes in diet consistency. Extraarticular manifestations include increased metabolic rate secondary to the inflammatory process, SS, and changes in the gastrointestinal mucosa.

Increased metabolic rate secondary to the inflammatory process leads to increased nutrient needs, often in the face of a diminishing nutrient intake. Taste alterations secondary to xerostomia and dryness of the nasal mucosa; dysphagia secondary to pharyngeal and esophageal dryness; and anorexia secondary to medications, fatigue, and pain may reduce dietary intake. Changes in the gastrointestinal mucosa affect intake, digestion, and absorption. The effect of RA and the medications used may be evident throughout the gastrointestinal tract. Based on the patient's unique profile, a registered dietitian can determine the most appropriate nutrition intervention, followed by monitoring and evaluation.

The association of foods with disease flares should be discussed. Whether food intake can modify the course of RA is an issue of continued scientific debate and interest. Dietary manipulation by either modifying food composition or reducing body weight may give some clinical benefit in improving RA symptoms. Some benefits may be related to a reduction in immunoreactivity to food antigens eliminated by a change in diet (Karatay et al., 2005) (see Chapter 27).

Some literature has suggested that fasting may be beneficial in reducing pain at the inflammation site; nevertheless fasting has never been shown as an effective treatment for RA symptoms (Smedslund et al., 2010). A vegan, gluten-free diet causes improvement in some patients, possibly because of the reduction of immunoreactivity to food antigens. See Chapter 27.

The anti-inflammatory diet described in Box 40-2 should be considered. The similar Mediterranean-style eating plan includes foods that almost everyone should aim to consume on a daily basis, such as moderate amounts of lean meat, unsaturated fats instead of saturated fats, plenty of fruits and vegetables, and fish. See Fig. 34-6. These diets are also nutritionally adequate and cover all of the food groups (Smedslund et al., 2010).

If food does play a role in RA, it most likely does so a few years before clinical diagnosis (Pedersen et al., 2005). Red meat has been identified as having proinflammatory properties as a source of ARA (see Box 40-1); no link has been identified between RA and coffee or tea consumption (Choi and Curhan, 2010).

Energy

Objective measures of actual energy needs for this population have not been determined. It is important to remember that the actual effect of the inflammatory response on the metabolic rate is unknown and may vary from individual to individual. In addition, activity levels vary greatly. Although traditional measures to assess energy requirements can be used, weight should be monitored and energy intake modified as needed to achieve desirable or usual body weight. Methods to determine energy requirements are noted in Chapter 2. For patients who are totally sedentary, calculations should be estimated at the resting energy expenditure and adjusted for weight changes that occur over time. When intakes are poor, enteral or parenteral supplementation may be required, and home nutrition support is beneficial for chronic cases. See Chapter 14.

Protein

Well-nourished individuals require protein at levels comparable to the DRIs for age and sex. Patients with RA tend to have increased whole-body protein breakdown (regardless of age) from growth hormone factor, glucagon, and TNF-α production. Protein may be needed at levels of 1.5 to 2 g/kg/day.

Lipids

Low-fat diets (including use of low-fat substitutes) lead to low serum levels of vitamins A and E and actually stimulate lipid peroxidation and eicosanoid production, thus aggravating RA. Therefore low-fat or fat-free dieting may actually be counterproductive for patients susceptible to or afflicted by RA. Rather than eliminating fat, changing the type of fat in the diet is useful and likely offers advantages for both the arthritis and cardiovascular systems. The anti-inflammatory diet (Box 40-2) with higher ω-3 fatty acids can reduce inflammatory activity, increase physical function, and improve vitality for RA patients.

Omega-3 fatty acids have increased in popularity in the management of RA because of their role in inflammatory pathways. Some other oils of marine origin and a range of vegetable oils (olive and evening primrose oil) have indirect antiinflammatory actions probably mediated via PG E_1 (see *Focus On:* Fatty Acids and the Inflammatory Process). Fish oil alleviates RA symptoms and reduces the use of NSAIDS in RA patients The beneficial effects are generally delayed for up to 12 weeks after they are started but last up to 6 weeks after discontinuing therapy (Bhangle and Kolasinski, 2011). See Appendix 40 for ω-3 and ω-6 fatty acid content of foods.

Minerals, Vitamins, and Antioxidants

Several vitamins and minerals function as antioxidants and therefore affect inflammation. Vitamin E is just such a vitamin, and along with ω-3 and ω-6 fatty acids, may affect cytokine and eicosanoid production by decreasing proinflammatory cytokines and lipid mediators. Synovial fluid and plasma trace element concentrations, excluding Zn, change in inflammatory RA. Altered trace element concentrations in inflammatory RA may result from changes of the immunoregulatory cytokines (Yazar et al., 2005). Degradation of collagen and eicosanoid stimulation are associated with oxidative damage. However, there are not significant data to support routine supplementation with vitamin C, vitamin A, or β-carotene unless patients are shown to have inadequate concentrations of antioxidants.

RA patients often have nutritional intakes below the DRIs for folic acid, calcium, vitamin D, vitamin E, zinc, vitamin B, and selenium. In addition the often used drug MTX is known to decrease serum folate levels with the result of elevated homocysteine levels. Thus in these patients, adequate intakes of folate and vitamins B_6 and B_{12} should be encouraged. Calcium and vitamin D malabsorption and bone demineralization are characteristic of advanced stages of the disease, leading to osteoporosis or fractures. Prolonged use of glucocorticoids can also lead to osteoporosis. Therefore supplementation with calcium and vitamin D should be considered. Indeed, vitamin D is a

FOCUS ON

Fatty Acids and the Inflammatory Process

Two classes of polyunsaturated fatty acids—ω-6 and ω-3—are metabolized competitively, including conversion to their corresponding eicosanoids: prostanoids (prostaglandin [PG] and thromboxane [Tx]) and leukotrienes (LTs). Eicosapentaenoic acid (EPA, 20:5) and docosahexaenoic acid (DHA, 22:6) are ω-3 polyunsaturated fatty acids (PUFAs) that are abundant in cold-water fish such as salmon, sardines, mackerel, herring, tuna, fish oils and some algae. α-Linolenic acid (ALA, 18:3) is also an ω-3 PUFA found in abundance in flaxseed, walnuts, and soy and canola (rapeseed) oils. EPA, DHA, and ALA have all been shown to replace the synthesis of inflammatory eicosanoids by competing with the conversion of arachidonic acid (ARA, 20:4 ω-6) to the series 2 of PG and Tx. ARA comes exclusively from animal foods. Linoleic acid (LA, 18:2), an ω-6 PUFA found in safflower and other oils, is a precursor of ARA; therefore its consumption should be limited in rheumatic patients.

The type of mediator that is produced is determined by the type of PUFAs present in the phospholipids of the cell membrane, which in turn is influenced by the type of PUFAs in the diet. Theoretically, a person can replace ω-6 PUFAs with ω-3 PUFAs by increasing their consumption. This in turn, will result in the synthesis of prostanoids (PG and Tx) with antiinflammatory effects. Similarly, reducing the amount of ARA minimizes inflammation and can enhance the benefits of fish oil supplementation.

Studies during the last 20 years have clearly shown beneficial changes in eicosanoid metabolism with fish oil supplementation in patients with rheumatoid arthritis (Calder et al., 2009; Galli et al., 2009), even when administered parenterally (Bahadori et al., 2010). Although fish oil seems to exert an antiinflammatory effect in short-term studies, these effects may vanish during long-term treatment because of decreased numbers of autoreactive T cells via apoptosis. In already existing disease increased consumption might not be beneficial. (Calder et al., 2009).

Lowered intake of ω-6 fatty acids and increased intake of ω-3 oils should not replace conventional drug therapies. These oils should be used in conjunction with improved eating habits. A diet that includes baked or broiled fish one to two times per week, or an ω-3 supplement (approximate daily dose up to: EPA-50 mg/kg/day, DHA-30 mg/kg/day) can be recommended for rheumatoid arthritis patients. However, the Food and Drug Administration (FDA) has identified shark, swordfish, king mackerel, and tilefish as high-mercury fish that should be avoided. Although the quality of fish oil supplements is steadily improving, these supplements are not without their own side effects, such as their fishy taste or odor, causing increased bleeding time or gastrointestinal distress; although these manifestations are usually dose dependent (Bhangle and Kolasinski, 2011).

Additional benefits may come from a combination of fish oils and olive oil (Berbert et al., 2005). A component of olive oil has been shown to inhibit cyclooxygenase enzyme in the synthesis of prostaglandins just as ibuprofen can. This action has been attributed to oleocanthal, a compound in newly pressed extra virgin olive oil that has natural antiinflammatory activity (Beauchamp et al., 2005). More studies are needed to determine an effective dose and identify any limits to its use for patients with rheumatic disease. The addition of an antioxidant is required to improve the oxidative stability of olive oil (Lee et al., 2006).

selective immunosuppressant and greater intakes of vitamin D may be beneficial. Because of drug-induced alterations in specific vitamin or mineral levels, mounting evidence supports supplementation beyond the minimum levels for vitamins D and E, folic acid and vitamins B_6 and B_{12}.

Elevated levels of copper and ceruloplasmin in serum and joint fluid are seen in RA. Plasma copper levels correlate with the degree of joint inflammation, decreasing as the inflammation is diminished. Elevated plasma levels of ceruloplasmin, the carrier protein for copper, may have a protective role because of its antioxidant activity.

Alternative Therapies

The increasing popularity of the use of alternative treatments appears to be particularly evident with people afflicted with RA. Herbal therapy is popular; however, concerns of toxicity must also be addressed because the Food and Drug Administration (FDA) provides relatively little regulation of herbal therapies.

Gamma-linolenic acid (GLA) is an ω-6 fatty acid found in the oils of black currant, borage, and evening primrose that can be converted into the antiinflammatory PG E_1 or into ARA, a precursor of the inflammatory PG E_2. Because of competition between ω-3 and ω-6 fatty acids for the same enzymes, the relative dietary contribution of these fats appears to affect which pathways are favored. The enzyme delta-5 desaturase converts GLA into ARA, but a diet high in ω-3 fats will pull more of this enzyme to the ω-3 pathway, allowing the body to use GLA to produce PGE_1. This antiinflammatory PGE_1 may relieve pain, morning stiffness, and joint tenderness with no serious side effects. Further studies are required to establish optimum dosage and duration.

Thunder god vine (*Tripterygium wilfordii*) has been used in China to treat patients with a number of autoimmune diseases. There are no consistent, high-quality thunder god vine preparations being manufactured in the United States. High doses and long-term use of thunder god vine may suppress the immune system and reduce bone density (NCCAM, 2009).

SJÖGREN'S SYNDROME

Sjögren's syndrome (SS) is a chronic autoimmune disease characterized by lymphocytic infiltration of the exocrine glands, particularly the salivary and lacrimal glands, leading to dryness of the mouth (xerostomia) and of the eyes (xerophthalmia).

Pathophysiology

Common signs include thirst, burning sensation in the oral mucosa, inflammation of the tongue (glossitis), and lips (cheilitis), cracking of the corners of the lips (cheilosis), difficulties in chewing and swallowing (dysphagia), severe dental caries, progressive dental decay, and nocturnal oral discomfort. SS can be present alone (primary SS) or as secondary SS, as a result of another rheumatic disorder (RA, lupus). Patients may also suffer from disorders of the skin, lung, kidney, nerve, connective tissue, and digestive system because of more extensive glandular damage.

SS patients frequently develop disturbances in smell perception (dysosmia) and in taste acuity (dysgeusia) (Gomez et al., 2004; Kamel et al., 2009), as well as in their dietary habits because of difficulties in biting, chewing, or swallowing.

Nutrient insufficiency may play a role in the development or progression of SS. Altered consumption of several nutrients has been noted in SS patients including higher intake of supplemental calcium and lower intake of nonsupplemental vitamin C, PUFAs, linoleic acid, and ω-3 fatty acids. Biochemical deficiency of vitamin B_6 (pyridoxine) has also been observed (Tovar et al., 2002). That can be corrected by pyridoxine supplementation.

Medical Management

Medications for SS address the issues of dry eyes and dry mouth. These include artificial tears and immunosuppressant drops such as cevimeline (Evoxac) and pilocarpine (Salagen), respectively (AF, 2005b).

Medical Nutrition Therapy

The goal of dietary management in patients with SS is to relieve symptoms and reduce eating discomfort, which can result in lack of appetite, weight loss, fatigue, difficulty chewing and swallowing, mouth infections, and anemia. Management of xerostomia should also include strategies for reducing the risk of dental decay, including frequent rinsing with water, toothbrushing, using topical fluorides, or chewing sugar-free gum. Because of the lack of saliva (and the protective substances normally present in it), sugary foods should be reduced or eliminated from the diet to minimize cavities. If sugary foods or beverages are consumed, the teeth should be brushed and rinsed with water immediately.

Because swallowing is a problem, ready-to-eat foods may be useful. Foods should all be moist, and extremes in temperature should be avoided. The most common modifications include soaking or overcooking certain foods to make them softer; chopping and cutting meats and fruits to make them smaller; and limiting consumption of citrus fruits, irritant foods, and spices. The tartness of artificially sweetened, sour-flavored hard candy may help to stimulate salivary flow. Artificial saliva or products such as lemon glycerin may also be recommended by dental or dietetic professionals.

Malnutrition does not seem to be more common in this population. Iron and vitamin deficiencies such as vitamin C, vitamin B_{12}, vitamin B_6 and folate are possible, but these can be easily avoided with a well-balanced diet or appropriate vitamin supplementation.

TEMPOROMANDIBULAR DISORDERS

Temporomandibular disorders (TMDs) affect the temporomandibular joint, which connects the lower jaw (mandible) to the temporal bone. TMDs can be classified as myofascial pain, internal derangement of the joint, or degenerative joint disease. One or more of these conditions may be present at the same time, causing pain or discomfort in the muscles or joint that control jaw function.

Pathophysiology

Besides experiencing a severe jaw injury, there is little scientific evidence to suggest a cause for TMD. It is generally agreed that physical or mental stress may aggravate this condition.

Medical Nutrition Therapy

The goal of dietary management is to alter food consistency to reduce pain while chewing. According to the National Institute of Dental and Craniofacial Research, diet should be mechanically soft in consistency; all foods should be cut into bite-size pieces to minimize the need to chew or open the jaw widely; and chewing gum, sticky foods, and biting hard foods such as raw vegetables, candy, and nuts should be avoided (National Institutes of Health, 2010). Nutrient intake of TMD patients appears to be the same as for the general population with regard to total calories, protein, fat, carbohydrates, vitamins, and minerals. However, during times of acute pain, intake of fiber is often reduced.

CHRONIC FATIGUE SYNDROME AND FIBROMYALGIA

Disorders such as **chronic fatigue syndrome (CFS)** and **fibromyalgia** have rheumatic symptoms. Some experts believe that CFS and fibromyalgia are variations of the same pain and fatigue syndrome. In fact, 50% to 70% of people with a diagnosis of fibromyalgia also meet the criteria for CFS and vice versa (Davis, 2005). In the US, fibromyalgia affects between 2% to 4% of the population or 12 million people (Lawrence, 2008); and CFS affects 0.007% to 2% of the general population (Avellaneda Fernández et al., 2009). Women are affected two to four times more often than men (Mayo Clinic, 2009). The etiology and pathogenic mechanisms of fibromyalgia and CFS are to date not fully understood.

CFS and fibromyalgia mimic autoimmune disorders such as SLE or hypothyroidism. Viral pathogens, immune dysregulation, central nervous system dysfunction, clinical depression, musculoskeletal disorders, and allergies have been proposed as contributing factors in CSF. In fibromyalgia, central nervous system dysfunction, mitochondrial dysfunction, nutrient deficiencies, and other systemic abnormalities have been suggested.

Mitochondrial dysfunction can result in lack of energy (ATP) for muscular work. Some symptoms include poor growth, loss of muscle coordination and muscle weakness. This can have effects on several organs and result in visual and hearing problems, learning disabilities, mental retardation, heart disease, liver disease, kidney disease, gastrointestinal disorders, respiratory disorders, neurological problems, autonomic dysfunction, and dementia (Hassani A et al., 2010).

Pathophysiology

In fibromyalgia, nonarticular aches at specific pressure points (See Fig 40-5) and fatigue cause disabling symptoms including muscle tenderness, sleep disturbances, fatigue, morning stiffness, numbness and tingling, symptoms of anxiety and depression, chronic headaches, irritable bowel, and irritable bladder. In 2009, new diagnostic criteria for fibromyalgia were introduced (Wolfe et al., 2011) that do not require examination for specific tender points. Rather, diagnosis is based on the combination of chronic widespread pain and a symptom severity score based on the amount of fatigue, sleep disturbances, cognitive dysfunction, and other somatic symptoms. The diagnosis of fibromyalgia often overlaps with other chronic pain syndromes, including irritable bowel syndrome, temporo-mandibular disorders, and idiopathic low back pain (Staud, 2009). In CFS, chronic fatigue is the major symptom. It lasts 6 months or longer and is accompanied by hypotension, sore throat, multiple joint pains, headaches, postexertion lethargy, muscle pain, and impaired concentration (Avellaneda Fernández et al, 2009).

Medical Management

A treatment program for CFS should be multidisciplinary and include exercise, MNT, appropriate sleep hygiene, low-dose tricyclic antidepressants or selective serotonin reuptake inhibitors (SSRIs), and cognitive behavior therapy (Iversen et al., 2010; Lucas, 2006).

Management of concomitant disorders, including irritable bowel syndrome, depression, and migraine headaches, can improve quality of life for these patients.

Tricyclic antidepressants and SSRIs are commonly used with CFS patients although they are not FDA approved for fibromyalgia. They may be helpful in treating depression and sleep disturbances. Side effects may include agitation, dry mouth, drowsiness, and weight gain. Analgesics such as tramadol (Ultram) may be an option for treating patients with fibromyalgia. More recently, serotonin norepinephrine reuptake inhibitors (SNRIs) such as duloxetine (Cymbalta) and milnacipran (Savella) and the anticonvulsant pregabalin (Lyrica) have been suggested for fibromyalgia patients and are FDA approved for this purpose (Mease P, 2009, Argoff CE, 2010).

Exercise

Exercise is helpful; supervised moderate-intensity graded aerobic exercise, or water aerobics (minimum 12 weeks, 3×/week) is suggested (Busch et al., 2007; Williams DA, 2009). Similarly a multidisciplinary rehabilitation program consisting of supervised exercise therapy, group pain and stress management lectures, massage therapy sessions, and a nutrition information was found to improve self-perceived health status and pain intensity (Lemstra and Olszynski, 2005).

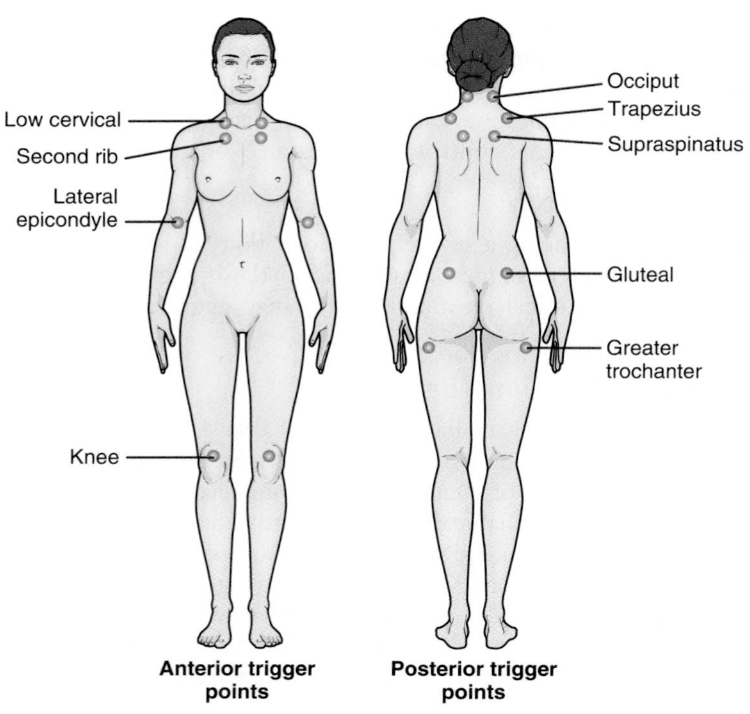

FIGURE 40-5 Pressure points of fibromyalgia pain. *(From the Clinical Slide Collection on the Rheumatic Diseases, copyright 1991, 1995, 1997. Used by permission of the American College of Rheumatology, Atlanta.)*

Medical Nutrition Therapy

Data regarding MNT for CFS are extremely limited. When hypotension is identified medically in CFS patients, increases in sodium and fluid intakes have been suggested. Evidence is not strong for elimination diets, or for the use of nutritional supplements (Häuser et al., 2008); however, vegetarian diets could have some beneficial effects probably due to the increase in antioxidant intake (Arranz LI, 2010). The vegan "living food" diet of berries, fruits, vegetables and roots, nuts, germinated seeds, and sprouts rich in carotenoids and vitamins C and E has shown anecdotal benefits. The natural antiinflammatory quercetin also shows promise (Lucas et al., 2006), as does intake of ω-3 fatty acids (Maes et al., 2005). Weight control seems to be an effective tool to improve the symptoms in these patients (Arranz LI, 2010, Ursini F, 2011). There is no specific treatment for any of the mitochondrial myopathies, physical therapy may extend the range of movement of muscles and improve dexterity. Vitamin therapies such as riboflavin, coenzyme Q, and carnitine (a specialized amino acid) may provide subjective improvement in fatigue and energy levels in some patients (Hassani A et al., 2010).

Alternative Therapies

Patients often seek complementary and alternative medicine treatments for relief. A survey of fibromyalgia patients found that 98% had used some type of CAM, including massage therapy, chiropractic therapy, and vitamin or mineral supplements (Wahner-Roedler et al., 2005). A recent systematic review with meta-analysis concluded that acupuncture may have a small analgesic effect but cannot be recommended as single therapy for management of fibromyalgia (Langhorst J et al, 2010). Homeopathy has also proven ineffective. (Perry R, 2010). The usual treatment options appear to be limited and generally unsatisfactory. However, cognitive behavioral therapy has been shown useful in both fibromyalgia and CFS (Williams DA, 2009, Avellaneda Fernández et al., 2009).

GOUT

Gout, one of the oldest diseases in recorded medical history, is a disorder of **purine** metabolism in which abnormally high levels of uric acid accumulate in the blood (hyperuricemia). Renal disease is common, and uric acid nephrolithiasis can occur. As the disease advances, symptoms occur more frequently and are more prolonged. Unfortunately, the prevalence of gout is increasing (Hak and Choi, 2008; Lawrence et al., 2008). In the past few decades gout has approximately doubled in prevalence in the United States, and has increased in other countries. The disease usually occurs after the age of 35 years and predominantly affects men. However, it becomes equally distributed in both sexes with age (Saag and Choi, 2006).

Pathophysiology

Gout is characterized by the sudden and acute onset of localized arthritic pain that usually begins in the big toe and continues up the leg. The urate deposits can destroy joint tissues, leading to chronic symptoms of arthritis (Figure 40-6). As a consequence, sodium urates are formed and deposited as tophi in the small joints and surrounding tissues.

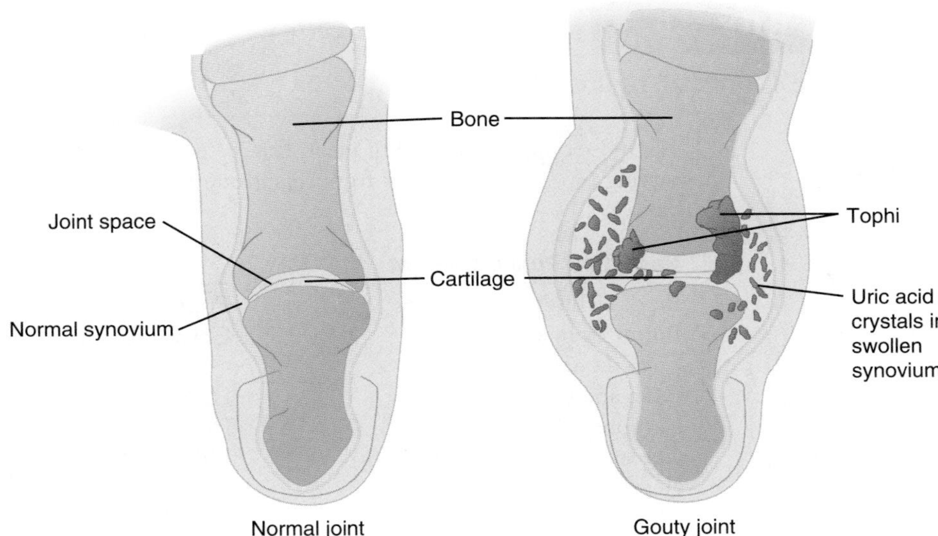

FIGURE 40-6 Comparison of a gouty joint and a normal joint in the toe. *(From Black JM et al: Medical surgical nursing, ed 7, Philadelphia, 2005, Saunders.)*

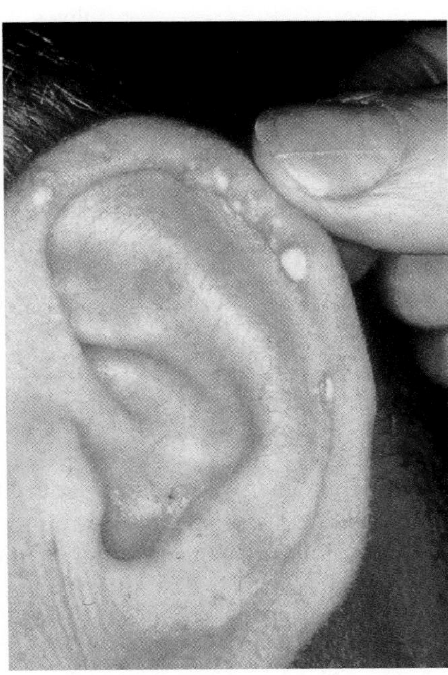

FIGURE 40-7 Tophi on the ear of a patient who has had gout for many years. *(Courtesy American College of Rheumatology, Atlanta.)*

In chronic gout a classic site is the helix of the ear (Figure 40-7); a more common site is the large toe or the elbow.

Genetic factors play an important role in the pathogenesis of gout and regulation of serum uric acid levels (Riches et al., 2009). One comorbidity of gout is obesity. Although weight loss appears to be protective (Choi et al., 2005a), ketosis associated with fasting or a low-carbohydrate diet can also precipitate an attack of gout. Occasionally the disturbance follows surgery. Hypertension and use of diuretics are also risk factors (Choi et al., 2005b). Epidemiologic studies suggest an association between gout and dyslipidemia, diabetes mellitus, and insulin resistance syndrome (Fam, 2005).

Medical Management

The goals of treatment are to reduce the pain associated with acute attacks, to prevent future attacks, and to avoid the formation of tophi and nephrolithiasis. The primary treatment for gout involves pharmacologic therapy (colchicine, allopurinol, NSAIDs, and others depending on the acute or chronic condition and renal function). Maintaining a serum urate level of less than 6 mg/dL may reduce the risk of recurrent gout attacks.

Gout is treated with drugs that inhibit uric acid synthesis. Probenecid (Benemid) and sulfinpyrazone decrease the blood uric acid level by increasing elimination through the kidneys. Allopurinol inhibits uric acid production. Both probenecid and sulfinpyrazone are often used in conjunction with colchicine, a drug that has no effect on uric acid metabolism but has been shown to relieve the joint pain of gouty arthritis. Colchicine is most valuable during the acute stage but may be needed during symptom-free periods as a preventive measure. Other antiinflammatory agents such as indomethacin or phenylbutazone are sometimes used in the acute stage of gout.

Medical Nutrition Therapy

Uric acid, derived from the metabolism of purines, constitutes a part of nucleoproteins. It appears that approximately two thirds of the daily purine load results from endogenous cell turnover, with just one third supplied by the diet (Fam, 2005). Although gout has traditionally been treated with a low-purine diet, drugs have largely replaced the need for rigid restriction of the diet. However, the patient can take an active role by adhering to the nutrition guidelines for the management of gout as well (Zhang et al., 2006).

The third National Health and Nutrition Examination Survey found that higher levels of meat and seafood consumption were associated with increased serum uric acid

BOX 40-3

Purine Content of Foods

High Purine Content (100 to 1000 mg of Purine Nitrogen per 100 g of Food)

Anchovies	Meat extracts
Bouillon	Mincemeat
Brains	Mussels
Broth	Partridge
Consommé	Roe
Goose	Sardines
Gravy	Scallops
Heart	Sweetbreads
Herring	Yeast (baker's and brewer's), taken as supplement
Kidney	
Mackerel	

Foods in this list should be omitted from the diet of patients who have gout (acute and remission stages).

Moderate Purine Content (9 to 100 mg of Purine Nitrogen per 100 g of Food)

Meat and Fish	Vegetables
Fish	Asparagus
Poultry	Beans, dried
Meat	Lentils
Shellfish	Mushrooms
	Peas, dried
	Spinach

One serving (2 to 3 oz) of meat, fish, or poultry or 1 serving (½ C) of vegetables from this group is allowed daily.

Negligible Purine Content

Bread (white) and crackers	Fruit
Butter or margarine (in moderation)*	Gelatin desserts
Cake and cookies	Herbs
Carbonated beverages[†]	Ice cream
Cereal beverage (e.g., Postum)	Milk
Cereals and cereal products	Macaroni products
Cheese	Noodles
Chocolate	Nuts
Coffee	Oil
Condiments	Olives
Cornbread	Pickles
Cream (in moderation)*	Popcorn
Custard	Puddings
Eggs	Relishes
Fats (in moderation)*	Rennet desserts
Vegetables (except those in group 2)	Rice
	Salt
	Sugar and sweets[†]
	Tea
	Vinegar

levels in adults, but total protein intake was not (Choi et al., 2005a). It is prudent to advise patients to consume a balanced meal plan with limited intake of animal foods and alcohol, avoidance of high purine foods (see Box 40-3), limited consumption of sources of fructose (sweetened soft drinks and juices, candies and sweet pastries) (Li and Micheletti, 2011), and controlled food portion size, and reduced noncomplex carbohydrate intake to achieve weight loss and improve insulin sensitivity (Hayman and Marcason, 2009). High intake of fluids (8 to 16 cups of fluid/day, at least half as water) should be encouraged to assist with the excretion of uric acid and to minimize the possibility of renal calculi formation (Hayman and Marcasom, 2009). Dairy products (milk, or cheese), eggs, vegetable protein, cherries, and coffee (Choi and Curhan, 2010; Li and Micheletti, 2011) appear to be protective, possibly because of the alkaline ash effect of these foods. See *Clinical Insight*: Urine pH—How Does Diet Affect It? in Chapter 36.

SCLERODERMA

Scleroderma is a chronic, systemic sclerosis or hardening of the skin and visceral organs characterized by deposition of fibrous connective tissue. Women tend to be afflicted four times more often than men. **Raynaud's syndrome** occurs, with ischemia or coldness in the small extremities, causing difficulty in preparation and consumption of meals. SS is often also present, but there is variability among patients.

Pathophysiology

Scleroderma is considered an autoimmune rheumatic disease with a genetic component. Free-radical, oxidative damage from cytokines, in which fibroblast proteins are modified, is involved (Kurien et al., 2006). Gastrointestinal symptoms include gastroesophageal reflux, nausea and vomiting, dysphagia, diarrhea, constipation, fecal incontinence, and small intestine bacterial overgrowth (SIBO). Joint stiffness and pain, renal dysfunction, hypertension, pulmonary fibrosis, and pulmonary arterial hypertension are also common (Scleroderma Research Foundation, 2005).

Medical Management

The disease is usually, but not always progressive, and no current treatment corrects the overproduction of collagen; therefore treatment is aimed at relieving symptoms and limiting damage. Pharmacologic therapy is often involved. Some studies have been undertaken with the use of anti-TNF therapies with some promising results (Alexis and

Strober, 2005). Treatments for the pulmonary hypertension and renal crises have shown good results overall (Charles et al., 2006). The 5-year survival rate after diagnosis is 80% to 85%.

Medical Nutrition Therapy

Dysphagia requires nutrition intervention (see Appendix 35). Dry mouth with resultant tooth decay, loose teeth, and tightening facial skin can make eating difficult (Figure 40-8). Consuming adequate fluids, choosing moist foods, chewing sugarless gum, and using saliva substitutes help moisten the mouth and may offer some relief. If gastroesophageal reflux is a concern, small, frequent meals are recommended along with avoidance of late-night eating, alcohol, caffeine, and spicy or fatty foods (see Chapter 28).

Malabsorption of lactose, vitamins, fatty acids, and minerals can cause further nutrition problems; supplementation may be required. A high-energy, high-protein supplement or enteral feeding may prevent or correct weight loss. Home enteral or parenteral nutrition is often required when problems such as chronic diarrhea persist (see Chapter 14).

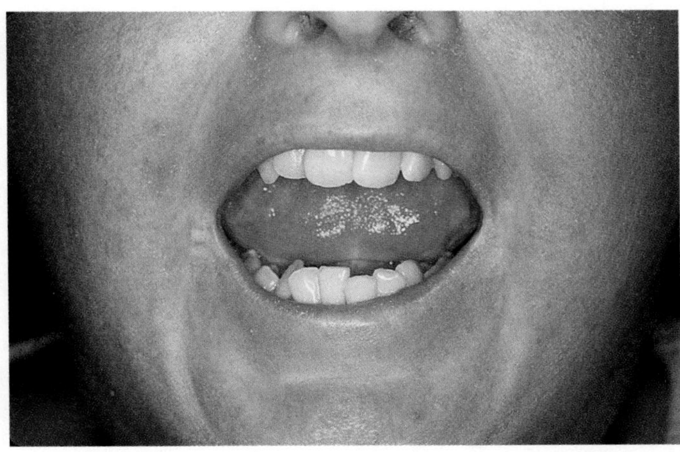

FIGURE 40-8 Facial scleroderma. Taut smooth skin over the face and reduced oral aperture of a woman with long-standing disease. *(From Wigley FM, Hummers LK: Clinical features of systemic sclerosis. In Hochberg MC et al., editors:* Practical rheumatology, *ed 3, Toronto, 2004, Mosby.)*

SYSTEMIC LUPUS ERYTHEMATOSUS

Systemic lupus erythematosus (SLE) is commonly known as *lupus*. Lupus is most prevalent in women of childbearing age and is more common in blacks and women of Hispanic, Asian, and Native American descent than in whites. Common symptoms include extreme fatigue, painful or swollen joints, unexplained fever, skin rashes, mouth ulcers, and kidney problems (NIAMS, 2009).

Pathophysiology

SLE has a genetic predisposition and overproduction of type 1 interferon and other cytotoxic cells (Banchereau and Pascual, 2006). SLE is considered to be an autoimmune disease that affects all organ systems. Renal function is deranged in lupus, thus causing excessive excretion of protein and often renal failure.

Medical Management

Lupus itself and the medications used (corticosteroids, NSAIDs, immunosuppressants, antimalarials) affect nutrient metabolism, needs, and excretion. Recent therapies include rituximab, a drug also used in cancer chemotherapy which causes depletion of the immune B cells. B cell depletion helps promote remission while maintaining normal levels of IgG and IgM (Smith et al., 2006).

Plaquenil, an antimalarial drug, appears to be effective in clearing up skin lesions for some individuals with lupus but has side effects that include nausea, abdominal cramping, and diarrhea. Immunosuppressives such as cyclophosphamide may be useful when there is renal involvement, but gastrointestinal and fertility problems may occur.

Medical Nutrition Therapy

No specific dietary guidelines for managing SLE exist. Rather, the diet needs to be tailored to the individual needs of the patient. Priorities include addressing the sequelae of the disease and the pharmacologic effects on organ function and nutrient metabolism. Protein, fluid, and sodium requirements are altered as a result of disordered renal function and steroid-induced side effects. See Chapter 36. Energy needs should be tailored to the individual's dry weight. The goal should be to attain and maintain the usual body weight. Enteral nutrition support may be required in chronic cases. Yet, because there appears to be significant crossover of symptoms among several autoimmune diseases, specific MNT guidelines prove to be a challenge.

CLINICAL SCENARIO

Beth is a 47-year-old woman who now lives with her husband after her two daughters left home to attend college. About 5 years ago, Beth noted that some of the foods she usually enjoyed preparing and eating were getting stuck in her hard palate, so she started to drink increasing amounts of water to dislodge them. Among those foods were pasta (i.e., linguini, lasagna), rice (fried, parboiled), cereals (breakfast cereals, granola, high-fiber content cereals), cookies, and soda crackers. The drier the meal, the more difficult it was to dislodge the foods from her palate.

Although she was very conscientious about her oral hygiene, Beth noted an increase in cavities and displacement

Continued

CLINICAL SCENARIO—cont'd

of her front teeth, as well as difficulties in swallowing. Soon she started to experience difficulties in biting hard fruits and vegetables (apples, peaches, carrots, cucumbers) and some cuts of meats. She also started to complain about a burning sensation in her tongue, cheeks, and gums when she ate spicy "ethnic" foods (Mexican, Asian), or drank fruit juices (orange, grapefruit, pineapple). She also presents geographic tongue, cheilitis, and cheilosis. She cannot eat a sourdough turkey sandwich without the corners of her mouth cracking and bleeding. Additionally, Beth had problems resting at night because of dryness of her nose and oral mucosa, and her eyelids were stuck together upon awakening.

Beth's history suggests a decrease in the production of saliva and tears, and she most likely has Sjögren's syndrome. Whether it is primary or secondary to systemic lupus erythematosus remains to be determined. Beth's diet seems to be low in protein, dietary fiber, vitamins (particularly of the B complex), and zinc. Due to her signs and symptoms, Beth could easily be misdiagnosed as having severe riboflavin (B_2) deficiency.

Nutrition Diagnostic Statements

1. Difficulty Chewing
2. Inadequate Oral Intake

Nutrition Care Questions

1. If these are Beth's nutrition diagnoses, write statements using the problem-etiology-signs and symptoms format.
2. What type of nutrition education and counseling would help Beth cope with the difficulties she experiences when eating?
3. What vitamin and mineral supplements may be needed?
4. How would you suggest use of artificial saliva?
5. What questions would you ask about her diet recall to determine compliance with your recommendations?
6. Would you consider consultation with a rheumatologist?

USEFUL WEBSITES

American College of Rheumatology
http://www.rheumatology.org

Arthritis Foundation
http://www.arthritis.org

Lupus Foundation of America
http://www.lupus.org

National Center for Complementary and Alternative Medicine
http://nccam.nih.gov/

National Fibromyalgia Association
http://www.fmaware.org

National Institute of Arthritis and Musculoskeletal and Skin Diseases
http://www.nih.gov/niams

Scleroderma Foundation
http://www.scleroderma.org

Scleroderma Research Foundation
http://www.srfcure.org

Sjögren's Syndrome Foundation
http://www.sjogrens.org

REFERENCES

Alexis AF, Strober BE: Off-label dermatologic uses of anti-TNF-*a* therapies, *J Cutan Med Surg* 9:296, 2005.

American College of Rheumatology: *Biologic agents for rheumatic disease*, 2006. Accessed 18 March 2011 from http://www.rheumatology.org/practice/clinical/position/biologics.pdf.

Anderson JW, et al: Glucosamine effects in humans: a review of effects on glucose metabolism, side effects, safety considerations and efficacy, *Food Chem Toxicol* 43:187, 2005.

Argoff CE: Fibromyalgia: Overview of Etiology, Pathophysiology, Treatment, and Management, *Pain Medicine News 2010* Dec:46, 2010.

Arranz LI, et al: Fibromyalgia and nutrition, what do we know, *Rheumatol Int* 30:1417, 2010.

Arthritis Foundation: *Arthritis today: 2007 drug guide*, 2007. Accessed 9 April 2007 from www.arthritis.org/conditions/drugguide/.

Arthritis Foundation: *Arthritis today, supplements and vitamins*, 2005a. Accessed 20 March 2011 from http://www.arthritistoday.org/treatments/supplement-guide/facts-about-supplements.php.

Arthritis Foundation: *Herbs and supplements and their uses*, 2005b. Accessed 20 March 2011 from http://www.arthritistoday.org/treatments/supplement-guide/index.php.

Avellaneda Fernández A, et al: Chronic fatigue syndrome: etiology, diagnosis and treatment, *BMC Psychiatry* Oct 23:9(Suppl 1):S1, 2009.

Bahadori B, et al: Omega-3 fatty acids infusions as adjuvant therapy in rheumatoid arthritis, *J Parent Enter Nutr* 34:151, 2010.

Banchereau J, Pascual V: Type I interferon in systemic lupus erythematosus and other autoimmune diseases, *Immunity* 25:383, 2006.

Beauchamp GK, et al: Phytochemistry: ibuprofen-like activity in extra-virgin olive oil, *Nature* 437:7055, 2005.

Berbert AA, et al: Supplementation of fish oil and olive oil in patients with rheumatoid arthritis, *Nutrition* 21:2, 2005.

Bhangle S, Kolasinski S: Fish oil in rheumatic diseases, *Rheum Dis Clin N Am* 37:77, 2011.

Busch AJ, et al: Exercise for treating fibromyalgia syndrome, *Cochrane Database Syst Rev* 4:CD003786, 2007.

Calder PC, et al: Inflammatory disease processes and interactions with nutrition, *Br J Nutr* 101:S1, 2009.

Cannon M: *Minocycline*, 2009. Accessed 20 March 2011 from http://www.rheumatology.org/practice/clinical/patients/medications/minocycline.pdf.

Canter PH, et al: The antioxidant vitamins A, C, E and selenium in the treatment of arthritis: a systematic review of randomized clinical trials, *Rheumatology (Oxford)* 46(8):1223, 2007.

Centers for Disease Control and Prevention (CDC): National and state medical expenditures and lost earnings attributable to arthritis and other rheumatic conditions—United States, 2003, *MMWR* 56:4, 2007.

Charles C, et al: Systemic sclerosis: hypothesis-driven treatment strategies, *Lancet* 367(9523):1683, 2006.

Choi HK, et al: Intake of purine-rich foods, protein, and dairy products and relationship to serum levels of uric acid: the Third National Health and Nutrition Examination Survey, *Arthritis Rheum* 52:1, 2005a.

Choi HK, et al: Obesity, weight change, hypertension, diuretic use, and risk of gout in men: the health professionals' follow-up study, *Arch Intern Med* 165:7, 2005b.

Choi HK, Curhan G: Coffee consumption and risk of incident gout in women: the Nurses' Health Study, *Am J Clin Nutr* 92:922, 2010.

Colgazier CL, Sutej PG: Laboratory testing in the rheumatic diseases: a practical review, *South Med J* 98:2, 2005.

Davis C: *What's in a name: fibro vs. CFS*, Arthritis Foundation, 2005. Accessed 24 July 2005 from www.arthritis.org.

Egan BA, Mentes JC: Benefits of physical activity for knee osteoarthritis: a brief review, *J Gerontol Nurs* 36:9, 2010.

Fam AG: Gout: excess calories, purines and alcohol intake and beyond: response to a urate-lowering diet, *J Rheumatol* 32:5, 2005.

Food and Drug Administration: FDA announces important changes and additional warnings for COX-2 selective and non-selective nonsteroidal anti-inflammatory drugs (NSAIDs), 2005. Accessed 20 March 2011 from http://www.fda.gov/Drugs/DrugSafety/PostmarketDrugSafetyInformationforPatientsandProviders/ucm150314.htm.

Fukuda W, et al: Malnutrition and disease progression in patients with rheumatoid arthritis, *Mod Rheumatol* 15:2, 2005.

Galli C, et al: Effects of fat and fatty acid intake on inflammatory and immune responses: a critical review, *Ann Nutr Metab* 55:123, 2009.

Gomez FE, et al: Detection and recognition thresholds to the 4 basic tastes in Mexican patients with primary Sjögren's syndrome, *Eur J Clin Nutr* 58:629, 2004.

Hak AE, Choi HK: Lifestyle and gout, *Curr Opin Rheumatol* 20:179, 2008.

Hassani A, et al: Mitochondrial myopathies: developments in treatment, *Curr Opin Neurol* 23:459, 2010.

Häuser W, et al: Management of fibromyalgia syndrome—an interdisciplinary evidence-based guideline, *Ger Med Sci* 6:14, 2008.

Hayman S, Marcason W: Gout: is a purine-restricted diet still recommended? *J Am Diet Assoc* 109:1652, 2009.

Helmick CG, et al: Estimates of the prevalence of arthritis and other rheumatic conditions in the United States. Part I, *Arthritis and Rheumatism* 58:15, 2008.

Holliday KL, et al: Lifetime body mass index, other anthropometric measures of obesity and risk of knee or hip osteoarthritis in the GOAL case-control study, *Osteoarthritis Cartilage* PubMed PMID: 21044695, 31 October 2010. [Epub ahead of print.]

Huskisson EC: Glucosamine and chondroitin for osteoarthritis, *J Int Med Res* 36:1161, 2008.

Huskisson EC: Modern management of mild-to-moderate joint pain due to osteoarthritis: a holistic approach, *J Int Med Res* 38:1175, 2010.

Iversen MD, et al: Self-management of rheumatic diseases: state of the art and future perspectives, *Ann Rheum Dis* 69:955, 2010.

Kamel UF, et al: Impact of primary Sjögren's syndrome on smell and taste: effect on quality of life, *Rheumatology* 48:1512, 2009.

Karatay S, et al: General or personal diet: the individualized model for diet challenges in patients with rheumatoid arthritis, *Rheumatol Int* 26:556, 2005.

Kosuwon W, et al: Efficacy of symptomatic control of knee osteoarthritis with 0.0125% of capsaicin versus placebo, *J Med Assoc Thai* 93:1188, 2010.

Kurien BT, et al: Oxidatively modified autoantigens in autoimmune diseases, *Free Radic Biol Med* 41:549, 2006.

Kwon YD, et al: Acupuncture for peripheral joint osteoarthritis: a systematic review and meta-analysis, *Rheumatology (Oxford)* 45:1331, 2006.

Langhorst J, et al: Efficacy of acupuncture in fibromyalgia syndrome–a systematic review with a meta-analysis of controlled clinical trials, *Rheumatology (Oxford)* 49:778, 2010.

Lawrence RC, et al: National Arthritis Data Workgroup. Estimates of the prevalence of arthritis and other rheumatic conditions in the United States: Part II, *Arthritis Rheum* 58:26, 2008.

Lee JH, et al: Antioxidant evaluation and oxidative stability of structured lipids from extra virgin olive oil and conjugated linoleic acid, *J Agric Food Chem* 54:5416, 2006.

Lemstra M, Olszynski WP: The effectiveness of multidisciplinary rehabilitation in the treatment of fibromyalgia: a randomized controlled trial, *Clin J Pain* 21:2, 2005.

Li S, Michelleti R: Role of diet in rheumatic diseases, *Rheum Dis Clin N Am* 37:119, 2011.

Lucas HJ: Fibromyalgia—new concepts of pathogenesis and treatment, *Int J Immunopathol Pharmacol* 19:5, 2006.

Maes M, et al: In chronic fatigue syndrome, the decreased levels of omega-3 poly-unsaturated fatty acids are related to lowered serum zinc and defects in T cell activation, *Neuro Endocrinol Lett* 26:745, 2005.

Manek NJ, et al: What rheumatologists in the United States think of complementary and alternative medicine: results of a national survey, *BMC Complement Altern Med* 10:5, 2010.

Marcason W: What is the anti-inflammatory diet? *J Am Diet Assoc* 110:1780, 2010.

Marcus D: *Herbal and Natural Remedies*, 2005. Accessed 2005 from www.rheumatology.org.

Mayo Clinic Staff: Chronic fatigue syndrome, overview, 2009. Accessed 20 March 2011 from http://www.mayoclinic.com/health/chronic-fatigue-syndrome/DS00395.

McAlindon TE, Biggee BA: Nutritional factors and osteoarthritis: recent developments, *Curr Opin Rheumatol* 17:5, 2005.

Mease PJ: Fibromyalgia: key clinical domains, comorbidities, assessment and treatment, *CNS Spectr* 14:12(Suppl 16):6, 2009.

National Center for Complementary and Alternative Medicine (NCCAM): *Rheumatoid arthritis and alternative medicine*, 2009. Accessed 20 March 2011 from http://nccam.nih.gov/health/RA/getthefacts.htm.

National Institute of Arthritis and Musculoskeletal and Skin Diseases (NIAMS): *Osteoarthritis, handout on health*, 2010. Accessed 20 March 2011 from National Institute of Arthritis and Musculoskeletal and Skin Diseases (NIAMS): *Osteoarthritis, handout on health*, 2006. Accessed 2006 from http://www.niams.nih.gov/Health_Info/Osteoarthritis/.

National Institute of Arthritis and Musculoskeletal and Skin Diseases: *Systemic lupus erythematosus, handout on health*, 2009.

Accessed 20 March 2011 from http://www.niams.nih.gov/Health_Info/Lupus.

National Institutes of Health: *TMJ disorders*, NIH Publication No. 10-3487. Accessed October 2010 from www.nidcr.nih.gov/NR/rdonlyres/39C75C9B-1795-4A87-8B46-8F77DDE639CA/0/TMJ_Disorders.pdf.

National Institutes of Health: *Questions and answers: NIH glucosamine/chondroitin arthritis intervention trial (GAIT)*, 2008. Accessed 20 March 2011 from http://nccam.nih.gov/research/results/gait/qa.htm.

Pedersen M, et al: Diet and risk of rheumatoid arthritis in a prospective cohort, *J Rheumatol* 32:7, 2005.

Perry R, et al: A systematic review of homoeopathy for the treatment of fibromyalgia, *Clin Rheumatol* 29:457, 2010.

Pittler MH, et al: Static magnets for reducing pain: systematic review and meta-analysis of randomized trials, *CMAJ* 25(177):736, 2007.

Riches PL, et al: Recent insights into the pathogenesis of hyperuricaemia and gout, *Hum Mol Genet* 18:R177, 2009.

Rosenbaum CC, et al: Antioxidants and antiinflammatory dietary supplements for osteoarthritis and rheumatoid arthritis, *Altern Ther Health Med* 16:32, 2010.

Saag KG, Choi H: Epidemiology, risk factors, and lifestyle modifications for gout, *Arthritis Res Ther* 8:S2, 2006.

Scleroderma Research Foundation: *Treatment information*, 2005. Accessed 8 October 2005 from www.srfcure.org.

Smedslund G, et al: Effectiveness and safety of dietary interventions for rheumatoid arthritis: a systematic review of randomized controlled trials, *J Am Diet Assoc* 110:727, 2010.

Smith KG, et al: Long-term comparison of rituximab treatment for refractory systemic lupus erythematosus and vasculitis: remission, relapse, and re-treatment, *Arthritis Rheum* 54:2970, 2006.

Snow MH, Mikuls TR: Rheumatoid arthritis and cardiovascular disease: the role of systemic inflammation and evolving strategies for prevention, *Curr Opin Rheumatol* 17:3, 2005.

Staud R: Mechanisms of fibromyalgia pain, *CNS Spectr* 14(12 Suppl 16):4, 2009.

Tovar AR, et al: Biochemical deficiency of pyridoxine does not affect interleukin-2 production of lymphocytes from patients with Sjögren's syndrome, *Eur J Clin Nutr* 56:1087, 2002.

Ursini F, et al: Fibromyalgia and obesity: the hidden link, *Rheumatol Int 2011* Apr 8 2011. [Epub ahead of print]

Wahner-Roedler DL, et al: Use of complementary and alternative medical therapies by patients referred to a fibromyalgia treatment program at a tertiary care center, *Mayo Clin Proc* 80:6, 2005.

Walitt B, et al: Coffee and tea consumption and method of coffee preparation in relation to risk of rheumatoid arthritis and systemic lupus erythematosus in postmenopausal women, *Ann Rheum Dis* 69(Suppl 3):350, 2010.

Williams DA: The role of non-pharmacologic approaches in the management of fibromyalgia, *CNS Spectr* 14(12 Suppl 16):10, 2009.

Wolfe F et al: Fibromyalgia criteria and severity scales for clinical and epidemiological studies: a modification of the ACR preliminary diagnostic criteria for fibromyalgia, J Rheum Feb 1, 2011. [e-pub ahead of print.]

Yazar M, et al: Synovial fluid and plasma selenium, copper, zinc and iron concentrations in patients with rheumatoid arthritis and osteoarthritis, *Biol Trace Elem Res* 106:2, 2005.

Zhang W, et al: EULAR evidence based recommendations for gout. Part II: management. Report of a task force of the EULAR Standing Committee for International Clinical Studies Including Therapeutics (ESCISIT), *Ann Rheum Dis* 65:1312, 2006.

Zhang W, et al: EULAR evidence based recommendations for the management of hand osteoarthritis: report of a Task Force of the EULAR Standing Committee for International Clinical Studies Including Therapeutics (ESCISIT), *Ann Rheum Dis* 66:377, 2007.

Zhang W, et al: OARSI recommendations for the management of hip and knee osteoarthritis, Part II: OARSI evidence-based, expert consensus guidelines, *Osteoarthritis Cartilage* 16:137, 2008.

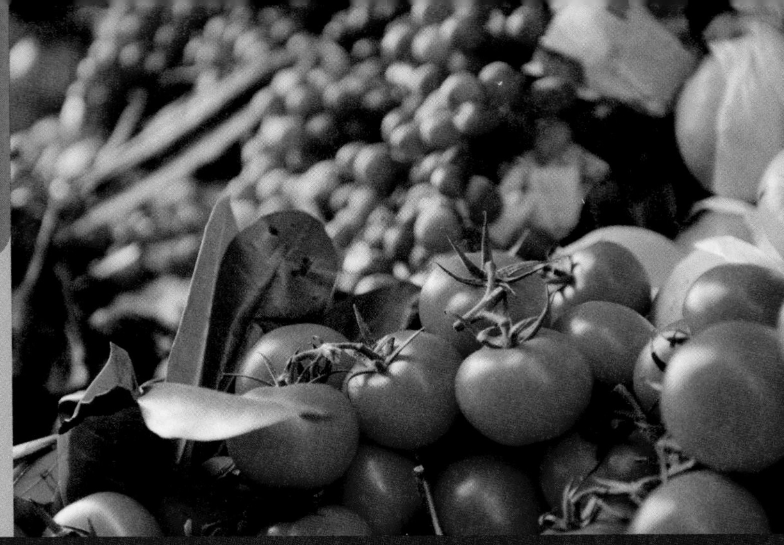

CHAPTER 41

Valentina M. Remig, PhD, RD, LD, FADA
Allisha Weeden, PhD, RD, LD

Medical Nutrition Therapy for Neurologic Disorders

KEY TERMS

absence seizure (petit mal)
adrenomyeloleukodystrophy (ALD)
agnosia
Alzheimer's disease (AD)
amyloid beta (Aβ)
amyotrophic lateral sclerosis (ALS)
anomia
anosmia
aphasia
apraxia
cortical blindness
deglutitory dysfunction
diffuse axonal injury
dysarthria
dysomia
dysphagia
echolalia
embolic stroke
epidural hematoma
epilepsy
Guillain-Barré syndrome (GBS)
hemiparesis
hemianopsia
hydrocephalus
hyperosmia
intracranial pressure (ICP)
ketogenic diet
migraine syndrome
multiple sclerosis (MS)
myasthenia gravis (MG)
myelopathy
neglect
otorrhea
paraplegia
paresthesia
Parkinson's disease (PD)
peripheral neuropathy
rhinorrhea
seizure
spinal cord injury (SCI)
subarachnoid hemorrhage (SAH)
subdural hematoma
syrinx
tetraplegia
thromboembolic event
thrombotic stroke
tonic-clonic (grand mal) seizure
transient ischemic attack (TIA)
traumatic brain injury (TBI)
Wernicke-Korsakoff syndrome (WKS)

Neurologic diseases arise from causes that vary in complexity. Some neurologic diseases result from a simple deficiency or excess of a nutrient, whereas others have more complex causes like diabetic neuropathy, stroke, or trauma. More complicated conditions arise with the interaction of genetics with other factors, as is the case with multiple sclerosis (MS), Parkinson's disease (PD), Alzheimer's disease (AD), and alcoholism. The medical and health history is often the most important part of a neurologic evaluation.

Numerous symptoms and malnutrition often accompany neurologic diseases. Complaints of even minor symptoms such as headaches, dizziness, insomnia, fatigue, weakness, pain, or discomfort must be skillfully evaluated for the presence of a nutrition component in their cause and treatment. Although not all neurologic diseases have a nutritional cause, nutritional considerations are integral to effective medical and clinical management (Table 41-1). Some neurologic dysfunctions such as **peripheral neuropathy** occur secondary to disease or a deficiency of a single or several vitamins, whereas other diseases of the nervous system may be attributed to dietary deficiency or excess (Table 41-2). This chapter emphasizes conditions with nutritionally significant dysfunction.

In those neurologic diseases with a nonnutritional cause, nutrition therapies are important adjuncts to effective medical management. Traumatic head, brain, and spinal cord injuries are of increasing interest to some researchers secondary to athletic or sports trauma as well as injuries to military personnel, especially during war. Many elements of nutrition care for neurologic diseases and conditions are similar, regardless of the origin of the disease process.

THE CENTRAL NERVOUS SYSTEM

The central nervous system (CNS) in mammals is differentiated functionally into three components so that lesions in the nervous system leave a unique "calling card" for localized dysfunction. Localizing the defect (lesion) to muscle, nerve, spinal cord, or brain is part of the medical diagnosis. Nerve tracts coming to and from the brain cross to opposite sides in the CNS (Figure 41-1). Therefore a lesion in the

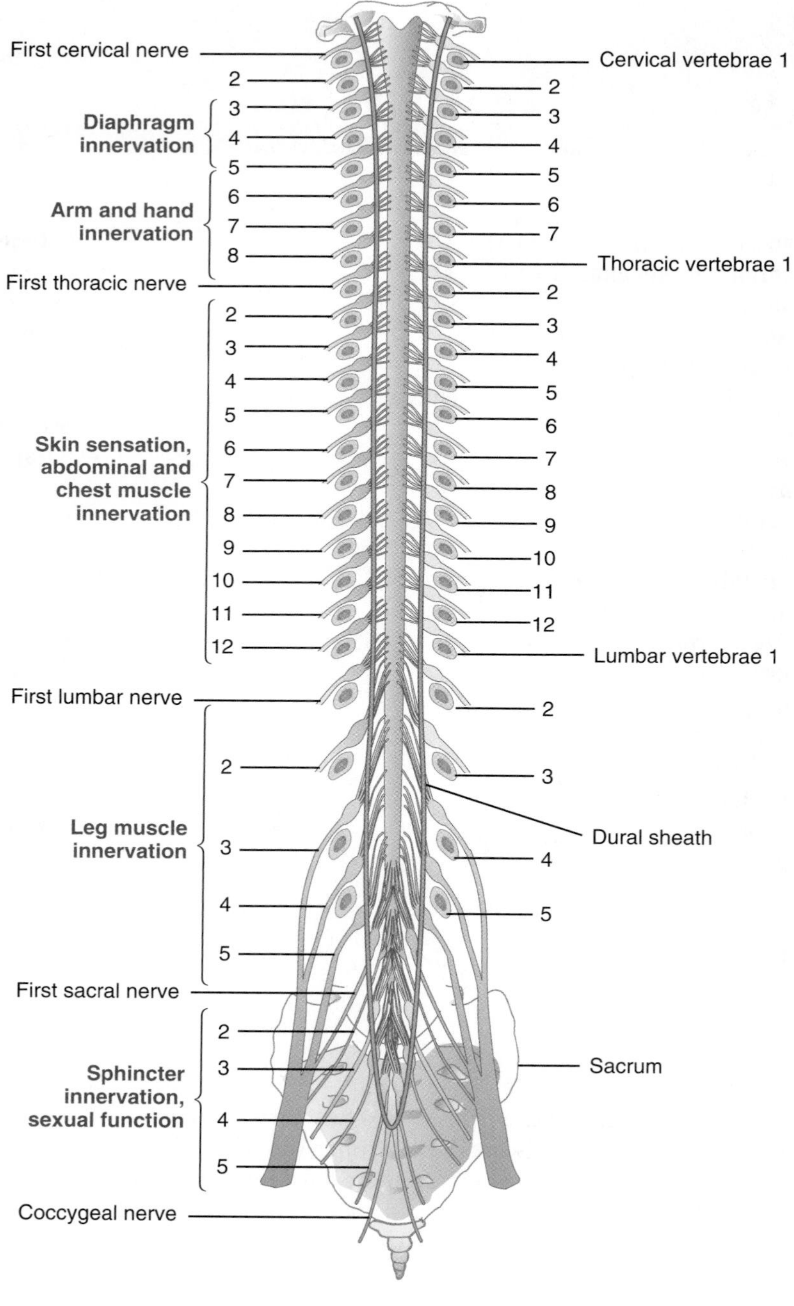

FIGURE 41-1 Spinal cord lying within the vertebral canal. Spinal nerves are numbered on the left side; vertebrae are numbered on the right side; body areas supplied by various levels are in blue.

TABLE 41-1

Nutritional Considerations for Neurologic Conditions

Medical Condition	Relevant Nutrition Therapy
Adrenoleukodystrophy	Dietary avoidance of VLCFAs has not been proven. Lorenzo's oil may lower VLCFA levels.
Alzheimer's disease (see Table 41-7)	Recommend antioxidants and antiinflammatory diet. Minimize distractions at mealtime. Initiate smell or touch of food. Guide hand to initiate eating. Provide nutrient-dense foods and ω-3 fatty acids.
Amyotrophic lateral sclerosis (see Table 41-9)	Intervene to prevent malnutrition and dehydration. Monitor dysphagia. Antioxidant use (vitamins C, E, selenium, methionine) is well tolerated, but not proven.
Epilepsy	Provide ketogenic diet (see Table 41-10).
Guillain-Barré	Attain positive energy balance with high-energy, high-protein tube feedings. Assess dysphagia.
Migraine headache	Follow general recommendations for food avoidance. Maintain adequate dietary and fluid intake. Keep extensive records of symptoms and foods.
Myasthenia gravis	Provide nutritionally dense foods at beginning of meal. Small, frequent meals are recommended. Limit physical activity before meals. Place temporary feeding tube.
Multiple sclerosis	Recommend antioxidants and antiinflammatory diet. Possibly recommend linoleic acid supplement. Evaluate health and especially vitamin D status of patient. Nutrition support may be needed in advanced stages. Distribute fluids throughout waking hours; limit before bed.
Neurotrauma	Enteral or parenteral nutrition support needed.
Parkinson's disease (see Table 41-11)	Focus on drug-nutrient interactions. Minimize dietary protein at breakfast and lunch. Recommend antioxidants and antiinflammatory diet.
Pernicious anemia	Administer vitamin B_{12} injections. Provide diet liberal in HBV protein. Provide diet supplemented with Fe^+, vitamin C, and B complex vitamins.
Spinal trauma	Provide enteral or parenteral nutrition support. Provide high-fiber diet, adequate hydration to minimize constipation. Provide dietary intake to maintain nutrition health and adequate weight.
Stroke	Dietary alterations for primary prevention. Maintain good nutrition status. Assess possible dysphagia. Enteral or parenteral nutrition support may be needed.
Wernicke-Korsakoff syndrome	Provide thiamin supplementation. Provide adequate hydration. Provide diet liberal in high-thiamin foods. Eliminate alcohol. Dietary protein may need to be restricted.

Fe^+, Iron; *HBV*, high biologic value; *VLCFA*, very-long-chain fatty acid.

TABLE 41-2

Neurologic Syndromes Attributed to Nutritional Deficiency or Excess

Nutritional Deficiency	
Site of Major Syndrome	**Name**
Encephalon	Hypocalcemia and tetany seizures from lack of vitamin D
	Impaired intellectual and cognitive function (protein-calorie deprivation)
	Cretinism (iodine deficiency)
	Wernicke-Korsakoff syndrome (thiamin deficiency)
Optic nerve	Nutritional deficiency optic neuropathy ("tobacco-alcohol amblyopia")
Brainstem	Central pontine myelinolysis (sodium)
Cerebellum	Alcoholic cerebellar degeneration
	Vitamin E deficiency caused by bowel disease
Spinal cord	Combined system disease (B_{12} deficiency)
	Tropical spastic paraparesis
Peripheral nerves	Beriberi (thiamin deficiency), pellagra (nicotinic acid deficiency)
	Hypophosphatemia
	Tetany (vitamin D deficiency)
Muscle	Myopathy of osteomalacia

Nutritional Excess		
Syndrome	**Condition**	**Agent**
Increased intracranial pressure	Self-medication	Vitamin A
Encephalopathy	Phenylketonuria	Phenylalanine
	Water intoxication	Water
	Hepatic encephalopathy	Protein (and NH_3)
	Ketotic or nonketotic coma in diabetes	Glucose, insulin
Stroke	Hyperlipidemia	Lipid
Peripheral neuropathy	Hypochondriasis	Pyridoxine
	Insomnia, anxiety	Tryptophan
Myopathy	Anorexia nervosa, bulimia	Emetine, ipecac
Myoglobinuria	Constipation	Licorice

brain that affects the right arm is found on the left side of the brain. Figure 41-2 shows the segments of the brain.

Signs of weakness are the most quantifiable clinical signs of nervous system disease. The neurons in the motor strip (upper motor neurons) receive input from all parts of the brain and project their axons all the way to their destinations in the spinal cord. Axons connect to the spinal cord motor neurons (lower motor neurons). These neurons extend from the spinal cord to muscles without interruption. The location of a lesion in the nervous system can often be deduced clinically by observing stereotypical abnormalities and function of either upper or lower motor neurons (Table 41-3).

Pathophysiology and Signs of Mass Lesions

The frontal lobes in the brain are the source of the most complex activities and commonly offer the most complex presentations. Psychiatric manifestations such as depression, mania, or personality change may herald a tumor or other frontal lobe mass, either right or left. With a lesion or tumor near the skull base, one may lose the sense of smell or have visual changes because olfactory and optic nerves track along the bottom of these frontal lobes. Chemosensory losses of smell have been described as **anosmia** (absence of smell), **hyperosmia** (increased sensitivity of smell), or **dysomia** (distortion of normal smell).

Frontal lobes are larger, and the posterior portions of the frontal lobes contain the motor strips. Lesions in the central portion of the frontal lobes may present as a motor apraxia. A person with **apraxia** cannot properly execute a complex activity, although he or she may understand a request to perform the activity.

Temporal lobes control memory and speech; lesions there may affect these abilities, as seen with AD and stroke. Although any lesion of cerebral gray matter may produce seizures, the temporal lobes are particularly prone to seizures. A right parietal lobe mass may result in chronic inability to focus attention, thus completely ignoring the body's left side. Because speech centers are located near the junction of the left temporal, parietal, and frontal lobes, pathologic conditions in this region may cause speech problems.

The occipital lobes are reserved for vision, and dysfunction here may bring about **cortical blindness** of varying degrees. In this condition the person is unaware that he or

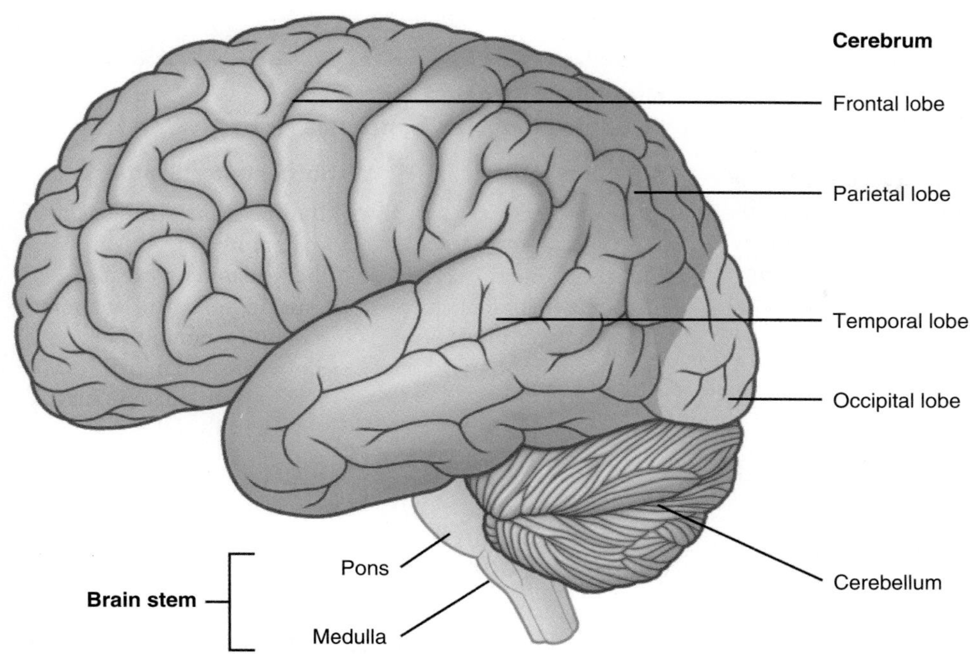

FIGURE 41-2 Parts of the brain. Trauma or disease in one area may affect speech, vision, movement or eating ability. *(From http://projectflexner.sites.medinfo.ufl.edu/files/2009/04/brain-regions.jpg. From Scully C: Medical problems in dentistry, ed 6, 2010, Churchill Livingstone.)*

TABLE 41-3

Basic Functions of Cranial Nerves

Number	Nerve Function
Olfactory (I)	Smell
Optic (II)	Vision
Oculomotor (III)	1. Eye movement 2. Pupil constriction
Trochlear (IV)	Eye movement
Trigeminal (V)	1. Mastication 2. Facial heat, cold, touch 3. Noxious odors 4. Input for corneal reflex
Abducens (VI)	Eye movement
Facial (VII)	1. All muscles of facial expression 2. Corneal reflex 3. Facial pain 4. Taste on anterior two thirds of tongue
Vestibulocochlear (VIII)	Hearing and head acceleration and input for oculocephalic reflex
Glossopharyngeal (IX)	1. Swallowing 2 Gag reflex 3. Palatal, glossal, and oral sensation
Vagus (X)	1. Heart rate, gastrointestinal activity, sexual function 2. Cough reflex 3. Taste on posterior third of tongue
Spinal accessory (XI)	1. Trapezius 2. Sternocleidomastoid muscle
Hypoglossal (XII)	Tongue movement

she cannot see. Lesions at other points along the visual pathway can cause several different types of visual field deficits.

Lesions of the cerebellum and brainstem may obstruct the ventricular system where it is the narrowest. This obstruction may precipitate life-threatening **hydrocephalus**, a condition of increased **intracranial pressure (ICP)** that may quickly result in death. Other signs of hydrocephalus include trouble with balance, walking and coordination abnormalities, marked sleepiness, and complaints of a headache that is worse on awakening. Lesions in the brainstem may infiltrate any of the cranial nerves that enervate structures of the face and head, including the eyes, ears, jaw, tongue, pharynx, and facial muscles (see Table 41-3). These lesions have consequences for nutrition because the patient is often unable to eat without risking aspiration of food or liquids into the lung. Tumors or other lesions in the medulla may infiltrate respiratory and cardiac centers, and dysregulation of these centers has grim consequences.

Lesions in the spinal cord are much less common than brain tumors and ordinarily cause lower motor neuron signs at the level of the lesion and upper motor signs in segments below the level of the lesion. Spinal cord injury (SCI) is the most common pathologic condition in this region. Other examples of spinal cord abnormalities are MS, amyotrophic lateral sclerosis (ALS), tumor, syrinx (fluid-filled neurologic cavity), chronic meningitis, vascular insufficiency, and mass lesions of the epidural space.

Lesions of the pituitary gland and hypothalamus are often heralded by systemic manifestations that may include electrolyte and metabolic abnormalities secondary to adrenocortical, thyroid, and antidiuretic hormone dysregulation. Because of the proximity to the visual pathways, changes may occur in visual field or acuity. The syndrome of inappropriate antidiuretic hormone secretion (SIADH) is often a complication; volume status and hyponatremia are part of the medical diagnosis (see Chapter 7). Because the hypothalamus is the regulatory center for hunger and satiety, lesions here may present as anorexia or overeating.

Finally, disorders of peripheral nerves and the neuromuscular junction affect one's ability to maintain proper nutrition. Disorders such as Guillain-Barré syndrome (GBS) or myasthenia gravis (MG) may counteract the efforts to maintain nutritional balance. To eat and drink effectively, many parts of the nervous system are required. A problem at any step along the way can result in an inability to meet metabolic demands.

ISSUES COMPLICATING NUTRITION THERAPY

The nutritional management of patients with neurologic disease is complex. Severe neurologic impairments often compromise the mechanisms and cognitive abilities needed for adequate nourishment. Many patients have **dysphagia** (difficulty swallowing), and the ability to obtain, prepare, and present food to the mouth can be compromised. As a result, all patients with neurologic disease are at risk for malnutrition. Early recognition of signs and symptoms, implementation of an appropriate care plan to meet the nutritional requirements of the individual, and counseling for the patient and family members on dietary choices are essential. Regular evaluation of the patient's nutrition status and disease management are priorities, with the ultimate goal of improving outcomes and the patient's nutritional quality of life.

Nutrition assessment requires detailed histories. The diet history and mealtime observations are used to assess patterns of normal chewing, swallowing, and rate of ingestion. Weight loss history establishes a baseline weight; a weight loss of 10% or more is indicative of nutritional risk. Assessment for nutrients involved in neurotransmitter synthesis is particularly important in these patients (Table 41-4). Nutrition diagnoses common in the neurologic patient population include:

- Chewing difficulty
- Increased energy expenditure
- Inadequate energy intake
- Inadequate oral food and beverage intake
- Physical inactivity
- Poor nutrition quality of life
- Self-feeding difficulty
- Swallowing difficulty
- Underweight
- Inadequate access to food
- Inadequate access to fluid

Meal Preparation

Confusion, dementia, impaired vision, or poor ambulation may contribute to difficulty with meal preparation, thus hindering oral food and beverage intake. Assistance with shopping and meal planning are frequently necessary.

TABLE 41-4

Nutrients Involved with Neurotransmitter Synthesis

Neurotransmitter	Nutrients for Synthesis
Acetylcholine	Choline, pantothenic acid, vitamin C
Catecholamines (dopamine, epinephrine, norepinephrine)	Phenylalanine, tyrosine, niacin, folic acid, vitamin B_6 and vitamin C
Gamma aminobutyric acid	Glutamate, vitamin B_6
Serotonin	Tryptophan, thiamin, niacin, vitamin B_6, folic acid

Self-Feeding Difficulties and Inadequate Access to Food or Fluid

With chronic neurologic diseases, a decline in function may hinder the ability for self-care and nourishment. Access to food and satisfying basic needs may depend on the involvement of family, friends, or professionals. With acute neurologic situations such as trauma, stroke, or GBS, the entire process of eating can be interrupted abruptly. The patient may require enteral nutrition for a time until overall function improves and adequate oral intake is resumed.

Feeding Issues: Presentation of Food to the Mouth

The patient with neurologic disease may be unable to feed himself or herself because of limb weakness, poor body positioning, hemianopsia, apraxia, confusion, or neglect. Tremors in PD, spastic movements, or involuntary movements that occur with cerebral palsy, Huntington's disease, or tardive dyskinesia may further restrict dietary intake. The affected region of the CNS determines the resulting disability (Table 41-5).

If limb weakness or paralysis occurs on the dominant side of the body, poor coordination resulting from a new reliance on the nondominant side may make eating difficult and unpleasant. The patient may have to adjust to eating with one hand and also to using the nondominant hand. **Hemiparesis** is weakness on one side of the body that causes the body to slump toward the affected side; it may increase a patient's risk of aspiration.

Hemianopsia is blindness for one half of the field of vision. The patient must learn to recognize that he or she no longer has a normal field of vision and must compensate by turning the head. **Neglect** is inattention to a weakened or paralyzed side of the body; this occurs when the nondominant (right) parietal side of the brain is affected. The patient ignores the affected body part, and his or her perception of the body's midline is shifted. Hemianopsia and neglect can occur together and severely impair the patient's function. A patient may eat only half of the contents of a meal because he or she recognizes only half of it (Figure 41-3).

TABLE 41-5

Common Impairments with Neurologic Diseases

Site in the Brain	Impairment	Results
Cortical lesions of the parietal lobe (perception of sensory stimuli)	Sensory deficits	Fine regulation of muscle activities impossible if the patient is unable to perceive joint position and motion and tension of contracting muscles.
Lesions of the nondominant hemisphere	Hemi inattention syndrome (neglect)	Patient neglects that side of the body.
Optic tract lesions (usually of the middle cerebral artery or the artery near the internal capsule)	Visual field cuts	Patient reads one half of a page, eats from only half of the plate, etc. (see Figure 41-3).
Loss of subcortically stored pattern of motor skills	Apraxia	Inability to perform a previously learned task (e.g., walking, rising from a chair), but paralysis, sensory loss, spasticity, and incoordination are not present.
No identification with a particular brain disorder or a specifically located lesion	Language apraxia	Inability to produce meaningful speech, even though oral muscle function is intact and language production has not been affected.
Lesion of Broca area	Nonfluent aphasia	Thought and language formulation are intact, but the patient is unable to connect them into fluent speech production.
Lesion of Wernicke area	Fluent aphasia	Flow of speech and articulation seem normal, but language output makes little or no sense.
Extensive brain damage	Global aphasia	Both expression and speech perception are severely impaired.
Brainstem lesions, bilateral hemispheric lesions, cerebellar disorders	Dysarthria	Inability to produce intelligible words with proper articulation.

From Steinberg FU: Rehabilitating the older stroke patient: what's possible? Geriatrics 41:85, 1986.

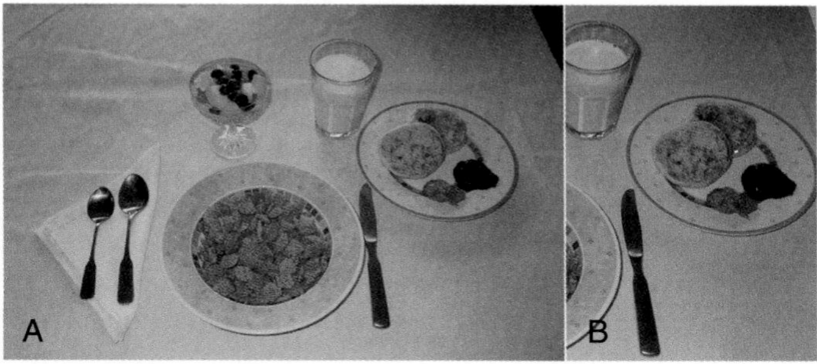

FIGURE 41-3 A, Normal vision. **B,** Vision with hemianopsia.

Another potential interference with self-feeding is apraxia because the person is unable to carry out an action and follow directions. Demonstration may make it possible to do the action; however, judgment may be affected as well and can result in the performance of dangerous tasks. This makes it unsafe to leave the patient alone.

DYSPHAGIA

Dysphagia often leads to malnutrition because of inadequate intake. Symptoms of dysphagia may include drooling, choking, or coughing during or following meals; inability to suck from a straw; a gurgly voice quality; holding pockets of food in the buccal recesses (of which the patient may be unaware); absent gag reflex; and chronic upper respiratory infections. Patients with intermediate or late-stage PD, MS, ALS, dementia, or stroke are likely to have dysphagia.

A swallowing evaluation by a speech-language pathologist (SLP) is important in assessing and treating swallowing disorders. The SLP is often consulted for individual patients following traumatic brain injury (TBI), stroke, or cancers of the head and neck, and for those at risk of aspiration or with other conditions that result in a lack of coordination in swallowing. Many registered dietitians (RDs) have acquired additional training in swallowing therapies to help coordinate this evaluative process.

Phases of Swallowing

Proper position for effective swallowing should be encouraged (i.e., sitting bolt upright with the head in a chin-down position). Concentrating on the swallowing process can also help reduce choking. Initiation of the swallow begins voluntarily but is completed reflexively. Normal swallowing allows for safe and easy passage of food from the oral cavity through the pharynx and esophagus into the stomach by propulsive muscular force, with some benefit from gravity. The process of swallowing can be organized into three phases, as shown in Figure 41-4.

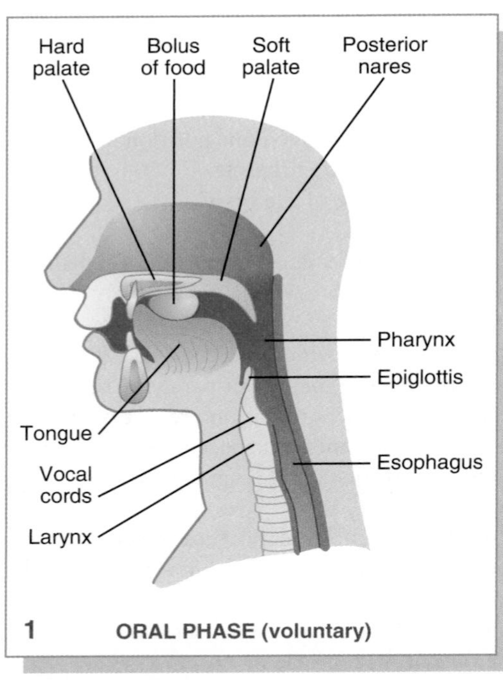

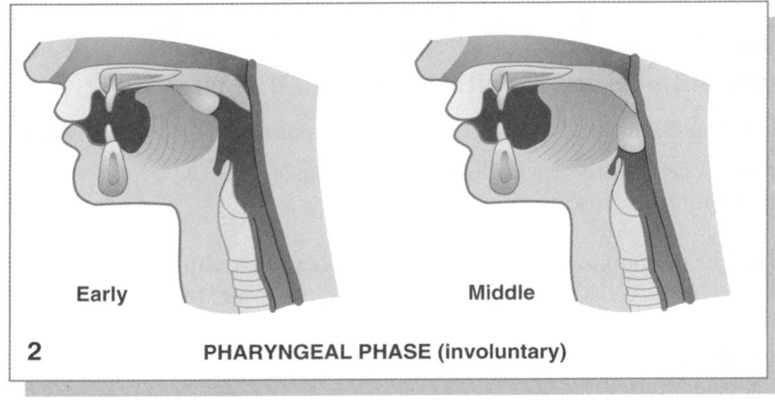

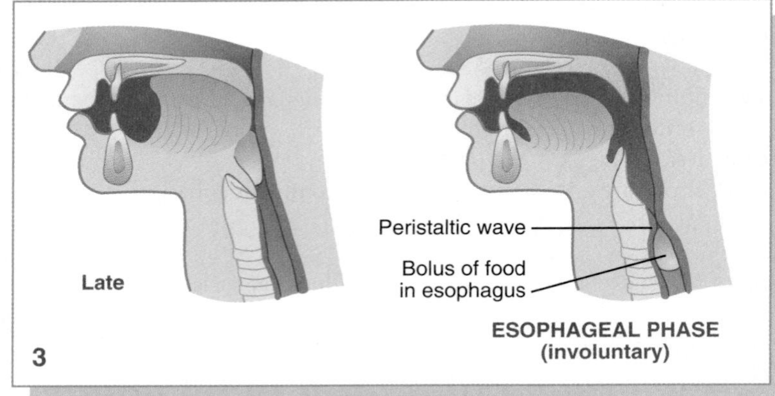

FIGURE 41-4 Swallowing occurs in three phases:
1. Voluntary or oral phase: Tongue presses food against the hard palate, forcing it toward the pharynx.
2. Involuntary, pharyngeal phase: Early: wave of peristalsis forces a bolus between the tonsillar pillars. Middle: soft palate draws upward to close posterior nares, and respirations cease momentarily. Late: vocal cords approximate, and the larynx pulls upward, covering the airway and stretching the esophagus open.
3. Involuntary, esophageal phase: Relaxation of the upper esophageal (hypopharyngeal) sphincter allows the peristaltic wave to move the bolus down the esophagus.

Oral Phase

During the preparatory and oral phases of swallowing, food is placed in the mouth, where it is combined with saliva, chewed if necessary, and formed into a bolus by the tongue. The tongue pushes the food to the rear of the oral cavity by gradually squeezing it backward against the hard and soft palate. Increased ICP or intracranial nerve damage may result in weakened or poorly coordinated tongue movements and lead to problems in completing the oral phase of swallowing. Weakened lip muscles result in the inability to completely seal the lips, form a seal around a cup, or suck through a straw. Patients are often embarrassed by drooling and may not want to eat in front of others. The patient may have difficulty forming a cohesive bolus and moving it through the oral cavity. Food can become pocketed in the buccal recesses, especially if sensation in the cheek is lost or facial weakness exists.

Pharyngeal Phase

The pharyngeal phase is initiated when the bolus is propelled past the faucial arches. Four events must occur in rapid succession during this phase. The soft palate elevates to close off the nasopharynx and prevent oropharyngeal regurgitation. The hyoid and larynx elevate, and the vocal cords adduct to protect the airway. The pharynx sequentially contracts while the cricopharyngeal sphincter relaxes, allowing the food to pass into the esophagus. Breathing resumes at the end of the pharyngeal phase. Symptoms of poor coordination during this phase include gagging, choking, and nasopharyngeal regurgitation.

Esophageal Phase

The final or esophageal phase, during which the bolus continues through the esophagus into the stomach, is completely involuntary. Difficulties that occur during this phase are generally the result of a mechanical obstruction, but neurologic disease cannot be ruled out. For example, impaired peristalsis can arise from a brainstem infarct.

Medical Nutrition Therapy

Weight loss and anorexia are key concerns with dysphagia. Observation during meals allows the nurse or RD to screen informally for signs of dysphagia and bring them to the attention of the health care team. Environmental distractions and conversations during mealtime increase the risk for aspiration and should be curtailed. Reports of coughing and unusually long mealtimes are associated with tongue, facial, and masticator muscle weakness. Changing the consistency of foods served may be beneficial. Keep the diet palatable and nutritionally adequate by recommending changes in food consistency. A mechanically soft or pureed consistency can reduce the need for oral manipulation and to conserve energy while eating (Box 41-1). Appendix 35 provides more detail for the National Dysphagia Diet.

BOX 41-1

Guidelines for Feeding the Dysphagic Patient

Nonoral Intake

Level 1: Severe Dysphagia: No Oral Feeding, Nothing by Mouth

May exhibit one or more of the following:

- Severe retention in pharynx; unable to clear
- Severe oral stage bolus loss or retention; unable to clear
- Silent aspiration with two or more consistencies; nonfunctional volitional cough or unable to achieve swallow

Level 2: Moderately Severe Dysphagia: Maximum Assistance or Maximum Use of Strategies With Partial Nutrition by Mouth Only

May exhibit one or more of the following:

- Severe retention in pharynx; unable to clear or needs multiple cues
- Severe oral stage bolus loss or retention; unable to clear or needs multiple cues
- Aspiration with two or more consistencies, no reflexive cough and weak volitional cough; or aspiration with one or more consistencies, no cough, and airway penetration to cords with one or more consistencies, no cough

Oral Diet: Modified Texture and Independence

Level 3: Moderate Dysphagia: Total Assist, Supervision, or Strategies; Two or More Diet Consistencies Restricted

May exhibit one or more of the following:

- Moderate retention in pharynx that is cleared with cue
- Moderate retention in oral cavity that is cleared with cue
- Airway penetration to the level of the vocal cords without cough with two or more consistencies or aspiration with two consistencies

Level 4: Mild-Moderate Dysphagia: Intermittent Supervision/Cueing; One to Two Diet Consistencies Restricted

May exhibit one or more of the following:

- Retention in pharynx that is cleared with cue
- Retention in oral cavity that is cleared with cue
- Aspiration with one consistency; airway penetration to the level of the vocal cords with cough with two consistencies, or airway penetration to the level of the vocal cords without cough with one consistency

Level 5: Mild Dysphagia: Distant Supervision; May Need One Diet Consistency Restricted

May exhibit one or more of the following:

- Aspiration of thin liquids only but with strong reflexive cough to clear completely
- Airway penetration midway to cords or to cords with one consistency but clears spontaneously
- Retention in pharynx that is cleared spontaneously
- Mild oral dysphagia with reduced mastication or oral retention that is cleared spontaneously

Full Oral Intake of a Normal Diet

Level 6: Within Functional Limits, Modified Independence

- Normal diet; functional swallow
- Mild oral or pharyngeal delay, retention, or trace epiglottal undercoating but independently and spontaneously compensates and clears
- May need extra time for meal
- No aspiration with different consistencies

Level 7: Normal Diet in All Situations

- Normal diet
- No strategies or extra time needed

Techniques for Improving Acceptance of Dysphagia Diets

Feeding individuals with dysphagia requires extra care and consideration. Food is enjoyed with all of the senses. Pureed meals need to look good, smell good, and taste good. Ideas to improve the sensory experience for those with dysphagia follow. Start simple and build a puree program to be creative; serve attractive meals.

Aroma

- Good-smelling food and a pleasant atmosphere may increase appetite and improve consumption.
- Serve foods seasoned with aromatic ingredients such as garlic, pepper, onions, and cinnamon.

Seasoning

- Individuals with dysphagia often have a dulled sense of taste.
- Taste all foods and enhance seasoning as needed.

Continued

BOX 41-1

Guidelines for Feeding the Dysphagic Patient—cont'd

- Serve foods that have stronger flavors such as chili, spaghetti, and apple pie.

Garnishing

- Garnishing has big visual effect, increasing the likelihood of better intake.
- Only garnish with foods appropriate for the diet consistency.
- Use sauces, gravies, and syrups. Put them in squeeze bottles to use for decorating the plates.
- Pipe garnishes around edges such as piping lettuce around the edge of a pureed sandwich.
- Cut shapes out of cranberry sauce and serve with turkey.

Molding

- To mold, use a thickener or a shaping or enhancing product.
- For hot foods: prepare per recipe, freeze and heat to temperature before serving.
- For cold foods: prepare per recipe, freeze, set on plate, and serve (they will thaw quickly).

Layering or Swirling

- Swirling vegetables together is simple and makes a great plate presentation; peas and carrots are striking together and taste great.
- Use standardized recipes to make attractive layered casseroles such as shepherd's pie, lasagna, or chicken á la king.

Piping

- Place pureed food into a pastry bag and pipe for a lovely plate presentation.
- Keep it simple and have fun; pureed pasta can be quite attractive, for example.

Slurries

- Prepare slurry with thickener and juice or milk.
- Prepare slurry with a liquid that goes well with the food being prepared.
- Slurry shortcake with juice and serve with pureed strawberries.
- Slurry sugar cookies with milk.
- Slurries work well with biscuits, cakes, graham crackers, muffins, and brownies.

These are a few simple ideas when serving modified-consistency foods. Beautiful plate presentations and good-tasting foods will help maintain good intake and positive nutrition status. Good-looking and good-tasting food can help people feel more dignified in spite of their neurologic condition.

Modified from the American Dietetic Association: National dysphagia diet: standardization for optimal care, Chicago, 2003, American Dietetic Association.

Liquids

Swallowing liquids of thin consistency such as juice or water requires the most coordination and control. Liquids are easily aspirated into the lungs and may pose a life-threatening event because aspiration pneumonia may ensue, even from sterile water in the lungs. Sterile water is no longer sterile once it is introduced to the bacterial load of the oral cavity.

If a patient has difficulty consuming thin liquids, fluid requirements must still be met. Liquids of all types can be thickened with nonfat dry milk powder, cornstarch, modular carbohydrate supplements, or commercial thickeners that contain a modified cornstarch thickener. Thick liquids that contain a high percentage of water are needed to maintain fluid balance. Fatigue and malaise are often associated with a "mild chronic dehydration" that results from decreased fluid intake. Fresh fruit is an additional source of free water.

Some long-term care facilities use the Frazier Water Protocol, which allows for drinking water in those who otherwise require thickened liquids. This protocol is based on the following assumptions:

1. Aspiration of water poses little risk to the patient if oral bacteria associated with the development of aspiration pneumonia can be minimized.
2. Allowing free water decreases the risk of dehydration.
3. Allowing free water increases patient compliance with swallowing precautions and improves quality of life.
4. Good oral hygiene is a key ingredient of the water protocol and offers other benefits to swallowing.

Liquid intake is a concern in those with neurogenic bladder and urinary retention, a common management issue in patients with a **myelopathy** (a pathologic condition of the spinal cord) or an SCI. This predisposes the individual to urinary tract infections (UTIs) and miscalculation of fluid balance. Alternately, myelopathy and SCI may result in urinary urgency, frequency, or incontinence. To minimize these problems, distributing fluids evenly throughout the waking hours and limiting them before bedtime may help. Some patients limit fluid intake severely to decrease urgency or frequent urination. This practice increases the risk of UTI and is not recommended.

One nontraumatic cause of myelopathy and neurogenic bladder is MS, an unpredictable and severe, progressive disease of the CNS. Individuals with MS have a higher incidence of UTIs. Increased intake of cranberry juice may reduce the frequency of UTIs (see Chapter 36).

Milk is considered a liquid with unique properties. Some people associate consumption of milk with symptoms of excess mucus production; however, no evidence shows an increase in mucus production. When the dysphagic patient reports increased phlegm after milk consumption, it may actually be a consequence of poor swallowing ability rather than mucus production. Patients are encouraged to "chase" the milk products with appropriately thickened liquids to help flush the throat rather than eliminate nutrient-rich dairy products.

Textures

As chronic neurologic disease progresses, cranial nerves become damaged, leading to neurologic deficits often manifested by dysphagia or elimination of entire food groups. Nutrition intervention should be individualized according to the type and extent of dysfunction. Vitamin and mineral supplementation may be necessary. If chewable supplements are not handled safely, liquid forms may be added to acceptable foods.

Presented with small, frequent meals, the patient may eat more. Swallowing can also be improved by carefully selecting various tastes, textures, and temperatures of foods. Juices can be substituted for water and provide flavor, nutrients, and calories. A cool temperature facilitates swallowing; therefore cold food items may be better tolerated. Carbonation may also be better tolerated because there is the beneficial effect of texture. Sauces and gravies lubricate foods for ease in swallowing and can help prevent fragmentation of foods in the oral cavity. Moist pastas, casseroles, and egg dishes are generally well tolerated. Avoid foods that crumble easily in the mouth, because they can increase choking risk.

Enteral Nutrition

Patients with acute and chronic neurologic diseases may benefit from nutrition support. In acute disease it may be required initially until a degree of function is regained, whereas in chronic neurologic disease it may be required in the late stages to meet changing metabolic demands. Well-managed nutrition support helps to prevent pneumonia and sepsis, which can complicate these diseases. Enteral tube feedings may be necessary if the risk of aspiration from oral intake is high, or if the patient cannot eat enough to meet his or her nutritional needs. In the latter case nocturnal tube feedings can bridge the gap between oral intake and actual nutritional requirements. This should allow the normal sensation of hunger to be generated and provide freedom from tube feeding during the day.

In most instances the gastrointestinal tract function remains intact, and enteral nutrition is the preferred method of administering nutrition support. One noted exception occurs after SCI, in which ileus is common for 7 to 10 days after the insult, and parenteral nutrition may be necessary. Although a nasogastric (NG) tube can be a short-term option, a percutaneous endoscopic gastrostomy (PEG) or gastrostomy-jejunostomy (PEG/J) tube is preferred for long-term management. These should be considered for patients whose swallowing is inadequate to ensure their nutritional health (see Chapter 14).

Malnutrition itself can produce neuromuscular weakness that negatively affects quality of life; it is a prognostic factor for poor survival. In the acutely ill but previously well-nourished individual who is unable to resume oral nourishment within 7 days, nutrition support is used to prevent decline in nutritional health and aid in recovery until oral intake can be resumed. Conversely, in the chronically ill, nutrition support is an issue that each patient must eventually address because it may result in prolonged therapy. However, adequate nutrition can promote health and may be a welcome relief to an overburdened patient.

Some patients may decline early placement of a feeding tube because of the emotional, economic, or physical effects of this choice. In advanced stages of disease the patient may refuse tube feedings, choosing not to prolong life. Nutrition support should be used when it can enhance quality of life. The health care team should alleviate patient and family concerns and support informed decisions. The patient needs to be fully informed about the effects of tube feeding on daily life. Discussion of both the advantages and disadvantages of nutrition support should be initiated with the patient and family well ahead of need. Options should include a description of feeding schedules, tube placement procedures, and appropriate training for on-going care.

NEUROLOGIC DISEASES OF NUTRITIONAL ORIGIN

Dietary deficiencies of thiamin and niacin can directly result in neurologic symptoms. With **Wernicke-Korsakoff syndrome (WKS)**, the neurologic effect occurs secondary to alcoholism. Most neurologic symptoms arising from nutritional deficiencies can be corrected with increased food intake or supplements. See Table 41-2 through Table 41-6.

NEUROLOGIC DISORDERS FROM TRAUMA

Cerebrovascular Accident (Stroke)

Stroke (cerebrovascular accident) is defined as an acute onset of focal or global neurologic deficit lasting more than 24 hours; it is attributable to diseases of the intracranial or extracranial neurovasculature. Severe strokes are often preceded by **transient ischemic attacks (TIAs)**, brief attacks of cerebral dysfunction of vascular origin with no persistent neurologic defect. Stroke is the third most common cause of death in the United States and the most common cause of disability in the United States (National Institutes of Health [NIH], 2006). Old age is the most significant risk

TABLE 41-6

Neurologic Diseases Arising From Nutritional Deficiencies

Disease	Nutrient	Physiologic Effect	Treatment
Wet beriberi	Thiamin	Peripheral or central neurologic dysfunction	Thiamin supplementation
Pellagra	Niacin	Memory loss, hallucinations, dementia	Niacin supplementation
Pernicious anemia	Vitamin B_{12}	Lesions occur in myelin sheaths of optic nerves, cerebral white matter, peripheral nerves	Monthly vitamin B_{12} injections Oral vitamin B_{12} supplements
Wernicke-Korsakoff syndrome	Thiamin	Encephalopathy, involuntary eye movements, impaired movement, amnesia	Eliminate alcohol, thiamin supplementation, adequate hydration

factor for stroke. Among modifiable risk factors, hypertension and smoking contribute most often. (See Chapter 33.) Other factors include obesity, coronary heart disease, diabetes, physical inactivity, and genetics (Goldstein et al., 2006). The high costs of stroke are attributed to the degree of disability imparted by these events.

Pathophysiology

Embolic stroke occurs when a cholesterol plaque is dislodged from a proximal vessel, travels to the brain, and blocks an artery, most commonly the middle cerebral artery (MCA). In patients with dysfunctional cardiac atria, clots may be dislodged from there and embolize. In **thrombotic stroke** a cholesterol plaque within an artery ruptures, and platelets subsequently aggregate to clog an already narrowed artery. Most strokes are incited by a **thromboembolic event**, which may be aggravated by atherosclerosis, hypertension, diabetes, and gout (*Pathophysiology and Care Management Algorithm:* Stroke).

Intracranial hemorrhage occurs in only 15% of strokes but is often fatal immediately. Intracranial hemorrhage occurs more commonly in individuals with hypertension. In intraparenchymal hemorrhage, a vessel inside the brain ruptures. A variation of intraparenchymal hemorrhage is a lacunar (deep pool) infarct. These smaller infarcts occur in the deep structures of the brain such as the internal capsule, basal ganglia, pons, thalamus, and cerebellum. Even a small lacunar infarct can produce significant disability because the brain tissue in the deep structures is so densely functional. A second type of intracranial hemorrhage is **subarachnoid hemorrhage (SAH)**. SAH occurs commonly as a result of head trauma but more often as a result of a ruptured aneurysm of a vessel in the subarachnoid space.

Medical Management

Hemorrhage is suspected when the patient presents with headache, decreased level of consciousness, and vomiting, all of which occur within minutes to hours. A thromboembolic stroke is more likely to occur when the patient is fully conscious, but onset of motor or sensory changes occurs suddenly. As with all neurologic disease, the clinical presentation depends on the location of the abnormality. An infarct of a particular cerebrovascular territory can be suspected by seeking out various neurologic deficits. An MCA occlusion produces paresis, with sensory deficits of limbs on the opposite side of the body because this artery supplies the motor and sensory strips. If the left MCA is occluded, **aphasia**, or loss of speech or expression may be present.

In the past, treatment for embolic stroke was supportive; it focused on prevention of further brain infarction and rehabilitation. Use of thrombolytic, "clot-busting" drugs reverses brain ischemia by lysing the clots. Initiation of therapy needs to occur within 6 hours of the onset of symptoms. Use of aspirin may be of some value in preventing further cerebrovascular events, but its effectiveness varies from one patient to another.

Controlling ICP while maintaining sufficient perfusion of the brain is the treatment for intracranial hemorrhage. This may include surgical evacuation of large volumes of intracranial blood, ventricular drainage, or other neurosurgical interventions. Rehabilitation is a key component. Hemorrhage, particularly SAH, has severe functional consequences and therefore has a longer period of convalescence than ischemic stroke.

Medical Nutrition Therapy

Primary prevention is the cornerstone for preventing stroke, in part by diet as well as by other lifestyle behaviors (Goldstein et al., 2006). Nutrition-related factors have been compiled from various large population-based prospective studies (Box 41-2).

Given the prevalence of stroke and its associated burden of disease, treatment for those afflicted with this disease cannot be ignored. In 2003 alone, strokes cost the United States an estimated $51 billion in lost productivity and health, including $12 billion in nursing home expenses (Centers for Disease Control and Prevention, 2006). Efforts should be directed toward maintaining the overall health of the patient. Omega-3 fatty acids may prevent some types of stroke, but should be avoided by anyone taking a blood thinner like warfarin or aspirin.

Feeding difficulties are determined by the extent of the stroke and the area of the brain affected. Dysphagia, an independent predictor of mortality, commonly accompanies stroke and contributes to complications and poor outcome from malnutrition, pulmonary infections, disability,

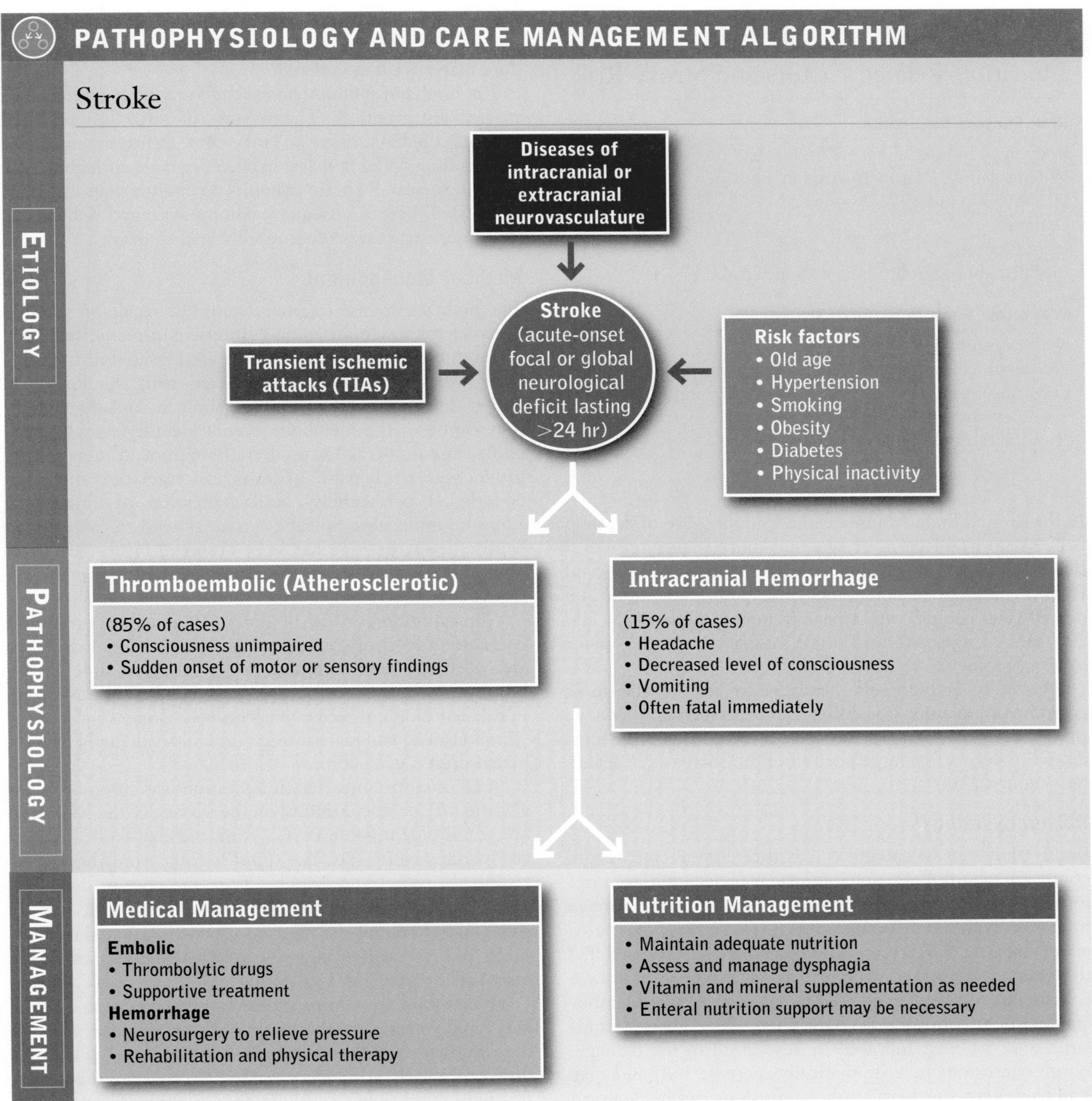

increased length of hospital stay, and institutional care. In some instances nutrition support is required to maintain nutritional health until oral alimentation can be resumed. As motor functions improve, eating and other activities of daily living are part of the patient's rehabilitation process and necessary for resuming independence. Malnutrition predicts a poor outcome and should be prevented.

HEAD TRAUMA OR NEUROTRAUMA

Traumatic brain injury (TBI) refers to any of the following, alone or in combination: brain injury, skull fractures, extraparenchymal hemorrhage—epidural, subdural, subarachnoid—or hemorrhage into the brain tissue itself, including intraparenchymal or intraventricular hemorrhage.

BOX 41-2

Nutrition-Related Factors and Stroke Risk

Risk Factors for Stroke

Body mass index >25 kg/m2 in women
Weight gain >11 kg in 16 years in women
Waist-to-hip ratio >0.92 in men
Diabetes
Hypertension
Elevated cholesterol in hemorrhagic stroke

Protective Factors against Stroke

Daily consumption of fresh fruit
Flavonoid consumption >4.7 cups green tea/daily
Fish consumption and fish oil use by white and black women and by black men
High HDL cholesterol in ischemic stroke

In the United States trauma is the leading cause of death in persons up to 44 years of age, and more than one half of these deaths are the result of head injuries (Victor and Ropper, 2005). The annual incidence is estimated to be 200 per 100,000 people, with a peak frequency between 15 and 24 years of age. Motor vehicle collisions are the major source of injury.

Morbidity is high and headache is one of the most common complaints. It is difficult to accurately predict neurologic recovery. Despite intensive intervention, long-term disability occurs in a large portion of the survivors of severe head injury.

Pathophysiology

Brain injury can be categorized as three types: concussion, contusion, and diffuse axonal injury. A concussion is a brief loss of consciousness, less than 6 hours, with no damage found on computed tomography (CT) or magnetic resonance imaging (MRI) scans. Microscopic studies have failed to find any evidence of structural damage in areas of known concussion, although evidence of change in cellular metabolism exists. A contusion is characterized by damaged capillaries and swelling, followed by resolution of the damage. Large contusions may dramatically increase ICP and may lead to ischemia or herniation. Contusions can be detected by CT or MRI scans. **Diffuse axonal injury** results from the shearing of axons by a rotational acceleration of the brain inside the skull. Damaged areas are often found in the corpus callosum (the bridge between the two hemispheres) and the upper, outer portion of the brainstem.

Skull fractures of the calvarium and the base are described in the same manner as other fractures. *Comminution* refers to splintering of bone into many fragments. *Displacement* refers to a condition in which bones are displaced from their original positions. *Open* or *closed* describes whether a fracture is exposed to air. Open fractures dramatically increase the risk of infection (osteomyelitis), and open skull fractures in particular carry an increased risk for meningitis because the dura mater is often violated.

Epidural and **subdural hematomas** are often corrected by surgical intervention. The volume of these lesions often displaces the brain tissue and may cause diffuse axonal injury and swelling. When the lesion becomes large enough, it may cause herniation of brain contents through various openings of the skull base. Consequent compression and ischemia of vital brain structures often rapidly lead to death.

Medical Management

The body's response to stress from TBI results in production of cytokines (interleukin-1, interleukin-6, interleukin-8, and tumor necrosis factor). These are elevated in the body after head injury and are associated with the hormonal milieu that negatively affects metabolism and organ function. Some of the metabolic events include fever, neutrophilia, muscle breakdown, altered amino acid metabolism, production of hepatic acute-phase reactants, increased endothelial permeability, and expression of endothelial adhesion molecules. Specific cytokines tend to cause organ demise; tissue damage has been observed in the gut, liver, lung, and brain. Overall, the molecular basis of functional recovery is poorly understood. (See Chapter 39.)

Clinical findings of brain injury often include a transient decrease in level of consciousness. Headache and dizziness are relatively common and not worrisome unless they become more intense or are accompanied by vomiting. Focal neurologic deficits, progressively decreasing level of consciousness, and penetrating brain injury demand prompt neurosurgical evaluation.

Skull fractures underneath lacerations can often be felt as a "drop off" or discontinuity on the surface of the skull, and are readily identifiable by CT scan. Basilar skull fractures are manifested by **otorrhea** (fluid leaking from the ear) or **rhinorrhea** (salty fluid dripping from the nose or down the pharynx). Other signs include raccoon eyes and Battle's sign—blood behind the mastoid process. Basilar skull fractures may precipitate injuries to cranial nerves, which are essential for chewing, swallowing, taste, and smell.

Hematomas are neurosurgical emergencies because they may rapidly progress to herniation of brain contents through the skull base and to subsequent death. These lesions may present similarly, with decreased level of consciousness, contralateral hemiparesis, and pupillary dilation. These lesions damage brain tissue by gross displacement and traction. Classically the **epidural hematoma** presents with progressively decreasing consciousness after an interval of several hours during which the patient had only a brief loss of consciousness. Subdural hematoma usually features progressively decreasing consciousness from the time of injury.

Sequelae most often include epilepsy and the postconcussive syndrome, a constellation of headache, vertigo, fatigue, and memory difficulties. Treatment for these patients can be highly complex, but the two goals of any therapeutic intervention are to maintain cerebral perfusion and to regulate ICP. Perfusion and pressure control have implications for nutrition therapy.

Medical Nutrition Therapy

The goal of nutrition therapy is to oppose the hypercatabolism and hypermetabolism associated with inflammation. Hypercatabolism is manifested by protein degradation, evidenced by profound urinary urea nitrogen excretion. Nitrogen catabolism in a fasting normal human is only 3 to 5 g of nitrogen per day, whereas nitrogen excretion is 14 to 25 g of nitrogen per day in the fasting patient with severe head injury. In the absence of nutritional intake, this degree of nitrogen loss can result in a 10% decrease in lean mass within 7 days. A 30% weight loss increases mortality rate (Brain Trauma Foundation, 2007).

Hypermetabolism contributes to increased energy expenditure. Correlations between the severity of brain injury as measured by the Glasgow Coma Scale and energy requirements have been shown. Replacement of 100% to 140% resting metabolism expenditure with 15% to 20% nitrogen calories reduces nitrogen loss (Brain Trauma Foundation, 2007). In patients medicated with barbiturates, metabolic expenditure may be decreased to 100% to 120% of basal metabolic rate. This decreased metabolic rate in pharmacologically paralyzed patients suggests that maintaining muscle tone is an important part of metabolic expenditure.

Nourishing the neurologically critically ill patient is accomplished by administering either enteral or parenteral nutrition support. Nutrition support is usually begun within 72 hours after injury and is necessary to achieve nutritional replacement by 7 days after injury (Brain Trauma Foundation, 2007). Both modes of therapy must be initiated at levels below actual requirements and increased gradually to meet nutritional requirements. For more guidelines, refer to Chapter 39.

Research in this area is exciting. An experimental dietary intervention based on a pyrazole curcumin derivative reestablishes membrane integrity and homeostasis following TBI (Sharma et al., 2010). The ω-3 fatty acids docosahexaenoic acid (DHA) and eicosapentaenoic acid (EPA) have antioxidative, anti-inflammatory, and antiapoptosis effects, leading to neuron protection in the damaged brain (Su, 2010). Clearly, more nutrient trials are needed in this population.

SPINE TRAUMA AND SPINAL CORD INJURY

Spine trauma encompasses many types of injuries, ranging from stable fractures of the spinal column to catastrophic transsection of the spinal cord. A complete **spinal cord injury (SCI)** is defined as a lesion in which there is no preservation of motor or sensory function more than three segments below the level of the injury. With an incomplete injury there is some degree of residual motor or sensory function more than three segments below the lesion. SCI is somewhat less common than head injury; both are most often seen in the young. Motor vehicle collisions account for one third to one half of SCIs; athletic injuries and domestic and industrial accidents account for the remainder.

Pathophysiology

The spinal cord responds to insult in a manner similar to the brain. Bleeding, contusion, and shorn axons appear first, followed by a several-year remodeling process consisting of gliosis and fibrosis. Liquefactive necrosis may predispose to the formation of a **syrinx**, fluid collection in the center of the spinal cord; effects manifest as a slow but progressive neurologic deficit. SCIs are usually associated with spinal column fractures and ligament instability. Such processes may be amenable to either surgical or nonsurgical reduction and stabilization.

The location of the SCI and the disruption of the descending axons determines the extent of paralysis. **Tetraplegia** (formerly known as quadraplegia) exists when the injury to the spinal cord affects all 4 extremities. When the SCI location results in only lower extremity involvement it is called **paraplegia**.

Medical Management

Spinal cord injuries have numerous clinical manifestations, depending on the level of the injury. Complete transsection results in complete loss of function below the level of the lesion, including the bladder and sphincters. After the patient is stabilized hemodynamically, the doctor evaluates the degree of neurologic deficit. Patients with suspected SCI are usually immobilized promptly in the field. Complete radiographic evaluation of the spinal column is obligatory in multitrauma and unconscious patients.

In the awake patient, clinical evidence of spine compromise is usually sufficient to determine the need for further workup. CT and MRI are used to more accurately delineate bony damage and spinal cord compromise. A dismal 3% of patients with complete spinal cord insults recover some function after 24 hours. Failure to regain function after 24 hours predicts a 0% chance of reestablishment of function in the future. Incomplete spinal cord syndromes may have somewhat improved outcomes.

Morbidity and mortality rates associated with SCI have improved dramatically, particularly in the last two decades. Advances in acute-phase care have reduced early mortality and prevented complications frequently associated with early death, such as respiratory failure and pulmonary emboli. Today, fewer than 10% of patients with SCI die from the acute injury.

Medical Nutrition Therapy

Technologic advances in enteral and parenteral feeding techniques and formulas have played a role in maintaining nutrition status of these patients. Although the metabolic response to neurotrauma has been studied extensively, the acute metabolic response to SCI has not; but it is similar to other forms of neurotrauma during the acute phase. Initially paralytic ileus may occur but often resolves within 72 hours after injury. Because DHA and EPA have antioxidative, anti-inflammatory, antiapoptosis effects, patients may benefit from fish oil supplementation (Su, 2010).

For those who survive the injury but are disabled for life, there are significant alterations in lifestyle as well as the possibility of secondary complications. In general the number and frequency of complications, and the presence of constipation, pressure ulcers, obesity, and pain vary but will involve nutrition. Box 41-3 describes the rehabilitation potential based on the level of injury. Evidence-based practice guidelines for SCI were released in 2010 by the American Dietetic Association.

Individuals with SCI have significantly high fat mass and low lean mass. Loss of muscle tone caused by skeletal muscle paralysis below the level of injury contributes to decreased metabolic activity, initial weight loss, and predisposition to osteoporosis. Guidelines for accepted weights adjusted for paraplegia and tetraplegia are as follows: the paraplegic should weigh 10 to 15 lb less than the ideal body mass index (BMI) would indicate; the tetraplegic should weigh 15 to 20 lb less than ideal weight dictated by the BMI. The higher the injury, the lower the metabolic rate; a lower energy requirement occurs.

Tetraplegic patients have lower metabolic rates than paraplegic patients, proportional to the amount of denervated muscle in their arms and legs, caused in part by the loss of residual motor function. In the rehabilitation phase, tetraplegics may require approximately 25% to 50% fewer calories than conventional equations predict. Thus these patients have the potential to become overweight. It has been proposed that obesity may slow the eventual rehabilitation process by limiting functional outcome.

As a consequence of bone loss resulting from the loss of mineralization caused by immobilization, SCI is associated with osteopenia and osteoporosis, and the prevalence of long-bone fractures increases. Adequate intake of vitamin D and calcium should be planned without excessive daily intakes.

BOX 41-3

Key Guidelines for Managing Spinal Cord Injury

- If the patient with spinal cord injury (SCI) is in the acute phase, the registered dietitian (RD) should assess energy needs by indirect calorimetry (IC).
- Initial weight loss during the acute phase of injury may lead to weight gain in the chronic phase because of body mass redistribution.
- Patients with SCI have reduced metabolic activity because of denervated muscle. Actual energy needs are at least 10% below predicted needs.
- Because of decreased energy expenditure and caloric needs, secondary to lower levels of spontaneous physical activity and a lower thermic effect of food, adults in the chronic phase of SCI are often overweight or obese and therefore at risk for diabetes and cardiovascular disease.
- Persons of all ages with SCI appear to be at high risk for cardiovascular disease, atherogenesis, and undesirable blood lipid values. Modifiable risk factors such as obesity, inactivity, dietary factors, and smoking need to be addressed. Physical activity, including sports, swimming, electrically stimulated exercise, and body-weight supported treadmill training, may result in improvements in blood lipid parameters. Dietary intervention using the current evidence-based guide for lipid disorders should be provided by an RD.
- Nutrition care provided by the RD as part of a multidisciplinary team results in improved nutrition-related outcomes in the acute care, rehabilitation, and community settings. SCI patients experience improvements in nutrient deficiencies, nutrition problems associated with social isolation and mobility issues, overweight and obesity, bowel management, swallowing, and nutrition-related chronic diseases.
- Cranberry juice is somewhat beneficial for prevention of urinary tract infections. One cup (250 mL) three times daily can be recommended.
- A minimum of 1.5 L of fluid is recommended per day. Therapeutic diets of high fiber and adequate water intake alone often do not suffice for treatment of constipation; a routine bowel preparation program may be required. For chronic bowel dysfunction, 15 g of fiber seems more beneficial than higher levels (20-30 g).
- Maintenance of nutritional health is important because poor nutrition is a risk factor for infection and pressure ulcer development. Regular assessment of nutritional status, the provision of adequate nutritional intake, and the implementation of aggressive nutritional support measures are indicated. Reduced pressure ulcer development occurs in patients who maintain a normal weight, higher activity levels, and better serum levels of total protein, albumin, prealbumin, zinc, and vitamin D and vitamin A. Thus sufficient intake of calories, protein, zinc and vitamins C, A, and B-complex is warranted.
- When pressure ulcers are present, use 30-40 kcal/kg of body weight/day. Use 1.2 g to 1.5 g of protein/kg body weight/day in Stage II pressure ulcers and 1.5 g to 2 g of protein/kg body weight/day for Stage III or IV pressure ulcers. See Table 21-2 in Chapter 21. Fluid requirements should be at least 1 mL fluid per kcal provided; increase if air-fluidized beds are used and when losses are increased for any reason.

Data from American Dietetic Association: Evidence analysis library: spinal cord injury guidelines. Accessed 31 October 2010 from http://www.adaevidencelibrary.com/topic.cfm?cat=3486&auth=1.

NEUROLOGIC DISEASES

Adrenomyeloleukodystrophy

Pathophysiology

Adrenomyeloleukodystrophy (ALD) is a rare congenital enzyme deficiency that affects the metabolism of very-long-chain fatty acids (VLCFAs) in young men. This leads to accumulation of VLCFAs, particularly hexacosanoic acid (C26:0) and tetracosanoic acid (C24:0) in the brain and adrenal glands (Deon et al., 2006). The incidence is 1 in 21,000 male births and 1 in 14,000 female (Moser, 2006). It is an X-linked recessive disorder characterized by myelopathy, peripheral neuropathy, and cerebral demyelination. The adult variant, adrenomyeloneuropathy, has chronic distal axonopathy of spinal cord and peripheral nerves marked by cerebral inflammatory demyelination; head trauma is an environmental factor that is detrimental in those people genetically at risk (Raymond et al., 2010). The mental and physical deterioration progresses to dementia, aphasia, apraxia, dysarthria, and blindness.

Medical Management

Clinical manifestations usually occur before age 7 and may manifest as adrenal insufficiency or cerebral decompensation.

Dysarthria (impairment of the tongue or other muscles needed for speech) and dysphagia may interfere with oral alimentation. Bronzing of the skin is a late clinical sign. With adrenal insufficiency, replacement of steroids is indicated, which may improve neurologic symptoms and prolong life. Numerous therapies have been directed at the root of the disorder but have been disappointing. The selective use of bone marrow transplant is one current therapy; gene therapy holds promise for the future.

Medical Nutrition Therapy

Nutritional therapy by dietary avoidance of VLCFAs does not lead to biochemical change because of endogenous synthesis. A specialty altered fatty acid product, Lorenzo's oil (C18:1 oleic acid and C22:1 erucic acid), lowers the VLCFA level. Although the clinical course is not significantly improved, a slower decline in function may result.

Alzheimer's Disease

Alzheimer's Disease (AD) is the most common form of dementia, with varying patterns and rates of cognitive decline (Soto et al., 2005). It is named after Alois Alzheimer, who first described the clinical features and pathologic changes of this degenerative brain disease in 1907. The incidence rate of new cases of AD is similar for both sexes and throughout the world, but prevalence is three times higher in women (who tend to live longer than men). Age is the most important risk factor for AD; the number of people with the disease doubles every 5 years beyond age 65. More than 35 million people worldwide are estimated to have this disease (Querfurth, 2010). Given the increase in the number of adults living longer, the personal, familial, financial, and clinical effects of AD are staggering.

Etiology

At least three genes have been discovered that cause early-onset, familial AD; other genetic mutations have been associated with age-related, sporadic AD. Apolipoprotein-E4 (Apo-E4) is a protein located on chromosome 19; it binds β-amyloid and is involved in the transport of cholesterol. Thus, Apo-E4 has both cardiovascular and nutritional implications. Damage to key mitochondrial components (Kidd, 2005), oxidative stress, impaired insulin signaling, elevated homocysteine (Hcy), low folate, and high serum cholesterol may be causal factors.

Lead, iron, aluminum, copper and zinc have been implicated in AD pathogenesis because they catalyze the production of free radicals and induce dementia (Ramesh et al., 2010). With aging, changes occur in neurogenesis and Reelin signaling (Shetty, 2010). Inflammatory pathways have been implicated as well. Beclin 1 is a protein involved in the regulation of autophagy, a cellular degradation and maintenance pathway that is reduced in patients with AD (Jaeger and Wyss-Coray, 2010).

Pathophysiology

Alzheimer's disease (AD) is a progressive, neurodegenerative disease characterized in the brain by abnormal clumps of **amyloid beta (Aβ)** peptide and neurofibrillary tangles (NIH, 2006). The early symptoms of AD, forgetfulness and loss of concentration, are often missed because they are misinterpreted as natural signs of aging (see *Pathophysiology and Care Management Algorithm:* Alzheimer's Disease).

AD begins gradually; advances; and eventually leads to confusion, personality and behavior changes, and impaired judgment. Manifestations of AD result in a progressive dementia, with increasing loss of memory, intellectual function, disturbances in speech, loss of independence, disordered eating behavior, and weight change.

Persons with poor physical function seem to have a high risk for developing AD (Wang, 2006). Initially, day-to-day events are forgotten, possessions are misplaced, and appointments are missed but memories are retained. Cerebral function declines, mostly evident after pronounced memory loss. Names of objects are forgotten (**anomia**), words spoken by others are repeated (**echolalia**), and comprehension is mostly lost (**agnosia**). Over time, motor skills deteriorate, evidenced by changes in reflexes and a shuffling gait. When AD reaches the terminal stage, bowel and bladder controls are lost; limb weakness and contractures occur; intellectual activity ceases. The patient becomes completely incapacitated in a vegetative state as death approaches.

Medical Management

AD is diagnosed by histopathologic examination. The disease includes a preclinical disease stage, a mild cognitive impairment stage, and finally dementia. For the first time in decades, new diagnostic and treatment guidelines are being developed by the National Institute on Aging. Nonsteroidal antiinflammatory drugs (NSAIDs) or aspirin in combination with intake of food sources of vitamin E, other antioxidants,

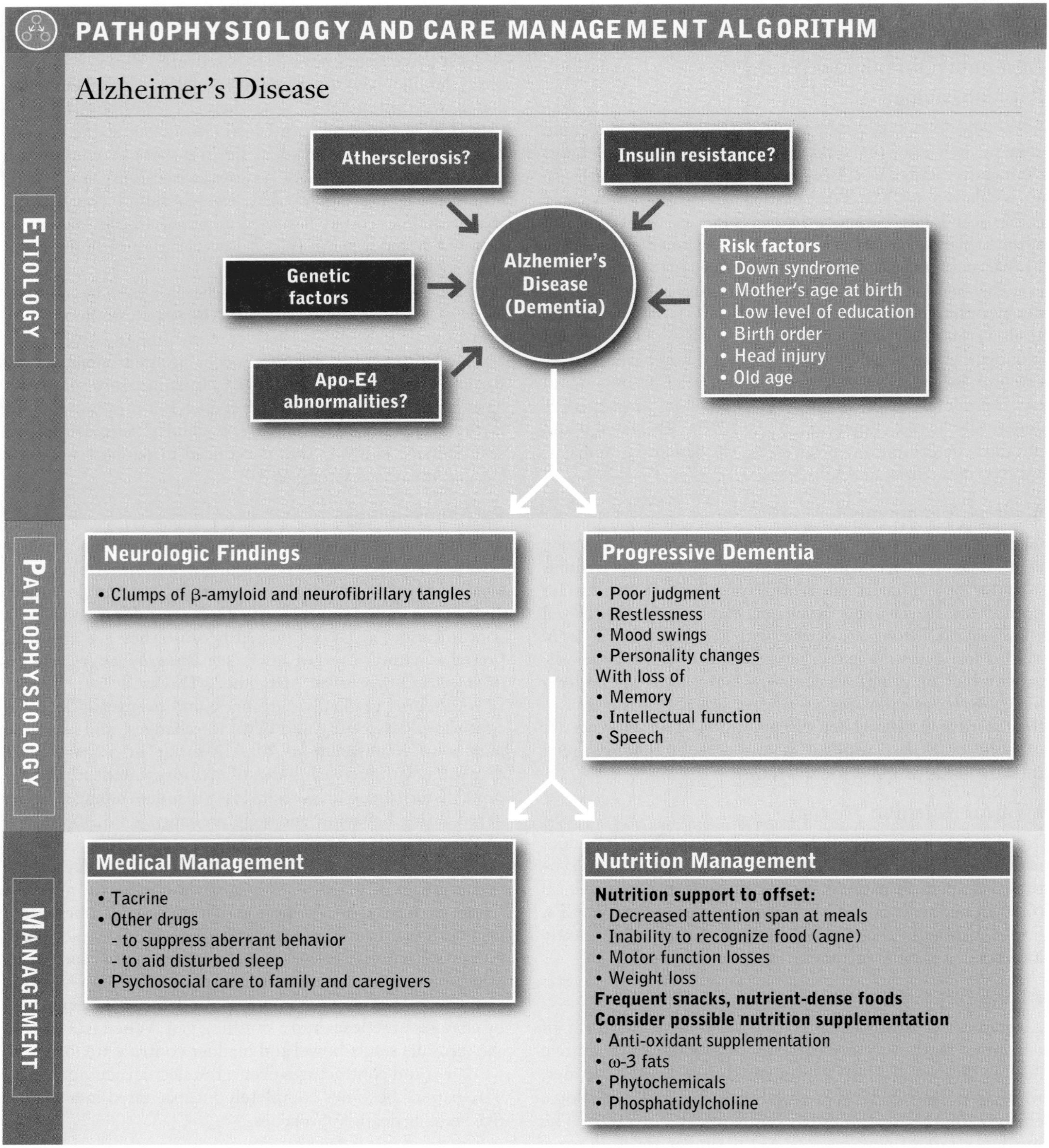

PATHOPHYSIOLOGY AND CARE MANAGEMENT ALGORITHM

Alzheimer's Disease

ETIOLOGY

- Athersclerosis?
- Insulin resistance?
- Genetic factors
- Apo-E4 abnormalities?

→ Alzhemier's Disease (Dementia)

Risk factors
- Down syndrome
- Mother's age at birth
- Low level of education
- Birth order
- Head injury
- Old age

PATHOPHYSIOLOGY

Neurologic Findings
- Clumps of β-amyloid and neurofibrillary tangles

Progressive Dementia
- Poor judgment
- Restlessness
- Mood swings
- Personality changes

With loss of
- Memory
- Intellectual function
- Speech

MANAGEMENT

Medical Management
- Tacrine
- Other drugs
  - to suppress aberrant behavior
  - to aid disturbed sleep
- Psychosocial care to family and caregivers

Nutrition Management

Nutrition support to offset:
- Decreased attention span at meals
- Inability to recognize food (agne)
- Motor function losses
- Weight loss

Frequent snacks, nutrient-dense foods

Consider possible nutrition supplementation
- Anti-oxidant supplementation
- ω-3 fats
- Phytochemicals
- Phosphatidylcholine

and ω-3 fatty acids are currently most effective (Shetty, 2010).

Cerebral vasodilators, stimulants, levodopa, and megadoses of vitamins remain unproven and drug treatment is experimental. Tacrine, the first cholinesterase inhibitor approved by the Food and Drug Administration (FDA) for treatment of AD, gives only modest improvement in function and cognition. Some other medications are used to suppress aberrant behavior, disturbed sleep, anxiety, or agitation. Collaborative interdisciplinary care may improve behavioral and psychological symptoms (Callahan et al., 2006). Stem cell transplantation may be tested for improving memory (Shetty, 2010). Other therapies are under development; see *New Directions:* Supplementation of Cell Membrane Phospholipids in Alzheimer's Disease?

Medical Nutrition Therapy

Diets rich in saturated fatty acids and alcohol, and deficient in antioxidants and vitamins promote the onset of the disease; diets rich in unsaturated fatty acids, vitamins, antioxidants, wine, curcumin and some spices suppress its onset by scavenging free radicals and preventing oxidative damage (Ramesh et al., 2010). Proper inclusion of antioxidants and specific nutrients may protect the AD patient. A 2010 report of a 4 year prospective cohort study of 2148 community-based adults (65+ years of age) found that persons with a diet characterized by higher intakes of salad dressing, nuts, fish, tomatoes, poultry, cruciferous vegetables, fruits, and dark and green leafy vegetables were less likely to acquire AD than those eating diets of high-fat dairy products, red meat, organ meats, and butter (Gu et al., 2010). Because several dietary polyphenols are known to chelate metals, their routine use may also be protective (Ramesh et al., 2010). Garlic may be neuroprotective (Chauhan, 2005) and resveratrol prevents neuronal decline with aging (Anekonda, 2006; Ramesh et al., 2010). See also Figure 41-5.

Problems with Self-Feeding, Oral Intake, and Weight Management. A wide range of neurologic functions are impaired that interfere with eating. Cognitive losses impair attention span, reasoning, and judgment; the ability to recognize feelings of hunger, thirst, and satiety decline. As the disease progresses, attention span decreases, and meals may be forgotten as soon as they are eaten or may not be eaten at all. Dehydration is also a problem; recognizing thirst and then seeking water is neglected.

Although a gluttonous appetite and weight gain may develop in some individuals with AD, generally weight loss is the norm. Whether increased resting metabolic rate or

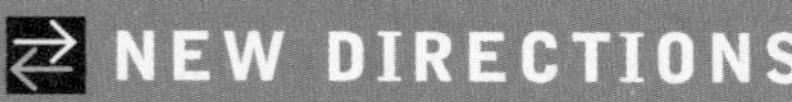

Supplementation of Cell Membrane Phospholipids in Alzheimer's Disease?

Choline, a B-vitamin, makes several metabolic contributions to cell membrane phospholipids. Because of this, it is gaining interest for its potential role in neurologic conditions. It is a precursor for phosphatidylserine and phosphatidylcholine, phospholipids located in the cell membrane of cells, including nerve cells (Tan, 1998; Zeisel, 2010).

Phosphatidylserine is located on the cytosol side of the lipid membrane of cells. It has been studied in brain health, and may offer neuro-protection by inhibiting the formation of beta amyloid fragments in those with AD. Early studies using bovine phosphatidylserine showed positive results in those with cognitive decline. Due to fears of mad cow disease, the compound was replaced in studies with a soy-based phosphatidylserine which is not exactly the same. Weak evidence supporting improvement in age-related memory impairment has been associated with the soy-based compound, but overall results are inconclusive and more research is needed (Wollen, 2010).

Because phosphatidylcholine may offer protection, it is noted that precursor CDP-choline shows promise. There may be positive effects on memory and behavior in patients with various forms of dementia, including AD. Longer term studies are needed to investigate full benefits (Fioravanti et al, 2010). Nonetheless, nutritional intake can be enhanced. Choline is found in eggs (especially yolks), beef (especially brains and liver), fish, pork, poultry, beans, nuts, peas, and soy products.

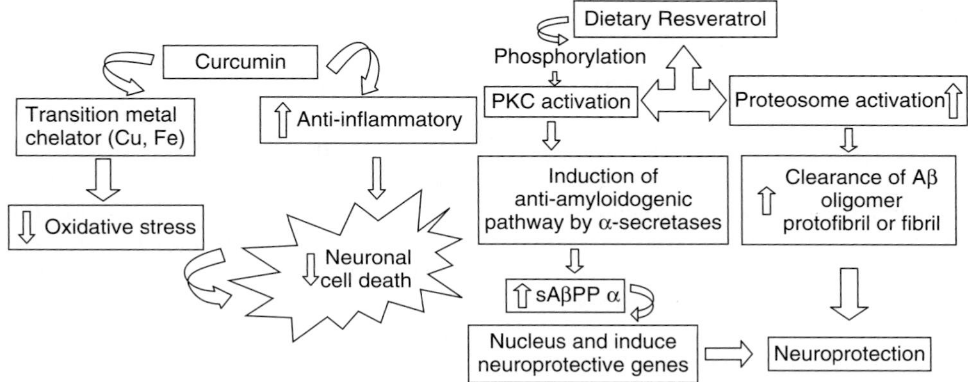

FIGURE 41-5 The role of curcumin and resveratrol in neuroprotection.
Left: Curcumin has multiple biologic effects: it chelates transition metals (iron and copper) and acts as an antioxidant and antiinflammatory molecule, protecting from oxidative stress.
Right: Resveratrol favors phosphorylation in protein kinase C, activating the nonamyloidogenic pathway of AβPP cleavage, and this leads to reduction in Aβ formation. sAβPPβ, a product of AβPP cleavage, gets translocated to the nucleus and modulates the genes. All these events favor neuronal cell survival. *(From Ramesh BN et al: Neuronutrition and Alzheimer's disease, J Alzheimer's Dis 19:1123, 2010. With permission from IOS Press.)*
Aβ, Amyloid beta; *PKC,* protein kinase C; *sAPPβ,* secreted fragment of amyloid protein precursor beta.

increased energy expenditure from constant pacing causes weight loss is unclear. For others, eating is neglected and inadequate oral intake results from impaired self-feeding. In still other cases weight loss may be secondary to frequent infections. Weight loss in turn increases the risk of skin ulcers and consequently decreases quality of life.

Mealtimes should be kept simple. Noise can be distracting; the radio or television should be turned off during mealtime. Food may need to be placed on small plates or bowls and served one at a time so as not to offer too many choices. As social inhibitions decrease, the patient may take another person's food, consume inedible items or spoiled foods, or drink hazardous fluids. AD patients should be closely supervised during meals.

With sensory losses, perception of the surrounding world and related auditory, visual, or tactile recognition are distorted; this is called *agnosia*. Visual agnosia, the inability to recognize food, is manifested by not eating. The touch or smell of food is needed to initiate eating responses. Another sensory loss is the inability to recognize food when it is served in a bowl the same color as the food item. Use of colored bowls and plates that are in contrast to the color of the food may be necessary so that food can be distinguished from the place setting. Patients may have difficulty using eating utensils, but may model behaviors when demonstrated by staff or caregivers.

Motor losses occur during the course of the illness. Some clients may need hand guidance to initiate eating, then verbal cues to continue. As motor skills decline, the patient may be able to use only a spoon. However, eating utensils should not be removed prematurely because this may contribute to agitation, excessive disability, inadequate oral intake, and eventual weight loss. In addition, motor skills should be assessed routinely. Finger foods may be used, but only if the patient has no difficulty with chewing or swallowing. If the patient is inclined to swallow large boluses of food, finger foods are not appropriate. Although adaptive equipment is sometimes useful, it may be unfamiliar to the patient. As end-stage disease approaches, swallowing often becomes impossible. Dysphagia should be managed to prevent aspiration.

Frequent snacks, nutrient-dense foods, and nutrition supplements are needed to combat weight loss. Behavior modification and the use of altered food choices can improve quality of life. Evaluation of nutrition status is needed throughout the stages of AD to ensure that objectives of nutrition therapy continue to be met. Table 41-7 lists additional interventions.

Further, a succinct listing of drugs commonly used in the treatment of various neurologic diseases is shown in Table 41-8.

Amyotrophic Lateral Sclerosis

Amyotrophic lateral sclerosis (ALS) is the most common motor system disease. ALS is also called *Lou Gehrig disease*, after the famous baseball player afflicted with the disease. The incidence is 2 in 100,000 (International Alliance of ALS, 2010). ALS involves a progressive denervation, atrophy, and weakness of muscles; hence the name *amyotrophy*. The prevalence is constant throughout the world, but men are affected more than women. The average age of onset is the mid-50s, and it is usually found in the 40- to 70-year age group.

Etiology

The cause of ALS is not clear. Genetic analysis of patients with familial, chromosome 21–linked ALS suggests that misfolding mutations in the copper-zinc superoxide dismutase (SOD1) gene may be involved (Nordlund and Oliveberg, 2006). Risk factors related to occupation, trauma, diet, or socioeconomic status are not consistent. However, it has been noted in several studies that elevated Hcy has neurotoxic effects. Because high Hcy levels induce oxidative stress and stimulate excitotoxic receptors, they damage motor neurons (Zoccolella et al., 2010).

Pathophysiology

The pathologic basis of weakness in ALS is the selective death of motor neurons in the ventral gray matter of the spinal cord, brainstem, and in the motor cortex. Clinical manifestations are characterized by generalized skeletal muscular weakness, atrophy, and hyperreflexia. The natural course for ALS is unpleasant. Decline is relentless and without remissions, relapses, or plateaus; it finally progresses to death usually in 2 to 6 years (Czaplinski, 2006).

The typical presentation is evidenced with both lower motor neuron (weakness, wasting, fasciculation) and upper motor neuron deficits (hyperactive tendon reflexes, Hoffman signs, Babinski signs, or clonus). Muscle weakness begins in the legs and hands and progresses to the proximal arms and oropharynx. As these motor nerves deteriorate, almost all of the voluntary skeletal muscles are at risk for atrophy and complete loss of function. The loss of spinal motor neurons causes the denervation of voluntary skeletal muscles of the neck, trunk, and limbs, resulting in muscle wasting, flaccid weakness, involuntary twitching (fasciculations) and loss of mobility.

Progressive loss of function in cortical motor neurons can lead to spasticity of jaw muscles, resulting in slurred speech and dysphagia. The onset of dysphagia is usually insidious. Swallowing difficulties usually follow speech difficulties. Although some weight loss is inevitable given the muscle atrophy, consistent or dramatic loss may be an indicator of chewing difficulties or dysphagia (Bulat and Orlando, 2005). Eye movement and eye blink are spared, as are the sphincter muscles of the bowel and bladder; thus incontinence is rare. Sensation remains intact and mental acuity is maintained.

Medical Management

No currently known therapy cures the disease. To lower high serum Hcy levels, short-term treatment with a high dose of methylcobalamin (B_{12}) shows promise (Zoccolella et al., 2010). Use of folate and antioxidant treatments should also be investigated. Although mechanical ventilation can extend the life of patients, most decline this option. Quality

TABLE 41-7

Practical Interventions for Eating-Related Behavioral Problems Common in Individuals with Dementia

Behavioral Problem	Intervention
Attention or concentration deficit	Verbally direct client through each step of eating process; place utensils in hand. Make food and fluids available and visible.
Combative, throws food	Identify provocative agent, remove. Feeder stands or sits on nondominant side. Provide nonbreakable dishes with suction holder. Give one food at a time. Reward appropriate mealtime behavior.
Chews constantly	Tell client to stop chewing after each bite. Serve soft foods to reduce the need to chew. Offer small bites.
Eats nonedible things	Remove nonedibles from reach; provide finger foods. Use edible centerpiece or table decorations.
Eats too quickly	Set utensils down between bites. Offer food items separately. Offer bulky foods that require chewing. Use a smaller spoon or cup.
Eats too slowly	Monitor eating place and provide verbal cues: "chew," "take a bite." Serve first to allow more time. Use insulated dishes to maintain proper temperatures.
Forgetful or disoriented	Follow simple routines. Provide constant environment. Provide assigned seating. Minimize distractions and limit choices.
Forgets to swallow	Tell client to swallow. Feel for swallow before offering next bite. Stroke upward on larynx.
Inappropriate emotional expression	Engage in conversation; ignore emotional display. Provide a quiet environment.
Paces	Sit beside client at table. Change dining location. Provide aerobic exercise before meals. Offer finger foods. Use cups with covers or spouts.
Plays in food	Serve one food at a time. Fill glass or plate half full at refill. Offer finger foods. Use cups with covers or spouts.
Shows paranoia	Provide structured routine. Present food in consistent manner. Serve foods in closed containers. Do not put medicine in food.
Spits	Evaluate chewing and swallowing ability. Tell client not to spit. Place client away from others who would be offended. Provide mealtime supervision.
Will not go into dining room	Ask why; change dining location. Provide a single dining partner versus a group. Serve meals in room if needed.

Modified from National Institute on Aging (NIA) at http://www.nia.nih.gov/nia.nih.gov/templates/ADEAR Accessed 3/22/2011

TABLE 41-8

Drugs Commonly Used in the Treatment of Neurologic Diseases

Disease or Condition	Drug	Basic Function	Nutrition-Related Side Effects
Adrenomyeloleukodystrophy	Adrenal hormones		Weight gain
Alzheimer's Disease	Donepezil	Supports nerve cell communication	Anorexia, weight loss
	Galantamine		
	Rivastigmine	Delays worsening of symptoms	
	Tacrine		
	Memantine	May help improve attention, reasoning, language	
Amyotrophic Lateral Sclerosis	Riluzole	Decreases motor neuron damage	Suggests decreased use of caffeine
Epilepsy	Valproate	Anticonvulsant	Increased appetite, weight
	Phenytoin	Anticonvulsant	Increased metabolism of vitamin D and K
	Gabapentin	Anticonvulsant	Weight gain
	Carbamazepine	Anticonvulsant	Possible increased need of calcium and vitamin D
	Phenobarbital	Sedative, hypnotic	Increased metabolism of vitamins D, K, & possibly folic acid
	Primidone	Anticonvulsant	
Guillain-Barré Syndrome	Immunoglobulins or plasmapheresis	Decreases immune attacks	
Migraine Headache	NSAIDS	Antiinflammatory	
	Sympathomimetics		
	Serotonin agonists		
	Sumatriptan	Serotonin 5-HT1 receptor agonist	Dehydration, anorexia
Myasthenia Gravis	Anticholinesterase inhibitors	Improve muscle contraction and strength	GI upset, increased urination
Multiple Sclerosis	Corticosteroids: Oral prednisone, IV methylprednisolone	Reduce inflammation	Increased appetite, weight gain
	Interferon: beta 1a –(Avonex, Rebif)	Slow rate of symptom development	Anorexia, increased or decreased weight
	beta 1b –(Betaseron)		
	Novantrone (Mitoxantrone)	Immunosuppressants, anticancer antibiotics	Anorexia, harmful to heart, leukemia
	Anthracenedione		
	Natalizumab (formerly Antegran)	Monotherapy	Risk of progressive multifocal leukoencephalopathy
	Glatiramer acetate	Immunomodulator drug for relapsing-remitting MS	Flushing, sweating
	Symptomatic therapies: Amantadine	Reduces fatigue,	Anorexia, weight loss
		Reduces spasticity	Increased appetite, weight
	Diazepam	Decreases paroxysmal dystonia, sensory symptoms	Anorexia, N/V, diarrhea
	Carbamazepine		
	Amitryptyline	Reduces pain	
Parkinson's Disease	Levodopa	Dopamine precursor	Anorexia
	COMT inhibitors:	Prolongs effectiveness of levodopa	
	Entacapone		
	Tolcapone		

TABLE 41-8

Drugs Commonly Used in the Treatment of Neurologic Diseases—cont'd

Disease or Condition	Drug	Basic Function	Nutrition-Related Side Effects
	Exelon	Acetylcholinesterase inhibitor	Anorexia, weight loss,
	MAO-B Inhibitors	Reduces breakdown of dopamine	
	Trihexyphenidyl Benztropine Ethopropazine	Anticholinergics	
Stroke	Anticoagulants Antiplatelet agents	Preventive	Bleeding, decreased platelets
	Thrombolitic therapy when acute: heparin	Dissolves clots	

Data from National Institute of Neurologic Disorders and Stroke: Disorders index. Accessed 15 July 2010 from http://www.ninds.nih.gov/disorders; Accessed 4 November 2010 from http://www.mayoclinic.com/health-information.

COMT (catechol-O-methyltransferase); *GI*, gastrointestinal; *IV*, intravenous; *MAO-B* (monoamine oxidase B); *MS*, multiple sclerosis; *NSAID*, nonsteroidal antiinflammatory drug; *N/V*, nausea and vomiting.

TABLE 41-9

Nutritional and Metabolic Changes During the Progression of Amyotrophic Lateral Sclerosis

	Early Phase	Late Phase
Pathophysiology	Cycles of muscle denervation, muscle catabolism and atrophy, reinnervation, and protein synthesis	Net muscle catabolism and atrophy
Functional status	Mild functional restriction of physical activity Mild impairment of respiration	Progressive limitation of physical activity Increased work of ventilation
Nutritional and metabolic changes	Positive nitrogen balance Normal resting energy expenditure Probable neutral energy balance	Negative nitrogen balance Increased resting energy expenditure Decrease in body fat

From Kasarskis EJ et al: Nutritional status of patients with amyotrophic lateral sclerosis: relation to the proximity of death, Am J Clin Nutr 63:130, 1996.

of life is poor in advanced ALS and supportive comfort measures are primarily used.

Medical Nutrition Therapy

There are decreases in body fat, lean body mass, muscle power, and nitrogen balance and an increase in resting energy expenditure as death approaches. Some of the nutritional changes during the different stages of ALS are noted in Table 41-9.

Hypermetabolic status and increased resting energy expenditure measurements have been noted. The relationship between dysphagia and respiratory status is important. As ALS progresses, a progressive loss of function in bulbar and respiratory muscles contributes to oral and pharyngeal dysphagia. In late stages, when the respiratory status is impaired, alternative tube placement besides PEG may be required.

The clinician should become familiar with common clinical findings in ALS to prevent secondary complications of malnutrition and dehydration. The functional status of each patient should be monitored closely so that timely intervention with the appropriate management techniques can be started. In particular, dysphagia should be monitored closely. Oropharyngeal weakness affects survival in ALS by placing the patient at continuous risk of aspiration, pneumonia, and sepsis and by curtailing the adequate intake of energy and protein. These problems can compound the deteriorating effects of the disease. The Amyotrophic Lateral Sclerosis Severity Scale is often used to assess the functional level of swallowing, speech, upper and lower extremities. Once the severity of deficits has been identified, appropriate interventions can be implemented (see *Focus On:* Dysphagia Intervention for Amyotrophic Lateral Sclerosis).

Epilepsy

Epilepsy is a chronic condition characterized by unprovoked, recurring seizures that disrupt the nervous system. **Seizures** (or convulsions) are intermittent derangements in brain function caused by abnormal electrical activity of a group of brain cells, and present with apparent clinical

FOCUS ON

Dysphagia Intervention for Amyotrophic Lateral Sclerosis

Strand and colleagues (1996) outlined dysphagia intervention on a continuum of five stages that correlate to the amyotrophic lateral sclerosis (ALS) severity scale. They include:

1. ***Normal Eating Habits (ALS Severity Scale Rating 10-9).*** Early assessment and intervention are critical for maintaining nutritional health in ALS. This is the appropriate time to begin educating the patient, before the development of speech or swallowing symptoms. Hydration and maintenance of nutritional health are critical at this stage. Fluid intake of at least 2 q/day is important. Dehydration contributes to fatigue and thickens saliva. For patients with spinal ALS, emphasis on fluids is important because they may intentionally limit fluid intake because of difficulties with toileting. The diet history is helpful to assess patterns of normal chewing, swallowing, and the rate of ingestion. Weight loss history establishes a baseline weight. A weight loss of 10% or more is indicative of nutritional risk.
2. ***Early Eating Problems (Severity Scale Rating 8-7).*** At this point patients begin to report difficulties eating; reports of coughing and unusually long mealtimes are associated with tongue, facial, and masticator muscle weakness. Dietary intervention begins to focus on modification of consistency, avoidance of thin liquids, and use of foods that are easier to chew and swallow.
3. ***Dietary Consistency Changes (Severity Scale Rating 6-5).*** As symptoms progress, the oral transport of food becomes difficult as dry, crumbly foods tend to break apart and cause choking. Foods that require more chewing (e.g., raw vegetables or steak) are typically avoided. As dysphagia progresses, ingestion of thin liquids, especially water, may become more problematic. Often the patient has fatigue and malaise, which may be associated with a mild chronic dehydration resulting from a decreased fluid intake. Dietary intervention should change food consistency to mechanically soft or pureed (see Appendix 35) to reduce the need for oral manipulation and to conserve energy. Small, frequent meals may also increase intake. Thick liquids that contain a high percentage of water, as well as attempts to increase fluid intake, need to be emphasized to maintain fluid balance. Popsicles, gelatin, ice, and fresh fruit are additional sources of free water. Liquids can be thickened with a modified cornstarch thickener. Swallowing can be improved by emphasizing taste, texture, and temperature. Juices can be substituted for water to provide taste, nutrients, and calories. A cool temperature facilitates the swallowing mechanism; therefore cold food items may be better tolerated; heat does not provide the same advantage. Carbonation may also be better tolerated because of the beneficial effect of texture. Instructions for preventing aspiration should be addressed: safe swallowing includes sitting bolt upright with the head in a chin-down position. Concentrating on the swallowing process can also help reduce choking. Avoid environmental distractions and conversation during mealtime; however, families should be encouraged to maintain a normal mealtime routine. As dysphagia progresses, the limitation of food consistencies may result in the exclusion of entire food groups. Vitamin and mineral supplementation may be necessary. If chewable supplements are not handled safely, liquid forms may be added to acceptable foods. Fiber may also need to be added along with fluids for constipation problems.
4. ***Tube Feeding (Severity Scale Rating 4-3).*** Dehydration will occur acutely before malnutrition, a more chronic state, is exhibited. This may be an early indication of the need for nutrition support. Weight loss from muscle wasting and dysphagia will eventually lead to placement of a percutaneous endoscopic gastrostomy (PEG) tube for nutrition and protection against aspiration caused by dysphagia. Enteral nutrition support is preferred because the gastrointestinal tract should be functioning properly. Given the progressive nature of ALS, placing feeding tubes with signs of dysphagia and dehydration is better than initiating this therapy later, after the patient has become overtly malnourished or when respiratory status is marginal. The decision of whether to place a feeding tube for nutrition support is part of the decision-making process each patient must face. Adequate nutriture can maintain health of the individual longer and may be a welcome relief for the patient. The purpose of nutrition support should be to enhance the quality of life. Long-term access should be considered via a PEG or percutaneous endoscope jejunostomy tube (see Chapter 14).
5. ***Nothing by Mouth (Severity Scale Rating 2-1).*** The final level of dysphagia is reached when the patient can neither eat orally nor manage his or her own oral secretions. Although saliva production is not increased, it tends to pool in the front of the mouth as a result of a declining swallow response. Once the swallowing mechanism is absent, mechanical ventilation is required to manage saliva flow. Tube feeding is permanent at this stage.

Data from Strand EA et al: Management of oral-pharyngeal dysphagia symptoms in amyotrophic lateral sclerosis, Dysphagia 11:129, 1996.

symptoms and findings. It is estimated that 2.3 million individuals in the United States have epilepsy; 45,000 children younger than age 15 develop epilepsy each year according to the Epilepsy Foundation (2006).

Pathophysiology

Most seizures begin in early life, but a resurgence of epileptic events occurs after age 60. The first occurrence of a seizure in adults should prompt investigation into a cause. A clinical workup usually reveals no anatomic abnormalities, and the cause of the seizure may remain unknown (idiopathic). Seizures before age 2 are usually caused by developmental defects, birth injuries, or a metabolic disease (see Chapters 44 and 45). The medical history is the key component for suggesting further avenues of diagnostic investigation and potential treatments, especially in children. An electroencephalogram can help to delineate seizure activity. It is most helpful in localizing partial complex seizures.

Medical Management

The dramatic **tonic-clonic (grand mal) seizure** is the most common image of a seizure (lasting 1 to 2 minutes), yet numerous classifications of seizures, each with a different and often less dramatic clinical presentation, exist. A generalized seizure involves or appears to involve the entire brain cortex from its beginning phases. The tonic-clonic seizure comes under this heading. After such a seizure the patient wakes up slowly after a time; he or she will be groggy and disoriented for minutes to hours after the event. This is termed the *postictal phase* and is characterized by deep sleep, headache, confusion, and muscle soreness.

The **absence seizure (petit mal)** is also generalized in nature. A patient with absence seizures may appear to be daydreaming during an episode, but he or she recovers consciousness within a few seconds and has no postictal fatigue or disorientation. Partial seizures occur when there is a discrete focus of epileptogenic brain tissue. A simple partial seizure involves no loss of consciousness, whereas a complex partial seizure is characterized by a change in consciousness. Failure of partial seizure control may prompt consideration of seizure surgery. A localized focus resected from nonessential brain renders a patient seizure free in 75% of cases.

Determining the seizure type is key to implementing effective therapy. Generalized seizures are ordinarily managed with valproate or phenytoin. Phenytoin metabolism has unusual kinetics; thus toxic levels may be attained with very small dosage adjustments. These drugs interact with other drugs metabolized in the liver and may cause liver damage. Liver enzymes and serum drug levels must be monitored periodically. Gabapentin is rapidly gaining popularity because of its safety and ease of use. Carbamazepine or phenytoin can usually control partial seizures. Use of just one antiseizure medication is recommended initially, resorting to combination therapies only when needed.

Medications used in anticonvulsant therapy may alter the nutrition status of the patient (see Chapter 9 and Appendix 31). Phenobarbital has been associated with decreased intelligence quotient when used in children. It is occasionally considered for use after failure of other antiepileptic drugs. Phenobarbital, phenytoin, and primidone interfere with intestinal absorption of calcium by increasing vitamin D metabolism in the liver. Long-term therapy with these drugs may lead to osteomalacia in adults or rickets in children, and vitamin D supplementation is recommended. Folic acid supplementation interferes with phenytoin metabolism; thus it contributes to difficulties in achieving therapeutic levels. If folic acid supplementation is necessary, it should be consistent, and medication adjusted accordingly.

Phenytoin and phenobarbital are bound primarily to albumin in the bloodstream. Decreased serum albumin levels in malnutrition or advanced cirrhosis limits the amount of drug that can be bound. This results in an increased free drug concentration and possible drug toxicity even with a standard dose.

Absorption of phenobarbital is delayed by the consumption of food; therefore administration of the drug must be staggered around mealtimes if it is used. Continuous enteral feeding slows the absorption of phenytoin, thus necessitating an increase in the dose to achieve a therapeutic level. Stopping the tube feeding 1 hour before and 1 hour after the phenytoin dose is generally recommended. Whenever tube feedings are stopped, the dose of phenytoin needs to be adjusted to avoid toxicity.

Medical Nutrition Therapy

A **ketogenic diet** can be used for treatment of all types of seizures in children with intractable epilepsy in whom drug therapies have failed. The ketogenic diet has minimal side effects, and risks of the diet are low blood sugar, upset stomach at first caused by the high amounts of fat, and constipation. The long-term risk of kidney stones is rare; elevated serum cholesterol is usually is temporary and disappears with discontinuation of the diet; and growth, which is sometimes slowed while on the diet, resumes at the child's normal rate (Patel et al., 2010). Although the diet is very demanding and requires continued effort even after the first phase, it completely controls epilepsy in one third of the children whose seizures are otherwise uncontrollable (Groomes et al., 2011). Practical guidelines for implementing the diet have been released by the American Academy of Neurology and the American Epilepsy Society and can be retrieved from the Epilepsy Foundation website (Kossoff et al., 2009).

The diet is designed to create and maintain a state of ketosis (Bough and Rho, 2007). The beneficial effect in epilepsy may be caused by a change in neuronal metabolism; ketones may inhibit neurotransmitters, thus producing an anticonvulsant effect in the body. To begin the diet the individual usually fasts in the hospital for 24 to 72 hours until ketonemia is produced as measured by the level of beta-hydroxybutyrate in the blood. For many patients, if the diet is going to work, it usually works during this initial period with a reduction in seizures; however, sometimes the child needs to follow the subsequent ketogenic diet for 3

TABLE 41-10

Typical Ketogenic Diet Pattern

	Amount (g)	Fat (g)	Protein (g)	Carbohydrates (g)	Energy (kcal)
Breakfast					
Keto waffles (made with ketocal powder 4:1)	72	27.5	6.12	2.92	284
Raspberries	29	0	0.29	2.9	13
Butter	12	9.73	0.1	0.01	88
Total		**37.23**	**6.51**	**5.83**	**385**
AM Snack					
36% heavy cream	14	5.04	0.28	0.42	48
Strawberry	9	0	0.09	0.9	4
Total		**5.04**	**0.37**	**1.32**	**52**
Lunch					
36% heavy cream	43	15.48	0.86	1.29	148
Broccoli	45	0	0.9	3.15	16
Chicken breast, no skin and cooked	14	0.5	4.34	0	22
Macadamia nuts	15	11.41	1.17	0.72	110
Olive oil	10	10	0	0	90
Total		**37.39**	**7.27**	**5.16**	**386**
PM Snack					
Avocado	19	2.93	0.37	0.35	29
Carrots	12	0.03	0.11	0.81	4
Olive oil	2	2	0	0	18
Total		**4.96**	**0.48**	**1.16**	**51**
Dinner					
36% heavy cream	35	12.6	0.7	1.05	120
Noodles: miracle shirataki, angel hair pasta	40	0	0.03	0.11	1
Peaches	30	0	0.3	3	13
Cheese, Kraft Cheddar	26	8.62	6.47	0.33	105
Butter	20	16.22	0.17	0.01	147
Total		**37.44**	**7.67**	**4.5**	**386**
DAILY TOTAL		**122.06**	**22.3**	**17.97**	**1260**

Created by Marta Mazzanti, RD, Seattle Children's Hospital, Seattle, WA.

months before there are any reductions in seizure activity. It should also be noted that antiepileptic drugs are not stopped when administering the ketogenic diet.

In the traditional approach, once ketosis is established, caloric intake is resumed in a ratio of 3:1 or 4:1, meaning that there are 3 or 4 g of fat for every 1 g of protein and carbohydrate combined in the diet. With a 4:1 ratio, the diet is calculated so that at least 80% of the kilocalories are from fat. Protein is calculated to provide appropriate intake for growth (approximately 1 g/kg/day). Carbohydrates are added to make up the remaining small portion of calories.

The majority of the diet is composed of fresh meats, eggs, cheese, fish, heavy whipping cream, butter, oils, nuts, and seeds. Vegetables and fruits are added in small amounts, within the current diet prescription (Table 41-10). Ketosis is monitored by regular measurements of serum β-hydroxybutyrate. Even though goal levels are patient specific, most individuals need to be in the range of 35-60 mg/L (4-7mmol/L) for seizure control. A carbohydrate-free multiple vitamin and mineral supplement is necessary to ensure that the diet is nutritionally complete. However, additional vitamins and minerals are often necessary, including calcium, vitamin D, and selenium.

Other nonfood items such as sugar-containing toothpaste, shampoo, and lotions need to be avoided. It is important that the diet be strictly followed; the smallest amount of extra carbohydrate can cause a breakthrough seizure. The child should be monitored, because too rapid a rate of weight gain can decrease ketosis and reduce effectiveness.

A variation of the ketogenic diet is the modified Atkins diet in which calories are not restricted, but carbohydrates are drastically limited to 10 to 20 g/day. The ratio of fat to protein and carbohydrate is usually 1:1. It appears that the best results are achieved when the diet begins with 10 g/day of carbohydrate and is then adjusted upward, always maintaining ketosis (Porta et al., 2009; Weber et al., 2009).

Another modification of the traditional ketogenic diet is the medium-chain triglyceride (MCT) oil–based ketogenic diet, used frequently in the United Kingdom and Canada, in which some of the long-chain fats of the traditional diet are replaced with MCTs. MCT oil is an odorless, colorless, tasteless oil and was originally used as a means of improving the palatability of the diet. A greater amount of nonketogenic foods such as fruits and vegetables and small amounts of bread and other starches can be allowed because ketosis from MCT can be more readily achieved with a lower percentage of fat in the diet. MCT can be added in to the classic ketogenic diet and modified Atkins diet to increase ketosis. Coconut oil can also be used as a source of MCT to increase palatability, but it contains only 45% to 50% MCT so more may be needed. MCT oil or coconut oils are also added if the serum triglycerides are too high with the use of the traditional ketogenic diet.

Initiating the ketogenic diet is intense. Further, the diet may be unpalatable as well as complex, requiring weighing and measuring of all foods, thus making compliance difficult to achieve. To be successful, children may benefit from behavioral techniques, whereas parents most often require substantial psychosocial support. Attention required during the fine-tuning phase varies and is affected by the patient's health status, growth, and development. For the child whose epilepsy is controlled by the diet, complying with the diet is much easier than dealing with devastating seizures and injuries.

Discontinuation of the diet can be considered after 2 to 3 years, especially if the child has been seizure free for a year, although seizure control medication may still be necessary. The person is "weaned" off the ketogenic diet over a period of several months to a year as small amounts of carbohydrates are added with observation for seizure reoccurrence.

Guillain-Barré Syndrome

Guillain-Barré syndrome (GBS) is an acute-onset, inflammatory, demyelinating polyneuropathy of the proximal motor nerves, including the cranial nerves and the diaphragm. The incidence is approximately 2 in 100,000.

Etiology

In 60% of cases the disorder follows an infection, surgery, or an immunization. Some of the more common organisms are *Campylobacter jejuni* and *Mycoplasma*. Several pathologic varieties exist, and the nature of the distinction is related to the segment of the immune system that is inflicting nerve damage. The clinical course of GBS is similar regardless of subtype, although GBS after a *Campylobacter* infection tends to be more severe.

Pathophysiology

Relatively symmetric weakness with **paresthesia** usually begins in the legs and progresses to the arms. The loss of function in affected nerves occurs because of demyelination. Myelin is the specialized fatty insulation that envelops the conducting part of the nerve, the axon. In GBS the immune system recognizes myelin and mounts an attack against it. Presumably myelin shares a common characteristic with the pathogen from the antecedent infection; thus the immune system cannot differentiate what is foreign (the pathogen) from what is native (myelin). When the nerve is demyelinated, its ability to conduct signals is severely impaired, resulting in neuropathy.

Medical Management

GBS reveals itself in a matter of days. The most common sequence of symptoms is areflexia (absence of reflexes), followed by proximal limb weakness, cranial nerve weakness and respiratory insufficiency. These symptoms normally peak by 2 weeks but may progress up to 1 month. Medical diagnosis is ordinarily made on clinical grounds, but nerve conduction studies are also beneficial. Before the clinical course is apparent, myelopathic disorders need to be considered.

Because of the precipitous progression of GBS, hospitalization is usually necessary. Vital capacity and swallowing function may rapidly deteriorate such that intensive care is sometimes necessary. Intubation and respiratory support should be instituted early in respiratory decline to avoid the need for resuscitation. Plasmapheresis, the exchange of the patient's plasma for albumin, is often helpful to reduce the load of circulating antibodies. Intravenous immunoglobulin or steroids have been shown to be of benefit.

Medical Nutrition Therapy

Guillain-Barré syndrome evolves quickly; during the acute stage, the metabolic response of GBS is similar to the stress response that occurs in neurotrauma. Energy needs assessed by indirect calorimetry may be as high as 40 to 45 kcal/kg and protein needs twice the usual amount. Supportive nutritional care should be offered to attenuate muscle wasting.

For a small percentage of patients, oropharyngeal muscles may be affected, leading to dysphagia and dysarthria. In this situation, a visit by the dietitian at mealtime can be a valuable way to observe difficulties the patient may have with chewing or swallowing. Specific difficulties warrant evaluation by a swallowing specialist. The speech therapist can evaluate the degree of dysphagia and make appropriate dietary recommendations pertaining to texture. As the patient recovers, it is important to discuss safe food handling and future prevention of *C. jejuni* infection.

Migraine Syndrome

The **migraine syndrome** is defined clinically as an episodic intense, throbbing head pain that lasts from 4 to 72 hours. It is usually on one side of the head and becomes worse with exertion. It may be accompanied by nausea and classically is associated with a prodrome of visual disturbances or unusual olfactory and gustatory perception. Most persons report an associated transient visual aura, including flashing lights. Migraines are more common between the ages 15 and 55 and affect women three times more often than men.

Pathophysiology

Although the cause is unknown, migraine headache is thought to be vascular in origin and follows a family history of migraines or of visual prodromata. The leading theory proposes that dural blood vessels become dilated and the pulsatile blood flow through these vessels distends and irritates the highly pain-sensitive dura mater. This would explain the throbbing quality of the headache. An inflammatory component to migraine headache is also present along with mitochondrial dysfunction (Gardner and Boles, 2010).

Medical Management

Treatment depends on the frequency of attacks and the presence of comorbid illness. A thorough history is the key to medical diagnosis. To qualify for a diagnosis of migraine headache, the headache must be throbbing, episodic, and supremely intense. A history of intercurrent nausea, vomiting, photophobia, and visual or olfactory auras should be present.

Numerous medicines are used to prevent or abort migraine, indicating a less than clear understanding of its pathophysiologic characteristics. NSAIDs are often the first line, followed by sympathomimetics and serotonin agonists such as sumatriptan. Prophylaxis can include calcium channel antagonists, β-adrenergic blockers, and serotonin antagonists.

Medical Nutrition Therapy

Migraine attacks are triggered by a variety of factors, including food, drugs, odors, and changes in sleep habits; they respond to a variety of treatments (Dowson et al., 2006). Because foods implicated in one individual may not trigger attacks in another and food intolerance thresholds vary over time, generalized recommendations about food avoidance are ill advised. There has been attention to biogenic amines such as tyramine or phenylethylamine in foods as triggers of migraine headaches. A trial of a tyramine- or phenylethylamine-restricted diet may be recommended for some clients (see Box 9-3 in Chapter 9 for biogenic amine–containing foods), but evidence is not clear on its success (Sun-Edelstein and Mauskop, 2009a). Because suspect food items or "trigger foods" can only be correctly identified if eliminated and then reintroduced into the diet, the dietitian can strategize on this approach. See Chapter 27 for a food diary form to record intake and timing of symptoms, and to determine which foods may be a problem. In some patients dehydration may be the instigator; one simple measure is to drink more water (at least 2-3 cups) to rehydrate (Blau, 2005; Spigt et al., 2005).

Many patients try herbs or botanical products or nutritional supplementation to manage their headaches. Feverfew is used by many migraine sufferers, even though a Cochrane Database Review has not proven its efficacy. Because of their roles in energy metabolism, two nutrients, riboflavin and coenzyme Q_{10}, have been suggested (Hershey et al., 2007; Schiapparelli et al., 2010). Magnesium has also been shown effective in treating migraine headaches (Sun-Edelstein and Mauskop, 2009b).

Myasthenia Gravis

Myasthenia gravis (MG) is the most well-known disorder of the neuromuscular junction. The neuromuscular junction is the site on the striated muscle membrane where a spinal motor neuron connects. Here the signal from the nerve is carried to the muscle via a submicron-size gap, a synapse. The molecule that carries the signal from the nerve ending to the muscle membrane is acetylcholine (Ach), and acetylcholine receptors (AchRs) populate the muscle membrane. These receptors translate the chemical signal of Ach into an electrical signal that is required for contraction of muscle fibers. MG is one of the most well-characterized autoimmune diseases, a class of disorders in which the body's immune system raises a response to AchRs. The incidence of MG is low, approximately 14 in 100,000 people.

Pathophysiology

In MG the body unwittingly makes antibodies to AchR. These antibodies are the same that fight off colds and give immunity. The AchR antibodies bind to AchR and make them unresponsive to Ach. There is no disorder of nerve conduction and no intrinsic disorder of muscle. The characteristic weakness in MG occurs because the signal of the nervous system to the muscle is garbled at the neuromuscular junction. Patients with MG commonly have an overactive thymus gland. This gland resides in the anterior thorax and plays a role in the maturation of B lymphocytes, the cells that are charged with synthesizing antibodies.

Medical Management

Relapsing and remitting weakness and fatigue, varying from minutes to days, characterize MG. The most common presentation is diplopia (double vision) caused by extraocular muscle weakness, followed by dysarthria, facial muscle weakness, and dysphagia. Dysphagia or swallowing disorders (resulting from fatigue following mastication) may cause malnutrition. Less commonly, proximal limb weakness in the hips and shoulders may be present. Severe diaphragmatic weakness can result in respiratory difficulty. No involvement of sensory nerves occurs.

Anticholinesterases are medicines that inhibit acetylcholinesterase, thus serving to increase the amount of Ach in the neuromuscular junction. Corticosteroids are immunosuppressive. Removal of the thymus results in symptomatic improvement in most patients.

Medical Nutrition Therapy

Chewing and swallowing are often compromised in MG. Because this compromise occurs with fatigue, it is important to provide nutritionally dense foods at the beginning of meals before the patient tires. Small, frequent meals that are easy to chew and swallow are helpful. Difficulties holding a bolus on the tongue have also been observed, suggesting that foods that do not fall apart easily may be better tolerated. For patients treated with anticholinesterase drugs, it is crucial to time medication with feeding to facilitate optimal swallowing.

Physical activity should be limited before mealtime to ensure maximum strength to eat a meal. It is also important not to encourage food consumption once the patient begins to tire because this may contribute to aspiration. If and when respiratory crisis occurs, it is usually temporary. Nutrition support via NG tube may be implemented in the interim to assist in maintaining vital functions of the patient until the crisis subsides. Once extubated, a swallow evaluation using cinefluoroscopy is appropriate to assess the degree of **deglutitory dysfunction** (swallowing irregularity) or risk of aspiration associated with an oral diet.

Multiple Sclerosis

Multiple sclerosis (MS) is a chronic disease that affects the CNS and is characterized by destruction of the myelin sheath, the function of which is transmission of electrical nerve impulses. Multiple areas of optic nerves, spinal cord, and brain undergo "sclerosis" whereby myelin is replaced with sclera or scar tissue. No single test can ascertain whether a patient has MS; however, diagnostic criteria (McDonald criteria) were developed for use by practicing clinicians (Polman et al., 2005).

The signs and symptoms of MS are easily distinguished, and they recur over the natural history of this disease. In the worst scenario MS can render a person unable to write, speak, or walk. Fortunately the majority of patients are only mildly affected. The prevalence is lower in equatorial areas, southern United States, and southern Europe; it is higher in Canada, northern Europe, and the northern United States. MS is the most common demyelinating disorder of the CNS, affecting 2.5 million people worldwide (Freedman, 2006).

Pathophysiology

The precise cause of MS remains undetermined. A familial predisposition to MS has been noted in a minority of cases. However, familial tendency is not well established and no consistent pattern of Mendelian inheritance has emerged (Victor and Ropper, 2005). Geographic latitude and diet are therefore implicated. Epidemiologic studies have linked the incidence of MS to geographic location and sunshine exposure. The degree of sunlight exposure catalyzes the production of vitamin D_3 in the skin. This form of vitamin D_3 is a selective immune system regulator and may inhibit MS progression (Mark and Carson, 2006). Further, in cross-sectional evaluations of MS and vitamin D, an increased prevalence of clinical vitamin D deficiency was associated with decreased bone density (Mark and Carson, 2006). Given the current evidence of the potential benefits of vitamin D, it appears to be reasonable and safe to consider vitamin D supplementation adequate to achieve normal levels in patients with MS (Solomon and Whitham, 2010).

Medical Management

Fluctuating symptoms and spontaneous remissions make treatments difficult to evaluate. Currently no proven treatment for changing the course of MS, preventing future attacks, or preventing deterioration exists. Initially recovery from relapses is nearly complete, but over time, neurologic deficits remain. Therefore measures to maximize recovery from initial attacks or exacerbations, prevent fatigue and infection, and use all of the available rehabilitative measures to postpone the bedridden stage of disease are imperative. Physical and occupational therapies are standard for weakness, spasticity, tremor, uncoordination, and other symptoms.

Drugs for spasticity can be initiated at a low dose and cautiously increased until the patient responds. Physical therapy for gait training and range-of-motion exercises helps. Steroid therapy is used in treating exacerbations; adrenocorticotropic hormone (ACTH) and prednisolone are the drugs of choice. However, treatment is not consistently effective and tends to be more useful in cases of less than 5 years' duration. Side effects of short-term steroid treatment include increased appetite, weight gain, fluid retention, nervousness, and insomnia. Reduced cerebrospinal fluid and serum levels of vitamin B_{12} and folate have been noted in MS patients who receive high-dose steroids. Methotrexate may also be used with ACTH, causing anorexia and nausea. Drug therapies may be a challenge (see Chapter 9 and Appendix 31).

Medical Nutrition Therapy

Several dietary regimens for managing MS have been studied, all of which have yielded equivocal results. Various diets such as allergen-free, gluten-free, pectin-free, fructose-restricted, raw food diet, megadoses of micronutrients, zinc phosphates with calcium, and other combinations have been ruled ineffective. The RD's evaluation of the patient to maximize nutritional intake is imperative. Vitamin D status should be assessed by measuring 25-hydroxy vitamin D and supplementation may be warranted; total intake should be monitored from multivitamin and mineral supplements and fortified foods (Brown, 2006).

As the disease progresses, neurologic deficits and dysphasia may occur as the result of damaged cranial nerves. Thus diet consistency may need to be modified from solids to mechanically soft or pureed items, even progressing to thick liquids to prevent aspiration. Impaired vision, dysarthria, and poor ambulation make meal preparation into a difficult task. In this situation reliance on comfort foods or prepackaged, single-serving, or convenience foods often permits independent preparation of meals. Given the chronic nature of this debilitating disease, patients may require enteral nutrition support.

Neurogenic bladder is common, causing urinary incontinence, urgency, and frequency. To minimize these problems, distributing fluids evenly throughout the waking hours and limiting them before bed is helpful. Some patients limit fluid intake severely to decrease frequency of urination but thereby increase the risk of UTIs. UTIs are common in patients with MS, and some patients increase their intake of cranberry juice as a form of self-treatment (see Chapter 36).

Neurogenic bowel can cause either constipation or diarrhea, and incidence of fecal impaction is increased in MS. A diet that is high in fiber with additional prunes and adequate fluid can moderate both problems.

Parkinson's Disease

Parkinson's disease (PD) is a progressive, disabling, neurodegenerative disease, first described by James Parkinson in 1817. PD is characterized by slow and decreased movement, muscular rigidity, resting tremor, postural instability, and decreased dopamine transmission to the basal ganglia. Although the natural history of this disease can be remarkably benign in some cases, approximately 66% of patients are disabled within 5 years, and 80% are disabled after 10 years (Victor and Ropper, 2005).

PD is one of the most common neurologic diseases in North America; it affects approximately 1% of the population older than 65 years of age. The incidence is similar across socioeconomic groups, although PD is less common in blacks and Asians in comparison with whites. It most commonly occurs between the ages of 40 and 70.

Pathophysiology

Although the cause of PD remains unclear, it is multifactorial and the pathogenesis is well described. It involves an interaction of inheritance with environmental factors. There is a marked loss of dopaminergic neurons (pigmented cells) in the substantia nigra, as well as tyrosine hydroxylase, the rate-limiting enzyme for dopamine.

In studying the brains of people with PD after they die, accumulations of protein called *Lewy bodies* (named after the doctor who first found them) are found. More than 10 genes causing familial PD have been identified. Genetic testing for PD is not warranted at this time, but continued investigations hold promise.

The role of endogenous toxins from cellular oxidative reactions has emerged because aging has been associated with a loss of neurons containing dopamine and an increase in monoamine oxidase. When metabolized (enzymatic oxidation and autooxidation), dopamine produces endogenous toxins (hydrogen peroxide and free radicals), causing peroxidation of membrane lipids and cell death. In the presence of an inherited or acquired predisposition, severe oxidative injury can lead to substantial loss of dopaminergic neurons similar to that observed in PD.

Several other environmental factors have also been implicated as causal factors of PD. The connection between smoking and a lowered risk for PD has been evaluated, but results are inconsistent (Zhang et al., 2006). In older patients, drug-induced PD may occur as a side effect of neuroleptics or metoclopramide (see Chapter 9 and Appendix 31).

Nutrient-related findings are biologically plausible and support the hypothesis that oxidative stress may contribute to the pathogenesis of PD (Czlonkowska et al, 2010). The relationships of folate, elevated plasma homocysteine levels, fiber and caloric deficits are being evaluated. Vitamin B_6 intake may also decrease the risk of PD (De Lau et al., 2006). The final environmental factor associated with the incidence of PD is exposure to chemicals and toxins, as in farming communities where pesticides are used. However, no one chemical toxin or heavy metal is known as the cause (Victor and Ropper, 2005).

Medical Management

The "classic triad" signs—tremor at rest, rigidity, and bradykinesia—remain the criterion for medical diagnosis. However, it was well over a century before l-dopa (a precursor to dopamine) was introduced for controlling symptoms. Exelon, a cholinesterase inhibitor, was approved by the FDA in 2006 for use in mild to moderate PD dementia. Pharmacotherapy agents, surgical interventions, and physical therapy are the best adjunctive therapies.

Medical Nutrition Therapy

The primary nutrition intervention should be to focus on drug-nutrient interactions, especially between dietary protein and l-dopa. Side effects of medications for PD include anorexia, nausea, reduced sense of smell, constipation, and dry mouth. To diminish the gastrointestinal side effects of l-dopa, it should be taken with meals. Avoid foods that contain natural l-dopa such as broad beans (fava beans). For some patients dyskinesia may be reduced by limiting dietary protein at breakfast and lunch and including it in the evening meal. Table 41-11 presents a sample menu for this diet.

Fiber and fluid adequacy lessen constipation, a common concern for persons with PD. Interactions between pyridoxine and aspartame should be considered as well. Pyridoxine has a possible interaction with l-dopa. Decarboxylase, the enzyme required to convert l-dopa to dopamine, depends on pyridoxine. If excessive amounts of the vitamin are present, l-dopa may be metabolized in the periphery and not in the CNS where its therapeutic activity occurs. Therefore vitamin preparations containing pyridoxine should not be taken with doses of l-dopa. In addition, manganese should be carefully monitored to avoid excesses above DRI levels.

The high demand for molecular oxygen, the enrichment of polyunsaturated fatty acids in membrane phospholipids, and the relatively low abundance of antioxidant defense enzymes are all relevant factors (Sun et al., 2008). Antiinflammatory and neuroprotective effects come from phenolic compounds, such as resveratrol from grapes and red wine, curcumin from turmeric, apocynin from Picrorhiza kurroa, and epigallocatechin from green tea (Sun et al., 2008). Sufficient intake of vitamin D_3 and ω-3 fatty acids can be suggested.

As the disease progresses, rigidity of the extremities can interfere with the patient's ability to perform self-feeding. Rigidity interferes with the ability to control the position of the head and trunk, necessary for eating. Eating is slowed; mealtimes can take up to an hour. Simultaneous movements such as those required to handle both a knife and fork

TABLE 41-11

Dietary Protein Redistribution with L-Dopa Therapy

	Amount of Protein (g)
Breakfast	
½ C oatmeal	2
1 orange	0.5
1 C Rice Dream beverage	0.5
Egg Replacer (unlimited)	0
Low-protein bread toast	0
Margarine or butter (unlimited)	0
Jelly or jam (unlimited)	0
Sugar or sugar substitute (unlimited)	0
Coffee or tea (unlimited)	0
Lunch	
½ C vegetable soup	2
1 C tossed salad	1
Salad dressing (unlimited)	0
1 banana	1
Low-protein pasta (unlimited)	0
Margarine or butter (unlimited)	0
Low-protein cookies (unlimited)	0
Juice, coffee, tea, or water	0
Afternoon Snack	
Gum drops or hard candy (unlimited)	0
Apple or cranberry juice (unlimited)	0
TOTAL	7
Dinner	
4 oz (at least) beef, pork, veal, chicken	28 or more
1 C stuffing	4
Gravy	0
½ C peas	2
¾ C yogurt	8
1 C milk	8
Evening Snack	
1 oz cheese or deli meat	7
4 crackers	2
Juice, herbal tea or water	0
DAILY TOTAL	66 or more

become difficult. Tremor in the arms and hands may make self-feeding of liquids impossible without spilling. Perception and spatial organization can become impaired.

Dysphagia is often a late complication. A large number of patients may be silent aspirators, which affects nutrition status.

Experimental treatment procedures are being tested and reported with increasing frequency. Deep brain penetration, other surgical interventions, and efforts with stem cell research continue in hopes that a "cure" is possible.

CLINICAL SCENARIO

Clarence is a 74-year-old white man hospitalized for evaluation of dementia progression and recent hearing difficulty. He was diagnosed with Alzheimer's disease 5 years ago and has been taking donepezil (Aricept) and furosemide (Lasix). He lives at home with his 68-year-old Italian wife who is his primary caregiver. Clarence is 5′10″ and currently weighs 155 lb. His medical chart indicates that his weight was 170 lb at his last hospital visit 6 months ago, following a fall. Clarence's wife notes that his appetite and hearing seem to have changed and he shows little interest in food at meal times. They don't talk much during home meals and nursing staff have observed his wife helping him eat and suspect some problems with feeding. His wife describes their meals as follows:

Breakfast: ½ C oatmeal, ½ C 2% milk, 1 orange ; food is usually consumed while watching the morning news

Lunch: ½ C vegetable beef soup, ½ turkey sandwich with white bread, light mayonnaise, lettuce, tomato slice, 10 baby carrots, water

Supper: frozen TV dinner (generally small meat serving, vegetable, and starch item;) TV is on in the background

Nutrition Diagnostic Statement

Increased energy expenditure
Inadequate fluid intake
Chewing (mastication) difficulty
Self-feeding difficulty

Nutrition Care Questions

1. What dietary advice do you have for Clarence and his caregiver?
2. What types of foods and eating environment are more appropriate for individuals with Alzheimer's disease?
3. Develop a plan for monitoring and evaluating Clarence.

USEFUL WEBSITES

Alzheimer's Disease Education and Referral Center
http://www.nia.nih.gov/Alzheimer's

American Stroke Association
http://www.strokeassociation.org

Epilepsy Foundation
http://www.epilepsyfoundation.org

Migraine Awareness Group
http://www.migraines.org

Myasthenia Gravis
http://www.myasthenia.org

National Headache Foundation
http://www.headaches.org

National Human Genome Research Institute
http://www.genome.gov
National Institute of Neurological Disorders and Stroke
http://www.ninds.nih.gov/
National Institutes of Health: Swallowing Disorders
http://www.ninds.nih.gov/disorders/swallowing_disorders/swallowing_disorders.htm
National Institute of Neurologic Disorders and Stroke: Stroke Page
http://www.ninds.nih.gov/disorders/stroke/stroke.htm
Parkinson's Disease Foundation
http://www.pdf.org/en/symptoms

REFERENCES

American Dietetic Association: Spinal cord injury and nutrition guideline. Accessed 30 October 2010 from http://www.adaevidencelibrary.com/category.cfm?cid=14&cat=0

Anekonda TS: Resveratrol—a boon for treating Alzheimer's disease? *Brain Res Rev* 52:316, 2006.

Blau JN: Water deprivation: a new migraine precipitant? *Headache* 45:757, 2005.

Brain Trauma Foundation: *Guidelines for the management of severe traumatic brain injury*, ed 3, New York, 2007, Brain Trauma Foundation. Accessed 30 October 2010 from http://www.braintrauma.org/pdf/protected/Guidelines_Management_2007w_bookmarks.pdf.

Bough KJ, Rho JM: Anticonvulsant mechanisms of the ketogenic diet, *Epilepsia* 48:43, 2007.

Brown SJ: The role of vitamin D in multiple sclerosis, *Ann Pharmacother* 40:1158, 2006.

Bulat RD, Orlando RC: Oropharyngeal dysphagia, *Curr Treat Options Gastroenterol* 8:269, 2005.

Callahan CM, et al: Effectiveness of collaborative care for older adults with Alzheimer's disease in primary care, *JAMA* 295:2148, 2006.

Centers for Disease Control and Prevention: *Heart disease and stroke*, 2006. Accessed 30 June 2006 from http://www.cdc.gov/nccdphp/scientific.htm.

Chauhan NB: Multiplicity of garlic health effects and Alzheimer's disease, *J Nutr Health Aging* 9:421, 2005.

Czaplinski A, et al: Amyotrophic lateral sclerosis: early predictors of prolonged survival, *J Neurol* 13 June:2226, 2006.

Czlonkowska A, Kurkowska-Jastrzebska I: Inflammation and gliosis in neurological diseases—clinical implications, *J Neuroimmunol* 231:78, 2011.

De Lau LM, et al: Dietary folate, vitamin B_{12}, and vitamin B_6 and the risk of Parkinson's disease, *Neurology* 67:315, 2006.

Deon M, et al: The effect of Lorenzo's oil on oxidative stress in X-linked adrenoleukodystrophy, *J Neurol Sci* 247(2):157, 2006.

Dowson AJ, et al: Review of clinical trials using acute intervention with oral triptans for migraine management, *Int J Clin Pract* 60:698, 2006.

Epilepsy Foundation: Statistics, 2006. Accessed 30 June 2006 from http://www.epilepsyfoundation.org/answerplace/statistics.cfm.

Freedman MS: Disease-modifying drugs for multiple sclerosis: current and future aspects, *Expert Opin Pharmacother* 7:S1, 2006.

Fioravanti M, Yangi M: Cytidinediphophocholine (CDP-choline) for cognitive and behavioral disturbances associated with chronic cerebral disorders in the elderly, Cochrane Database of Systematic Reviews 2010. Accessed 28 March 2011 from http://onlinelibrary.wiley.com/o/cochrane/clsysrev/articles/CD000269/pdf_fs.html.

Gardner A, Boles RG: Beyond the serotonin hypothesis: mitochondria, inflammation and neurodegeneration in major depression and affective spectrum disorders, *Prog Neuropsychopharmacol Biol Psychiatry* 35:730, 2011.

Goldstein LB, et al: Primary prevention of ischemic stroke: a guideline from the American Heart Association/American Stroke Association Stroke Council, *Stroke* 37:1583, 2006.

Groomes LB, et al: Do patients with absence epilepsy respond to ketogenic diets, *J Child Neurol* 26:160, 2011.

Gu Y, et al: Food combination and Alzheimer's disease risk, *Arch Neurol* 67:699, 2010.

Hershey AD, et al: Coenzyme Q_{10} deficiency and response to supplementation in pediatrics and adolescent migraine, *Headache* 47:73, 2007.

International Alliance of ALS: *What is ALS/MND?* Accessed 22 March 2010 from www.alsmndalliance.org/whatis.html.

Jaeger PA, Wyss-Coray T: Beclin 1 complex in autophagy and Alzheimer's disease, *Arch Neurol* 67:1181, 2010.

Kidd PM: Neurodegeneration from mitochondrial insufficiency: nutrients, stem cells, growth factors, and prospects for brain rebuilding using integrative management, *Altern Med Rev* 10:268, 2005.

Kossoff EH, et al: Optimal clinical management of children receiving the ketogenic diet: recommendations of the International Ketogenic Diet Study Group, *Epilepsia* 50:304, 2009.

Mark BL, Carson JA: Vitamin D and autoimmune disease—implications for practice from the multiple sclerosis literature, *J Am Diet Assoc* 106:418, 2006.

Moser HW: Therapy of X-linked adrenoleukodystrophy, *NeuroRx* 3:246, 2006.

National Institutes of Health: *Stroke*, 2006. Accessed 22 March 2011 from http://www.ninds.nih.gov/.

Nordlund A, Oliveberg M: Folding of Cu/Zn superoxide dismutase suggests structural hotspots for gain of neurotoxic function in ALS: parallels to precursors in amyloid disease, *Proc Natl Acad Sci USA* 103:10218, 2006.

Patel A, et al: Long-term outcomes of children treated with the ketogenic diet in the past, *Epilepsia* 51:1277, 2010.

Polman CH, et al: Diagnostic criteria for multiple sclerosis: 2005 revisions to the "McDonald" criteria, *Ann Neurol* 58:840, 2005.

Porta N, et al: The ketogenic diet and its variants: state of the art, *Rev Neurol* 165:430, 2009.

Querfurth HW, LaFerla FM: Alzheimer's disease, *N Engl J Med* 362:329, 2010.

Ramesh BN, et al: Neuronutrition and Alzheimer's disease, *J Alzheimer's Dis* 19:1123, 2010.

Raymond GV, et al: Head trauma can initiate the onset of adrenoleukodystrophy, *J Neurol Sci* 290:70, 2010.

Schiapparelli P, et al: Non-pharmacological approach to migraine prophylaxis: part II, *Neurol Sci* 31(Suppl 1):S137, 2010.

Sharma S, et al: A pyrazole curcumin derivative restores membrane homeostasis disrupted after brain trauma, *Exp Neurol* 226:191, 2010.

Shetty AK: Reelin signaling, hippocampal neurogenesis, and efficacy of aspirin intake & stem cell transplantation in aging and Alzheimer's disease, *Aging Dis* 1:2, 2010.

Solomon AJ, Whitham RH: Multiple sclerosis and vitamin D: a review and recommendations, *Curr Neurol Neurosci Rep* 10:389, 2010.

Soto ME, et al: Rapid cognitive decline: searching for a definition and predictive factors among elderly with Alzheimer's disease, *J Nutr Health Aging* 9:158, 2005.

Spigt MG, et al: Increasing the daily water intake for the prophylactic treatment of headache: a pilot trial, *Europ J Neurol* 12:715, 2005.

Strand EA, et al: Management of oral-pharyngeal dysphagia symptoms in amyotrophic lateral sclerosis, *Dysphagia* 11:129, 1996.

Su HM: Mechanisms of n-3 fatty acid-mediated development and maintenance of learning memory performance, *J Nutr Biochem* 21:364, 2010.

Sun AY, et al: Botanical phenolics and brain health, *Neuromolecular Med* 10:259, 2008.

Sun-Edelstein C, Mauskop A: Foods and supplements in the management of migraine headaches, *Clin J Pain* 25:446, 2009a.

Sun-Edelstein C, Mauskop A: Role of magnesium in the pathogenesis and treatment of migraine, *Expert Rev Neurother* 9:369, 2009b.

Tan J, et al: Lack of effect of oral choline supplement on the concentrations of choline metabolites in human brain, *Magn Reson Med* 39:1005, 1998

Victor M, Ropper AH: *Adams and Victor's principles of neurology*, ed 8, New York, 2005, McGraw-Hill, Health Professions Division.

Wang L, et al: Performance-based physical function and future dementia in older people, *Arch Intern Med* 166:1115, 2006.

Weber S, et al: Modified Atkins diet to children and adolescents with medical intractable epilepsy, *Seizure* 18:237, 2009.

Wollen KA: Alzheimer's Disease: the pros and cons of pharmaceutical, nutritional, botanical, and stimulatory therapies, with a discussion of treatment strategies from the perspective of patients and practitioners, *Altern Med Rev* 15:223, 2010.

Zeisel SH, Caudill MA: Choline, *Advances in Nutrition* 1:46, 2010.

Zhang ML, et al: Dietary factors and smoking as risk factors for PD in a rural population in China: a nested case-control study, *Acta Neurol Scand* 113:278, 2006.

Zoccolella S, et al: Homocysteine levels and amyotrophic lateral sclerosis: a possible link, *Amytroph Lateral Scler* 11:140, 2010.

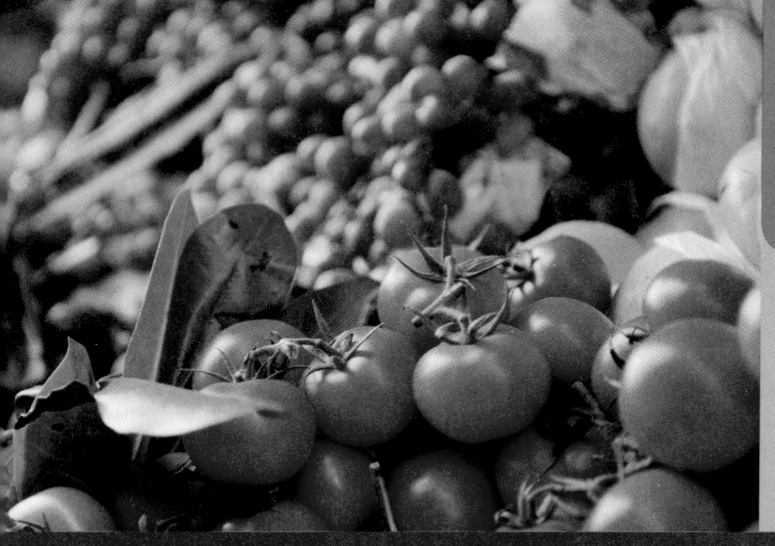

CHAPTER 42

Gretchen K. Vannice, MS, RD

Medical Nutrition Therapy for Psychiatric Conditions

KEY TERMS

alpha-linolenic acid (ALA)
arachidonic acid (ARA)
attention-deficit disorder (ADD)
axis I disorders
axis II disorders
borderline personality disorder
***Diagnostic and Statistical Manual,* IV (DSM-IV)**
depression
docosahexaenoic acid (DHA)
eicosapentaenoic acid (EPA)
Minnesota Multiphasic Personality Inventory
phytochemicals
post-partum depression
post-traumatic stress disorder (PTSD)

Psychiatric disorders (mental illnesses) involve altered brain or nervous system function that may result in altered perception and response to the environment. There are more than 450 million people with mental, neurologic, or behavioral problems throughout the world (World Health Organization, 2010). One in four individuals will suffer some type of mental illness during their lifetime. Indeed, many famous individuals have suffered from mental illnesses in the past (*Focus On:* Who Has Suffered from Mental Illness?)

CLASSIFICATION

The American Psychiatric Association classifies conditions into two different categories: *Axis I* and *Axis II disorders.* **Axis I disorders** often do not improve without medication. In fact, left unchecked, they can be degenerative and permanently destructive to brain and nervous system tissue. **Axis II disorders** are personality disorders. These disorders are primarily learned behaviors and do not respond to medication, with the possible exception of bipolar disorders, which may respond to very-long chain ω-3 fatty acids (e.g., fish oil) supplementation.

Axis I Disorders

The primary Axis I disorders include depression, anxiety disorder, obsessive-compulsive disorder, bipolar disorder, attention-deficit/hyperactivity disorder (ADHD), schizophrenia, and post-traumatic stress disorder (PTSD). The eating disorders (anorexia nervosa, bulimia nervosa, and binge eating disorder) are also classified as Axis I disorders. Thus eating disorders are not merely behavioral issues; they require medical, nutritional, and often pharmacologic treatment in addition to psychotherapy. See Chapter 23. These interventions can be the foundation for successful response to psychotherapy. Nutrition is crucial for the rehabilitation of every mental health issue, not just eating disorders. In 1990 the United States Congress voted to establish the first week of October as Mental Illness Awareness Week, and much progress has been made in the past several decades. Box 42-1 lists psychiatric disorders that can have nutritional implications.

Despite their strong physiologic component, Axis I disorders are diagnosed primarily through behavioral criteria and psychological testing (e.g., the **Minnesota Multiphasic**

Sections of this chapter were written by Monica Woolsey, MS, RD for the previous edition of this text.

FOCUS ON

Who Has Suffered from Mental Illness?

April 20, 1999, Littleton, Colorado: 13 students and 1 teacher were killed, 23 students and 1 teacher wounded in a shootout at Columbine High School.

December 7, 2005, Miami, Florida: A 44-year-old man was shot and killed by air marshals as he ran from a plane claiming he was carrying a bomb.

May 4, 2010, Los Angeles, California: A woman stabs four people at a Target in West Hollywood.

What do these news items have in common? Each of these tragedies involved a person with a mental illness. In addition, in each of the news stories cited, for various reasons, the individual was not using medications to help his or her condition at the time he was involved in the tragic event. Unfortunately, when mental health issues appear in the news, they are often related to tragedies such as these.

What is often overlooked is that some of history's most illustrious and creative individuals accomplished their greatest achievements while also managing the mental chaos, disruption in logical thinking, and hypersensitivity to stress that mental diagnoses can impose on the brain and nervous system. It is to the credit of all of these individuals and to the benefit of all of us who enjoy the outcomes of their labor that they persisted and created in spite of their struggles and emotional turmoil. Famous living and historical figures who had mental illness include Sir Isaac Newton, Ernest Hemingway, Charles Dickens, Michelangelo, Tennessee Williams, Ludwig van Beethoven, Terry Bradshaw, Brooke Shields, President Abraham Lincoln, Winston Churchill, and Vincent van Gogh.

Source: Mental Health Ministries. Accessed 2 November 2010 from http://www.mentalhealthministries.net/links_resources/other_resources/famouspeople.pdf.

BOX 42-1

Psychiatric Conditions with Nutritional Implications

- Autism spectrum disorders
- Attention-deficit/hyperactivity disorder
- Bipolar disorder
- Borderline personality disorder
- Dissociative disorders
- Dual diagnosis: mental illness and substance abuse disorder
- Eating disorders
- Major depression
- Obsessive-compulsive disorder
- Panic disorder
- Post-traumatic stress disorder
- Schizoaffective disorder
- Schizophrenia
- Seasonal affective disorder
- Suicide
- Tourette syndrome

Personality Inventory). Because there currently is no definitive diagnostic testing (e.g., blood tests, genetic tests, brain scans) for these disorders, it can be difficult to convince a person with such a diagnosis that he or she has a medical issue requiring treatment. It can also be difficult for friends, family members, and colleagues to understand that challenging behaviors affecting relationships and productivity are sometimes medical or biochemical in origin. For both parties, frustration, shame, and destructive behavior can result from attempting to willfully change behaviors that will not respond to anything less than intensive biologic intervention.

Altered food or eating behaviors can be the first indication that an Axis I disorder exists. For example, a person with obsessive-compulsive disorder may struggle making choices in grocery stores and restaurants, where a multitude of choices exist. They may seek help from a registered dietitian (RD) for specific direction (e.g., "just tell me what to eat") to lessen the stress that these daily activities can induce. A person with bipolar disorder may alternate between periods of mania and depression. During the manic phase consumption of sugar, caffeine, and large quantities of food can be extreme and during the depression phase food intake may cease completely. These mood fluctuations often manifest as weight fluctuations and can even be misidentified as hypoglycemia. Often the medical comorbidity, not the core mental health diagnosis, is the reason an individual seeks an initial nutrition consultation.

A nutritionist's job is to recognize unusual eating behaviors so that appropriate recommendations for treatment can be made. In general, when an individual seems to be genuinely trying to follow nutrition treatment recommendations or to change behavior, yet seems to be driven to behaviors that counter those intentions, the existence of an Axis I disorder should always be considered and the individual should be evaluated.

Axis II Disorders

The personality disorders listed in the American Psychological Association, **Diagnostic and Statistical Manual, IV (DSM-IV)** include antisocial, narcissistic, histrionic, schizoid, avoidant, dependent, and borderline behavior. Psychotherapy is required to achieve symptom relief. Axis II disorders differ from Axis I disorders because, to the individual who has an Axis II disorder, the personality change serves an important purpose. A person with low self-esteem or who knows from experience that he or she struggles with interpersonal relationships may develop an Axis II disorder to prevent abandonment. For a person who does not have alternative communication, conflict resolution or coping skills, the perceived potential loss of that connection to others can be traumatizing. Whereas treating an Axis I disorder can provide great relief and improved well-being, treating an Axis II disorder may actually temporarily *increase* distress and behavioral acting out as treatment progresses.

Comorbidity

Axis I and Axis II disorders are often comorbid conditions. When an Axis I diagnosis impairs an individual's ability to interact with his or her environment, an Axis II disorder may develop as a coping mechanism. For example, a person with **post-traumatic stress disorder (PTSD)** is likely to be easily overstimulated and fluctuate between periods of intense anxiety and depression. **Borderline personality disorder** is a common condition occurring comorbidly with PTSD. This person with this personality type often engages in extreme behaviors, including hypersexuality, emotional volatility, poor impulse control, manipulative behavior, and suicide attempts to (1) provide an emotional diversion from the physical wear and tear that the PTSD inflicts, and (2) maintain relationships with loved ones the individual perceives might otherwise abandon him or her.

NUTRITION FOR THE BRAIN AND NERVOUS SYSTEM

One of the most important contributions of nutrition to mental health is the maintenance of the structure and function of the neurons and brain centers coordinating communication within the body and between the body and the environment. See *Pathophysiology and Care Management Algorithm:* Psychiatric Disorders.

Omega-3 Fatty Acids

Omega-3 (ω-3) polyunsaturated fatty acids are preferred fatty acids in the brain and nervous system. From conception through maturity, eicosapentaenoic acid (EPA) and docosahexaenoic acid (DHA) ω-3 fatty acids make unique, important, and irreplaceable contributions to overall brain and nervous system functioning. Clinical research has shown effective and promising roles for EPA and DHA ω-3 fats in various psychiatric conditions.

Alpha-linolenic acid (ALA), another ω-3 fat with a chain length of 18 carbons and 3 double bonds (18:3 ω-3), is found in the oil of some seeds (e.g., flax, chia, sunflower) and some nuts (walnuts are the best source). **Eicosapentaenoic acid (EPA)** is a 20-carbon ω-3 fatty acid with 5 double bonds (20:5 ω-3), and **docosahexaenoic acid (DHA)** is a 22-carbon fatty acid with 6 double bonds (22:6 ω-3). EPA and DHA occur naturally in fatty fish and seafood.

Conversion Factors

ALA serves as a precursor for EPA and DHA. Research has shown that conversion of ALA to EPA and DHA in humans is low: conversion of ALA to EPA is approximately 5% to 10%, and conversion of ALA to DHA is even lower (<3%). Health status and other nutritional factors appear to influence conversion rates. There are also genetic variations in conversion (e.g., production of delta-6 desaturase enzyme), and recent studies have suggested possible differences in conversion rates between vegetarians and carnivores. Individuals with mental health conditions often have compromised nutritional intake or eating habits. Most nutrition and mental health experts do not recommend reliance on ALA as a source of EPA or DHA (Davis and Kris-Etherton, 2003; Harris et al, 2009; Kris-Etherton and Innis, 2007).

Omega-3s, Omega-6s and Mental Health

EPA works in balance with **arachidonic acid (ARA)**, a 20-carbon ω-6 fatty acid with 4 double bonds (20:4 ω-6). ARA and EPA are eicosanoids, that is, precursors to prostaglandins, thromboxanes, and leukotrienes, which are involved with inflammation, vasoconstriction, and a multitude of metabolic regulations. Although specific mechanisms remain unclear, clinical research has shown the importance of sufficient EPA intake for general mental health, and particularly for nutrition support in conditions such as depression, suicide ideation, and homicide. In general, EPA works better when ingested with DHA. They also occur together naturally in foods.

DHA is preferred and selectively stored in brain and nerve cells. Similar to EPA, DHA is involved with metabolic regulation. DHA is required for normal brain growth, development, and maturation. DHA is involved with neurotransmission (how brain cells communicate with each other), lipid messaging, genetic expression, and cell membrane synthesis. DHA also provides vital structural contributions; DHA is concentrated in the phospholipids of brain cell membranes. Box 42-2 lists conditions in which DHA and EPA play a role.

Diet Is First

Although deep-sea oily fish such as salmon and tuna contain more EPA and DHA per serving, all fish and seafood contain

BOX 42-2

Some Conditions for Which EPA and DHA have Benefit

Anxiety disorder
Attention-deficit/hyperactivity disorder
Autism
Bipolar disorders
Depression
Dyspraxia
Eating disorders
Postpartum depression
Schizophrenia
Suicide ideation

DHA, Docosahexaenoic acid; *EPA*, eicosapentaenoic acid.

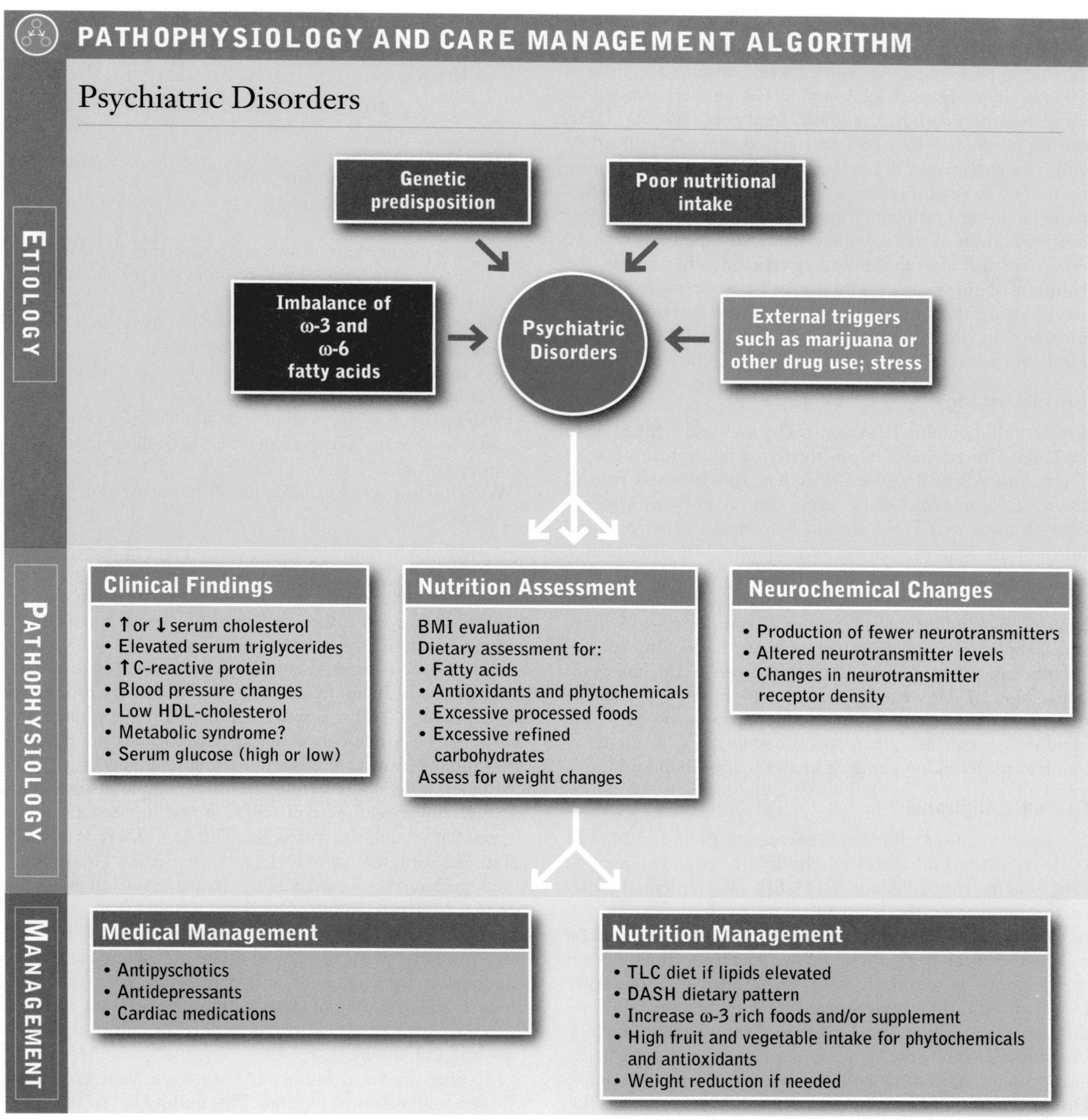

some ω-3 in varying amounts. Sardines, for example, are an excellent choice, whereas tilapia is low in ω-3 fatty acids. There are additional benefits of consuming fish in the diet; fish provides lean protein and trace minerals and can displace other less nutritious food choices. However, the white fish used in processed food fish fillets is lower in ω-3; and because of the added batter and frying, the caloric contribution of ω-3s may be less than the other fat calories in these convenience foods. See Appendix 40.

During Pregnancy and Lactation

Experts recommend that pregnant women consume at least 200-300 mg DHA during pregnancy for proper infant development (Koletzko, 2007). The role of DHA and EPA in pregnancy and lactation is discussed in Chapter 16.

Up to 10% of pregnant women can experience depression, and there is considerable interest in finding effective alternatives to prescription medication. Several pilot trials using EPA and DHA from fish oil have been conducted in depressed pregnant women and women with **postpartum depression**. One dose-ranging study reported measurable improvements in women who consumed as little as 500 mg of combined EPA and DHA. Experts have also recently suggested that a daily intake of 900 mg DHA during pregnancy may be necessary to support both infant and maternal needs. A landmark study that followed more than 9000 pregnant women and their children for 8 years reported lower intelligence quotient and social development in the children of those women who consumed less than 12 ounces of fish a week while pregnant. In other words, the children of the women who ate fish two or more times a week during their pregnancy fared better emotionally and mentally in their youth (Freeman et al, 2006a, 2006b; Hibbeln et al, 2007b, Hibbeln and Davis, 2009).

During Infancy

Breast milk contains EPA and DHA ω-3 and ARA ω-6. In 2002 the United States began fortifying infant formula with DHA and ARA. Because DHA has an identified role in infant development (brain, eyes, central nervous system), experts agree that DHA should be considered an essential nutrient in infancy, particularly among preterm infants. DHA accumulation in the brain begins in utero and continues into adolescence. It is important to remember that humans (including infants) cannot synthesize ω-3 fatty acids; the amount taken in depends on the feeding source. Infants can convert EPA and DHA from ALA, but again conversion of ALA to DHA has been shown to be inadequate for infant needs. A precise role for ω-3s in neurologic conditions, such as autism spectrum disorder, is currently being considered but remains unclear. See Chapter 45.

During Childhood

Depression among children is increasing. The few clinical trials conducted in depressed children have shown significant benefit from EPA and DHA fish oil supplementation. At the same time, the few studies measuring consumption of EPA and DHA in children report very low average intakes.

Most clinical trials using EPA and DHA from fish oil supplements in children with **attention-deficit disorder (ADD)** or ADHD have reported benefit, but not all. The difference in findings may be due to many variables, including study design, dose, age of supplementation, the background diet, genetics, and teacher or family dynamics. However, it has been shown that children with ADD, ADHD, behavior problems, or who are overweight tend to have lower levels of EPA and DHA in their blood (Antalis et al, 2006; Richardson, 2000, 2006). Box 42-3 lists questions about fatty acids and a person's early feeding history that may be useful in a nutrition assessment.

BOX 42-3

Questionnaire: Early Feeding History and Fatty Acid Intake

Were you born at term?
If you were born early, how early?
Did your premature birth affect how and what you were fed?
Did your mother have prolonged postpartum depression after you were born? If yes, how did this influence your feeding?
Were you nursed or bottle-fed? For how long? In what country? If formula-fed, which formula?
How many children did your mother have and nurse and for how long each time?
Where are you in the rank of your siblings? (Essential fatty acid availability may decrease with successive pregnancies).
Women: How many children have you nursed? For how long?

During Adulthood

According to the World Health Organization, major depression is the leading cause of disability around the world. **Depression** is a mental health condition; diagnosis and treatment by a mental health professional is recommended. A significant number of depressed individuals feel ashamed and do not seek treatment. Those who suffer from depression tend to report lower quality of life, social impairment, and problems in the workplace. Data from the National Health and Nutrition Examination Survey suggests that more than 1 in 20 adults in the United States are experiencing depression, and it is more common among women and the poor. Depression is often associated with poor health and higher health care costs.

Epidemiologic research has identified associations between lower seafood consumption and increased rates of depression around the world. See Fig. 42-1. Dozens of clinical studies using EPA and DHA ω-3 supplements for depression have been conducted, and results are mixed but generally positive (Martins, 2009). Questions remain regarding the dose of ω-3s, the form, and the duration of supplementation. In 2011 more than 30 clinical trials are investigating the relationship between ω-3s and depression. Omega-3s are often provided in conjunction with antidepressant medication and usually show additive benefit (Freeman et al, 2006a; Jazayeri et al, 2008).

Increases in homicide occurrence have been associated with less seafood consumption. This finding led to an article in the *New York Times* entitled "Does Eating Salmon Lower the Murder Rate?" (Mihm, 2006). When EPA and DHA ω-3s and multivitamins were given to prison inmates, antisocial behavior, including violence, fell significantly, compared with those on placebo. In another study, teens who had previously attempted suicide made fewer suicide attempts when given EPA and DHA (Hallahan et al, 2007; Hibbeln, 2001, 2007a).

During the Aging Years

Omega-3 fatty acids are also considered important in maintaining cognitive function with age. Research suggests

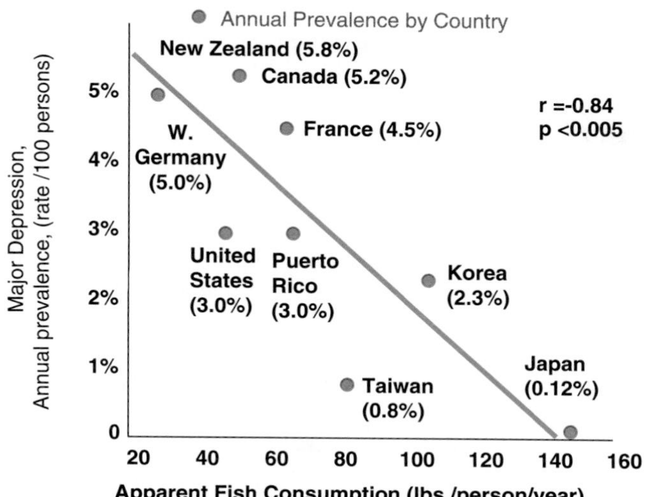

FIGURE 42-1 Fish Consumption and Major Depression This inverse relationship between the amount of fish consumed by a population and the incidence of depression in that population is thought to be related to amount of ω-3 fats contributed by fish in the diet, and resulting body and brain tissue levels of ω-3 fats. *(Hibbeln JR: Fish consumption and major depression, Lancet 351:1213, 1998.)*

that individuals who consume more fish and seafood during their lifetimes have better cognitive function as they age. Higher blood levels of DHA have been associated with better cognitive function in middle adulthood. Some studies have shown that eating fish or supplementing with EPA and DHA ω-3s improves cognition (e.g., delays cognitive decline) and the onset of dementia, but not all studies report positive findings and questions remain, including the role of genetics in risk factors for onset of cognitive difficulties. Researchers and dietitians question if EPA and DHA ω-3s have a greater effect in prevention or intervention for mental health (Dangour et al, 2010; Muldoon et al, 2010; Vannice, 2005; Whalley et al, 2004). Neurologic disorders are discussed in Chapter 41.

Although much focus is on DHA, it is interesting to note that research has generally shown that consuming both EPA and DHA, but more EPA relative to DHA is necessary for clinical benefit in many psychiatric conditions. To date clinical intervention studies in mental health using DHA alone have been generally disappointing. Researchers are actively seeking answers. Freeman et al, 2006; Marangell et al, 2003, Martins, 2009.

The American Dietetic Association recommends that children and adults eat fish at least twice a week. A minimum intake of 500 mg EPA and DHA is recommended for adults (Kris-Etherton and Innis, 2007). The International Society for the Study of Fatty Acids and Lipids also recommends a daily minimum of 500 mg combined of EPA and DHA (Cunnane, 2004). American Psychiatric Association recommendations for ω-3 intake are shown in Table 42-1.

TABLE 42-1

American Psychiatric Association Recommendations for Omega-3 Intake

Who	Recommendation
All adults	Eat fish two or more times per week.
Individuals with mood, impulse-control, or psychotic disorders	Consume 1 g (1000 mg) EPA and DHA per day.
Patients with mood disorders	Use a supplement providing 1-9 g of EPA and DHA. Use of more than 3 g/day should be monitored by a physician.

Source: Freeman MP et al: Omega-3 fatty acids: evidence base for treatment and future research in psychiatry, J Clin Psychiatry 67:1954, 2006.

DHA, Docosahexaenoic acid; *EPA*, eicosapentaenoic acid.

Omega-3 Supplements

As supplements, EPA and DHA ω-3 fatty acids are available from fish oil and cod liver oil. Other marine sources, such as krill and calamari, are coming to the market. An algal (vegetarian) source of DHA is also available. Omega-3 supplements are best absorbed when consumed with a fat-containing meal or snack. This practice also improves patient compliance, particularly with higher doses. Better ω-3 supplements include an antioxidant, such as vitamin E, in the formula. The purpose of adding an antioxidant is to stabilize and preserve the long-chain polyunsaturated fats. Fortification of foods with ω-3s is increasing, and as always, reading the label is imperative to know the form and dose of ω-3. Genetically modified forms of EPA and DHA are also coming to the market for use in fortified foods and supplements (Vannice, 2010). See *Focus On*: Genetically Modified (GM) Foods, in Chapter 27.

Vitamin D

Vitamin D affects hundreds of genes in the human body and is recognized as an important nutrient for brain health as well as for bone and skeletal health. Because vitamin D can be synthesized from sunlight, adequate sun exposure or vitamin D_3 intake can help maintain mental health. Clinical research has associated vitamin D deficiency with the presence of an active mood disorder, with aspects of cognitive disorder as well as increased risk for both major and minor depression in older adults (Hoogendijk et al, 2008; Stewart et al, 2010; Wilkins et al 2006).

In November 2010 the Institute of Medicine (IOM) of the National Academies published new dietary reference intakes for vitamin D. Focusing on vitamin D and physical health, specifically bone health, the IOM report established a recommended dietary allowance (RDA) of 600 IU/day of vitamin D, an increase of 50% from 1997 (Institute of

Medicine, 2010). The tolerable upper limit was increased to 4000 IU/day.

Serum levels of vitamin D are most often tested by assessing circulating levels of 25(OH)D, which is the combined product of skin synthesis from sun exposure and dietary sources (Calvo et al, 2005). Currently, no official agreement has been reached regarding blood levels of 25(OH)D that indicate deficiency, insufficiency, and sufficiency of vitamin D. Other biomarkers of nutritional vitamin D status include parathyroid hormone levels, intestinal calcium absorption, insulin sensitivity, beta cell function, and innate immune function.

The best sources of vitamin D are exposure to sunlight, foods such as oily fish and egg yolks, and fortified foods, such as cow, soy or other fortified milks, and cereals. Due to recent changes in lifestyle such as more time indoors and more use of sunscreens to protect against skin cancer, many people do not receive adequate exposure to sunlight. Similarly, many people do not eat egg yolks, oily fish, or fortified foods in sufficient quantity to meet the RDA for vitamin D. Therefore recommending supplements or ensuring regular consumption of fortified foods may be warranted.

B-Complex Vitamins

The B-complex vitamins are known for having an effect on neurologic and brain health and sufficient intake is important for individuals with psychiatric disorders. Recent human studies have identified genetic alterations that alter the production and function of serotonin, dopamine, and other neurotransmitters. These alterations may be identified by various biochemical or deoxyribonucleic acid (DNA) testing. For example, the methylenetetrahydrofolate reductase (MTHFR) test can reveal alleles (C > T and A > C) that decrease production of serotonin and dopamine, as well as increase homocysteine retention. Clients with these genetic SNPs (see Chapter 5) usually require folate supplementation in a methylated form. A methylmalonic acid test can reveal whether B_{12} levels are sufficient to maintain low serum homocysteine levels. See Chapters 3, 8, and 33 for further discussion of the B vitamins and brain function.

The best sources of folate are brewer's yeast, mushrooms, spinach, broccoli, brussels sprouts, asparagus, kale and other greens, legumes, liver, and orange juice. Vitamin B_{12} is found in animal sources only, such as beef, liver, clams, oysters, crab, tuna, and halibut. Thus, vegans must choose foods and supplements wisely. Pyridoxine (B_6) is found in beef liver, oatmeal, bananas, chicken, potatoes, avocado, sunflower seeds, brewer's yeast, halibut, pork, and brown rice.

Phytochemicals

New research suggests that plant-based foods rich in the bioactive chemicals, **phytochemicals**, make important nutritional and biochemical contributions to normal brain function and mental health. Foods such as berries, citrus fruits, green tea and some spices contain phytochemicals, as well as essential vitamins and minerals. The phytochemicals showing the most promise are 3 sub-classes of flavonoids: flavanols, anthocyanins and flavanones. These phytochemicals have antioxidant activity, but their more important contributions may be protecting and preserving brain cell structure and metabolism through a complex cascade of cellular mechanisms, including signaling, transcription, phosphorylation and gene expression (Williams et al, 2004; Dashwood, 2008; Spencer, 2010).

There is evidence that other plant-based foods have nutritional and possibly pharmacological effects in the brain, but the mechanisms are yet to be elucidated. These foods appear to impact brain health through antioxidant, anti-inflammatory and nutragenomic influences, and more mechanisms are plausible. Examples of these foods include onion, ginger, tumeric, oregano, sage, rosemary and garlic. This is an exciting area of research to watch in the 21st century (Jellin, 2011).

A summary of flavonoids and nutrients that support healthy brain and nervous system can be found in Table 42-2.

WEIGHT MANAGEMENT

Managing weight, eating behaviors and diet can be challenging for psychiatric patients. Depression and other mental health conditions are known to affect nutrition choices, interpersonal relationships, and lifestyle habits such as

TABLE 42-2

Phytochemicals and Nutrients that Support Brain and Mental Health

Flavonoid-Rich Foods
Apples
Berries, particularly red, blue, and purple
Chocolate
Citrus fruits, such as oranges, grapefruit and lemons
Grapes and grape juice
Teas, including green, black, white, and oolong
Nutrients
α-Lipoic acid
Choline
Docosahexaenoic acid
Eicosapentaenoic acid
Folate
Glutathione
Selenium
Thiamin
Vitamin A
Vitamin B_6
Vitamin B_{12}
Vitamin C
Vitamin D
Vitamin E

smoking, drinking, and self-care and each of these factors influence food choices and cooking practices. Individuals with psychiatric disorders who are taking psychotropic medicines may experience rapid or excessive weight gain. In fact, a commonly known side-effect of anti-depressant medications is weight gain, and many patients cite this reason to avoid or cease use of their medication. Depressed individuals can also experience loss of appetite and unintentional weight loss or anorectic behavior (Freeman et al, 2006; Jensen, 2008; Murphy et al, 2009).

Being proactive with patients is important. Keep in mind that eating behavior, appetite, focus, concentration, and even the circadian rhythm which affects the sleep/wake cycle can be altered. Individuals may lose or gain interest in food, shopping, and cooking, which affects their families as well as themselves. Working with patients to strategize healthy food choices, to practice supportive eating behaviors and meal planning is valuable. Knowing that one's loved ones are cared for through a difficult period can be rewarding and psychologically uplifting. Encouraging regular physical activity and eating plans that support healthy weight and alleviate stress in the home and workplace is helpful (Gouin et al, 2010; Kiecolt-Glaser, 2010).

ADDICTION AND SUBSTANCE ABUSE RECOVERY

Addiction is a chronic brain disorder that involves compulsive and relapsing behavior, with biochemical, psychological, and social vulnerabilities. A variety of behavioral and psychological anomalies result from ingestion of or exposure to a drug of abuse, medication, or toxin. The master "pleasure" molecule of addiction is dopamine; it is triggered by heroin, amphetamines, marijuana, alcohol, nicotine, and caffeine (Escott-Stump, 2012). In addition, poor diet and stress enhance the problems of the addicted individual and family members.

Alcohol dependence is a public health concern throughout the world. Event-related brain oscillations are seen, along with inherited neuroelectric deficits; for example, the serotonin receptor gene HTR7 is part of the biologic basis of alcohol dependence (Zlojutro et al., 2010). The addictive personality type is often perfectionistic and prone to depression; antidepressant medications may be useful for some individuals.

Eating disorders and substance abuse are similar; many clients have both. Eating disorders can arise from gene-environment interactions that alter genetic expression via epigenetic processes (Campbell et al., 2010). In most psychiatric disorders, either increased or decreased changes in appetite occur. It is important to be aware of the types of malnutrition and counseling techniques appropriate for this population. Counseling should include tips such as how a proper, nutritious diet can reduce cravings; how to choose a brain-healthy diet; maintaining physical activity; choosing nutrient-rich snacks; stress management; and tracking positive changes and successes (see Chapter 23).

NUTRITION INTERVENTIONS

The primary responsibility of a dietitian working with individuals who have a mental health diagnosis is to impart information and support for eating choices that minimize the negative effects of these illnesses on the client and their affected loved ones. Therapy for behavioral issues is primarily the responsibility of the psychotherapy team. Common nutrition diagnoses in this population may include:

- Deficit of food and nutrition knowledge
- Harmful food and nutrition attitudes and beliefs
- Poor food choices
- Nutrient deficiencies
- Imbalance of fats from foods
- Excessive carbohydrate intake
- Excessive intake of processed and refined foods
- Altered nutrition-related laboratory values
- Excessive or inadequate oral food and beverage intake
- Underweight, overweight or obesity
- Food-medication interactions

Individuals who have a psychiatric condition may not adapt readily to the fluctuations of life and changes in diet and lifestyle can exacerbate anxiety or depression. When working with the mentally ill, the dietitian should incorporate varying responses to diet, environment, genetics, behavior and stress and offer support and strategies to these individuals. See Fig. 42-2. For example, a primary goal of "behavioral change" in nutrition counseling is not usually easily embraced by members of this population. Although the long-term outcome of healthy food and lifestyle change is certainly positive, a person with a psychiatric condition, regardless of intelligence and life-stage, may find *any* change (e.g., food

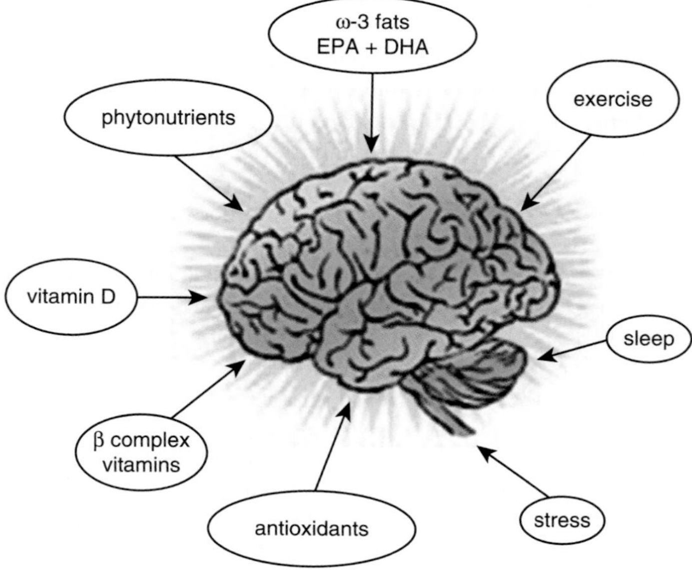

FIGURE 42-2 Brain function is affected by many more nutrients and lifestyle factors than previously thought, and research is rapidly revealing new connections. *(© 2011 Photos.com a division of Getty Images. All rights reserved.)*

choices, relationships, or any life situation) overwhelming or even frightening. However, even small improvements in nutritional status can lead to meaningful results. And a positive experience with a dietitian can build a foundation and motivation to attempt other positive changes long after nutrition counseling is finished.

For dietitians working in psychiatric units, suicide precautions are often needed. Therefore, those meals require special attention to prevent giving patients anything that they could use to do harm to themselves or others. Plastic utensils and paper goods may be a necessary precaution. A balanced, nutritious diet rich in ω-3 fatty acids and plant-based foods should be made available. Table 42-3 gives more specific guidance about nutrition in other psychiatric conditions.

Text continued on p. 968

TABLE 42-3

Nutrition for Specific Psychiatric Conditions

Mental Disorder	Explanation	Relevance to Nutrition
Acute stress disorder or posttraumatic stress disorder	Development of anxiety and dissociative and other symptoms within 1 month following exposure to an extremely traumatic event; the symptoms may include reexperiencing the event, nightmares, and avoidance of trauma-related stimuli.	May increase or decrease appetite. Overall nutrition status may decline, or obesity may result.
Adjustment disorder	Maladaptive reaction to identifiable stressful life events.	May increase or decrease appetite. Overall nutrition status may decline, or obesity may result.
Amnestic disorder	Mental disorder characterized by acquired impairment in the ability to learn and recall new information, sometimes accompanied by inability to recall previously learned information, and not coupled with dementia or delirium.	Impaired ability to retain new information from nutrition counseling.
Anxiety disorders	A group of mental disorders in which anxiety and avoidance behavior predominate, including panic disorder, agoraphobia, specific phobias, social phobia, obsessive-compulsive disorder, posttraumatic stress disorder, acute stress disorder, and generalized anxiety disorder.	May increase or decrease appetite. Overall nutrition status may decline, or obesity may result. May respond to increased intake of ω-3 fats to 1-3 g/day.
Attention deficit disorder and attention-deficit/hyperactivity disorder	Mental disorder characterized by inattention (such as distractibility, forgetfulness, not finishing tasks, and not appearing to listen), hyperactivity and impulsivity (such as fidgeting and squirming, difficulty in remaining seated, excessive running or climbing, feelings of restlessness, difficulty awaiting one's turn, interrupting others, and excessive talking) or both types of behavior	Impaired ability to retain and use new information after nutrition counseling. May respond to increased intake of ω-3 fats to 1-3 g/day.
Autistic disorder	Severe pervasive developmental disorder with onset usually before 3 years of age and a biologic basis related to neurologic or neurophysiologic factors. Characterized by qualitative impairment in reciprocal social interaction (e.g., lack of awareness of the existence of feelings of others, failure to seek comfort at times of distress, lack of imitation), verbal and nonverbal communication, and capacity for symbolic play and by restricted and unusual repertoire of activities and interests.	May affect appetite, with increased needs common. Overall nutrition status may decline. May respond to increased intake of ω-3 fats, especially DHA, to 1-3 g/day. Gluten-free, casein-free, or soy-free diet may be useful.
Binge eating disorder	An eating disorder characterized by repeated episodes of binge eating, as in bulimia nervosa, but not followed by inappropriate compensatory behavior such as purging, fasting, or excessive exercise.	May affect nutrition status; health may decline or obesity may result.

TABLE 42-3

Nutrition for Specific Psychiatric Conditions—cont'd

Mental Disorder	Explanation	Relevance to Nutrition
Bipolar disorders	Mood disorders characterized by a history of manic, mixed, or hypomanic episodes, usually with concurrent or previous history of one or more major depressive episodes.	May increase or decrease appetite. Overall nutrition status may decline, or obesity may result. May respond to increased intake of ω-3 fats to 1-3 g/day preferably in combination with standard mood stabilizers.
Body dysmorphic disorder	A mental disorder in which a normal-appearing person is either preoccupied with some imagined defect in appearance or is overly concerned about some very slight physical anomaly.	Likely to cause altered eating habits with potential for decline in intake. May lead to eating disorder. May be prone to food fads or use of herbs or steroids.
Catatonia	Immobilization caused by the physiologic effects of a general medical condition.	May decrease appetite. Overall nutrition status may decline.
Childhood disintegrative disorder	Pervasive developmental disorder characterized by marked regression in a variety of skills, including language, social skills or adaptive behavior, play, bowel or bladder control, and motor skills after at least 2, but less than 10 years of apparently normal development.	May increase or decrease appetite. Overall nutrition status may decline; or obesity may result.
Conduct disorder	A type of disruptive behavior disorder of childhood and adolescence characterized by a persistent pattern of conduct in which rights of others or age-appropriate societal norms or rules are violated.	No specific nutritional challenges except that mealtimes may be disrupted.
Conversion disorder	Mental disorder characterized by conversion symptoms (loss or alteration of voluntary motor or sensory functioning suggesting physical illness, such as seizures, paralysis, dyskinesia, anesthesia, blindness, or aphonia) having no demonstrable physiologic basis.	May increase or decrease appetite. Overall nutritional status may decline or obesity may result.
Delusional disorder	Mental disorder marked by well-organized, logically consistent delusions, but lacking other psychotic symptoms. Most functioning is not markedly impaired, the criteria for schizophrenia are not met; symptoms of a major mood disorder are present only briefly, but delusional disorder may coexist with other psychiatric conditions.	May increase or decrease appetite. Overall nutrition status may decline, or obesity may result.
Depersonalization disorder	Dissociative disorder characterized by one or more severe episodes of depersonalization (feelings of unreality and strangeness in one's perception of self or one's body image) not caused by another mental disorder such as schizophrenia. The perception of reality remains intact; patients are aware of their incapacitation. Episodes are usually accompanied by dizziness, anxiety, or fears of going insane.	May increase or decrease appetite. An eating disorder or obesity can result; overall nutrition status may decline.
Depressive disorders	Mood disorders, such as major depressive disorder, dysthymia, or minor depression, in which depression is unaccompanied by manic or hypomanic episodes.	May increase or decrease appetite. Nutrition status may decline. May respond to increased intake of ω-3 fats to 1-3 g/day.

Continued

TABLE 42-3

Nutrition for Specific Psychiatric Conditions—cont'd

Mental Disorder	Explanation	Relevance to Nutrition
Dissociative disorders	Mental disorders characterized by sudden, temporary alterations in identity, memory, or consciousness, segregating normally integrated memories or parts of the personality from the dominant identity of the individual.	May increase or decrease appetite. Overall nutrition status may decline, or obesity may result.
Dissociative identity disorder	A disorder characterized by the existence in an individual of two or more distinct personalities, each having unique memories, characteristic behavior, and social relationships. Also referred to as *multiple personality disorder*.	May increase or decrease appetite. Overall nutrition status may decline, or obesity may result.
Dysthymic disorder	Mood disorder characterized by depressed feeling (sad, blue, low), loss of interest or pleasure in one's usual activities, and by at least some of the following: altered appetite, disturbed sleep patterns, lack of energy, low self-esteem, poor concentration or decision-making skills, and feelings of hopelessness. Symptoms have persisted 2 years but are not severe enough to meet the criteria for major depressive disorder.	May increase or decrease appetite. Overall nutrition status may decline, or obesity may result. May coexist with an eating disorder. May respond to increased intake of ω-3 fats to 1-3 g/day.
Eating disorders	Any of several disorders in which abnormal feeding habits are associated with psychological factors; in DSM-IV these include anorexia nervosa, bulimia nervosa, pica and rumination disorder.	Overall nutrition status may decline, or obesity may result, depending on the specific condition. May respond to increased intake of ω-3 fats to 1-3 g/day. See Chapter 23.
Generalized anxiety disorder	Disorder characterized by the presence of excessive, uncontrollable anxiety and worry about two or more life circumstances for 6 months or longer, accompanied by some combination of restlessness, fatigue, muscle tension, irritability, disturbed concentration or sleep, and somatic symptoms.	May increase or decrease appetite. Overall nutrition status may decline, or obesity may result. May coexist with an eating disorder. May benefit from increased intake of ω-3 fats, especially DHA, 1-3 g/day.
Impulse control disorders	Group of mental disorders characterized by repeated failure to resist an impulse to perform some act harmful to oneself or others.	May increase or decrease appetite. Overall nutrition status may decline, but more likely obesity may result.
Motor skills disorder	Any disorder characterized by inadequate development of motor coordination severe enough to limit locomotion or restrict the ability to perform tasks, schoolwork, or other activities.	No specific nutritional changes, but may have difficulty preparing food.
Obsessive-compulsive disorder	Anxiety disorder characterized by recurrent obsessions (often about fear of contamination, disease, or other harm or punishment) or compulsions that are severe enough to interfere significantly with personal or social functioning. Performing compulsive rituals may release tension temporarily, and resisting them causes increased tension.	May increase or decrease appetite. May be avoidance of specific foods or food groups. Overall nutrition status may decline, or obesity may result.

TABLE 42-3

Nutrition for Specific Psychiatric Conditions—cont'd

Mental Disorder	Explanation	Relevance to Nutrition
Oppositional defiant disorder	A type of disruptive behavior disorder characterized by a recurrent pattern of defiant, hostile, disobedient, and negativistic behavior directed toward those in authority, including such actions such as defying the requests or rules of adults, deliberately annoying others, arguing, spitefulness, and vindictiveness that occur much more frequently than would be expected on the basis of age and developmental stage.	May increase or decrease appetite. Overall nutrition status may decline, or obesity may result. Mealtimes and thus quality of nutritional intake may be disrupted.
Pain disorder	A somatoform disorder characterized by a chief complaint of severe chronic pain that causes substantial distress or impairment in functioning; the pain is neither feigned nor intentionally produced, and psychological factors appear to play a major role in its onset, severity, exacerbation, or maintenance.	May increase or decrease appetite. Overall nutrition status may decline, or obesity may result. May benefit from increased intake of ω-3 fats, especially EPA, for their inflammatory effect, 1-3 g/day.
Panic disorder	Anxiety disorder characterized by recurrent panic (anxiety) attacks, episodes of intense apprehension; fear or terror associated with somatic symptoms such as dyspnea, palpitations, dizziness, vertigo, faintness, or shakiness, and with psychological symptoms such as feelings of unreality or fears of dying, going crazy, or losing control. There is usually chronic nervousness and tension between attacks; often, but not always associated with agoraphobia.	May increase or decrease appetite. Food may be used to soothe. Overall nutrition status may decline, or obesity may result.
Personality disorders	Mental disorders characterized by enduring, inflexible, and maladaptive personality traits that deviate markedly from cultural expectations; are self-perpetuating; pervade a broad range of situations, and either generate subjective distress or result in significant impairments in social, occupational, or other functioning. Onset in adolescence or early adulthood.	May increase or decrease appetite. Overall nutrition status may decline, or obesity may result. May respond to increased intake of ω-3 fats to 1-3 g/day.
Pervasive developmental disorders	Group of disorders characterized by impairment of development in multiple areas, including the acquisition of reciprocal social interaction, verbal and nonverbal communication skills, and imaginative activity, and by stereotyped interests and behaviors. Included are autism, Rett syndrome, childhood disintegrative disorder, and Asperger syndrome.	Comprehension of information shared during nutrition counseling may be affected. Autism and Asperger syndrome may benefit from dietary and nutrition changes.
Premenstrual dysphoric disorder	Premenstrual syndrome viewed as a psychiatric disorder. Often referred to as *PMS*.	May increase or decrease appetite. Overall nutrition status may decline, or obesity may result. May benefit from increasing intake of ω-3 fats to 1-3 g/day.
Rumination disorder	Eating disorder seen in infants younger than 1 year of age; after a period of normal eating habits, the child begins excessive regurgitation and rechewing of food, which is then ejected from the mouth or reswallowed.	If untreated, death from malnutrition may occur. May require enteral or parenteral nutrition.

Continued

TABLE 42-3

Nutrition for Specific Psychiatric Conditions—cont'd

Mental Disorder	Explanation	Relevance to Nutrition
Schizoaffective disorder	A mental disorder in which a major depressive episode, manic episode, or mixed episode occurs along with prominent psychotic symptoms characteristic of schizophrenia. Symptoms of the mood disorder are present for a substantial portion of the illness, and the disturbance is not the result of the effects of a psychoactive substance.	May increase or decrease appetite. Overall nutrition status may decline, or obesity may result. May respond to increased intake of ω-3 fats to 1-3 g/day, preferably in combination with antipsychotic drugs.
Seasonal affective disorder	A cyclic mood disorder characterized by depression, extreme lethargy, increased need for sleep, hyperphagia, and carbohydrate craving. It intensifies most commonly in winter months and is hypothesized to be related to melatonin levels. In DSM-IV terminology called "mood disorder with seasonal pattern." Often referred to as "winter blues" in common parlance.	May increase or decrease appetite. Overall nutrition status may decline, or obesity may result. May respond to increasing ω-3 fat intake to 1-3 g/day. May benefit from increasing protein intake to balance blood sugar levels.
Sleep disorder	Chronic disorders involving sleep. Primary sleep disorders comprise dyssomnias and parasomnias. Causes of secondary sleep disorders may include a general medical condition, mental disorder, or psychoactive substance.	May affect appetite, with increased intake common; night eating syndrome may present. Obesity may result.

Data from Merck manual of medical information. Accessed 23 October 2010 from http://www.mercksource.com/pp/us/cns/cns_home.jsp.

DHA, Docosahexaenoic acid; *DSM-IV*, *Diagnostic and Statistical Manual*, IV; *EPA*, eicosapentaenoic acid.

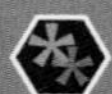

CLINICAL SCENARIO

Nels is a 20-year-old white man who was recently admitted to the adult psychiatric unit of your hospital. He has exhibited signs of psychosis, and his medical record indicates a family history of schizophrenia, diabetes, and bipolar disorder. He has been prescribed aripiprazole and bupropion; he is becoming more alert. His fasting blood glucose is normal at 100 mg/dL, but his serum low-density lipoprotein cholesterol is low at 70 mg/dL. His diet has been poor lately, and he has been consuming mostly snack foods and sweetened carbonated beverages. He seldom eats fish and eats fewer than three fruits and vegetables weekly.

Nutrition Diagnostic Statements

1. Inadequate intake of food fats (i.e., ω-3 fatty acids) related to poor diet as evidenced by low serum cholesterol and psychiatric symptoms.
2. Inadequate bioactive substance intake related to antioxidants and phytochemicals as evidenced by intake of fewer than three fruits and vegetables weekly.

Nutrition Care Questions

1. What information will you need to assess his nutritional history and patterns more thoroughly?
2. What dietary components will you suggest for Nels?
3. What are the nutritional side effects of the medications he is taking?
4. What long-term nutrition care will he need?

USEFUL WEBSITES

American Association on Mental Retardation
http://www.AAMR.org

American Academy of Child and Adolescent Psychiatry
http://www.aacap.org/

American Psychiatric Association
http://www.psych.org/

Internet Mental Health
www.mentalhealth.com

National Depressive & Manic-Depressive Association
http://www.ndmda.org/

National Alliance for the Mentally Ill
http://www.nami.org/

REFERENCES

Antalis CJ, et al: Omega-3 fatty acid status in attention-deficit/hyperactivity disorder, *Prostaglandins Leukot Essent Fatty Acids* 75:299, 2006.

Calvo MS, et al: Vitamin D intake: a global perspective of current status, *J Nutr* 135:310, 2005.

Campbell IC, et al: Eating disorders, gene-environment interactions and epigenetics, *Neurosci Biobehav Rev* 35:784, 2011.

Cunnane S: Report on Dietary Intake of Essential Fatty Acids, *International Society for the Study of Fatty Acids and Lipids* 2004.

Dangour AD, et al: Effect of 2-y n-3 long-chain polyunsaturated fatty acid supplementation on cognitive function in older people: a randomized, double-blind, controlled trial, *Am J Clin Nutr* 91:1725, 2010.

Dashwood RH: Flavonoids. Micronutrient Information Center, Linus Pauling Institute. 2008, Accessed April 25, 2011 from http://lpi.oregonstate.edu/infocenter/phytochemicals/flavonoids.

Davis BC, Kris-Etherton PM: Achieving optimal essential fatty acid status in vegetarians: current knowledge and practical implications, *Am J Clin Nutr* 78(Suppl):640S, 2003.

Escott-Stump S: *Nutrition and diagnosis-related care*, ed 7, Baltimore, 2012, Lippincott-Williams & Wilkins.

Freeman MP, et al: Omega-3 fatty acids: evidence base for treatment and future research in psychiatry, *J Clin Psychiatry* 67:1954, 2006a.

Freeman MP, et al: Randomized dose-ranging pilot trial of omega-3 fatty acids for postpartum depression, *Acta Psych Scand* 113:31, 2006b.

Gouin JP, et al: Altered expression of circadian rhythm genes among individuals with a history of depression. *J Affect Disord* 126:161, 2010.

Hallahan B, et al: Omega-3 fatty acid supplementation in patients with recurrent self-harm, *British J Psychiatry* 190:188, 2007.

Harris WS, et al: Towards establishing dietary reference intakes for eicosapentaenoic and docosahexaenoic acids, *J Nutr* 139:804S, 2009.

Hibbeln JR: From homicide to happiness: a commentary on omega-3 fatty acids in human society: Cleave Award Lecture, *Nutr Health* 19:9, 2007a.

Hibbeln JR: Seafood consumption and homicide mortality. A cross-national ecological analysis, *World Rev Nutr Diet* 88:41, 2001.

Hibbeln JR, Davis JM: Considerations regarding neuropsychiatric nutritional requirements for intakes of omega-3 highly unsaturated fatty acids, *Prostaglandins Leukot Essent Fatty Acids* 81:179, 2009.

Hibbeln JR, et al: Maternal seafood consumption in pregnancy and neurodevelopmental outcomes in childhood (ALSPAC study): an observational cohort study, *Lancet* 369:578, 2007b.

Hoogendijk WJ, et al: Depression is associated with decreased 25-hydroxyvitamin D and increased parathyroid hormone levels in older adults, *Arch Gen Psychiatry* 65:508, 2008.

Institute of Medicine: Dietary reference intakes for calcium and vitamin D, 2010. Accessed 22 December 2010 from www.iom.edu/vitamind

Jazayeri S, et al: Comparison of therapeutic effects of omega-3 fatty acid eicosapentaenoic acid and fluoxetine, separately and in combination, in major depressive disorder. *Aust New Zealand J Pysch* 42:192, 2008.

Jellin J: Natural Medicines Comprehensive Database. Therapeutic Research Faculty. Stockton, CA 2011, Accessed April 24, 2011 from http://naturaldatabase.therapeuticresearch.com.

Jensen GL: Drug-Induced Hyperphagia: What Can We Learn From Psychiatric Medications? *J Parenter Enteral Nutr* 32:578, 2008.

Kiecolt-Glaser JK: Stress, food, and inflammation: psychoneuroimmunology and nutrition at the cutting edge, *Psychosom Med* 72:365, 2010.

Koletzko B, et al, for the Perinatal Lipid Intake Working Group: Dietary fat intakes for pregnant and lactating women, *Br J Nutr* 98:873, 2007.

Kris-Etherton PM, Innis S: Position of the American Dietetic Association and Dietitians of Canada: dietary fatty acids, *J Am Diet Assoc* 107:1599, 2007.

Marangell LB, et al: A double-blind, placebo-controlled study of the omega-3 fatty acid docosahexaenoic acid in the treatment of major depression. *Am J Psychiatry* 160:996, 2003.

Martins JG: EPA but not DHA appears to be responsible for the efficacy of omega-3 long chain polyunsaturated fatty acid supplementation in depression: evidence from a meta-analysis of randomized controlled trials, *J Am Coll Nutr* 28:525, 2009.

Mihm S: Does Eating Salmon Lower the Murder Rate? *The New York Times Magazine* 2006, April 16. Accessed Mar 22, 2011 from http://www.nytimes.com/2006/04/16/magazine/16wwln_idealab.html.

Muldoon MF, et al: Serum phospholipid docosahexaenoic acid is associated with cognitive functioning during middle adulthood, *J Nutrition* 140:848, 2010.

Murphy JM, et al: Obesity and weight gain in relation to depression: findings from the Stirling County Study, *Int J Obes* 33:335, 2009.

Richardson AJ, Puri BK: The potential role of fatty acids in attention-deficit/hyperactivity disorder, *Prostaglandins Leukot Essent Fatty Acids* 63(1/2):79, 2000.

Richardson AJ, Montgomery P: Omega-3 fatty acids in ADHD and related neurodevelopmental disorders, *Int Rev Psychiatry* 18:155, 2006.

Spencer JP: The impact of fruit flavonoids on memory and cognition, *Br J Nutr* 104:40S, 2010.

Stewart R, et al: Relationship between vitamin D levels and depressive symptoms in older residents from a national survey population, *Psychosomatic Med* 72:608, 2010.

Vannice GK: Cognition, aging and omega-3 fatty acids, *J Applied Nutrition* 55(1):2, 2005.

Vannice GK: N-3s from fish and the risk of metabolic syndrome, *J Am Diet Assoc* 110:1014, 2010.

Williams RJ, et al: Flavonoids: antioxidants or signaling molecules? *Free Radic Biol Med* 36:838, 2004.

Whalley LJ, et al: Cognitive aging, childhood intelligence, and the use of food supplements: possible involvement of omega-3 fatty acids, *Am J Clin Nutr* 80:1650, 2004.

Wilkins CH, et al: Vitamin D deficiency is associated with low mood and worse cognitive performance in older adults, *Am J Geriatr Psychiatry* 14:1032, 2006.

World Health Organization: *Mental health*, 2010. Accessed 3 November 2010 from http://www.who.int/en/.

Zlojutro M, et al: Genome-wide association study of theta band event-related oscillations identifies serotonin receptor gene HTR7 influencing risk of alcohol dependence, *Am J Med Genet B Neuropsychiatr Genet* 2 November 2010. [Epub ahead of print.]

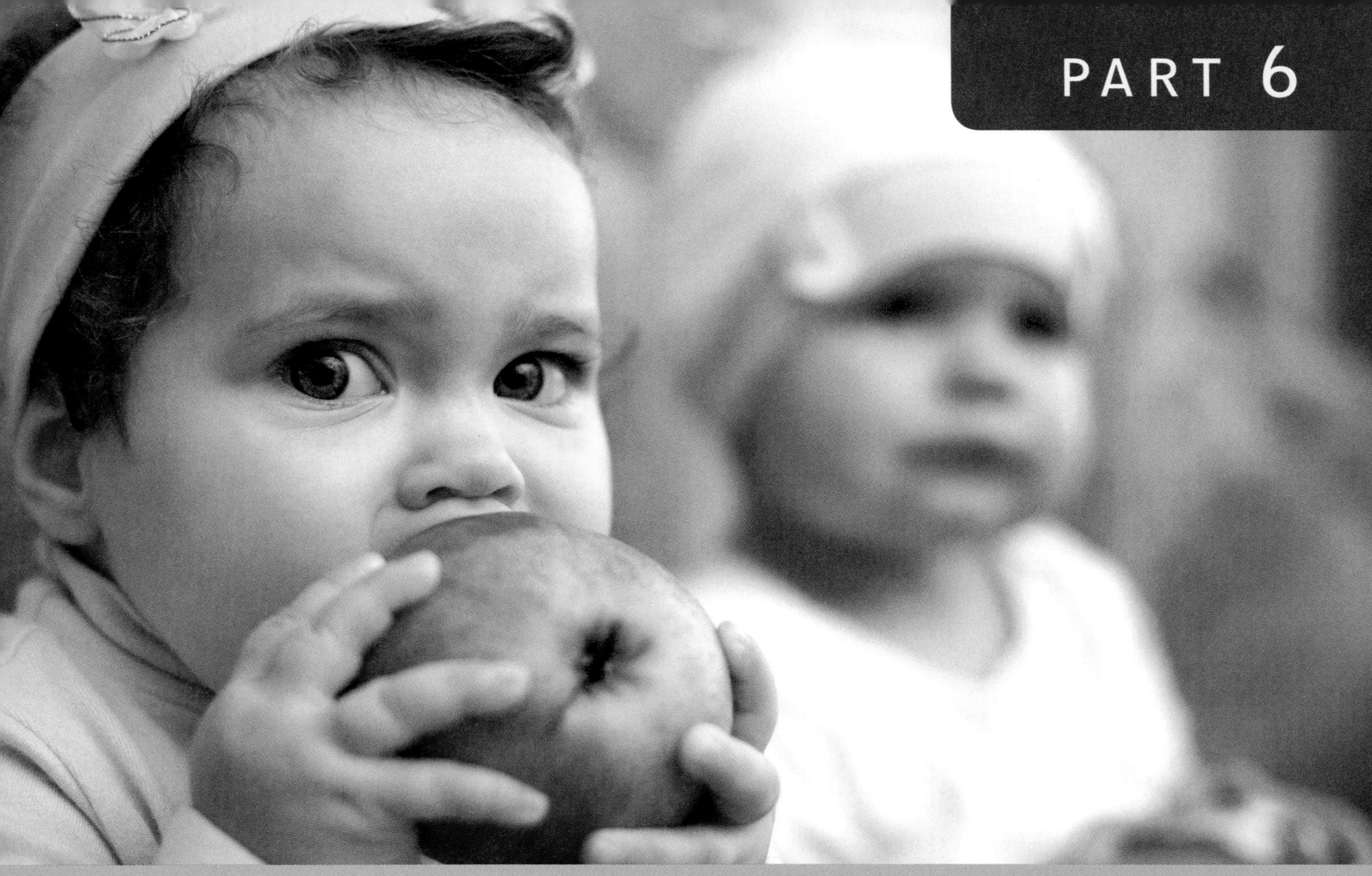

PART 6

Pediatric Specialties

The unique, special roles of nutrition in the pediatric population cannot be underestimated. Pediatricians, nurses, and dietitians all recognize that unusual feeding problems or disorders can negatively influence growth and health, especially in the very young. This section addresses the categories affecting the nutritional intake and growth velocity of infants and children. In some cases, adolescents are mentioned if relevant, but most of this section considers younger patients.

Whether in neonatal units, in hospital pediatric units, in out-patient clinics, in long-term care units, or in home care, children need to grow as well as cope with genetic or acquired disorders. More than ever, nutrition care in this specialty arena requires an understanding of the biochemical, physiological, social, and economic challenges that our youngest citizens face.

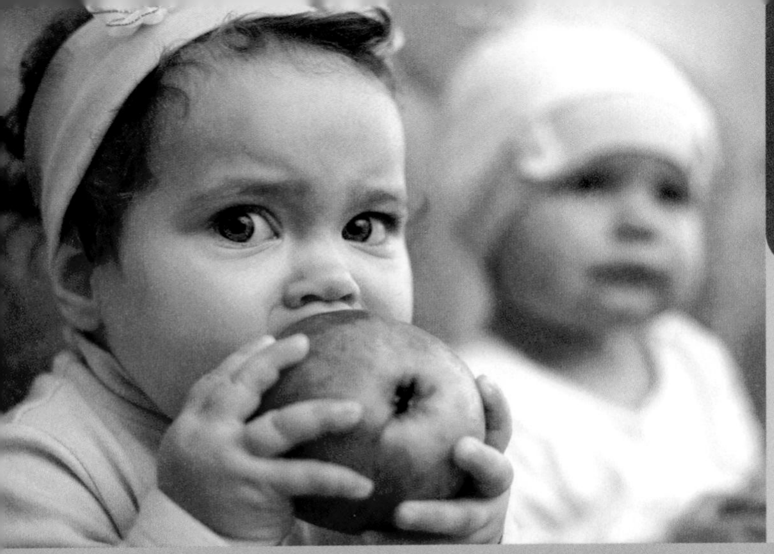

CHAPTER 43

Diane M. Anderson, PhD, RD, CSP, FADA

Medical Nutrition Therapy for Low-Birth-Weight Infants

KEY TERMS

appropriate for gestational age (AGA)
bronchopulmonary dysplasia (BPD)
carnitine
extrauterine growth restriction (EUGR)
extremely low birthweight (ELBW)
gastric gavage
gestational age
glucose load
hemolytic anemia
human milk fortifiers
infancy
infant mortality rate
intrauterine growth restriction (IUGR)
kangaroo care
large for gestational age (LGA)
low birthweight (LBW)
necrotizing enterocolitis (NEC)
neonatal period
neutral thermal environment
osteopenia of prematurity
perinatal period
premature (preterm) infant
respiratory distress syndrome (RDS)
small for gestational age (SGA)
surfactant
term infant
very low birthweight (VLBW)

The management of low birthweight (LBW) infants requiring intensive care is continually improving. With new technologies, enhanced understanding of pathophysiologic conditions of the **perinatal period** (from 28 weeks of gestation to 4 weeks after birth), current nutrition management principles, and regionalization of perinatal care, the mortality rate during **infancy**—that period from birth to 1 year of age—remains stable in the United States. In particular, the development and use of **surfactant**—a mixture of lipoproteins secreted by alveolar cells into the alveoli and respiratory air passages that contributes to the elastic properties of pulmonary tissue—has increased the survival of preterm infants, as has the use of antepartum corticosteroids. Most premature infants have the potential for long and productive lives (Hack, 2009).

Nutrition can be provided to LBW infants in many ways, each of which has certain benefits and limitations. The infant's size, age, and clinical condition dictate the nutrition requirements and the way they can be met. Because of the complexities involved in the neonatal intensive care setting, a team that includes a registered dietitian trained in neonatal nutrition should make the decisions necessary to facilitate optimal nutrition. In regionalized perinatal care systems, the neonatal nutritionist may also consult with health care providers in community hospitals and public health settings.

INFANT MORTALITY AND STATISTICS

In 2007 the **infant mortality rate** in the United States remains stable at 6.77 infant deaths per 1000 live births (Heron et al., 2010). More than 65% of these deaths occur in the neonatal period, with the leading causes being birth defects, prematurity, and LBW. The preterm birth rate was 12.7% and the incidence of LBW was 8.2%. Both rates are decreased from the 2006 rate and mark a change from the previous 20-year increase in premature and LBW infants.

The United States' infant mortality rate remains higher than that for many industrialized countries (Heron et al., 2010). This discrepancy may be attributable to the inconsistent collection of mortality data among nations, which may falsely lower mortality rates in other countries. However the high incidence of premature infants born in the United States contributes to this high infant mortality rate (MacDorman and Mathews, 2009).

PHYSIOLOGIC DEVELOPMENT

Gestational Age and Size

At birth an infant who weighs less than 2500 g (5½ lb) is classified as having a **low birthweight (LBW)**; an infant weighing less than 1500 g (3⅓ lb) has a **very low birthweight (VLBW)**; and an infant weighing less than 1000 g (2¼ lb) has an **extremely low birthweight (ELBW)**. LBW may be attributable to a shortened period of gestation, prematurity, or a restricted intrauterine growth rate, which makes the infant small for gestational age (SGA).

The **term infant** is born between the 37th and 42nd weeks of gestation. A **premature (preterm) infant** is born before 37 weeks of gestation, whereas a postterm infant is born after 42 weeks of gestation.

Antenatally, an estimate of the infant's **gestational age** is based on the date of the mother's last menstrual period, clinical parameters of uterine fundal height, the presence of quickening (the first movements of the fetus that can be felt by the mother), fetal heart tones, or ultrasound evaluations. After birth, gestational age is determined by clinical assessment. Clinical parameters fall into two groups: (1) a series of neurologic signs, which depend primarily on postures and tone; and (2) a series of external characteristics that reflect the physical maturity of the infant. The New Ballard Score (Ballard et al., 1991) examination is a frequently used clinical assessment tool. An accurate assessment of gestational age is important for establishing nutritional goals for individual infants and differentiating the premature infant from the term SGA infant.

An infant who is **small for gestational age (SGA)** has a birth weight that is lower than the 10th percentile of the standard weight for that gestational age. An SGA infant whose intrauterine weight gain is poor, but whose linear and head growth are between the 10th and 90th percentiles on the intrauterine growth grid, has experienced asymmetric **intrauterine growth restriction (IUGR)**. An SGA infant whose length and occipital frontal circumference are also below the 10th percentile of the standards has symmetric IUGR. Symmetric IUGR, which usually reflects early and prolonged intrauterine deficit, is apparently more detrimental to later growth and development. Some infants can be SGA because they are genetically small, and these infants usually do well.

An infant whose size is **appropriate for gestational age (AGA)** has a birth weight between the 10th and 90th percentiles on the intrauterine growth chart. The obstetrician diagnoses IUGR when the fetal growth rate decreases. Serial ultrasound measurements document this reduction in fetal anthropometric measurements, which may be caused by maternal, placental, or fetal abnormalities. The future growth and development of infants who have had IUGR is diverse, depending on the specific cause of the IUGR and treatment. Some infants who suffered from IUGR are SGA, but many may plot as AGA infants at birth. Decreased fetal growth does not always result in an infant who is SGA.

An infant whose birth weight is above the 90th percentile on the intrauterine growth chart is **large for gestational age (LGA)**. Box 43-1 summarizes the weight classifications. Figure 43-1 shows the classification of neonates based on maturity and intrauterine growth.

Characteristics of Immaturity

The premature or LBW infant has not had the chance to develop fully in utero and is physiologically different from the term infant (Figure 43-2). Because of this, LBW infants have various clinical problems in the early **neonatal period**, depending on their intrauterine environment, degree of prematurity, birth-related trauma, and function of immature or stressed organ systems. Certain problems occur with such frequency that they are considered typical of prematurity (Table 43-1). Premature infants are at high risk for poor nutrition status because of poor nutrient stores, physiologic immaturity, illness (which may interfere with nutritional management and needs), and the nutrient demands required for growth.

Most fetal nutrient stores are deposited during the last 3 months of gestation; therefore the premature infant begins life in a compromised nutritional state. Because metabolic (i.e., energy) stores are limited, nutrition support in the form of parenteral nutrition (PN), enteral nutrition (EN), or both should be initiated as soon as possible. In the preterm infant weighing 1000 g, fat constitutes only 1% of total body

BOX 43-1

Classification of Birth Weight and Intrauterine Growth

Low birth weight < 2500 g
Very low birth weight < 1500 g
Extremely low birth weight < 1000 g
Small for gestational age = Birth weight < 10th percentile of standard for gestational age
Appropriate for gestational age = Birth weight between the 10th and 90th percentile of standard for gestational age
Large for gestational age = Birth weight > 90th percentile of standard for gestational age

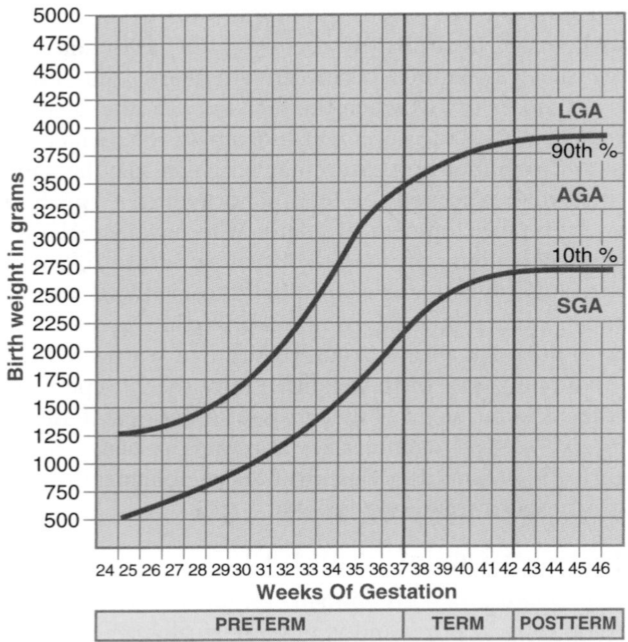

FIGURE 43-1 Classification of neonates based on maturity and intrauterine growth (small for gestational age [SGA], appropriate for gestational age [AGA], or large for gestational age [LGA]). *(From Battaglia FC, Lubchenco LO: A practical classification of newborn infants by weight and gestational age, J Pediatr 71:159, 1967.)*

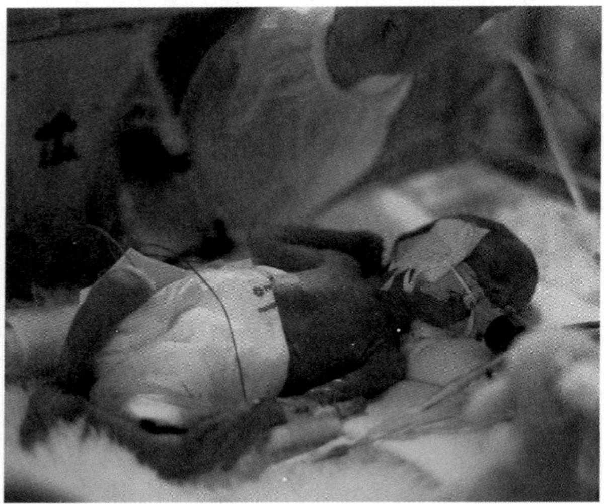

FIGURE 43-2 A.R., born at 27 weeks of gestation; birth weight of 870 g (1 lb, 14 oz).

weight; by contrast the term infant (3500 g) has a fat percentage of approximately 16%. For example, a 1000-g AGA premature infant has a glycogen and fat reserve equivalent to approximately 110 kcal/kg of body weight. With basal metabolic needs of approximately 50 kcal/kg/day, it is obvious that this infant will rapidly run out of fat and carbohydrate fuel unless adequate nutrition support is established. The depletion time is even shorter for preterm infants weighing less than 1000 g at birth. Nutrient reserves are also depleted most quickly by tiny infants who have IUGR as a result of their decreased nutrient stores.

TABLE 43-1

Common Problems Among Premature Infants

System	Problem
Respiratory	Respiratory distress syndrome, chronic lung disease (bronchopulmonary dysplasia)
Cardiovascular	Patent ductus arteriosus
Renal	Fluid and electrolyte imbalance
Neurologic	Intraventricular hemorrhage, periventricular leukomalacia (cerebral necrosis)
Metabolic	Hypoglycemia, hyperglycemia, hypocalcemia, metabolic acidosis
Gastrointestinal	Hyperbilirubinemia, feeding intolerance, necrotizing enterocolitis
Hematologic	Anemia
Immunologic	Sepsis, pneumonia, meningitis
Other	Apnea, bradycardia, cyanosis, osteopenia

From Cloherty JP et al., editors: Manual of neonatal care, ed 6, Philadelphia, 2008, Wolters Kluwer/Lippincott Williams & Wilkins.

TABLE 43-2

Expected Survival Time of Starved (H_2O Only) and Semistarved ($D_{10}W$) Infants

	Estimated Survival Time (Days)	
Birth Weight (g)	**H_2O**	**$D_{10}W$**
1000	4	11
2000	12	30
3500	32	80

Data from Heird WC et al: Intravenous alimentation in pediatric patients, J Pediatr 80:351, 1972.

$D_{10}W$, Dextrose 10% in water; *H_2O*, water.

Theoretic estimates of survival time of starved and semistarved infants are shown in Table 43-2. These estimates assume depletion of all glycogen and fat and approximately one third of body protein tissue at a rate of 50 kcal/kg/day. The effects of fluids such as intravenously provided water (which has no exogenous calories) and 10% dextrose solution ($D_{10}W$) are shown. Currently, PN fluids are started on the day of birth to provide energy and protein for the VLBW infant. Early protein intake promotes positive nitrogen balance, normal plasma amino acid levels, and glucose tolerance.

The small premature infant is particularly vulnerable to undernutrition. Malnutrition in premature infants may increase the risk of infection, prolong chronic illness, and adversely affect brain growth and function. In fact, Lucas and colleagues (1998) reported that the type of milk used for the neonatal diet may be directly linked to neurodevelopment at 18 months of age. Human milk or premature infant formula fed the first month of life resulted in improved development.

NUTRITION REQUIREMENTS: PARENTERAL FEEDING

Many critically ill preterm infants have difficulty progressing to full enteral feedings in the first several days or even weeks of life. The infant's small stomach capacity, immature gastrointestinal tract, and illness make the progression to full enteral feedings difficult (see *Pathophysiology and Care Management Algorithm:* Nutrition Support of Premature Infants). PN becomes essential for nutrition support, either as a supplement to enteral feedings or as the total source of nutrition. Chapter 14 offers a complete discussion of PN; only aspects related to feeding of the preterm infant are presented here.

Fluid

Because fluid needs vary widely for preterm infants, fluid balance must be monitored. Inadequate intake can lead to dehydration, electrolyte imbalances, and hypotension; excessive intake can lead to edema, congestive heart failure, and possible opening of the ductus arteriosus. Additional neonatal clinical complications reported with high fluid intakes include necrotizing enterocolitis (NEC) and bronchopulmonary dysplasia (BPD) (see Chapter 35).

The premature infant has a greater percentage of body water (especially extracellular water) than the term infant (see Chapter 7). The amount of extracellular water should decrease in all infants during the first few days of life. This reduction is accompanied by a normal loss of 10% to 15% of body weight and improved renal function. Failure of this transition in fluid dynamics and lack of diuresis may complicate the course of preterm infants with respiratory disease.

Water requirements are estimated by the sum of the predicted losses from the lungs and skin, urine, and stool, and the water needed for growth. A major route of water loss in preterm infants is evaporation through the skin and respiratory tract. This insensible water loss is highest in the smallest and least mature infants because of their larger body surface area relative to body weight, increased permeability of the skin epidermis to water, and greater skin blood flow relative to metabolic rate. Insensible water loss is increased by radiant warmers and phototherapy lights and decreased by heat shields, thermal blankets, and humidified incubators. Insensible water loss can vary from 50 to 100 mL/kg/day on the first day of life and increase up to 120 to 200 mL/kg/day, depending on the infant's size, gestational age, day of life, and environment. The use of humidified incubators can decrease insensible water losses and thereby reduce fluid requirements.

Excretion of urine, the other major route of water loss, varies from 24 to 72 mL/kg/day. This loss depends on the fluid volume and solute load presented to the kidneys. The infant's ability to concentrate urine increases with maturity. Stool water loss is generally 5 to 10 mL/kg/day, and 10 to 15 mL/kg/day is suggested as optimal for growth (Dell and Davis, 2006).

Because of the many variables affecting neonatal fluid losses, fluid needs must be determined on an individual basis. Usually fluid is administered at a rate of 80 to 105 mL/kg/day the first day of life to meet insensible losses and urine output. Fluid needs are then evaluated by assessing fluid intake and comparing it with the clinical parameters of urine output volume; urine specific gravity; and serum electrolyte, creatinine, and urea nitrogen levels. Assessments of weight, blood pressure, peripheral perfusion, skin turgor, and mucous membrane moisture are performed daily. Daily fluid administration generally increases by 10 to 20 mL/kg/day. By the end of the second week of life, preterm infants may receive fluids at a rate of 140 to 160 mL/kg/day. Fluid restriction may be necessary in preterm infants with patent ductus arteriosus, congestive heart failure, renal failure, or cerebral edema. However, more fluids are needed by preterm infants who are placed under phototherapy lights or a radiant warmer or when the environmental or body temperature is elevated.

Energy

The energy needs of preterm infants fed parenterally are less than those of enterally fed infants because absorption loss does not occur when nutritional intake bypasses the intestinal tract. Enterally fed preterm infants usually require 105 to 130 kcal/kg/day to grow, whereas parenterally fed premature neonates can grow well if they receive 90 to 100 kcal/kg/day (American Academy of Pediatrics [AAP], 2009b). Minimum maintenance energy needs and adequate protein should be provided as soon as possible to prevent tissue catabolism. Providing VLBW infants with 1.5 to 2 g of protein and 30 to 50 kcal/kg/day promotes nitrogen balance during the first 3 days of life (AAP, 2004; AAP, 2009b). Up to 3 g/kg/day of protein is tolerated (Thureen et al., 2003).

Energy and protein intake should be increased as the infant's condition stabilizes and growth becomes the goal (Table 43-3). Many VLBW infants are born AGA but at discharge from the hospital weigh less than the 10th percentile for their postmenstrual age. This new SGA status is called **extrauterine growth restriction (EUGR)**. EUGR may occur as a result of poor energy and protein intakes, and the decreased growth associated with illness (Ehrenkranz, 2010).

Glucose

Glucose or dextrose is the principal energy source (3.4 kcal/g). However, glucose tolerance is limited in premature infants, especially in VLBW infants, because of inadequate insulin production, insulin resistance, and

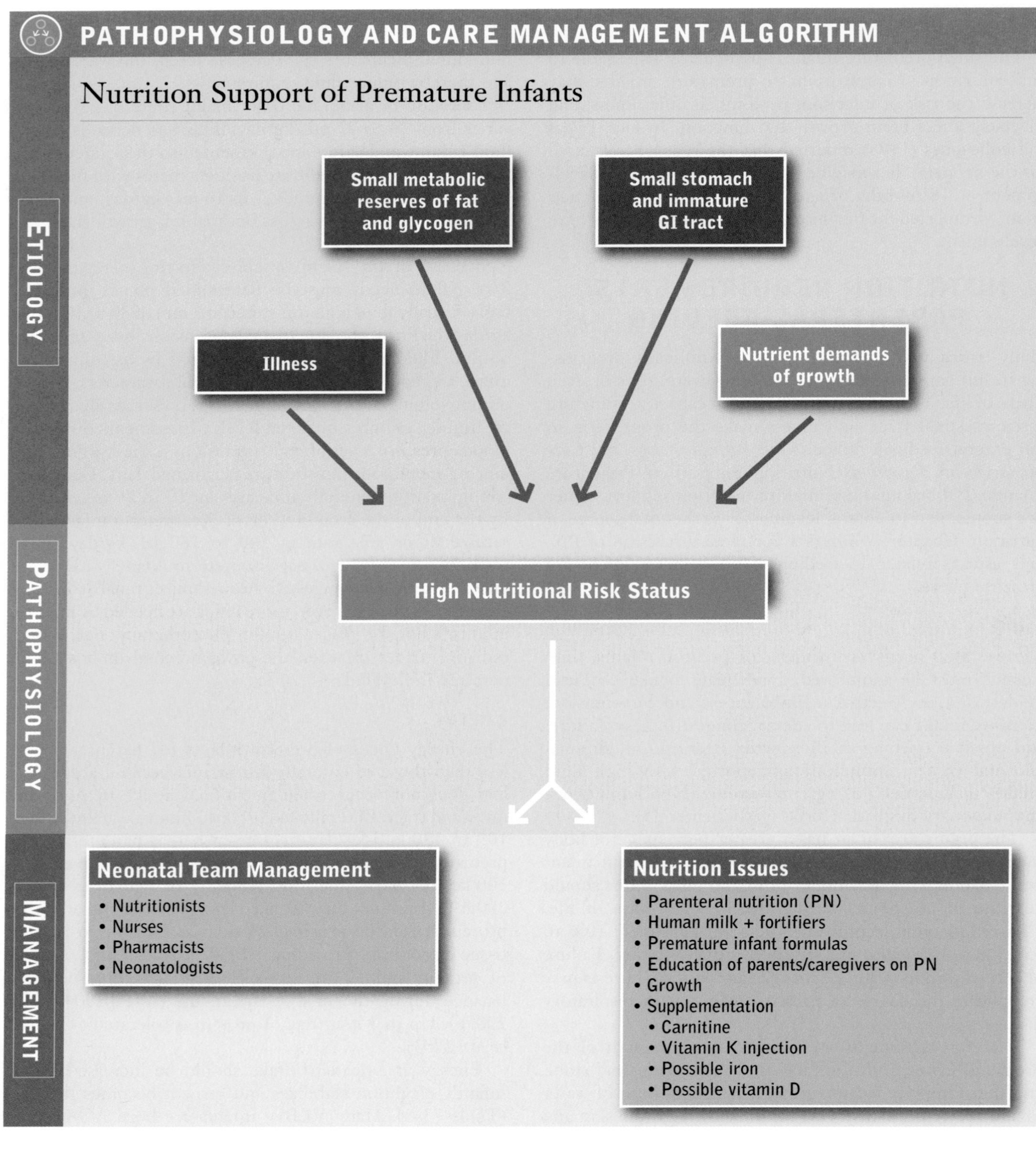

TABLE 43-3

Comparison of Parenteral and Enteral Energy Needs of Premature Infants

	Parenteral	Enteral
Maintenance		
Gradually increase intake to meet energy needs by the end of the first week	30-50 cal/kg/day	50 kcal/kg/day
Growth		
Meet energy needs as soon as the infant's condition is stable	90-100 cal/kg/day	105-130 kcal/kg/day

continued hepatic glucose release while intravenous glucose is infusing. Hyperglycemia is less likely when glucose is administered with amino acids than when it is infused alone. Amino acids exert a stimulatory effect on insulin release. Prevention of hyperglycemia is important because it can lead to diuresis and dehydration.

To prevent hyperglycemia in VLBW infants, glucose should be administered in small amounts. The **glucose load** is a function of the concentration of the dextrose infusion and the rate at which it is administered (Table 43-4). The administration of exogenous insulin may be necessary for infants with persistent or very high glycemia, but changes in the infant's blood glucose level are common problems associated with its use. In addition, protein synthesis may be inhibited by insulin administration in premature infants (Denne, 2007).

In general, preterm infants should receive an initial glucose load of less than 6 mg/kg/min, with a gradual increase to 11 to 12 mg/kg/min. The glucose load can be advanced by 1 to 2 mg/kg/min/day. Hypoglycemia is not as common a problem as hyperglycemia, but it may occur if the glucose infusion is abruptly decreased or interrupted.

Amino Acids

Protein guidelines range from 2.7 to 3.5 g/kg/day (AAP, 2009b). Some ELBW infants need as much as 3.5 to 4 g/kg/day (AAP, 2009b; Tsang et al., 2005). Protein in excess of these parenteral requirements should not be administered because additional protein offers no apparent advantage, and increases the risk of metabolic problems. In practice preterm infants are usually given 1.5 to 3 g/kg/day of protein for the first few days of life, and then protein is provided as tolerated. Many nurseries stock starter PN, which is water, glucose, protein, and perhaps calcium and is available 24 hours a day. Infants can then be provided with protein immediately on admission to the nursery.

In the United States several pediatric PN solutions are available. The use of pediatric PN solutions results in plasma amino acid profiles similar to those of fetal and cord blood or to those of healthy infants fed breast milk (Schanler and Anderson, 2008). These solutions promote adequate weight gain and nitrogen retention. Standard amino acid solutions were not designed to meet the particular needs of immature infants and may provoke imbalances in plasma amino acid levels. For example, cysteine, tyrosine, and taurine levels in these solutions are low relative to the needs of the preterm infant; but the methionine and glycine levels are relatively high. Because premature infants do not effectively synthesize cysteine from methionine because of decreased concentrations of the hepatic enzyme cystathionase, a cysteine supplement has been suggested. Cysteine is insoluble and unstable in solution; thus it is added as cysteine hydrochloride when the PN solution is prepared.

In addition to plasma amino acid imbalances, other metabolic problems associated with amino acid infusions in preterm infants include metabolic acidosis, hyperammonemia, and azotemia. These problems can be minimized by using the crystalline amino acid products that are available and by keeping the protein load within the recommended guidelines (Table 43-5).

Lipids

Intravenous fat emulsions are used for two reasons: (1) to meet essential fatty acid (EFA) requirements and (2 to provide a concentrated source of energy. EFA needs can be met by providing 0.5 to 1 g/kg/day of lipids. Biochemical evidence of EFA deficiency has been noted during the first week of life in VLBW infants fed parenterally without fat. The clinical consequences of EFA deficiency may include coagulation abnormalities, abnormal pulmonary surfactant, and adverse effects on lung metabolism.

Lipids can be initiated at 1 to 2 g/kg/day and should be provided over 24 hours (AAP, 2009b). Lipids can be advanced by 1 to 2 g/kg/day until a rate of 3 g/kg/day is reached (Table 43-6). Plasma triglycerides should be monitored because elevated triglyceride levels may develop in infants with a decreased ability to hydrolyze triglycerides. These infants usually have lower gestational age, SGA status, infection, surgical stress, or liver disease. Monitoring of serum

TABLE 43-4

Guidelines for Glucose Load in Premature Infants

Initial Load (mg/kg/min)*	Daily Increments (mg/kg/min)	Maximum Load (mg/kg/min)
4-6	1-2	11-12

*Use the following formula to calculate glucose load: (% Glucose × mL/kg/day) × (1000 mg/g glucose) ÷ (1440 min/day). For example, (0.10 × 150 mL/kg/day) × (1000 mg/g glucose) ÷ (1440 min/day) = 10.4 mg/kg/min.

TABLE 43-5

Guidelines for Administration of Parenteral Amino Acids for Premature Infants

Initial Rate (g/kg/day)*	Increments (g/kg/day)	Maximum Rate (g/kg/day)
1.5-3	Advance to meet needs	3.5-4†

Data from American Academy of Pediatrics, Committee on Nutrition: Nutritional needs of preterm infants. In Kleinman RE, editor: Pediatric nutrition handbook, ed 6, Elk Grove, IL, 2009, American Academy of Pediatrics.

*Use the following formula to calculate protein load: % Protein × mL/kg/day = Protein g/kg/day.

For example: 2% amino acid parenteral solution provided at 150 mL/kg/day *is* × 0.02 × 150 mL/kg/day = 3 g/kg/day.

†From Tsang RC et al: Summary of reasonable nutrient intakes. In Tsang RC: Nutrition of the preterm infant, ed 2, Cincinnati, OH, 2005, Digital Educational Publishing, Inc. 4 g/kg/day is recommended for infants weighing less than 1000 g.

TABLE 43-6

Guidelines for Administration of Parenteral Lipids for Premature Infants

Initial Rate (g/kg/day)*	Increments (g/kg/day)	Maximum Rate (g/kg/day)
1-2	1	3

Data from American Academy of Pediatrics, Committee on Nutrition: Nutritional needs of preterm infants. In Kleinman RE, editor: Pediatric nutrition handbook, ed 6, Elk Grove, IL, 2009, American Academy of Pediatrics.

*Use the following formula to calculate lipid load: % Lipid × mL/kg/day = Lipid g/kg/day. For example, 0.20 × 15 mL/kg = 3 g/kg/day.

triglyceride levels is indicated, and a rate of less than 3 g/kg/day of fat may be required to keep serum triglyceride levels under 200 mg/dL (AAP, 2009b). Once the infant is medically stable and additional energy is needed for growth, lipid loads can slowly be increased. Intralipids can be given to the infant with hyperbilirubinemia. At the present recommendation of 3 g/kg/day, given during 24 hours, the displacement of bilirubin from albumin-binding sites does not occur (AAP, 2009b).

The total lipid load is usually less than 30% to 40% of nonprotein calories, but it should not exceed 60% of nonprotein calories. (The lipid emulsions currently in use are described in Chapter 14). In preterm infants 20% solutions providing 2 kcal/mL are recommended because plasma triglyceride, cholesterol, and phospholipid levels are generally lower with these than with the 10% emulsions. The lower plasma fat levels may be attributable to a decreased phospholipid load per gram of fat in the 20% emulsion.

Intravenous fat emulsions are made from soybean oil and contain ω-6 fatty acids, linoleic acid and arachidonic acid (ARA). These EFAs increase the production of inflammatory mediators and increase the infant's inflammatory state (Gura, 2010). There is a fish-oil base intravenous fat and it contains ω-3 fatty acids: eicosapentaenoic acid and docosahexaenoic acid (DHA). These ω-3 fatty acids are antiinflammatory and are helpful in the treatment of PN-associated liver disease (Gura, 2010). This fish-oil product is produced in Europe and requires approval for compassionate use by the Food and Drug Administration for patients in the United States. Investigations are ongoing to determine if this product can be used to prevent PN-associated liver disease, which presents with an elevated conjugated bilirubin.

Carnitine is frequently added to PN solutions provided to premature infants. **Carnitine** facilitates the mechanism by which fatty acids are transported across the mitochondrial membrane, allowing their oxidation to provide energy. Intravenous lipid does not contain carnitine and premature infants have limited ability to produce carnitine (Hay, 2008). Carnitine supplementation may be helpful for preterm infants who are receiving only PN for 2 to 4 weeks.

TABLE 43-7

Guidelines for Administration of Parenteral Electrolytes for Premature Infants

Electrolyte	Amount (mEq/kg/day)
Sodium	2-4
Chloride	2-4
Potassium	1.5-2

Electrolytes

After the first few days of life, sodium, potassium, and chloride are added to parenteral solutions to compensate for the loss of extracellular fluid. To prevent hyperkalemia and cardiac arrhythmia, potassium should be withheld until renal flow is demonstrated. In general, the preterm infant has the same electrolyte requirements as the term infant, but actual requirements vary, depending on factors such as renal function, state of hydration, and the use of diuretics (Table 43-7). Very immature infants may have a limited ability to conserve sodium and thus may require increased amounts of sodium to maintain a normal serum sodium concentration. Serum electrolyte levels should be monitored periodically.

Minerals

Calcium and phosphorus are important components of the PN solution. Premature infants who receive PN with low calcium and phosphorus concentrations are at risk for developing osteopenia of prematurity. This poor bone mineralization is most likely to develop in VLBW infants who receive PN for prolonged periods. Calcium and phosphorus status should be monitored using serum calcium, phosphorus, and alkaline phosphatase activity levels (see Appendix 30 for normal range). Alkaline phosphatase activity levels in premature infants are greater than the levels seen with adults. It is common to see levels up to 600 IU/L, which may reflect rapid bone growth (Mitchell et al., 2009). When alkaline phosphatase activity levels of 800 IU/L or more persist, knee or wrist radiographs should be examined for rickets (Mitchell et al., 2009). Elevation in alkaline phosphatase activity may also be seen with liver disease.

Preterm infants have higher calcium and phosphorus needs than term infants. However, it is difficult to add enough calcium and phosphorus to parenteral solutions to meet these higher requirements without causing precipitation of the minerals. Calcium and phosphorus should be provided simultaneously in separate PN solutions. Alternate-day infusions are not recommended because abnormal serum mineral levels and decreased mineral retention develop.

Current recommendations for parenteral administration of additional calcium, phosphorus, and magnesium are presented in Table 43-8. The intakes are expressed at a volume intake of 120 to 150 mL/kg/day, with 2.5 g/100 mL of amino acids or protein. Lower fluid volumes or lower protein concentrations may cause the minerals to precipitate

TABLE 43-8

Guidelines for Administration of Parenteral Minerals for Premature Infants

Minerals	Amount (mg/kg/day)*
Calcium	60-80
Phosphorus	39-67
Magnesium	4.3-7.2

From American Academy of Pediatrics, Committee on Nutrition: Nutritional needs of preterm infants. In Kleinman RE, editor: Pediatric nutrition handbook, ed 6, Elk Grove, IL, 2009, American Academy of Pediatrics.

*These recommendations assume an average fluid intake of 120 to 150 mL/kg/day with 2.5 g of amino acids per 100 mL. The amino acid concentration prevents the precipitation of these minerals.

TABLE 43-9

Guidelines for Administration of Parenteral Trace Elements for Premature Infants

Trace Elements	Amount (mcg/kg/day)
Zinc	400
Copper	20*
Manganese	1*
Selenium	2†
Chromium	0.2†
Molybdenum	0.25†
Iodine	1

From American Academy of Pediatrics, Committee on Nutrition: Parenteral nutrition. In Kleinman RE, editor: Pediatric nutrition handbook, ed 6, Elk Grove, IL, 2009, AAP.

*Reduced or not provided for infants with obstructive jaundice.

†Reduced or not provided for infants with renal dysfunction.

out of solution. The addition of cysteine hydrochloride increases the acidity of the fluid, which inhibits precipitation of calcium and phosphorus.

Trace Elements

Zinc should be given to all preterm infants receiving PN. If enteral feedings cannot be started by 2 weeks of age, additional trace elements should be added. However, the amounts of copper and manganese should be reduced for infants with obstructive jaundice; and the amounts of selenium, chromium, and molybdenum should be reduced in infants with renal dysfunction. Parenteral iron is not routinely provided because infants often receive blood transfusions soon after birth, and enteral feedings, which provide a source of iron, can often be initiated. If necessary, the dosage for parenteral iron is approximately 10% of the enteral dosage; guidelines range from 0.1 to 0.2 mg/kg/day (Rao and Georgieff, 2005). Recommended guidelines have not yet been established for parenteral administration of fluoride to preterm infants (Table 43-9).

TABLE 43-10

Guidelines for Administration of Parenteral Vitamins for Premature Infants

	Preterm
Percentage of one 5-mL vial of MVI-Pediatric/ INFUVITE*	40%/kg

MVI, multivitamin for infusion.

Maximum volume intake is 5 mL/day, which is achieved at 2.5 kg body weight.

Data from American Academy of Pediatrics, Committee on Nutrition: Nutritional needs of preterm infants. In Kleinman RE, editor: Pediatric nutrition handbook, ed 6, Elk Grove, IL, 2009, American Academy of Pediatrics.

*MVI-Pediatric/INFUVITE (5 mL) contains the following vitamins: 80 mg of ascorbic acid, 2300 USP units of vitamin A, 400 USP units of vitamin D, 1.2 mg of thiamin, 1.4 mg of riboflavin, 1 mg of vitamin B_6, 17 mg of niacin, 5 mg of pantothenic acid, 7 USP units of vitamin E, 20 mcg of biotin, 140 mcg of folic acid, 1 mcg of vitamin B_{12}, and 200 mcg of vitamin K.

Vitamins

Shortly after birth all newborn infants receive an intramuscular (IM) injection of 0.5 to 1 mg of vitamin K to prevent hemorrhagic disease of the newborn from vitamin K deficiency. Stores of vitamin K are low in newborn infants, and there is little intestinal bacterial production of vitamin K until bacterial colonization takes place. Because initial dietary intake of vitamin K is limited, neonates are at nutritional risk if they do not receive this IM supplement.

Only intravenous multivitamin preparations currently approved and designed for use in infants should be given to provide the appropriate vitamin intake and prevent toxicity from additives used in adult multivitamin injections. The American Academy of Pediatrics (AAP, 2009b) recommends 40% of the multivitamin for infusion (MVI)-pediatric 5-mL vial per kilogram of weight. The maximum dose of 5 mL is given to an infant with a weight of 2.5 kg (Table 43-10).

Respiratory distress syndrome (RDS) is a disease that occurs in premature infants shortly after birth because these infants are deficient in the lung substance surfactant. Surfactant is responsible for keeping the lung elastic while breathing; thus surfactant supplements are given to the infant to prevent RDS or to lessen the illness. Lipids and proteins are components of surfactant, and phospholipids are the major lipid. Choline is required for phospholipid synthesis, but choline supplementation does not increase the production of phospholipids (van Aerde and Narvey, 2006). Choline is a conditionally essential nutrient because the infant can synthesize choline (see Chapter 16 for a discussion of requirement for choline in pregnancy). Choline is added to premature infant formulas at the level contained in human milk. The upper level is extrapolated from the adult safe level of intake (Klein, 2002).

Bronchopulmonary dysplasia (BPD) is a chronic lung disease that commonly develops in the premature infant as a result of RDS and the mechanical ventilation and oxygen used to treat it. Because of the role of vitamin A in facilitating tissue repair, and because of reports of preterm infants having low vitamin A stores, large supplemental doses of vitamin A have been suggested for the prevention of BPD. One report suggests that providing ELBW premature infants with IM injections of vitamin A at 5000 units/day three times per week during the first month of life decreases the incidence of BPD (Tyson et al., 1999). Physicians may or may not use this supplementation. The decision will be based on the incidence of BPD in their nursery, the lack of proven additional benefits and the acceptability of using IM injections (Darlow and Graham, 2008). See Chapter 35 for discussion of BPD.

TRANSITION FROM PARENTERAL TO ENTERAL FEEDING

It is beneficial to begin enteral feedings for preterm infants as early as possible because the feedings stimulate gastrointestinal enzymatic development and activity, promote bile flow, increase villous growth in the small intestine, and promote mature gastrointestinal motility. These initial enteral feedings can also decrease the incidence of cholestatic jaundice and the duration of physiologic jaundice and can improve subsequent feeding tolerance in preterm infants. At times small, initial feedings are used only to prime the gut and are not intended to optimize enteral nutrient intake until the infant demonstrates feeding tolerance or is clinically stable.

When making the transition from parenteral to enteral feeding, it is important to maintain parenteral feeding until enteral feeding is well established to maintain adequate net intake of fluid and nutrients. In VLBW infants it may take 7 to 14 days to provide a full enteral feeding, and it may take longer for infants with feeding intolerances or illness. The smallest, sickest infants usually receive increments of only 10 mL/kg/day. Larger, more stable preterm infants may tolerate increments of 20 to 30 mL/kg/day (see Chapter 14 for a more detailed discussion of transitional feeding).

NUTRITION REQUIREMENTS: ENTERAL FEEDING

Enteral alimentation is preferred for preterm infants because it is more physiologic than parenteral alimentation and is nutritionally superior. Initiating a tiny amount of an appropriate breast milk feeding whenever possible is beneficial (Sisk et al., 2007). However, determining when and how to provide enteral feedings is often difficult and involves consideration of the degree of prematurity, history of perinatal insults, current medical condition, function of the gastrointestinal tract, respiratory status, and several other individual concerns (Table 43-11).

TABLE 43-11

Factors to Consider Before Initiating or Increasing the Volume of Enteral Feedings

Category	Factors
Perinatal	Cardiorespiratory depression
Respiratory	Stability of ventilation, blood gases, apnea, bradycardia, cyanosis
Medical	Vital signs (heart rate, respiratory rate, blood pressure, temperature)
Gastrointestinal	Anomalies (gastroschisis, omphalocele), patency, gastrointestinal tract function (bowel sounds present, passage of stool), risk of necrotizing enterocolitis
Infection	Sepsis or suspect sepsis

Data from Adamkin DH: Nutritional strategies for the very low birthweight infant, Cambridge, 2009,Cambridge University Press; Hay WW: Strategies for feeding the preterm infant, *Neonatol* 94:245, 2008.

Preterm infants should be fed enough to promote growth similar to that of a fetus at the same gestational age, but not so much that nutrient toxicity develops. Although the exact nutrient requirements are unknown for preterm infants, several useful guidelines exist. In general the requirements of premature infants are higher than those of term infants because the preterm infant has smaller nutrient stores, decreased digestion and absorption capabilities, and a rapid growth rate. Stress, illness, and certain therapies for illness may further influence nutrient requirements. It is also important to remember that, in general, enteral nutrient requirements are different from parenteral requirements.

Energy

The energy requirements of premature infants vary with individual biologic and environmental factors. It is estimated that an intake of 50 kcal/kg/day is required to meet maintenance energy needs, compared with 105 to 130 kcal/kg/day for growth (Table 43-12). However, energy needs may be increased by stress, illness, and rapid growth. Likewise, energy needs may be decreased if the infant is placed in a **neutral thermal environment** (the environmental temperature at which an infant expends the least amount of energy to maintain body temperature). It is important to consider the infant's rate of growth in relation to average energy intakes. Some premature infants may need greater than 130 kg/day to sustain an appropriate rate of growth. ELBW infants or those with BPD often require such increased amounts. To provide such a large number of calories to infants with a limited ability to tolerate large fluid volumes, it may be necessary to concentrate the feedings to a level of more than 24 kcal/oz (Box 43-2).

Protein

The amount and quality of protein must be considered when establishing protein requirements for the preterm infant. Amino acids should be provided at a level that meets demands without inducing amino acid or protein toxicity.

TABLE 43-12

Estimation of Energy Requirements of the Low-Birth-Weight Infant

Activity	Average Estimation (kcal/kg/day)
Energy expended	40-60
Resting metabolic rate	40-50*
Activity	0-5*
Thermoregulation	0-5*
Synthesis	15†
Energy stored	20-30†
Energy excreted	15
Energy intake	90-120

Modified from American Academy of Pediatrics, Committee on Nutrition: Nutritional needs of preterm infants. In Kleinman RE, editor: Pediatric nutrition handbook, ed 6, Elk Grove, IL, 2009, AAP; Committee on Nutrition of the Preterm Infant, European Society of Paediatric Gastroenterology and Nutrition (ESPGAN): Nutrition and feeding of preterm infants, Oxford, 1987, Blackwell Scientific.

*Energy for maintenance.

†Energy cost of growth.

BOX 43-2

Recipes for Preparing 90 mL (3 oz) of Concentrated Premature Infant Formula

Kcal/oz RTF* Formula	Ratio 24/30 kcal oz RTF Formula	Volume (mL) RTF* Premature 24	Volume RTF* (mL) Premature 30
24	1/0	90	0
26	2/1	60	30
27	1/1	45	45
28	1/2	30	60
30	0/1	0	90

RTF, Ready-to-Feed formula.

*RTF (at 24 and 30 kcal/oz).

Example: Recipe for Making a 26 kcal/oz formula:

Goal = 90 mL (3 oz) of formula

2 parts of 24 kcal/oz formula + 1 part of 30 kcal/oz formula = 3 parts of formula

90 mL ÷ 3 parts = 30 mL per part

30 mL × 2 parts = 60 mL of RTF Premature 24 kcal/oz formula + 30 mL × 1 part = 30 mL of Premature 30 kcal/oz = 90 mL (3 parts) of 26 kcal/oz formula

A reference fetus model has been used to determine the amount of protein that needs to be ingested to match the quantity of protein deposited into newly formed fetal tissue (Ziegler, 2007). To achieve these fetal accretion rates, additional protein must be supplied to compensate for intestinal losses and obligatory losses in the urine and skin. Based on this method for determining protein needs, the advisable protein intake is 3.5 to 4 g/kg/day. This amount of protein is well tolerated.

The quality or type of protein is an important consideration because premature infants have different amino acid needs than term infants because of immature hepatic enzyme pathways. The amino acid composition of whey protein, which differs from that of casein, is more appropriate for premature infants. The essential amino acid cysteine is more highly concentrated in whey protein, and premature infants do not synthesize cysteine well. In addition, the amino acids phenylalanine and tyrosine are lower, and the preterm infant has difficulty oxidizing them. Furthermore, metabolic acidosis decreases with consumption of whey-predominant formulas. Because of the advantages of whey protein for premature infants, breast milk or formulas containing predominately whey proteins should be chosen whenever possible.

Taurine is a sulfonic amino acid that may be important for preterm infants. Human milk is a rich source of taurine, and taurine is added to most infant formulas. Term and preterm infants develop low plasma and urine concentrations of taurine without a dietary supply. The premature infant may have difficulty with synthesizing taurine from cysteine. Although no overt disease has been reported in infants fed low taurine formulas, low taurine may affect the development of vision and hearing (Klein, 2002).

Energy must be provided at sufficient levels to allow protein to be used for growth and not merely for energy expenditure. A range of 10.2% to 12.4% of calories from protein has been suggested. Inadequate protein intake is growth limiting, whereas excessive intake causes elevated plasma amino acid levels, azotemia, and acidosis.

Lipids

The growing preterm infant needs an adequate intake of well-absorbed dietary fat to help meet the high energy needs of growth, provide EFAs, and facilitate absorption of other important nutrients such as the fat soluble vitamins and calcium. However, neonates in general, and premature and SGA infants in particular, digest and absorb lipids inefficiently.

Fat should constitute 40% to 50% of total calories. Furthermore, a diet that is high in fat and low in protein may yield more fat deposition than is desirable for the growing preterm infant. To meet EFA needs, linoleic acid should compose 3% of the total calories, and α-linolenic acid should be added in small amounts (AAP, 2009b). Additional longer-chain fatty acids—ARA and DHA—are present in human milk and are added to infant formulas for term and premature infants to meet federal guidelines.

The premature infant has a greater need than the term infant for ARA and DHA supplementation. These fatty acids accumulate in fatty tissue and the brain during the last 3 months of gestation; thus the premature infant has decreased stores. Premature infants fed formulas supplemented with ARA and DHA from birth to 92 weeks' postmenstrual age (12 months after term) demonstrate greater gain in weight and length and higher psychomotor development scores than premature infants not receiving the fatty acid supplementation (Clandinin et al., 2005).

Preterm infants have low levels of pancreatic lipase and bile salts, and this decreases their ability to digest and absorb fat. Lipases are needed for triglyceride breakdown, and bile salts solubilize fat for ease of digestion and absorption. Because medium-chain triglycerides (MCTs) do not require pancreatic lipase and bile acids for digestion and absorption, they have been added to the fat mixture in premature infant formulas. Human milk and vegetable oils contain the EFA linoleic acid, but MCT oil does not. Premature infant formulas must contain vegetable oil and MCT oil to provide the essential long-chain fatty acids.

The composition of dietary fat also plays a role in the digestion and absorption of lipid. In general, infants absorb vegetable oils more efficiently than saturated animal fats, although one exception is the saturated fat in human milk. Infants digest and absorb human milk fat better than the saturated fat in cow's milk or the vegetable oil in standard infant formulas. Human milk contains two lipases that facilitate fat digestion and has a special fatty acid composition that aids absorption.

Carbohydrates

Carbohydrates are an important source of energy, and the enzymes for endogenous production of glucose from carbohydrate and protein are present in preterm infants. Approximately 40% of the total calories in human milk and standard infant formulas are derived from carbohydrates. Too little carbohydrate may lead to hypoglycemia, whereas too much may provoke osmotic diuresis or loose stools. The recommended range for carbohydrate intake is 40% to 50% of total calories.

Lactose, a disaccharide composed of glucose and galactose, is the predominant carbohydrate in almost all mammalian milks and may be important to the neonate for glucose homeostasis, perhaps because galactose can be used for either glucose production or glycogen storage. Generally galactose is used for glycogen formation first, and then it becomes available for glucose production as blood glucose levels decrease. Because infants born before 28 to 34 weeks of gestation have low lactase activity, the premature infant's ability to digest lactose may be marginal. In practice, malabsorption is not a clinical problem because lactose is hydrolyzed in the intestine or fermented in the colon and absorbed. Sucrose is another disaccharide that is commonly found in commercial infant formula products. Because sucrase activity early in the third trimester is at 70% of newborn levels, sucrose is well tolerated by most premature infants. Sucrase and lactase are sensitive to changes in the intestinal milieu. Infants who have diarrhea, are undergoing antibiotic therapy, or are undernourished, may develop temporary intolerances to lactose and sucrose.

Glucose polymers are common carbohydrates in the preterm infant's diet. These polymers, consisting mainly of chains of five to nine glucose units linked together, are used to achieve the isoosmolality of certain specialized formulas. Glucosidase enzymes for digesting glucose polymers are active in small preterm infants.

TABLE 43-13

Recommendations for Enteral Administration of Vitamins for the Premature Infant

Vitamin	Amount (kg/day)
Vitamin A	700-1500 IU
Vitamin D	150-400 IU*
Vitamin E	6-12 IU
Vitamin K	8-10 mcg
Ascorbic acid	18-24 mg
Thiamin	180-240 mcg
Riboflavin	250-360 mcg
Pyridoxine	150-210 mcg
Niacin	3.6-4.8 mg
Pantothenate	1.2-1.7 mg
Biotin	3.6-6 mcg
Folate	25-50 mcg
Vitamin B_{12}	0.3 mcg

Data from American Academy of Pediatrics, Committee on Nutrition: Nutritional needs of preterm infants. In Kleinman RE, editor: Pediatric nutrition handbook, ed 6, Elk Grove, IL, 2009, American Academy of Pediatrics.

*Maximum of 400 IU/day.

Minerals and Vitamins

Premature infants require greater amounts of vitamins and minerals than term infants because they have poor body stores, are physiologically immature, are frequently ill, and will grow rapidly. Formulas and **human milk fortifiers** that are developed especially for preterm infants contain higher vitamin and mineral concentrations to meet the needs of the infant, obviating the need for additional supplementation in most cases (Table 43-13). One major exception is infants receiving human milk with a fortifier that does not contain iron. An iron supplement of 2 mg/kg/day should be sufficient to meet their needs (AAP, 2009b). The other exception is the use of donor human milk fortifier, which requires the addition of a multiple vitamin and an iron supplement.

Calcium and Phosphorus

Calcium and phosphorus are just two of many nutrients that growing premature infants require for optimal bone mineralization. Intake guidelines have been established at levels that promote the bone mineralization rate that occur in the fetus. An intake of 100-220 mg/kg/day of calcium and 60-140 mg/kg/day of phosphorus is recommended. Two thirds of the calcium and phosphorus body content of the term neonate is accumulated through active transport mechanisms during the last trimester of pregnancy. Infants who are born prematurely are deprived of this important intrauterine mineral deposition. With poor mineral stores and low dietary intake, preterm infants can develop **osteopenia of prematurity**, a disease characterized by demineralization of growing bones and documented by radiologic evidence of "washed-out" or thin bones. Very immature babies are particularly susceptible to osteopenia and may develop bone fractures or florid rickets with a prolonged dietary deficiency. Osteopenia of prematurity is most likely to develop in preterm infants who are (1) fed infant formula that is not specifically formulated for preterm infants, (2) fed human milk that is not supplemented with calcium and phosphorus, or (3) receiving long-term PN without enteral feedings.

Vitamin D

Human milk with human milk fortifier or infant formula for preterm infants provides adequate vitamin D when infants consume the entire calorie intake suggested. The current recommendations for intake range from 150 to 400 IU/day for preterm infants.

Vitamin E

Preterm infants require more vitamin E than term infants because of their limited tissue stores, decreased absorption of fat-soluble vitamins, and rapid growth. Vitamin E protects biologic membranes against oxidative lipid breakdown. Because iron is a biologic oxidant, a diet high in either iron or polyunsaturated fatty acids (PUFAs) increases the risk of vitamin E deficiency. The PUFAs are incorporated into the red blood cell membranes and are more susceptible to oxidative damage than when saturated fatty acids compose the membranes.

A premature infant with vitamin E deficiency may experience **hemolytic anemia** (oxidative destruction of red blood cells). However, this anemia is now uncommon today because of improvements in human milk fortifiers and infant formula composition. The human milk fortifiers and premature infant formulas now contain appropriate vitamin E/PUFA ratios for preventing hemolytic anemia.

Because the dietary requirement for vitamin E depends on the PUFA content of the diet, the recommended intake of vitamin E is commonly expressed as a ratio of vitamin E to PUFA. The recommendation for vitamin E is 0.7 IU (0.5 mg of d-α-tocopherol) per 100 kcal, and at least 1 IU of vitamin E per gram of linoleic acid.

Pharmacologic dosing of vitamin E (50 to 100 mg/kg/day) has not proven to be helpful in preventing BPD or retinopathy of prematurity by reducing the toxic effects of oxygen. Furthermore, high doses of vitamin E have been associated with intraventricular hemorrhage, sepsis, NEC, liver and renal failure, and death.

Iron

Preterm infants are at risk for iron deficiency anemia because of the reduced iron stores associated with early birth. At birth most of the available iron is in the circulating hemoglobin. Thus frequent blood sampling further depletes the amount of iron available for erythropoiesis. Transfusions of red blood cells are often needed to treat the early physiologic anemia of prematurity. Recombinant erythropoietin (EPO) therapy has been used to prevent anemia. Iron supplementation is indicated to facilitate red blood cell production, and a dosage of 6 mg/kg/day of enteral iron has been used (AAP, 2009b). This therapy has not consistently prevented anemia and the need for blood transfusions (AAP, 2009b).

In general the recommendation for iron intake is 2 to 4 mg/kg/day (AAP, 2009b). Infants fed human milk should be given ferrous sulfate drops beginning at 1 month of age (Baker and Greer, 2010). Formulas fortified with iron usually contain sufficient iron for preterm infants (AAP, 2009b).

Folic Acid

Premature infants seem to have higher folic acid needs than infants born at term. Although serum folate levels are high at birth, they decrease dramatically, probably as a result of high folic acid use by the premature infant for deoxyribonucleic acid and tissue synthesis needed for rapid growth.

A mild form of folic acid deficiency causing low serum folate concentrations and hypersegmentation of neutrophils is not unusual in premature infants. Megaloblastic anemia is much less common. A daily folic acid intake of 25 to 50 mcg/kg effectively maintains normal serum folate concentrations. Fortified human milk and formulas for premature infants meet these guidelines when full enteral feedings are established.

Sodium

Preterm infants, especially those with VLBW, are susceptible to hyponatremia during the neonatal period. These infants may have excessive urinary sodium losses because of renal immaturity and an inability to conserve adequate sodium. Furthermore, their sodium needs are high because of their rapid growth rate.

Daily sodium intakes of 4 to 8 mEq/kg or more may be required by some infants to prevent hyponatremia. Routine sodium supplementation of fortified human milk and infant formulas is not necessary. However, it is important to consider the possibility of hyponatremia and monitor infants by assessing serum sodium until the blood level is normal. Milk can be supplemented with sodium if repletion is necessary.

FEEDING METHODS

Decisions about breast-feeding, bottle-feeding, or tube-feeding depend on the gestational age and the clinical condition of the preterm infant. The goal is to feed the infant via the most physiologic method possible and supply nutrients for growth without creating clinical complications.

Gastric Gavage

Gastric gavage by the oral route is often chosen for infants who are unable to suck because of immaturity or problems with the central nervous system. Infants less than 32 to 34 weeks of gestational age, regardless of birth weight have poorly coordinated sucking, swallowing, and breathing abilities because of their developmental immaturity. Consequently they have difficulty with nipple-feeding.

With the oral **gastric gavage** method, a soft feeding tube is inserted through the infant's mouth and into the stomach. The major risks of this technique include aspiration and gastric distention. Because of weak or absent cough reflexes and poorly developed respiratory muscles, the tiny infant may not be able to dislodge milk from the upper airway, which can cause reflex bradycardia or airway obstruction. However, electronic monitoring of vital functions and proper positioning of the infant during feeding minimize the risk of aspiration from regurgitation of stomach contents. Tiny, immature infants whose small gastric capacity and slow intestinal motility can impede the tolerance of large-volume bolus feeds may need bolus feedings provided with a pump for a 30 to 60 minute infusion to aid in feeding tolerance.

Occasionally elimination of the distention and vagal bradycardia requires the use of an indwelling tube for continuous gastric gavage feedings rather than intermittent administration of boluses. Continuous feedings may lead to loss of milk fat, calcium, and phosphorus, which deposit in the feeding tubing so that the infant does not receive the total amount of nutrition provided. Bolus feedings provided with the use of the pump infusion can decrease nutrient loss and promote better weight gain. (Hay, 2008; Rogers et al., 2010).

Nasal gastric gavage is sometimes better tolerated than oral tube-feeding. However, because neonates must breathe through the nose, this technique may compromise the nasal airway in preterm infants and cause an associated deterioration in respiratory function. This method is helpful for infants who are learning to nipple-feed. An infant with a nasal gastric tube can still form a tight seal on the bottle nipple, but it can be difficult if an oral feeding tube is in place during feedings (see Chapter 14).

Transpyloric Feeding

Transpyloric tube-feeding is indicated for infants who are at risk for aspirating milk into the lungs or who have slow gastric emptying. The goal of this method is to circumvent the often slow gastric emptying of the immature infant by passing the feeding tube through the stomach and pylorus and placing its tip within the duodenum or jejunum. Infants with severe gastrointestinal reflux do well with this method, which prevents aspiration of feedings into the lungs. This method is also used for infants whose respiratory function is compromised and who are at risk for milk aspiration. The possible disadvantages of transpyloric feedings include decreased fat absorption, diarrhea, dumping syndrome, alterations of the intestinal microflora, intestinal perforation, and bilious fluid in the stomach. In addition, the placement of transpyloric tubes also requires considerable expertise and radiographic confirmation of the catheter tip location. Although associated with many possible complications, transpyloric feedings are used when gastric feeding is not successful.

Nipple-Feeding

Nipple-feeding may be attempted with infants whose gestational age is greater than 32 weeks and whose ability to feed from a nipple is indicated by evidence of an established sucking reflex and sucking motion. Before this time they are unable to coordinate sucking, swallowing, and breathing. Because sucking requires effort by the infant, any stress from other causes such as hypothermia or hypoxemia diminishes the sucking ability. Therefore nipple-feeding should be initiated only when the infant is under minimum stress and is sufficiently mature and strong to sustain the sucking effort. Initial oral feedings may be limited to one to three times per day to prevent undue fatigue or too much energy expenditure, either of which can slow the infant's rate of weight gain. Before oral feedings begin, a standardized oral stimulation program can help infants successfully nipple-feed more quickly (Fucile et al., 2005).

Breast-Feeding

When the mother of a premature infant chooses to breastfeed, nursing at the breast should begin as soon as the infant is ready. Before this time the mother must express her milk so that it can be tube-fed to her infant. These mothers need emotional and educational support for successful lactation. Studies report that premature breast-fed infants have better sucking, swallowing, and breathing coordination and fewer breathing disruptions than bottle-fed infants (Hurst, 2007). **Kangaroo care**—allowing the mother to maintain skin-to-skin contact while holding her infant—facilitates her lactation. In addition, this type of contact promotes continuation of breast-feeding and enhances the mother's confidence in caring for her high-risk infant. The latter benefit may also apply to fathers who engage in kangaroo care with their infants (Stevens et al., 2010).

Feeding infants with cups instead of bottles to supplement breast-feeding has been suggested for preterm infants based on the rationale that it may prevent infant "nipple confusion" (i.e., confusion between nursing at the breast and from a bottle). Complications such as milk aspiration and low volume intakes need to be monitored. Cup feeding has been associated with successful breast-feeding at discharge, but increased length of stay in the hospital for the premature infant (Collins et al., 2008).

Tolerance of Feedings

All preterm babies receiving EN should be monitored for signs of feeding intolerance. Vomiting of feedings usually signals the infant's inability to retain the provided amount of milk. When not associated with other signs of a systemic illness, vomiting may indicate that feeding volumes were increased too quickly or are excessive for the infant's size and maturity. Simply reducing the feeding volume may resolve the problem. If not, or if the infant has signs of a systemic illness, feedings may need to be interrupted until the infant's condition has stabilized.

Abdominal distention may be caused by excessive feeding, organic obstruction, excessive swallowing of air, resuscitation, sepsis (i.e., systemic infection), or NEC. Observing infants for abdominal distention should be a routine practice for nurses. Abdominal distention often indicates the need to interrupt feeding until its cause is determined and resolved.

Gastric residuals, measured by aspiration of the stomach contents, may be determined routinely before each bolus gavage feeding and intermittently in all continuous drip feedings. Whether a residual amount is significant depends partly on its volume in relation to the total volume of the feeding. For example, a residual volume of more than 50% of a bolus feeding or equal to the continuous infusion rate might be a sign of feeding intolerance. However, when interpreting the significance of a gastric residual measurement, it is important to consider other concurrent signs of feeding intolerance and the previous pattern of residual volumes established for a particular infant. Residuals are frequently present before feedings are initiated and as small volume feedings are started. As long as no signs of illness are present, feedings should not be held.

Bile-stained emesis or residuals frequently may be due to overdistention of the stomach with reflux of bile from the intestine or to a feeding tube that has slipped into the intestine, or may indicate that the infant has an intestinal blockage and needs additional evaluation (Schanler and Anderson, 2008). Bloody or bilious gastric residuals are more alarming than those that seem to be undigested milk.

The frequency and consistency of bowel movements should be constantly monitored when feeding preterm infants. Simple inspections can detect the presence of gross blood. All feeding methods for preterm infants have associated complications. Unless close attention is paid to symptoms that indicate poor feeding tolerance, serious complications may ensue. Certain diseases can be recognized by recognizing signs of feeding intolerance. For example, **necrotizing enterocolitis (NEC)** is a serious and potentially fatal disease associated with specific symptoms such as abdominal distention and tenderness, abnormal gastric residuals, and grossly bloody stools.

SELECTION OF ENTERAL FEEDING

During the initial feeding period premature infants often require additional time to adjust to EN and may experience concurrent stress, weight loss, and diuresis. The primary goal of enteral feeding during this initial period is to establish tolerance to the milk. Infants seem to need a period of adjustment to be able to assimilate a large volume and concentration of nutrients. Thus parenteral fluids may be necessary until infants can tolerate adequate amounts of feedings by mouth.

After the initial period of adjustment, the goal of enteral feeding changes from establishing milk tolerance to providing complete nutrition support for growth and rapid organ development. All essential nutrients should be provided in quantities that support sustained growth. The following feeding choices are appropriate: (1) human milk supplemented with human milk fortifier and iron and vitamins as indicated by fortifier used, (2) iron-fortified premature infant formula for infants who weigh less than 2 kg, or (3) iron-fortified standard infant formula for infants who weigh more than 2 kg.

Premature infants who are discharged from the hospital can be given a transitional formula. Additional vitamin D may be indicated to provide 400 IU per day (Wagner and Greer, 2008). Iron supplements may be needed for some infants with the use of this enriched formula (Baker and Greer, 2010). Breast-fed infants may be provided with two to three bottles of transitional formula daily to meet needs. The breast-fed premature infant should also receive 2 mg /kg/day of iron and a multiple vitamin for the first year of life (AAP, 2009b). Premature infants discharged home on standard formula should receive a multivitamin until the infant reaches 3 kg in weight (AAP, 2009b).

Human Milk

Human milk is the ideal food for healthy term infants and premature infants. Although human milk requires nutrient supplementation to meet the needs of premature infants, its benefits for the infant are numerous. During the first month of lactation, the composition of milk from mothers of premature infants differs from that of mothers who have given birth to term infants; the protein and sodium concentrations of breast milk are higher in mothers with preterm infants (Klein, 2002). When premature infants are fed their own mother's milk, they grow more rapidly than infants fed banked, mature breast milk (Schanler et al., 2005).

In addition to its nutrient concentration, human milk offers nutritional benefits because of its unique mix of amino acids and long-chain fatty acids. The zinc and iron in human milk are more readily absorbed, and fat is more easily digested because of the presence of lipases. Moreover, human milk contains factors that are not present in formulas. These components include (1) macrophages and T and B lymphocytes; (2) antimicrobial factors - secretory immunoglobulin A, lactoferrin, and others; (3) hormones; (4) enzymes; and (5) growth factors. It has been reported that human milk as compared with premature infant formula fed to preterm infants reduces the incidence of NEC and sepsis, improves neurodevelopment, facilitates a more rapid advancement of enteral feedings, and leads to an earlier discharge (Sisk et al., 2007; Sisk et al., 2008). The use of mother's own milk for her infant supplemented with liquid donor human milk fortifier and donor human milk is linked to decreased incidence of NEC (Sullivan et al., 2010).

However, one well-documented problem is associated with feeding human milk to preterm infants. Whether it is preterm, term, or mature, human milk does not meet the calcium and phosphorus needs for normal bone mineralization in premature infants. Therefore calcium and phosphorus supplements are recommended for rapidly growing preterm infants who are fed predominantly human milk. Currently three human milk fortifiers are available: powder bovine milk base, liquid bovine milk base, and liquid donor human milk base. The bovine products contain calcium and phosphorus, as well as protein, carbohydrates, fat, vitamins, and minerals, and are designed to be added to expressed breast milk fed to premature infants (Table 43-14). Vitamin supplements are not needed. One bovine fortifier is iron fortified and the other requires the addition of iron. The human-milk base product is made from donor human milk that has been pasteurized, concentrated, and supplemented with calcium, phosphorous, zinc, and electrolytes. A multivitamin and an iron supplement is needed with the use of the human-milk base fortifier.

Providing human milk to a premature infant can be a very positive experience for the mother, one that promotes involvement and interaction. Because many preterm infants are neither strong enough nor mature enough to nurse at their mother's breast in the early neonatal period, their mothers usually express their milk for several days (and occasionally for several weeks) before nursing can be established. The proper technique of expression, storage, and transport of milk should be reviewed with the mother (see Chapter 16). Many summaries of the special considerations for nursing a preterm infant have been published (AAP and the American College of Obstetricians and Gynecologists, 2006; Hurst, 2007).

Premature Infant Formulas

Formula preparations have been developed to meet the unique nutritional and physiologic needs of growing preterm infants. The quantity and quality of nutrients in these products promote growth at intrauterine rates. These formulas, which have caloric densities of 20, 24, and 30 kcal/oz, are available only in a ready-to-feed form. These premature formulas differ in many respects from standard cow's milk–based formulas (see Table 43-14). The types of carbohydrate, protein, and fat differ to facilitate digestion and absorption of nutrients. These formulas also have higher concentrations of protein, minerals, and vitamins.

Transitional Infant Formulas

Formulas containing 22 kcal/oz have been designed as transition formulas for the premature infant. Their nutrient content is less than that of the nutrient-dense premature infant formulas and more than that of the standard infant formula (see Table 43-14). These formulas can be introduced when the infant reaches a weight of 2000 g or more, and they can be used throughout the first year of life. Not all premature infants need these formulas to grow appropriately. The AAP (2009a) suggests that the transitional formulas be continued until the infant's weight for length is maintained at greater than the 25th percentile, or up to 9 or 12 months corrected age. It is not clear which premature infants need this specialized formula as studies have not always demonstrated improved growth with the use of transitional formula (AAP, 2009b). Transitional formulas are available in powder form and in ready-to-feed form.

Formula Adjustments

Occasionally it may be necessary to increase the energy content of the formulas fed to small infants. This may be appropriate when the infant is not growing quickly enough and is already consuming as much as possible during feedings.

Concentration

One approach to providing hypercaloric formula is to prepare the formula with less water, thus concentrating all its nutrients, including energy. Concentrated infant formulas with energy contents of 24 kcal/oz are available to hospitals as ready-to-feed nursettes. However, when using these concentrated formulas, it is important to consider the infant's fluid intake and losses in relation to the renal solute load of the concentrated feeding to ensure that a positive water balance is maintained. This method of increasing formula density is often preferred because the nutrient balance remains the same; infants who need more energy also need additional nutrients. As mentioned, the transitional formulas are available in ready-to-feed and powder form and can be concentrated from 24 to 30 kcal/oz. However, this formula is still inadequate for infants who need additional calcium (e.g., infants with osteopenia).

A ready-to-feed 30 kcal/oz premature infant formula is available. It meets the nutritional needs for premature infants who must be fluid restricted because of illness. This 30 kcal/oz formula can be diluted with premature infant formula 24 kcal/oz to make 26, 27, or 28 kcal/oz milks (see Box 43-2). These milks are sterile and are the preferred source of providing concentrated milks to premature infants in the neonatal intensive care unit (NICU). Infant formula powder is not sterile and is not to be used with high-risk infants when a nutritionally adequate liquid, sterile product is available (Robbins and Beker, 2004).

Caloric Supplements

Another approach to increasing the energy content of a formula involves the use of caloric supplements such as vegetable oil, MCT oil, or glucose polymers. These supplements increase the caloric density of the formula without markedly altering solute load or osmolality. However, they do alter the relative distribution of total calories derived from protein, carbohydrate, and fat. Because even small amounts of oil or carbohydrate dilute the percentage of calories derived from protein, adding these supplements to human milk or standard (20 kcal/oz) formulas is not advised. Caloric supplements should be used only when a formula already meets all nutrient requirements other than energy or when the renal solute load is a concern.

When a high-energy formula is needed, glucose polymers can be added to a base that has a concentration of 24 kcal/oz or greater (either full-strength premature formula or a concentrated standard formula), with a maximum of 50% of total calories from fat and a minimum of 9% of total calories from protein. Vegetable oil may be added

TABLE 43-14

Comparison of the Nutritional Content of Human Milk and Formulas

	Human Milk	Human Milk + Powder Bovine–Based Fortifier*	Human Milk + Liquid Bovine–Based Fortifier**	Human Milk + Liquid Donor Human Milk–Based Fortifier[†]	Standard Formula[‡]	Transitional Formula[§]	Premature Formula[¶]
Caloric density (kcal/oz)	20	24	24	24	20	22	20, 24, 30
Protein whey/casein ratio	70:30	Whey predominates	Whey predominates	Whey predominates	60:40, 48:52; 100:0	60:40, 50:50	60:40;100:0
Protein(g/L)	9	19-20	30	19	14-15	21	20, 24 & 27, 28 &30
Carbohydrate	Lactose	Lactose, glucose polymers	Lactose, citrate, pectin	Lactose	Lactose or lactose and glucose polymers	Lactose, glucose polymers	Lactose, glucose polymers
Carbohydrate (g/L)	80	80-95	70	82	75-78	75-77	72, 83, 78
Fat	Human fat	Human fat, MCT oil	Human fat, MCT, vegetable oil, DHA, ARA	Human fat	Vegetable oil	Vegetable oil, MCT oil	Vegetable oil, MCT oil
Fat (g/L)	35	38-44	51	46	34-37	39-41	36, 43, 67
Calcium (mg/L)	230	1110-1360	1340	1360	450-530	780-890	1170, 1395, 1826
Phosphorus (mg/L)	130	610-780	736	800	260-290	460-490	620, 740, 1014
Vitamin D (units/L)	10	1180-1470	1891	270	400-410	520-590	1315, 1580, 1522
Vitamin E (units/L)	5.5	38-52	60	8	10-13	26-29	34, 41, 41
Folic acid (mcg/L)	110	340-360	396	142	101-107	183-190	274, 328, 375
Sodium (mEq/L)	8	14-15	18	23	7-8	11	15, 18, 19

Data from American Academy of Pediatrics, Committee on Nutrition: Appendix C. Table C-1 Representative values for constituents of human milk. In Kleinman RE, editor: Pediatric nutrition handbook, ed 6, Elk Grove, Ill, 2009, American Academy of Pediatrics.

ARA, Arachidonic acid; *DHA*, docosahexaenoic acid; *MCT*, medium-chain triglyceride.

*Based on the composition of term human milk fortified with either powder Enfamil or Similac Human Milk Fortifiers at four packets per 100 mL.

**Based on the composition of term human milk fortified with liquid Enfamil Human Milk Fortifier at 1 vial + 25 mL milk.

[†]Based on the composition of term human milk fortified with Prolact +4.

[‡]Based on the composition of Enfamil Premium, Similac Advance, and Good Start Gentle Plus formulas.

[§]Based on the composition of Similac NeoSure, and Enfamil EnfaCare formulas.

[¶]Based on the composition of Enfamil Premature Lipil, Good Start Premature, and Similac Special Care formulas.

to a feeding or given as a oral medication. Vegetable oil added to a day's supply of formula will separate out from the milk and cling to the milk storage container, and will not be in the feeding to the infant. See Table 45-6.

NUTRITION ASSESSMENT AND GROWTH

Dietary Intake

Dietary intake needs to be evaluated to ensure that the nutrition provided meets the infant's needs. Parenteral fluids and milk feedings are advanced as tolerated, and the nutrient intakes must be reviewed to ensure that they are within the guidelines for premature infants and that the infant is thriving on the nutrition provided. Appropriate growth and growth charts are reviewed in the following paragraphs.

Laboratory Indices

Laboratory assessments usually involve measuring the following parameters: (1) fluid and electrolyte balance, (2) PN or EN tolerance, (3) bone mineralization status, and (4) hematologic status (Table 43-15). Hemoglobin and hematocrit will be monitored as medically indicated. The early decrease in hematocrit reflects the physiologic drop in hemoglobin after birth and blood drawings for laboratory assessments. Early low hemoglobins are treated with blood transfusions if needed. Dietary supplementation will not change this early physiologic drop in hemoglobin.

Growth Rates and Growth Charts

All neonates typically lose some weight after birth. Preterm infants are born with more extracellular water than term infants and thus tend to lose more weight than term infants. However, the postnatal weight loss should not be excessive. Preterm infants who lose more than 15% of their birth weight may become dehydrated from the inadequate fluid intake or experience tissue wasting from poor energy intake. An infant's birth weight should be regained by the second or third week of life. The smallest and sickest infants take the longest time to regain their birth weights.

During the first 98 days of life the Ehrenkranz growth chart is commonly used to assess weight progress (Ehrenkranz et al., 1999) (Figure 43-3). This chart longitudinally depicts daily weight changes and actual growth curves for 1660 infants who were born with a weight of 501 to 1500 g (1⅒ to 3⅓ lb). These infants received care in 12 different NICUs for various neonatal medical problems. Charts are also available for length, head circumference, and midarm circumference (see Useful Websites for a source to create a growth curve for an individual infant). These charts reflect how premature infants grow, and do not allow for the assessment of catch-up growth by the premature infant.

Intrauterine growth curves have been developed using birth weight, birth length, and birth head circumference data of infants born at several successive weeks of gestation. The intrauterine growth curves are the standard of growth recommended for premature infants. During the first week of life premature infants fall away from their birth weight percentile, which reflects the normal postnatal weight loss of newborn infants. After an infant's condition stabilizes and the infant begins consuming all needed nutrients, the infant may be able to grow at a rate that parallels these curves. An intrauterine weight gain of 15 g/kg/day can be achieved.

Although weight is an important anthropometric parameter, measurements of length and head circumference can also be helpful. A growth curve can be used to evaluate the

TABLE 43-15

Monitoring of the Feeding of the Premature Infant

Monitor	Parenteral Nutrition	Enteral Nutrition
Fluid & electrolyte balance	Fluid intake Urine output Daily weights Serum sodium, potassium and chloride Serum creatinine BUN	Fluid intake Urine output Daily weights
Glucose homeostasis	Serum glucose	Not routine
Fat tolerance	Serum triglycerides	Not indicated
Protein nutriture: BUN	Not helpful	Low levels with human milk–fed infants may indicate need for more protein
Osteopenia	Serum calcium Serum phosphorous Serum alkaline phosphatase activity	Serum calcium Serum phosphorous Serum alkaline phosphatase activity
Parenteral nutrition toxicity	Cholestasis: conjugated bilirubin Liver function: ALT	Not indicated

ALT, Alanine aminotransferase; *BUN,* blood urea nitrogen.

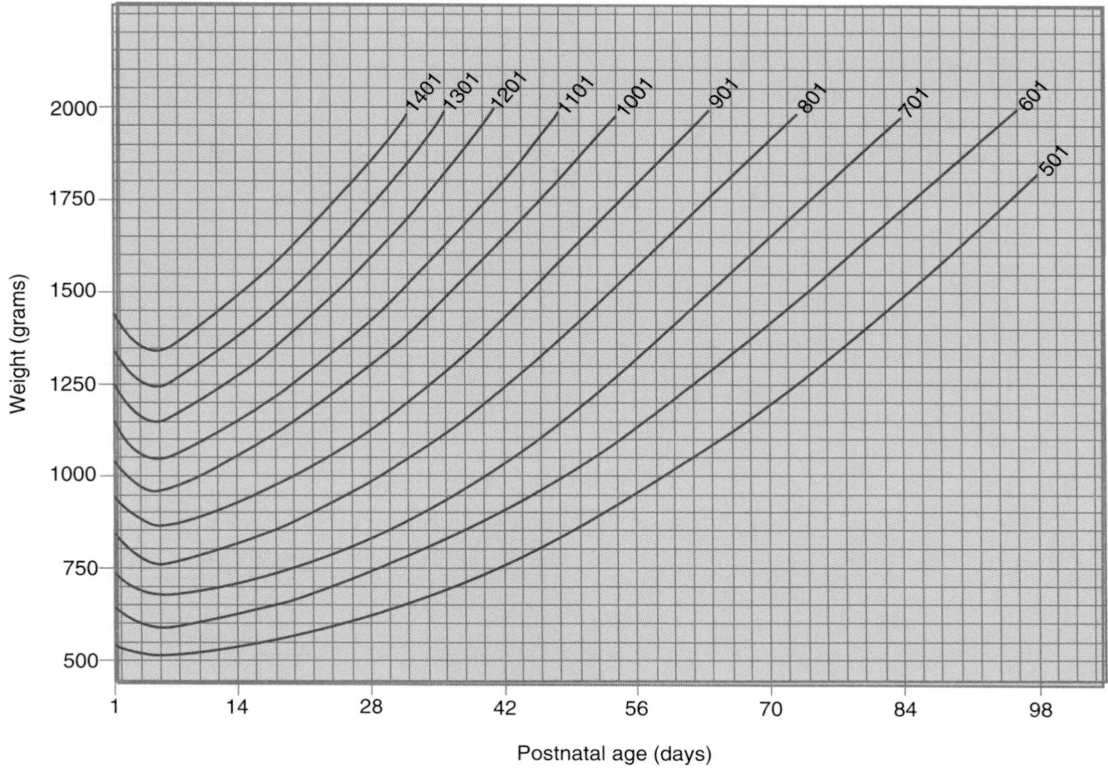

FIGURE 43-3 Weight chart for premature infants based on actual growth data. *(From Ehrenkranz RA et al: Longitudinal growth of hospitalized very-low-birth-weight infants, Pediatrics 104:283, 1999.)*

adequacy of growth in all three areas (Figure 43-4). This chart has a built-in correction factor for prematurity; the infant's growth can be followed from 22 to 50 weeks of gestation and it represents cross-sectional data from Canada, Sweden, Australia, and the United States (Fenton, 2003).

Additional intrauterine growth charts based on the birth-weight, birth length, and head circumferences of infants born in the United States have been developed (Olsen et al., 2010). Separate charts for male and female infants are available and infants can be plotted from 23 to 41 weeks' gestation.

The 2006 World Health Organization Growth Charts designed for children from birth to 2 years of age should also be used for preterm infants once they reach 40 weeks' gestation, as long as the age is adjusted (see *Focus On:* Long-Term Outcome for Premature Infants). For example, an infant born at 28 weeks of gestation is 12 weeks premature (40 weeks of term gestation minus 28 weeks of birth gestational age). Four months after birth, the growth parameters of a premature infant born at 28 weeks of gestation can be compared with those of a 1-month-old infant born at term (Box 43-3). When using growth grids, age should be adjusted for prematurity until at least 2½ to 3 years of corrected age. In Figure 43-5 A.R.'s pattern of growth is shown through 18 years of age. These charts are based on term, healthy infants who were breast-fed the first year of life (Grummer-Strawn et al., 2010). By using this chart, the infant's growth can be compared with the term infant to assess catch-up growth.

BOX 43-3

Steps for Adjusting Age for Prematurity on Growth Charts

Calculate the number of weeks the infant was premature:

- 40 weeks (term) – birth gestational age = number of weeks premature
- The resulting number of weeks is the correction factor.

Calculate the adjusted age for prematurity:

- Chronologic age – Correction factor = Adjusted age for prematurity

For example:

40 weeks – 28 weeks of gestation = 12 weeks premature
Therefore 12 weeks (3 months) is the correction factor.
4 months (chronologic age) – 3 months (correction factor) = 1 month adjusted age

DISCHARGE CARE

Establishment of successful feeding is a pivotal factor determining whether a preterm infant can be discharged from the hospital nursery. Preterm infants must be able to (1) tolerate their feedings and usually obtain all of their feedings from the breast or bottle, (2) grow adequately

FIGURE 43-4 Example of a growth record of weight, length, and head circumference for infants from 22 to 50 weeks of gestation. This chart has a built-in correction factor for prematurity. http://members.shaw.ca/growthchart/ *(From Fenton TR: A new growth chart for preterm babies: Babson and Benda's chart updated with recent data and a new format, BMC Pediatr 3:13, 2003.)*

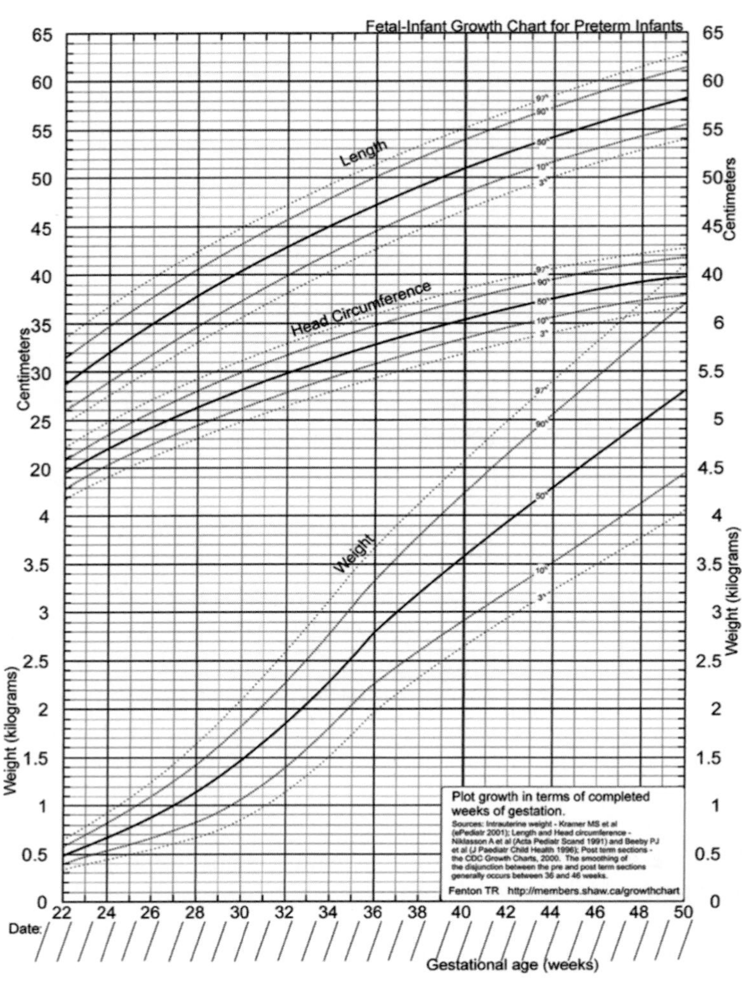

FOCUS ON

Long-Term Outcome for Premature Infants

As the survival of premature infants continues to improve, their physical growth, mental development, health, and quality of life are being evaluated and investigated. Previously it was believed that, if premature infants experienced catch-up growth, it would occur only during the first few years of life. However, catch-up growth for weight, length, and head circumference can continue throughout childhood. As adults, premature infants tend to be shorter and weigh more than infants born at term (Doyle and Anderson, 2010). However, premature infants have normal heights and their heights may reflect their genetic potential.

The premature infants' increase in body mass index may be a risk factor for type 2 diabetes. In adulthood, very low birthweight infants often have decreased glucose regulation as compared with infants born at term. Higher fasting insulin levels, impaired glucose tolerance, and increased insulin resistance may occur (Hovi et al., 2007). The extremely low birthweight (ELBW) infants have been reported to have higher blood pressures than infants born at term and normal weight (Doyle and Anderson, 2010).

Only recently have tools been developed and validated that assess how adults report their health status and quality of life. Saigal and colleagues (2006a, 2006b) compared two groups of adults at 23 years of age. The first group included 143 adults who were born prematurely with ELBW. The second group consisted of 130 adults who were born at term and were not low birthweight infants. All adults were interviewed in the same way except for seven adults who were severely neurologically impaired. Parents completed the evaluations for their children. The adults born ELBW reported more functional limitations in cognition, sensation, mobility, and self-care. However, there was no difference between the two groups in their mean self-reported, health-related quality of life. The two groups were similar in their level of education attainment, living on their own or with parents, martial status, and employment.

Therefore not only are more premature infants surviving, but they also are growing into adults who are enjoying and living productive lives (Doyle and Anderson, 2010; Hack, 2009). The medical and nutrition care in the hospital nursery continues to progress, which improves outcome in the nursery and sets the stage for later development.

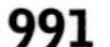

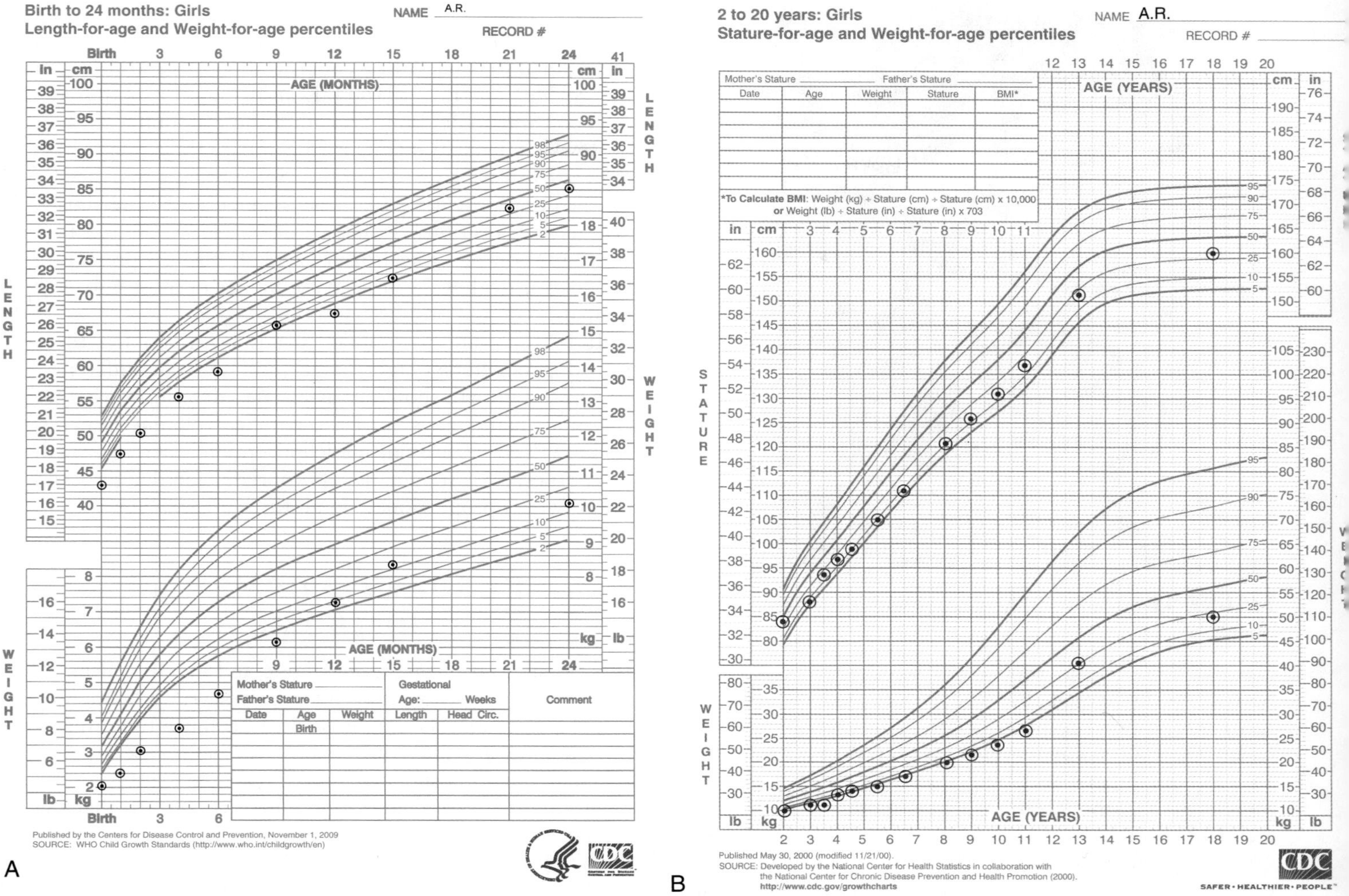

FIGURE 43-5 A, Graphs showing how A.R. (from Figure 43-2), who was born at 27 weeks of gestation, grew after leaving the neonatal unit 1 day before her due date at a weight of 4½ lb. Heights and weights until age of 24 months are plotted on the grid at "corrected age" points. A.R. experienced catch-up growth during the first 12 months. **B,** A.R.'s growth pattern from the age of 2 to 18 years. During the first 10 years she grew at the 5th percentile for weight and the 10th percentile for height. She followed her channel of growth but did not experience catch-up growth. However, between the ages of 10 and 13 she began to change growth channels and moved to the 25th percentile for weight and the 25th percentile for height (catch-up growth). At 18 years she crossed the 25th percentile for height and fell slightly below the 25th percentile for weight.

on a modified-demand feeding schedule (usually every 3 to 4 hours during the day for bottle-fed infants or every 2 to 3 hours for breast-fed infants), and (3) maintain their body temperature without the help of an incubator. Medically stable premature infants who have delayed feeding development will go home on gavage feedings for a short period. In addition, it is important that any ongoing chronic illnesses, including nutrition problems, be manageable at home.

Most important, the parents must be ready to care for their infant. In hospitals that allow parents to visit their infants in the nursery 24 hours a day, staff can help parents develop their caregiving skills and learn to care for their infant at home. Often, parents are permitted to "room in" with their infant (i.e., stay with the infant all day and night) before discharge, which helps build confidence in their ability to care for a high-risk infant (Figure 43-6).

Many preterm infants who are discharged from the hospital weigh less than 5½ lb. Although these infants must meet certain discharge criteria before they can go home, the stress of a new environment may lead to setbacks. Small preterm infants should be followed very closely during the first month after discharge, and parents should be given as much information and support as possible. Within the first week of discharge, a home visit by a nurse, dietitian, or both and a visit to the pediatrician can be extremely helpful educationally; and they can provide opportunity for early intervention for developing problems.

Factors that affect the feeding skills and behavior of preterm infants are particularly important after the infants

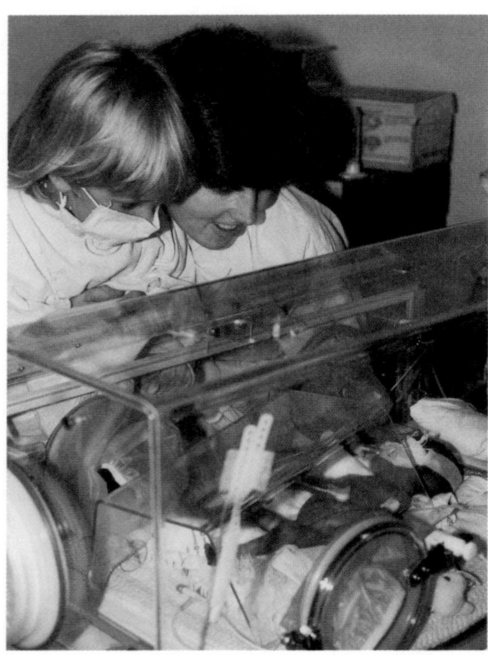

FIGURE 43-6 Family in the nursery with their premature infant.

have been discharged. Physical factors such as a variable heart rate, a rapid respiratory rate, and tremulousness are examples of physiologic events that interfere with feeding. In addition, infants weighing less than 5½ lb have poor muscle tone. Although muscle tone gradually improves as an infant becomes larger and more mature, it can deteriorate quickly in infants who are tired or weak. Feeding is often difficult for infants who have limited muscle flexion and strength and poor head and neck control, which are needed to maintain a good feeding posture. Positioning these infants in a manner that supports normal body flexion and ensures proper alignment of the head and neck during feedings is helpful. Premature infants may also need their chin and cheeks supported while bottle-feeding.

Small infants tend to sleep more than larger and term infants. It is much easier for preterm infants to feed effectively if they are fully awake. To awaken a preterm infant, the caregiver should provide one type of gentle stimulation for a few minutes and then change to a different type, repeating this pattern until the infant is fully awake. Lightly swaddling of the infant and then placing him or her in a semiupright position may also help.

The feeding environment should be as quiet as possible. Preterm infants are easily distracted and have difficulty focusing on feeding when noises or movements interrupt their attention. They also tire quickly and are easily overstimulated. When they are overstimulated, they may show only subtle signs of distress. It is important to teach parents of premature infants to recognize the subtle cues that indicate the need for rest or comfort and to respond to them appropriately.

After discharge, most preterm infants need approximately 180 mL/kg/day (2¾ oz/lb/day) of breast milk or standard infant formula containing 20 kcal/oz. This amount of milk provides 120 kcal/kg/day (55 kcal/lb/day). Alternatively, transitional formula with a concentration of 22 kcal/oz can be provided at a rate of 160 mL/kg/day (or 2½ oz/lb/day). The best way to determine whether these amounts are adequate for individual infants is to compare their intake with their growth progress over time. Some infants may need a formula that provides 24 kcal/oz. As mentioned previously, powdered transitional formula can be readily altered to a concentration of 24 kcal/oz. The ready-to-feed premature formulas providing 24 kcal/oz are higher in most nutrients than are required postdischarge.

It is important to evaluate needs based on the three growth parameters: weight, length, and head circumference. Patterns of growth should be assessed to determine whether (1) individual curves at least parallel reference curves, (2) growth curves are shifting inappropriately across growth percentiles, (3) weight is appropriate for length, and (4) growth is proportionate in all three areas.

NEURODEVELOPMENTAL OUTCOME

It is possible to meet the metabolic and nutritional needs of premature infants sufficiently to sustain life and promote growth and development. In fact, more tiny premature infants are surviving than ever before because of adequate nutrition support and the recent advances in neonatal intensive care technology. There is concern that the ELBW infant is often smaller at discharge than the infant of the same postmenstrual age who was not born prematurely. One report suggests that providing appropriate protein intake during week 1 of life to ELBW infants leads to improved growth of weight, length and head circumference at 36 weeks' gestation, and improved head circumference in male infants at 18 months' corrected age (Poindexter et al., 2006). Improved neurodevelopment and growth at 18 months has been reported with ELBW infants who gained more weight and had greater head circumference growth during their stay in the nursery (Ehrenkranz et al., 2006). The developmental outcome scores for ELBW infants have been higher as the intakes of human milk increase (Vohr et al., 2007).

The increased survival rate of ELBW infants has increased concerns about their short- and long-term neurodevelopmental outcomes. Many questions have been raised about the quality of life awaiting infants who receive neonatal intensive care. As a rule, VLBW infants should be referred to a follow-up clinic to evaluate their development and growth and begin early interventions (Wilson-Costello and Hack, 2006). The survival of ELBW infants has increased, with an increase in the number of children with neurodevelopmental disabilities, but also with an increase in the number of children who are developmentally normal (Wilson-Costello and Hack, 2006). Many of these premature infants reach adulthood with no evidence of any disability (Figure 43-7).

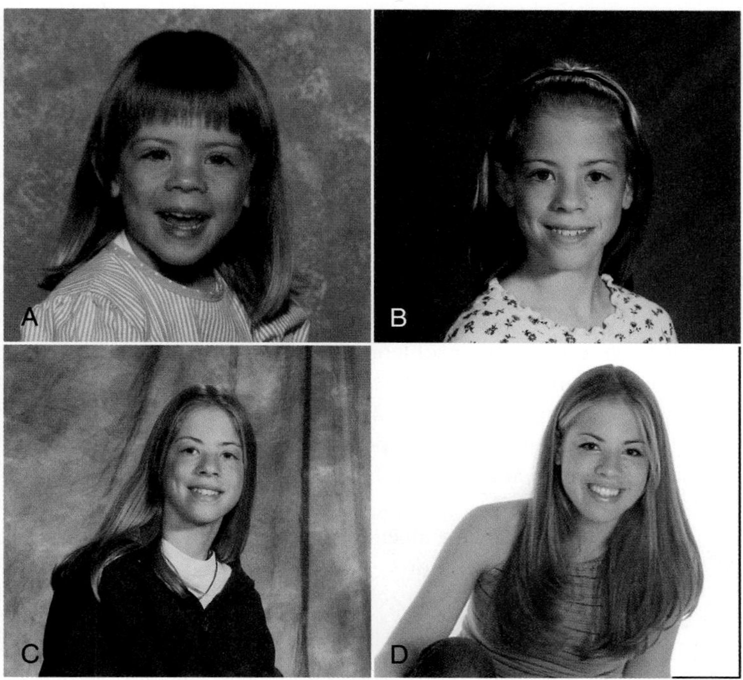

FIGURE 43-7 The premature infant A.R. (see Figures 43-2 and 43-6) as she grows up. **A,** 3½ years. **B,** 10 years. **C,** 14 years. **D,** 18 years. *(D Courtesy Yuen Lui Studio, Seattle, Wash.)*

CLINICAL SCENARIO 1

Sara, an infant born at 26 weeks of gestation, was admitted to the neonatal intensive care unit. Her birth weight was 850 g (appropriate for gestational age). Sara had respiratory distress syndrome and had to receive a tube for mechanical ventilation. During the first few hours of her life, she was given surfactant, and her ventilator settings were lowered. She was also placed in a humidified incubator and given 100 mL/kg/day of starter parenteral nutrition (dextrose 10% in water with amino acids) intravenously.

On the second day after her birth, she had gained 20 g, and her serum sodium concentration and urine volume output were low. She was diagnosed with a patent ductus arteriosus and was given indomethacin to close the ductus arteriosus.

On the fourth day after birth, her body weight had decreased 50 g—6% of her birth weight—and her serum electrolyte levels were normal. The protein concentration of her parenteral fluids was increased, as was the volume of intravenous fat being provided.

By the sixth day, Sara was clinically stable. She began receiving feedings of milk from her mother—0.7 mL every 2 hours (10 mL/kg of her birth weight)—via bolus oral gastric tube. The feedings were tolerated well. She then began receiving daily a larger volume of her mother's breast milk and less parenteral fluids. Full enteral feedings were established, and following extubation Sara was successfully breathing on her own.

Nutrition Diagnostic Statement, Day 2

Excessive fluid intake related to intravenous fluids as evidenced by gain of 20 g and low serum sodium level.

Nutrition Diagnostic Statement, Day 6

Inadequate intake of protein and minerals related to need for human milk fortifier as evidenced by feeding only expressed breast milk.

Nutrition Care Questions

1. On the second day after birth, should Sara's intravenous fluid volume have been (1) increased because she needed more calories, (2) decreased because she was overhydrated, or (3) changed to enteral feedings because she was clinically stable?
2. How should the intravenous fat that was given to Sara have been administered?
3. The breast milk from Sara's mother may have inadequate amounts of which nutrients? What do you recommend to resolve this?

CLINICAL SCENARIO 2

Baby Jones was born at 29 weeks of gestation, and his birthweight was 1400 g. He is now 1 week old or 30 weeks' postmenstrual age and weighs 1375 g. He is receiving parenteral nutrition at 130 mL/kg/day that contains 12.5% dextrose and 3.5% amino acids and a 20% intravenous fat emulsion at 15 mL/kg per day. The registered dietitian assesses the nutrient intake, and calculations are given in the following table. The patient's intakes are compared with the parenteral guidelines of the American Academy of Pediatrics (AAP) (2009b) for premature infants.

NUTRIENT	NUTRIENT (KG/DAY)	GUIDELINES (KG/DAY)
Kilocalories kcal/kg/day	103	90-100
Glucose mg/kg/min	11.3	11-12
Protein g/kg	4.6	2.7-3.5
Fat g/kg	3	1-3

Nutrition Diagnostic Statement

Excessive protein intake related to protein intake 4.6 g/kg/day as evidenced by intake greater than recommendation of 3.5 g of protein per kilogram established by the AAP in 2009.

Nutrition Care Questions

1. The registered dietitian chooses the nutrition diagnosis and writes the problem-etiology-signs and symptoms statement. Interventions include decreasing the amino acid concentration to 2.7%, which will provide 3.5 g of protein per kilogram per day.
2. Monitor and evaluate infant's nutrition status in how many days?
3. What guidance is needed for the staff to evaluate for signs of dehydration?

USEFUL WEBSITES

American Academy of Pediatrics
www.aap.org

Ehrenkranz Growth Charts—National Institute of Child Health and Human Development, Neonatal Research Network
http://neonatal.rti.org

Fenton Growth Chart
http://members.shaw.ca/growthchart/

Human Milk Banking Association of North American
www.hmbana.org

March of Dimes
www.marchofdimes.org

Olsen Growth Chart
http://www.nursing.upenn.edu/media/infantgrowthcurves/Documents/Olsen-NewIUGrowthCurves_2010permission.pdf

World Health Organization Growth Curves
http://www.cdc.gov/growthcharts/who_charts.htm

National Center for Education in Maternal and Child Health
www.ncemch.org

REFERENCES

American Academy of Pediatrics (AAP) and the American College of Obstetricians and Gynecologists (ACOG): Breastfeeding infants with special needs. In Schanler RJ, et al, editors: *Breastfeeding handbook for physicians*, Evanston, IL, 2006, American Academy of Pediatrics.

American Academy of Pediatrics (AAP), Committee on Nutrition: Nutritional needs of preterm infants. In Kleinman RE, editor: *Pediatric nutrition handbook*, ed 5, Elk Grove, IL, 2004, American Academy of Pediatrics.

American Academy of Pediatrics (AAP), Committee on Nutrition: Failure to thrive. In Kleinman RE, editor: *Pediatric nutrition handbook*, ed 6, Elk Grove, IL, 2009a, American Academy of Pediatrics.

American Academy of Pediatrics (AAP), Committee on Nutrition: Nutritional needs of preterm infants. In Kleinman RE, editor: *Pediatric nutrition handbook*, ed 6, Elk Grove, IL, 2009b, American Academy of Pediatrics.

Baker RD, Greer FR, American Academy of Pediatrics (AAP), Committee on Nutrition: Clinical report-diagnosis and prevention of iron deficiency and iron-deficiency anemia in infants and young children (0-3 years of age), *Pediatrics* 126, 2010. Accessed January 5, 2011 from www.pediatrics.org/cgi/doi/10.1542/peds.2010-2576.

Ballard JL, et al: New Ballard score, expanded to include extremely premature infants, *J Pediatr* 119:417, 1991.

Clandinin MT, et al: Growth and development of preterm infants fed infant formulas containing docosahexaenoic acid and arachidonic acid, *J Pediatr* 146:461, 2005.

Collins CT, et al: Avoidance of bottles during the establishment of breast feeds in preterm infants (Review). *Cochrane Database Syst Rev* 2008, Issue 4. Art.No.:CD005252. DOI: 10.1002/14651858.CD005252.pub.2.

Darlow BA, Graham PJ: Vitamin A supplementation for preventing morbidity and mortality in very low birthweight infants, 2008. Accessed 1 June 2010 from www.nichd.nih.gov/cochraneneonatal/.

Dell KM, Davis ID: Fluid, electrolyte, and acid-base homeostasis. In Martin RJ, et al, editors: *Neonatal-perinatal medicine diseases of the fetus and infant*, ed 8, Philadelphia, 2006, Mosby.

Denne SC: Regulation of proteolysis and optimal protein accretion in extremely premature newborns, *Am J Clin Nutr* 85(Suppl): 621S, 2007.

Doyle LW, Anderson PJ: Adult outcome of extremely preterm infants, *Pediatrics* 126:342, 2010.

Ehrenkranz RA, et al: Longitudinal growth of hospitalized very low birth weight infants, *Pediatrics* 104:280, 1999.

Ehrenkranz RA, et al: Growth in the neonatal intensive care unit influences neurodevelopment and growth outcomes of extremely low birth weight infants, *Pediatrics* 117:1253,2006.

Ehrenkranz RA: Early nutritional support and outcomes in ELBW infants, *Ear Hum Dev* 86:S21, 2010.

Fenton TR: A new growth chart for preterm babies: Babson and Benda's chart updated with recent data and a new format, *BMC Pediatrics* 3:13, 2003.

Fucile S, et al: Effect of an oral stimulation program on sucking skill maturation of preterm infants, *Dev Med Child Neurology* 47:158, 2005.

Grummer-Strawn LM, et al: Centers for Disease Control and Prevention, Use of World Health Organization and CDC growth charts for children aged 0-59 months in United States, *MMWR* 59(No. RR-9):1, 2010. Erratum in *MMWR Recomm Rep.* 59(36):1184, 2010.

Gura KM: Potential benefits of parenteral fish oil lipid emulsions in parenteral nutrition-associated liver disease, *ICAN: Infant, Child, & Adolescent Nutrition* 2:251, 2010.

Hack M: Adult outcomes of preterm children, *J Dev Behavioral Pediatr* 30:460, 2009.

Hay WW: Strategies for feeding the premature infant, *Neonatology* 94:245, 2008.

Heron M, et al: Annual summary of vital statistics: 2007, *Pediatrics* 125:4, 2010.

Hovi P, et al: Glucose regulation in young adults with very low birth weight, *N Engl J Med* 356:20, 2007.

Hurst NM: The 3M's of breast-feeding the preterm infant, *J Perinat Neonat Nurs* 21:234, 2007.

Klein CJ, editor: Nutrient requirements for preterm infant formula, *J Nutr* 132:1395S, 2002.

Lucas A, et al: Randomised trial of early diet in preterm babies and later intelligence quotients, *Br Med J* 317:1481, 1998.

MacDorman MF, Mathews TJ: *Behind international rankings of infant mortality: how the United States Compares with Europe. NCHS Data Brief* No. 23. 1-8. Hyattsville, MD, 2009, National Center for Health Statistics.

Mitchell SM, et al: High frequencies of elevated alkaline phosphatase activity and rickets exist in extremely low birth weight infants despite current nutrition support, *BMC Pediatrics* 9:47, 2009.

Olsen IE, et al: New intrauterine growth curves based on United States data, *Pediatrics* 125:e214, 2010.

Poindexter BB, et al: Early provision of parenteral amino acids in extremely low birth weight infants: relation to growth and neurodevelopmental outcome, *J Pediatr* 148:300, 2006.

Rao R, Georgieff M: Microminerals. In Tsang RC, et al, editors: *Nutrition of the preterm infant*, ed 2, Cincinnati, OH, 2005, Digital Educational Publishing, Inc.

Robbins ST, Beker LT, editors: *Infant feedings: guidelines for preparation of formula and breastmilk in health care facilities*, Chicago, 2004, American Dietetic Association.

Rogers SP, et al: Continuous feedings of fortified human milk lead to nutrient losses of fat, calcium and phosphorous, *Nutrients* 2:230, 2010.

Saigal S, et al: Comparison of current health, functional limitations, and health care use of young adults who were born with extremely low birth weight and normal weight, *Pediatrics* 119:e562, 2006a.

Saigal S, et al: Self-perceived health-related quality of life of former extremely low birth weight infants at young adulthood, *Pediatrics* 118:1140, 2006b.

Schanler RJ, et al: Randomized trial of donor human milk versus preterm formula as substitutes for mothers' own milk in feeding of extremely premature infants, *Pediatrics* 116:400, 2005.

Schanler RJ, Anderson DM: The low-birth-weight infant: inpatient care. In Duggan C, et al., editors: *Nutrition in pediatrics*, ed 4, Hamilton, Ontario, 2008, BC Decker Publishers.

Sisk PM, et al: Early human milk feeding is associated with a lower risk of necrotizing enterocolitis in very low birth weight infants, *J Peri* 27:428, 2007.

Sisk PM, et al: Human milk consumption and full enteral feeding among infants who weigh ≦ 1250 grams, *Pediatrics* 121:e1528, 2008.

Stevens DC, et al: Achieving success in supporting parents and families in the neonatal intensive care unit. In McGrath J, Kenner C, editors: *Developmental care newborns and infants: a guide for health professionals*, ed 2, Glenview, IL, 2010, National Association of Neonatal Nurses.

Sullivan S, et al: An exclusively human milk-based diet is associated with a lower rate of necrotizing enterocolitis than a diet of human milk and bovine milk-based products, *J Pediatr* 156:562, 2010.

Thureen PJ, et al: Effect of low versus high intravenous amino acid intake on very low birth weight infants in the early neonatal period, *Pediatr Res* 53:24, 2003.

Tsang RC, et al: Summary of reasonable nutrient intakes. In Tsang RC, editor: *Nutrition of the preterm infant*, ed 2, Cincinnati, OH, 2005, Digital Educational Publishing, Inc.

Tyson JE, et al: Vitamin A supplementation for extremely-low-birth-weight infants, *N Engl J Med* 340:1962, 1999.

van Aerde JE, Narvey M: Acute respiratory failure. In Thureen PJ, Hay WW, editors: *Neonatal nutrition and metabolism*, ed 2, Cambridge, 2006, Cambridge University Press.

Wagner CL, Greer FR; American Academy of Pediatrics, Section on Breastfeeding; American Academy of Pediatrics, Committee on Nutrition: Prevention of rickets and vitamin D deficiency in infants, children, and adolescents, *Pediatrics* 122(5):1142, 2008 (published correction appears in *Pediatrics* 123(1):197, 2009).

Wilson-Costello DE, Hack M: Follow-up for high-risk neonates. In Fanaroff AA, Martin RJ, editors: Neonatal-perinatal medicine diseases of the fetus and infant, vol 2, ed 8, Philadelphia, 2006, Mosby.

Vohr BR, et al: Persistent beneficial effects of breast milk ingested in the neonatal intensive care unit on outcomes of extremely low birth weight infants at 30 months of age, *Pediatrics* 120:e953, 2007.

Ziegler EE: Protein requirements of very low birth weight infants, *J Pediatr Gastroenterology and Nutrition* 45:170, 2007.

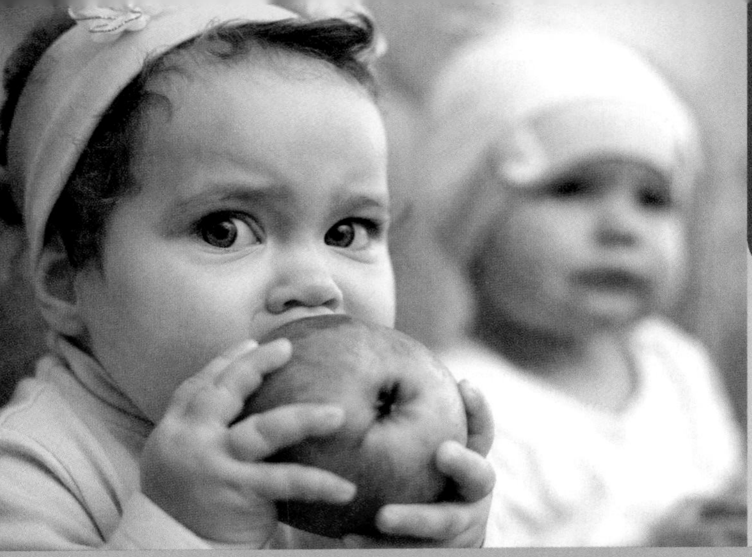

CHAPTER 44

Cristine M. Trahms, MS, RD, CD, FADA
Beth N. Ogata, MS, RD, CD, CSP

Medical Nutrition Therapy for Genetic Metabolic Disorders

KEY TERMS

argininosuccinic aciduria (ASA)
autosomal-recessive
branched-chain ketoaciduria or maple syrup urine disease (MSUD)
carbamyl-phosphate synthetase (CPS) deficiency
citrullinemia
galactosemia
genetic metabolic disorders
gluconeogenesis
glycogen storage diseases (GSDs)
glycogenolysis
ketone utilization disorder
L-carnitine
long-chain 3-hydroxyacyl-CoA dehydrogenase deficiency (LCHAD)
medium-chain acyl-CoA dehydrogenase deficiency (MCAD)
methylmalonic acidemia
ornithine transcarbamylase (OTC) deficiency
phenylketonuria (PKU)
propionic acidemia

Genetic metabolic disorders are inherited traits that result in the absence or reduced activity of a specific enzyme or cofactor. Most genetic metabolic disorders are inherited as **autosomal-recessive** traits; *autosomal* means that the gene is located on a chromosome other than the X or Y chromosomes. The treatment for many metabolic disorders is medical nutrition therapy (MNT), with medications specific to the disorder (e.g., phenylketonuria PKU). Here, the goals of MNT are to maintain biochemical equilibrium for the affected pathway, provide adequate nutrients to support typical growth and development, and support social and emotional development. Nutrition interventions are designed to circumvent the missing or inactive enzyme by (1) restricting the amount of substrate available, (2) supplementing the amount of product, (3) supplementing the enzymatic cofactor, or (4) combining any or all of these approaches. This chapter describes the primary conditions found more commonly in the United States. Table 44-1 outlines other disorders by the enzymatic defects, distinctive clinical and biochemical features, and current approaches to dietary therapy.

In some instances, when treatment is initiated early in the newborn period and meticulously continued for a lifetime, the affected individual can be cognitively and physically normal. In conditions such as galactosemia, cognitive and physical damage can occur despite early and meticulous treatment. Biochemical disorders range from variations in enzyme activity that are benign, to severe manifestations that are incompatible with life. For many of them, significant questions related to diagnosis and treatment remain.

NEWBORN SCREENING

Most inherited metabolic disorders are associated with severe clinical illness that often appears soon after birth. Intellectual disability and severe neurologic involvement

Text continued on p. 1001

TABLE 44-1

Selected Genetic Metabolic Disorders That Respond To Dietary Treatment

Disorder	Affected Enzyme	Prevalence	Clinical and Biochemical Features	Medical Nutrition Therapy	Adjunct Treatment
Urea Cycle Disorders (UCDs)					
Carbamyl-phosphate synthetase deficiency	Carbamyl-phosphate synthetase	1:30,000 (all UCDs)	Vomiting, seizures, sometimes coma → death Survivors usually have ID ↑ plasma ammonia and glutamine	Food: low protein Formula: without nonessential amino acids	L-carnitine, phenylbutyrate,* L-citrulline, L-arginine Hemodialysis or peritoneal dialysis during acute episodes
Ornithine transcarbamylase deficiency	Ornithine transcarbamylase (x-linked)	1:30,000 (all UCDs)	Vomiting, seizures, coma → death as a newborn ↑ plasma ammonia, glutamine, glutamic acid and alanine	Food: low protein Formula: without nonessential amino acids	L-carnitine, phenylbutyrate,* L-citrulline, L-arginine
Citrullinemia	Argininosuccinate synthetase	1:30,000 (all UCDs)	*Neonatal:* vomiting, seizures, coma → death *Infantile:* vomiting, seizures, progressive developmental delay ↑ plasma citrulline and ammonia, alanine	Food: low protein Formula: without nonessential amino acids	L-carnitine, phenylbutyrate,* L-arginine
Argininosuccinic aciduria	Argininosuccinate lyase	1:30,000 (all UCDs)	*Neonatal:* hypotonia, seizures *Subacute:* vomiting, FTT, progressive developmental delay ↑ plasma argininosuccinic acid, citrulline and ammonia	Food: low protein Formula: lower protein SF (without nonessential amino acids)	L-carnitine, phenylbutyrate*
Argininemia	Arginase	1:30,000 (all UCDs)	Periodic vomiting, seizures, coma Progressive spastic diplegia, developmental delay ↑ arginine and ammonia related to protein intake	Food: low protein Formula: lower protein SF (without nonessential amino acids)	L-carnitine, phenylbutyrate*

Continued

TABLE 44-1

Selected Genetic Metabolic Disorders That Respond To Dietary Treatment—cont'd

Disorder	Affected Enzyme	Prevalence	Clinical and Biochemical Features	Medical Nutrition Therapy	Adjunct Treatment
Organic Acidemias					
Methylmalonic acidemia	Methylmalonyl-CoA mutase or similar	1:80,000	Metabolic acidosis, vomiting, seizures, coma, often death ↑ organic urine acid and plasma ammonia levels	Food: low protein Formula: lower protein SF (without isoleucine, methionine, threonine, valine)	L-carnitine, vitamin B_{12} IV fluids, bicarbonate during acute episodes
Propionic acidemia	Propionyl-CoA carboxylase or similar	1:80,000	Metabolic acidosis, ↑ plasma ammonia and propionic acid, ↑ urine methylcitric acid	Food: low protein Formula: lower protein SF (without isoleucine, methionine, threonine, valine)	L-carnitine, biotin IV fluids, bicarbonate during acute episodes
Isovaleric acidemia	Isovaleryl-CoA dehydrogenase	1:80,000	Poor feeding, lethargy, seizures, metabolic ketoacidosis, hyperammonemia	Food: low protein Formula: SF (without leucine)	L-carnitine, L-glycine
Ketone utilization disorder	2-methylacetoacetyl-CoA-thiolase or similar	Unknown	Vomiting, dehydration, metabolic ketoacidosis	Food: low protein Formula: SF (without isoleucine) Avoid fasting, high complex carbohydrates	L-carnitine, Bicitra
Biotinidase deficiency	Biotinidase or similar	1:60,000	In infancy, seizures, hypotonia, rash, stridor, apnea; in older children, also see alopecia, ataxia, developmental delay, hearing loss		Supplemental oral biotin
Carbohydrate Disorders					
Galactosemia	Galactose-1-phosphate uridyltransferase	1:50,000	Vomiting, hepatomegaly, FTT, cataracts, ID, often early sepsis ↑ urine and blood galactose	Eliminate lactose, low galactose, use soy protein isolate formula	
Hereditary fructose intolerance	Fructose-1-phosphate aldolase	estimated: 1:20,000	Vomiting; hepatomegaly; hypoglycemia, FTT, renal tubular defects after fructose introduction ↑ blood and urine fructose after fructose feeding	No sucrose, fructose	
Fructose 1,6-diphosphatase deficiency	Fructose 1,6-diphosphatase	Unknown	Hypoglycemia, hepatomegaly, hypotonia, metabolic acidosis upon fructose introduction No ↑ blood/urine fructose	No sucrose, fructose	

Glycogen storage disease, type Ia	Glucose-6-phosphatase	1:60,000	Profound hypoglycemia, hepatomegaly	Low lactose, fructose, sucrose; low fat; high complex carbohydrate; avoid fasting	Raw cornstarch, iron supplements
Amino Acid Disorders					
Hyperphenylalaninemias					
Phenylketonuria	Phenylalanine hydroxylase	1:15,000		Food: low protein Formula: SF (without Phe, supplemented with tyrosine)	
Mild phenylketonuria	Phenylalanine hydroxylase	1:24,000	↑ blood Phe	Food: low protein Formula: SF (without Phe, supplemented with tyrosine)	
Dihydropteridine reductase deficiency	Dihydropteridine reductase	Rare	↑ blood Phe Irritability, developmental delay, seizures	Food: low protein Formula: SF (without Phe, supplemented with tyrosine)	Biopterin, 5-hydroxytryptophan, L-dopa, folinic acid
Biopterin synthase defect	Biopterin synthase	Rare	Mild ↑ blood Phe, irritability, developmental delay, seizures	None	L-dopa, tetrahydrobiopterin, 5-hydroxytryptophan
Tyrosinemia, type I	Fumarylacetoacetate hydrolase	<1:120,000	Vomiting, acidosis, diarrhea, FTT, hepatomegaly, rickets ↑ blood and urine tyrosine, methionine; ↑ urine parahydroxy derivatives of tyrosine; liver cancer	Food: low protein Formula: SF (without tyrosine, Phe, methionine)	Nitisinone[†]
Maple Syrup Urine Disease					
MSUD	Branched-chain ketoacid decarboxylase complex (<2% activity)	1:200,000	Seizures, acidosis Plasma leucine, isoleucine, valine 10× normal	Food: low protein Formula: SF (without leucine, isoleucine, valine)	Thiamin[‡]
Intermittent MSUD	Branched-chain ketoacid decarboxylase complex (<20% activity between episodes)	Rare	Intermittent symptoms Plasma leucine, isoleucine, valine 10× normal during illness	Food: low protein Formula: SF (without leucine, isoleucine, valine)	
Homocystinuria	Cystathionine synthase or similar	1:200,000	Detached retinas; thromboembolic and cardiac disease; mild to moderate ID; bony abnormalities; fair hair and skin; ↑ methionine, homocysteine	Food: low protein Formula: SF (without methionine, supplemented with L-cystine)	Betaine, folate, vitamin B_{12}, vitamin B_6[‡] if folate levels are normal

Continued

TABLE 44-1

Selected Genetic Metabolic Disorders That Respond To Dietary Treatment—cont'd

Disorder	Affected Enzyme	Prevalence	Clinical and Biochemical Features	Medical Nutrition Therapy	Adjunct Treatment
Fatty Acid Oxidation Disorders					
Long chain acyl-CoA dehydrogenase deficiency	Long-chain acyl-CoA dehydrogenase	Rare	Vomiting, lethargy, hypoglycemia	Low fat, low long-chain fatty acids; avoid fasting	MCT oil, L-carnitine[§]
Long-chain 3-hydroxy-acyl-CoA dehydrogenase deficiency	Long-chain 3-hydroxy-acyl-CoA dehydrogenase	Rare	Vomiting, lethargy, hypoglycemia	Low fat, low long-chain fatty acids; avoid fasting	MCT oil, L-carnitine[§]
Medium chain acyl-CoA dehydrogenase deficiency	Medium-chain acyl-CoA dehydrogenase	1:20,000	Vomiting, lethargy, hypoglycemia	Low fat, low medium-chain fatty acids, avoid fasting	L-carnitine[§]
Short chain acyl-CoA dehydrogenase deficiency	Short-chain acyl-CoA dehydrogenase	Rare	Vomiting, lethargy, hypoglycemia	Low fat, low short-chain fatty acids, avoid fasting	L-carnitine[§]
Very long chain acyl-CoA dehydrogenase deficiency	Very-long-chain acyl-CoA dehydrogenase	Rare	Vomiting, lethargy, hypoglycemia	Low fat, low long-chain fatty acids, avoid fasting	L-carnitine,[§] MCT oil

CoA, Coenzyme A; *FTT*, failure to thrive; *ID*, intellectual disability; *IV*, intravenous; *MCT*, medium-chain triglyceride; *MSUD*, maple syrup urine disease; *Phe*, phenylalanine; *SF*, specialized formulas are available for medical nutrition therapy for this disorder; *UCD*, urea cycle disorder.

*Phenylbutyrate is a chemical administered to enhance waste ammonia excretion; other compounds producing the same effect are also used.

†*Nitisinone*, formerly *NTBC*, 2-(2-nitro-4-trifluoro-methyl-benzoyl-1,3-cyclohexanedione, commercially available as Orfadin.®

‡Patient may or may not respond to the compound.

§Use depends on clinic.

may be immediately apparent. Diagnosis of a specific disorder may be difficult, and appropriate treatment measures may be uncertain. Prenatal diagnosis is available for many metabolic disorders, but it usually requires the identification of a family at risk, which can be done only after the birth of an affected child. Effective newborn screening programs, as well as advanced diagnostic techniques and treatment modalities have improved the outcome for many of these infants.

Infants suspected of having a metabolic disorder should be afforded access to care offered by centers with expertise in treating these disorders. Infants who are afebrile for no apparent reason, lethargic, vomiting, in respiratory distress, or having seizures should be evaluated for an undiagnosed metabolic disorder. The initial assessment should include blood gas measurements, electrolyte values, glucose and ammonia tests, and a urine test for ketones.

Advances in newborn screening technology offer opportunities for earlier diagnosis, prevention of neurologic crisis, and improved intellectual and physical outcomes. When tandem mass spectrometry techniques are used in newborn screening laboratories, infants with a broader range of metabolic disorders can be identified, and the disorder can be identified earlier (see *Focus On:* Newborn Screening). See Fig. 44-1.

DISORDERS OF AMINO ACID METABOLISM

Nutrition therapy for amino acid disorders most commonly consists of substrate restriction, which involves limiting one or more essential amino acids to the minimum requirement while providing adequate energy and nutrients to promote typical growth and development (e.g., restricting phenylalanine [Phe] in phenylketonuria PKU). An inadequate intake of an essential amino acid is often as detrimental as excess. Supplementation of the product of the specific enzymatic reaction is usually required in nutrition therapy for amino acid disorders; for example, tyrosine (Tyr) is supplemented in formulas for treatment of PKU.

Requirements for individual amino acids are difficult to determine because typical growth and development can be achieved over a wide range of intake. The data of Holt and Snyderman (1967) are often used as the basis for prescribing

FOCUS ON

Newborn Screening (NBS)

Since the 1960s, states across the United States have adopted mandatory newborn screening (NBS) as law (Waisbren, 2006). These programs were developed as a result of the efficacy of the Guthrie bacterial inhibition assay, in which dried blood spots were assayed. This simple, sensitive, and inexpensive screening test became the basis for population-based screening systems for newborns. Hemoglobinopathies, endocrine disorders, metabolic disorders, and some infectious disorders can be effectively identified in this way.

In the 1990s tandem mass spectrometry began to be used in NBS and is now used across the United States (Therrell, 2006). This technology makes it possible to identify multiple disorders from dried blood spots. The number of disorders screened for varies widely by state, and expanded screening is also offered by private, for-profit companies. Follow-up programs also vary; some states have a centralized program, whereas follow-up in other states is less coordinated. Successful early NBS programs include screening for congenital hypothyroidism, phenylketonuria, congenital adrenal hyperplasia, galactosemia, sickle cell disease, and maple syrup urine disease (Brosco et al., 2006).

The Maternal and Child Health Bureau (MCHB) of the U.S. Health Resources and Services Administration commissioned a report from the American College of Medical Genetics (ACMG). This expert panel identified 29 conditions for which newborn screening should be mandated and 25 secondary conditions that may be detected incidentally (MCHB, 2007). The ACMG developed a series of ACTion (ACT) sheets and confirmatory algorithms for disorders that are identified by NBS screening. The ACT sheets describe the steps health professionals should follow in communicating with the family and determining follow-up. They are available at http://www.acmg.net/AM/Template.cfm?Section=NBS_ACT_Sheets_and_Algorithms_Table&Template=/CM/HTMLDisplay.cfm&ContentID=5649.

Other groups, including the World Health Organization, March of Dimes, and Massachusetts Newborn Screening Advisory Committee, have also issued recommendations.

Providers who may be involved in the care and follow-up of families identified by NBS should have a good understanding of their state's system, as well as the factors that may affect results. Communication among families, primary health care providers, and tertiary clinics is critical to timely identification and treatment. Follow-up, including referral to the appropriate specialists, is important for any family who receives NBS test results. NBS fact sheets from the Committee on Genetics of the American Academy of Pediatrics describe (1) newborn testing; (2) follow-up of abnormal screening results to facilitate timely diagnostic testing and management; (3) diagnostic testing; (4) disease management, which requires coordination with the medical home and genetic counseling; and (5) continuous evaluation and improvement of the NBS system (Kaye et al., 2006).

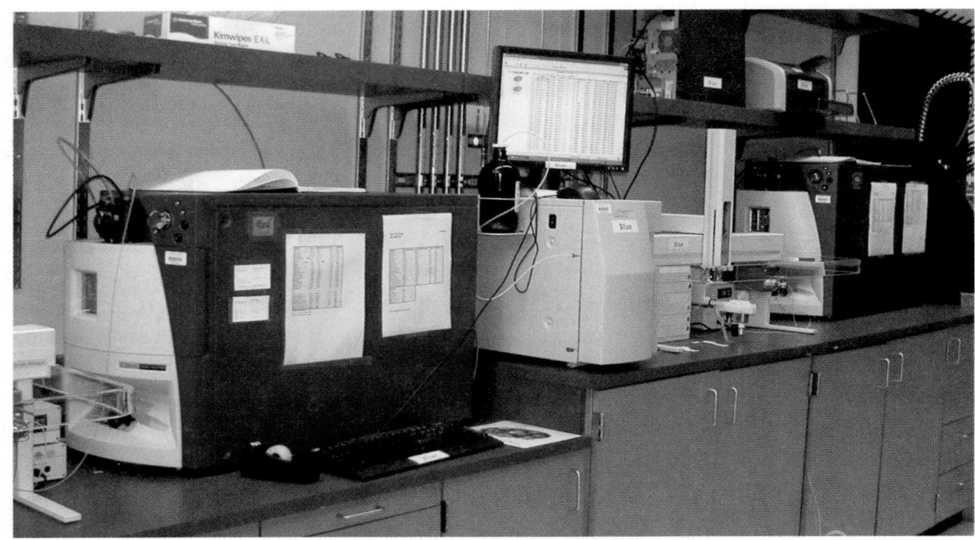

FIGURE 44-1 Tandem mass spectrometer. This technology makes screening for a broad range of metabolic disorders feasible. Blood levels of a number of organic acids are measured. *(Courtesy Washington State Newborn Screening Program.)*

amino acid intakes (Table 44-2). Careful and frequent monitoring is required to ensure the adequacy of the nutritional prescription. Although nitrogen studies are the most precise, weight gain in infants is a sensitive and easily monitored index of well being and nutrition adequacy.

Phenylketonuria

Phenylketonuria (PKU) is the most common of the hyperphenylalaninemias. In this disorder phenylalanine is not metabolized to Tyr because of a deficiency or inactivity of phenylalanine hydroxylase as shown in Figure 44-2. Of the amino acid disorders, PKU provides a reasonable model for detailed discussion because it (1) occurs relatively frequently and most neonates are screened for it; (2) has a successful MNT treatment; and (3) has a predictable course, with available documentation of "natural" and "intervention" history (see *Focus On:* Time Line of Events in the Diagnosis and Treatment of Phenylketonuria).

Nutritional treatment involves restricting the substrate (Phe) and supplementing the product (Tyr) (see *Pathophysiology and Care Management Algorithm:* Phenylketonuria). Most affected infants exhibit phenylalanine hydroxylase deficiency; the remainder (less than 3%) have defects in associated pathways. Low phenylalanine nutrition therapy does not prevent the neurologic deterioration present in the disorders of associated pathways.

Medical Treatment

All states have newborn screening programs for PKU and other metabolic disorders. Diagnostic criteria for PKU include blood concentrations of Phe that consistently exceed 6 to 10 mg/dL (360 to 600 mmol/L) and Tyr concentrations of less than 3 mg/dL (165 mmol/L). The diagnostic process should also include evaluation for hyperphenylalaninemia that results from the deficiency of enzymes other than phenylalanine hydroxylase. An effective newborn screening program and access to an organized follow-up program are critical to early identification and treatment of infants with PKU.

The advantage of rigorous nutrition therapy has been demonstrated by measurements of intellectual function. Individuals who do not receive diet therapy have severe intellectual disability (mean intelligence quotient [IQ] of approximately 40), whereas individuals who are on therapy from the early neonatal period have normal IQs. Outcome, measured as intellectual function, depends on the age of the infant at diagnosis and start of nutrition therapy, as well as the individual's biochemical control over time.

Tetrahydrobiopterin (BH_4) has been studied to evaluate its effectiveness as an alternative treatment to severe dietary Phe restriction. BH_4 is a cofactor needed for proper activity of the enzyme. Although supplementation with BH_4 holds promise as an adjunct therapy for some milder mutations, observations on long-term outcome are needed (Lee et al., 2005). Those individuals who respond have what is called *BH4-responsive PKU.* Other studies have examined the possibility of enzyme substitution with phenylalanine ammonia lyase to degrade Phe, or gene therapy to restore phenylalanine hydroxylase activity (Blau et al., 2010).

Blood Phenylalanine Control. Blood Phe concentration must be checked regularly, depending on the age and health status of the child, to be sure it remains within the range of 2 to 6 mg/dL or 120 to 360 mmol/L. Phe-containing foods are offered as tolerated as long as the blood concentration of Phe remains in the range of good biochemical control. The child's rate of growth and mental development must be carefully monitored.

Effective management requires a team approach in which the child, parents, registered dietitian, pediatrician, psychologist, social worker, and nurse work together to achieve and maintain biochemical control in an atmosphere promoting normal mental and emotional development. An essential

TABLE 44-2

Approximate Daily Requirements for Selected Dietary Components and Amino Acids in Infancy and Childhood

Dietary Component or Amino Acid	Age and Requirement	
	Birth to 12 mo (mg/kg)	**1 to 10 yr (mg/day)**
Phenylalanine	1-5 mo: 47-90 6-12 mo: 25-47	200-500*
Histidine	16-34	
Tyrosine†	1-5 mo: 60-80 6-12 mo: 40-60	25-85 (mg/kg)
Leucine	76-150	1000
Isoleucine	1-5 mo: 79-110 6-12 mo: 50-75	1000
Valine	1-5 mo: 65-105 6-12 mo: 50-80	400-600
Methionine‡	20-45	400-800
Cyst(e)ine§	15-50	400-800
Lysine	90-120	1200-1600
Threonine	45-87	800-1000
Tryptophan	13-22	60-120
Energy	1-5 mo: 108 kcal/kg 6-12 mo: 98 kcal/kg	70-102 kcal/kg
Water	100 ml/kg	1000 ml
Carbohydrate	kcal × 0.5 ÷ 4 = g/day	kcal × 0.5 ÷ 4 = g/day
Total protein	1-5 mo: 2.2 g/kg 6-12 mo: 1.6 g/kg	16-18
Fat	kcal × 0.35 ÷ 9 = g/day	kcal × 0.35 ÷ 9 = g/day

Modified from Committee on Nutrition, American Academy of Pediatrics: Special diets for infants with inborn errors of metabolism, Pediatrics 57:783, 1976. Compiled from amino acid data of Holt and Snyderman. Information on amino acid requirements of infants and children at different ages is limited; the figures given here are in excess of minimum requirements. Consequently, this table should be used only as a guide and should not be regarded as an authoritative statement to which individual patients must conform.

*More phenylalanine (>800 mg) is required in the absence of tyrosine.

†Total phenylalanine plus tyrosine should be considered in the prescription because most phenylalanine is converted to tyrosine.

‡More methionine is required in the absence of cyst(e)ine.

§More cyst(e)ine is required in presence of a blocked *trans*-sulfuration outflow pathway for methionine metabolism.

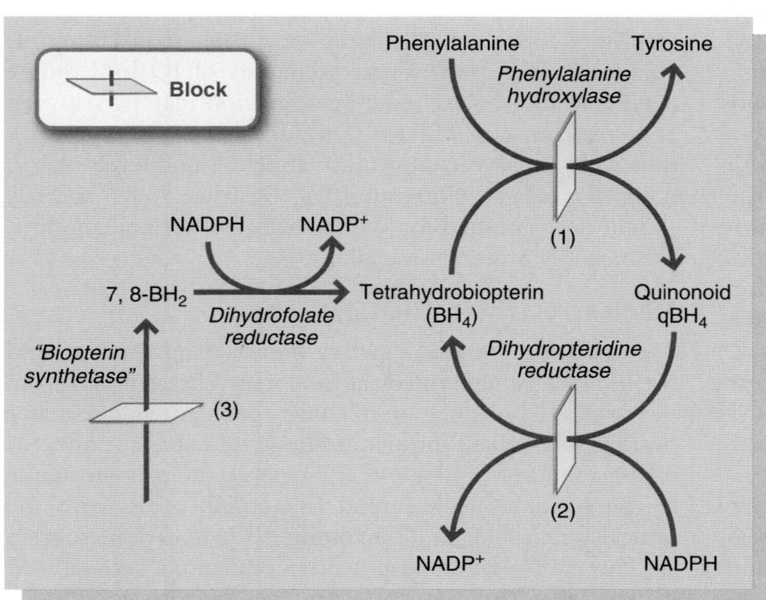

FIGURE 44-2 Hyperphenylalaninemias. **1,** Phenylalanine hydroxylase deficiency; **2,** Dihydropteridine reductase deficiency; **3,** Biopterin synthetase deficiency. *NADPH,* Nicotinamide-adenine dinucleotide phosphate (reduced form); *NADP+,* nicotinamide-adenine dinucleotide phosphate (oxidized form).

FOCUS ON

Time Line of Events in the Diagnosis and Treatment of Phenylketonuria

1934: A. Folling identifies phenylpyruvic acid in the urine of mentally retarded siblings.

1950s: G. Jervis demonstrates a deficiency of phenylalanine oxidation in the liver tissue of an affected patient. H. Bickel demonstrates that dietary phenylalanine restrictions lower the blood concentration of phenylalanine.

1960s: R. Guthrie develops a bacterial inhibition assay for measuring blood phenylalanine levels.

Mid-1960s: Semisynthetic formulas restricted in phenylalanine content become commercially available.

1965-1970: States adopt newborn screening programs to detect phenylketonuria (PKU).

1967-1980: Collaborative Study of Children Treated for Phenylketonuria is conducted. Data from this study form the basis for treatment protocols for PKU clinics in the United States.

Late-1970s: Detrimental effects of maternal PKU are recognized as a significant public health problem.

1980s: Lifelong restriction of phenylalanine intake becomes the standard of care in PKU clinics in the United States.

1983: The Maternal PKU Collaborative Study begins to study the effects of treatment on the pregnancy outcome of women with phenylketonuria.

1987: Techniques for carrier detection and prenatal diagnosis of PKU are developed.

Late-1980s: The gene for phenylalanine hydroxylase deficiency (MIM No. 261600) is located on chromosome 12q22-q24.1. Deoxyribonucleic acid mutation analysis can be accomplished with peripheral leukocytes.

1990s: Phenylalanine level of 1-6 mg/dL (60-360 mmol/L), lower than the previous level of less than 10 mg/dL (600 mmol/L), becomes the new standard of care for treatment of PKU.

2000: Tetrahydrobiopterin-responsive forms of PKU are recognized, especially those with mild mutations.

2010: Continued research into alternative and adjunct therapies such as the use of large neutral amino acids, BH4 supplementation, enzyme substitution, and somatic gene therapy.

Data from Maternal Child Health Bureau: Newborn screening: toward a uniform screening panel and system, Genet Med 8(Suppl1):1S, 2006; Saugstad LF: From genetics to epigenetics, Nutr Health, 18:285, 2006; Mitchell JJ, Scriver CR: Phenylalanine hydroxylase deficiency. In Pago RA et al., editors: GeneReviews [Internet]. Seattle, 1993-2000, University of Washington, Seattle [updated November 5, 2010].

management tool for parents, children, and clinicians is the food diary used to monitor Phe intake. Daily record keeping supports compliance with treatment and builds self-management skills. An accurate record of food and formula intake for at least the 3 days before a laboratory specimen is obtained is mandatory for accurate interpretation of the results and subsequent adjustment of the Phe prescription.

Elevations in blood Phe concentration are generally caused by either excessive Phe intake or tissue catabolism. Intake of Phe in excess of the amount required for growth accumulates in the blood. Deficient energy intake or the stress of illness or infection can result in protein breakdown and the release of amino acids, including Phe, into the blood. In general, the anorexia of illness limits energy intake. Preventing tissue catabolism by maintaining intake of the formula/medical food as much as possible is essential. Although it may occasionally be necessary to offer only clear liquids during an illness, the Phe-free formula/medical food should be reintroduced as soon as it is feasible. It can be used as a tube feeding if oral intake is not possible.

The necessity of continuing the restricted-Phe dietary therapy beyond adolescence is a consideration. Progressively decreasing IQs, learning difficulties, poor attention span, and behavioral difficulties have been reported in children who have discontinued the dietary regimen. Children who maintain well-controlled blood Phe levels demonstrate comparatively higher intellectual achievement than those who do not. Good dietary control of blood Phe concentrations is the best predictor of IQ, whereas "off-diet" blood Phe concentrations of greater than 20 mg/dL (1200 mmol/L) are the best predictors of IQ loss. Subtle deficits in higher-level cognitive function may persist even at blood Phe levels of 6 to 10 mg/dL (360 to 600 mmol/L); thus most clinics recommend treatment blood levels of 1 to 6 mg/dL (60 to 360 mmol/L). Restricted-Phe therapy should be continued for life to maintain normal cognitive function (Waisbren et al., 2007).

Medical Nutrition Therapy

Formula. For PKU dietary therapy is planned around the use of a formula/medical food with Phe removed from the protein. Formulas or medical foods provide a major portion of the daily protein and energy needs for affected infants, children, and adults. In general, the protein source in the formula/medical food is L-amino acids, with the critical amino acid (i.e., Phe) omitted. Carbohydrate sources are corn syrup solids, modified tapioca starch, sucrose, and hydrolyzed cornstarch. Fat is provided by a variety of oils.

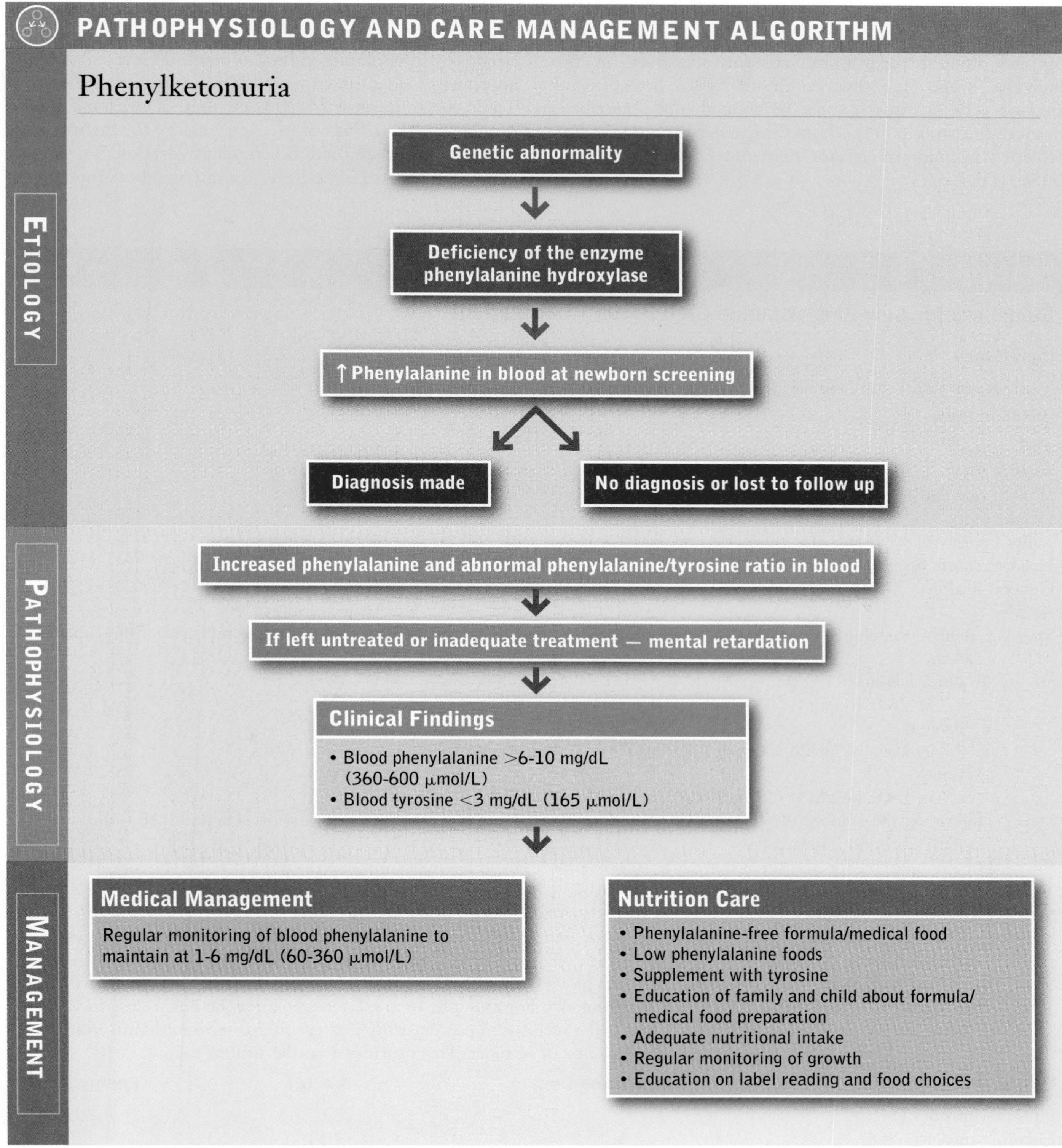

Some formula/medical foods contain no fat or carbohydrate; therefore these components must be provided from other sources. If prescribing formulas without fat, sources of essential fatty acids must be provided. Essential fatty acid deficiencies have been noted among individuals consuming fat-free formulas (Cleary et al., 2006; Rose, et al., 2005). Most formulas and medical foods contain calcium, iron, and all other necessary vitamins and minerals and are a reliable source of these nutrients. When others are devoid of these nutrients, supplementation is needed to ensure nutritional adequacy.

Phe-free formula is supplemented with regular infant formula or breast milk during infancy and cow's milk in early childhood to provide high–biologic value protein, nonessential amino acids, and sufficient Phe to meet the individualized requirements of the growing child. The optimal amount of protein substitute depends on the individual's age (and thus requirements for growth) and enzyme activity; thus it must be individually prescribed. Because the protein in specialized formulas is synthetic, it is provided in amounts greater than the Dietary Reference Intake (DRI).

The Phe-free formula and milk mixture should provide approximately 90% of the protein and 80% of the energy needed by infants and toddlers. A method for calculating the appropriate quantities of a Phe-free formula is shown in Table 44-3. It must be stressed that calculations should provide adequate but not excessive energy for the infant, as well as appropriate fluid to maintain hydration. To support metabolic control effectively, formula/medical foods must

TABLE 44-3

Guidelines for Low-Phenylalanine Food Pattern Calculations

Case Study

Molly is a 6-month-old infant with phenylketonuria.

Baseline Data

Age	6 mo
Weight (kg)	7.7
Weight percentile	50th
Height (cm)	67.8
Length percentile	50th
Head circumference (cm)	43.3
General health	Good
Activity	Very active

Step 1 Calculate the child's requirement for phenylalanine, protein, and energy (kcal) by using the information in Table 44-2.

A. Phenylalanine

7.7 kg body weight × 60* mg phenylalanine/kg/day = 462 mg phenylalanine/day

B. Protein

7.7 kg body weight × 3.3† g protein/kg/day = 25.4 g protein/day

C. Energy

7.7 kg body weight × 115† kcal/kg/day = 885 kcal/day

Step 2 Determine the amount of phenylalanine-free formula required per day. This information is determined from the infant's protein requirement.

For example, 25.4 g of protein per day × 90% of protein from phenylalanine-free formula powder (Phenex-1) = 23 g of protein = 145 g of formula powder per day.

Step 3 Determine the amount of standard infant formula to be included in the formula.

Step 4 Determine the amounts of phenylalanine, protein, and energy in the phenylalanine-free and infant formulas as shown in the following examples.

Step 5 Determine the amount of water to mix with the phenylalanine-free formula. The consistency of the formula will vary according to the infant's age and fluid requirements. For example, to prepare formula for the infant described in the case study, mix 145 g of Phenex-1 and 120 g of Enfamil powder with 4 oz of water to prevent lumps from forming. Then add water to make a total of 32 oz of formula. This provides 4 bottles of 8 oz each.

Formula	Phenylalanine (mg)	Protein (g)	Energy (kcal)
Phenex-1 powder (145 g)		23.0	695
Enfamil powder (120 g)	410	4.8	120
TOTAL	410	27.8	815

Step 6 Determine the amount of phenylalanine, protein, and energy to be obtained from foods other than the formula mixture.

Total phenylalanine	462 mg/day
Phenylalanine in formula	410 mg/day
Phenylalanine from other foods	52 mg/day
Total protein	25.4 g/day
Protein in formula	27.8 g/day

TABLE 44-3

Guidelines for Low-Phenylalanine Food Pattern Calculations—cont'd

Formula	Phenylalanine (mg)	Protein (g)	Energy (kcal)
Protein from other foods		1-2 g/day	
Total energy		885 kcal/day	
Energy in formula		815 kcal/day	
Energy from other foods		70 kcal/day	
Step 7 Determine the amount of foods other than formula to be included in the dietary plan[‡]			
	Phenylalanine (mg)	**Protein (g)**	**kcal**
Baby rice cereal, 1 Tbsp	9	0.2	9
Green beans, strained, 1 Tbsp	9	0.2	4
Banana, mashed, 50 g	22	0.6	44
Carrots, strained, 3 Tbsp	9	0.3	12
TOTAL	49	1.3	69

Step 8 Determine the actual amounts of phenylalanine, protein, and energy per kilogram of body weight by dividing the total available nutrients by the body weight (in kg).

Phenylalanine (mg)

460 mg of phenylalanine ÷ 7.7 kg body weight = 60 mg of phenylalanine per kilogram per day

Protein29.1 g of protein ÷ 7.7 kg body weight = 3.8 g protein per kilogram per day

Energy

885 kcal ÷ 7.7 kg of body weight = 115 kcal per kilogram per day

*A phenylalanine intake of 60 mg/kg/day is chosen as a moderate intake level. The prescription for phenylalanine must be adapted to individual needs as judged by growth and blood levels.

[†]Although these intakes are higher than the recommended dietary allowance, they are the intakes found by the Collaborative Study to promote normal growth with consumption of protein hydrolysate-based formula (Acosta, 1996).

[‡]Total energy intake must be adjusted to meet individual needs, and an excess must be avoided.

be consumed in three or four nearly equal portions throughout the day.

Low-Phenylalanine Foods. Foods of moderate- or low-Phe content are used as a supplement to the formula or medical food mixture. These foods are offered at the appropriate ages to support developmental readiness and to meet energy needs. Puréed foods from a spoon might be introduced at 5 to 6 months of age, finger foods at 7 to 8 months, and the cup at 8 to 9 months, using the same timing and progression of texture recommended for typical children. Table 44-4 suggests typical low-Phe food patterns for young children.

Low-protein pastas, breads, and baked goods made from wheat starch add variety to the food pattern and allow children to eat some foods "to appetite." A variety of low-protein pastas, rice, baked goods, egg replacers, and other foods are available. Wheat starch and a variety of low-protein baking mixes for breads, cakes, and cookies are also available. Table 44-5 compares low-protein and regular food items.

In many cases parents create recipes or adapt family favorites to meet the needs of their children. These recipes offer the children a variety of textures and food choices, allowing them to participate in family meals. Families are also able to meet the energy and Phe needs of their children without resorting to excessive intakes of sugars and concentrated sweets.

A formula or medical food that is free of Phe and has a more appropriate amino acid, vitamin, and mineral composition for an older child is generally introduced in the toddler or preschool period. The criteria for introduction of the "next-step" formulas are that the child accept the food pattern and formula well and reliably consume a wide variety of foods from the low-Phe food list. Successful management with consistently low blood Phe levels is based on habit (i.e., the formula/medical food is offered and consumed without negotiation or threat). Children respond favorably to the regularity of the time of ingestion of the formula/medical food and the familiarity of its taste and presentation. Table 44-6 compares a restricted Phe food pattern with a typical food pattern for a child of the same age.

Education about Therapy Management. The energy needs and amino acid requirements of children with PKU do not differ appreciably from those of children in general. With proper management, typical growth can be expected (Figure 44-3). However, parents may tend to offer excessive energy as sweets because they feel the child is being deprived of food experiences. Health care providers should support families in recognizing that children with PKU are healthy children who must make careful food

TABLE 44-4

Typical Menus for a 3-Year-Old With Phenylketonuria

Tolerance: 300 mg of phenylalanine/day Formula/medical food for 24 hours: 100 g of Phenyl-Free-2, 125 g of 2% milk, water to 34 oz This formula mixture provides 25.8 g of protein, 670 kcal of energy, 200 mg of phenylalanine.		Tolerance: 400 mg of phenylalanine/ day Formula/medical food for 24 hours: 100 g of Phenyl-Free-2, 125 g of 2% milk, water to 34 oz This formula mixture provides 25.8 g of protein, 670 kcal of energy, 200 mg of phenylalanine.	
Menu for 100 mg of Phenylalanine from Food	**Amount of Phenylalanine**	**Menu for 200 mg of Phenylalanine from Food**	**Amount of Phenylalanine**
Breakfast		**Breakfast**	
Formula mixture, 10 oz		Formula mixture, 10 oz	
Kix cereal, 4 g (3 Tbsp)	15 mg	Rice Krispies, 20 g (¼ C)	22 mg
Peaches, canned, 60 g (¼ C)	9 mg	Nondairy creamer, ¼ C	19 mg
Lunch		**Lunch**	
Formula mixture, 8 oz		Formula mixture, 8 oz	
Low protein bread, ½ slice	7 mg	Vegetable soup (¼ C soup plus ¼ C water)	52 mg
Jelly, 1 tsp	0	Grapes, 50 g (10)	9 mg
Carrots, cooked, 40 g (¼ C)	13 mg	Low-protein crackers, 5	3 mg
Apricots, canned, 25 g (½ C)	6 mg	Low-protein cookie, 2	2 mg
Snack		**Snack**	
Apple slice, peeled, 4	4 mg	Rice cakes, 6 g (2 mini)	18 mg
Goldfish crackers, 10	18 mg	Jelly, 1 tsp	0
Formula mixture, 8 oz		Formula mixture, 8 oz	
Dinner		**Dinner**	
Formula mixture, 8 oz		Formula mixture, 8 oz	
Low-protein pasta, ½ C, cooked	5 mg	Potato, diced, 50 g (5 Tbsp)	50 mg
Tomato sauce, 2 Tbsp	16 mg	Dairy-free margarine, 1 tsp	0 mg

TABLE 44-5

Comparison of Protein and Energy Content of Foods Used in Low-Protein Diets

Food Item	Energy (kcal)	Protein (g)
Pasta, ½ C, cooked		
Low-protein	107	0.15
Regular	72	2.4
Bread, 1 slice		
Low-protein	135	0.2
Regular	74	2.4
Cereal, ½ C, cooked		
Low-protein	45	0.0
Regular	80	1.0
Egg, 1		
Low-protein egg replacer	30	0.0
Regular	67	5.6

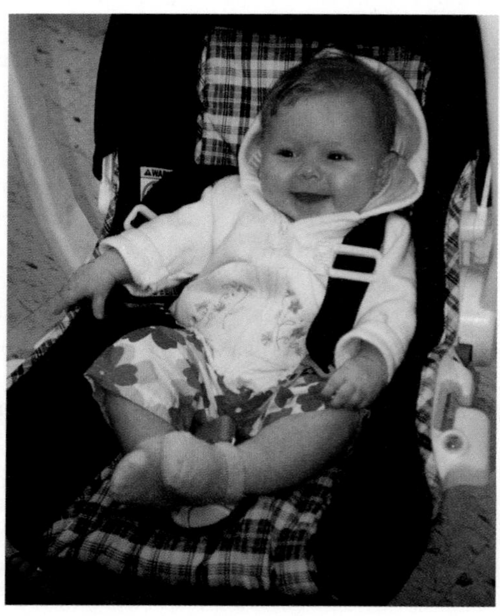

FIGURE 44-3 Infant with phenylketonuria, who was identified by a newborn screening program and started on treatment by 7 days of age, demonstrates typical growth and development. *(Courtesy Cristine M. Trahms, Seattle.)*

TABLE 44-6

Comparison of Menus Appropriate for Children with and without Phenylketonuria

Meal	Menu for PKU	Phenylalanine (mg)	Regular menu	Phenylalanine (mg)
Breakfast	Phenylalanine-free formula	0	Milk	450
	Puffed rice cereal		Puffed rice cereal	
	Orange juice		Orange juice	
Lunch	Jelly sandwich with low-protein bread	18	Peanut butter and jelly sandwich with regular bread	625
	Banana		Banana	
	Carrot and celery sticks		Carrot and celery sticks	
	Low-protein chocolate chip cookies	4	Chocolate chip cookies	60
	Juice		Juice	
Snack	Phenylalanine-free formula	0	Milk	450
	Orange		Orange	
	Potato chips (small bag)		Potato chips	
Dinner	Phenylalanine-free formula	0	Milk	450
	Salad		Salad	
	Low-protein spaghetti with tomato sauce	8	Spaghetti with tomato sauce and meatballs	240 600
	Sorbet	10	Ice cream	120
ESTIMATED INTAKE		40		2995

PKU, Phenylketonuria.

choices for themselves, not chronically ill children who require food indulgences.

Appropriate clinical interaction with family members provides them with the information and skills to differentiate between food behaviors that are typical for the age and developmental level of the child and those related specifically to PKU (Ievers-Landis et al., 2005). To avoid power struggles and conflicts over food, it is advisable to involve the child in choosing appropriate foods at an early age. Children who are 2 to 3 years old can master the concept of appropriate choices when foods are categorized as "yes foods" and "no foods." The concept of an appropriate quantity of a food can be introduced to a 3- or 4-year-old child in terms of "how many" by counting crackers or raisins and then in terms of "how much" by weighing or measuring foods such as cereal or fruit. The child then moves to more complex tasks (e.g., formula and food preparation) and planning of meals (e.g., breakfast or a packed lunch). Responsibility for planning a full day's menu by calculating the quantity of Phe in portions of food and compiling the daily total is the ultimate goal. These age-related tasks are shown in Table 44-7.

Psychosocial Development. The necessity of carefully controlling food intake may prompt parents to overprotect their children and perhaps to restrict their social activities. The children, in turn, may react negatively to their parents and to their nutrition therapy. The ability of the family to respond to the stresses of PKU, as reflected by adaptability and cohesion scores, is demonstrated by improved blood Phe concentrations and the positive coping behaviors of older children with PKU. Thus continuing nutrition therapy beyond early childhood requires that children become knowledgeable about and responsible for managing their own food choices. The health care team becomes responsible for working with families and children to provide strategies that enable children and adolescents to participate in social and school activities, interact with peers, and progress through the typical developmental stages with self-confidence and self-esteem (Ievers-Landis et al., 2005).

Children require parental and professional support as they assume responsibility for their food management. Self-management of food choices is a strategy to prevent the child using dietary noncompliance as a wedge against parental restrictions. Normal intellectual development is a laudable goal of management of PKU, but to be entirely successful children with PKU concomitantly need to develop self-assurance and a strong self-image. This can be achieved in part by fostering self-management, problem-solving skills, independence, and a typical lifestyle.

Maternal PKU

A pregnant woman with elevated blood Phe concentrations endangers her fetus because of the amplified transport of amino acids across the placenta. The fetus is exposed to approximately twice the Phe level contained in normal maternal blood. Babies whose mothers have elevated blood

TABLE 44-7

Tasks Expected of Children with Phenylketonuria by Age Level

Age (yr)	School Level	Task
2-3	Preschool	Distinguishing between "yes" and "no" foods
3-4	Preschool	Counting: how many?
4-5	Preschool	Measuring: how much?
5-6	Kindergarten	Preparing own formula; using scale
6-7	Grade 1-2	Writing basic notes in food diary
7-8	Grade 2	Making some decisions on after-school snack
8-9	Grade 3	Preparing breakfast
9-10	Grade 4	Packing lunches
10-14	Middle school	Managing food choices with increasing independence
14-18	High school	Independently managing phenylketonuria

TABLE 44-8

Frequency of Abnormalities in Children Born to Mothers with Phenylketonuria

	Maternal Phenylalanine Levels (mg/dL)				
Complication (% of Offspring)	20	16-19	11-15	3-10	Non-PKU Mother
Mental retardation	92	73	22	21	5.0
Microcephaly	73	68	35	24	4.8
Congenital heart disease	12	15	6	0	0.8
Low birth weight	40	52	56	13	9.6

Modified from Lenke RR, Levy HL: Maternal phenylketonuria and hyper-phenylalaninemia: an international survey of the outcome of untreated and treated pregnancies, N Engl J Med 303:1202, 1980.

PKU, Phenylketonuria

Phe concentrations have an increased occurrence of cardiac defects, retarded growth, microcephaly, and intellectual disability, as presented in Table 44-8. The fetus appears to be at risk of damage even with minor elevations in maternal blood Phe levels, and the higher the level, the more severe the effect. Strict control of maternal Phe levels before conception and throughout pregnancy offers the best opportunity for normal fetal development (Koch et al., 2010).

Nutrition management for pregnant women with hyperphenylalaninemia is complex. The changing physiology of pregnancy and fluctuating nutritional needs are difficult to monitor with the precision required to maintain appropriately low blood-Phe concentrations. Even with meticulous attention to Phe intake, blood concentrations, and the nutritional requirements of pregnancy, a woman cannot be assured of a normal infant (Lee et al., 2005). The risks of abnormal development of the fetus, even with therapeutic dietary management and maintenance of blood Phe concentrations at 1 to 5 mg/dL (60 to 300 mmol/L), are an important consideration for young women with PKU considering pregnancy (Waisbren and Azen, 2003).

Nutritional management during pregnancy is challenging, even for women who have consistently followed a low-Phe dietary regimen since infancy. Women who have discontinued Phe dietary treatment find that reinstituting medical food consumption and limiting food choices can be difficult and overwhelming. Inadequate maternal nourishment (i.e., inadequate intakes of total protein, fat, and energy) may contribute to poor fetal development and should be avoided. Adherence to nutrition therapy during pregnancy for even the well-motivated woman requires family and professional support, as well as frequent monitoring of biochemical and nutritional aspects of both pregnancy and PKU.

Adults Living with Phenylketonuria

Many adults with PKU have had the benefits of early diagnosis and treatment and are less likely to be affected by neurologic damage. However, among those who have had some degree of intellectual disability, hyperactivity and self-abuse are often major concerns. Not all patients have responded to late initiation of treatment with improved behavioral or intellectual function. For the difficult-to-manage older patient, a trial of a low-Phe food pattern is recommended. If successful, continued Phe restriction therapy may facilitate behavioral management.

Reinstituting a Phe-restricted food pattern is difficult after the eating pattern has been liberalized. However, the current recommendation of most clinics is effective management of blood Phe concentration throughout a lifetime. This recommendation is based on reports of declining intellectual capabilities and changes in the brain after prolonged, significant elevation of Phe concentrations (Waisbren and Azen, 2003). The efficacy of continued treatment throughout adulthood has been documented by reports of improved intellectual performance and problem-solving abilities when blood Phe levels are kept low. Dietary management of PKU throughout the life span is similar to that of other chronic disorders, and prudent MNT results in a normal quality of life (Bosch et al., 2006).

Maple Syrup Urine Disease

Maple syrup urine disease (MSUD), or **branched-chain ketoaciduria**, results from a defect in enzymatic activity, specifically the branched chain α-ketoacid dehydrogenase complex. It is an autosomal-recessive disorder. Infants appear normal at birth, but by 4 or 5 days of age they demonstrate poor feeding, vomiting, lethargy, and periodic hypertonia. A characteristic sweet, malty odor from the urine and perspiration can be noted toward the end of the first week of life.

Pathophysiology

The decarboxylation defect of MSUD prevents metabolism of the branched-chain amino acids (BCAAs) leucine, isoleucine, and valine (Figure 44-4). Leucine tends to be more problematic than the others. The precise mechanism for the complete decarboxylase reaction and the resultant neurologic damage is not known. Neither is the reason why leucine metabolism is significantly more abnormal than that of the other two BCAAs.

Medical Treatment

Failure to treat this condition leads to acidosis, neurologic deterioration, seizures, and coma, proceeding eventually to death. Management of acute disease often requires peritoneal dialysis and hydration (see Chapter 36).

Depending on the severity of the enzyme defect, early intervention and meticulous biochemical control can provide a more hopeful prognosis for infants and children with MSUD. Reasonable growth and intellectual development in the normal-to-low-normal range have been described. Diagnosis before 7 days of age and long-term metabolic control are critical factors in long-term normalization of intellectual development. Maintenance of plasma leucine concentrations in infants and preschool children should be

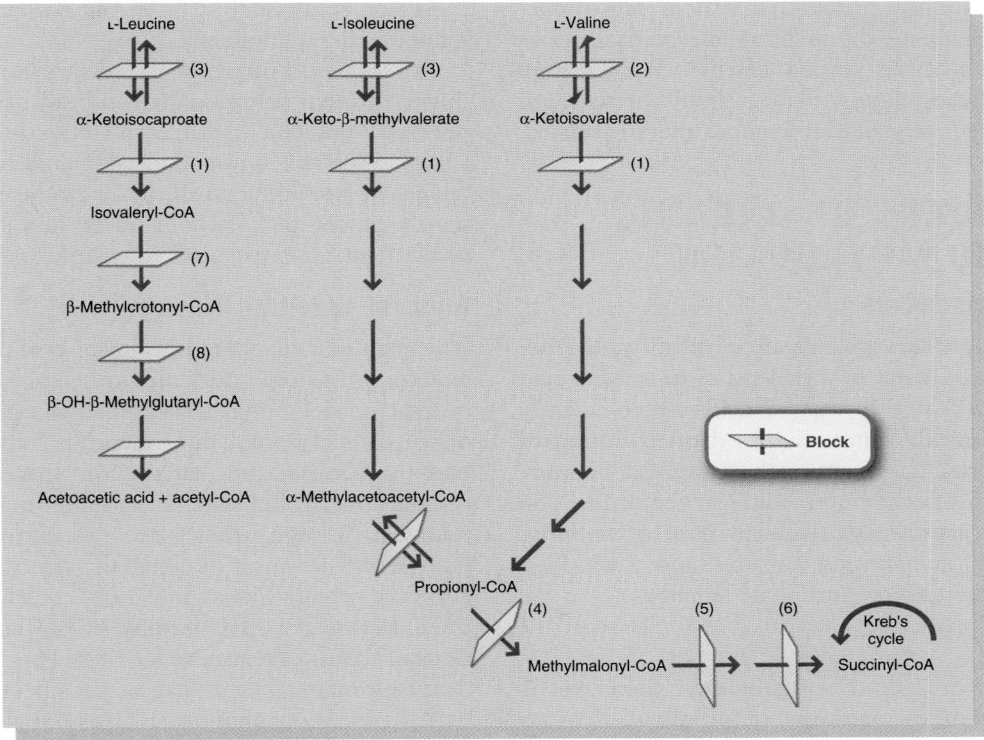

FIGURE 44-4 Organic acidemias and maple syrup urine disease (MSUD). **1,** Branched-chain ketoacid decarboxylase (MSUD); **2,** Valine aminotransferase; **3,** Leucine-isoleucine aminotransferase; **4,** Propionyl-CoA carboxylase (propionic acidemia); **5,** Methylmalonyl-CoA racemase (methylmalonic aciduria); **6,** Methylmalonyl-CoA mutase (methylmalonic aciduria); **7,** Isovaleryl-CoA dehydrogenase (isovaleric acidemia); **8,** β-methylcrotonyl-CoA carboxylase (biotin-responsive multiple carboxylase deficiency). *CoA,* Coenzyme A.

as close to physiologically normal as possible (Hoffman, 2006). Concentrations above 10 mg/dL (760 mmol/L) are often associated with α-ketoacidemia and neurologic symptoms.

Because the liver is the central site of metabolic control for amino acids and other compounds that cause acute degeneration of the brain during illness, therapeutic liver transplantation has been proposed as an option in MSUD. Studies are underway to assess the long-term effects of this procedure on stabilization of biochemical and neurologic status (Strauss et al., 2006).

Medical Nutrition Therapy

Nutrition therapy requires very careful monitoring of blood concentrations of leucine, isoleucine, and valine as well as growth and general nutritional adequacy. Several formulas specifically designed for the treatment of this disorder are available to provide a reasonable amino acid and vitamin mixture. These are generally supplemented with a small quantity of standard infant formula or cow's milk to provide the BCAAs needed to support growth and development. Some infants and children may require additional supplementation with L-valine or L-isoleucine to maintain biochemical balance.

BCAAs may be introduced gradually into the diet when plasma leucine concentrations are sufficiently decreased (Chuang and Shih, 2010). Clinical relapse is most often related to the degree of elevation of leucine concentrations, and these relapses often are related to infection. Acute infections represent life-threatening medical emergencies in this group of children. If the plasma leucine concentration increases rapidly during illness, BCAAs should be removed from the diet immediately and intravenous therapy started.

DISORDERS OF ORGANIC ACID METABOLISM

Organic Acid Disorders

The organic acid disorders are a group of disorders characterized by the accumulation in the blood of nonamino acid organic acids. Most of the organic acids are efficiently excreted in the urine. Diagnosis is based on excretion of compounds not normally present or the presence of abnormally high amounts of other compounds in the urine. The clinical course can vary but is generally marked by vomiting, lethargy, hypotonia, dehydration, seizures, and coma. Survivors often have permanent neurologic damage.

Pathophysiology

Propionic acidemia is a defect of propionyl–coenzyme A (CoA) carboxylase in the pathway of propionyl-CoA to methylmalonyl-CoA, as illustrated in Figure 44-4. Metabolic acidosis with a marked anion gap and hyperammonemia is characteristic. Long-chain ketonuria may also be present.

At least five separate enzyme deficiencies have been identified that result in **methylmalonic acidemia** or aciduria. The defect of methylmalonyl-CoA mutase apoenzyme is the most frequently identified. In methylmalonic academia, the clinical features are similar to those of propionic acidemia. Acidosis is common, and diagnosis is confirmed by the presence of large amounts of methylmalonic acid in blood and urine. Other findings include hypoglycemia, ketonuria, and elevation of plasma ammonia and lactate levels.

Ketone utilization disorders (mitochondrial 2-methylacetoacetyl-CoA thiolase deficiency or similar enzyme defect) are disorders of isoleucine and ketone body metabolism. Affected individuals are usually older infants or toddlers who present with ketoacidosis, vomiting, and lethargy with secondary dehydration and sometimes coma. This event often is preceded by febrile illness or fasting.

Medical Treatment

Some patients with propionic acidemia may respond to pharmacologic doses of biotin. Long-term outcome in propionic acidemia is variable; hypotonia and cognitive delay may result even in children who are diagnosed early and who receive rigorous treatment. Liver damage and cardiomyopathy are possible sequelae. Liver transplantation may limit intellectual disability and cardiac changes (de Baulny et al., 2005).

Methylmalonic acidemia patients may respond to pharmacologic doses of vitamin B_{12}. Responsiveness should be determined as part of the diagnostic process (Venditti, 2007). Progressive renal insufficiency is often a long-term outcome. Developmental delay is often caused by early and or prolonged hyperammonemia.

For ketone utilization use disorders, the treatment is dietary protein restriction (usually 1.5 g/kg of body weight per day); supplementation with **L-carnitine**, a carrier of fatty acids across the mitochondrial membranes; avoidance of fasting by providing small, frequent meals that consist primarily of complex carbohydrates; and the use of Bicitra (sodium citrate-citric acid) to treat ketoacidosis.

Medical Nutrition Therapy

The goals of managing acute episodes of propionic acidemia and methylmalonic acidemia are to achieve and maintain normal nutrient intake and biochemical balance. Maintenance of energy and fluid intake is important to prevent tissue catabolism and dehydration. Intravenous fluids correct electrolyte imbalances, and abnormal metabolites are removed through urinary excretion, promoted by a high fluid intake. Relapses of metabolic acidosis may result from excessive protein intake, infection, constipation, or unidentified factors. Parents become skilled at identifying early signs of illness. Treatment for these episodes must be rapid because coma and death can occur quickly.

Restricted protein intake is an essential component of the treatment of organic acid disorders. A daily protein intake of 1 to 1.5 g/kg of body weight is often an effective treatment modality for infants who have a mild form of the disorder. This can be supplied by diluting standard infant formula to decrease the protein content and adding a protein-free formula to meet nutrient needs. Specialized formulas that limit threonine and isoleucine and omit methionine and valine are used, as clinically indicated, to support an adequate protein intake and growth.

Requirements for the limited amino acids may vary widely. Growth rate, state of health, residual enzyme activity, and overall protein and energy intakes must be monitored carefully and correlated with plasma amino acid levels. Adequate hydration is critical to maintain metabolic equilibrium. Food refusal and lack of appetite may complicate nutrition therapy, which compromises medical management.

DISORDERS OF UREA CYCLE METABOLISM

All urea cycle defects result in an accumulation of ammonia in the blood. The clinical signs of elevated ammonia are vomiting and lethargy, which may progress to seizures, coma, and ultimately death. In infants the adverse effects of elevated ammonia levels are rapid and devastating. In older children symptoms of elevated ammonia may be preceded by hyperactivity and irritability. Neurologic damage may result from frequent and severe episodes of hyperammonemia. The severity and variation of the clinical courses of some urea cycle defects may be related to the degree of residual enzyme activity (Brusilow and Horwich, 2010). The common urea cycle defects are discussed in a progression that proceeds around the urea cycle, as shown in Figure 44-5.

Pathophysiology

Ornithine transcarbamylase (OTC) deficiency is an X-linked recessive disorder marked by blockage in the conversion of ornithine and carbamyl phosphate to citrulline. OTC deficiency is identified by hyperammonemia and increased urinary orotic acid, with normal levels of citrulline, argininosuccinic acid, and arginine. Severe OTC deficiency is usually lethal in males. Heterozygous females with various degrees of enzyme activity may not demonstrate symptoms until they are induced by stress, as from an infection, or a significant increase in protein intake.

Citrullinemia is the result of a deficiency of argininosuccinic acid synthetase in the metabolism of citrulline to argininosuccinic acid. Citrullinemia is identified by markedly elevated citrulline levels in the urine and blood. Symptoms may be present in the neonatal period, or they may develop gradually in early infancy. Poor feeding and recurrent vomiting occur which, without immediate treatment, progress to seizures, neurologic abnormalities, and coma.

Argininosuccinic aciduria (ASA) results from deficiency of argininosuccinate lyase, which is involved in the metabolism of argininosuccinic acid to arginine. ASA is identified by the presence of argininosuccinic acid in urine and blood. L-Arginine must be supplemented to provide an alternative pathway for waste nitrogen excretion.

Carbamyl-phosphate synthetase (CPS) deficiency is the result of deficient activity of CPS. The onset is usually in the early neonatal period, with vomiting, irritability, marked hyperammonemia, respiratory distress, altered muscle tone, lethargy, and often coma. Specific laboratory findings usually include low plasma levels of citrulline and arginine and normal orotic acid levels in urine.

Medical Treatment

Acute episodes of illness are managed by discontinuing protein intake and administering intravenous fluids and glucose to correct dehydration and provide energy. If hyperammonemia is severe, peritoneal dialysis, hemodialysis, or exchange transfusion may be required. Intravenous sodium benzoate or other alternative pathway compounds have been beneficial in reducing the hyperammonemia.

Neurologic outcome and intellectual development in individuals with urea cycle disorders vary, with a range from

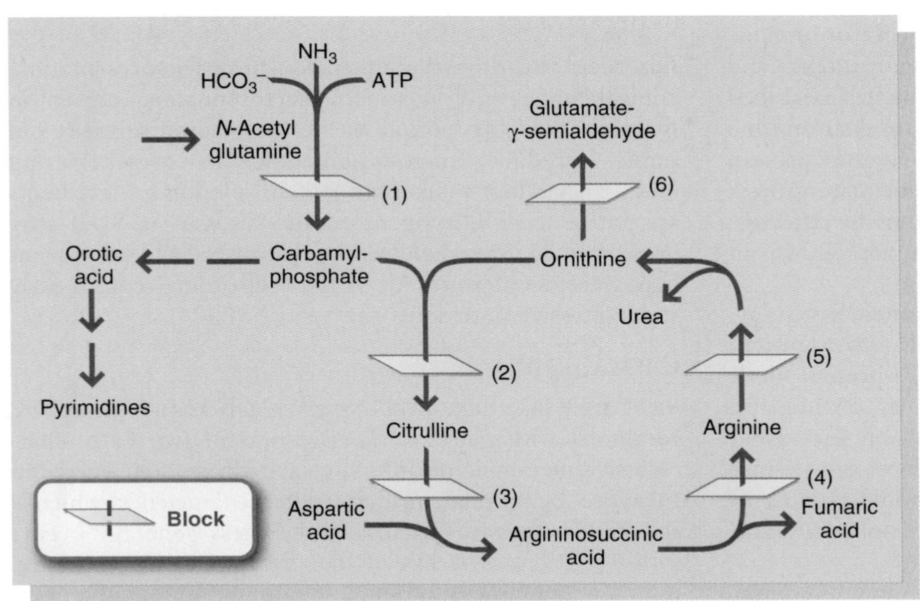

FIGURE 44-5 Urea cycle disorders. **1,** Carbamyl-phosphate synthetase deficiency; **2,** Ornithine carbamyl transferase deficiency; **3,** Argininosuccinic acid synthetase (citrullinemia); **4,** Argininosuccinic acid lyase (argininosuccinic aciduria); **5,** Arginase deficiency (arginemia); **6,** Adenosine triphosphate.

normal IQ and motor function to severe intellectual disability and cerebral palsy. Although information on long-term follow-up is limited, the use of alternative pathways for waste nitrogen excretion and a protein-restricted food pattern may improve the outcome.

Medical Nutrition Therapy

Nutritional management of patients who have urea cycle disorders is a challenging task (Singh et al., 2005). The aim of therapy for the urea cycle disorders is to prevent or decrease hyperammonemia and the detrimental neurologic consequences associated with it. Treatment is similar for all of the disorders. For mildly affected infants a standard infant formula can be diluted to provide protein at 1 to 1.5 g/kg body weight per day. The energy, vitamin, and mineral concentrations can be brought up to recommended intake levels with the addition of a protein-free formula. However, for most individuals, specialized formulas are needed to adjust protein composition in an effort to limit ammonia production.

The amount of protein tolerated is affected by variables such as specific enzyme defect, age-related growth rate, health status, level of physical activity, amount of free amino acids administered, energy needs, residual enzyme function, and the use of nitrogen-scavenging medications. Recommendations must take family lifestyle and the individual's eating behaviors into consideration (Singh et al., 2005). Long-term therapy consists of restricting dietary protein to 1 to 2 g/kg/day, depending on individual tolerance. For most infants and children with these disorders, except for arginase deficiency, L-arginine supplements are required to prevent arginine deficiency and assist in waste nitrogen excretion. L-Arginine is supplemented based on individual needs, except in the case of arginase deficiency (Brusilow and Howich, 2010). Phenylbutyrate or other compounds that enhance alternative metabolic pathways are usually required to normalize ammonia levels.

Protein-Restricted Diets

Infants and children with urea cycle defects or organic acidemias generally require restricted-protein intakes and specialized formulas. The amount of protein prescribed is based on the individual's tolerance or residual enzyme activity, age, and projected growth rate. The highest protein level tolerated should be given to ensure adequate growth and a margin of nutritional safety. The steps for effective planning of a low-protein food pattern are shown in Box 44-1.

In general, low-protein or restricted-protein food patterns can be formulated from readily available, lower-protein infant, toddler, and table foods. Special low-protein foods (see Table 44-5) can be used to provide energy, texture, and variety in the food pattern without appreciably increasing the protein load. The prescribed protein level can be met by adding a protein-free or specialized formula product to standard infant formula. Supplementing carbohydrate and fat makes up the resultant energy deficit.

BOX 44-1

Steps in Designing a Low-Protein Eating Plan

1. Determine the protein tolerance of the individual based on (1) diagnosis, (2) age, and (3) growth. Consider the metabolic stability and total protein intake required for the infant's or child's weight.
2. Calculate the protein and energy needs of the individual based on age, activity, and weight.
3. Provide at least 70% of total protein as high–biologic value protein from formula for infants and from milk or dairy foods for older children. Use a specialized formula if the infant or child cannot tolerate the entire protein intake from intact protein.
4. Provide energy and nutrient sources to meet basic needs.
5. Add water to meet fluid requirements and maintain appropriate concentration of formula mixture.
6. For the older infant and child, provide foods to meet food variety, texture, and energy needs.
7. Provide adequate intake of calcium, iron, zinc and all other vitamins and minerals for age.

Specialty formulas are available when needed. The appropriate choice depends on the level of protein restriction, age, and condition of the child. The usual recommendations for energy density and vitamin and mineral composition are generally appropriate to support growth for the infant or child. Osmolarity of the formula must be considered; feedings of no more than 400 mOsm/L of solution have been recommended.

DISORDERS OF CARBOHYDRATE METABOLISM

Disorders of carbohydrate metabolism vary in presentation, clinical course, and outcome. Galactosemia may present in the early newborn period as life-threatening seizures and sepsis. Hereditary fructose intolerance may present during midinfancy when solids that contain offending ingredients are introduced. Glycogen storage diseases (GSDs) may present at the time when feedings are spaced and subsequent hypoglycemia appears. All of these disorders require early and aggressive nutritional therapy.

Galactosemia

Galactosemia, a high level of plasma galactose-1-phosphate combined with galactosuria, is found in two autosomal-recessive metabolic disorders: galactokinase deficiency and galactose-1-phosphate uridyltransferase deficiency, which is also called "classic galactosemia." Illness generally occurs within the first 2 weeks of life. Symptoms are vomiting,

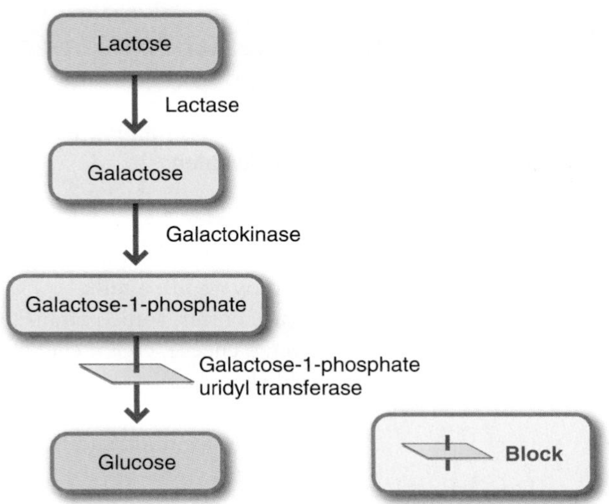

FIGURE 44-6 Schematic diagram of the metabolism of galactose in galactosemia.

diarrhea, lethargy, failure to thrive, jaundice, hepatomegaly, and cataracts. Infants with galactosemia may be hypoglycemic and susceptible to infection from gram-negative organisms. If the condition is not treated, death frequently ensues secondarily to septicemia.

Pathophysiology

Galactosemia results from a disturbance in the conversion of galactose to glucose because of the absence or inactivity of one of the enzymes shown in Figure 44-6. The enzyme deficiency causes an accumulation of galactose, or galactose and galactose-1-phosphate, in body tissues. In addition, expanded newborn screening programs have identified many newborns with Duarte galactosemia. These infants have one allele for galactosemia and one for "Duarte" galactosemia and are often said to have "DG/G galactosemia." The Duarte allele produces approximately 5% to 20% of the GALT enzyme. Little is known about the natural history of DG galactosemia; apparently infants and children develop normally without medical complications.

Medical Treatment

When diagnosis and therapy are delayed, intellectual disability can result (Waisbren, 2006). With early diagnosis and treatment, physical and motor development should proceed normally. However, intellectual achievement may be depressed. Patients often have IQs of 85 to 100; visual-perceptual and speech difficulties are common (Kaufman et al., 1995). Ovarian failure affects approximately 95% of women with galactosemia (Forges et al., 2006).

Medical Nutrition Therapy

Galactosemia is treated by lifelong galactose restriction. Although galactose is required for the production of galactolipids and cerebrosides, it can be produced by an alternative pathway if galactose is omitted from the diet. Galactose restriction mandates strict avoidance of all milk and milk products and lactose-containing foods because lactose is hydrolyzed into galactose and glucose. Effective galactose restriction requires careful reading of food product labels. Milk is added to many products, and lactose often appears in the coating of the tablet form of medications. Infants are fed soy-based formula. Some fruits and vegetables contain significant amounts of galactose. Whether these sources of galactose contribute to the pathophysiology characteristics of the disorder is unclear. Table 44-9 presents a low-galactose food pattern.

Medical opinions differ about the intensity and duration of treatment for Duarte galactosemia. Many centers eliminate galactose from the diets of these children for the first year of life; other centers do not.

Glycogen Storage Diseases

Glycogen storage diseases (GSDs) reflect an inability to metabolize glycogen to glucose. There are a number of possible enzyme defects along the pathway. The most common of the GSD disorders are types I and III. Their symptoms are poor physical growth, hypoglycemia, hepatomegaly, and abnormal biochemical parameters, especially for cholesterol and triglycerides. Advances in the treatment of GSDs may improve the quality of life for affected children (Bali and Chen, 2010).

Pathophysiology

GSD type Ia is a defect in the enzyme glucose-1-6-phosphatase, which impairs the formation of new glucose (**gluconeogenesis**) and the breakdown of glycogen from storage (**glycogenolysis**). The affected person is unable to metabolize glycogen stored in the liver. Severe hypoglycemia can result and cause irreparable damage.

Amylo-1, 6-glucosidase deficiency (GSD III or debrancher enzyme deficiency) prevents glycogen breakdown beyond branch points. This disorder is similar to GSD I in that glycogenolysis is inefficient but gluconeogenesis is amplified to help maintain glucose production. The symptoms of GSD III are usually less severe and range from hepatomegaly to severe hypoglycemia (Dagli et al., 2010).

Medical Treatment

The outcome of treatment has been good. The hazard of severe hypoglycemic episodes is diminished, physical growth is improved, and liver size is decreased. The risk of progressive renal dysfunction is not entirely eliminated by current treatment, but liver transplantation for some types of GSD (e.g., type Ib) is sometimes an option. Treatment protocols for the GSDs are still evolving. The protocols include various kinds of carbohydrates at various doses during the day and night. Individual tolerance, body weight, state of health, ambient temperature, and physical activity all play important roles in designing the specific pattern of carbohydrate administration. The goal for all of the protocols remains the same: normalization of blood glucose levels.

TABLE 44-9

Food Lists for Low-Galactose Food Pattern

Allowable Foods	Galactose-Containing Foods to Be Avoided*
Milk and Milk Substitutes	
Similac Sensitive Isomil Soy Enfamil Prosobee Gerber Good Start Soy Plus	All forms of animal milk Imitation or filled milk Cream, butter, some margarines Cottage cheese, cream cheese Hard cheeses Yogurt Ice cream, ice milk, sherbet Breast milk
Fruits	
All fresh, frozen, canned, or dried fruits except those processed with unsafe ingredients†	
Vegetables	
All fresh, frozen, canned, or dried vegetables except those processed with unsafe ingredients,† seasoned with butter or margarine, breaded, or creamed	
Meat, Poultry, Fish, Eggs, Nuts	
Plain beef, lamb, veal, pork, ham, fish, turkey, chicken, game, fowl, Kosher frankfurters, eggs, nut butters, nuts	
Breads and Cereals	
Cooked and dry cereals, bread or crackers without milk or unsafe ingredients,† macaroni, spaghetti, noodles, rice, tortillas	
Fats	
All vegetable oils; all shortening, lard, margarines, and salad dressings except those made with unsafe ingredients†; mayonnaise; olives	

*Lactose is often used as a pharmaceutical bulking agent, filler, or excipient; thus tablets, tinctures, and vitamin and mineral mixtures should be evaluated carefully for galactose content. The *Physician's Desk Reference* now lists active and inactive ingredients in medications, as well as manufacturers' telephone numbers.

†Unsafe ingredients include milk, buttermilk, cream, lactose, galactose, casein, caseinate, whey, dry milk solids, or curds. Labels should be checked regularly and carefully because formulations of products change often.

Medical Nutrition Therapy

The rationale for intervention is to maintain plasma glucose in a normal range and prevent hypoglycemia by providing a constant supply of exogenous glucose. Administration of raw cornstarch at regular intervals and a high–complex carbohydrate, low-fat dietary pattern are advocated to prevent hypoglycemia. Some infants and children do very well with oral cornstarch administration, whereas others require glucose polymers administered via continuous-drip gastric feedings to prevent hypoglycemic episodes during the night (Bali and Chen, 2010; Dagli et al., 2010). The dose of cornstarch should be individualized; doses of 1.6 to 2.5 g/kg at 4- to 6-hour intervals are generally effective for young children with GSD I (Bali and Chen, 2010. The glucose vehicle suggested is a lactose-free formula. Iron supplementation is required to maintain adequate hematologic status because cornstarch interferes with iron absorption.

DISORDERS OF FATTY ACID OXIDATION

Recent laboratory advancements have enabled identification of fatty acid oxidation disorders such as **medium-chain acyl-CoA dehydrogenase deficiency (MCAD)** and **long-chain 3-hydroxyacyl-CoA dehydrogenase deficiency (LCHAD)** (Figure 44-7). Children who are not identified by newborn screening usually present during periods of fasting or clinical illness with symptoms of variable severity, including failure to thrive, episodic vomiting, and hypotonia.

Pathophysiology

Children with MCAD who present clinically typically have hypoglycemia without urine ketones, lethargy, seizures, and coma. Children with LCHAD become hypoglycemic and demonstrate abnormal liver function, reduced or absent ketones in the urine, and often secondary carnitine deficiency. They may also have hepatomegaly and acute liver disease. Hypoglycemia can progress quickly and be fatal (Matern and Rinaldo, 2005; Roe and Ding, 2010).

Medical Nutrition Therapy

The concept underlying effective treatment for fatty acid oxidation disorders is straightforward: avoidance of fasting. This is accomplished by the regularly spaced intake of foods that provide an adequate energy intake and are high in carbohydrates. A low-fat diet is advocated because fats are not effectively metabolized. Consumption of not more than 30% of energy as fat has been recommended; some individuals require more restriction. Supplementation with L-carnitine, a substance that functions as a carrier of fatty acids across the mitochondrial membranes, is recommended by some centers. Children often do very well with three meals and three snacks offered at regular intervals. Most children may require additional carbohydrate, either a complex carbohydrate snack or uncooked cornstarch before bed, based on individual ability to maintain blood glucose levels throughout the night (Matern and Rinaldo, 2005). Depending on the disorder, supplementation with specific fatty acids (e.g., medium-chain fats for disorders that involve blocks of long-chain metabolism) may be indicated.

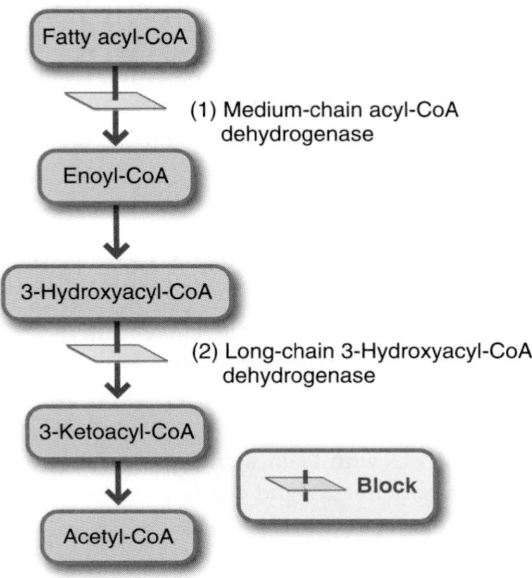

FIGURE 44-7 Mitochondrial fatty acid oxidation disorders: **1,** Medium-chain acyl-Coenzyme A dehydrogenase deficiency, the most common fatty acid oxidation disorder. **2,** Long-chain 3-hydroxyacyl-CoA dehydrogenase deficiency.

ROLE OF THE NUTRITIONIST IN GENETIC METABOLIC DISORDERS

The role of the pediatric nutrition specialist in the treatment of metabolic disorders is a complex one that requires expertise in MNT for the specific disorder. Preparation and competency requires access to detailed information about the disorders and treatment modalities. A family-centered counseling approach, knowledge of feeding-skill development, and understanding of behavior modification techniques, as well as the support and counsel of a team of health care providers involved in the care of the patient, are also required. Nutrition intervention is often a lifelong consideration. Specific objectives of nutrition care are shown in Box 44-2.

BOX 44-2

Intervention Objectives for the Nutritionist Involved in the Treatment of Genetic Metabolic Disorders

In the clinic the registered dietitian (RD) has a major role in ongoing therapy and planning for each child. These responsibilities include gathering of objective food intake data from the family, assessing the adequacy of the child's intake, and working with the family to teach its members appropriate ways to monitor the restricted food intake pattern. The child with a metabolic disorder often presents with a wide range of concerns, which may include unstable biochemical levels, failure to gain weight, excessive weight gain, difficulty adhering to the diet, and behaviors that cause an adverse feeding situation. Thus managing a child with a metabolic disorder requires input from the entire health care team. The nutritionist uses skills and a basic knowledge of foods as sources of nutrients, parent-child relationships, growth, development, and interviewing to obtain the necessary information for assessing and planning for the child with a genetic metabolic disorder.

I. The RD functions as an effective interdisciplinary team member by doing the following:
- **A.** Becoming familiar with the background and current status of the child by reviewing the medical record
- **B.** Recognizing and accepting the responsibility as the nutritionist by doing the following:
  - **1.** Identifying appropriate intake of nutrients for growth, activity, and biochemical balance
  - **2.** Identifying developmental stages of feeding behavior
  - **3.** Understanding the concept of food as a support of developmental progress
  - **4.** Identifying behavior as it affects nutrient intake
- **C.** Understanding, respecting, and using the expertise of the team disciplines in providing care for the child

Continued

BOX 44-2

Intervention Objectives for the Nutritionist Involved in the Treatment of Genetic Metabolic Disorders—cont'd

II. The RD provides adequate and supportive patient services by doing the following:
  A. Establishing a positive, cooperative working relationship with the parent and child
  B. Interviewing the parents about dietary intake and the feeding situation in a nonjudgmental manner
  C. Assessing the parent-child relationship as it relates to dietary management and control of the disorder
  D. Developing a plan for appropriate dietary management based on growth, biochemical levels, nutrient needs, developmental progress and nutrition diagnosis, such as:
  - Excessive protein intake
  - Altered nutrition-related laboratory values
  - Intake of inappropriate amino acids
  - Inadequate vitamin intake
  - Inadequate mineral intake
  - Food medication interaction
  - Food- and nutrition-related knowledge deficit
  - Limited adherence to nutrition-related recommendations

  E. Developing a plan that includes appropriate foods and recognizes the parents' skills in food preparation, as well as family routines
  F. Working with the parents to establish a method to deal effectively with negative feeding behaviors, if necessary
  G. Contacting the family after receiving laboratory results and calculating food records to make necessary and appropriate changes in diet prescription
  H. Supporting parents in their efforts at effective dietary and behavior management

III. The RD develops a professional database by doing the following:
  A. Becoming familiar with the current literature on the treatment of metabolic disorders
  B. Understanding the genetic basis of metabolic disorders

IV. The RD works with team members to understand the long-term patient care and create a written care plan for the patient.

CLINICAL SCENARIO

The 1-day newborn screening test result for phenylalanine for a 7-lb, 4-oz male child was 3 mg/dL (180 mmol/L). The infant was breast-fed with no supplemental formula. A repeat sample was requested to further document the phenylalanine concentration in the infant's blood. The result from this sample, collected on day 5 of life, was 24 mg/dL (1440 mmol/L). To confirm the diagnosis for this child, which was considered to be "presumptive positive," a quantitative sample was obtained, and phenylalanine and tyrosine levels were measured. On day 9 of life the serum phenylalanine concentration was 25.5 mg/dL (1530 mmol/L), and the tyrosine level was 1.1 mg/dL (60.5 mmol/L); phenylalanine to tyrosine ratio was 23 : 2.

To provide adequate protein and energy intake and at the same time decrease the serum phenylalanine concentration, a phenylalanine-free formula was introduced at standard dilution without a phenylalanine supplement. Within 24 hours the infant's serum phenylalanine concentration had decreased to 16.5 mg/dL (990 mmol/L) while the infant was being provided an intake of 16 oz of formula. Within 48 hours the level was 8.8 mg/dL (528 mmol/L), with an intake of 18 oz of formula. At this point, standard infant formula was added to bring the calculated phenylalanine intake to approximately 60 mg/kg and to maintain a generous protein and energy intake for this 3.6-kg infant.

Phenylalanine concentrations were measured on alternate days for 4 days, and the levels were 7.6 mg/dL (456 mmol/L) and 5.6 mg/dL (336 mmol/L), respectively. In subsequent weeks growth and serum phenylalanine concentrations continued to be monitored carefully, and energy and phenylalanine intakes were adjusted as necessary to maintain blood phenylalanine concentrations between 1 and 6 mg/dL (60-360 mmol/L) and to maintain growth in appropriate channels. The parents are apprehensive about preparing formula.

Nutrition Diagnostic Statement

Nutrition-related knowledge deficit related to the need for and preparation of a specialized formula (used for treatment of phenylketonuria in infants), as evidenced by a new diagnosis and the parents' asking for information

Nutrition Care Questions

1. What is the expected energy requirement for this infant with phenylketonuria?
2. What baseline formula would you use for this infant to provide phenylalanine at 60 mg/kg, formula at 20 kcal/oz, and protein and energy intakes at recommended levels?
3. What are the growth expectations for this infant?
4. What steps would you take if the plasma phenylalanine concentration exceeded 6 mg/dL (360 mmol/L) on subsequent measurements?

USEFUL WEBSITES

American College of Medical Genetics (ACMG)
http://www.acmg.net
Gene Reviews
http://www.geneclinics.org
Genetics Home Reference
http://ghr.nlm.nih.gov
Genetic Metabolic Dietitians International (GMDI)
http://www.gmdi.org
MedlinePlus: Metabolic Disorders
http://www.nlm.nih.gov/medlineplus/metabolicdisorders.html
National Newborn Screening and Genetics Resource Center
http://genes-r-us.uthscsa.edu/
National PKU News
http://www.pkunews.org

REFERENCES

Acosta PB: Recommendations for protein and energy intakes by patients with phenylketonuria, *Eur J Pediatr* 155:S121, 1996.

Bali S, Chen YT: *Glycogen storage disease type 1. Gene reviews*, 2010 Accessed 17 March 2011 from http://www.geneclinics.org.

Blau N, et al: Optimizing the use of sapropterin (BH4) in the management of phenylketonuria, *Molec Genet Metab* 96:158, 2010.

Bosch AM, et al: The course of life and quality of life of early and continuously treated Dutch patients with phenylketonuria, *J Inherit Metab Dis* 29:576, 2006.

Brosco JP, et al: Universal newborn screening and adverse medical outcomes: a historical note, *Ment Retard Dev Disabil Res Rev* 12:262, 2006.

Brusilow SW, Horwich AL: Urea cycle enzymes. In Valle D, et al, editors: *The online metabolic and molecular bases of inherited disease*, New York, 2010, McGraw Hill.

Chuang DT, Shih VE: Maple syrup urine disease (branched-chain ketoaciduria). In Valle D, et al, editors: *The online metabolic and molecular bases of inherited disease*, New York, 2010, McGraw Hill.

Cleary MA, et al: Randomised controlled trial of essential fatty acid supplementation in phenylketonuria, *Eur J Clin Nutr* 60:915, 2006.

Dagli A, et al: Glycogen storage disease type III. GeneReviews, 2010. Accessed 1 August 2010 from http://www.geneclinics.org.

de Baulny HO, et al: Methylmalonic and propionic acidaemias: management and outcome, *J Inherit Metab Dis* 28:415, 2005.

Forges T, et al: Pathophysiology of impaired ovarian function in galactosaemia, *Human Reprod Update* 12:573, 2006.

Hoffman B: Impact of longitudinal plasma leucine levels on the intellectual outcome in patients with classic MSUD, *Pediatr Res* 59:17, 2006.

Holt LE, Snyderman SE: The amino acid requirements of children. In Nyhan WL, editor: *Amino acid metabolism and genetic variation*, New York, 1967, McGraw-Hill.

Ievers-Landis CE, et al: Situational analysis of dietary challenges of the treatment regimen for children and adolescents with phenylketonuria and their primary caregivers, *J Dev Behav Pediatr* 26:186, 2005.

Kaufman FR, et al: Cognitive functioning, neurologic status and brain imaging in classical galacotsemia, *Eur J Pediatr* 154(7 Suppl 2):S2, 1995.

Kaye CI, et al: Newborn screening fact sheets, *Pediatrics* 118:e934, 2006.

Koch R, et al: Psychosocial issues and outcomes in maternal PKU, *Mol Genet Metab* 99:S68, 2010.

Lee PJ, et al: Maternal phenylketonuria: report from the United Kingdom Registry 1978-1997, *Arch Dis Child* 90:143, 2005.

Matern D, Rinaldo P: Medium-chain acyl-coenzyme A dehydrogenase deficiency. GeneReviews, 2005. Accessed 1 August 2010 from http://www.geneclinics.org.

Maternal Child Health Bureau (MCHB): Advisory Committee on Heritable Disorders and Genetic Diseases in Newborns and Children, 2007. Accessed 1 August 2010 from http://www.hrsa.gov/heritabledisorderscommittee/default.htm.

Maternal Child Health Bureau: Newborn screening: toward a uniform screening panel and system, *Genet Med* 8(suppl 1):1S, 2006.

Roe CR, Ding J: Mitochondrial fatty acid oxidation disorders. In Valle D, et al, editors: *The online metabolic and molecular bases of inherited disease*, New York, 2010, McGraw Hill.

Rose HJ, et al: Fat intakes of children with PKU on low phenylalanine diets, *J Hum Nutr Diet* 18:395, 2005.

Saugstad LF: From genetics to epigenetics, *Nutr Health*, 18:285, 2006.

Singh RH, et al: Nutritional management of urea cycle disorders, *Crit Care Clin* 21:S27, 2005.

Strauss KA, et al: Elective liver transplantation for the treatment of classical maple syrup urine disease, *Am J Transplant* 6:557, 2006.

Therrell BL, et al: Status of newborn screening programs in the United States, *Pediatrics* 117:S212, 2006.

Venditti CP: Methylmalonic acidemia. GeneReviews, 2007. Accessed 1 August 2010 from http://www.geneclinics.org.

Waisbren SE: Newborn screening for metabolic disorders, *JAMA* 296:993, 2006.

Waisbren SE, Azen C: Cognitive and behavioral development in maternal phenylketonuria offspring, *Pediatrics* 112:1544, 2003.

Waisbren SE, et al: Phenylalanine blood levels and clinical outcomes in phenylketonuria: a systemic literature review and meta-analyisis, *Mol Genet Metab* 92:63, 2007.

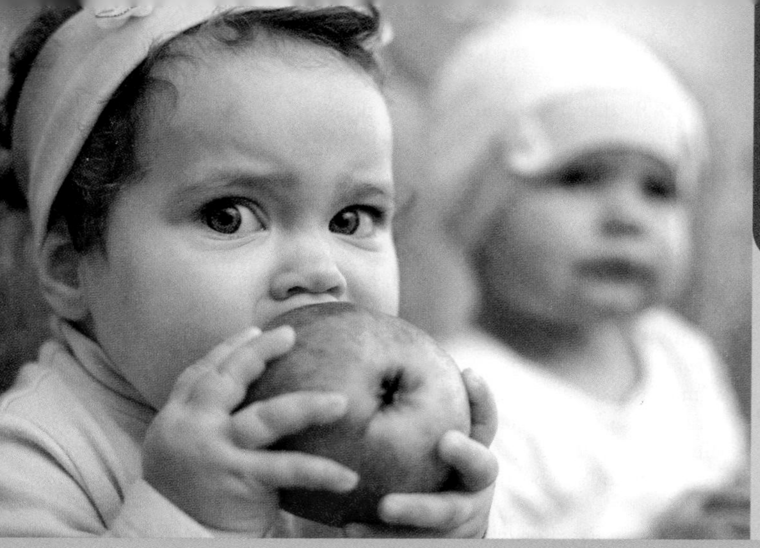

CHAPTER 45

Harriet Cloud, MS, RD, FADA

Medical Nutrition Therapy for Intellectual and Developmental Disabilities

KEY TERMS

Arnold Chiari malformation of the brain
Asperger syndrome
attention-deficit/hyperactivity disorder (ADHD)
autism spectrum disorders (ASDs)
cerebral palsy (CP)
cleft lip and cleft palate (CL/CP)
developmental disability
Down syndrome (DS)
fetal alcohol syndrome (FAS)
hypotonia
individualized education plan (IEP)
individualized family plan
intellectual disability
midfacial hypoplasia
mosaicism
myelomeningocele (MM)
nondysjunction
oral-motor problems
pervasive developmental disorder (PDD)
Prader-Willi syndrome (PWS)
spina bifida
translocation

Individuals with developmental disabilities were generally housed in institutions for the first half of the 20th century. Little attention was paid to their education or medical or nutritional care. In 1963 the Developmental Disabilities Assistance and Bill of Rights Act was passed. Through this Act federal funds supported the development and operation of state councils, protection and advocacy systems, university centers, and projects of national significance. This Act provided the structure to assist people with developmental disabilities to pursue meaningful and productive lives. The institutions that housed these individuals were gradually closed or reduced in size. By 1975 these individuals were cared for at home, in schools, or in small residential facilities. In 1975 Public Law (P.L.) 94-142 was passed, opening public schools to children with developmental disabilities. In 1985 P.L. 99-487 (102-119 in 1992), the Early Intervention Act, was passed, bringing services to children from birth to school age.

A **developmental disability** is defined as a severe chronic disability that is attributable to a mental or physical impairment or combination of mental and physical impairments. It is manifested before the person attains age 22; is likely to continue indefinitely; results in substantial functional limitations in three or more areas of major life activity (self-care, receptive and expressive language, learning, mobility, self-direction, capacity for independent living, and economic self-sufficiency); and reflects the person's need for a combination of generic or specialized interdisciplinary care, treatments, or other services that are lifelong or of extended duration and individually planned and coordinated. Developmental disabilities affect individuals of all ages and are not a disease state. They are conditions that are caused by fetal abnormalities, birth defects, and metabolic and chromosomal disorders.

Intellectual disability replaced the term *mental retardation* in the 11th edition of the Definition Manual of the American Association on Intellectual and Developmental Disabilities (AAIDD, 2011). **Intellectual disability** is the most common developmental disability, characterized by significantly below-average intellectual functioning along with related limitations in areas such as communication, self-care, functional academics, home living, self-direction, health and safety, leisure, or work and social skills. It is estimated that 1% to 3% of the population have this diagnosis.

Developmental disabilities have been traced to many causes: chromosomal aberrations, congenital anomalies, specific syndromes, neuromuscular dysfunction, neurologic disorders, prematurity, cerebral palsy (CP), untreated inborn errors of metabolism, toxins in the environment, and nutrient deficiencies. The Centers for Disease Control and Prevention (CDC) reports that 3% of all live births have a birth defect (CDC, 2010) and there are 4.5 million Americans living with developmental disabilities (American Dietetic Association [ADA], 2010).

MEDICAL NUTRITION THERAPY

Medical nutrition therapy (MNT) services vary depending on the individual's physical or mental problem, and much has been learned about the role of nutrition in both the prevention of disabilities and intervention when a nutrition problem exists. The role of the registered dietitian (RD) is essential. Because there is an abundance of information that parents and caretakers use from support groups and websites that are untested scientifically, RDs are often providing evidence-based counseling to counteract misinformation.

Numerous nutrition problems have been identified in the individual with developmental disabilities. Growth retardation, obesity, failure to thrive, feeding problems, metabolic disorders, medication-nutrient interactions, constipation, and renal problems may be present. Other health problems exist, depending on the disorder. Table 45-1 lists the most common developmental disabilities and their associated nutrition problems.

The ADA confirmed that nutrition services provided by RDs are essential components of comprehensive care for infants, children, and adults with intellectual and developmental disabilities. Nutrition services should be provided throughout the life cycle. Educational and vocational programs should provide MNT in a manner that is interdisciplinary, family centered, community based, and culturally competent (ADA, 2010).

Nutrition Assessment

Anthropometric Measures

Anthropometric measures are altered when an individual is unable to stand, suffers from contractions, or has other gross motor problems. Measuring body weight may require special equipment such as chair scales or bucket scales. Wheelchair scales are used in some clinics but require that the wheelchair weight be known. Obtaining height for the nonambulatory individual requires either a recumbent board that can be purchased or constructed. Other measures of height include arm span, knee-to-ankle height, or sitting height (Figure 45-1; see Appendixes 19 and 20).

Although growth charts for children with various syndromes do exist, most clinicians recommend using the general CDC charts (Appendixes 9 to 16) because the information in the specialized charts is often based on small numbers, mixed populations, and old data (CDC, 2010). See Chapter 6.

Other measures that can be used to explore weight issues include arm circumference, triceps skinfold measures, and body mass index (BMI). BMI is a part of the CDC growth charts and can also be found in Appendixes 12, 16, and 23. Using the BMI for age can be controversial. For example, BMI is limited for identifying overweight in children who are overly fat because of decreased muscle mass and short stature.

Biochemical Measures

Laboratory assessment for the child and adult with developmental disabilities is generally the same as that discussed in Chapter 8 and Appendix 30. Additional tests may be indicated for the individual with epilepsy or seizures who is receiving an anticonvulsant medication such as phenytoin, divalproex sodium, topiramate, or carbamazepine. Use of these medications can lead to low blood levels of folic acid, carnitine, ascorbic acid, calcium, vitamin D, alkaline phosphatase, phosphorus, and pyridoxine. Assessment of thyroid status is part of the protocol for children with Down syndrome (DS), and a glucose tolerance test is recommended for evaluation of the child with Prader-Willi syndrome (PWS). As appropriate, genetic testing may be encouraged for both affected individuals and their biological family members.

Dietary Intake and Feeding Problems

Dietary information should be obtained for the child with a developmental disability through a diet history. However, there are difficulties in obtaining an accurate recall when the child is in a day-care center. Written diaries are also difficult to obtain when the child has multiple caretakers or when he or she is in school. When working with an adult with developmental disabilities, it is often difficult to obtain accurate information unless the individual has supervision, such as in special residential housing. Use of pictures and food models can often help in obtaining an estimate of the individual's intake.

Many children and adults with developmental disabilities display feeding problems that seriously decrease their ability to eat an adequate diet. Feeding problems are defined as the inability or refusal to eat certain foods because of neuromotor dysfunction, obstructive lesions such as strictures, and psychosocial factors (Cloud et al., 2005). Other causes of feeding problems in this population include oral-motor

TABLE 45-1

Selected Syndromes and Developmental Disabilities: Frequent Nutrition Diagnoses

Syndrome or Disability	Underweight or Overweight/ Obesity	Altered Energy Requirements	Altered GI function	Feeding Problems	Other Issues
Cerebral Palsy					
A disorder of muscle control or coordination resulting from injury to the brain during its early (fetal, perinatal, and early childhood) development; there may be associated problems with intellectual, visual, or other functions.	Growth problems	Failure to thrive	Constipation	Oral/motor problems	Central nervous system involvement; orthopedic problems; medication-nutrient interactions related to seizure disorder treatment
Down Syndrome (Genetic Disorder)					
Results from an extra chromosome 21, causing developmental problems such as congenital heart disease, intellectual disability, small stature, and decreased muscle tone.	Risk for obesity	Related to short stature and limited activity	Constipation	Poor suck in infancy	Gum disease; increased risk of heart disease; osteoporosis; Alzheimer's disease risk
Prader-Willi Syndrome (Genetic Disorder)					
A disorder characterized by uncontrollable eating habits, inability to distinguish hunger from appetite; severe obesity; poorly developed genitalia; and moderate to severe intellectual disability.	Risk for obesity	Failure to thrive in infancy	N/A	Weak suck in infancy; abnormal food related activities	Risk of diabetes mellitus
Autism					
Classified as a type of pervasive developmental disorder; diagnostic criteria include communication problems, ritualistic behaviors, and inappropriate social interactions	N/A	N/A	Possible dysfunction	Limited food selections; strong food dislikes	Pica; medication-nutrient interactions
Spina Bifida (Myelomeningocele)					
Results from a midline defect of the skin, spinal column, and spinal cord; characterized by hydrocephalus, intellectual disability, and lack of muscular control.	Risk for obesity	Altered energy needs based on short stature and limited mobility	Constipation	Swallowing problems caused by Arnold Chiari malformation of the brain	Urinary tract infections

Data from American Dietetic Association: Position of the American Dietetic Association: providing nutrition services for people with developmental disabilities and special health care needs, J Am Diet Assoc 110:297, 2010.

GI, Gastrointestinal; *N/A*, not applicable.

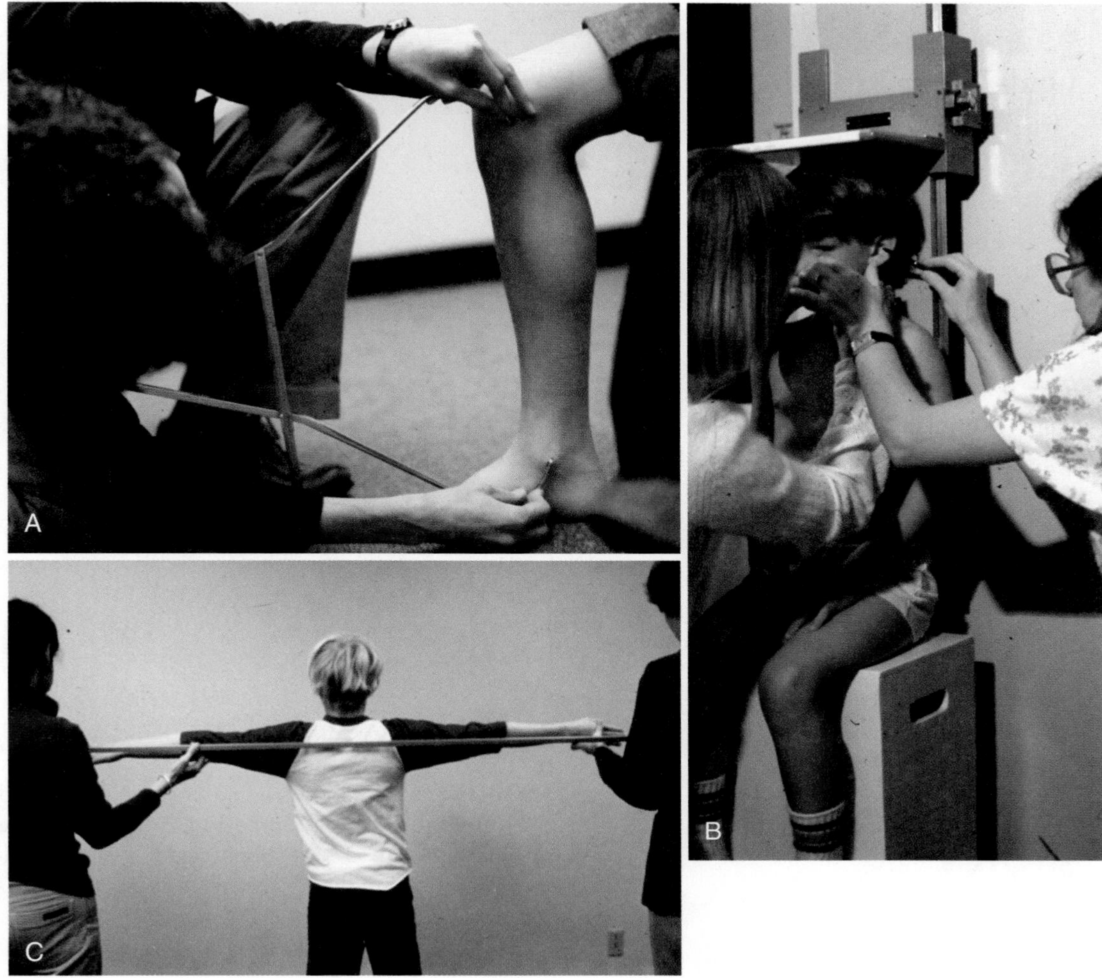

FIGURE 45-1 **A,** Knee height measure. **B,** Sitting height measure. **C,** Arm span measure. *(Courtesy Cristine M. Trahms, 2002.)*

difficulties, positioning problems, conflict in parent-child relationships, sensory issues, and tactile resistance from previous intubation (Tobin et al., 2005). The nutritional consequences of feeding problems include inadequate weight gain, poor growth in length, lowered immunity, anemia, vitamin and mineral deficiencies, dental caries, and psychosocial problems. Feeding problems should be assessed with an understanding of the normal development of feeding and the physical makeup of the mouth and pharynx (see Chapters 17-19 and Chapter 41).

Estimates are that feeding problems are found in 40% to 70% of children with special health care needs and 80% of children with developmental delays. Feeding problems are classified as oral motor, positioning, behavioral, and self-feeding. **Oral-motor problems** include difficulty with suckling, sucking, swallowing, and chewing. They also include sensory motor integration and problems with self-feeding and are described as exaggerations of normal neuromotor mechanisms that disrupt the rhythm and organization of oral-motor function and interfere with the feeding process (Box 45-1).

Children with developmental disabilities such as DS, CP, or cleft lip and palate often have oral-motor feeding problems that may be related to the cleft, muscle tone, and inability to accept texture changes. The oral-motor problem can also be related to the developmental level, which may be delayed.

Positioning a child for feeding relates to his or her motor development, head control, trunk stability, and ability to have hips and legs at a right angle (Figures 45-2 and 45-3). This is frequently a problem for individuals with CP, spina bifida, and DS. However, without proper positioning, oral-motor problems are difficult to correct. The ability to self-feed may be delayed in the child with developmental disabilities and requires training by a feeding specialist. A feeding evaluation is best completed with actual observation by a team composed of a speech therapist, a dentist, a physical therapist, an occupational therapist, and an RD. An excellent interdisciplinary feeding evaluation form is the Developmental Feeding Tool shown in Figure 45-4. Frequently, adaptive feeding equipment is needed.

Behavioral issues may result from oral-motor or sensory problems, medical problems, certain medications, and the amount of emphasis placed on feeding. Issues such as control of the feeding process along with lack of autonomy in the

BOX 45-1

Oral-Motor Problems

Problem	Description
Tonic bite reflex	Strong jaw closure when teeth and gums are stimulated
Tongue thrust	Forceful and often repetitive protrusion of an often bunched or thick tongue in response to oral stimulation
Jaw thrust	Forceful opening of the jaw to the maximum extent during eating, drinking, attempting to speak, or general excitement
Tongue retraction	Pulling back the tongue within the oral cavity at the presentation of food, spoon, or cup
Lip retraction	Pulling back the lips in a very tight smile like pattern at the approach of the spoon or cup toward the face
Sensory defensiveness	A strong adverse reaction to sensory input (touch, sound, light)

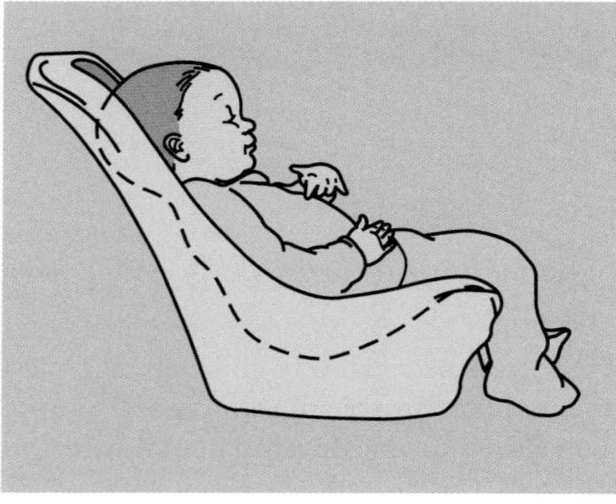

FIGURE 45-2 Proper feeding position for the infant. *(From Cloud H: Team approach to pediatric feeding problems, Chicago, 1987, American Dietetic Association. © American Dietetic Association. Reprinted with permission.)*

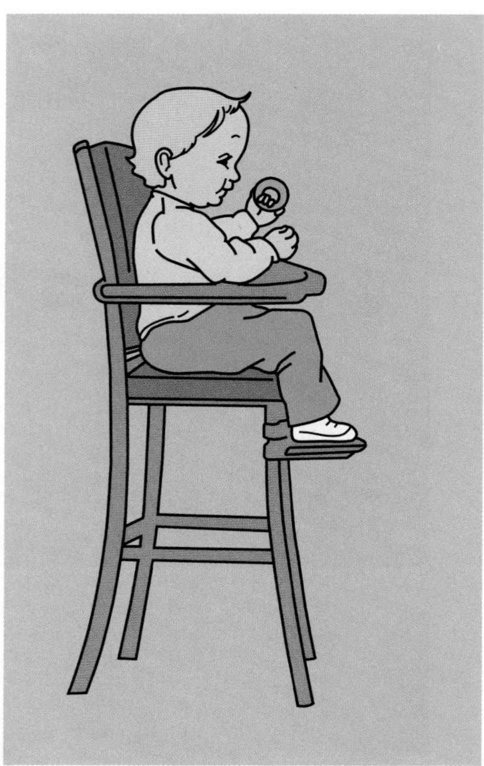

FIGURE 45-3 Good feeding position for a child ages 6 to 24 months, showing hip flexion, trunk in midline, and head in midline. Good foot support with a stool should continue throughout childhood. *(From Cloud H: Team approach to pediatric feeding problems, Chicago, 1987, American Dietetic Association. © American Dietetic Association. Reprinted with permission.)*

child may create negative behavior. Environmental factors also influence the eating behavior of the child. Examples include where the child is fed, distractibility, serving sizes, delayed weaning, and frequency of feeding.

Nutrition Diagnosis

Once the nutrition assessment has been completed, problems should be identified related to growth. Excessive or inadequate weights; inadequate dietary intake; excessive or inadequate fluid intake; altered gastrointestinal problems such as constipation, vomiting, and diarrhea; intake of foods that are unsafe because of contamination or food allergies; food-medication interactions; chewing and swallowing difficulties; and problems with self-feeding may be issues. The nutrition diagnoses should be listed and priorities established. When possible, this information is shared with the parent, caregiver, or the adult client before the intervention process begins.

Interventions

Once the nutrition diagnoses are identified and prioritized, short- and long-term goals should be set. Consideration must be given to the motivational level of the parent or client, his or her cultural background, and how the therapy can be community based and family centered. This means that consideration must be given to where the client will be served so that it becomes a part of the **individualized education plan (IEP)** or the **individualized family plan**.

Intervention plans should include all aspects of an individual's treatment program to avoid issuing an isolated set of instructions relevant to only one treatment goal. In some cases MNT may not be the family's first priority in the care of the child or adult, making it important for the RD to recognize the family's cues (see Chapter 15). Even when the family is ready for an intervention, such as weight management for a child with spina bifida, many factors require consideration. The parent or caregiver's educational level and income, language barriers, access to safe and

Developmental Feeding Tool (DFT)

Parent/Guardian____________________ Date____________
Address____________________ Staff member____________
City__________ State______ Zip______ Child's name____________________
County__________ Telephone__________ Birth date__________ Age______ Sex______ Race______
Referrer____________________ Head circumference (cm)___ (%ile NCHS)___ Hand dominance____
Height (cm)____ (%ile NCHS)____ Weight (kg)____ (%ile NCHS)____
Weight for height (%ile NCHS)____ Hematocrit____ Urine screen____

PHYSICAL (Yes ____ No ____)

Size
1. Weight (avg. %ile NCHS)
2. Underweight
3. Overweight
4. Stature (avg. %ile NCHS)
5. Short (below 5th %ile for ht. NCHS)
6. Tall (above 95th %ile for ht. NCHS)
7. Abnormal body proportions*
8. Head circumference (avg. %ile NCHS)
9. Microcephalic
10. Macrocephalic

Laboratory
11. Hematocrit (normal)
12. Urine screen (normal)*

Health Status
13. Bowel problems*
14. Diabetes
15. Vomiting
16. Dental caries
17. Anemia
18. Food allergies/intolerance*
19. Medications*
20. Vitamin/mineral supplements*
21. Ingests non-food items
22. Therapeutic diet*
23. General appearance (normal)*
24. Head (normal)*
25. Eyes (normal)*
26. Ears (normal)*
27. Nose (normal)*
28. Teeth/gums (normal)*
29. Palate (normal)*
30. Skin (normal)*
31. Muscles (normal)*
32. Arms/hands (normal)*
33. Legs/feet (normal)*

NEUROMOTOR/MUSCULAR (Yes ____ No ____)

Tonicity
34. Body tone (normal)*

Head and Trunk Control
35. Head control (normal)*
36. Lifts head in prone
37. Head lags when pulled to sitting
38. Head drops forward
39. Head drops backward
40. Trunk control (normal)*

Upper Extremity Control
41. Range of motion (normal)*
42. Approach to object (normal)*
43. Grasp of object (normal)*
44. Release of object (normal)*
45. Brings hand to mouth
46. Dominance established

Reflexes
47. Grossly normal
48. Asymmetrical tonic neck reflex*
49. Symmetical tonic neck reflex*
50. Moro reflex*
51. Grasp reflex*

Body Alignment
52. Scoliosis
53. Kyphosis
54. Lordosis
55. Hip subluxation or dislocation, suspected

Position in Feeding
56. Mother's lap
57. Infant seat
58. High chair
59. Table and chair
60. Wheelchair
61. Other adaptive chair*

ORAL/MOTOR (Yes ____ No ____)

Facial Expression
62. Symmetrical structure/function*
63. Muscle tone lips/cheeks (normal)
64. Hypertonic muscle tone of lips
65. Hypotonic muscle tone of lips

Oral Reflexes
66. Gag (normal)*
67. Bite (normal)*
68. Rooting (normal)*
69. Suck/swallow (normal)*

Respiration
70. Mouth
71. Nose
72. Thoracic
73. Abdominal
74. Regular rhythm*

Oral Sensitivity
75. Inside mouth (normal)*
76. Outside mouth (normal)*
77. Hypersensitivity*
78. Hyposensitivity*
79. Intolerance to brushing teeth

FEEDING PATTERNS (Yes ____ No ____)

Bottle-feeding
80. Suckling tongue movements
81. Sucking tongue movements
82. Firm lip seal*
83. Coordinated suck-swallow-breathing
84. Difficulty swallowing*

Cup-drinking
85. Adequate lip closure*
86. Loses less than 1/2 total amount*

(Yes ____ No ____)

87. Wide up-and-down jaw movements
88. Stabilizes jaw by biting edge of cup
89. Stabilizes jaw through muscle control
90. Drinks through a straw

Feeding Patterns—Spoon-feeding
91. Suckles as food approaches
92. Cleans food off lower lip
93. Cleans food off spoon with upper lip
94. Munching pattern

Lateralizes Tongue:
95. When food placed between molars
96. When food placed in center of tongue
97. To move food from side to side
98. Vertical jaw movements
99. Rotary jaw movements

Feeding Patterns—Chewing
100. Lip closure during chewing*

FIGURE 45-4 Developmental feeding tool. *(Smith MAH et al: Feeding management for a child with a handicap: a guide for professionals, Memphis, 1982, University of Tennessee: The Boling Child Development Center, University of Tennessee Center for Health Sciences).*

Continued

Developmental Feeding Tool (Cont'd)

Yes No Isolated, Voluntary Tongue Movements

_____ _____ 101. Protrudes/retracts tongue
_____ _____ 102. Elevates tongue outside mouth
_____ _____ 103. Elevates tongue inside mouth
_____ _____ 104. Depresses tongue outside mouth
_____ _____ 105. Depresses tongue inside mouth
_____ _____ 106. Lateralizes tongue outside mouth
_____ _____ 107. Lateralizes tongue inside mouth

Special Oral Problems

_____ _____ 108. Drools*
_____ _____ 109. Thrusts tongue when utensil placed in mouth*
_____ _____ 110. Thrusts tongue during chewing/swallowing*
_____ _____ 111. Other oral-motor problem*

NUTRITION HISTORY

Yes No Past Status

_____ _____ 112. Feeding problems birth—1 year*
_____ _____ 113. Breast fed
_____ _____ 114. Bottle fed
_____ _____ 115. Weaned

Current Status

_____ _____ 116. Eats blended food
_____ _____ 117. Eats limited texture
_____ _____ 118. Eats chopped table foods
_____ _____ 119. Eats table foods
_____ _____ 120. Feeds unassisted
_____ _____ 121. Feeds with partial guidance
_____ _____ 122. Feeds with complete guidance
_____ _____ 123. Drinks from a cup unassisted
_____ _____ 124. Drinks from a cup assisted
_____ _____ 125. Finger-feeds
_____ _____ 126. Uses a spoon
_____ _____ 127. Uses a fork
_____ _____ 128. Uses a knife

Yes No

_____ _____ 129. Average rate of eating
_____ _____ 130. Fast rate of eating
_____ _____ 131. Slow rate of eating

Diet Review

_____ _____ 132. Appetite normal
_____ _____ 133. Eats 3 meals/day
_____ _____ 134. Snacks daily

Dietary Intake, Current

_____ _____ 135. Milk/dairy products, 3-4/day
_____ _____ 136. Vegetables, 2-3/day
_____ _____ 137. Fruit, 2-3/day
_____ _____ 138. Meat/meat substitute, 2-3/day
_____ _____ 139. Bread/cereal, 3-4/day
_____ _____ 140. Sweets/snacks, 1-2/day
_____ _____ 141. Liquids, 2 cups/day

SOCIAL/BEHAVIORAL

Yes No Child-Caregiver Relationship

_____ _____ 142. Child responds to caregiver
_____ _____ 143. Caregiver affectionate to child

Social Skills

_____ _____ 144. Eye contact
_____ _____ 145. Smiles
_____ _____ 146. Gestures, i.e. waves byebye
_____ _____ 147. Clings to caregiver
_____ _____ 148. Interacts with examiner
_____ _____ 149. Responds to simple directions
_____ _____ 150. Seeks approval
_____ _____ 151. Toilet trained
_____ _____ 152. Knows own sex

Behavior Problems

_____ _____ 153. Self abusive
_____ _____ 154. Hyperactive
_____ _____ 155. Aggressive
_____ _____ 156. Withdrawn
_____ _____ 157. Other*

Play

_____ _____ 158. Plays infant games, i.e., pat-a-cake
_____ _____ 159. Solitary play
_____ _____ 160. Parallel play
_____ _____ 161. Cooperative play
_____ _____ 162. Additional comments*

Number COMMENTS

FIGURE 45-4, cont'd

appropriate food, and family coping strategies should always be identified (see Chapter 15).

Monitoring and Evaluation

Once MNT has been initiated, the need for follow-up evaluation and monitoring either by the RD or another health care professional is important. Giving information in writing, followed by a phone call, gives the chance to repeat some of the discussion and to answer any questions not asked during the initial session. Clarification of suggestions is often needed when monitoring nutrition changes that affect growth and development; a follow-up visit may also be needed.

A case manager may be involved who communicates with the adult with the disability. The RD may need to find appropriate resources to pay for supplemental nutrition products, tube feedings, and special food products as a part of the follow-up process. Community and agency resources will be discussed.

CHROMOSOMAL ABERRATIONS

Down Syndrome

Down syndrome (DS) is a chromosomal aberration of chromosome 21 (trisomy 21). It has an incidence of 1 in 700 live births and results from the presence of an extra chromosome in each cell of the body. This anomaly causes the physical and developmental features of short stature; congenital heart disease; mental retardation; decreased muscle tone; hyperflexibility of joints; speckling of the iris (Brushfield spots); upward slant of the eyes; epicanthal folds; small oral cavity; short, broad hands with the single palmar crease; and a wide gap between the first and second toes (Capone et al., 2005).

Pathophysiology

Normally every cell of the human body except for the gametes (sperm or ova) contains 46 chromosomes, which are arranged in pairs (see Chapter 5). With DS there is one extra chromosome for a total of 47. There are three processes by which this anomaly can occur: nondysjunction, translocation, and mosaicism. In **nondysjunction**, chromosome 21 fails to separate before conception and the abnormal gamete joins with a normal gamete at conception to form a fertilized egg with three of chromosome 21. This may also occur during the first cell division after conception. This type of DS is usually sporadic and has a recurrence rate of 0.5% to 1%. In **translocation**, the extra chromosome is attached to another chromosome (usually 14, 15, or 22). Approximately half the time, this type of DS is inherited from a parent who is a carrier; it has a much higher risk of recurrence in another pregnancy. In **mosaicism** the abnormal separation of chromosome 21 occurs sometime after conception. All future divisions of the affected cell result in cells with an extra chromosome. Therefore the child has some cells with the normal number of chromosomes and other cells with an extra chromosome. Frequently the child with this type of DS lacks some of the more distinctive features of the syndrome (Capone et al., 2005) (see *Pathophysiology and Care Management Algorithm:* Down Syndrome).

Medical Treatment

The National Down Syndrome Congress has published a listing of the health concerns for individuals with DS; many have nutrition implications (Table 45-2).

Medical Nutrition Therapy

Anthropometric Measures. Height, weight, head circumference, triceps skinfold, and arm circumference are obtained for the child with DS with the usual measurements. See Chapter 6. BMI can be taken but may be higher than normal because of short stature. Growth measures are an important part of the assessment and ongoing nutrition therapy because these individuals tend to be short. Muscle tone is low and gross motor ability is often delayed, leading to the possibility of the individual becoming overweight. Monitoring should be frequent, and growth plotted on the CDC charts (see Appendixes 9 through 16).

Biochemical Measures. Numerous studies have shown biochemical and metabolic abnormalities in individuals with DS; however, many have involved small samples and were difficult to interpret (Capone et al., 2005). Although serum concentrations of albumin have been found to be low, the guidelines from the Down Syndrome Medical Congress do not list serum albumin assessment as routine. Increased glucose levels have been reported, with an increased incidence of diabetes mellitus.

Current guidelines for the treatment of infants and children with DS include evaluation of thyroid function at birth and thereafter annually.

TABLE 45-2

Health Concerns of Children with Down Syndrome

Health Concern	Implications	Treatment
Congenital heart disease	40%-50% of population	Medication or surgical repair
Hypotonia	Reduced muscle tone, increased range of joints	
Motor function problem	Poor physical function	Early intervention for physical therapy, occupational therapy
Delayed growth	Short stature	In some cases growth hormone
Developmental delays	Poor physical, emotional function	Early intervention
Hearing concerns	Small ear canals, otitis media, conductive impairment	Early intervention
Dental problems	Decreased saliva, reflux, and vomiting	Low sucrose intake
Ocular problems	Refractive errors, strabismus, cataracts	Corrective glasses
Cervical spine abnormality		None
Thyroid disease	Hypothyroidism	Thyroid supplement, tests repeated annually
Overweight	Excessive weight gain, inactivity	Decrease energy, increase activity
Seizure disorders	Variable nutrient intake	Medications
Emotional disorders	May occur late in childhood	Medication, counseling

Updated from Saenz RB: Primary care of infants and young children with Down syndrome, Am Fam Phys 59:381, 1999.

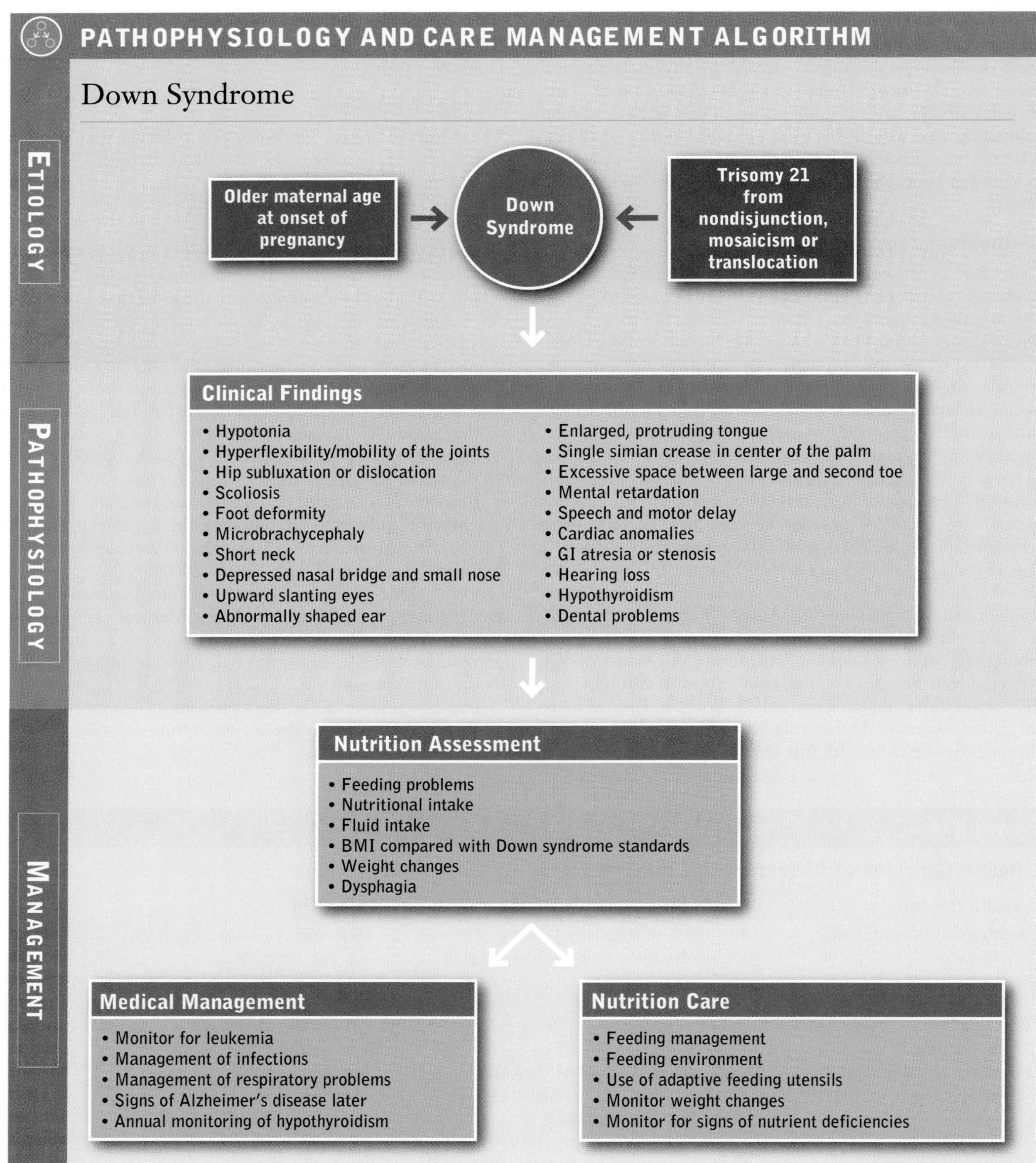

Dietary Intake. During infancy the food intake of the infant with DS may differ from that of the normal infant. Although human breast milk is recommended, many infants with DS are formula fed. Infant illnesses, admission to the neonatal unit, frustration, depression, perceived milk insufficiency, and difficulty in suckling by the infant are reasons why formula feeding is used.

Progression to solid food has been found to be delayed in children with DS, mostly as a result of delays in feeding and motor development. Introduction of solid food may not be

TABLE 45-3

Estimated Caloric Needs for Special Conditions

Condition	kcal/cm	Comments
Normal child	Average 16	
Prader-Willi	Maintain growth: 10-11 Promote weight loss: 8.5	For all children and adolescents
Cerebral palsy		
Mild	14	Reliable for ages 5-11 yr
Severe, limited mobility	11	Reliable for ages 5-11 yr
Down syndrome	Girls: 14.3 Boys: 16.1	Reliable for ages 5-11 yr
Motor dysfunction		
Nonambulatory	7-11	Reliable for ages 5-12 yr
Ambulatory	14	Reliable for ages 5-12 yr
Spina bifida	Maintain weight: 9-11 Promote weight loss: 7	For all children older than 8 years of age and minimally active

Modified from Rokusek C, Heindicles E: Nutrition and feeding for persons with special needs, with permission of the South Dakota University Affiliated Program, Interdisciplinary Center for Disabilities, 1992.

offered at 6 months if the infant has poor head control or is not yet sitting. Low tone and sucking problems also delay weaning from the breast or bottle to the cup. IEPs include feeding and feeding progression instruction and practice.

An important part of evaluating the dietary intake is determining energy and fluid needs, because children with DS have a high prevalence of obesity. Studies have indicated that the resting energy expenditure (REE) of the child with DS is lower than for controls without DS—and may be as much as 10% lower than the dietary reference intake (DRI) for energy. For the child older than the age of 5, calculations for energy requirements may need to be based on height rather than weight (Table 45-3) (see Chapter 2).

Feeding Skills. Feeding skills are delayed in the infant and child with DS. Some parents find difficulty in initiating oral motor skills such as suckling and sucking. The infant with DS often has difficulty in coordinating sucking, swallowing, and breathing, which are the foundations for early feeding. When the infant has a congenital heart defect, which occurs in 40% to 60% of the DS infants, sucking is weakened, and fatigue interferes with the feeding process. Gastrointestinal anomalies are found in 8% to 12% of infants with DS, and these infants often require nasogastric or gastrostomy feedings.

Other physical factors that make feeding difficult in the first years of life include a **midfacial hypoplasia** (a craniofacial deformity common in cleft palate), a small oral cavity, a small mandible, delayed or abnormal dentition, malocclusion, nasal congestion, small hands, and short fingers. Weaning and self-feeding are usually late when compared with the normal infant, and frequently do not emerge until 15 to 18 months of age. The DS infant strives for independence and autonomy approximately 6 months later than the child without DS.

Intervention Strategies

Overweight. The most effective intervention for the overweight child with DS is to design a calorie-controlled eating plan based on kilocalories per centimeter of height (see Table 45-3). Dietary management includes assessing the feeding developmental level of the child, working with a physical therapist related to gross motor skills to determine possible activity levels, and making environmental changes. Environmental changes should include following a regular eating schedule that includes three meals at regular times with the child sitting either in a high chair or at the table. Planned snacks should be low in fat and sugar. Soft drinks should be eliminated, and milk should be low fat (after age 2). Physical activity should be encouraged. Counseling in which the parent helps determine a realistic plan should focus on serving sizes and food preparation and decreasing the number of times meals are purchased in fast-food restaurants. If the child or adolescent is school age, a prescription for a special meal at school can be obtained by using the school food service prescription (to be discussed later in the chapter).

Feeding Skills. Often parents wrongly expect different feeding development for the child with DS. Behavioral problems related to feeding usually develop based on what happens between the parent and child at mealtime. An example of this is the unnecessary delay of weaning to a cup or progression of food textures because of inadequate effort or education. During intervention programs the feeding team can guide the parent in positioning the child and working toward attainable feeding skills related to the developmental level of the child.

Constipation. This is a frequent problem for the child with DS because of overall low tone followed by lack of fiber and fluid in the diet. Treatment should involve increasing fiber and fluid, with water consumption emphasized. Fiber content of the diet for children after age 3, is 5 to 6 g per year of age per day. For adults the recommendation is for 25 to 30 g of dietary fiber daily.

Prader-Willi Syndrome

Prader-Willi syndrome (PWS) was first described in 1956 by Doctors Prader, Willi, and Lambert. It is a genetic condition caused by the absence of chromosomal material. PWS occurs with a frequency of 1 in 10,000 to 1 in 25,000 live births. Characteristics of the syndrome include developmental delays, poor muscle tone, short stature, small hands and feet, incomplete sexual development, and unique facial features. Insatiable appetite leading to obesity is the classic feature of PWS; however, in infancy the problem of **hypotonia** (low muscle tone) interferes with feeding and leads to failure to thrive (McCune and Driscoll, 2005). Developmental delays (affecting 50% of the population), learning disabilities, and mental retardation (affecting 10%) are associated with PWS.

The genetic basis of PWS is complex. Individuals with PWS have a portion of genetic material deleted from chromosome 15 received from the father. Of the cases of PWS, 70% are caused from the paternal deletion, occurring in a specific region on the q arm of the chromosome. PWS can also develop if a child receives both chromosome 15s from the mother. This is seen in approximately 25% of the cases of PWS and is called *maternal uniparental disomy*. Early detection of PWS is now possible because of the use of deoxyribonucleic acid methylation analysis, which correctly diagnoses 99% of the cases (McCune and Driscoll, 2005). This is an important development in the early identification and subsequent treatment of these children to prevent obesity and growth retardation and is used to identify the infant born with features and characteristics described previously

Pathophysiology

Metabolic Abnormalities. Short stature in the individual with PWS has been attributed to growth hormone deficiency. In addition to decreased growth hormone release, children have low serum insulin-like growth factor (IGF)-1, low IGF-binding protein-1, and low insulin compared with normal obese children. Growth hormone therapy was approved by the Food and Drug Administration in 2000, and in one 5-year study in Japan 37 patients from age 3 to 21 years experienced significant increase in height gain velocity when given growth hormone (Obata et al., 2003). A more recent study (Carrel et al., 2010) found that GH therapy of infants and toddlers for 12 months significantly improved body composition and mobility skill acquisition.

In addition to the growth hormone deficiency, individuals have a deficiency in the hypothalamic-pituitary-gonadal axis, causing delayed and incomplete sexual development. Finally there is a decreased insulin response to a glucose load in children with PWS compared with age-matched non-PWS obese children (Talebizadeh and Butler, 2005).

Appetite and Obesity. Appetite control and obesity are common problems for individuals with PWS. After the initial period of failure to thrive, children begin to gain excessively between the ages of 1 and 4, and appetite slowly becomes excessive. Based on longitudinal study, Miller et al describe this gradual and complex progression in terms of 7 nutritional phases based on levels of appetite, metabolic changes and growth. In fact, some adults with PWS may progress to the last stage - one, with no insatiable appetite and the person is able to feel full (Miller et al, 2011).

This uncontrollable appetite, a classic feature of PWS, when combined with overeating, a low basal metabolic rate, and decreased activity, leads to the characteristic obesity. The cause of the uncontrollable appetite is suspected to involve the hypothalamus and altered levels of satiety hormones and peptides such as ghrelin (Scerif et al, 2011).

Body composition is an important consideration in the evaluation of individuals with PWS. They have decreased lean body mass and increased body fat, even in infancy (Reus et al, 2011). Body fat is generally deposited in the thighs, buttocks, and abdominal area. The lowered energy expenditure is found in young children, adolescents, and adults with PWS, with one study showing adolescents with PWS having a total energy expenditure (TEE) 53% of that of normal obese adolescents (McCune and Driscoll, 2005). The low muscle tone contributes greatly to the lack of interest in physical activity.

Nutrition Assessment

Anthropometric Measures. Height measurements tend to be lower in PWS infants and young children, with the rate of height gain tapering off between the ages of 1 and 4. The usual measurements of length or height, weight, and head circumference should be taken and plotted on the CDC growth curves. Other measures of interest include arm circumference and triceps skinfold measures. BMI may be distorted for the individual with PWS because of the short stature; however, plotting the BMI over time is useful in determining unusual changes (see Appendixes 12 and 16). It is important that anthropometric measures be taken frequently and reported to the parents or caregiver.

Biochemical Measures. Biochemical studies are generally the same for the PWS individual, with the exception of either fasting blood glucose tests or glucose tolerance tests. These are added because of the risk for diabetes mellitus, possibly related to the decreased insulin response and obesity that usually accompanies PWS.

Dietary Intake. Dietary information varies for individuals with PWS, depending on their age. In infancy the dietary information should be obtained with a careful dietary history and analyzed for energy and nutrient intake. Infants are commonly difficult to feed because of their hypotonia, poor suck, and delayed motor skills. Generally their feeding development is slower than in the normal infant, and transitioning to food at 4 to 6 months of age may be difficult. Many of these infants have gastroesophageal reflux requiring medication or thickening of their formula.

During the toddler years weight gain may increase rapidly as dietary intake increases. This requires careful assessment of portion sizes, frequency of feeding, and types of foods served. Although some parents may report that the child with PWS does not eat more than other children in the family, they need to be educated that the energy needs of the child are lower because of the reduced lean muscle mass and slow development of motor skills and activity. As the child gets older, interest in food increases; and, starting around ages 5 through 12, the child may be hungry all the time and display difficult behaviors such as tantrums, stubbornness, and food stealing. Many parents have found it necessary to lock cabinets, refrigerators, and the kitchen door to control food intake. Information gathered during the dietary interview should include asking about environmental control techniques.

Determination of energy needs for the infant with PWS is the same as for a normal infant. However, as the child enters the toddler years, he or she will need fewer calories to maintain weight gain along the growth curve. This will apply in adulthood when fewer calories are needed to maintain weight. Energy needs have been calculated according to centimeters of height from 2 years on. It has been recommended that the macronutrient intake of the diet be 25% protein, 50% carbohydrate, and 25% fat (see Table 45-3).

Feeding Skills. The infant with PWS often presents with weak oral skills and poor sucking skills in the first year of life. As the child matures, feeding skills are not a problem, but they may be delayed. Chewing and swallowing problems are not usually seen, although they may be associated with the low muscle tone. Behavioral feeding issues are associated with an insatiable appetite and not being provided with food. This can bring about tantrums.

Intervention Strategies

Intervention for PWS should occur at each developmental stage: infancy, toddler, preschool age, school age, and adult.

Infancy. Providing adequate nutrition as established by the American Academy of Pediatrics (AAP) related to breastfeeding or formula feeding is recommended. Because feeding may be difficult related to sucking, concentrating the formula or breast milk may be necessary to promote adequate weight gain. Feeding intervention will assist in improving the sucking problems caused by hypotonia. As the infant matures, a concentrated formula is not necessary, and foods can be added when head control and trunk stability are achieved, usually at approximately ages 4 to 6 months.

Toddler and Preschool Age. Most children begin to gain excessive weight between 1 and 4 years of age. Beginning a structured dietary protocol for the child and the family is important so that the toddler learns that meals are provided at specified times so that a pattern of grazing doesn't develop. Parents should be taught to provide small servings of meats, vegetables, grains, and fruits and limited amounts of sweets. Early intervention for these children in the preschool years is very important in working with feeding issues and intake control as they grow older. Weight, height, and nutrient intake should be monitored monthly, and energy needs adjusted if weight gain becomes excessive. Concurrently physical activity must be encouraged as a part of the IEP, and physical therapy services made available if necessary.

School Age. For the school-age child, collaboration with the school food service program becomes important. Energy needs should be calculated per centimeter of height (see Table 45-3) and are generally 50% to 75% of the energy needs of unaffected children. This may require using the prescription for special meals through the school food service program. At home environmental controls may be required, with cupboards and refrigerators being locked, because the child and adolescent have limited satiety, and will search for food away from mealtime. Some parents say that growth hormone therapy for their child helps, but it doesn't seem to change the child's lack of satiety. Appetite-suppressing medications have been used but are largely unsuccessful.

Adulthood. Prevention of obesity is truly the key for successful treatment of PWS; however, many adults who are not identified early become very obese. Weight management programs providing a very low 6 to 8 kcal per centimeter of height may be required. Nutrient values should be calculated, and vitamin-mineral supplements added, as well as essential fatty acids (EFAs) if indicated. Many dietary treatments have been tried such as the ketogenic diet and the protein-sparing modified-fast diets. However, with any approach strict supervision is usually required, and great emphasis must be placed on physical activity. A behavior management approach has also been recommended to implement both the dietary management and physical activity plans. In many states there are group homes for adults with PWS where supervised independent living is possible and meals can be very structured and exercise programs implemented.

MNT of children and adults with PWS requires follow-up with many health care providers and schools. Fortunately parents of the individual with PWS now have access to a number of support groups and organizations dedicated to education, research, and establishing treatment programs.

NEUROLOGIC DISORDERS

Spina Bifida

Spina bifida is a neurologic tube defect that presents in a number of ways: meningocele, **myelomeningocele (MM)**, and spina bifida occulta. MM is the most common derangement in the formation of the spinal cord and generally occurs between 26 to 30 days of gestation, with the date of occurrence affecting the location of the lesion. The lesion may occur in the thoracic, lumbar, or sacral area and will influence the amount of paralysis. The higher the lesion, the greater is the paralysis. Manifestations range from weakness in the lower extremities to complete paralysis and loss of sensation. Other manifestations include incontinence and hydrocephalus. The incidence of spina bifida is about 1 in 1430 births in the United States (CDC, 2010).

Prevention of spina bifida is now possible. In the 1980s, studies reported a positive effect from supplementation of mothers with folic acid plus multivitamins (Smithells et al, 1983). This reduced the risk of a second pregnancy with spina bifida as an outcome. As a result of numerous studies showing folic acid supplementation before conception to be effective, the national recommendation is 400 mcg/day for all women of childbearing age. Folic acid has been added to many flours and other cereal and grain products in the food supply since 1996 (CDC, 2010). These public health measures have resulted in increased folic acid blood levels in U.S. women of childbearing age and a decrease of 20% in the national rate of spina bifida (Robbins et al., 2006) (see Chapter 16).

Pathophysiology

The spinal lesion may be open and can be surgically repaired shortly after birth, usually within 24 hours to prevent infection. Although the spinal opening can be surgically repaired, the nerve damage is permanent, resulting in the varying degrees of paralysis of the lower limbs. In addition to physical and mobility issues, most individuals have some form of learning disability.

The spinal lesion affects many systems of the body and can result in weakness in the lower extremities, paralysis, and nonambulation; poor skin condition caused by pressure sores; loss of sensation and bladder incontinence; hydrocephalus; urinary tract infections; constipation; and obesity. Seizures also occur in approximately 20% of children with MM and require medication. Chronic medication is required for prevention and treatment of urinary tract infections and for bladder control. The resultant nutrition problems include obesity, feeding problems, constipation, and drug-nutrient interaction problems. Children with spina bifida may be allergic to latex. It has been recommended that they avoid certain foods such as bananas, kiwi, and avocados. Mild reactions can occur from apples, carrots, celery, tomatoes, papaya, and melons (Cloud et al., 2005) (see Box 27-3 in Chapter 27).

Nutrition Assessment

Anthropometric Measures. Infants and children with neural tube defects are usually shorter because of reduced length and atrophy of the lower extremities, although other problems such as hydrocephalus, scoliosis, renal disease, and malnutrition may contribute. The level of the lesions can also affect the length and height of the individual.

Obtaining accurate length and height measures can be difficult, especially as the child grows older. An alternate measure for determining height, the arm span/height ratio, is used and modified, depending on leg muscle mass. Arm span can be used directly as a height measure (arm span × 1) if there is no leg muscle mass loss, as in a sacral lesion. Arm span × 0.95 can be used to determine height if there is partial leg muscle loss, and arm span × 0.90 is used for a height measurement when there is complete leg muscle loss such as with a thoracic spinal lesion (Ekvall and Cerniglia, 2005). See Fig. 45-1 and Appendix 20.

Weight measures can be obtained for the child unable to stand by using chair scales, bucket scales, and wheelchair scales. To monitor the weight accurately, it should be obtained in a consistent manner, with the person in light clothing or undressed. Triceps skinfold measures can also be used, along with subscapular measures and abdominal and thorax measures, to determine the amount of body fat. See Chapter 6.

Head circumference should be measured in infants and toddlers up to age 3. A high percentage of children with spina bifida have head shunts as a result of their hydrocephalus. Unusual changes in the size of the head may indicate a problem with the shunt.

Biochemical Measures. Most protocols in the treatment of spina bifida include iron status tests, measurements of vitamin C and zinc levels, and other tests related to the nutritional consequences of medications needed for seizures and urinary tract infection control (see Chapter 9 and Appendix 31).

Dietary Intake. Many children with spina bifida eat a limited variety of foods, and they are frequently described as a "picky eaters" by the parents. When doing a dietary history, it is important to ask about the variety of foods, particularly of high-fiber foods. The school-age child may be prone to skipping breakfast because early morning preparations for school require more time than for the nonaffected child.

Energy needs are lower for the child with spina bifida (see Table 45-3), and calorie requirements must be determined carefully to prevent the obesity to which many are prone. Ekvall and Cerniglia (2005) found that for MM children 8 years or older, the caloric need is 7 cal/cm of height for weight loss and 9 to 11 cal/cm of height to maintain weight. It is important to evaluate how the mother or caretaker perceives food for the child since it represents sympathy and love for many parents.

It is important to evaluate fluid intake because so many children have urinary tract infections and may be drinking inadequate amounts of water and excessive amounts of soft drinks or tea. Cranberry juice can be offered. Physical activity must also be evaluated and may be found to be very limited, particularly when the child is nonambulatory. Ambulatory individuals with a shunt may be restricted from contact sports but can be involved in walking and running.

Feeding skills need to be evaluated, along with oral motor function in particular. Many children with spina bifida are born with **Arnold Chiari malformation of the brain**, which affects the brainstem and swallowing. See Appendix 35 for dietary recommendations for dysphagia. Difficulty in swallowing may contribute to the child avoiding certain foods later in life. Because of this there may be delays in weaning from the breast or bottle to the cup, but there should be no delays in gaining self-feeding skills.

Clinical Evaluation. Evaluation should include looking for pressure sores and signs of dehydration, along with asking about the amount and type of fluids consumed. Constipation may be caused by the neurogenic bowel combined with a diet low in fiber and fluids. The evaluation should include a review of food intake, fiber content, and fluids.

Intervention Strategies

Many children with spina bifida are overweight. It usually occurs when ambulation is a problem leading to decreased energy needs. Refusal to accept a wide variety of foods is common. Frequent feeding is both an oral-motor and a behavioral problem. Counseling should include introducing foods around age 6 months, limiting the intake of high-sucrose infant jar foods, and training the child to accept a wide variety of flavors and textures.

Obesity prevention should include addressing the problems of limited physical activity, increasing fluids and fiber and calculating the appropriate amount of calories. Once the child is in school, the food service manager should be provided with a prescription for a low-calorie breakfast and lunch, and weight management program should be listed as a part of the IEP. Enrollment in a group weight management program has been used successfully with modification of the accompanying physical exercise. The ideal program uses a team approach with involvement of the RD, nurse, occupational therapist, physical therapist, educator, and psychologist.

In many clinics the child or adult with spina bifida is seen on a semiannual or annual basis. This frequent follow-up is necessary and should include monitoring of growth, particularly weight; food and fluid intake; and medication use. School programs and IEPs are excellent follow-up tools; however, the school often lacks appropriate scales for weighing a nonambulatory student. In this situation the parent should be encouraged to bring the child to the clinic for weight checks or, if distance is a problem, find a long-term care facility that will permit use of its scales. Follow-up by phone contact or e-mail can be done for evaluating dietary intake and fluid management.

Cerebral Palsy

Cerebral palsy (CP) is a disorder of motor control or coordination resulting from injury to the brain during its early development. Among the causative agents of CP are prematurity; blood-type incompatibility; placental insufficiency; maternal infection that includes German measles; other viral diseases; neonatal jaundice; anoxia at birth; and other bacterial infections of the mother, fetus, or infant that affect the central nervous system.

The problem in CP lies in the inability of the brain to control the muscles, even though the muscles themselves and the nerves connecting them to the spinal cord are normal. The extent and location of the brain injury determine the type and distribution of CP. The incidence of CP varies with different studies, but the most commonly used rate is 2 to 3 in 1000 live births. The prevalence of premature births has contributed to maintenance of this figure despite electro-fetal monitoring.

Pathophysiology

There are various types of CP, which are classified according to the neurologic signs involving muscle tone and abnormal motor patterns and postures. The diagnosis of CP is generally made between 9 to 12 months of age and as late as 2 years with some types (Box 45-2).

BOX 45-2

Different Types of Cerebral Palsy

Spastic CP: Increased muscle tone, persistent infant reflexes, increased deep tendon reflexes in one of three patterns: hemiplegia (arm and leg on one side of the body), diplegia (involving the lower extremities), and quadriplegia (all four extremities and may include the trunk, head, and neck)

Dyskinetic CP: Abnormalities in muscle tone that affect the entire body; includes athetoid CP, which includes uncontrolled and continuous involuntary movements

Mixed CP: A condition in which both athetosis and spasticity are present

Ataxic CP: Abnormalities of voluntary movement and balance such as unsteady gait

Athetoid dyskinetic CP: Normal intelligence but difficulty walking, sitting, speaking clearly

Data from 4MYCHILD: What type of cerebral palsy does my child have? Accessed 8 November 2010 from http://www.cerebralpalsy.org/types-of-cerebral-palsy/.

CP, Cerebral palsy.

Poor nutrition status and growth failure, often related to feeding problems, are common in children with CP. Meeting energy and nutrient needs is particularly difficult in children and adults with more severe forms of CP such as spastic quadriplegia and athetoid CP. For example, bone mineral density of children and adolescents with moderate to severe CP is reduced in those with gross motor function and feeding difficulties (Henderson et al., 2005).

Other health problems include constipation, usually caused by inactivity and lack of fiber and fluids, often connected to feeding problems. Dental problems occur and are often related to malocclusion, dental irregularities, and fractured teeth. Lengthy and prolonged bottle-feedings of milk and juice promote the decay of the primary upper front teeth and molars (see Chapter 26). Hearing problems and especially visual impairments, mental retardation, respiratory problems, and seizures affect nutrition status. Seizures are controlled with anticonvulsants, and a number of drug-nutrient interaction problems occur (see Chapter 9 and Appendix 31).

Nutrition Assessment

Anthropometric Measures. This is an important area of assessment because of the growth failure of the more severely involved child or adult with CP. Children with CP are often shorter, and, depending on the level of severity, some children with CP may need to be measured for length using recumbent length boards or standing boards even as they grow older. See Appendix 20. However, some of the measuring devices are inappropriate for the child with contractures and inability to be stretched out full length.

Arm span can be used when the individual's arms are stretchable, as well as upper arm and lower leg length. Stevenson (2005) has recommended lower leg length or knee height as a possible measure for determining height for both children and adults with lower-leg CP (Fig. 45-1). The CDC recommends using the CDC curves designed for nonaffected children, plotting sequentially for indications of malnutrition rather than using the disease-specific curves.

Weight measures should be collected over time. Scales may require modifications, with positioning devices for the individual with CP who has developed scoliosis, contractures, and spasticity. Working with a physical therapist to find a positioning device that can be placed in a chair scale or using a bucket scale often works well. Mid–upper arm circumference and triceps skinfold measures are recommended reliable ways to screen for fat stores in children with CP. Head circumference should be measured regularly from birth to 36 months and plotted on the CDC growth curves.

Biochemical Measures. Although there are no specific laboratory tests indicated for the child with CP, a complete blood count, including hemoglobin and hematocrit, should be done when food intake is limited and malnutrition is a possibility. Because bone fractures are a significant problem for many children and adults with spastic quadriplegia, bone mineral density may need evaluating. Medications for seizures may be given; many have nutrition interaction problems (see Appendix 31). Evaluation of vitamin D, calcium, carnitine, and vitamin K levels is recommended.

Dietary Intake. Feeding methods can result in limiting the intake of food and fluid; caretakers may not provide sufficient food to meet nutritional needs. The energy needs of the individual with CP vary according to the type of CP. Studies show that the REE and TEE are lower in those with spastic quadriplegic CP than in normal controls (see Table 45-3).

Intervention Strategies

A high percentage of children with CP have feeding problems that are largely the result of oral-motor, positioning, and behavioral factors. As infants they have difficulty swallowing and coordinating swallowing and chewing, so that the normal progression to solid foods is later than usual. All this may lead to inadequate intake and growth limitations. For those infants and children with IEPs, the team of dietitian, speech therapist, occupational therapist, and physical therapist should evaluate the problem and work together in planning therapy.

Gastroesophageal reflux is frequently seen in these infants and toddlers. A tube feeding may be required if a modified barium swallow reveals aspiration. Alternative techniques in feeding should be considered, which could include thickening all beverages or placing a gastrostomy tube (Sullivan, 2005). RDs should evaluate gastrostomy feedings for caloric and nutritional value, volume required, and osmolality; and offer directions for inclusion of solid foods in addition to the formula if necessary.

Usual problems identified in the evaluation will be altered growth, inadequate energy or fluid intakes, drug-nutrient interaction problems, constipation, and feeding problems. Working out an intervention plan is most successful when it involves the parent as part of the team, addresses cultural issues, and recognizes the importance of the feeding problem. Children with CP have complex problems that require continuing follow-up with the family in the community and will take time to correct. There are state agencies that provide tube-feeding formulas and special wheelchairs and equipment to assist with feeding problems. These agencies vary from state to state.

Autism

Autism is one of five disorders under the category **pervasive developmental disorder (PDD)**. PDD was first used in the 1980s to describe a class of disorders as shown in Table 45-4. All types of PDD are neurologic disorders that are usually evident by age 3. In general, children who have a type of PDD have difficulty in talking, playing with other children, and relating to others, including their families.

Pathophysiology

Autism spectrum disorders (ASDs) are diagnosed by the presence of qualitatively impaired reciprocal social interaction; impaired communication skills; and restricted, repetitive, stereotypical interests and behaviors. Many children with autism also have intellectual compromise. ASD is four times more common in boys than in girls.

Asperger syndrome describes children with the problems of ASD but who have normal to high cognitive levels. These children have a difficult time socializing, but may otherwise be able to attend school successfully.

ASDs may occur with other developmental or physical disabilities. They have been associated with tuberous sclerosis and maternal rubella. Macrocephaly has been a common finding in large surveys of individuals with autism and also among their relatives. Overall growth is usually normal, and medical problems nonexistent. However, with the limited variety of foods usually eaten by these children, vitamin and mineral intake could be inadequate.

Efforts to find the cause of ASD have led to many studies looking at a possible toxic environment or food, a nutritionally deficient diet, immune system problems, oxidative stress, and pesticide exposure as important factors. Other studies have studied neurotransmitters such as elevated serotonin levels and disturbances in gamma-amino butyric acid (GABA) receptors, glutamate transmitters, and cholinergic activity. A number of prenatal causes have been evaluated, including pesticides. In one California study (Roberts et al., 2007) women in the first 8 weeks of pregnancy who lived near farm fields sprayed with dicofol and endosulfan were several times more likely to give birth to children with autism. More research is needed with greater numbers of mothers included.

Some treatment and research programs are using genomic panels to identify specific intervention protocols. The genomic panel identifies single-nucleotide polymorphisms,

TABLE 45-4

Pervasive Developmental Disorders (PDD)

Disorder	Characteristics
Autistic disorder	Impairment in social interaction Poor communication skills Repetitive and stereotypical behavior
Rett syndrome	Normal until 6-18 months Loss of motor skill abilities Loss of social interaction Deceleration of head growth between 5 and 48 months
Childhood disintegrative disorder	Before age 10 years Loss of expressive language, social skills, bowel or bladder control, play motor skills
Asperger syndrome	Impairment in social interaction Restricted repetitive or stereotypical behavior Normal language development Normal cognitive development
Pervasive developmental disorder not otherwise specified	Deficits in social behavior Impairment in understanding speech and in speech development Does not meet the criteria for the other four disorders

which are identified from blood samples or cell cultures (see Chapter 5). This work has revealed that the child with autism may need additional ω-3 or EFAs; nutrients with antioxidants qualities such as vitamins A, C, E, and selenium; mineral supplementation with zinc, calcium, and magnesium; a mercury-free diet; or an allergy-elimination diet (see Chapter 27).

Interest in a neurochemical cause of ASD has noted gluten and casein as the suspected sources. Intestinal inflammation has been reported in children with ASD and has improved with dietary restriction of gluten and casein (Reichelt and Knivsberg, 2003). Antibodies to casein, gluten, and soy have been noted in some children with ASD.

Nutrition Assessment

Anthropometric Measures. Height and weight are determined for the child and adult with ASD using the equipment and growth charts for nonaffected individuals. Head circumference has been found to be larger than that of the non-ASD individual.

Biochemical Measures. There is no standard pattern of tests that should be given other than the regular blood work for health monitoring. However, amino acid screening shortly after birth, thyroid testing, and allergy testing may be indicated (see Chapter 27).

Dietary Intake. Evaluations are sometimes difficult to complete for the child with a very limited intake. An effective measure may be provided by having the parents and caregivers keep a food diary for several days to determine the macronutrient intake in addition to the vitamin and mineral intake. See Chapter 4. Obtaining information related to when food is presented and the amount eaten is important, along with fluid consumption. Often excessive fluids are provided to compensate for limited food consumption.

Evaluations should include an observation of the child during mealtime. Some children are slow in arriving at developmental milestones for self-feeding and require feeding. Others finger feed or insist on self-feeding. The texture of the food presented should be recorded because sensory integration is difficult for children with ASD, and they may be very resistant to texture progression or variety. This is reflected in their fixation on one food (e.g., crackers, dry cereal, or chips). Food jags and picky eating are common. Evaluation should include a description of the feeding environment, whether there is a high chair or age-appropriate toddler chair, the timing of meals, and the location for meals.

Intervention Strategies

No one therapy or method will work for all individuals with ASD. Many professionals and families use a range of treatments simultaneously, including behavior modification, structured educational approaches, medication, speech therapy, occupational therapy, and counseling. Popular nutrition interventions include mineral and vitamin therapy and elimination diets such as a gluten-free (see Chapter 29), casein-free diet (see Chapter 27); allergy diets (see Chapter 27); supplementation with essential fatty acids (EFAs) and megavitamins.

There are anecdotal reports of success. The exclusion diets are now used in some treatment centers and are publicized on various websites (http://www.autismndi.com). Table 45-5 describes some exclusion diets. It is important for the RD to understand these various forms of therapy in order to counsel the parent effectively. Because of the increasing prevalence of ASD, research on potential MNT

TABLE 45-5

Comparison of Foods Allowed in the Gluten-Free and Casein-Free Diet, Specific Carbohydrate Diet, and Body Ecology Diet

Food	Gluten- and Casein-Free	Specific Carbohydrate Diet	Body Ecology Diet
Gluten-containing grains (wheat, rye, barley, spelt, kamut, possibly oats) and any products from those grains	Not allowed	Not allowed	Not recommended
Rice	Unlimited	Not allowed	Not recommended
Corn	Unlimited	Not allowed	Some OK if tolerated
Millet, quinoa, amaranth, buckwheat	Unlimited	Not allowed	Unlimited (80/20 rule)*, presoaked
Eggs and meat (beef, fish, lamb, chicken, turkey)	Unlimited	Allowed, processed not permitted	Recommended, organic free range or wild caught preferred, use 80/20 rule*
Vegetables	Unlimited	Fresh or frozen allowed, no canned, no potatoes and yams	Unlimited, fermented vegetables highly recommended
Fruits	Unlimited	Allowed, cooked in initial phase, no canned	Not recommended except lemon, lime, cranberry or black currants; no tomatoes
Milk products	Not allowed	Not initially; then 24-hr goat yogurt, dry curd cottage cheese, specific cheeses and butter	Raw butter and cream initially, kefir in 1 month
Sweeteners	Unlimited	Honey and saccharin	Stevia only
Vinegar	Unlimited	White or apple cider	Raw apple cider only
Juice	Unlimited	Those with no added sugar	Only those from fruits listed previously
Oils	Unlimited	Unlimited	Olive, coconut, pumpkin seed
Condiments	Unlimited	No added sugars, spices	Wheat-free tamari, herbs and spices, Celtic sea salt
Nuts and seeds	Unlimited	Most nuts, no seeds for 3 months	Unlimited raw and soaked
Seaweed	Unlimited	Not allowed	Highly recommended
Beans	Unlimited	After 3 months and soaked 12 hr	Not recommended
Coffee and tea	Unlimited	Allowed weak	Only herb tea or green tea
Coconut products	Unlimited	Fresh only	All recommended
Gelatin	Unlimited	Allowed	Not recommended. Use agar-agar instead

Developed by G. A. Houston-Ludlam. Reprinted with permission from The ANDI News, Autism Network for Dietary Intervention, 2005.

*80/20 = meal contains: 1) 80% land and ocean vegetables and 20% either protein or a grain and 2) 80% alkaline-forming foods and 20% acid forming foods.

should be promoted. One of the problems with the gluten-, casein-free diet is cost, because special foods needed to provide sufficient food choices are expensive and sometimes difficult to find (see Chapter 27).

When MNT is used, taking a team approach and working with the occupational therapist, speech therapist, and others is important for success. Parents also should be members of the team and counseled that changes will take time. Unfortunately, there have been no double-blind, randomized, controlled studies.

Follow-up is an important component of all therapy. From a nutritional standpoint, routine measures of height and weight should be scheduled, and there should be regular evaluation of eating and feeding behavior related to increasing ability to self-feed and accept new and different foods.

Attention-Deficit/Hyperactivity Disorder

Attention-deficit/hyperactivity disorder (ADHD) is a neurobehavioral problem seen in children with increasing frequency. It has been associated with learning disorders, inappropriate degrees of impulsiveness, hyperactivity, and attention deficit. Diagnostic criteria were developed by the American Psychiatric Association and have designated three types: (1) combined type of hyperactivity and attention deficit, (2) predominately inattentive type, and (3) predominately hyperactive-impulse type. ADHD affects the child at home, in school, and in social situations.

Nutrition Assessment

Many factors should be considered, along with the usual anthropometric measures, particularly when the individual is on medication.

Anthropometric Measures. Measurements of height and weight should be taken and recorded on a regular basis because the medications used in treatment may cause anorexia if given at inappropriate times, resulting in inadequate energy intake and potential slowing of growth. A 10 year prospective study of over 250 children with and without ADHD, treated or not treated with medication, found no evidence of limited growth in height over time. (Biederman J et al, 2010).

Biochemical Measures. These measurements should include a complete blood count and blood and tissue levels of vitamin and minerals if megavitamin therapy is used.

Dietary Intake. A detailed dietary history would include infant feeding history, food likes and dislikes, behavior at mealtimes, snacking behavior, presence of food allergies or food intolerances, or use of special diets. If the individual is on medications, the time of administration in relation to mealtime is important. Information should be obtained regarding any specific diet for the child or individual and how closely it is being followed.

Feeding evaluations should include observing the individual at mealtime. Generally the problems around feeding will be behavioral and will not include oral-motor or positioning peculiarities. Evaluating the environment around mealtime is important because distractions can be problematic.

Intervention Strategies

Current treatment may include psychotropic medications and the use of consistent behavioral management techniques. The timing and type of medication must be adjusted so that there is minimum influence on the child's dietary intake.

Specific diets have been used for many years, but they are not based on scientific research. For example, parents have been advised to use the Feingold diet, which states that foods containing synthetic food colors and naturally occurring salicylates be removed from the diet because of their neurologic effect.

Recently there has been renewed interest in the role of artificial food colorings (previously advised by Feingold) in exacerbating hyperactivity in selective children. Eight dyes are included: FD&C Blue 1 and 2, FD&C green 3, Orange B, FD&C Red 3, Red 40, FD&C Yellow 5 and 6. The outcome of current interest involves the Food and Drug Administration and committee discussion related to removing food coloring from the food supply (Pelsser LM et al, 2011).

Other recommendations have included the elimination of sugar, the elimination of caffeine, or the addition of large doses of vitamins (megavitamin therapy). A series of well-designed studies to evaluate the effectiveness of these recommendations have generally had negative results, and successful outcomes are largely anecdotal (see Chapter 18).

For the child or adult who is up and down throughout the meal, behavior modification may be indicated, and it should be a part of the overall behavioral management program. Distractions should be eliminated.

The most effective treatment for the individual with ADHD is a diet based on wholesome foods as outlined in the Dietary Guidelines or MyPlate and in Chapter 12. The food should be served at regular times, with small servings followed by refills. This is an important concept because of the tendency of the child or individual to eat very small amounts and leave the table, planning to return or graze throughout the day. Some programs recommend removing the food and returning it only once after explaining why this is being done. The intervention requires that the child or individual sit at the table in the high chair away from television or other distractions. These suggestions are most applicable to children in preschool settings and in the school cafeteria or classroom.

It has been suggested that a lack of EFAs is a possible cause of hyperactivity in children. It is more likely the result of varying biochemical influences. These children have a deficiency of EFAs because they cannot metabolize linoleic acid normally, they cannot absorb EFAs effectively from the intestine, or their EFA requirements are higher than normal. A recent study in Germany of 810 children ages 5-12 provided a food supplement containing ω-3 and ω-6 fatty acids plus zinc and magnesium resulting in considerable reduction in attention deficit and hyperactivity after 12 weeks of supplementation (Huss et al., 2010). This type of supplementation can be considered.

Cleft Lip and Palate

Cleft lip and cleft palate (CL/CP) are the most commonly occurring craniofacial birth defects (Merritt, 2005). **Cleft lip** is a condition that creates an opening of the upper lip. It can range from a slight notch to complete separation in one or both sides of the lips, and extending upward. If it occurs on one side of the lip, it is called a *unilateral cleft lip;* if it occurs on both sides, it is called a *bilateral cleft lip*. The **cleft palate** occurs when the roof of the mouth has not joined completely; it can be either unilateral or bilateral. Cleft palate can range from just an opening at the back of the soft palate or separation of the roof of the mouth with both soft and hard palate involved. CL/CP result from incomplete merging and fusion of embryonic processes during formation of the face. There is also a condition called *submucous cleft palate* in which there is incomplete fusion of the muscular layers of the soft palate with fusion of the overlying mucosa (Figures 45-5 and 45-6).

Lip and palate development occur between 5 and 12 weeks of gestation. Lip development begins first, usually at 5 weeks of gestation, followed by the development of the maxilla prominences and the primary palate. Fusion of the hard palate is completed by 10 weeks of gestation and the soft palate by 12 weeks.

The incidence of CL/CP varies but is generally 1 in 700 live births. CL/CP have multiple causes and are often associated with underlying syndromes such as Pierre Robin sequence. The Pierre Robin syndrome or complex is a birth condition that involves the lower jaw being either small in size (micrognathia) or set back from the upper jaw (retrognathia) (Cleft Palate Foundation, 2006). As a result, the tongue tends to be displaced back toward the throat, where it can fall back and obstruct the airway. Most infants will have a cleft palate, but none will have a cleft lip. The incidence of Pierre Robin ranges from 1 in 2000 to 30,000 births, based on how strictly the diagnosis is made. The basic cause appears to be the failure of the lower jaw to develop normally before birth.

Approximately 50% of children with cleft palate have an underlying syndrome or multiple anomalies. Wide ranges of studies in developmental biology have shown that both genetics and environmental factors are involved in causing oral clefts. Some of the risk factors from the environment include maternal folic acid deficiency, smoking, alcohol use, anticonvulsant use, and some maternal illnesses. Genetic counseling can now identify high-risk families.

Nutrition Assessment

Nutrition assessment for CL/CP includes the usual anthropometric measures for all infants and children. Biochemical measures are also those used with nonaffected children, and dietary intake information depends on the feeding problems that exist. Other problems include dental abnormalities and missing teeth, speech difficulties, and increased incidence of middle ear infections. The feeding evaluation is a major part of the assessment and is best accomplished with a team approach, including the parents. Because the major problem in CL/CP is feeding and providing adequate intake, growth can be jeopardized and needs to be assessed regularly.

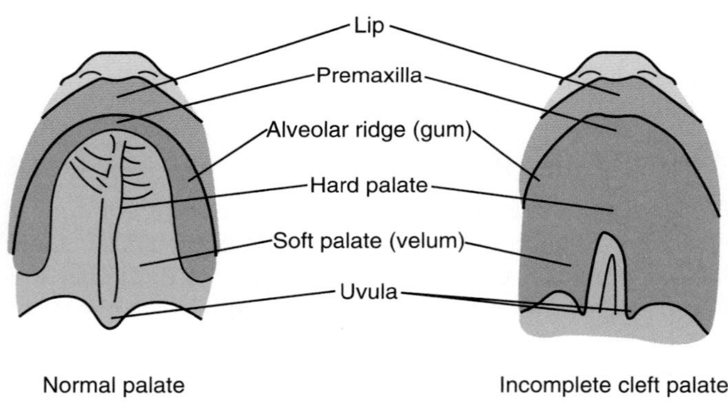

FIGURE 45-5 Cleft palate. *(From the Cleft Palate Foundation. Accessed 28 December 2006 from www.cleftline.org.)*

Intervention Strategies

Surgical repair of the cleft lip is generally done at 2 to 3 months of age, and cleft palate repair at 9 months. Other operations may involve minor improvements to the lip or nose and are usually completed before the child starts school.

Breast-feeding is difficult for these infants because of problems with sucking, although those infants with just the cleft lip may be successful. It is generally recommended that the mother who wishes to breast-feed express her milk and give it to her baby from a specialized bottle and nipple. Parents and caregivers need to be educated in the positioning of the child for feeding, nipple selection, bottle selection, and monitoring of intake.

Energy needs are generally the same as for a nonaffected infant or child, but, if the feeding process is too difficult, the energy needs may not be met. Strategies for solving that problem vary, with some professionals advising tube feeding, whereas others recommend continuing with appropriate bottles and nipples but using more concentrated formula or breast milk; see Chapter 43 and Table 45-6.

Effective feeding requires that the infant be able to form a vacuum inside the mouth and form a seal around the nipple with the lips. This is achieved through the proper bottle, nipple, and position for feeding. Some of the acceptable nipples and bottles include a regular newborn nipple with enlarged holes, a lamb's nipple, a Ross cleft palate assembly, an obturator nipple, and the orthodontic vented nipple. Bottles can vary from a very soft bottle with a cross-cut nipple to a Haberman feeder, squeeze bottle, or an Asepto feeder.

Individuals with CL/CP are different; thus it is extremely important that the feeding team evaluate various types of equipment and carefully educate the parent in their use.

FIGURE 45-6 Cleft lip. *(From the Cleft Palate Foundation. Accessed 28 December 2006 from www.cleftline.org.)*

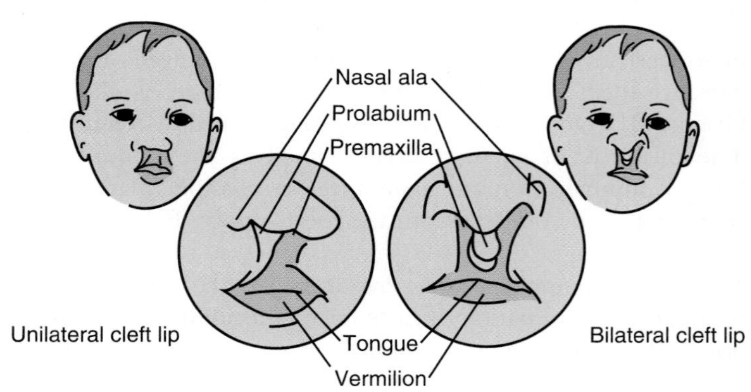

TABLE 45-6

Increasing Calories through Concentration of Formulas and Addition of Oils and Carbohydrates

Using 20 cal/oz Formula Caloric Density Required Per Ounce	Measures of Powder	Water Added
20 calories	1 scoop	2 oz
22 calories	2 scoops	3.5 fl oz
24 calories	3 scoops	5 fl oz
27 calories	3 scoops	4.25 fl oz
Using 22 cal/oz Formula		
22 cal	1 scoop	2 fl oz
24 cal	3 scoops	5.5 fl oz
27 cal	5 scoops	8 fl oz

Adding Oil or Carbohydrates

Product	kcal	Source
Corn oil or safflower oil	9/g or 8.3/mL	Corn or safflower oil
Microlipid	4.5/mL	Safflower oil
MCT oil	8.3/g or 7.6/mL	Fractionated coconut oil
Karo syrup	1 Tbsp = 58 kcal	Polysaccharides
Polycose liquid	2/mL or 60/fl oz	Glucose polymers
Polycose powder	3.8/g; 8/tsp; 23/Tbsp	Glucose polymers
Modulcal powder	30/Tbsp	Glucose polymers

MCT, Medium-chain triglyceride.

Palate obturators have been used to cover the cleft palate until the child can have surgery to close it; their use results in improved intake, better feeding skills, increased weight gain, and growth of the dental arches. Disadvantages include cost and the inconvenience of refabricating the devices as the infant grows to maintain effectiveness. One study (Prahl et al., 2005) measured growth and the length of feeding between two groups, one using the obturator and one without, and found no significant difference in growth, leading the researchers to conclude that the obturator could be abandoned. Positioning in an upright position, choosing the appropriate nipple, and directing the liquid flow to the side or back of the mouth seem to be just as effective in promoting optimal feeding and are recommended. The baby should be given ample opportunities for frequent burping in an upright position.

Introduction of solid foods for the CL/CP infant can follow the usual protocol at 4 to 6 months of age. By this time the cleft lip should have been repaired, and the child has achieved good head control and trunk stability. Care needs to be taken that the food is presented slowly, allowing the infant to control each bite while gradually learning how to direct the food around the cleft until it is repaired. Following the repair and healing of the cleft palate, feeding along the developmental pathway should progress slowly but normally. See Chapter 17.

FETAL ALCOHOL SYNDROME

Fetal alcohol syndrome (FAS) is a pattern of mental and physical defects that can develop in the fetus of a woman who drinks alcohol during pregnancy. The effects of the alcohol consumption include growth retardation and usually characteristic facial stigmata, damaged neurons and brain structures which can result in psychological or behavioral problems and other physical problems. The prevalence rate in the US and Europe is estimated to be between 0.2-1.5 in every 1000 live births. FAS was named in 1973 by Drs. Kenneth Jones and David Smith at the University of Washington School of Medicine after identifying a pattern of craniofacial, limb and cardiovascular defects in eight unrelated children of three ethnic groups all born to women who were alcoholics (Jones, KL, et al, 1973).

Diagnosis of fetal alcohol syndrome requires that the following criteria are fully met: 1) growth deficiency, 2) FAS facial features, 3) central nervous system damage, and 4) prenatal alcohol exposure. The three facial features include smooth filtrum (the groove between the upper lip and the nose; thin upper lip; small palpebral (between the upper and lower eyelid) fissures. See Fig. 16-4 on p. 361.

Nutrition Assessment

Anthropometric measures are very important in the assessment of the FAS child since growth deficiency is part of the diagnosis. In severe growth deficiency both the height and weight are below the 3rd percentile, while in moderate cases of growth deficiency, either the height or weight is below the 3rd percentile, but not both. Growth should be evaluated frequently and plotted on the CDC and WHO growth curves. Studies have shown that the prenatal growth retardation of the infant may persist postnatally and some infants have failure to thrive. (Huber A, Ekvall S. 2005). Feeding problems have also been associated with FAS, including having a week suck and oral motor problems, making these babies difficult to feed. This would contribute to failure to thrive.

Intervention Strategies

Nutritional intervention for the child with FAS is focused on the specific nutrition problem that exists for that child. Working with growth deficiency, failure to thrive and feeding problems requires the usual evaluation and intervention used in other infants and children with developmental disabilities. Energy and nutrient needs are the same as for non-affected children, although strategies for increasing calories would be required for those who have failure to thrive. For some children ADHD has been reported, and the treatment should be the same as already described.

CONTROVERSIAL NUTRITION THERAPY

An important factor in providing MNT for children and adults with developmental disabilities is realizing that counseling may have been inadequate in helping the parent accept the limitations of the disorder, limitations such as growth, feeding problems, and cognitive ability. As a result, many parents look for unusual medical or nutrition therapies. Major sources of information are often the Internet and parent support groups. Recent media coverage has promoted the use of antioxidant vitamins (A, C, and E) and minerals (zinc, copper, manganese, and selenium) along with the amino acids glucosamine, tyrosine, and tryptophan. The expected outcomes are improved growth; increased cognition, alertness, and attention span; and changed facial features.

There is little scientific information to back up these therapies. Research studies have addressed the vitamin needs of children with DS, spina bifida, fragile X syndrome, and autism, and findings do not indicate that the vitamin and mineral needs of these children with developmental disabilities are higher than normal. Numerous historical studies have searched for nutritional deficiencies as causative factors in DS. Traditionally, the studies have included numerous vitamins, minerals, fatty acids, digestive enzymes, lipotropic nutrients, and numerous drugs, with no definitive results.

The key concept in the proposed nutrition interventions for DS is metabolic correction of genetic overexpression. It is postulated that presence of the third chromosome 21 causes overproduction of superoxide dismutase and cystathionine *b*-synthase, which disrupts active methylation pathways. Vitamin supplements of folic acid and antioxidants counteract this and are considered key to the treatment. However, these are just theories, and at this point nutrition supplements are considered an expensive, questionable approach.

Parents of children with ADHD report that omitting sugar from the children's diets decreases hyperactivity, but there is no scientific evidence to support this. However, it probably is a good idea to eliminate or at least reduce the sugar intake in any child's diet to promote better nutritional intake. Blue-green algae has been promoted for children with DS and other developmental disabilities, purportedly to increase attention span and concentration. High-dose supplementation of vitamin B_6 and magnesium has been proposed for autism to diminish tantrums and self-stimulation activities and improve attention and speech. Another proposed treatment is dimethyl glycine. Limited research is available.

COMMUNITY RESOURCES

For many types of nutrition problems and MNT, the school system is an excellent resource through the school lunch and school breakfast programs. Children and adolescents may receive modified meals at school. Child and adult care food programs must provide meals at no extra cost for children and adolescents with special needs and developmental disabilities. School food service is required to offer special

Name of student for whom special meals at school are requested:

____

Disability or medical condition that requires the student to have a special diet. Include a brief description of the major life activity affected by the student's condition.

____

____

Foods omitted and substitutions (Please check food groups to be omitted. List specific foods to be omitted and suggest substitutions using the back of this form or attach information.)

- Meat and meat alternatives
- Milk and milk products
- Bread and cereal products
- Fruits and vegetables

Textures allowed: Please check the allowed texture

☐ Regular ☐ Chopped ☐ Ground ☐ Pureed

Other information regarding diet or feeding:

I certify that the above named student needs special school meals prepared as described above because of the student's disability or chronic medical condition.

______________________________ ______________________________

Physician/Recognized Medical Authority Signature — Office Phone Number/Date

FIGURE 45-7 Diet prescription for meals at school. *(Reprinted with permission from CARE: special nutrition for kids, Birmingham, AL, 1999, Alabama Department of Education.)*

meals at no additional cost to children whose disabilities restrict their diets as defined in the U.S. Department of Agriculture's nondiscrimination regulations.

The term "child with a disability" under Part B of the Individuals with Disabilities Education Act (IDEA) refers to a child evaluated in accordance with IDEA as having one of the 13 recognized disability categories: (1) autism; (2) deaf-blindness; (3) deafness; (4) mental retardation; (5) orthopedic impairments; (6) other health impairments caused by chronic or acute health problems such as asthma, nephritis, diabetes, sickle cell anemia, a heart condition, epilepsy, rheumatic fever, hemophilia, leukemia, lead poisoning, or tuberculosis; (7) emotional disturbances; (8) specific learning disabilities; (9) speech or language impairment; (10) traumatic brain injury; (11) visual impairment; (12) multiple disabilities; and (13) developmental delays. Attention deficit disorder may fall under 1 of the 13 categories.

When a referral is made to the school system for a special meal related to a developmental disability, it must be accompanied by a medical statement for a child with special dietary needs (Figure 45-7). The request requires an identification of the medical or other special dietary condition, the food or foods to be omitted, and the food or choice of foods to be substituted. The statement requires the signature of the physician or recognized medical authority. The school food service may make food substitutions for individual children

CLINICAL SCENARIO 1

Mitchell is a 2-month-old boy with Down syndrome. He was born prematurely (30 weeks of gestation) and was started on gastrostomy tube feeding at 10 days of age because of his poor weight gain and severe gastroesophageal reflux. The poor weight gain was caused by a poor suck, although swallowing was not a problem. He was first seen by a nutritionist in an early intervention program at 4 months of age when he was 22.5 in long and weighed 10 lb 7 oz.

At 16 months he started eating table foods, and his tube-feeding formula was PediaSure. By 21 months his height was 28 inches, and his weight 18.5 lb. He was at the 5th percentile for length and weight using the CDC growth curves, but at the 25th percentile when the Down syndrome curves were used. He had been taking oral feeds since 7 months of age, but his total oral consumption was one jar of baby food a day in addition to his gastrostomy feeds. He was crawling but not yet walking, and he had very limited self-feeding skills. Now at age 21 months his mother's highest priority is to stop the tube feeding and have Mitchell continue to grow well; she is concerned about his rate of weight gain. She is also concerned that constipation has become a problem requiring medication.

Nutrition Diagnostic Statement

Self-feeding difficulty related to developmental delays as evidenced by inability to feed self most foods offered.

Nutrition Care Questions

1. What would be your approach in working with this mother and the other team members?
2. What do you think would be his nutritional needs, starting with energy?
3. How many ounces of a 30 cal/oz tube-feeding formula would you recommend for Mitchell to promote weight gain?
4. What steps should be taken to increase his oral intake and decrease the tube feeding?
5. What would you recommend for management of his constipation?

CLINICAL SCENARIO 2

Luke is a 2-year-old boy with Prader-Willi syndrome. He was born weighing 7 lb and was 18 in long. A test done in the nursery determined that he had Prader-Willi syndrome. Typical of Prader-Willi syndrome, Luke was a very hypotonic infant with a very poor suck. Mom wanted to breast-feed, but Luke was unable to latch on at the breast, so she pumped her milk. Also it was recommended that human milk fortifier (HMF) be added to the breast milk. She was very concerned about adding the HMF because she had read about potential obesity as Luke grew older. After discharge from the hospital Luke entered an early intervention program with nutrition services. Eventually the mother changed Luke to an infant formula, but Luke continued to have a weak suck, and feeding services were needed.

Nutrition Diagnostic Statement

Inability to feed self related to weak suck and hypotonia as evidenced by need for feeding services.

Nutrition Care Questions

1. What would be a good plan for continuing nutrition care for Luke?
2. What kind of information should the nutritionist provide to the mother related to her fear of eventual obesity for Luke?
3. As Luke grows older, what would be a good way to determine the number of calories he should receive to prevent obesity?

who do not have a disability but who are medically certified as having a special medical or dietary need. An example is the child with severe allergies or an inborn error of metabolism. The availability of school food service for children with developmental disabilities is an important resource in the long-term implementation of MNT.

USEFUL WEBSITES

Centers for Disease Control and Prevention Birth Defects Research
http://www.cdc.gov/ncbddd/birthdefects/research.html
March of Dimes
http://www.modimes.org
National Center for Education in Maternal and Child Health
http://www.ncemch.org/
National Dissemination Center for Children with Disabilities
http://www.nichcy.org
National Folic Acid Campaign
http://www.cdc.gov/folicacid/promote.htm

REFERENCES

American Dietetic Association (ADA): Position of the American Dietetic Association: providing nutrition services for people with developmental disabilities and special health care needs, *J Am Diet Assoc* 110:297, 2010.

AAIDD: American Association on Intellectual and Developmental Disabilities. Definitions. Accessed April 10, 2011 from http://www.aaidd.org/content_100.cfm?navID=21.

Biederman J, et al: A naturalistic 10-year prospective study of height and weight in children with attention-deficit hyperactivity disorder grown up: sex and treatment effects, *J Pediatr* 157:635, 2010.

Carrel AL, et al: Long-term growth hormone therapy changes the natural history of body composition and motor function in children with Prader-Willi syndrome, *J Clin Endo Met* 95:1131, 2010.

Capone G, et al: Down syndrome. In Ekvall SW, Ekvall VK, editors: *Pediatric nutrition in chronic disease and developmental disorders*, New York, 2005, Oxford University Press.

Centers for Disease Control and Prevention: CDC Grand Rounds: additional opportunities to prevent neural tube detects, *MMWR Morb Mortal Wkly Rep* 59(31):980, 2010.

Centers for Disease Control and Prevention: Updated national birth prevalence estimates for selected birth defects in the United States, 2004-2006, 2010. Atlanta, Ga. Accessed 28 October 2010 from http://www.cdc.gov/ncbdddfeatures/birthdefects.

Cleft Palate Foundation: Information about Pierre Robin sequence/complex, 2006, Accessed 21 April 2011 from http://www.cleftline.org/publications/pierre_robin

Cloud HH, et al: Feeding problems of the child with special health care needs. In Ekvall SV, Ekvall VK, editors: *Pediatric nutrition in chronic disease and developmental disorders*, ed 2, New York, 2005, Oxford University Press.

Ekvall SW, Cerniglia F: Myelomeningocele. In Ekvall SW, Ekvall VK, editors: *Pediatric nutrition in developmental disabilities and chronic disorders*, ed 2, New York, 2005, Oxford University Press.

Henderson RC, et al: Longitudinal changes in bone density in children and adolescents with moderate to severe cerebral palsy, *J Pediatr* 146:769, 2005.

Huber A, Ekvall SW: Fetal Alcohol Syndrome. In Ekvall SV, Ekvall VK, editors: *Pediatric nutrition in chronic disease and developmental disorders*, ed 2, New York, 2005, Oxford University Press.

Huss M, et al: Supplementation of polyunsaturated fatty acids, magnesium and zinc in children seeking medical advice for attention-deficit/hyperactivity problems-an observational cohort study, *Lipids Health Dis* 9:105, 2010.

Jones KL, et al: Pattern of malformation in offspring of chronic alcoholic mothers, *Lancet* 1(7815):1267, 1973.

McCune H, Driscoll D: Prader-Willi syndrome. In Ekvall SW, Ekvall VK, editors: *Pediatric nutrition in chronic disease and developmental disorders*, ed 2, New York, 2005, Oxford University Press.

Merritt L: Physical assessment of the infant with cleft lip and/or palate, *Adv Neonatal Care* 5:125, 2005.

Miller JL, et al: Nutritional phases in Prader-Willi syndrome, *Am J Med Genet A* 155:1040, 2011.

Obata K, et al: Effects of 5 years growth hormone treatment in patients with Prader-Willi syndrome, *J Pediatr Endocrinol Metab* 16:155, 2003.

Pelsser LM, et al: Effects of a restricted elimination diet on the behavior of children with attention-deficit hyperactivity disorder (INCA study): a randomised controlled trial, *Lancet* 377(9764):494, 2011.

Prahl C, et al: Infant orthopedics in UCLP: effect on feeding, weight, and length: a randomized clinical trial (Dutch cleft), *Cleft Palate Craniofac J* 42:171, 2005.

Reichelt K, Knivsberg AM: Why use the gluten free and casein-free diet? What the results have shown so far. Autism Research Institute, 2003. www.autismwebsite.com/ARI/fsn/reicvhelt.htm. accessed April 14, 2007.

Reus L, et al: Motor problems in Prader-Willi syndrome: a systematic review on body composition and neuromuscular functioning, *Neurosci Biobehav Rev* 35:956, 2011.

Robbins JM, et al: Hospitalizations of newborns with folate-sensitive birth defects before and after fortification of foods with folic acid, *Pediatrics* 118:906, 2006.

Roberts EM, et al: Maternal residence near agricultural pesticide applications and autism spectrum disorders among children in the Californiat Central valley, *Environ Health Perspect* 115:1482, 2007.

Scerif M, et al: Ghrelin in obesity and endocrine diseases, *Mol Cell Endocrinol* [Feb 21, 2011, e-pub ahead of print].

Smithells RN, et al: Further experience of vitamin supplementation for prevention of neural tube defect recurrences, *Lancet* 1:1027, 1983.

Stevenson RD: Use of segmental measures to estimate stature in children with cerebral palsy, *Arch Paediatr Adolesc Med* 149:658, 2005.

Sullivan PB, et al: Gastrostomy tube feeding in children with cerebral palsy: a prospective longitudinal study, *Dev Med Child Neurol* 47:77, 2005.

Talebizadeh Z, Butler MG: Insulin resistance and obesity-related factors in Prader-Willi syndrome: comparison with obese subjects, *Clin Genet* 67:230, 2005.

Tobin SP, et al: The role of an interdisciplinary feeding team in the assessment and treatment of feeding problems: building blocks for life: Pediatric Nutrition Practice Group, *J Am Diet Assoc* 28:3, 2005.

Appendixes

GENERAL INFORMATION

NUTRITION CARE PROCESS

PHYSICAL ASSESSMENT

LABORATORY TESTS AND MEDICATIONS

NUTRITION INTERVENTION

Nutrient Delivery: Enteral Formulary

Nutrition Education and Counseling

*Nutritional Facts**

Nutritional Facts* (Appendixes 38-58) unless otherwise noted created from the North Carolina Dietetic Association: Nutrition care manual, 2011, Raleigh, North Carolina; USDA Agricultural Research Service, Nutrient Data Laboratory, accessed March 2011 from http://www.nal.usda.gov/fnic/foodcomp/search/. Compiled by Maria Balance, MS, RD, LDN.

APPENDIX 1. Medical Abbreviations

ABGs	arterial blood gases
ACTH	adrenocorticotropic hormone
AD	Alzheimer's disease
ADH	antidiuretic hormone
ADI	adequate daily intake
ADIME	assessment, diagnosis, intervention, monitoring, evaluation
ADLs	activities of daily living
AI	adequate intake
AIDS	acquired immunodeficiency syndrome
ALA	α-linolenic acid
ALS	amyotrophic lateral sclerosis
AP	angina pectoris
ARF	acute renal failure
ASHD	atherosclerotic heart disease
ATP	adenosine triphosphate
BCAA	branched-chain amino acid
BEE	basal energy expenditure
BHA	butylated hydroxyanisole
BHT	butylated hydroxytoluene
BMI	body mass index
BMR	basal metabolic rate
BMT	bone marrow transplantation
BPD	bronchopulmonary dysplasia
BSA	body surface area
BV	biologic value
CA	cancer
CAD	coronary artery disease
CAPD	continuous ambulatory peritoneal dialysis
CAVH	continuous arteriovenous hemofiltration
CCK	cholecystokinin
CCU	coronary care unit
CDC	Centers for Disease Control and Prevention
CHD	coronary heart disease
CHI	closed head injury
CKD	chronic kidney disease
CNS	central nervous system
COPD	chronic obstructive pulmonary disease
CPN	central parenteral nutrition
CSII	continuous subcutaneous insulin infusion
CSF	cerebrospinal fluid
CVA	cerebrovascular accident
DCCT	Diabetes Control and Complications Trial
DHA	docosahexaenoic acid
DHHS	Department of Health and Human Services
DJD	degenerative joint disease
DKA	diabetic ketoacidosis
DM	diabetes mellitus
DNA	deoxyribonucleic acid
DRI	dietary reference intake
ECG/EKG	electrocardiogram
EDTA	ethylenediaminetetraacetate
EFA	essential fatty acid
EPA	eicosapentaenoic acid
EPO	erythropoietin
ERT	estrogen replacement therapy
ESR	erythrocyte sedimentation rate
ESRD	end-stage renal disease
FAD	flavin adenine dinucleotide
FBG	fasting blood glucose
FBS	fasting blood sugar
FFA	free fatty acid
FIGLU	formimino glutamic acid
FMN	flavin mononucleotide
FPG	fasting plasma glucose
FTT	failure to thrive
Fx	fracture
GB	gallbladder
GFR	glomerular filtration rate
GI	gastrointestinal
GIP	gastric inhibitory polypeptide
GTF	glucose tolerance factor
GTT	glucose tolerance test
GVHD	graft-versus-host disease
HAV	hepatitis A virus
Hgb	hemoglobin
HBV	hepatitis B virus
HCT	hematocrit
HDL	high-density lipoprotein
HE	hepatic encephalopathy
HF	heart failure
Hgb	hemoglobin
H&D	history and physical
HIV	human immunodeficiency virus
HPN	home parenteral nutrition
HSL	hormone-sensitive lipase
HTN	hypertension
Hx	history
IBD	inflammatory bowel disease
IBS	irritable bowel syndrome
IBW	ideal body weight
ICU	intensive care unit
IF	intrinsic factor
IgE	immunoglobulin E
IGT	impaired glucose tolerance
IL-2	interleukin-2
IM	intramuscular
INH	isonicotinic acid hydrazide
INR	international normalized ratio
I&O	intake and output
IV	intravenous
J	joule
kcal (Cal)	kilocalorie
kJ	kilojoule
KUB	kidney, ureter, bladder
LBM	lean body mass
LCT	long-chain triglyceride
LDL	low-density lipoprotein
LES	lower esophageal sphincter
LFT	liver function test
LPL	lipoprotein lipase
MAOI	monoamine oxidase inhibitor
MCH	mean corpuscular hemoglobin
MCT	medium-chain triglyceride
MCV	mean corpuscular volume
MDS	minimum data set
MET	metabolic equivalent
MFOS	mixed-function oxidase system
MI	myocardial infarction
MSG	monosodium glutamate
MSUD	maple syrup urine disease
NANB	non-A, non-B hepatitis virus
NCEP	National Cholesterol Education Program
NCP	Nutrition Care Process
NG	nasogastric
NPO	nothing by mouth
NPU	net protein utilization
NSAID	nonsteroidal antiinflammatory drug
NSP	nonstarch polysaccharide
N&V	nausea and vomiting

Continued

APPENDIX 1. Medical Abbreviations—cont'd

OCA	oral contraceptive agent	ROS	review of systems
OGTT	oral glucose tolerance test	RQ	respiratory quotient
OHA	oral hypoglycemic agent	RTA	renal tubular acidosis
PBI	protein-bound iodine	SCA	sickle cell anemia
PCM	protein-calorie malnutrition	SCT	short-chain triglycerides
PEG	percutaneous endoscopic gastrostomy	SFA	saturated fatty acid
PEM	protein-energy malnutrition	SLE	systemic lupus erythematosus
PER	protein efficiency ratio	SMBG	self-monitoring of blood glucose
PG	prostaglandin	SOB	shortness of breath
PHE	phenylalanine	S/P	status post
PKU	phenylketonuria	TBSA	total body surface area
PLP	pyridoxal phosphate	TC	total cholesterol
PN	parenteral nutrition	TEE	total energy expenditure
PPN	peripheral parenteral nutrition	TEF	thermic effect of food
PRN	as needed	TG	triglyceride or triacylglycerol
PT	patient	THF	tetrahydrofolate
PTA	prior to admission	TIA	transient ischemic attack
PTT	partial thromboplastin time	TIBC	total iron-binding capacity
PUD	peptic ulcer disease	TNF	tumor necrosis factor
PUFA	polyunsaturated fatty acid	TS	transferrin saturation
RAST	radioallergosorbent test	UL	upper intake level
RBC	red blood cell	URI	upper respiratory infection
RDA	recommended dietary allowance	UTI	urinary tract infection
RDS	respiratory distress syndrome	VLCD	very-low-calorie diet
REE	resting energy expenditure	VLDL	very-low-density lipoprotein
RMR	resting metabolic rate	VOD	venous occlusive disease
RNA	ribonucleic acid	VS	vital signs
R/O	rule out	WNL	within normal limits

APPENDIX 2. Unit Abbreviations

Along with the specialized vocabulary that is used in the medical, dietetic, and nursing fields, there are acceptable forms of abbreviations. The following is a list of abbreviations commonly used.

aa: Gr. *ana*; of each
ac: L. *ante cibum;* before meals
ad, add: L. *adde*, *addatus*, or *addantur;* add or added
ad lib: L. *ad libitum;* at pleasure, as desired
aq: L. *aqua;* water
aq dest: L. *aqua destillata;* distilled water
bid, bis in d: L. *bis in die;* twice a day
c̄: L. *cum;* with
c: cup
Cent; cent; C: centigrade, Celsius
cm: centimeter
dilut: L. *dilutus;* dilute
div: L. *divide;* divide
fac: make
g: gram
gr: L. *granum;* grain
gtt: L. *guttae;* drops
hs: L. *hora somni;* at hour of sleep
IU: international unit
kcal: kilocalorie
kg: kilogram
kJ: kilojoule
lb: pound
mcg: microgram
mEq: milliequivalent
mg: milligram
mil or mL: milliliter
mM: millimole
µmol: micromol
mOsm: milliosmole
oz: ounce
prn: L. *pro re nata;* may be repeated according to instructions
pt: pint
pulv: L. *pulvis;* powder
qd: L. *quaque die;* every day
QID, qid: L. *quater in die;* four times daily
q3h: every 3 hours
qs: L. *quantum satis;* a sufficient quantity
qt: quart
RE: retinal equivalent
s̄: L. *sine;* without
sol: solution
ss: L. *semis;* half
stat: L. *statim;* immediately
T, tsp: teaspoon
T, Tbsp: tablespoon
tid: L. *ter in die:* three times a day

APPENDIX 3. Milliequivalents and Milligrams of Electrolytes

To Convert Milligrams to Milliequivalents: Divide milligrams by atomic weight and then multiply by the valence.

$$\text{Example: } \frac{\text{Milligrams}}{\text{Atomic weight}} \times \text{Valence} = \text{Milliequivalents}$$

Mineral Element	Chemical Symbol	Atomic Weight (mg)	Valence
Calcium	Ca	40	2
Chlorine	Cl	35	1
Magnesium	Mg	24	2
Phosphorus	P	31	2
Potassium	K	39	1
Sodium	Na	23	1
Sulfate	SO_4	96	2
Sulfur	S	32	

To Convert Specific Weight of Sodium to Sodium Chloride: Multiply by 2.54.

$$\text{Example: } 1000 \text{ mg Sodium} = 1000 \times 2.54$$
$$= 2540 \text{ mg Sodium chloride (2.5 g)}$$

To Convert Specific Weight of Sodium Chloride to Sodium: Multiply by 0.393.

$$\text{Example: } 2.5 \text{ g Sodium chloride} = 2.5 \times 0.393$$
$$= 1000 \text{ mg sodium}$$

Milligrams	Sodium in Milliequivalents (mEq)	Grams of Sodium Chloride
500	21.8	1.3
1000	43.5	2.5
1500	75.3	3.8
2000	87.0	5.0

Modified from Merck Manual, Ready Reference Guide. Accessed 22 March 2011 from http://www.merckmanuals.com/professional/print/appendixes/ap1/ap1a.html; Nelson JK et al: Mayo Clinic diet manual, ed 7, St Louis, 1994, Mosby.

APPENDIX 4. Equivalents, Conversions,* and Portion (Scoop) Sizes

Liquid Measure—Volume Equivalents

1 tsp = 1/3 Tbsp = 5 mL or cc
1 Tbsp = 3 tsp = 15 mL or cc
2 Tbsp = 1 fluid oz = 1/8 cup = 30 mL or cc
2 Tbsp + 2 tsp = 1/6 cup = 40 mL or cc
4 Tbsp = 1/4 cup = 2 fluid oz = 60 mL or cc
5 Tbsp + 1 tsp = 1/3 cup = 80 mL or cc
6 Tbsp = 3 fluid oz = 3/8 cup = 90 mL or cc
8 Tbsp = 1/2 cup = 120 mL or cc
10 Tbsp + 2 tsp = 2/3 cup = 160 mL or cc
12 Tbsp = 3/4 cup = 180 mL or cc
48 tsp = 16 Tbsp = 1 cup (8 fluid ounces) = 1/2 pint = 240 mL or cc
2 cups = 1 pint (16 fluid oz) = 0.4732 L
4 cups = 2 pints = 1 quart (32 fluid oz) = 0.9462 L
1.06 quarts = 34 fluid oz = 1000 mL or cc
4 quarts = 1 gallon = 3785 mL or cc

Dry Measure

1 quart = 2 pints = 1.101 L
Dry measure and quarts are approximately 1/6 larger than liquid measure pints and quarts.

Weights

English (Avoirdupois)	Metric
1 oz	Approx 30 g
1 lb (16 oz)	454 g
2.2 lb	1 kg

Scoop Sizes

It is important to use the proper scoop size when portioning out foods to serve to patients. The dietitian will be expected to know and guide staff accordingly.

Number	Approximate Liquid Volume
6	2/3 cup (5 fluid oz)
8	1/2 cup (4 fluid oz)
10	3/8 cup (3 1/4 fluid oz)
12	1/3 cup (2 2/3 fluid oz)
16	1/4 cup (2 fluid oz)
20	3 1/5 Tbsp (1 3/5 fluid oz)
24	2 2/3 Tbsp (1 1/3 fluid oz)
30	2 1/5 Tbsp (1 fluid oz)
40	1 3/5 Tbsp (0.8 fluid oz)
60	1 Tbsp (0.5 fluid oz)

Metric Conversion Factors

Multiply	By	To Get
Fluid ounces	29.57	Grams
Ounces (dry)	28.35	Grams
Grams	0.0353	Ounces
Grams	0.0022	Pounds
Kilograms	2.21	Pounds
Pounds	453.6	Grams
Pounds	0.4536	Kilograms
Quarts	0.946	Liters
Quarts (dry)	67.2	Cubic inches
Quarts (liquid)	57.7	Cubic inches
Liters	1.0567	Quarts
Gallons	3.785	Cubic centimeters
Gallons	3.785	Liters

From North Carolina Dietetic Association: Nutrition care manual, 2011, Raleigh, NC, The Association.

*Note: In the U.S. measuring systems the same word may have two meanings. For example, an ounce may mean 1/16 of a pound and 1/16 of a pint; but the former is strictly a weight measure, and the latter is a volume measure. Except in the case of water, milk, or other liquids of the same density, a fluid ounce and an ounce of weight are two completely different quantities. These measures are not to be used interchangeably.

APPENDIX 5. Focus on Nutrition Care Process: Nutrition Assessment

Step 1. Nutrition assessment is designed to identify nutrition-related problems and their causes. A nutrition assessment matrix links nutrition assessment parameters with nutrition diagnoses.

Nutrition Assessment and Monitoring and Evaluation Terminology

This is a combined list of Nutrition Assessment and Monitoring and Evaluation terms. Indicators that are shaded are used ONLY for nutrition assessment. The rest of the indicators are used for assessment and monitoring and evaluation.

FOOD/NUTRITION-RELATED HISTORY (FH)

Food and nutrient intake, food and nutrient administration, medication/herbal supplement use, knowledge/beliefs/attitudes, behavior, food and supply availability, physical activity and function, nutrition-related patient/client-centered measures.

Food and Nutrient Intake (1)

Composition and adequacy of food and nutrient intake, and meal and snack patterns.

Energy Intake (1.1)

Total energy intake from all sources, including food, beverages, supplements, and via enteral and parenteral routes.

Energy intake (1.1.1)

- ❑ Total energy intake FH-1.1.1.1

Food and Beverage Intake (1.2)

Type, amount, and pattern of intake of foods and food groups, indices of diet quality, intake of fluids, breast milk and infant formula

Fluid/beverage intake (1.2.1)

- ❑ Oral fluids FH-1.2.1.1
- ❑ Food-derived fluids FH-1.2.1.2
- ❑ Liquid meal replacement or supplement FH-1.2.1.3

Food intake (1.2.2)

- ❑ Amount of food FH-1.2.2.1
- ❑ Types of food/meals FH-1.2.2.2
- ❑ Meal/snack pattern FH-1.2.2.3
- ❑ Diet quality index FH-1.2.2.4
- ❑ Food variety FH-1.2.2.5

Breast milk/infant formula intake (1.2.3)

- ❑ Breast milk intake FH-1.2.3.1
- ❑ Infant formula intake FH-1.2.3.2

Enteral and Parenteral Nutrition Intake (1.3)

Specialized nutrition support intake from all sources, e.g., enteral and parenteral routes.

Enteral nutrition intake (1.3.1)

- ❑ Formula/solution FH-1.3.1.1
- ❑ Feeding tube flush FH-1.3.1.2

Parenteral nutrition intake (1.3.2)

- ❑ Formula/solution FH-1.3.2.1
- ❑ IV fluids FH-1.3.2.2

Bioactive Substance Intake (1.4)

Alcohol, plant stanol and sterol esters, soy protein, psyllium and β-glucan, and caffeine intake from all sources, e.g., food, beverages, supplements, and via enteral and parenteral routes.

Alcohol intake (1.4.1)

- ❑ Drink size/volume FH-1.4.1.1
- ❑ Frequency FH-1.4.1.2
- ❑ Pattern of alcohol consumption FH-1.4.1.3

Bioactive substance intake (1.4.2)

- ❑ Plant sterol and stanol esters FH-1.4.2.1
- ❑ Soy protein FH-1.4.2.2
- ❑ Psyllium and β-glucan FH-1.4.2.3
- ❑ Food additives *(specify)* FH-1.4.2.4
- ❑ Other *(specify)* FH-1.4.2.5

Caffeine intake (1.4.3)

- ❑ Total caffeine FH-1.4.3.1

Macronutrient Intake (1.5)

Fat and cholesterol, protein, carbohydrate, and fiber intake from all sources including food, beverages, supplements, and via enteral and parenteral routes.

Fat and cholesterol intake (1.5.1)

- ❑ Total fat FH-1.5.1.1
- ❑ Saturated fat FH-1.5.1.2
- ❑ Trans fatty acids FH-1.5.1.3
- ❑ Polyunsaturated fat FH-1.5.1.4
- ❑ Monounsaturated fat FH-1.5.1.5
- ❑ Omega-3 fatty acids FH-1.5.1.6
- ❑ Dietary cholesterol FH-1.5.1.7
- ❑ Essential fatty acids FH-1.5.1.8

Protein intake (1.5.2)

- ❑ Total protein FH-1.5.2.1
- ❑ High biological value protein FH-1.5.2.2
- ❑ Casein FH-1.5.2.3
- ❑ Whey FH-1.5.2.4
- ❑ Amino acids FH-1.5.2.5
- ❑ Essential amino acids FH-1.5.2.6

Carbohydrate intake (1.5.3)

- ❑ Total carbohydrate FH-1.5.3.1
- ❑ Sugar FH-1.5.3.2
- ❑ Starch FH-1.5.3.3
- ❑ Glycemic index FH-1.5.3.4
- ❑ Glycemic load FH-1.5.3.5
- ❑ Source of carbohydrate FH-1.5.3.6
- ❑ Insulin-to-carbohydrate ratio FH-1.5.3.7

Fiber intake (1.5.4)

- ❑ Total fiber FH-1.5.4.1
- ❑ Soluble fiber FH-1.5.4.2
- ❑ Insoluble fiber FH-1.5.4.3

Micronutrient Intake (1.6)

Vitamin and mineral intake from all sources, e.g., food, beverages, supplements, and via enteral and parenteral routes.

Vitamin intake (1.6.1)

- ❑ A (1)
- ❑ C (2)
- ❑ D (3)
- ❑ E (4)
- ❑ K (5)
- ❑ Thiamin (6)
- ❑ Riboflavin (7)
- ❑ Niacin (8)
- ❑ Folate (9)
- ❑ B6 (10)
- ❑ B12 (11)
- ❑ Multivitamin (12)
- ❑ Other *(specify)* ________________ (13)

Mineral/element intake (1.6.2)

- ❑ Calcium (1)
- ❑ Chloride (2)
- ❑ Iron (3)
- ❑ Magnesium (4)
- ❑ Potassium (5)
- ❑ Phosphorus (6)
- ❑ Sodium (7)
- ❑ Zinc (8)
- ❑ Multi-mineral (9)
- ❑ Multi-trace element (10)
- ❑ Other, *(specify)* ________________ (11)

Food and Nutrient Administration (2)

Current and previous diets and/or food modifications, eating environment, and enteral and parenteral nutrition administration.

Diet History (2.1)

Description of food and drink regularly provided or consumed, past diets followed or prescribed and counseling received, and the eating environment.

Diet order (2.1.1)

- ❑ General, healthful diet FH-2.1.1.1
- ❑ Modified diet *(specify)* ________________ FH-2.1.1.2
- ❑ Enteral nutrition order *(specify)* ________________ FH-2.1.1.3
- ❑ Parenteral nutrition order *(specify)* ________________ FH-2.1.1.4

Diet experience (2.1.2)

- ❑ Previously prescribed diets FH-2.1.2.1
- ❑ Previous diet/nutrition education/counseling FH-2.1.2.2
- ❑ Self-selected diet/s followed FH-2.1.2.3
- ❑ Dieting attempts FH-2.1.2.4

Eating environment (2.1.3)

- ❑ Location FH-2.1.3.1
- ❑ Atmosphere FH-2.1.3.2
- ❑ Caregiver/companion FH-2.1.3.3
- ❑ Appropriate breastfeeding accommodations/facility FH-2.1.3.4
- ❑ Eats alone FH-2.1.3.5

Enteral and parenteral nutrition administration (2.1.4)

- ❑ Enteral access FH-2.1.4.1
- ❑ Parenteral access FH-2.1.4.2

Medication and Herbal Supplement Use (3)

Prescription and over-the counter medications, including herbal preparations and complementary medicine products used.

Medication and herbal supplements (3.1)

- ❑ Medications, specify prescription or OTC FH-3.1.1
- ❑ Herbal/complementary products *(specify)* FH-3.1.2
- ❑ Misuse of medication *(specify)* FH-3.1.3

Knowledge/Beliefs/Attitudes (4)

Understanding of nutrition-related concepts and conviction of the truth and feelings/emotions toward some nutrition-related statement or phenomenon, along with readiness to change nutrition-related behaviors.

Food and nutrition knowledge (4.1)

- ❑ Area(s) and level of knowledge FH-4.1.1
- ❑ Diagnosis specific or global nutrition-related knowledge score FH-4.1.2

Beliefs and attitudes (4.2)

- ❑ Conflict with personal/family value system FH-4.2.1
- ❑ Distorted body image FH-4.2.2
- ❑ End-of-life decisions FH-4.2.3
- ❑ Motivation FH-4.2.4
- ❑ Preoccupation with food/nutrients FH-4.2.5
- ❑ Preoccupation with weight FH-4.2.6
- ❑ Readiness to change nutrition-related behaviors FH-4.2.7
- ❑ Self-efficacy FH-4.2.8
- ❑ Self-talk/cognitions FH-4.2.9
- ❑ Unrealistic nutrition-related goals FH-4.2.10
- ❑ Unscientific beliefs/attitudes FH-4.2.11
- ❑ Food preferences *(specify)* FH-4.2.12
- ❑ Emotions *(specify)* FH-4.2.13

Behavior (5)

Patient/client activities and actions, which influence achievement of nutrition-related goals.

Adherence (5.1)

- ❑ Self-reported adherence score FH-5.1.1
- ❑ Nutrition visit attendance FH-5.1.2
- ❑ Ability to recall nutrition goals FH-5.1.3
- ❑ Self-monitoring at agreed upon rate FH-5.1.4
- ❑ Self-management as agreed upon FH-5.1.5

Avoidance behavior (5.2)

- ❑ Avoidance FH-5.2.1
- ❑ Restrictive eating FH-5.2.2
- ❑ Cause of avoidance behavior FH-5.2.3

3rd Edition

APPENDIX 5. Focus on Nutrition Care Process: Nutrition Assessment—cont'd

Nutrition Assessment and Monitoring and Evaluation Terminology, cont'd

Bingeing and purging behavior (5.3)
- ❑ Binge eating behavior FH-5.3.1
- ❑ Purging behavior FH-5.3.2

Mealtime behavior (5.4)
- ❑ Meal duration FH-5.4.1
- ❑ Percent of meal time spent eating FH-5.4.2
- ❑ Preference to drink rather than eat FH-5.4.3
- ❑ Refusal to eat/chew FH-5.4.4
- ❑ Spitting food out FH-5.4.5
- ❑ Rumination FH-5.4.6
- ❑ Patient/client/caregiver fatigue during feeding process resulting in inadequate intake FH-5.4.7
- ❑ Willingness to try new foods FH-5.4.8
- ❑ Limited number of accepted foods FH-5.4.9
- ❑ Rigid sensory preferences FH-5.4.10

Social network (5.5)
- ❑ Ability to build and utilize social network FH-5.5.1

Factors Affecting Access to Food and Food/Nutrition-Related Supplies (6)
Factors that affect intake and availability of a sufficient quantity of safe, healthful food as well as food/nutrition-related supplies.

Food/nutrition program participation (6.1)
- ❑ Eligibility for government programs FH-6.1.1
- ❑ Participation in government programs FH-6.1.2
- ❑ Eligibility for community programs FH-6.1.3
- ❑ Participation in community programs FH-6.1.4

Safe food/meal availability (6.2)
- ❑ Availability of shopping facilities FH-6.2.1
- ❑ Procurement, identification of safe food FH-6.2.2
- ❑ Appropriate meal preparation facilities FH-6.2.3
- ❑ Availability of safe food storage FH-6.2.4
- ❑ Appropriate storage technique FH-6.2.5

Safe water availability (6.3)
- ❑ Availability of potable water FH-6.3.1
- ❑ Appropriate water decontamination FH-6.3.2

Food and nutrition-related supplies availability (6.4)
- ❑ Access to food and nutrition-related supplies FH-6.4.1
- ❑ Access to assistive eating devices FH-6.4.2
- ❑ Access to assistive food preparation devices FH 6.4.3

Physical Activity and Function (7)
Physical activity, cognitive and physical ability to engage in specific tasks, e.g., breastfeeding, self-feeding.

Breastfeeding (7.1)
- ❑ Initiation of breastfeeding FH-7.1.1
- ❑ Duration of breastfeeding FH-7.1.2
- ❑ Exclusive breastfeeding FH-7.1.3
- ❑ Breastfeeding problems FH-7.1.4

Nutrition-related ADLs and IADLs (7.2)
- ❑ Physical ability to complete tasks for meal preparation FH-7.2.1
- ❑ Physical ability to self-feed FH-7.2.2
- ❑ Ability to position self in relation to plate FH-7.2.3
- ❑ Receives assistance with intake FH 7.2.4
- ❑ Ability to use adaptive eating devices FH 7.2.5
- ❑ Cognitive ability to complete tasks for meal preparation FH-7.2.6
- ❑ Remembers to eat, recalls eating FH-7.2.7
- ❑ Mini Mental State Examination Score FH-7.2.8
- ❑ Nutrition-related activities of daily living (ADL) score FH-7.2.9
- ❑ Nutrition-related instrumental activities of daily living (IADL) score FH-7.2.10

Physical activity (7.3)
- ❑ Physical activity history FH-7.3.1
- ❑ Consistency FH-7.3.2
- ❑ Frequency FH-7.3.3
- ❑ Duration FH-7.3.4
- ❑ Intensity FH-7.3.5
- ❑ Type of physical activity FH-7.3.6
- ❑ Strength FH-7.3.7
- ❑ TV/screen time FH-7.3.8
- ❑ Other sedentary activity time FH-7.3.9
- ❑ Involuntary physical movement FH-7.3.10
- ❑ NEAT FH-7.3.11

Nutrition-Related Patient/Client-Centered Measures (8)
Patient/client's perception of his or her nutrition intervention and its impact on life.

Nutrition quality of life (8.1)
- ❑ Nutrition quality of life responses FH-8.1.1

ANTHROPOMETRIC MEASUREMENTS (AD)
Height, weight, body mass index (BMI), growth pattern indices/percentile ranks, and weight history.

Body composition/growth/weight history (1.1)
- ❑ Height/length AD-1.1.1
- ❑ Weight AD-1.1.2
- ❑ Frame size AD-1.1.3
- ❑ Weight change AD-1.1.4
- ❑ Body mass index AD-1.1.5
- ❑ Growth pattern indices/percentile ranks AD-1.1.6
- ❑ Body compartment estimates AD-1.1.7

BIOCHEMICAL DATA, MEDICAL TESTS AND PROCEDURES (BD)
Laboratory data, (e.g., electrolytes, glucose, and lipid panel) and tests (e.g., gastric emptying time, resting metabolic rate).

Acid-base balance (1.1)
- ❑ Arterial pH BD-1.1.1
- ❑ Arterial bicarbonate BD-1.1.2
- ❑ Partial pressure of carbon dioxide in arterial blood, $PaCO_2$ BD-1.1.3
- ❑ Partial pressure of oxygen in arterial blood, PaO_2 BD-1.1.4
- ❑ Venous pH BD-1.1.5
- ❑ Venous bicarbonate BD-1.1.6

Electrolyte and renal profile (1.2)
- ❑ BUN BD-1.2.1
- ❑ Creatinine BD-1.2.2
- ❑ BUN:creatinine ratio BD-1.2.3
- ❑ Glomerular filtration rate BD-1.2.4
- ❑ Sodium BD-1.2.5
- ❑ Chloride BD-1.2.6
- ❑ Potassium BD-1.2.7
- ❑ Magnesium BD-1.2.8
- ❑ Calcium, serum BD-1.2.9
- ❑ Calcium, ionized BD-1.2.10
- ❑ Phosphorus BD-1.2.11
- ❑ Serum osmolality BD-1.2.12
- ❑ Parathyroid hormone BD-1.2.13

Essential fatty acid profile (1.3)
- ❑ Triene:Tetraene ratio BD-1.3.1

Gastrointestinal profile (1.4)
- ❑ Alkaline phophatase BD-1.4.1
- ❑ Alanine aminotransferase, ALT BD-1.4.2
- ❑ Aspartate aminotransferase, AST BD-1.4.3
- ❑ Gamma glutamyl transferase, GGT BD-1.4.4
- ❑ Gastric residual volume BD-1.4.5
- ❑ Bilirubin, total BD-1.4.6
- ❑ Ammonia, serum BD-1.4.7
- ❑ Toxicology report, including alcohol BD-1.4.8
- ❑ Prothrombin time, PT BD-1.4.9
- ❑ Partial thromboplastin time, PTT BD-1.4.10
- ❑ INR (ratio) BD-1.4.11
- ❑ Fecal fat BD-1.4.12
- ❑ Amylase BD-1.4.13
- ❑ Lipase BD-1.4.14
- ❑ Other digestive enzymes (*specify*) BD-1.4.15
- ❑ D-xylose BD-1.4.16
- ❑ Hydrogen breath test BD-1.4.17
- ❑ Intestinal biopsy BD-1.4.18
- ❑ Stool culture BD-1.4.19
- ❑ Gastric emptying time BD-1.4.20
- ❑ Small bowel transit time BD-1.4.21
- ❑ Abdominal films BD-1.4.22
- ❑ Swallow study BD-1.4.23

Glucose/endocrine profile (1.5)
- ❑ Glucose, fasting BD-1.5.1
- ❑ Glucose, casual BD-1.5.2
- ❑ HgbA1c BD-1.5.3
- ❑ Preprandial capillary plasma glucose BD-1.5.4
- ❑ Peak postprandial capillary plasma glucose BD-1.5.5
- ❑ Glucose tolerance test BD-1.5.6
- ❑ Cortisol level BD-1.5.7
- ❑ IGF-binding protein BD-1.5.8
- ❑ Thyroid function tests (TSH, T4, T3) BD-1.5.9

Inflammatory profile (1.6)
- ❑ C-reactive protein BD-1.6.1

Lipid profile (1.7)
- ❑ Cholesterol, serum BD-1.7.1
- ❑ Cholesterol, HDL BD-1.7.2
- ❑ Cholesterol, LDL BD-1.7.3
- ❑ Cholesterol, non-HDL BD-1.7.4
- ❑ Total cholesterol:HDL cholesterol BD-1.7.5
- ❑ LDL:HDL BD-1.7.6
- ❑ Triglycerides, serum BD-1.7.7

Metabolic rate profile (1.8)
- ❑ Resting metabolic rate, measured BD-1.8.1
- ❑ RQ BD-1.8.2

Mineral profile (1.9)
- ❑ Copper, serum or plasma BD-1.9.1
- ❑ Iodine, urinary excretion BD-1.9.2
- ❑ Zinc, serum or plasma BD-1.9.3
- ❑ Other BD-1.9.4

Nutritional anemia profile (1.10)
- ❑ Hemoglobin BD-1.10.1
- ❑ Hematocrit BD-1.10.2
- ❑ Mean corpuscular volume BD-1.10.3
- ❑ Red blood cell folate BD-1.10.4
- ❑ Red cell distribution width BD-1.10.5
- ❑ B12, serum BD-1.10.6
- ❑ Methylmalonic acid, serum BD-1.10.7
- ❑ Folate, serum BD-1.10.8
- ❑ Homocysteine, serum BD-1.10.9
- ❑ Ferritin, serum BD-1.10.10
- ❑ Iron, serum BD-1.10.11
- ❑ Total iron-binding capacity BD-1.10.12
- ❑ Transferrin saturation BD-1.10.13

3rd Edition

Assessment & Montioring & Evaluation

Continued

APPENDIX 5. Focus on Nutrition Care Process: Nutrition Assessment—cont'd

Nutrition Assessment and Monitoring and Evaluation Terminology, cont'd

Protein profile (1.11)

❑ Albumin	BD-1.11.1
❑ Prealbumin	BD-1.11.2
❑ Transferrin	BD-1.11.3
❑ Phenylalanine, plasma	BD-1.11.4
❑ Tyrosine, plasma	BD-1.11.5
❑ Amino acid, other, specify	BD-1.11.6
❑ Antibody level, specify	BD-1.11.7

Urine profile (1.12)

❑ Urine color	BD-1.12.1
❑ Urine osmolality	BD-1.12.2
❑ Urine specific gravity	BD-1.12.3
❑ Urine test, specify	BD-1.12.4
❑ Urine volume	BD-1.12.5

Vitamin profile (1.13)

❑ Vitamin A, serum or plasma retinol	BD-1.13.1
❑ Vitamin C, plasma or serum	BD-1.13.2
❑ Vitamin D, 25-hydroxy	BD-1.13.3
❑ Vitamin E, plasma alpha-tocopherol	BD-1.13.4
❑ Thiamin, activity coefficient for erythrocyte transketolase activity	BD-1.13.5
❑ Riboflavin, activity coefficient for erythrocyte glutathione reductase activity	BD-1.13.6
❑ Niacin, urinary N'methyl-nicotinamide concentration	BD-1.13.7
❑ Vitamin B6, plasma or serum pyridoxal 5'phosphate concentration	BD-1.13.8
❑ Other	BD-1.13.9

NUTRITION-FOCUSED PHYSICAL FINDINGS (PD)

Findings from an evaluation of body systems, muscle and subcutaneous fat wasting, oral health, suck/swallow/breathe ability, appetite, and affect.

Nutrition-focused physical findings (1.1)

❑ Overall appearance (*specify*) ________	PD-1.1.1
❑ Body language (*specify*) ________	PD-1.1.2
❑ Cardiovascular-pulmonary (*specify*) ________	PD-1.1.3
❑ Extremities, muscles and bones (*specify*) ________	PD-1.1.4
❑ Digestive system (mouth to rectum) (*specify*) ________	PD-1.1.5
❑ Head and eyes (*specify*) ________	PD-1.1.6
❑ Nerves and cognition (*specify*) ________	PD-1.1.7
❑ Skin (*specify*) ________	PD-1.1.8
❑ Vital signs (*specify*) ________	PD-1.1.9

CLIENT HISTORY (CH)

Current and past information related to personal, medical, family, and social history.

Personal History (1)

General patient/client information such as age, gender, race/ethnicity, language, education, and role in family.

Personal data (1.1)

❑ Age	CH-1.1.1
❑ Gender	CH-1.1.2
❑ Race/Ethnicity	CH-1.1.3
❑ Language	CH-1.1.4
❑ Literacy factors	CH-1.1.5
❑ Education	CH-1.1.6
❑ Role in family	CH-1.1.7
❑ Tobacco use	CH-1.1.8

Personal data (1.1), cont'd

❑ Physical disability	CH-1.1.9
❑ Mobility	CH-1.1.10

Patient/Client/Family Medical/Health History (2)

Patient/client or family disease states, conditions, and illnesses that may have nutritional impact.

Patient/client OR family nutrition-oriented medical/health history (2.1)

Specify issue(s) and whether it is patient/client history (P) or family history (F)

❑ Patient/client chief nutrition complaint (*specify*) ________	CH-2.1.1	P or F
❑ Cardiovascular (*specify*) ________	CH-2.1.2	P or F
❑ Endocrine/metabolism (*specify*) ________	CH-2.1.3	P or F
❑ Excretory (*specify*) ________	CH-2.1.4	P or F
❑ Gastrointestinal (*specify*) ________	CH-2.1.5	P or F
❑ Gynecological (*specify*) ________	CH-2.1.6	P or F
❑ Hematology/oncology (*specify*) ________	CH-2.1.7	P or F
❑ Immune (e.g., food allergies) (*specify*) ________	CH-2.1.8	P or F
❑ Integumentary (*specify*) ________	CH-2.1.9	P or F
❑ Musculoskeletal (*specify*) ________	CH-2.1.10	P or F
❑ Neurological (*specify*) ________	CH-2.1.11	P or F
❑ Psychological (*specify*) ________	CH-2.1.12	P or F
❑ Respiratory (*specify*) ________	CH-2.1.13	P or F
❑ Other (*specify*) ________	CH-2.1.14	P or F

Treatments/therapy/complementary/alternative medicine (2.2)

Documented medical or surgical treatments, complementary and alternative medicine that may impact nutritional status of the patient

❑ Medical treatment/therapy (*specify*) ________	CH-2.2.1
❑ Surgical treatment (*specify*) ________	CH-2.2.2
❑ Complementary/alternative medicine (*specify*) ________	CH-2.2.3
❑ Palliative/end-of-life care (*specify*) ________	CH-2.2.4

Social History (3)

Patient/client socioeconomic status, housing situation, medical care support and involvement in social groups.

Social history (3.1)

❑ Socioeconomic factors (*specify*) ________	CH-3.1.1
❑ Living/housing situation (*specify*) ________	CH-3.1.2
❑ Domestic issues (*specify*) ________	CH-3.1.3
❑ Social and medical support (*specify*) ________	CH-3.1.4
❑ Geographic location of home (*specify*) ________	CH-3.1.5
❑ Occupation (*specify*) ________	CH-3.1.6
❑ Religion (*specify*) ________	CH-3.1.7

Social history (3.1), cont'd

❑ History of recent crisis (*specify*) ________	CH-3.1.8
❑ Daily stress level	CH-3.1.9

COMPARATIVE STANDARDS (CS)

Energy Needs (1)

Estimated energy needs (1.1)

❑ Total energy estimated needs	CS-1.1.1
❑ Method for estimating needs	CS-1.1.2

Macronutrient Needs (2)

Estimated fat needs (2.1)

❑ Total fat estimated needs	CS-2.1.1
❑ Type of fat needed	CS-2.1.2
❑ Method for estimating needs	CS-2.1.3

Estimated protein needs (2.2)

❑ Total protein estimated needs	CS-2.2.1
❑ Type of protein needed	CS-2.2.2
❑ Method for estimating needs	CS-2.2.3

Estimated carbohydrate needs (2.3)

❑ Total carbohydrate estimated needs	CS-2.3.1
❑ Type of carbohydrate needed	CS-2.3.2
❑ Method for estimating needs	CS-2.3.3

Estimated fiber needs (2.4)

❑ Total fiber estimated needs	CS-2.4.1
❑ Type of fiber needed	CS-2.4.2
❑ Method for estimating needs	CS-2.4.3

Fluid Needs (3)

Estimated fluid needs (3.1)

❑ Total fluid estimated needs	CS-3.1.1
❑ Method for estimating needs	CS-3.1.2

Micronutrient Needs (4)

Estimated vitamin needs (4.1)

❑ A (1)	❑ Riboflavin (7)
❑ C (2)	❑ Niacin (8)
❑ D (3)	❑ Folate (9)
❑ E (4)	❑ B6 (10)
❑ K (5)	❑ B12 (11)
❑ Thiamin (6)	

❑ Other (*specify*) (12)
❑ Method for estimating needs (13)

Estimated mineral needs (4.2)

❑ Calcium (1)	❑ Potassium (5)
❑ Chloride (2)	❑ Phosphorus (6)
❑ Iron (3)	❑ Sodium (7)
❑ Magnesium (4)	❑ Zinc (8)

❑ Other (*specify*) (9)
❑ Method for estimating needs (10)

Weight and Growth Recommendation (5)

Recommended body weight/body mass Index/growth (5.1)

❑ Ideal/reference body weight (IBW)	CS-5.1.1
❑ Recommended body mass index (BMI)	CS-5.1.2
❑ Desired growth pattern	CS-5.1.3

Assessment & Montioring & Evaluation

3rd Edition

APPENDIX 6. Focus on Nutrition Care Process: Nutrition Diagnosis

Step 2. Nutrition diagnosis is designed to identify and describe a specific nutrition problem that can be resolved or improved through intervention by a registered dietitian (RD). Unlike a medical diagnosis, a nutrition diagnosis often can be resolved. RDs use the data collected in the nutrition assessment to identify the patient's or client's nutrition diagnosis using standard terminology. The specific definition, possible causes, and common signs or symptoms are identified in this care process step. Nutrition diagnoses are organized into three categories:

Intake	Clinical	Behavioral-Environmental
Too much or too little of a food or nutrient compared with actual or estimated needs	Nutrition problems that relate to medical or physical conditions	Knowledge, attitudes, beliefs, physical environment, access to food, or food safety

The nutrition diagnosis is written as a problem, etiology, and sign and symptoms (PES) statement to describe the problem, its root cause, and the signs and symptoms (assessment data) that provide evidence for that nutrition diagnosis. The PES statement is "Nutrition problem label related to ___________ as evidenced by ____________."

(P) Problem (nutrition diagnosis)	(E) Etiology: Cause and Contributing Risk Factors	(S) Signs and Symptoms
Describes alterations in the patient's or client's nutrition status.	Linked to the nutrition diagnosis label by the words "related to."	Data used to determine that the patient or client has the nutrition diagnosis specified; linked to the etiology by the words "as evidenced by."

APPENDIX 6. Focus on Nutrition Care Process: Nutrition Diagnosis—cont'd

Nutrition DiagnosticTerminology

INTAKE NI

Defined as "actual problems related to intake of energy, nutrients, fluids, bioactive substances through oral diet or nutrition support"

Energy Balance (1)

Defined as "actual or estimated changes in energy (kcal) balance"

- ❑ Unused NI-1.1
- ❑ Increased energy expenditure NI-1.2
- ❑ Unused NI-1.3
- ❑ Inadequate energy intake NI-1.4
- ❑ Excessive energy intake NI-1.5
- ❑ Predicted suboptimal energy intake NI-1.6
- ❑ Predicted excessive energy intake NI-1.7

Oral or Nutrition Support Intake (2)

Defined as "actual or estimated food and beverage intake from oral diet or nutrition support compared with patient goal"

- ❑ Inadequate oral intake NI-2.1
- ❑ Excessive oral intake NI-2.2
- ❑ Inadequate enteral nutrition infusion NI-2.3
- ❑ Excessive enteral nutrition infusion NI-2.4
- ❑ Less than optimal enteral nutrition NI-2.5
- ❑ Inadequate parenteral nutrition infusion NI-2.6
- ❑ Excessive parenteral nutrition infusion NI-2.7
- ❑ Less than optimal parenteral nutrition NI-2.8
- ❑ Limited food acceptance NI-2.9

Fluid Intake (3)

Defined as "actual or estimated fluid intake compared with patient goal"

- ❑ Inadequate fluid intake NI-3.1
- ❑ Excessive fluid intake NI-3.2

Bioactive Substances (4)

Defined as "actual or observed intake of bioactive substances, including single or multiple functional food components, ingredients, dietary supplements, alcohol"

- ❑ Inadequate bioactive substance intake NI-4.1
- ❑ Excessive bioactive substance intake NI-4.2
- ❑ Excessive alcohol intake NI-4.3

Nutrient (5)

Defined as "actual or estimated intake of specific nutrient groups or single nutrients as compared with desired levels"

- ❑ Increased nutrient needs (*specify*) ____________ NI-5.1
- ❑ Malnutrition NI-5.2
- ❑ Inadequate protein-energy intake NI-5.3
- ❑ Decreased nutrient needs (*specify*) ____________ NI-5.4
- ❑ Imbalance of nutrients NI-5.5

Fat and Cholesterol (5.6)

- ❑ Inadequate fat intake NI-5.6.1
- ❑ Excessive fat intake NI-5.6.2
- ❑ Inappropriate intake of fats (*specify*) ____________ NI-5.6.3

Protein (5.7)

- ❑ Inadequate protein intake NI-5.7.1
- ❑ Excessive protein intake NI-5.7.2
- ❑ Inappropriate intake of protein or amino acids (*specify*) ____________ NI-5.7.3

Carbohydrate and Fiber (5.8)

- ❑ Inadequate carbohydrate intake NI-5.8.1
- ❑ Excessive carbohydrate intake NI-5.8.2
- ❑ Inappropriate intake of types of carbohydrate (*specify*) ____________ NI-5.8.3
- ❑ Inconsistent carbohydrate intake NI-5.8.4
- ❑ Inadequate fiber intake NI-5.8.5
- ❑ Excessive fiber intake NI-5.8.6

Vitamin (5.9)

- ❑ Inadequate vitamin intake (*specify*) ____________ NI-5.9.1
  - ❑ A (1) ❑ Riboflavin (7)
  - ❑ C (2) ❑ Niacin (8)
  - ❑ D (3) ❑ Folate (9)
  - ❑ E (4) ❑ B6 (10)
  - ❑ K (5) ❑ B12 (11)
  - ❑ Thiamin (6)
  - ❑ Other (*specify*) ____________ (12)
- ❑ Excessive vitamin intake (*specify*) ____________ NI-5.9.2
  - ❑ A (1) ❑ Riboflavin (7)
  - ❑ C (2) ❑ Niacin (8)
  - ❑ D (3) ❑ Folate (9)
  - ❑ E (4) ❑ B6 (10)
  - ❑ K (5) ❑ B12 (11)
  - ❑ Thiamin (6)
  - ❑ Other (*specify*) ____________ (12)

Mineral (5.10)

- ❑ Inadequate mineral intake (*specify*) ____________ NI-5.10.1
  - ❑ Calcium (1) ❑ Potassium (5)
  - ❑ Chloride (2) ❑ Phosphorus (6)
  - ❑ Iron (3) ❑ Sodium (7)
  - ❑ Magnesium (4) ❑ Zinc (8)
  - ❑ Other (*specify*) ____________ (9)
- ❑ Excessive mineral intake (*specify*) ____________ NI-5.10.2
  - ❑ Calcium (1) ❑ Potassium (5)
  - ❑ Chloride (2) ❑ Phosphorus (6)
  - ❑ Iron (3) ❑ Sodium (7)
  - ❑ Magnesium (4) ❑ Zinc (8)
  - ❑ Other (*specify*) ____________ (9)

Multi-nutrient (5.11)

- ❑ Predicted suboptimal nutrient intake NI-5.11.1
- ❑ Predicted excessive nutrient intake NI-5.11.2

CLINICAL NC

Defined as "nutritional findings/problems identified that relate to medical or physical conditions"

Functional (1)

Defined as "change in physical or mechanical functioning that interferes with or prevents desired nutritional consequences"

- ❑ Swallowing difficulty NC-1.1
- ❑ Biting/Chewing (masticatory) difficulty NC-1.2
- ❑ Breastfeeding difficulty NC-1.3
- ❑ Altered GI function NC-1.4

Biochemical (2)

Defined as "change in capacity to metabolize nutrients as a result of medications, surgery, or as indicated by altered lab values"

- ❑ Impaired nutrient utilization NC-2.1
- ❑ Altered nutrition-related laboratory values (specify) ____________ NC-2.2
- ❑ Food–medication interaction NC-2.3
- ❑ Predicted food–medication interaction NC-2.4

Weight (3)

Defined as "chronic weight or changed weight status when compared with usual or desired body weight"

- ❑ Underweight NC-3.1
- ❑ Unintended weight loss NC-3.2
- ❑ Overweight/obesity NC-3.3
- ❑ Unintended weight gain NC-3.4

BEHAVIORAL-ENVIRONMENTAL NB

Defined as "nutritional findings/problems identified that relate to knowledge, attitudes/beliefs, physical environment, access to food, or food safety"

Knowledge and Beliefs (1)

Defined as "actual knowledge and beliefs as related, observed, or documented"

- ❑ Food- and nutrition-related knowledge deficit NB-1.1
- ❑ Harmful beliefs/attitudes about food- or nutrition-related topics (use with caution) NB-1.2
- ❑ Not ready for diet/lifestyle change NB-1.3
- ❑ Self-monitoring deficit NB-1.4
- ❑ Disordered eating pattern NB-1.5
- ❑ Limited adherence to nutrition-related recommendations NB-1.6
- ❑ Undesirable food choices NB-1.7

Physical Activity and Function (2)

Defined as "actual physical activity, self-care, and quality-of-life problems as reported, observed, or documented"

- ❑ Physical inactivity NB-2.1
- ❑ Excessive physical activity NB-2.2
- ❑ Inability or lack of desire to manage self-care NB-2.3
- ❑ Impaired ability to prepare foods/meals NB-2.4
- ❑ Poor nutrition quality of life NB-2.5
- ❑ Self-feeding difficulty NB-2.6

Food Safety and Access (3)

Defined as "actual problems with food safety or access to food, water, or nutrition-related supplies"

- ❑ Intake of unsafe food NB-3.1
- ❑ Limited access to food or water NB-3.2
- ❑ Limited access to nutrition-related supplies NB-3.3

APPENDIX 7. Focus on Nutrition Care Process: Nutrition Intervention

Step 3. Nutrition interventions are designed for the registered dietitian and team members to resolve or improve the identified nutrition diagnosis by planning and implementing appropriately tailored actions. Selection of a nutrition intervention is related to the **cause** of the nutrition problem. Intervention strategies are purposefully selected to change nutritional intake, nutrition-related knowledge or behavior, risk factors, environmental conditions, or access to supportive care and services. Intervention goals provide the basis for monitoring progress and measuring outcomes. Interventions are organized into four categories:

Food and Nutrient Delivery	Nutrition Education	Nutrition Counseling	Coordination of Nutrition Care
An individualized approach for food and nutrient provision, including meals and snacks, enteral and parenteral feeding, and supplements	A formal process to instruct or train a patient or client in a skill or to impart knowledge to help them voluntarily manage or modify food choices and eating behavior to maintain or improve health	A supportive process, characterized by a collaborative counselor-patient relationship, to set priorities, establish goals, and create individualized action plans that acknowledge and foster responsibility for self-care to treat an existing condition and promote health	Consultation with, referral to, or coordination of nutrition care with other health care providers, institutions, or agencies that can assist in treating or managing nutrition-related problems

The two distinct and interrelated processes of intervention include:

Planning: Prioritizing nutrition diagnoses; consulting the American Dietetic Association's medical nutrition therapy evidence-based guides and other practice guides; determining patient-focused expected outcomes for each nutrition diagnosis; conferring with patient or client and caregivers; defining an intervention plan and strategies; defining time and frequency of care; identifying resources needed.

Implementation: Communicating the nutrition care plan; carrying out the plan; collecting data, documenting, and modifying the plan based on goals and progress.

APPENDIX 7. Focus on Nutrition Care Process: Nutrition Intervention—cont'd

Nutrition Intervention Terminology

Nutrition Prescription
The patient/client's individualized recommended dietary intake of energy and/or selected foods or nutrients based on current reference standards and dietary guidelines and the patient/client's health condition and nutrition diagnosis (*specify*).

____
____
____

FOOD AND/OR NUTRIENT DELIVERY — ND

Meal and Snacks (1)
Regular eating event (meal); food served between regular meals (snack).
- ❑ General/healthful diet — ND-1.1
- ❑ Modify distribution, type, or amount of food and nutrients within meals or at specified time — ND-1.2
- ❑ Specific foods/beverages or groups — ND-1.3
- ❑ Other — ND-1.4
  (*specify*) ______________

Enteral and Parenteral Nutrition (2)
Nutrition provided through the GI tract via tube, catheter, or stoma (enteral) or intravenously (centrally or peripherally) (parenteral).

Enteral Nutrition (2.1)
Nutrition provided through the GI tract.
- ❑ Formula/solution — ND-2.1.1
- ❑ Insert enteral feeding tube — ND-2.1.2
- ❑ Site care — ND-2.1.3
- ❑ Feeding tube flush — ND-2.1.4

Parenteral Nutrition/IV Fluids (2.2)
Nutrition and fluids provided intravenously.
- ❑ Formula/solution — ND-2.2.1
- ❑ Site care — ND-2.2.2
- ❑ IV fluids — ND-2.2.3

Supplements (3)

Medical Food Supplements (3.1)
Commercial or prepared foods or beverages that supplement energy, protein, carbohydrate, fiber, fat intake.
Type
- ❑ Commercial beverage — ND-3.1.1
- ❑ Commercial food — ND-3.1.2
- ❑ Modified beverage — ND-3.1.3
- ❑ Modified food — ND-3.1.4
- ❑ Purpose — ND-3.1.5
  (*specify*) ______________

Vitamin and Mineral Supplements (3.2)
Supplemental vitamins or minerals.
- ❑ Multivitamin/mineral — ND-3.2.1
- ❑ Multi-trace elements — ND-3.2.2
- ❑ Vitamin — ND-3.2.3
  - ❑ A (1)
  - ❑ C (2)
  - ❑ D (3)
  - ❑ E (4)
  - ❑ K (5)
  - ❑ Thiamin (6)
  - ❑ Riboflavin (7)
  - ❑ Niacin (8)
  - ❑ Folate (9)
  - ❑ B6 (10)
  - ❑ B12 (11)
  - ❑ Other (*specify*) ______________ (12)
- ❑ Mineral — ND-3.2.4
  - ❑ Calcium (1)
  - ❑ Chloride (2)
  - ❑ Iron (3)
  - ❑ Magnesium (4)
  - ❑ Potassium (5)
  - ❑ Phosphorus (6)
  - ❑ Sodium (7)
  - ❑ Zinc (8)
  - ❑ Other (*specify*) ______________ (9)

Bioactive Substance Management (3.3)
Addition or change in provision of bioactive substances.
- ❑ Plant sterol and stanol esters — ND-3.3.1
- ❑ Soy protein — ND-3.3.2
- ❑ Psyllium and β-glucan — ND-3.3.3
- ❑ Food additives — ND-3.3.4
- ❑ Other — ND-3.3.5
  (*specify*) ______________

Feeding Assistance (4)
Accommodation or assistance in eating.
- ❑ Adaptive equipment — ND-4.1
- ❑ Feeding position — ND-4.2
- ❑ Meal set-up — ND-4.3
- ❑ Mouth care — ND-4.4
- ❑ Other — ND-4.5
  (*specify*) ______________

Feeding Environment (5)
Adjustment of the factors where food is served that impact food consumption.
- ❑ Lighting — ND-5.1
- ❑ Odors — ND-5.2
- ❑ Distractions — ND-5.3
- ❑ Table height — ND-5.4
- ❑ Table service/set up — ND-5.5
- ❑ Room temperature — ND-5.6
- ❑ Other — ND-5.7
  (*specify*) ______________

Nutrition-Related Medication Management (6)
Modification of a medication or herbal to optimize patient/client nutritional or health status.
- ❑ Medications — ND-6.1
  (*specify prescription or OTC*) ______________
- ❑ Herbal/complementary products — ND-6.2
  (*specify*) ______________

NUTRITION EDUCATION — E

Nutrition Education–Content (1)
Instruction or training intended to lead to nutrition-related knowledge.
- ❑ Purpose of the nutrition education — E-1.1
- ❑ Priority modifications — E-1.2
- ❑ Survival information — E-1.3
- ❑ Nutrition relationship to health/disease — E-1.4
- ❑ Recommended modifications — E-1.5
- ❑ Other or related topics — E-1.6
- ❑ Other — E-1.7
  (*specify*) ______________

Nutrition Education–Application (2)
Instruction or training leading to nutrition-related result interpretation or skills.
- ❑ Result interpretation — E-2.1
- ❑ Skill development — E-2.2
- ❑ Other — E-2.3
  (*specify*) ______________

NUTRITION COUNSELING — C

Theoretical Basis/Approach (1)
The theories or models used to design and implement an intervention.
- ❑ Cognitive-Behavioral Theory — C-1.1
- ❑ Health Belief Model — C-1.2
- ❑ Social Learning Theory — C-1.3
- ❑ Transtheoretical Model/ Stages of Change — C-1.4
- ❑ Other — C-1.5
  (*specify*) ______________

Strategies (2)
Selectively applied evidence-based methods or plans of action designed to achieve a particular goal.
- ❑ Motivational interviewing — C-2.1
- ❑ Goal setting — C-2.2
- ❑ Self-monitoring — C-2.3
- ❑ Problem solving — C-2.4
- ❑ Social support — C-2.5
- ❑ Stress management — C-2.6
- ❑ Stimulus control — C-2.7
- ❑ Cognitive restructuring — C-2.8
- ❑ Relapse prevention — C-2.9
- ❑ Rewards/contingency management — C-2.10
- ❑ Other — C-2.11
  (*specify*) ______________

COORDINATION OF NUTRITION CARE — RC

Coordination of Other Care During Nutrition Care (1)
Facilitating services with other professionals, institutions, or agencies during nutrition care.
- ❑ Team meeting — RC-1.1
- ❑ Referral to RD with different expertise — RC-1.2
- ❑ Collaboration/referral to other providers — RC-1.3
- ❑ Referral to community agencies/ programs (*specify*) ______________ — RC-1.4

Discharge and Transfer of Nutrition Care to New Setting or Provider (2)
Discharge planning and transfer of nutrition care from one level or location of care to another.
- ❑ Collaboration/referral to other providers — RC-2.1
- ❑ Referral to community agencies/ programs (*specify*) ______________ — RC-2.2

APPENDIX 8. Focus on Nutrition Care Process: Nutrition Monitoring and Evaluation

Step 4. Nutrition monitoring and evaluation is the step designed to determine the amount of progress made and whether goals are being met. Nutrition monitoring and evaluation tracks patient or client outcomes relevant to the nutrition diagnosis and intervention plans and goals. Nutrition care outcomes—the desired results of nutrition care—have been defined, and specific indicators that can be measured and with reference standards or norms have been identified. The aim is to promote uniformity in assessing the effectiveness of nutrition intervention.

What to Measure

Selection of the appropriate nutrition care indicators is determined by the nutrition diagnosis, its causes and signs or symptoms, and the nutrition intervention used. The medical diagnosis and health care outcome goals and quality management goals for nutrition also influence which nutrition care outcome indicators are chosen. Other factors such as practice setting, patient or client population, and disease state and severity also affect the indicator selection. Outcomes for nutrition monitoring and evaluation are organized into four categories.

Food/Nutrition-Related History Outcomes	Anthropometric Measurement Outcomes	Biochemical Data, Medical Tests, and Procedure Outcomes	Nutrition-Focused Physical Finding Outcomes
Patient's or client's food and nutrient intake	Patient's or client's anthropometric, biochemical, and physical examination parameters	Patient's or client's lab data (e.g., electrolytes, glucose) and tests (e.g., gastric emptying time, resting metabolic rate)	Patient's or client's physical appearance, muscle and fat wasting, swallow function, appetite, and affect

Monitor, Measure, and Evaluate: Monitor the patient's or client's progress: determine whether the nutrition intervention is being implemented and provide evidence that the nutrition intervention is or is not changing the client's behavior or status. Measure the outcomes by selecting the appropriate nutrition care outcome indicators. Evaluate and compare the patient's current findings or indicator with previous status, nutrition intervention goals, and reference standards (i.e., criteria). See Appendix 5 for terms used in monitoring and evaluation.

APPENDIX 9. Birth to 24 Months: Boys Length-for-Age and Weight-for-Age Percentiles

Birth to 24 months: Boys
Length-for-age and Weight-for-age percentiles

NAME ______________________

RECORD # ______________

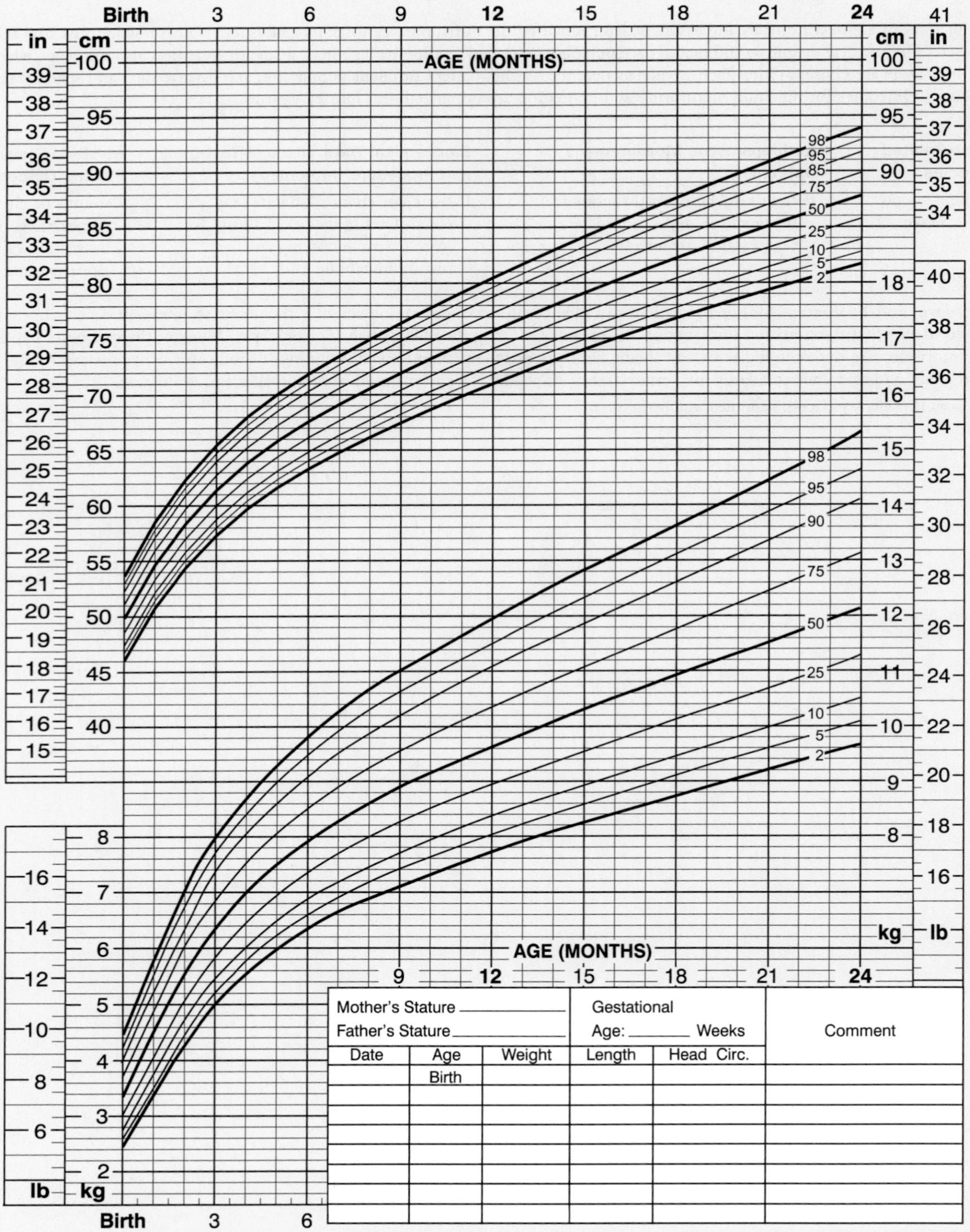

AGE (MONTHS): Birth, 3, 6, 9, 12, 15, 18, 21, 24

LENGTH (cm): 40–100; (in): 15–41

Length percentiles: 98, 95, 85, 75, 50, 25, 10, 5, 2

WEIGHT (kg): 2–18; (lb): 6–40

Weight percentiles: 98, 95, 90, 75, 50, 25, 10, 5, 2

Mother's Stature ______			Gestational		Comment
Father's Stature ______			Age: ______ Weeks		
Date	Age	Weight	Length	Head Circ.	
	Birth				

Published by the Centers for Disease Control and Prevention, November 1, 2009
SOURCE: WHO Child Growth Standards (http://www.who.int/childgrowth/en)

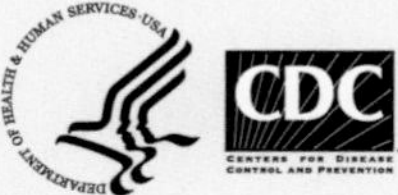

APPENDIX 10. Birth to 24 Months: Boys Head Circumference-for-Age and Weight-for-Length Percentiles

Birth to 24 months: Boys Head circumference-for-age and Weight-for-length percentiles

NAME ______________________

RECORD # ____________

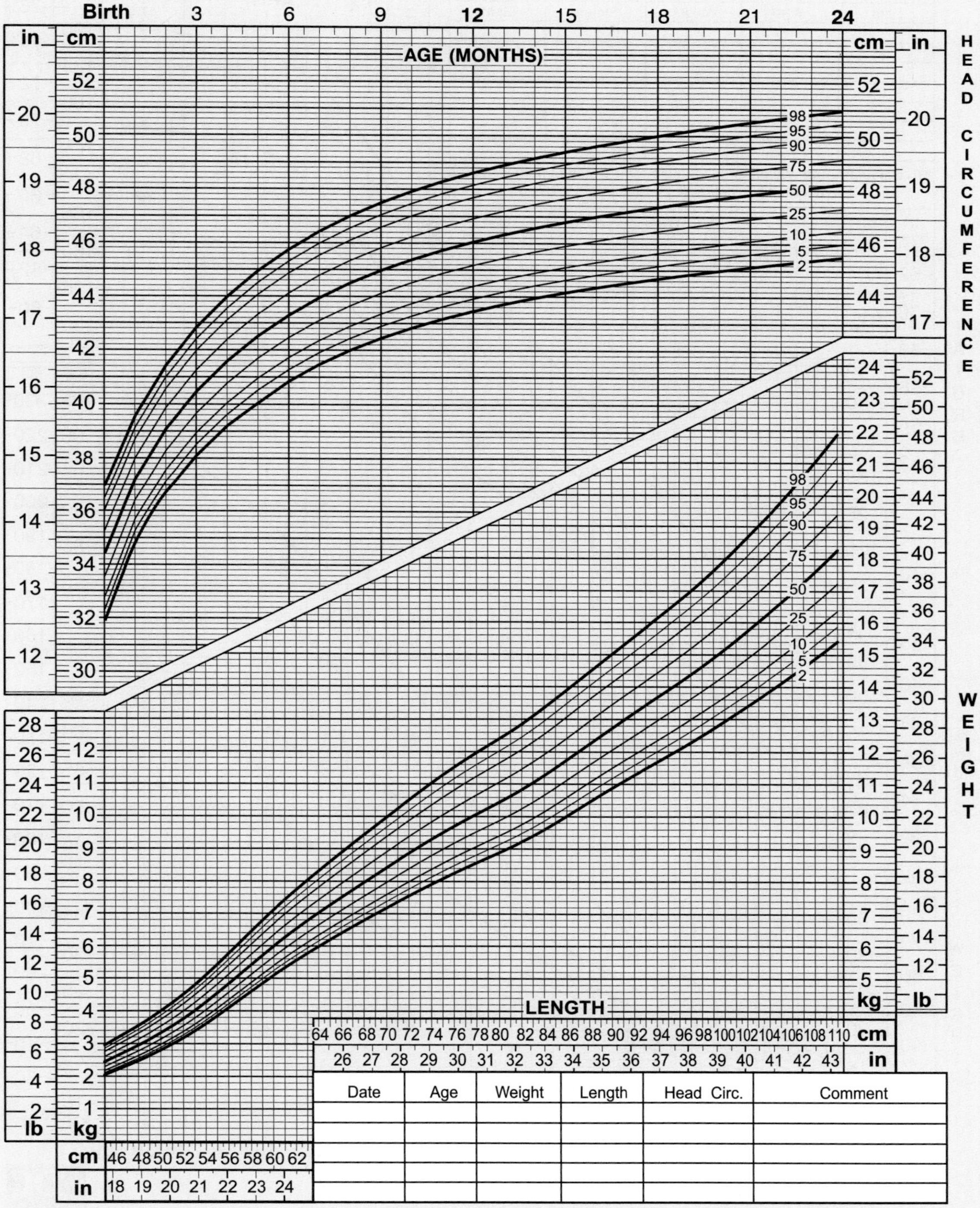

AGE (MONTHS): Birth, 3, 6, 9, 12, 15, 18, 21, 24

HEAD CIRCUMFERENCE (cm): 30, 32, 34, 36, 38, 40, 42, 44, 46, 48, 50, 52

HEAD CIRCUMFERENCE (in): 12, 13, 14, 15, 16, 17, 18, 19, 20

Percentiles: 98, 95, 90, 75, 50, 25, 10, 5, 2

WEIGHT (kg): 1, 2, 3, 4, 5, 6, 7, 8, 9, 10, 11, 12, 13, 14, 15, 16, 17, 18, 19, 20, 21, 22, 23, 24

WEIGHT (lb): 2, 4, 6, 8, 10, 12, 14, 16, 18, 20, 22, 24, 26, 28, 30, 32, 34, 36, 38, 40, 42, 44, 46, 48, 50, 52

LENGTH (cm): 46, 48, 50, 52, 54, 56, 58, 60, 62, 64, 66, 68, 70, 72, 74, 76, 78, 80, 82, 84, 86, 88, 90, 92, 94, 96, 98, 100, 102, 104, 106, 108, 110

LENGTH (in): 18, 19, 20, 21, 22, 23, 24, 26, 27, 28, 29, 30, 31, 32, 33, 34, 35, 36, 37, 38, 39, 40, 41, 42, 43

Date	Age	Weight	Length	Head Circ.	Comment

Published by the Centers for Disease Control and Prevention, November 1, 2009
SOURCE: WHO Child Growth Standards (http://www.who.int/childgrowth/en)

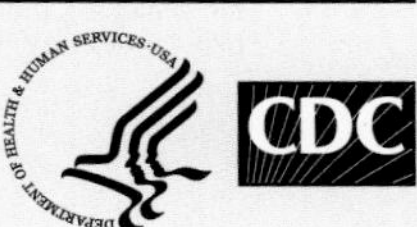

APPENDIX 11. 2 to 20 Years: Boys Stature-for-Age and Weight-for-Age Percentiles

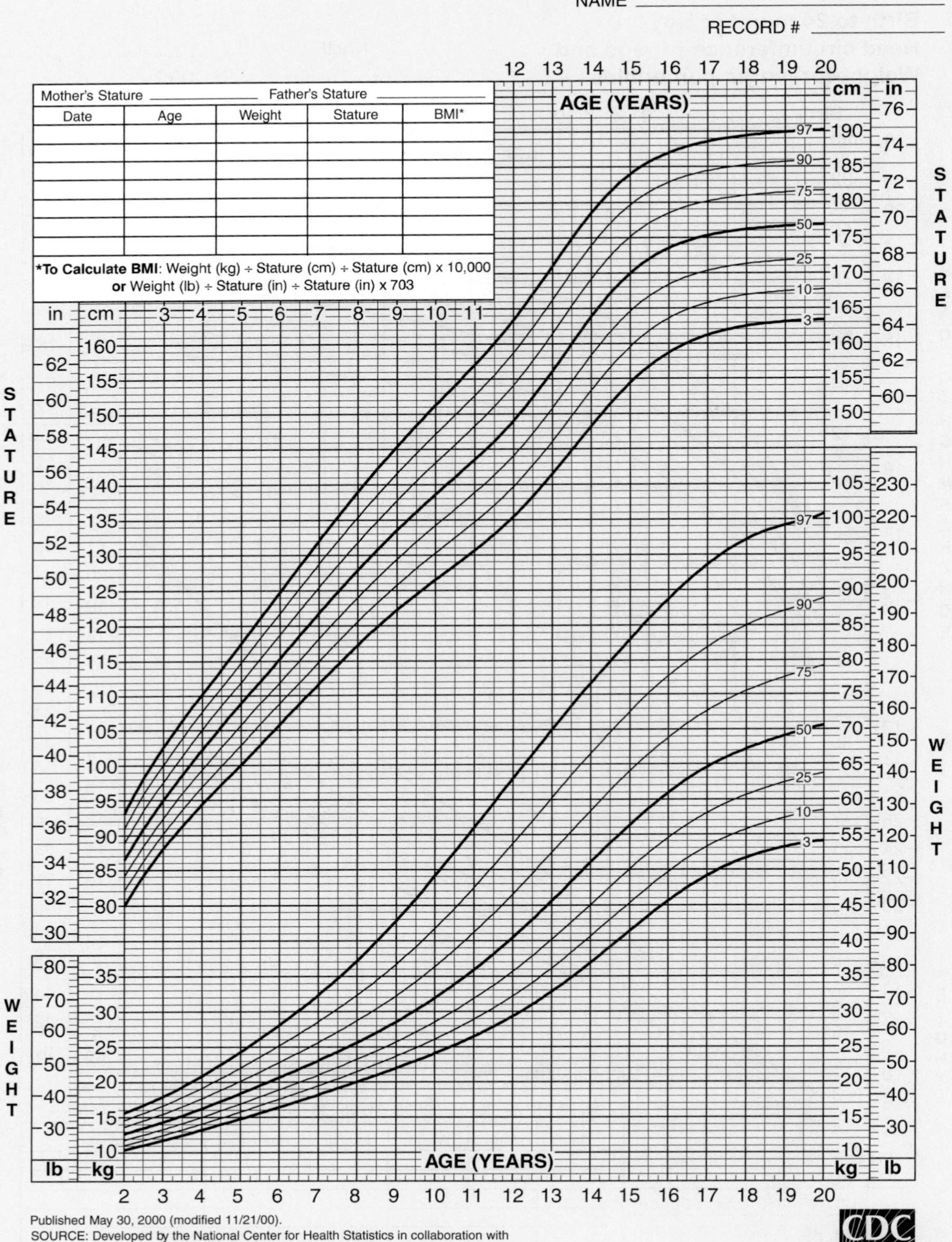

Published May 30, 2000 (modified 11/21/00).
SOURCE: Developed by the National Center for Health Statistics in collaboration with the National Center for Chronic Disease Prevention and Health Promotion (2000).
http://www.cdc.gov/growthcharts

CDC
SAFER•HEALTHIER•PEOPLE

APPENDIX 12. Body Mass Index-for-Age Percentiles: Boys, 2 to 20 Years

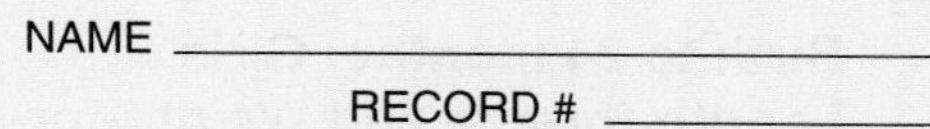

Date	Age	Weight	Stature	BMI*	Comments

***To Calculate BMI**: Weight (kg) ÷ Stature (cm) ÷ Stature (cm) x 10,000
or Weight (lb) ÷ Stature (in) ÷ Stature (in) x 703

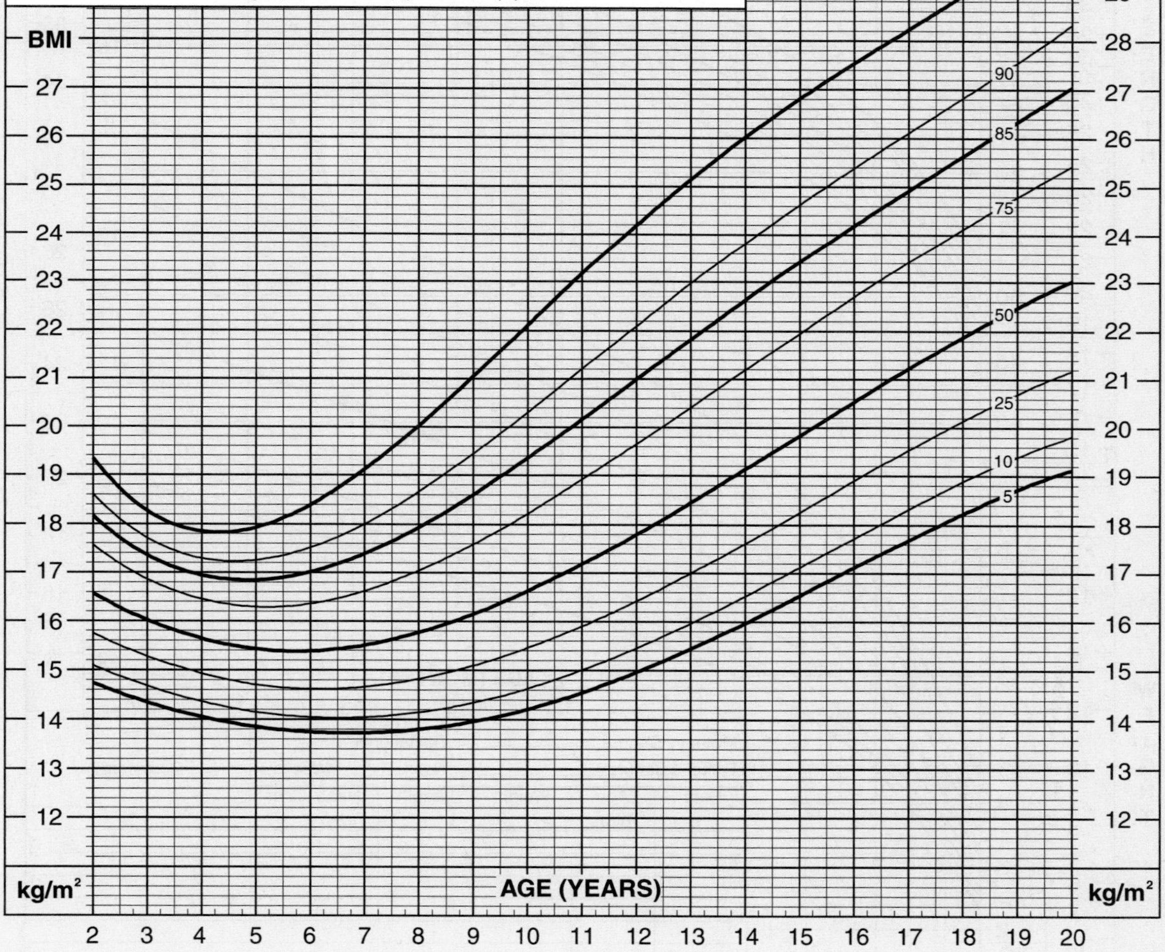

BMI
35
34
33
32
31
30
29
28
27
26
25
24
23
22
21
20
19
18
17
16
15
14
13
12
kg/m²

95
90
85
75
50
25
10
5

AGE (YEARS)
2 3 4 5 6 7 8 9 10 11 12 13 14 15 16 17 18 19 20

Published May 30, 2000 (modified 10/16/00).
SOURCE: Developed by the National Center for Health Statistics in collaboration with the National Center for Chronic Disease Prevention and Health Promotion (2000).
http://www.cdc.gov/growthcharts

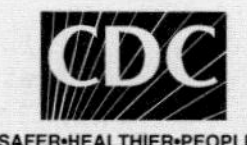

APPENDIX 13. Birth to 24 Months: Girls Length-for-Age and Weight-for-Age Percentiles

Birth to 24 months: Girls
Length-for-age and Weight-for-age percentiles

NAME ______________________

RECORD #

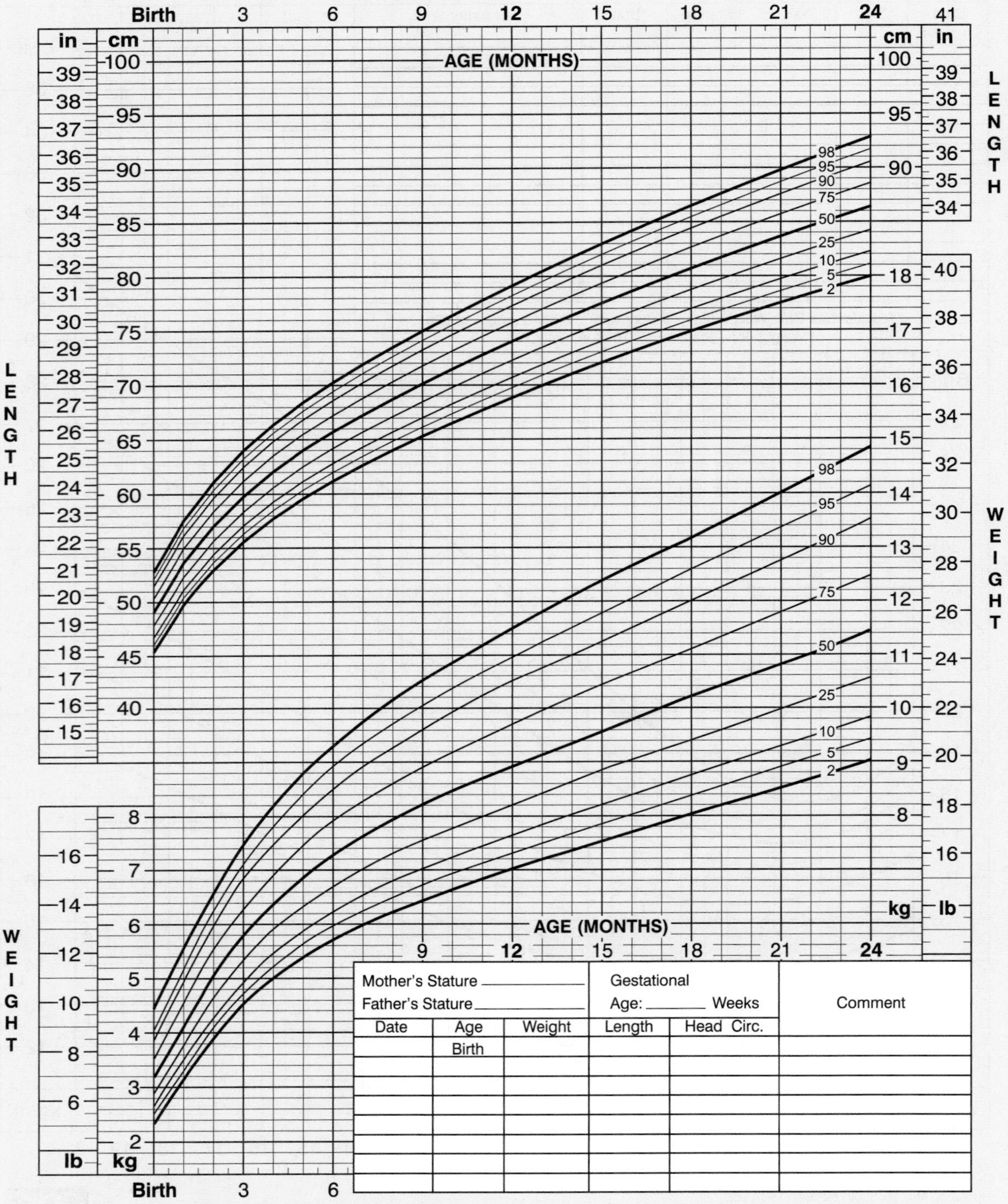

Birth 3 6 9 12 15 18 21 24

AGE (MONTHS)

LENGTH: in 15 16 17 18 19 20 21 22 23 24 25 26 27 28 29 30 31 32 33 34 35 36 37 38 39 41; cm 40 45 50 55 60 65 70 75 80 85 90 95 100

Length percentiles: 98 95 90 75 50 25 10 5 2

Weight percentiles: 98 95 90 75 50 25 10 5 2

WEIGHT: kg 2 3 4 5 6 7 8 9 10 11 12 13 14 15 16 17 18; lb 6 8 10 12 14 16 18 20 22 24 26 28 30 32 34 36 38 40

AGE (MONTHS)

Mother's Stature ______ Father's Stature ______			Gestational Age: ______ Weeks		Comment
Date	Age	Weight	Length	Head Circ.	
	Birth				

Published by the Centers for Disease Control and Prevention, November 1, 2009
SOURCE: WHO Child Growth Standards (http://www.who.int/childgrowth/en)

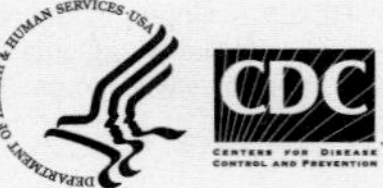

APPENDIX 14. Birth to 24 Months: Girls Head Circumference-for-Age and Weight-for-Length Percentiles

Birth to 24 months: Girls
Head circumference-for-age and
Weight-for-length percentiles

NAME ______________________

RECORD # __________

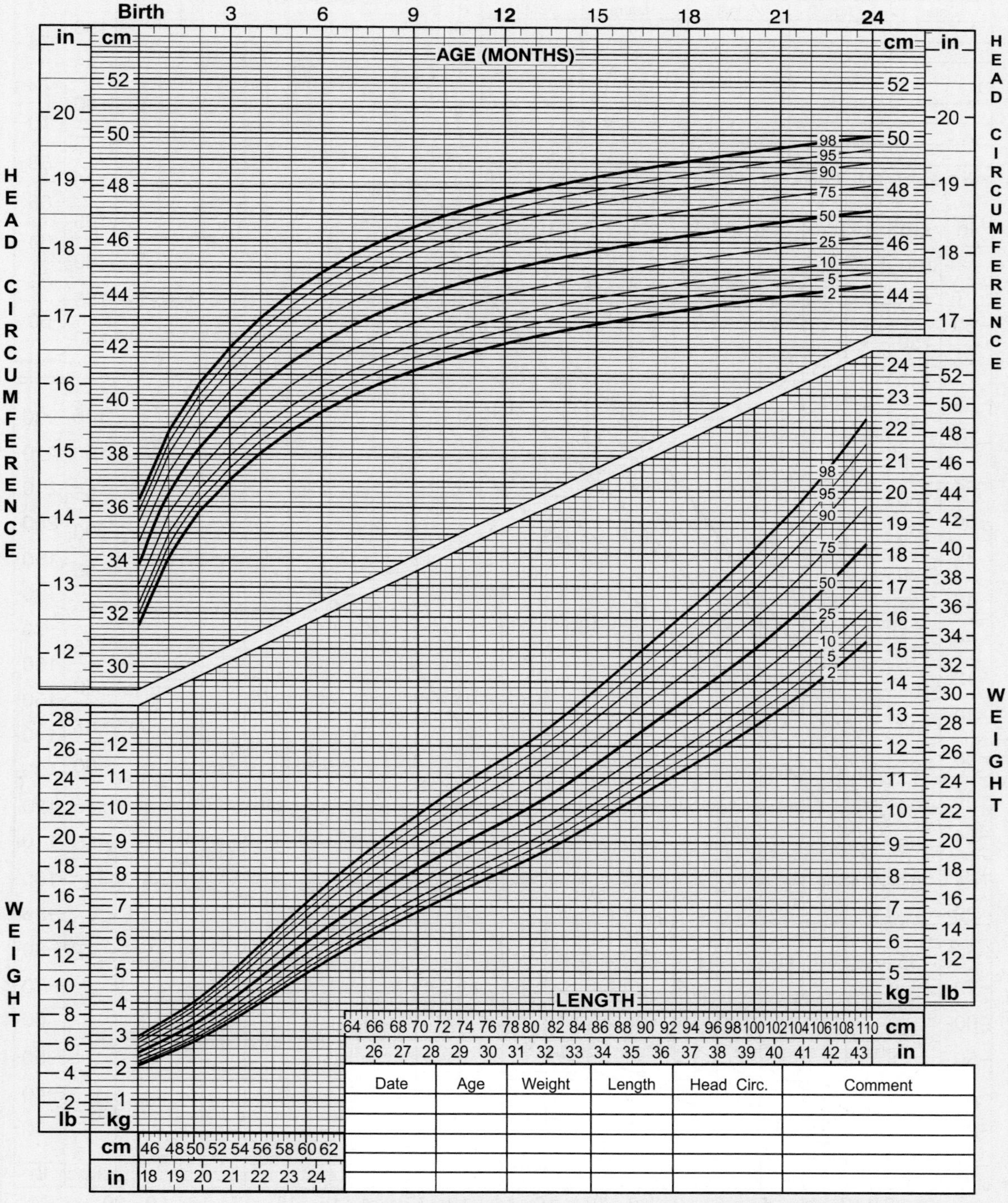

HEAD CIRCUMFERENCE — AGE (MONTHS): Birth, 3, 6, 9, 12, 15, 18, 21, 24

WEIGHT — LENGTH

Date	Age	Weight	Length	Head Circ.	Comment

Published by the Centers for Disease Control and Prevention, November 1, 2009
SOURCE: WHO Child Growth Standards (http://www.who.int/childgrowth/en)

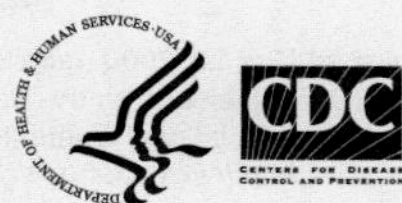

APPENDIX 15. 2 to 20 Years: Girls Stature-for-Age and Weight-for-Age Percentiles

NAME ______________________

RECORD # ______________

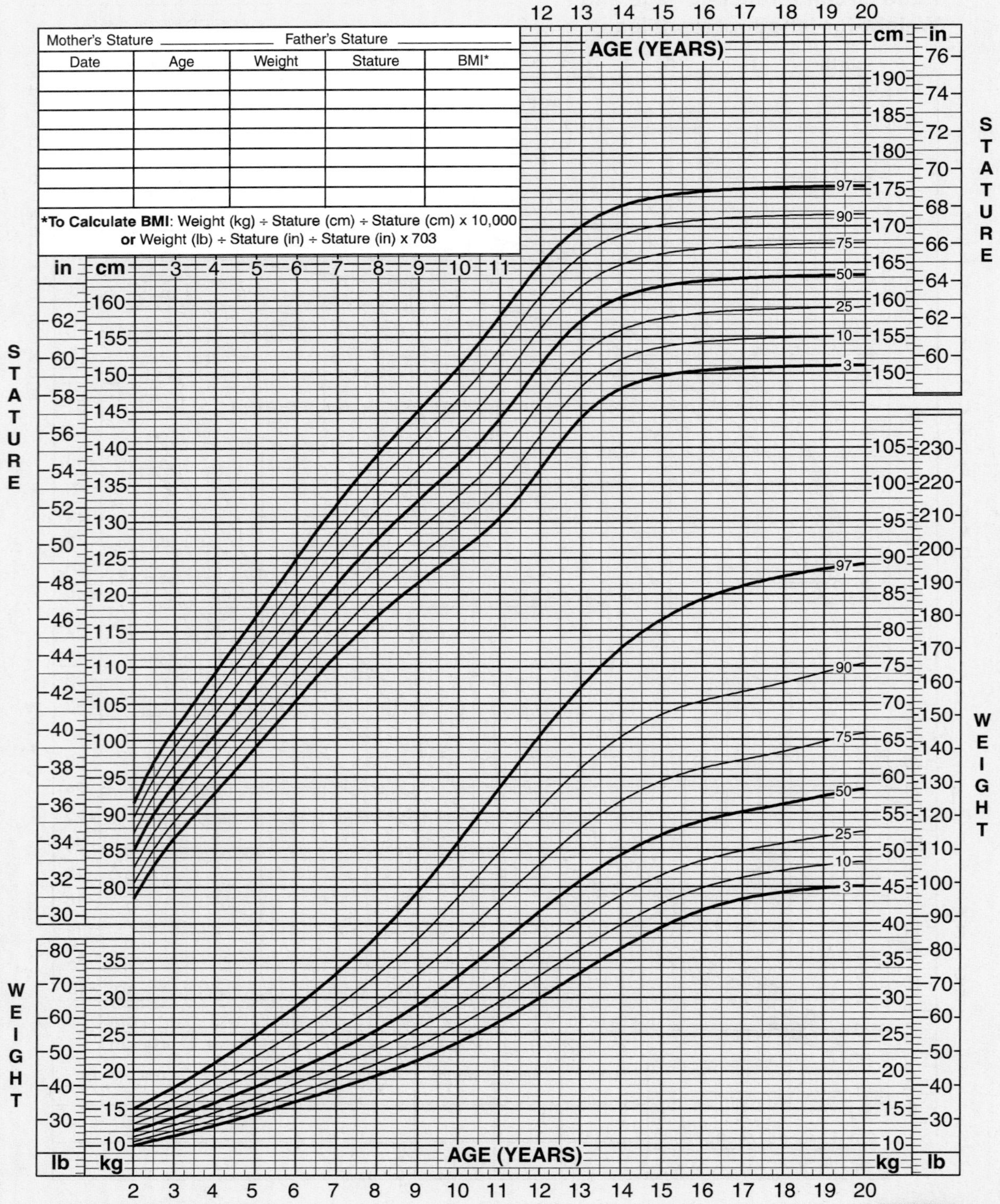

Mother's Stature ______________ Father's Stature ______________

Date	Age	Weight	Stature	BMI*

***To Calculate BMI**: Weight (kg) ÷ Stature (cm) ÷ Stature (cm) x 10,000
or Weight (lb) ÷ Stature (in) ÷ Stature (in) x 703

Published May 30, 2000 (modified 11/21/00).
SOURCE: Developed by the National Center for Health Statistics in collaboration with the National Center for Chronic Disease Prevention and Health Promotion (2000).
http://www.cdc.gov/growthcharts

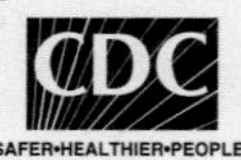

APPENDIX 16. Body Mass Index-for-Age Percentiles: Girls, 2 to 20 Years

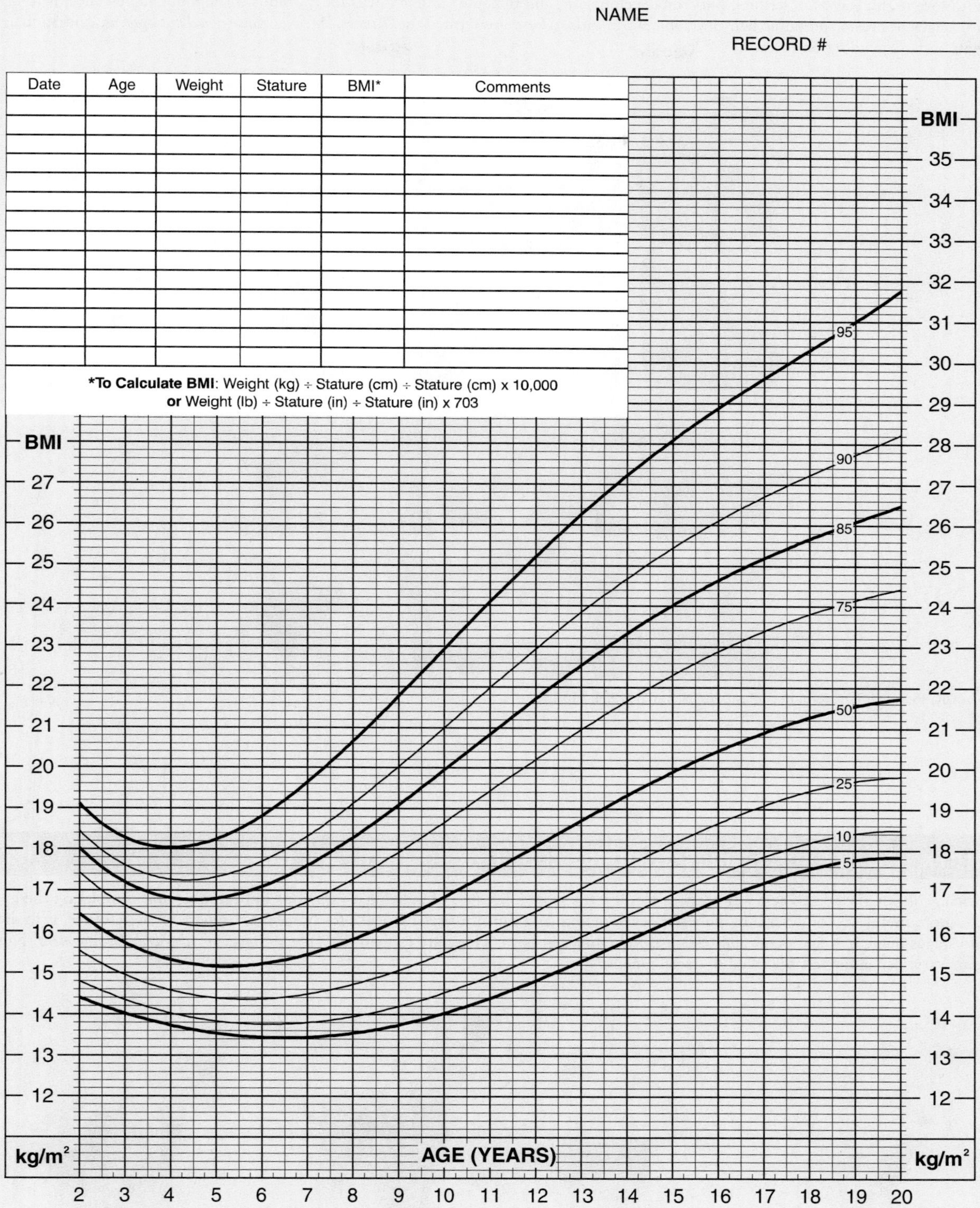

NAME ______________________

RECORD # ______________

Date	Age	Weight	Stature	BMI*	Comments

***To Calculate BMI**: Weight (kg) ÷ Stature (cm) ÷ Stature (cm) x 10,000
or Weight (lb) ÷ Stature (in) ÷ Stature (in) x 703

BMI

35
34
33
32
31
30
29
28
27
26
25
24
23
22
21
20
19
18
17
16
15
14
13
12

95
90
85
75
50
25
10
5

kg/m²

AGE (YEARS)

2 3 4 5 6 7 8 9 10 11 12 13 14 15 16 17 18 19 20

Published May 30, 2000 (modified 10/16/00).
SOURCE: Developed by the National Center for Health Statistics in collaboration with the National Center for Chronic Disease Prevention and Health Promotion (2000).
http://www.cdc.gov/growthcharts

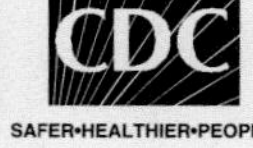

APPENDIX 17. Tanner Stages of Adolescent Development for Girls

Chronologic age is not always the best way to assess adolescent growth because of individual variations in beginning and completing the growth sequence. A more useful way of describing pubertal development, and thus the varying needs for nutrients throughout adolescence, is to divide growth into stages of breast and pubic hair development in girls. These are termed the *Tanner Stages of Adolescent Development.* Nutritional requirements vary, depending on the stage of development.

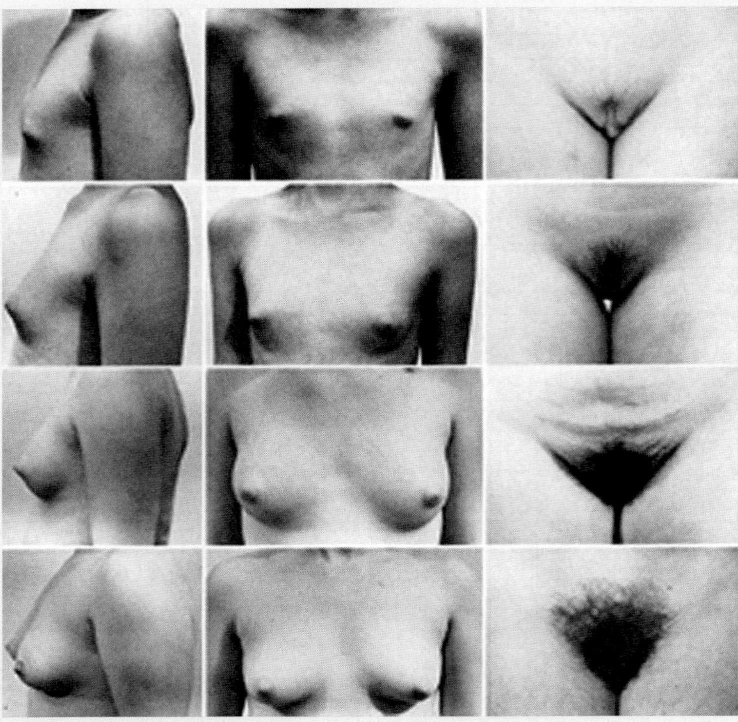

From Mahan LK, Rees JM: Nutrition in adolescence, St Louis, 1984, Mosby.

APPENDIX 18. Tanner Stages of Adolescent Development for Boys

Chronologic age is not always the best way to assess adolescent growth because of individual variations in beginning and completing the growth sequence. A more useful way of describing pubertal development, and thus the varying needs for nutrients throughout adolescence, is to divide growth into stages pubic hair and penis and testicle development in boys. These are termed the *Tanner Stages of Adolescent Development.* Nutritional requirements vary, depending on the stage of development.

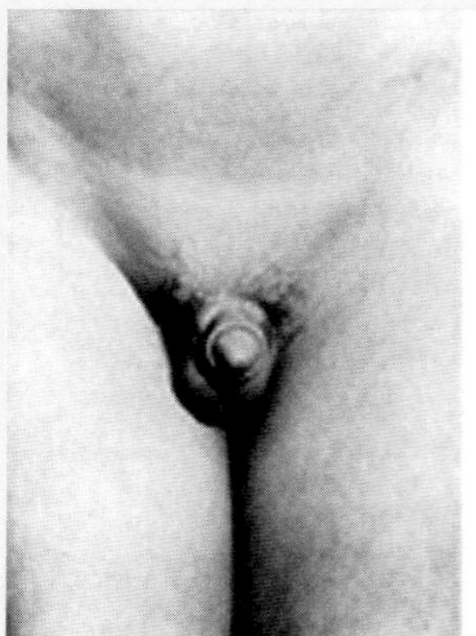

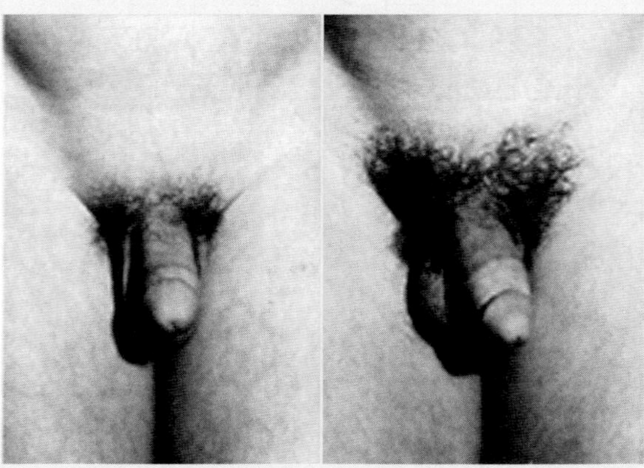

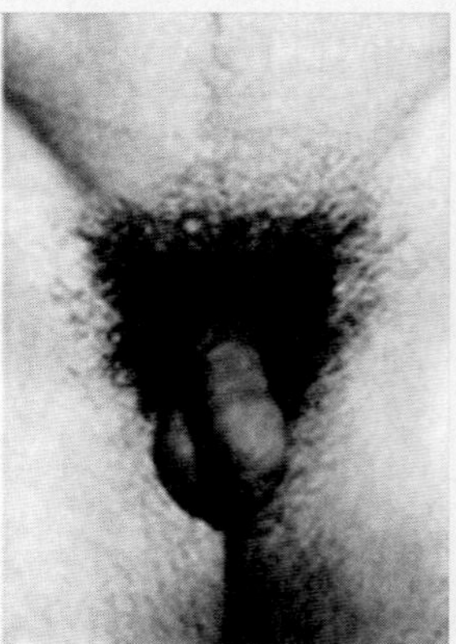

From Mahan LK, Rees JM: *Nutrition in adolescence*, St. Louis, 1984, Mosby.

APPENDIX 19. Direct Methods for Measuring Height and Weight

Height

1. Height should be measured without shoes.
2. The individual's feet should be together, with the heels against the wall or measuring board.
3. The individual should stand erect, neither slumped nor stretching, looking straight ahead, without tipping the head up or down. The top of the ear and outer corner of the eye should be in a line parallel to the floor (the "Frankfort plane").
4. A horizontal bar, a rectangular block of wood, or the top of the statiometer should be lowered to rest flat on the top of the head.
5. Height should be read to the nearest ¼ inch or 0.5 cm.

Weight

1. Use a beam balance scale, not a spring scale, whenever possible.
2. Periodically calibrate the scale for accuracy, using known weights.
3. Weigh the subject in light clothing without shoes.
4. Record weight to the nearest ½ lb or 0.2 kg for adults and ¼ lb or 0.1 kg for infants. Measurements above the 90th percentile or below the 10th percentile warrant further evaluation.

APPENDIX 20. Indirect Methods for Measuring Height

Measuring Arm Span

Steps:

1. The arms are extended straight out to the sides at a 90-degree angle from the body.
2. The distance from the longest fingertip of one hand to the longest finger of the other hand is measured.

Adult Recumbent

Steps:

1. Stand on right side of the body.
2. Align body so that the lower extremities, trunk, shoulders, and head are straight.
3. Place a mark at the top of the sheet in line with the crown of the head and one at the bottom of the sheet in line with the base of the heels.
4. Measure length between marks with measuring tape.

Knee Height

Knee height measurement is highly correlated with upright height. It is useful in those who cannot stand and in those who may have curvatures of the spine.

Steps:

1. Use the left leg for measurements.
2. Bend the left knee and the left ankle to 90-degree angles. A triangle may be used if available.
3. Using knee height calipers, open the caliper and place the fixed part under the heel. Place the sliding blade down against the thigh (approximately 2 inches behind the patella).
4. Measure from the heel to the anterior surface of the thigh, using a cloth measuring tape.
5. Obtain the measurement and convert it to centimeters by multiplying by 2.54.
6. Formulas to use to calculate estimated height from knee height:

$$\text{Men (height in centimeters)} = 64.19 - (0.04 \times \text{Age}) + (2.02 \times \text{Knee height in centimeters})$$

$$\text{Women (height in centimeters)} = 84.8 - (0.24 \times \text{Age}) + (1.83 \times \text{Knee height in centimeters})$$

Predicting Stature From Knee Height: Recommended Equations for Predicting Stature from Knee Height in Adults (18 to 60 years) and Children (6 to 18 years)

Group	Equations
White men	Stature = 71.85 + (1.88 knee height) R^2 = 0.65; RMSE = 3.97; SEI = 3.97 cm; CV = 2.28
Black men	Stature = 73.42 + (1.79 knee height) R^2 = 0.69; RMSE = 3.60; SEI = 3.60 cm; CV = 2.08
White women	Stature = 70.25 + (1.87 knee height) − (0.06 age) R^2 = 0.66; RMSE = 3.60; SEI = 3.60 cm; CV = 2.23
Black women	Stature = 68.10 + (1.86 knee height) − (0.06 age) R^2 = 0.69; RMSE = 3.80; SEI = 3.80 cm; CV = 2.36
White boys	Stature = 40.54 + (2.22 knee height) R^2 = 0.96; RMSE = 4.16; SEI = 4.21 cm; CV = 2.79
Black boys	Stature = 39.60 + (2.18 knee height) R^2 50.95; RMSE = 4.44; SEI = 4.58 cm; CV = 2.99
White girls	Stature = 43.21 + (2.15 knee height) R^2 = 0.95; RMSE = 3.84; SEI = 3.90 cm; CV = 2.63
Black girls	Stature = 46.59 + (2.02 knee height) R^2 = 0.94; RMSE = 4.25; SEI = 4.39 cm; CV = 2.91

Data from Chumlea WC et al: Nutritional assessment of the elderly through anthropometry, Columbus, OH, 1984, Ross Laboratories.

CV, Coefficient of variation; *RMSE*, root mean square error; *SEI*, standard error for an individual.

APPENDIX 21. Determination of Frame Size

Method 1: Height is recorded without shoes. Wrist circumference is measured just distal to the styloid process at the wrist crease on the right arm, using a tape measure. The following formula is used (From Grant JP: Handbook of total parenteral nutrition, Philadelphia, 1980, Saunders):

$$r = \frac{\text{Height (cm)}}{\text{Wrist circumference (cm)}}$$

Frame size can be determined as follows:

Males	Females
r >10.4 small	r >11.0 small
r = 9.6-10.4 medium	r = 10.1-11.0 medium
r < 9.6 large	r <10.1 large

Method 2: The patient's right arm is extended forward perpendicular to the body, with the arm bent so the angle at the elbow forms 90 degrees with the fingers pointing up and the palm turned away from the body. The greatest breadth across the elbow joint is measured with a sliding caliper along the axis of the upper arm on the two prominent bones on either side of the elbow. This is recorded as the elbow breadth. The following tables give the elbow breadth measurements for medium-framed men and women of various heights (from Metropolitan Life Insurance Co., 1983). Measurements lower than those listed indicate a small frame size; higher measurements indicate a large frame size.

Men		Women	
Height in 1″ Heels	**Elbow Breadth (inches)**	**Height in 1″ Heels**	**Elbow Breadth (inches)**
5′2″-5′3″	2½-2⅞	4′10″-4′11″	2¼-2½
5′4″-5′7″	2⅝-2⅞	5′0″-5′3″	2¼-2½
5′8″-5′11″	2¾-3	5′4″-5′7″	2⅜-2⅝
6′0″-6′3″	2¾-3⅛	5′8″5′11″	2⅜-2⅝
6′4″	2⅞-3¼	6′0″	

APPENDIX 22. Adjustment of Desirable Body Weight for Amputees

The percentages listed here are estimates because body proportions vary in individuals. Use of these percentages provides an approximation of desirable body weight, which is more accurate than a comparison with the standards for normal adults. Ideal body weight (IBW) must be adjusted downward to compensate for missing limbs or paralysis. It is estimated that 5% to 10% should be subtracted from IBW for a paraplegic and from 10% to 15% subtracted for a tetraplegic (quadriplegic.)

Adjustment of Ideal Body Weight for Amputees

Body Segment	Average % of Total Weight
Lower arm and hand	2.3
Trunk without extremities	50.0
Entire arm	5.0
Hand	0.7
Entire lower leg	16.0
Below knee including foot	5.9
Foot	1.5

Data from Brunnstrom S: *Clinical kinesiology*, Philadelphia, 1972, FA Davis.

$$\text{Estimated IBW} = \frac{100 - \%\text{ amputation}}{100} \times \text{IBW for original height}$$

To use this information, determine the patient's approximate height before the amputation. Span measurement is a rough estimate of height at maturity and is calculated as follows: with the upper extremities, including the hands, fully extended and parallel to the ground, measure the distance between the tip of one middle finger and the tip of the other middle finger. Use this height or actual measurement to calculate the desirable body weight for the normal body size; then adjust the figures according to the type of amputation performed.

Example: To determine the desirable body weight for a 5′10″ male with a below-the-knee amputation:

1. Calculate desirable body weight for a 5′10″ male:	166 lb
2. Subtract weight of amputated limb (6%) = 166 × 0.06:	– 9.96 (approx. 10 lb)
3. Desirable weight of a 5′10″ male with a below-knee amputation:	156 lb

From North Carolina Dietetic Association: Nutrition care manual, 2011, Raleigh, NC, The Association.

APPENDIX 23. Body Mass Index Table

	Normal Weight						Overweight					Obese					
BMI	**19**	**20**	**21**	**22**	**23**	**24**	**25**	**26**	**27**	**28**	**29**	**30**	**31**	**32**	**33**	**34**	**35**
Height	**Weight (in pounds)**																
4′10″ (58″)	91	96	100	105	110	115	119	124	129	134	138	143	148	153	158	162	167
4′11″ (59″)	94	99	104	109	114	119	124	128	133	138	143	148	153	158	163	168	173
5′ (60″)	97	102	107	112	118	123	128	133	138	143	148	153	158	163	168	174	179
5′1″ (61″)	100	106	111	116	122	127	132	137	143	148	153	158	164	169	174	180	185
5′2″ (62″)	104	109	115	120	126	131	136	142	147	153	158	164	169	175	180	186	191
5′3″ (63″	107	113	118	124	130	135	141	146	152	158	163	169	175	180	186	191	197
5′4″ (64″)	110	116	122	128	134	140	145	151	157	163	169	174	180	186	192	197	204
5′5″ (65″	114	120	126	132	138	144	150	156	162	168	174	180	186	192	198	204	210
5′6″ (66″	118	124	130	136	142	148	155	161	167	173	179	186	192	198	204	210	216
5′7″ (67″	121	127	134	140	146	153	159	166	172	178	185	191	198	204	211	217	223
5′8″ (68″)	125	131	138	144	151	158	164	171	177	184	190	197	203	210	216	223	230
5′9″ (69″)	128	135	142	149	155	162	169	176	182	189	196	203	209	216	223	230	236
5′10″ (70″)	132	139	146	153	160	167	174	181	188	195	202	209	216	222	229	236	243
5′11″ (71″)	136	143	150	157	165	172	179	186	193	200	208	215	222	229	236	243	250
6′ (72″)	140	147	154	162	169	177	184	191	199	206	213	221	228	235	242	250	258
6′1″ (73″)	144	151	159	166	174	182	189	197	204	212	219	227	235	242	250	257	265
6′2″ (74″)	148	155	163	171	179	186	194	202	210	218	225	233	241	249	256	264	272
6′3″ (75″)	152	160	168	176	184	192	200	208	216	224	232	240	248	256	264	272	279

Data from National Institutes of Health and National Heart, Lung, and Blood Institute: Evidence report of clinical guidelines on the identification, evaluation, and treatment of overweight and obesity in adults, Bethesda, MD, 1998, NIH/NHLBI. For a BMI of greater than 30, please go to http://www.nhlbi.nih.gov/guidelines/obesity/bmi_tbl.pdf.

BMI, Body mass index.

APPENDIX 24. Percentage of Body Fat Based on Four Skinfold Measurements*

	Males (Age in Years)				Females (Age in Years)			
Sum of Skinfolds (mm)	**17-29**	**30-39**	**40-49**	**50+**	**16-29**	**30-39**	**40-49**	**50+**
15	4.8	—	—	—	10.5	—	—	—
20	8.1	12.2	12.2	12.6	14.1	17.0	19.8	21.4
25	10.5	14.2	15.0	15.6	16.8	19.4	22.2	24.0
30	12.9	16.2	17.7	18.6	19.5	21.8	24.5	26.6
35	14.7	17.7	19.6	20.8	21.5	23.7	26.4	28.5
40	16.4	19.2	21.4	22.9	23.4	25.5	28.2	30.3
45	17.7	20.4	23.0	24.7	25.0	26.9	29.6	31.9
50	19.0	21.5	24.6	26.5	26.5	28.2	31.0	33.4
55	20.1	22.5	25.9	27.9	27.8	29.4	32.1	34.6
60	21.2	23.5	27.1	29.2	29.1	30.6	33.2	35.7
65	22.2	24.3	28.2	30.4	30.2	31.6	34.1	36.7
70	23.1	25.1	29.3	31.6	31.2	32.5	35.0	37.7
75	24.0	25.9	30.3	32.7	32.2	33.4	35.9	38.7
80	24.8	26.6	31.2	33.8	33.1	34.3	36.7	39.6
85	25.5	27.2	32.1	34.8	34.0	35.1	37.5	40.4
90	26.2	27.8	33.0	35.8	34.8	35.8	38.3	41.2
95	26.9	28.4	33.7	36.6	35.6	36.5	39.0	41.9
100	27.6	29.0	34.4	37.4	36.4	37.2	39.7	42.6
105	28.2	29.6	35.1	38.2	37.1	37.9	40.4	43.3
110	28.8	30.1	35.8	39.0	37.8	38.6	41.0	43.9
115	29.4	30.6	36.4	39.7	38.4	39.1	41.5	44.5
120	30.0	31.1	37.0	40.4	39.0	39.6	42.0	45.1
125	30.5	31.5	37.6	41.1	39.6	40.1	42.5	45.7
130	31.0	31.9	38.2	41.8	40.2	40.6	43.0	46.2
135	31.5	32.3	38.7	42.4	40.8	41.1	43.5	46.7
140	32.0	32.7	39.2	43.0	41.3	41.6	44.0	47.2
145	32.5	33.1	39.7	43.6	41.8	42.1	44.5	47.7
150	32.9	33.5	40.2	44.1	42.3	42.6	45.0	48.2
155	33.3	33.9	40.7	44.6	42.8	43.1	45.4	48.7
160	33.7	34.3	41.2	45.1	43.3	43.6	45.8	49.2
165	34.1	34.6	41.6	45.6	43.7	44.0	46.2	49.6
170	34.5	34.8	42.0	46.1	44.1	44.4	46.6	50.0
175	34.9	—	—	—	—	44.8	47.0	50.4
180	35.3	—	—	—	—	45.2	47.4	50.8
185	35.6	—	—	—	—	45.6	47.8	51.2
190	35.9	—	—	—	—	45.9	48.2	51.6
195	—	—	—	—	—	46.2	48.5	52.0
200	—	—	—	—	—	46.5	48.8	52.4
205	—	—	—	—	—	—	49.1	52.7
210	—	—	—	—	—	—	49.4	53.0

From Durnin JVGA, Wormersley J: Body fat assessed from total body density and its estimation from skinfold thickness: measurements on 481 men and women ages 16-72 years, Br J Nutr 32:77, 1974.

*Measurements made on the right side of the body, using biceps, triceps, subscapular, and suprailiac skinfolds.

APPENDIX 25. Arm Anthropometry for Children

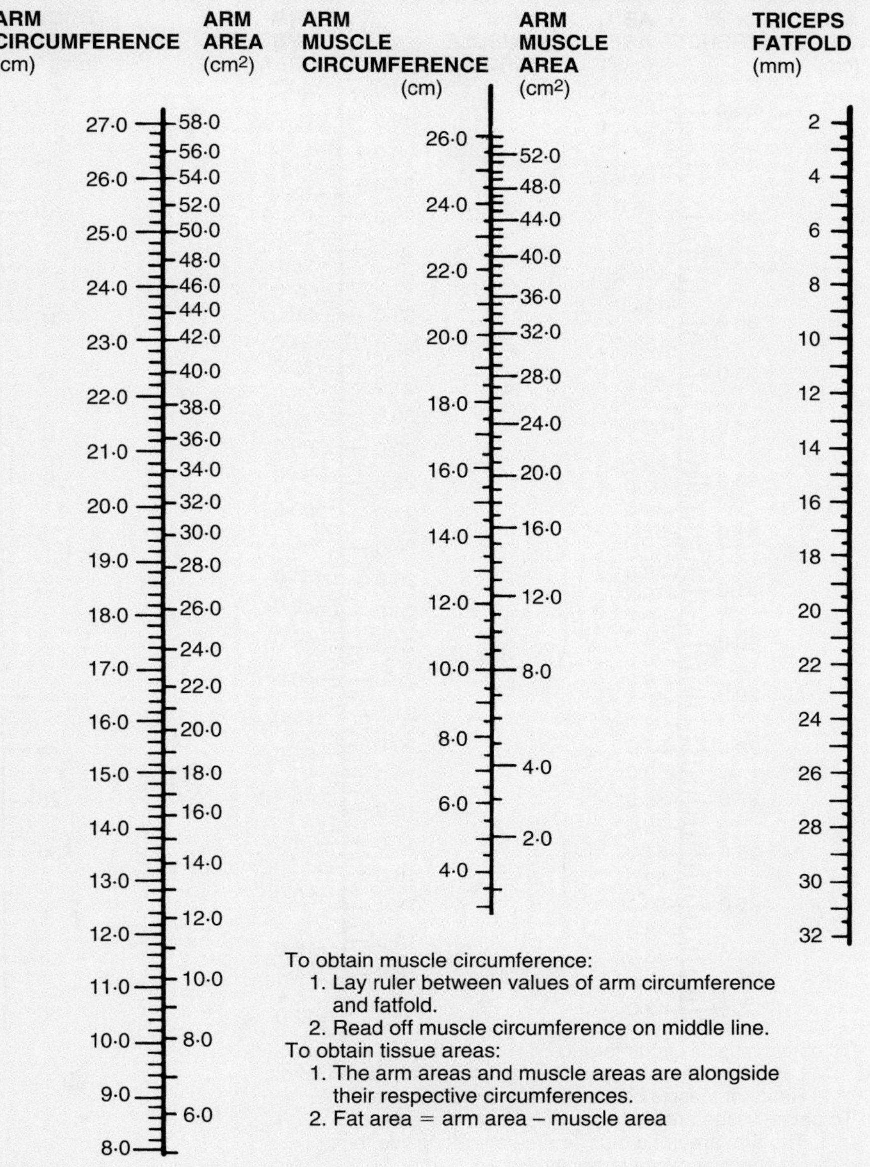

From Gurney JM, Jelliffe DB: Arm anthropometry in nutritional assessment: nomogram for rapid calculation of muscle circumference and cross-sectional muscle fat areas, Am J Clin Nutr 26:913, 1973.

APPENDIX 26. Arm Anthropometry for Adults

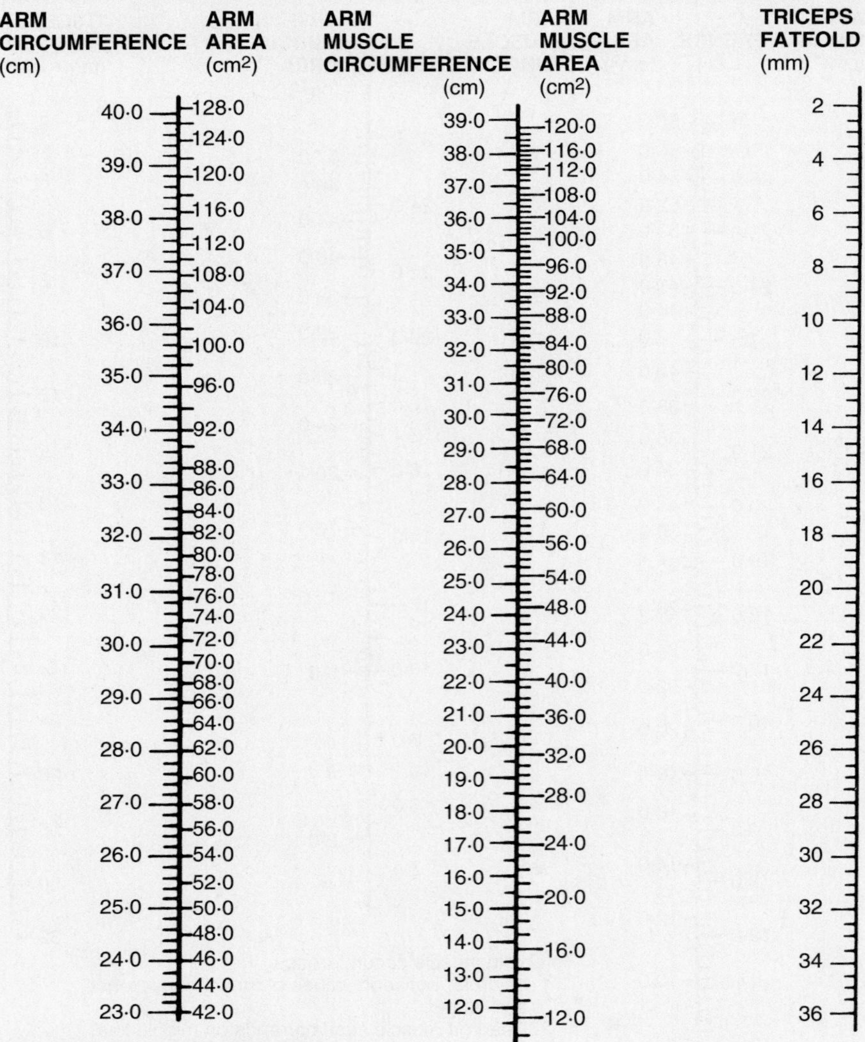

To obtain muscle circumference:

1. Lay ruler between value of arm circumference and fatfold.
2. Read off muscle circumference on middle line.

To obtain tissue areas:

1. The arm area and muscle area are alongside their respective circumferences.
2. Fat area = arm area – muscle area

From Gurney JM, Jelliffe DB: Arm anthropometry in nutritional assessment: nomogram for rapid calculation of muscle circumference and cross-sectional muscle fat areas, Am J Clin Nutr 26:913, 1973.

APPENDIX 27. Recommendations for Clinical Application of Bioelectrical Impedance Analysis

Instruments, Material	Definition, Comments	Recommendations
Statiometer	Calibrated to 0.5 cm	Use tape measure for subjects who are unable to stand and for knee height or arm span.
Scale	Calibrated to 0.1 kg	Regularly cross-calibrate with other scales.
Subjects		
Height and weight	Measure height (0.5 cm) and weight (0.1 kg) at time of BIA measurement.	Self-reported height and weight not valid.
Food, drink, alcohol	Fasting, no alcohol for >8 h recommended	Shorter periods of fasting may be acceptable for clinical practice (vs. research).
Bladder voided		Subject has voided before measurement.
Physical exercise		No exercise for >8 h.
Timing	Note time of measurement.	For longitudinal follow-up, perform measurement at the same time of day; note menstrual cycle.
Skin condition	Temperature	Record ambient temperature.
	Integrity	No skin lesions at site of electrodes; change site of electrodes.
	Cleaning	Clean with alcohol.
Electrode position	Note body site of measurement; distance between electrodes.	Always measure same body side. Minimum of 5 cm between electrodes; if needed, move proximal electrode.
Limb position	Abduction of limbs	Separate arms from trunk by approximately 30 degrees; separate legs by approximately 45 degrees.
Body position	Supine, except for "scale" type BIA instruments	Ambulatory subjects supine for 5 to 10 min; for research protocol, standardize time that subjects are supine before measurement; note if subject is confined to bed (patients).
Environment	Electrical interference	Ensure noncontact with metal frame of bed; neutral environment (no strong electrical or magnetic fields).
Body shape	Note body abnormalities.	Note measurement validity (e.g., R or Xc outside of expected range for subject). Consider validity of measurement when interpreting results (e.g., abnormally low R suggests edema).
	Amputation	Measure nonaffected limb; not valid for research but permits determination of body compartment because measurement error is consistent. Measure nonaffected side.
	Atrophy and hemiplegia	Note abnormal condition.
	Abnormal limb or trunk (e.g., scoliosis dystrophy (e.g., HIV, Cushing's syndrome)	Limited validity exists in conditions of abnormal body compartment distribution.
	Obesity	Use electricity-isolating material (e.g., towel) between arm and trunk and between thighs.
Ethnic group		Note race; use race-specific BIA equation, if applicable.
Disease Conditions		
Cardiac insufficiency	Edema interferes with measurement.	Measure patient in stable condition.
Liver failure	Ascites and edema interfere with measurement accuracy.	Consider segmental BIA measurement.
Kidney failure	Edema and altered ion balance interfere with measurement.	
Abnormal serum electrolyte concentrations	Electrolyte concentration affects BIA measurement.	Perform BIA when serum electrolytes are within normal range. Compare BIA results when serum electrolyte concentrations are similar.
Hypothyroid	Pachyderma	May invalidate measurement because of high skin resistance.
Treatments		
Intravenous and electrolyte infusions	Peripheral edema interferes with measurement.	Measurements are invalid if patient is abnormally hydrated.
Drugs that affect water balance	Steroids, growth hormone, diuretics	If patient is in stable condition, measurement should be taken at same time after medication administration.
Dialysis	Hemo-1 peritoneal dialysis	Use special protocols; standardize measurement procedure (i.e., measurement should be performed 20 to 30 minutes after dialysis).
Ascites puncture		Use special protocols; standardize measurement procedure.
Orthopedic prostheses and implants (metal)	Hip prosthesis, for example	Measure nonaffected body side; note prostheses and implants.
Pacemakers, defibrillators	Implanted cardiac defibrillator	No interference with pacemakers or defibrillators is anticipated; although there are no known incidents reported as a result of BIA measurement, the possibility cannot be eliminated that the induced field of current during the measurement could alter the pacemaker or defibrillator activity; therefore the patient should be monitored for cardiac activity.

Reprinted from Kyle UG, Bosaeus I, et al. Bioelectrical impedance analysis—Part II: Utilization in clinical practice, Clin Nutr 23:1430, 2004.

BIA, Bioelectrical impedance analysis; *HIV*, human immunodeficiency virus; *R*, resistance; *Xc*, reactance.

APPENDIX 28. Physical Activity and Calories Expended per Hour

Activity	Type	Body Weight							
		(110 lb)	(130 lb)	(150 lb)	(170 lb)	(190 lb)	(210 lb)	(230 lb)	(250 lb)
Aerobics class	Water	210	248	286	325	364	401	439	477
Aerobics class	Low impact	263	310	358	406	455	501	549	596
Aerobics class	High impact	368	434	501	568	637	702	768	835
Aerobics class	Step with 6- to 8-inch step	446	527	609	690	774	852	933	1014
Aerobics class	Step with 10- to 12-inch step	525	621	716	812	910	1003	1097	1193
Backpack	General	368	434	501	568	637	702	768	835
Badminton	Singles and doubles	236	279	322	365	410	451	494	537
Badminton	Competitive	368	434	501	568	637	702	768	835
Baseball	Throw, catch	131	155	179	203	228	251	274	298
Baseball	Fast or slow pitch	263	310	358	406	455	501	549	596
Basketball	Shooting baskets	236	279	322	365	410	451	494	537
Basketball	Wheelchair	341	403	465	528	592	652	713	775
Basketball	Game	420	496	573	649	728	802	878	954
Bike	10-11.9 mph, slow	315	372	430	487	546	602	658	716
Bike	12-13.9 mph, moderate	420	496	573	649	728	802	878	954
Bike	14-15.9 mph, fast	525	621	716	812	910	1003	1097	1193
Bike	16-19.9 mph, very fast	630	745	859	974	1092	1203	1317	1431
Bike	>20 mph, racing	840	993	1146	1299	1457	1604	1756	1908
Bike	50 watts, stationary, very light	158	133	215	243	273	301	329	358
Bike	100 watts, stationary, light	289	341	394	446	501	552	603	656
Bike	150 watts, stationary, moderate	368	434	501	568	637	702	768	835
Bike	200 watts, stationary, vigorous	551	652	752	852	956	1053	1152	1252
Bike	250 watts, stationary, very vigorous	656	776	895	1015	1138	1253	1372	1491
Bike	BMX or mountain	446	527	609	690	774	852	933	1014
Boxing	Punching bag	315	372	430	487	546	602	658	716
Boxing	Sparring	473	558	644	730	819	902	988	1074
Calisthenics	Back exercises	184	217	251	284	319	351	384	417
Calisthenics	Pull-ups, jumping jacks	420	496	573	649	728	802	878	954
Calisthenics	Push-ups or sit-ups	420	496	573	649	728	802	878	954
Circuit training	General	420	496	573	649	728	802	878	954
Football	Flag or touch	420	496	573	649	728	802	878	954
Football	Competitive	473	558	644	730	819	902	988	1074
Frisbee	General	158	133	215	243	273	301	329	358
Frisbee	Ultimate	420	496	573	649	728	802	878	954
Golf	Power cart	184	217	251	284	319	351	384	417
Golf	Pull clubs	226	267	308	349	391	431	472	513
Golf	Carry clubs	236	279	322	365	410	451	494	537
Handball	General	630	745	859	974	1092	1203	1317	1431
Hike	General	315	372	460	487	546	602	658	716
Hockey	Ice, field hockey	420	496	573	649	728	802	878	954
Jog	General	368	434	501	568	637	702	768	835
Jog	Jog-walk combination	315	372	430	487	546	602	658	716
Jump rope	Slow	420	496	573	649	728	802	878	954
Jump rope	Moderate	525	621	716	812	910	1003	1097	1193
Jump rope	Fast	630	745	859	974	1092	1203	1317	1431
Kayak	General	263	310	358	406	455	501	549	596
Martial arts	General	525	621	716	812	910	1003	1097	1193
Racquetball	Casual	368	434	501	568	637	702	768	835
Racquetball	Competition	525	621	716	812	910	1003	1097	1193
Rafting	Whitewater	263	310	358	406	455	501	549	596
Rock climb	General	420	496	573	649	728	802	878	954
Rugby	General	525	621	716	812	910	1003	1097	1193
Run	5 mph, 12 min/mile	420	496	573	649	728	802	878	954
Run	5.2 mph, 11.5 min/mile	473	558	644	730	819	902	988	1074
Run	6 mph, 10 min/mile	525	621	716	812	910	1003	1097	1193
Run	6.7 mph, 9 min/mile	578	683	788	893	1001	1103	1207	1312

APPENDIX 28. Physical Activity and Calories Expended per Hour—cont'd

Activity	Type	Body Weight (110 lb)	(130 lb)	(150 lb)	(170 lb)	(190 lb)	(210 lb)	(230 lb)	(250 lb)
Run	7 mph, 8.5 min/mile	604	714	824	933	1047	1153	1262	1372
Run	7.5 mph, 8 min/mile	656	776	895	1015	1138	1253	1372	1491
Run	8 mph, 7.5 min/mile	709	838	967	1096	1229	1354	1481	1610
Run	8.6 mph, 7 min/mile	735	869	1003	1136	1274	1404	1536	1670
Run	9 mph, 6.5 min/mile	788	931	1074	1217	1366	1504	1646	1789
Run	10 mph, 6 min/mile	840	993	1146	1299	1457	1604	1756	1908
Run	10.9 mph, 5.5 min/mile	945	1117	1289	1461	1639	1805	1975	2147
Run	Cross country	473	558	644	730	819	902	988	1074
Skate, ice	General	368	434	501	568	637	702	768	835
Skate, inline	Inline, general	656	776	895	1015	1138	1253	1372	1491
Skateboard	General	263	310	358	406	455	501	549	596
Ski, downhill	Light	263	310	358	406	455	501	549	596
Ski, downhill	Moderate	315	372	430	487	546	602	658	716
Ski, downhill	Vigorous, race	420	496	573	649	728	802	878	954
Ski machine	General	368	434	501	568	637	702	768	835
Ski, cross-country	2.5 mph, slow	368	434	501	568	637	702	768	835
Ski, cross-country	4-4.9 mph, moderate	420	496	573	649	728	802	878	954
Ski, cross-country	5-7.9 mph, brisk	473	558	644	730	819	902	988	1074
Snowboard	General	394	465	537	609	683	752	823	895
Snowshoe	General	420	496	573	649	728	802	878	954
Soccer	Casual	368	434	501	568	637	702	768	835
Soccer	Competitive	525	621	716	812	910	1003	1097	1193
Softball	General	263	310	358	406	455	501	549	596
Stair stepper	General	473	558	644	730	819	902	988	1074
Stationary rower	50 watts, light	184	217	251	284	319	351	384	417
Stationary rower	100 watts, moderate	368	434	501	568	637	702	768	835
Stationary rower	150 watts, vigorous	446	527	609	690	774	852	933	1014
Stationary rower	200 watts, very vigorous	630	745	859	974	1092	1203	1317	1431
Stretch, yoga	General, Hatha	131	155	179	203	228	251	274	298
Swim	Lake, ocean, or river	315	372	430	487	546	602	658	716
Swim	Laps freestyle, slow or moderate	368	434	501	568	637	702	768	835
Swim	Laps freestyle, fast	525	621	716	812	910	1003	1097	1193
Swim	Backstroke	368	434	501	568	637	702	768	835
Swim	Sidestroke	420	496	573	649	728	802	878	954
Swim	Breaststroke	525	621	716	812	910	1003	1097	1193
Swim	Butterfly	578	683	788	893	1001	1103	1207	1312
Tennis	Doubles	315	372	430	487	546	602	658	716
Tennis	Singles	420	496	573	649	728	802	878	954
Treadmill, run	6 mph, 10 min/mile, 0% incline	525	621	716	812	910	1003	1097	1193
Treadmill, run	6 mph, 10 min/mile, 2% incline	578	683	788	893	1001	1103	1207	1312
Treadmill, run	6 mph, 10 min/mile, 4% incline	620	732	845	958	1074	1183	1295	1408
Treadmill, run	6 mph, 10 min/mile, 6% incline	667	788	909	1031	1156	1273	1394	1515
Treadmill, run	7 mph, 8.5 min/mile, 0% incline	604	714	824	933	1047	1153	1262	1372
Treadmill, run	7 mph, 8.5 min/mile, 2% incline	667	788	909	1031	1156	1273	1394	1515
Treadmill, run	7 mph, 8.5 min/mile, 4% incline	719	850	981	1112	1247	1374	1503	1634
Treadmill, run	7 mph, 8.5 min/mile, 6% incline	767	906	1046	1185	1329	1464	1602	1741
Treadmill, run	8 mph, 7.5 min/mile, 0% incline	709	838	967	1096	1229	1354	1481	1610
Treadmill, run	8 mph, 7.5 min/mile, 2% incline	756	894	1031	1169	1311	1444	1580	1718
Treadmill, run	8 mph, 7.5 min/mile, 4% incline	814	962	1110	1258	1411	1554	1701	1849

Continued

APPENDIX 28. Physical Activity and Calories Expended per Hour—cont'd

		Body Weight							
Activity	**Type**	**(110 lb)**	**(130 lb)**	**(150 lb)**	**(170 lb)**	**(190 lb)**	**(210 lb)**	**(230 lb)**	**(250 lb)**
Treadmill, run	8 mph, 7.5 min/mile, 6% incline	872	1030	1189	1347	1511	1665	1821	1980
Treadmill, run	3 mph, 20 min/mile, 0% incline	173	205	236	268	300	331	362	394
Treadmill, run	3 mph, 20 min/mile, 2% incline	194	230	265	300	337	371	406	441
Treadmill, run	3 mph, 20 min/mile, 4% incline	215	254	293	333	373	411	450	489
Treadmill, run	3 mph, 20 min/mile, 6% incline	236	279	322	365	410	451	494	537
Treadmill, run	4 mph, 15 min/mile, 0% incline	263	310	358	406	455	501	549	596
Treadmill, run	4 mph, 15 min/mile, 2% incline	294	348	401	455	510	562	614	668
Treadmill, run	4 mph, 15 min/mile, 4% incline	326	385	444	503	564	622	680	740
Treadmill, run	4 mph, 15 min/mile, 6% incline	352	416	480	544	610	672	735	799
Tread water	Moderate	210	248	286	325	364	401	439	477
Tread water	Vigorous	525	621	716	812	910	1003	1097	1193
Volleyball	Noncompetitive	158	133	215	243	273	301	329	358
Volleyball	Competitive	420	496	573	649	728	802	878	954
Walk	<2 mph	105	124	143	162	182	201	219	239
Walk	2 mph, 30 min/mile	131	155	179	203	228	251	274	298
Walk	2.5 mph, 24 min/mile	158	133	215	243	273	301	329	358
Walk	3 mph, 20 min/mile	173	205	236	268	300	331	362	394
Walk	3.5 mph, 17 min/mile	200	236	272	308	346	381	417	453
Walk	4 mph, 15 min/mile	263	310	358	406	455	501	549	596
Walk	4.5 mph, 13 min/mile	331	391	451	511	574	632	691	751
Walk	Race walking	341	403	465	528	592	652	713	775
Water polo	General	525	621	716	812	910	1003	1097	1193
Weight training	Free, nautilus, light/moderate	158	133	215	243	273	301	329	358
Weight training	Free, nautilus, vigorous	315	372	430	487	546	602	658	716
Wind surf	Casual	158	133	215	243	273	301	329	358

NOTE: This chart is not intended to be a comprehensive list for all nutritional or metabolic deficiencies or nonnutrition examples.

From Hammond K: Physical assessment: a nutritional perspective, Nurs Clin North Am 32(4):779, 1997.

APPENDIX 29. Nutrition-Focused Physical Assessment

Kathleen A. Hammond, MS, RN, BSN, BSHE, RD, LD

System	Normal Findings	Physical Findings	Possible Nutrition and Metabolic Associations	Nonnutritional Examples
General survey	Weight for height appropriate, well-nourished, alert, and cooperative	Loss of weight, muscle mass and fat stores, skeletal muscle wasting (especially in quadriceps, and deltoids), subcutaneous fat loss (face, triceps, thighs, waist) or overall weight loss, growth retardation, sarcopenia (loss of lean body mass in older adults)	Protein-energy deficiency Decreased food intake	Endocrine disorders, osteogenic disorders, menopausal disorders secondary to estrogen depletion Sarcopenia related to decreased physical activity, increased cytokine (interleukin-6) and decreased levels of growth hormone and insulin-like growth factor
Skin	Pink, soft, moist turgor with instant recoil, smooth appearance	Excess fat stores	Excess energy intake	Diabetes, steroids
		Poor or delayed wound healing, pressure ulcers	Protein, vitamin C, or zinc deficiency	
		Dry with fine lines and shedding, scaly (xerosis)	Essential fat or vitamin A deficiency	Environmental or hygiene factors
		Spinelike plaques around hair follicles on buttocks, thighs, or knees (follicular hyperkeratosis)	Vitamin A or essential fat deficiency	
		Pellagrous dermatitis (hyperpigmentation of skin exposed to sunlight)	Niacin or tryptophan deficiency	Thermal, sun, or chemical burns; Addison's disease
		Pallor	Iron or folic acid deficiency	Skin pigmentation disorders, hemorrhage, low volume, low perfusion state
		Generalized dermatitis	Zinc, essential fatty acid deficiency	Atopic dermatitis, contact dermatitis, allergic or medication rash, psoriasis, connective tissue disease
		Yellow pigmentation	Carotene excess	Jaundice
		Poor skin turgor	Fluid loss	Aging process
		Petechiae, ecchymoses	Vitamin K or C deficiency	Aspirin overdose, liver disease, or trauma
Nails	Smooth, translucent, slightly curved nail surface and firmly attached to nail bed; nail beds with brisk capillary refill	Spoon-shaped (koilonychia)	Iron deficiency	COPD, heart disease, aortic stenosis
		Dull, lackluster	Protein or iron deficiency	Chemical effects
		Pale, mottled, poor blanching	Vitamin A or C deficiency	Infection, chemical effects
		Ridging, transverse-more than one extremity	Protein	Beau's lines, grooves caused by trauma, coronary occlusion, skin disease, transient illness
Scalp	Pink, no lesions, tenderness; fontanels without softening, bulging	Softening or craniotabes	Vitamin D deficiency	
		Open anterior fontanel (usually closes by ≈18 months of age)	Vitamin D deficiency	Hydrocephalus
Hair	Natural shine, consistency in color and quantity, fine to coarse texture	Lack of shine and luster, thin, sparse	Protein, zinc, or linoleic acid deficiency	Hypothyroidism, chemotherapy, psoriasis, color treatment
		Easily pluckable	Protein deficiency	Hypothyroidism, chemotherapy, psoriasis, color treatment

Continued

APPENDIX 29. Nutrition-Focused Physical Assessment—cont'd

System	Normal Findings	Physical Findings	Possible Nutrition and Metabolic Associations	Nonnutritional Examples
		Alternating bands of light and dark hair in young children (flag sign)	Protein deficiency	Chemically processed or bleached hair
		"Corkscrew" hair	Copper (Menkes disease)	Chemical alteration
Face	Skin warm, smooth, dry, soft, moist with instant recoil	Diffuse depigmentation, swollen	Protein deficiency	Steroids and other medications
		Pallor	Iron, folate, or B_{12} deficiency	Low-perfusion, low-volume states
		Moon face	Protein, calorie	Cushing's disease
		Bilateral temporal wasting	Protein, calorie	Neuromuscular disorders
Eyes	Evenly distributed brows, lids, lashes; conjunctiva pink without discharge sclerae, without spots; cornea clear; skin without cracks or lesions	Pale conjunctiva	Iron, folate, or B_{12} deficiency	Low output states
		Night blindness	Vitamin A deficiency	
		Dry, grayish, yellow or white foamy spots on whites of eyes (Bitot's spots)	Vitamin A deficiency	Pterygium, Gaucher's disease
		Dull, milky, or opaque cornea (corneal xerosis)	Vitamin A deficiency	
		Dull, dry, rough appearance to whites of eyes and inner lids (conjunctival xerosis)	Vitamin A deficiency	Chemical, environmental
		Softening of cornea (keratomalacia)	Vitamin A deficiency	
		Cracked and reddened corners of eyes (angular palpebritis)	Riboflavin, niacin deficiency	Infection, foreign objects
Nose	Uniform shape, septum slightly to left of midline, nares patent bilaterally, mucosa pink and moist, able to identify smells	Scaly, greasy, with gray or yellowish material around nares (nasolabial seborrhea)	Riboflavin, niacin, pyridoxine deficiency	
		Inflammation, redness of sinus tract, discharge, obstruction or polyps	Irritation of skin membranes	Need to reconsider if placing nasoenteric feeding tube; evaluate for nonfood allergies
Oral Cavity				
Lips, mouth	Pink, symmetric, smooth intact	Bilateral cracks, redness of lips (angular stomatitis)	Riboflavin, niacin, pyridoxine deficiency	Poor-fitting dentures, herpes, syphilis
		Vertical cracks of lips (cheilosis)	Riboflavin, niacin deficiency	Acquired immune deficiency syndrome (Kaposi's sarcoma), environmental exposure
Tongue	Pink, moist, midline, symmetric with rough texture	Magenta (purplish-red color), inflammation of the tongue (glossitis)	Riboflavin deficiency, B_6, niacin, folate, B_{12}, B_2	Crohn's Disease, uremia, Infectious disease state, antibiotics, malignancy, Irritants (excess tobacco, alcohol, spices), generalized skin disorder
		Smooth, slick, loss of papillae (atrophic filiform papillae)	Folate, niacin, riboflavin, iron, or B_{12} deficiency	
		Beefy red color, atrophied taste buds, mucosa red and swollen	Niacin, folate, riboflavin, iron, B_{12} or pyridoxine deficiency	Crohn's disease, infection
		Decreased taste (hypogeusia) Distorted taste (dysgeusia)	Zinc deficiency	Cancer therapy, advanced age

Gums	Pink, moist without sponginess	Spongy, bleeding, receding	Vitamin C deficiency	Dilantin and other medication, poor hygiene, lymphoma, polycythemia, thrombocytopenia
Teeth	Repaired, no loose teeth; color may be various shades of white	Missing, poor repair, caries, loose	Excess sugar	Trauma, syphilis, aging, poor dental hygiene
		White or brownish patches (mottled)	Excess fluoride	Enamel hypoplasia, erosion
Cranial nerves	Intact	Abnormal	Feeding route	
Gag reflex	Intact	Absent	Route of feeding	
Jaw	Proper alignment, movement from side to side	Improper alignment and movement	Ability to chew properly	
Parotid gland	Located anterior to earlobe, no enlargement	Bilateral enlargement	Protein deficiency	Bulimia, cysts, tumors, hyperparathyroidism
Neck nodules	Trachea midline, freely movable without enlargement or nodules	Enlarged thyroid	Iodine deficiency	Cancer, allergy, cold infection
Cardiopulmonary				
Chest, lungs	Anterior and posterior thorax; adequate muscle and fat stores, respirations even and unlabored, symmetric rise and fall of chest during inspiration and expiration, lung sounds clear	Somatic muscle- and fat-wasting; labored respirations; breath sounds such as crackles, rhonchi, and wheezing: evaluate for fluid status vs. tenacious secretions that may labor breathing and increase energy expenditure; also consider increased rate and depth, decreased rate and depth	Protein-energy deficiency Metabolic acidosis Metabolic alkalosis	Respiratory disease (e.g., COPD)
Heart	Rhythm regular and rate within normal range; S_1 and S_2 heart sounds	Irregular rhythm	Potassium deficiency or excess calcium deficiency	Cardiopulmonary disease states
			Magnesium deficiency or excess phosphorus deficiency	
		Enlarged heart	Thiamin deficiency associated with anemia and beriberi	
		Pitting edema	Retention of sodium chloride, which causes the body to retain water Edema-associated disease of heart, liver, kidneys Fluid leaking into the interstitial tissue spaces	
Vascular access devices intact	No swelling, redness, drainage	Purulent drainage, swelling, excessive redness	Nutrition effects if device has to be removed	
Abdomen	Soft, nondistended, symmetric, bilateral without masses, umbilicus in midline, no ascites, bowel sounds present and normoactive; tympanic on percussion; feeding device intact without redness, swelling	Generalized symmetric distention	Obesity	Enlarged organs, fluid, or gas, ileus
		Protruding, everted umbilicus; tight glistening appearance (ascites)	Effects on protein, fluid, sodium concerns of feeding	
		Scaphoid appearance	Protein-calorie deficiency	
		Increased bowel sounds	Nutrition effects in gastroenteritis (normal if hunger pains)	

Continued

APPENDIX 29. Nutrition-Focused Physical Assessment—cont'd

System	Normal Findings	Physical Findings	Possible Nutrition and Metabolic Associations	Nonnutritional Examples
		High-pitched tinkling	Nutrition effects if intestinal fluid and air present, indicating early obstruction	
		Decreased bowel sounds	Nutrition effects if peritonitis or paralytic ileus present	
Kidney, ureter, bladder	Urine golden yellow (ranges from pale yellow to deep gold), clear without cloudiness, adequate output	Decreased output, extremely dark, concentrated	Dehydration	
Musculoskeletal	Full range of motion without joint swelling or pain, adequate muscle strength	Inability to flex, extend, and rotate neck adequately	Interference with ability to feed or make hand-to-mouth contact	
		Decreased range of motion, swelling, impaired joint mobility of upper extremities; muscle wasting on arms, legs; skin folding on buttocks	Protein-calorie deficiency	
		Swollen, painful joints	Vitamin C deficiency	Connective tissue disease
		Enlargement of epiphyses at wrist, ankle, or knees	Vitamins D or C deficiency	Trauma, deformity, or congenital cause
		Bowed legs	Vitamin D deficiency, calcium deficiency	
		Beading of ribs	Vitamin D deficiency, calcium deficiency	Renal rickets, malabsorption
		Pain in calves, thighs	Thiamin deficiency	Deep vein thrombosis, other neuropathy or other
Neurologic	Alert, oriented, hand-to-mouth coordination; no weakness or tremors	Decreased or absent mental alertness; inadequate or absent hand-to-mouth coordination	Interference with the ability to feed or make hand-to-mouth contact	
		Psychomotor changes, confusion, peripheral neuropathy	Protein deficiency; thiamin, pyridoxine, vitamin B_{12} deficiency	Trauma, neurologic disease
		Tetany	Calcium, magnesium deficiency	
	Cranial nerves intact: primary nutritionally focused ones include trigeminal, facial, glossopharyngeal, vagus, and hypoglossal			
	Reflexes (biceps, brachioradialis patella, and Achilles common in examination), functioning within normal range of 2^{++}	Hyperactive reflexes	Hypocalcemia	Tetany, upper motor neuron disease
	Hypoactive reflexes	Hypokalemia	Associated with metabolic diseases such as diabetes mellitus and hypothyroidism	
		Hypoactive Achilles, patellar reflex	Thiamin, vitamin B_{12}	Neurologic disorder

From Hammond K: Physical assessment: a nutritional perspective, Nurs Clin North Am 32(4):779, 1997. Modified, 2010; Hammond K: History and physical examination. In Matarese LE and Gottschlich M., editors: Contemporary Nutrition Support Practice, Philadelphia, 2003, Saunders Company; Porter RS, Kaplan JL (eds.): Nutrition disorders, Merck Manual Online. Accessed March 2010 from http://www.merckmanuals.com/professional/sec01/ch002/ch002a.html.

This chart is not intended to be a comprehensive list for all nutritional or metabolic deficiencies or nonnutrition examples.

APPENDIX 30. Laboratory Values for Nutritional Assessment and Monitoring

Diana Noland, MPH, RD, CCN

I. Principles of Nutritional Laboratory Testing

A. Purpose

Laboratory-based nutritional testing, used to estimate nutrient availability in biologic fluids and tissues, is critical for assessment of both clinical and subclinical nutrient deficiencies. Laboratory data are the only objective data used in nutrition assessment that are "controlled"—that is, the validity of the method of its measurement is checked each time a specimen is assayed by also assaying a sample with a known value. The known sample is called a *control,* and if the value obtained for the sample is outside the range of normal analytic variability, both the specimen and control are measured again. The nutrition professional can use laboratory data to support subjective data and clinical assessment findings. Furthermore, because numeric values do not themselves connote personal judgment, this kind of data can often be passed on to a patient or client without implicit or perceived blame.

B. Specimen Types

Ideally the specimen to be tested reflects the total body content of the nutrient to be assessed. However, often the best specimen is not readily available. The most common specimens for analysis are the following:

Whole blood—Must be collected with an anticoagulant if entire content of the blood is to be evaluated. The two common anticoagulants for whole blood analyses are ethylenediaminetetraacetic acid, a calcium chelator used in hematologic analyses, and heparin (maintains the blood in its most natural state).*

Blood cells—Separated from anticoagulated whole blood for measurement of cellular analyte content.

Plasma—The uncoagulated fluid that bathes the formed elements (blood cells).

Serum—The fluid that remains after whole blood or plasma has coagulated. Coagulation proteins and related substances are missing or significantly reduced.

Urine—Contains a concentrate of excreted metabolites.

Feces—Important in nutritional analyses when nutrients are not absorbed and therefore are present in fecal material.

Hair—An easy-to-collect tissue; usually a poor indicator of actual body levels.

Other tissues—Buccal cells and solid organ biopsy specimens are rarely used in nutrition laboratory assessment.

C. Interpretation of Laboratory Data

As with all data, nutrition data may be quantitative (e.g., how much, how often, how fast), semiquantitative (e.g., many, most, few, a lot, usually, majority, several), or qualitative (e.g., color, shape, species). The advantage of quantitative data is that they are less ambiguous or more objective than other types of observations. Although objective laboratory data are extremely important resources in nutrition assessment, one should be extremely cautious about using a single isolated laboratory test value to make an assessment. One value is often misleading, especially when taken out of the context of an individual's habits, clinical status, and dietary and medical histories. The best data are obtained from analysis of changes in laboratory values. When monitoring patients for changes in nutrition test values, one must consider how much change is necessary to give confidence that a difference is significant. The change required for statistical significance has been called the *critical difference.* It is calculated from measurement of the variances calculated from repeated measurements of an analyte: (1) specimens that have been obtained, at several different times, from each of several healthy persons (intrasubject variation); and (2) separate samples from a large specimen pool (analytic variation).

The critical differences for some plasma proteins of nutritional significance are the following:[†]

Protein	Critical Difference
Albumin	8%
Prealbumin/transthyretin	32%

The statistical probability that two consecutive albumin measurements are statistically different requires that the concentration change by 8% or more. Therefore an albumin increase, for example, from 30 g/L to 32.4 g/L indicates that a statistically significant change has occurred. For prealbumin, an increase from 30 mg/dL to 39.6 mg/dL would be significant. There are two reasons for the large discrepancy in the critical differences for these three proteins. The major reason is that the albumin level is very stable in healthy persons, whereas prealbumin concentrations vary considerably. Also contributing to these differences is the fact that the currently available methods measure albumin more precisely than prealbumin. In practice, assessments are not based on the measurement of a single analyte at one point in time. Changes in laboratory tests may have biologic significance (e.g., patient's condition is improving) long before statistical significance is achieved. The changes in laboratory data may precede changes in other nutritional indices, but generally, although not always, the data available should point to the same conclusion.

D. Reference Ranges

To determine whether a particular laboratory value is abnormal, particularly when serial data are not available, the value is generally compared to a reference range. The reference range is constructed from a large number of test values (20 to >1000). The average value and the standard deviation for these data are determined, and the reference range is calculated from the mean ±2 standard deviations. If the sample group is representative of the reference population, the reference range will include values that reflect those found in approximately 95% of the reference population. Approximately 2.5% of this normal population will have values greater than the upper end of the reference range, and 2.5% will have values less than the lower end. This means that one normal individual in 20 would have a value below or above the reference range.

Reference ranges can be made for different populations. For example, reference ranges based on gender, age, race, and so forth, can be developed. In practice, the differences between populations are often ignored because the importance of small differences in a nutrient analyte is not usually significant. However, in the event of borderline values, the possible influence differences between the population of which the patient is a member and the reference population may need to be taken into account. Reference ranges often are determined by obtaining blood from personnel working in or near the clinical laboratory. This population is often skewed toward younger persons, has few minorities, and is overrepresented by women.

Continued

APPENDIX 30. Laboratory Values for Nutritional Assessment and Monitoring—cont'd

E. Units

Many types of units are used in reporting nutrient-dependent laboratory values. Two basic systems of units are in common use: the conventional system and the Système Internationale d'Unités (SI) system.[‡] The conventional system sometimes lacks convention; thus different laboratories adopt different units to report the same analyte. For example, the conventional report of an ionized calcium value could be 2.3 mEq/L, 46 mg/L or 4.6 mg/dL. However, in the SI system only 1.15 mmol/L is allowed.

F. Nature of Nutritional Testing and Types of Tests

Typically laboratory tests are static assays (i.e., the concentration of an analyte is measured in a biologic fluid [e.g., a fasting blood specimen] at a point in time). Assessment of nutrient status made by this approach is often inaccurate or distorted. Some nutrients can be assessed by tests that are based on measurements that reflect the endogenous availability of a nutrient to a measurable biologic function (e.g., biochemical, tissue, or organ). Most often, functional assessment of nutrient status may be done by measurement of a biochemical marker (i.e., a normal or abnormal metabolite) of function. The results of this type of testing can be reliably considered to reflect the adequacy of a nutrient pool.

*Samples obtained for blood coagulation tests are diluted with solutions containing sodium citrate (a calcium chelator). Because of the dilutional effect of the anticoagulant solutions, citrated samples are not suitable for measurement of the concentrations of analytes.

†Clark GH, Fraser CG: Biological variation of acute phase proteins, *Ann Clin Biochem* 30:373, 1993.

‡Monsen ER: The *Journal* adopts SI units for clinical laboratory values, *J Am Diet Assoc* 37:356, 1987.

Sections of this appendix were written by Mary Litchford, RD, PhD, for the previous edition of this text.

 **NEW DIRECTIONS**

Bioelectrical Impedance Analysis (BIA)—A New Functional Test?

Nutrition assessment is taking on a new level of specificity with the explosion of technology and discoveries of the pathophysiology of disease and functions of the human body. These breakthroughs assist in molecular level identification of nutrition status. Bioelectrical Impedance Analysis (BIA) has a credible history of use in research, but recently has found an increasing use as a clinical tool in nutrition assessment.

BIA estimates body composition and cellular activity by measuring the bulk electrical impedance of the body. The testing procedure involves application of conductors (electrodes) to a person's hand and foot, and sending a small alternating electric current through the body. The different electrical conductive properties of various body tissues (adipose, muscular and skeletal) affect the impedance measurement. An algorithm derived from statistical analysis of BIA measurements is used to calculate the various parameters that can be measured by this technique. Normal hydration is critical for results to be valid, with guidelines prior to testing: drink water (16-24 oz during 4 hours prior to test), and no alcohol (12 hours), food or caffeine drinks (4 hours), or exercise (12 hours) prior to test. Contraindications to BIA testing are pregnancy, or the presence of implants like pacemakers or defibrillators. Follow-up monitoring testing should attempt to be near the same time of day.

There are commercially available BIA devices that measure only body fat % and weight. But professional BIA instruments are available that provide reliable, more comprehensive data, and automatically calculate total body water, intracellular & extracellular water, fat-free mass, percent body fat, phase angle, capacitance and body cell mass. They are very useful in being to track changes in an individual's progress over time.

The multiple parameters measured in a BIA test provide three categories of data:

1. *Anthropometric:* BMI, BMR, Body Fat %, and Lean Body Mass %. These measurements are used with weight management, monitoring wasting syndromes, and acute care formulation of dietary prescriptions. Weight/height/age/gender date must be entered to obtain these results.
2. *Cellular metabolism*: Phase angle (cell membrane fluidity/prognostic marker of mortality), Capacitance (electrical resistance cell membrane), Body Cell Mass (metabolically active cells). Using these three measurements provide an easy-to-use, non-invasive, and reproducible technique to evaluate changes in body composition and nutritional status. Phase angle (BIA) detects changes in tissue electrical properties and is hypothesized as a marker of malnutrition for investigating various diseases in the clinical setting. Lower phase angles suggest cell death or decreased cell integrity, while higher phase angles suggest large quantities of intact cell membranes (Selberg).
3. *Hydration*: Total Body Water (lb. & %), Intracellular water (lb. & %), Extracellular water (lb. & %) Examples for clinical use: general health management, wound care, prevention of pressure ulcers.

NEW DIRECTIONS

Bioelectrical Impedance Analysis (BIA)—A New Functional Test?—cont'd

Every professional practicing nutrition therapy can now consider adding a reasonably priced BIA instrument to their nutritional assessment tool box so as to assist their management of a client or patient. The three companies from which professional BIA instruments can be obtained are:

www.biodynamics.com
www.impedimed.com
www.rjlsystems.com

These companies also provide informative education on the technology and operation of their bioimpedance instruments.

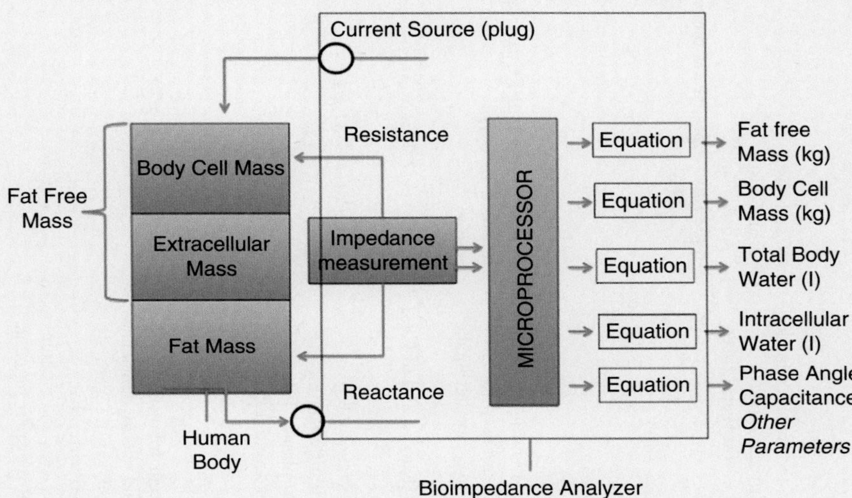

Bauer JM, et al: The Mini Nutritional Assessment (R)—its history, today's practice, and future perspectives, *Nutr Clin Pract* 23:388-396, 2008.

Davis MP, et al: Bioelectrical impedance phase angle changes during hydration and prognosis in advanced cancer, *Am J Hosp Palliat Care* June/July 26(3):180-187, 2009.

Gupta D, et al: The relationship between bioelectrical impedance phase angle and subjective global assessment in advanced colorectal cancer, *Nutrition Journal* 7:19, 2008.

Gupta D, et al: Bioelectrical impedance phase angle as a prognostic indicator in breast cancer, *BMC Cancer* 8:249, 2008.

Hengstermann S, et al: Nutrition status and pressure ulcer: what we need for nutrition screening, *JPEN J Parenter Enteral Nut* 31:288-294, 2007.

Kyle UG: Bioelectrical impedance analysis-part II: utilization in clinical practice, *The American Journal of Clinical Nutrition* 23:1226-1243, 2004.

Methods of Body Composition Tutorials (Interactive). Dept. of Nutrition and Food Sciences, University of Vermont. http://nutrition.uvm.edu/bodycomp/ Accessed May 19, 2011.

Norman K, et al: Cutoff percentiles of bioelectrical phase angle predict functionality, quality of life, and mortality in patients with cancer, *Am J Clin Nutr* 92:612-619, 2010.

Selberg O, Selberg D: Norms and correlates of bioimpedance phase angle in healthy human subjects, hospitalized patients, and patients with liver cirrhosis, *Eur J Appl Physiol* 86:509-516, 2002.

Van Loan MD, et al: Use of bioimpedance spectroscopy (BIS) to determine extracellular fluid (ECF), intracellular fluid (ICF), total body water (TBW), and fat free mass (FFM). In Ellis K, editor: *Human Body Composition: In Vivo Measurement and Studies*, New York, 1993, Plenum Publishing Co., pp 6770.

APPENDIX 30. Laboratory Values for Nutritional Assessment and Monitoring—cont'd

II. Clinical Chemistry Panels

A. Protein Status

Test	Principles	Interpretation	Reference Range	Limitations and Implications
Urea Urinary Nitrogen (UUN)	The protein pool (visceral and somatic) N is catabolized to urea; urine urea represents ~80% of N catabolized; requires accurate estimate of protein intake; thus usually used only for TPN or tube-feeding patients.	UUN is compared with the actual N intake. Nitrogen Balance = Nitrogen intake (Protein g/day÷6.25) – Nitrogen Losses (UUN (g)+ 4)[a]	– = Catabolism 0 = Catabolism + = Anabolism (3-6 g/24 hr = optimal use range)	24 hour urine collection must be quantitative (complete); UUN not appropriate in renal insufficiency; does not account for wound leakage, cell losses, or diarrhea; inaccurate in metabolically stressed patients.
Total Urinary Nitrogen (TUN)	Some N is excreted as non-urea N (e.g., ammonia and creatinine); 24-hour TUN reflects total protein catabolism, accounting for all sources of urinary N; as for UUN, requires accurate protein intake. Used primarily to accurately follow the protein catabolic response during disease and response to nutritional support.	TUN is compared with the actual N intake; Nitrogen Balance = Nitrogen intake (Protein g/day÷6.25) – Nitrogen Losses (TUN (g)+ 2)[b]	– = Catabolism 0 = Catabolism + = Anabolism (3-6 g/24 hr = optimal use range)	Urine 24 hour collection must be quantitative (complete); TUN not appropriate in renal insufficiency; not done in many institutions; does not account for wound leakage, cell losses, or diarrhea.
Urea Kinetic Modeling (UKM)	Formulas used to estimate nPCR from changes in BUN concentration in patients with impaired renal function.	Urinary urea (KrU) and BUN levels (urea generation rate—GU) are used to determine nPCR; 1- to 3-day diet intake compared with nPCR. Urea kinetic Modeling (Kt/V_{urea} and nPCR)	In protein balance, nPRC = protein intake (g/kg/day)	Urea lost in dialysis must be accounted for in calculating urea nitrogen appearance. Dietary protein intake hard to estimate.
Visceral Proteins				
Total protein (TP)	Protein concentration in serum is easily measured colorimetrically; largely reflects albumin (~50% of TP) and globulin (~50%).	TP levels parallel clinical signs of malnutrition if significant inflammatory condition not present; plasma TP is 0.4 g/dL greater than serum TP.	6.4-8.3 g/dL (64-83 g/L)	Total protein measurements can reflect nutritional status and may be used to screen for kidney and liver disease; does not reflect protein status during inflammatory (acute-phase) response; monitor other inflammatory markers when evaluating TP.
Albumin (ALB)	Easily and quickly measured colorimetrically; large body pool (3-5 g/kg body weight), ~60% is outside the plasma in the extravascular pool; long half-life of 3 weeks.	Decreased levels can occur following short-term protein and energy deficiency or protein exudates such as in severe burns; often associated with other deficiencies (i.e., zinc, iron, and vitamin A) reflecting the ALB transport function of many small molecules.	3.5-5 g/dL) (35-50 g/L)	Stable half life ~3 weeks. Preserved in the presence of starvation (marasmus). Significance confounded by being a negative phase reactant, liver disease, protein-losing enteropathy, nephrotic syndrome, pregnancy, oral contraceptive use, strenuous exercise, and hemodilution. Hepatic proteins are indicators of morbidity and mortality: help identify patients who are at increased nutritional risk because of trauma or illness.[1]
Globulin (GLOB)	Large body pool (3-5 g/kg body weight), ~35% is outside the plasma in the extravascular pool; long half-life averages 23 days, but varies with particular globulins.	Globulin proteins include enzymes and carriers that transport proteins including antibodies that primarily assist in immune function and fight infection.	2.3-3.4 g/dL (23-34 g/L)	Significance confounded by acute stress reaction, infection, inflammatory conditions.

A/G Ratio	Calculated from ALB and GLOB values by direct measurement of TP and ALB.	It represents the relative amounts of ALB and GLOB	A/G Ratio 1:1 - normal <1:1 - disease state	
Normalized Protein Catabolic Rate (nPCR)	nPCR is determined by measuring the intradialytic appearance of urea in body fluids plus any urea lost in the urine in patients with residual renal function. nPCR = 0.22 + (0.036 x *intradialytic rise in BUN x × 24)/(intradialytic interval). (also called: Protein Nitrogen Appearance rate (PNA) (g/day) = 13 + 7.31 UNA (mmol/day) [UNA (mmol/day) = Vd(ml) x Cd (mmol/L) + Vu (ml) + Cu (mmol/L)]	Useful in assessing Dietary Protein Intake (DPI) in patients who are in a steady state on hemodialysis, as a means toward determining adequate nutrition status.	0.81-1.02 g UN/kg per day	nPCR considered superior to sAlb for monitoring nutrition protein status due to sAlb influence by processes other than nutrition status..[2] During hemodialysis the PCR can also reflect inadequate dialysis. For CAPD patients the nPCR value has not been consistently predictive of outcome.[3]
Transferrin (Tf or TFN)	The iron bound globulin protein that responds to the need for iron. Can be calculated from TIBC and serum iron; half-life ~9 days. See Chapter 8	Tf increased with low iron stores, and prevents build up of highly toxic excess unbound iron in circulation. In iron overload states Tf levels decrease. Because B6 is required for iron to bind to Hgb, B6 deficiency promotes ↑ Tf from the ↑ circulating iron that binds to Tf; smaller extravascular pool than albumin.	Adult male: 215-365 mg/dL (2.15-3.65 g/L) Adult female: 250-380 mg/dL (2.50-3.80 g/L) Newborn: 130-275 mg/dL (1.3-2.75 g/L) Child: 203-360 mg/dL (2.03-3.6 g/L) Pregnancy and estrogen HRT associated with ↑ Tf.	Lead can biologically mimic and displace iron thus releasing Fe into circulation and ↑ Tf. Tf is a negative acute phase reactant diminished in chronic illness and hypoproteinemia.
Transferrin Saturation (Tf-sat or TSAT)	Tf-sat (%) = Serum iron level÷TIBC x 100%	Tf-sat decreases to <15% in Fe deficiency; useful in diagnosis of iron toxicity or Fe overload (hemochromatosis).	M: 20%-50% F: 15%-50% Chronic illness: normal Tf-sat%. Late pregnancy: low Tf-sat%.	Increased Tf-sat when low vitamin B_6 as in aplastic anemia.
PreAlbumin (PAB)/ Transthyretin (TTR)	Transports T_4 and acts as a carrier for retinol-binding protein; PAB also called *thyroxin-binding protein*; half-life 2 days.	More sensitive protein-energy balance indicator than ALB or transferrin even during inflammatory conditions; responds rapidly to nutrition intervention; reportedly more sensitive to energy intake than to protein intake. Zinc deficiency reduces PAB levels.	15-36 mg/dL or 150-360 mg/L (1.5-3.6 g/L) Malnutrition: <8 mg/dL (<0.8 g/L or <80 mg/L)	Very sensitive to stress response, also ↓ in liver disease, protein-losing enteropathy, nephrotic syndrome, hemodilution, acute zinc deficiency and acute stress reaction. PAB shown not to be a good marker of protein status, but continues as a prognostic index for mortality and morbidity.[4]
Retinol-binding protein (RBP)	Transport retinol; because of low molecular weight, RBP is filtered by glomerulus and catabolized by the kidney tubule; half-life = 12 hours	More sensitive protein-energy balance indicator than ALB or PAB; responds rapidly to nutritional intervention; reportedly more sensitive to protein intake than to energy intake.	2.6-7.6 mg/dL (1.43-2.86 mmol/L)	Very sensitive to stress response; also decreased in liver disease, protein-losing enteropathy, nephrotic syndrome, vitamin A and zinc deficiencies, and hemodilution; increased in chronic renal disease, regardless of PEM status.
Insulin-like growth factor-1 (IGF-1) (Somatomedin C)	The peptide mediator of growth hormone activity produced by the liver; half-life of a few hours; much less sensitive to stress response than other proteins.	Low in chronic undernutrition; increases rapidly during nutrition repletion; TSAT, PAB, and RBP are not affected. Elevated levels associated with elevated GH in acromegaly and neoplastic activity.	Adult: 42-110 ng/mL Children age 0-19: can vary with age and gender Tanner Stages (Appendices 17 & 18) used for references per age	Reduced levels seen in hypopituitarism, hypothyroidism, liver disease, and with estrogen use. Growing evidence of elevated IGF-1 as a prognostic biomarker of neoplastic activity.[5,6]

Continued

APPENDIX 30. Laboratory Values for Nutritional Assessment and Monitoring—cont'd

Test	Principles	Interpretation	Reference Range	Limitations and Implications
B. Tests of Metabolic Indicators				
Urine creatinine (U:Cr)	U:Cr concentration in fasting, first-void urine used to compare amino acid catabolism (BUN) with muscle mass (creatinine).	Urine concentration (mg/dL) U:Cr = Urine area (mg/dL) ÷ Urine creatinine (mg/dL). The U:Cr is used in comparing other markers like microablbumin, albumin, GFR ratios. Can be used in uncomplicated protein-energy deficiency to approximate status.	*Risk* / *Ratio* Low >12.0 Medium 6.0-12.0 High <6.0	Affected by recent protein intake; therefore not useful for estimating long-term status; not used for accurate assessment or monitoring of catabolism.
Hemoglobin A1C (HgbA1C)	Glycosylated hemoglobin; dependent on blood glucose level over life span of RBC (120 days); the more glucose the GHb is exposed, the greater the % HgbA1C.	Assessment of the mean glycemic blood level and of chronic diabetic control detecting for the previous 2-3 months.[7]	Non-diabetic adult/child: 4%-5.9% Controlled diabetes (DM): 4-7% Fair DM control: 7-8% Poor DM control: >8%	HbgA1 measurement is a simple, rapid, and objective procedure. Home testing available.
Insulin, fasting	Pancreatic hormone signaling cell membrane insulin receptors to initiate glucose transport into cell; Test fasting 7 hours, or 1 or 2 hours post prandial; usually ordered with blood glucose test.	Elevated levels associated with hyperinsulinemia related to metabolic syndrome; diagnosis of insulin-producing neoplasms; excess insulin associated with inflammatory conditions.	Adult values: Fasting 6-27 μ IU/mL 1 or 2 hour PP: see lab reference	Good test and retest reliability, and covariance is stable over time.[8] Insulin antibodies may invalidate the test.
Triglycerides (TG)	TG molecule of glycerol with three fatty acids; Blood test fasting 12-14 hours.	TG increase following a meal, sugar or alcohol. Accurate CVD risk with calculation of LDL/VLDL; TG >1000 associated with pancreatitis. One of five parameters for diagnosis of metabolic syndrome.	Age adjusted normal: <150 mg/dL (<1.7 (mmol/L) Borderline High: 150-199 mg/dL (1.8 to 2.2 mmol/L) High: 200-499 mg/dL (2.3 to 5.6 mmol/L) Very high—500 mg/dL or above (5.7 mmol/L or above)	Good test and retest reliability, and covariance is stable over time. Avoid alcohol and high-sugar foods for 24 hours prior to test, or may reflect abnormal TG elevation.
Low Density Lipoproteins (LDL-C)	12-14 hour fasting sample	LDL-C indicating cardiovascular risk.	Normal: 100-130 mg/dL If high risk CVD patient: <100 mg/dL If very high risk CVD patient: <70 mg/dL	Good test and retest reliability, and covariance is stable over time.
Fibrinogen	Acute-phase reactant protein essential to blood-clotting mechanism/ coagulation system.	Decreased fibrinogen related to prolonged PT and PTT; produced in liver; rises sharply during tissue inflammation or necrosis; association with CHD, stroke, myocardial infarction and peripheral arterial disease.	200-400 mg/dL If <100 mg/dL, increased risk of bleed ing. Should be monitored in conjunction with blood platelet levels involved with coagulation status.	Good test and retest reliability, and covariance is stable over time; diets rich in Omega 3/6 fatty acids reduce fibrinogen blood levels.
C-Reactive Protein high sensitivity (hs-CRP)	A nonspecific acute phase reactant; short half life 5-7 hr; CRP responds to inflammation in 6-10 hours. (also called CRP-ultra sensitivity and CRP-cardio)	A sensitive marker of bacterial disease and systemic inflammation; associated with periodontitis, trauma, cardiovascular disease, neoplastic proliferation and bacterial infections.	Low Risk for CVD = Less than 1.0 mg/L Intermediate Risk for CVD = 2.9 mg/L High Risk for CVD = Greater than 3.0 mg/L Seek inflammatory cause >10 mg/L	Useful metabolic indicator for adults.[9] Acute-phase reactant; relates mostly to bacterial infection, central adiposity, trauma and neoplastic activity.

C. Immune Dysregulation Tests *Allergies/Sensitivity*				
Immunoglobulins (IgE, IgG, IgM, IgA)	Serologic antibody screening tests; testing of Immunoglobulins; Total IgE ELISA; RAST (radioallergosorbent-blood IgE); Bloodspot: IgG Provocative specific antigen skin prick: (IgE related skin response) used to diagnose allergy and identify the allergen.	Used to determine immunodeficiency states; measurement of +IgE = allergic disorders; (see Table 27-3) +IgG = delayed immunologic sensitivity or intolerance response (see Table 27-3). IgA = largest % Ig primarily made in GI lymphoid tissue and marker of immune strength and response.	Total IgA: Adults = 85-385 mg/dL Children = 1-350 mg/dL Total IgG: Adults = 565-1765 mg/dL Total IgE = <10 IU/L RAST IgE = <1 low allergic risk Total IgM: Adults 55-375 mg/dL Children 20-200 mg/dL Total IgD = minimal	NSAIDS, glucocorticosteroids, vitamin C, bioflavonoids can suppress the immunologic response and promote a false negative. IgA used as a biomarker reference of adequate immune response to enable measurement of IgG, IgE, IgM.
Innate Immune Factors				
Total Leukocyte Count (TLC)	Calculated from the percentage of lymphocytes reported in the hemogram and the WBC count. Units = cells/µl or cells/mm^3	Decreased in protein-energy malnutrition and immunocompromised state.	Normal: >2700 Moderate depletion: 900-1800 Severe depletion: <900	
Delayed cutaneous hypersensitivity	Anergy for antigens, such as mumps and *Candida;* occurs in malnutrition; antigens injected intradermally; redness (erythema) and hardness (induration) read 1, 2, or 3 days later.	Response affected by protein-energy status and vitamin A, iron, zinc, and vitamin B_6 deficiencies.	*Induration* 1+: <5 mm 2+: 6-10 mm 3+: 11-20 mm 4+: >20 mm Erythema present or absent	Usefulness in acute care limited by drugs, effect of aging and disease (metabolic, malignant, and infectious diseases); difficult to administer and interpret results; semiquantitative.
Cytokines	Serum or joint fluid proteins tested from venous blood. They include lymphocytes, (T & B cells), monocytes, leukocytes (interleukins), eosinophils, interferon and growth factors. (See Chapter 8)	A group of immune reactant proteins that have many functions even from one cell to another. They respond to the environmental influences to communicate and orchestrate the immune response to protect from cancer, infection and inflammation.	Cytokine examples: IL-1 IL-6 IL-8 IL-10 TNF-α TH-1 TH-2 (per lab references)	
Adaptive Immune Factors				
Eosinophils (Eosinophil leukocyte)	Blood: BAL fluid CSF specimen to rule out eosinophilic meningitis.	Blood: Wide range of clinical conditions reflect nonspecific eosinophilia; elevated related to possible allergies, asthma, sensitivities, or cancers; particularly elevated eosinophils are found with intestinal parasites; noninfectious conditions.	Blood: 1% to 3% 50-500/mm^3 BAL negative for infection CSF < 10 mm^3	Because of the nonspecific nature of blood eosinophilia, it can require further clinical investigation to determine the causal agent.
Food Intolerance/Sensitivity Panels				
Antigen Leucocyte Cellular Antibody Test (ALCAT)	Measurement of leukocyte cellular reactivity in whole blood, measures levels of mediators by blood cells presented with food or chemical antigens; measures relative changes in cell size (see Table 27-3)	Food and chemical non-IgE sensitivity (intolerance) testing for up to 350 foods plus gliadin/gluten, casein/whey, and candida albicans; food additives, molds, environmental chemicals, pharmacoactive agents, and other suspected items upon request.	350 Foods: Acceptable Foods Mild Intolerance Moderate Intolerance Severe Intolerance Candida/gluten-gliadin/casein-whey, chemicals/molds: No Reaction Mild, Moderate or Severe Reaction	NSAIDS, glucocorticosteroids, vitamin C, bioflavonoids can suppress the immunologic response and promote a false negative. IgA used as a biomarker reference of adequate immune response.

Continued

APPENDIX 30. Laboratory Values for Nutritional Assessment and Monitoring—cont'd

Test	Principles	Interpretation	Reference Range	Limitations and Implications
Mediator Release Test (MRT) (immunologic food reaction test)	Untreated whole blood assay; sample is divided into 150 aliquots plus control samples and incubated with a precise dilution of pure extract of a specific food or food additive[c] (see Chapter 27)	Non IgE-mediated reactions; measurement of blood components; blood speciman checked against the specific signs of cell-mediated reactivity to the antigen challenged (imminent or actual mediator release). See Table 27-3.	Normal = negative Mild, moderate or severe reactions are delineated.	NSAIDS, glucocorticosteroids, vitamin C, bioflavonoids can suppress the immunologic response and promote a false negative. IgA used as a biomarker reference of adequate immune response to measure.
Celiac Panel/Gluten Sensitivity Panel	1. Immunologic and genomic for celiac or gluten sensitivity–related genes.	Measurements to identify a possible genetic or immunologic disease of the small bowel in response to exposure to gluten or gliadin molecules in diet. Continued long-term exposure to gluten or gliadin molecules promotes nutrient deficiencies and insufficiencies.	See celiac tests 2.- 10.	Any of the celiac tests 2-10 tests should be compared with baseline IgA serum levels and presence of immune suppressive medications to rule out IgA deficiency, which can skew test results to false negative because of compromised or suppressed immune response. Undiagnosed celiac is associated with increased incidence of all chronic diseases and shortened lifespan[10,11,12]
	2. Endomysial antibodies (EMA)	High specificity for celiac disease; may obviate need for small bowel biopsy for diagnosis; become negative on gluten-free diet;	EMA negative	Sensitivity/Specificity 90+%/95%
	3. TissueTransglutaminase (tTG-IgA, tTG-IgG)	Autoantigen of Celiac disease, tTG is indicative of villous atrophy secondary to gluten exposure causing damage to GI small intestine villi. tTG negative test results indicate gluten-free diet compliance; marker of restoration of GI villi tight junctions and small bowel villi integrity.	tTG IgA negative tTG IgG negative	Sensitivity/specificity 98%/95% in adults; 96%/99% in children. Best age to begin measuring tTG is age 2-3 years.[13]
	4. Antigliadin antibodies (AGA IgA, AGA IgG))	Positive results are evidence of immune response to the gliadin proteins in gluten-containing foods.	AGA IgA negative AGA IgG negative	Lowest sensitivity among celiac panel (70%-85%) and specificity (70%-90%) for celiac. Also useful for non-celiac gluten sensitivity.
	5. Deamidated gliadin peptide (DGP)	DGP antibodies improves[14] diagnostic accuracy for diagnosis of CD when tested with tTG; proteins present in the submucosa of affected person's bond to deamidated peptides to form molecular complexes that stimulate the immune system.	DGP negative	Specificity varied between 97.3% and 99.3%. Sensitivity of IgG anti-DGP significantly better than that of IgG anti-tTG ($p < 0.05$). Specificity was significantly better than IgA and IgG AGA[15]
	6. Celiac genetic HLA haplotype HLA-DQ2 HLA-DQ8 Cellular assay/MLC to test HLA class II types	HLA-DQ2 and HLA-DQ8 positive indicates a low positive predictive value but a very high negative predictive value for celiac disease. Higher prevalence of CD in patients with Type 1 DM or autoimmune thyroid disease (2%-4%) than in general population	Genotype: HLA DQ2 negative HLA DQ8 negative	More than 97% of individuals with celiac disease share the two HLA markers DQ2 and DQ8, which have high sensitivity and poor specificity. One of the markers can increase possible non-celiac gluten sensitivity (e.g., Type 1 DM DQA1*0501:DQB1*0201 haplotype).[14,15,16]

	7. Wheat/Gluten Proteome Reactivity & Autoimmunity	Functional medicine serum lab tests to broaden the view of celiac and gluten sensitivity by assessing antibody production against an array of protein, enzyme and peptide antigens; includes *glutens, lectins, opioids* and the enzyme *glutamic decarboxylase* (GAD65) IgG, IgA. Available from www.cyrexlabs.com.	ELISA Index Wheat IgG 0.30-1.30 IgA 0.40-2.40 Agglutinin IgG 0.30-1.50 IgA 0.90-1.90 Alpha Gliadin 17 MER IgG 0.30-1.50 IgA 0.60-2.00 Alpha Gliadin 33 MER IgG 0.30-1.40 IgA 0.60-1.80 Gamma Gliadin 15 MER Omega Gliadin IgG 0.50-1.60 IgA 0.60-1.80 Glutenin IgG 0.20-1.50 IgA 0.50-1.70 Gluteomorphin IgG 0.30-1.50 IgA 0.60-1.80 Prodynorphin IgG 0.40-1.70 IgA 0.60-1.80 GAD65 IgG 0.40-1.30 IgA 0.80-1.50	Enhances clinical sensitivity and specificity in detection of celiac and gluten sensitivity reactions
	8. Gluten-Associated Cross-Reactive Foods and Foods Sensitivity IgG + IgA Combined Cow's Milk Alpha-Casein & Beta-Casein Casomorphin Milk Butyrophilin American Cheese Chocolate (Others available)	Functional medicine serum lab tests to assess IgG and IgA immune antibody reactions to known cross-reactive food antigens, with the most common being casein. Other foods included are: sesame, hemp, rye, barley, polish wheat, buckwheat, sorghum, millet, spelt, amaranth, quinoa, yeast, tapioca, oats, coffee, corn, rice, potato.	ELISA Index: IgG & IgA combined 0.20/0.40-1.80/2.00	Assists further dietary evaluation for celiac or gluten sensitive individuals that are non-responsive to a gluten-free diet; can relate to gut dysbiosis and continued GI inflammation. Available from cyrexlabs.com.
	9. Biopsy, small bowel/jejunal	Gold standard for diagnosis of celiac disease. Recommended to correlate with positive serology.	Negative	Current tendency to rely on serologic examination and genetic testing for therapeutic recommendations and monitoring of individual because of invasive nature of biopsy.
III. Tests of Carbohydrate Absorption **Lactose Intolerance**				
Hydrogen Breath Test for Lactose (HBT-lactose)	Lactose loading (2 g/kg) in lactase deficiency allows bacterial metabolism of lactose with production of H_2 gas. Breath analyzed for H_2 by gas chromatography.	Breath H_2 measured fasting and 0.5 and 2 hours after dosing with lactose; a significant increase is associated with malabsorption.	Normal increase: <50 parts/million (i.e., <50 ppm)	Bacterial overgrowth can cause false-positive results; consumption of soluble fiber or legumes and smoking are associated with H_2 production; false-negative results caused by antibiotics.

Continued

APPENDIX 30. Laboratory Values for Nutritional Assessment and Monitoring—cont'd

Test	Principles	Interpretation	Reference Range	Limitations and Implications
Lactose tolerance test	Lactose loading (50 g) followed by blood sampling at 5, 10, 30, 60, 90, and 120 min after dose; glucose produced from lactose is assayed.	Lactase deficiency associated with <20 mg/dL increase in glucose.	Normal glucose increase >20 mg/dL	Test is not specific (many false positives) or sensitive (many false negatives).
Fructose Intolerance				
Hydrogen Breath Test-Fructose (HBT-fructose)	An assessment for the change in the level of hydrogen and/or methane gas is diagnostic for fructose malabsorption.	HBT-fructose can be used to diagnose a mutation in the adlolase B gene. If hereditary fructose intolerance, may result in gastrointestinal symptoms and hypoglycemia. (Guery 2007)	Normal increase <20 parts/million (<20 ppm) Positive BHT-fructose >20 parts per million (>20 ppm)	Positive test results indicate probable benefit of a fructose-restricted diet; research supports use in abdominal pain, IBS, gout, and unexplained liver disease.
Fructose Sensitivity	Blood lymphocyte speciman grown with a mitogen to measure growth by incorporating tritiated radioactive thymidine into the DNA of the cells A functional test of fructose metabolism.	Functional intracelluar metabolic test of possible in-born errors compromising fructose metabolism like fructose-6-phospate (Vantygmhem 2009)	> 34% (valid for male and female of 12 years or older)	Rule out fructose sensitivity in hypoglycemia of unknown etiology, overweight, obesity.
IV. Tests of Lipid Status				
Lipids				
Cholesterol, Total serum or plasma (CHOL)	CHOL is enzymatically released from cholesterol esters; fasting test	Total CHOL correlated with risk for cardiovascular diseases but not as good an indicator as HDL-c and LDL-c. See NCEP guidelines.	Desirable: <200 mg/dL (<5.2 mmol/L) Borderline: 200-239 mg/dL (5.2-6.2 mmol/L) High risk: 240 mg/dL (6.2 mmol/L) Lower limit: 120 mg/dL (3.0 mmol/dL)	Cholesterol measurements have considerable within-subject variability. May partly result from variability in specimen collection or handling.
High Density Lipoproteins (HDL-c)	LDL-c (and VLDL-c) are precipitated from the serum before measurement of residual of particle size HDL-c; direct measurement of HDL-c is now done in some laboratories.	HDL-c is called "good cholesterol" to indicate that it is protective against atherosclerotic vascular development, or a negative risk factor	Desirable: Men >40 mg/dL (>1 mmol/L) Women >50 mg/dL (>1.25 mmol/L)	Some precipitation methods cause underestimation of HDL. HDL can be divided into classes: HDL_1, HDL_2, and HDL_3; Elevated HDL_3 correlates with risk of CVD.
Low Density Lipoproteins (LDL-c)	LDL-c is estimated by the Friedewald formula, LDL-c = total cholesterol – HDL-c – TG/5, or by new direct assays. Available lipid particle size testing examples: www.privateMDLab.com(VAP(tm) Lipid Profile) www.BerkeleyHeartLab.com	LDL-c is called "bad cholesterol" to indicate that it is a postive risk factor for CVD. See NCEP guidelines. Pattern B (small, dense LDL-C) is associated with increased risk of CHD and is responsive to diet. Pattern A (larger, buoyant LDL) is not associated with risk.	Desirable: <100 mg/dL (<2.59 mmol/L) Borderline: 130-159 mg/dL(3.4-4.1 mmol/L) High risk: >160 mg/dL (>4.1 mmol/L) Women: 40-160 mg/dL (0.45-1.81 mmol/L) Men: 35-135 mg/dL (0.40-1.55 mmol/L)	Calculation only valid when TG concentration is <400 mg/dL, cannot be determined in nonfasting serum or plasma. Direct assay methods preferred.
Triglycerides (TGs)	Lipases release glycerol and fatty acids from TGs;	The association of TGs and CHD has been shown. Elevated TG increases blood viscosity.	<150 mg/dL normal 150-199 mg/dL Borderline high 200-399 mg/dL High >500 mg/dL very high	Fasting specimen is essential; sugar concentrated foods and alcohol ingestion can increase; some anticoagulants may affect TG level.
Fat Malabsorption				
Fecal fat screening	Microscopic inspection of fat-stained (Sudan stain) specimens for the presence of lipid droplets.	Trained observers are able to identify excessive fat in ~80% of persons with fat malabsorption.	Qualitative results	Patient must be consuming sufficient fat for analysis to reveal malabsorption. Semiquantitative.

Prothrombin time (PT)	Fat malabsorption decreases absorption of fat-soluble vitamins A,E,D,K,Beta-Carotene; low vitamin K levels impair coagulation, causing a prolonged PT. (also can be called INR (international normalized ratio))	A prolonged PT is a relatively sensitive but nonspecific indicator of the fat-soluble vitamin K from fat malabsorption.	10-15 sec INR: 0.8-1.1 Possible critical value: > 20 sec. INR: > 5.5	Tests effected by oral anticoagulants and other drugs, reduced platelet count, acquired and hereditary bleeding diseases, and liver disease PT.
Quantitative fecal fat determination	Patient must consume 100 g fat/day (4-8 oz whole milk/day, and 2 Tbsp vegetable oil/meal) during and for 2 days before collection	Quantitative 72-hour stool collection required for accurate assessment; average daily discharge used for interpretation.	Normal: <5 g fat/24 hr Malabsorption: >10 g/24 hr	Failure to adhere to the diet invalidates the results.
Carotene, Serum Total) (CARO)	Carotenoids, fat-soluble pigments in plant foods, poorly absorbed in fat malabsorption; light sensitive; transport specimen in amber transport tube; Quantitative Spectrophotometry testing. See Raman Spectroscopy, Chapter 27.	A CARO level of less than 50 mg/dL is seen in ~85% of patients with fat malabsorption.	50-200 mcg/dL (0.74-3.72 mmol/L)	Decreased CARO levels or Low spectrophotometry score are also seen in those with low vegetable and fruit diets (e.g., in TPN or tube feeding), liver failure, celiac disease, cystic fibrosis, human immunodeficiency virus, and some lipoprotein disorders.
Vitamin A, D, E, K	See V. Tests of Micronutrient Status.			
Fatty acid analysis	Whole blood or RBC levels of ALA (C18:3n3) and LA (C18:2*n*6) reflect essential fatty acid status; Also, complex relationships regarding fatty acid analysis are known in lipid biochemistry-related to neurological and inflammatory diseases, cell membrane dysfunction and genetic disorders [17,18]	RBC fatty acid shown to associate with fatty acid tissue composition. Plasma fatty acid is associated with fat dietary or supplement intake or fat digestion and absorption. Endogenous synthesis assessed by eicosapentaenoic (EPA (C20:3*n*9): DHA(C22:4n3): DGLA (C20:3n6) Ratio supports neurologic integrity and inflammation control; plasma phospholipid C20:3*n*9/C18:2*n*6 ratio used to assess status.	C20:3*n*9/C18:2*n*6 ratio >0.2 confirms imbalance of EPA:DHA general Reference 1:1. Omega 6:3 between 1:1 and 4:1.	Is not specific for risk of atherosclerotic disease; inflammation influences this fatty acid test. Likely causes are minor injuries, trauma, and other. Bacterial infections, periodontal/cavitations, orodental disease,[19] *chlamydia pneumoniae,*[20] and central adiposity[21]
V. Tests of Micronutrient Status				
A. Vitamins				
Thiamin (B_1)[c]	Thiamin status is usually assessed by measuring the amount of TPP needed to fully activate the RBC enzyme transketolase.	The TPP needed to fully activate transketolase is inversely related to B_1 status; percent stimulation by TTP.	Normal: 70-200 nmol/L (for individuals not taking thiamine (B1)) Stimulation >20% (index >1.2) indicates deficiency	Amount (and activity) of enzyme affected by drugs, iron, folate, or vitamin B_{12} status, malignant or GI diseases, and diabetes.
Riboflavin (B_2)	Riboflavin status is assessed by measuring the amount of FAD needed to fully activate RBC enzyme GR	The FAD needed to fully activate GR is inversely related to B_2 status; percent stimulation.	% Stimulation >40% (index >1.4) indicates deficiency	Amount or activity of enzyme may change with age, iron status, liver disease, and glucose-6-phosphate dehydrogenase deficiency.
Niacin (B_3)[d]	No tests have been developed.[d]			
Pyridoxine (B_6)[e] PLP compounds	1. RBC enzymes, ALT (SGPT) or AST (SGOT),[e] are assayed for the presence of PLP as the enzymes' cofactor. 2. Plasma PLP can be directly measured by chromatography.	1. Difference between enzyme activities before and after addition of PLP is inversely related to B_6 status. 2. PLP is major transport form of B_6; therefore serum levels reflect body stores.	1. % ALT stimulation of >25% or AST activity of >50% in deficiency 2. Normal: 0.50-3.0 mcg/dL (20-120 nmol/L)	1. Disease and drugs that affect the liver and heart and pregnancy confound interpretation. 2. Deficiency may be seen clinically before plasma PLP levels decrease.

Continued

APPENDIX 30. Laboratory Values for Nutritional Assessment and Monitoring—cont'd

Test	Principles	Interpretation	Reference Range	Limitations and Implications
	3. Trp load test, measures excretion of the PLP-dependent metabolite xanthurenate acid (XA). 24 hour urine collection required.	3. In this functional test the levels of urinary XA should decrease significantly when 3-5 g of L-Trp is ingested if marginal vitamin B_6 status	3. Marginal status: >50 mg/24 hr	3. Steroid drugs and estrogen enzyme activity; some drugs cause analytic errors. Trp load test most sensitive and responsive to functional adequacy of B6.
Folate[g]	1. Because of ↓ DNA synthesis, large RBCs are produced.	1. Deficiency leads to increase in MCV (macrocytic sized RBCs)	1. Normal: MCV <100	1. Not sensitive or specific for folate. Possible involvement with B_6, B_{12}, SAMe and other cofactors in the methionine pathway.
	2. Shape of neutrophil nucleus affected by folate deficiency.	2. Neutrophil lobe count seen in folate deficiency.	2. Normal: < or equal 4 lobes per neutrophil	2. Lobe count sensitive but not specific.
	3. Blood folate levels can be directly measured by radioimmunoassay.	3. Both RBC and serum folate are indicators of body stores.	3. 2-10 mcg/L serum; 140-960 ng/L RBC (3.2-22 nmol/L)	3. Plasma from nonfasted subjects may reflect recent intake; RBC folate is not measured accurately.
	4. Functional folate status assayed by FIGLU in 24-hour urine or after oral histidine loading.	4. After 2-15 g loading dose, 10-50 mg of FIGLU should be excreted in 8 hours.	4. Normal: <7.4 mg/24 hours (<42.6 mmol/24 hr) without loading	4. FIGLU affected by vitamin B_{12}, drugs, liver disease, cancer, tuberculosis, and pregnancy.
	5. Single Nucleotide Polymorphisms (SNPs) MTHFR 677C MTHFR1298C	5. SNPs of compromised methylation (transfer of methyl groups in metabolism) potential in use and conversion of folate or folic acid intracellularly. See Chapter 5.	MTHF 677C/1298C Normal = Wild type –/–	Other SNPs are known that affect methylation metabolism: COMT, CYP1B1, and other cytochrome enzymes. See Chapter 5.
Cobalamin (B_{12})	1. Because of low B12 resulting in decreased DNA synthesis, large RBCs are produced.	1. Deficiency leads to increase in MCV	1. Normal: MCV <100	1. Not sensitive or specific for B_{12}.
	2. Shape of neutrophil nucleus is affected by B_{12} deficiency.	2. Increased neutrophil lobe count in B_{12} deficiency.	2. Normal: < or equal 4 lobes per neutrophil	2. Lobe count sensitive but not specific.
	3. B_{12} can be directly measured by radioimmunoassay.	3. Levels <150 ng/L indicate deficiency (age affects level).	3. 160-950 pg/mL (118-701 pmol/L)	3. Marginal deficiency not corolated with level.
	4. Methylmalonic acid excretion reflects a functional test of B_{12} availability for BCAA metabolism.	4. Methylmalonic acid (MMA) excretion >300 mg/24 hr in B_{12} deficiency. Sensitive test without being overly specific.	4. Normal excretion: 5 mg/24 hr (42 mmol/24 hr) Serum MMA -0.08-0.56 mmol/L (Normal < 105 ng/mL)	4. Specific for B_{12} but requires normal BCAA levels; available at most laboratories.
	5. Schilling test for intrinsic factor and B_{12} absorption assesses radiolabeled B_{12} absorption as reflected by urinary excretion.	5. Abnormal B_{12} absorption indicated by excretion <3% of B_{12} radioactivity per 24 hours.	5. Normal excretion: ~8% of radioactivity per 24 hours	5. Test must be repeated with oral administration of intrinsic factor (IF) to differentiate IF deficiency and malabsorption.
	6. Homocysteine (Hcy)	Hcy level is an independent risk factor for CVD, venous thrombotic disease, and other diseases; folic acid and vitamins B_{12} and B_6 reduce plasma Hcy levels. Total Hcy (oxidized + reduced forms) is an intermediate amino acid in methionine metabolism.	4-14 mmol/L Optimum levels suggested 4-7 mmol/L	Hcy and LDL cholesterol risk is increased even at slightly elevated levels. Hcy has a strong association with degenerative neurologic conditions like Parkinson's disease and dementias. Hcy suggests poor methylating capacity of client with need for increased intake of folic acid, B_6, B_{12}, and SAMe.
Ascorbic acid (C)	Plasma or leukocyte C measured by (1) chromatography; (2) by ascorbate oxidase; (3) spectrophotometrically by reaction with 2,4-dinitrophenylhydrazine.	Leukocyte C is less affected by recent intake, but well-fasted plasma levels parallel leukocyte levels; plasma preferred for acutely ill patients because leukocyte level is affected by infection,[22] some drugs, and hyperglycemia; <0.2 mg/dL (<10 mcg/10^8 WBC)	Plasma:0.5-1.4 mg/dL (30-80 mmol/L) Leukocyte deficiency: 20-50 mcg/10^8 WBCs (1.1-3 fmol/cell)	Blood samples must be carefully prepared for assay to prevent C breakdown. Oxalate, glucose, and proteins interfere with some assays; recent intake can mask deficiency.

Retinols (A)	Serum retinol and retinol esters; functional tests (e.g., dark adaptation) only detect severe deficiency; Age and sex important determining factors for normal retinol levels.	Retinol levels <20 mcg/dL (<0.7 mmol/L) indicate severe deficiency; specific levels are being determined for placental/ newborn deficiency serum levels.	Normal: 20 to 100 mcg/dL (0.7-3.5 mmol/L) Suboptimum (NHANES II/Gibson): Age 3-11 y: < 0.35 mmol/L Age 12-17 y <0.70 mmol/L Age 18-74 mmol/L 0.70-1.05 mmol/L Pregnancy 0.79-1.91 mmol/L Upper Limit: 3.5 mmol\L	Exposure of serum to bright light or oxygen destroys vitamin A; low RBP level is associated with low vitamin A, zinc and iron (see protein-energy section). Vitamin A's gene transcription is on the nuclear RXR;[22] the vitamin D receptor forms a heterodimer, requiring balance between vitamins A& D for optimum function.
Tocopherols (E)	Serum alpha- and beta-gamma-tocopherols serve different antioxidant functions. Growing evidence beta-gamma tocopherol may be more important than alpha-tocopherol for human vitamin E nutrition.	Lower values found in infants. Interpretation requires monitoring lipid levels; if hyperlipidemia calculate plasma alpha-tocopherol: cholesterol mmol/L ratio <2.2 or alpha-tocopherol <5 mg/L indicates risk of vitamin E deficiency[23]	Normal: alpha-tocopherol 5.7-20 mg/L beta-gamma-tocopherol 4.3 or less mg/L	Plasma level depends on recent intake and level of lipids, especially TGs, in blood. Smoking and BMI also negatively effect tocopherol levels.
Cholecalciferol / (D_3) (D_2) Ergocalciferol	1. Alkaline phosphatase activity reflects level of bone activity and indirectly vitamin D status. (see further discussion of ALP in Liver Enzymes section).		Adult: 25-100 U/L Child 1-12 yr: <350 U/L	1. Not specific, but a sensitive indicator; serum Ca and PO_4 should also be evaluated. Zinc and B_{12} are rate-limiting co-cofactors for production of alkaline phosphatase;, therefore low levels < 40 U/L suggest possible zinc or B_{12} or intrinsic factor insufficiencies.
	2. CholeCalcidiol (D3 25OH-D) and ergocalciferol (D2 25OH-D).	2. <20 ng/mL (7.4 nmol/L) indicates deficiency; >200 ng/mL (500 nmol/L) indicates hypervitaminosis D.	2. 15-80 mcg/L summer (37-200 nmol/L) 14-42 mcg/L winter (35-105 nmol/L)	2. Best indicator of status (liver stores), but marginal levels hard to interpret.[24] Increased BMI and body fat% may reduce serum D3 25OHD.
	3. Calcitriol (1,25-[OH]2-D_3)	3. Used to show that vitamin D metabolism is occurring normally; Active vitamin D to signal nuclear RXR receptor.	3. 2.5-4.5 ng/dL (60-108 pmol/L) (little seasonal change)	3. Poor indicator of status because of tight control of synthesis independent of body stores.
25-hydroxyvitamin D (25OHD) / Calcifediol/ Calcidiol	Prohormone Vitamin D malabsorption can lead to secondary malabsorption of calcium. Vitamin D supplementation can lead to increased absorption of calcium and phosphorus; contraindiations of supplementation for individuals with kidney or gall stones, sarcoidosis, tuberculosis, lymphoma, or when become hypercalcemic with vitamin D supplementation.	Vitamin D insufficiency is defined as the lowest threshold value for plasma 25OHD that prevents secondary hyperparathyroidism, bone turnover, bone mineral loss, or seasonal variations in plasma PTH.	25OHD: 30-100 ng/mL (85-160 nmol/L) Deficiency: <20 ng/mL (<57 nmol/L (lab references vary per individual laboratory)	Available at all laboratories. If elevated serum calcium, further evaluation recommended by testing vitamin 1,25 DOH, PTH, ionized or free calcium, vitamin A retinol and osteocalcin (as a vitamin K2 marker) before supplementation.
Phylloquinone (K_1) and Menaquinoneione (K_2) Menadione (K_3)	Normal coagulation factor synthesis requires K1; PT assesses coagulation status. K2 primarily involved with calcium metabolism, including bone health.	In K1 deficiency, PT increases with increasing production of abnormal coagulation factors.[h] K1 vegetable plant source; drug-nutrient interaction with blood thinners. K2 animal and bacterial fermented sources. K3 synthetic form of Vitamin K; vitamin precursor to Vitamin K2 known as a provitamin.	K1: 0.13-1,19 ng/mL (0.29-2.64 nmol/L K2: (not commercially available—see K2 marker, Osteocalcin, below)	The level of vitamin K available for vitamin K–dependent bone proteins may not be reflected by the PT; test references variy significantly with method.

Continued

APPENDIX 30. Laboratory Values for Nutritional Assessment and Monitoring—cont'd

Test	Principles	Interpretation	Reference Range	Limitations and Implications
Osteocalcin (OC) / undercarboxylated osteocalcin (ucOC) (K2 marker)	Serum noncollagenous protein specific for bone and dentin formation and turnover. Functional marker of vitamin K2, a rate-limiting cofactor of formation of osteocalcin. (Also known as Bone Gla Protein). One of the osteocalcin fragments, undercarboxylated osteocalcin, is most sensitive K2 marker and associated with risk of fracture.	Can be used as a marker of metabolic trend, suggesting low or high vitamin K2; useful in assessing need for a vitamin K2 rich diet or K2 supplementation to optimize formation of intracellular bone osteocalcin; inhibit soft tissue calcification, and other uses for K2. OC/ucOC considered more sensitive markers of bone activity than alkaline phosphatase during corticosteroid therapy.	O: 11-50 ng/mL ucOC: Normal < 1.65 ng/mL High > 1.65 ng/mL NOTE: Elevated levels associated with low Vitamin D25OH levels	Vitamin K2 is not as involved with coagulation as K1. Vitamin K2 is important in calcium metabolism and therefore calcium and vitamin D status. There is a synthetic vitamin K3 that has similar actions as K2 being used as adjunctive to integrative cancer therapy usually administered IV.
B. Minerals *Electrolytes*				
Sodium (Na^+) Potassium (K^+) Chloride (Cl^-) Bicarbonate or total CO_2	Serum electrolytes, including bicarbonate, are usually measured together by ion-specific electrodes in autoanalyzers; sometimes Na and K are measured by flame emission spectrophotometry.[i]	Elevated serum Na seen in water loss; decreased serum Na and K occurs in diarrhea and poor dietary intake or cellular uptake. Ddecreased chloride levels with changes with in cation and osmotic changes in the body; Bicarbonate levels reflect acid-base balance.	135-145 mEq/L (135-145 mmol/L) 3.5-5 mEq/L (3.5-5 mmol/L) 100-110 mEq/L (100-110 mmol/L) 21-30 mEq/L (21-30 mmol/L)	Electrolytes change rapidly in response to changes in physiology (e.g., hormonal stimulus, renal and other organ dysfunction, acid-base balance changes, and drug action); serum electrolytes are minimally affected by diet.
Major Minerals				
Calcium (Ca^{2+})	1. Total serum Ca^{2+} (bound and unbound)	Usually slightly more than half of the serum Ca^{2+} is bound to albumin or complexed with other molecules; the remaining Ca^{2+} is called *ionized Ca (ICA)*; ICA is available physiologically. Elevated IgE and mast cell release increases intracellular calcium ion levels and negatively distributes ICA.	1. 8.6-10 mg/dL (2.15-2.5 mmol/L)	Calcium status is related to many factors, including vitamin D, vitamin K2, phosphate, parathyroid function, malignancy, and renal function; medications (thiazide diuretics, lithium, vitamin A toxicity).
	2. Ionized (free) Ca^{2+}	When interpreting ionized calcium, important to consider other related markers: osteocalcin, vitamin D25 and D1,25OH, and vitamin A retinol.	2. 4.64-5.28 mg/dL (1.16-1.32 mmol/L)	Ionized calcium depends on vitamin K2 to enter the bone matrix and to prevent calcification of soft tissue. If phosphate <3.0 mg/dL, check intake of phosphate-binding medications.
Phosphate (H_2PO_4, PO_4^{2}, and PO_4^{3-}) (Phosphorus)	Phosphorus in body as phosphate form; Test measures inorganic phosphate (Most phosphate part of organic compounds; small part is inorganic).	Abnormal P level is most closely associated with disturbed intake, distribution, or renal function.	2.7-4.5 mg/dL (0.87-1.45 mmol/L) (higher in children)	Reported as phosphorus (P), not phosphate; hemolyzed blood cannot be used because of high RBC phosphate levels.
Magnesium (Mg^{2+})	1. Total serum Mg^{2+} measured after reaction to form chromogenic or fluorescent complexes.	Neuromuscular function (hyperirritability, tetany, convulsion, and electrocardiographic changes) affected when levels of total serum $Mg2^+$ fall to <1 mEq/L.	1. 1.3-2.5 mEq/L (0.65-1.25 mmol/L)	Usually 45% of the serum Mg^{2+} is complexed with other molecules; the remaining Mg^{2+} is called ionized magnesium; serum levels remain constant until body stores are nearly depleted.
	2. Ionized (free) Mg^{2+}		2. 0.7-1.2 mEq/L (0.35-0.60 mmol/L)	

Trace Minerals				
Iron CBC[k] and RBC indices	1. HCT = % RBC in whole blood 2. Hgb = blood hemoglobin concentration 3. MCV = mean RBC volume	A CBC with RBC indices is one of the first set of tests that a patient receives; although CBC data are not specific for nutrition status, their universal and repeated presence in the patient's record make them very important.	1. F: 35%-47% (0.35-0.47)[l] M: 42%-52% (0.42-0.52) 2. F: 12-15 g/dL (7.45-9.31 mmol/L) M: 14-17 g/dL (8.44-10.6 mmol/L) 3. 82-99 mm^3 (82-99 fL)	These tests are affected only when iron stores are essentially depleted, and HCT and Hgb are sensitive to hydration status; low MCV also occurs in thalassemias and lead poisoning as well as iron and copper deficiencies; high MCV suggests macrocytic RBCs and possible inadequate folate, vitamins B_6, or B_{12}.
Serum iron (Fe)	Serum Fe^{3+} reduced to Fe^{2+} and then complexed with chromogen.	Slightly higher in males than in premenopausal females; reflects recent Fe intake.	F: 40-150 mcg/dL (7.2-26.9 mmol/L) M: 50-160 mg/dL (8.9-28.7 mmol/L)	Very insensitive index of total Fe stores; extremely variable (day-to-day and diurnal).
Total Iron Binding Capacity (TIBC)	TIBC determined by saturating serum transferrin with Fe and then remeasuring serum Fe.	Reflects transferrin concentration.	250-400 mcg/dL (45-71 mmol/L)	TIBC does not increase until Fe stores are essentially completely depleted. TIBC decreases with increased Fe stores needing to rule out excess iron intake or hemochromatosis.
Transferrin (Tf or TFN)	The iron bound globulin protein that responds to the need for iron; half-life ~9 days. (see Chapter 8)	(see Section I:A. Protein Status: Tf)	Adult male: 215-365 mg/dL (2.15-3.65 g/L) Adult female: 250-380 mg/dL (2.15-3.80 g/L) Newborn: 130-275 mg/dL Child: 203-360 mg/dL	
Transferrin Saturation (Tf-sat or TSAT)	Tf-sat (%) = Serum iron level÷TIBC x 100%	(see Section I:A. Protein Status: Tf-sat)	M: 20%-50% F: 15%-50% Chronic illness normal Tf-sat%. Late pregnancy low Tf-sat%.	↓ when Fe stores essentially depleted; low vitamin B_6 and low Tf-sat in aplastic anemia.
RBC Distribution Width (RDW)	Measurement of variation in RBC diameter (anisocytosis); reported to be helpful in distinguishing Fe deficiency and anemia associated with chronic inflammation.	Very sensitive indicator of Fe status; normal RDW reportedly rules out anemia caused by chronic inflammatory diseases.[m] Thalassemia (low MCV, normal RDW) differentiated from iron-deficiency (low MCV, high RDW)	Normal value: 11.0-14.5% Microscopic electronic interpretation required.	Specificity of RDW for Fe deficiency is relatively low; interpretation confounded by red cell transfusion; measurement usually not reported.
Ferritin	The primary intracellular Fe-storage protein; stored mostly in liver; serum levels parallel iron stores;	Best biochemical index of uncomplicated iron deficiency or overload (iron toxicity) and excess storage. Rule out hemochromatosis or pancreatitis if Ferritin >1000 ng/dL (>1000 mcg/L).	Iron overload: >400 ng/mL (mcg/L) With anemia of chronic disease: <100 ng/mL (<100 mcg/L) M: 12-300 ng/mL (12-300 mcg/L) F: 10-150 ng/mL (10-150 mcg/L) Females with anemia of chronic disease: <20 ng/mL(<20 mcg/L) 6 mos.-15 yr: 7-142 ng/mL (7-142 mcg/L) <1 mo.-5 mos.: 50-200 ng/mL (50-200 mcg/L) Newborn: 25-200 ng/mL (25-200 mcg/L)	A positive acute phase reactant increases during metabolic response to injury, even when Fe stores are adequate; not useful in anemia of chronic and inflammation diseases.
Zinc (Zn)[n]	Serum levels measured by atomic absorption spectrophotometry.	Serum levels affected by diet and the inflammatory response. Zinc deficiency associated with many diseases and trauma.	0.7-1.2 mg/L (11-18 mmol/L)	Serum levels detect frank—but not marginal—deficiency; blood must be collected in zinc-free tubes.

Continued

APPENDIX 30. Laboratory Values for Nutritional Assessment and Monitoring—cont'd

Test	Principles	Interpretation	Reference Range	Limitations and Implications
Copper (Cu)	1. Serum levels measured by flame emission atomic absorption spectrophotometry. 2. Ceruloplasmin is the major Cu-containing plasma protein; measured by immunoassay (e.g., nephelometry).	1. Cu deficiency is associated with neutropenia, anemia, and scurvy-like bone disease and megadoses of zinc. 2. Ceruloplasmin is required for conversion of Fe^{3+} to Fe^{2+} during cellular Fe uptake; anemia can result from low ceruloplasmin; useful marker to follow tetrathiomolybdate ™ copper chelation for Wilson's Disease and cancer anti-angiogenesis therapy.[25]	M: 70-140 mcg/dL (11-22 mmol/L) F: 80-155 mcg/dL (13-24 mmol/L) 20 to 35 mg/dL (1-4 mmol/L)	1. Serum levels detect frank but not marginal deficiency; use of oral contraceptives serum Cu. 2. Ceruloplasmin not a useful marker of Cu status but can be used to assess changes in status after supplementation; useful to calculate free copper index with serum zinc and copper as a cancer biomarker.[26,28,29]
Selenium (Se)	1. Serum Selenium test 2. Whole blood levels better reflect long-term status.	Margin between deficiency and toxicity is narrower for Se than any other trace component of the antioxidant enzyme element; important in glutathione peroxidase.	(1) 80-320 mcg/L (1-4 mmol/L) (2) 60-340 mcg/L (0.75-4.3 mmol/L)	Cutoff points for deficiency or toxicity are not well established.
Iodine (I)	Urinary excretion is best indicator of I status, either mcg/24 hr or mcg/g creatinine; thyroid hormone level related to I status. Urine test can use 50 mg I/KI challenge.	Excretion should be >DRT for 24-hour urine or >50 mcg/g creatinine; it can be beneficial to test thyroid hormone and antibodies (TSH, T_3-free, T_4-free, thyroid peroxidase and thyroglobulin antibodies) for improved interpretation; iodine important for other metabolic functions.	No urinary I reference range; T_4 reference range: F: 5-12 mcg/dL (64-154 mmol/L) M: 4-12 mcg/dL (51-154 mmol/L)	Thyroid hormone levels are affected by many factors besides iodine status. Other halogen elements are known antagonists to iodine metabolism; when completing the iodine urine testing, some laboratories will also test for bromine, fluorine, and chlorine.
Creatinine (Cr)	Urinary excretion usually tested by atomic absorption spectrophotometry.	Excretion should be greater or equal to DRI; deficiency reported in patients on long-term TPN; decreased levels in diabetes mellitus.	10-200 ng/dL (1.9-38 nmol/L)	Test not available in most clinical laboratories; special handling required to prevent specimen contamination during collection.
VI. Blood Gases and Hydration Status				
pH	pH = –log [H^+]; H^+ depends mainly on the CO_2 from respiration: CO_2 +. $H_2O \Leftrightarrow H_2CO_3 \Leftrightarrow HCO_3 + H^+$. Measured by ion-selective electrodes (like those found in common pH meters)	In: Acidosis pH <7.35Alkalosis pH >7.45 pH compatible with life 6.80-7.80.	Whole blood: Arterial: 7.35-7.45 Venous: 7.32-7.42	Blood must not be exposed to air before or during measurement.
Po_2 and O_2 saturation (SaO_2)	Whole blood O_2 measured by oxygen electrode; Po_2 = "pressure" contributed by O_2 to the total "pressure" of all the gases dissolved in blood O_2 Content (CaO2) = O_2/gm SaO_2 x Hgb (gm/dl) x 1.34 ml + PaO_2 x (.003 ml O_2/mm Hg/dl) Capacity $PaO_2 = FIO_2(PB\text{-}47) - 1.2(PaCO_2)$	Affected by alveolar gas exchange, ventilation-perfusion inequalities, and generalized alveolar hypoventilation.	Arterial blood: PaO_2: 83-108 mm Hg <40 mm Hg = critical value (gravely dangerous) O_2 saturation:0.95-0.98 (95%-98%) Elderly = 95% Newborn = 40-90%	Blood must not be exposed to air before or during measurement.
PCO_2	Measured by ion-selective electrode; "pressure" contributed by CO_2 to the total "pressure" of all the gases dissolved in blood.	Increased in respiratory acidosis (increased CO_2 in inspired air or decreased in alveolar ventilation) and decreased in respiratory alkalosis (e.g., in hyperventilation from anxiety, mechanical ventilator, or closed head injury [damaged respiratory center]).	Whole blood: Arterial M: 35-48 mm Hg F: 32-45 mm Hg Venous 6-7 mm Hg higher	Blood must not be exposed to air before or during measurement.

Bicarbonate (HCO_3^-) and total CO_2 (tCO_2)	For whole blood (HCO_3^-) is calculated from the equation given in pH section.	Increased in compensated respiratory acidosis and in metabolic acidosis; decreased in metabolic acidosis and in compensated respiratory alkalosis.	Whole blood, arterial: 21-28 mEq/L (21-28 mmol/L)	Blood must not be exposed to air before or during measurement.
Osmolality (Osmol)	Osmol depends on amount of particles (solutes) dissolved in a solution; measurement based on relationship between solute concentration and freezing point; serum osmol assesses hydration status and solute load.	Osmol increases in dehydration, diabetic coma, diabetic ketoacidosis; also estimated from the formula: mOsmol/L = 1.86 a(Na^+) + (Glucose)/18 + (BUN)/2.8	282-300 mOsmol/kg H_2O (1 Osmol = 1 mol of solute particles; 1 kg serum/L)	Freezing point depression gives a more accurate estimate of osmol than the calculated value (e.g., in ketoacidosis).
Urinalysis: Specific Gravity (Sp.Gr.)	Specimen midstream clean-catch if infection suspected, or regular collection. Dip Stick or laboratory testing for Specific Gravity.	One of a multiple of tests on a urine specimen. Sp.Gr. a measure of concentration of particle, electrolytes in the urine; weight of urine: distilled water.	Adult: 1.005-1.030 (usual 1.010-1.025) Newborn: 1.001-1.020	Appearance can also give subjective indication of fluid concentration-high concentration darker in color.
VII. Tests of Antioxidant Status and Oxidative Stress				
Water-soluble compounds	See Vitamin C.			
Lipid-soluble compounds: see Vitamin E Carotenoids Coenzyme Q_{10}	The carotenoids: lutein, xanthine zeaxanthin, alpha- and beta-carotene, and lycopene; carotenoids and coenzyme Q_{10} (ubiquinone-10) are measured chromatographically.	Reference ranges for these compounds vary greatly, depending on the method used for their assay.	See reference for carotenoid range under fat malabsorption	Tests for carotenoids and coenzyme Q are not yet available for routine clinical use.
Total antioxidant capacity (e.g., ORAC, TEAC, FRAP)	ORAC: Oxygen radical absorbance capacity TEAC: Trolox-equivalent antioxidant capacity FRAP: Ferric-reducing ability of plasma. See Raman Spectroscopy, Chapter 27.	These assays reflect the presence of all of plasma or serum antioxidants, including vitamins C and E, carotenoids, coenzyme Q_10, glutathione, uric acid, bilirubin, superoxide dismutase, catalase, glutathione peroxidase, and albumin.		These assays are now commercially available but are currently performed only in specialized laboratories. Testing botanicals also available.
Oxidative stress markers:	Free radical oxidation products of lipids	8-Isoprostane (also called 8-epiprostaglandin F_{2a}) increases in plasma or urine of patients with lung disease, hypercholesterolemia, or diabetes mellitus. 8HDG represents whole-body cytosolic and nuclear free radical activity, including status of DNA. Lipid peroxides is a marker of membrane oxidative damage by ROS to PUFAs of cell membranes.	Examples: *o*-tyrosine nitro-tyrosine 8-isoprostane 4-hydroxynonenal malondialdehyde Lipid Peroxides 8-hydroxy-2-deoxyguanosine (8-OHDG) (refer to Laboratory references)	8-Isoprostane assays are now commercially available. Markers of oxidative stress are currently assayed only in specialized laboratories.
VIII. Tests for Monitoring Nutrition Support				
CRP (see section V. hs-CRP)	CRP is an acute-phase protein used to assess inflammatory status.	Large increases in CRP are associated with development of a catabolic state during the stress response; CRP levels begin to fall when the anabolic phase is entered.	CRP <10 mg/L	Serial values rather than a single value must be used to specify the stage of the stress response.
Chemistry panel with phosphate and Mg^{2+}	Panel includes electrolytes, glucose, creatinine, BUN, and total CO_2 (bicarbonate); see earlier discussion for additional test information.	Used to monitor carbohydrate tolerance, hydration status, and major organ system function.	See earlier discussion on phosphate and magnesium.	Very frequently ordered test panel.
Osmolality	(see discussion in VII. Blood Gases and Hydration Status)			

Continued

APPENDIX 30. Laboratory Values for Nutritional Assessment and Monitoring—cont'd

Test	Principles	Interpretation	Reference Range	Limitations and Implications
Protein-Energy Balance	(see earlier discussion on PAB, RBP, Tf, ALB, nPCR, Nitrogen Balance, UUN and TUN)			
Minerals: Zn, Cu, Se, Cr	(see earlier discussion of serum zinc, serum copper, ceruloplasmin, and lymphocyte micronutrient testing)			
Vitamins C, D and A	(see earlier discussion of vitamins C, D and A) Because vitamins C, D25OH, and A are important in immune function and wound healing, they should be assessed regularly.	Note regarding TPN nutritional monitoring: Vitamin C levels can ↓ sharply in response to stress. Vitamin D and A nuclear receptors share the same connection with the RXR receptor which have synergistic function and should be monitored congruently.[27,28]		Note regarding TPN nutritional monitoring: Systematic, regular monitoring protocol should be followed. Vitamin D25-hydroxy is produced in the liver and can be suppressed with hepatic stress conditions.[29]
Vitamin K1 & K2 status	(TPN only) (see earlier discussion) Contribution of the gut flora to vitamin K status is absent during TPN, and basic TPN formulas are devoid of it.			Important to differentiate between vitamin K1 and K2.
IX. Liver Function Tests				
Bilirubin (BILI T/D) (Direct and Indirect)	Total serum bilirubin represents both the conjugated or direct and unconjugated or indirect bilirubin. Elevated levels suggest medical problem.	Conjugated bilirubin levels elevated with cancer of pancreas or liver and bile duct obstruction; unconjugated bilirubin level elevated with hepatitis, jaundice anemias	Total bilirubin: 0.3-1 mg/dL (5.1-17 mmol/L) Indirect bilirubin: 0.2-0.8 mg/dL (3.4-12 mmol/L) Direct bilirubin: 0.1-0.3 mg/dL; (1.7-5.1 mmol/L)	Many medications are associated with elevated bilirubin levels.
Alanine Amino Transferase (ALT)	Enzyme found primarily in the liver. (also called serum glutamic pyruvic transaminase (SGPT)	Injury to the liver results in elevated levels of ALT. Depressed in malnutrition.	4-36 U/L Infant: 2 x adult levels	Many medications and alcohol intake are associated with elevated ALT levels. ALT levels are often compared with AST for differential diagnosis.
Gamma-glutamyl transferase (GGT)	Biliary excretory enzyme involved in transfer of amino acids across cell membranes.	Used to evaluate progression of liver disease and screening for alcoholism	F: 4-25 UL M: 12-38 UL	Many medications are associated with elevated GGT levels.
Alkaline phosphatase (ALP)	Enzyme found primarily in the bone, liver, and biliary tract; increased in an alkaline environment.	Elevated levels noted in liver and bone disorders.	30-120 U/L	Nonspecific test; other tests need to confirm diagnosis. Many medications are associated with elevated ALP levels.
Aspartate Amino Transferase (AST)	Enzyme primarily found in the heart, liver, and skeletal muscle cells. (also called serum glutamic oxaloacetic transaminase (SGOT))	Diagnostic tool when coronary occlusive heart disease or hepatocellular disease is suspected.	0-35 U/L	Many medications are associated with elevated AST levels. AST levels are often compared with ALT for differential diagnosis.
Alpha 1 Antitrypsin (A1AT)	A1AT is a serine protease inhibitor secreted primarily by hepatocytes.; Most common genetic A1AT variants are ZZ, SS, MZ, SZ. (see Table 30-1)	Serum electrophoresis decreased or absent Alpha-1-band. A1AT is an acute-phase reactant associated with emphysema, COPD and cirrhosis of the liver; A1AT elevated with states of inflammation, infection or malignancy.	85-213 mg/dL (0.85-2.13 g/L) Homozygous + + variants: severe disease early in life. 80 known variants of A1AT gene: Heterozygous ZZ and SS gene variants: majority have hepatic or pulmonary symptoms MZ and SZ milder gene variants: rarely have symptoms.[o,p]	There are 100 known variants of the A1AT gene.[o,p] If a person is not diagnosed with a severe form as a child, an individual may not be identified until an adult with end-stage lung and liver conditions.

X. Thyroid Function Tests				
Thyroxine T_4, Total and T_4, Free	Measures the total amount of T_4 in the blood; free T_4 active form. (see Chapter 32)	T_4 increased in Hyperthyroidism; T_4 decreased in hypothyroidism and malnutrition	T_4, Total F: 5-12 mcg/dL; (64-154 nmol/L) M: 4-12 mcg/dL (51-154 nmol/L) T_4, Free 0.7-1.9 ng/dl (10-23 pmol/L)	Tests are ordered to distinguish between euthyroidism, or hyperthyroidism and hypothyroidism. Can be related to iodine deficiencies.
Triiodothyronine T_3, Total and T_3, Free	Measures the total amount of T_3 in the blood; free T_3 active form. (see Chapter 32)	Hyperthyroidism-usally elevated; hypothyroidism-usually decreased and can show low function of thyroid peroxidase enzyme when T_4 normal or high and T_3 low (poor conversion).	T_3, Total 20-50 yr: 70-205 ng/dL (1.2-3.4 nmol/L) >50 yr: 40-180 ng/dL (0.6-2.8 nmol/L) T_3, Free 230-619 pg/mL	Tests are ordered to distinguish between euthyroidism, or hyperthyroidism and hypothyroidism. If low T_3 levels, consider insufficient nutrient cofactors (selenium, vitamin E) for thyroid peroxidase enzyme conversion of T_4 to T_3.
Thyroid-stimulating hormone (TSH)	Used to monitor exogenous thyroid replacement or thyroid suppression. (see Chapter 32)	Decreased TSH in Hyperthyroidism; Elevated TSH in hypothyroidism	0.5-5 mIU/L AACE Standards: Target TSH: 0.3-3.0 μIU/mL[o]	Tests are ordered to distinguish between euthyroidism, hyperthyroidism and hypothyroidism. If depressed, use caution with iodine intake. If elevated, consider assessing nutrient cofactors: iodine, selenium, vitamin E, A.
Antithyroglobulin antibody (anti-TG)	Anti-TG blood test used as a marker for autoimmune thyroiditis and related diseases.[30] High prevelance of thyroid autoantibodies in celiac and rheumatoid arthritis patients	Anti-TG autoantibodies bind to thyroglobulin affecting thyroid hormone synthesis, storage and release. Recommend investigation of gluten intolerance if elevated Anti-TG.	Titer <4 IU/mL Anti-TG often tested in conjunction with Anti-TPO test.	Resulting disordered thyroid function most common related conditions: Hashimoto's thyroiditis and autoimmune hypothyroid.
Antithyroid peroxidase antibody (Anti-TPO or TPO-Ab)	Anti-TPO blood test used in the diagnosis of thyroid diseases, such as Hashimoto's thyroiditis or chronic lympocytic thyroiditis (in children). High prevelance of thyroid autoantibodies in celiac and rheumatoid arthritis patients	Thryoid microsomal antibodies action on a section of microsome in the thyroid cell initiating inflammatory and cytotoxic effects on the thyroid follicle. Recommend investigation of gluten intolerance if elevated Anti-TPO.	Titer <9 IU/mL Anti-TPO often tested in conjunction with Anti-TG test.	Most sensitive assay for antimicrosomal antibody. Nutritional considerations are vitamin E and selenium co-factors for production of TPO enzyme.
XI. Tests for Metabolic Disease				
Amino acidurias	Dietary treatment is the major therapy for many of these genetic diseases: phenylketonuria, cystinuria, maple syrup urine disease, tyrosinemia, homocystinuria, Hartnup disease. See Chapter 44. Urine or plasma amino acid testing.	Monitoring amino acid level in urine or serum is necessary to assess adequacy of treatment.	Examples: Phe: 2-6 g/L (120-360 mmol/L) Phe (during pregnancy): 2-6 mg/dL(120-360 mmol/L) Cys: 2-22 g/L (10-90 mmol/L) Val: 17-37 g/L (145-315 mmol/L) Tyr: 4-16 g/L (20-90 mmol/L)	There are several methods used to measure (e.g., phenylalanine); these usually do not have exactly equivalent reference ranges.
Organic Acids Panel	Urine organic acids panel; home collection of 10 ml sample of nocturnal and first morning urine, frozen, shipped to lab.[q]	Sensitive, broad range test that evaluates comprehensive functional markers for metabolic nutrient pathway functions that can suggest early markers for risk of disease or metabolic imbalances.	(see particular lab references)	Excellent for overview of metabolic function and non-invasive pediatric testing.
Diabetes Mellitus (See Chapter 31)				
Prediabetes diagnosis	FBG: 100-125 mg/dL (impaired fasting glucose)	Prediabetes, blood glucose levels are higher than normal but not high enough for a diagnosis of diabetes.	Nondiabetic FBG = < 99 mg/dL	American Diabetes Association recommends testing for prediabetes in adults without symptoms who are overweight or obese, and one or more additional risk factors for diabetes.

Continued

APPENDIX 30. Laboratory Values for Nutritional Assessment and Monitoring—cont'd

Test	Principles	Interpretation	Reference Range	Limitations and Implications
Diabetes diagnosis	1. Serum or whole blood glucose: after fasting 8-16 hours or on a casual blood sample.	1. Two or more fasting levels FBG >126 mg/dL are diagnostic; casual level >200 mg/dL followed by fasting level >126 mg/dL are diagnostic. Fasting levels of 110 to 126 mg/dL indicate IGT.	2. Serum: Fasting: <110 mg/dL (<6.1 mmol/L) 30 min: <200 mg/dL (<11.1 mmol/L) 1 hour: <200 mg/dL (<11.1 mmol/L) 2 hours: <140 mg/dL (<7.8 mmol/L) 3 hours: 70-115 mg/dL (<6.4 mmol/L) 4 hours: 70-115 mg/dL (<6.4 mmol/L) Urine: glucose negative	1. Elevated glucose levels are normal in physiologic stress; whole blood gives slightly lower values.
	2. Glucose tolerance test (GGT); 75 g glucose (100 g during pregnancy) given after fasting; serum glucose measured by before and five times during the next 3 hours after oral dosing. Glucose measured by automated chemistry procedure.	2. Serum levels FBG >200 mg/dL at 2-hour point is diagnostic; 2-hour level <140 and all 0- to 2-hour levels <200 are normal; 140-199 at 2 hours indicates IGT. Gestational diabetes: fasting >105; 1-hour GGT >190; 2 hour GGT >165; and 3-hour GGT >145 mg/dL.	2. Serum: Fasting: <110 mg/dL (<6.1 mmol/L) 30 min: <200 mg/dL (<11.1 mmol/L) 1 hour: <200 mg/dL (<11.1 mmol/L) 2 hours: <140 mg/dL (<7.8 mmol/L) 3 hours: 70-115 mg/dL (<6.4 mmol/L) 4 hours: 70-115 mg/dL (<6.4 mmol/L) Urine: glucose negative	2. Often used for confirmation; ambulatory patient only; bed rest or stress impairs GGT; inadequate carbohydrate consumption before test invalidates results.
Diabetes monitoring	1. Blood glucose—monitoring requires that *the patient* monitor blood glucose level.	1. Tight diabetes control requires frequent monitoring of glucose levels.	1. 70-99 mg/dL (3.9-5.5 mmol/L)	A combination of glucose monitoring (by patient) and laboratory measurement of glycated proteins are needed to effectively monitor glucose control; fructosamine must be interpreted in light of plasma protein half-lives, and HgbA1C must be interpreted in light of RBC half-life.
	2. Serum fructosamine—assesses medium-term glucose control by measured glycated serum proteins; currently testing available in the laboratory and home tests.	2. Allows assessment of average glucose levels for previous 2-3 weeks.	2. Normal levels: 1%-2% of total protein Ranges vary according to method used.	
	3. Serum glycated hemoglobin or HgbA1C—assesses longer-term glucose control. 4. Porphyrin urine or whole blood testing for dioxin,[31] a toxin with significant association with promoting diabetes	3. Allows assessment of average glucose levels for previous 2-3 months and verification of patient's serum glucose log.	3. Normal levels: Nondiabetic: 4-5.9% Good diabetic control: 4-7% Fair diabetic control: 6%-8% Poor diabetic control: >8%; Mean blood sugar 205 mg/dL or greater is associated with increased risk of side effects	Department of Defense study (July 2005) 47% percent increase in diabetes among veterans with the highest levels of dioxin.[31]

1. Parrish CR, Series Ed: Serum proteins as markers of nutrition: what are we treating? Nutr Issues in Gastroenterology, Series 43, *Prac Gastroenterol* October, 2006.
2. Juarez-Congelosi M et al: Normalized protein catabolic rate versus serum albumin as a nutrition status marker in pediatric patients receiving hemodialysis, *J Renal Nutr* 17 (4):269, 2007.
3. Harty JC et al: The normalized protein catabolic rate is a flawed marker of nutrition in CAPD patients, *Kidney Int* 45:103, 1994.
4. Beck FK, Rosenthal TC: Prealbumin: a marker for nutritional evaluation, *Am Fam Physician* 65:1575, 2002.
5. Wu X et al: Joint effect of insulin-like growth factors and mutagen sensitivity in lung cancer risk, *J Natl Cancer Inst* 92:737, 2000.
6. Rowlands MA: Circulating insulin-like growth factor peptides and prostate cancer risk: a systematic review and meta-analysis, *Int J Cancer* 124:2416, 2009.
7. Gonen B et al: Haemoglobin A1: An indicator of the metabolic control of diabetic patients, *Lancet* 2(8041):734, 1977.
8. Riese H et al: Covariance of metabolic and hemostatic risk indicators in men and women, *Fibrinolysis Proteolysis* 15(1):9, 2001.
9. Bo S et al: Dietary magnesium and fiber intakes and inflammatory and metabolic indicators in middle-aged subjects from a population-based cohort 1,2,3, *Am J Clin Nutr* 84:1062, 2006.
10. Douglas D: MedScape Today News. Improved Diagnosis Does Not Change Celiac Mortality, Reuters Health Information, Feb 1, 2011.
11. Grainge MJ et al: Causes of Death in People With Celiac Disease Spanning the Pre- and Post-Serology Era: A Population-Based Cohort Study From Derby, UK, *Am J of Gastroenterol* 106:933, 2011.
12. Lewis NR: Risk of Morbidity in Contemporary Celiac Disease, *Expert Rev Gastroenterol and Hepatol* 4:767, 2010.
13. Donaldson MR et al: Strongly positive tissue transglutaminase antibodies are assodciated with Marsh 3 histopathology in adult and pediatric celiac disease. *J Clin Gastroenterol* 42:256, 2008.

14. Vermeersch P et al: Use of likelihood ratios improves clinical interpretation of IgG and IgA anti-DGP antibody testing for celiac disease in adults and children, *Clin Biochem* 44:248, 2011.
15. Vermeersch P et al: Diagnostic performance of IgG anti-deamidated gliadin peptide antibody assays is comparable to IgA anti-tTG in celiac disease, *Clin ChimActa* 411:931, 2010.
16. Sharifi N et al: Celiac disease in patients with type-1 diabetes mellitus screened by tissue transglutaminase antibodies in northwest of Iran, *Int J Diab Dev Ctries* 28:95, 2008.
17. Lampasona V et al: Antibodies to tissue transglutaminase C in type I diabetes, *Diabetologia* 42:1195, 1999.
18. Holopainena P et al: Candidate gene regions and genetic heterogeneity in gluten sensitivity, *Gut* 48:696, 2001.
19. Feingold KR et al: Infection decreases fatty acid oxidation and nuclear hormone receptors in the diaphragm, *J Lipid Res* 50:2055, 2009.
20. Lord R, Bralley JA, editors: *Laboratory evaluations for integrative and functional medicine*, ed 2, Duluth, GA, 2008, MetaMetrix Institute.
21. Sypniewska G: Pro-inflammatory and prothrombotic factors and metabolic syndrome, Department of Laboratory Medicine, Collegium Medicum, Nicolae Copernicus University, Bydgoszcz, Poland, 2007.
22. Ng KY et al: Vitamin D and vitamin A receptor expression and the proliferative effects of ligand activation of these receptors on the development of pancreatic progenitor cells derived from human fetal pancreas, *Stem Cell Rev* 7:53, 2011.
23. Aslam A et al: Vitamin E deficiency induced neurological disease in common variable immunodeficiency: two cases and a review of the literature of vitamin E deficiency, *Clin Immunol* 112(1):24, 2004.
24. Kim K et al: Associations of visceral adiposity and exercise participation with C-reactive protein, insulin resistance, and endothelial dysfunction in Korean healthy adults, *Metabolism* 57:1181, 2008.
25. Finney L et al: Copper and angiogenesis: unravelling a relationship key to cancer progression, *Clin Exp Pharmacol Physiol* 36:88, 2009.
26. Charney P, Malone AM: *ADA pocket guide to nutrition assessment*, ed 2, Chicago, IL, 2009, American Dietetic Association.
27. Snellman G et al: Determining vitamin D status: a comparison between commercially available assays, *PLoS One* 5(7):e11555, 2010.
28. Katz K et al: Suspected Nonalcoholic Fatty Liver Disease Is Not Associated with Vitamin D Status in Adolescents after Adjustment for Obesity, *J Obes* 2010; 2010. Published online Feb. 2011.
29. Ahmed A: The role of 11b-hydroxysteroid dehydrogenase type 1 and hepatic glucocorticoid metabolism in the metabolic syndrome, Doctoral thesis to College of Medical and Dental Sciences, University of Birmingham, 2010.
30. Yu W et al: RXR: a coregulator that enhances binding of retinoic acid, thyroid hormone, and vitamin D receptors to their cognate response elements, *Cell* 67:1251, 1991.
31. Longnecker MP, Michalek JE: Serum dioxin level in relation to diabetes mellitus among Air Force veterans with background levels of exposure, *Epidemiol* 11:44, 2000.

A1AT, alpha 1 antitypsin; *AACE*, American Association of Clinical Endocrinologists; *A/C ratio*, albumin/globulin ratio; *AGA*, antigliadian antibodies; *ALA*, alpha linolenic acid; *ALB*, albumin; *ALP*, alkaline phosphatase; *ALT*, alanine amino transferase; *Anti-TG*, antithyroglobulin antibody; *Anti-TPO*, antithyroid peroxidase antibody; *AST*, aspartate aminotransferase; *BAL*, bronchoalveolar lavage; *BCAA*, branched-chain amino acid; *BILI T/D*, Bilirubin Total/Direct: *BUN*, blood urea nitrogen; *CAPD*, continuous ambulatory peritoneal dialysis; *CBC*, complete blood count; *CD*, cardiac disease; *CHD*, coronary heart disease; *Cr*, chromium; *CRP*, C-reactive protein; *CSF*, cerebrospinal fluid; *CVD*, cardiovascular disease; *DGLA*, dihomo-gammalinolenic acid; *DGP*, deamidated gliadin peptide antibody; *DHA*, docosahexaenoic acid; *DNA*, deoxyribonucleic acid; *DRI*, dietary reference intake; *DRT*, diet readiness test; *EDTA*, ethylenediaminetetraacetic acid; *EFA*, essential fatty acid; *EMA*, endomysium antibody; *EPA*, eicosapentaenoic acid; *FAD*, flavin adenine dinucleotide; *FIGLU*, formiminoglutamic acid; *FBG*, fasting blood glucose; *FBS*, fasting blood sugar; *FPG*, fasting plasma glucose; *FRAP*, ferric-reducing ability of plasma; *GGT*, gamma glutamyl transferase; *GH*, growth hormone; *GI*, gastrointestinal; *GLOB*, globulin; *GOT*, glutamic-oxalacetic transaminase; *GPT*, glutamic-pyruvate transaminase; *GR*, glutathione reductase; *GU*, urea generation rate; *HBT-lactose*, hydrogen breath test-lactose; *HBT-fructose*, hydrogen breath test-fructose; *HCT*, hematocrit; *Hcy*, homocysteine; *Hgb*, hemoglobin; *HLA*, human leukocyte antigen; *HPLC*, high performance liquid chromotography; *hs-CRP*, high-sensitivity C-reactive protein; *I*, iodine; *ICA*, ionized calcium; *Ig*, immunoglobulin; *IGF*, insulin-like growth factor; *IGT*, impaired glucose tolerance; *IV*, intravenously; *KrU*, residual renal urea clearance; Kt/V_{urea}, urea kinetics(kinetic dialyzer) x time(min)/volume urea(ml); *LA*, linoleic acid; *LDL*, low-density lipoprotein; *MCV*, mean cell volume; *MLC*, mixed lymphocyte culture; *N*, nitrogen; *NCEP*, National Cholesterol Education Program; *NSAID*, nonsteroidal antiinflammatory disease; *nPCR*, normalized protein catabolic rate; *ORAC*, oxygen radical absorbance capacity; *PAB*, prealbumin; *PCR*, protein catabolic rate; *PEM*, protein-energy malnutriton; *PLP*, pyridoxal phosphate; *PNA*, protein equivalent of nitrogen appearance; *PT*, prothrombin time; *PTH*, parathyroid hormone; *PTT*, partial thromboplastin time; *PUFA*, polyunsaturated fatty acid; *RBC*, red blood cell; *RBP*, retinol-binding protein; *RDW*, RBC distribution width; *ROS*, reaction oxygen species; *RXR*, retinoid X receptor; *SAMe*, s-adenosylmethionine; *SNP*, single nucleotide polymorphism; T_3, triiodothyronine; T_4, thyroxine; *T1DM*, type 1 diabetes mellitus; *TEAC*, trolox-equivalent antioxidant capacity; *Tf-sat*, transferrin saturation; *TG*, triglyceride; *TIBC*, total iron-binding capacity; *TLC*, total lymphocyte count; *TP*, total protein; *TPN*, total parenteral nutrition; *TPP*, thiamin pyrophosphate; *Trp*, tryptophan; *TSAT*, transferrin saturation; *tTG*, tissue transglutaminase; *TUN*, total urinary nitrogen; *U:Cr*, urea/creatine ratio; *UUN*, urea urinary nitrogen; *VLDL*, very-low-density lipoprotein; *WBC*, white blood cell; *XA*, xanthuric acid.

[a]Factor = 5.95 for TPN; reflects severity of metabolic stress.

[b]Factor = 5.95 for TPN; reflects severity of metabolic stress; TUN gives the most accurate estimation of total protein catabolism.

[c]Red blood cells are separated from plasma by centrifugation and washed with saline; after hemolyzing the cells, the intracellular material is analyzed for vitamin availability.

[d]No biochemical tests have been developed to assess B_3 status; the fraction of whole blood niacin as NAD is a potentially useful test (see Powers HJ: Current knowledge concerning optimum nutritional status of riboflavin, niacin, and pyridoxine, *Proc Nutr Soc* 58:435, 1999).

[e]ALT and GPT are the same enzyme; AST and GOT are the same enzyme.

[f]PLP is a rate-limiting co-enzyme in the transamination of amino acids (ALT and AST). PLP found primarily in liver and muscles.

[g]Microbiologic growth assays, the deoxyuridine suppression test, and recently developed research tests for folate and vitamin B_{12} are not generally offered in the contemporary clinical laboratory.

[h]More sensitive procedures for measurement of vitamin K include serum chromatography and determination of the serum level of vitamin K–dependent bone protein called osteocalcin. Deficiency significantly increases the amount of abnormal forms of this protein. These tests are not yet widely available.

[i]These substances are measured by similar techniques when the concentration in urine or other body fluids is determined.

[j]These tests are combined with serum glucose, creatinine, and BUN on a test battery or panel. This set of tests is among the first and most frequently administered laboratory tests.

[k]The CBC includes the red cell count, the red cell indices, Hb concentration, HCT, MCV, mean cell hemoglobin (MCH), mean cell hemoglobin concentration (MCHC), and white cell and platelet counts. Only HCT, Hb, and MCV are discussed here (see Savage RA: The red cell indices: yesterday, today, and tomorrow, *Clin Lab Med* 13:773-785, 1993).

[l]Ranges are for adult men and premenopausal women. Pregnant women, infants, and children have different reference ranges.

[m]See van Zeben D et al: Evaluation of microcytosis using serum ferritin and red cell distribution width, *Eur J Haematol* 44:106-109, 1990.

[n]Taste acuity tests can be used to supplement laboratory methods (see, e.g., Gibson RS et al: A growth limiting mild zinc deficiency syndrome in some Southern Ontario boys with low growth percentiles, *Am J Clin Nutr* 49:1266,1989)

[o]AACE supports target TSH level between 0.3- and 3.0 mIU/mL to reduce the incidence of risks associated with subclinical hypothyroidism. AACE Task Force Thyroid Guidelines, *Endocr Pract.* 8:466, 2002.

[p]More recent awareness of the highly undiagnosed common disease of A1AT is improving education of healthcare providers regarding this condition. Kohnlein, T, Welte T: alpha-1 antitrypsin deficiency: pathogenesis, clinical presentation, diagnosis, and treatment, *The Am J of Med* 121:3, 2008.

[q]organic acid functional markers for metabolic effects of micronutrient inadequacies, toxic exposure, neuroendocrine activity and intestinal bacterial overgrowth. Lord R, Bralley J: Organics in urine: assessment of gut dysbiosis, nutrient deficiencies and toxemia. *Nutr Pers* 1997:20:25.

APPENDIX 31. Nutritional Implications of Selected Drugs

Sr. Jeanne P. Crowe, PharmD, RPh, RPI

Drug	Category	Drug Effect	Nutritional Implications and Cautions
Selected Antiinfective Agents			
Penicillins	Antibacterial agents	Long-term use may lead to oral candidiasis, diarrhea, epigastric distress. Some products contain high amounts of potassium or sodium. May cause *Clostridium difficile* pseudomembranous colitis.	Use caution with low-sodium diet or potassium supplements. Take most oral forms 1 hour before or 2 hours after food to improve absorption. Take amoxicillin/potassium clavulanate with food to decrease GI distress. Focus on fluid and electrolyte replacement for diarrhea.
Selected Macrolides			
Azithromycin (Zithromax) Clarithromycin (Biaxin) Erythromycin (Ery-Tab)	Macrolide antibacterial agent Macrolide antibacterial agent Macrolide antibacterial agent	May cause GI distress, anorexia, stomatitis, bad taste in the mouth, or diarrhea. May increase sedative effect of alcohol. May cause *Clostridium difficile* pseudomembranous colitis.	Take with food to decrease GI distress. Eat frequent, small, appealing meals to counteract anorexia. Use mouth rinses, sugarless gum, or lemon water for abnormal taste in mouth. Focus on fluid and electrolyte replacement for diarrhea. Avoid alcohol.
Sulfamethoxazole/ trimethoprim (Bactrim, Bactrim DS)	Sulfonamide combination antibacterial agent	May interfere with folate metabolism, especially with long-term use. May cause stomatitis, anorexia, nausea and vomiting, severe allergic reactions. May cause *Clostridium difficile* pseudomembranous colitis.	Take with food and 8 oz of fluid to lessen nausea, vomiting, and anorexia. Folate supplement may be necessary. Discontinue drug and consult physician at first sign of allergic reaction. Focus on fluid and electrolyte replacement for diarrhea.
Selected Cephalosporins			
Cephalexin (Keflex) Cefprozil (Cefzil)	Cephalosporin antibacterial agent Cephalosporin antibacterial agent	May cause stomatitis, sore mouth and tongue and interfere with eating. May cause diarrhea. May cause *Clostridium difficile* pseudomembranous colitis.	Focus on fluid and electrolyte replacement for diarrhea. Eat moist, soft, low-salt foods as well as cold foods such as ice chips, sherbet, and yogurt for stomatitis and sore mouth.
Cefuroxime axetil (Ceftin)	Cephalosporin antibacterial agent	Food increases bioavailability of tablets and suspension. Antacids, calcium, and magnesium supplements may decrease bioavailability.	Take with a meal for optimal bioavailability. Take separately from antacids, calcium, or magnesium supplements
Selected Fluoroquinolones			
Ciprofloxacin (Cipro) Levofloxacin (Levaquin) Gatifloxacin (Tequin) Moxifloxacin (Avelox)	Fluoroquinolone antibacterial agents	Drug may rarely precipitate in renal tubules. Drug will bind to magnesium, calcium, zinc, and iron, forming an insoluble, unabsorbable complex. Ciprofloxacin inhibits the metabolism of caffeine, causing increased central nervous system stimulation. May cause *Clostridium difficile* pseudomembranous colitis.	Take drug with 8 oz of fluid; maintain adequate fluid intake. Limit caffeine intake. Take drug at least 2 hours before or 6 hours after antacids, magnesium, calcium, iron, or zinc supplements or multivitamin with minerals. Focus on fluid and electrolyte replacement for diarrhea.
Selected Antimicrobial Agents			
Linezolid (Zyvox)	Oxazolidinone antibacterial agent	Drug exhibits mild monoamine oxidase inhibition. May cause taste change, oral candidiasis, and pseudomembranous colitis.	Avoid significant amounts (>100 mg) of high tyramine/ pressor foods. See chart in 16th edition of *Food Medication Interactions*. Eat multiple small meals of appealing foods if taste changes become a problem. Focus on fluid and electrolyte replacement for diarrhea.

Tetracycline (Sumycin)	Antibacterial agent	Drug may cause anorexia. Drug will bind to Mg^{+}, Ca^{++}, Zn^{++}, and Fe^{++}, forming an insoluble unabsorbable complex. May decrease bacterial production of vitamin K in intestinal tract. May cause vitamin B deficiency with long-term use. Drug combined with vitamin A may increase the risk of benign intracranial hypertension. May cause *Clostridium difficile* pseudomembranous colitis.	Take supplements separately by 3 hours. Eat frequent, small, appealing meals to decrease anorexia. Avoid excessive vitamin A while taking drug. Vitamins K and B supplements may be necessary with long-term use. Focus on fluid and electrolyte replacement for diarrhea.
Metronidazole (Flagyl)	Antibacterial agent/antiprotozoal agent	May cause anorexia, GI distress, stomatitis, and metallic taste in mouth. May cause disulfiram-like reaction when ingested with alcohol.	Take with food to avoid GI distress. Eat frequent, small, appealing meals to decrease anorexia. Avoid all alcohol during use and for 3 days after discontinuation.
Nitrofurantoin (Macrobid)	Nitrofuran Antibacterial agent	Drug may cause peripheral neuropathy, muscle weakness, and muscle wasting, especially in individuals with preexisting anemia, vitamin B deficiency, and electrolyte abnormalities. May cause *Clostridium difficile* pseudomembranous colitis.	Drug should be taken with adequate calories, protein, and vitamin B complex. Avoid in G-6-PD deficiency because of increased risk of hemolytic anemia. Focus on fluid and electrolyte replacement for diarrhea.
Gentamicin (Garamycin) Amikacin (Amikin)	Aminoglycoside Antibacterial agent Aminoglycoside Antibacterial agent	Drug may be ototoxic and nephrotoxic. Dehydration increases risk of toxicity.	Adequate fluid intake and hydration necessary to lower risk of toxicity.
Isoniazid (Nydrazid)	Antitubercular agent	Drug may cause pyridoxine (vitamin B_6) and niacin (vitamin B_3) deficiency resulting in peripheral neuropathy and pellagra. Drug may affect vitamin D metabolism and decrease calcium and phosphate absorption. Drug processes MAO inhibitor–like activity.	Avoid use in malnourished individuals and others at increased risk for peripheral neuropathy. Supplement with 25 to 50 mg of pyridoxine and possibly B-complex if skin changes occur. Avoid foods high in tyramine (e.g., aged cheeses). Maintain adequate calcium and vitamin D intake.
Rifampin (Rifadin)	Antitubercular agent	Drug may increase metabolism of vitamin D. Rare cases of osteomalacia have been reported.	May need vitamin D supplement with long-term use.
Ethambutol (Myambutol)	Antitubercular agent	Drug may decrease body copper and zinc. Drug may decrease the excretion of uric acid, leading to hyperuricemia and gout.	Increase intake of foods high in copper and zinc; take daily multivitamin with minerals when drug is used long term. Maintain adequate hydration and purine-restricted diet.
Pyrazinamide	Antitubercular agent	Drug may decrease the excretion of uric acid, leading hyperuricemia and gout.	Maintain adequate hydration and purine-restricted diet.
Selected Antifungal Agents			
Amphotericin B (Fungizone)	Antifungal agent	Drug may cause anorexia and weight loss. Drug causes loss of potassium, magnesium, and calcium.	Eat frequent, small, appealing meals high in magnesium, potassium, calcium. Ensure adequate hydration.
Ketoconazole (Nizoral)	Antifungal agent	Drug does not dissolve at pH >5.	Take with food to increase absorption. Take with acidic liquid (e.g., cola), especially individuals with achlorhydria.
Hematologic Agents			
Warfarin (Coumadin)	Anticoagulant	Prevents the conversion of oxidized vitamin K to the active form. Produces a state of systemic anticoagulation. May inhibit mineralization of newly formed bone.	Consistent intake of dietary supplements (i.e., in vitamins) must be consistent to achieve desired state of anticoagulation. Monitor bone mineral density in individuals on long-term therapy.
Aspirin (Bayer Ecotrin)	Salicylate platelet inhibitor	Drug may cause GI irritation and bleeding. Drug may decrease uptake of vitamin C by leukocytes and increase urinary loss; decreases systemic levels of iron, folic acid, sodium, and potassium, especially with high dose and long-term use.	Incorporate foods high in vitamin C and folic acid into diet. Monitor electrolytes, hemoglobin to determine need for potassium or iron supplements. Avoid alcohol consumption. See new recommendation for use of low dose aspirin (81 mg) in 16th edition of *Food Medication Interaction*.

Continued

APPENDIX 31. Nutritional Implications of Selected Drugs—cont'd

Drug	Category	Drug Effect	Nutritional Implications and Cautions
Hormonal and Metabolic Agents			
Metformin (Glucophage)	Biguanide	Drug may decrease absorption of vitamin B_{12}, folic acid. May cause lactic acidosis.	Maintain prescribed diabetic diet. Increase foods high in vitamin B_{12} and folic acid or supplement if necessary. Avoid alcohol to decrease risk of lactic acidosis.
Prednisone Methylprednisolone (Medrol)	Corticosteroid Corticosteroid	Drug induces protein catabolism, resulting in muscle wasting, atrophy of bone protein matrix, delayed wound healing. Drug decreases intestinal absorption of calcium; promotes urinary loss of calcium, potassium, zinc, vitamin C, nitrogen; causes sodium retention.	Maintain diet high in calcium, vitamin D, protein, potassium, zinc, and vitamin C, and low in sodium. Calcium and vitamin D supplements recommended for prevention of osteoporosis with long-term use of drug.
Alendronate (Fosamax) Risedronate (Actonel) Ibandronate (Boniva)	Bisphosphonates	Drug may induce mild decrease in serum calcium.	Diet high in calcium or calcium and vitamin D supplement. Drug must be taken 30 minutes (alendronate and risedronate) or 1 hour (ibandronate) before first food or medication of the day on completely empty stomach with plain water only.
Oxandrolone (Oxandrin)	Anabolic steroid	Drug is used to promote weight gain and muscle mass after surgery, trauma, infection. May increase blood glucose and lipids.	Diet must consist of adequate calories and protein to promote anabolic effect. Monitor weight, blood glucose, lipids, and hepatic function.
Estrogen (Premarin) Oral contraceptives	Sex hormones	Drug may decrease absorption and tissue uptake of vitamin C. Drug may increase absorption of vitamin A. May inhibit folate conjugate and decrease serum folic acid levels. Drug may decrease serum levels vitamin B_6, B_{12}, riboflavin, magnesium, zinc.	Maintain diet with adequate magnesium, folic acid, vitamin B_6 and B_{12}, riboflavin, and zinc. Calcium and vitamin D supplements may be recommended with estrogen as hormone replacement for postmenopausal women.
Cardiovascular Agents			
Digoxin (Lanoxin)	Cardiac glycoside	Drug may increase urinary loss of magnesium and decrease serum levels of potassium.	Hypokalemia, hypomagnesemia, and hypercalcemia increase drug toxicity. Maintain diet high in potassium and magnesium. Caution with calcium supplements and antacids.
Propranolol (Inderal LA, InnoPran LA) Metoprolol (Lopressor, Toprol XL) Atenolol (Tenormin)	β-Adrenergic antagonist β-Adrenergic antagonist β-Adrenergic antagonist	Drug may mask sympathetic signs of hypoglycemia. Drug may prolong hypoglycemia. Drug may decrease insulin release in response to hyperglycemia.	Maintain prescribed diabetic diet. Monitor blood glucose for hyperglycemia. Monitor for nonsympathetic signs of hypoglycemia.
Benazepril (Lotensin) Enalapril (Vasotec) Fosinopril (Monopril) Lisinopril (Zestril, Prinivil)	ACE inhibitor ACE inhibitor ACE inhibitor ACE inhibitor	Drug may increase serum potassium levels.	Caution with high potassium diet or potassium supplements. Avoid salt substitutes. Ensure adequate fluid intake and hydration. Check recommendation for each agent as regards ingestion with food. See monograph in 16th edition of *Food Medication Interactions.*
Candesartan (Atacand) Irbesartan (Avapro) Losartan (Cozaar) Olmesartan (Benicar) Telmisartan (Micardis) Valsartan (Diovan)	Angiotensin II receptor antagonist Angiotensin II receptor antagonist Angiotensin II receptor antagonist Angiotensin II receptor antagonist Angiotensin II receptor antagonist Angiotensin II receptor antagonist	Drug may increase serum potassium levels.	Caution with high-potassium diet or potassium supplements. Avoid salt substitutes. Ensure adequate fluid intake and hydration. Avoid natural licorice. Avoid grapefruit and related citrus with losartan.

Clonidine (Catapres)	Alpha-adrenergic agonist	Drug commonly causes dizziness, drowsiness, sedation.	Avoid alcohol and alcohol products. Drug increases sensitivity to alcohol, which may increase sedation caused by drug alone.
Hydralazine (Apresoline)	Peripheral vasodilator	Drug interferes with pyridoxine (vitamin B_6) metabolism. May result in pyridoxine deficiency.	Maintain a diet high in pyridoxine. Supplementation may be necessary.
Quinidine (Quinaglute)	Antiarrhythmic agent	Cardiac toxicity of drug is increased in the presence of hypokalemia, hypomagnesemia, and hypocalcemia.	Provide diet adequate in potassium, magnesium, calcium to maintain normal serum levels. Supplementation may be necessary.
Antihyperlipidemic Agents			
Atorvastatin (Lipitor) Fluvastatin (Lescol) Lovastatin (Mevacor) Pravastatin (Pravachol) Rosuvastatin (Crestor) Simvastatin (Zocor)	HMG Co-A reductase inhibitor HMG Co-A reductase inhibitor HMG Co-A reductase inhibitor HMG Co-A reductase inhibitor HMG Co-A reductase inhibitor HMG Co-A reductase inhibitor	Drug may cause significant reduction in coenzyme Q_{10}. Drug lowers low-density lipoprotein- cholesterol; raises high-density lipoprotein cholesterol.	Supplementation with coenzyme Q_{10} is controversial. Drug is adjunct to diet therapy. Maintain low-fat, low-cholesterol diet for optimal drug effect. Avoid grapefruit and related citrus with atorvastatin, lovastatin, or simvastatin.
Gemfibrozil (Lopid) Fenofibrate (Tricor)	Fibric acid derivative Fibric acid derivative	Drug decreases serum triglycerides.	Maintain low-fat, low-sucrose diet; avoid alcohol for optimal therapeutic effect.
Cholestyramine (Questran)	Bile acid sequestrant	Drug binds fat-soluble vitamins (A, E, D, K), β-carotene, calcium, magnesium, iron, zinc, and folic acid.	Take fat-soluble vitamins in water-miscible form or take vitamin supplement at least 1 hour before first dose of drug daily. Maintain diet high in folic acid, magnesium, calcium, iron, zinc, or supplements when necessary. Monitor serum nutrient levels with long-term use of drug.
Niacin (Niaspan)	Nicotinic acid	High dose may elevate blood glucose and uric acid.	Maintain diabetic, low-purine diet if necessary.
Diuretics			
Furosemide (Lasix) Bumetanide (Bumex)	Loop diuretic Loop diuretic	Drug increases urinary excretion of sodium, potassium, magnesium, calcium.	Maintain diet high in potassium, magnesium, and calcium. Avoid natural licorice, which may counteract the diuretic effect of the drug. Monitor electrolytes; supplementation may be necessary.
Hydrochlorothiazide (HydroDIURIL)	Thiazide diuretic	Drug increases urinary excretion of sodium, potassium, magnesium. Drug increases renal resorption of calcium.	Maintain diet high in potassium and magnesium. Avoid natural licorice, which may counteract the diuretic effect of the drug. Monitor electrolytes; supplementation may be necessary. Use caution with calcium supplements.
Triamterene (Dyrenium) Spironolactone (Aldactone)	Potassium-sparing diuretic Potassium-sparing diuretic	Drug increases renal resorption of potassium.	Avoid salt substitutes. Use caution with potassium supplements. Avoid excessive potassium intake in diet.
Analgesics			
Acetaminophen (Tylenol) NSAIDs such as ibuprofen (Motrin), naproxen (Naprosyn), meloxicam (Mobic)		Drug may cause hepatotoxicity at high dose. Chronic alcohol ingestion increases the risk of hepatotoxicity. **Standard warning with all NSAIDs**: **GI:** NSAIDS cause an increased risk of serious GI adverse events, including bleeding, ulceration, and perforation of the stomach and intestines, which can be fatal. These events can occur at anytime during use and without prior symptoms. The elderly are at greater risk for serious GI events. **Cardiovascular:** NSAIDs may cause increased risk of serious cardiovascular thrombotic events, myocardial infarction, and stroke, which can be fatal.	Maximum safe adult dose is <4 g/day. Avoid alcohol or limit to <2 drinks/day. Take drug with food or milk to decrease risk of GI toxicity. Avoid use in the elderly. Avoid use in individuals with severe cardiovascular disease.

Continued

APPENDIX 31. Nutritional Implications of Selected Drugs—cont'd

Drug	Category	Drug Effect	Nutritional Implications and Cautions
Selected Narcotic Analgesics			
Morphine (MS Contin, Avinza) Oxycodone (OxyContin) Fentanyl (Duragesic, Onsolis)	Narcotic analgesic Narcotic analgesic Narcotic analgesic	All narcotics may cause dose-related sedation, respiratory depression, dry mouth, constipation. May be severe. Heat causes faster absorption of transdermal fentanyl.	Monitor respiratory function and bowel function (not with paralytic ileus). Do not crush or chew sustained-released formulas. Do not use with heating pad, hot tub, sunbathing. Use caution with high fever.
Antidepressants			
Fluoxetine (Prozac) Paroxetine (Paxil) Sertraline (Zoloft)	Selective serotonin reuptake inhibitor Selective serotonin reuptake inhibitor Selective serotonin reuptake inhibitor	Fluoxetine may cause anorexia and weight loss. Fluoxetine may decrease the absorption of leucine. Some herbal and natural products may increase toxicity.	Monitor weight and caloric intake if necessary. Avoid tryptophan, St. John's wort. Additive effects may produce adverse effects or serotonin syndrome.
Trazodone (Desyrel) Venlafaxine (Effexor XR) Mirtazapine (Remeron)	Unclassified antidepressant Unclassified antidepressant Unclassified antidepressant	Some herbal and natural products may increase toxicity. Mirtazapine may cause significant increase in appetite and weight gain.	Avoid tryptophan, St. John's wort. Additive effects may produce adverse effects or serotonin syndrome.
Amitriptyline (Elavil)	Tricyclic antidepressant	Drug may cause increased appetite (especially for carbohydrates and sweets) and weight gain. High fiber may decrease drug absorption.	Monitor caloric intake. Maintain consistent amount of fiber in diet.
Phenelzine (Nardil)	MAO inhibitor	Drug may cause increased appetite (especially for carbohydrates and sweets) and weight gain. Risk for severe reaction with dietary tyramine.	Avoid foods high in tyramine during drug use and for 2 weeks after discontinuation to prevent hypertensive crisis. Monitor caloric intake to avoid weight gain.
Lithium carbonate (Lithobid)	Antimanic and antidepressant	Sodium intake affects drug levels. Low-sodium diet, dehydration, increased drug toxicity. Drug may cause GI irritation.	Drink 2 to 3 L of fluid daily to avoid dehydration. Maintain consistent dietary sodium intake. Take with food to decrease GI irritation.
Antipsychotic Agents			
Clozapine (Clozaril)	Second generation antipsychotic	Drug may cause increased appetite and weight gain. Drug may cause life-threatening toxic agranulocytosis.	Monitor for weight gain and calorie count. Individual must be enrolled in and adhere to requirements of Clozaril program, including a weekly white blood cell count.
Olanzapine (Zyprexa) Risperidone (Risperdal) Quetiapine (Seroquel)	Second generation antipsychotics	Drugs may cause increased appetite and weight gain. May cause increased blood sugar and HbA1c. May increase lipids and triglycerides.	Monitor weight and food intake. Monitor fasting blood sugar and HbA1c. Monitor lipids and triglycerides. Do not use in elderly dementia patients. May increase risk of stroke.
Chlorpromazine (Theorizing)	First-generation antipsychotic, low potency	Drug may impair glucose tolerance and insulin release. May cause increased appetite and weight gain. Risk for tardive dyskinesia.	Closer monitoring of blood glucose in the diagnosed diabetic individual. Periodic check of blood glucose in the "at-risk" nondiabetic individual. Monitor weight and calorie count. Tardive dyskinesia may interfere with biting, chewing, swallowing.
Haloperidol (Haldol)	First-generation antipsychotic, high potency	May cause increased appetite and weight gain. Risk for tardive dyskinesia.	Monitor weight and calorie count. Tardive dyskinesia may interfere with biting, chewing, swallowing.

Antianxiety and Hypnotic Agents			
Lorazepam (Ativan)	Benzodiazepine	Drugs may cause significant sedation.	Avoid concurrent ingestion of alcohol, which will produce CNS depression. Limit or avoid caffeine, which may decrease the therapeutic effect of the drug. Use caution with herbal and natural products that cause CNS stimulation or sedation.
Diazepam (Valium)	Benzodiazepine		
Alprazolam (Xanax)	Benzodiazepine		
Clonazepam (Klonopin)	Benzodiazepine		
Temazepam (Restoril)	Benzodiazepine hypnotic		
Zolpidem (Ambien)	Nonbenzodiazepine hypnotic		
Selected Anticonvulsant Agents			
Carbamazepine (Tegretol)		Drug may decrease biotin, folic acid, and vitamin D levels.	Maintain diet high in folic acid and vitamin D. Calcium and vitamin D supplementation may be necessary for long-term therapy to prevent loss of bone mineral density.
Phenytoin (Dilantin)	Hydantoin	Drug may decrease serum levels of folic acid, calcium, vitamin D, biotin, and thiamin.	Folic acid, calcium, and vitamin D supplement may be recommended with long-term use.
Phenobarbital	Barbiturate	Drug may induce rapid metabolism of vitamin D and produce deficiency of vitamin D and calcium. Drug may increase the metabolism of vitamin K, decrease serum folic acid and vitamin B_{12} levels.	Increase dietary intake of calcium, vitamin D, and folic acid. May need calcium, vitamin D, folic acid, and vitamin B_{12} supplementation with long-term use of drug.
Lamotrigine (Lamictal)	Anticonvulsant and adjunct mood stabilizer in bipolar disorder	Dose must be titrated slowly to avoid rash which may be fatal. Increased incidence of rash in children	Avoid alcohol. Monitor for rash. Monitor renal and hepatic function.
Lacosamide (Vimpat)		Drug may cause dizziness, ataxia, dry mouth, nausea and vomiting.	May cause hepatotoxicity. Do not use in individual with mild hepatic dysfunction. Monitor hepatic function.
Anti-Alzheimer's Agents			
Donepezil (A1icept)	Cholinesterase inhibitor	Drug is highly cholinergic; may cause anorexia, nausea and vomiting, diarrhea, increased gastric acid secretion, GI bleeding.	Take drug with food to prevent GI irritation. Monitor food intake and weight.
Rivastigmine (Exelon)	Cholinesterase inhibitor		
Galantamine (Razadyne)	Cholinesterase inhibitor		Avoid diet that alkalinizes the urine to avoid drug toxicity.
Memantine (Namenda)	NMDA receptor antagonist	Drug is cleared from the body almost exclusively by renal excretion. Urine pH >8 decreases renal excretion by 80%.	
Gastrointestinal Agents			
Famotidine (Pepcid)	H_2 receptor antagonist	Drug may reduce the absorption of vitamin B_{12} and iron.	Monitor iron studies, vitamin B_{12} level while on long-term therapy. Supplement if necessary.
Nizatidine (Axid)	H_2 receptor antagonist		
Ranitidine (Zantac)	H_2 receptor antagonist		
Omeprazole (Prilosec)	Proton pump inhibitor	Inhibition of acid secretion may inhibit the absorption of iron and vitamin B_{12}.	Monitor iron studies and vitamin B_{12} levels with long-term use of drug. Supplement if necessary.
Lansoprazole (Prevacid)	Proton pump inhibitor		
Pantoprazole (Protonix)	Proton pump inhibitor	Long-term calcium absorption leading to osteoporosis.	Monitor bone density with long-term use.
Rabeprazole (Aciphex)	Proton pump inhibitor	Long-term inhibition of acid secretion may increase the risk of *Clostridium difficile* pseudomembranous colitis.	
Dexlansoprozole	Proton pump inhibitor		
Metoclopramide (Reglan)	Prokinetic agent	Metoclopramide increases gastric emptying; may change insulin requirements in persons with diabetes; may increase CNS depressant effects of alcohol. Drug may cause tardive dyskinesia with extended use.	Monitor blood glucose in persons with diabetes carefully when drug is initiated. Avoid alcohol. Tardive dyskinesia may interfere with biting, chewing, swallowing.

Continued

APPENDIX 31. Nutritional Implications of Selected Drugs—cont'd

Drug	Category	Drug Effect	Nutritional Implications and Cautions
Selected Antineoplastic Agents			
Methotrexate	Folate antagonist	Drug inhibits dihydrofolate reductase; decreased formation of active folate. Drug may cause GI irritation or injury.	Maintain diet high in folic acid and vitamin B_{12}. Daily folic acid supplement recommended with antirheumatic doses. Leucovorin rescue may be necessary with antineoplastic doses.
Cyclophosphamide (Cytoxan)	Alkylating agent	Drug metabolite causes bladder irritation, acute hemorrhagic cystitis.	Maintain high fluid intake (2-3 L daily) to induce frequent voiding.
All antineoplastic agents		All agents are cytotoxic; potential to damage intestinal mucosal.	Extensive effects discussed in Chapter 16.
Selected Anti-Parkinson Agents			
Carbidopa/levodopa (Sinemet)	Dopamine precursor	Carbidopa protects levodopa against pyridoxine-enhanced peripheral decarboxylation to dopamine.	Pyridoxine supplements in excess of 10-25 mg daily may increase carbidopa requirements and increase adverse effects of levodopa.
Bromocriptine (Parlodel)	Dopamine agonist	Drug may cause GI irritation, nausea, vomiting, and GI bleeding.	Take drug with food to prevent GI irritation. Take drug at bedtime to decrease nausea.
Selegiline (Eldepryl)	MAO-B inhibitor	Drug selectively inhibits MAO-B at 10 mg or less per day. Drug loses selectivity at higher doses.	Avoid high-tyramine foods at doses greater than 10 mg/day. May precipitate hypertension.
Entacapone (Comtan)	COMT inhibitor	Drug chelates iron; may decrease serum iron levels.	Take iron supplement separately from drug.
CNS Stimulants			
Methylphenidate (Ritalin, Concerta)	CNS stimulant	Drug may cause anorexia, weight loss, and decreased growth.	Ensure adequate calorie intake. Limit ingestion of caffeine; avoid alcohol and herbal products. Monitor children's weight and growth.
Amphetamine (Adderall, Dexedrine)	CNS stimulant	Drug may cause anorexia, decreased weight loss, and decreased growth.	Ensure adequate calorie intake. Limit ingestion of caffeine; avoid alcohol and herbal products. High-dose vitamin C may decrease drug absorption, increase drug excretion, and decrease half-life of drug. Monitor children's weight and growth.
Miscellaneous			
Sapropterin (Kuvan)	Hyper – PKU treatment Enzyme enhancer in BH4 responsive PKU	Patient must have sufficient residual PAH.	Take with food to increase absorption. Drug is an adjunct to low phenylalanine diet. Monitor phenylalanine level.

Appendix created by Sr. Jeanne P. Crowe, PharmD, Rph. Adapted from Pronsky ZM and Crowe JP: Food medication interactions, ed 16, 2010.

ACE, Angiotensin-converting enzyme; *CNS*, central nervous system; *Co-A*, coenzyme A; *COMT*, catechol-o-methyl transferase; *G-6-PD*, glucose-6-phosphate dehydrogenase; *GI*, gastrointestinal; *HbA1c*, hemoglobin A1c; *HMG*, 3-hydroxy-3-methyl-glutaryl; *MAO*, monoamine oxidase; *NSAID*, nonsteroidal antiinflammatory drug; *PKU*, phenylketonuria.

APPENDIX 32. Enteral Formulas and Their Indications for Use

General information on formula types and their use is presented here. For more detailed information on formulas consult: Abbott Nutrition, www.abbottnutrition.com and Nestlé Nutrition, www.nestle-nutrition.com.

Enteral Formulas	kcal/mL	Protein (g/L)	CHO (g/L)	Fat (g/L)	mOsm	Free H_2O (mL/L)	Notes
Standard	1-1.2	44-53	144-160	35-39	300-450	800-1260	For patients without malabsorption, hypermetabolism, or major organ failure; available with or without fiber
Calorie-dense	1.5	63-68	170-203	49-65	525-650	762-778	For patients requiring less volume; available with or without fiber
High-protein	1-1.2	53-63	130-160	26-39	340-490	818-839	For patients with healing needs or low kcal:protein needs; available with or without fiber
Renal	1.8-2	45-81	167-205	96-100	700-960	709-736	For patients with compromised renal function; formulas differ based on if patient is on dialysis or if diabetes present
Glucose-control	1-1.2	45-60	96-100	48-59	280-470	805-840	Low carbohydrate, high fat, fiber containing
*Peptide-based	1-1.5	40-68	127-188	39-56	380-585	771-832	Formulated to promote maximal intestinal absorption of protein; contains di- and tri-peptides from whey protein; increased MCT:LCT fat ratio; available with higher levels of protein
Critical Care	1.5	94	134-172	51-68	480-595	759-772	High calorie, high protein formulated to support immune function and support healing; increased omega-3 fat; some with fiber
Pulmonary	1.5	63-68	100-106	93-95	330-785	535-785	Low carbohydrate; aimed at decreasing respiratory quotient and decreasing inflammation
Modular Additives	**kcal**	**Protein (g)**	**CHO (g)**	**Fat (g)**			
Protein/100 g	357	6	0	0			Whey protein aimed at increasing protein content of food and formulas
Glucose/100 g	380	0	94	0			Glucose polymer powder for adding carbohydrate calories
Lipid/15 mL	68	0	0	7.5			Safflower oil for adding fat calories

*Available in pediatric formulas

APPENDIX 33. DASH Diet

The DASH diet is an eating pattern that reduces high blood pressure. It is not the traditional low-salt diet. DASH uses foods high in the minerals calcium, potassium, and magnesium, which, when combined, help lower blood pressure. It is also low in fat and high in fiber, an eating style recommended for everyone.

The Healthy Eating Pattern is the template for the DASH eating pattern, with inclusion of ½ to 1 serving of nuts, seeds, and legumes daily, limited fats and oils, and use of nonfat or low-fat milk. The eating pattern is reduced in saturated fat, total fat, cholesterol, and sweet and sugar-containing beverages; and provides abundant servings of fruits and vegetables.

Although the DASH eating plan is naturally lower in salt because of the emphasis on fruits and vegetables, all adults should still make an effort to reduce packaged and processed foods and high-sodium snacks (such as salted chips, pretzels, and crackers) and use less or no salt at the table.

DASH can be an excellent way to lose weight. Because weight loss can help lower blood pressure, it is often suggested. In addition to following DASH, try adding in daily physical activity such as walking or other exercise. You may want to check with your doctor first.

Current recommendations include:

The Dash Diet

Food Group	1600 kcal Servings/Day	2000 kcal Servings/Day	2600 kcal Servings/Day	3100 kcal Servings/Day
Grains (whole grains)	6	7-8	10-11	12-13
Vegetables	3-4	4-5	5-6	6
Fruits and juices	4	4-5	5-6	6
Milk, nonfat or low-fat	2-3	2-3	3	3-4
Meats, poultry, and fish	1-2	2 or less	6	2-3
Nuts, seeds, and legumes	3/week	½-1	1	1
Fats and oils	2	2-3	3	4
Sweets	0	5/week	Less than 2	2

Dietary Guidelines

Food Group	Servings/Day	Serving Sizes	Examples	Significance of Each Food Group
Grains	6-13	1 slice bread ½ cup (1 oz) dry cereal* ½ cup cooked rice, pasta, or cereal and fiber	Whole-wheat bread, English muffin, pita bread, bagel, cereals, grits, oatmeal, crackers, unsalted pretzels, and popcorn	Major sources of energy
Vegetables	3-6	1 cup raw, leafy veg ½ cup cooked veg 6 oz veg juice	Tomatoes, potatoes, carrots, peas, kale, squash, broccoli, turnip greens, collards, spinach, artichokes, beans, sweet potatoes	Rich sources of potassium, magnesium, antioxidants, and fiber
Fruits	4-6	6 oz fruit juice 1 medium fruit ¼ cup dried fruit ½ cup fresh, frozen, or canned fruit	Apricots, bananas, dates, grapes, oranges and juice, tangerines, strawberries, mangoes, melons, peaches, pineapples, prunes, raisins, grapefruit and juice	Important sources of energy, potassium, magnesium, and fiber
Low-fat dairy	2-4	8 oz milk, 1 cup yogurt, or 1.5 oz cheese	Fat-free or 1% milk, fat-free or low-fat buttermilk, yogurt, or cheese	Major sources of calcium, vitamin D, and protein
Meat, poultry, fish	1-3	3 oz cooked meats, poultry, or fish 1 egg white†	Select only lean meats; trim away visible fats, broil, roast, boil, instead of frying; remove skin from poultry	Rich sources of protein, zinc, and magnesium
Nuts, seeds, legumes	3/wk–1/day	1.5 oz (½ cup) nuts, ½ oz or 2 tbsp seeds, ½ cup cooked legumes	Almonds, filberts, mixed nuts, walnuts, sunflower seeds, kidney beans, lentils	Rich sources of energy, magnesium, protein, monounsaturated fats, and fiber
Fat	2-4	1 tsp soft margarine, veg oil, 1 Tbsp low-fat mayo or salad dressing, or 2 Tbsp light salad dressing‡	Soft margarine, low fat mayo, veg oil, light salad dressing	The DASH study had 27% of calories as fat, including fat in or added to foods Sweets should be low in fat

National Institutes of Health, National Heart, Lung, and Blood Institute: YOUR GUIDE TO Lowering Your Blood Pressure With DASH, U.S. Department of Health and Human Services, NIH Publication No. 06-4082, 2006.

*Serving sizes vary between ½ cup and 1¼ cup, depending on cereal type. Check the product's Nutrition Facts label.

†Because eggs are high in cholesterol, limit egg yolk intake to no more than four per week; two egg whites have the same protein content as 1 oz of meat.

‡Fat content changes serving amount for fats and oils. For example, 1 Tbsp of regular salad dressing equals one serving; 1 Tbsp of a low-fat dressing equals one-half serving; 1 Tbsp of a fat-free dressing equals zero servings.

APPENDIX 33. DASH Diet—cont'd

Sample Menu

Breakfast	Lunch	Dinner
1 cup calcium-fortified orange juice ¾ cup Raisin Bran 1 cup skim milk Mini –whole-wheat bagel 1½ tsp soft margarine 1 cup coffee 2 tsp sugar	3-oz boneless skinless chicken breast 2 slices reduced-fat cheese 2 large leaves lettuce 2 slices tomato 1 Tbsp light mayonnaise 2 slices whole wheat bread 1 medium apple ½ cup raw carrot sticks 1 cup iced tea	1 cup spaghetti with vegetarian/low-sodium tomato sauce 3 Tbsp Parmesan cheese ½ cup green beans 1 cup spinach, raw ½ cup mushrooms, raw 2 Tbsp croutons 2 Tbsp low-fat Italian dressing 1 slice Italian bread ½ cup frozen yogurt
Midmorning Snack	**Midafternoon Snack**	
1 cup apple juice 2 oz walnuts	1 large banana	
Nutritional Analysis:	Kilocalories: 1980 Protein: 78 g Fat: 56 g Saturated fat: 13 g Carbohydrates: 314 g	Sodium: 2377 mg Potassium: 4129 mg Fiber: 32 g Magnesium: 517 g

APPENDIX 34. Exchange Lists for Meal Planning

Menu Plan

Meal Plan for: ______________________ Date: ______________________

Dietitian: ______________________ Phone: ______________________

	Grams	Percent
Carbohydrate	______	______
Protein	______	______
Fat	______	______
Calories	______	______

Time	Number of Exchanges and Choices	Menu Ideas	Menu Ideas
	________ Carbohydrate group ________ Starch ________ Fruit ________ Milk ________ ________ Meat group ________ ________ Fat group ________		
	________ ________ ________ ________ ________ ________ ________ Carbohydrate group ________ Starch ________ Fruit ________ Milk ________ ________ Vegetables ________Meat group ________Fat group		
	________ ________ ________ ________ ________ ________ ________ Carbohydrate group ________ Starch ________ Fruit ________ Milk ________ ________ Vegetables ________ Meat group ________ Fat group		

Continued

APPENDIX 34. Exchange Lists for Meal Planning—cont'd

How This Exchange List Works With Meal Planning

There are three main groups of foods in this exchange list. They are based on the three major nutrients: carbohydrates, protein (meat and meat substitutes), and fat. Each food list contains foods grouped together because they have similar nutrient content and serving sizes. Each serving of a food has about the same amount of carbohydrate, protein, fat, and calories as the other foods on the same list.

- Foods on the **Starch** list, **Fruits** list, **Milk** list, and **Sweets, Desserts, and Other Carbohydrates** list are similar because they contain 12 to 15 grams of carbohydrate per serving.
- Foods on the **Fat** list and **Meat and Meat Substitutes** list usually do not have carbohydrate (except for the plant-based meat substitutes such as beans and lentils).
- Foods on the Starchy Vegetables list (part of the **Starch** list and including foods (such as potatoes, corn, and peas) contain 15 grams of carbohydrate per serving.
- Foods on the **Nonstarchy Vegetables** list (such as green beans, tomatoes, and carrots) contain 5 grams of carbohydrate per serving.
- Some foods have so little carbohydrate and calories that they are considered "free," if eaten in small amounts. You can find these foods on the **Free Foods** list.
- Foods that have different amounts of carbohydrates and calories are listed as **Combination Foods** (such as lasagna) or **Fast Foods.**

Foods are listed with their serving sizes, which are usually measured after cooking. When you begin, measuring the size of each serving will help you learn to "eyeball" correct serving sizes. The following chart shows the amount of nutrients in one serving from each list:

Food List	Carbohydrate (grams)	Protein (grams)	Fat (grams)	Calories
Carbohydrates				
Starch: breads, cereals and grains, starchy vegetables, crackers and snacks, and beans, peas, and lentils	15	0-3	0-1	80
Fruits	15	—	—	60
Milk				
Fat-free, low-fat, 1%	12	8	0-3	100
Reduced fat, 2%	12	8	5	120
Whole	12	8	8	160
Sweets, desserts, and other carbohydrates	15	Varies	Varies	Varies
Nonstarchy Vegetables	5	2	—	25
Meat and Meat Substitutes				
Lean	—	7	0-3	45
Medium-fat	—	7	4-7	75
High-fat	—	7	8+	100
Plant-based proteins	Varies	7	Varies	Varies
Fats	—	—	5	45
Alcohol	Varies	—	—	100

Starch

Cereals, grains, pasta, breads, crackers, snacks, starchy vegetables, and cooked beans, peas, and lentils are starches. In general, 1 starch is:

- ½ cup of cooked cereal, grain, or starchy vegetable
- ½ cup of cooked rice or pasta
- 1 oz of a bread product, such as 1 slice of bread
- ¾ oz to 1 oz of most snack foods (some snack foods may also have extra fat)

Nutrition Tips

1. A choice on the **Starch** list has 15 grams of carbohydrate, 0-3 grams of protein, 0-1 grams of fat, and 80 calories.
2. For maximum health benefits, eat three or more servings of whole grains each day. A serving of whole grain is about ½ cup of cooked cereal or grain, 1 slice of whole-grain bread, or 1 cup of whole-grain cold breakfast cereal.

Selection Tips

1. Choose low-fat starches as often as you can.
2. Starchy vegetables, baked goods, and grains prepared with fat count as 1 starch and 1 fat.
3. For many starchy foods (bagels, muffins, dinner rolls, buns), a general rule of thumb is 1 oz equals 1 serving. Always check the size you eat. Because of their large size, some foods have a lot more carbohydrate (and calories) than you might think. For example, a large bagel may weigh 4 oz and equal 4 carbohydrate servings.
4. For specific information, read the Nutrition Facts panel on the food label.

Food	Serving Size
Bread	
Bagel, large (about 4 oz)	¼ (1 oz)
Biscuit, 2½ inches across†	1
Bread	
Reduced-calorie*	2 slices (1½ oz)
White, whole-grain, pumpernickel, rye, unfrosted raisin	1 slice (1 oz)
Chapatti, small, 6 inches across	1
Cornbread, 1¾ inch cube†	1 (1½ oz)
English muffin	½
Hot dog bun or hamburger bun	½ (1 oz)
Naan, 8 inches by 2 inches	¼
Pancake, 4 inches across, ¼ inch thick	1
Pita, 6 inches across	½
Roll, plain, small	1 (1 oz)
Stuffing, bread†	⅓ cup
Taco shell, 5 inches across†	2
Tortilla, corn, 6 inches across	1

APPENDIX 34. Exchange Lists for Meal Planning—cont'd

Food	Serving Size
Tortilla, flour, 6 inches across	1
Tortilla, flour, 10 inches across	⅓ tortilla
Waffle, 4-inch square or 4 inches across†	1
Cereals and Grains	
Barley, cooked	⅓ cup
Bran, dry	
Oat*	¼ cup
Wheat*	½ cup
Bulgar (cooked)*	½ cup
Cereals	
Bran*	½ cup
Cooked (oats, oatmeal)	½ cup
Puffed	1½ cup
Shredded wheat, plain	½ cup
Sugar-coated	½ cup
Unsweetened, ready-to-eat	¾ cup
Couscous	⅓ cup
Granola	
Low-fat	¼ cup
Regular†	¼ cup
Grits, cooked	½ cup
Kasha	½ cup
Millet, cooked	⅓ cup
Muesli	¼ cup
Pasta, cooked	⅓ cup
Polenta, cooked	⅓ cup
Quinoa, cooked	⅓ cup
Rice, white or brown, cooked	⅓ cup
Tabbouleh (tabouli), prepared	½ cup
Wheat germ, dry	3 Tbsp
Wild rice, cooked	½ cup
Starchy Vegetables	
Cassava	⅓ cup
Corn	½ cup
On cob, large	½ cob (5 oz)
Hominy, canned*	¾ cup
Mixed vegetables with corn, peas, or pasta*	1 cup
Parsnips*	½ cup
Peas, green*	½ cup
Plantain, ripe	⅓ cup
Potato	
Baked with skin	¼ large (3 oz)
Boiled, all kinds	½ cup or ½ medium (3 oz)
Mashed, with milk and fat†	½ cup
French fried (oven-baked)	1 cup (2 oz)
Pumpkin, canned, no sugar added*	1 cup
Spaghetti/pasta sauce	½ cup
Squash, winter (acorn, butternut)*	1 cup
Succotash*	½ cup
Yam, sweet potato, plain	½ cup
Crackers and Snacks	
Animal crackers	8
Crackers	
Round-butter type†	6
Saltine-type	6
Sandwich-style, cheese or peanut butter filling†	3
Whole-wheat regular†	2-5 (¾ oz)
Whole-wheat lower fat or crispbreads*	2-5 (¾ oz)
Graham cracker, 2½ -inch square	3
Matzoh	¾ oz
Melba toast, about 2-inch by 4-inch piece	4 pieces
Oyster crackers	20
Popcorn (microwave popped)	3 cups
With butter†*	3 cups
No fat added*	3 cups
Lower fat*	3 cups
Pretzels	¾ oz
Rice cakes, 4 inches across	2
Snack chips	
Fat-free or baked (tortilla, potato), baked pita chips	15-20 (¾ oz)
Regular (tortilla, potato)†	9-13 (¾ oz)
Beans, Peas, and Lentils	
The choices on this list count as 1 starch + 1 lean meat.	
Baked beans*	⅓ cup
Beans, cooked (black, garbanzo, kidney, lima, navy, pinto, white)*	½ cup
Lentils, cooked (brown, green, yellow)*	½ cup
Peas, cooked (black-eyed, split)*	½ cup
Refried beans, canned‡*	½ cup

*More than 3 grams of dietary fiber per serving.
†Extra fat, or prepared with added fat. (Count as 1 starch + 1 fat.)
‡480 milligrams or more of sodium per serving.

Fruits

Fresh, frozen, canned, and dried fruits and fruit juices are on this list. In general, 1 fruit choice is:

- ½ cup of canned or fresh fruit or unsweetened fruit juice
- 1 small fresh fruit (4 oz)
- 2 tablespoons of dried fruit

Nutrition Tips

1. A choice on the **Fruits** list has 15 grants of carbohydrate, 0 grants of protein, 0 grants of fat, and 60 calories.
2. Fresh, frozen, and dried fruits are good sources of fiber. Fruit juices contain very little fiber. Choose fruits instead of juices whenever possible.
3. Citrus fruits, berries, and melons are good sources of vitamin C.

Selection Tips

1. Use a food scale to weigh fresh fruits. Practice builds portion skills.
2. The weight listed includes skin, core, seeds, and rind.
3. Read the Nutrition Facts on the food label. If 1 serving has more than 15 g of carbohydrate, you may need to adjust the size of the serving.
4. Portion sizes for canned fruits are for the fruit and a small amount of juice (1 to 2 tablespoons).
5. Food labels for fruits may contain the words *no sugar added* or *unsweetened.* This means that no sucrose (table sugar) has been added; it *does not* mean the food contains no sugar.
6. Fruit canned in *extra light syrup* has the same amount of carbohydrate per serving as the *no sugar added* or the *juice pack.* All canned fruits on the **Fruits** list are based on one of these three types of pack. Avoid fruit canned in heavy syrup.

Continued

APPENDIX 34. Exchange Lists for Meal Planning—cont'd

The weight listed includes skin, core, seeds, and rind.

Food	Serving Size
Fruit	
Apple, unpeeled, small	1 (4 oz)
Apples, dried	4 rings
Applesauce, unsweetened	½ cup
Apricots	
Canned	½ cup
Dried	8 halves
Fresh*	4 whole (5½ oz)
Banana, extra small	1 (4 oz)
Blackberries*	¾ cup
Blueberries	¾ cup
Cantaloupe, small	⅓ melon or 1 cup cubed (11 oz)
Cherries	
Sweet, canned	½ cup
Sweet fresh	12 (3 oz)
Dates	3
Dried fruits (blueberries, cherries, cranberries, mixed fruit, raisins)	2 Tbsp
Figs	
Dried	1½
Fresh*	1½ large or 2 medium (3½ oz)
Fruit cocktail	½ cup
Grapefruit	
Large	½ (11 oz)
Sections, canned	¾ cup
Grapes, small	17 (3 oz)
Honeydew melon	1 slice or 1 cup cubed (10 oz)
Kiwi*	1 (3½ oz)
Mandarin oranges, canned	¾ cup
Mango, small	½ fruit (5½ oz) or ½ cup
Nectarine, small	1 (5 oz)
Orange, small*	1 (6½ oz)
Papaya	½ fruit or 1 cup cubed (8 oz)
Peaches	
Canned	½ cup
Fresh, medium	1 (6 oz)
Pears	
Canned	½ cup
Fresh, large	½ (4 oz)
Pineapple	
Canned	½ cup
Fresh	¾ cup
Plums	
Canned	½ cup
Dried (prunes)	3
Small	2 (5 oz)
Raspberries*	1 cup
Strawberries*	1¼ cup whole berries
Tangerines, small*	2 (8 oz)
Watermelon	1 slice or 1¼ cups cubes (13½ oz)
Fruit Juice	
Apple juice/cider	½ cup
Fruit juice blends, 100% juice	⅓ cup
Grape juice	⅓ cup
Grapefruit juice	½ cup
Orange juice	½ cup
Pineapple juice	½ cup
Prune juice	⅓ cup

*More than 3 grams of dietary fiber per serving.

Milk

Different types of milk and milk products are on this list. However, 2 types of milk products are found in other lists:

- Cheeses are on the **Meat and Meat Substitutes** list (because they are rich in protein).
- Cream and other dairy fats are on the **Fats** list.

Milks and yogurts are grouped in 3 categories (fat-free/low-fat, reduced-fat, or whole) based on the amount of fat they have. The following chart shows you what 1 milk choice contains:

	Carbohydrate (grams)	Protein (grams)	Fat (grams)	Calories
Fat-free (skim), low-fat (1%)	12	8	0-3	100
Reduced-fat (2%)	12	8	5	120
Whole	12	8	8	160

Nutrition Tips

1. Milk and yogurt are good sources of calcium and protein.
2. The higher the fat content of milk and yogurt, the more saturated fat and cholesterol it has.
3. Children over the age of 2 and adults should choose lower-fat varieties such as skim, 1%, or 2% milks or yogurts.

Selection Tips

1. 1 cup equals 8 fluid oz or ½ pint.
2. If you choose 2%, or whole-milk foods, be aware of the extra fat.

APPENDIX 34. Exchange Lists for Meal Planning—cont'd

Food	Serving Size	Count As
Milk and Yogurts		
Fat-free or low-fat (1%)		
Milk, buttermilk, acidophilus milk, Lactaid	1 cup	1 fat-free milk
Evaporated milk	½ cup	1 fat-free milk
Yogurt, plain or flavored with an artificial sweetener	⅔ cup (6 oz)	1 fat-free milk
Reduced-fat (2%)		
Milk, acidophilus milk, kefir, Lactaid	1 cup	1 reduced-fat milk
Yogurt, plain	⅔ cup (6 oz)	1 reduced-fat milk
Whole		
Milk, buttermilk, goat's milk	1 cup	1 whole milk
Evaporated milk	½ cup	1 whole milk
Yogurt, plain	8 oz	1 whole milk
Dairy-Like Foods		
Chocolate milk		
Fat-free	1 cup	1 fat-free milk + 1 carbohydrate
Whole	1 cup	1 whole milk + 1 carbohydrate
Eggnog, whole milk	½ cup	1 carbohydrate + 2 fats
Rice drink		
Flavored, low-fat	1 cup	2 carbohydrates
Plain, fat-free	1 cup	1 carbohydrate
Smoothies, flavored, regular	10 oz	1 fat-free milk + 2½ carbohydrates
Soy milk		
Light	1 cup	1 carbohydrate + ½ fat
Regular, plain	1 cup	1 carbohydrate + 1 fat
Yogurt		
And juice blends	1 cup	1 fat-free milk + 1 carbohydrate
Low carbohydrate (less than 6 grams carbohydrate per choice)	⅔ cup (6 oz)	½ fat-free milk
With fruit, low-fat	⅔ cup (6 oz)	1 fat-free milk + 1 carbohydrate

Sweets, Desserts, and Other Carbohydrates

You can substitute food choices from this list for other carbohydrate-containing foods (such as those found on the **Starch, Fruit,** or **Milk** lists) in your meal plan, even though these foods have added sugars or fat.

Common Measurements

Dry:
3 tsp = 1 Tbsp
4 oz = ½ cup
8 oz = 1 cup

Liquid:
4 Tbsp = ¼ cup
8 oz = ½ pint

Nutrition Tips

1. A carbohydrate choice has 15 grams of carbohydrate, variable grams of protein, variable grams of fat, and variable calories.
2. The foods on this list do not have as many vitamins, minerals, and fiber as the choices on the **Starch, Fruits,** or **Milk** lists. When choosing sweets, desserts, and other carbodrate foods, you should also eat foods from other food lists to balance out your meals.
3. Many of these foods don't equal a single choice. Some will also count as one or more fat choices.
4. If you are trying to lose weight, choose foods from this list less often.
5. The serving sizes for these foods are small because of their fat content.

Selection Tips

1. Read the Nutrition facts on the food label to find the serving size and nutrient information.
2. Many sugar-free, fat-free, or reduced-fat products are made with ingredients that contain carbohydrate. These types of food usually have the same amount of carbohydrate as the regular foods they are replacing. Talk with your RD and find out how to fit these foods into your meal plan.

Food	Serving Size	Count As
Beverages, Soda, and Energy/Sports Drinks		
Cranberry juice cocktail	½ cup	1 carbohydrate
Energy drink	1 can (8.3 oz)	2 carbohydrates
Fruit drink or lemonade	1 cup (8 oz)	2 carbohydrates
Hot chocolate		
Regular	1 envelope added to 8 oz water	1 carbohydrate + 1 fat
Sugar-free or light	1 envelope added to 8 oz water	1 carbohydrate
Soft drink (soda), regular	1 can (12 oz)	2½ carbohydrates
Sports drink	1 cup (8 oz)	1 carbohydrate

Continued

APPENDIX 34. Exchange Lists for Meal Planning—cont'd

Food	Serving Size	Count As
Brownies, Cake, Cookies, Gelatin, Pie, and Pudding		
Brownie, small, unfrosted	1¼ -inch square, ⅞ inch high (about 1 oz)	1 carbohydrate + 1 fat
Cake		
Angel food, unfrosted	1/12 of cake (about 2 oz)	2 carbohydrates
Frosted	2-inch square (about 2 oz)	2 carbohydrates + 1 fat
Unfrosted	2-inch square (about 2 oz)	1 carbohydrate + 1 fat
Cookies		
Chocolate chip	2 cookies (2¼ inches across)	1 carbohydrate + 2 fats
Gingersnap	3 cookies	1 carbohydrate
Sandwich, with creme filling	2 small (about ⅔ oz)	1 carbohydrate + 1 fat
Sugar-free	3 small or 1 large (¾-1 oz)	1 carbohydrate + 1-2 fats
Vanilla wafer	5 cookies	1 carbohydrate + 1 fat
Cupcake, frosted	1 small (about 1¾ oz)	2 carbohydrates + 1-1½ fats
Fruit cobbler	½ cup (3½ oz)	3 carbohydrates + 1 fat
Gelatin, regular	½ cup	1 carbohydrate
Pie		
Commercially prepared fruit, 2 crusts	⅙ of 8-inch pie	3 carbohydrates + 2 fats
Pumpkin or custard	⅛ of 8-inch pie	1½ carbohydrates + 1½ fats
Pudding		
Regular (made with reduced-fat milk)	½ cup	2 carbohydrates
Sugar-free or sugar- and fat-free (made with fat-free milk)	½ cup	1 carbohydrate
Candy, Spreads, Sweets, Sweeteners, Syrups, and Toppings		
Candy bar, chocolate/peanut	2 "fun size" bars (1 oz)	1½ carbohydrates + 1½ fats
Candy, hard	3 pieces	1 carbohydrate
Chocolate "kisses"	5 pieces	1 carbohydrate + 1 fat
Coffee creamer		
Dry, flavored	4 tsp	½ carbohydrate + ½ fat
Liquid, flavored	2 Tbsp	1 carbohydrate
Fruit snacks, chewy (pureed fruit concentrate)	1 roll (¾ oz)	1 carbohydrate
Fruit spreads, 100% fruit	1½ Tbsp	1 carbohydrate
Honey	1 Tbsp	1 carbohydrate
Jam or jelly, regular	1 Tbsp	1 carbohydrate
Sugar	1 Tbsp	1 carbohydrate
Syrup		
Chocolate	2 Tbsp	2 carbohydrates
Light (pancake type)	2 Tbsp	1 carbohydrate
Regular (pancake type)	1 Tbsp	1 carbohydrate
Condiments and Sauces		
Barbeque sauce	3 Tbsp	1 carbohydrate
Cranberry sauce, jellied	¼ cup	1½ carbohydrates
Gravy, mushroom, canned[‡]	½ cup	½ carbohydrate + ½ fat
Salad dressing, fat-free, low fat, cream-based	3 Tbsp	1 carbohydrate
Sweet and sour sauce	3 Tbsp	1 carbohydrate
Doughnuts, Muffins, Pastries, and Sweet Breads		
Banana nut bread	1-inch slice (1 oz)	2 carbohydrates + 1 fat
Doughnut		
Cake, plain	1 medium (1½ oz)	1½ carbohydrates + 2 fats
Glazed	3¾ inches across (2 oz)	2 carbohydrates + 2 fats
Muffin (4 oz)	¼ muffin (1 oz)	1 carbohydrate + ½ fat
Sweet roll or Danish	1 (2½ oz)	2½ carbohydrates + 2 fats
Frozen Bars, Frozen Desserts, Frozen Yogurt, and Ice Cream		
Frozen pops	1	½ carbohydrate
Fruit juice bars, frozen, 100% juice	1 bar (3 oz)	1 carbohydrate
Ice cream		
Fat-free	½ cup	1½ carbohydrates
Light	½ cup	1 carbohydrate + 1 fat
No sugar added	½ cup	1 carbohydrate + 1 fat
Regular	½ cup	1 carbohydrate + 2 fats
Sherbet, sorbet	½ cup	2 carbohydrates
Yogurt, frozen		
Fat-free	⅓ cup	1 carbohydrate
Regular	½ cup	1 carbohydrate + 0-1 fat

APPENDIX 34. Exchange Lists for Meal Planning—cont'd

Food	Serving Size	Count As
Granola Bars, Meal Replacement Bars/Shakes, and Trail Mix		
Granola or snack bar, regular or low-fat	1 bar (1 oz)	1½ carbohydrates
Meal replacement bar	1 bar (1⅓ oz)	1½ carbohydrates + 0-1 fat
Meal replacement bar	1 bar (2 oz)	2 carbohydrates + 1 fat
Meal replacement shake, reduced calorie	1 can (10-11 oz)	1½ carbohydrates + 0-1 fat
Trail mix		
Candy/nut-based	1 oz	1 carbohydrate + 2 fats
Dried fruit-based	1 oz	1 carbohydrate + 1 fat

‡480 mg or more of sodium per serving.

Nonstarchy Vegetables

Vegetable choices include vegetables in this **Nonstarchy Vegetables** list and the Starchy Vegetables list found within the **Starch** list. Vegetables with small amounts of carbohydrate and calories are on the **Nonstarchy Vegetables** list. Vegetables contain important nutrients. Try to eat at least 2 to 3 nonstarchy vegetable choices each day (as well as choices from the Starchy Vegetables list). In general, 1 nonstarchy vegetable choice is:

- ½ cup of cooked vegetables or vegetable juice
- 1 cup of raw vegetables

If you eat 3 cups or more of raw vegetables or 1½ cups of cooked vegetables in a meal, count them as 1 carbohydrate choice.

Nutrition Tips

1. A choice on this list (½ cup cooked or 1 cup raw) equals 5 grams of carbohydrate, 2 grams of protein, 0 grams of fat, and 25 calories.
2. Fresh and frozen vegetables have less added salt than canned vegetables. Drain and rinse canned vegetables to remove some salt.
3. Choose dark green and dark yellow vegetables each day. Spinach, broccoli, romaine, carrots, chilies, squash, and peppers are great choices.
4. Brussels sprouts, broccoli, cauliflower, greens, peppers, spinach, and tomatoes are good sources of vitamin C.
5. Eat vegetables from the cruciferous family several times each week. Cruciferous vegetables include bok choy, broccoli, brussels sprouts, cabbage, cauliflower, collards, kale, kohlrabi, radishes, rutabaga, turnip, and watercress.

Selection Tips

1. Canned vegetables and juices are also available without added salt.
2. A 1-cup portion of broccoli is a portion about the size of a regular light bulb.
3. Starchy vegetables such as corn, peas, winter squash, and potatoes that have more calories and carbohydrates are on the Starchy Vegetables section in the **Starch** list.
4. The tomato sauce referred to in this list is different from spaghetti/pasta sauce, which is on the Starchy Vegetables list.

Nonstarchy Vegetables

Amaranth or Chinese spinach
Artichoke
Artichoke hearts
Asparagus
Baby corn
Bamboo shoots
Beans (green, wax, Italian)
Bean sprouts
Beets
Borscht‡
Broccoli
Brussels sprouts*
Cabbage (green, bok choy, Chinese)
Carrots*
Cauliflower
Celery
Chayote*
Coleslaw, packaged, no dressing
Cucumber
Eggplant
Gourds (bitter, bottle, luffa, bitter melon)
Green onions or scallions
Greens (collard, kale, mustard, turnip)
Hearts of palm
Jicama
Kohlrabi
Leeks
Mixed vegetables (without corn, peas, or pasta)
Mung bean sprouts
Mushrooms, all kinds, fresh
Okra
Onions
Oriental radish or daikon
Pea pods
Peppers (all varieties)*
Radishes
Rutabaga
Sauerkraut‡
Soybean sprouts
Spinach
Squash (summer, crookneck, zucchini)
Sugar pea snaps
Swiss chard*
Tomato
Tomatoes, canned
Tomato sauce‡
Tomato/vegetable juice‡
Turnips
Water chestnuts
Yard-long beans

*More than 3 grams of dietary fiber per serving.
‡480 milligrams or more of sodium per serving.

Meat and Meat Substitutes

Meat and meat substitutes are rich in protein. Foods from this list are divided into 4 groups based on the amount of fat they contain. These groups are lean meat, medium-fat meat, high-fat meat, and plant-based proteins. The following chart shows you what one choice includes:

	Carbohydrate (grams)	Protein (grams)	Fat (grams)	Calories
Lean meat	—	7	0-3	45
Medium-fat meat	—	7	4-7	75
High-fat meat	—	7	8+	100
Plant-based protein	Varies	7	Varies	Varies

Continued

APPENDIX 34. Exchange Lists for Meal Planning—cont'd

Nutrition Tips

1. Read labels to find foods low in fat and cholesterol. Try for 3 grams of fat or less per serving.
2. Read labels to find "hidden" carbohydrate. For example, hot dogs actually contain a lot of carbohydrate. Most hot dogs are also high in fat, but are often sold in lower-fat versions.
3. Whenever possible, choose lean meats.
   a. Select grades of meat that are the leanest.
   b. Choice grades have a moderate amount of fat.
   c. Prime cuts of meat have the highest amount of fat.
4. Fish such as herring, mackerel, salmon, sardines, halibut, trout, and tuna are rich in omega-3 fats, which may help reduce risk for heart disease. Choose fish (not conimercially fried fish fillets) two or more times each week.
5. Bake, roast, broil, grill, poach, steam, or boil instead of frying.

Selection Tips

1. Trim off visible fat or skin.
2. Roast, broil, or grill meat on a rack so that the fat will drain off during; cooking.
3. Use a nonstick spray and a nonstick pan to brown or fry foods.
4. Some processed meats, seafood, and soy products contain carbohydrate. Read the food label to see if the amount of carbohydrate in the serving size you plan to eat is close to 13 grams. If so, count it as 1 carbohydrate choice and 1 or more meat choice.
5. Meat or fish that is breaded with cornmeal, flour, or dried bread crumbs contain carbohydrate. Count 3 Tbsp of one of these dry grains as 15 grams of carbohydrate.

Food	Amount
Lean Meats and Meat Substitutes	
Beef: Select or Choice grades trimmed of fat: ground round, roast (chuck, rib, rump), round, sirloin, steak (cubed, flank, porterhouse, T-bone), tenderloin	1 oz
Beef jerky‡	1 oz
Cheeses with 3 grams of fat or less per oz	1 oz
Cottage cheese	¼ cup
Egg substitutes, plain	¼ cup
Egg whites	2
Fish, fresh or frozen, plain: catfish, cod, flounder, haddock, halibut, orange roughy, salmon, tilapia, trout, tuna	1 oz
Fish, smoked: herring or salmon (lox)‡	1 oz
Game: buffalo, ostrich, rabbit, venison	1 oz
Hot dog with 3 grams of fat or less per oz‡ (8 dogs per 14 oz package) *(Note: Maybe high in carbohydrate)*	1
Lamb: chop, leg, or roast	1 oz
Organ meats: heart, kidney, liver *(Note: Maybe high in cholesterol)*	1 oz
Oysters, fresh or frozen	6 medium
Pork, lean	
Canadian bacont‡	1 oz
Rib or loin chop/roast, ham, tenderloin	1 oz
Poultry, without skin: Cornish hen, chicken, domestic duck or goose (well-drained of fat), turkey	1 oz
Processed sandwich meats with 3 grams of fat or less per oz: chipped beef, deli thin-sliced meats, turkey ham, turkey kielbasa, turkey pastrami	1 oz
Salmon, canned	1 oz
Sardines, canned	2 medium
Sausage with 3 grams of fat or less per oz‡	1 oz
Shellfish: clams, crab, imitation shellfish, lobster, scallops, shrimp	1 oz
Tuna, canned in water or oil, drained	1 oz
Veal, loin chop, roast	1 oz

‡480 milligrams or more of sodium per serving.

Food	Amount
Medium-Fat Meat and Meat Substitutes	
Beef: corned beef, ground beef, meatloaf, Prime grades trimmed of fat (prime rib), short ribs, tongue	1 oz
Cheeses with 4-7 grams of fat per oz: feta, mozzarella, pasteurized processed cheese spread, reduced-fat cheeses, string	1 oz
Egg *(Note: High in cholesterol, so limit to 3 per week)*	1
Fish, any fried product	1 oz
Lamb: ground, rib roast	1 oz
Pork: cutlet, shoulder roast	1 oz
Poultry: chicken with skin; dove, pheasant, wild duck, or goose; fried chicken; ground turkey	1 oz
Ricotta cheese	2 oz or ¼ cup
Sausage with 4-7 grams of fat per oz‡	1 oz
Veal, cutlet (no breading)	1 oz

‡480 milligrams or more of sodium per serving.

The following foods are high in saturated fat, cholesterol, and calories and may raise blood cholesterol levels if eaten on a regular basis. Try to eat 3 or fewer servings from this group per week.

High-Fat Meat and Meat Substitutes

Food	Amount
Bacon	
Pork‡	2 slices (16 slices per lb or 1 oz each, before cooking)
Turkey‡	3 slices (½ oz each before cooking)
Cheese, regular: American, bleu, brie, cheddar, hard goat, Monterey jack, queso, and Swiss	1 oz
Hot dog: beef, pork, or combination (10 per lb-sized package)†‡	1
Hot dog: turkey or chicken (10 per lb-sized package)‡	1
Pork: ground, sausage, spareribs	1 oz
Processed sandwich meats with 8 grams of fat or more per oz: bologna, pastrami, hard salami	1 oz
Sausage with 8 grams fat or more per oz: bratwurst, chorizo, Italian, knockwurst, Polish, smoked, summer†‡	1 oz

†Extra fat, or prepared with added fat. (Add an additional fat choice to this food.)
‡480 milligrams or more of sodium per serving.

APPENDIX 34. Exchange Lists for Meal Planning—cont'd

Because carbohydrate content varies among; plant-based proteins, you should read the food label.

Food	Amount	Countas
Plant-Based Proteins		
"Bacon" strips, soy-based	3 strips	1 medium-fat meat
Baked beans*	⅓ cup	1 starch + 1 lean meat
Beans, cooked: black, garbanzo, kidney, lima, navy, pinto, white*	½ cup	1 starch + 1 lean meat
"Beef" or "sausage" crumbles, soy-based*	2 oz	½ carbohydrate + 1 lean meat
"Chicken" nuggets, soy-based	2 nuggets (1½ oz)	½ carbohydrate + 1 medium-fat meat
Edamame*	½ cup	½ carbohydrate + 1 lean meat
Falafel (spiced chickpea and wheat patties)	3 patties (about 2 inches across)	1 carbohydrate + 1 high-fat meat
Hot dog, soy-based	1 (1½ oz)	½ carbohydrate + 1 lean meat
Hummus*	⅓ cup	1 carbohydrate + 1 high-fat meat
Lentils, brown, green, or yellow*	½ cup	1 carbohydrate + 1 lean meat
Meatless burger, soy-based*	3 oz	½ carbohydrate + 2 lean meats
Meatless burger, vegetable- and starch-based*	1 patty (about 2½ oz)	1 carbohydrate + 2 lean meats
Nut spreads: almond butter, cashew butter, peanut butter, soy nut butter	1 Tbsp	1 high-fat meat
Peas, cooked: black-eyed and split peas*	½ cup	1 starch + 1 lean meat
Refried beans, canned[‡]*	½ cup	1 starch + 1 lean meat
"Sausage" patties, soy-based	1 (1½ oz)	1 medium-fat meat
Soy nuts, unsalted	¾ oz	½ carbohydrate + 1 medium-fat meat
Tempeh	¼ cup	1 medium-fat meat
Tofu	4 oz (½ oz)	1 medium-fat meat
Tofu, light	4 oz (½ oz)	1 lean meat

*More than 3 grams of dietary fiber per serving.
[‡]480 milligrams or more of sodium per serving.

Fats

Fats are divided into 3 groups, based on the main type of fat they contain:

- **Unsaturated fats** (omega-3, monounsaturated, and polyunsaturated) are primarily vegetable and are liquid at room temperature. These fats have good health benefits.
  - **Omega-3 fats** are a type of polyunsaturated fat and can help lower triglyceride levels and the risk of heart disease.
  - **Monounsaturated fats** also help lower cholesterol levels and may help raise HDL (good) cholesterol levels.
  - **Polyunsaturated fats** can help lower cholesterol levels.
- **Saturated fats** have been linked with heart disease. They can raise LDL (bad) cholesterol levels and should be eaten in small amounts. Saturated fats are solid at room temperature.
- ***Trans* fats** are made in a process that changes vegetable oils into semi-solid fats. These fats can raise blood cholesterol levels and should be eaten in small amounts. Partially hydrogenated and hydrogenated fats are types of man-made *trans* fats and should be avoided. *Trans* fats are also found naturally occurring in some animal products such as meat, cheese, butter, and dairy products.

Nutrition Tips

1. A choice on the **Fats** list contains 5 grams of fat and 45 calories.
2. All fats are high in calories. Limit serving sizes for good nutrition and health.
3. Limit the amount of fried foods you eat.
4. Nuts and seeds are good sources of unsaturated fats if eaten in moderation. They have small amounts of fiber, protein, and magnesium.
5. Good sources of omega-3 fatty acids include:
   a. Fish such as albacore tuna, halibut, herring, mackerel, salmon, sardines, and trout
   b. Flaxseeds and English walnuts
   c. Oils such as canola, soybean, flaxseed, and walnut.

Selection Tips

1. Read the Nutrition Facts on food labels for serving sizes. One fat choice is based on a serving size that has 5 grams of fat.
2. The food label also lists total fat grams, saturated fat, and *trans* fat grams per serving. When most of the calories come from saturated fat, the food is part of the Saturated Fats list.
3. When selecting fats, consider replacing saturated fats with monounsaturated fats and omega-3 fats. Talk with your RD about the best choices for you.
4. When selecting regular margarine, choose those that list liquid vegetable oil as the first ingredient. Soft or tub margarines have less saturated fat than stick margarines and are a healthier choice. Look for *trans* fat-free soft margarines.
5. When selecting reduced-fat or lower-fat margarines, look for liquid vegetable oil (*trans* fat-free). Water is usually the first ingredient.

Fats and oils have mixtures of unsaturated (polyunsaturated and monounsaturated) and saturated fats. Foods on the Fats list are grouped together based on the major type of fat they contain. In general, 1 fat choice equals:

- 1 teaspoon of regular margarine, vegetable oil, or butter
- 1 tablespoon of regular salad dressing

Food	Serving Size
Unsaturated Fats—Monounsaturated Fats	
Avocado, medium	2 Tbsp (1 oz)
Nut butters (*trans* fat-free): almond butter, cashew butter, peanut butter (smooth or crunchy)	1½ tsp

Food	Serving Size
Nuts	
Almonds	6 nuts
Brazil	2 nuts
Cashews	6 nuts
Filberts (hazelnuts)	5 nuts

Continued

APPENDIX 34. Exchange Lists for Meal Planning—cont'd

Food	Serving Size
Macadamia	3 nuts
Mixed (50% peanuts)	6 nuts
Peanuts	10 nuts
Pecans	4 halves
Pistachios	16 nuts
Oil: canola, olive, peanut	1 tsp
Olives	
Black (ripe)	8 large
Green, stuffed	10 large
Polyunsaturated Fats	
Margarine: lower-fat spread (30%-50% vegetable oil, *trans* fat-free)	1 Tbsp
Margarine: stick, tub (*trans* fat-free), or squeeze (*trans* fat-free)	1 tsp
Mayonnaise	
Reduced-fat	1 Tbsp
Regular	1 tsp
Mayonnaise-style salad dressing	
Reduced-fat	1 Tbsp
Regular	2 tsp
Nuts	
Walnuts, English	4 halves
Pignolia (pine nuts)	1 Tbsp
Oil: corn, cottonseed, flaxseed. grape seed, safflower, soybean, sunflower	1 tsp
Oil: made from soybean and canola oil—Enova	1 tsp
Plant stanol esters	
Light	1 Tbsp
Regular	2 tsp
Salad dressing	
Reduced-fat (Note: May be high in carbohydrate)‡	2 Tbsp
Regular‡	1 Tbsp
Seeds	
Flaxseed, whole	1 Tbsp
Pumpkin, sunflower	1 Tbsp
Sesame seeds	1 Tbsp
Tahini or sesame paste	2 tsp

‡480 milligrams or more of sodium per serving.

Food	Serving Size
Saturated Fats	
Bacon, cooked, regular or turkey	1 slice
Butter	
Reduced-fat	1 Tbsp
Stick	1 tsp
Whipped	2 tsp
Butter blends made with oil	
Reduced-fat or light	1 Tbsp
Regular	1½ tsp
Chitterlings, boiled	2 Tbsp (½ oz)
Coconut, sweetened, shredded	2 Tbsp
Coconut milk	
Light	⅓ cup
Regular	1½ Tbsp
Cream	
Half and half	2 Tbsp
Heavy	1 Tbsp
Light	1½ Tbsp
Whipped	2 Tbsp
Whipped, pressurized	¼ cup
Cream cheese	
Reduced-fat	1½ Tbsp (¾ oz)
Regular	1 Tbsp (½ oz)
Lard	1 tsp
Oil: coconut, palm, palm kernel	1 tsp
Salt pork	¼ oz
Shortening, solid	1 tsp
Sour cream	
Reduced-fat or light	3 Tbsp
Regular	2 Tbsp

Free Foods

A "free" food is any food or drink choice that has less than 20 calories and 5 grams or less of carbohydrate per serving.

Selection Tips

1. Most foods on this list should be limited to 3 servings (as listed here) per day. Spread out the servings throughout the day. If you eat all 3 servings at once, it could raise your blood glucose level.
2. Food and drink choices listed here without a serving size can be eaten whenever you like.

Food	Serving Size
Low Carbohydrate Foods	
Cabbage, raw	½ cup
Candy, hard (regular or sugar-free)	1 piece
Carrots, cauliflower, or green beans, cooked	¼ cup
Cranberries, sweetened with sugar substitute	½ cup
Cucumber, sliced	½ cup
Gelatin	
Dessert, sugar-free	
Unflavored	
Gum	
Jam or jelly, light or no sugar added	2 tsp
Rhubarb, sweetened with sugar substitute	½ cup
Salad greens	
Sugar substitutes (artificial sweeteners)	
Syrup, sugar-free	2 Tbsp
Modified Fat Foods with Carbohydrate	
Cream cheese, fat-free	1 Tbsp (½ oz)
Creamers	
Nondairy, liquid	1 Tbsp
Nondairy, powdered	2 tsp

APPENDIX 34. Exchange Lists for Meal Planning—cont'd

Food	Serving Size
Margarine spread	
Fat-free	1 Tbsp
Reduced-fat	1 tsp
Mayonnaise	
Fat-free	1 Tbsp
Reduced-fat	1 tsp
Mayonnaise-style salad dressing	
Fat-free	1 Tbsp
Reduced-fat	1 tsp
Salad dressing	
Fat-free or low-fat	1 Tbsp
Fat-free, Italian	2 Tbsp
Sour cream, fat-free or reduced-fat	1 Tbsp
Whipped topping	
Light or fat-free	2 Tbsp
Regular	1 Tbsp
Condiments	
Barbecue sauce	2 tsp
Catsup (ketchup)	1 Tbsp
Honey mustard	1 Tbsp
Horseradish	
Lemon juice	
Miso	1½ tsp
Mustard	
Parmesan cheese, freshly grated	1 Tbsp
Pickle relish	1 Tbsp
Pickles	
Dill[‡]	1½ medium
Sweet, bread and butter	2 slices
Sweet, gherkin	¾ oz
Salsa	¼ cup
Soy sauce, light or regular[‡]	1 Tbsp
Sweet and sour sauce	2 tsp
Sweet chili sauce	2 tsp
Taco sauce	1 Tbsp
Vinegar	
Yogurt, any type	2 Tbsp

[‡]480 milligrams or more of sodium per serving.

Free Snacks

These foods in these serving sizes are perfect free-food snacks:
- 5 baby carrots and celery sticks
- ¼ cup blueberries
- ½ oz sliced cheese, fat-free
- 10 goldfish-style crackers
- 2 saltine-type crackers
- 1 frozen cream pop, sugar-free
- ½ oz lean meat
- 1 cup light popcorn
- 1 vanilla wafer

Drinks/Mixes

Any food on this list—without a serving size listed—can be consumed in any moderate amount:
- Bouillon, broth, consommé[‡]
- Bouillon or broth, low-sodium
- Carbonated or mineral water
- Club soda
- Cocoa powder, unsweetened (1 Tbsp)
- Coffee, unsweetened or with sugar substitute
- Diet soft drinks, sugar-free
- Drink mixes, sugar-free
- Tea, unsweetened or with sugar substitute
- Tonic water, diet
- Water
- Water, flavored, carbohydrate free

Seasonings

Any food on this list can be consumed in any moderate amount:
- Flavoring extracts (for example, vanilla, almond, peppermint)
- Garlic
- Herbs, fresh or dried
- Nonstick cooking spray
- Pimento
- Spices
- Hot pepper sauce
- Wine, used in cooking
- Worcestershire sauce

Combination Foods

Many of the foods you eat are mixed together in various combinations, such as casseroles. These "combination" foods do not fit into any one choice list. This is a list of choices for some typical combination foods. This list will help you fit these foods into your meal plan. Ask your RD for nutrient information about other combination foods you would like to eat, including your own recipes.

Food	Serving Size	Count As
Entrees		
Casserole type (tuna noodle, lasagna, spaghetti with meatballs, chili with beans, macaroni and cheese)[‡]	1 cup (8 oz)	2 carbohydrates + 2 medium-fat meats
Stews (beef/other meats and vegetables)[‡]	1 cup (8 oz)	1 carbohydrate + 1 medium-fat meat + 0-3 fats
Tuna salad or chicken salad	½ cup (3½ oz)	½ carbohydrate + 2 lean meats + 1 fat
Frozen Meals/Entrees		
Burrito (beef and bean)[‡*]	1 (5 oz)	3 carbohydrates + 1 lean meat + 2 fats
Dinner-type meal[‡]	Generally 14-17 oz	3 carbohydrates + 3 medium-fat meats + 3 fats
Entree or meal with less than 340 calories[‡]	About 8-11 oz	2-3 carbohydrates + 1-2 lean meats

Continued

APPENDIX 34. Exchange Lists for Meal Planning—cont'd

Food	Serving Size	Count As
Pizza		
Cheese/vegetarian, thin crust‡	¼ of a 12 inch (4½-5 oz)	2 carbohydrates + 2 medium-fat meats
Meat topping, thin crust‡	¼ of a 12 inch (5 oz)	2 carbohydrates + 2 medium-fat meats + 1½ fats
Pocket sandwich‡	1 (4½ oz)	3 carbohydrates + 1 lean meat + 1-2 fats
Pot pie‡	1 (7 oz)	2½ carbohydrates + 1 medium-fat meat + 3 fats
Salads (Deli-Style)		
Coleslaw	½ cup	1 carbohydrate + 1½ fats
Macaroni/pasta salad	½ cup	2 carbohydrates + 3 fats
Potato salad‡	½ cup	1½-2 carbohydrates + 1-2 fats
Soups		
Bean, lentil, or split pea‡	1 cup	1 carbohydrate + 1 lean meat
Chowder (made with milk)‡	1 cup (8 oz)	1 carbohydrate + 1 lean meat + 1½ fats
Cream (made with water)‡	1 cup (8 oz)	1 carbohydrate + 1 fat
Instant‡	6 oz prepared	1 carbohydrate
With beans or lentils‡	8 oz prepared	2½ carbohydrates + 1 lean meat
Miso soup‡	1 cup	½ carbohydrate + 1 fat
Oriental noodle‡	1 cup	2 carbohydrates + 2 fats
Rice (congee)	1 cup	1 carbohydrate
Tomato (made with water)‡	1 cup (8 oz)	1 carbohydrate
Vegetable beef, chicken noodle, or other broth-type‡	1 cup (8 oz)	1 carbohydrate

*More than 3 grams of dietary fiber per serving.
‡600 milligrams or more of sodium per serving (for combination food main dishes/meals).

Fast Foods

The choices in the **Fast Foods** list are not specific fast food meals or items, but are estimates based on popular foods. You can get specific nutrition information for almost every fast food or restaurant chain. Ask the restaurant or check its website for nutrition information about your favorite fast foods.

Food	Serving Size	Count As
Breakfast Sandwiches		
Egg, cheese, meat, English muffin‡	1 sandwich	2 carbohydrates + 2 medium-fat meats
Sausage biscuit sandwich‡	1 sandwich	2 carbohydrates + 2 high-fat meats + 3½ fats
Main Dishes/Entrees		
Burrito (beef and beans)‡*	1 (about 8 oz)	3 carbohydrates + 3 medium-fat meats + 3 fats
Chicken breast, breaded and fried‡	1 (about 5 oz)	1 carbohydrate + 4 medium-fat meats
Chicken drumstick, breaded and fried	1 (about 2 oz)	2 medium-fat meats
Chicken nuggets‡	6 (about 3½ oz)	1 carbohydrate + 2 medium-fat meats + 1 fat
Chicken thigh, breaded and fried‡	1 (about 4 oz)	½ carbohydrate + 3 medium-fat meats + 1½ fats
Chicken wings, hot‡	6 (5 oz)	5 medium-fat meats + 1½ fats
Oriental		
Beef/chicken/shrimp with vegetables in sauce‡	1 cup (about 5 oz)	1 carbohydrate + 1 lean meat + 1 fat
Egg roll, meat‡	1 (about 3 oz)	1 carbohydrate + 1 lean meat + 1 fat
Fried rice, meatless	½ cup	1½ carbohydrates + 1½ fats
Meat and sweet sauce (orange chicken)‡	1 cup	3 carbohydrates + 3 medium-fat meats + 2 fats
Noodles and vegetables in sauce (chow mein, lo mein)‡*	1 cup	2 carbohydrates + 1 fat
Pizza		
Cheese, pepperoni, regular crust‡	⅛ of a 14 inch (about 4 oz)	2½ carbohydrates + 1 medium-fat meat + 1½ fats
Cheese/vegetarian, thin crust‡	¼ of a 12 inch (about 6 oz)	2½ carbohydrates + 2 medium-fat meats + 1½ fats
Sandwiches		
Chicken sandwich, grilled‡	1	3 carbohydrates + 4 lean meats
Chicken sandwich, crispy‡	1	3½ carbohydrates + 3 medium-fat meats + 1 fat

APPENDIX 34. Exchange Lists for Meal Planning—cont'd

Food	Serving Size	Count As
Fish sandwich with tartar sauce	1	2½ carbohydrates + 2 medium-fat meats + 2 fats
Hamburger		
Large with cheese‡	1	2½ carbohydrates + 4 medium-fat meats + 1 fat
Regular	1	2 carbohydrates + 1 medium-fat meat + 1 fat
Hot dog with bun‡	1	1 carbohydrate + 1 high-fat meat + 1 fat
Submarine sandwich		
Less than 6 grams fat‡	6-inch sub	3 carbohydrates + 2 lean meats
Regular‡	6-inch sub	3½ carbohydrates + 2 medium-fat meats + 1 fat
Taco, hard or soft shell (meat and cheese)	1 small	1 carbohydrate + 1 medium-fat meat + 1½ fats
Salads		
Salad, main dish (grilled chicken type, no dressing or croutons)‡*	Salad	1 carbohydrate + 4 lean meats
Salad, side, no dressing or cheese	Small (about 5 oz)	1 vegetable
Sides/Appetizers		
French fries, restaurant style†	Small	3 carbohydrates + 3 fats
	Medium	4 carbohydrates + 4 fats
	Large	5 carbohydrates + 6 fats
Nachos with cheese‡	Small (about 4½ oz)	2½ carbohydrates + 4 fats
Onion rings‡	1 serving (about 3 oz)	2½ carbohydrates + 3 fats
Desserts		
Milkshake, any flavor	12 oz	6 carbohydrates + 2 fats
Soft-serve ice cream cone	1 small	2½ carbohydrates + 1 fat

*More than 3 grams of dietary fiber per serving.
†Extra fat, or prepared with extra fat.
‡600 milligrams or more of sodium per serving (for fast food main dishes/meals).

Alcohol

Nutrition Tips

1. In general, 1 alcohol choice (½ oz absolute alcohol) has about 100 calories.

Selection Tips

1. If you choose to drink alcohol, you should limit it to 1 drink or less per day for women, and 2 drinks or less per day for men.
2. To reduce your risk of low blood glucose (hypoglycemia), especially if you take insulin or a diabetes pill that increases insulin, always drink alcohol with food.
3. While alcohol, by itself, does not directly affect blood glucose, be aware of the carbohydrate (for example, in mixed drinks, beer, and wine) that may raise your blood glucose.
4. Check with your RD if you would like to fit alcohol into your meal plan.

Alcoholic Beverage	Serving Size	Count As
Beer		
Light (4.2%)	12 fl oz	1 alcohol equivalent + ½ carbohydrate
Regular (4.9%)	12 fl oz	1 alcohol equivalent + 1 carbohydrate
Distilled spirits: vodka, rum, gin, whiskey 80 or 86 proof	1½ fl oz	1 alcohol equivalent
Liqueur, coffee (53 proof)	1 fl oz	1 alcohol equivalent + 1 carbohydrate
Sake	1 fl oz	½ alcohol equivalent
Wine		
Dessert (sherry)	3½ fl oz	1 alcohol equivalent + 1 carbohydrate
Dry, red or white (10%)	5 fl oz	1 alcohol equivalent

APPENDIX 35. National Dysphagia Diets

The following solid food texture levels have been recommended based on the food properties on the food texture scales.

Level 1: Dysphagia: Pureed

Description: This diet consists of pureed, homogenous, and cohesive foods. Food should be "puddinglike." No coarse textures, raw fruits or vegetables, nuts, and so forth are allowed. Any foods that require bolus formation, controlled manipulation, or mastication are excluded.

Rationale: This diet is designed for people who have moderate to severe dysphagia, with poor oral phase abilities and reduced ability to protect their airway. Close or complete supervision and alternate feeding methods may be required.

Liquid Consistency (circle one)

Thin (includes all unthickened beverages and supplements)	Nectarlike	Honeylike	Spoon-thick

Food Textures for NDD Level 1: Dysphagia: Pureed

Food Groups	Recommended	Avoid	If Thin Liquids Are Allowed, Also May Have
Beverages	Any smooth, homogenous beverages without lumps, chunks, or pulp; beverages may need to be thickened to appropriate consistency	Any beverages with lumps, chunks, seeds, pulp, etc.	Milk, juices, coffee, tea, sodas, carbonated beverages, alcoholic beverages, nutritional supplements, ice chips
Breads	Commercially or facility-prepared pureed bread mixes, pregelled slurried breads, pancakes, sweet rolls, Danish pastries, French toast, etc., that are gelled through entire thickness of product	All other breads, rolls, crackers, biscuits, pancakes, waffles, French toast, muffins, etc.	
Cereals *(Cereals may have just enough milk to moisten)*	Smooth, homogenous, cooked cereals such as farina-type cereals Cereals should have a "puddinglike" consistency	All dry cereals and any cooked cereals with lumps, seeds, chunks Oatmeal	Enough milk or cream with cereals to moisten; they should be blended in well
Desserts	Smooth puddings, custards, yogurt, pureed desserts, and soufflés	Ices, gelatins, frozen juice bars, cookies, cakes, pies, pastry, coarse or textured puddings, bread and rice pudding, fruited yogurt *These foods are considered thin liquids and should be avoided if thin liquids are restricted:* Frozen malts, milk shakes, frozen yogurt, eggnog, nutritional supplements, ice cream, sherbet, regular or sugar-free gelatin, or any foods that become thin liquid at either room (70° F) or body temperature (98° F)	Frozen malts, yogurt, milk shakes, eggnog, nutritional supplements, ice cream, sherbet, plain regular or sugar-free gelatin
Fats	Butter, margarine, strained gravy, sour cream, mayonnaise, cream cheese, whipped topping Smooth sauces such as white sauce, cheese sauce, or hollandaise sauce	All fats with coarse or chunky additives	
Fruits	Pureed fruits or well-mashed fresh bananas Fruit juices without pulp, seeds, or chunks (may need to be thickened to appropriate consistency if thin liquids are restricted)	Whole fruits (fresh, frozen, canned, dried)	Unthickened fruit juices
Meats and meat substitutes	Pureed meats Braunschweiger Soufflés that are smooth and homogenous Softened tofu mixed with moisture Hummus or other pureed legume spread	Whole or ground meats, fish, or poultry Nonpureed lentils or legumes Cheese, cottage cheese Peanut butter, unless pureed into foods correctly Nonpureed, fried, scrambled, or hard-cooked eggs	
Potatoes and starches	Mashed potatoes or sauce; pureed potatoes with gravy, butter, margarine, or sour cream Well-cooked pasta, noodles, bread dressing, or rice that has been pureed in a blender to smooth, homogenous consistency	All other potatoes, rice, noodles Plain mashed potatoes, cooked grains Nonpureed bread dressing	
Soups	Soups that have been pureed in a blender or strained; may need to be thickened to appropriate viscosity	Soups that have chunks, lumps, etc.	Broth and other thin, strained soups

APPENDIX 35. National Dysphagia Diets—cont'd

Food Groups	Recommended	Avoid	If Thin Liquids Are Allowed, Also May Have
Vegetables	Pureed vegetables without chunks, lumps, pulp, or seeds Tomato paste or sauce without seeds Tomato or vegetables juice (may need to be thickened to appropriate consistency if juice is thinner than prescribed liquid consistency)	All other vegetables that have not been pureed Tomato sauce with seeds, thin tomato juice	Thin tomato or vegetable juices
Miscellaneous	Sugar, artificial sweetener, salt, finely ground pepper, and spices Ketchup, mustard, barbecue sauce, and other smooth sauces Honey, smooth jellies Very soft, smooth candy such as truffles	Coarsely ground pepper and herbs Chunky fruit preserves and seedy jams Seeds, nuts, sticky foods Chewy candies such as caramels or licorice	Smooth chocolate candy with no nuts, sprinkles, etc.

Level 2: Dysphagia: Mechanically Altered Characteristics

Description: This level consists of foods that are moist, soft-textured, and easily formed into a bolus. Meats are ground or are minced no larger than ¼-inch pieces; they are still moist, with some cohesion. All foods from NDD Level 1 are acceptable at this level.

Rationale: This diet is a transition from the pureed textures to more solid textures. Chewing ability is required. The textures on this level are appropriate for individuals with mild to moderate oral or pharyngeal dysphagia. Patients should be assessed for tolerance to mixed textures. It is expected that some mixed textures are tolerated on this diet.

Liquid Consistency (circle one)

Thin (includes all unthickened beverages and supplements)	Nectarlike	Honeylike	Spoon-thick

Food Textures for NDD Level 2: Dysphagia: Mechanically Altered (includes all foods on NDD Level 1: Dysphagia: Pureed in addition to the foods listed below)

Food Groups	Recommended	Avoid	If Thin Liquids Are Allowed, Also May Have
Beverages	All beverages with minimum amounts of texture, pulp, etc.; any texture should be suspended in the liquid and should not precipitate out; may need to be thickened, depending on liquid consistency recommended		Milk, juices, coffee, tea, sodas, carbonated beverages, alcoholic beverages If allowed, nutritional supplements Ice chips
Breads	Soft pancakes, well moistened with syrup or sauce Pureed bread mixes, pregelled or slurried breads that are gelled through entire thickness	All others	
Cereals *(Cereals may have ¼ cup milk or just enough milk to moisten if thin liquids are restricted. The moisture should be well-blended into food.)*	Cooked cereals with little texture, including oatmeal Slightly moistened dry cereals with little texture such as corn flakes, Rice Krispies, Wheaties Unprocessed wheat bran stirred into cereals for bulk *Note:* If thin liquids are restricted, it is important that all of the liquid is absorbed into the cereal	Very coarse cooked cereals that may contain flaxseed or other seeds or nuts Whole grain dry or coarse cereals Cereals with nuts, seeds, dried fruit, or coconut	Milk or cream for cereals
Desserts	Pudding, custard Soft fruit pies with bottom crust only Crisps and cobblers without seeds or nuts and with soft breading or crumb mixture Canned fruit (excluding pineapple) Soft, moist cakes with icing or slurried cakes Pregelled cookies or soft, moist cookies that have been dunked in milk, coffee, or other liquid	Dry, coarse cakes and cookies Anything with nuts, seeds, coconut, pineapple, or dried fruit Breakfast yogurt with nuts Rice or bread pudding *These foods are considered thin liquids and should be avoided if thin liquids are restricted:* Frozen malts, milk shakes, frozen yogurt, eggnog, nutritional supplements, ice cream, sherbet, regular or sugar-free gelatin, or any foods that become thin liquid at either room (70° F) or body temperature (98° F)	Ice cream, sherbet, malts, nutritional supplements, frozen yogurt, and other ices Plain gelatin or gelatin with canned fruit, excluding pineapple

Continued

APPENDIX 35. National Dysphagia Diets—cont'd

Food Groups	Recommended	Avoid	If Thin Liquids Are Allowed, Also May Have
Fats	Butter, margarine, cream for cereal (depending on liquid consistency recommendations), gravy, cream sauces, mayonnaise, salad dressings, cream cheese, cream cheese spreads with soft additives, sour cream, sour cream dips with soft additives, whipped toppings	All fats with coarse or chunky additives	Cream for cereal
Fruits	Soft, drained canned or cooked fruits without seeds or skin Fresh soft, ripe banana Fruit juices with small amount of pulp If thin liquids are restricted, fruit juices should be thickened to appropriate viscosity	Fresh or frozen fruits Cooked fruit with skin or seeds Dried fruits Fresh, canned, or cooked pineapple	Thin fruit juices Watermelon without seeds
Meats, meat substitutes, entrees *(Meat pieces should not exceed ¼ -inch cube and should be tender.)*	Moistened ground or cooked meat, poultry, or fish; moist ground or tender meat may be served with gravy or sauce Casseroles without rice Moist macaroni and cheese, well-cooked pasta with meat sauce, tuna-noodle casserole, soft, moist lasagna Moist meatballs, meatloaf, or fish loaf Protein salads such as tuna or egg without large chunks, celery, or onion Cottage cheese, smooth quiche without large chunks Poached, scrambled, or soft-cooked eggs (egg yolks should not be runny but should be moist and mashable with butter, margarine, or other moisture added to them) (cook eggs to 160° F or use pasteurized eggs for safety) Soufflés may have small soft chunks Tofu Well-cooked, slightly mashed, moist legumes such as baked beans All meats or protein substitutes should be served with sauces or moistened to help maintain cohesiveness in the oral cavity	Dry meats, tough meats such as bacon, sausage, hot dogs, bratwurst Dry casseroles or casseroles with rice or large chunks Cheese slices and cubes Peanut butter Hard-cooked or crisp fried eggs Sandwiches Pizza	
Potatoes and starches	Well-cooked, moistened, boiled, baked, or mashed potatoes Well-cooked shredded hash brown potatoes that are not crisp (all potatoes need to be moist and in sauces) Well-cooked noodles in sauce Spaetzel or soft dumplings that have been moistened with butter or gravy	Potato skins and chips Fried or French-fried potatoes Rice	
Soups	Soups with easy-to-chew or easy-to-swallow meats or vegetables; particle sizes in soups should be <½ inch (soups may need to be thickened to appropriate consistency, if soup is thinner than prescribed liquid consistency)	Soups with large chunks of meat and vegetables Soups with rice, corn, peas	All soups except those noted in **Avoid** list
Vegetables	All soft, well-cooked vegetables Vegetables should be <½ inch; should be easily mashed with a fork	Cooked corn and peas Broccoli, cabbage, Brussels sprouts, asparagus, or other fibrous, nontender, or rubbery cooked vegetables	
Miscellaneous	Jams and preserves without seeds, jelly Sauces, salsas, etc., that may have small tender chunks <½ inch Soft, smooth chocolate bars that are easily chewed	Seeds, nuts, coconut, sticky foods Chewy candies such as caramel and licorice	

APPENDIX 35. National Dysphagia Diets—cont'd

Food Groups	Recommended	Avoid	If Thin Liquids Are Allowed, Also May Have
Level 3: Dysphagia: Transition to Regular Diet			

Description: This level consists of food of nearly regular textures with the exception of very hard, sticky, or crunchy foods. Foods still need to be moist and should be in bite-size pieces at the oral phase of the swallow.

Rationale: This diet is a transition to a regular diet. Adequate dentition and mastication are required. The textures of this diet are appropriate for individuals with mild oral or pharyngeal phase dysphagia. Patients should be assessed for tolerance of mixed textures. Mixed textures are expected to be tolerated on this diet.

Liquid Consistency (circle one)

Thin (unthickened)
Nectarlike
Honeylike
Spoon-thick

Food Textures for NDD Level 3: Dysphagia: Advanced

Food Groups	Recommended	Avoid	If Thin Liquids Are Allowed, Also May Have
Beverages	Any beverages, depending on recommendations for liquid consistency		Milk, juices, coffee, tea, sodas, carbonated beverages, alcoholic beverages, nutritional supplements Ice chips
Breads	Any well-moistened breads, biscuits, muffins, pancakes, waffles, etc.; need to add adequate syrup, jelly, margarine, butter, etc., to moisten well	Dry bread, toast, crackers, etc. Tough, crusty breads such as French bread or baguettes	
Cereals *(Cereals may have ¼ cup milk or just enough milk to moisten if thin liquids are restricted.)*	All well-moistened cereals	Coarse or dry cereals such as shredded wheat or All Bran	
Desserts	All others except those on **Avoid** list	Dry cakes, cookies that are chewy or very dry Anything with nuts, seeds, dry fruits, coconut, pineapple *These foods are considered thin liquids and should be avoided if thin liquids are restricted:* Frozen malts, milk shakes, frozen yogurt, eggnog, nutritional supplements, ice cream, sherbet, regular or sugar-free gelatin or any foods that become thin liquid at either room (70° F) or body temperature (98° F)	Malts, milk shakes, frozen yogurts, ice cream, and other frozen desserts Nutritional supplements, gelatin, and any other desserts of thin liquid consistency when in the mouth
Fats	All other fats except those on **Avoid** list	All fats with coarse, difficult-to-chew, or chunky additives such as cream-cheese spread with nuts or pineapple	
Fruits	All canned and cooked fruits Soft, peeled fresh fruits such as peaches, nectarines, kiwi, mangos, cantaloupe, honeydew, watermelon (without seeds) Soft berries with small seeds such as strawberries	Difficult-to-chew fresh fruits such as apples or pears Stringy, high-pulp fruits such as papaya, pineapple, or mango Fresh fruits with difficult-to-chew peels such as grapes Uncooked dried fruits such as prunes and apricots Fruit leather, fruit roll-ups, fruit snacks, dried fruits	Any fruit juices
Meats, meat substitutes, entrees	Thin-sliced, tender, or ground meats and poultry Well-moistened fish Eggs prepared any way Yogurt without nuts or coconut Casseroles with small chunks of meat, ground meats, or tender meats	Tough, dry meats and poultry Dry fish or fish with bones Chunky peanut butter Yogurt with nuts or coconut	

Continued

APPENDIX 35. National Dysphagia Diets—cont'd

Food Groups	Recommended	Avoid	If Thin Liquids Are Allowed, Also May Have
Potatoes and starches	All, including rice, wild rice, moist bread dressing, and tender, fried potatoes	Tough, crisp-fried potatoes Potato skins Dry bread dressing	
Soups	All soups except those in the **Avoid** list Strained corn or clam chowder (may need to be thickened to appropriate consistency if soup is thinner than prescribed liquid consistency)	Soups with tough meats Corn or clam chowders Soups that have large chunks of meat or vegetables >1 inch	All thin soups except those in **Avoid** list Broth and bouillon
Vegetables	All cooked, tender vegetables Shredded lettuce	All raw vegetables except shredded lettuce Cooked corn Nontender or rubbery cooked vegetables	
Miscellaneous	All seasonings and sweeteners All sauces Nonchewy candies without nuts, seeds, or coconut Jams, jellies, honey, preserves	Nuts, seeds, or coconut Chewy caramel or taffy-type candies Candies with nuts, seeds, or coconut	

From American Dietetic Association: National dysphagia diet: standardization for optimal care, Chicago, 2003, ADA.

APPENDIX 36. Renal Diet for Dialysis

Your diet depends on your kidney function. Most of the information here relates to people on dialysis. What is right for others is not always right for you. As your kidney function changes, your diet may change as well. This guide will help you do two things: plan nutritious meals you enjoy and keep your body working at its best. Your renal dietitian will work with you to make any changes needed to your usual meal plan, but this appendix contains helpful guidelines.

1. Increase Protein

   You will need to eat a high-protein diet. Beef, pork, lamb, fish, shellfish, chicken, eggs, and other animal foods provide most of the protein in your diet. Your protein needs are based on your weight. Most people need at least 6 to 8 oz of protein per day. A deck of cards is about the size of a 3-oz serving of protein.

2. Limit Potassium

   Most foods contain some potassium, but fruits and vegetables are the easiest to control. Limit fruits, vegetables, and juices to 6 servings per day. A serving is usually ½ cup.

   Do not use salt substitute or "lite" salt because they are made with potassium.

3. Limit Salt

   Limit the salt you eat. Don't add salt during cooking or at the table. Avoid high-salt foods such as frozen meals; canned or dried foods; "fast foods"; and salted meats such as ham, sausage, and luncheon meats. Use salt-free spices or spice mixes such as Mrs. Dash instead of salt to add flavor to your food.

4. Limit Phosphorus

   Use only 1 serving of milk or dairy food per day. A serving is usually ½ to 1 cup. Take phosphate binders such as Tums, PhosLo, Renagel, or Fosrenol with your meals as prescribed by your doctor.

5. Fluid

   A safe amount of fluid to drink is different for everyone. It depends on how much urine you are making. Try not to drink more than 3 cups (24 oz) of fluid each day plus the amount equal to your urine output. If you are limiting your salt intake, you should not feel thirsty.

   Fluids include all beverages and foods that are liquid at room temperature such as Jell-O, ice cream, ice, and soup.

6. Poor Appetite and Weight Loss

   It is common to have a poor appetite if you are new to dialysis. If your appetite has been poor, try eating small frequent meals and extra snacks.

   Try adding high-calorie fats such as butter, margarine, and oils; sauces and gravies; and sour cream, cream cheese, or whipped cream for extra calories. Adding rice, pasta, bread, and rolls to meals also adds calories.

   Sugar and sweets such as cakes, candies, and pastries are also a good source of calories if you are not following a diabetic diet.

   Talk to your nutritionist about trying a nutritional supplement.

Protein

When on dialysis, you need to eat a high-protein diet. This is because you lose protein during each dialysis treatment. To stay healthy, you need to eat enough protein for your daily needs and also make up for the amount lost during dialysis. Meat, fish, poultry, eggs, and other animal foods provide most of the protein in your diet. Your body uses protein to build and repair muscles, skin, blood, and other tissues.

Albumin

Albumin is a protein found in blood. Each month a laboratory test measures your albumin. It is a good way to know how healthy you are. Your albumin level should be more than 3.4 mg/dL.

APPENDIX 36. Renal Diet for Dialysis—cont'd

Keeping a Healthy Albumin Level

Make sure that you eat enough protein every day. How much protein you need daily depends on how much you weigh.

Find your weight on the chart below to see how many protein servings you need each day.

Protein Servings for You

If you weigh:	You need:
40 kg	4-5 servings
50 kg	5-6 servings
60 kg	6-7 servings
70 kg	7-8 servings
80 kg	8-9 servings
90 kg	9-10 servings

Your weight: ________________ kg

You need: ________________ protein servings each day

One Serving of Protein Is:

1 egg
1 oz cooked meat, fish, poultry
¼ cup cooked or canned fish, seafood
½ cup tofu
1 cup milk
1 oz cheese
¼ cup cottage cheese
¾ cup pudding or custard
2 Tbsp peanut butter
1 scoop protein powder
½ protein bar

Common Serving Sizes

Most people eat protein foods in portions larger than 1 serving. Here are some examples:

Average hamburger patty (3 oz) = 3 protein servings
Small beefsteak (3 in × 4 in) = 4 protein servings
Half chicken breast (3 oz) = 3 protein servings
Chicken drumstick or thigh (2 oz) = 2 protein servings
Average pork chop (3 oz) = 3 protein servings
Fish fillet (3 in × 3 in) = 3 protein servings

Estimating Serving Sizes

Here are some other easy ways to estimate protein serving sizes:

- Your whole thumb is about the size of 1 oz.
- Three stacked dice are about the size of 1 oz.
- A deck of cards is about the size of 3 oz.
- The palm of your hand is about the size of 3 to 4 oz.
- Your clenched fist is about the size of 1 cup.

Tips for Eating More Protein

Some people on dialysis dislike the taste of protein. Some people find cooking smells unpleasant. Still others are not able to eat enough protein each day.

The following tips will be helpful:

- Use gravy, sauces, seasonings, or spices to improve or hide flavors.
- Prepare meals ahead of time, or stay away from kitchen smells if they spoil your appetite.
- Eat cooked protein foods cold. Try cold fried chicken, a roast beef sandwich, or shrimp salad.
- Add cut-up meats or beans to soups or salads.
- Use more eggs. Try hardboiled eggs, egg salad sandwiches, custards, or quiches. Stir beaten eggs into casseroles and soups.
- Try other protein foods such as angel food cake, peanut butter, or bean salads.
- Eat a protein bar. Your nutritionist can help you choose one.
- Use a protein powder. Your nutritionist can help you choose one and give you ideas for using it.

Nutritional Supplements

Nutritional supplements provide extra calories and protein. In general, use one can of supplement as a snack each day. Add one extra can for each meal you miss.

Not all nutritional supplements are safe for dialysis patients. Check with your nutritionist before using any supplement. Here are some of the supplements that are used by people on dialysis:

Malnutrition

If you are not eating enough meat, fish, poultry, eggs, and other high-protein foods, your albumin level will drop below the recommended level.

If your albumin level is low, the cells in your body cannot hold fluid well. This leads to swelling (edema) and low blood pressure during dialysis. Low albumin increases your risk of death. Patients with albumin levels above 4 have the lowest death rate.

It is also important to eat enough calories. Your nutritionist can help you make sure you are getting plenty of protein and calories.

Exercise

Try to be active in some way each day (e.g., walk, swim, garden, stretch). Using your muscles helps keep them strong. Protein that is stored in your muscles helps support your albumin level.

Potassium for People on Hemodialysis

- Most foods have some potassium, but fruits and vegetables are the easiest form to control in your diet. The following list groups vegetables and fruits by the amount of potassium in one serving.
- Remember, there are no foods that you cannot eat on your diet. What is important is the amount of foods you eat and how often you eat them. Keep this list handy for shopping or eating out.
- If there are fruits and vegetables you enjoy that are not on the list, ask your nutritionist about them.

Most People on Hemodialysis May Have

- 1 serving per day from the high-potassium group
- 2 servings per day from the medium-potassium group
- 2 to 3 servings per day from the low-potassium group

This is approximately 2000 to 3000 mg of potassium per day with the other foods you eat. Check the serving size for each food, listed in parentheses next to the item.

Soaking Vegetables and Beans

Soaking works well for high-potassium foods such as potatoes, parsnips, sweet potatoes, winter squash, and beans. The procedure for soaking follows.

1. Peel vegetables and slice thinly (⅛ inch). Rinse well. Place them in a bowl of warm water, using four times more water than vegetable. For example, soak 1 cup of sliced vegetables in 4 cups of water. Soak at least 1 hour. Drain and rinse again.
2. Vegetables that have been soaked this way can then be fried, mashed, scalloped, put in soups or stews, or served fresh. If you are boiling the food, use four times more water than food and cook as usual.
3. Dried beans should be cooked and then chopped and soaked, using the preceding directions. Canned beans can simply be chopped, rinsed, and soaked.

Continued

APPENDIX 36. Renal Diet for Dialysis—cont'd

Food Category	Low-Potassium Foods 5-150 mg	Medium-Potassium Foods 150-250 mg	High-Potassium Foods 250-500 mg
Fruits	Applesauce (½ cup) Blackberries (½ cup) Blueberries (1 cup) Grapefruit (½ cup) Pears, canned (½ cup) Pineapple (½ cup) Plums, canned (½ cup) Raspberries (½ cup) Rhubarb, cooked (½ cup Strawberries (½ cup) Tangerine (1)	Apple (1 medium), cherries (8-10) Fruit cocktail (½ cup) Grapes (10-15) Mango (½ medium) Melons: cantaloupe, honeydew (½ cup), papaya (½ cup) Peaches, canned (½ cup) Pear, fresh (1 medium) Plums (2) Watermelon (1 cup)	Apricots (3) Avocados (¼) Banana (1 medium) Dates (5) Figs (3) Kiwi (1) Nectarine (1 medium) Orange (1 medium) Peach, fresh (1 medium) Prunes (5) Raisins and dried fruit (¼ cup)
Vegetables	Asparagus (4 spears) Bean sprouts (½ cup) Cabbage (½ cup) Cauliflower (½ cup) Corn (½ cup) Cucumber (½) Green and wax beans (½ cup) Lettuce (1 cup) Okra (3 pods) Onions (½ cup) Peas (½ cup) Radishes (5) Rutabagas (½ cup) Summer squash (½ cup) Turnips (½ cup) Water chestnuts (4)	Broccoli (½ cup) Brussels sprouts (4-6) Beets (½ cup) Carrots (½ cup) Celery (½ cup) Eggplant (½ cup) Mixed vegetables (½ cup) Mushrooms (½ cup) Peanut butter (2 Tbsp) Pepper, green (1) Potato chips (10) Soaked potatoes (½ cup)	Artichoke (1 medium) Beans: lima, kidney, navy, pinto (½ cup) Greens: beet, collard, mustard, spinach, turnip (½ cup) Lentils, split peas, chickpeas, black-eyed peas (½ cup) Nuts: all kinds (½ cup) Parsnips (½ cup) Potatoes (½ cup or 1 small) Pumpkin (½ cup) Spinach (½ cup) Tomato (1 medium) Tomato sauce, tomato salsa (¼ cup) Winter squash (½ cup) Yams, sweet potatoes (½ cup)
Juices	Apple juice (½ cup) Cranberry juices (1 cup) Grape juice, frozen (1 cup) Tang, Hi-C and other fruit drinks (1 cup), Kool-Aid (1 cup) Lemonade and limeade (1 cup) Peach or pear nectar (½ cup)	Apricot nectar (½ cup) Grape juice, canned (½ cup) Grapefruit juice (½ cup) Pineapple juice (½ cup)	Pomegranate juice (½ cup) Prune juice (½ cup) Tomato juice (½ cup) V-8 juice (½ cup)

Other High-Potassium Foods

- Milk is high in potassium. Limit milk to 1 cup per day unless you are told to do otherwise.
- Supplements such as Ensure Plus and Enhancer Plus also contain a lot of potassium. Always speak to your nutritionist before using supplements.
- Most salt substitutes and "lite" salt products are made with potassium. Do not use these products. If you are unsure, ask your nutritionist.

Shaking the Salt Habit

Salt, or "sodium chloride," is found in convenience and preserved foods. Foods that do not spoil easily are usually high in sodium. The more sodium you eat, the thirstier you will be. The following list of foods is grouped by sodium levels.

Following a low-sodium diet can be challenging. This list of sodium levels of foods is meant to help you learn what foods and how much of them you can enjoy.

Remember, there are no foods that you cannot eat on your diet. What is important is the amount of foods you eat and how often you eat them. Keep this list handy for shopping or dining.

Most People on Dialysis May Have

- 1 serving per day from the high group
- 1 serving per day from the medium group
- As many servings as desired from the low group
- 3 servings per day from the medium group
- As many servings as you want from the low group

This is 2000 to 3000 mg of sodium per day. Check the serving size for each food, listed in parentheses next to the item.

Rinsing Canned Foods to Lower Sodium (Canned Vegetables, Chunk or Flaked Fish or Shellfish, Poultry or Meats)

1. Empty can into colander or sieve.
2. Drain brine and discard.
3. Break up chunks into flakes or smaller pieces.
4. Rinse under running water for 1 min.
5. Drain food until most moisture is gone.

APPENDIX 36. Renal Diet for Dialysis—cont'd

Food Category	Low-Sodium Foods 1-150 mg	Medium-Sodium Foods 150-250 mg	High-Sodium Foods 250-700 mg
Breads and cereals	Breads, white, whole grain Cakes, cookies, crepes, doughnuts Cereals: cooked, granola, puffed rice, puffed wheat, Shredded Wheat, Sugar Pops, Sugar Smacks, Sugar Crisps Crackers: graham, low salt, melba toast Macaroni, noodles, spaghetti, rice	Biscuits, rolls, muffins: homemade (1) Pancakes (1) "Ready-to-eat" cereals (¾ cup) Saltine crackers (6) Sweet roll (1)	All Bran (¼ cup) Instant mixes: noodles, potatoes, rice (½ cup) Instant mixes: biscuits, breads, muffins, rolls (1 serving) Waffles (1)
Condiments	Butter, margarine, oil Horseradish, mustard, spices, herbs, sugar, syrup, Tabasco, vinegar, Worcestershire	Bacon (2 slices) Catsup, steak sauce (1 Tbsp) Commercial salad dressing (1 Tbsp) Gravy (2 Tbsp) Low-sodium soy sauce (2 tsp) Mayonnaise (2 Tbsp) Pickle relish (2 Tbsp) Sweet pickles (2 small)	Salt (¼ tsp)
Dairy products	Cheeses: cream, Monterey, Mozzarella, Ricotta, low-salt types Cream: half-and-half, sour, whipping Custard, ice cream, sherbet Milk: all kinds, yogurt Nondairy creamer	Cheeses (1-oz slice) Cottage cheese (½ cup) Pudding (¾ cup)	Buttermilk (1 cup) Processed cheeses and cheese spreads (1 slice or 2 Tbsp)
Main dishes	All unprocessed meats, fish, poultry Eggs Peanut butter Tuna: low-sodium or rinsed		Broth (½ cup) Canned fish, meat (¼ cup) Canned soups (½ cup) Hot dog (1) Luncheon meat (1 slice) Canned entrees (e.g., pork and beans, spaghetti, stew) (1 cup) Sausage (1 oz)
Fruits and vegetables	All fresh or frozen vegetables All fruits and juices Canned tomatoes, tomato paste Canned vegetables: low-sodium or rinsed	Vegetables (½ cup) Juices: tomato, vegetable (½ cup)	Canned tomato sauce or puree (¼ cup) Frozen vegetables with special sauce (½ cup) Sauerkraut (¼ cup)
Beverages and snacks	Beer, wine, coffee, tea Candy: all kinds Fruit drinks, Popsicles, soda pop, Kool-Aid, Tang Low-salt products: without potassium substitutes Unsalted nuts, unsalted popcorn	Potato and corn chips (1 cup) Snack crackers (5-10)	Commercial dips (¼ cup) Dill pickle chips (3 slices) Olives (5) Salted nuts (½ cup)

Phosphorus

Low-Phosphorus Diet

When phosphorus is high for too long, bones become brittle and weak. You may have joint and bone pain. Extra phosphorus may go into your soft tissue, causing hard or soft lumps. Also, you may have severe itching.

The good news is that with diet, binders, and good dialysis, you can keep your phosphorus level under control.

Phosphorus is a mineral found in most foods. Dialysis does not remove it easily. Your phosphorus level depends on the foods you eat and your medications. Keeping your phosphorus at a safe level will help keep your bones healthy.

Each month your phosphorus level will be measured. High phosphorus is a common problem for people on dialysis. A good phosphorus level in your blood is between 3 and 6 g/dL.

High-Phosphorus Foods

Phosphorus is found in most foods you eat, especially protein foods. The foods that are highest in phosphorus are milk and things made from milk (dairy foods).

By limiting these foods you can cut down on the phosphorus you are eating. Most people on dialysis can have one serving daily from this list of dairy foods. The serving size is also noted.

You can also eat part of a serving of different foods to add up to 1 serving.

Milk (1 cup)
Cheese (2 oz)
Cottage cheese (⅔ cup)
Yogurt (1 cup)
Ice cream (1½ cup)
Frozen yogurt (1½ cup)
Milkshake (1 cup)
Hot chocolate (1 cup)
Pudding or custard (1 cup)

Other High-Phosphorus Foods

When your phosphorus level is high, you may need to limit these foods to once a week.

Bran cereals (1 oz)

Continued

APPENDIX 36. Renal Diet for Dialysis—cont'd

Dried beans or peas (½ cup cooked)
Chili (½ cup)
Nuts (½ cup)
Frozen waffles (1)

Phosphorus and Potassium

High-phosphorus foods are often high in potassium as well. This is another reason to limit dairy foods and other high-phosphorus foods.

Phosphate Binders

Phosphate binders are pills you take when you eat. Binders help keep phosphorus in your food from going into your blood.

Your doctor will decide which binder is best for you and how many you should take each time you eat.

It is important to take all your binders planned for each day.

You can take your binders just before you start a meal, during the meal, or right after eating.

If you forget to take them or skip a meal, it may be difficult to get your full binder dose. Ask your doctor what to do if this happens.

It may take some hard work to remember to take binders each time you eat. Try these ideas:

- Each morning take out the number of binders you need that day. Put them in a small container to carry with you. It should be empty at the end of the day.
- Carry a spare container of binders for when you travel or eat out.
- Take your binders with high-protein snacks such as sandwiches or dairy foods.
- Binders may cause constipation. Talk with your nutritionist about ideas to help with bowel movements.
- There are many types of binders. If you don't like the kind you are taking, talk with your doctor, pharmacist, or nutritionist about other kinds.

Lower-Phosphorus Ideas

Following are some lower-phosphorus choices you can make in the place of milk and other creamy dairy products. Check those you will try.

- Use nondairy creamer such as Mocha Mix or Coffee Rich on cereal, for creamy sauces or soups, and in shakes.
- Try rice milk or soymilk. They are lower in potassium too.
- Try soy cheese or soy yogurt. They are available in a variety of flavors.
- Use cream cheese in the place of regular cheese or cottage cheese.
- Use sour cream or imitation sour cream on fruits or to replace yogurt in dips.
- Try a nondairy frozen ice cream made from soy, rice, or nondairy creamer such as Mocha Mix.
- Enjoy sorbet or sherbet instead of ice cream.

High Phosphorus Levels

Following are some reasons for a high phosphorus level. Check the ones that you think may apply to you:

- Eating too many high-phosphorus foods
- Forgetting to take your binders
- Not taking all the phosphate binders ordered for you
- Not taking your phosphate binders at the right times

Even if you follow your diet and take your binders, your phosphorus level may be high. When calcium and phosphorus are out of balance, your parathyroid gland becomes overactive. High levels of parathyroid hormone damage your bones. Your doctor can test for this problem and recommend treatment.

Appendix created by Katy G. Wilkens, MS, RD.

NOTE: Some foods are very high in sodium and should be used only once a week. These include Chinese, Oriental foods; corned beef, ham, pastrami; fast foods (e.g., commercial hamburgers, pizza, tacos); pickles; soy sauce; and TV dinners and frozen entrees.

APPENDIX 37. Sodium-Restricted Diets

Sodium restriction is used in the management of essential hypertension and for cardiovascular disease, severe cardiac failure, impaired liver function, renal disease, and chronic renal failure. The goal of the sodium-restricted meal plan is to manage hypertension in sodium-sensitive persons and promote the loss of excess fluids in edema and ascites. Sodium is restricted to various degrees to meet the requirement.

Adequacy

Depending on individual food choices, sodium-restricted meal plans are adequate in all nutrients based on the Dietary Reference Intakes. When sodium is restricted to 1000 mg or less, a calcium supplement may be needed.

Special Considerations

A large volume of research has assessed the relationship of dietary sodium intake to prevention and treatment of high blood pressure. One result of this research is that sodium in combination with chloride (table salt) may aggravate hypertension is some people who are sensitive to salt. Numerous health agencies agree that sodium intake should be limited to 2.4 g (2400 mg) or less per day for healthy people. 1 tsp salt contains 2300 mg sodium.

A therapeutic sodium-restricted meal plan should be prescribed in terms of milligrams of sodium desired on a daily basis. The following are the commonly used levels of sodium restrictions:

No Added Salt (NAS): This is the least restrictive of the sodium-restricted diets. Table salt should not be used, and salt should be limited in cooking. When high-sodium foods such as smoked, cured, or dried meats and cheeses; condiments and seasonings, salted snacks, and canned and dried soups and bouillon are also limited, the NAS diet provides approximately 4000 mg of sodium daily.

3000 mg sodium (7.5 g NaCl or 130 mEq Na): This diet *restricts* foods and beverages that have been highly processed with sodium such as fast foods; salad dressings; soy sauce; salty snack foods; smoked, salted, and kosher meats; regular canned foods; pickled vegetables; luncheon meats; and commercially softened water. Up to ¼ tsp salt per day may be used in cooking or at the table.

2000 mg sodium (5 g NaCl or 87 mEq Na): This diet *eliminates* processed and prepared foods and beverages that are high in sodium. Salt should not be used in cooking or at the table. Milk and milk products are limited to 16 oz daily. Only salt-free commercially prepared foods should be used.

1000 mg sodium (2.5 g NaCl or 45 mEq Na): Processed and prepared foods and beverages that are high in sodium are eliminated. Regular canned foods, many frozen foods, deli foods, fast foods, cheeses, margarines, and regular salad dressings are also eliminated (low-sodium or sodium-free versions should be

APPENDIX 37. Sodium-Restricted Diets—cont'd

substituted). Regular breads are limited to two servings/day. Milk and milk products are limited to 16 oz/day. Salt should not be used in cooking or at the table. Note: Most medical professionals no longer recommend eating patterns with less than 1000 mg sodium. In addition to being unpalatable, they are very restrictive and could result in nutritional deficiencies if followed for an extended period.

Guidelines for Sodium Restriction

- Obtain and evaluate a diet history before prescribing or instructing on a sodium restriction.
- Recommend salt substitutes containing potassium chloride only if approved by a physician. Salt-free seasoning products are readily available in most grocery stores and should be suggested instead.
- Instruct patients on reading the Nutrition Facts food label for sodium content of foods.
- Recommend potassium replacement if diuretics are used. If potassium intake from foods is not sufficient, potassium supplements may be necessary.
- Provide information on choosing low-sodium foods at restaurants.
- Recommend baked products, using sodium-free baking powder, potassium bicarbonate (instead of sodium bicarbonate or baking soda), and salt-free shortening in place of those containing sodium.
- Avoid obviously salted foods such as bouillon, soup and gravy bases, canned soups and stews; bread and rolls with salt toppings, salted crackers; salted nuts or popcorn, potato chips, pretzels, and other salted snack foods.
- Avoid smoked or cured meats, such as bacon, bologna, cold cuts, other processed meats, chipped or corned beef, frankfurters, ham, koshered or kosher style meats, and canned meat poultry.
- Avoid salted and smoked fish such as cod, herring, and sardines.
- Avoid sauerkraut, olives, pickles, relishes, and other vegetables prepared in brine, tomato, and vegetable cocktail juices.
- Avoid seasonings such as celery salt, garlic, Worcestershire sauce, and soy sauce.
- Serve cheeses (e.g., Swiss, American, and other processed cheeses) in limited amounts (approximately two times a week).
- Include sodium-containing medications, seltzer waters, toothpaste, and chewing tobacco in total sodium allotment if the restriction is below 2000 mg.
- Monitor the sodium content of various medications, including over-the-counter brands.

Sodium Content of Selected Over-the-Counter Medications

Medication	Trade Name	Sodium Content	
		Milligrams per Dose	Milligrams per 100 mL
Analgesic	Aspirin (various others)	49	—
Antacid analgesic	Bromo-Seltzer	717	—
Antacid laxative	Alka-Seltzer (blue box)	521	—
Antacids	Sal Hepatica	1000	—
	Rolaids	53	—
	Soda Mint	89	—
	Alka-Seltzer (gold box)	276	—
	Brioschi	710	—
Laxatives	Metamucil Instant Mix	250	—
	Fleet's Enema	250-300	—
Sleep aids	Miles Nervine Effervescent	544	—
Antacid suspensions	Milk of Magnesia	—	10
	Amphojel	—	14
	Basaljel	—	36
	Maalox	—	50
	Riopan	—	14
	Mylanta I	—	76
	Mylanta II	—	160
	Digel	—	170
	Titralac	—	220

Seasoning without salt: Flavorings or seasonings will make food more appetizing. For example:

- Lemon or vinegar is excellent with fish or meat and with many vegetables such as broccoli, asparagus, green beans, or salads.
- Meat may be seasoned with onion, garlic, green pepper, nutmeg, ginger, dry mustard, sage and marjoram. It may be cooked with fresh mushrooms or unsalted tomato juice.
- Cranberry sauce, applesauce, or jellies make appetizing accompaniments to meats and poultry.
- Vegetables may be flavored by the addition of onion, mint, ginger, mace, dill seed, parsley, green pepper, or fresh mushrooms.
- Unsalted cottage cheese may be flavored with minced onion, chopped chives, raw green pepper, grated carrots, chopped parsley, or crushed pineapple.
- A number of salt-free seasonings for use in cooking are available in the spice section of most supermarkets.

Continued

APPENDIX 37. Sodium-Restricted Diets—cont'd

3000-mg Sodium Diet

Food Category	Recommended	Not Recommended
Beverages	Milk, buttermilk (limit to 1 cup daily); eggnog; all fruit juices; low sodium, salt-free vegetable juices; regular vegetable or tomato juices (limit to ½ cup daily); coffee, tea, low-sodium carbonated beverages	Regular vegetable or tomato juices used in excessive amounts
Breads and cereals	Enriched white, wheat, rye, and pumpernickel bread, hard rolls, and dinner rolls; biscuits, muffins, cornbread, pancakes, and waffles; most dry and hot cereals; unsalted crackers and breadsticks	Breads, rolls, and crackers with salted tops; instant hot cereals
Desserts and sweets	All	None
Fats	Butter or margarine; vegetable oils; low-sodium salad dressing, other salad dressings in limited amounts; light, sour, and heavy cream	Salad dressings containing bacon fat, bacon bits, and salt pork; snack dips made with instant soup mixes or processed cheese
Fruits	All	None
Meats and meat substitutes	Any fresh or frozen beef, lamb, pork, poultry, fish and most shellfish; canned tuna or salmon, rinsed; eggs and egg substitutes; regular cheese, ricotta, and cream cheese (2 oz daily); low-sodium cheese as desired; cottage cheese, drained; regular yogurt; regular peanut butter (3 times weekly); dried peas and beans; frozen dinners (<600 mg sodium)	Any smoked, cured, salted, kosher, commercially prepared meat, fish, or poultry, including bacon, chipped beef, cold cuts, ham, hot dogs, sausage, sardines, anchovies, marinated herring, and pickled meats; frozen breaded meats; pickled eggs; processed cheese, cheese spreads and sauces; salted nuts
Potatoes and potato substitutes	White or sweet potatoes; winter squash; enriched rice, barley, noodles, spaghetti, macaroni, and other pastas; homemade bread stuffing	Commercially prepared potato, rice, or pasta mixes; commercial bread stuffing
Soups	Commercially prepared and dehydrated soups, broths, and bouillons (once per week); homemade broth, soups without added salt and made with allowed vegetables; reduced-sodium commercially prepared soups and broths	Commercially prepared or dehydrated regular soups (more than once per week)
Vegetables	All fresh and frozen vegetables, commercially prepared, drained vegetables	Sauerkraut, pickled vegetables, and others prepared in brine; vegetables seasoned with ham, bacon, or salt pork
Miscellaneous	Limit added salt to ¼ tsp/day used at the table or in cooking; salt substitute with physician's approval; pepper, herbs, spices; vinegar, lemon, or lime juice; hot pepper sauce; low-sodium soy sauce (1 tsp); unsalted tortilla chips, pretzels, potato chips, popcorn; salsa (2 Tbsp), catsup and mustard (1 Tbsp), low-sodium baking powder	Any seasoning made with salt, including garlic salt, celery salt, onion salt, and seasoned salt; sea salt, rock salt, kosher salt; meat tenderizers; monosodium glutamate; regular soy sauce, teriyaki sauce, most flavored vinegars; regular snack chips, olives

Sample Menu for 3000-mg Sodium Diet

Breakfast	Lunch	Dinner
½ cup calcium-fortified orange juice	3-oz boneless, skinless chicken breast	1 cup spaghetti with meat sauce
¾ cup Raisin Bran	½ cup white rice	1 cup tossed salad with assorted vegetables
2 slices whole wheat toast	½ cup broccoli	1 Tbsp low-fat Italian dressing
2 tsp margarine	½ cup coleslaw	1 slice Italian bread
1 Tbsp jelly	1 whole wheat roll	½ cup apple crisp
1 cup skim milk	1 tsp margarine	2 tsp margarine
1 cup coffee	1 cup iced tea	1 cup skim milk
2 tsp sugar	½ cup chocolate pudding	1 cup coffee
	½ Tbsp whipped topping	¼ tsp pepper
	¼ tsp pepper	2 tsp sugar
	2 tsp sugar	

Nutritional Analysis

Kilocalories: 2038
Protein: 79 g
Fat: 49 g
Carbohydrate: 337 g
Sodium: 3050 mg
Potassium: 3534 mg
Fiber: 21g

APPENDIX 37. Sodium-Restricted Diets—cont'd

2000-mg Sodium Diet

Food Category	Recommended	Not Recommended
Beverages	Milk (limit to 2 cup daily), buttermilk (limit to 1 cup daily), eggnog, all fruit juices, low-sodium, salt-free vegetable juices, coffee, tea, low-sodium carbonated beverages	Malted milk, milkshakes, chocolate milk, regular vegetable or tomato juices, commercially softened water used for drinking or cooking
Breads and cereals	Enriched, white, wheat, rye, and pumpernickel bread, hard rolls, and dinner rolls; muffins, cornbread, waffles; most dry cereals, cooked cereal without added salt; unsalted crackers and breadsticks; low-sodium or homemade bread crumbs	Breads, rolls, and crackers with salted tops; quick breads; instant hot cereals; commercial bread stuffing; self-rising flour and biscuit mixes; regular bread crumbs or cracker crumbs; pancakes
Desserts and sweets	All; desserts and sweets made with milk should be within allowance	Instant pudding mixes and cake mixes
Fats	Butter or margarine; vegetable oils; unsalted salad dressings; light, sour, and heavy cream; regular salad dressing limited to 1 Tbsp	Regular salad dressings containing bacon fat, bacon bits, and salt pork; snack dips made with instant soup mixes or processed cheese
Fruits	Most fresh, frozen, and canned fruits	Fruits processed with salt or sodium-containing compounds (i.e., some dried fruits)
Meats and meat substitutes	Any fresh or frozen beef, lamb, pork, poultry, fish; some shellfish; canned tuna or salmon, rinsed; eggs and egg substitutes; low-sodium cheese, including low-sodium ricotta and cream cheese; low-sodium cottage cheese; regular yogurt; low-sodium peanut butter; dried peas and beans; frozen dinners (<500 mg sodium)	Any smoked, cured, salted, kosher, commercially prepared meat, fish, or poultry, including bacon, chipped beef, cold cuts, ham, hot dogs, sausage, sardines, anchovies, marinated herring, and pickled meats; crab, lobster, frozen, breaded meats, pickled eggs, regular hard and processed cheese; cheese spreads and sauces; salted nuts
Potatoes and potato substitutes	White or sweet potatoes; winter squash; enriched rice, barley, noodles, spaghetti, macaroni, and other pastas cooked without salt; homemade bread stuffing	Commercially prepared potato, rice, or pasta mixes; commercial bread stuffing
Soups	Low-sodium commercially prepared and dehydrated soups, broth, and bouillon; homemade broth soups made without added salt and with allowed vegetables; cream soups within milk allowance	Regular commercially prepared or dehydrated soups, broth, or bouillon
Vegetables	Fresh, frozen vegetables and low-sodium commercially prepared vegetables	Regular commercially prepared vegetables, sauerkraut, pickled vegetables, and others prepared in brine; frozen vegetables in sauces; vegetables seasoned with ham, bacon, or salt pork
Miscellaneous	Salt substitute with physician's approval; pepper, herbs, spices; vinegar, lemon or lime juice; low-sodium soy sauce (1 tsp); hot pepper sauce; low-sodium condiments (catsup, chili sauce, mustard); fresh ground horseradish; unsalted tortilla chips, pretzels, potato chips, popcorn, salsa (2 Tbsp)	Any seasoning made with salt, including garlic salt, celery salt, onion salt, and seasoned salt; sea salt, rock salt, kosher salt; meat tenderizers, monosodium glutamate; regular soy sauce, barbecue sauce, teriyaki sauce, steak sauce, Worcestershire sauce, most flavored vinegars; canned gravy and mixes; regular condiments; salted snack foods, olives

Sample Menu for 2000-mg Sodium Diet

Breakfast	Lunch	Dinner
½ cup calcium-fortified orange juice	3-oz boneless, skinless chicken breast	1 cup spaghetti with low-sodium tomato or meat sauce
¾ cup raisin bran	½ cup white rice	1 cup tossed salad with assorted vegetables
2 slices whole-wheat toast	½ cup broccoli	1 slice Italian bread
2 tsp margarine	½ cup coleslaw	1 tsp margarine
1 Tbsp jelly	1 whole-wheat roll	½ cup apple crisp
1 cup skim milk	1 tsp margarine	1 cup coffee
1 cup coffee	½ cup homemade pudding	¼ tsp pepper
2 tsp sugar	½ Tbsp whipped cream	2 tsp sugar
	1 cup iced tea	
	¼ tsp pepper	
	2 tsp sugar	

Nutritional Analysis

Kilocalories: 1972
Protein: 78 g
Fat: 42 g
Saturated fat: 8 g
Carbohydrate: 348 g
Sodium: 2061 mg
Potassium: 3154 mg
Fiber: 26 g

Continued

APPENDIX 37. Sodium-Restricted Diets—cont'd

1000-mg Sodium Diet

Food Category	Recommended	Not Recommended
Beverages	Milk (limited to 2 cup daily); eggnog; all fruit juices; low-sodium, salt-free vegetable juices; low-sodium carbonated beverages, coffee, tea	Malted milk; milkshake, buttermilk, chocolate milk; regular vegetable or tomato juices; commercially softened water used for drinking or cooking
Breads and cereals	Enriched white, wheat, rye and pumpernickel bread, hard rolls, and dinner rolls (2 servings/day); low-sodium bread, crackers, matzo, and Melba toast; muffins, cornbread, pancakes, and waffles made with low-sodium baking powder; cooked cereal without added salt; low-sodium dry cereals, including puffed rice, puffed wheat, and shredded wheat; unsalted crackers and breadsticks; low-sodium bread crumbs and cracker crumbs	Breads, rolls, and crackers with salted tops or made with regular baking powder; quick breads; instant hot cereals; self-rising flour and biscuit mixes; regular bread crumbs and cracker crumbs, graham crackers
Desserts and sweets	Ice cream, pudding, and custard made with milk should be within allowance; fruit ice; unsalted bakery goods, homemade or commercial; sherbet and flavored gelatin (not to exceed ½ cup/day), low-salt baking powder	All candies made with sweet chocolate, nuts, or coconut; desserts made with rennin or rennin tablets; instant pudding mixes, commercial cakes, cookies, and brownie mixes
Fats	Unsalted butter or margarine; vegetable oils; unsalted salad dressings; low-sodium mayonnaise; nondairy cream (up to 1 oz daily)	Salted butter and margarine; all regular salad dressings; snack dips made with instant soup mixes or processed cheese
Fruits	Most fresh, frozen, and other commercially prepared fruits	Fruits processed with salt or sodium-containing compounds
Meat and meat substitutes	Any fresh or frozen beef, lamb, pork, poultry, fish; low-sodium canned tuna or salmon; eggs; low-sodium cheese, cottage cheese, ricotta, and cream cheese; regular yogurt; low-sodium peanut butter; dried peas and beans; frozen dinners (<150 mg sodium)	Any smoked, cured, salted, kosher, commercially prepared meat, fish, or poultry including bacon, chipped beef, cold cuts, ham, hot dogs, sausage, sardines, anchovies, marinated herring, and pickled meats; all shellfish; frozen breaded meats; pickled eggs, egg substitutes; regular hard and processed cheese; cheese spreads and sauces; salted nuts
Potatoes and potato substitutes	White or sweet potatoes; winter squash; unsalted enriched rice, barley, noodles, spaghetti, macaroni, and other pasta cooked without salt; homemade bread stuffing	Commercially prepared potato, rice, or pasta mixes; instant potatoes; commercial bread stuffing
Soups	Low-sodium commercially prepared and dehydrated soups, broths, and bouillon; homemade broth, soups without added salt and made with allowed vegetables; low-sodium cream soups within milk allowance	Regular commercially prepared or dehydrated soups, broths, or bouillon
Vegetables	Fresh, unsalted frozen vegetables, and low-sodium commercially prepared vegetables	Regular commercially prepared vegetables; sauerkraut, pickled vegetables, and others prepared in brine; frozen peas, lima beans, and mixed vegetables; all frozen vegetables in sauces; vegetables seasoned with ham, bacon, or salt pork
Miscellaneous	Salt substitute with physician's approval; pepper, herbs, spices; vinegar, lemon, or lime juice; low-sodium soy sauce; hot pepper sauce; low-sodium condiments (catsup, chili sauce, mustard); fresh ground horseradish; unsalted tortilla chips, pretzels, potato chips, popcorn	Salt and any seasoning made with salt, including garlic salt, celery salt, onion salt, seasoned salt; sea salt, rock salt, kosher salt; meat tenderizers; monosodium glutamate; regular soy sauce, barbecue sauce, teriyaki sauce, steak sauce, Worcestershire sauce, most flavored vinegars; canned gravy and mixes; regular olives, horseradish, pickles, relish, catsup, and mustard, commercial salsa

APPENDIX 37. Sodium-Restricted Diets—cont'd

Sample Menu for 1000-mg Sodium Diet

Breakfast	Lunch	Dinner
½ cup calcium-fortified orange juice	3-oz boneless, skinless chicken breast	1 cup spaghetti (unsalted) with unsalted tomato and meat sauce
¾ cup shredded wheat	½ cup white rice prepared without salt	1 cup tossed salad with vegetables
2 slices low-sodium whole wheat toast	½ cup salt-free steamed broccoli	1 Tbsp low-sodium salad dressing
2 tsp unsalted margarine	½ cup low-sodium coleslaw	1 slice low-sodium bread
1 Tbsp jelly	1 slice low-sodium whole wheat bread	2 tsp unsalted margarine
1 cup skim milk	1 tsp unsalted margarine	1 apple
1 cup coffee	½ cup homemade pudding	½ cup skim milk
1 tsp sugar	1 cup tea	1 cup coffee
	¼ tsp pepper	¼ tsp pepper
	2 tsp sugar	2 tsp sugar

Nutritional Analysis

Kilocalories: 1907
Protein: 78g
Fat: 45 g
Saturated fat: 10 g
Carbohydrate: 307 g
Sodium: 1070 mg
Potassium: 2956 mg
Fiber: 23 g

From the North Carolina Dietetic Association: Nutrition care manual, Raleigh, NC, 2005, The Association.

APPENDIX 38. Nutritional Facts on Alcoholic Beverages

Alcohol may have beneficial effects when consumed in moderation. The lowest all-cause mortality occurs at an intake of one to two drinks per day. The lowest coronary heart disease mortality also occurs at an intake of one to two drinks per day. Morbidity and mortality are highest among those drinking large amounts of alcohol.

Guidelines:

- Alcoholic beverages should not be consumed by some individuals, including those who cannot restrict their alcohol intake, women of childbearing age who may become pregnant, pregnant and lactating women, children and adolescents, individuals taking medications that can interact with alcohol, and those with specific medical conditions.
- Those who choose to drink alcoholic beverages should do so sensibly and in moderation—defined as the consumption of up to one drink per day for women and up to two drinks per day for men.
- Alcoholic beverages should be avoided by individuals engaging in activities that require attention, skill, or coordination, such as driving or operating machinery.

Calories in Selected Alcoholic Beverages*

This table is a guide to estimate the caloric intake from various alcoholic beverages. A sample serving volume and the calories in that drink are shown for beer, wine, and distilled spirits. Higher alcohol content (higher percent alcohol or higher proof) and mixing alcohol with other beverages such as sweetened soft drinks, tonic water, fruit juice, or cream increase the amount of calories in the beverage. Alcoholic beverages supply calories but provide few essential nutrients.

Beverage	Serving (oz)	Alcohol (g)	Carbohydrate (g)	Calories	Exchanges for Calorie or Diabetes Control
Beer					
Regular	12	13	13	150	1 starch, 2 fat
Light	12	11	5	100	2 fat
Near beer	12	1.5	12	60	1 starch
Distilled spirits					
80-Proof (gin, rum, vodka, whiskey, scotch)	1.5	14	Trace	100	2 fat
Dry brandy, cognac	1	11	Trace	75	1.5 fat
Table wines					
Dry white	4	11	Trace	80	2 fat
Red or rose	4	12	2	85	2 fat
Sweet wine	4	12	5	105	⅓ starch, 2 fat
Light wine	4	6	1	50	1 fat
Wine cooler	12	13	30	215	2 fruit, 2 fat
Dealcoholized wines	4	Trace	6-7	25-35	0.5 fruit
Sparkling wines					
Champagne	4	12	4	100	2 fat
Sweet kosher wine	4	12	12	132	1 starch, 2 fat
Appetizer and dessert wines					
Sherry	2	9	2	74	1.5 fat
Sweet sherry, port, muscatel	2	9	7	90	0.5 starch, 1.5 fat
Cordials, liqueurs	1	13	18	160	1 starch, 2 fat
Vermouth					
Dry	3	13	4	105	2 fat
Sweet	3	13	14	140	1 starch, 2 fat
Cocktails					
Bloody Mary	5	14	5	116	1 vegetable, 2 fat
Daiquiri	2	14	2	111	2 fat
Manhattan	2	17	2	178	2.5 fat
Martini	2.5	22	Trace	156	3.5 fat
Old-fashioned	4	26	Trace	180	4 fat
Tom Collins	7.5	16	3	120	2.5 fat
Mixes					
Mineral water	Any	0	0	0	Free
Sugar-free tonic	Any	0	0	0	Free
Club soda	Any	0	0	0	Free
Diet soda	Any	0	0	0	Free
Tomato juice	4	0	5	25	1 vegetable
Bloody Mary mix	4	0	5	25	1 vegetable
Orange juice	4	0	15	60	1 fruit
Grapefruit juice	4	0	15	60	1 fruit
Pineapple juice	4	0	15	60	1 fruit

From Franz MJ: Alcohol and diabetes: its metabolism and guidelines for its occasional use. Part TI, Diabetes Spectrum 3(4):210-216, 1990.

*The caloric contribution from alcohol of an alcoholic beverage can be estimated by multiplying the number of ounces by the proof and then again by the factor 0.8. For beers and wines, kilocalories from alcohol can be estimated by multiplying ounces by percentage of alcohol (by volume) and then by the factor 1.6.

APPENDIX 39. Nutritional Facts on Caffeine-Containing Products

Caffeine is similar in structure to adenosine, a chemical found in the brain that slows down its activity. Because the two compete, the more caffeine that is consumed, the less adenosine that is available up to a point. Caffeine temporarily heightens concentration and wards off fatigue. Within 30 to 60 minutes of drinking a cup of coffee, caffeine reaches peak concentrations in the bloodstream and takes 4 to 6 hours for its effects to wear off. The average American adult consumes about 200 mg of caffeine a day, and many may consume twice that level. It is generally safe to consume no more than the equivalent amount of caffeine in 1 to 2 cups of coffee daily during pregnancy or lactation. Individuals with heart disease and hypertension may benefit from a reduction in caffeine consumption. To reduce caffeine and its stimulant effects, monitor intake from foods and beverages listed below.

Selected Food and Beverage Sources of Caffeine

Caffeine-Containing Products	Serving (mg)
Coffee	
Starbucks coffee (in store), 16 oz.	330
Starbucks coffee (at home), 16 oz.	260
Brewed, drip method, 6 oz	103
Brewed, percolator method, 6 oz	75
Instant, 1 rounded tsp	57
Flavored, regular and sugar-free, 6 oz	26-75
Espresso, 1 oz	40
Café Latte, short (8 oz) or tall (12 oz) (Starbucks)	35
Decaffeinated, 6 oz	2
Tea	
Black or green tea, 16 oz	60-100
3-minute brew, 12-oz	72
Lipton, Arizona, or Snapple tea, 16 oz	30-60
Instant, 1 rounded tsp in 8 oz of water	25-35
Tea, green brewed, 8 oz	30
Tea, bottles (12 oz) or from instant mix, 8 oz	14
Decaffeinated, 5- minute brew, 6-oz cup	1
Carbonated Beverages	
7-Eleven Big Gulp cola, 64 oz	190
Mountain Dew MDX or Vault, 12 oz	120
Diet Pepsi Max, 20 oz	70
Mountain Dew, 12 oz, regular or diet	54
Mellow Yellow, 12 oz, regular or diet	52
Regular or diet cola, cherry colas, Dr. Pepper, Mr. Pibb, 12 oz	35-50
Decaffeinated drinks, 12 oz	Trace
Cocoa and Chocolate	
Chocolate, baking, unsweetened, 1 oz	58
Chocolate, sweet, semisweet, dark, milk, 1 oz	8-20
Milk chocolate bar , 1.5 oz	10
Chocolate milk, 8 oz	8
Cocoa beverage, 6-oz cup	4
Chocolate-flavored syrup, 1 oz	5
Chocolate pudding, ½ cup	4-8
Miscellaneous	
Powershot (8 oz)	800
Rock Star, 16 oz	240
NoDoz, Maximum Strength (1), or Vivarin (1)	200
Pit Bull Energy Bar, 2 oz	165
Excedrin (2)	130
NoDoz, Regular Strength (1)	100
Red Bull (8.3 oz)	80
Water, caffeinated (Edge 2 O), (8 oz)	70
Anacin (2)	65
Bud Extra Beer, 10 oz	55
Propel Invigorating water	50
Jolt (8 oz)	48

APPENDIX 40. Nutritional Facts on Essential (Omega) Fatty Acids

Essential fatty acids (EFAs) are fatty acids that are required in the human diet. They must be obtained from food because human cells have no biochemical pathways capable of producing them internally. There are two closely related families of EFAs: **omega-3 (Ω-3 or ω-3)** and **omega-6 (Ω-6 or ω-6)**. Only one substance in each of these families is truly essential, because, for example, the body can convert one ω-3 to another ω-3 but cannot create an ω-3 from scratch.

In the body essential fatty acids serve multiple functions. In each of these the balance between dietary ω-3 and ω-6 strongly affects function. They are modified to make the eicosanoids (affecting inflammation and many other cellular functions); the endogenous cannabinoids (affecting mood, behavior, and inflammation); the lipoxins from ω-6 EFAs and resolvins from ω-3 (in the presence of aspirin, down-regulating inflammation); the isofurans, isoprostanes, hepoxilins, epoxyeicosatrienoic acids, and neuroprotectin D; and the lipid rafts (affecting cellular signaling). They also act on deoxyribonucleic acid (activating or inhibiting transcription factors for nuclear factor–κ-B [NFκB], a proinflammatory cytokine).

Between 1930 and 1950 arachidonic and linolenic acids were termed *essential* because each was more or less able to meet the growth requirements of rats given fat-free diets. Further research has shown that **human metabolism requires both fatty acids.** To some extent any ω-3 and any ω-6 can relieve the worst symptoms of fatty acid deficiency. However, in many people the ability to convert the ω-3 α-linolenic acid (ALA) to the ω-3 eicosapentaenoic (EPA) and docosahexaenoic acid (DHA) is only 5% efficient. Therefore it is important to incorporate the EPA and DHA directly into the diet usually as fish or a fish oil supplement. Particular fatty acids such as DHA are needed at critical life stages (e.g., infancy and lactation) and in some disease states.

The essential fatty acids are:

- ALA (18:3)-ω-3
- Linoleic acid (18:2)- ω-6

These two fatty acids cannot be synthesized by humans because humans lack the desaturase enzymes required for their production. They form the starting point for the creation of longer and more desaturated fatty acids, which are also referred to as long-chain polyunsaturates:

ω-3 Fatty acids:

- EPA (20:5)
- DHA (22:6)
- ALA (18:)

ω-6 Fatty acids:

- γ-Linolenic acid (GLA) (18:3)
- Dihomo-γ-linolenic acid (DGLA) (20:3)
- Arachidonic acid (AA) (20:4)

ω-9 Fatty acids are not essential in humans, because humans possess all the enzymes required for their synthesis.

Adequate Intakes for ω-3 Fatty Acids for Children and Adults

Age (years)	Males and Females (g/day)	Pregnancy (g/day)	Lactation (g/day)
1-3	0.7	N/A	N/A
4-8	0.9	N/A	N/A
9-13	1.2 for boys; 1 for girls	N/A	N/A
14-18	1.6 for boys;1.1 for girls	1.4	1.3
19+	1.6 for men; 1.1 for women	1.4	1.3

N/A, Not applicable.

Adequate Intakes for ω-6 Fatty Acids for Children and Adults

Age (years)	Males and Females (g/day)	Pregnancy (g/day)	Lactation (g/day)
1-3	7	N/A	N/A
4-8	10	N/A	N/A
9-13	12 for boys; 10 for girls	N/A	N/A
14-18	16 for boys; 11 for girls	13	13
19+	17 for men; 12 for women	13	13

Dietary Sources

Some of the food sources of ω-3 and ω-6 fatty acids are fish and shellfish, flaxseed (linseed), soya oil, canola (rapeseed) oil, hemp oil, chia seeds, pumpkin seeds, sunflower seeds, leafy vegetables, and walnuts.

EFAs play a part in many metabolic processes, and there is evidence to suggest that low levels of EFAs or the wrong balance of types among the EFAs may be a factor in a number of illnesses.

Plant sources of ω-3s do not contain EPA and DHA. This is thought to be the reason that absorption of EFAs is much greater from animal rather than plant sources.

EFA content of vegetable sources varies with cultivation conditions. Animal sources vary widely, both with the animal's feed and that the EFA makeup varies markedly with fats from different body parts.

Omega-3 Fatty Acids

There is some evidence that suggests that ω-3s may:

- Help lower elevated triglyceride levels. High triglyceride levels can contribute to coronary heart disease.
- Reduce the blood's tendency to clot, which may relate to the clogging that occurs with atherosclerosis.
- Reduce the inflammation involved in conditions such as rheumatoid arthritis.
- Improve symptoms of depression and other mental health disorders in some individuals.

Dietary sources of ω-3 fatty acids include fish oil and certain plant and nut oils. Fish oil contains both DHA and EPA, whereas some nuts (English walnuts) and vegetable oils (canola, soybean, flaxseed and linseed, olive) contain only the ω-3 ALA.

There is evidence from multiple large-scale population (epidemiologic) studies and randomized controlled trials that intake of recommended amounts of DHA and EPA in the form of fish or fish oil supplements lowers triglycerides; reduces the risk of death, heart attack, dangerous abnormal heart rhythms, and strokes in people with known cardiovascular disease; slows the buildup of atherosclerotic plaques ("hardening of the arteries"); and lowers blood pressure slightly. However, high doses may have harmful effects such as an increased risk of bleeding. Some species of fish carry a higher risk of environmental contamination such as with methyl mercury.

APPENDIX 40. Nutritional Facts on Essential (Omega) Fatty Acids—cont'd

Common Food Sources of Omega-3 Fats

Omega-3 Fat	Food Source
ALA	Ground flaxseed and walnuts and soybeans Flaxseed, walnut, soybean and canola oils, and nonhydrogenated canola and soy margarines
DHA and EPA	Mackerel, salmon, herring, trout and sardines, and other fish and shellfish Marine algae supplements

Fish or Other Food Source	Omega-3 Content in a 4-oz Serving
English walnuts	6.8 g
Chinook salmon	3.6 g
Sockeye salmon	2.3 g
Mackerel	1.8-2.6 g
Herring	1.2-2.7 g
Rainbow trout	1.0 g
Wheat germ and oat germ	0.7-1.4 g
Halibut	0.5-1.3 g
White tuna	0.97 g
Light tuna	0.35 g
Whiting	0.9 g
Spinach	0.9 g
Flounder	0.6 g
King crab	0.6 g
Shrimp	0.5 g
Tofu	0.4 g (probably much less in "lite" tofu)
Clam	0.32 g
Cod	0.3 g
Scallop	0.23 g
Supplements*	
Cod liver oil	800-100 mg/tsp
Fish body oil	1200-1800 mg/tsp
Omega-3 fatty acid concentrate	250 mg/capsule

*Exact omega-3 content varies per manufacturer. Check label.

Enhancing Intake of Omega-3 Fats

- Eat fish at least two times each week.
- Include canned fish in your diet (examples: salmon, sardines, light tuna). Try sardines on toast.
- Add ground flaxseed to foods such as hot or cold cereal or yogurt. NOTE: Pregnant women should limit their intake of ground flaxseed to occasional use (not daily). Ground flaxseeds contain lignans. There is not enough information about their safety in pregnancy.
- Eat walnuts. Add walnuts to salads, cereals, baking (examples, muffins, cookies, breads) and pancakes.
- Have fresh or frozen soybeans (edamame) as a vegetable at meals.
- Use soybean oil or canola oil in salad dressings and recipes.
- Use nonhydrogenated margarine made from canola or soybean as a spread or in baking.
- Cook with ω-3 liquid eggs or eggs in the shell. Enjoy scrambled eggs or try a homemade egg sandwich.
- Use other ω-3 fortified products such as milk, yogurt, bread, and pasta.
- Substitute ¼ cup ground flaxseed for ¼ cup flour in bread, pizza dough, muffin, cookie, or meatloaf recipes.
- Replace 1 egg with 1 Tbsp ground flaxseed and 3 Tbsp water in recipes.

APPENDIX 41. Nutritional Facts on a High-Fiber Diet

This diet is a modification of the regular diet. The purpose of this diet is to decrease transit time through the intestine, promote more frequent bowel movements, and softer stools. This diet may be prescribed as a treatment for diverticulosis, irritable bowel syndrome, hemorrhoids, or constipation. It includes all the foods on a regular diet, with emphasis on the proper planning and selection of foods to increase the daily intake of fiber. Fluid intake should be increased. The American Dietetic Association recommends that the average adult have a daily fiber intake of 20 to 35 g from a variety of sources. For children the child's age plus 5 g of fiber is recommended daily. In cases of severe constipation more fiber is recommended. Because of possible interactions with absorption of nutrients, regular intake of greater than 50 g of fiber per day is not recommended.

Dietary Reference Intakes for Fiber for Children and Adults

Age (years)	Males and Females (g/day)	Pregnancy (g/day)	Lactation (g/day)
1-3	19	N/A	N/A
4-8	25	N/A	N/A
9-13	31 for boys; 26 for girls	N/A	N/A
14-18	38 for boys; 26 for girls	28	29
19+	38 for men; 25 for women	28	29

N/A, Not applicable.

Although numerous over-the-counter fiber supplements are available, food sources provide other nutrients and are the preferred method of increasing dietary fiber. Adequate liquid consumption (at least eight 8-oz glasses per day) is recommended. Fiber should be added to the diet slowly because of possible cramps, bloating, and diarrhea with a sudden fiber increase. Maximum therapeutic benefits of fiber are obtained after several months of compliance. There are two components of dietary fiber, each providing health benefits: insoluble and soluble.

Continued

APPENDIX 41. Nutritional Facts on a High-Fiber Diet—cont'd

Types of Dietary Fiber

Type of Fiber	Components of Cells	Food Sources	Health Benefits
Soluble fibers	Gums, mucilages, pectin, certain hemicelluloses	Vegetables, fruits, barley; legumes, oats, and oat-bran	Decrease total blood cholesterol. Guard against diabetes. Prevent constipation. May help manage irritable bowel syndrome. May protect against colon cancer and gallstones.
Insoluble fibers	Cellulose, lignin, some hemicelluloses	Whole-wheat products, wheat and corn bran, and many vegetables (including cauliflower, green beans, potatoes, and skins of root vegetables)	May prevent diverticular disease. Prevents constipation. May delay glucose absorption (probably insignificant). May increase satiety and therefore assist with weight loss. Lower cholesterol. May protect against colon cancer.

Guidelines for High-Fiber Diet

1. Increase consumption of whole-grain breads, cereals, flours, and other whole-grain productions to 6 to 11 servings daily.
2. Increase consumption of vegetables, legumes and fruits, nuts, and edible seeds to 5 to 8 servings daily.
3. Consume high-fiber cereals, granolas, and legumes as needed to bring fiber intake to 25 g or more daily.
4. Increase consumption of fluids to at least 2 L (or approximately 2 qt) daily.
5. For a high-fiber diet of approximately 24 g of dietary fiber: use 12 or more servings of the foods from the groups below (each food contains approximately 2 g of dietary fiber). For example, ½ cup of baked beans (8 Tbsp) would count as 4 servings.

Each of these foods in this amount contains 2 g of dietary fiber:

Apple, 1 small
Orange, 1 small
Banana, 1 small
Peach, 1 medium
Strawberries, ½ cup
Pear, ½ small
Cherries, 10 large
Plums, 2 small

Whole-wheat bread, 1 slice
All Bran, 1 Tbsp
Rye bread, 1 slice
Corn flakes, ⅔ cup
Cracked wheat bread, 1 slice
Oatmeal, dry, 3 Tbsp
Shredded wheat, ½ biscuit
Wheat bran, 1 tsp
Grape-nuts, 3 Tbsp
Puffed wheat, 1⅓ cup

Broccoli, ½ stalk
Lettuce, raw, 2 cups
Brussels sprouts, 4
Green beans, ½ cup
Carrots, ⅔ cup
Potato, 2-in diameter
Celery, 1 cup
Tomato, raw, 1 medium
Corn on the cob, 2 in
Baked beans, canned, 2 Tbsp

Selected Food Sources of Fiber

Food	Grams per Serving	% Daily Value*
Navy beans, cooked, ½ cup	9.5	38
Bran ready-to-eat cereal (100%), ½ cup	8.8	35
Kidney beans, canned, ½ cup	8.2	33
Split peas, cooked, ½ cup	8.1	32
Lentils, cooked, ½ cup	7.8	31
Black beans, cooked, ½ cup	7.5	30
Pinto beans, cooked, ½ cup	7.7	31
Lima beans, cooked, ½ cup	6.6	26
Artichoke, globe, cooked, 1 each	6.5	26
White beans, canned, ½ cup	6.3	25
Chickpeas, cooked, ½ cup	6.2	24
Great northern beans, cooked, ½ cup	6.2	24
Cowpeas, cooked, ½ cup	5.6	22
Soybeans, mature, cooked, ½ cup	5.2	21
Bran ready-to-eat cereals, various, 1 oz	2.6-5.0	10-20
Crackers, rye wafers, plain, 2 wafers	5.0	20
Sweet potato, baked, with peel, l medium (146 g)	4.8	19
Asian pear, raw, 1 small	4.4	18
Green peas, cooked, ½ cup	4.4	18
Whole-wheat English muffin, 1 each	4.4	18
Pear, raw, 1 small	4.3	17
Bulgur, cooked, ½ cup	4.1	16

*Daily values (DVs) are reference numbers based on the recommended dietary allowance. They were developed to help consumers determine if a food contains a lot or a little of a specific nutrient. The DV for fiber is 25 g. The percent DV (%DV) listed on the Nutrition Facts panel of food labels states the percentage of the DV provided in 1 serving. %DVs are based on a 2000-calorie diet.

Food Sources of Dietary Fiber ranked by grams of dietary fiber per standard amount. (All are ≥10% of adequate intake for adult women, which is 25 g/day.)

APPENDIX 41. Nutritional Facts on a High-Fiber Diet—cont'd

Selected Food Sources of Fiber

Food	Grams per Serving	% Daily Value*
Mixed vegetables, cooked, ½ cup	4.0	16
Raspberries, raw, ½ cup	4.0	16
Sweet potato, boiled, no peel, 1 medium (156 g)	3.9	15.5
Blackberries, raw, ½ cup	3.8	15
Potato, baked, with skin, 1 medium	3.8	15
Soybeans, green, cooked, ½ cup	3.8	15
Stewed prunes, ½ cup	3.8	15
Figs, dried, ¼ cup	3.7	14.5
Dates, ¼ cup	3.6	14
Oat bran, raw, ¼ cup	3.6	14
Pumpkin, canned, ½ cup	3.6	14
Spinach, frozen, cooked, ½ cup	3.5	14
Shredded wheat ready-to-eat cereals, various, ≈1 oz	2.8-3.4	11-13
Almonds, 1 oz	3.3	13
Apple with skin, raw, 1 medium	3.3	13
Brussels sprouts, frozen, cooked, ½ cup	3.2	13
Whole-wheat spaghetti, cooked, ½ cup	3.1	12
Banana, 1 medium	3.1	12
Orange, raw, 1 medium	3.1	12
Oat bran muffin, 1 small	3.0	12
Guava, 1 medium	3.0	12
Pearled barley, cooked, ½ cup	3.0	12
Sauerkraut, canned, solids, and liquids, ½ cup	3.0	12
Tomato paste, ¼ cup	2.9	11.5
Winter squash, cooked, ½ cup	2.9	11.5
Broccoli, cooked, ½ cup	2.8	11
Parsnips, cooked, chopped, ½ cup	2.8	11
Turnip greens, cooked, ½ cup	2.5	10
Collards, cooked, ½ cup	2.7	11
Okra, frozen, cooked, ½ cup	2.6	10
Peas, edible-podded, cooked, ½ cup	2.5	10

High-Fiber Meal Plan

Breakfast	Lunch	Dinner
1 orange	3-oz boneless, skinless chicken breast	1 cup spaghetti with meat sauce
¾ cup raisin bran	½ cup broccoli	1 cup tossed salad with assorted vegetables and ¼ cup chickpeas*
2 slices whole wheat toast	½ cup long grain and wild rice	1 slice Italian bread
2 tsp margarine	1 whole wheat roll	½ cup apple crisp
1 cup skim milk	½ cup chocolate pudding	2 tsp margarine
1 cup coffee	½ Tbsp whipped topping	1 cup skim milk
2 tsp sugar	2 tsp margarine	1 cup coffee
	1 cup iced tea	¼ tsp salt
	¼ tsp salt	¼ tsp pepper
	¼ tsp pepper	2 tsp sugar
	2 tsp sugar	

Nutritional Analysis

Kilocalories: 2074
Protein: 84 g
Fat: 52 g
Carbohydrate: 313 g
Sodium: 4647 mg
Potassium: 3706 mg
Fiber: 28 g

*Fiber content may be higher, depending on vegetables selected for salad.

APPENDIX 42. Nutritional Facts on Fluid and Hydration

Adequate **hydration** is essential for life. Body water is necessary to regulate body temperature, transport nutrients, moisten body tissues, compose body fluids, and make waste products soluble for excretion. **Principles:** As the most plentiful substance in the human body, water is also the most plentiful nutrient in the diet. The amount of water recommended for an individual varies with age, activity, medical condition, and physical condition. The water in juice, tea, milk, decaffeinated coffee, and carbonated beverages contributes the majority of water in the diet. Solid foods also contribute water to the diet but usually are not counted in the amount of water provided per day.

Water deficiency, or **dehydration,** is characterized by dark urine; decreased skin turgor; dry mouth, lips, and mucous membranes; headache; a coated, wrinkled tongue; dry or sunken eyes; weight loss; a lowered body temperature; and increased serum sodium, albumin, blood urea nitrogen (BUN), and creatinine values. Dehydration may be caused by inadequate intake in relation to fluid requirements or excessive fluid losses caused by fever, increased urine output, diarrhea, draining wounds, ostomy output, fistulas, environmental temperature, or vomiting. Concentrated or high-protein tube feeding formulas may increase the water requirement.

Thirst is often the first noticed sign of the need for more water. However, athletes or workers exercising or working hard in hot climates may be significantly dehydrated before they realize they are thirsty. In these situations they should be drinking at regular intervals; they may not be able to rely on thirst to determine their need to drink.

Water excess or **overhydration** is rare and may be the result of inadequate output or excessive intake. Overhydration is characterized by increased blood pressure; decreased pulse rate; edema; and decreased serum sodium, potassium, albumin, BUN, and creatinine values. Fluid restrictions may be necessary for certain medical conditions such as kidney or cardiac disease. For those on fluid restrictions, the fluid needs should be calculated on an individual basis. The usual diet provides approximately 1080 mL (36 oz), a little more than a quart of fluid per day.

Approximate Fluid Content of Common Foods

Food	Fluid Ounces	Household Measure	Metric Measure
Juice	2	¼ cup	60 mL
	3	⅓ cup	90 mL
	4	½ cup	120 mL
	8	1 cup	240 mL
Coffee, tea, decaffeinated coffee	6	⅔ cup	180 mL
Gelatin	4	½ cup	120 mL
Ice cream, sherbet	3	⅓ cup	90 mL
Soup	6	⅔ cup	180 mL
Liquid coffee creamer	1	2 Tbsp	30 mL

Estimating Daily Fluid Requirements for Healthy Individuals

Children	Body Weight	Daily Fluid Requirement
Infants		140 to 150 mL/kg
Children		
Method 1		50 to 60 mL/kg
Method 2	3 to 10 kg of body weight	100 mL/kg
	11 to 20 kg of body weight	1000 mL + 50 mL/kg >10
	More than 20 kg	1500 mL + 20 mL/kg >20
Adults*		
Method 1	30 to 35 mL per weight in kilograms	
Method 2	1 mL fluid per calorie consumed	
Method 3	First 10 kg of body weight	100 mL/kg
	Second 10 kg of body weight	+50 mL/kg
	Remaining kg of body weight (age <50)	+20 mL/kg
	Remaining kg of body weight (age >50)	+15 mL/kg
Method 4	Age in years	
	16-30 (active)	40 mL/kg
	20-55	35 mL/kg
	55-75	30 mL/kg
	>75	25 mL/kg

From the California Diet Manual, ©2003, State of California Department of Developmental Services, revised 2004.

*The 1 mL of fluid per calorie method should be used with caution because it will underestimate the fluid needs of those with low-calorie needs. Persons who are significantly obese may best be evaluated by Method 3 because it adjusts for high body weight.

Note: 3 oz is approximately ⅓ cup; 6 oz is approximately ⅔ cup.

APPENDIX 43. Glycemic Index and Glycemic Load of Selected Foods*

Food	GI	GL
Breakfast Cereals		
Kellogg's All-Bran	30	4
Kellogg's Cocoa Puffs	77	20
Kellogg's Corn Flakes	92	24
Kellogg's MiniWheats	58	12
Kellogg's Nutrigrain	66	10
Old-fashioned oatmeal	42	9
Kellogg's Rice Krispies	82	22
Kellogg's Special K	69	14
Kellogg's Raisin Bran	61	12
Grains and Pastas		
Buckwheat	54	16
Bulgur	48	12
Rice		
Basmati	58	22
Brown	50	16
Instant	87	36
Uncle Ben's	39	14
Converted, white	4	
Noodles—instant	7	19
Pasta		
Egg fettuccine (avg)	40	18
Spaghetti (avg)	38	18
Vermicelli	35	16
Tortellini, Stouffer's	50	1
Bread		
Bagel	72	25
Croissant[†]	67	17
Crumpet	69	13
"Grainy" breads (avg)	49	6
Pita bread	57	10
Pumpernickel (avg)	50	6
Rye bread (avg)	58	8
White bread (avg)	70	10
Whole-wheat bread (avg)	77	9
Crackers and Crispbread		
Kavli	71	12
Puffed crisp bread	81	15
Ryvita	69	11
Water cracker	78	14
Cookies		
Oatmeal	55	12
Milk Arrowroot	69	12
Shortbread (commercial)[†]	64	10
Cake		
Chocolate, frosted, Betty Crocker	38	20
Oat bran muffin	69	24
Sponge cake	46	17
Waffles	76	10
Vegetables		
Beets, canned	64	5
Carrots (avg)	47	3
Parsnip	97	12
Peas (green, avg)	48	3
Potato		
Baked (avg)	85	26
Boiled	88	16
French fries	75	22
Microwaved	82	27
Pumpkin	75	3
Sweet corn	60	11
Sweet potato (avg)	61	17
Rutabaga	72	7
Yam (avg)	37	13
Legumes		
Baked beans (avg)	48	7
Broad beans	79	9
Butter beans	31	6
Chickpeas (avg)	28	8
Cannellini beans (avg)	38	12
Kidney beans (avg)	28	7
Lentils (avg)	29	5
Soy beans (avg)	18	1
Fruit		
Apple (avg)	38	6
Apricot (dried)	31	9
Banana (avg)	51	13
Cherries	22	3
Grapefruit	25	3
Grapes (avg)	46	8
Kiwi fruit (avg)	53	6
Mango	51	8
Orange (avg)	48	5
Papaya	59	10
Peach (avg)		
Canned (natural juice)	38	4
Fresh (avg)	42	5
Pear (avg)	38	4
Pineapple	59	7
Plum	39	5
Raisins	64	28
Cantaloupe	65	4
Watermelon	72	4
Dairy Foods		
Milk		
Full-fat	27	3
Skim	32	4
Chocolate-flavored	42	13
Condensed	61	33
Custard	43	7
Ice cream		
Regular (avg)	61	8
Low-fat	50	3
Yogurt, low-fat	33	10
Beverages		
Apple juice	40	12
Coca Cola	63	16
Lemonade	66	13
Fanta	68	23
Orange juice (avg)	52	12
Snack Foods		
Tortilla chips[†] (avg)	63	17
Fish sticks	38	7
Peanuts[†] (avg)	14	1
Popcorn	72	8
Potato chips[†]	57	10
Convenience Foods		
Macaroni and cheese	64	32
Soup		
Lentil	44	9
Split-pea	60	16
Tomato	38	6
Sushi (avg)	52	19
Pizza, cheese	60	16
Sweets		
Chocolate[†]	44	13
Jelly beans (avg)	78	22
Life Savers	70	21
Mars Bar	68	27
Kudo whole-grain chocolate-chip bar	62	20
Sugars		
Honey (avg)	55	10
Fructose (avg)	19	2
Glucose*	100	10
Lactose (avg)	46	5
Sucrose (avg)	68	7
Sports Bars		
Clif bar (cookies and cream)	101	3
PowerBar (chocolate)	83	35
METRx bar (vanilla)	74	37

From Brand Miller J et al: The new glucose revolution, New York, 2003, Avalon/Marlowe & Company.

*Glucose = 100.

[†]These foods are high in saturated fat.

APPENDIX 44. Nutritional Facts on a High-Protein Diet

The high-protein diet is designed for individuals requiring increased protein in addition to their normal diet. This diet provides additional high-quality protein, primarily from milk, eggs, cheese, soy, and meat sources. An individual's protein intake may be increased to 100 g of protein per day, or 1.25 up to 2 g/kg. Indications for use are the presence of pressure ulcers, surgery, infection, or malnutrition. Contraindications include hepatic coma and renal insufficiency. Patients on this diet may have loss of or poor appetite; therefore six feedings per day may improve patient adherence.

Adequacy: The high-protein diet is adequate in all nutrients and exceeds the dietary reference intake for protein.

Minimum Portions to Achieve 100 g of Protein

2-3 Cups or more (8 oz each) fortified milk or substitute
3-4 Servings (2-3 oz servings) meat or meat substitute
3-4 Servings fruits and vegetables (1 vitamin C–rich source daily such as 1 citrus fruit, 1 carotenoid source such as 1 dark green or yellow vegetable)
3-4 Servings or more of whole grain or enriched breads and cereals
Other foods are included to provide adequate calories.

Special Notes

1. Nonfat dry milk may be added to cooked foods to increase protein intake. One quarter cup powdered milk is equivalent to 1 cup fluid milk. Nonfat dry milk can be added to hot cereal, cream soups, and casseroles.
2. Supplemental high-protein feedings may be required if the patient has a poor appetite.
3. One fluid cup (8 oz) commercial eggnog contains 15 g of protein, almost twice as much protein as 1 fluid cup (8 oz) of milk. This is a very good snack for use in a high-protein diet.

Suggested Meal Pattern: High-Protein

Breakfast	Noon Meal	Evening Meal
½ cup fruit or juice	3 oz meat or substitute	3 oz meat or substitute
½ cup cereal	½ cup potato or substitute	½ cup potato or substitute
2 eggs	½ cup veg and/or	½ cup veg and/or
1 serving bread	½ cup veg and/or	½ cup veg and/or
1 tsp margarine	½-¾ cup salad	½-¾ cup salad
1 cup (8 oz) milk	Salad dressing	Salad dressing
Coffee or tea	1 serving bread	1 serving bread
	1 tsp margarine	1 tsp margarine
	½ cup fruit or dessert	½ cup fruit or dessert
	1 cup (8 oz) milk	1 cup (8 oz) milk
AM Snack	**PM Snack**	**Bedtime Snack**
8 oz. eggnog	Cheese or crackers	Milk and sandwich

APPENDIX 45. Nutritional Facts on Vegetarian Eating

These diets are designed for those who prefer vegetarian eating for religious, ecologic, or personal reasons. Because of the variations in vegetarian diets, it is recommended that the dietitian work closely with the patient and his or her family in establishing a diet pattern. Vegetarian diets are usually classified into one of the following three types:

1. Lacto-ovo-vegetarian is a modification of the diet, which restricts all dietary sources of animal protein except dairy products and eggs. This is the most common type of vegetarian diet and is the easiest of the vegetarian diets to prepare.
2. Lacto-vegetarian is a modification of the diet, which restricts all dietary sources of animal protein except dairy products.
3. Strict vegetarian (vegan diet) is a modification of the diet, which restricts all dietary sources of animal protein.

Adequacy: the lacto-ovo and lacto-vegetarian diets require careful planning to be adequate in all nutrients to meet the dietary reference intakes. The strict vegetarian diet (vegan diet) may be deficient in protein, zinc, calcium, and vitamins D and vitamin B_{12}; therefore supplements or fortified foods are recommended.

Protein: No foods are prepared with meat-based broth. Substitute soy-based and vegetable broths.

The following foods provide approximately the same amount of protein as does 1 oz of meat (7 g of protein):

¼ cup cottage cheese	½ cup legumes, cooked
1 cup regular or soy milk	¼ cup soy beans
1 oz cheese	1 oz processed soy protein
⅓ cup mixed nuts	¼ cup tofu (soy cheese)
1 egg	¾ cup yogurt
2 Tbsp peanut butter	

Proper protein combinations combine the essential amino acids to provide high-quality proteins, but they do not have to be at the same meal. The following list provides some of the combinations:

Grains

Rice with legumes
Rice cooked in milk
Corn with legumes
Macaroni and cheese
Whole-wheat bread and cheese
Whole-grain breakfast cereal with milk
Whole-wheat toast with poached egg

Nuts and Seeds

Peanut butter sandwich with milk
Sesame seeds with beans as in hummus

Legumes

Baked beans with whole-wheat bread
Legumes with rice
Split pea soup and whole-wheat bread
Soy beans with rice and wheat
Soy beans with corn and milk
Soy yogurt with granola

Vegetables

Lima beans, peas, Brussels sprouts, cauliflower or broccoli with sesame seeds, Brazil nuts, or mushrooms

Calcium: All vegetarians, especially young women, should ensure adequate calcium intake for development and maintenance of strong bones. In place of dairy products, choose abundant amounts of dark, leafy greens (e.g., kale, mustard and turnip greens, collards); bok choy; broccoli; legumes; tofu processed with calcium; dried figs; sunflower seeds; and calcium-fortified cereals and juice. The following foods provide approximately the same amount of calcium as 1 cup of milk (approximately 300 mg).

1 cup calcium-fortified soy milk	3 cups cooked dried beans
1⅓ cups sunflower seeds	1 cup almonds
1 cup collards, cooked	3 pieces enriched cornbread

APPENDIX 45. Nutritional Facts on Vegetarian Eating—cont'd

Iron: Iron deficiency rates are similar between vegetarians and nonvegetarians. When consumed along with foods rich in vitamin C, plant sources of iron are better absorbed. High-iron foods include legumes, dark green vegetables (i.e., spinach and beet greens), dried fruits; prune juice, blackstrap molasses, pumpkin seeds, soy nuts, and iron-fortified breads and cereals.

Vitamin B12: Found only in animal foods, vitamin B12 is not a nutrient of great concern for vegetarians who regularly consume eggs or dairy products (lacto-ovo-vegetarians). Vegans should include vitamin B12–fortified foods such as fortified soy milk and commercial breakfast cereals, or a B12 supplement in their diets. Vitamin B12 is also found in Brewer's yeast.

Vitamin D: In the United States the primary source of vitamin D is dairy products, most of which are fortified with vitamin D. However, cheese and yogurt do not have to be made from vitamin D–fortified milk. The other main source results from sunlight exposure, causing vitamin D to be synthesized in the skin. If dairy products are not consumed and direct sunlight exposure is limited, supplementation is warranted. Foods containing vitamin D include fortified cow's milk, soy milk, rice milk, or nut milk. Supplementation is needed for individuals who do not consume milk products or who spend little time in the sun.

Zinc: Because zinc is found in animal foods, the vegetarian diet may be limited. The following foods can be included in the diet to increase the needed amount of zinc:

- Wheat germ
- Nuts
- Dried beans

Minimum Portions to Be Included Daily

Food Categories	Recommended Daily Servings	Recommended Serving Sizes
Breads, cereals, rice, and pasta	6 or more	1 slice bread 1 oz ready to eat cereal, calcium fortified* ½ cup cooked cereal, rice, or pasta
Vegetables	4 or more	1 cup raw leafy vegetables, ½ cup cooked vegetables, calcium rich—1 cup cooked, 2 cups raw: bok choy,* okra,* broccoli,* collards,* kale,* Chinese cabbage,* mustard greens* ½ cup vegetable juice fortified*
Fruits	2 or more	1 medium piece of fruit ½ cup chopped, cooked, or canned fruit, figs (5)* ½ cup fruit juice, fortified*
Calcium-rich foods	8 or more	1 cup milk, yogurt, ½ cup fortified soy milk ¾ oz natural cheese 2 oz process cheese
Legumes and meat substitutes	5	½ cup cooked dry beans, soybeans* or peas, ½ cup soy nuts* 1 egg or 2 egg whites (optional) ¼ cup nuts or seeds, ¼ cup almonds* ½ cup Tempeh or calcium-set tofu* 2 Tbsp almond butter or sesame tahini,* 2 Tbsp peanut butter
Fats, sweets, and alcohol	Use sparingly	

*Calcium-rich foods.

Special Notes

Pregnancy and Lactation: Well-planned vegan and lacto-ovo-vegetarian eating patterns adequately provide for the nutritional needs of pregnant and lactating women (American Dietetic Association, 2003). Folate supplements are recommended for all pregnant women, including vegetarians. Vegans must ensure daily intake of 2 mcg of vitamin B12 daily during pregnancy and 2.6 mcg during lactation, whether through supplements or fortified foods. Women with limited sun exposure should include vitamin D–fortified foods. Caution should be used with vitamin D supplementation because excess vitamin D can cause fetal abnormalities.

Infants, Children, and Adolescents: According to the American Dietetic Association (2003), well-planned vegan and lacto-ovo-vegetarian eating patterns adequately provide for the nutritional needs of infants, children, and adolescents. Because of the high bulk of low-fat vegetarian eating patterns, it may be difficult for children and adolescents to consume enough food to provide for their energy needs. Frequent meals and snacks with nutrient-dense foods can help meet energy and nutrient needs. If sun exposure is limited, vitamin D fortified–foods or supplements may be used. Vegan children should include a reliable source of vitamin B12 in their diets. To provide for growth, calcium, iron, and zinc intakes deserve special attention. It is recommended that parents of vegetarian infants and youth consult a registered dietitian with expertise in the vegetarian eating pattern.

Continued

APPENDIX 45. Nutritional Facts on Vegetarian Eating—cont'd

Meal Pattern: Lacto-Ovo-Vegetarian

Breakfast	Lunch	Dinner	Snack
½ cup orange juice (calcium fortified)	2-3 oz meat alt	2-3 oz meat alt	½ cup soy nuts
½ cup cereal	½ cup potato or substitute	½ cup rice or substitute	½ cup fortified tomato juice
1 egg	½ cup vegetable	½ cup vegetable	
1 serving bread	½-¾ cup salad	½-¾ cup salad	
1 tsp margarine	Salad dressing	Salad dressing	
1 cup (8 oz) milk	1 serving bread	1 serving bread	
Coffee or tea	1 tsp margarine	1 tsp margarine	
2 tsp sugar	½ cup fruit	½ cup fruit	
	½ cup (4 oz) milk	½ cup (4 oz) milk	
	Coffee/tea	Coffee or tea	
	¼ tsp salt	½ tsp salt	
	½ tsp pepper	½ tsp pepper	

Meal Pattern: Lacto-Vegetarian

Breakfast	Lunch	Dinner	Snack
½ cup orange juice (calcium fortified)	2-3 oz meat alt	2-3 oz meat alt	½ cup soy nuts
½ cup cereal	½ cup pasta or substitute	½ cup brown rice or substitute	½ cup fortified tomato juice
1 egg	½ cup vegetable	½ cup vegetable	
1 serving bread	½-¾ cup salad	½-¾ cup salad	
1 tsp margarine	Salad dressing	Salad dressing	
1 cup (8 oz) milk	1 serving bread	1 serving bread	
Coffee or tea	1 tsp margarine	1 tsp margarine	
2 tsp sugar	½ cup fruit	½ cup fruit	
	½ cup (4 oz) milk	½ cup (4 oz) milk	
	Coffee or tea	Coffee or tea	
	¼ tsp salt	¼ tsp salt	
	¼ tsp pepper	¼ tsp pepper	

Meal Pattern: Vegan

Breakfast	Lunch	Dinner	Snack
½ cup orange juice (calcium fortified)	6 oz lentil soup with ½ cup brown rice	2 burritos:	¼ cup soy nuts
½ cup oatmeal	4 sesame seed crackers	2- to 6-in soft corn tortillas	½ cup fortified tomato juice
2 slices whole wheat bread	Spinach salad:	1 cup pinto beans	
2 Tbsp peanut butter*	1 cup raw spinach	¾ cup shredded lettuce	
1 cup fortified soy milk	¼ cup shredded carrot	½ cup diced tomato	
2 Tbsp raisins	2 Tbsp chopped mushrooms	2 Tbsp diced onions	
2 tsp sugar	2 oz tofu (calcium set)	¼ cup salsa	
	2 Tbsp low calorie Italian dressing	½ cup broccoli and cauliflower mix	
	1 fresh apple	1 Tbsp margarine	
	1 cup fortified soy milk	½ cup fruit cocktail	
	¼ tsp salt	1 cup fortified soy milk	
	¼ tsp pepper	¼ tsp salt	
		¼ tsp pepper	

Nutritional Analysis

Kilocalories: 2395
Protein: 93 g
Total fat: 90 g
Monounsaturated fat: 33.2 g
Polyunsaturated fat: 30.8 g
Carbohydrates: 323 g
Sodium: 5762 mg*
Potassium: 4690 mg
Fiber: 45 g

*Use unsalted peanut butter, tomato juice, and soup to reduce sodium content.

Data from National Center for Nutrition and Dietetics, Food guide pyramid for vegetarian meal planning. Chicago, 1997, American Dietetic Association Foundation; American Dietetic Association: Position of the American Dietetic Association: vegetarian diets, J Am Diet Assoc 103:748-765, 2003.

APPENDIX 46. Nutritional Facts on Folic Acid, Vitamin B_6, and Vitamin B_{12}

Folate is a water-soluble B vitamin that occurs naturally in food. Folic acid is the synthetic form of folate that is found in supplements and added to fortified foods. Folate or folic acid helps produce and maintain new cells, which is especially important during periods of rapid cell division and growth such as infancy, adolescence, and pregnancy. Folate is needed to make deoxyribonucleic acid (DNA) and ribonucleic acid, the building blocks of cells. It also helps prevent changes to DNA that may lead to cancer. Both adults and children need folate to make normal red blood cells and prevent anemia. Folate is also essential for the metabolism of homocysteine and helps maintain normal levels of this amino acid.

Dietary Reference Intakes for Folate for Children and Adults

Age (years)	Males and Females (mcg/day)	Pregnancy (mcg/day)	Lactation (mcg/day)
1-3	150	N/A	N/A
4-8	200	N/A	N/A
9-13	300	N/A	N/A
14-18	400	600	500
19+	400	600	500

N/A, Not applicable.

Selected Food Sources of Folate and Folic Acid

Food	Micrograms per Serving	% Daily Value*
Breakfast cereals fortified with 100% of the DV, ¾ cup†	400	100
Beef liver, cooked, braised, 3 oz	185	45
Cowpeas (blackeyes), immature, cooked, boiled, ½ cup	105	25
Breakfast cereals, fortified with 25% of the DV, ¾ cup†	100	25
Spinach, frozen, cooked, boiled, ½ cup	100	25
Great Northern beans, boiled, ½ cup	90	20
Asparagus, boiled, 4 spears	85	20
Rice, white, long-grain, parboiled, enriched, cooked, ½ cup†	65	15
Vegetarian baked beans, canned, 1 cup	60	15
Spinach, raw, 1 cup	60	15
Green peas, frozen, boiled, ½ cup	50	15
Broccoli, chopped, frozen, cooked, ½ cup	50	15
Egg noodles, cooked, enriched, ½ cup†	50	15
Broccoli, raw, 2 spears (each 5 in long)	45	10
Avocado, raw, all varieties, sliced, ½ cup sliced	45	10
Peanuts, all types, dry roasted, 1 oz	40	10
Lettuce, Romaine, shredded, ½ cup	40	10
Wheat germ, crude, 2 Tbsp	40	10
Tomato juice, canned, 6 oz	35	10
Orange juice, chilled, includes concentrate, ¾ cup	35	10
Turnip greens, frozen, cooked, boiled, ½ cup	30	8
Orange, all commercial varieties, fresh, 1 small	30	8
Bread, white, 1 slice†	25	6
Bread, whole wheat, 1 slice†	25	6
Egg, whole, raw, fresh, 1 large	25	6
Cantaloupe, raw, ¼ medium	25	6
Papaya, raw, ½ cup cubes	25	6
Banana, raw, 1 medium	20	6

DV, Daily value.

*DVs are reference numbers based on the recommended dietary allowance. They were developed to help consumers determine if a food contains a lot or a little of a specific nutrient. The DV for folate is 400 mcg. The %DV listed on the Nutrition Facts panel of food labels states the percentage of the DV provided in one serving.

†Fortified with folic acid as part of the Folate Fortification Program.

Vitamin B_6

Vitamin B_6 is a water-soluble vitamin that exists in three major chemical forms: pyridoxine, pyridoxal, and pyridoxamine and performs a wide variety of functions in the body. It is needed for more than 100 enzymes involved in protein metabolism and is essential for red blood cell metabolism. The nervous and immune systems need vitamin B_6 to function efficiently, and it is also needed for the conversion of tryptophan (an amino acid) to niacin. A vitamin B_6 deficiency can result in a form of anemia that is similar to iron deficiency anemia.

Through its involvement in protein metabolism and cellular growth, vitamin B_6 is important to the immune system. It helps maintain the health of lymphoid organs (thymus, spleen, and lymph nodes) that make white blood cells. It is also important for maintaining normal blood glucose levels.

Continued

APPENDIX 46. Nutritional Facts on Folic Acid, Vitamin B_6, and Vitamin B_{12}—cont'd

Dietary Reference Intakes for Vitamin B_6 for Children and Adults

Age (years)	Males and Females (mg/day)	Pregnancy (mg/day)	Lactation (mg/day)
1-3	0.5	N/A	N/A
4-8	0.6	N/A	N/A
9-13	1.0	N/A	N/A
14-18	1.3	1.9	2.0
19+	1.3	1.9	2.0

N/A, Not applicable.

Selected Food Sources of Vitamin B_6

Food	Milligrams per serving	% Daily Value*
Ready-to-eat cereal, 100% fortified, ¾ cup	2.00	100%
Potato, baked, flesh and skin, 1 medium	0.70	35%
Banana, raw, 1 medium	0.68	34%
Garbanzo beans, canned, ½ cup	0.57	30%
Chicken breast, meat only, cooked, ½ breast	0.52	25%
Ready-to-eat cereal, 25% fortified, ¾ cup	0.50	25%
Oatmeal, instant, fortified, 1 packet	0.42	20%
Pork loin, lean only, cooked, 3 oz	0.42	20%
Roast beef, eye of round, lean only, cooked, 3 oz	0.32	15%
Trout, rainbow, cooked, 3 oz	0.29	15%
Sunflower seeds, kernels, dry roasted, 1 oz	0.23	10%
Spinach, frozen, cooked, ½ cup	0.14	8%
Tomato juice, canned, 6 oz	0.20	10%
Avocado, raw, sliced, ½ cup	0.20	10%
Salmon, Sockeye, cooked, 3 oz	0.19	10%
Tuna, canned in water, drained solids, 3 oz	0.18	10%
Wheat bran, crude or unprocessed, ¼ cup	0.18	10%
Peanut butter, smooth, 2 Tbsp	0.15	8%
Walnuts, English or Persian, 1 oz	0.15	8%
Soybeans, green, boiled, drained, ½ cup	0.05	2%
Lima beans, frozen, cooked, drained, ½ cup	0.10	6%

*Daily values (DVs) are reference numbers based on the recommended dietary allowance. They were developed to help consumers determine if a food contains a lot or a little of a specific nutrient. The DV for vitamin B_6 is 2 mg. The %DV listed on the Nutrition Facts panel of food labels states the percentage of the DV provided in one serving.

Vitamin B_{12}

Along with folate and vitamin B_6, vitamin B_{12} is helpful in lowering the level of the amino acid homocysteine in the blood. It has been hypothesized that at high levels homocysteine might damage coronary arteries or make it easier for blood-clotting cells to clump together and form a clot. This could increase risks for a heart attack or stroke.

Vitamin B_{12} is a member of the vitamin B complex. It contains cobalt; thus it is also known as cobalamin. It is exclusively synthesized by bacteria and is found primarily in meat, eggs, and dairy products. There has been considerable research into proposed plant sources of vitamin B_{12}. Fermented soy products, seaweeds, and algae (spirulina) have all been suggested as containing significant B_{12}. However, the present consensus is that any B_{12} present in plant foods is likely to be unavailable to humans; thus these foods should not be relied on as safe sources. Many vegan foods are supplemented with B_{12}.

Vitamin B_{12} is necessary for the synthesis of red blood cells, the maintenance of the nervous system, and growth and development in children. Deficiency can cause anemia. Vitamin B_{12} neuropathy, involving the degeneration of nerve fibers and irreversible neurologic damage, can also occur. Vitamin B_{12} can be stored in small amounts by the body. Proper vitamin B_{12} absorption requires the presence of intrinsic factor, which tends to diminish with aging. Total body store is 2 to 5 mg in adults. Approximately 80% of this is stored in the liver.

Dietary Reference Intakes for Vitamin B_{12} for Children and Adults

Age (years)	Males and Females (mcg/day)	Pregnancy (mcg/day)	Lactation (mcg/day)
1-3	0.9	N/A	N/A
4-8	1.2	N/A	N/A
9-13	1.8	N/A	N/A
14-18	2.4	2.6	2.8
19 and older	2.4	2.6	2.8

N/A, Not applicable.

APPENDIX 46. Nutritional Facts on Folic Acid, Vitamin B_6, and Vitamin B_{12}—cont'd

Selected Food Sources of Vitamin B_{12}

Food	Micrograms per Serving	% Daily Value*
Mollusks, clam, mixed species, cooked, 3 oz	84.1	1400
Liver, beef, braised, 1 slice	47.9	780
Fortified breakfast cereals (100% fortified), ¾ cup	6.0	100
Trout, rainbow, wild, cooked, 3 oz	5.4	90
Salmon, sockeye, cooked, 3 oz	4.9	80
Trout, rainbow, farmed, cooked, 3 oz	4.2	50
Beef, top sirloin, lean, choice, broiled, 3 oz	2.4	40
Fast food, cheeseburger, regular, double patty and bun, 1 sandwich	1.9	30
Fast food, taco, 1 large	1.6	25
Fortified breakfast cereals (25% fortified), ¾ cup	1.5	25
Yogurt, plain, skim, with 13 g of protein per cup, 1 cup	1.4	25
Haddock, cooked, 3 oz	1.2	20
Clams, breaded and fried, ¾ cup	1.1	20
Tuna, white, canned in water, drained solids, 3 oz	1.0	15
Milk, 1 cup	0.9	15
Pork, cured, ham, lean only, canned, roasted, 3 oz	0.6	10
Egg, whole, hard boiled, 1	0.6	10
American pasteurized cheese food, 1 oz	0.3	6
Chicken, breast, meat only, roasted, ½ breast	0.3	6

*Daily values (DVs) are reference numbers based on the recommended dietary allowance. They were developed to help consumers determine if a food contains a lot or a little of a specific nutrient. The DV for vitamin B_{12} is 6 mcg. The %DV listed on the Nutrition Facts panel of food labels states the percentage of the DV provided in one serving.

APPENDIX 47. Nutritional Facts on Vitamin A and Carotenoids

Vitamin A includes a group of compounds that affect vision, bone growth, reproduction, cell division, immunity, healthy surface linings of the respiratory tract, and mucous membranes. There are two categories of vitamin A, depending on whether the food source is an animal or a plant. Vitamin A found in foods that come from animals is called *preformed vitamin A* and is absorbed as retinol. Sources include liver, whole milk, and some fortified food products. In the body retinol can be made into retinal and retinoic acid (other active forms of vitamin A). Vitamin A deficiency rarely occurs in the United States, but vitamin A is needed for children with measles, infection, or eye disease in communities where vitamin A deficiency is a serious problem. Fat malabsorption can result in diarrhea and prevent normal absorption of vitamin A; this may result in vitamin A deficiency in celiac disease, Crohn's disease, and pancreatic disorders. The best absorbed form of vitamin A is in the oil form such as in cod liver oil.

Plant sources of vitamin A provide the provitamin A, called *carotenoids.* They can be made into retinol in the body and then to the other active forms of vitamin A. In the United States approximately 26% to 34% of vitamin A consumed is in the form of provitamin A carotenoids. Common provitamin A carotenoids found in plants give them color and are β-carotene, α-carotene, and β-cryptoxanthin. Among these, β-carotene is most efficiently made into retinol. The darker the color of a fruit or vegetable, the greater is its carotenoid content.

Dietary Reference Intakes for Vitamin A for Children and Adults

Age (years)	Males and Females (mcg RAEs/day)	Pregnancy (mcg RAEs/day)	Lactation (mcg RAEs/day)
1-3	300	N/A	N/A
4-8	400	N/A	N/A
9-13	600	N/A	N/A
14-18	900 for boys; 700 for girls	1200	750
19+	900 for men; 700 for women	770	1300

N/A, Not applicable; *RAE,* Retinol activity equivalent.

1 RAE = 1 mcg of retinol = 12 mg of β-carotene = 3.33 IU of vitamin A on a label.

Food Sources of Vitamin A

Vitamin A in foods is expressed as micrograms of retinol activity equivalents (RAEs) of vitamin A per standard amount, but it is also stated as IU = 0.33 mcg RAEs. (All are ≥20% of the recommended dietary allowance for adult men, which is 900 mcg RAE/day.)

Selected Animal Sources of Vitamin A

Food	Vitamin A (IU)	% Daily Value
Liver, beef, cooked, 3 oz	27,185	545
Liver, chicken, cooked, 3 oz	12,325	245
Milk, fortified skim, 1 cup	500	10
Cheese, cheddar, 1 oz	284	6
Milk, whole (3.25% fat), 1 cup	249	5
Egg substitute, ¼ cup	226	5

Continued

APPENDIX 47. Nutritional Facts on Vitamin A and Carotenoids—cont'd

Selected Plant Sources of Vitamin A (from β-Carotene)

Food	Vitamin A (IU)	% Daily Value*
Carrot juice, canned, ½ cup	22,567	450
Carrots, boiled, ½ cup slices	13,418	270
Spinach, frozen, boiled, ½ cup	11,458	230
Kale, frozen, boiled, ½ cup	9558	190
Carrots, 1 raw (7½ in)	8666	175
Vegetable soup, canned, chunky, ready-to-serve, 1 cup	5820	115
Cantaloupe, 1 cup cubes	5411	110
Spinach, raw, 1 cup	2813	55
Apricots with skin, juice pack, ½ cup	2063	40
Apricot nectar, canned, ½ cup	1651	35
Papaya, 1 cup cubes	1532	30
Mango, 1 cup sliced	1262	25
Oatmeal, instant, fortified, plain, prepared with water, 1 cup	1252	25
Peas, frozen, boiled, ½ cup	1050	20
Tomato juice, canned, 6 oz	819	15
Peaches, canned, juice pack, ½ cup halves or slices	473	10
Peach, 1 medium	319	6
Pepper, sweet, red, raw, 1 ring (3 inches diameter by ¼ inch thick)	313	6

*Daily values (DVs) are reference numbers based on the recommended dietary allowances. They were developed to help consumers determine if a food contains a lot or a little of a nutrient. The DV for vitamin A is 5000 IU. Most food labels do not list vitamin A content. The %DV column in this table indicates the percentage of the DV provided in one serving. A food providing 5% or less of the DV is a low source, whereas a food that provides 10% to 19% of the DV is a good source. A food that provides 20% or more of the DV is high in that nutrient. It is important to remember that foods that provide lower percentages of the DV also contribute to a healthful diet.

Another way to summarize important foods is through **retinol equivalents.**

Food	Vitamin A (mcg RAEs)	Calories
Organ meats (liver, giblets), various, cooked, 3 oz†	1490-9126	134-235
Carrot juice, ¾ cup	1692	71
Sweet potato with peel, baked, 1 medium	1096	103
Pumpkin, canned, ½ cup	953	42
Carrots, cooked from fresh, ½ cup	671	27
Spinach, cooked from frozen, ½ cup	573	30
Collards, cooked from frozen, ½ cup	489	31
Kale, cooked from frozen, ½ cup	478	20
Mixed vegetables, canned, ½ cup	474	40
Turnip greens, cooked from frozen, ½ cup	441	24
Instant cooked cereals, fortified, prepared, 1 packet	285-376	75-97
Various ready-to-eat cereals, with added vitamin A, ≈1 oz	180-376	100-117
Carrot, raw, 1 small	301	20
Beet greens, cooked, ½ cup	276	19
Winter squash, cooked, ½ cup	268	38
Dandelion greens, cooked, ½ cup	260	18
Cantaloupe, raw, ¼ medium melon	233	46
Mustard greens, cooked, ½ cup	221	11
Pickled herring, 3 oz	219	222
Red sweet pepper, cooked, ½ cup	186	19
Chinese cabbage, cooked, ½ cup	180	10

RAE, Retinol activity equivalent.

Note: Mixed dishes and multiple preparations of the same food item have been omitted from this table.

†High in cholesterol.

Carotenoids in Fruits and Vegetables

	Neoxanthins and Violaxanthins	Lutein and zeaxanthin	Lutein	Zeaxanthin	Cryptoxanthins	Lycopenes	β-carotene	β-carotene
Egg yolk	8	89	54	35	4	0	0	0
Maize (corn)	9	86	60	26	5	0	0	0
Kiwi	38	54	54	0	0	0	0	8
Red seedless grapes	23	53	43	10	4	5	3	16
Zucchini squash	19	52	47	5	24	0	0	5
Pumpkin	30	49	49	0	0	0	0	21
Spinach	14	47	47	0	19	4	0	16
Orange pepper	4	45	8	37	22	0	8	21
Yellow squash	19	44	44	0	0	0	28	9
Cucumber	16	42	38	4	38	0	0	4
Pea	33	41	41	0	21	0	0	5
Green pepper	29	39	36	3	20	0	0	12
Red grape	27	37	33	4	29	0	1	6
Butternut squash	24	37	37	0	34	0	5	0
Orange juice	28	35	15	20	25	0	3	8
Honeydew	18	35	17	18	0	0	0	48
Celery (stalks, leaves)	12	34	32	2	40	1	13	0
Green grapes	10	31	25	6	52	0	0	7
Brussels sprouts	20	29	27	2	39	0	0	11
Scallions	32	29	27	2	35	4	0	0
Green beans	27	25	22	3	42	0	1	5

APPENDIX 47. Nutritional Facts on Vitamin A and Carotenoids—cont'd

	Neoxanthins and Violaxanthins	Lutein and zeaxanthin	Lutein	Zeaxanthin	Cryptoxanthins	Lycopenes	β-carotene	β-carotene
Orange	36	22	7	15	12	11	8	11
Broccoli	3	22	22	0	49	0	0	27
Apple (red delicious)	22	20	19	1	23	13	5	17
Mango	52	18	2	16	4	6	0	20
Green lettuce	33	15	15	0	36	0	16	0
Tomato juice	0	13	11	2	2	57	12	16
Peach	20	13	5	8	8	0	10	50
Yellow pepper	86	12	12	0	1	0	1	0
Nectarine	18	11	6	5	23	0	0	48
Red pepper	56	7	7	0	2	8	24	3
Tomato (fruit)	0	6	6	0	0	82	0	12
Carrots	0	2	2	0	0	0	43	55
Cantaloupe	9	1	1	0	0	3	0	87
Dried apricots	2	1	1	0	9	0	0	87
Green kidney beans	72	0	0	0	28	0	0	0

Table from Sommerburg O et al: Fruits and vegetables that are sources for lutein and zeaxanthin: the macular pigment in human eyes, Br J Ophthalmol 82:907, 1998.

The content of the major carotenoids are given in mole%. The amounts of the carotenoids were shown in seven major groups, as neoxanthins and violaxanthins (neoxanthin, violaxanthin, and their related isomers, lutein 5, 6 epoxide), lutein, zeaxanthin, cryptoxanthins (α-cryptoxanthin, β-cryptoxanthins, and related isomers), lycopenes (lycopene and related isomers), β-carotene (all *trans* β-carotene and *cis* isomers), and β-carotene (all *trans* β-carotene and *cis* isomers). Lutein and zeaxanthin are given combined and as single amounts. The data are sorted by the combined amount of lutein and zeaxanthin.

APPENDIX 48. Nutritional Facts on Vitamin C

Vitamin C is a nutrient required in very small amounts to allow a range of essential metabolic reactions in the body. Vitamin C is principally known as a water-soluble antioxidant, and it prevents scurvy. It is also known by the chemical name of its principal form, L-ascorbic acid or simply ascorbic acid. The dietary reference intakes range from 15 to 90 mg/day as shown in the following table, with a tolerable upper intake of no more than 2 g/day (2000 mg/day).

Dietary Reference Intakes for Vitamin C for Children and Adults

Age (years)	Males and Females (mg/day)	Pregnancy (mg/day)	Lactation (mg/day)
1-3	15	N/A	N/A
4-8	25	N/A	N/A
9-13	45	N/A	N/A
14-18	75 for boys; 65 for girls	80	115
19+	90 for men; 75 for women	85	120

N/A, Not applicable.

Continued

APPENDIX 48. Nutritional Facts on Vitamin C—cont'd

Selected Food Sources of Vitamin C

Food	Milligrams per Serving	% Daily Value*
Guava, raw, ½ cup	188	209
Red sweet pepper, raw, ½ cup	142	158
Red sweet pepper, cooked, ½ cup	116	129
Kiwi fruit, 1 medium	70	78
Orange, raw, 1 medium	70	78
Orange juice, ¾ cup	61-93	68-103
Green pepper, sweet, raw, ½ cup	60	67
Green pepper, sweet, cooked, ½ cup	51	56.6
Grapefruit juice, ¾ cup	50-70	55.5-78
Vegetable juice cocktail, ¾ cup	50	55.5
Strawberries, raw, ½ cup	49	54
Brussels sprouts, cooked, ½ cup	48	53
Cantaloupe, ¼ medium	47	52
Papaya, raw, ¼ medium	47	52
Kohlrabi, cooked, ½ cup	45	50
Broccoli, raw, ½ cup	39	43
Edible pod peas, cooked, ½ cup	38	42
Broccoli, cooked, ½ cup	37	41
Sweet potato, canned, ½ cup	34	38
Tomato juice, ¾ cup	33	36.5
Cauliflower, cooked, ½ cup	28	31
Pineapple, raw, ½ cup	28	31
Kale, cooked, ½ cup	27	30
Mango, ½ cup	23	25.5

*Daily values (DVs) are reference numbers based on the recommended dietary allowance. They were developed to help consumers determine if a food contains a lot or a little of a specific nutrient. The DV for vitamin C is 90 mg. The %DV listed on the Nutrition Facts panel of food labels states the percentage of the DV provided in one serving.

APPENDIX 49. Nutritional Facts on Vitamin E

Vitamin E is a fat-soluble vitamin that exists in eight different forms. Each form has its own biologic activity, which is the measure of potency or functional use in the body. α-Tocopherol is the name of the most active form; it is a powerful biologic antioxidant. Vitamin E in supplements is usually sold as α-tocopheryl acetate, a form of α-tocopherol that protects its ability to function as an antioxidant. The synthetic form is labeled *dl*, whereas the natural form is labeled *d*. The synthetic form is only half as active as the natural form. It is important to include foods high in vitamin E on a daily basis to get enough vitamin E from foods alone. Vegetable oils, nuts, green leafy vegetables, and fortified cereals are common food sources of vitamin E.

Vitamin E deficiency is usually characterized by neurologic problems in the hands and feet, as well as peroxidation of cellular lipid membranes. Although vitamin E deficiency is rare in humans, it is likely to occur in specific situations:

1. In persons who cannot absorb dietary fat because of an inability to secrete bile or those who have rare disorders of fat metabolism
2. In individuals with rare genetic abnormalities in the α-tocopherol transfer protein
3. In premature, very-low-birth weight infants (birth weights less than 1500 g, or 3 lb, 4 oz)

Most food labels do not list a the vitamin E content of food. The percent daily value (%DV) listed on the table indicates the percentage of the DV provided in one serving. The DV for vitamin E is 30 IU. A food providing 5% of the DV or less is a low source, whereas a food that provides 10% to 19% of the DV is a good source. A food that provides 20% or more of the DV provides 6 units and is considered high in vitamin E. Vitamin E content of food is stated as milligrams of α-tocopherol, milligrams of α-tocopherol equivalents (mg α-TE), or as units on supplement labels. 1 unit = 0.67 α-TE in the *d* form and approximately ½ of that in the *dl* or synthetic form.

Dietary Reference Intakes for Vitamin E (in milligrams) of α-TE for Children and Adults

Age (years)	Males and Females (mg/day)	Pregnancy (mg/day)	Lactation (mg/day)
1-3	6	N/A	N/A
4-8	7	N/A	N/A
9-13	11	N/A	N/A
14-18	15	15	19
19+	15	15	19

N/A, Not applicable.

APPENDIX 49. Nutritional Facts on Vitamin E—cont'd

Selected Food Sources of Vitamin E

Food	Milligrams per Serving	% Daily Value*
Fortified ready-to-eat cereals, ≈1 oz	1.6-12.8	11-85
Sunflower seeds, dry roasted, 1 oz	7.4	49
Almonds, 1 oz	7.3	
Sunflower oil, high linoleic, 1 Tbsp	5.6	37
Cottonseed oil, 1 Tbsp	4.8	32
Safflower oil, high oleic, 1 Tbsp	4.6	31
Hazelnuts (filberts), 1 oz	4.3	29
Mixed nuts, dry roasted, 1 oz	3.1	21
Turnip greens, frozen, cooked, ½ cup	2.9	19
Tomato paste, ¼ cup	2.8	18
Pine nuts, 1 oz	2.6	17
Peanut butter, 2 Tbsp	2.5	16.5
Tomato puree, ½ cup	2.5	16.5
Tomato sauce, ½ cup	2.5	16.5
Canola oil, 1 Tbsp	2.4	16
Wheat germ, toasted, plain, 2 Tbsp	2.3	15
Peanuts, 1 oz	2.2	14.5
Avocado, raw, ½ avocado	2.1	14
Carrot juice, canned, ¾ cup	2.1	14
Peanut oil, 1 Tbsp	2.1	14
Corn oil, 1 Tbsp	1.9	12.5
Olive oil, 1 Tbsp	1.9	12.5
Spinach, cooked, ½ cup	1.9	12.5
Dandelion greens, cooked, ½ cup	1.8	12
Sardine, Atlantic, in oil, drained, 3 oz	1.7	11
Blue crab, cooked or canned, 3 oz	1.6	10.5
Brazil nuts, 1 oz	1.6	10.5
Herring, Atlantic, pickled, 3 oz	1.5	10

*Daily values (DVs) are reference numbers based on the recommended dietary allowance. They were developed to help consumers determine if a food contains a lot or a little of a specific nutrient. The DV for vitamin E is 15 mg α-TE. The %DV listed on the Nutrition Facts panel of food labels states the percentage of the DV provided in one serving.

Sample Meal Plan

Breakfast

¾ cup ready-to-eat cereal
½ cup low-fat or fat-free milk
1 red delicious apple
2 Tbsp peanut butter (2.5 mg vitamin E)

Lunch

1 cup mixed salad greens
3 oz tuna steak
2 slices multigrain bread
½ cup fruit salad

Dinner

3 oz grilled chicken breast
½ cup fresh steamed spinach (1.9 mg vitamin E)
½ cup whole grain rice
Side salad

Snack

1 oz sliced almonds (7.3 mg vitamin E)
1 Tbsp low-fat granola
½ cup low-fat or fat-free yogurt

Note: Take one multivitamin or multimineral supplement daily.

APPENDIX 50. Nutritional Facts on Vitamin K

Vitamin K comes from the foods that we eat and the bacteria that normally reside in the intestines, which are able to make vitamin K. Antibiotics may interfere with this normal production. Other circumstances that may lead to vitamin K deficiency include liver disease, serious burns, health problems that can prevent the absorption of vitamin K (such as gallbladder or biliary disease, which may alter the absorption of fat), cystic fibrosis, celiac disease, Crohn's disease, and chronic antibiotic therapy. Excess vitamin E can inhibit vitamin K activity and precipitate signs of deficiency. The classic sign of a vitamin K deficiency is a prolonged prothrombin time, which increases the risk of spontaneous hemorrhage. Because vitamin K is stored in the liver, clinical deficiencies are rare.

Vitamin K is needed to make clotting factors that help the blood to clot and prevent bleeding. The amount of vitamin K in food may affect drug therapy, such as that from warfarin or other anticoagulants. When taking these medications, it is necessary to eat a normal, balanced diet, maintaining a consistent amount of vitamin K, and avoiding drastic changes in dietary habits.

In general, leafy green vegetables and certain legumes and vegetable oils contain high amounts of vitamin K. Foods that contain a significant amount of vitamin K include beef liver, green tea, turnip greens, broccoli, kale, spinach, cabbage, asparagus, and dark green lettuce. Chlorophyll, which is water soluble, is the substance in plants that gives them their green color and provides vitamin K; thus chlorophyll supplements need to be considered when assessing vitamin K intake. Foods that appear to contain low amounts of vitamin K include roots, bulbs, tubers, the fleshy portion of fruits, fruit juices and other beverages, and cereal grains and their milled products.

Dietary Reference Intakes for Vitamin K for Children and Adults

Age (years)	Males and Females (mcg/day)	Pregnancy (mcg/day)	Lactation (mcg/day)
1-3	30	N/A	N/A
4-8	55	N/A	N/A
9-13	60	N/A	N/A
14-18	75	75	75
19+	120 for men; 90 for women	90	90

N/A, Not applicable.

Continued

APPENDIX 50. Nutritional Facts on Vitamin K—cont'd

Selected Food Sources of Vitamin K

Food	Micrograms per Serving
Brussels sprouts, ½ cup	460
Turnip greens, raw, chopped, 1 cup	364
Broccoli, ½ cup	248
Lentils, dry, ½ cup	214
Cauliflower, ½ cup	150
Kale, ½ cup cooked	150
Spinach, raw, chopped, ½ cup	149
Garbanzo beans, dry, ½ cup	132
Swiss chard, ½ cup	123
Beef, 3.5 oz	104
Pork, 3.5 oz	88
Soybean oil, 1 Tbsp	68
Lettuce, chopped, ½ cup	63
Asparagus, 1 cup, cooked	49
Eggs, whole	25
Strawberries, 1 cup	23
Oats, 1 oz	18
Milk, 8 oz	10

Dietary reference intake of vitamin K = 90-120 mcg.

APPENDIX 51. Nutritional Facts on Calcium and Vitamin D

Calcium

Any dietary source of calcium counts toward the daily intake, but low-fat milk or yogurt or fortified substitutes are the most efficient and readily available. Lactose-free milk and soy nut and rice drinks fortified with calcium and vitamin D are now available. In addition to milk, a variety of foods and calcium-fortified juices contain calcium and can help children, teens, and adults get sufficient levels of calcium in their diets. If it is difficult to get the recommended amounts of calcium and vitamin D from foods, a combination of food sources and supplements may be needed. Recommended dietary allowances (RDAs) were established in 2011.

Dietary Reference Intakes for Calcium for Children and Adults

Age (years)	Males and Females (mg/day)	Pregnancy (mg/day)	Lactation (mg/day)
1-3	700	N/A	N/A
4-8	1000	N/A	N/A
9-13	1300	N/A	N/A
14-18	1300	1300	1300
19+	1000	1000	1000
51-70 women	1200	N/A	N/A
51-70 men	1000	N/A	N/A
71+ men and women	1200	N/A	N/A

N/A, Not applicable.

Selected Food Sources of Calcium

Food	Milligrams per Serving
Dairy Foods	
Milk, with added calcium, 1 cup	420
Milk, whole, 2%, 1% skim, 1 cup	300
Yogurt, low fat, plain, ¾ cup	300
Cheese, processed slices, 2 slices	265
Yogurt, fruit bottom, ¾ cup	250
Processed cheese spread, 3 Tbsp	250
Cheese, hard, 1 oz	240
Milk, evaporated, ¼ cup	165
Cottage cheese, ¾ cup	120
Frozen yogurt, soft serve, ½ cup	100
Ice cream, ½ cup	85
Beans and Bean Products	
Soy cheese substitutes, 1 oz	0-200
Tofu, firm, made with calcium sulfate, 3½ oz	125
White beans, ½ cup	100
Navy beans, ½ cup	60
Black turtle beans, ½ cup	50
Pinto beans, chickpeas, ½ cup	40
Nuts and Seeds	
Almonds, dry roast, ¼ cup	95
Whole sesame seeds (black or white), 1 Tbsp	90
Tahini (sesame seed butter), 1 Tbsp	63
Brazil, hazelnuts, ¼ cup	55
Almond butter, 1 Tbsp	43
Meats, Fish, and Poultry	
Sardines, canned, 3½ oz (8 med)	370
Salmon, canned with bones, 3 oz	180
Oysters, canned, ½ cup	60
Shrimp, canned, ½ cup	40
Turnip greens, ½ cup	95
Okra, frozen, ½ cup	75
Chinese cabbage or bok choy, ½ cup	75
Kale, ½ cup	50
Mustard greens, ½ cup	50
Chinese broccoli (gai lan), ½ cup	44
Rutabaga, ½ cup	40
Broccoli, ½ cup	35

APPENDIX 51. Nutritional Facts on Calcium and Vitamin D—cont'd

Food	Milligrams per Serving
Fruit	
Orange, 1 med	55
Dried figs, 2 med	54
Nondairy Drinks	
Calcium enriched orange juice, 1 cup	300
Fortified rice beverage, 1 cup	300
Fortified soy beverage, 1 cup	300
Regular soy beverage, 1 cup	20
Grains	
Amaranth, raw, ½ cup	150
Whole wheat flour, 1 cup	40
Other	
Brown sugar, 1 cup	180
Blackstrap molasses, 1 Tbsp	170
Regular molasses, 1 Tbsp	40
Asian Foods	
Sea cucumber, fresh, 3 oz	285
Soy bean curd slab, spiced, semisoft, 3 oz	269
Shrimp, small, dried, 1 oz	167
Dried fish, smelt, 2 Tbsp	140
Seaweed, dry (hijiki), 10 g	140
Seaweed, dry (agar), 10 g	76
Lily flower, dried, ¼ cup	70
Soy bean milk film, stick shape, 3 oz	69
Fat-choy, dried, ¼ cup	50
Oyster, dried, 3	45
Soy bean milk film, dried, 3 oz	43
Boiled bone soup, ½ cup	Negligible
Laver, nori, and wakame seaweeds are low in calcium.	
Native Foods	
Oolichan, salted, cooked, 3 oz	210
Fish head soup, 1 cup	150
Indian ice cream (whipped soapberries), ½ cup	130

Calcium Supplements

Calcium carbonate is the most common and least expensive calcium supplement. It can be difficult to digest and causes gas in some people. Taking magnesium with it can help to prevent constipation. Calcium carbonate is 40% elemental calcium; 1000 mg will provide 400 mg of calcium. Take this supplement with food to aid in absorption.

Calcium citrate is more easily absorbed (bioavailability is 2.5 times higher than calcium carbonate), easier to digest, and less likely to cause constipation and gas than calcium carbonate. It also has a lower risk of contributing to the formation of kidney stones. Calcium citrate is approximately 21% elemental calcium; 1000 mg will provide 210 mg of calcium. It is more expensive than calcium carbonate, and more of it must be taken to get the same amount of calcium.

Calcium phosphate costs more than calcium carbonate but less than calcium citrate. It is easily absorbed and is less likely to cause constipation and gas.

Calcium lactate and calcium aspartate are both more easily digested but more expensive than calcium carbonate.

Vitamin D

Vitamin D is needed for the absorption of calcium from the stomach and for the functioning of calcium in the body. It also acts like a hormone in the body and has many functions throughout the body unrelated to its co-functions with calcium that are continuing to be discovered. Besides being in bone, receptors for vitamin D have been identified in the gastrointestinal tract, brain, breast, nerves, and many other tissues. The vitamin D in foods are micrograms of calciferol.

IU are used on supplement labels and in the 2011 RDA levels in the following table. 1 mcg = 40 IU of vitamin D or calciferol.

Dietary Reference Intakes for Vitamin D for Children and Adults

Age (years)	Males and Females	Pregnancy	Lactation
1-3	600 IU (15 mcg)	N/A	N/A
4-8	600 IU (15 mcg)	N/A	N/A
9-13	600 IU (15 mcg)	N/A	N/A
14-18	600 IU (15 mcg)	600 IU (15 mcg)	600 IU (15 mcg)
19-70	600 IU (15 mcg)	600 IU (15 mcg)	600 IU (15 mcg)
71+	800 IU (20 mcg)	N/A	N/A

Continued

APPENDIX 51. Nutritional Facts on Calcium and Vitamin D—cont'd

There are only a few food sources of vitamin D. Good sources of vitamin D are fortified foods and beverages such as milk, fortified soy, rice and nut beverages, and margarine (check the labels on these foods). Fish, liver, and egg yolks are the only foods that naturally contain vitamin D. If you do not eat vitamin D–rich foods often, you may want to consider taking a vitamin D supplement. Most multiple vitamin supplements contain vitamin D. In addition to dietary sources, sunlight can provide the body with vitamin D because it is synthesized through the skin. Natural food sources include those listed in the following table.

Selected Food Sources of Vitamin D

Food	Micrograms per Serving
Natural Sources	
Herring, 3 oz	13.83
Herring, pickled, 3 oz	5.78
Salmon, pink, canned, 3 oz	5.30
Halibut, 3 oz	5.10
Cod liver oil, 1 tsp	4.50
Catfish, 3 oz	4.25
Mackerel, Atlantic, 3 oz	3.06
Oyster, 3 oz	2.72
Shitake mushrooms, dried, 4	2.49
Sardines, Pacific, canned in tomato sauce	2.13 per ½ cup, 1.82 per sardine
Sardines, Atlantic, canned in oil	2.03 per ½ cup, 0.33 per sardine
Tuna, light meat, canned in oil, 3 oz	2
Shrimp, 3 oz	1.29
Egg, cooked	0.26 per whole egg, 0.25 per yolk
Fortified Sources	
Tofu, fortified, ⅕ block	1.20
Cow's milk, all types, 8 oz	1
Milk, canned evaporated, 4 oz	1
Rice milk, fortified, 8 oz	1
Soy milk, fortified, 8 oz	1
Orange juice, fortified, 8 oz	1
Pudding, made with fortified milk, ½ cup	0.50
Cereal, fortified, ¾ cup	0.40
Yogurt, fortified, ½ cup	0.40
Supplemental Sources	
Most multivitamins for adults	Usually 10
Calcium with vitamin D	Amount varies
Vitamin D only	Amount varies

APPENDIX 52. Nutritional Facts on Chromium

Chromium is known to enhance the action of insulin; chromium was identified as the active ingredient in the "glucose tolerance factor" many years ago. Chromium also appears to be directly involved in carbohydrate, fat, and protein metabolism; but more research is needed to determine the full range of its roles in the body. Chromium is widely distributed in the food supply, but most foods provide only small amounts (less than 2 mcg per serving). Meat and whole-grain products, as well as some fruits, vegetables, and spices, are relatively good sources, but Brewer's yeast is by far the most concentrated food source. Foods high in simple sugars (such as sucrose and fructose) are low in chromium. Dietary intakes of chromium cannot be reliably determined because the content of the mineral in foods is substantially affected by agricultural and manufacturing processes and food-composition databases are inadequate. Chromium values in foods are approximate and should only serve as a guide. It appears that chromium picolinate and chromium nicotinate used in supplements are more bioavailable than chromic chloride.

Dietary Reference Intakes for Chromium for Children and Adults

Age (years)	Males and Females (mcg/day)	Pregnancy (mcg/day)	Lactation (mcg/day)
1-3	11	N/A	N/A
4-8	15	N/A	N/A
9-13	25 for boys, 21 for women	N/A	N/A
14-18	35 for boys, 24 for women	29	44
19+	35 for men, 25 for women	30	45

N/A, Not applicable.

Selected Food Sources of Chromium

Food	Micrograms per Serving
Brewer's yeast, 1 Tbsp or 15 g	60
Broccoli, ½ cup	11
Grape juice, 1 cup	8
English muffin, whole wheat, 1	4
Potatoes, mashed, 1 cup	3
Garlic, dried, 1 tsp	3
Basil, dried, 1 Tbsp	2
Beef cubes, 3 oz	2
Orange juice, 1 cup	2
Turkey breast, 3 oz	2
Whole wheat bread, 2 slices	2
Red wine, 5 oz	1-13
Apple, unpeeled, 1 med	1
Banana, 1 med	1
Green beans, ½ cup	1

Interactions Between Chromium and Medications

Medications	Nature of Interaction
Antacids Corticosteroids H_2 blockers (e.g., cimetidine, famotidine, nizatidine, and ranitidine) Proton-pump inhibitors (e.g., omeprazole, lansoprazole, rabeprazole, pantoprazole, and esomeprazole)	These medications alter stomach acidity and may impair chromium absorption or enhance excretion.
β-blockers (such as atenolol or propranolol) Corticosteroids Insulin Nicotinic acid Nonsteroidal antiinflammatory drugs Prostaglandin inhibitors (e.g., ibuprofen, indomethacin, naproxen, piroxicam, and aspirin)	These medications may have their effects enhanced if taken together with chromium, or they may increase chromium absorption.

APPENDIX 53. Nutritional Facts on Iodine

Iodine is an important mineral that is found in a variety of foods, but it is most concentrated in foods from the ocean. It is mainly used to make thyroid hormones, which help to regulate metabolic rate, body temperature, growth, reproduction, blood cell production, muscle function, nerve function, and even gene expression. The most useful clinical tool for measuring thyroid function and thus iodine sufficiency is to measure thyroid-stimulating hormone (TSH), which is released from the pituitary gland and stimulates thyroid hormone production and release. If the TSH is high, thyroid function should be evaluated further. Selenium-dependent enzymes are also required for the conversion of thyroxine (T4) to the biologically active thyroid hormone, triiodothyronine (T3); thus deficiencies of selenium, vitamin A, or iron may also affect iodine status.

Deficiency

Iodine deficiency is an important health problem throughout much of the world. Most of the earth's iodine is found in its oceans; thus parts of the world away from the oceans and exposed for millions of years longer have iodine-deficient soils, and large percentages of people living there can be iodine deficient unless public health measures are taken. Iodine deficiency can cause mental retardation, hypothyroidism, goiter, and varying degrees of other growth and developmental abnormalities. Iodine is now recognized as the most common cause of preventable brain damage in the world, with millions living in iodine-deficient areas.

The major source of dietary iodine in the United States is "iodized" salt, which has been fortified with iodine. In the United States assume that any salt in prepared foods is iodized unless the product label shows that it is *not iodized.* In the United States and Canada iodized salt contains 77 mcg of iodine per gram of salt. Iodine is also added in the diet because it is used in the feed of animals and in many processed or preserved foods as a stabilizer and a component of red food dyes. Vegetarian and nonvegetarian diets that exclude iodized salt, fish, and seaweed have been found to contain very little iodine. Urinary iodine excretion studies suggest that iodine intakes are declining in the United States, possibly as a result of increased adherence to dietary recommendations to reduce salt intake.

Goitrogens

Substances that interfere with iodine use or thyroid hormone production are known as goitrogens and occur in some foods. Some species of millet and cruciferous vegetables (e.g., cabbage, broccoli, cauliflower, and Brussels sprouts) contain goitrogens; and the soybean isoflavones genistein and daidzein have also been found to inhibit thyroid hormone synthesis. Most of these goitrogens are not of clinical importance unless they are consumed in large amounts or there is coexisting iodine deficiency.

Dietary Reference Intakes for Iodine

Life Stage	Age	Males (mcg/day)	Females (mcg/day)
Infants	0-6 months	110 (AI)	110 (AI)
Infants	7-12 months	130 (AI)	130 (AI)
Children	1-3 years	90	90
Children	4-8 years	90	90
Children	9-13 years	120	120
Adolescents	14-18 years	150	150
Adults	19 years and older	150	150
Pregnancy	All ages	—	220
Breast-feeding	All ages	—	290

AI, Adequate intake.

The iodine contents of some common foods containing iodine are given in the following table. The iodine content of fruits and vegetables depends on the soil in which they were grown; the iodine content of animal foods, outside of those from the ocean, depends on where they were raised and which plants they consumed. Therefore these values are average approximations.

Selected Food Sources of Iodine

Food	Serving	Micrograms per Serving	% Daily Value*
Salt (iodized)	1 g	77	51
Cod	3 oz	99	66
Shrimp	3 oz	35	23
Fish sticks	2 fish sticks	35	23
Tuna, canned in oil	3 ounces (½ can)	17	11
Milk (cow's)	1 cup (8 fluid oz)	56	37
Egg, boiled	1 large	29	19
Navy beans, cooked	½ cup	35	23
Potato with peel, baked	1 medium	63	42
Turkey breast, baked	3 ounces	34	22
Seaweed	1 oz, dried	Variable; may be greater than 18,000 mcg (18 mg)	12

*Daily values (DVs) are reference numbers based on the recommended dietary allowance. They were developed to help consumers determine if a food contains a lot or a little of a specific nutrient. The DV for iodine is 150 mcg. The %DV listed on the Nutrition Facts panel of food labels states the percentage of the DV provided in one serving.

APPENDIX 54. Nutritional Facts on Iron

Iron is a nutrient found in trace amounts in every cell of the body. Iron is part of hemoglobin in red blood cells and myoglobin in muscles. The role of both of these molecules is to carry oxygen. Iron also makes up part of many proteins and enzymes in the body. Iron deficiency anemia is common in children, adolescent girls, and women of childbearing age. It is usually treated with an iron-rich diet as well as iron supplements. Iron exists in foods in two forms: heme iron and nonheme iron. Vitamin C enhances the absorption of nonheme iron and should be consumed at the same time as an iron-rich food or meal. Substances that decrease the absorption of nonheme iron are:

- Oxalic acid, found in raw spinach and chocolate
- Phytic acid, found in wheat bran and beans (legumes)
- Tannins, found in commercial black or pekoe teas
- Polyphenols, found in coffee
- Calcium carbonate supplements

Heme iron is absorbed more efficiently than nonheme iron. Heme iron enhances the absorption of nonheme iron. The richest dietary sources of iron are from:

- Oysters
- Liver
- Lean red meat (especially beef)
- Poultry, dark red meat
- Tuna
- Salmon
- Iron-fortified cereals
- Dried beans
- Whole grains
- Eggs (especially egg yolks)
- Dried fruits
- Reasonable amounts: lamb, pork, and shellfish

Iron from **nonheme sources** (as in vegetables, fruits, grains, and supplements) is harder for the body to absorb. These sources include:

- Whole grains
  - Wheat
  - Millet
  - Oats
  - Brown rice
- Legumes
  - Lima beans
  - Soybeans
  - Dried beans and peas
  - Kidney beans
- Nuts
  - Almonds
  - Brazil nuts
- Dried fruits
  - Prunes
  - Raisins
  - Apricots
- Vegetables and Greens
  - Broccoli
  - Spinach
  - Kale
  - Collards
  - Asparagus
  - Dandelion greens

Dietary Reference Intakes for Iron for Children and Adults

Age (years)	Males and Females (mg/day)	Pregnancy (mg/day)	Lactation (mg/day)
1-3	7	N/A	N/A
4-8	10	N/A	N/A
9-13	8	N/A	N/A
14-18	11 for boys; 15 for girls	27	10
19+	8 for men; 18 for women	27	9

N/A, Not applicable.

Selected Food Sources of Iron

Food	Milligrams Per Serving	% Daily Value*
Clams, canned, drained, 3 oz	23.8	132
Fortified ready-to-eat cereals (various), ≈1 oz	1.8-21.1	10-12
Oysters, eastern, wild, cooked, moist heat, 3 oz	10.2	57
Organ meats (liver, giblets), various, cooked, 3 oz†	5.2-9.9	29-55
Fortified instant cooked cereals (various), 1 packet	4.9-8.1	27-45
Soybeans, mature, cooked, ½ cup	4.4	24
Pumpkin and squash seed kernels, roasted, 1 oz	4.2	23
White beans, canned, ½ cup	3.9	22
Blackstrap molasses, 1 Tbsp	3.5	19
Lentils, cooked, ½ cup	3.3	18
Spinach, cooked from fresh, ½ cup	3.2	18
Beef, chuck, blade roast, lean, cooked, 3 oz	3.1	17
Beef, bottom round, lean, 0 in fat, all rades, cooked, 3 oz	2.8	15.5
Kidney beans, cooked, ½ cup	2.6	14
Sardines, canned in oil, drained, 3 oz	2.5	14
Beef, rib, lean, ¼ in. fat, all grades, 3 oz	2.4	13
Chickpeas, cooked, ½ cup	2.4	13
Duck, meat only, roasted, 3 oz	2.3	13
Lamb, shoulder, arm, lean, ¼ in fat, choice, cooked, 3 oz	2.3	13
Prune juice, ¾ cup	2.3	13
Shrimp, canned, 3 oz	2.3	13
Cowpeas, cooked, ½ cup	2.2	12
Ground beef, 15% fat, cooked, 3 oz	2.2	12
Tomato puree, ½ cup	2.2	12
Lima beans, cooked, ½ cup	2.2	12
Soybeans, green, cooked, ½ cup	2.2	12
Navy beans, cooked, ½ cup	2.1	11.5
Refried beans, ½ cup	2.1	11.5
Beef, top sirloin, lean, 0 in fat, all grades, cooked, 3 oz	2.0	11
Tomato paste, ¼ cup	2.0	11

*Daily values (DVs) are reference numbers based on the recommended dietary allowance. They were developed to help consumers determine if a food contains a lot or a little of a specific nutrient. The DV for iron is 18 mg. The %DV listed on the Nutrition Facts panel of food labels states the percentage of the DV provided in one serving.

†High in cholesterol.

Continued

APPENDIX 54. Nutritional Facts on Iron—cont'd

Tips For Increasing Iron Intake

The amount of iron the body absorbs varies, depending on several factors. For example, the body will absorb more iron from foods when iron stores are low and will absorb less when stores are sufficient. In addition, certain dietary factors affect absorption.

Combine heme and nonheme sources of iron. Eat foods rich in vitamin C with nonheme iron sources:

Bell peppers
Papayas
Oranges and orange juice
Broccoli
Strawberries
Grapefruit
Cantaloupe
Tomatoes and tomato juice
Potatoes
Cabbage
Spinach and collard greens

Drink coffee or tea between meals rather than with a meal.

Cook acidic foods in cast iron pots, which can increase iron content up to 30 times.

What About Too Much Iron?

It is unlikely that a person would take iron at toxic (too high) levels. However, children can sometimes develop iron toxicity by eating iron supplements, mistaking them for candy. Symptoms include the following: fatigue, anorexia, dizziness, nausea, vomiting, headache, weight loss, shortness of breath, and grayish color to the skin.

Hemochromatosis is a genetic disorder that affects the regulation of iron absorption. Treatment consists of a low-iron diet, no iron supplements, and phlebotomy (blood removal) on a regular basis.

Excess storage of iron in the body is known as hemosiderosis. The high iron stores come from eating excessive iron supplements or from receiving frequent blood transfusions, not from increased iron intake in the diet.

To reduce the iron from dietary sources, review the list of foods and exclude or severely limit their intake until the iron overload is alleviated. Pay particular attention to sports drinks, energy bars, and fortified cereals that have significant amounts of added iron.

Sample Meal Plan

Breakfast

½ cup low-fat or fat-free yogurt
1 whole wheat English muffin
1 Tbsp whipped cream cheese
½ cup cantaloupe

Lunch

2 grilled steak fajitas (with mixed peppers)
1 oz shredded low-fat pepper jack cheese
½ cup black refried beans
Side salad with low-fat dressing

Dinner

3 oz grilled turkey breast
½ cup mashed potatoes
½ cup fresh steamed green beans topped with almonds
1 small whole wheat dinner roll
½ cup fresh strawberries

Snack

1 med orange
¼ cup mixed nuts

APPENDIX 55. Nutritional Facts on Magnesium

The mineral magnesium is important for every organ in the body, particularly the heart, muscles, and kidneys. It also contributes to the composition of teeth and bones. Most important, it activates enzymes, contributes to energy production, and helps regulate calcium levels, as well as copper, zinc, potassium, vitamin D, and other important nutrients in the body.

Dietary Sources

Rich sources of magnesium include tofu, legumes, whole grains, green leafy vegetables, wheat bran, Brazil nuts, soybean flour, almonds, cashews, blackstrap molasses, pumpkin and squash seeds, pine nuts, and black walnuts. Other good dietary sources of this mineral include peanuts, whole-wheat flour, oat flour, beet greens, spinach, pistachio nuts, shredded wheat, bran cereals, oatmeal, bananas, baked potatoes (with skin), chocolate, and cocoa powder. Many herbs, spices, and seaweeds supply magnesium, such as agar seaweed, coriander, dill weed, celery seed, sage, dried mustard, basil, cocoa powder, fennel seed, savory, cumin seed, tarragon, marjoram, and poppy seed.

Dietary Reference Intakes for Magnesium for Children and Adults

Age (years)	Males and Females (mg/day)	Pregnancy (mg/day)	Lactation (mg/day)
1-3	80	N/A	N/A
4-8	130	N/A	N/A
9-13	240	N/A	N/A
14-18	410 for boys, 360 for girls	400	360
19+	400 for men, 310 for women	350	310

N/A, Not applicable.

APPENDIX 55. Nutritional Facts on Magnesium—cont'd

Selected Food Sources of Magnesium

Food	Milligram per Serving	% Daily Value*
Pumpkin and squash seed kernels, roasted, 1 oz	151	38
Brazil nuts, 1 oz	107	27
Bran ready-to-eat cereal (100%), ≈1 oz	103	25.5
Mackerel, baked, 3 oz	97	24
Halibut, cooked, 3 oz	91	23
Quinoa, dry, ¼ cup	89	22
Spinach, canned, ½ cup	81	20
Almonds, 1 oz	78	19.5
Spinach, cooked from fresh, ½ cup	78	19.5
Buckwheat flour, ¼ cup	75	19
Cashews, dry roasted, 1 oz	74	18.5
Soybeans, mature, cooked, ½ cup	74	18.5
Pine nuts, dried, 1 oz	71	17.5
Mixed nuts, oil roasted, with peanuts, 1 oz	67	17
White beans, canned, ½ cup	67	17
Pollock, walleye, cooked, 3 oz	62	15.5
Black beans, cooked, ½ cup	60	15
Bulgur, dry, ¼ cup	57	14
Oat bran, raw, ¼ cup	55	13.5
Soybeans, green, cooked, ½ cup	54	13.7
Tuna, yellowfin, cooked, 3 oz	54	13.5
Artichokes (hearts), cooked, ½ cup	50	12.5
Peanuts, dry roasted, 1 oz	50	12.5
Lima beans, baby, cooked from frozen, ½ cup	50	12.5
Beet greens, cooked, ½ cup	49	12
Navy beans, cooked, ½ cup	48	12
Tofu, firm, prepared with nigari,† ½ cup	47	11.7
Okra, cooked from frozen, ½ cup	47	11.7
Soy beverage, 1 cup	47	11.7
Cowpeas, cooked, ½ cup	46	11.5
Hazelnuts, 1 oz	46	11.5
Oat bran muffin, 1 oz	45	11.3
Great northern beans, cooked, ½ cup	44	11
Oat bran, cooked, ½ cup	44	11
Buckwheat groats, roasted, cooked, ½ cup	43	10.7
Cod, baked, 3 oz	42	10.5
Brown rice, cooked, ½ cup	42	10.5
Haddock, cooked, 3 oz	42	10.5
Chicken, cooked, 3 oz	38	9.5
T-bone steak, broiled, lean only, 3 oz	25	6.5
Turkey, roasted, white meat, 3 oz	24	6
Veal, cutlet, cooked, 3 oz	24	6
Beef, ground, cooked, extra lean, 17% fat, 3 oz	17	4

*Daily values (DVs) are reference numbers based on the recommended dietary allowance. They were developed to help consumers determine if a food contains a lot or a little of a specific nutrient. The DV for magnesium is 400 mg. The %DV listed on the Nutrition Facts panel of food labels states the percentage of the DV provided in one serving.

†Calcium sulfate and magnesium chloride.

Common and Important Magnesium-Drug Interactions

Drug	Potential Interaction
Loop and thiazide diuretics (e.g., Lasix, Bumex, edecrin, and hydrochlorothiazide Antineoplastic drugs (e.g., cisplatin) Antibiotics (e.g., gentamicin and amphotericin)	These drugs may increase the loss of magnesium in urine; thus taking these medications for long periods may contribute to magnesium depletion.
Tetracycline antibiotics	Magnesium binds tetracycline in the gut and decreases the absorption of tetracycline.
Magnesium-containing antacids and laxatives	Many antacids and laxatives contain magnesium. When frequently taken in large doses, these drugs can inadvertently lead to excessive magnesium consumption and hypermagnesemia, which refers to elevated levels of magnesium in blood.

Sample Meal Plan

Breakfast

1 med oat bran muffin (45 mg magnesium)
1 small banana
½ cup low-fat or fat-free milk

Lunch

½ cup penne pasta with the following:
- 3 oz grilled chicken breast
- ½ cup fresh cooked spinach (81 mg magnesium)
- Toasted pine nuts (71 mg magnesium)
- 1 cup mixed salad greens topped with spinach leaves, tomatoes, shredded lettuce
- 1 oz shredded low-fat mozzarella cheese

Dinner

2 Cajun shrimp skewers
½ cup fresh steamed green beans
½ cup brown rice (42 mg magnesium)
½ cup fresh pineapple

Snack

1 cup soy fruit smoothie (47 mg magnesium)
1 oz Brazil nuts (107 mg magnesium)

APPENDIX 56. Nutritional Facts on Potassium

A potassium-rich diet is useful for cardiac patients who are trying to lower their blood pressure using diet. If diuretics are also used, it is important to know if potassium is retained or depleted, and it should be monitored. Most patients with chronic kidney disease or on renal dialysis need to be aware of the potassium in their diets. Athletes who sweat a great deal may also need attention to the potassium in their diet.

Dietary Reference Intakes for Potassium for Children and Adults

Age (years)	Males and Females (mg/day)	Pregnancy (mg/day)	Lactation (mg/day)
1-3	3000	N/A	N/A
4-8	3800	N/A	N/A
9-13	4500	N/A	N/A
14-18	4700	4700	5100
19+	4700	4700	5100

N/A, Not applicable.

Selected Food Sources of Potassium

Food	Milligrams per Serving	% Daily Value*
Sweet potato, baked, 1 potato (146 g)	694	19.8
Tomato paste, ¼ cup	664	18.9
Beet greens, cooked, ½ cup	655	18.7
Potato, baked, flesh, 1 potato (156 g)	610	17.4
White beans, canned, ½ cup	595	17
Yogurt, plain, non-fat, 8-oz container	579	16.5
Tomato puree, ½ cup	549	15.7
Clams, canned, 3 oz	534	15.3
Yogurt, plain, low-fat, 8-oz container	531	15.2
Prune juice, ¾ cup	530	15.1
Carrot juice, ¾ cup	517	14.8
Blackstrap molasses, 1 Tbsp	498	14.2
Halibut, cooked, 3 oz	490	14
Soybeans, green, cooked, ½ cup	485	13.9
Tuna, yellow fin, cooked, 3 oz	484	13.8
Lima beans, cooked, ½ cup	484	13.8
Winter squash, cooked, ½ cup	448	9.5
Soybeans, mature, cooked, ½ cup	443	12.8
Rockfish, Pacific, cooked, 3 oz	442	12.6
Cod, Pacific, cooked, 3 oz	439	12.5
Bananas, 1 med	422	12.1
Spinach, cooked, ½ cup	419	12
Tomato juice, ¾ cup	417	11.9
Tomato sauce, ½ cup	405	11.6
Peaches, dried, uncooked, ¼ cup	398	11.4
Prunes, stewed, ½ cup	398	11.4
Milk, nonfat, 1 cup	382	10.9
Pork chop, center loin, cooked, 3 oz	382	10.9
Apricots, dried, uncooked, ¼ cup	378	10.8
Rainbow trout, farmed, cooked, 3 oz	375	10.7
Pork loin, center rib (roasts), lean, roasted, 3 oz	371	10.6
Buttermilk, cultured, low-fat, 1 cup	370	10.5
Cantaloupe, ¼ med	368	10.5
1%-2% milk, 1 cup	366	10.4
Honeydew melon, ⅛ med	365	10.4
Lentils, cooked, ½ cup	365	10.4
Plantains, cooked, ½ cup slices	358	10.2
Kidney beans, cooked, ½ cup	358	10.2
Orange juice, ¾ cup	355	10.1
Split peas, cooked, ½ cup	355	10.1
Yogurt, plain, whole milk, 8-oz container	352	10.0

*Daily values (DVs) are reference numbers based on the recommended dietary allowance. They were developed to help consumers determine if a food contains a lot or a little of a specific nutrient. The DV for potassium is 3500 mg. The %DV listed on the Nutrition Facts panel of food labels states the percentage of the DV provided in one serving. Percent DVs are based on a 2000-calorie diet.

APPENDIX 57. Nutritional Facts on Selenium

Selenium is incorporated into proteins to make selenoproteins, which are important antioxidant enzymes. The antioxidant properties of selenoproteins prevent cellular damage from free radicals. Other selenoproteins help regulate thyroid function and play a role in the immune system. Selenium, as a nutrient that functions as an antioxidant, may be protective against some types of cancer. Its role in heart disease is not clear, but it may have a preventive role.

Plant foods are the major dietary sources of selenium. The content of selenium in food depends on the selenium content of the soil where plants are grown or animals are raised. Soil in Nebraska and the Dakotas has very high levels of selenium. The southeast coastal areas in the United States have very low levels; selenium deficiency is often reported in these regions. Selenium is also found in some meats and seafood. Animals that eat grains or plants that were grown in selenium-rich soil have higher levels of selenium in their muscle. In the United States meats, bread, and Brazil nuts are common sources of dietary selenium.

Most food labels do not list the selenium content of a food. The % Daily Value (DV) listed on the label indicates the percentage of the DV provided in one serving. A food providing 5% of the DV or less is a source, whereas a food that provides 10% to 19% of the DV is a good source. A food that provides 20% or more of the DV is high in that nutrient. It is important to remember that foods that provide lower percentages of the DV also contribute to a healthful diet.

Dietary Reference Intakes for Selenium for Children and Adults

Age (years)	Males and Females (mcg/day)	Pregnancy (mcg/day)	Lactation (mcg/day)
1-3	20	N/A	N/A
4-8	30	N/A	N/A
9-13	40	N/A	N/A
14-18	55	60	70
19+	55	60	70

N/A, Not applicable.

Selected Food Sources of Selenium

Food	Micrograms per Serving
Brazil nuts, dried, unblanched, 1 oz	544
Tuna, light, canned in oil, drained, 3 oz	63
Beef, cooked, 3½ oz	35
Spaghetti with meat sauce, frozen entrée, 1 serving	34
Cod, cooked, 3 oz	32
Turkey, light meat, roasted, 3½ oz	32
Beef chuck roast, lean only, roasted, 3 oz	23
Chicken breast, meat only, roasted, 3½ oz	20
Noodles, enriched, boiled, ½ cup	17
Macaroni, elbow, enriched, boiled, ½ cup	15
Egg, whole, 1 med	14
Cottage cheese, low fat 2%, ½ cup	12
Oatmeal, instant, fortified, cooked, 1 cup	12
Rice, white, enriched, long grain, cooked, ½ cup	12
Rice, brown, long-grained, cooked, ½ cup	10
Bread, enriched, whole wheat, commercially prepared, 1 slice	10
Walnuts, black, dried, 1 oz	5
Bread, enriched, white, commercially prepared, 1 slice	4
Cheddar cheese, 1 oz	4

The dietary reference intakes for selenium are 20-70 mcg.

Sample Meal Plan

Breakfast

½ cup oatmeal (6 mcg selenium)
1 medium scrambled egg (14 mcg selenium)
1 small banana
½ cup low-fat or fat-free milk

Lunch

1 turkey sandwich (36 mcg selenium)
½ cup carrot sticks
1 bag baked chips

Dinner

3 oz meatloaf
½ cup macaroni and cheese (20 mcg selenium)
½ cup fresh steamed green beans

Snack

½ cup cottage cheese (12 mcg selenium)
½ cup fresh sliced peaches

Note: Take one multivitamin or multimineral supplement daily.

APPENDIX 58. Nutritional Facts on Zinc

Zinc is an essential mineral that is found in almost every cell. It stimulates the activity of approximately 100 enzymes, which are substances that promote biochemical reactions in the body. Zinc supports immunity; is needed for wound healing; helps maintain the sense of taste and smell; is needed for deoxyribonucleic acid synthesis; and supports normal growth and development during pregnancy, childhood, and adolescence.

Zinc is found in a wide variety of foods. Atlantic oysters contain more zinc per serving than any other food, but red meat and poultry provide the majority of zinc in the American diet. Other good food sources include beans, nuts, certain seafood, whole grains, fortified breakfast cereals, and dairy products. Because zinc absorption is greater from a diet high in animal protein than a diet rich in plant proteins, vegetarians may become deficient if they are not monitored carefully. Phytates from whole-grain breads, cereals, legumes, and other products can decrease zinc absorption.

Dietary Reference Intakes for Zinc for Children and Adults

Age (years)	Males and Females (mg/day)	Pregnancy (mg/day)	Lactation (mg/day)
1-3	3	N/A	N/A
4-8	5	N/A	N/A
9-13	8	N/A	N/A
14-18	11 for boys, 9 for girls	12	13
19+	11 for men, 8 for women	11	12

N/A, Not applicable.

Selected Food Sources of Zinc

Food	Milligrams per Serving	% Daily Value*
Oysters, battered and fried, 6 med	16.0	100
RTE breakfast cereal, fortified with 100% of the DV for zinc per serving, ¾ cup serving	15.0	100
Beef shank, lean only, cooked 3 oz	8.9	60
Beef chuck, arm pot roast, lean only, cooked, 3 oz	7.4	50
Beef tenderloin, lean only, cooked, 3 oz	4.8	30
Pork shoulder, arm picnic, lean only, cooked, 3 oz	4.2	30
Beef, eye of round, lean only, cooked, 3 oz	4.0	25
RTE breakfast cereal, fortified with 25% of the DV for zinc per serving, ¾ cup	3.8	25
RTE breakfast cereal, complete wheat bran flakes, ¾ cup serving	3.7	25
Chicken leg, meat only, roasted, 1 leg	2.7	20
Pork tenderloin, lean only, cooked, 3 oz	2.5	15
Pork loin, sirloin roast, lean only, cooked, 3 oz	2.2	15
Yogurt, plain, low fat, 1 cup	2.2	15
Baked beans, canned, with pork, ½ cup	1.8	10
Baked beans, canned, plain or vegetarian, ½ cup	1.7	10
Cashews, dry roasted without salt, 1 oz	1.6	10
Yogurt, fruit, low fat, 1 cup	1.6	10
Pecans, dry roasted without salt, 1 oz	1.4	10
Raisin bran, ¾ cup	1.3	8
Chickpeas, mature seeds, canned, ½ cup	1.3	8
Mixed nuts, dry roasted with peanuts, without salt, 1 oz	1.1	8
Cheese, Swiss, 1 oz	1.1	8
Almonds, dry roasted, without salt, 1 oz	1.0	6
Walnuts, black, dried, 1 oz	1.0	6
Milk, fluid, any kind, 1 cup	0.9	6
Chicken breast, meat only, roasted, ½ breast with bone and skin removed	0.9	6
Cheese, cheddar, 1 oz	0.9	6
Cheese, mozzarella, part skim, low moisture, 1 oz	0.9	6
Beans, kidney, California red, cooked, ½ cup	0.8	6
Peas, green, frozen, boiled, ½ cup	0.8	6
Oatmeal, instant, low sodium, 1 packet	0.8	6
Flounder or sole, cooked, 3 oz	0.5	4

RTE, Ready to eat.

*Daily values (DVs) are reference numbers based on the recommended dietary allowance. They were developed to help consumers determine if a food contains a lot or a little of a specific nutrient. The DV for zinc is 15 mg. The %DV listed on the Nutrition Facts panel of food labels states the percentage of the DV provided in one serving.

Sample Meal Plan

Breakfast

¼ cup scrambled eggs
¾ cup ready-to-eat breakfast cereal with 25% DV (3.8 mg zinc)
½ cup sliced peaches
½ cup low-fat or fat-free milk

Lunch

1 chicken salad sandwich
½ cup carrot sticks
2 Tbsp Ranch dressing
1 bag baked chips

Snack

Yogurt, plain (2.2 mg zinc)

Dinner

3 oz grilled beef shank (8.9 mg zinc)
½ cup fresh steamed peas (0.8 mg zinc)

Side salad

1 small sweet potato
½ cup fresh pineapple

Snack

½ cup Trail mix (raisins, pecans, cashews, dried cranberries)

Index

Page numbers followed by "f" indicate figures, "t" indicate tables, and "b" indicate boxes.

I

P

Dietary Reference Intakes (DRIs): ACCEPTABLE MACRONUTRIENT DISTRIBUTION RANGES
Food and Nutrition Board, Institute of Medicine, National Academies

Macronutrient	Range (percent of energy)		
	Children, 1-3 y	Children, 4-18 y	Adults
Fat	30-40	25-35	20-35
n-6 polyunsaturated fatty acids[a] (linoleic acid)	5-10	5-10	5-10
n-3 polyunsaturated fatty acids[a] (α-linolenic acid)	0.6-1.2	0.6-1.2	0.6-1.2
Carbohydrate	45-65	45-65	45-65
Protein	5-20	10-30	10-35

[a]Approximately 10 percent of the total can come from longer-chain *n*-3 or *n*-6 fatty acids.

SOURCE: *Dietary Reference Intakes for Energy, Carbohydrate, Fiber, Fat, Fatty Acids, Cholesterol, Protein, and Amino Acids* (2002/2005). The report may be accessed via www.nap.edu.

Dietary Reference Intakes (DRIs): ACCEPTABLE MACRONUTRIENT DISTRIBUTION RANGES
Food and Nutrition Board, Institute of Medicine, National Academies

Macronutrient	Recommendation
Dietary cholesterol	As low as possible while consuming a nutritionally adequate diet
Trans fatty Acids	As low as possible while consuming a nutritionally adequate diet
Saturated fatty acids	As low as possible while consuming a nutritionally adequate diet
Added sugars[a]	Limit to no more than 25 % of total energy

[a]Not a recommended intake. A daily intake of added sugars that individuals should aim for to achieve a healthful diet was not set.

SOURCE: *Dietary Reference Intakes for Enemy, Carbohydrate, Fiber, Fat, Fatty Acids, Cholesterol, Protein, and Amino Acids* (2002/2005). The report may be accessed via www.nap.edu.

Dietary Reference Intakes (DRIs): TOLERABLE UPPER INTAKE LEVELS, VITAMINS
Food and Nutrition Board, Institute of Medicine, National Academies

Life Stage Group	Vitamin A (μg/d)[a]	Vitamin C (mg/d)	Vitamin D (μg/d)	Vitamin E (mg/d)[b,c]	Vitamin K	Thiamin	Riboflavin	Niacin (mg/d)[c]	Vitamin B_6 (mg/d)	Folate (μg/d)[c]	Vitamin B_{12}	Pantothenic Acid	Biotin	Choline (g/d)	Carotenoids[d]
Infants															
0 to 6 mo	600	ND[e]	25	ND	ND	ND	ND	ND	ND	ND	ND	ND	ND	ND	ND
6 to 12 mo	600	ND	38	ND	ND	ND	ND	ND	ND	ND	ND	ND	ND	ND	ND
Children															
1-3 y	600	400	63	200	ND	ND	ND	10	30	300	ND	ND	ND	1.0	ND
4-8 y	900	650	75	300	ND	ND	ND	15	40	400	ND	ND	ND	1.0	ND
Males															
9-13 y	1,700	1,200	100	600	ND	ND	ND	20	60	600	ND	ND	ND	2.0	ND
14-18 y	2,800	1,800	100	800	ND	ND	ND	30	80	800	ND	ND	ND	3.0	ND
19-30 y	3,000	2,000	100	1,000	ND	ND	ND	35	100	1,000	ND	ND	ND	3.5	ND
31-50 y	3,000	2,000	100	1,000	ND	ND	ND	35	100	1,000	ND	ND	ND	3.5	ND
51-70 y	3,000	2,000	100	1,000	ND	ND	ND	35	100	1,000	ND	ND	ND	3.5	ND
>70 y	3,000	2,000	100	1,000	ND	ND	ND	35	100	1,000	ND	ND	ND	3.5	ND
Females															
9-13 y	1,700	1,200	100	600	ND	ND	ND	20	60	600	ND	ND	ND	2.0	ND
14-18 y	2,800	1,800	100	800	ND	ND	ND	30	80	800	ND	ND	ND	3.0	ND
19-30 y	3,000	2,000	100	1,000	ND	ND	ND	35	100	1,000	ND	ND	ND	3.5	ND
31-50 y	3,000	2,000	100	1,000	ND	ND	ND	35	100	1,000	ND	ND	ND	3.5	ND
51-70 y	3,000	2,000	100	1,000	ND	ND	ND	35	100	1,000	ND	ND	ND	3.5	ND
>70 y	3,000	2,000	100	1,000	ND	ND	ND	35	100	1,000	ND	ND	ND	3.5	ND
Pregnancy															
14 18 y	2,800	1,800	100	800	ND	ND	ND	30	80	800	ND	ND	ND	3.0	ND
19-30 y	3,000	2,000	100	1,000	ND	ND	ND	35	100	1,000	ND	ND	ND	3.5	ND
31-50 y	3,000	2,000	100	1,000	ND	ND	ND	35	100	1,000	ND	ND	ND	3.5	ND
Lactation															
14-18 y	2,800	1,800	100	800	ND	ND	ND	30	80	800	ND	ND	ND	3.0	ND
19-30 y	3,000	2,000	100	1,000	ND	ND	ND	35	100	1,000	ND	ND	ND	3.5	ND
31-50 y	3,000	2,000	100	1,000	ND	ND	ND	35	100	1,000	ND	ND	ND	3.5	ND

NOTE: A Tolerable Upper Intake Level (UL) is the highest level of daily nutrient intake that is likely to pose no risk of adverse health effects to almost all individuals in the general population. Unless otherwise specified, the UL represents total intake from food, water, and supplements. Due to a lack of suitable data, ULs could not be established for vitamin K, thiamin, riboflavin, vitamin B_{12}, pantothenic acid, biotin, and carotenoids. In the absence of a UL, extra caution may be warranted in consuming levels above recommended intakes. Members of the general population should be advised not to routinely exceed the UL. The UL is not meant to apply to individuals who are treated with the nutrient under medical supervision or to individuals with predisposing conditions that modify their sensitivity to the nutrient.

[a]As preformed vitamin A only.

[b]As α-tocopherol; applies to any form of supplemental α-tocopherol.

[c]The ULs for vitamin E, niacin, and folate apply to synthetic forms obtained from supplements, fortified foods, or a combination of the two.

[d]β-Carotene supplements are advised only to serve as a provitamin A source for individuals at risk of vitamin A deficiency.

[e]ND = Not determinable due to lack of data of adverse effects in this age group and concern with regard to lack of ability to handle excess amounts. Source of intake should be from food only to prevent high levels of intake.

SOURCES: *Dietary Reference Intakes for Calcium, Phosphorous, Magnesium, Vitamin D, and Fluoride* (1997); *Dietary Reference Intakes for Thiamin, Riboflavin, Niacin, Vitamin B_6, Folate, Vitamin B_{12}, Pantothenic Acid, Biotin, and Choline* (1998); *Dietary Reference Intakes for Vitamin C, Vitamine E, Selenium, and Carotenoids* (2000); *Dietary Reference Intakes for Vitamin A, Vitamin K, Arsenic, Boron, Chromium, Copper, Iodine, Iron, Manganese, Molybdenum, Nickel, Silicon, Vanadium, and Zinc* (2001); and *Dietary Reference Intakes for Calcium and Vitamin D* (2011). These reports may be accessed via www.nap.edu.